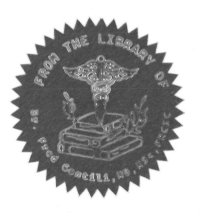

PRINCIPLES OF
SURGERY

PRINCIPLES OF SURGERY

SECOND EDITION

Volume 1, Pages 1–966

EDITOR-IN-CHIEF

SEYMOUR I. SCHWARTZ, M.D.
Professor of Surgery
University of Rochester School of Medicine and Dentistry

ASSOCIATE EDITORS

RICHARD C. LILLEHEI, M.D., Ph.D.
Professor of Surgery
University of Minnesota Medical School

G. THOMAS SHIRES, M.D.
Professor and Chairman
Department of Surgery
University of Texas Southwestern Medical School

FRANK C. SPENCER, M.D.
Professor and Director
Department of Surgery
New York University School of Medicine

EDWARD H. STORER, M.D.
Professor of Surgery
Yale University School of Medicine

McGRAW-HILL BOOK COMPANY   **A Blakiston Publication**

New York   St. Louis   San Francisco   Düsseldorf   Johannesburg   Kuala Lumpur
London   Mexico   Montreal   New Delhi   Panama   Paris   São Paulo
Singapore   Sydney   Tokyo   Toronto

NOTICE

Medicine is an ever-changing science. As new research and clinical experience broaden our knowledge, changes in treatment and drug therapy are required. The editors and the publisher of this work have made every effort to ensure that the drug dosage schedules herein are accurate and in accord with the standards accepted at the time of publication. The reader is advised, however, to check the product information sheet included in the package of each drug he plans to administer to be certain that changes have not been made in the recommended dose or in the contraindications for administration. This recommendation is of particular importance in regard to new or infrequently used drugs.

PRINCIPLES OF
SURGERY

1 2 3 4 5 6 7 8 9 0   DODO   7 9 8 7 6 5 4

Library of Congress Cataloging in Publication Data
Main entry under title:

Principles of surgery.

 "A Blakiston publication."
 Includes bibliographies.
 1. Surgery. I. Schwartz, Seymour I., ed.
II. Lillehei, Richard C., ed. [DNLM: 1. Surgery.
W0100 P957 1974]
RD31.P88 1974b   617   73-21797 (1 vol.)
                             73-20491 (2 vols.)

ISBN 0-07-055723-3 (1 vol.)
ISBN 0-07-055724-1 (2 vols.)

This book was set in Times Roman by York Graphic Services, Inc. The editors were Paul K. Schneider and Andrea Stryker-Rodda; the designer was Barbara Ellwood; the production supervisor was Sam Ratkewitch.
R. R. Donnelley & Sons Company was printer and binder.

Sources for cover drawings from Bettman Archives.

DEDICATION

To students of surgery,
at all levels,
in their quest for knowledge

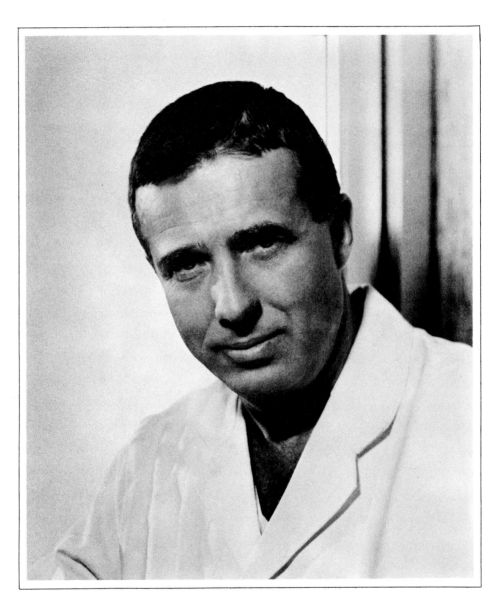

DAVID M. HUME

Whose contributions to surgery have been and will continue to be appreciated by the entire profession.

Whose contributions to Principles of Surgery *were particularly meaningful both to the Editors, for the opportunity to cement a friendship with an esteemed colleague, and to all the readers, for whom his expressed thoughts and recorded experiences represent a legacy.*

Contents

List of Contributors   xi

Preface to the Second Edition   xvii

Acknowledgments   xix

Preface to the First Edition   xxi

Part I. Basic Considerations

1. Endocrine and Metabolic Responses to Injury   *David M. Hume*   1

2. Fluid, Electrolyte, and Nutritional Management of the Surgical Patient   *G. Thomas Shires* and *Peter C. Canizaro*   65

3. Hemostasis, Surgical Bleeding, and Transfusion   *Seymour I. Schwartz* and *Stanley B. Troup*   97

4. Circulatory Collapse and Shock   *Richard C. Lillehei* and *Ronald H. Dietzman*   133

5. Infections   *Isidore Cohn, Jr.,* and *George H. Bornside*   165

6. Trauma   *G. Thomas Shires, Ronald C. Jones, Malcolm O. Perry, Adolph H. Giesecke, Jr., Edward R. Johnson, Robert F. Jones, William H. Snyder, III, Robert N. McClelland,* and *Erwin R. Thal*   195

7. Burns   *John A. Moncrief*   253

8. Wound Healing and Wound Care   *Erle E. Peacock, Jr.*   275

9. Oncology   *Donald L. Morton, Frank C. Sparks,* and *Charles M. Haskell*   297

10. Transplantation   *Richard L. Simmons, John E. Foker, Richard R. Lower,* and *John S. Najarian*   349

11. Anesthesia   *Nicholas M. Greene*   443

12. Complications   *Seymour I. Schwartz*   461

13. Physiologic Monitoring of the Surgical Patient   *Louis R. M. Del Guercio*   491

Part II. Specific Organ Systems

14. Skin and Subcutaneous Tissue   *Seymour I. Schwartz*   513

15. Breast   *Benjamin F. Rush, Jr.*   527

16. Tumors of the Head and Neck   *Benjamin F. Rush, Jr.*   555

17. Chest Wall, Pleura, Lung, and Mediastinum   *Herbert C. Maier* and *Seymour I. Schwartz*   595

18. Congenital Heart Disease   *Frank C. Spencer*   677

19. Acquired Heart Disease   *Frank C. Spencer*   749

20. Diseases of Great Vessels   *Frank C. Spencer*   815

21. Peripheral Arterial Disease   *Frank C. Spencer* and *Anthony M. Imparato*   839

22. Venous and Lymphatic Disease   *James A. DeWeese*   913

23. Surgically Correctible Hypertension   *John H. Foster*   939

24. Manifestations of Gastrointestinal Disease   *Seymour I. Schwartz* and *Edward H. Storer*   967

25. Esophagus and Diaphragmatic Hernias   *W. Spencer Payne* and *F. Henry Ellis, Jr.*   1009

26. Stomach   *René B. Menguy*   1049

27. Small Intestine   *Edward H. Storer*   1089

28. Colon, Rectum, and Anus   *Edward H. Storer, Stanley M. Goldberg,* and *Santhat Nivatvongs*   1109

29. Appendix   *Edward H. Storer*   1167

30. Liver   *Seymour I. Schwartz*   1177

31. Gallbladder and Extrahepatic Biliary System   *Seymour I. Schwartz*   1221

32. Pancreas   *William Silen*   1225

33. Spleen   *Seymour I. Schwartz*   1281

34. Peritonitis and Intraabdominal Abscesses   *Edward H. Storer*   1297

35. Abdominal Wall, Omentum, Mesentery, and Retroperitoneum   *James T. Adams*   1313

36. Abdominal Wall Hernias   *John H. Morton*   1345

37. Pituitary and Adrenal   *David M. Hume* and *Timothy S. Harrison*   1363

38. Thyroid and Parathyroid   *Seymour I. Schwartz, David M. Hume,* and *Edwin L. Kaplan*   1429

39. Pediatric Surgery   *J. Alex Haller, Jr.*   1513

40. Urology   *Donald F. McDonald*   1547

41. Gynecology   *Arthur L. Herbst* and *Howard Ulfelder*   1589

42. Neurologic Surgery   *William F. Collins, Jr., John C. VanGilder, Joan L. Venes,*
                                               and *Joseph H. Galicich*   1631

43. Manifestations of Musculoskeletal Disease   *Robert B. Duthie* and *Franklin T. Hoaglund*   1675

44. Congenital Orthopedic Deformities   *Robert B. Duthie* and *Franklin T. Hoaglund*   1725

45. Generalized Bone Disorders   *Robert B. Duthie* and *Franklin T. Hoaglund*   1741

46. Tumors of the Musculoskeletal System   *Robert B. Duthie* and *Franklin T. Hoaglund*   1775

47. Fractures and Joint Injuries   *Franklin T. Hoaglund* and *Robert B. Duthie*   1791

48. Diseases of Joints   *Franklin T. Hoaglund* and *Robert B. Duthie*   1845

49. Amputations   *Seymour I. Schwartz* and *Franklin T. Hoaglund*   1879

50. Hand   *Lester M. Cramer* and *Robert A. Chase*   1895

51. Plastic and Reconstructive Surgery   *Lester M. Cramer* and *Robert A. Chase*   1919

52. Rehabilitation   *Howard A. Rusk* and *J. Herbert Dietz, Jr.*   1967

Indexes

   Name Index   1
   Subject Index   9

List of Contributors

ADAMS, JAMES T., M.D.
Associate Professor of Surgery
University of Rochester School of Medicine and Dentistry

BORNSIDE, GEORGE H., Ph.D.
Professor of Surgical Research
Professor of Microbiology
Louisiana State University School of Medicine

CANIZARO, PETER C., M.D.
Associate Professor of Surgery
The University of Texas Southwestern Medical School at Dallas

CHASE, ROBERT A., M.D.
Professor and Executive
Department of Surgery
Stanford University School of Medicine

COHN, ISIDORE, JR., M.D.
Professor and Chairman
Department of Surgery
Louisiana State University School of Medicine

COLLINS, WILLIAM F., JR., M.D.
Professor and Chairman
Section of Neurological Surgery
Yale University School of Medicine

CRAMER, LESTER M., M.D.
Professor and Chairman
Section of Plastic Surgery and Surgery of the Hand
Temple University Health Sciences Center

DeWEESE, JAMES A., M.D.
Professor of Surgery
University of Rochester School of Medicine and Dentistry

DIETZ, J. HERBERT, JR., M.D.
Assistant Professor of Rehabilitation Medicine
New York University School of Medicine

DIETZMAN, RONALD H., M.D., Ph.D.
Assistant Professor of Surgery
University of Minnesota Health Sciences Center

DUTHIE, ROBERT B., M.D., M.B.
Nuffield Professor of Orthopedic Surgery
Nuffield Orthopedic Center, Oxford, England

Del GUERCIO, LOUIS R. M., M.D.
Director of Surgery, Saint Barnabas Medical Center
(Livingston, New Jersey)
Clinical Professor of Surgery
College of Medicine and Dentistry of New Jersey at Newark

ELLIS, F. HENRY, JR., M.D., Ph.D.
Lecturer in Surgery, Harvard Medical School
Chief, Cardiovascular Surgery, Lahey Clinic Foundation

FOKER, JOHN E., M.D.
Instructor, Department of Surgery
University of Minnesota Health Sciences Center

FOSTER, JOHN H., M.D.
Professor of Surgery
Vanderbilt University School of Medicine

GALICICH, JOSEPH H., M.D.
Associate Professor of Neurosurgery
Cornell University School of Medicine, New York, N.Y.

GIESECKE, ADOLPH H., JR., M.D.
Professor and Chairman
Department of Anesthesiology
University of Texas Medical School at Houston

GOLDBERG, STANLEY M., M.D.
Clinical Professor of Surgery
Director and Head, Division of Colon and Rectal
Surgery
Department of Surgery
University of Minnesota Health Sciences Center

GREENE, NICHOLAS M., M.D.
Professor of Anesthesiology
Yale University School of Medicine

HALLER, J. ALEX, JR., M.D.
Professor of Pediatric Surgery
The Johns Hopkins University School of Medicine

HARRISON, TIMOTHY S., M.D.
Professor of Surgery
University of Michigan Medical School

HASKELL, CHARLES M., M.D.
Assistant Professor of Surgery and Medicine
Division of Oncology
Center for the Health Sciences, University of California at Los Angeles

HERBST, ARTHUR L., M.D.
Assistant Clinical Professor of Obstetrics and Gynecology
Harvard Medical School

HOAGLUND, FRANKLIN T., M.D.
Professor and Chairman
Department of Orthopedic Surgery
University of Vermont College of Medicine

HUME, DAVID M., M.D.
Professor and Chairman
Department of Surgery
Medical College of Virginia

IMPARATO, ANTHONY M., M.D.
Professor of Clinical Surgery
New York University School of Medicine

JOHNSON, EDWARD R., M.D.
Assistant Professor of Anesthesiology
The University of Texas Southwestern Medical School at Dallas

JONES, ROBERT F., M.D.
Associate Professor of Surgery
The University of Texas Southwestern Medical School at Dallas

JONES, RONALD C., M.D.
Associate Professor of Surgery
The University of Texas Southwestern Medical School at Dallas

KAPLAN, EDWIN L., M.D.
Associate Professor of Surgery
Pritzker School of Medicine, University of Chicago
LILLEHEI, RICHARD C., M.D., Ph.D.
Professor of Surgery
University of Minnesota Health Sciences Center
LOWER, RICHARD R., M.D.
Professor and Chairman
Division of Thoracic and Cardiac Surgery
Medical College of Virginia
McCLELLAND, ROBERT N., M.D.
Professor of Surgery
The University of Texas Southwestern Medical School at Dallas
McDONALD, DONALD F., M.D.
Professor and Chief,
Division of Urology
University of Texas Medical Branch at Galveston
MAIER, HERBERT C., M.D.
Associate Clinical Professor of Surgery
Columbia University College of Physicians and Surgeons
MENGUY, RENÉ B., M.D.
Professor of Surgery, University of Rochester School
of Medicine and Dentistry
Chief of Surgery, Genesee Hospital
MONCRIEF, JOHN A., M.D.
Professor of Surgery
University of South Carolina Medical School
MORTON, DONALD L., M.D.
Professor of Surgery
Chief, Division of Oncology
Center for the Health Sciences, University of
California at Los Angeles
MORTON, JOHN H., M.D.
Professor of Surgery
University of Rochester School of Medicine and Dentistry

NAJARIAN, JOHN S., M.D.
Professor and Chairman
Department of Surgery
University of Minnesota Health Sciences Center

NIVATVONGS, SANTHAT, M.D.
Instructor, Division of Colon and Rectal Surgery
Department of Surgery
University of Minnesota Health Sciences Center

PAYNE, W. SPENCER, M.D.
Associate Professor of Surgery in the Mayo
Foundation Graduate School,
University of Minnesota Health Sciences Center

PEACOCK, ERLE E., JR., M.D.
Professor and Chairman
Department of Surgery
University of Arizona College of Medicine

PERRY, MALCOLM O., M.D.
Professor of Surgery
The University of Texas Southwestern Medical School at Dallas

RUSH, BENJAMIN F., JR., M.D.
Professor and Chairman
Department of Surgery
College of Medicine and Dentistry of New Jersey at Newark

RUSK, HOWARD A., M.D.
Professor of Rehabilitation Medicine
New York University School of Medicine

SCHWARTZ, SEYMOUR I., M.D.
Professor of Surgery
University of Rochester School of Medicine and Dentistry

SHIRES, G. THOMAS, M.D.
Professor and Chairman
Department of Surgery
The University of Texas Southwestern Medical School at Dallas

SILEN, WILLIAM, M.D.
Chief of Surgery, Beth Israel Hospital
Professor of Surgery, Harvard Medical School

SIMMONS, RICHARD L., M.D.
Associate Professor of Surgery and Microbiology
Department of Surgery
University of Minnesota Health Sciences Center

SNYDER, WILLIAM H., III, M.D.
Assistant Professor of Surgery
The University of Texas Southwestern Medical School at Dallas

SPARKS, FRANK C., M.D.
Assistant Professor of Surgery
Center for the Health Sciences
University of California at Los Angeles

SPENCER, FRANK C., M.D.
Professor and Director
Department of Surgery
New York University School of Medicine

STORER, EDWARD H., M.D.
Professor of Surgery
Yale University School of Medicine

THAL, ERWIN R., M.D.
Assistant Professor of Surgery
The University of Texas Southwestern Medical School at Dallas

TROUP, STANLEY B., M.D.
Professor of Medicine
University of Rochester School of Medicine and Dentistry

ULFELDER, HOWARD, M.D.
Joe V. Meigs Professor of Gynecology
Harvard Medical School

VanGILDER, JOHN C., M.D.
Assistant Professor, Section of Neurological Surgery
Yale University School of Medicine

VENES, JOAN L., M.D.
Associate Professor
Neurosurgery and Pediatrics
Yale University School of Medicine

Preface to the Second Edition

Unlike literature, which if meaningful has an intrinsic permanence, only the title of a textbook of surgery may be considered immutable. The explosion of factual knowledge has persisted and increased. Therefore, the expressed ultimate goal of the Editorial Board to create a book which is deserving of the adjective "modern" required a significant revision. The second edition of *Principles of Surgery* is a "modern" textbook which maintains its identifiable format of logic and consistency but reflects the changes of the past five years.

The most legitimate question to be answered is "What is new?" There are 21 new authors, who were selected in appreciation of their active contributions to their fields. Several chapters, including Fluid and Electrolyte Therapy in Surgery, Circulatory Collapse and Shock, Infections, Oncology, Transplantation, and Spleen, have been rewritten in their entirety, as have the sections on Rectum and Anus, Adrenal, and Parathyroid. A timely chapter focusing on Physiologic Monitoring of Surgical Patients has been added. Representative additions to other chapters include: Metabolic changes associated with trauma and new considerations regarding nutritional supplements, new concepts of fluid therapy for burn patients, postoperative and post-traumatic respiratory failure, modern regimens for treatment of melanoma, description of total and partial laryngectomy, new approaches to the management of congenital heart disease plus an appropriate emphasis on the correction of coronary occlusive disease, noninvasive techniques to diagnose thromboembolic disease, ex vivo reconstruction of arterial lesions associated with renovascular hypertension, new consideration of pain theories, acute gastric mucosal lesions and concepts of back diffusion, present status of intestinal bypass procedures for obesity, ischemic colitis, early detection of colon cancer, evaluation of the new shunts to manage portal hypertension, treatment of fulminant hepatic failure, formation of gallstones, new considerations regarding intracranial vascular diseases and cerebral ischemia, orthopedic management of stroke patients, radiographic diagnosis of orthopedic disorders, new methods of detecting and managing metastatic tumors in bone, hip and knee replacements, and several new considerations in reconstructive surgery.

SEYMOUR I. SCHWARTZ

Acknowledgments

The Editors wish to express their appreciation to Ms. Frances Sargent whose helpful efforts persisted throughout the development of this second edition. *Principles of Surgery* represents the combined efforts of many contributors; the Editors are most appreciative of their cooperation, promptness, and continued interest. We wish to convey special thanks to Drs. John E. Foker, Timothy S. Harrison, Edwin L. Kaplan, John S. Najarian, and Richard L. Simmons who, at short notice and in the face of a markedly compressed time allotment, provided their excellent contributions. Finally, in view of the extreme demands on time which this book imposed upon the Editorial Board, we would like to acknowledge the patience, cooperation, and sacrifice on the part of our families throughout the gestational period.

Preface to the First Edition

The raison d'etre for a new textbook in a discipline which has been served by standard works for many years was the Editorial Board's initial conviction that a distinct need for a modern approach in the dissemination of surgical knowledge existed. As incoming chapters were reviewed, both the need and satisfaction became increasingly apparent and, at the completion, we felt a sense of excitement at having the opportunity to contribute to the education of modern and future students concerned with the care of surgical patients.

The recent explosion of factual knowledge has emphasized the need for a presentation which would provide the student an opportunity to assimilate pertinent facts in a logical fashion. This would then permit correlation, synthesis of concepts, and eventual extrapolation to specific situations. The physiologic bases for diseases are therefore emphasized and the manifestations and diagnostic studies are considered as a reflection of pathophysiology. Therapy then becomes logical in this schema and the necessity to regurgitate facts is minimized. In appreciation of the impact which Harrison's PRINCIPLES OF INTERNAL MEDICINE has had, the clinical manifestations of the disease processes are considered in detail for each area. Since the operative procedure represents the one element in the therapeutic armentarium unique to the surgeon, the indications, important technical considerations, and complications receive appropriate emphasis. While we appreciate that a textbook cannot hope to incorporate an atlas of surgical procedures, we have provided the student a single book which will satisfy the sequential demands in the care and considerations of surgical patients.

The ultimate goal of the Editorial Board has been to collate a book which is deserving of the adjective "modern." We have therefore selected as authors dynamic and active contributors to their particular fields. The *au courant* concept is hopefully apparent throughout the entire work and is exemplified by appropriate emphasis on diseases of modern surgical interest, such as trauma, transplantation, and the recently appreciated importance of rehabilitation. Cardiovascular surgery is presented in keeping with the exponential strides recently achieved.

There are two major subdivisions to the text. In the first twelve chapters, subjects that transcend several organ systems are presented. The second portion of the book represents a consideration of specific organ systems and surgical specialties.

Throughout the text, the authors have addressed themselves to a sophisticated audience, regarding the medical student as a graduate student, incorporating material generally sought after by the surgeon in training and presenting information appropriate for the continuing education of the practicing surgeon. The need for a text such as we have envisioned is great and the goal admittedly high. It is our hope that this effort fulfills the expressed demands.

SEYMOUR I. SCHWARTZ

PRINCIPLES OF
SURGERY

Endocrine and Metabolic Responses to Injury

by **David M. Hume**

Stimuli Inducing Change

Central Nervous System and Endocrine Changes

Hormones with Generally Increased Secretion in Trauma
Hormones with Unaltered or Decreased Secretion in Trauma
    Goals of Endocrine Changes

Metabolic Changes

Energy Metabolism
Starvation
    Role of the Hormones in Altered Metabolism of Starvation
Metabolic Effects of Injury
Carbohydrate Metabolism
Fat Metabolism
Protein Metabolism
Blood Coagulation
Wound Healing
Therapeutic Considerations
    Nutritional Supplementation
    Component Therapy

Acid-Base Balance and Water and Electrolyte Metabolism

Alkalosis
Acidosis
Water and Electrolyte Metabolism

Oxygen Transport

Immunologic Protective Mechanisms

Organ System Changes

Cardiovascular Function
Pulmonary Function
Hepatic Function
Gastrointestinal Function
Renal Function

General Considerations

Injury comes in so many variegated forms that it is no small wonder that response to injury may also be quite variable. There are, however, endocrine and metabolic changes that are common to many kinds of injury and that when taken together constitute the body's response to trauma on an elemental and nonspecific plane. These responses are sometimes greatly modified by anesthesia, fluid and electrolyte replacement, transfusion, and other surgical and anesthetic iatrogens, so that identical injuries produced, on the one hand, by an automobile accident and, on the other, during a planned and controlled operation under general anesthesia may lead to courses which vary considerably either in magnitude or direction of response.

Furthermore, adaptation to certain kinds of injury may occur—e.g., to Noble-Collip drum shock or hemorrhagic shock in the rat, altitude hypoxia and poisons in man—thus increasing an already marked individual variation in response.

In this initial chapter consideration will be given to some of the factors producing the changes consequent upon injury, the mechanisms through which they are known or speculated to act, and the changes themselves. Some specific examples will be given to illustrate patient management problems related to trauma, together with their suggested solutions.

STIMULI INDUCING CHANGE

Once an injury has been incurred, a series of endocrine and metabolic events follow. Some of the factors directly responsible for inciting these changes will be briefly discussed.

AFFERENT NERVE STIMULI FROM THE INJURED AREA. This is a tremendously important factor in the initiation of many of the endocrine changes that follow injury, particularly those related to increased ACTH and cortisol secretion. We have shown that in dogs abdominal laparotomy, burns, or severe trauma failed to produce an increased ACTH release if the traumatized area had been denervated so that afferent impulses from it failed to reach the brain. Trauma to the area which remained innervated continued to produce a normal response. This absence of increased ACTH release was also shown to be true for paraplegic or quadriplegic patients undergoing traumatic plastic or orthopedic procedures in the denervated area, or abdominal laparotomy for gastric resection (Figs. 1-1 and 1-2). Egdahl performed an ingenious experiment which confirmed these observations. In a series of dogs

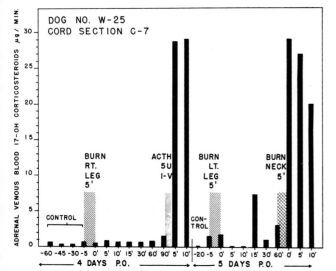

Fig. 1-1. Adrenocortical response to a burn following section of the cord at the level of C_7. A burn below the level of section produced no increase in the adrenocorticosteroid secretion over the control values. Five units of ACTH given intravenously produced an immediate marked rise in adrenocortical output. With the patient under Nembutal anesthesia a burn of the left hind leg produced no significant increase in adrenocorticosteroid output. In contrast, a burn of the neck above the level of cord section produced a marked and immediate increase in adrenocortical secretion. (*From D. M. Hume and R. H. Egdahl, Ann Surg, 150:697, 1959.*)

he divided the skin, muscle, and bone of one hind leg, thus isolating it from the body except for the femoral artery, vein, and nerve. Trauma to the innervated portion of the leg continued to evoke an increased secretion of ACTH and cortisol. The nerve was then divided, leaving the artery and vein intact. Following this, trauma no longer produced an increased secretion of ACTH (Fig. 1-3).

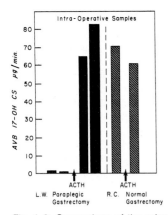

Fig. 1-2. Comparison of the adrenal venous blood 17-hydroxy-corticosteroid (17-OHCS) response to a gastric operation in a patient with spinal cord transection at T_4 with that seen in a normal patient. The paraplegic patient fails to release endogenous ACTH in response to the operation but shows a marked rise in adrenal 17-OHCS secretion following ACTH. The normal patient shows a maximal secretion of 17-OHCS in response to the operation, and no further increase is seen with ACTH. (*From D. M. Hume et al., Surgery, 52:174, 1962.*)

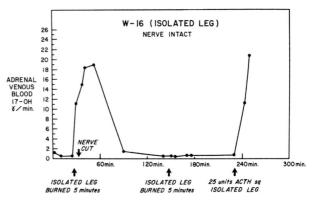

Fig. 1-3. Effect of limb denervation on ACTH secretion following trauma. The hind leg has been isolated so that it is attached to the body only by one artery, one vein, and one nerve. The burn of the isolated leg produces a marked and immediate response in adrenal venous blood corticosteroid secretion. During the height of the response the nerve was cut, and the secretion dropped rather promptly to control levels. A second burn of the same leg now produced no adrenocortical response. ACTH injected subcutaneously into the isolated leg produced a prompt and marked increase in adrenocorticosteroid secretion. (*From D. M. Hume and R. H. Egdahl, Ann Surg, 150:697, 1959.*)

HEMORRHAGE AND HYPOVOLEMIA. Many severe injuries are accompanied by hemorrhage and hypovolemia. This in itself is a strong stimulus to the secretion of renin, aldosterone, antidiuretic hormone (ADH), epinephrine, norepinephrine, cortisol, growth hormone (GH), and glucagon. The effect of hypovolemia is felt in various pressure-sensitive systems, including the aortic arch, carotid sinus, juxtaglomerular apparatus in the kidney, volume sensors in the hypothalamus, and presumably also a pressure-sensitive system in the hypothalamus the stimulation of which leads to the release of epinephrine and norepinephrine via impulses passing down the cord from these areas and out into the sympathetic nerves. Thus ADH, epinephrine, norepinephrine, cortisol, GH, renin, and aldosterone secretion occur in response to hypovolemia. Glucagon secretion is increased also, but the mechanism is unknown. In addition to this, changes in renal perfusion lead to alterations in water and salt retention, while changes in carotid sinus pressure lead to alterations in the cardiovascular system.

LOCAL WOUND FACTORS. From the discussion of the importance of afferent nerve impulses in the release of some of the hormones following injury it might appear that none of the other wound factors is an important initiator of the metabolic response to injury. This is not the case, however. Although it is true that ACTH and cortisol secretion do not increase following even rather severe trauma to a denervated area and, at least in the acute injury, wound toxins which could have a remote effect do not seem to be formed, the wound does nevertheless produce metabolic change in spite of denervation. This generally proceeds at a slower pace than that due to nerve stimulation. It is brought about in part by the collection of edema fluid, which in extensive burns and crush injury can produce hypovolemia, the loss of blood or fluid from the wound's surface, the collection of large amounts of sequestered blood in the wound (as in severe fractures), the development of sepsis and endotoxin release, and sometimes the production of chemical inflammation such as may be seen with gastric perforation, or when bile, blood, or pancreatic fluid are lost into the peritoneal cavity. The sequestration of blood may give rise to potassium absorption, hyperkalemia, and interference with cardiac action. Wound factors may be more important if the wound is located in a particularly critical area—the heart or head, for example.

SHOCK. When, as a consequence of severe hypovolemia, bacterial toxins, or myocardial infarction, or for any other reason, tissue perfusion drops to shock levels, profound metabolic disturbances occur. The decrease in tissue perfusion is made worse by direct damage to vital organs, particularly the brain, liver, heart, lungs, and kidneys. Until shock becomes profound, the chain of events set in motion by hypovolemia may appear first, followed then by changes due to organ failure and acidosis.

CHANGES IN BLOOD pH. Severe acidosis may be produced by some types of trauma including bacterial infection, prolonged shock, open heart surgical procedures with the pump-oxygenator, operations on diabetics who are out of control, temporary respiratory and cardiac arrest, and ingestion of acid, to name but a few. Acidosis itself interferes further with cellular function, and if compensatory mechanisms are blocked out or the change occurs too rapidly, death may supervene. Alkalosis may occur with trauma, particularly in patients who are on gastric suction or those with cirrhosis, who are frequently alkalotic when they go to the operating room. The development of marked alkalosis is sometimes seen in patients who are hyperventilated or those overtreated with bicarbonate. A marked change of pH in either direction from normal may be hazardous or even fatal to the patient.

INFECTION. Bacterial endotoxin is capable of providing direct hypothalamic stimulation with attendant release of ACTH, epinephrine, norepinephrine, ADH, and GH (Fig. 1-4). In additon to this, of course, severe infection has profound influences on the cardiovascular system and can, if unchecked, lead to shock and ultimately to renal, hepatic, cardiac, and cerebral failure and death.

ANESTHESIA AND OTHER DRUGS. Anesthesia has an effect upon the endocrine system, the cardiovascular system, the pulmonary and renal systems, the brain, and in fact the entire metabolism of the body. Depending upon the anesthetic agent employed, it may depress or abolish certain of the endocrine responses or stimulate or augment them. It may produce a relative hypoxia or improve oxygenation. It may produce vasodilatation or vasoconstriction, stimulate the heart or depress it. Almost all anesthetic agents, however, depress hepatic function to a greater or lesser degree. No operative trauma ought to be thought of without a consideration of the particular anesthetic agent employed, as well as the depth and duration of anesthesia.

Morphine and Nembutal tend to depress hypothalamic stimulation of ACTH release, but this depression can be overcome by operative trauma. They also depress respiration and gastrointestinal motility. Atropine produces tach-

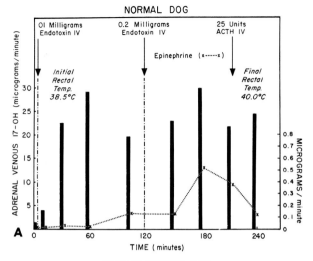

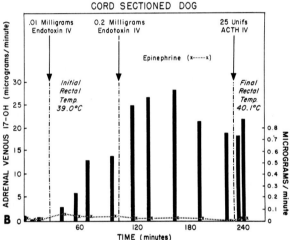

Fig. 1-4. Effects of endotoxin on 17-OHCS and epinephrine secretion. *A.* In the normal dog, a small dose of endotoxin produces a marked increase in the adrenal venous blood secretion of 17-OHCS, with almost no increase in the adrenal medullary output of epinephrine. A larger dose of endotoxin produces an increase both in 17-OHCS and epinephrine secretion in the adrenal venous blood. *B.* When the same experiment is repeated in the dog with section of the spinal cord, the endotoxin again produces a marked increase in the secretion of adrenal venous blood 17-OHCS, but now there is no increase at all in epinephrine secretion.

The experiments in *A* and *B* demonstrate that endotoxin acts at the level of the hypothalamus to stimulate the release of ACTH and also to stimulate the cells controlling the secretion of epinephrine via the spinal cord and sympathetic nerves. When the cord is cut, although the hypothalamic effect of endotoxin on ACTH release is retained, impulses can no longer pass down the cord and into the sympathetic nerves to bring about a release of epinephrine. (*From R. H. Egdahl, J Clin Invest, 38:1120, 1959.*)

ycardia and decreases salivary gland activity. Penicillin given intravenously in large doses may add a considerable potassium load. Antihypertensive drugs may lead to a marked hypotension with the induction of anesthesia, and many other commonly used drugs may have important effects in altering the response to injury.

CENTRAL NERVOUS SYSTEM INJURY. The endocrine and metabolic responses to injury may be greatly altered if the central nervous system itself is injured. Thus the patient who is in a coma from a head injury may respond very differently to a severe injury elsewhere in his body than he would if he had not had an associated head injury. Head injury can produce diabetus insipidus, abnormal salt metabolism, inappropriate secretion of ADH, depressed pulmonary and cardiac action, or arrest, shock, and death. The patient whose spinal cord is transected may have tremendous vasodilatation of the vessels in the lower part of the body and may respond very poorly to blood loss, in addition to which he will not respond with an increased ACTH secretion to severe trauma below the level of cord section.

EMOTIONAL TRAUMA. The emotional trauma of an injury may either inhibit or stimulate the endocrine response, although it usually does the latter. The effect of emotional trauma on endocrine secretion was originally demonstrated by Harris, who showed indirect evidence for an increased adrenocortical secretion in rabbits who were restrained. It was subsequently demonstrated by Ganong et al. that a tremendous rise in adrenal venous blood corticosteroid output accompanied restraint in nervous dogs (Fig. 1-5).

Everyone is familiar with the effect which emotional factors have on epinephrine release (sweating, tachycardia, dry mouth, pallor, intestinal motility, blood pressure, etc.). This factor may contribute to some of the differences between the effects of injury in the conscious state versus those of the same type of injury in the anesthetized patient.

An example of the effect of a psychic stimulus on epinephrine and corticosteroid secretion is shown in Fig. 1-12. The magnitude of the response is greater than that seen with an acute loss of 24 percent of the blood volume. Further examples are shown in Fig. 1-28.

ANOXIA. Anoxia caused, for example, by a pneumothorax due to a penetrating wound or a flail chest with rib fractures may produce profound change through tissue hypoxia. It is a strong stimulant to catecholamine release. Anoxia may be a primary trauma in itself, as it is in high altitudes or carbon monoxide poisoning.

IMMOBILIZATION. Immobilization leads to metabolic change by muscle wasting and mobilization of skeletal calcium and phosphorus. Bed rest alters the secretion of renin, aldosterone, and to some extent epinephrine and norepinephrine. It promotes thrombosis in the deep veins of the pelvis and lower extremities.

STARVATION. Many types of severe trauma are accompanied by a negative nitrogen balance brought about by starvation, at least on a temporary basis. Inadequate intake of vitamins and calories may produce considerable metabolic change, particularly if starvation is present over a long period of time.

HYPOGLYCEMIA. Hypoglycemia is a potent stimulus to the hypothalamic centers controlling the secretion of ACTH, GH, epinephrine, and norepinephrine. If it is persistent and profound, it will produce marked interference with central nervous system activity.

ENVIRONMENTAL TEMPERATURE CHANGES AND FEVER. If the trauma has a thermal component, profound general changes can be brought about by this agent alone. A hot or cold environment produces striking change in skin circulation with concomitant compensatory changes in other parts of the body. Heat and cold by themselves can each produce changes in the output of many hormones, including ACTH, cortisol, aldosterone, ADH, epinephrine, norepinephrine, thyroxin, and others. Respiration may be increased, fluid and electrolyte losses occur, and many other changes may ensue (Fig. 1-6). Fever increases catabolism, oxygen consumption, cardiac work, and water and salt loss. Ambient temperature alterations were recently shown by Redding and Mueller to have a profound effect on survival following tourniquet shock.

POISONS. Some injuries are accompanied by the addition of poisons, which may act locally or systemically. The bite of a poisonous snake is an example in which the local and general changes wrought by the injury itself are minor compared with those caused by the poison. Crush injury may be accompanied by the release of methemoglobin. Toxic bacterial products occur in injury associated with infections. Pancreatitis is accompanied by the release of pancreatic enzymes which, by virtue of their action on bile or the contents of the abdominal cavity, may produce highly toxic end products. Various other poisons, such as methyl alcohol, may have been ingested prior to the injury, giving rise to widespread metabolic changes.

WITHDRAWAL SYMPTOMS. The injured patient may be an alcoholic, and the early postoperative course may be complicated by the severe withdrawal symptoms of delirium tremens with its profound metabolic complications. The same may be said of narcotic withdrawal, or even

Fig. 1-5. Effect of forced immobilization on adrenal venous blood 17-OHCS secretion. This is shown in two groups of control dogs. Fifteen minutes after the introduction of the restraint there is an output of adrenal venous blood 17-OHCS secretion equivalent to that seen during major operative trauma as a consequence of the emotional stress of forced immobilization in untrained dogs. Lesions of the median eminence abolish this response, indicating that it is mediated by the hypothalamus. (*From W. F. Ganong et al., Fed Proc, 14:54, 1955.*)

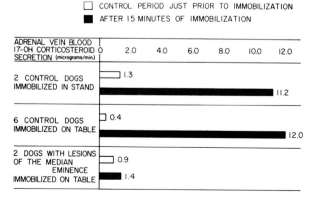

☐ CONTROL PERIOD JUST PRIOR TO IMMOBILIZATION
■ AFTER 15 MINUTES OF IMMOBILIZATION

ADRENAL VEIN BLOOD 17-OH CORTICOSTEROID SECRETION (micrograms/min.)	0 2.0 4.0 6.0 8.0 10.0 12.0
2 CONTROL DOGS IMMOBILIZED IN STAND	1.3 / 11.2
6 CONTROL DOGS IMMOBILIZED ON TABLE	0.4 / 12.0
2 DOGS WITH LESIONS OF THE MEDIAN EMINENCE IMMOBILIZED ON TABLE	0.9 / 1.4

ADRENAL CORTICOSTEROID OUTPUT AND BLOOD ACTH LEVELS
IN HYPOTHERMIA

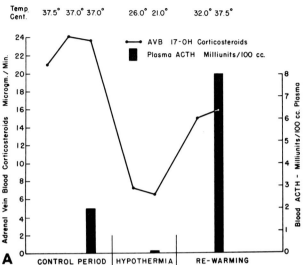

A

ADRENAL SYMPATHIN AND CORTICOSTEROID OUTPUT
IN HYPOTHERMIA

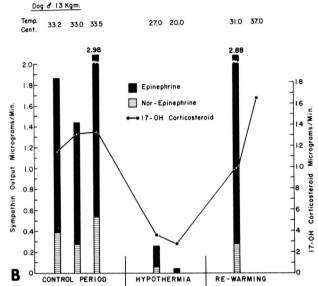

B

Fig. 1-6. Effects of hypothermia on ACTH and 17-OHCS secretion. *A.* The plasma ACTH levels and adrenal venous blood 17-OHCS output in a dog traumatized under ether anesthesia and then subjected to hypothermia. There is a marked depression of corticosteroid secretion during hypothermia with an increase again after rewarming. Blood ACTH, which is elevated before the induction of hypothermia, becomes too low to measure during hypothermia and is again easily detected after rewarming. *B.* Epinephrine, norepinephrine, and corticosteroid secretion in the adrenal venous blood of a dog traumatized under ether anesthesia before, during, and after induction of hypothermia. A marked decrease in epinephrine and norepinephrine output occurs during hypothermia, while a marked increase in the secretion of these substances is seen on rewarming. The output of 17-OHCS follows a similar pattern. (*From D. M. Hume and R. H. Egdahl, Ann NY Acad Sci, 80:435, 1959.*)

withdrawal of commonly used drugs, such as insulin—for example, in patients who are unconscious and not known to be diabetics. If the traumatic event happens to be an operation in which an adrenal tumor was removed for Cushing's disease, a large pheochromocytoma for hypertension, a parathyroid adenoma in a patient with hyperparathyroidism, an insulinoma, or the thyroid in a patient with thyrotoxicosis, severe withdrawal symptoms may complicate the metabolic response to the trauma.

ANAPHYLAXIS. Under some circumstances the overreactive response of the body to the injury can be much more devastating than the injury itself. A typical example of this is a bee sting in a patient who is hypersensitive to bee stings. Under these circumstances a bee sting may produce shock, coma, and death, the devastating chain of events occurring because of the body's pathologic hypersensitivity response to the antigen.

Thus it may be seen that there are many stimuli producing their effects through many different pathways in different kinds of trauma. Very frequently there are several stimuli to endocrine and metabolic change working simultaneously in the same patient.

CENTRAL NERVOUS SYSTEM AND ENDOCRINE CHANGES

In response to the stimuli discussed above rather profound changes occur in the endocrine system, in metabolism in general, and in certain organs in particular. Some of these changes and the mechanisms by which they are brought about will be described briefly.

The initial stimulus for the release of ACTH, cortisol, GH, epinephrine and norepinephrine, and to some extent ADH and aldosterone depends upon afferent nerve impulses emanating in the injured area and transmitted up the cord to the brain (Fig. 1-7). These impulses travel along pain pathways and in the reticular formation and terminate both in cortical stimulation and in hypothalamic stimulation. Cortical stimulation may lead either to enhancing or inhibiting effects (Fig. 1-8).

Control of the secretion of several hormones, anterior pituitary and others, lies in the hypothalamus. These general control areas are shown in Fig. 1-9. ADH is manufactured in the supraoptic nucleus and stored in the posterior lobe, while oxytocin is made in the paraventricular nucleus and stored in the posterior lobe. Long fiber tracts from these nuclei course down the lateral side of the median eminence and terminate in the posterior pituitary. A group

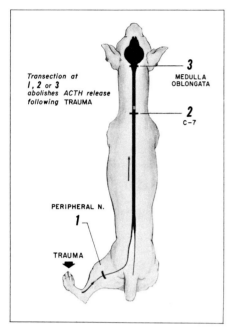

Fig. 1-7. Effects of cord transection on ACTH release following trauma. Trauma to the hind leg no longer leads to pituitary adrenocortical activation after transection at any of the three locations indicated in the diagram. It is thus apparent that an afferent nerve impulse has to reach the brain in order to produce ACTH release in response to peripheral trauma. (*From D. M. Hume and R. H. Egdahl, Ann Surg, 150:697, 1959.*)

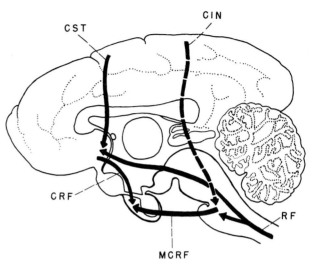

Fig. 1-8. Cortical enhancing and inhibiting effects on ACTH release following trauma. Following peripheral trauma afferent impulses ascend from the injured area, probably via the reticular formation (RF). These impulses stimulate cells in the lower brain stem and in the hypothalamus. Descending stimulatory psychic impulses from the cortex of the brain (CST) are also capable of exciting the hypothalamic control centers. As a consequence of these and other stimuli the ACTH control center in the hypothalamus secretes a corticotropin-releasing factor (CRF), which leads to ACTH release from the anterior pituitary. Cortical inhibitory influences (CIN) are also present, and these normally totally inhibit the release of the lower brainstem corticotropin-releasing factor (MCRF). In the absence of the cortex of the brain the inhibitory mechanism is gone and MCRF is released, causing ACTH secretion from the pituitary even the absence of the hypothalamus. (*From D. M. Hume and R. H. Egdahl, Ann Surg, 150:697, 1959.*)

of cells at the posterior part of the supraoptic nucleus lying more mediad than the others (Fig. 1-10) elaborate a hormone known as CRF (corticotropin-releasing factor). This substance is responsible for the release of corticosteroidogenic ACTH from the anterior pituitary. CRF is a polypeptide very similar to ADH and oxytocin in composition but distinctly separate from them in action, site of production, and area of maximal concentration. While ADH travels down the nerve axons to be stored in the posterior lobe and released into the bloodstreams from this organ, CRF is released directly into the capillary loops of the hypophyseoportal system, whence it is carried into the substance of the anterior lobe, where it stimulates the cells manufacturing ACTH (Fig. 1-11). This system is more fully discussed in Chap. 37.

Slightly above the CRF area but overlapping it is an area which releases a hormone (thyrotropin-releasing factor), which helps to regulate the secretion of TSH (thyroid-stimulating hormone) to control thyroid activity. This system is much more loosely put together than the one controlling ACTH secretion, however, and does not exert the autonomy over TSH release seen for the CRF-ACTH system.

An area which has some control over the release of GH is said to lie generally in the area shown in the diagram. Here again the control is not as absolute as that seen for ACTH release.

Farther back in the median eminence just anterior to the mammillary bodies is the area for the control of follicle-stimulating hormone (FSH) and luteinizing hormone (LH) secretion. This area exerts very strict control over the release of the gonadotropins from the pituitary, and small lesions here exert as profound an effect as hypophysectomy. Scattered throughout the hypothalamus are areas for the control of epinephrine and norepinephrine secretion. These are somewhat more generally concentrated in the posterior part of the hypothalamus, while areas for the control of the vagus nerve are located generally in the anterior part of the hypothalamus. When the nerve impulses reach the hypothalamus, they stimulate the control centers for some of the anterior pituitary hormones, and this is followed very promptly by the release of that hormone and a secondary alteration of the activity of its target organ.

Apart from its neuroendocrine functions, the hypothalamus also exerts an influence over heat production and temperature regulation in injury.

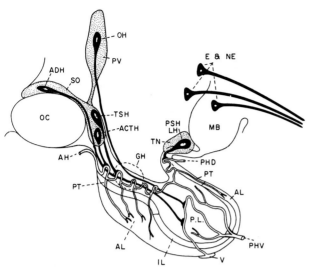

Fig. 1-9. Hypothalamic centers for the control of various endocrine secretions. The cells for the control of ADH secretion are located in the supraoptic (SO) nucleus, and their axons extend all the way down into the posterior lobe of the pituitary, whence ADH is released into the bloodstream. Cells for the control of the release of the oxytocic hormone (OH) are located in the paraventricular (PV) nucleus, and their axons likewise extend down into the posterior lobe, where their hormones can be released into the bloodstream. The center controlling the release of ACTH is located in the posterior part of the supraoptic nucleus, and its axons end in foot plates which are applied to the hypophyseoportal system of capillary loops. The hormone produced by the cells, corticotropin-releasing factor (CRF), is released into the capillary loops, whence it makes its way to the anterior lobe to stimulate the release of ACTH. A similar system obtains for the release of thyroid-stimulating hormone (TSH), and these cell groups are located in close proximity to those for ACTH control but slightly above and anterior to them. The control of TSH secretion is much more casual and less complete than that for ACTH secretion. The cells controlling the release of the gonadotropic hormones are located in the tuberal nucleus (TN). The control of follicle-stimulating hormone (FSH) and luteinizing hormone (LH) is brought about by hypophyseoportal system of capillary loops coming into the posterior part of the median eminence. Cells for the control of epinephrine (E) and norepinephrine (NE) secretion are located in the posterior part of the hypothalamus, and their axons run down the spinal cord, where they are transmitted to sympathetic nerves controlling the adrenal medulla and the peripheral sympathetics. Other structures on the diagram are the optic chiasm (OC); the mammillary body (MB); the control center for the release of growth hormone (GH), about which relatively little is known; the anterior hypophyseal artery (AH); the dorsal branch of the posterior hypophyseal artery (PHD) and the ventral branch of the same artery (PHV); a vein (V) draining the posterior lobe (PL); the intermediate lobe (IL), the anterior lobe (AL); and the pars tuberalis (PT).

Hormones with Generally Increased Secretion in Trauma

ACTH—CORTISOL

Most types of trauma are characterized by an increased secretion of ACTH and thus of cortisol. A more profound response is seen when the magnitude of the trauma is great, when infection, hemorrhage, and emotional trauma are present, and when stimulating anesthetic agents such as ether are used. The response is diminished or abolished by cord section, preexisting pituitary or adrenal disease, and certain inhibitory anesthetic agents, such as Nembutal and Pentothal (Figs. 1-12 through 1-18).

EFFECTS OF EXOGENOUS CORTICOSTEROIDS. The exogenous administration of corticosteroids partially inhibits ACTH, apparently at a hypothalamic level, and leads to decreased adrenal stimulation, atrophy, and finally very little production of corticosteroid. Even large doses of corticosteroids may not completely inhibit the release of ACTH customarily seen in response to trauma, but if the adrenal is sufficiently atrophic, even a large dose of ACTH will fail to arouse the adrenal cortex acutely to produce an increased output of corticosteroids. Continued trauma or continued ACTH administration will again

Fig. 1-10. Horizontal view through the median eminence. This indicates some of the relationships of the supraoptic nucleus (SON) and the tuberal nucleus to the hypophyseoportal blood vessels. The laterally placed axons of the supraoptic nucleus concerned with the production and release of ADH travel down into the posterior lobe (PL), as shown in the diagram. The more mediad placed cells of the postoptic (PO) part of the nucleus terminate in the anterior portion of the median eminence on the hypophyseoportal capillaries. A lesion made at the point indicated by A will abolish the ACTH response to trauma without producing diabetes insipidus. A lesion made at the point indicated by B will produce diabetes insipidus without interfering with ACTH release. If a lesion is made at the level indicated by A but is somewhat larger, extending laterally, it will produce both diabetes insipidus and a failure of ACTH release in response to trauma. The cells of the tuberal nucleus which control gonadotropin release terminate in the posterior part of the median eminence on capillary loops of the posterior portion of the hypophyseoportal system. Their action is unaffected by lesions located either at A or B.

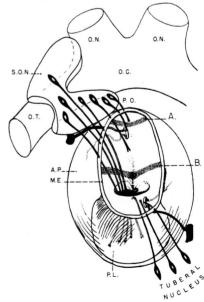

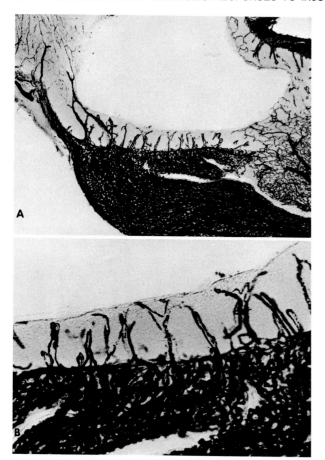

Fig. 1-11. Sagittal section of the hypothalamus and pituitary of the dog. A. The brain has been injected with India ink to show the vascular supply. The open area above is the third ventricle, while the clear area with the capillary loops is the median eminence. A portion of the posterior lobe is shown to the right, and the anterior lobe is the dark area to the left and below. At the extreme left, superiorly, is the optic chiasm. Connections can be seen between the vessels of the posterior lobe of the pituitary and the capillary loops in the median eminence. The capillary loops transmitting the hormones controlling gonadotropin secretion to the anterior lobe are in the extreme upper right hand corner of the picture, while those controlling ACTH and TSH secretion are in the anterior portion of the median eminence. B. High-powered view of the median eminence superiorly and the anterior lobe below. The optic chiasm is to the right, but out of view. The capillary loops may be seen projecting up into the median eminence and then descending down into the anterior pituitary.

stimulate corticosteroidogenesis in the adrenal cortex, with the production of cortisol. Patients who have been on steroid administration for long periods of time, whose adrenal has become atrophic, and who are not given corticosteroids to support them during an operation have sometimes died because of the failure of cortisol release from an adrenal rendered temporarily inactive by atrophy.

ADRENAL INSUFFICIENCY. If a patient with unsuspected adrenal insufficiency is inadvertently operated upon without being supported with exogenous corticosteroids, death

is likely to ensue. Thus cortisol is necessary for the normal response in trauma. Severe adrenal insufficiency (Addison's disease) is more fully discussed in the section on the adrenal (see Chap. 37). For purposes of the present discussion it is important to recognize that severe insufficiency may be seen in several forms. It may first be noted in the immediate newborn period, when it occurs as part of the adrenogenital syndrome. It is particularly hard to recognize in males, who, unlike females, do not show any physical stigmata of the syndrome. In females, the syndrome may be suspected because of enlargement of the clitoris. It is manifested by fever, weight loss, vomiting, hyponatremia, shock, and marked salt loss in the urine. These symptoms usually appear in the first week after birth but sometimes do not become manifest for 5 or 6 weeks. The disease is caused by an enzymatic defect in the adrenal cortex which leads to failure of hydroxylation at the C_{11}, C_{20}, or C_{21} positions. Addison's disease is particularly apt to occur when the defect is in C_{20} or C_{21} hydroxylation. A C_{20} block produces a general deficiency of corticosteroids. No survivals have ever been reported. A C_{21} defect with Addison's disease can be successfully treated if recognized (Fig. 1-19).

If chronic adrenal insufficiency is present prior to the time of surgical treatment and is unrecognized, death is likely to occur within a matter of hours after operation has begun. Typically adrenal insufficiency is characterized by pigmentation, weakness, weight loss, hypotension, easy fatigability, nausea, vomiting, abdominal pain, hypoglycemia, hyponatremia, and hyperkalemia. Operative intervention will precipitate an acute Addisonian crisis leading to death if treatment is not promptly instituted.

The most common kind of adrenal insufficiency is seen in patients who have been on corticosteroid medication for some period of time. Patients should always be questioned preoperatively to determine whether they have been on corticosteroid medication either in pill form or in an ointment.

A semiacute type of adrenal insufficiency occurs when the adrenal damage takes place at the time of, or shortly after, the operative event. This has occasionally been seen in patients who were given heparin and developed bilateral adrenal hemorrhages in the postoperative period, and of course it occurs automatically when the operation is a bilateral adrenalectomy. Here, however, exogenous corticosteroids are administered to compensate for the failure of endogenous secretion. If the condition is unrecognized, the patients tend to get along fairly well for 3 or 4 days, after which increasing difficulties develop which may lead to severe hyponatremia, hypoglycemia, and death if untreated.

The hormones secreted by the adrenal cortex are shown in Fig. 1-20, and their relative secretion rates are shown in Table 1-1 and Fig. 1-21. The adrenal androgens and estrogens seem relatively unimportant in the response to trauma, but cortisol and aldosterone are of the utmost importance. A diagram showing the pathways for the secretion of cortisol may be seen in Fig. 1-22. The degradation of cortisol takes place by reduction to tetrahydrocortisol and conjugation with glucuronic acid or sulfuric acid. When these steps have taken place, the cortisol becomes highly water-soluble and can be readily excreted in urine. Since the liver is responsible for reduction and conjugation of corticosteroids, severe liver disease may interfere with this step, and the level of blood conjugates may be very low. The kidney is responsible for excreting the vast majority of the conjugated cortisol, so that the presence of kidney disease permits extremely high levels of the conjugates to build up in the bloodstream. The reduced and conjugated corticosteroid is no longer biologically effective.

Despite the obvious demonstration that an increased secretion of cortisol occurs in response to almost all types of trauma, that cortisol is necessary for the organism to withstand trauma successfully, and that patients with unrecognized adrenal insufficiency die following trauma whereas patients with bilateral adrenalectomy can tolerate trauma if given exogenous cortisol, adrenal insufficiency is rarely the cause of death after injury.

It was demonstrated by Ingle that adrenalectomized animals traumatized while on a constant dose of corticosteroids showed some of the metabolic changes formerly ascribed to an *increased* secretion of these hormones, and this effect has been termed by him the "permissive" action of corticosteroids. Furthermore paraplegic patients, who fail to respond to operative trauma with an increased secretion of cortisol, generally tolerate the operative procedure well. These seeming paradoxes may be explained, at least in part, in the following ways:

In severe trauma hepatic conjugation of corticosteroids into the inactive form may be reduced, so that larger amounts of unconjugated (active) corticosteroids are suddenly available even though the rate of infusion or secretion remains constant. The secretion of cortisol in the paraplegic remains low despite trauma because of the absence of afferent nerve impulses, but it can still increase if uncompensated hemorrhage or infection supervenes or if hypothalamic stimulation results from hypoglycemia or an excitatory anesthetic agent. The secretion of aldosterone is increased in trauma despite the absence of increased ACTH release (Fig. 1-23), and this hormone helps to

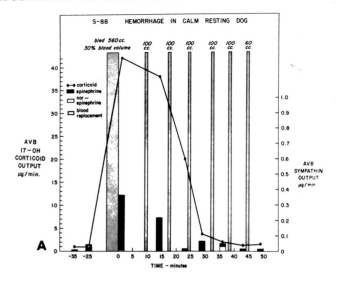

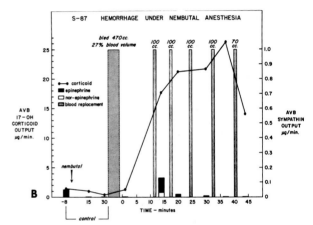

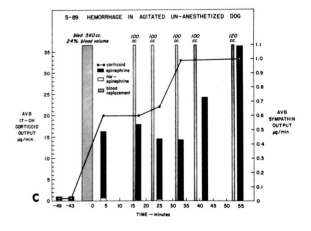

Fig. 1-12. Effects of anesthesia and agitation on 17-OHCS, epinephrine, and norepinephrine secretion in response to bleeding. *A.* Adrenal venous blood 17-OHCS, epinephrine, and norepinephrine secretion in the conscious dog during blood withdrawal and replacement. There is a marked increase in the secretion of 17-OHCS and epinephrine in response to the withdrawal of blood, and this secretion gradually returns to the base-line levels as the blood is replaced. *B.* When the same experiment is conducted under Nembutal anesthesia, there is still an increase in adrenal venous blood 17-OHCS output, but the epinephrine response to bleeding is now almost absent. *C.* The experiment shown in *A* is repeated, but an untrained agitated dog is used. There is again an increase in 17-OHCS and epinephrine secretion in response to bleeding, but this time, as the blood is replaced, there is a continued increase in the output of both hormones as a result of the emotional stimulus of restraint, and this persists even when all the blood has been replaced. (*From D. M. Hume. Fed Proc, 20 [Suppl 9]: 1, 1961.*)

support the response to injury through sodium retention and maintenance of blood pressure, although its effects on carbohydrate metabolism are negligible. Finally, an operative trauma is far better tolerated in patients whose body cells have not been deprived of the adrenal corticosteroids

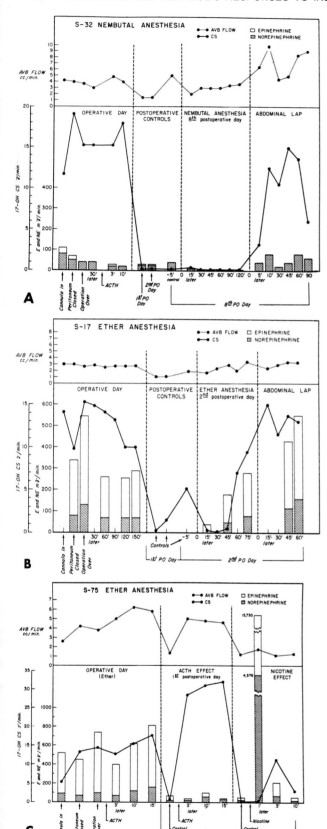

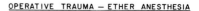

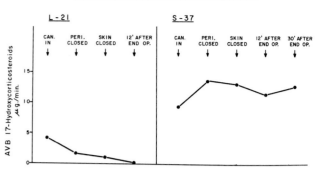

Fig. 1-14. Effects of anterior median eminence lesion on 17-OHCS secretion with operative trauma. Adrenal venous blood corticosteroid secretion in response to operative trauma. At the left are the values obtained in a dog with a lesion of the anterior median eminence. At the right are the values obtained in a normal control animal. A very minimal response was seen in the animal with the hypothalamic lesion, and the values declined during the course of the operation. In contrast, there was an excellent response in the normal animal which continued throughout the operative and immediate postoperative period. This illustrates the importance of the hypothalamus to the release of ACTH in response to trauma. (*From D. M. Hume, "Reticular Formation of the Brain," p. 231, Little, Brown and Company, Boston, 1958.*)

preoperatively than one in whom preexisting deficiency is present. For this reason the patient who has adrenal insufficiency because of Addison's disease will tolerate the immediate operative event less well than a normal patient whose adrenals are removed without his being given corti-

Fig. 1-13. Effects of Nembutal and ether anesthesia on 17-OHCS, epinephrine, and norepinephrine in dogs undergoing laparotomy. *A.* Adrenal venous blood 17-OHCS, epinephrine, and norepinephrine secretion in a dog undergoing abdominal laparotomy under Nembutal anesthesia, in the postoperative period, during Nembutal anesthesia alone, and with a second abdominal laparotomy under Nembutal anesthesia. The adrenal venous blood flow in milliliters per minute is given in the top portion of the chart. It may be seen that a very good response of 17-OHCS secretion occurs with the operative trauma and that this drops to low levels in the immediate postoperative period. Nembutal anesthesia itself has no effect on the secretion of 17-OHCS, but a second abdominal laparotomy again produces a marked increase in the secretion of this substance. There is no increase in the secretion of epinephrine or norepinephrine in response to Nembutal anesthesia and only a very modest increase in the secretion of these substances in response to operative trauma. *B.* The same experiment performed under ether anesthesia. Here there is not only a marked increase in 17-OHCS secretion in response to operation, but there is also a marked increase in the secretion of epinephrine and norepinephrine. Epinephrine, norepinephrine, and 17-OHCS secretion are stimulated by ether anesthesia alone, and further stimulation occurs as a consequence of a second abdominal laparotomy. *C.* A similar experiment but with ACTH given on the first postoperative day, producing a marked increase in 17-OHCS secretion without any significant change in epinephrine or norepinephrine secretion. By contrast an injection of nicotine produces a tremendous increase in epinephrine and norepinephrine secretion with only a very slight increase in the output of 17-OHCS. (*From D. M. Hume, Fed Proc, 20 [Suppl 9]: 1, 1961.*)

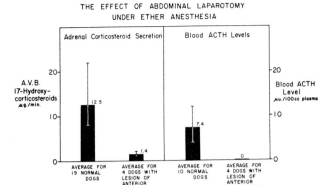

Fig. 1-15. Effect of anterior median eminence lesion on 17-OHCS and ACTH secretion during laparotomy: the adrenal venous blood 17-OHCS secretion and the blood ACTH level in response to operative trauma in normal dogs contrasted to dogs with lesions of the anterior median eminence. The solid bars represent mean values and the vertical lines the range of values. It may be seen that the animals with hypothalamic lesions show a markedly reduced pituitary and adrenal response to trauma. (*From D. M. Hume, "Reticular Formation of the Brain," p. 231, Little, Brown and Company, Boston, 1958.*)

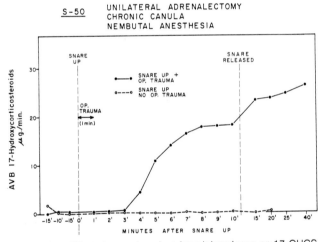

Fig. 1-16. Effect of nerve impulses from injured area on 17-OHCS secretion. This experiment was performed on an animal with a unilateral adrenalectomy and a cannula placed in the adrenal vein of the opposite side. The animal was put to sleep under Nembutal anesthesia, and after a series of base-line measurements a snare around the medial end of the adrenal view was pulled up so that all of the secretion of the only remaining adrenal drained to the outside over a period of 20 minutes. This had the effect of suddenly stopping all adrenal secretion into the blood of the animal, but this sudden hypoadrenalism did not produce a stimulus to ACTH release or increase in the secretion of 17-OHCS. After releasing the snare again, and following a suitable control period, the experiment was repeated exactly as before except that this time after the control period and the pulling up of the snare the animal was suddenly severely traumatized. Within 2 minutes there was a marked increase in adrenal venous blood 17-OHCS secretion. This indicates that the release of ACTH in response to trauma is not brought about as a consequence of a sudden diminution in blood levels of 17-OHCS but is instead stimulated by nervous impulses originating in the injured area.

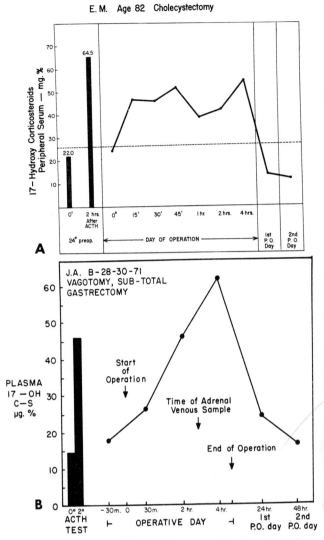

Fig. 1-17. Comparison of 17-OHCS increases following surgical procedures and ACTH injection. *A.* The response to cholecystectomy in an eighty-two-year-old patient. There is a marked increase in the level of plasma 17-OHCS during the operative procedure which rapidly returns to normal levels on the day after operation. The response to operative trauma is not quite as high as the response to an injection of ACTH. *B.* The plasma 17-OHCS response to a vagotomy and subtotal gastrectomy. There is a marked increase in the levels of 17-OHCS on the operative day, the values returning to normal the day after operation. The peak response was even greater than that seen with ACTH. This operation was of somewhat greater magnitude than the cholecystectomy shown in *A.*

sol or one whose adrenals are suppressed by prolonged corticosteroid administration which is stopped abruptly at operation. Nevertheless it should be emphasized that when in the past bilateral adrenalectomy was attempted in patients prior to the availability of cortisone, it was universally fatal, and hypophysectomy without corticosteroid support was likewise accompanied by an increased mortality, though hypophysectomy was far better tolerated than

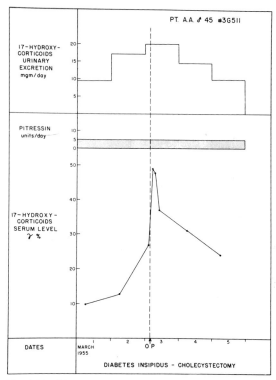

Fig. 1-18. Urinary and plasma 17-OHCS values in a patient with diabetes insipidus undergoing cholecystectomy. The patient was maintained on a constant dose of Pitressin before and after the operation. In spite of the absence of endogenous ADH production, the patient showed a very normal increase in 17-OHCS secretion in response to the operative trauma. This indicates the fact that, although CRF is very similar to ADH, it is not ADH. It is possible to have a lesion which will prevent the production of ADH without interfering with the production of CRF. (See also Fig. 1-10.)

adrenalectomy in the absence of corticosteroid administration.

Adrenal exhaustion, which was once thought to occur following prolonged trauma, probably never occurs. Most patients who die following injury, sepsis, burns, infection and other forms of severe prolonged trauma die with very high blood levels of corticosteroids (Fig. 1-24). In fact the very existence of continued high levels of plasma corticosteroids in the severely burned patient is usually a bad prognostic sign, suggesting that the trauma of burns is continuing and severe (Figs. 1-24 and 1-25). Nonetheless there is an occasional burned patient who shows evidences of adrenal insufficiency; there is an occasional patient in whom it develops in response to bilateral adrenal hemorrhage due to anticoagulant therapy; and there is an occasional patient in whom prolonged corticosteroid administration or preexisting Addison's disease has been unrecognized at the time of operation. Since the operative event is so apt to be fatal under these circumstances and since excellent replacement therapy is now available, adrenal insufficiency becomes an important and preventable cause of postoperative demise, despite its rarity. The causes and manifestations of adrenal insufficiency are dealt with further in the chapter on the adrenal (Chap. 37).

The Waterhouse-Friderichsen syndrome, which consists of bilateral adrenal hemorrhage in patients, usually children, with meningococcal septicemia, was originally thought to produce death as a consequence of adrenal failure. When death occurs in this condition, however, it occurs very rapidly and is due to the meningococcal septicemia—the adrenal hemorrhage occurring as a terminal complication and an almost incidental finding. These patients die with elevated blood cortisol levels.

When the patient has been found to have adrenal insufficiency, replacement therapy is given. While orally or intravenously administered cortisol is effective almost at once, intramuscularly administered cortisol acetate is slowly absorbed and does not become maximally effective until 12 to 18 hours after administration. Initial therapy therefore always should be intravenous.

RENIN

Most traumatic events are accompanied by an increased secretion of renin, presumed to be brought about by a fall in perfusion pressure of the afferent arterioles in the renal cortex. The juxtaglomerular apparatus, whose cells are in close proximity to the afferent arteriole, is presumed to be responsive to changes in the afferent arteriolar perfusion pressure, so that its cells secrete renin into the renal venous blood and lymph (see Chap. 23). The renin in turn activates angiotensinogen (made in the liver) into angiotensin I, which is then converted in the bloodstream into angiotensin II. Angiotensin II stimulates the adrenal cortex to secrete aldosterone. Angiotensin II (hypertensin) has a hypertensive effect of its own and is sometimes used to treat hypotension.

ALDOSTERONE

The increased secretion of aldosterone seen in response to injury emanates principally from the renin-angiotensin stimulus. However, its secretion is further enhanced by the increased ACTH secretion that routinely accompanies trauma and by the falling sodium and rising potassium values which occur in some types of injury. While the effect of ACTH on increased cortisol production is an essential

Fig. 1-19. Steroid nucleus showing, in the circles, three of the defects which may be seen with congenital adrenal hyperplasia. A defect located at A produces hypertension, one located at B produces severe salt wasting and hypotension, and one located at C is usually fatal.

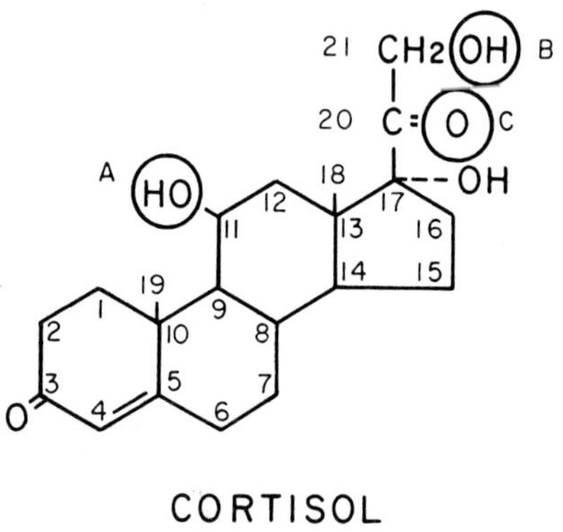

CORTISOL

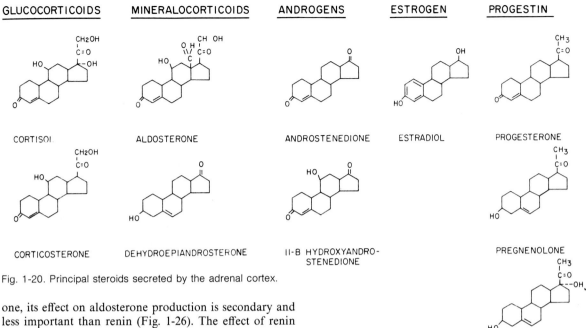

Fig. 1-20. Principal steroids secreted by the adrenal cortex.

one, its effect on aldosterone production is secondary and less important than renin (Fig. 1-26). The effect of renin and aldosterone is to maintain the blood pressure and conserve sodium as a compensatory mechanism for combating hypovolemia.

EPINEPHRINE AND NOREPINEPHRINE

Epinephrine and norepinephrine are both secreted in response to trauma, although the amounts of these substances secreted during operative trauma depend to a considerable extent on the anesthesia employed. Ether, for example, is a strong stimulus to epinephrine release, whereas Nembutal inhibits it almost entirely (see Fig. 1-13). The increased secretion of epinephrine and norepi-

nephrine is quite short-lived and is usually limited to the day of trauma unless the injury is a very severe and continuing one. During operative trauma, with the anesthetic agents commonly employed, there is a greater total secretion of norepinephrine than of epinephrine. This is probably because the entire source of epinephrine is from the adrenal medulla whereas norepinephrine is also secreted from the sympathetic nerve endings (Figs. 1-27 and 1-28). There is a greater secretion of epinephrine in the adrenal venous blood than of norepinephrine, though this is not striking (Fig. 1-29).

The effect of epinephrine and norepinephrine secretion is to increase cardiac output and elevate the blood pressure. It is brought about both by changes in blood volume

Fig. 1-21. Adrenal venous blood glucocorticoid secretion in man during operative trauma, at rest, and after an injection of ACTH. The principal glucocorticoid is cortisol (compound F), and the second is corticosterone (compound B). Only small amounts of cortisone (compound E and compound S) are secreted. (*From D. M. Hume et al., Surgery, 52:174, 1962.*)

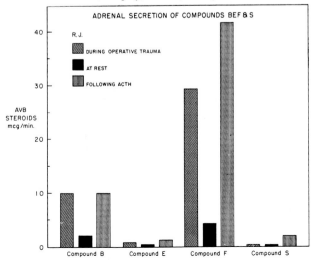

Table 1-1. DAILY SECRETION RATES OF HORMONES

Compound	Mean 24-hr secretion rate
Cortisol, mg	15–30
Corticosterone, mg	2–5
Aldosterone, μg	50–150
Dehydroepiandrosterone, mg.	15–30
Androstenedione, mg	0–10
Hydroxyandrostenedione, mg	0–10
Progesterone, mg	0.4–0.8
Pregnenolone, mg	0.5–0.8
17-OH pregnenolone, mg.	0.2–0.4
Estradiol, mg	Trace

SOURCE: From P. H. Forsham, The Adrenal Cortex, in R. H. Williams (ed.); "Textbook of Endocrinology," p. 287, W. B. Saunders Company, Philadelphia, 1968.

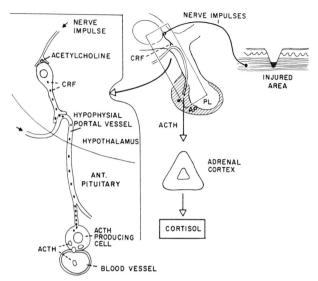

Fig. 1-22. Pathways for secretion of cortisol. The increased secretion of cortisol in response to injury comes about as a consequence of nerve impulses from the injured area to the hypothalamus where CRF is released and carried to the anterior lobe of the pituitary via the hypophyseoportal system. Here the CRF stimulates the ACTH-producing cells to release ACTH into the bloodstream, and this substance in turn stimulates the adrenal cortex to secrete cortisol. Hypotension, endotoxin, emotional stress, and various other factors can affect the hypothalamus directly to bring about the secretion of cortisol.

Fig. 1-23. Effect of ACTH on adrenal venous blood aldosterone secretion. No further increase in aldosterone secretion is seen in patient I. P. when ACTH is injected intraoperatively. This patient had an adequate endogenous release of ACTH. An increase in aldosterone secretion is seen in patient L. W., who had virtually no ACTH release during operation as a consequence of paraplegia. ACTH produced an increased aldosterone secretion in two of three patients to whom it was administered in the resting state. (*From D. M. Hume et al., Surgery, 52:174, 1962.*)

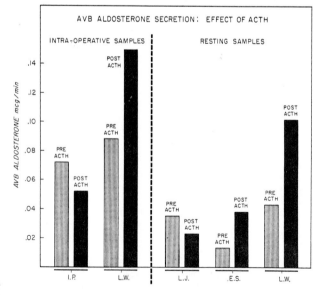

(see Fig. 1-12) and by afferent sensory impulses impinging on the hypothalamus (Fig. 1-9). Cells in the posterior part of the hypothalamus are stimulated, sending impulses down the cord to the intermediolateral cell columns and out into the sympathetic efferents. Adrenal medullary secretory activity is brought about through the splanchnic sympathetics. Denervation of the adrenal stops the secretion of catecholamines in the adrenal venous blood. Some noxious stimuli, such as endotoxin, can act directly upon the hypothalamic sympathetic control centers producing epinephrine and norepinephrine release (see Fig. 1-4). Hypoglycemia is also a stimulus to epinephrine and norepinephrine release. This apparently acts at a hypothalamic level. While histamine in large doses is a potent stimulus to epinephrine release, it is doubtful whether the amounts of histamine released physiologically play any role in the increased secretion of catecholamines seen in response to trauma.

ANTIDIURETIC HORMONE (ADH)

Most trauma is accompanied by an increased secretion of ADH brought about by afferent neural stimuli impinging upon the hypothalamus. Stimulation of the supraoptic nucleus leads to a release of ADH from the posterior pituitary. Hypovolemia is also a potent stimulus to ADH release, presumably through the mediation of pressor receptors located in the hypothalamus. The pressor receptors are homeostatic mechanisms for the maintenance of normovolemia. The role of ADH in trauma is to conserve water, which is a worthwhile goal. There are, however, ways in which the secretion of ADH in trauma may be detrimental to the patient. If, for example, hypotension and shock are prolonged so that renal blood flow is severely compromised, the secretion of ADH tends to compound the renal injury. It is possible experimentally to select a degree of renal ischemia which will invariably lead to acute tubular necrosis when ADH is administered and which will not be damaging when ADH secretion is prevented. Furthermore ADH secretion contributes to the production of dilutional hyponatremia in the postoperative state by prompting water retention.

With head injury two additional peculiarities in ADH secretion sometimes occur. The first of these is called *inappropriate ADH secretion.* This is a term given to excessive secretion of ADH beyond that needed to promote homeostasis. The ADH secretion continues after the initial period of damage and produces a low urinary output with high osmolarity and a profound dilutional hyponatremia (see Chap. 42). The converse phenomenon of diabetes insipidus is sometimes seen with head injury, particularly basilar skull fractures. This may be either temporary or permanent and results from damage to the supraopticohypophyseal system. It may cause severe dehydration or even death in patients with head injury and coma who are given tube feedings. Since the patient is comatose, he cannot express thirst, and a continued excessive polyuria dehydrates him, leading to hypernatremia. This is compounded by the use of tube feedings high in sodium, small protein fractions, and glucose, which thus combines an

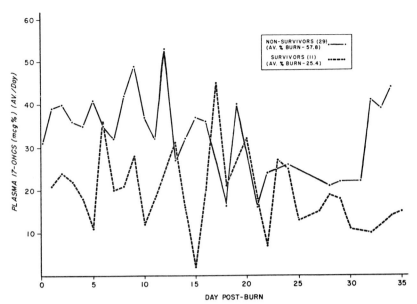

Fig. 1-24. Plasma 17-OHCS values in burn patients. It may be seen that the values in those patients who ultimately recovered gradually declined during the postburn period, whereas those patients who did not survive had higher values at first and later showed gradually increasing values up to the time of death.

excessive sodium load with an osmotic diuresis, further dehydrating the patient.

GH

There is a hypothalamic center which helps to control the release of GH (see Fig. 1-9). This center is sensitive to hypoglycemia, and GH release can be easily triggered by insulin administration. This center is activated in trauma both by neural impulses and by blood loss. Meyer and Knobil have found hemorrhage to be a potent stimulus to GH release in monkeys, and Carey et al. have found war wounds to be strong stimuli to GH release in man.

Hypoglycemia has long been known to be the strongest stimulus to GH release, but this is certainly not the stimulus to the secretion of GH in most injury, which is characterized by hyperglycemia to which GH contributes. Certain

amino acids stimulate GH release as well, and Carey et al. postulate that elevated plasma amino acid levels seen in injury are responsible for the increase in GH secretion. Again, this seems unlikely, as plasma amino acid levels usually are not elevated in injury, and arginine concentration, which is the best stimulus to GH release, decreases.

Fig. 1-25. Relationship between plasma 17-OHCS and percentage of burn. It may be seen that the more severe the burn, the higher in general were the plasma 17-OHCS values.

Fig. 1-26. Stimuli to the secretion of aldosterone. The principal stimulus to the secretion of aldosterone is a decrease in intravascular volume. This produces a decreased tension on the afferent arteriole in the kidney, which in turn stimulates the juxtaglomerular cells to release renin into the bloodstream. Renin combines with angiotensinogen from the liver to form angiotensin I. This substance is converted by a special enzyme into angiotensin II in the peripheral bloodstream. Angiotensin II stimulates the adrenal cortex to release aldosterone. ACTH from the anterior pituitary also has some effect on aldosterone production but considerably less than angiotensin II. An increased blood level of potassium likewise stimulates aldosterone release.

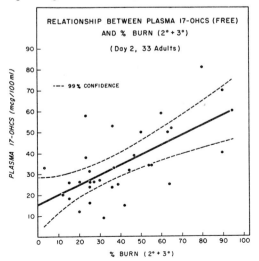

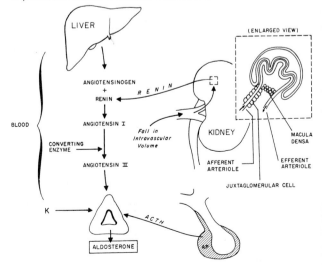

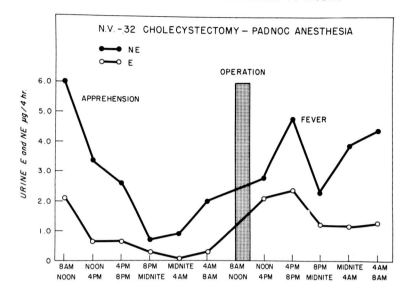

Fig. 1-27. Urinary epinephrine and norepinephrine values before, during, and after a cholecystectomy under Pentothal, Anectine, Demerol, nitrous oxide, oxygen, and curare anesthesia. Rather high levels of norepinephrine and epinephrine were seen preoperatively when the patient was apprehensive, and a slight rise was noted as a consequence of the operative trauma, as well. A further rise was noted in the postoperative period when the patient became febrile.

The major roles of GH in trauma are to help promote hyperglycemia by stimulating gluconeogenesis and antagonizing insulin, and to aid the catecholamines and glucagon in the mobilization of fatty acids.

GLUCAGON

Glucagon is a diabetogenic hormone made by the alpha cells of the pancreatic islets. A glucagonlike substance is also made in the upper small intestine. Glucagon secretion is stimulated by hypoglycemia. There is increasing interest in the role of glucagon in the metabolism of injury. Some of its effects are listed in Tables 1-2 and 1-3.

Glucagon is a marked stimulus to lipolysis, increasing cyclic adenosine monophosphate (cyclic AMP) in fat which in turn increases the activity of the lipolytic enzyme which hydrolyzes triglyceride to fatty acid and glycerol. The elevated free fatty acid levels stimulate gluconeogenesis, but glucagon has a direct effect on gluconeogenesis as well. Another important effect of glucagon is to promote glycogenolysis.

The main results of increased glucagon secretion in trauma are to produce increases in blood glucose through stimulation of glycogenolysis and gluconeogenesis and

through an anti-insulin effect, and to produce energy through lipolysis. Glucagon also promotes ketogenesis and ureagenesis and decreases lipoprotein release, but these effects are less striking than those relating to glucose and fat mobilization.

Glucagon also has been said to produce ionotropic cardiovascular effects when given to patients or animals in shock. These effects consist of an increase in cardiac output and stroke volume, and a decrease in peripheral vascular resistance despite β-receptor blockade. To what degree these effects are part of the physiologic response to injury is unknown.

Hormones with Unaltered or Decreased Secretion in Trauma

TSH—THYROXIN

Because there is a hypermetabolic state in the immediate postoperative or posttraumatic period, it was originally thought that TSH secretion led to increased thyroid activity. More recent studies seem to indicate that this is not so. Although the presence of thyroid hormone is necessary

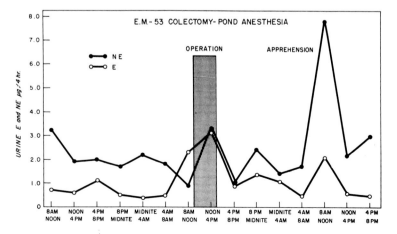

Fig. 1-28. Urinary epinephrine and norepinephrine values before, during, and after colectomy under Pentothal, oxygen, nitrous oxide, and Demerol anesthesia. Again a slight rise in norepinephrine and epinephrine secretion was seen in operative trauma, but a much greater rise was noted in the postoperative period when the patient suddenly became quite apprehensive.

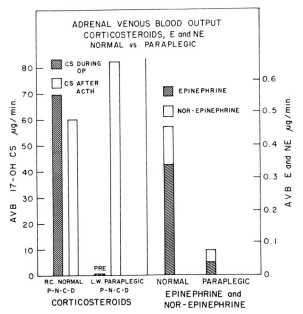

Fig. 1-29. Adrenal venous blood corticosteroids, epinephrine, and norepinephrine in normal versus paraplegic patients. It may be seen that the intraoperative production of 17-OHCS in the paraplegic patient was so low as to be nearly unmeasurable whereas after the injection of ACTH it rose promptly to a very high level. The secretion of epinephrine and norepinephrine too was greatly reduced in paraplegic patients.

for the normal functioning of organs in response to a traumatic stress, an increased secretion is apparently not necessary to meet this challenge.

INSULIN

Insulin secretion is not usually increased in response to trauma. Epinephrine, which is, tends to inhibit the release of insulin, and many factors are working to produce an elevation of the blood sugar level and to make carbohydrate available. The administration of glucose intravenously may call forth an insulin secretion, but there is a relatively diabetic glucose tolerance curve in the immediate posttraumatic period.

FSH-LH AND OVARIAN HORMONE SECRETION

No increased secretion of FSH or LH occurs in response to trauma, and there is some evidence to indicate that the secretion of these substances may even be inhibited somewhat during this period. Although menstrual periods may be missed in the immediate postoperative period, they more commonly occur on schedule. The emotional response to the trauma may to some extent influence cyclic activity. It is much more common to note amenorrhea in patients with chronic renal failure, however, than in the otherwise healthy woman who undergoes a severe trauma.

FSH-LH AND TESTICULAR HORMONES

There are relatively little data on the secretion of androgens either of testicular or adrenal origin in the posttraumatic period. From a purely logical viewpoint the androgens should be helpful in the rebuilding process, since they

are anabolic agents and help to lay down protein. Whether they actually are secreted in increased amounts during this phase of recovery has not, however, been demonstrated unequivocally.

ADRENAL ANDROGENS

There are no very good data available to indicate whether or not adrenal androgens are present in increased amounts following trauma. In the immediate posttrauma period there is only a very modest increase in urinary 17-ketosteroids.

Goals of Endocrine Changes

One may summarize the endocrine changes which occur in response to injury by saying that they seem to be directed toward water and salt conservation, blood pressure maintenance, gluconeogenesis, glycolysis, general mobilization of carbohydrate, lipolysis, the outpouring of hormones essential for cell life, and the providing of ready energy to the muscles, heart, and brain. The effects of these hormones on metabolism are shown in Table 1-3.

METABOLIC CHANGES

Following a severe injury there is marked tissue wasting and weight loss. This is partly due to semistarvation and partly to the extreme catabolism which occurs in the immediate postinjury period. The intensity and duration of the catabolic period depends upon the severity of the

Table 1-2. REPORTED EFFECTS OF
GLUCAGON ON ISOLATED LIVER

Process	Change	Involvement of Cyclic AMP
Glycogenolysis	Increase	Yes
Phosphorylase	Increase	Yes
Gluconeogenesis	Increase	Yes
Glycogen synthesis	Decrease	Yes
Glycogen synthetase	Decrease	Yes
Ureogenesis.	Increase	Yes
Protein synthesis	Decrease (?)	?
Protein breakdown	Increase (?)	?
Ketogenesis.	Increase	Yes
Lipolysis	Increase	Yes
Amino acid uptake	Increase	Yes
Tyrosine aminotransferase	Increase	Yes
p-Pyruvate carboxykinase.	Increase	Yes
Lysosome activation	Increase	?
K^+ release	Increase	Yes
Ca^{++} release	Increase	Yes
Mitochondrial pyruvate uptake .	Increase	?
Krebs cycle.	Increase	?
Transamination	Increase	?
Lipoprotein release	Decrease	Yes

SOURCE: J. H. Exton, M. Vi, S. B. Lewis, and C. R. Park, Mechanism of Glucagon Activation of Gluconeogenesis, in H. D. Soling and B. Willms (eds.), "Regulation of Gluconeogenesis," p. 160, Academic Press, Inc., New York, 1971.

Table 1-3. SOME METABOLIC EFFECTS OF HORMONES WITH GENERALLY INCREASED SECRETION IN TRAUMA

	Proteolysis (in muscle)	Gluconeogenesis (in liver & kidney)	Glycolysis Muscle	Glycolysis Adipose tissue	Glycogenolysis Liver	Glycogenolysis Muscle	Lipolysis (adipose tissue, liver, muscle)	Insulin antagonism	Insulin secretion	Plasma sodium	Plasma potassium	Water retention
ACTH-cortisol	+++	+++	0	0	. . . . . .	0	++	++	++	+	0	0
Renin-aldosterone .	. . . . . .	. . . . . .	. .	. . . .	. . . . . .	. . . .	. . . . . .	. . . . . .	. . . . . .	++	00	
Epinephrine, norepinephrine .	+	++*	0	++	++++	++	++++*	+++	0	+	0	
ADH	. . . . . .	. . . . . .	. .	. .	. . . . . .	. .	. . . . . .	. . . . . .	+++	. .	0	++++
Growth hormone .	0	+	0	++	. .	. .	++*	+	+++			
Glucagon	+	+++*	0	. .	++†	. .	+++*	++	+++	. .	. .	

*Only in the presence of the adrenal corticosteroids.

†By stimulating catecholamine secretion.

injury and on whether or not the injury is protracted by sepsis and other serious complications. The protein loss is far greater in healthy young men than in elderly patients, women, or children (Fig. 1-30), but it can be greatly decreased by the administration of amino acids and calories intravenously.

The metabolic changes which accompany trauma depend not only upon the intensity and duration of the injury but upon the presence or absence of shock, the degree of anoxia, the type of repair solutions administered to the patient, and the success or failure of the body in adapting itself to the injury. In order to understand the metabolic response to injury it becomes necessary to examine the energy sources available to the body, the effect of starvation and hyperalimentation, the changes produced by increased hormone secretion, and the adaptive mechanisms essential to recovery from profound injury.

Energy Metabolism

Energy is stored in the body in the form of carbohydrate (glycogen), protein, and fat (triglycerides). Glycogen is stored in muscle and liver in combination with water and electrolytes, so that 1 Gm of glycogen yields only 1 or 2 kcal instead of the 4 kcal found in 1 Gm of dry carbohydrate. Protein is stored primarily in muscle, and, like carbohydrate, in combination with water. Therefore, muscles are only one-quarter to one-fifth protein. Furthermore, body protein is not designed primarily as a source of fuel, but performs other important functions in the form of enzymes, plasma protein, structural protein, cardiac and skeletal muscle, etc. Ingested protein beyond that needed to replenish body stores is metabolized, the nitrogen is excreted as urea, and the calories thus created are expended or, if unneeded, stored as fat.

Lipid is not stored in combination with water, and body fat therefore yields lipid contents as high as 90 percent of total weight. One gram of body fat thus provides nearly the full 9.4 kcal present in one gram of pure triglyceride.

Table 1-4 is modified from a concise and lucid review by Cahill on the metabolic effects of starvation in man. It may be seen that extracellular fluids and muscle and liver glycogen make very small contributions to the body energy pool when compared to muscle protein, and especially to fat—the major energy depot. During starvation man attempts to conserve protein by burning fat instead, and to preserve muscle and liver glycogen by accelerating gluconeogenesis. Cahill did not list plasma protein as a potential source of fuel, because in simple, short-term starvation the body is able to replenish plasma protein at a rate equal to its degradation. Plasma protein can probably be used as fuel, however, as demonstrated by the experiments of Allen et al., in which puppies were maintained and grew while receiving protein only in the form of intravenous plasma. With prolonged fasting in the face of trauma and marked catabolism, endogenous plasma proteins are burned, and the liver is incapable of synthesizing albumin at a rate equal to its loss, necessitating the replacement of plasma proteins from exogenous sources. Red blood cells probably are consumed as well. It is ex-

tremely important, therefore, to administer amino acids, albumin, plasma, or whole blood to surgical patients who are in a catabolic state and unable to eat, not only to replace plasma protein and blood lost externally or to the third space but also that which is burned as fuel.

With acute trauma, anoxia, and exercise muscle and liver glycogen are used as emergency fuels, and with severe or prolonged injury muscle protein is used as well, unless attempts are made to conserve it by the vigorous intravenous administration of protein or amino acids, and calories.

Starvation

An understanding of the metabolic changes seen following injury in man requires a consideration of the effects of starvation, which accompanies most injury, especially that of a progressive or long-term nature. These are shown in Figs. 1-31 and 1-32. Glucose is derived from glycogenolysis of liver glycogen and from gluconeogenesis. The new glucose formed from gluconeogenesis derives in part from amino acids and in part from glycerol, which comes from the triglycerides of body fat. In the early fasting state, shown in Fig. 1-31 and in Table 1-5, a 70-kg man would be expected to make about 16 Gm of new glucose from glycerol and about 43 Gm from muscle protein for a total of 59 Gm a day. In addition to this he would obtain 85 Gm of glucose from glycogen breakdown and 36 Gm from recycled glucose, for a total of 180 Gm a day. While the brain normally completely metabolizes glucose to carbon dioxide and water, other glycolytic tissues such as peripheral nerve, erythrocytes, leukocytes, bone marrow, renal medulla, and to a lesser extent normal muscle metabolize glucose mainly by converting it to lactate and pyruvate. These substances are released into the bloodstream and carried back to the liver and kidney, where they are remade into glucose, thus contributing to the total available glucose without creating any net gain of glucose. This process is known as the *Cori cycle*; its effect is to provide energy for the peripheral tissues by the anaerobic glycolysis of glucose, while the energy thus given up is regained in the liver by the reconversion of lactate into glucose utilizing energy derived from the oxidation of fat (Fig. 1-33). The entire process of gluconeogenesis requires energy, and this energy is supplied by the oxidation of fatty acids. By means of the Cori cycle the amount of glucose that has to be supplied from protein breakdown is limited.

While the brain and the other glycolytic tissues depend directly upon glucose for their energy, the rest of the organism derives its energy from fat, in the form of either fatty acids or ketone bodies created by the partial oxidation of fatty acids to acetoacetate or β-hydroxybutyrate. While these tissues, especially muscle, readily utilize glucose in the presence of insulin in the nonfasting state or with vigorous exercise or anoxia, they completely abandon glucose metabolism during starvation, thus helping to conserve body protein.

The liver derives its energy from fatty acid oxidation in two stages: The partial oxidation of fatty acids to acetyl coenzyme A (acetyl CoA), and the terminal combustion

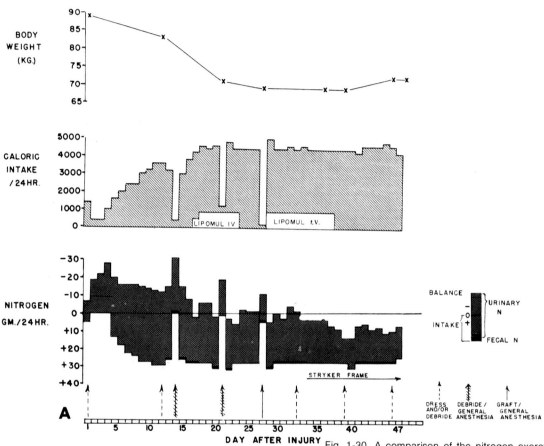

Fig. 1-30. A comparison of the nitrogen excretion in a burned woman and a burned man illustrating the far greater catabolism and nitrogen loss in the man. *A.* Twenty-eight-year-old white man with 55 percent burn. *B.* Thirty-one-year-old white woman with 55 percent burn.

Table 1-4. FUEL COMPOSITION OF NORMAL 70-kg MAN

Fuel	Kilograms	Calories
Tissues:		
Fat (adipose triglyceride)	15.0	141,000
Protein (mainly muscle)	6.0	24,000
Glycogen (muscle)	0.150	600
Glycogen (liver)	0.075	300
Total	. . . . . .	165,900
Circulating fuels:		
Glucose (extracellular fluid) . . .	0.020	80
Free fatty acids (plasma)	0.0003	3
Triglycerides (plasma)	0.003	30
Plasma proteins	0.210	840
Total	. . . . . .	953

SOURCE: Adapted from G. F. Cahill, Jr., *N Eng J Med,* **282**:668, 1970.

of the acetate in the tricarboxylic acid cycle (Krebs cycle). About one-third of the total energy in fat is ordinarily derived from the first stage, but in starvation ketosis the first stage provides the major portion of the liver's energy, since the function of the tricarboxylic acid cycle is diminished and acetyl CoA is disposed of in the circulation as acetoacetate and β-hydroxybutyrate. Ketogenesis generally, though not always, parallels the rate of gluconeogenesis.

In prolonged fasting rather profound changes in metabolism occur, as shown in Table 1-6 and in Fig. 1-32. It is apparent that liver and muscle glycogen cannot continue to supply glucose at all, since the total body store is only 225 Gm and this would be exhausted in a few days. Furthermore, body protein cannot continue to be converted to glucose at the rate of 75 Gm a day, since in about a month this would deplete the total body protein beyond the level which would permit survival. It thus becomes

NITROGEN METABOLISM FOLLOWING THERMAL INJURY

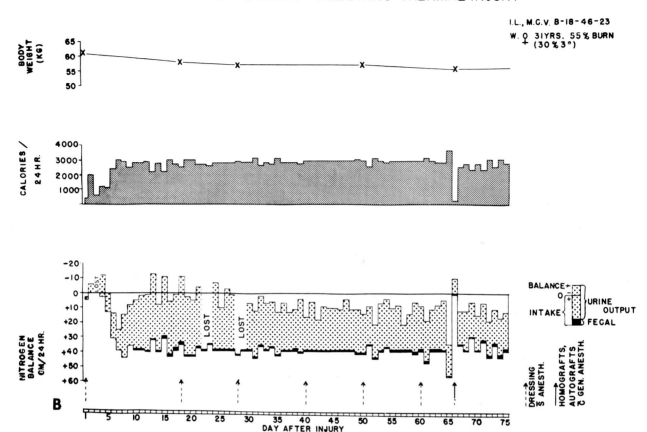

Fig. 1-30B. Continued.

apparent that diminished utilization of glucose and sparing of body protein is essential for the survival of prolonged starvation.

If the brain is the one organ which needs glucose normally, it must either reduce its fuel consumption or substitute another fuel, or the body must make glucose directly from fatty acids, which it cannot do, since the enzymes required for this are not found in animals.

Owen and coworkers found that on prolonged fasting the ketone bodies, acetoacetate and β-hydroxybutyrate, replaced glucose as the predominate fuel for brain metabolism. This change of fuels by the brain did not produce

any deficits in the function of the brain or change in the electroencephalogram. The amount of glucose completely utilized by the brain drops from 144 Gm to 30 Gm a day, 14 of the 44 Gm presented to the brain being recycled through the Cori cycle. The blood ketones are capable of being utilized by the brain in part because they, like glucose, are water-soluble and readily penetrate the blood-brain barrier.

The body not only manages to conserve protein, but also maintains almost normal levels of blood glucose, glycerol, amino acids, lactate, and pyruvate. The blood levels of free fatty acids and ketones are of course markedly increased.

Table 1-5. GLUCOSE AVAILABLE IN EARLY STARVATION STATE IN A 70-kg MAN

Origin	Amount of glucose, Gm/24 hr
New glucose (gluconeogenesis):	
Fat (glycerol)	16
Protein	43
Stored or recycled glucose:	
Glycogen	85
Recycled glucose	36
Total	180

Table 1-6. GLUCOSE AVAILABLE IN LATE STARVATION STATE IN A 70-kg MAN

Origin	Amount of glucose, Gm/24 hr
New glucose (gluconeogenesis):	
Fat (glycerol)	18
Protein	12
Stored or recycled glucose:	
Glycogen	0
Recycled glucose	50
Total	80

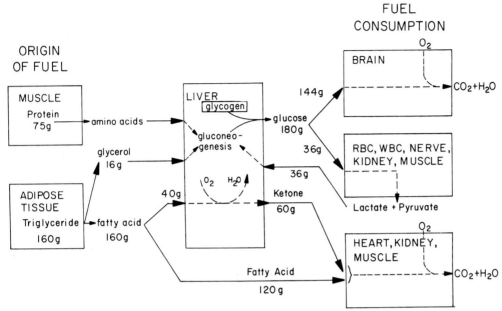

FASTING MAN
(24 hours, basal : ~1800 calories)

Fig. 1-31. Scheme of fuel metabolism in a normal, fasted man. The two primary fuel sources are muscle protein and fat. The brain oxidizes glucose completely, the glycolyzers break down glucose by anaerobic metabolism into lactate and pyruvate, which are remade in the liver into glucose, and the rest of the body burns fatty acids and ketones. (*Adapted from G. F. Cahill, N Engl J Med, 282:668, 1970.*)

One other striking change that occurs in prolonged fasting is a shift from the liver to the kidney of gluconeogenesis from protein sources. The liver continues to make glucose by recycling lactate and pyruvate, and it also continues gluconeogenesis from glycerol. Almost all of the gluconeogenesis from amino acids, however, takes place in the kidney, where there is a stoichiometric relation between ammoniogenesis and gluconeogenesis. The ammoniogenesis is required to maintain acid homoeostasis by titrating the ketone acids lost in the urine.

While there is only a slight change in concentration of total amino acids during starvation, there are striking changes in the values for individual amino acids. Glycine increases during starvation; valine, leucine, and isoleucine increase briefly and then decrease; arginine falls progressively; and lysine does not change at all. Alanine falls progressively, decreasing to less than one-third of the fed level. Alanine is the principle amino acid utilized by the liver for gluconeogenesis, and it is the decrease of alanine during fasting which limits gluconeogenesis in the liver. Alanine comes from muscle protein and also may be synthesized from pyruvate, as shown in Fig. 1-33.

ROLE OF THE HORMONES IN ALTERED METABOLISM OF STARVATION

The presence of the adrenal glucocorticoids, particularly cortisol, is essential for a normal rate of gluconeogenesis, and this hormone participates in the hyperglycemia which occurs in the early posttraumatic period. The administration of large doses of glucorticoids to fasting subjects did not result in an increased rate of nitrogen excretion, however.

GH likewise fails to increase daily nitrogen excretion in fasting subjects, but appears to be responsible for the level of insulin and blood glucose. Dwarfs having a congenital lack of growth hormones were found to be capable of mobilizing fatty acids and excreting nitrogen at rates similar to those observed in normal persons of the same size.

There is a marked rise in circulating glucagon in patients fasting for 2 or 3 days. Glucagon not only increases glycogenolysis in the liver but also increases gluconeogenesis, directly opposing insulin in this regard. Glucagon appears to have a role in regulating the level of circulating amino acids. The near absence of glucagon in a totally pancreatectomized subject may be the reason that such patients require less insulin to affect homeostasis than most severely ill diabetics.

Insulin has at least two important effects on the regulation of fuel sources: it inhibits the rate of release of free fatty acids from adipose tissue, in which it opposes the catecholamines and glucagon, and it increases amino acid uptake by muscle and protein synthesis in which it appears to be opposed by glucagon and cortisol. Insulin, therefore, not only impedes fatty acid release but impedes amino acid release from muscle as well.

The hypothalamus controls all the hormones regulating glucose production, except glucagon and insulin. In addition, it contains an appetite-satiety center which is presumably responsive to the blood glucose level, and has been said by Conway et al. to regulate lipolysis in response to changes in glucose levels.

Gamble demonstrated many years ago that small

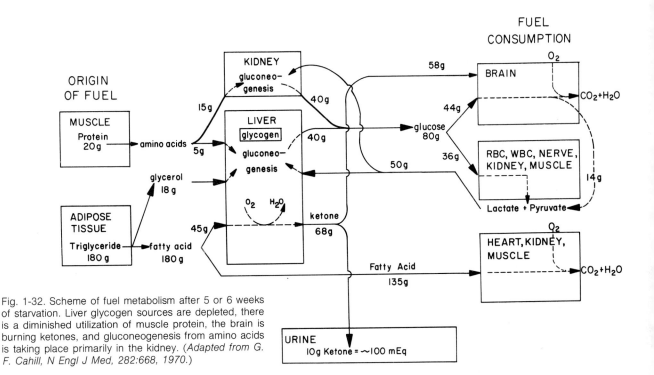

Fig. 1-32. Scheme of fuel metabolism after 5 or 6 weeks of starvation. Liver glycogen sources are depleted, there is a diminished utilization of muscle protein, the brain is burning ketones, and gluconeogenesis from amino acids is taking place primarily in the kidney. (*Adapted from G. F. Cahill, N Engl J Med, 282:668, 1970.*)

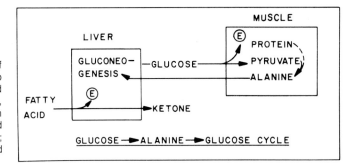

Fig. 1-33. The Cori cycle (top) provides for a transfer of energy from the liver to the periphery. Glucose gives up energy in the periphery by anaerobic glycolysis to lactate and pyruvate. The latter are then remade into glucose in the liver, utilizing energy derived by the metabolism of fatty acids. In the glucose-to-alanine-to-glucose cycle (bottom) described by Felig et al., glucose is metabolized to pyruvate in muscle; pyruvate is then converted to alanine, which is transported to the liver, where it is remade into glucose.

amounts of administered glucose were capable of decreasing the excretion of nitrogen in the urine; this concept has recently been challenged by Blackburn et al. The classic concept is to maintain that the daily administration of 100 Gm of glucose given intravenously spares the proteolysis of about 50 Gm of protein. This effect presumably results from the increased secretion of insulin brought about by the elevated glucose level which in turn inhibits muscle proteolysis. The need for gluconeogenesis by the liver is no longer present, since the administered glucose takes care of the brain's need. Ketogenesis also ceases, and the rest of the body continues to utilize free fatty acids.

Clearly it is important to spare protein breakdown in the starved injured patient, since protein breakdown leads to muscle wasting, ineffective coughing, pneumonia, impaired wound repair, poor resistance to infection, and diminished synthesis of enzymes and plasma proteins. Blackburn et al. contend that they were unable to achieve nitrogen balance in fasting patients given an amino acid solution intravenously in combination with 100 Gm of glucose every 24 hours whereas they were able to achieve nitrogen balance in those patients given the same amount of amino acids without any added glucose. Their explanation is that the administration of glucose increases the output of insulin, which in turn exerts an antilipolytic effect which decreases the mobilization of fatty acids and makes it necessary to continue using muscle protein as a source of energy. By giving protein without glucose the insulin level remained low, and there was an increased mobilization of body fat with an associated ketosis, thus

leading to a use of body fat as the energy source and sparing protein. Positive nitrogen balance could be achieved by administering 90 Gm of amino acid/day without any other caloric source.

While it may be true that small amounts of glucose even in the presence of protein administration may not lead to optimal utilization of body fat as an energy source, it is certainly true that the administration of hyperalimentation mixtures containing protein hydrolysates or amino acids in conjunction with an adequate caloric intake supplied by hypertonic glucose provides optimal protein sparing, and improves wound healing and resistance to infection.

Metabolic Effects of Injury

The effects of trauma and sepsis on body metabolism are summarized in Table 1-7 and Fig. 1-34. In contrast to starvation, injury produces (1) hyperglycemia, unless the injury is overwhelming and fatal; (2) marked fatty acid mobilization and elevation of plasma free fatty acids; (3) a striking catabolism of muscle protein beyond that needed as a source for energy, in contrast to late starvation, where protein conservation is seen; and (4) an increase in the synthesis of urea and the so-called "acute-phase reactants" (AP reactants) (Table 1-8).

Oxygen consumption is not increased in ordinary elective operations, but it is increased by as much as 25 percent after multiple fractures, and with severe sepsis may increase by 50 percent. Burns increase oxygen consumption by as much as 100 percent, partly because of sepsis and

Table 1-7. EFFECT OF TRAUMA ON CARBOHYDRATE, FAT, AND PROTEIN METABOLISM

Charge	Cause	Charge	Cause
Carbohydrate: Early hyperglycemia	Increased glycogenolysis produced principally by CA* and to lesser extent by glucagon. Increased gluconeogenesis produced by increased fatty acid level and by 17-OHCS and GH. Insulin inhibition produced by CA, glucagon, 17-OHCS and GH.	Triglycerides: no change	In trauma there is an increased ability to remove excess lipids from bloodstream, thus compensating for increased fat mobilization.
		Rise in β-hydroxybutyrate/ acetoacetate ratio blood, liver, kidney, etc., in profound shock or sepsis	Hypoxia.
		Protein: Muscle:	
Hyperglycemia and glucose intolerance during convalescence	Moderate injury: insulin intolerance with decreased ability to oxidize glucose and block of conversion of pyruvate to two-carbon fragments. Severe injury: no change or an increase in rate oxidation glucose, but marked increase in glucose production.	Markedly increased catabolism Decreased protein synthesis	17-OHCS and glucagon promote catabolism muscle proteins to amino acids and inhibit protein synthesis. Starvation also leads to protein breakdown. Some breakdown due direct trauma, wound loss, etc. Protein catabolism above that needed for energy alone supplies carbohydrate intermediates, and is required to maintain level of circulating amino acids. Inhibition of increased insulin secretion. Insulin has an anabolic effect.
Hypoglycemia seen in profound shock or sepsis	Glycogen depletion. Utilization of glucose at rate faster than gluconeogenesis can provide it. Defect in gluconeogenesis.		

Table 1-7. Continued

Charge	Cause	Charge	Cause
Rise in lactate/pyruvate ratio in blood and tissue in profound shock or sepsis	Hypoxia, producing a block in conversion of pyruvate to acetyl CoA, rise in lactic acid level, and progressive tissue deficit of ATP.	Liver and kidney proteins: Increased turnover of protein, but no protein depletion	Increased protein synthesis involves largely "export" proteins like albumin and acute-phase (AP) reactants but probably involves intrinsic protein as well. Whereas in starvation there may be a decrease in liver and kidney protein, in injury the 17-OHCS produces a preferential increase in catabolism of muscle protein, which leads to an increased synthesis of protein in liver and kidney—mainly through alanine release from muscle protein.
Fat: Fatty acid mobilization Elevated FFA plasma	CA and glucagon increase cyclic AMP in fat, thus increasing activity of lipolytic enzyme which hydrolyzes triglyceride to fatty acids and glycerol. GH and 17-OHCS have similar but much weaker effect. Insulin especially, and prostaglandins and metabolites (glucose, lactate, pyruvate, ketone bodies) to a lesser extent have opposite effect.		
Elevation liver ketones	Moderate injury: FFA mobilization produces an increase in hepatic fatty acid oxidation to ketones. Glucagon stimulates this. Severe injury: Inhibition of liver citrate synthase due to ischemia, prevents acetyl CoA from entering tricarboxylic acid cycle, thus diverting it to synthesis of ketone bodies.	Plasma proteins: Increased catabolism Probably increased synthesis of albumin as well, but masked by catabolism γ-Globulin increased	Plasma proteins participate in protein catabolism seen in trauma. Liver increases synthesis of "export" proteins. γ-globulin increased by antibody production in response to sepsis.
Blood ketones unchanged or slightly elevated	Ketone metabolism unimpaired, some excess excreted urine.	Plasma amino acids: Decreased somewhat as gluconeogenesis uses up substrates; subsequently total kept fairly constant, although some glucogenic amino acids (such as alanine) tend to fail while lysine does not change at all and glycine rises	Exact mechanism unknown, though balance between insulin (which decreases amino acid release from muscle and decreases glucaneogenesis) and glucagon and 17-OHCS (which increase amino acid release from muscle and increase gluconeogenesis) plays an important regulatory role. If amino acids are infused at rates in excess of energy needs, the excess will be converted to fat and the nitrogen excreted in the urine, while the plasma level remains constant.
Lipoproteins: cholesterol falls	Cause unknown; related to albumin level; may be due to starvation, or to glucagon.		
		Urea: Urea synthesis greatly increased Urea excretion in urine greatly increased Plasma urea increased due to increased production; further increased if renal failure present	Increased deamination of alanine in liver to provide substrate for increased gluconeogenesis makes nitrogen available to the liver for synthesis into urea.
		AP reactants: Increased synthesis	Reason unknown.

*CA: catecholamines (epinephrine and norepinephrine).
17-OHCS: glucocorticoids (cortisol and corticosterone principally).
GH: growth hormone.
FFA: free fatty acids.

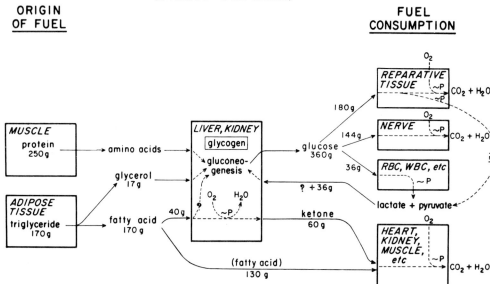

TRAUMATIZED MAN

(24 hours : −2400 calories)

ORIGIN OF FUEL

FUEL CONSUMPTION

Fig. 1-34. Hypothetic scheme of rates of substrate flow in a traumatized individual excreting 40 Gm of nitrogen/day. Presumably reparative tissues are glucose utilizers, but the amount of glucose terminally combusted to carbon dioxide and that metabolized to lactate would depend both on the maturity of the tissue (presence of mitochondria) and on adequate perfusion and oxygenation. Fat still provides the bulk of the calories. (*From G. F. Cahill et al., in C. L. Fox, Jr., and G. G. Nahas (eds.): "Body Fluid Replacement in the Surgical Patient," p. 286, Grune & Stratton, Inc., New York, 1970.*)

partly because of the break in the epidermis producing evaporative water loss which requires enormous expenditures of energy.

Carbohydrate Metabolism

The early elevation of blood glucose level after most types of injury is brought about primarily by the catecholamines and to a lesser extent by glucagon. These hormones produce an increase in hepatic glycogenolysis and an inhibition of insulin production. The elevated blood levels are also a consequence of enhancement of gluconeogenesis, brought about by the glucocorticoids and glucagon, and to a lesser extent by the catecholamines and GH. The increased plasma fatty acid concentrations also stimulate gluconeogenesis, and the presence of available substrate, especially alanine, provides an additional stimulus to this reaction.

The presence of hyperglycemia provides a ready source of energy for the injured organism and is important to early survival. Starvation reduces the ability of the body to tolerate shock, by depleting the energy substrate and leading to acidosis and hypoglycemia. The administration of glucose prolongs survival after shock, as shown by Drucker and his colleagues in hypovolemic dogs and Berk and his associates in endotoxin shock. McNamara and his

Table 1-8. ACUTE-PHASE (AP) REACTANTS

Haptoglobin
Fibrinogen
Ceruloplasmin
Seromucoid fraction
C-reactive protein
α_2-AP globulin
α_1-Acid glycoprotein
α_1-Antitrypsin

colleagues demonstrated that patients in hypovolemic shock who were resuscitated in the usual manner and at the same time received either 50% glucose, 25% mannitol, or 3% saline solution in equal osmolar doses had a much greater increase in blood pressure and pulse pressure when they received glucose than with either of the other two agents.

While hemorrhagic shock has been found by some workers to be associated both with hyperglycemia and an elevated insulin level, others have claimed that insulin levels are low. All agree, however, that there are elevated levels of anti-insulin hormones and that there is both a glucose intolerance and insulin resistance after injury.

During the recovery phase there continues to be a diabeticlike glucose tolerance curve which is more marked after severe injury. There is an insulin intolerance and a decrease in the ability to oxidize glucose. Drucker has demonstrated a partial block in the metabolic conversion of pyruvate to two-carbon fragments.

Glucagon plays a major role in the hyperglycemia of injury through stimulation of gluconeogenesis. This results not only from the effect of increased fatty acids, to which glucagon contributes, but also from a direct effect of glucagon. The effects of glucagon on the liver are summarized in Table 1-2.

In profound shock or sepsis hypoglycemia may be present. This is due to depletion of glycogen stores and the utilization of glucose at a rate faster than gluconeogenesis can provide it. It is also due to a defect in gluconeogenesis. There may be a rise in the lactate/pyruvate ratio due to hypoxia, which produces a block in the conversion of pyruvate to acetyl CoA, a rise in the lactic acid level, and a progressive tissue deficit of adenosine triphosphate (ATP).

Fat Metabolism

Fat is the main energy source in trauma, as in starvation. The catecholamines and glucagon increase cyclic AMP in fat, thus increasing the activity of the lipolytic enzyme which hydrolyzes triglyceride to fatty acid and glycerol. GH and the glucocorticoids have a similar though much weaker effect.

The glycerol provides substrate for gluconeogenesis. The fatty acids are burned in the liver to supply energy for gluconeogenesis, and in the periphery to supply energy directly.

Liver ketones are elevated due to the increase in free fatty acids and the influence of glucagon. In very severe injury the level of ketones is further increased because of inhibition of liver citrate synthase, which prevents acetyl CoA from entering the tricarboxylic acid cycle, thus diverting it to the synthesis of ketone bodies.

In very profound shock and sepsis there is a rise in the ratio of β-hydroxybutyrate to acetoacetate in blood, liver, kidney and other tissues as a consequence of hypoxia.

Protein Metabolism

The daily intake of protein for a healthy young adult is usually about 80 to 120 Gm, or 13 to 20 Gm of nitrogen. Of this quantity of nitrogen about 2 to 3 Gm/day is lost in the stool and 11 to 17 Gm in the urine. Urinary nitrogen excretion increases greatly after injury, rising to as much as 30 to 50 Gm/day following severe trauma. This is nearly all in the form of urea nitrogen. In the patient with anuria or one whose kidneys have been removed preparatory to transplantation, operative trauma produces a very rapid rise in blood urea nitrogen (BUN) in comparison to that seen between dialyses in the nontraumatized state (Fig. 1-35).

The increase in nitrogen excretion begins shortly after injury, reaches a peak about the first week, and may continue for 3 to 7 weeks. In elective operative procedures the negative nitrogen balance is rapidly reversed, but in the burned patient the negative balance may be prolonged for a very considerable period of time. During this time the patient may lose 50 to 75 lb of weight. In the early postinjury period protein may be lost from the body surface if there is a large open or burned area, into the peritoneal cavity if there is peritonitis or ascites, into edema fluid if there is an extensive crush injury or burn, in tissue slough and necrotic muscle, and into areas where blood has been sequestered, or lost to the body economy.

The source of the great urinary protein loss is still not

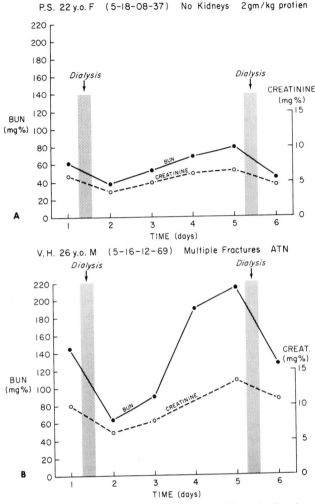

Fig. 1-35. Comparison of dialysis in patients with minimal and severe catabolism. *A.* Chronic dialysis in an anephric patient with very little catabolism, taking 2 Gm of protein/kg body weight daily. Note the slow rise in BUN and creatinine levels between dialyses despite high protein intakes. *B.* Dialysis in a patient with multiple fractures and acute tubular necrosis on no protein intake. Note the rapid rise in BUN and creatinine levels associated with marked catabolism. The patient recovered completely.

entirely certain. In studies of burned rats Levenson and his colleagues have demonstrated that the incorporation of labeled nitrogen in tissue protein was equal to, or greater than, that seen in the control animals, which means that they were synthesizing protein at the same time that they were losing large quantities of nitrogen in the urine. Therefore simple catabolism of body protein was not the only source for urinary nitrogen loss.

In a subsequent series of experiments it was found that the protein content of the liver and other active organs changed very little after burns whereas the muscle, which had a rather slow turnover rate, lost enough protein to account for most of the urinary nitrogen loss. These experiments suggested that the integrity of the vital organs was maintained at the expense of skeletal muscle. Munro and Chalmers found that in rats fed on a protein-free diet until

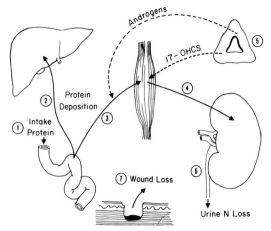

Fig. 1-36. Protein storage and catabolism. Protein may be preferentially deposited in the liver while it is being catabolized from muscle stores. Its catabolism is increased by glucocorticoids and decreased by insulin and adrenal androgens.

they were depleted negative nitrogen balance failed to develop after injury, and they hypothesized that the protein lost after injury was storage protein. If storage protein is largely muscle protein, this would account for the far greater protein loss seen in muscular young men than in women or debilitated elderly patients (see Fig. 1-30). It has also been noted by Browne and Schenker and by Howard et al. that if the patient has repeated injuries in close succession, the protein loss is less with each succeeding injury, perhaps because the storage protein has been wiped out by the previous trauma (Fig. 1-36).

The striking muscle protein catabolism seen in trauma is far in excess of that needed to supply energy. The magnitude of this response is related to the magnitude of the injury.

Protein contribution to the normal caloric requirement is in the range of 12 to 15 percent of the total, while Duke observed that this remained approximately 15 percent in most surgical conditions and did not rise much above 20 percent even with major increases in nitrogen excretion after extensive injury. Thus the major weight loss seen after surgery is not primarily the result of protein breakdown as a means of obtaining extra fuel. Although it has been claimed by Blackburn et al. that injury inhibits the mobilization and oxidation of fat from adipose tissue as a fuel source, Carlson and other investigators have shown that free fatty acids are readily mobilized in injury. They have even raised the question of whether excessive mobilization of fatty acids may sometimes occur.

The protein loss after injury is not due to impaired protein synthesis. Furthermore the protein loss occurs primarily from muscle, there being no decrease in the protein content of the liver and kidneys. As mentioned earlier, alanine is the principal amino acid released from muscle, and this amino acid is the principal gluconeogenic precursor in the liver. Felig et al. have suggested that a cycle similar to the Cori cycle of glucose to lactate to glucose may be achieved through glucose to alanine to

glucose, which serves as a mechanism for transferring energy to the periphery from the liver by the consumption of energy from ketone bodies. One of the other effects of severe injury is to decrease the activity of citrate synthase, which slows down the tricarboxylic acid cycle and increases the production of ketone bodies. During the early response to injury there is an increased proportion of fatty acids oxidized to ketone bodies in the liver, and the uptake of ketone bodies by the extrahepatic tissues is increased.

There is some evidence that the increased nitrogen metabolism may be related to the need for carbohydrate intermediates via gluconeogenesis, rather than to the total energy needs of the body as indicated by its oxygen consumption. This evidence as summarized by Kinney et al. is as follows: (1) the caloric contribution of protein to the fuel mixture of normal and injured man is rather small; (2) two-carbon fragments are readily available from adipose tissue and are utilized as the major energy source in most tissues after injury; (3) the body has a continuous requirement for carbohydrate intermediates for synthetic purposes, for which deamination of amino acids is the primary endogenous source; and (4) fatty acids cannot directly yield a net gain of carbohydrate intermediates, glucose, or glycogen.

Carbohydrate intermediates are used for the synthesis of nonessential amino acids, glycogen, glucose, and tricarboxylic acid cycle intermediates.

As a by-product of the increased gluconeogenesis of trauma, there is an increased synthesis of urea, which is made from nitrogen stripped from alanine and other glucogenic amino acids as their carbon remains are used in the formation of glucose (Fig. 1-35).

The plasma proteins undergo increased catabolism, but there is an increased synthesis of albumin as well. γ-Globulin is likewise increased, presumably by antibody production against microorganisms. The total plasma amino acids decrease somewhat, but individual amino acids may increase or decrease depending on their utility as gluconeogenic substrates.

Acute-phase-reactant proteins (AP reactants) (Table 1-8) are those protein components of plasma whose concentration is significantly increased in the acute phase of trauma or inflammation. All these contain 5 to 20 percent carbohydrate in the molecule, and all are synthesized exclusively in the liver. A recent article by Koj summarizes our current knowledge of them.

Although most of the AP reactants are present normally and show an increased response to trauma, at least two of them, C-reactive protein in man and rabbit and α_2-AP globulin in the rat, do not appear to be present in healthy animals but appear only after injury. In some forms of trauma there may be an increase in the rate of synthesis of albumin as well as AP reactants, but because in severe trauma there is a marked increase in catabolism of albumin, the increased synthesis is not apparent.

The AP-reactant glycoproteins appear at different time intervals after injury. C-Reactive protein in man and α_2-AP globulin in rats respond most promptly, appearing in plasma soon after injury, while haptoglobin and fibrinogen appear 4 to 6 hours after, and seromucoid and ceruloplasmin reach maximal value several days after injury. The response of the various AP reactants to repeated injuries or to adrenalectomy or the administration of corticosteroids is very variable. Some of the AP reactants are inhibited and others are stimulated by adrenalectomy.

Presumably the AP reactants are of some benefit to the injured organism. Fibrinogen apparently improves clotting, and haptoglobins may help to prevent damage to the kidneys by binding hemoglobin released as a consequence of the injury. Other AP reactants may bind toxic products or inactivate lyzosomal enzymes whose release triggers production of toxins.

Blood Coagulation

Trauma, infection, operation, or measures taken by the surgeon during these events may produce either hypercoagulation or a bleeding tendency, or both simultaneously. Some of the factors responsible for these changes are listed below.

HYPERCOAGULATION

Normal pregnancy produces a state of hypercoagulation. This is particularly evident as parturition approaches and is manifest by an increase in fibrinogen, prothrombin, and stable factor (VII), with a decrease in fibrinolysin. The antithrombin factor may be low, and placental thromboplastin may seep into the circulation. Birth control pills also produce a state of hypercoagulation to such an extent that fatal pulmonary emboli are seven times as common in women taking the pills as in women of the same age group not taking the pills. Estrogen produces hypercoagulation by increasing labile factor (V) and prothrombin and by decreasing plasma antithrombin activity. These factors should be taken into account when operations are necessary during pregnancy or immediately after delivery.

The increased secretion of ACTH and cortisol which accompanies most types of trauma produces hypercoagulation by increasing platelets and decreasing capillary fragility. Epinephrine is said to produce hypercoagulation at first, followed by hypocoagulation.

Attar and his associates determined the clotting time at intervals after hemorrhagic shock in 33 patients and found hypercoagulability reaching its peak 7 hours after the onset of hemorrhage, after which blood coagulation became normal, at 24 hours. This was followed by a hypocoagulable state which peaked at 36 hours, and a final return to normal again at about 63 hours. After this the curve oscillated between hypercoagulability and hypocoagulability with diminishing amplitude and frequency, gradually becoming normal again. The more severe the shock, the greater the swings.

Similar studies were carried out in 23 patients in septic shock. A similar cyclic swing between hypercoagulability and hypocoagulability was found. Fibrinogen levels were measured in 42 patients with septic shock. Although there were individual variations in the pattern, there generally was either very little change or a slight elevation at first

followed by a marked and sustained increase. The surviving patients then had a gradual return to normal, while in the fatal cases there was an abrupt fall to normal or hypofibrinogenemic levels.

Some of the coagulation changes said to occur in shock are artifacts due to the reservoir technique employed or are species-specific and not applicable to man. Hemorrhagic shock in baboons was said by Herman and his colleagues not to produce any coagulation defect although the euglobulin lysis time decreased somewhat, and resuscitation by crystalloids produced only a prolongation of prothrombin time, partially reversed by fresh heparinized blood.

Thus, although there are many references to hypercoagulation occurring in trauma (pulmonary embolus would seem to be a manifestation of this), it has not been unequivocally documented in man.

HYPOCOAGULATION

Coagulation changes have been reported in combat casualties by Attar et al., by Simonds et al., and by Hirsch et al., among others. Attar reported a prolongation of prothrombin and partial thromboplastin times (PTT) and a transient decrease in fibrinogen followed by an increase. Simonds found no change in prothrombin time or PTT. Hirsch found increases in clotting time and PTT (more pronounced in those patients who ultimately succumbed). Fibrinolytic activity as demonstrated by fibrin-split products was usually associated with metabolic acidosis and hypotension, and when these three conditions coexisted, there was a uniformly fatal prognosis. Disseminated intravascular coagulation (DIC) was seen in only one patient as a near-terminal event in the presence of overwhelming sepsis.

Ljungqvist and Bergentz found no change in platelet quality with trauma in dogs but suggested that there is an irreversible aggregation of platelets that occurs with trauma.

Sepsis has a more profound effect on coagulation mechanisms than hemorrhage or trauma. Horwitz and his colleagues found that intravenous injections of *Escherichia Coli* in baboons produced marked prolongation of prothrombin and PTT times, decreased fibrinogen, and a fall in platelet counts. There was also evidence of increased fibrinolysis. These changes were due to the bacteremia and not to hypoperfusion or acidosis.

Dextran produces a hemostatic defect that can lead to serious bleeding problems in patients. The defect has been shown by Howard et al. to be more severe the greater the molecular weight of the dextran. The causes of the defect include (1) complexes of dextran and fibrinogen producing hypofibrinogenemia, first shown by Richetts; (2) a decrease in platelets, shown by Adelson et al.; (3) an aberration in the electrophoretic properties of platelets caused by fibrin on the platelet surface; (4) a decline of platelet factor III; (5) an increase in antithrombin III; and (6) a delay in prothrombin consumption.

Apart from the hypocoagulable states just mentioned there are several causes for failure of normal coagulation in surgical patients. The detection of most of these conditions has been outlined by Wilson. A brief description of the most common coagulation defects seen in surgical patients is given below (see also Chap. 3).

MULTIPLE TRANSFUSION SYNDROME. The hemorrhagic tendency which accompanies multiple transfusions of banked blood is primarily due to a deficit in platelets and, secondarily, to decreases in fibrinogen and prothrombin (primarily labile factor V) factors, and to increases in fibrinolytic activity. A high antithrombin level may also be occasionally observed. A hemolytic transfusion reaction can further increase the production of fibrinolysin. The defects can usually be prevented by the administration of fresh "walking donor" blood for every six transfusions of bank blood. When the condition has already developed, it is best treated by superfresh blood, fibrinogen (1 Gm to start, then additional amounts until the fibrinogen assay is normal), and 500 mg of cortisol given intravenously. A calcium lack will not usually give rise to a coagulation defect until the blood level is so low that tetany has occurred. The calcium level may occasionally get so low in patients with multiple transfusions, however, that ECG changes of a prolonged Q-T interval can be noted and calcium may have to be administered.

EXTRACORPOREAL CIRCULATION (ECC). This may produce the same defects noted in the multiple transfusion syndrome plus the addition of anticoagulants (heparin and dextran), blood diluents (dextran), and increased capillary fragility. The treatment is fresh blood, fibrinogen, cortisol, and protamine to neutralize the heparin.

DISSEMINATED CARCINOMA. This may produce hypocoagulation in a number of different ways. Invasion of bone marrow or liver tissue may interfere with the production of platelets or coagulation factors. Substances from the tumor may escape into the bloodstream and by their thromboplastic activity produce intravascular clotting and fibrinolysis. Abnormal proteins may be released from the tumor and are capable of interfering with the activity of coagulation factors. Platelet antibodies are sometimes present, producing thrombocytopenia. Occasionally tumor emboli will produce thrombosis of small vessels.

ACUTE FIBRINOGENOPENIA. Fibrinogenopenia is perhaps the most common cause of coagulation abnormalities in surgical patients. It may be due to a whole variety of different situations that pertain to injury and operative trauma. Either a depletion of circulating fibrinogen, brought about by diffuse intravascular thrombosis, or increased fibrinolysis, or occasionally both, may be responsible for the fibrinogenopenia. It occurs with disseminated carcinoma, multiple transfusions, transfusion reactions, and extracorporeal circulation as already mentioned, and in addition in trauma, shock, acquired hemolytic anemia, extensive liver disease, and polycythemia (particularly that seen in congenital heart disease); during surgical treatment of the lungs, pancreas, uterus, or prostate; with severe infections; and with obstetric accidents such as premature separation of the placenta, miscarriage, toxemia, septic abortion, or bilateral cortical necrosis of the kidneys. There is some debate as to whether hypothermia can also pro-

duce fibrinolysis; apparently it can under some circumstances, even though it usually does not do so when combined with extracorporeal circulation. Snakebites by poisonous snakes produce fibrinogenopenia both by intravascular deposition of fibrin and by activation of fibrinolysin.

The treatment of this hemorrhagic diathesis is the administration of ACTH and cortisone intravenously; fibrinogen, beginning with an intravenous dose of 1 Gm and continuing until the defect is corrected; fresh blood (to add platelets, which may be depleted by intravascular clotting); and, if necessary, ϵ-aminocaproic acid intravenously in doses of 1 to 6 Gm or more. Fibrinogen may carry the virus of homologous serum hepatitis, and the use of γ-globulin apparently does not offer protection against posttransfusion or fibrinogen-carried hepatitis, although γ-globulin made from donors who have recovered from hepatitis may help.

HYPOPROTHROMBINEMIA AND UNSUSPECTED ANTICOAGULANT THERAPY. Patients with severe liver disease or those who have been taking anticoagulants from whom no history can be obtained may have to be operated upon in an emergency situation. Although the administration of vitamin K_1 is capable of reversing the defect created by the coumarin-type drugs, this process usually takes several hours. Furthermore these drugs usually have very little if any effect in patients with severe liver disease. The defect can best be reversed by the utilization of fresh blood. The clotting mechanisms can be returned to the normal range by an exchange transfusion of 10 to 15 pt of fresh blood, and we have occasionally used this technique in patients with severe liver disease to stop the bleeding from esophageal varices. A prothrombin time should be obtained on patients suspected of having liver disease prior to surgical treatment.

OTHER UNSUSPECTED BLEEDING DISORDERS. Mild hemophilia may be difficult to detect prior to surgical treatment, and the first evidence of it may be severe bleeding during operative intervention. Classic hemophilia should be suspected when the patient is a male, particularly a child, and when no evidence for fibrinogen or prothrombin deficiencies or thrombocytopenia have been detected in laboratory tests. The PTT will strengthen the suspicion, and a factor VIII determination will confirm the diagnosis. Antihemophilic globulin (factor VIII) should be administered, and the operation should be terminated as quickly as possible. Factor VIII–rich fibrinogen is also useful. If the deficiency is in either factor IX or factor XI instead of factor VIII, fresh whole blood or platelet-rich plasma will correct the defect.

A rather spectacular example of the production of fibrinolysin occurred in a patient operated upon by us some years ago. This patient had an acute dissecting aneurysm of the thoracic aorta and was taken to the operating room for a thoracic fenestration procedure about 3 hours after the onset of symptoms. The patient was anesthetized and placed on an ice mattress. Because of a short, thick neck and a peculiar angulation of the larynx it was impossible to intubate the trachea, and repeated attempts produced edema of the vocal cords, partial airway obstruction, and some hypoxia. Because of respiratory embarrassment an immediate tracheostomy was performed. Anesthesia was then administered via tracheostomy tube. Almost immediately after completion of the tracheostomy the patient began to lose blood copiously from the tracheostomy wound. The wound was reexplored four times, was sutured and resutured, coagulated with the cautery, and packed with hemostatic agents but continued to ooze considerable quantities of blood, which ran out of the wound and down on the floor.

As attempts were made to control bleeding, generalized hypothermia was gradually being induced. Samples of blood were taken to identify the bleeding defect, and the patient was found to have great quantities of fibrinolysin. He was intravenously given fibrinogen up to a total of 12 Gm, 50 units of ACTH, and 500 mg of hydrocortisone. Fresh blood was administered. These events all took a period of nearly 6 hours, at the end of which time the defect was corrected and coagulation in the tracheostomy wound finally took place. All this time the patient was under generalized anesthesia and, for the last half, hypothermia as well. We then carried out the operation as planned without difficulty and without any abnormal bleeding. The patient made an uneventful recovery.

Coagulation factors are discussed in more detail in Chap. 3.

Wound Healing

Wound healing is discussed in detail in Chap. 8. Many factors affect wound healing, chief among them being local factors of hematoma, dehiscence, infection, edema, blood supply, location, and extent. The administration of antibiotics can improve wound healing by decreasing sepsis, and the correction of clotting defects can promote healing by preventing hemorrhage in the wound. Various systemic metabolic factors are involved in wound healing.

Ascorbic acid is essential for collagen synthesis, and thus plays an important role in the healing of wounds. Cognizance is customarily taken of this by the intravenous administration of large doses of ascorbic acid after operation. It has been demonstrated by Levenson and his associates that injuries are accompanied by a decrease in plasma ascorbic acid concentration and by similar changes in thiamine and nicotinamide. This is associated with a decrease in urinary excretion of these substances. A decrease in the urinary excretion of riboflavin is also seen. It was found that the decrease in plasma ascorbic acid constituted a true physiologic scurvy and that this could be reversed by the administration of large doses of ascorbic acid, 500 to 2,000 mg daily. Sullivan and Eisenstein have noted ascorbic acid depletion during hemodialysis corrected by adding ascorbate to the dialysate concentrate.

There are considerable recent data on the effects of the fat-soluble vitamins on wound healing. Certain types of trauma are accompanied by a decrease in blood and hepatic concentrations of vitamin A. Chernov et al. reported

that vitamin A depletion following thermal injury is associated with stress ulcers. Restoration of serum vitamin A levels markedly reduced the risk of ulceration. Hutcher et al. showed that vitamin A reduced the incidence of steroid-induced gastric ulcers. Collagen synthesis and wound healing are suppressed by corticosteroids, but collagen synthesis and tensile strength can be returned to normal by vitamin A administration, as shown by Hunt and his colleagues, and by Stein and Keiser. When steroids are used for immunosuppression, it was shown by Cohen and Cohen that vitamin A must be used with caution because it exerts an adjuvant-like effect and antagonizes steroid-induced immunosuppression.

It may be necessary to administer vitamin K in prolonged starvation, mild liver damage, biliary fistulas, or other circumstances in which intestinal absorption of this vitamin is chronically reduced. In the absence of preexisting vitamin K deficiency its acute depletion in trauma is not generally a problem. The same may be said for vitamin D, which is stored in the body for long periods of time.

Although the role of trace metals in wound repair and metabolism awaits clearer definition, there is increasing evidence that zinc and copper are essential for normal healing. Hsu and Hsu have shown that zinc is necessary for both epithelialization and collagen synthesis. Cohen et al. have recently noted that zinc-depleted burned patients have decreased taste acuity and an associated anorexia, which is corrected by zinc repletion. While zinc depletion interferes with wound healing, this process cannot be speeded up by giving zinc to individuals with normal levels.

Abnormal wound healing in copper deficiency is detailed in Carnes' review. Copper is essential for lysyl oxidase, the enzyme that cross-links collagen. Drugs such as D-penicillamine which bind copper and block aldehyde cross-link sites will subsequently diminish collage cross linking and inhibit wound healing. They may be clinically useful in the treatment of diseases characterized by overabundant collagen deposition, such as cirrhosis, esophageal stricture, or keloids. D-Penicillamine has been clinically used by Harris and Sjoerdama for patients with scleroderma to inhibit skin collagen deposition.

Although various substances have been claimed to accelerate normal wound healing, there are no scientific data to show that cartilage extracts, vitamins, or metals accelerate healing in a normal healing wound.

The oxygen tension of the healing wound is said by Hunt and others to be directly related to the rate of healing. In the wound the oxygen reaches the area of injury by diffusion, and as the blood P_{O_2} is increased by breathing oxygen, the oxygen available in the wound is greater, and wound healing is accelerated. This is said to be because increases in wound P_{O_2} levels have three effects: (1) to increase the rate at which fibroblasts reproduce, (2) to increase the rate at which fibroblasts synthesize collagen, and (3) to increase the rate at which epithelial cells reproduce.

The studies of wound oxygen concentrations seem to give validity to the use of hyperbaric oxygen in the treatment of chronically unhealed wounds, supporting the claims that it improves wound healing.

Therapeutic Considerations

NUTRITIONAL SUPPLEMENTATION

The parenteral nutritional supplementation of the surgical patient has for many years included glucose solutions and blood and blood products, with abortive attempts to introduce amino acids intravenously to produce a positive nitrogen balance, and fat solutions to provide concentrated calories. In recent years, with the advent of parenteral "hyperalimentation" utilizing concentrated glucose and amino acid solutions introduced through an intraatrial catheter via the subclavian vein, there has been a plethora of papers devoted to the advantages and hazards of such therapy. Intravenous fat (Intralipid) was developed in Sweden and has received extensive experimental trial in this country. It seems to be a useful source of calories and essential fatty acids.

Greenstein and his colleagues in 1960 produced a nutritionally complete water-soluble liquid diet which when administered orally to rats maintained them for long periods without any detectable deficiencies. The diet contained 18 crystalline amino acids (9 essential and 9 nonessential), the water-soluble vitamins, the trace metals (Mg, Fe, Mn, Cu, Co, Zn) Na, K, Ca, ethyl linoleate, and sometimes vitamins A and D. Diets which did not include a linoleic acid source produced signs of essential fatty acid deficiency (scaling of skin, failure to grow well, occasionally cachexia).

Terry and his colleagues in 1948 first demonstrated that it was possible to maintain dogs for prolonged periods of time solely on oral glucose and parenteral plasma. The plasma proteins contributed to body tissue protein and did not produce a urinary nitrogen loss, but in fact decreased the urinary nitrogen loss seen in fasting.

Total parenteral alimentation in dogs was described by Meng and Early in 1949. Allen et al. in 1956 used intravenously given plasma as the only protein source for littermate puppies and were able to obtain growth rates equivalent to those seen when the same amount of protein was given orally. Stemmer et al. republished these results 10 years later.

To Dudrick and his colleagues belongs the credit for pushing studies on parenteral hyperalimentation with amino acid and concentrated carbohydrate mixtures. In 1967–1968 these investigators demonstrated that it was possible to achieve normal growth in puppies supported entirely by intravenous feedings. The feedings consisted of amino acids, glucose, vitamins, Na, K, Ca, Cl, HPO_4, and trace metals with or without the addition of fat. They also reported 30 patients fed exclusively by vein for 10 to 200 days, using amino acids, 20% glucose, electrolytes, trace metals, and vitamins. Positive nitrogen balance was achieved, and the patients demonstrated better wound healing, weight gain, and increased strength and activity.

It seems clear that parenteral hyperalimentation is unnecessary for short-term surgical problems but is of great

Table 1-9. REQUIREMENTS FOR PROLONGED INTRAVENOUS TOTAL ALIMENTATION

Essential amino acids
Possibly alanine and some other nonessential amino acids
Glucose
Na, K, Ca
Vitamins
Trace metals (Zn, Cu, Cr, Co, Mg, Mn, I, Fe)
Cl and HPO_4
Plasma or albumin
Linoleic acid

value for patients with long-term problems or for malnourished patients prior to surgery. It has also proved useful for putting the bowel at rest in severe diarrheal states such as ulcerative colitis and granulomatous colitis, and for maintaining patients with the short bowel syndrome.

The requirements for total parenteral alimentation solutions are given in Table 1-9. The amino acids may be supplied by any of the solutions shown in Table 1-10. Protein hydrolysates differ from mixtures of crystalline amino acids primarily by virtue of their contamination with trace elements and peptides, and (except for Aminosol) their content of phosphate (Table 1-11). The essential amino acids are listed in Table 1-12. The amino acid content of two of the commonly used commercial solutions are shown in Table 1-13, and a composition in which they are often administered is shown in Table 1-14.

Mixtures containing only the essential amino acids are used for patients with uremia or hepatic failure. In 1956 Rose and Dekker showed in rats that urea could be used for synthesis of nonessential amino acids when essential amino acids were supplied in the diet. This led to the clinical use by Giordano and by Giovannetti and Maggiore of similar diets for patients with uremia. The use of a parenteral essential amino acid–hypertonic glucose mixture has been described by Dudrick and his coworkers and others for surgical patients with renal failure and inability to eat. The blood urea nitrogen level falls, or remains stable after dialysis, and hyperphosphatemia, hypocalcemia, and acidosis are spontaneously reversed. Protein synthesis occurs, presumably from the metabolism of urea nitrogen.

In liver failure the administration of protein hydrolysates is contraindicated because of their high ammonia content. Concentrated glucose solutions can be adminis-

Table 1-10. AMINO ACID SOURCES FOR INTRAVENOUS ALIMENTATION

Protein hydrolysates
Crystalline amino acid mixtures
Essential amino acids only
Plasma
Plasmanate
Albumin
Whole blood

Table 1-11. PHOSPHATE CONTENT OF AMINO ACID SOLUTIONS

Amino acid solution	Percent	Phosphate, mEq/L
Protein hydrolysate:		
Amigen	5	30
CPH	5	14
Hyprotigen	5	25
Aminosol	5	0
Crystalline amino acid:		
Cutter	8	0
Freamine	8.5	0
Freamine-E	5.25	0

tered using the techniques of hyperalimentation. While mixtures containing only essential amino acids can sometimes be used, their effect on hepatic encephalopathy is unpredictable. It is preferable to use albumin, which is capable of directly entering into body protein tissues without deamination or increasing ammonia levels. Furthermore the albumin exerts an osmotic force which helps to mobilize and excrete ascitic and edema fluid.

There are various well-known complications that occur with intravenous hyperalimentation. These can be divided into catheter problems—which include pneumothorax, sepsis, subclavian artery injury, or air or fat embolization—and metabolic problems. Chief among the metabolic problems is hyperglycemic, hyperosmolar dehydration usually due either to too rapid administration, too concentrated glucose solutions, latent diabetes, or administration during a state of glucose intolerance such as one sees soon after severe trauma or during continued sepsis. Reactive hypoglycemia also can be seen if the fluid is suddenly stopped, particularly if insulin has been used.

Five other metabolic complications are seen occasionally with long-term hyperalimentation. The first of these is an excessive plasma level of amino acids beyond that which the body can metabolize. This produces impairment of brain function, and stimulation of insulin secretion. The effect of excess aminoacidemia can be ameliorated in part by the concomitant administration of large amounts of carbohydrate.

The second complication is a metabolic hyperchloremic acidosis produced only by the synthetic amino acid mixtures. Heird and his colleagues ascribe this to the catabolism of positively charged amino acids. This problem is not seen with the hydrolysates because they have sufficient negatively charged amino acids and peptides to offset the hydrogen ion release by the cationic amino acids.

The third complication is hypophosphatemia, which

Table 1-12. ESSENTIAL AMINO ACIDS

Leucine	Threonine
Valine	Methionine
Lysine	Histidine
Isoleucine	Tryptophan
Phenylalanine	

Table 1-13. AMINO ACID CONTENT OF TWO COMMONLY USED PARENTERAL AMINO ACID SOLUTIONS

Amigen (casein hydrolysate)

Essential	Nonessential
Leucine	Glutamic acid
Valine	Proline
Lysine	Serine
Isoleucine	Aspartic acid
Phenylalanine	Alanine
Threonine	Arginine
Methionine	Tyrosine
Histidine	Hydroxyproline
Tryptophan	Glycine
	Cystine

Freamine (synthetic amino acids)

Essential	Nonessential
Leucine	Alanine
Valine	Arginine
Lysine	Proline
Isoleucine	Serine
Phenylalanine	Cysteine
Threonine	Glycine
Methionine	
Histidine	
Tryptophan	

Table 1-14. COMPOSITION OF AMINO ACID–SUGAR SOLUTIONS COMMONLY ADMINISTERED

Amigen, 800 (5% Amigen; 12.5% fructose, 2.4% alcohol)

Protein, Gm	37.4
Nitrogen, Gm	5.54
Calories	800
Na, mEq	35
K, mEq	19
Ca, mEq	5
Mg, mEq	2
Cl, mEq	20
HPO_4, mEq	30

Freamine

Dextrose, Gm	250
Nitrogen, Gm	4.17
Calories	900
Na, mEq	23.6
K, mEq	40
Mg, mEq	5
Cl, mEq	35
Acetate, mEq	52
$ZnSO_4$, mEq	2.5

Table 1-15. ESSENTIAL FATTY ACID
DEFICIENCY

Fall in:
   Linoleic
   Arachidonic
   8,11,14-Eicosatetraenaic
Rise in:
   Palmitoleic
   Oleic
   5,8,11-Eicosatetraenoic

occurs when fibrin hydrolysates or crystalline amino acids are used without added phosphate (Table 1-11). This can be corrected by adding Ca and P to the solutions. Hyperphosphatemia can occur from administration of the casein hydrolysate solutions, especially if phosphate is added.

The fourth complication is essential fatty acid deficiency. Fatty acid deficiency was first described in animals by Burr and Burr in 1929. Pensler and his colleagues described the first clinical case in 1971. The essential defect is a decrease in plasma linoleic, arachidonic, and linolenic acids, with an increase in oleic, palmitoleic, and 5,8,11-eicosatetraenoic acids. It is characterized clinically by scaly skin, itching, poor wound healing, weakness, lethargy, and thrombocytopenia. The thrombocytopenia appears to be due to a failure of separation of megakaryocyte buds.

Linoleic acid is the key essential acid, since arachidonic acid can be synthesized from it, and it has not been established whether linolenic acid is essential (Table 1-15). Although it has been recommended that patients on long-term hyperalimentation receive plasma on a weekly basis for its essential fatty acid content, it is doubtful whether this supplies enough linoleic acid to prevent the development of fatty acid deficiency. Intravenous fat in the form of Intralipid will correct the defect, but this substance is still available in this country only on an experimental basis.

The fifth complication is trace element deficiency. While trace elements have often been added to pediatric hyperalimentation mixtures, they are not routinely added to mixtures for adults. The trace elements thought to be important are listed in Table 1-16. The administration of amino acid mixtures without trace elements led to the

Table 1-16. TRACE METALS PRESENT IN
ENZYMES

Metal	*Enzymes*
Iron	Cytochromes, peroxidases
Copper	Tyrosinase, ascorbic oxidase
Zinc	Peptidase, carbonic anhydrase
Magnesium	Phosphatases, kinases
Maganese	Kinases, peptidases, arginase
Molybdenum	Xanthine oxidase, nitrate reductase
Cobalt	Vitamin B_{12} coenzyme complexes
Potassium	Pyruvic kinase, β-methyl aspartase

SOURCE: Conn and Stumpf, "Outlines of Biochemistry," 3d ed., p. 233, John Wiley & Sons, Inc., New York, 1972.

development of copper deficiency in one of our patients. This was characterized by dryness of the skin, weakness, and anemia, associated with a very low serum copper level. The symptoms were corrected by the intravenous administration of copper. As plasma and plasmanate contain trace elements, the periodic administration of plasma may prevent the development of deficiencies.

Alcohol, which is a component of some hyperalimentation solutions, probably should not be used. It potentiates ketosis, increases metabolic acidosis, uncouples oxidative phosphorylation (thus increasing oxygen consumption without energy production), depolarizes nerves, and may produce sedation and mild inebriation in children.

Fructose, also a component of some solutions, appears definitely inferior to glucose. It increases uric acid, lactic acid, amino acids, and bilirubin. The latter effect is apparently due to hepatic cell injury by fructose, which also increases the serum glutamic oxaloacetic transaminase (SGOT).

The elements are now available for the production of an ideal parenteral alimentation solution tailored to the individual patient. Long-term home hyperalimentation has been started, and a completely closed portable system has been devised. Provided the use of hyperalimentation solutions is not extended to patients who could do better without them and precautions are taken to avoid the complications, it will provide an exciting and important contribution to the care of the surgical patient.

COMPONENT THERAPY

Component therapy is a term for the intravenous administration of blood components, or substitutes for these components, instead of whole blood in order to create an intravenous mixture that offers some particular advantage over whole blood. To some extent this advantage may simply be that of greater availability, as for example reconstituted blood over fresh blood, but in some circumstances it may actually do a better job.

OXYGEN TRANSPORT. Traumatized patients may develop a shift of the oxygen dissociation curve to the left as a consequence primarily of alkalosis and lowered erythrocyte 2,3-diphosphoglycerate (2,3-DPG) levels. The reduced DPG level interferes with the ability of the red cell to give up its oxygen to the tissues. Old banked blood contains red cells with low 2,3-DPG content, and multiple transfusions of such blood tend to contribute to tissue anoxia. One may improve tissue oxygenation by correcting alkalosis or by providing erythrocytes high in 2,3-DPG content. Experiments have been made with free hemoglobin solutions and with chemical substitutes for hemoglobin.

Frozen erythrocytes are high in 2,3-DPG, in contrast to blood banked in the usual fashion, and have the advantage over fresh whole blood of not containing white cells (which are antigenic) and being far less likely to transmit hepatitis virus.

Free hemoglobin can also be used as an oxygen carrier. Although myoglobin produces renal damage, hemoglobin does not. Hemoglobin contaminated with red cell stroma produces a consumption coagulopathy, and pure hemoglobin produces anticoagulation as a result of reduced plasma factor VIII and factor V activity. Absorption with aluminum hydroxide was shown by Moss and his colleagues to remove the anticoagulant activity.

Fluorocarbons have been under investigation as an oxygen transport system, and there has been a recent symposium published on this subject. Clark and Galan first demonstrated that mice could be given liquid ventilation with an oxygenated fluorocarbon fluid at atmospheric pressure. Modell and his colleagues were able to ventilate dogs for 8 hours on liquid fluorocarbons with survival. Acidosis tends to develop because of poor CO_2 diffusion; however, mechanical hyperventilation produces pulmonary edema, and the chemicals themselves produce alveolitis, atelectasis, perivascular hemorrhage, and other lung changes.

Geyer and his coworkers have been able to replace almost all the erythrocytes in rats with emulsified fluorochemicals and keep them alive on 100% oxygen for 8 hours. It was found by Sloviter and his colleagues, however, that these substances produced a progressive anoxia and death in most laboratory animals, although frogs and mice could live several days with their erythrocytes replaced by circulating fluorocarbons. At least part of the damage caused by the fluorochemicals is related to the fact that they produce pronounced platelet agglutination and microemboli, not prevented by heparin.

While hemoglobin substitutes are an intriguing possibility, they do not yet seem to be serious contenders with red cells, or even free hemoglobin, for the honor of carrying the oxygen around the body.

CLOTTING COMPONENTS. The clinically useful clotting components consist of fresh frozen plasma, cryoprecipitate, concentrates of factors II, VII, IX, X, antihemophilic globulin, platelet packs, and fibrinogen.

Fresh frozen plasma can be used to replenish the factors contributing to the prothrombin time and in bleeding patients in hepatic failure whose prothrombin times are low. It has the advantage over banked blood that it contains some labile factor V, which is characteristically low in liver failure and absent from banked blood, and the disadvantage that it contains no platelets. It is used in plasmapheresis for hepatic coma, where it is combined with the patient's own erythrocytes, and therefore it can be used for patients with rare blood types for whom the acquisition of multiple units of fresh whole blood might be difficult. Fresh frozen plasma is also useful for patients undergoing operations who develop bleeding tendencies secondary to deficiencies of clotting factors.

Cryoprecipitate contains factor VIII and some fibrinogen, while antihemophilic globulin contains only concentrated factor VIII. Both are used for hemophiliacs with factor VIII deficiency for whom replacement is desired.

Preparations containing factors II, VII, IX, and X (Konyne, Proplex) are used to treat Christmas disease.

Platelet packs are used to administer platelets to patients with hypersplenism, thrombocytopenic purpura, massive transfusions, and other deficiency states where thrombocytopenia can be demonstrated to be contributing to the bleeding disorder.

Fibrinogen is the specific therapy for patients with bleeding due to the presence of excessive amounts of fibrinolysin. It may be combined with steroids and EACA (ε-amino caproic acid).

PLASMA SUBSTITUTES. The risk of hepatitis from pooled plasma is so great that most hospitals have stopped using this preparation entirely. There is, of course, a significant risk from single blood or plasma transfusions, too, and for this reason transfusions or plasma infusions should never be given without a specific important indication. Apart from the administration of fresh frozen plasma discussed above, there is almost never a reason to administer plasma.

Ringer's lactate solution is, more or less, plasma without the plasma proteins, i.e., the immunoglobulins (IgG, IgA, IgM), albumin, fibrinogen, and the prothrombin-related clotting factors. The combination of Ringer's lactate solution (sometimes with modifications of the electrolyte content) and albumin makes a very satisfactory plasma substitute. Albumin itself is the therapy of choice in cirrhosis, not only because it replaces a specific loss, provides oncotic pull, and helps to promote diuresis, but also because its amino acids can enter muscle protein without deamination to create toxic nitrogen fragments. Furthermore hepatitis is not transmitted by albumin preparations.

Plasmanate is plasma with the clotting factors removed. It is made up as 5% protein in saline solution, and contains 88% albumin and 12% globulins. It is nearly free of hepatitis transmission.

The administration of fibrinogen to traumatized patients is seldom necessary, because there is an increased hepatic synthesis of fibrinogen in response to injury. It may be necessary, however, in patients with increased fibrinolysin.

ALIMENTATION MIXTURES. Special alimentation mixtures, discussed earlier in this chapter, offer a variety of combinations to fit the circumstances. Apart from hyperalimentation in severe, sustained, or septic trauma, the single most dramatic effect is that of essential amino acid mixtures in renal failure. This type of therapy makes possible the administration of amino acids which are not metabolized to release nitrogen but which are used in muscle synthesis—thus not contributing to urea formation—and in the presence of hypertonic glucose, even inducing the body to burn urea.

COMPONENT BLOOD. Frozen red cells are at present the best oxygen carrier available. Added to Ringer's lactate solution and albumin, they make a very acceptable blood substitute for patients not requiring clotting factors. Fresh frozen plasma is the best source of clotting factors but is the first component to introduce a risk of hepatitis. Platelet packs complete the clotting constituents, with the exception of fibrinogen which is needed only in the presence of excess fibrinolysins.

Apart from the leukocytes, which are specifically contraindicated in patients awaiting renal transplantation, and the ready availability of the constituents, there is no advantage attributable to component blood over fresh blood, which itself has the advantage of being cheaper and easier to prepare.

ACID-BASE BALANCE AND WATER AND ELECTROLYTE METABOLISM

Alkalosis

Attention has been directed to the development of alkalosis after trauma or operative insult. Some of the mechanisms involved have been summarized by Lyons and Moore, who find that alkalosis is observed more frequently than acidosis in patients with mild to moderate trauma who have not deteriorated to the point of severe renal circulatory or pulmonary decompensation. The criteria used by these writers to describe changes in acid-base balance are reproduced in Table 1-17, since they provide a handy guide for discussion of this subject. It was found that 64 percent of 105 patients operated upon developed alkalosis on at least one determination in the postoperative period. Of the 67 patients in whom alkalosis developed, 29 demonstrated this change after open heart operations,

19 after ventilatory assistance, 8 had alkalosis from chronic pulmonary disease, 5 had so-called "residual posttraumatic alkalosis," and 6 had miscellaneous forms of alkalosis. It is of significance that the open heart surgical patients received 9 to 18 Gm of tris buffer routinely in the first few hours after bypass and were hyperventilated after operation. These pH changes were not, therefore, so much the consequence of trauma as of overenthusiastic use of the measures taken for the prevention of acidosis. Among the patients with ventilatory alkalosis only those with pulmonary disease had elevated buffer base values. Extreme hypocapnic alkalosis occasionally developed in patients with normal lungs.

Lyons and Moore point out that it is important to prevent severe alkalosis in the surgical patient because of its potential hazards and that by the same token it might be well to avoid creating it by the injudicious use of administered base or hyperventilation. Among the dangers listed by these writers was the production of tissue hypoxia through the effect of alkalosis on the oxygen-hemoglobin dissociation curve and on vasomotor tone. The rise in blood lactate level which accompanies respiratory alkalosis sets the stage for severe metabolic acidosis should hypo-

Table 1-17. COMPARISON OF SYSTEMS OF NOMENCLATURE USED TO DESCRIBE DISTURBANCES OF NEUTRALITY REGULATION*

Disturbance in conventional terms	pH (units)	$[H^+]$ (mEq/L)	P_{CO_2} (mm Hg)	Standard HCO_3^- (mM/L)	Actual HCO_3^- (mM/L)	CO_2 content (mM/L)	CO_2 combining power† (mM/L)	Buffer base (mM/L) Hemoglobin (Gm %) 10	15	20	Buffer base deviation (mM/L) Hemoglobin (Gm %) 10	15	20
Normal	7.40	39.8	40.0	23.9	23.9	25.1	25.1	45.7	48.0	50.1	0.0	0.0	0.0
Uncompensated respiratory alkalosis	7.53	29.5	25.0	23.9	20.2	20.9	22.9	45.0	48.0	50.9	− 0.7	0.0	+ 0.8
Uncompensated metabolic alkalosis	7.53	29.3	40.0	32.5	32.5	33.7	33.7	55.7	58.0	60.1	+10.0	+10.0	+10.0
Mixed respiratory and metabolic alkalosis	7.68	24.0	25.0	32.5	28.5	29.3	31.2	55.1	58.0	61.0	+ 9.4	+10.0	+10.9
Uncompensated respiratory acidosis	7.31	48.9	55.0	23.9	26.8	28.4	26.7	46.5	48.0	49.4	+ 0.8	0.0	− 0.7
Uncompensated metabolic acidosis	7.24	57.2	40.0	16.7	16.7	17.9	17.7	36.1	38.0	39.7	− 9.6	−10.0	−10.4
Mixed respiratory and metabolic acidosis	7.16	68.4	55.0	16.7	19.2	20.8	19.2	36.7	38.0	39.1	− 9.0	−10.0	−11.0
Mixed respiratory alkalosis and metabolic acidosis	7.40	39.8	25.0	18.4	15.0	15.7	17.5	37.7	41.5	43.1	− 8.0	− 7.5	− 7.0
Mixed respiratory acidosis and metabolic alkalosis	7.40	39.8	55.0	30.0	32.9	34.6	32.7	53.3	55.0	56.5	+ 7.6	+ 7.0	+ 6.4
Respiratory alkalosis with metabolic compensation	7.47	34.2	25.0	21.0	17.4	18.2	20.2	41.4	44.2	47.0	− 4.3	− 3.8	− 3.1
Metabolic alkalosis with respiratory compensation‡	7.47	34.2	50.0	32.5	34.8	36.3	35.0	56.2	58.0	59.7	+10.5	+10.0	+ 9.6
Respiratory acidosis with metabolic compensation	7.35	44.3	55.0	26.5	29.5	31.3	29.7	49.7	51.3	52.8	+ 4.0	+ 3.3	+ 2.7
Metabolic acidosis with respiratory compensation	7.35	44.3	25.0	16.7	13.5	14.2	16.0	35.4	38.0	40.4	−10.3	−10.0	− 9.7

*Actual bicarbonate obtained from Henderson-Hasselbalch equation with $pK^1 = 6.10$. Buffer base, buffer base deviation, standard bicarbonate, and CO_2 combining power obtained from Siggaard-Andersen blood acid-base curve and alignment nomograms. Equilibration temperature = 38°C, oxyhemoglobin saturation = 100 percent and hemoglobin = 15 Gm percent unless otherwise indicated.

†Expressed as total CO_2 of anaerobically collected separated plasma or serum.

‡Some deny the clinical existence of this disturbance. Other studies indicate that respiratory compensation does occur but is weaker than the compensation accompanying metabolic acidosis.

SOURCE: (J. H. Lyons, Jr., and F. D. Moore, *Surgery*, **60**:93, 1966.)

capnia suddenly yield to hypoventilation or hypoperfusion. Alkalosis tends to produce hypocalcemia and hypokalemia, and the latter may be extremely dangerous to the patient receiving digitalis or to patients who already have hypokalemia. Hypocapnic vasoconstriction tends to produce a reduced cerebral blood flow.

One of the mechanisms for the development of alkalosis is pulmonary arteriovenous shunting, which occurs in patients with cirrhosis or in atelectasis. Patients with cirrhosis frequently have hypokalemia and a metabolic alkalosis to begin with, and this is further complicated by the respiratory alkalosis which develops as a consequence of the shunting. The shunting that occurs in atelectasis also permits venous blood to traverse the pulmonary bed unoxygenated. By producing hypoxia this increases ventilation, thereby blowing off carbon dioxide and producing respiratory alkalosis.

Atelectasis can produce hyperventilation even in the absence of hypoxia by stimulation of the Hering-Breuer reflexes, while hypoxemia produces hyperventilation by stimulating the aortic and carotid body chemoreceptors. Furthermore a reduction in blood supply to the chemoreceptor bodies will stimulate hyperventilation. Thus respiration may be stimulated during hypotension and decreased cardiac output even though the arterial blood is adequately oxygenated. This, then, may be another mechanism for the production of respiratory alkalosis in surgical patients. Three of the patients described by Lyons and Moore had a metabolic alkalosis, one from overtreatment of diabetic acidosis and the others from gastrointestinal obstruction and vomiting.

Lactic acid accumulation occurs with hyperventilation and can be prevented by adding carbon dioxide to the inspired gas mixture. It is apparently dependent upon the reduction of carbon dioxide tension P_{CO_2} rather than the associated change in pH. Its exact mechanism is not known but may be related to the effect of hypocapnia on carbohydrate metabolism. If hyperventilation is suddenly stopped, the P_{CO_2} may rise more rapidly than the accumulated lactate can be cleared from the blood, leading to an acute metabolic acidosis. This is worsened by the accumulation of lactic acid of hypoxic origin.

The effects of alkalosis on ionized calcium and on potassium are important to myocardial irritability. It is claimed by Lyons and Moore that alkalosis generally promotes the renal excretion of sodium bicarbonate and an alkaline urine but that in the posttraumatic period this mechanism is blocked by adrenal cortical activity. This produces an increased renal potassium loss and paradoxic aciduria. Potassium chloride is said to restore the renal ability to conserve hydrogen ion and thus initiate the correction of the acid-base disorder. This statement is a little hard to reconcile with the findings that in primary aldosteronism, where there may be marked hypokalemia of a degree seldom seen in surgical patients combined with an alkalosis, there is an alkaline, not an acid, urine. Furthermore, the writers state that alkalosis and hypokalemia secondary to pyloric obstruction are aggravated by sodium chloride and ammonium chloride and can be corrected only by potassium chloride. While potassium chloride is undeni-

ably useful, corrections of the alkalosis can be brought about by the administration of sodium chloride and ammonium chloride.

Acidosis

Many articles have called attention to the development of acidosis in response to injury or operative trauma. Some of the patients alluded to above would have been acidotic had it not been for their vigorous treatment pushing them over into alkalosis.

BLOOD TRANSFUSION. Blood transfusion may produce either alkalosis or acidosis. Since citrated blood is intrinsically acid by virtue of the citric acid anticoagulant, it produces a metabolic acidosis upon rapid, massive infusion that persists until the fixed acid is metabolized. A standard acid citrate dextrose (ACD) solution also contains about 17 mEq of trisodium citrate per unit of blood, however. As the citrate is catabolized, sodium ions are released to the cation pool of the body and are balanced by newly formed bicarbonate. If renal bicarbonate excretion is inhibited, as it is following trauma, an "addition" metabolic alkalosis results. It takes about 135 mEq of sodium citrate, or the amount contained in 8 units of blood, to produce a discernible alkalosis. In the presence of hepatic impairment, whether brought about by preexisting disease, hypotension, hypoxia, or hypothermia, citrate metabolism is delayed, and transfusion acidosis then becomes more prominent. Transfusion alkalosis is postponed or never appears.

SHOCK. Shock, whether bacterial or hypovolemic, when severe tends to produce acidosis. The mechanism for this is decreased tissue perfusion due to hypotension compounded by the release of catecholamines in response to hemorrhage, which further produces tissue anoxia by vasospasm. Acidosis also increases coagulability of the blood and may produce capillary thrombosis. If the condition is allowed to persist, cellular death and terminal acidosis result. Hardaway and others have suggested that this condition can be reversed by the administration of vasodilators to open up the arterioles together with the simultaneous administration of blood or other fluid to maintain circulating blood volume. The increased blood flow to the organs improves tissue oxygenation and decreases the likelihood of capillary thrombosis. The acidosis can be further corrected by the administration of bicarbonate or other base.

Wilson et al. have used Dibenzyline, a vasodilator, in 19 patients with shock refractory to conventional treatment. The patients received doses varying between 0.2 and 2 mg/kg of body weight. This was administered over a 5-minute period in patients who were in pulmonary edema and over a 60-minute period in patients who were less severely ill. Large volumes of fluid were needed to maintain blood pressure, and attempts were made to correct acid-base changes when needed. The cardiac output increased in 8 of 9 patients studied, and urine output increased in 7 of 19. The use of vasodilators or of vasoactive drugs of any kind, in patients with shock is waning in popularity, although Dibenzyline unquestionably improves renal cortical blood flow. Fluid and blood replacement, monitoring of venous pressure and blood gases, adequate ventilation, and treatment of sepsis remain the primary modalities for the treatment of shock.

The accumulation of lactic acid accounts in part for the progressive acidosis of shock, as shown by Broder and Weil. Likelihood of survival of patients in profound shock could be estimated by the levels of excess lactate in the blood. When it was less than 1 mM/liter, 82 percent survived; when it was 2 mM/liter, 60 percent survived; and when it was 2 to 4 mM/liter, only 26 percent survived. If the excess lactate was ever over 3 mM/liter, a fatal outcome could not be averted.

Boyd et al. have shown that nonlactate solutes may also accumulate in shock and that their accumulation indicates a poor prognosis. These substances are demonstrated by measuring serum osmolality and then calculating by a formula using sodium, glucose, and blood urea nitrogen levels. The difference between the measured and calculated osmolality is called the *osmolal discriminant,* and it is only partly accounted for by lactic acid levels. If the osmolality and the osmolal discriminant remain high after treatment, the prognosis is grave. The lactic acid concentration is also high in this group, of course.

MacLean and his coworkers reported studies on 56 patients in shock. These patients were divided into two groups according to whether the central venous pressure was above or below normal prior to treatment and were further subdivided into those patients who were alkalotic or normal and those who were frankly acidotic. The patients were treated with isoproterenol (2 μg/minute) combined with blood and saline solution, which produced an increase in cardiac output and blood pressure with a decline in central venous pressure and in arterial blood lactate.

If the patient was normovolemic before the onset of septic shock, the manifestations included hyperventilation, respiratory alkalosis, high cardiac index, elevated central venous pressure, low peripheral resistance, increased blood volume, hypotension, oliguria, warm, dry extremities, and arterial blood lactate accumulation. If this syndrome was recognized while the patient was still alkalotic, he responded to therapy which was designed to maintain the cardiac output at even higher levels. In contrast, if the patient was hypovolemic at the onset of sepsis, the clinical picture consisted of low central venous pressure, low cardiac output, high peripheral resistance, and cold, cyanotic extremities. These patients were also initially alkalotic and responded to treatment consisting of volume replacement and surgical procedures. If, however, they were not seen until they were acidotic, a low fixed output persisted and a high mortality rate ensued.

Acidosis is the result of shock, not the cause of it. Prevention or correction of acidosis seldom influences survival in hypovolemic shock. On the other hand, restoring fluid volume without correcting the acidosis does favorably influence the outcome. Severe acidosis (pH below 7.1) occurs in exhaustive exercise and in diabetic acidosis without producing shock, with good cardiac performance and

ultimate recovery. The important thing is to remove the cause of the acidosis, not to treat the acidosis per se.

More patients with a normal or alkalotic pH survived than those with acidosis. In fact, of 18 patients with acidosis only 1 survived the shock episode, and none survived subsequently, whereas 33 of 48 who were normal or alkalotic survived the shock episode. It is postulated that in bacteremic shock hyperventilation occurs, leading to respiratory alkalosis. If the patient does not respond to treatment, a continued depression of tissue perfusion leads to the accumulation of large amounts of lactate with acidosis and death.

Bergentz and Brief showed that the development of refractory oligemic shock in dogs was accompanied by the production of acidosis and that the administration of a buffer prevented acidosis as well as the development of refractory shock. An identical volume of a concentrated sodium chloride solution also usually prevented the development of refractory shock without correcting the acidosis. It was felt that the improvement noted with hypertonic solutions was due to a redistribution of fluids from the intracellular to the extracellular space, thus perhaps preventing cellular swelling and promoting an expansion of the extracellular fluid volume.

CARDIAC ARREST. Chazan and his coworkers studied 22 patients during cardiac arrest and found that 10 had predominantly respiratory acidosis and 8 had metabolic acidosis. Most patients with a metabolic acidosis had had a myocardial infarction and had an arterial pH of 7.15 to 7.35. These patients appeared to be benefited by sodium bicarbonate with or without hyperventilation. In the 10 patients with respiratory acidosis, who were chiefly patients with pulmonary problems, the pH was 6.86 to 7.09 in 8. Hypercapnia was prevalent, alkalitherapy seemed less effective, and improved ventilation appeared to be the major therapeutic objective. Acidosis tends to develop during cardiac arrest, because the cardiac index is markedly reduced during resuscitation by closed-chest massage, and this results in decreased tissue perfusion, hypoxia, anaerobic metabolism, and the production of lactic acid. In addition, many of the patients may be inadequately ventilated, causing a rise in P_{CO_2} and the development of respiratory acidosis. Only 2 patients in the group of 22 survived and left the hospital, although several others recovered temporarily, only to die later. In 4 patients, the acidosis could not be definitely classified as either metabolic or respiratory.

BURNS. Peaston demonstrated that although there is a paucity of information on acid-base disturbances in burn patients, acidosis is a frequent finding in these patients. He studied 14 consecutive unselected patients admitted to a regional burn unit and expressed the severity of acidosis in terms of the base deficit, after the method of Siggaard-Andersen et al., obtained by interpolation from the Siggaard-Andersen nomogram. Significant respiratory alkalosis was assumed when the arterial P_{CO_2} was below 30 mm Hg. Uncompensated acidosis was said to be present when the arterial pH fell below 7.35. It was found that 12 of the 14 patients had a base deficit at some stage after thermal injury and that in 7 of these the metabolic acidosis was maximal on admission and in 3 others within 24 hours of admission. The maximal degree of acidosis was found to correlate closely with the total extent of the body burn surface area. The severe degrees of base deficit observed were usually compensated by respiratory alkalosis. Acidosis was treated by the administration of sodium bicarbonate in doses as great as 400 mEq over 24 hours, or 2,750 mEq over a period of 11 days. The acidosis could not be attributed to the liberal use of normal saline solution, because in many patients it was maximal on admission before the patients had received any saline solution. It was felt that because of the unfavorable effect of acidosis on renal function the prompt correction of acidosis in the burn patient would help to prevent acute renal failure.

EFFECTS OF ACIDOSIS. Acidosis has profound effects on the cardiovascular system, producing a decreased myocardial contractility, a decreased response of the myocardium and peripheral vasculature to catecholamines, and a predisposition to cardiac arrhythmias. Acidosis predisposes to acute renal failure. Furthermore, it increases respiratory work.

Greenberg and Kittle have studied the effect of pH and P_{CO_2} changes on coronary blood flow and cardiac output, and find that both are increased by elevations of P_{CO_2} and that they are further increased by an elevation of pH. Thus both are increased in respiratory acidosis and metabolic alkalosis (particularly the latter), and both are reduced in metabolic acidosis and respiratory alkalosis.

Huckabee reported a series of 9 patients who had a syndrome of hyperpnea, tachypnea, and dyspnea with weakness and fatigue progressing to stupor and finally death. All these patients had acidosis characterized by a low serum bicarbonate level and a high value of unmeasured anion in the serum electrolyte pattern which turned out to be lactate. This group of patients had nothing else in common except for a very high level of lactic acidosis, which appeared to be due to widespread tissue hypoxia. This again illustrates the lethal nature of uncorrected acidosis.

A Problem in Acid-Base Balance. Figure 1-37 presents some of the findings from a very interesting patient who progressed from presumed metabolic acidosis to respiratory acidosis to respiratory alkalosis to metabolic alkalosis, all within a 24-hour period. This fourteen-year-old boy who had a large pheochromocytoma of the left adrenal was operated upon under general anesthesia, and the pheochromocytoma was removed. Within minutes after the last vein was tied off, the patient's blood pressure fell precipitously, and a severe bradycardia, hypotension, pulmonary edema, and cardiac arrest developed despite the administration of norepinephrine and all other attempts to support his blood pressure and cardiac action. It became necessary to open his chest in order to restore a cardiac beat, and there was a considerable period of hypotension and hypoxia, which almost certainly must have led to metabolic acidosis, although no measurements were made at this precise time.

When the operation was completed, the patient was removed to the recovery room, where because of continued poor ventilation and pulmonary edema he was placed on a respirator. He failed to regain consciousness, and it was then discovered that the respirator was defective. A blood pH taken at this time was 7.02, and the patient was found to have a profound respiratory acidosis. When the respirator was noted to be defective, the patient was placed on a manual bag and breathed vigorously. His respiration was further improved by placing him on a volume respirator, which lowered his P_{CO_2} from 72 to 26 and raised his pH to 7.54. A profound respiratory alkalosis then developed with a pH of 7.74, a P_{CO_2} of 33, and a potassium level of 2.3 mEq/L. At this point carpopedal spasm developed, and the respirator was stopped. Because of the alkalosis and because he had been receiving Decadron, large amounts of urinary potassium were lost. A spot check showed 83 mEq/L of potassium in the urine, while the sodium concentration was 11 mEq/L. The marked potassium loss continued, and an acid urine developed. The pH, which had fallen to 7.42, rose to 7.51, with a P_{O_2} of 250 (on oxygen), a P_{CO_2} of 41, a carbon dioxide level of 30, and a potassium level of 2.5 mEq/L in spite of the administration of large amounts of potassium intravenously. At this point an uncompensated metabolic alkalosis appeared to have developed. Still larger amounts of potassium were administered, and the dose of Decadron was reduced. He went on to make an uneventful recovery.

It is important to note that at times it may be necessary to administer very much larger doses of potassium than one is accustomed to give. Several cases of this type, all of them diabetics, were collected by Pullen et al., in which potassium was administered in doses of up to 860 mEq in 24 hours.

Water and Electrolyte Metabolism

Although it is axiomatic that the response to injury or operation depends upon the utilization and type of anesthetic agent, the preinjury state of the patient, the type of injury, and the particular fluid and electrolyte solutions used in the patient's treatment, nevertheless some generalizations can be made to serve as a frame of reference for the infinite variations produced by the factors just mentioned.

One of the most constant responses to injury of all types is the release of ADH. This hormone produces oliguria unless specific steps are taken to overcome it. It was originally suggested that oliguria was a normal accompaniment of surgical trauma and that it did no particular harm. It is certainly reasonably well tolerated in most types of mild to moderate surgical trauma, but it is a potentially harmful condition in two ways: the first is that it predisposes to acute tubular necrosis in patients with severe trauma in whom hypovolemia and hypotension are apt to occur, and the second is that it sets the stage for the development of water intoxication if large amounts of non-solute-containing fluids are given to the patient before, during, or immediately after the operative event.

The increased ADH activity persists for 3 to 5 days

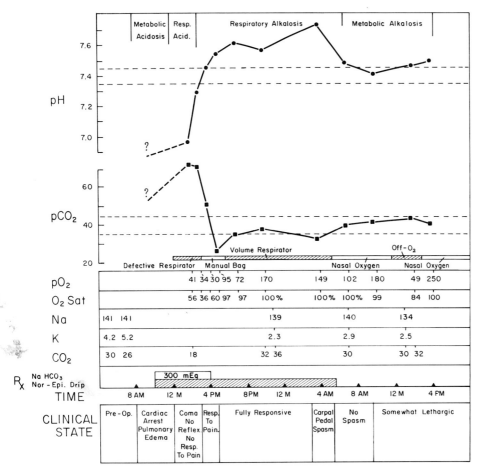

Fig. 1-37. Acid-base abnormalities in a patient with pheochromo-cytoma. The patient had a cardiac arrest on the operating table associated with peripheral vasoconstriction, overtransfusion with blood, tissue hypoxia, and pulmonary edema. It was necessary to open his chest to restore effective cardiac activity. During this time a severe metabolic acidosis was presumed to have developed, and the patient was given sodium bicarbonate intravenously. After getting his heart started again, the patient was maintained on intravenously administered norepinephrine and was returned to the recovery room and placed on a respirator. The respirator proved to be defective, producing a very severe hypoxia and a marked respiratory acidosis with a P_{CO_2} of 72. The patient's pH at this time was 7.02. When it was discovered that the respirator was defective, the patient was shifted to a manual bag, and this quickly brought the P_{CO_2} down, at which time the patient was placed on a volume respirator. This ventilated him so well that a rather marked respiratory alkalosis developed, with a pH of 7.74. Carpopedal spasm developed, and the respirator was discontinued. Subsequent to this a mild metabolic alkalosis developed, partly as a consequence of the administration of corticosteroids, and large amounts of potassium were lost in the urine, a rather significant hypokalemia developing. This was corrected by the administration of large amounts of potassium chloride intravenously, and the patient ultimately recovered completely.

postoperatively, depending upon the severity of the trauma, and it is a very common event to see patients who have undergone rather severe operative trauma eliminate their water load with a very brisk diuresis, sometimes ranging up to 200 or 300 ml/hour on the third or fourth postoperative day.

Measurements of ADH levels in surgical patients were made by Moran et al.; they found that the night before the operation the blood level of ADH was 0.6 μU/ml of whole blood, while just prior to the induction of anesthesia the value had risen to 1.7 μU, apparently as a consequence of the standard practice of withholding fluids the night before the surgical procedure. The rise was greatest in those patients who had been placed on nasogastric suction. Adequate fluid replacement prior to the induction of anesthesia reduced these values to 0.7 μU/ml. The start of the operation was delayed for up to 40 minutes to note the effect of anesthesia per se on ADH levels. Anesthesia produced a slight increase in ADH levels, but this could be completely offset by the rapid administration of parenteral fluid, which led instead of falling ADH levels. The value for the anesthetic period was therefore 1.4 μU/ml, which was similar to that of the preinduction period.

The anesthetic agents used were halothane, Pentothal, methoxyflurane, and nitrous oxide. If the operation was performed under epidural anesthesia, no response to the

abdominal incision was noted. In patients operated on under general anesthesia an increased output of ADH occurred within 5 minutes, and in all patients this increase occurred once traction was applied to the viscera innervated outside the area of effective block. A very minor response to skin incision alone took place, but a tenfold increase occurred when the incision was rapidly carried through all layers of the abdominal wall and traction was applied to the viscera.

The responses occurring during the intermediate portion of the operation were very variable. Sometimes the ADH level rose to a plateau which was maintained throughout the procedure, and at other times it simply rose and fell according to visceral traction. Levels as high as 40 to 150 μU/ml occurred during visceral traction. The magnitude of response was related generally to the magnitude of the procedure. Levels of the sort observed are capable of producing a temporary complete cessation of urine flow. In two patients with high ADH values the creatinine clearance decreased 50 percent, whereas in a patient with a much smaller response there was no change in the creatinine clearance.

The postoperative period was characterized by two phases: the first phase began shortly after skin closure, lasted 6 to 12 hours, and was characterized by a plateau of moderately increased ADH output; this period was followed by a gradual decrease of ADH levels until normal levels were reached on the fourth or fifth postoperative day. In cases of lesser magnitude the return to normal levels occurred by the second postoperative day. The high levels of ADH could be correlated very well with a low urinary output, while the falloff in ADH levels corresponded with diuresis. While hydration was capable of suppressing the increased output of ADH preoperatively and during anesthesia alone, it was not capable of suppressing the elevated levels of ADH seen during operation and in the postoperative period.

The unopposed ADH output produces water retention, oliguria, and hyponatremia. These changes are compounded by the administration of solute-free water and to some extent by water released through fat oxidation.

Insensible Water Loss

Insensible water losses have been said by Hayes to be about the same after as before injury and of the order of 750 ml/m²/day. This would be an insensible water loss of about 1,300 ml/day, which seems excessively high. Gump and Kinney report a loss of about 2 ml/m²/hour, which comes to about 860 ml/day. Actually it is more frequently in the order of 500 ml/day. We have had an opportunity to carry a large number of patients through operative procedures in the complete absence of all renal tissue. Unless there are excessive losses into the wound or an exceptionally high fever, the patients are maintained in equilibrium on about 500 ml/day. Increased losses can occur in the presence of hyperventilation or fever, and huge losses occur from the skin wounds of burned patients.

HYDRATION. It was shown by Hume and Egdahl that acute anuria after kidney transplantation in dogs could be prevented by sufficient hydration of the donor prior to and during operation in order to provide a brisk diuresis of the donor kidney before its removal. The same principle has been applied to renal homotransplantation in man. Barry and Malloy have stressed the value of preventing

oliguria in the surgical patient by means of substained hydration. These writers showed that at all concentrations of halothane anesthesia studied renal plasma flow, glomerular filtration rate, and urine flow were significantly depressed in fluid-restricted subjects. In contrast these measurements were normal in hydrated subjects, except when very high concentrations of halothane were used. The hydrated group was given a 0.3% saline solution. Sodium excretion in the hydrated and dehydrated groups were the same, but urine osmolality exceeded serum osmolality in all dehydrated subjects, whereas urine osmolality was considerably lower in the hydrated subjects.

During surgical procedures some sequestration of fluid occurs in the operative area (the so-called "third space"), and this produces a reduction in central circulatory volume which leads to a fall in renal blood flow. Renal blood flow can be restored to normal by the prompt administration of fluid, but if the deficit in central circulatory volume is allowed to persist beyond certain critical limits, the ability of renal circulation to respond promptly to restoration is lost. This reduction in central circulatory volume produces stimulation of the volume receptors, thus leading to the release of vasoconstrictor substances such as angiotensin and catecholamines. This produces a further decrease in renal blood flow which may be resistant to change. Oliguria can be prevented by the routine administration of 1,000 to 1,500 ml of a balanced salt solution in the 2- to 3-hour period prior to the beginning of anesthesia, and the administration of mannitol during the operative event. It is very important that the diuresis be established before the introduction of anesthesia.

Postoperative Patterns

The two patterns that are perhaps most frequently seen in the postoperative patient are illustrated in Figs. 1-38 and 1-39. The first is that of a mild to moderate dilutional hyponatremia with hyperkalemia. This is primarily brought about by ADH secretion plus overhydration of the patient with non-solute-containing fluids. The potassium level may be somewhat elevated, because potassium is lost from cells as a consequence of corticosteroid-induced injury and starvation catabolism, is infused in the form of high-potassium old blood, is absorbed from blood left in the peritoneal cavity or wound, and is not well excreted because of impaired renal perfusion.

This response is made much worse if the trauma is severe and prolonged or if the patient has had a chronic wasting illness prior to operation. Other factors which make the response worse are starvation, which in itself can produce hyponatremia, preexisting renal impairment, which predisposes to a further elevation of potassium level and depression of sodium level, cardiac disease with edema, preexisting hyponatremia, a pronounced shift of sodium into the cell with severe trauma, and episodes of hypotension during the operation which may further impair renal function. If a marked diuresis is induced by mannitol, this may produce considerable sodium diuresis and add to the hyponatremia if non-sodium-containing repair solutions are used. The cardiac patient may still need sodium therapy postoperatively, even though he has

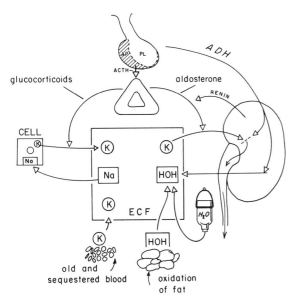

Fig. 1-38. Mechanism for the development of hyponatremia in the postoperative period. Under the influence of ADH the kidney retains water which dilutes sodium in the extracellular fluid (ECF) volume. In severe trauma there is a shift of sodium into the cell, further adding to the hyponatremia. The use of bank blood and the absorption of potassium from sequestered blood may produce a mild to moderate hyperkalemia. This is contributed to by the glucocorticoids, which through catabolism release potassium from the cells. Aldosterone would ordinarily increase the secretion of potassium by the kidney, but since there is a relative oliguria due to the action of ADH, there is a limited secretion of potassium and a net gain of this cation in the ECF space. The administration of solute-free water intravenously contributes to the expansion of the ECF and hyponatremia.

an elevated total body sodium level. Calcium can also be used but may potentiate digitalis effect if the potassium level remains high. These changes can be prevented or minimized by the use of sodium chloride–containing solutions in the preoperative, operative, and postoperative periods, and with the avoidance of potassium-containing solutions in the first 3 days postoperatively unless the patient has unusual potassium losses or is manifesting a declining blood potassium level. In most instances potassium supplementation will be unnecessary, since the patient can take potassium-containing solutions by mouth by the third day.

The second pattern is one of hypokalemic alkalosis. This is classically seen in the patient with an obstructing duodenal ulcer on gastric suction. The alkalosis created by the loss of hydrogen ion from the stomach produces marked potassium loss in the urine. This condition is made worse by starvation; the intravenous administration of fluids without potassium; the administration of chlorothiazide diuretics; the administration of corticosteroids; the presence of diarrhea or a fistula; hyperventilation alkalosis; the preoperative existence of certain diseases, such as severe liver disease, where hypokalemia may frequently be present; the administration of sodium bicarbonate or tris buffer, particularly to open heart patients on extracorporeal circulation; or the presence of chronic pulmonary

disease, where pulmonary arteriovenous shunts produce hypoxia and a secondary stimulus to hypocapnia. These changes can be prevented by avoidance of the factors listed above, which intensify the response, and by the administration of potassium-containing fluids as needed in the postoperative period. In particular the restoration of acquired deficits prior to operation when possible helps to prevent development of these changes.

OXYGEN TRANSPORT

Certain organic phosphates in erythrocytes interact with deoxygenated hemoglobin, thereby altering the affinity of hemoglobin for oxygen. The most abundant of these phosphates in man is 2,3-DPG, the erythrocyte concentration of which has an inverse relationship to the affinity of hemoglobin for oxygen.

Blood stored in ACD at 4°C shows a progressive loss of 2,3-DPG, and after 15 days there is almost none at all. This shifts the oxyhemoglobin dissociation curve strikingly to the left. If such blood is infused into patients, it has a diminished ability to give up oxygen to the tissues.

There are other factors which lower erythrocyte 2,3-DPG levels and produce tissue anoxia. These include (1) acidosis, (2) alkalosis, (3) hypophosphatemia (especially seen with hyperalimentation with synthetic amino acids without added phosphate), (4) septic shock, and (5) trauma without hypotension.

Hemorrhagic shock in patients or baboons usually does not alter red cell 2,3-DPG levels, but resuscitation with old banked blood does. Less severe trauma is usually associated with respiratory alkalosis, and this may depress 2,3-DPG levels and reduce tissue oxygenation. Severe shock with acidosis or septic shock reduces 2,3-DPG and interferes with tissue oxygenation.

Hyperalimentation with essential amino acid solutions not containing added phosphate leads to severe hypophosphatemia, which in turn reduces erythrocyte 2,3-DPG and ATP levels and increases red cell avidity for oxygen, leading to tissue hypoxia.

Increases in erythrocyte 2,3-DPG occurs at high altitudes, with chronic anemia, and in congestive heart failure.

Changes in erythrocyte 2,3-DPG levels were not observed by Naylor and his colleagues in rhesus monkeys subjected either to endotoxin or hypovolemic shock.

In clinical settings, the use of old banked blood, marked alkalosis, septic shock, and hyperalimentation are the circumstances in which depressed erythrocyte 2,3-DPG levels are usually seen. All these except septic shock are easily reversed. The administration of fresh or frozen blood, correction of alkalosis, and addition of phosphate to hyperalimentation mixtures solve the other problems.

IMMUNOLOGIC PROTECTIVE MECHANISMS

After injury there is an acute fall in lymphocytes, an increase in polymorphonuclear leukocytes, and a transient suppression of the reticuloendothelial system (RES). All these events are due in whole or in part to increased corticosteroid (17-OHCS) secretion. While the absence or severe diminution of corticosteroid secretion (Addison's disease) leads to an increased susceptibility to infection, the administration of pharmacologic doses of corticosteroids also interferes with defense mechanisms.

Immediately after a severe trauma there is a surge of neuroendocrine activity designed to counteract the early effects of the injury, an event obviously of paramount importance to the survival of the organism. If the individual survives, this surge diminishes in favor of the mechanisms of orderly repair, and protein and fat repletion. If the injury is complicated by sepsis or repeated traumatic insult, there will be a continuous neuroendocrine stimulus, and cortisol levels will generally remain elevated right up to the point of death. The lymphocyte and eosinophil counts remain low, and cellular immunity is suppressed.

The suppression of cellular immunity produced by the corticosteroids is the basis for the use of these substances in organ homotransplantation and hypersensitivity states —such as beesting and snakebites.

The corticosteroids may also interfere with the action of complement, and this may account for the beneficial effects claimed for the use of large doses of steroids in endotoxin shock. Many explanations have been advanced to explain this effect, including (1) a mildly positive inotrophic and vasodilating action; (2) a metabolic effect which increases lactic acid metabolism, decreases serum fatty acid and amino acid concentration, reduces acidosis, improves citric acid cycling, and increases energy production; (3) a stabilization of lysosomal membranes; (4) an inhibition of the production of myocardial depressant factor (MDF) by lysosomal enzymes of the pancreas; (5) a permissive support of catecholamine function; and (6) a corticosteroid binding of endotoxin. These explanations, however, either seem inadequate to account for the benefits claimed or could not be corroborated by other workers.

Stetson showed that most of the effects of endotoxin could be produced by antigen-antibody complexes, and Pillemer and his colleagues showed that gram-negative bacterial endotoxins could activate complement. Weil and Spink noted a marked resemblance between endotoxin shock and anaphylactic shock. Schumer and his colleagues investigated the thesis that endotoxin shock was produced by antigen-antibody complexes and complement, which combined to produce an anaphylactic reaction, and found that corticosteroids exerted a protective effect by decreasing either complement or complement fixation. While this may not be the sole explanation for the production of endotoxin shock or the beneficial effect of pharmacologic doses of corticosteroids, it seems likely that antigen-antibody complexes and complement play an important role in the production of this type of shock.

Polymorphonuclear leukocytes and platelets are increased in numbers by cortisol, so that although the lymphatic system is suppressed by the glucocorticoids, the bone marrow is generally stimulated. The RES, like the lymphatic system, is suppressed early after severe injury, at which time there is an increased susceptibility to shock and infection. Later there is a recovery and even hyper-

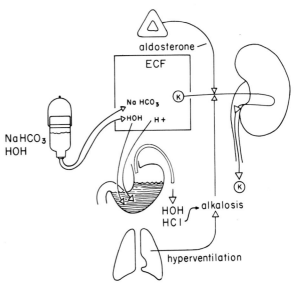

Fig. 1-39. Pattern of hypokalemic alkalosis in the postoperative patient. This is most commonly seen in patients who have been on gastric suction and who are alkalotic at the time of operation. The alkalosis produces an additional potassium loss in the urine. Hyperventilation increases the alkalosis and promotes further potassium loss. The administration of sodium bicarbonate, sometimes given in circumstances thought likely to produce acidosis, may further increase the alkalosis. These events then conspire to produce a severe hypokalemic alkalosis which, if renal function is good, may be made worse by the action of the corticosteroids in promoting potassium excretion.

activity of the RES. These patterns of activity appear to correlate with the level of corticosteroid secretion, and RES function is inversely related to corticosteroid levels.

The RES plays a role in resistance to certain types of shock which is quite apart from its antibacterial role. Stimulation of the RES by estrogen, choline, or zymosan increases phagocytic function and also increases the resistance to trauma. Adaptation to repeated trauma is accompanied by a marked hypertrophy and hyperfunction of the RES.

The RES aids in clearing away fibrin and other coagulation debris, and RES blockade leads to intravascular fibrin deposition and renal corticol necrosis. It also leads to increased susceptibility to shock.

In hemorrhagic shock the RES cell is said by Bell and his colleagues to undergo lysosomal disruption, a change which may lead to autolysis and RES failure.

Distant trauma increases the rate of wound or peritoneal infection in response to a bacterial inoculum. This is said by Hawley to be counteracted by dextran, which works by diminishing blood viscosity. The increased blood viscosity which normally accompanies trauma interferes with tissue perfusion and oxygenation, and thus increases susceptibility to infection.

Thus while there are obvious effects of trauma upon the immune system, the effects vary with the time after injury, the type of trauma, and the particular segment of the immune system which is studied. There are still many gaps in our knowledge of the response of the immune defense mechanisms to injury, and further work needs to be done to clarify this relationship.

ORGAN SYSTEM CHANGES

Cardiovascular Function

SURGERY. Many of the cardiovascular changes in severe trauma and shock have already been described. Clowes and Del Guercio followed the cardiac response in a series of patients before, during, and after operation. During operation the cardiac output fell an average of 33 percent from the preoperative level, mainly because of a decrease in stroke volume. This was accompanied by an elevation of central venous pressure. Immediately after the operation, following endotracheal extubation, the cardiac output rose on the average to 130 percent of the preoperative

Fig. 1-40. Effect of phenoxybenzamine in septicemic shock. After raising the central venous pressure with colloids and after the failure of other modalities of treatment, phenoxybenzamine produced a rise of blood pressure, a fall in central venous pressure, a fall in peripheral resistance, an increase in cardiac index, a fall in pulse, an increase in stroke volume, and a marked increase in urinary output. (*From R. M. Hardaway et al., JAMA, 199:779, 1967.*)

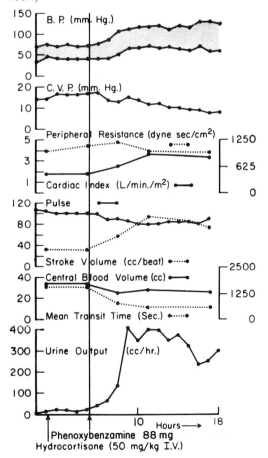

value and remained at somewhat elevated levels for the first postoperative week. This elevation of cardiac output after the end of the operation was characteristic of thoracic procedures but was not seen following abdominal laparotomy. Patients who died during the postoperative period never achieved circulatory flows comparable to their preoperative levels.

BURNS. Berk and his colleagues studied eight severely burned patients and found a characteristic pattern consisting of a decrease in cardiac output with normal blood pressure and increased total peripheral resistance. The oxygen consumption was increased with a high arteriovenous oxygen difference, resulting from the low total cardiac flows. The central blood volume was increased, and central venous pressure showed no evidence of hypovolemia.

SHOCK. MacLean and Duff found that septic shock in dogs and man was accompanied by a fall in cardiac output, blood pressure, and central venous pressure. In dogs, treatment with isoproterenol, blood, and hyperbaric oxygen restored cardiac output and decreased peripheral resistance but did not improve survival. In patients there was generally an increased peripheral resistance associated with hemorrhagic shock. Transfusion and isoproterenol restored venous pressure, cardiac output, and blood pressure to or toward normal and decreased peripheral resistance. Survival seems to have been favorably influenced by this treatment.

Wilson and coworkers evaluated the data in 31 patients in shock. Those in septic shock had a higher cardiac output and lower peripheral resistance than those in hypovolemic or cardiac shock, where the peripheral resistance was always high. No survival was noted in the septic shock group unless cardiac output was at least 2 liters/m²/minute. It was stressed that while vasodilators, such as phenoxybenzamine, might be of value when peripheral resistance was increased, their use in patients with decreased peripheral resistance was of no definite benefit and might be deleterious.

Severe trauma is thus characterized by a decreased cardiac output and often an increased peripheral resistance. Tissue arteriovenous shunts may open up, partly as a consequence of epinephrine release, thus increasing venous oxygenation and further intensifying tissue anoxia. This increases acidosis and additionally reduces cardiac output.

The use of phenoxybenzamine in certain patients in septic shock to overcome some of the unfavorable cardiovascular changes has been championed by Hardaway and his associates. Before administering phenoxybenzamine the patients had been treated with volume replacement, antibiotics, correction of acid-base imbalances, corticosteroids, and vasopressors, with progressive deterioration on this regimen. It is emphasized that vasodilators should be used only when preceded by fluid volume replacement to the point of an elevated central venous or pulmonary artery pressure. At this time, when the cardiac index is low and peripheral resistance high, phenoxybenzamine may produce a dramatic increase in cardiac index, fall in peripheral resistance, and brisk diuresis (Fig. 1-40). Respiratory insufficiency, which is usually present, must be corrected and treatment instituted for sepsis and defects in coagulation. Apart from its peripheral effect of vasodilatation and improved tissue perfusion, phenoxybenzamine is believed to improve cardiac performance by direct inotropic action on the myocardium, vasodilating effect on the coronary vessels and myocardial microvasculature, and relief of postcapillary pulmonary vasoconstriction with increased venous return to the left side of the heart. Most patients in septic shock, however, have peripheral vasodilatation, at least in the early and intermediate stages, and a hyperdynamic state. Therefore, the popularity of vasodilators has declined.

The cause of cardiac failure in shock, particularly in septic shock, is still being hotly debated. However, there is general agreement that septic shock induces initially a hyperdynamic state with a high cardiac output and a low peripheral resistance, unless the patient has previously had a reduced blood volume. Although those findings might be explained by arteriovenous shunting in the peripheral tissues or by defective oxygen transfer to the tissues as a consequence of the low erythrocyte 2,3-DPG levels known to be present in septic shock, Wright and his coworkers have developed evidence to suggest that there is instead a primary failure of the peripheral tissues in septic shock to extract oxygen, and that the hyperdynamic state results as a compensatory mechanism.

After a period of time the hyperdynamic state gives way to deterioration of cardiac function and ultimately cardiac failure and death. During the period of deterioration of function Cann and his coworkers found that ouabain was the only agent they tested which was capable of improving myocardial function. Coalson and her colleagues, however, found that digoxin treatment provided functional protection for the heart and prevented the mitochondrial changes produced in the myocardium by endotoxin.

Interest has recently been renewed in the concept that there is a circulatory factor present in shock, particularly endotoxin shock, which is a specific myocardial depressant, and that this agent is responsible for the failure of the heart in septic shock. Attar et al. believe that plasma kallikreins are partly responsible for this effect. These are proteolytic enzymes activated by Hageman factor which release bradykinin from its precursor. The kallikreins were found to be increased in shock, and were assumed to release bradykinin, thus producing hypotension.

Solis and Downing, Lefer et al., Glenn and Lefer, and Wagensteen and his colleagues have written a series of papers reviving the concept that MDF is the primary agent producing myocardial depression in shock, particularly septic shock. MDF is a small peptide produced in the pancreas by the action of lysosomal proteases released during shock. They feel that the primary event in any type of shock is splanchnic hypoperfusion which then releases lysosomal hydrolases, primarily from the pancreas, giving rise to MDF, which in turn exerts strong negative inotropic effect on the heart.

Goodyer and his colleagues have shown that the canine myocardium, which usually extracts pyruvate from coronary blood, produces pyruvate in hemorrhagic shock, even when the ventricular function is still well preserved. The coronary sinus oxygen falls below 20 percent at a time when the cardiac function is still quite good, and this may be responsible for the early abnormality in pyruvate metabolism, and the late impairment in contractile function. They feel that some factor present in the blood after 1 hour of shock may give rise to this change in oxygenation and in pyruvate metabolism and that their data generally support the concept of an MDF of some type. Low norepinephrine levels have been observed in the myocardium in shock by Hiott and Richardson, but the reduced myocardial effort could not be related to the levels of norepinephrine.

In the later stages of endotoxin shock there is universal agreement that cardiac failure supervenes. Hinshaw and his coworkers have noted a characteristic elevation of left ventricular end-diastolic pressure, decreased maximal change in the left ventricular pressure, and the need for a positive inotropic agent to drive the heart through an imposed after-load performance curve. Only slight improvement was noted with beta-adrenergic stimulatory agents.

Greenfield et al. and Hinshaw et al. have demonstrated normal myocardial performance in the early phases of endotoxin shock, and no adverse effects on cardiac work or metabolism during cross circulation with animals in the intermediate or late stages. These experiments did not, therefore, substantiate a primary role for MDF in endotoxin shock.

Levinson and Hume carried out exchange transfusions in animals and four patients in refractory shock. In the animal experiments this procedure proved to be much more effective than administration of corticosteroids, isoproterenol, or Ringer's lactate solution. The four patients showed improvement in cardiac output, mean arterial pressure, urine output, and arterial pH—although all ultimately died. It was postulated that the exchange transfusions might have washed out substances interfering with cardiac function, including vasoactive polypeptides, histamine, serotonin, catecholamines, or MDF. The exchange also added erythrocytes containing normal amounts of 2,3-DPG to replace those with the depressed 2,3-DPG levels seen in septic shock, thus perhaps improving tissue oxygenation.

It is obvious that the question of the primary of MDFs in septic shock has not yet been answered.

ANESTHESIA. Baez and Orkin studied the effect of various anesthetic agents on microcirculation and concluded that with cyclopropane anesthesia the compensatory mechanisms of vasomotion, epinephrine reactivity, and overall blood flow are well maintained whereas with ether these compensatory reactions, initially enhanced, are then depressed below normal. Halothane sustained compensatory vascular patterns until late in the course of observation. Methoxyflurane depressed compensatory mechanisms early. It was felt that these experiments confirmed the clinical observations of the utility of cyclopropane and halothane in shock.

Pulmonary Function

ANESTHESIA AND SURGERY. Hypoxia and hypercapnia following operation may be due to the continuing effects of anesthesia and muscle relaxants, together with the development of atelectasis. Significant decreases in pulmonary diffusion have been found following all types of operations, lasting as long as 5 days following operation. The ventilation perfusion defect or pulmonary arteriovenous shunting may involve 25 percent of the total pulmonary blood flow. This produces a considerable degree of hypoxia.

The work of breathing, which normally requires 1 to 2 percent of the cardiac output, may require as much as 30 to 50 percent of the total cardiac output after operation or trauma. Assisted respiration produces a decrease in oxygen consumption and cardiac output.

Anesthesia and surgical procedures alter respiration by depressing the pulmonary reflexes and the central nervous system response, thus depressing the patient's desire to breathe. This is true of both preoperative and postoperative medications, the general anesthetic agent, and of course the muscle relaxants. The patients may occasionally have very severe reactions to a muscle relaxant, so that they will not breathe on their own for several hours after the end of the operation. Respiratory excursion is also interfered with by spinal and epidural anesthesia and by disruption of the thorax, abdomen, or the respiratory tract itself. Secretions collect in the bronchial tree because of difficulty in coughing and moving, and this gives rise to atelectasis. Pulmonary arteriovenous shunts may be operative in atelectasis and in patients with cirrhosis, and profound acid-base changes may result as a consequence of hyperventilation or prolonged cardiopulmonary bypass.

Peters and Hedgpeth have shown that an increase in airway resistance and pulmonary vascular resistance both cause increased respiratory work. They also lead to ventilation perfusion incoordination by changing the time constant to the various areas of the lung. This causes more work. The increased respiratory work then leads to further acidosis in a vicious cycle, since acidosis leads to pulmonary vasoconstriction and further sensitizes the lung to vasoconstriction due to hypoxia. Metabolic acidosis superimposed on respiratory acidosis retards the increased cardiac output associated ordinarily with respiratory acidosis. Metabolic acidosis increases pulmonary vascular resistance, thus increasing respiratory work.

Prophylaxis. In an attempt to determine whether postoperative pulmonary complications can be prevented by the use of isoproterenol and intermittent positive pressure breathing (IPPB), Anderson and his colleagues studied 160 control patients and 42 patients receiving IPPB and isoproterenol. A very significant reduction in postoperative complications was encountered in the treated group. Roe has also urged the wider use of airway moisture, expectorants, tracheal aspiration, bronchoscopy, and tracheostomy as prophylaxis against pulmonary complications in postoperative patients.

High-Output Respiratory Failure. Burke and his coworkers have described the syndrome of high-output respiratory failure as that type of respiratory failure characterized by inability to produce adequate tissue oxygenation, and later carbon dioxide excretion, despite an initially increased gas exchange. In a study of 21 patients this type of failure frequently was associated with severe peritonitis or ileus. No deaths were directly attributable to the high-output failure. The syndrome of high-output respiratory failure may be suspected by persistent elevation of pulse and respiration with a normal blood pressure in an anxious exhausted patient. It is confirmed by a depressed arterial oxygen saturation. Previous lung disease, obesity, smoking, or severe debility predispose to it. Tracheostomy and assisted respiration may have to be used to treat it.

Nash and his coworkers have described a pulmonary lesion associated with oxygen therapy and artificial ventilation in 70 patients who died after prolonged artificial ventilation. These patients all showed characteristic pulmonary changes consisting of heavy, beefy, and edematous lungs. Microscopically these showed an early exudative phase characterized by congestion, alveolar edema, intraalveolar hemorrhage, and a fibrin exudate, with formation of prominent hyaline membranes without any associated inflammatory component. A late proliferative phase was characterized by marked aveolar and interlobular septal edema, fibroblastic proliferation with early fibrosis, and prominent hyperplasia of the lining cells. These changes were not related to the duration of the ventilation but to high concentrations of inspired oxygen. It was felt that patients should receive inspired oxygen concentration sufficient to ensure normal or nearly normal arterial oxygen tension and that this should be reduced as soon as blood-gas measurements show that reduction can be accomplished safely.

SHOCK. Cook and Webb have studied the pulmonary changes in shock and found that there was a rise in transpulmonary vascular pressure and a great increase in pulmonary vascular resistance which persisted for several hours after the shock was corrected. There was congestive atelectasis, recruitment of pulmonary vascular segments, and alveolar capillary dilatation, suggesting venous constriction. Ventilation increased while compliance decreased, indicating a diminished gas exchange with increased ventilatory work. Veith and his coworkers found that shock and transfusion produced an initial active arteriolar vasoconstriction followed by secondary vasodilatation, congestion, hemorrhage, and edema. These changes may help to explain the frequent pulmonary complications accompanying hemorrhagic shock.

POSTTRAUMATIC PULMONARY INSUFFICIENCY. There has been a great deal of interest recently in the lung changes that occur in severe trauma not involving the thorax. The condition has often been called "shock lung," but as shock alone does not actually produce it, it is probably best called the *posttraumatic pulmonary insufficiency syndrome*. There are several different etiologic factors—some or all of them operative in each case. Among the factors most frequently incriminated in the syndrome are (1) oxygen therapy, (2) loss of pulmonary surfactant, (3) alveolar collapse, (4) platelet aggregate emboli induced by trauma, (5) platelet aggregates and other debris in infused blood, (6) viable immunologically competent leukocytes in fresh blood, (7) pump oxygenators, (8) fat emboli, (9) pulmonary arteriovenous shunting, (10) sepsis, endotoxin, (11) vomiting and aspirating, and (12) fluid overloading.

Microemboli of various types are probably a factor in most patients with the pulmonary insufficiency syndrome. Platelet microemboli tend to develop in vivo after hemorrhage and as a consequence of endotoxemia. They also develop in banked blood and increase as the storage period is extended, and in pump-oxygenator systems. They are caused by an increase in platelet adhesiveness. Micropore filters have been developed to remove the emboli from infused blood.

Nahas and his colleagues have claimed that viable leukocytes infused in fresh blood can mount a graft versus host reaction in the lung. This can be avoided by the use of frozen red cells. Fat emboli occur not only from bone marrow injury, but also from the reesterification of fatty acids mobilized by the catecholamines and glucagon.

Oxygen toxicity is capable of producing fatal pulmonary damage. When oxygen concentrations of 70 to 100% are used with respirators for prolonged periods of time (giving P_{O_2} values above 350 mm Hg), there is damage to the endothelial cells, with interstitial edema, hyaline membrane deposition, alveolar epithelial cell hypertrophy and desquamation, and alveolar hemorrhage. Arteriovenous shunting and hypoxemia result from this. These are similar to changes seen in the posttraumatic lung.

Sepsis is a major factor in the lung changes seen after trauma. The bacteria may be filtered out by the lung following their embolization from a distant site, they may enter directly through the airway, or they may affect the lungs by means of endotoxins. Endotoxin produces damage to pulmonary capillaries, thus initiating the changes of the pulmonary insufficiency syndrome.

Probably the most important cause of the lung changes of trauma is the loss of pulmonary surfactant with alveolar collapse, focal atelectases, decreased compliance, arteriovenous shunting, and interstitial edema.

Hypothalamic hypoxia is thought to contribute to the development of the syndrome by producing autonomically mediated pulmonary venular spasms leading to interstitial edema, intraalveolar hemorrhage, surfactant neutralization by plasma, hyaline membranes, and alveolar atelectasis.

The hypocapnia that normally develops as a consequence of the postinjury hyperventilation is thought by Trimble and associates to be an important etiologic agent in the production of pulmonary insufficiency. Hypocapnia is said to induce bronchoconstriction, and the alkalosis produced by blowing off carbon dioxide affects blood flow to the lung and unfavorably affects oxyhemoglobin dissociation. The addition of carbon dioxide to the inspired air is said to improve oxygenation and other parameters of pulmonary physiology.

Vomiting and aspirating stomach contents or blood, and fluid overloading are contributing factors to the development of lung lesions after trauma.

The treatment and/or prevention of the pulmonary insufficiency syndrome consists of (1) the use of micropore filters for infused blood, (2) the avoidance of blood with viable leukocytes, (3) treatment of sepsis, (4) the avoidance of aspiration or fluid overloading by administering corticosteroids if aspiration occurs and diuretics for fluid overloads, (5) the use of corticosteroids for massive fat embolization, (6) the use of oxygen mixtures of 45% or less, (7) the determination of serial blood gases, (8) the use of a volume respirator which "sighs" periodically, and especially (9) the application of continuous positive pressure to provide 6 cm water pressure at the end of expiration. This helps to correct the alveolar collapse brought about by loss of surfactant.

The question whether resuscitation with noncolloidal fluids is more damaging to the lung than if colloids had been used is still largely unresolved. While the functional differences between these two repair solutions is slight, there are more ultrastructural lung changes when noncolloids are used than when albumin is used.

The use of a membrane oxygenator and extracorporeal heart-lung machine for a severe case of pulmonary failure has been said by Hill and his colleagues to have resulted in survival. This may be an important therapeutic modality in the future.

The effects of the pulmonary insufficiency syndrome are to produce a progressive hypoxemia with arteriovenous shunting, acidosis, hypercapnia, interstitial edema, and sepsis, with stiff, beefy, heavy, wet lungs and, after, death.

Hepatic Function

DRUGS AND ANESTHETIC AGENTS. Hepatic function may be depressed by many drugs and anesthetic agents administered to the patient prior to or during surgical procedures. If the liver is not diseased and the degree of trauma not too severe, these minor changes in function usually pass unnoticed and do not prove to be of any clinical significance. If the patient has cirrhosis or other liver damage, some of the commonly used drugs and virtually all the anesthetic agents may produce a depression of hepatic function which, because of inability of the damaged liver to detoxify them, leads to a profound generalized effect. Among these drugs are morphine, which may precipitate coma in patients with cirrhosis, and paraldehyde, which may produce a profound sleep or even death in such patients. This is also true of the barbiturates which are metabolized by the liver. Other drugs may interfere with bilirubin metabolism, such as the sulfonamides, which inhibit plasma binding; flavaspidic acid, which interferes with bilirubin transport through the cell; novobiocin, which interferes with glucuronide conjugation; cholecystographic media, which compete with the conjugated bilirubin for excretion into the biliary canaliculus; and methyltestosterone or chlorpromazine, which interfere with the excretion of the bilirubin into the canaliculus. In most instances these reactions are reversible. Direct hepatic toxicity sometimes results from the tetracyclines, particularly in malnutrition or pregnancy, ferrous sulfate, 6-mercaptopurine, methotrexate, and 5-fluoro-2-deoxyuridine. Cinchophen and iproniazid may cause a hepatitis-like reaction.

A great deal of debate has occurred over the effect of

the anesthetic agent halothane as a hepatotoxin. Severe reactions and even death can occur occasionally with halothane anesthesia, although fortunately these reactions are rare. They usually depend upon a personal individual sensitivity and almost always occur only when anesthesia has been administered twice for separate operations. It is therefore probably not wise to repeat halothane anesthesia within 6 months. Some of the antituberculosis drugs may cause a hypersensitivity reaction; chief among this group is para-aminosalicylate. Chlorpropamide and tolbutamide can also cause this reaction.

If hepatic reserve is decreased, as it may be in severe cirrhosis, very minor trauma or brief anesthesia can precipitate hepatic failure, coma, and even death.

SHOCK. In severe trauma and shock there is an increased Bromsulphalein (BSP) retention, increased serum bilirubin, increased prothrombin time, decreased fibrinogen, increased SGOT, increased blood ammonia, and decreased urea formation. Glycogen stores are depleted, and lactate acid accumulates. Ketonemia follows and ultimately gives way to low blood ketone levels as hepatic function is further impaired. Blood amino acid nitrogen level rises. Impairment of enzyme systems occurs, and the liver content of high-energy stores such as ATP, ADP, thiamine pyrophosphate (TPP), and flavin adenine dinucleotide (FAD) as well as phosphocreatinine becomes depleted. CoA and succinate oxidase are reduced. There is a reduced capacity for aerobic metabolism.

The liver has been implicated as one of the causes of irreversibility in shock. It has been postulated that the inability of the liver to detoxify injurious agents released in shock is responsible for the trend toward irreversibility. Actually most of the experiments suggesting this possibility have been carried out in the dog, in which differences in the splanchnic circulation and regular hepatic infection with microorganisms make this animal a poor model for the human system. The liver does seem to protect somewhat against intestinal ischemic shock. There is some depression of the RES of the liver in profound shock.

Holden and his coworkers carried out an electron microscopic study of the liver of the rat in shock. After 2 hours of shock there was a distortion of the endoplasmic reticulum, depletion of the glycogen granules, disorganization and swelling of the mitochondria, and in some cells an increase in the number and size of bodies thought to be lysosomes. Hypoxia produced by an atmosphere of 93% nitrous oxide and 7% oxygen for 1 hour failed to produce similar changes. It was concluded that the ultrastructural and biochemical changes observed in hypovolemic shock were not solely the result of cellular hypoxia but rather the result of the combined effects of cellular hypoxia, the neuroendocrine response to hypovolemia, and the altered physiochemical composition of extracellular fluid (ECF) resulting from diminished capillary perfusion.

A study of liver cell lysosomes in traumatic, ischemic, and endotoxin shock by Janoff showed that there was a disruption of lysosomes and the release of their contained enzymes in free active form in the liver of shocked animals. It was felt that the activation of lysosomal hydrolases within cells and their release into the circulation might play an important role in exacerbating tissue injury and accelerating the development of irreversible shock. In those animals rendered tolerant of shock or pretreated with cortisone there was a stabilization of lysosomes, and it was felt that this effect might constitute an important component of the resistance of such animals to shock. The exacerbating effect of reticuloendothelial blocking colloids on the lethality of shock procedures may be due in part to a direct action of these agents on lysosomes.

Blair and his colleagues have performed electron microscopic studies of the liver in shock and found that there was progressive hepatocellular damage during the first hour, characterized by reduction in glycogen, increased prominence of smooth endoplasmic reticulum, swelling of mitochondria, and a disarrangement of the rough endoplasmic reticulum. After 3 hours of shock there was a progressive increase in secondary lysosomes, and by $4\frac{1}{2}$ hours there was a marked prominence of secondary lysosomes which was related to the irreversible shock state. Clermont et al. demonstrated an increase in lysosomal enzyme acid phosphatase content of hepatic blood, lymph, and bile after the second hour of shock.

In addition to the changes in lysosomes, there is a decrease in cell transmembrane potential difference, a decrease in cyclic AMP, and a decrease in the energy-producing capabilities of mitochondria. The energy availability of the cell is dependent upon mitochondrial respiration, which in turn may be controlled by ATP-dependent membrane transport. Baue and his coworkers demonstrated that hepatic ATP-dependent membrane transport was progressively activated in shock, leading to increased sodium and decreased potassium in the mitochondria, with decreased mitochondrial respiration and energy depletion.

Patients with hepatic failure may have a buildup in the blood of substances profoundly toxic to cells throughout the body. Thus hepatic coma eventuates from the effect of these substances on the brain, oliguria appears as a consequence of their action on the kidney, and hypotension results from a depressed cardiac output as a consequence of a toxic effect on the myocardium. Further depression of hepatic function itself may also take place. These effects sometimes can be dramatically reversed by exchange transfusion, in which the toxic substances are washed out of the bloodstream as the patient's blood is replaced by large quantities of fresh donor blood. Fortunately, hepatic reserve in the normal patient is so great that liver failure is seldom a problem in severe trauma.

Gastrointestinal Function

The gastrointestinal changes in trauma range from the mild syndrome of ileus and temporary loss of appetite following intestinal operations, and mucosal changes in the intestinal tract brought about by shock, to stress ulcers of the stomach and duodenum.

SHOCK. Gurd has studied the metabolic and functional changes in the intestine in shock. He found that in dogs with irreversible shock there was a profound depression of oxygen uptake by the intestine after retransfusion, despite a return of mesenteric blood flow to normal. This was in spite of the fact that oxygen consumption in the liver and limbs returned for a time to normal, as did the cardiac output. Studies with ^{32}P showed a depression of oxidative phosphorylation and nucleotide synthesis in the mucosa of the small intestine of these animals after retransfusion, while full recovery of these processes was noted in the liver. Hemorrhagic necrosis of the bowel was often seen in dogs and could be protected against by the injection of Trasylol, a trypsin inhibitor, into the lumen of the bowel. Hemorrhagic necrosis of this sort is seldom seen in man, where the amount of trypsin present in the intestinal chyme is far less than in dogs.

A higher metabolic activity was observed in bowel washed free of its fecal content, suggesting that contact with feces has a deleterious effect on cellular metabolism in ischemic anoxia. After curare was placed in the lumen, the bowel demonstrated an increased permeability in the metabolically depressed mucosa. If the pancreatic ducts were ligated 48 hours before the shock state was induced, hemorrhagic necrosis was prevented.

It could be demonstrated that the mucin coat over the villi was lost at the moment when signs of irreversibility appeared in hypovolemia. In time mucin production ceased. The first areas to lose the mucin coat were the tips of the villi. The loss of mucin permitted damage to the cells by trypsin and led to the development of hemorrhagic necrosis.

There is a striking species difference between the intestinal changes seen in shock in dogs when compared with primates. In dogs endotoxin shock produces mesenteric vasoconstriction, intestinal ischemia, and epithelial necrosis, while in primates Barton and his colleagues found that endotoxemia was associated with a normal mesenteric blood flow, a fall in mesenteric vascular resistance, and no gross changes in the intestine. Hypovolemic shock in dogs characteristically produces intense mesenteric vasoconstriction, with diffuse necrosis of the epithelium. In primates mesenteric blood flow was decreased and vascular resistance was increased, but no lesions of the intestine were produced. Vyden and Corday, however, showed that in man gastrointestinal necrosis was sometimes seen in acute myocardial infarction, and that superior mesenteric artery blood flow fell under these circumstances.

Intraluminal mucosal nutrients were shown to protect the mucosa of the ischemic bowel from necrosis. Chiu et al. achieved protection by using intraluminal glucose, and Bounous et al. by an elemental diet. This protection was thought to be afforded by direct utilization of the substrate by the mucosa.

In hypovolemic shock Cook and associates have shown that the intestine becomes a secretory rather than absorptive organ and that there can be huge fluid losses into the intestinal lumen.

In experiments on dogs in hemorrhagic shock the intestine has often been implicated as the cause of irreversibility due to the absorption of toxins from the ischemic intestine. This was first thought to be due to bacteria which escaped from the bowel lumen into the circulation as a consequence of ischemic destruction of the intestinal mucosal barrier. However, bacteremia is not found in standard irreversible shock, and Lillehei and coworkers have shown that pretreatment of the dogs with oral neomycin and other antibiotics to the point of sterilization of the stool cultures does not influence the result of hemorrhagic shock. The course prior to death and the hemorrhagic necrosis of the intestinal mucosa at autopsy do not differ in treated dogs from other dogs not receiving oral antibiotics.

Moreover, Zweifach and coworkers found no increased survival from shock in germ-free rats, and Carter and Einheber have shown that intestinal ischemia produced by occluding the superior mesenteric artery in germ-free rats was acutely lethal and there was no significant difference in survival times of germ-free, contaminated germ-free, and normal control rats. The mucosal destruction in dogs is considerably greater than in man, and this is apparently related in part to loss of protecting mucin and the presence of trypsin and other proteolytic enzymes.

Goodman and Osborn have discussed the problem of acute gastric ulceration and its diverse origins. In the neurogenic ulcer seen after head injury there is frequent perforation from esophagogastromalacia, whereas stress ulcers seen with shock rarely perforate. Corticosteroid ulcers are usually antral and respond to antacids, while stress ulcers are superficial linear fundic erosions unaffected by antacids and not associated with increased acid production. Postburn ulcers are located in the depths of rugal folds of the fundus as well as the duodenum, are round and deep, and may show bacterial colonies in the base.

Robert and coworkers and Menguy and Masters have shown that steroid ulcers are due to a loss of mucin protection of the epithelium, and Hutcher and his colleagues found that vitamin A prevented steroid ulcers by restoring mucin production. Stress ulcers show relatively little deficit in mucin, however, although Lev and his coworkers found some reduction. The main etiologic factor in stress ulcers is probably mucosal ischemia. Sepsis, in some unknown way, greatly increases the likelihood of the development of stress ulcers.

Intraluminal nutrients protect against stress ulceration, as shown by Voitk, and hyperalimentation does also; hypoglycemia and starvation increase the likelihood of ulceration.

Renal Function

As mentioned earlier in this section, renal function is generally depressed in operative trauma as a result of the effect of ADH on the renal tubule, the usual dehydration of the patient prior to operation, the cardiac depression produced by some anesthetic agents, and the hypotension that may occur with blood loss. Renal function can usually be preserved at normal levels during operative trauma with proper hydration of the patient prior to operation, the avoidance of hypotension by the prompt replacement of blood loss, the monitoring of venous pressure, and the administration of mannitol to maintain an osmotic diuresis.

SHOCK. Severe shock may produce acute tubular necrosis or even cortical necrosis, with temporary or permanent renal failure. The treatment of this condition is considered in Chap. 40. It is now generally felt that the severely injured patient with acute tubular necrosis and severe oliguria or anuria should be treated with repetitive hemodialysis or peritoneal dialysis very early in the course of the renal insufficiency in order to ensure a smoother convalescence and to help prevent death from the complications of anuria. It is recognized that hyperkalemia is not the only indication for dialysis in renal shutdown, and the severely injured patient generally catabolizes tissue at such a rapid rate that early dialysis is mandatory to prevent demise. We have had occasion to dialyze patients in the recovery room within 48 hours of severe injury.

When cardiac output and aortic pressure are reduced experimentally by cardiogenic shock to 50 percent of normal, renal blood flow is 75 percent of normal, whereas similar conditions of cardiac function produced by hemorrhagic shock lead to renal blood flow that is 10 percent of normal. Gorfinkel and his colleagues conclude that this is a reflection of the intense renal vasoconstriction seen with hemorrhagic shock.

Severe oliguria and renal failure may occur in shock due to gram-negative septicemia. Under these circumstances renal function can often be restored by the administration of plasma until the venous pressure is at the upper limits of normal, of phenoxybenzamine to overcome peripheral vasoconstriction and improve renal plasma flow, and of mannitol to induce diuresis. In the traumatized patient who has become overly treated with fluids and who is edematous or in pulmonary edema, ethacrynic acid has been extremely valuable in promoting diuresis.

Staphylococcal toxin can produce shock and a profound depression of renal function consisting of reduction in total and effective renal plasma flow with congestion and secondary ischemia of the peripheral cortical zone. The free-water clearance falls, and the percentage of filtered sodium in the urine increases.

The depression of renal function in patients with severe shock differed in the survivors and nonsurvivors in a study by Strauch and coworkers in that the sodium and chloride clearances of the survivors reached levels of 1.2 to 1.4 ml/minute, whereas the values never exceeded 0.4 ml/minute in the nonsurvivors. There was a severe depression of glomerular filtration rate and urea clearance in all patients, but whereas this was transient in survivors, it was progressive in nonsurvivors.

Other aspects of renal function in trauma and shock have been considered in the preceding sections.

GENERAL CONSIDERATIONS

The aforegoing discussion of the endocrine and metabolic response to injury has perhaps demonstrated that there are many gaps in our knowledge and that many areas of controversy still remain. The degree to which the body is able to compensate for injury is astonishing, although at times the compensating mechanisms may work to the patient's disadvantage.

Therapeutic trends which have perhaps excited the most interest among surgeons recently include the protection of renal function by hydration and osmotic diuresis; the monitoring of central venous pressure as an aid in the assessment of fluid replacement and cardiac action; the swing away from the use of vasoconstrictors in shock to the use of blood volume replacement, maintenance of normal venous pressure, and control of sepsis; the use of intravenously administered bicarbonate to correct situations in which acidosis is known to occur; the correction of clotting defects with specific coagulation agents and fresh blood; an appreciation of the lung problems associated with injury and their correction with proper respirators; the electronic monitoring of blood pressure and other vital parameters; the more exact determination of antibiotic sensitivity of microorganisms; the realization that complete intravenous therapy can be given to patients who are forced to undergo long periods of starvation by the administration of protein and calories; and the frequent measurement of blood gases and fluid and electrolyte flux to determine the pattern of the endocrine and metabolic response to injury. This chapter simply serves as an introduction to some of these subjects, most of which will be covered in more detail in other portions of the book.

References

Stimuli Inducing Change

Brown, R. S., Mohr, P. A., Carey, J. S., and Shoemaker, W. C.: Cardiovascular Changes after Cranial Cerebral Injury and Increased Intracranial Pressure, *Surg Gynecol Obstet,* **125:** 1205, 1967.

Bursten, B., and Russ, J. J.: Preoperative Psychological State and Corticosteroid Levels of Surgical Patients, *Psychosom Med,* **27:**309, 1965.

Davis, J., Morrill, R., Fawcett, J., Upton, V., Bondy, P. K., and Spiro, H. M.: Apprehension and Elevated Serum Cortisol Levels, *J Psychosom Res,* **6:**83, 1962.

Ganong, W. F., Gold, N. I., and Hume, D. M.: The Effect of Hypothalamic Lesions on the Plasma 17-Hydroxycorticosteroid Response to Immobilization in the Dog, *Fed Proc,* **14:**54, 1955.

Harris, G. W.: "Neural Control of the Pituitary Gland," Edward Arnold (Publishers) Ltd., London, 1955.

Hume, D. M.: The Method of Hypothalamic Regulation of Pituitary and Adrenal Secretion in Response to Trauma, in S. Curri and L. Martini (eds.), "Pathophysiologia Diencephalica," p. 217, Springer-Verlag OHG, Vienna, 1958.

Noble, R. L.: The Development of Resistance by Rats and Guinea-pigs to Amounts of Trauma Usually Fatal, *Am J Physiol,* **138:**346, 1943.

——— and Collip, J. B.: A Quantitative Method for the Production of Experimental Traumatic Shock without Hemorrhage in Unanaesthetized Animals, *Q J Exp Physiol,* **31:**187, 1942.

Redding, M., and Mueller, C. B.: Effect of Ambient Temperature upon Responses to Hypovolemic Insult in the Unanesthetized, Unrestrained Albino Rat. *Surgery,* **64:**110, 1968.

Central Nervous System and Endocrine Changes

Bowman, H. M., Cowan, D., Kovach, G., Jr., and Hook, J. B.: Renal Effects of Glucagon in Rhesus Monkeys during Hypovolemia, *Surg Gynecol Obstet,* **134:**937, 1972.

Carey, L. C., Cloutier, C. T., and Lowery, B. D.: Growth Hormone and Adrenal Cortical Response to Shock and Trauma in the Human, *Ann Surg,* **174:**451, 1971.

———, Lowery, B. D., and Cloutier, C. T.: Blood Sugar and Insulin Response of Humans in Shock, *Ann Surg,* **172:**342, 1970.

Cerchio, G. M., Moss, G. S., Popovich, P. A., Butler, E., and Siegel, D. C.: Serum Insulin and Growth Hormone Response to Hemorrhagic Shock, *Endocrinology,* **88:**138, 1971.

Dyck, W. P.: Influence of Intrajejunal Glucose on Pancreatic Exocrine Function in Man, *Gastroenterology,* **60:**864, 1971.

Cooper, C. E., and Nelson, D. H.: ACTH Levels in Plasma in Preoperative and Surgically Stressed Patients, *J Clin Invest,* **41:**1599, 1962.

Egdahl, R. H.: Pituitary-Adrenal Response following Trauma to the Isolated Leg, *Surgery,* **46:**9, 1959.

———: Cerebral Cortical Inhibition of Pituitary Adrenal Secretion, *Endocrinology,* **68:**574, 1961.

Exton, J. H., Ui, M., Lewis, S. B., and Park, C. R.: Mechanism of Glucagon Activation of Gluconeogenesis, in H. D. Soling and B. Willms eds. , "Regulation of Gluconeogenesis," p. 160, Academic Press, Inc., New York, 1971.

Frohlich, J., and Wieland, O.: Dissociation of Gluconeogenic and Ketogenic Action of Glucagon in the Perfused Rat Liver, in H. D. Soling and B. Willms (eds.), "Regulation of Gluconeogenesis," p. 179, Academic Press, Inc., New York, 1971.

Genuth, P., and Lebovitz, H. E.: Stimulation of Insulin Release by Corticotropin, *Endocrinology,* **76:**1093, 1965.

Guillen, J., and Pappas, G.: Improved Cardiovascular Effects of Glucagon in Dogs with Endotoxin Shock, *Ann Surg,* **175:**535, 1972.

Halmagyi, D. F. J., Gillett, D. J., Lazarus, L., and Young, J. D.: Blood Glucose and Serum Insulin in Reversible Post Hemorrhagic Shock, *J Trauma,* **6:**623, 1966.

Henneman, D. H., and Henneman, P. H.: Effects of Human Growth Hormone on Levels of Blood and Urinary Carbohydrate and Fat Metabolites in Man, *J Clin Invest,* **39:**1239, 1960.

Herman, A. H., Mack, E., and Egdahl, R. H.: Adrenal Cortical Secretion following Prolonged Hemorrhagic Shock, *Surg Forum,* **20:**5, 1969.

———, ———, and ———: The Relationship of Adrenal Perfusion to Corticosteroid Secretion in Prolonged Hemorrhagic Shock, *Surg Gynecol Obstet,* **132:**795, 1971.

Hiebert, J. M., Soeldner, J. S., and Egdahl, R. H.: Altered Insulin and Glucose Metabolism Produced by Epinephrine during Hemorrhagic Shock in the Primate, *Surgery,* **74,** 1973.

Hume, D. M.: The Relationship of the Hypothalamus to Pituitary Secretion of ACTH, in *Ciba Found Colloq Endocrinol,* **4:**87, 1952.

———: Hypothalamic Localization for the Control of Various Endocrine Secretions, in H. H. Jasper et al. (eds.), "International Symposium: Reticular Formation of the Brain," p. 231, Little, Brown and Company, Boston, 1958.

———: Discussion of Neurohumeral and Endocrine Aspects of Shock, in Proceedings of a Conference on Recent Progress and Present Problems in the Field of Shock, *Fed Proc,* **20**(*Suppl* 9):1, 1961.

———: The Regulation of ACTH and Corticosteroid Secretion, *Proc 1st Int Cong Hormonal Steroids Milan 1962,* **1:**185, 1964.

——— and Bell, C. C., Jr.: The Secretion of Epinephrine, Norepinephrine, and Corticosteroid in the Adrenal Venous Blood of the Human, *Surg Forum,* **9:**6, 1959.

———, ———, and Bartter, F.: Direct Measurement of Adrenal Secretion during Operative Trauma and Convalescence, *Surgery,* **52:**174, 1962.

——— and Egdahl, R. H.: Effect of Hypothermia and of Cold Exposure on Adrenal Cortical and Medullary Secretion, *Ann NY Acad Sci,* **80:**435, 1959.

——— and ———: The Importance of the Brain in the Endocrine Response to Injury, *Ann Surg,* **150:**697, 1959.

——— and Nelson, D. H.: Adrenal Cortical Function in Surgical Shock, *Surg Forum,* **5:**568, 1955.

———, ———, and Miller, D. W.: Blood and Urinary 17-Hydroxycorticosteroids in Patients with Severe Burns, *Ann Surg,* **143:**316, 1956.

Ingle, D. J.: Permissive Action of Hormones, *J Clin Endocrinol Metab,* **14:**1272, 1954.

Krulich, L., and McCann, S. M.: Influence of Stress on the Growth Hormone (GH) Content of the Pituitary of the Rat, *Proc Soc Exp Biol Med,* **122:**612, 1966.

Lvoff, R., and Wilcken, D. E. L.: Glucagon in Heart Failure and in Cardiogenic Shock, *Circulation,* **45:**534, 1972.

Madden, J. J., Jr., Ludewig, R. M., and Wangensteen, S. L.: Failure of Glucagon in Experimental Hemorrhagic Shock, *Am J Surg,* **122:**502, 1971.

Martini, L., and Ganong, W. F. (eds.): "Neuroendocrinology," vols. I and II, Academic Press, Inc., New York, 1966, 1967.

Meyer, W., and Knobil, E.: Growth Hormone Secretion in the Unanesthetized Rhesus Monkey in Response to Noxious Stimuli, *Endocrinology,* **80:**163, 1967.

Moran, W. H., Jr., Miltenberger, F. W., Shuayb, W. A., and Zimmerman, B.: Relationship of Antidiuretic Hormone Secretion to Surgical Stress, *Surgery,* **56:**99, 1964.

Moss, G. S., Cerchio, G., Siegel, D. C., Reed, P. C., Cochin, A., and Fresquez, V.: Decline in Pancreatic Insulin Release during Hemorrhagic Shock in the Baboon, *Ann Surg,* **175:**210, 1972.

Newsome, H. H., Jr.: Pituitary-Adrenal Responsiveness in Surgical Patients on Acute and Chronic Corticosteroid Therapy, *Surgery,* **74,** 1973.

——— and Manalan, S. A.: Plasma Cortisol and Cortisone Concentrations following Postoperative Adrenal Steroid Replacement, *Surgery,* **73:**429, 1973.

Page, I. H.: Some Neurohumoral and Endocrine Aspects of Shock, in Proceedings of a Conference on Recent Progress and Present Problems in the Field of Shock, *Fed Proc,* **20**(*Suppl* 9):1, 1961.

Parmley, W. W., Gleck, G., and Sonnenblick, E. H.: Cardiovascular Effects of Glucagon in Man, *N Engl J Med,* **279:**12, 1968.

Price, H. L., Linde, H. W., Jones, R. E., Black, G. W., and Price,

M. L.: Sympatho-adrenal Responses to General Anesthesia in Man and Their Relation to Hemodynamics, *Anesthesiology*, **20:**563, 1959.

Samols, E., Tyler, J., Megyesi, C., and Marks, V.: Immunochemical Glucagon in Human Pancreas, Gut, and Plasma, *Lancet*, **2:**727, 1966.

Share, L., and Stadler, J. B.: Alterations in Sodium and Potassium Metabolism following Hind Leg Fracture in the Rat: Role of the Adrenal Cortex, *Endocrinology*, **62:**119, 1958.

Unger, R. H., Ohneda, A., Valverde, I., Eisentraut, A. M., and Exton, J.: Characterization of the Responses of Circulating Glucagon-like Immunoreactivity to Intraduodenal and Intravenous Administration of Glucose, *J Clin Invest*, **47:**48, 1968.

VanderWall, D. A., Stowe, N. T., Spangenberg, R., and Hook, J. B.: Effect of Glucagon in Hemorrhagic Shock, *J Surg Oncol*, **2:**177, 1970.

Von Euler, U. S.: Adrenal Medullary Secretion and Its Neural Control, in L. Martini and W. F. Ganong (eds.), "Neuroendocrinology," vol. II, Academic Press, Inc., New York, 1967.

Webb, W. R., Degerli, I. U., Hardy, J. D., and Unal, M.: Cardiovascular Responses in Adrenal Insufficiency, *Surgery*, **58:**273, 1965.

Metabolic Changes: General

Balegno, H. F., and Neuhaus, O. W.: Effect of Insulin on the Injury-stimulated Synthesis of Serum Albumin in the Rat, *Life Sci (II)*, **9:**1039, 1970.

Bauer, W. E., Vigas, S. N. M., Haist, R. E., and Drucker, W. R.: Insulin Response during Hypovolemic Shock, *Surgery*, **66:**80, 1969.

Blackburn, G. L., Flatt, J. P., Clowes, G. H. A., O'Donnell, T. F., and Hensle, T. E.: Protein Sparing Therapy during Periods of Starvation with Sepsis or Trauma, *Ann Surg*, **177:**588, 1973.

Cahill, G. F., Jr.: Starvation in Man, *N Engl J Med*, **282:**668, 1970.

Carey, L. C., Cloutier, C. T., and Lowery, B. D.: Growth Hormone and Adrenal Cortical Response to Shock and Trauma in the Human, *Ann Surg*, **174:**451, 1971.

Conway, M. J., Goodner, C. J., and Werrbach, J. H.: Studies of Substrate Regulation in Fasting: II. Effect of Infusion of Glucose into the Carotid Artery upon Fasting Lipolysis in the Baboon, *J Clin Invest*, **48:**1349, 1969.

Drucker, W. R., Craig, J., Kingsbury, B., Hofmann, N., and Woodward, H.: Citrate Metabolism during Surgery, *Arch Surg*, **85:**557, 1962.

Duke, J. H., Jr., Jorgensen, S. B., Broell, J. R., Long, C. L., and Kinney, J. M.: Contribution of Protein to Caloric Expenditure following Injury, *Surgery*, **68:**168, 1970.

Exton, J. H., Lewis, S. B., and Park, C. R.: Mechanism of Glucagon Activation of Gluconeogenesis, in H. D. Soling and B. Willms (eds.), "Regulation of Gluconeogenesis," p. 160, Academic Press, Inc., New York, 1971.

Felig, P., Marliss, E., Owen, O. E., and Cahill, G. F., Jr.: Role of Substrate in the Regulation of Hepatic Gluconeogenesis in Fasting Man, *Adv Enzyme Regul*, **7:**41, 1969.

————, Owen, O. E., Wahren, J., and Cahill, G. F., Jr.: Amino Acid Metabolism during Prolonged Starvation, *J Clin Invest*, **48:**584, 1969.

Frohlich, J., and Wieland, O.: Dissociation of Gluconeogenic and Ketogenic Action of Glucagon in the Perfused Rat Liver, in

H. D. Soling and B. Willms (eds.), "Regulation of Gluconeogenesis," p. 179, Academic Press, Inc., New York, 1971.

Guder, W., and Wieland, O.: The Effect of 3′,5′-cyclic AMP on Glucose Synthesis in Isolated Rat Kidney Tubules, in H. D. Soling and B. Willms (eds.), "Regulation of Gluconeogenesis," p. 226, Academic Press, Inc., New York, 1971.

Halmagyi, D. F. J., Neering, I. R., Lazarus, L., Young, J. D., and Pullin, J.: Plasma Glucagon in Experimental Posthemorrhagic Shock. *J Trauma*, **9:**320, 1969.

Hanson, R. W., Patel, M. S., Reshef, L., and Ballard, F. J.: The Role of Pyruvate Carboxylase and P-Enolpyruvate Carboxykinase in Rat Adipose Tissue, in H. D. Soling and B. Willms (eds.), "Regulation of Gluconeogenesis," p. 255, Academic Press, Inc., New York, 1971.

Hasselblatt, A., Panten, U., and Poser, W.: Stimulation of Amino Acid Metabolism and Gluconeogenesis from Amino Acids in the Liver of Fasting Rats Treated with Antilipolytic Agents, in H. D. Soling and B. Willms (eds.), "Regulation of Gluconeogenesis," p. 276, Academic Press, Inc., New York. 1971.

Heath, D. F., and Threlfall, C. J.: The Interaction of Glycolysis, Gluconeogenesis and the Tricarboxylic Acid Cycle in Rat Liver in Vivo, *Biochem J*, **110:**337, 1968.

Howard, J. M.: Studies of the Absorption and Metabolism of Glucose following Injury: The Systemic Response to Injury, *Ann Surg*, **141:**321, 1955.

Kinney, J. M., Long, C. L., and Duke, J. H.: Carbohydrate and Nitrogen Metabolism after Injury, in R. Porter and J. Knight (eds.), "Energy: Metabolism in Trauma," p. 123, J. & A. Churchill, London, 1970.

Koj, A.: Synthesis and Turnover of Acute-Phase Reactants, in R. Porter and J. Knight (eds.), "Energy: Metabolism in Trauma," p. 79, J. & A. Churchill, London, 1970.

Levenson, S. M., Nagler, A. L., and Einheber, A.: Some Metabolic Consequences of Shock, in S. G. Hershey (ed.), "Shock," p. 79, Little, Brown and Company, Boston, 1964.

————, Pulaski, E. J., and Del Guercio, L. R. M.: Metabolic Changes Associated with Injury, in Zimmerman, L. M., and Levine, R. (eds.), "Physiologic Principles of Surgery," W. B. Saunders Company, Philadelphia, 1964.

McNamara, J. J., Molot, M. D., Dunn, R. A., and Stremple, J. F.: Effect of Hypertonic Glucose in Hypovolemic Shock in Man, *Ann Surg*, **176:**247, 1972.

Mallette, L. E., Exton, J. H., and Park, C. R.: Control of Gluconeogenesis from Amino Acids in the Perfused Rat Liver, *J Biol Chem*, **244:**5713, 1969.

Moss, G. S., Cerchio, G. M., Siegel, D. C., Popovich, P. A., and Butler, E.: Serum Insulin Response in Hemorrhagic Shock in Baboons, *Surgery*, **68:**34, 1970.

Owen, O. E., Morgan, A. P., Kemp, H. G., Sullivan, J. M., Herrera, M. G., and Cahill, G. F., Jr.: Brain Metabolism during Fasting, *J Clin Invest*, **46:**1589, 1967.

Schumer, W., and Sperling, R.: Shock and Its Effect on the Cell, *JAMA*, **205:**215, 1968.

Siegel, D. B., Moss, G. S., Reed, P. C., Cochin, A., and Fresquez, V.: Decline in Pancreatic Insulin Release during Hemorrhagic Shock in the Baboon, *Rev Surg*, **29:**144, 1972.

Soling, H. D., Willms, B., and Kleineke, J.: Regulation of Gluconeogenesis in Rat and Guinea Pig Liver, in H. D. Soling and B. Willms (eds.), "Regulation of Gluconeogenesis," p. 210, Academic Press, Inc., New York, 1971.

Stoner, H. B., and Threlfall, C. J. (eds.): "The Biochemical Response to Injury," Charles C Thomas, Publisher, Springfield, Ill., 1960.

Threlfall, C. J., and Stoner, H. B.: Carbohydrate Metabolism in Ischemic Shock, *Q J Exp Physiol,* **39:**1, 1954.

Protein Metabolism

Browne, J. S. L., and Schenker, V.: "Conferences on Metabolic Aspects of Convalescence Including Bone and Wound Healing: Transactions of Third Meeting," p. 162, Josiah Macy, Jr. Foundation Publications, New York, 1943.

Cannon, P. R., Wissler, R. W., Woolride, R. L., and Benditt, E. P.: Relationship of Protein Deficiency to Surgical Infection, *Ann Surg,* **120:**514, 1944.

Clarke, H. C. M., Freeman, T., and Pryse-Phillips, W.: Serum Protein Changes after Injury, *Clin Sci,* **40:**337, 1971.

Costa, G., Ullrich, L., Kantor, F., and Holland, J. F.: Production of Elemental Nitrogen by Certain Mammals including Man, *Nature (Lond),* **218:**546, 1968.

Cuthbertson, D. P.: Further Observations on Disturbance of Metabolism Caused by Injury, with Particular Reference to Dietary Requirements of Fracture Cases, *Br J Surg,* **23:**505, 1936.

Davies, J. W. L., Bull, J. P., and Ricketts, C. R.: Catabolic Response to Injury, *Lancet,* **2:**320, 1971.

Fleck, A.: Protein Metabolism after Injury, *Proc Nutr Soc,* **30:**152, 1971.

Hinton, P., Allison, S. P., Littlejohn, S., and Lloyd, J.: Insulin and Glucose to Reduce Catabolic Response to Injury in Burned Patients, *Lancet,* **1:**767, 1971.

Howard, J. E., Bingham, R. S., Jr., and Mason, R. E.: Studies on Convalescence: IV. Nitrogen and Mineral Balances during Starvation and Graduated Feeding in Healthy Young Males at Bed Rest, *Trans Assoc Am Physicians,* **59:**242, 1946.

Kekomaki, M., and Louhimo, I.: Observations on Plasma Amino Acid Concentrations during Haemorrhagic Shock in the Rabbit, *Ann Chir Gynaecol Fenn,* **60:**214, 1971.

Kukral, J. C., Riveron, E., Tiffany, J. C., Vaitys, S., and Barrett, B.: Plasma Protein Metabolism in Patients with Acute Surgical Peritonitis, *Am J Surg,* **113:**173, 1967.

Levenson, S. M., Howard, J. M., and Rosen, I. T.: Studies of the Plasma Amino Acids and Amino Conjugates in Patients with Severe Battle Wounds, *Surg Gynecol Obstet,* **101:**35, 1955.

—— and Watkin, D. M.: Protein Requirements in Injury and Certain Acute and Chronic Diseases, *Fed Proc,* **18:**1155, 1959.

Munro, H. N., and Allison, J. B. (eds.): "Mammalian Protein Metabolism," Academic Press, Inc., New York, 1964.

—— and Chalmers, M. I.: Fracture Metabolism at Different Levels of Protein Intake, *Br J Exp Pathol,* **26:**396, 1945.

Blood Coagulation

Adelson, E., Crosby, W. H., and Roeder, W. H.: Further Studies of a Hemostatic Defect Caused by Intravenous Dextran, *J Lab Clin Med,* **45:**441, 1955.

Attar, S., Boyd, D., Layne, E., McLaughlin, J., Mansberger, A., and Cowley, R. A.: Alterations in the Coagulation and Fibrinolytic System in Acute Trauma, *J Trauma,* **9:**939, 1969.

Attar, S., Kirby, W. H., Jr., Masaitis, C., Mansberger, A. R., Jr., and Cowley, R. A.: Coagulation Changes in Clinical Shock: I. Effect of Hemorrhagic Shock on Clotting Time in Humans, *Ann Surg,* **164:**34, 1966.

——, Mansberger, A. R., Jr., Irani, B., Kirby, W., Jr., Masaitis, C., and Cowley, R. A.: Coagulation Changes in Clinical Shock: II. Effect of Septic Shock on Clotting Times and Fibrinogen in Humans, *Ann Surg,* **164:**41, 1966.

Carbone, J. V., Furth, F. W., Scott, R., Jr., and Crosby, W. H.: An Hemostatic Defect Associated with Dextran Infusion, *Proc Soc Exp Biol,* **85:**101, 1954.

Crowell, J. W., and Read, W. L.: In Vivo Coagulation: A Probable Cause of Irreversible Shock, *Am J Physiol,* **183:**565, 1955.

Deykin, D.: Thrombogenesis, *N Engl J Med.,* **276:**622, 1967.

Dhall, D. P., McKenzie, F. N., Arfors, K.-E., and Matheson, N. A.: Platelet Behavior in Dogs During and After Moderate and Severe Haemorrhage, *Eur Surg Res,* **1:**282, 1969.

Dinbar, A., Rapaport, S. I., Patch, M. J., Grant, W., and Fonkalsrud, E. W.: Hematologic Effects of Endotoxin on the Macaque Monkey, *Surgery,* **70:**596, 1971.

Ehrlich, E. W., Gollub, S., and Ulin, A. W.: Effects of Graded Hypovolemia on the Coagulation Mechanism, *Ann NY Acad Sci,* **115:**97, 1964.

Gans, H., Hanson, M., and Krivit, W.: Effect of Endotoxin on Clotting Mechanism, *Surgery,* **53:**792, 1963.

Gelin, L. E.: Reaction of the Body as a Whole to Injury, *J Trauma,* **10:**932, 1970.

Greene, G. R., and Sartwell, P. E.: Oral Contraceptive Use in Patients with Thromboembolism following Surgery, Trauma, or Infection, *Am J Public Health,* **62:**680, 1972.

Gruner, O. P. N.: Platelets, Fibrinogen, and Fat Embolism after Trauma in Rabbits, *Acta Chir Scand,* **138:**125, 1972.

Harada, Y.: A Hemostatic Defect and Delayed Healing of the Wound Caused by Dextran Preparation, *Hiroshima J Med Sci,* **20:**27, 1971.

Energy Metabolism

Kinney, J. M.: Energy Significance of Weight Loss, in G. S. M. Cowan, Jr., and W. L. Scheetz (eds.), "Intravenous Hyperalimentation" p. 84, Lea & Febiger, Philadelphia, 1972.

Kinney, J. M., Long, C. L., and Duke, J. H.: Carbohydrate and Nitrogen Metabolism after Injury, in R. Porter and J. Knight (eds.), "Energy Metabolism in Trauma," p. 103, J. & A. Churchill, London, 1970.

——, ——, and ——: Energy Demands in the Surgical Patient, in C. L. Fox, Jr., and G. G. Nahos (eds.), "Body Fluid Replacement in Surgical Patient," Grune & Stratton, Inc., New York, 1970.

Mehlman, M. A., and Hanson, R. W., (eds.): "Energy Metabolism and the Regulation of Metabolic Processes in Mitochondria," Academic Press, Inc., New York, 1972.

Porter, R., and Knight, J. (eds.): "Energy Metabolism in Trauma," J. & A. Churchill, London, 1970.

Soling, H. D., and Willms, B. (eds.): "Regulation of Gluconeogenesis," Academic Press, Inc., New York, 1971.

Wilmore, D. W.: Energy Requirements of Seriously Burned Patients and the Influence of Caloric Intake in Their Metabolic Rate, in G. S. M. Cowan, Jr., and W. L. Scheetz (eds.), "Intravenous Hyperalimentation," p. 96, Lea & Febiger, Philadelphia, 1972.

Starvation

Cahill, G. F., Jr.: Starvation in Man, *N Engl J Med,* **282:**668, 1970.

——— and Aoki, T. T.: The Starvation State and Requirements of the Deficit Economy, in G. S. M. Cowan, Jr. and W. L. Scheetz (eds.), "Intravenous Hyperalimentation," p. 21, Lea & Febiger, Philadelphia, 1972.

———, Felig, P., and Marliss, E. B.: Some Physiological Principles of Parenteral Nutrition, in C. L. Fox, Jr., and G. G. Nahas (eds.), "Body Fluid Replacement in the Surgical Patient," p. 286, Grune & Stratton, New York, 1970.

Owen, O. E., Felig, P., Morgan, A. P., Wahren, J., and Cahill, G. F., Jr.: Liver and Kidney Metabolism during Prolonged Starvation, *J Clin Invest,* **48:**574, 1969.

———, Morgan, A. P., Kemp, H. G., Sullivan, J. M., Herrera, M. G., and Cahill, G. F., Jr.: Brain Metabolism during Fasting, *J Clin Invest,* **46:**1589, 1967.

Hardaway, R. M.: The Role of Intravascular Clotting in the Etiology of Shock, *Ann Surg,* **155:**325, 1962.

———, Elovitz, M. J., Brewster, W. R., Jr., Houchin, D. N., Renzi, N. L., and Jackson, D. R.: Influence of Vasoconstrictors and Vasodilators on Disseminated Intravascular Coagulation in Irreversible Hemorrhagic Shock, *Surg Gynecol Obstet,* **119:**1053, 1964.

——— and Johnson, D.: Clotting Mechanism in Endotoxin Shock, *Arch Intern Med,* **112:**775, 1963.

Herman, C. M., Moquin, R. B., and Horwitz, D. L.: Coagulation Changes of Hemorrhagic Shock in Baboons, *Ann Surg,* **175:**197, 1972.

Hirsch, E. F., Fletcher, J. R., Moquin, R., Dostalek, R., and Lucas, S.: Coagulation Changes after Combat Trauma and Sepsis, *Surg Gynecol Obstet,* **133:**393, 1971.

Hissen, W., Fleming, J. S., Bierwagen, M. E., and Pindell, M. H.: Effect of Prostaglandin E_1 on Platelet Aggregation In Vitro and in Hemorrhagic Shock, *Microvasc Res,* **1:**374, 1969.

Holland, P. V., Rubinson, R. M., Morrow, A. G., and Schmidt, P. J.: γ-Globulin in the Prophylaxis of Posttransfusion Hepatitis, *JAMA,* **196:**471, 1966.

Horwitz, D. L., Moquin, R. B., and Herman, C. M.: Coagulation Changes of Septic Shock in the Sub-human Primate and Their Relationship to Hemodynamic Changes, *Ann Surg,* **175:**417, 1972.

Howard, J. M., Teng, C. T., and Loeffler, R. K.: Studies of Dextrans of Various Molecular Sizes, *Ann Surg,* **143:**369, 1956.

Ljungqvist, U., and Bergentz, S. E.: The Effect of Experimental Trauma on the Platelets, *Acta Chir Scand,* **136:**271, 1970.

———, ———, and Lewis, D. H.: The Distribution of Platelets Fibrin and Erythrocytes in Various Organs following Experimental Trauma, *Eur Surg Res,* **3:**293, 1971.

Long, D. M., Jr., Rosen, A. L., Malone, L. V. W., and Meier, M. A.: Blood Rheology in Trauma Patients, *Surg Clin North Am,* **52:**19, 1972.

McKay, D. G., and Shapiro, S. S.: Alterations in the Blood Coagulation System Induced by Bacterial Endotoxin. I. In Vivo (Generalized Schwartzman Reaction), *J Exp Med,* **107:**353, 1958.

Mosesson, M. W., Colman, R. W., and Sherry, S.: Chronic Intravascular Coagulation Syndrome, *N Engl J Med,* **278:**815, 1968.

Richetts, C. R.: Interaction of Dextran and Fibrinogen, *Nature (Lond),* **169:**970, 1952.

Simonds, R. L., Collins, J., Heisterkamp, C., Mills, D., Andren, R., and Phillips, L.: Coagulation Disorders in Combat Casualties, *Ann Surg,* **169:**455, 1969.

Stefanini, M., and Dameshek, W.: "The Hemorrhagic Disorders," Grune & Stratton, Inc., New York, 1962.

Turpini, R., and Stefanini, M.: The Nature and Mechanism of the Hemostatic Breakdown in the Course of Experimental Shock, *J Clin Invest,* **38:**53, 1959.

Ulin, A. W., and Gollub, S. S. (eds.): "Surgical Bleeding," McGraw-Hill Book Company, New York, 1966.

Von Kaulla, K. N., and Swan, H.: Clotting Deviations in Man Associated with Open Heart Surgery during Hypothermia, *J Thorac Cardiovasc Surg,* **36:**857, 1958.

——— and ———: Clotting Deviations in Man during Cardiac Bypass: Fibrinolysis and Circulating Anticoagulant, *J Thorac Cardiovasc Surg,* **36:**519, 1958.

Weil, P. G., and Webster, D. R.: Studies on the Bleeding Tendency following Dextran Infusion, *Surg Forum,* **6:**88, 1955.

Wilson, W. B.: Emergency Management of Unexpected Defects of Hemostatic Function in Surgical Patients, *JAMA,* **201:**123, 1967.

Carbohydrate Metabolism

Berk, J. L., Hagen, J. F., Beyer, W. H., and Gerber, M. J.: Hypoglycemia of Shock, *Ann Surg,* **171:**400, 1970.

Drucker, W. R., Schlatter, J. E., and Drucker, R. P.: Metabolic Factors Associated with Endotoxin-induced Tolerance for Hemorrhagic Shock, *Surgery,* **64:**75, 1968.

———: Carbohydrate metabolism: The Traumatized versus Normal States, in G. S. M. Cowan and W. L. Scheetz (eds.), "Intravenous Hyperalimentation," p. 55, Lea & Febiger, Philadelphia, 1972.

Green, H. N., and Stoner, H. B.: Effects of Injury on Carbohydrate Metabolism and Energy Transformation, *Br Med J,* **10:**38, 1955.

Jordan, G. L., Jr., Fischer, E. P., and Lefrak, E. A.: Glucose Metabolism in Traumatic Shock in the Human, *Ann Surg,* **175:**685, 1972.

Pappova, E., Urbaschek, B., Heitmann, L., Oroz, M., Streit, O. E., Lemeunier, A., and Lundsgaard-Hansen, P.: Energy-rich Phosphates and Glucose Metabolism in Early Endotoxin Shock. *J Surg Res,* **11:**506, 1971.

Schumer, W.: Metabolic Considerations in the Preoperative Evaluation of the Surgical Patient, *Surg Gynecol Obstet,* **121:**611, 1965.

———: Localization of the Energy Pathway Block in Shock, *Surgery,* 1974.

Taylor, F. H. L., Levenson, S. M., and Adams, M. A.: Abnormal Carbohydrate Metabolism in Human Thermal Burns, *N Engl J Med,* **231:**437, 1944.

Fat Metabolism

Barton, R. N. Ketone Body Metabolism after Trauma, in R. Porter and J. Knight (eds.), *Ciba Found Symp Energy Metab Trauma,* 1970, p. 173.

Carlson, L. A.: Mobilization and Utilization of Lipids after Trauma: Relation to Caloric Homeostasis, in R. Porter and J. Knight (eds), *Ciba Found Symp Energy Metab Trauma,* 1970, p. 155.

———: Fat Metabolism, in G. S. M. Cowan and W. L. Scheetz,

(eds.), "Intravenous Hyperalimentation," p. 68, Lea & Febiger, Philadelphia, 1972.

Coran, A. G., Cryer, P. E., Horwitz, D. L., and Herman, C. M.: Fat and Carbohydrate Metabolism during Hemorrhagic Shock in the Unanesthetized Baboon, *Surg Forum,* **22:**9, 1971.

——, ——, ——, and ——: The Metabolism of Fat and Carbohydrate during Hemorrhagic Shock in the Unanesthetized Subhuman Primate: Changes in Serum Levels of Free Fatty Acids, Total Lipids, Insulin, and Glucose, *Surgery,* **71:**465, 1972.

Evarts, C. M.: The Fat Embolism Syndrome: A Review, *Surg Clin North Am,* **50:**493, 1970.

Farago, G., Levene, R. A., Lau, T. S., and Drucker, W. R.: Availability of Lipid for Energy Metabolism during Hypovolemia, *Surg Forum,* **22:**7, 1971.

Hansen, O. H.: Fat Embolism and Post-traumatic Diabetes Insipidus, *Acta Chir Scand,* **136:**161, 1970.

Johnson, S. R., and Svanborg, A.: Investigations with Regard to the Pathogenesis of So-called Fat Metabolism, *Ann Surg,* **144:**145, 1956.

—— and Wadström, L. B.: Serum Fat in Tourniquet Shock: An Experimental Study in Rabbits, with Special Reference to the Action of Heparin, *Scand J Clin Lab Invest,* **8:**323, 1956.

Lyman, R. L.: Endocrine Influences on the Metabolism of Polyunsaturated Fatty Acids, *Prog Chem,* **9:**193, 1968.

McNamara, J. J., Molot, M., Dunn, R., Burran, E. L., and Stremple, J. F.: Lipid Metabolism after Trauma: Role in the Pathogenesis of Fat Embolism, *J Thorac Cardiovasc Surg,* **63:**968, 1972.

Masoro, E. J.: The Effect of Physical Injury on Lipid Metabolism, in H. B. Stoner and C. J. Threlfall (eds.), "The Biochemical Response to Injury," p. 175, Charles C Thomas, Publisher, Springfield, Ill., 1960.

Moore, F. D., Haley, H. B., Bering, E. A., Jr., Brooks, L., and Edelman, I. S.: Further Observations on Total Body Water: II. Changes of Body Composition in Disease, *Surg Gynecol Obstet,* **95:**155, 1952.

Shafrir, E., and Steinberg, D.: The Essential Role of the Adrenal Cortex in the Response of Plasma Free Fatty Acids, Cholesterol, and Phospholipids to Epinephrine Injection, *J Clin Invest,* **39:**310, 1960.

Spergel, G., Bleicher, S. J., and Ertel, N. H.: Carbohydrate and Fat Metabolism in Patients with Pheochromocytoma, *N Engl J Med,* **278:**803, 1968.

Symbas, P. N., Abbott, O. A., and Ende, N.: Surgical Stress and Its Effects on Serum Cholesterol, *Surgery,* **61:**221, 1967.

Wadström, L. B.: Effect of Glucose Infusion on Plasma Lipids in Newly Operated Patients, *Acta Chir Scand,* **116:**395, 1958.

Wound Healing

Azar, M. M., and Good, R. A.: The Inhibitory Effect of Vitamin A on Complement Levels and Tolerance Production, *J Immunol,* **106:**241, 1971.

Calloway, D. H., Grossman, M. I., Bowman, J., and Calhoun, W. K.: Effect of Previous Level of Protein Feeding on Wound Healing and on Metabolic Response to Injury, *Surgery,* **37:**935, 1955.

Carnes, W. H.: Role of Copper in Connective Tissue Metabolism, *Fed Proc,* **30:**995, 1971.

Chernov, M. S., Hale, H. W., and Wood, M.: Prevention of Stress Ulcers, *Am J Surg,* **122:**674, 1971.

Cohen, B., and Cohen, I. K.: "Vitamin A: Adjuvant and Steroid Antagonist in the Immune Response," Plastic Surgery Research Council, St. Louis, May, 1973.

Cohen, I. K., Schechter, P. J., and Henkin, R. I.: Hypogeusia, Anorexia, and Altered Zinc Metabolism following Thermal Burn, *JAMA,* **223:**914, 1973.

Harris, E. D., and Sjoerdsma, A.: Effect of Penicillamine on Human Collagen and Its Possible Application in Treatment of Scleroderma, *Lancet,* **2:**996, 1966.

Hsu, T. H. S., and Hsu, J. M.: Zinc Deficiency and Epithelial Wound Repair: An Autoradiographic Study of 3H-Thymidine Incorporation, *Proc Soc Exp Biol Med,* **140:**157, 1972.

Hunt, T. K., Ehrlich, H. P., Garcia, J. A., and Dunphy, J. E.: Effect of Vitamin A on Reversing the Inhibitory Effect of Cortisone on Healing of Open Wounds in Animals and Man, *Ann Surg,* **170:**633, 1969.

——, Niinikoski, J., and Zederfeldt, B.: Role of Oxygen in Repair Processes, *Acta Chir Scand,* **138:**109, 1972.

Hutcher, N., Silverberg, S. G., and Lee, H. M.: The Effect of Vitamin A on the Formation of Steroid Induced Gastric Ulcers, *Surg Forum,* **22:**322, 1971.

Levenson, S. M., Green, R. W., Taylor, F. H. L., Robinson, P., Page, R. C., Johnson, R. E., and Lund, C. C.: Ascorbic Acid, Riboflavin, Thiamine, and Nicotinic Acid in Relation to Severe Injury, Hemorrhage and Infection in the Human, *Ann Surg,* **124:**840, 1946.

Levenson, S. M., Pirani, C. L., Braasch, J. W., and Waterman, D. F.: The Effect of Thermal Burns on Wound Healing, *Surg Gynecol Obstet,* **99:**74, 1954.

——, Upjohn, H. L., Preston, J. A., and Steer, A.: Effect of Thermal Burns on Wound Healing, *Ann Surg,* **146:**357, 1957.

Niinikoski, J., Henghan, C., and Hunt, T. K.: Oxygen Tensions in Human Wounds, *J Surg Res,* **12:**77, 1972.

Quarantillo, E. P., Jr.: Effect of Supplemental Zinc on Wound Healing in Rats, *Am J Surg,* **121:**661, 1971.

Siegel, R. C., Pinnell, S. R., and Martin, G.: Cross-linking of Collagen and Elastin: Properties of Lysyl Oxidase, *Biochemistry,* **9:**4486, 1970.

Stein, H. D., and Keiser, H. R.: Collagen Metabolism in Granulating Wounds, *J Surg Res,* **11:**277, 1971.

Stephens, F. P., Hunt, T. K., Jawetz, E., Sonne, M., and Duphy, J. E.: Effect of Cortisone and Vitamin A on Wound Infection, *Am J Surg,* **121:**569, 1971.

Sullivan, J. F., and Eisenstein, A. B.: Ascorbic Acid Depletion during Hemodialysis. *JAMA,* **220:**1697, 1972.

Williamson, M. B., McCarthy, T. H., and Fromm, H. J.: Relation of Protein Nutrition to the Healing of Experimental Wounds, *Proc Soc Exp Biol Med,* **77:**302, 1951.

Udupa, K. N., Woessner, J. F., and Dunphy, J. E.: The Effect of Methionine on the Production of Mucopolysaccharides and Collagen in Healing Wounds of Protein-depleted Animals, *Surg Gynecol Obstet,* **102:**639, 1956.

Nutritional Supplementation

Abbott, W. E., Krieger, H., and Levey, S.: Postoperative Metabolic Changes in Relation to Nutritional Regimen, *Lancet,* **1:**704, 1958.

Abel, R. M., Abbott, W. M., and Fisher, J. E.: Intravenous Essential L-Amino Acids and Hypertonic Dextrose in Patients with Acute Renal Failure, *Am J Surg,* **123:**632, 1972.

———, Beck, C. H., Jr., Abbott, W. M., Ryan, J. A., Jr., Barnett, G. O., and Fischer, J. E.: Improved Survival from Acute Renal Failure after Treatment with Intravenous Essential L-Amino Acids and Glucose, *N Engl J Med,* **288:**695, 1973.

Allen, J. G., Stemmer, E. A., and Head, L. R.: Similar Growth Rates of Littermate Puppies Maintained on Oral Protein with Those on the Same Quantity of Protein as Daily Intravenous Plasma for 99 Days as Only Protein Source, *Ann Surg,* **144:** 349, 1956.

Brennan, M. F., Goldman, M. H., O'Connell, R. C., Kundsin, R. B., and Moore, F. D.: Prolonged Parenteral Alimentation: Candida Growth and the Prevention of Candidemia by Amphotericin Installation, *Ann Surg,* **176:**265, 1972.

Burr, A. O. and Burr, M. M.: A New Deficiency Disease Produced by the Rigid Exclusion of Fat from the Diet, *J Biol Chem,* **82:**345, 1929.

Cahill, G. F., Jr., and Aoki, T. T.: The Starvation State and Requirements of the Deficit Economy, in G. S. M. Cowan, Jr., and W. L. Scheetz (eds.), "Intravenous Hyperalimentation," p. 20, Lea & Febiger, Philadelphia, 1972.

———, Felig, P., and Marliss, E. B.: Some Physiological Principles of Parenteral Nutrition, in C. L. Fox, Jr. and G. G. Nahas (eds.), "Body Fluid Replacement in the Surgical Patient," p. 286, Grune & Stratton, Inc., New York, 1970.

Caldwell, M. D., Jonnsson, H. T., and Othersen, H. B., Jr.: Essential Fatty Acid Deficiency in an Infant Receiving Prolonged Parenteral Alimentation, *J Pediatr,* **81:**894, 1972.

Collins, F. D., Sinclair, A. J., and Royle, J. P.: Plasma Lipids in Human Linoleic Acid Deficiency, *Nutr Metabol,* **13:**150, 1971.

Cowan, G. S. M., Jr., and Scheetz, W. L. (eds.): "Intravenous Hyperalimentation," Lea & Febiger, Philadelphia, 1972.

Deitrick, J. E., Whedun, G. D., and Shorr, E.: Effects of Immobilization upon Various Metabolic and Physiologic Functions of Normal Men, *Am J Med,* **4:**3, 1948.

Dudrick, S. J., Wilmore, D. W., Vars, H. M., and Rhoads, J. E.: Long Term Total Parenteral Nutrition with Growth, Development and Positive Nitrogen Balance, *Surgery,* **64:**134, 1968.

———, MacFadyen, B. V., VanBuren, C. T., Ruberg, R. L., and Maynard, A. T.: Parenteral Hyperalimentation: Metabolic Problems and Solutions, *Ann Surg,* **176:**259, 1972.

———, Steiger, E., and Long, J. M.: Renal Failure in Surgical Patients: Treatment with Intravenous Essential Amino Acids and Hypertonic Glucose, *Surgery,* **68:**180, 1970.

———, ———, ———, Ruberg, R. L., Allen, T. R., Vars, H. M., and Rhoads, J. E.: General principles and techniques of intravenous hyperalimentation, in G. S. M. Cowan, Jr., and W. L. Scheetz (eds.), "Intravenous Hyperalimentation," p. 2, Lea & Febiger, Philadelphia, 1972.

Feller, I.: The Use of Plasma and Albumin in the Burned Patient, in C. L. Fox, Jr., and G. G. Nahas (eds.), "Body Fluid Replacement in the Surgical Patient," p. 153. Grune & Stratton, Inc., New York, 1970.

Fox, C. L., Jr., and Nahas, G. G. (eds.): "Body Fluid Replacement in the Surgical Patient," Grune & Stratton, Inc., New York, 1970.

Giordano, C.: Use of Exogenous and Endogenous Urea for Pro-

tein Synthesis in Normal and Uremic Subjects, *J Lab Clin Med,* **62:**321, 1963.

Giovannetti, S., and Maggiore, Q.: A Low Nitrogen Diet with Protein of High Biological Value for Severe Chronic Uremia, *Lancet,* **1:**1000, 1964.

Greenstein, J. P., Otey, M. C., Birnbaum, S. M., and Winitz, M.: Quantitative Nutritional Studies with Water-Soluble, Chemically Defined Diets: X. Formulation of a Nutritionally Complete Liquid Diet, *J Natl Cancer Inst,* **24:**211, 1960.

Hamilton, R. F., Davis, W. T., Stephenson, D. V., and McGee, D. F.: Effects of Parenteral Hyperalimentation on Upper Gastrointestinal Tract Secretions, *Arch Surg,* **102:**348, 1971.

Heird, W. C., Dell, R. B., Driscoll, J. M., Jr., Grebin, B., and Winters, R. W.: Metabolic Acidosis Resulting from Intravenous Alimentation Mixtures Containing Synthetic Amino Acids, *N Engl J Med,* **287:**943, 1972.

Holden, W. D., Krieger, H., Levey, S., and Abbott, W. E.: The Effect of Nutrition on Nitrogen Metabolism in the Surgical Patient, *Ann Surg,* **146:**563, 1957.

Holman, R. T.: Essential Fatty Acid Deficiency, *Prog Chem Toxicol,* **9:**279, 1968.

Host, W. H., Serlin, O., and Rush, B. F., Jr.: Hyperalimentation in Cirrhotic Patients, *Am J Surg,* **123:**57, 1972.

Jacobson, S., and Wretling, A.: The Use of Fat Emulsions for Complete Intravenous Nutrition, in C. L. Fox, Jr., and G. G. Nahas (eds.), "Body Fluid Replacement in the Surgical Patient," p. 334, Grune & Stratton, Inc., New York, 1970.

Kekomaki, M., Louhimo, I., Rahiala, E. L., and Suutarinen, T.: Comparison of Fructose and Glucose Solutions in the Treatment of Hypovolemic Shock in Rabbits, *Acta Chir Scand,* **138:**239, 1972.

Kinney, J. M., Long, C. L., and Duke, J. H., Jr.: Energy Demands in the Surgical Patient, in C. L. Fox and G. G. Nahas (eds.), "Body Fluid Replacement in the Surgical Patient," p. 296, Grune & Stratton, Inc., New York, 1970.

Long, J. M., Dudrick, S. J., Steiger, E., Ruberg, R. L., and Allen, T. R.: Use of Intravenous Hyperalimentation in Patients with Renal or Liver Failure, in G. S. M. Cowan, Jr., and W. L. Scheetz (eds.), "Intravenous Hyperalimentation," p. 147, Lea & Febiger, Philadelphia, 1972.

Meng, H. C., and Early, F.: Study of Complete Parenteral Alimentation on Dogs, *J Lab Clin Med,* **34:**1121, 1949.

Munro, H. N.: Adaptation of Mammalian Protein Metabolism to Hyperalimentation, in G. S. M. Cowan, Jr., and W. L. Scheetz (eds.), "Intravenous Hyperalimentation," p. 34, Lea & Febiger, Philadelphia, 1972.

Pensler, L., Whitten, C., Paulsund, J., and Holman, R.: Serum Fatty Acid Changes during Fat-free Intravenous Therapy, *J Pediatr,* **78:**1067, 1971.

Ravdin, I. S., McNamee, H. G., Kamholz, J. H., and Rhoads, J. E.: Effect of Hypoproteinemia on Susceptibility to Shock Resulting from Hemorrhage, *Arch Surg,* **48:**491, 1944.

Rose, W. C., and Dekker, E. E.: Urea as a Source of Nitrogen for the Biosynthesis of Amino Acids, *J Biol Chem,* **223:**107, 1956.

Schumer, W.: High Calorie Solutions in Traumatized Patients, in C. L. Fox, Jr. and G. G. Nahas (eds.), "Body Fluid Replacement in the Surgical Patient, p. 326, Grune & Stratton, Inc., New York, 1970.

Scribbner, B. H., Cole, J. J., Christopher, P. H., Vizzo, J. E., Atkins, R. C., and Blagg, C. R.: Long Term Total Parenteral Nutrition: The Concept of an Artificial Gut, *JAMA,* **212:**457, 1970.

Stemmer, E. A., Allen, J. G., and Connolly, J. E.: Nutritional Value of Blood Plasma Protein: Growth in Puppies on Intravenous Diets of Plasma, Red Cells and Amino Acid, *Am Surg,* **32:**665, 1966.

———, ———, and ———: Value of Blood Plasma in Restoring Plasma Proteins in the Depleted Surgical Patient, *Am J Surg,* **112:**251, 1966.

Terry, R., Sandrock, W. E., Nye, R. E., and Whipple, G. H.: Parenteral Plasma Protein Maintains Nitrogen Equilibrium over Long Periods, *J Exp Med,* **87:**547, 1948.

Whedon, G. D., Deitrick, J. E., and Shorr, E.: Modification of the Effects of Immobilization upon Metabolic Physiologic Functions of Normal Men by the Use of an Oscillating Bed, *Am J Med,* **6:**684, 1949.

Wilkinson, A. W.: Restriction of Fluid Intake after Partial Gastrectomy, *Lancet,* **2:**428, 1956.

Wilmore, D. W., Curreri, W., Spitzer, K. W., Spitzer, M. E., and Pruitt, B. A.: Supra-normal Dietary Intake in Thermally Injured Hypermetabolic Patients, *Surg Gynecol Obstet,* **132:**881, 1971.

Yuile, C. L., O'Dea, A. E., Lucas, F. V., and Whipple, G. H.: Plasma Protein Labeled with Lysine-E-D$_{14}$: Its Oral Feeding and Relating Protein Metabolism in the Dog, *J Exp Med,* **96:**247, 1952.

Component Therapy

Clark, I. C., Jr.: Symposium on Inert Organic Liquids for Biological Oxygen Transport, *Atlantic City, New Jersey, April 13, 1969, Fed Proc,* **29:**1698, 1970.

——— and Gollan, F.: Survival of Mammals Breathing Organic Liquids Equilibrated with Oxygen at Atmospheric Pressure, *Science,* **152:**1755, 1966.

Geyer, R. P.: Whole Animal Perfusion with Fluorocarbon Dispersions, *Fed Proc,* **29:**1758, 1970.

———, Monroe, R. G., and Taylor, K.: Survival of Rats Totally Perfused with a Fluorocarbon-Detergent Preparation, in J. Folkman, W. G. Hardison, L. E. Rudolf, and F. J. Veith (eds.), "Organ Perfusion and Preservation," p. 85, Appleton-Century-Crofts, New York, 1968.

Modell, J. H., Newby, E. J., and Ruiz, B. C.: Long Term Survival of Dogs after Breathing Oxygenated Fluorocarbon Liquid, *Fed Proc,* **29:**1731, 1970.

Moss, G. S.: Massive Transfusion of Frozen Processed Red Cells in Combat Casualties: Report of Three Cases, *Surgery,* **66:**1008, 1969.

———, Cochin, A., and DeWoskin, R.: "Pure" Hemoglobin Solution: Coagulability Changes Produced In Vitro, *Surgery,* **74,** 1973.

Patel, M. M., Patel, M. K., Szanto, P., Alrenga, D. P., and Long, D. M.: Ventilation with Synthetic Fluids, *Surg Clin North Am,* **51:**25, 1971.

Sloviter, H. A.: Erythrocyte Substitutes, *Med Clin North Am,* **54:**787, 1970.

———, Petkovic, M., Ogoshi, S., and Yamada, H.: Dispersed Fluorochemicals as Substitutes for Erythrocytes in Intact Animals, *J Appl Physiol,* **27:**666, 1969.

———, Yamada, H., and Ogoshi, S.: Some Effects of Intravenously Administered Dispersed Fluorochemicals in Animals, *Fed Proc,* **29:**1755, 1970.

Acid-Base Balance

Astrup, P., Jorgensen, K., Siggaard-Andersen, O., and Engel, K.: The Acid-Base Metabolism: A New Approach, *Lancet,* **1:**1035, 1960.

Barry, K. G., and Malloy, J. P.: Oliguric Renal Failure: Evaluation and Therapy by Intravenous Infusion of Mannitol, *JAMA,* **179:**510, 1962.

Bergentz, S.-E., and Brief, D. K.: The Effect of pH and Osmolality on the Production of Canine Hemorrhagic Shock, *Surgery,* **58:**412, 1965.

Blackburn, G. L., and Schloerb, P. R.: Intracellular Acid-Base Regulation in Hypoxia, *Arch Surg,* **93:**573, 1966.

Boyd, D. R., Howard, C. M., and Addis, C.: Solute Aberrations in Traumatic Shock, *Rev Surg,* **28:**449, 1971.

Bradley, M. N.: Profound Shock Associated with Acidosis: Occurrence and Treatment, *Am Surg,* **30:**589, 1964.

Broder, G., and Weil, M. H.: Excess Lactate: Index of Reversibility of Shock in Human Patients, *Science,* **143:**1457, 1964.

Broido, P. W., Butcher, H. R., Jr., and Moyer, C. A.: A Bioassay of Treatment of Hemorrhagic Shock: II. The Expansion of Volume Distribution of Extracellular Ions during Hemorrhagic Hypotension and Its Possible Relationship to Change in Physical-Chemical Properties of Extravascular-Extracellular Tissue, *Arch Surg,* **93:**556, 1966.

Chazan, J. A., Stenson, R., and Kurland, G. S.: Acidosis of Cardiac Arrest, *N Engl J Med,* **278:**360, 1968.

Collins, J. A.: Effect of Massive Blood Transfusions on Acid-Base Status of Combat Casualties in Vietnam, in C. L. Fox, Jr., and G. G. Nahas (eds.), "Body Fluid Replacement in the Surgical Patient," p. 72, Grune & Stratton, Inc., New York, 1970.

———, Simmons, R. L., James, P. M., Bredenberg, C. E., Anderson, R. W., and Heisterkamp, C. A.: Acid-Base Status of Seriously Wounded Combat Casualties: II. Resuscitation with Stored Blood, *Ann Surg,* **173:**6, 1971.

Crandall, W. B.: Respiratory Alkalosis in Surgical Patients: An Analysis of the Role of Hypoxia, *Trans N Engl Surg Soc,* **45:**172, 1964.

——— and Stueck, G. H., Jr.: Acid-Base Balance in Surgical Patients: I. A Survey of 62 Selected Cases, *Ann Surg,* **149:**342, 1959.

Cunningham, J. N., Shires, G. T., and Wagner, Y.: Changes in Intracellular Sodium and Potassium Content of Red Blood Cells in Trauma and Shock, *Am J Surg,* **122:**650, 1971.

Dillion, J., Lynch, L. J., Jr., Myers, R., Butcher, H. R., Jr., and Moyer, C. A.: Bioassay of Treatment of Hemorrhagic Shock, *Arch Surg,* **93:**537, 1966.

Dudley, H. F., Boling, E. A., LeQuesne, L. P., and Moore, F. D.: Studies on Antidiuresis in Surgery: Effects of Anesthesia, Surgery and Posterior Pituitary Antidiuretic Hormone on Water Metabolism in Man, *Ann Surg,* **140:**354, 1954.

Eichenholz, A., Mulhausen, R. O., Anderson, W. E., and Mac-

Donald, F. M.: Primary Hypocapnia: A Cause of Metabolic Acidosis, *J Appl Physiol,* **17:**283, 1962.

Flemma, R. J., and Young, W. G., Jr.: The Metabolic Effects of Mechanical Ventilation and Respiratory Alkalosis in Postoperative Patients, *Surgery,* **56:**36, 1964.

Greenberg, A. G., and Kittle, C. F.: The Effects of Acute Changes in Acid-Base Status on Coronary Blood Flow, *Surgery,* **64:**315, 1968.

Gruber, U. F., Smith, L. L., and Moore, F. D.: The Effect of Acute Addition Metabolic Alkalosis on the Cardiovascular Response of the Dog to Hemorrhage, *J Surg Res,* **3:**21, 1963.

Gump, F. E., and Kinney, J. M.: Measurement of Water Balance: A Guide to Surgical Care, *Surgery,* **64:**154, 1968.

Hardaway, R. M., James, P. M., Jr., Anderson, R. W., Bredenberg, C. E., and West, R. L.: Intensive Study and Treatment of Shock in Man, *JAMA,* **199:**779, 1967.

Hayes, M. A.: Current Concepts: Water and Electrolyte Therapy after Operation, *N Engl J Med,* **278:**1054, 1968.

Heaton, F. W., Clark, C. G., and Coligher, J. C.: Magnesium Deficiency Complicating Intestinal Surgery, *Br J Surg,* **54:**41, 1967.

Howland, W. S., and Ryan, G. M.: Massive Transfusion: A Reassessment, in C. L. Fox, Jr., and G. G. Nahas (eds.), "Body Fluid Replacement in the Surgical Patient," p. 57, Grune & Stratton, Inc., New York, 1970.

Hoye, R. C., Ketcham, A. S., and Berlin, N. I.: Total Red Cell and Plasma Volume Alterations Occurring with Extensive Surgery in Humans, *Surg Gynecol Obstet,* **123:**27, 1966.

Huckabee, W. E.: Abnormal Resting Blood Lactate: I. The Significance of Hyperlactalemia in Hospitalized Patients, *Am J Med.,* **30:**833, 1961.

Hume, D. M., and Egdahl, R. H.: Progressive Destruction of Renal Homografts Isolated from the Regional Lymphatics of the Host, *Surgery,* **28:**194, 1955.

Litwin, M. S., Smith, L. L., and Moore, F. D.: Metabolic Alkalosis following Massive Transfusion, *Surgery,* **45:**805, 1959.

Lyons, J. H., Jr., and Moore, F. D.: Posttraumatic Alkalosis: Incidence and Pathophysiology of Alkalosis in Surgery, *Surgery,* **60:**93, 1966.

MacLean, L. D., Mulligan, W. G., McLean, A. P. H., and Duff, J. H.: Patterns of Septic Shock in Man: A Detailed Study of 56 Patients, *Ann Surg,* **166:**543, 1967.

Peaston, M. J. T.: Metabolic Acidosis in Burns, *Br Med J,* **1:**809, 1968.

Pullen, H., Doig, A., and Lambie, A. T.: Intensive Intravenous Potassium Replacement Therapy, *Lancet,* **2:**809, 1967.

Robbins, H. S., and Dufrene, J. H.: Hyperkalemia in Anesthesia, *Pa Med,* **75:**77, 1972.

Schlobohm, R. M., and Holaday, D. A.: Prevention and Correction of Acidosis, in C. L. Fox, Jr., and G. G. Nahas (eds.), "Body Fluid Replacement in the Surgical Patient," p. 246, Grune & Stratton, Inc., New York, 1970.

Shoemaker, W. C., and Iida, F.: Studies on the Equilibration of Labeled Red Cells and T-1824 in Hemorrhagic Shock, *Surg Gynecol Obstet,* **114:**539, 1962.

Siggaard-Andersen, O.: The Acid-Base Status of Blood, *Scand J Clin Lab Invest,* **15**(Suppl 70):1, 1963.

———: Blood Acid-Base Alignment Homogram, *Scand J Clin Lab Invest,* **15:**211, 1963.

———, Engel, K., Jørgensen, K., and Astrup, P.: A Micro Method

for Determination of pH, Carbondioxide Tension, Base Excess and Standard Bicarbonate in Capillary Blood, *Scand J Clin Lab Invest,* **12:**172, 1960.

Suzuki, F., Baker, R. J., and Shoemaker, W. C.: Red Cell and Plasma Volume Alterations after Hemorrhage and Trauma, *Ann Surg,* **160:**262, 1964.

Wacker, W. E. C., and Parisi, A. F.: Magnesium Metabolism, *N Engl J Med,* **278:**712, 1968.

Oxygen Transport

Benesch, R., and Benesch, R.: Intracellular Organic Phosphates as Regulators of Oxygen Release by Haemoglobin, *Nature,* (*Lond*), **221:**618, 1969.

Naylor, B. A., Welch, M. H., Shafer, A. W., and Cuenter, C. A.: Blood Affinity for Oxygen in Hemorrhagic and Endotoxic Shock, *J Appl Physiol,* **32:**829, 1972.

Plzak, L. F.: Hyperalimentation and the Oxy-hemoglobin Dissociation Curve, in G. S. M. Cowan, Jr., and W. L. Scheetz, (eds.) "Intravenous Hyperalimentation," p. 196, Lea & Febiger, Philadelphia, 1972.

Proctor, H. J., Lentz, R. R., and Johnson, G., Jr.: Alterations in Baboon Erythrocyte 2,3-Diphosphoglycerate Concentration Associated with Hemorrhagic Shock and Resuscitation, *Ann Surg,* **174:**923, 1971.

Shoemaker, W. C., Boyd, D. R., Kim, S. I., Brown, R. S., Dreiling, D. A., and Kark, A. E.: Sequential Oxygen Transport and Acid-Base Changes after Trauma to the Unanesthetized Patient, *Surg Gynecol Obstet,* **132:**1033, 1971.

Sugerman, H., Miller, L. D., Oski, F. A., Diaco, J., Delivoria-Papadopoulos, M., and Davidson, D.: Decreased 2,3-Diphosphoglycerate (DPG) and Reduced Oxygen (O_2) Consumption in Septic Shock, *Clin Res,* **18:**418, 1970.

Travis, S. F., Sugerman, H. J., Ruberg, R. L., Dudrick, S. J., Delivoria-Papadopoulos, M. D., Miller, L. D., and Oski, F. A.: Alterations of Red Cell Poikilitic Intermediates and Oxygen Transport as a Consequence of Hypophosphatemia in Patients Receiving Intravenous Hyperalimentation, *N Engl J Med,* **285:**763, 1971.

Immunologic Protective Mechanisms

Bell, M. L., Herman, A. H., Egdahl, R. H., Smith, E. E., and Rutenburg, A. M.: Role of Lysosomal Disruption in the Development of Refractory Shock, *Surg Forum,* **21:**10, 1970.

Greyson, N. D., Rhodes, B. A., Buchanan, J. W., and Wagner, H. N., Jr.: Local Increases in Reticuloendothelial Function during Healing, *J Reticuloendothel Soc,* **11:**293, 1972.

Hawley, P. R.: The Role of Trauma in the Development of Peritonitis and the Protection Afforded by Intravenous Dextran Solutions, *Br J Surg,* **58:**305, 1971.

Liedberg, C. F.: Antibacterial Resistance in Burns: II. The Effect on Unspecific Humoral Defense Mechanisms, Phagocytosis and the Development of Bacteremia, *Acta Chir Scand,* **121:**351, 1961.

Munster, A. M., Eurenius, K., Mortensen, R. F., and Mason, A. D.: Ability of Splenic Lymphocytes from Injured Rats to Induce a Graft-versus-Host Reaction, *Transplantation,* **14:**106, 1972.

Palmerio, C., and Fine, J.: The Nature of Resistance to Shock, *Arch Surg,* **98:**679, 1969.

Pillemer, L., Schoenberg, M. D., Blum, L., and Wurz, L.: Properdin System and Immunity: II. Interaction of the Properdin System with Polysaccharides, *Science,* **122:**545, 1955.

Rittenburg, M. S., and Hanback, L. D.: Phagocytic Depression in Thermal Injuries, *J Trauma,* **7:**523, 1967.

Schildt, B. E.: Function of the RES after Thermal and Mechanical Trauma in Mice, *Acta Chir Scand,* **136:**359, 1970.

———— and Low, H.: Relationship between Trauma, Plasma Corticosterone and Reticuloendothelial Function in Anaesthetized Mice, *Acta Endocrinol (Kbh),* **67:**141, 1971.

Schumer, W., Erve, P. R., and Obernolte, R. P.: Mechanisms of Steroid Protection in Septic Shock, *Surgery,* **72:**119, 1972.

Stetson, C. A., Jr.: Studies on the Mechanism of the Shwartzman Phenomenon: Similarities between Reactions to Endotoxins and Certain Reactions of Bacterial Allergy, *J Exp Med,* **101:** 421, 1955.

Weil, M. H. and Spink, W. W.: A Comparison of Shock Due to Endotoxin with Anaphylactic Shock, *J Lab Clin Med,* **50:**501, 1957.

Zweifach, B. W.: Relation of the RES to Natural and Acquired Resistance to Shock, in S. G. Hershey (ed.), "Shock," Little, Brown and Company, Boston, 1964.

————, Benacerraf, B., and Thomas, L.: The Relationship Between the Vascular Manifestations of Shock Produced by Endotoxin, Trauma, and Hemorrhage, *J Exp Med,* **106:**403, 1957.

Organ Systems Changes: General

Bock, K. D. (ed.): "Shock: Pathogenesis and Therapy: An Internation Symposium, Stockholm, 27th-30th June, 1961," Ciba Symposium, Springer-Verlag OHG, Berlin, 1962.

Hardaway, R. M.: The Problem of Acute Severe Trauma and Shock, *Surg Gynecol Obstet,* **133:**799, 1971.

Hershey, S. G. (ed.): "Shock," Little, Brown and Company, Boston, 1964.

Jacobson, E. D.: A Physiologic Approach to Shock, *N Engl J Med,* **278:**834, 1968.

Landy, M., and Braun, W. (eds.): Bacterial Endotoxins, *Proc Symp Inst Microbiol Rutgers State Univ,* New Brunswick, N.J., 1964.

Mills, L. C., and Moyer, J. H. (eds.): "Shock and Hypotension: Pathogenesis and Treatment: The 12th Hahnemann Symposium," Grune & Stratton, Inc., New York, 1965.

Proceedings of a Conference on Recent Progress and Present Problems in the Field of Shock. Held at Walter Reed Army Institute of Research, Washington, D.C., December 14-17, 1960, *Fed Proc,* 20 (*Suppl* 9):1, 1961.

Shires, G. T.: Shock and Metabolism, *Surg Gynecol Obstet,* **124:** 284, 1967.

Cardiovascular Function

Anderson, R. W., James, P. M., Bredenberg, C. E., and Hardaway, R. M.: Phenoxybenzamine in Septic Shock, *Ann Surg,* **165:** 341, 1967.

Attar, S., McLaughlin, J., Hanashiro, P., and Cowley, R. A.: The Kallikreins in Human Shock and Trauma, *Surg Forum,* **22:**11, 1971.

Baez, S., and Orkin, L. R.: Microcirculatory Effects of Anesthesia in Shock, in S. G. Hershey (ed.), "Shock," p. 207, Little, Brown and Company, Boston, 1964.

Baue, A.: Shock and Metabolism, *Surg Gynecol Obstet,* **134:**276, 1972.

Berk, J. L., Hagen, J. F., Beyer, W. H., and Niazmand, R.: Effect of Epinephrine on Arteriovenous Shunts in Pathogenesis of Shock, *Surg Gynecol Obstet,* **124:**347, 1967.

Cann, M. S., Stevenson, T., Fiallos, E. E., and Thal, A. P.: Effect of Digitalis on Myocardial Contractility in Sepsis, *Surg Forum,* **22:**1, 1971.

Clowes, G. H. A., Jr., and Del Guercio, L. R. M.: Circulatory Response to Trauma of Surgical Operations, *Metabolism,* **9:**67, 1960.

Coalson, J. J., Woodruff, H. K., Greenfield, L. J., Guemter, C. A., and Hinshaw, L. B.: Effects of Digoxin on Myocardial Ultrastructure in Endotoxin Shock, *Surg Gynecol Obstet,* **135:**908, 1972.

Cohn, J. N.: Central Venous Pressure as Guide to Volume Expansion, *Ann Intern Med,* **66:**1283, 1967.

Duff, J. H., Malave, G., Peretz, D. I., Scott, H. M., and MacLean, L. D.: Hemodynamics of Septic Shock in Man and in the Dog, *Ann Surg,* **162:**161, 1965.

Glenn, T. M., Herlihy, B. L., Ferguson, W. W., and Lefer, A. M.: Protective Effect of Pancreatic Duct Ligation in Splanchnic Ischemia Shock, *Am J Physiol,* **222:**1278, 1972.

———— and Lefer, A. M.: Protective Effect of Thoracic Lymph Diversion in Hemorrhagic Shock, *Am J Physiol,* **219:**1305, 1970.

———— and ————: Significance of Splanchnic Proteases in the Production of a Toxic Factor in Hemorrhagic Shock, *Circ Res,* **29:**338, 1971.

Goodyer, A. V. N., Hammond, G. L., Gross, C. C., and Kabimba, J.: Myocardial Production of Pyruvate in Hemorrhagic Shock, *J Surg Res,* **11:**501, 1971.

Greenfield, L. J., McCurdy, J. R., Hinshaw, L. B., and Elkins, R. C.: Preservation of Myocardial Function during Cross-Circulation in Terminal Endotoxin Shock, *Surgery,* **72:**111, 1972.

Hardaway, R. M., James, P. M., Jr., Anderson, R. W., Bredenberg, C. E., and West, R. L.: Intensive Study and Treatment of Shock in Man, *JAMA,* **199:**779, 1967.

Hermreck, A. S., and Thal, A. P.: Mechanisms for the High Circulatory Requirements in Sepsis and Septic Shock, *Ann Surg,* **170:**677, 1969.

Hinshaw, L. B., Greenfield, L. J., Archer, L. T., and Guenter, C. A.: Effects of Endotoxin on Myocardial Hemodynamics, Performance, and Metabolism during Beta Adrenergic Blockade, *Proc Soc Exp Biol Med,* **137:**1217, 1971.

————, ————, Owen, S. E., Black, M. R., and Guenter, C. A.: Precipitation of Cardiac Failure in Endotoxin Shock, *Surg Gynecol Obstet,* **135:**39, 1972.

Hiott, D. W., and Richardson, J. A.: Cardiac Norepinephrine Levels and Contractile Force Responses with Hemorrhagic Shock, Acidosis and Sympathetic Stimulation, *Res Comm Chem Pathol Pharmacol,* **2:**429, 1971.

Huberty, J. R., Schwarz, R. H., and Emich, J. P., Jr.: Central Venous Pressure Monitoring, *Obstet Gynecol,* **30:**842, 1967.

Lefer, A. M., Cowgill, R., Marshall, F. F., Hall, L. M., and Brank, E. D.: Characterization of a Myocardial Depressant Factor Present in Hemorrhagic Shock, *Am J Physiol,* **213:**492, 1967.

Levinson, S. A., and Hume, D. M.: Effect of Exchange Transfusion with Fresh Whole Blood on Refractory Septic Shock, *Am Surg,* **38:**49, 1972.

Longerbeam, J. K., Vannix, R., Wagner, W., and Joergenson, E.:

Central Venous Pressure Monitoring: Useful Guide to Fluid Therapy during Shock and Other Forms of Cardiovascular Stress, *Am J Surg,* **110**:220, 1965.

MacLean, L. D., and Duff, J. H.: Use of Central Venous Pressure as Guide to Volume Replacement in Shock, *Dis Chest,* **48**:199, 1965.

Martin, A. M., Jr., Hackel, D. B., Entman, M. L., Capp, M. P., and Spach, M. S.: Mechanisms in the Development of Myocardial Lesions in Hemorrhagic Shock, *Ann NY Acad Sci,* **156**:79, 1969.

Mundth, E. D., Wright, J. E. C., Wanibuchi, Y., and Austen, W. G.: Effect of Varying After-load and Epinephrine Levels on the Ischemic Survival Time of the Dog Heart, *Surg Forum,* **22**:133, 1971.

Rush, B. F., Jr., Rosenberg, J. C., and Spencer, F. C.: Effect of Dibenzyline Treatment on Cardiac Dynamics and Oxidative Metabolism in Hemorrhagic Shock, *Ann Surg,* **162**:1013, 1965.

Schumer, W.: Microcirculatory and Metabolic Effects of Dibenzyline in Oligemic Shock, *Surg Gynecol Obstet,* **123**:787, 1966.

Solis, R. T. and Downing, S. E.: Effects of *E. Coli* Endotoxemia on Ventricular Performance, *Am J Physiol,* **211**:307, 1966.

Thal, A. P.: Shock and Metabolism, *Surg Gynecol Obstet,* **122**:283, 1966.

Wangensteen, S. L., Geissinger, W. T., Lovett, W. L., Glenn, T. M., and Lefer, A. W.: Relationship between Splanchnic Blood Flow and a Myocardial Depressant Factor in Endotoxin Shock, *Surgery,* **69**:410, 1971.

Weil, M. H., Schubin, H., and Rusoff, L.: Fluid Repletion in Circulatory Shock: Central Venous Pressure and Other Practical Guides, *JAMA,* **192**:688, 1965.

Weinstein, L., and Klainer, A. S.: Septic Shock: Pathogenesis and Treatment: IV. Management of Emergencies, *N Engl J Med,* **274**:950, 1966.

Wilson, R. F., Jablonski, D. V., and Thal, A. P.: Usage of Dibenzyline in Clinical Shock, *Surgery,* **56**:172, 1964.

———, Thal, A. P., Kindling, P. H., Grifka, T., and Ackerman, E.: Hemodynamic Measurements in Septic Shock, *Arch Surg,* **91**:121, 1965.

Wright, C. J., Duff, J. H., McLean, A. P. H., and MacLean, L. D.: Regional Capillary Blood Flow and Oxygen Uptake in Severe Sepsis, *Surg Gynecol Obstet,* **132**:637, 1971.

Pulmonary Function

Alho, A., Motsay, G. J., and Lillehei, R. C.: Comparison of Lung Changes in Haemmorrhagic and Endotoxin Shock, *Ann Chir Gynaecol Fenn,* **60**:202, 1971.

Anderson, W. H., Dossett, B. E., Jr., and Hamilton, G. L.: Prevention of Postoperative Pulmonary Complications: Use of Isoproterenol and Intermittant Positive Pressure Breathing on Inspiration, *JAMA,* **186**:763, 1963.

Ashbaugh, D. G., and Petty, T. L.: The Use of Corticosteroids in the Treatment of Respiratory Failure Associated with Massive Fat Embolism, *Surg Gynecol Obstet,* **123**:493, 1966.

———, ———, Bigelow, D. B., and Harris, T. M.: Continuous Positive-Pressure Breathing (CPPB) in Adult Respiratory Distress Syndrome, *J Thorac Cardiovasc Surg,* **57**:31, 1969.

———, Svitek, V., and Ambrose, P.: The Incidence and Effects of Particulate Aggregation and Microembolism in Pump-Oxygenator Systems, *J Thorac Cardiovasc Surg,* **55**:691, 1968.

Ayres, S. M., Mueller, H., Giannelli, S., Jr., Fleming, P., and

Grace, W. J.: The Lung in Shock: Alveolar-Capillary Gas Exchange in the Shock Syndrome, *Am J Cardiol,* **26**:588, 1970.

Barber, R. E., Lee, J., and Hamilton, W. K.: Oxygen Toxicity in Man: Study in Patients with Irreversible Brain Damage, *N Engl J Med,* **283**:1498, 1970.

Barnes, R. W., and Merendino, K. A.: Post-traumatic Pulmonary Insufficiency Syndrome, *Surg Clin North Am,* **52**:625, 1972.

Bendixen, H. H., Hedley-Whyte, J., and Layer, M. B.: Impaired Oxygenation in Surgical Patients during General Anesthesia with Controlled Ventilation, *N Engl J Med,* **269**:991, 1963.

Bergofsky, E. H.: The Adult Acute Respiratory Insufficiency Syndrome following Nonthoracic Trauma: The Lung in Shock, *Am J Cardiol,* **26**:619, 1970.

Burke, J. F., Pontoppidan, H., and Welch, C. E.: High Output Respiratory Failure: An Important Cause of Death Ascribed to Peritonitis or Ileus, *Ann Surg,* **158**:581, 1963.

Calabresi, P., and Abelmann, W. H.: Porto-caval and Portopulmonary Anastomoses in Laennec's Cirrhosis and in Heart Failure, *J Clin Invest,* **36**:1257, 1957.

Carlson, L. A.: Lipid Mobilization in Trauma: Friend or Foe?, in A. P. Morgan (ed.), "Proceedings of Conference on Energy Metabolism and Body Fuel Utilization," p. 50, Harvard University Press, Cambridge, Mass., 1966.

Comroe, J. H., Jr., Forster, R. E., II, Du-Bois, A. B., Briscoe, W. A., and Carlsen, E.: "The Lung," Year Book Medical Publishers, Inc., Chicago, 1962.

Cook, W. A., and Webb, W. R.: Pulmonary Changes in Hemorrhagic Shock, *Surgery,* **64**:85, 1968.

Dowd, J., and Jenkins, L. C.: The Lung in Shock: A Review, *Can Anaesth Soc J,* **19**:309, 1972.

Eltringham, W. K., Schroder, R., Jenny, M., Matloff, J. M., and Zollinger, R. M., Jr.: Pulmonary Arteriovenous Admixture in Cardiac Surgical Patients, *Circulation,* **37, 38** (*Suppl* 2):207, 1968.

Geiger, J. P., and Gleichinsky, L.: Acute Pulmonary Insufficiency: Treatment in Vietnam Casualties, *Arch Surg,* **102**:400, 1971.

Hamilton, W. K.: Alterations in Pulmonary Functions, *JAMA,* **202**:116, 1967.

Hechtman, H. B., Weisel, R. D., and Berger, R. L.: Independence of Pulmonary Shunting and Pulmonary Edema, *Surgery,* **74**, 1973.

Hill, J. D., O'Brien, T. G., Murray, J. J., Dontigny, L., Bramson, M. L., Osborn, J. J., and Gerbode, F.: Prolonged Extracorporeal Oxygenation for Acute Post-traumatic Respiratory Failure (Shock-Lung Syndrome), *N Engl J Med,* **286**:629, 1972.

Hillen, G. P., Gaisford, W. D., and Jensen, C. G.: Pulmonary Changes in Treated and Untreated Hemorrhagic Shock, *Am J Surg,* **122**:639, 1971.

Hirsch, E. F., Fletcher, R., and Lucas, S.: Hemodynamic and Respiratory Changes Associated with Sepsis following Combat Trauma, *Ann Surg,* **174**:211, 1971.

Kumar, A., Falke, K. J., Gettin, B., Aldredge, C. F., Laver, M. B., Lowenstein, E., and Pontoppidan, H.: Continuous Positive-Pressure Ventilation in Acute Respiratory Failure: Effects on Hemodynamics and Lung Function, *N Engl J Med,* **283**:1430, 1970.

Lahdensuu, M.: Studies on Phospholipid Metabolism in the Lung and Alveolar Surfactant in Experimental Traumatic and Haemorrhagic Shock, *Ann Chir Gynaecol Fenn,* **60**:245, 1971.

Lawson, D. W., Defalco, A. J., Phelps, J. A., Bradley, B. E., and

McClenathan, J. E.: Corticosteroids as Treatment for Aspiration of Gastric Contents: An Experimental Study, *Surgery,* **59:**845, 1966.

Levitsky, S., Annable, C. A., Park, B. S., Davis, A. L., and Thomas, P. A.: Depletion of Alveolar Surface Active Material by Transbronchial Plasma Irrigation of the Lung, *Ann Surg,* **173:**107, 1971.

McNamara, J. J., Melot, M. D., and Stremple, F. J.: Screen Filtration Pressure in Combat Casualties, *Ann Surg,* **172:**334, 1970.

Magilligan, D. J., Jr., Oleksyn, T. W., and Schwartz, S. I.: Pulmonary Intravascular and Extravascular Volumes in Hemorrhagic Shock and Fluid Replacement, *Surgery,* **72:**780, 1972.

Meagher, D. M., Piermattei, D. L., and Swan, H.: Platelet Aggregation during Progressive Hemorrhagic Shock in Pigs, *J Thorac Cardiovasc Surg,* **62:**823, 1971.

Moore, F. D., Lyons, J. H., Jr., Pierce, E. C., Morgan, A. P., Jr., Drinker, P. A., MacArthur, J. D., and Dammin, G. J.: "Post-traumatic Pulmonary Insufficiency," W. B. Saunders Company, Philadelphia, 1969.

Moseley, R. V., and Doty, D. B.: Physiologic Changes Due to Aspiration Pneumonitis, *Ann Surg,* **171:**73, 1970.

Moss, G., Staunton, C., and Stein, A. A.: Cerebral Hypoxia as the Primary Event in the Pathogenesis of the "Shock Lung Syndrome," *Surg Forum,* **22:**211, 1971.

Nahas, R. A., Melrose, D. G., Sykes, M. K., and Robinson, B.: Post-perfusion Lung Syndrome: Effect of Homologous Blood, *Lancet,* **2:**254, 1965.

———, ———, ———, and ———: Post-perfusion Lung Syndrome: Role of Circulatory Exclusion, *Lancet,* **2:**251, 1965.

Nash, G., Blennerhassett, J. B., and Pontoppidan, H.: Pulmonary Lesions Associated with Oxygen Therapy and Artificial Ventilation, *N Engl J Med,* **276:**368, 1967.

Pelter, L. F.: Fat Embolism: A Pulmonary Disease, *Surgery,* **62:** 756, 1967.

Peters, R. M., and Hedgpeth, E. McG., Jr.: Acid-Base Balance and Respiratory Work, *J Thorac Cardiovasc Surg,* **52:**649, 1966.

Ratliff, N. B., Wilson, J. W., Mikat, E., Hackel, D. B., and Graham, T. C.: The Lung in Hemorrhagic Shock: IV. The Role of Neutrophilic Polymorphonuclear Leukocytes, *Am J Pathol,* **65:**325, 1971.

Robb, H. J., Margulis, R. R., and Jabs, C. M.: Role of Pulmonary Microembolism in the Hemodynamics of Endotoxin Shock, *Surg Gynecol Obstet,* **135:**777, 1972.

Robin, E. D.: Abnormalities of Acid-Base Regulation in Chronic Pulmonary Disease, with Special Reference to Hypercapnia and Extracellular Alkalosis, *N Engl J Med,* **268:**917, 1963.

Roe, B. B.: Prevention and Treatment of Respiratory Complications in Surgery, *N Engl J Med,* **163:**547, 1960.

Siegel, D. C., Cochin, A., and Moss, G. S. The Ventilatory Response to Hemorrhagic Shock and Resuscitation, *Surgery,* **72:**451, 1972.

———, Moss, G. S., Cochin, A., and DasGupta, T. K.: Pulmonary Changes following Treatment for Hemorrhagic Shock: Saline versus Colloid Infusion, *Surg Forum,* **21:**17, 1970.

Trimble, C., Smith, D. E., Rosenthal, M. H., and Fosburg, R. G.: Pathophysiologic Role of Hypocarbia in Post-Traumatic Pulmonary Insufficiency, *Am J Surg,* **122:**633, 1971.

Veith, F. J., Hagstrom, J. W. C., Panossian, A., Nehlsen, S. L., and Wilson, J. W.: Pulmonary Microcirculatory Response to Shock, Transfusion, and Pump-Oxygenator Procedures: A Unified Mechanism Underlying Pulmonary Damage, *Surgery,* **64:**95, 1968.

Hepatic Function

Ballinger, W. F., Vollenweider, H., and Montgomery, E. H.: The Response of the Canine Liver to Anaerobic Metabolism Induced by Hemorrhagic Shock, *Surg Gynecol Obstet,* **112:**19, 1961.

Baue, A. E., Wurth, M. A., and Sayeed, M. M.: The Dynamics of Altered ATP-dependent and ATP-yielding Cell Processes in Shock, *Surgery,* **72:**94, 1972.

Blair, O. M., Stenger, R. J., Hopkins, R. W., and Simeone, F. A.: Hepatocellular Ultrastructure in Dogs with Hypovolemic Shock, *Lab Invest,* **18:**172, 1968.

Bloom, W. L.: Changes in Blood Ketones during Hemorrhagic Shock in Rats, *Metabolism,* **10:**171, 1961.

——— and Ward, J. A.: Changes in Carbohydrate Metabolism during Blood Loss, Shock, and Anoxia, *Metabolism,* **10:**379, 1961.

Buxton, R. W., Haines, B. W., and Michaelis, M.: Effects of Hemorrhagic Shock upon Succinic Oxidation in Dog, Liver and Brain Slices, *Bull School Med Univ Maryland,* **46:**3, 1961.

Clermont, H. G., Williams, J. S., and Adams, J. T.: Liver Acid Phosphatase as a Measure of Hepatocyte Resistance to Hemorrhagic Shock, *Surgery,* **71:**868, 1972.

DePalma, R. G., Holden, W. D., and Robinson, A. V.: Fluid Therapy in Experimental Hemorrhagic Shock: Ultrastructural Effects in Liver and Muscle, *Ann Surg,* **175:**539, 1972.

Holden, W. D., DePalma, R. G., Drucker, W. R., and McKalen, A.: Ultrastructural Changes in Hemorrhagic Shock: Electron Microscopic Study of Liver, Kidney, and Striated Muscle, *Ann Surg,* **162:**517, 1965.

Janoff, A.: Alterations in Lysosomes (Intracellular Enzymes) during Shock: Effects of Preconditioning (Tolerance) and Protective Drugs, in S. G. Hershey (ed.), "Shock," p. 93, Little, Brown and Company, Boston, 1964.

Kekomaki, M., and Louhimo, I.: Blood Ammonium Concentration during Hemorrhagic Shock in the Rabbit, *Acta Chir Scand,* **137:**745, 1971.

Lavine, L., Harano, Y., and DePalma, R. G.: ATPase Activity and Palmitate Oxidation of Hepatic Mitochondria in Energy Production in Endotoxemia, *Surg Forum,* **22:**5, 1971.

Murray, J. F., Dawson, A. M., and Sherlock, S.: Circulatory Changes in Chronic Liver Disease, *Am J Med,* **24:**358, 1958.

Rutenburg, A. M., Bell, M. L., Butcher, R. W., Polgar, P., Dorn, B. D., and Egdahl, R. H.: Adenosine 3',5'-Monophosphate Levels in Hemorrhagic Shock, *Ann Surg,* **174:**461, 1971.

Selkurt, E. E.: Role of Liver and Toxic Factors in Shock, in S. G. Hershey (ed.), "Shock," p. 34, Little, Brown and Company, Boston, 1964.

Sherlock, S.: Disease of the Digestive System. Drugs and the Liver, *Br Med J,* **1:**227, 1968.

Shoemaker, W. C., and Fitch, L. B.: Hepatic Lesions of Hemorrhagic Shock, *Arch Surg,* **85:**492, 1962.

Smart, C. J., and Rowlands, S. D.: Oxygen Consumption and Hepatic Metabolism in Experimental Posthemorrhagic Shock, *Trauma,* **12:**327, 1972.

Wurth, M. A., Sayeed, M. M., and Baue, A. E.: $(Na^+ + K^+)$-

ATPase Activity in the Liver with Hemorrhagic Shock, *Proc Soc Exp Biol Med,* **139:**1238, 1972.

Gastrointestinal Function

Abe, H., Carballo, J., Appert, H. E., and Howard, J. M.: The Release and Fate of the Intestinal Lysosomal Enzymes after Acute Ischemic Injury of the Intestine, *Surg Gynecol Obstet,* **135:**581, 1972.

Bacalzo, L. V., Jr., Parkins, F. M., Miller, L. D., and Parkins, W. M.: Effects of Prolonged Hypovolemic Shock on Jejunal Fluid and Sodium Transport, *Surg Gynecol Obstet,* **134:**399, 1972.

Barton, R. W., Reynolds, D. G., and Swan, K. G.: Mesenteric Circulatory Responses to Hemorrhagic Shock in the Baboon, *Ann Surg,* **175:**204, 1972.

Bounous, G.: Metabolic Changes in Intestinal Mucosa during Hemorrhagic Shock, *Can J Surg,* **8:**332, 1965.

———, McArdle, A. H., Hodges, D. M., Hampson, L. G., and Gurd, F. N.: Biosynthesis of Intestinal Mucin in Shock: Relationship to Tryptic Hemorrhagic Enteritis and Permeability to Curare, *Ann Surg,* **164:**13, 1966.

———, Sutherland, N. G., McArdle, A. H., and Gurd, F. N.: The Prophylactic Use of an "Elemental" Diet in Experimental Hemorrhagic Shock and Intestinal Ischemia, *Ann Surg,* **166:**312, 1967.

Carter, D., and Einheber, A.: Intestinal Ischemic Shock in Germ-free Animals, *Surg Gynecol Obstet,* **122:**66, 1966.

Chiu, C. J., Scott, H. J., and Gurd, F. N.: Volume Deficit Versus Toxic Absorption: A Study of Canine Shock after Mesenteric Arterial Occlusion, *Ann Surg,* **175:**479, 1972.

Clermont, H. G., and Williams, J. S.: Lymph Lysosomal Enzyme Acid Phosphatase in Hemorrhagic Shock, *Ann Surg,* **176:**90, 1972.

Cook, B. H., Wilson, E. R., Jr., and Taylor, A. E.: Intestinal Fluid Loss in Hemorrhagic Shock, *Am J Physiol,* **221:**1494, 1971.

DenBesten, L., and Hamza, K. N.: Effect of Bile Salts on Ionic Premeability of Canine Gastric Mucosa during Experimental Shock, *Gastroenterology,* **62:**417, 1972.

Fine, J.: Intestinal Circulation in Shock, *Gastroenterology,* **52:**454, 1967.

Fischer, R. P., and Stremple, J. F.: Stress Ulcers in Post-traumatic Renal Insufficiency in Patients from Vietnam, *Surg Gynecol Obstet,* **134:**790, 1972.

Goodier, T. E. W., Horwich, L., and Galloway, R. W.: Morphological Observations on Gastric Ulcers Treated with Carbonoxolone Sodium. *Gut,* **8:**544, 1967.

Goodman, A. A., and Osborne, M. P.: An Experimental Model and Clinical Definition of Stress Ulceration, *Surg Gynecol Obstet,* **134:**563, 1972.

Gurd, F. N.: Metabolic and Functional Changes in Intestine in Shock, *Am J Surg,* **110:**333, 1965.

——— and McClelland, R. N.: Trauma Workshop Report: The Gastrointestinal Tract in Trauma, *J Trauma,* **11:**1089, 1970.

Howerton, E. E., and Kolmen, S. N.: The Intestinal Tract as a Portal of Entry of Pseudomonas in Burned Rats, *J Trauma,* **12:**335, 1972.

Hutcher, N., Silverberg, S. G., and Lee, H. M.: The Effect of Vitamin A on the Formation of Steroid Induced Gastric Ulcers, *Surg Forum,* **22:**322, 1971.

Lev, R., Molot, M. D., McNamara, J., and Stremple, J. F.: "Stress" Ulcers following War Wounds in Vietnam: A Morphologic and Histochemical Study, *Lab Invest,* **25:**491, 1971.

Lillehei, R. C., Longerbeam, J. K., Bloch, J. H., and Manax, W. G.: The Nature of Experimental Irreversible Shock with Its Clinical Application, in S. G. Hershey (ed.), "Shock," p. 139, Little, Brown and Company, Boston, 1964.

Menguy, R., and Masters, Y. F.: Effect of Cortisone on Mucoprotein Secretion by Gastric Antrum of Dogs: Pathogenesis of Steroid Ulcer, *Surgery,* **54:**19, 1963.

——— and ———: Influence of Parathyroid Extract on Gastric Mucosal Content of Mucus, *Gastroenterology,* **48:**342, 1965.

Ritchie, W. P., and Fischer, R. P.: Studies on the Pathogenesis of "Stress Ulcer": Electrical Potential Difference and Ionic Fluxes across Canine Gastric Mucosa during Hemorrhagic Shock, *J Surg Res,* **12:**173, 1972.

———, Roth, R. R., and Fischer, R. P.: Studies on the Pathogenesis of "Stress Ulcer": Effect of Hemorrhage, Transfusion, and Vagotomy in the Restrained Rat, *Surgery,* **71:**445, 1972.

Robert, A., Bayer, R. B., and Nezamis, J. E.: Gastric Mucus Content during Development of Ulcers in Fasting Rats, *Gastroenterology,* **45:**740, 1963.

——— and Nezamis, J. E.: Effect of Prednisolone on Gastric Mucus Content and on Ulcer Formation, *Proc Soc Exp Biol Med,* **114:**545, 1943.

Shirazi, S. S., DenBesten, L., and Hamza, K. N.: Absorption of Bile Salts from the Gastric Mucosa during Hemorrhagic Shock, *Proc Soc Exp Biol Med,* **140:**924, 1972.

Swan, K. G., Barton, R. W., and Reynolds, D. G.: Mesenteric Hemodynamics during Endotoxemia in the Baboon, *Gastroenterology,* **61:**872, 1971.

——— and Reynolds, D. G.: Blood Flow to the Liver and Spleen during Endotoxin Shock in the Baboon, *Surgery,* **72:**388, 1972.

Voitk, A. J., Chiu, C. J., and Gurd, F. N.: Prevention of Porcine Stress Ulcer following Hemorrhagic Shock with Elemental Diet, *Arch Surg,* **105:**473, 1972.

Vyden, J. K., and Corday, E.: The Effect of Cardiogenic Shock on the Superior Mesenteric Circulation, *Geriatrics,* **26:**85, 1971.

Wilmore, D. W., Dudrick, S. J., Dailey, J. M., and Vars, H. M.: The Role of Nutrition in the Adaptation of the Small Intestine after Massive Resection, *Surg Gynecol Obstet,* **132:**673, 1971.

Zweifach, W. B., Gordon, H. A., Wagner, M., and Reyniers, J. A.: Irreversible Shock in Germ-free Rats, *J Exp Med,* **107:**437, 1958.

Renal Function

Barry, K. G., Mazze, R. I., and Schwartz, F. D.: Prevention of Surgical Oliguria and Renal-Hemodynamic Suppression by Sustained Hydration, *N Engl J Med,* **270:**1371, 1964.

Baxter, C., and Powers, S. R., Trauma Workshop Report: Kidney Response to Trauma, *J Trauma,* **10:**1072, 1970.

Blagg, C. R., and Parsons, F. M.: Earlier Dialysis and Anabolic Steroids in Acute Renal Failure, *Am Heart J,* **61:**287, 1961.

Boba, A., and Landmesser, C. M.: Renal Complications after Anesthesia and Operation, *Anesthesiology,* **22:**781, 1961.

Gorfinkel, H. J., Szidon, J. P., Hirsch, L. J., and Fishman, A. P.: Renal Performance in Experimental Cardiogenic Shock, *Am J Physiol,* **222:**1260, 1972.

Habif, D. V., Paper, E. M., Fitzpatrick, H. F., Lowrance, P., Smythe, C. McC., and Bradley, S. E.: Renal and Hepatic

Blood Flow, Glomerular Filtration Rate, and Urinary Output of Electrolytes during Cyclopropane, Ether, and Thiopental Anesthesia, Operation, and Immediate Postoperative Period, *Surgery,* **30:**241, 1951.

Hatcher, C. R., Jr., Gagnon, J. A., and Clark, R. W.: Effects of Hydration on Epinephrine-induced Renal Shut Down in Dogs, *Surg Forum,* **9:**106, 1958.

Jones, L. W., and Weil, M. H.: Water, Creatinine and Sodium Excretion following Circulatory Shock with Renal Failure, *Am J Med,* **51:**314, 1971.

Knuth, O. E., Wagenknecht, L. V., and Madsen, P. O.: The Effect of Various Treatments on Renal Function during Endotoxin Shock, *Invest Urol,* **9:**304, 1972.

Logan, A., Jose, P., Eisner, G., Lilienfield, L., and Slotkoff, L.: Intracortical Distribution of Renal Blood Flow in Hemorrhagic Shock in Dogs, *Circ Res,* **29:**257, 1971.

Mazze, R. I., Schwartz, F. D., Slocum, H. C., and Barry, K. G.: Renal Function during Anesthesia and Surgery. I. Effects of Halothane Anesthesia, *Anesthesiology,* **24:**279, 1963.

Merrill, J. P.: "The Treatment of Renal Failure," Grune & Stratton, Inc., New York, 1965.

Moyer, C. A.: Acute Temporary Changes in Renal Function Associated with Major Surgical Procedures, *Surgery,* **27:**198, 1950.

Mueller, C. G.: Mechanism and Use of Mannitol Diuresis in Major Surgery and in Trauma, *South Med J,* **59:**408, 1966.

Nagy, Z., Bencsath, P., Tornyai, K., and Vaslaki, L.: Arterio-venous Anastomoses in the Kidney: IX. Intrarenal Circulation During Tourniquet Shock, *Acta Physiol Acad Sci Hung,* **40:**121, 1971.

———, Meszaros, A., and Vaslaki, L.: Arterio-venous Anastomoses in the Kidney: X. Effect of Phenoxybenzamine on Intrarenal Circulation of Dogs in Tourniquet Shock, *Acta Physiol Acad Sci Hung,* **40:**129, 1971.

Parry, W. L., Schaefer, J. A., and Mueller, C. B.: Experimental Studies of Acute Renal Failure. I. Protective Effect of Mannitol, *J Urol,* **89:**1, 1963.

Selkurt, E. E.: Atropine Influence on Altered Hemodynamics of the Primate Kidney in Hemorrhagic Shock, *Proc Soc Exp Biol Med,* **138:**497, 1971.

———: Influence of Aortic Constriction on the Positive Free-Water Clearance of Primate Hemorrhagic Shock, *Proc Soc Exp Biol Med,* **140:**221, 1972.

Skinner, D. G., and Hayes, M. A.: Effect of Staphylococcic Toxin on Renal Function: Irreversible Shock, *Ann Surg,* **162:**161, 1965.

Strauch, M., McLaughlin, J. S., Mansberger, A., Young, J., Mendonca, P., Gray, K., and Cowley, R. A.: Effects of Septic Shock on Renal Function in Humans, *Ann Surg,* **165:**536, 1967.

Stremple, J. F., Ellison, E. H., and Carey, L. C.: Osmolar Diuresis: Success and/or Failure: A Collective Review, *Surgery,* **60:**924, 1966.

Tobian, L.: Renin-Angiotensin Mechanisms in Shock, in L. C. Mills and J. H. Moyer (eds.), "Shock and Hypotension: Pathogenesis and Treatment, The 12th Hahnemann Symposium," Grune & Stratton, Inc., New York, 1965.

Uldall, P. R., and Kerr, D. N. S., Post-traumatic Acute Renal Failure, *Br J Anaesth,* **44:**283, 1972.

Chapter 2

Fluid, Electrolyte, and Nutritional Management of the Surgical Patient

by G. Tom Shires and Peter C. Canizaro

Anatomy of Body Fluids

Total Body Water
Intracellular Fluid
Extracellular Fluid
Osmotic Pressure

Classification of Body Fluid Changes

Volume Changes
Concentration Changes
Mixed Volume and Concentration Abnormalities
Composition Changes
    Acid-Base Balance
    Potassium Abnormalities
    Calcium Abnormalities
    Magnesium Abnormalities

Normal Exchange of Fluid and Electrolytes

Water Exchange
Salt Gain and Losses

Fluid and Electrolyte Therapy

Parenteral Solutions
Preoperative Fluid Therapy
    Correction of Volume Changes
    Correction of Concentration Changes
    Composition and Miscellaneous Considerations
Intraoperative Management of Fluids
Postoperative Management of Fluids
    Immediate Postoperative Period
    Later Postoperative Period
    Special Considerations in the Postoperative Patient

Nutrition in the Surgical Patient

Body Fuel Reserves
Starvation
Surgery, Trauma, Sepsis
Base-Line Requirements
Indications and Methods for Nutritional Support

One of the most critical aspects of patient care is management of the body composition of fluid and electrolytes. Most diseases, many injuries, and even operative trauma impose a great impact on the physiology of fluid and electrolytes within the body. These changes often exceed those brought about by acute lack of alimentation. There-fore, a thorough understanding of the metabolism of salt, water, and electrolytes and of certain metabolic responses is essential to the care of surgical patients.

An attempt will be made here to define the anatomy of body fluids and the physiologic principles governing function of fluids and electrolytes. In addition to these normal functions, a classification of derangements will be developed so that rational therapy may be described.

ANATOMY OF BODY FLUIDS

A prerequisite to the understanding of fluid and elec-trolyte management is knowledge of the extent and com-position of the various body fluid compartments. Early attempts to define these compartments were relatively accurate, but a more precise definition has been obtained recently by many investigators through the use of isotope tracer techniques. The wide range of normal values is a function of body size, weight, and sex, but these com-partments are relatively constant in size in the individual patient in the normal steady state. The figures used in this section, therefore, are approximate and presented as a percentage of body weight.

Total Body Water

Water constitutes between 50 and 70 percent of total body weight. Using deuterium oxide or tritiated water for measurement of total body water (TBW), the average normal value for young adult males is 60 percent of body weight and 50 percent for young adult females. A normal variation of ± 15 percent applies to both groups. The actual figure for each healthy individual is remarkably constant and is a function of several variables, including lean body mass and age. Since fat contains little water, the lean individual has a greater proportion of water to total body weight than the obese person. Thus, an ex-tremely obese individual may have 25 to 30 percent less body water than a lean individual of the same weight. The lower percentage of total body water in females correlates well with a relatively large amount of subcutaneous adi-pose tissue and small muscle mass. Moore et al. have shown that total body water, as a percentage of total body weight, decreases steadily and significantly with age to a low of 52 and 47 percent in males and females respectively. Conversely, the highest proportion of total body water to

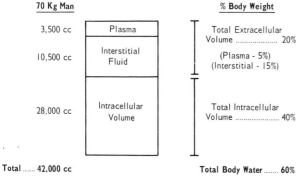

70 Kg Man .... **% Body Weight**

3,500 cc — Plasma — Total Extracellular Volume 20%

10,500 cc — Interstitial Fluid — (Plasma - 5%) (Interstitial - 15%)

28,000 cc — Intracellular Volume — Total Intracellular Volume 40%

Total ...... 42,000 cc .... Total Body Water 60%

Fig. 2-1. Functional compartments of body fluids.

body weight is found in newborn infants, with a maximum of 75 to 80 percent. During the first several months following birth there is a gradual "physiologic" loss of body water as the infant adjusts to his environment. At one year of age, the total body water averages approximately 65 percent of the body weight and remains relatively constant throughout the remainder of infancy and childhood.

The water of the body is divided into three functional compartments (Fig. 2-1). The fluid within the body's diverse cell population, intracellular water, represents between 30 and 40 percent of the body weight. The ex-

tracellular water represents 20 percent of the body weight and is divided between the intravascular fluid, or plasma (5 percent of body weight), and the interstitial, or extra-vascular, extracellular fluid (15 percent of body weight).

Intracellular Fluid

Measurement of intracellular fluid is determined indirectly by subtraction of the measured extracellular fluid from the measured total body water. The intracellular water is between 30 and 40 percent of the body weight, with the largest proportion in the skeletal muscle mass. Because of the smaller muscle mass in the female, the percentage of intracellular water is lower than in the male.

The chemical composition of the intracellular fluid is shown in Fig. 2-2, with potassium and magnesium the principal cations, and phosphates and proteins the principal anions. This is an approximation, since so few data concerning the intracellular fluid are available.

Extracellular Fluid

The total extracellular fluid volume represents approximately 20 percent of the body weight. The extracellular fluid compartment has two major subdivisions. The plasma volume comprises approximately 5 percent of the body weight in the normal adult. The interstitial, or extravas-

Fig. 2-2. Chemical composition of body fluid compartments.

PLASMA — 154 mEq/l / 154 mEq/l

CATIONS		ANIONS	
Na⁺	142	Cl⁻	103
		HCO₃⁻	27
		SO₄⁻⁻	3
		PO₄⁻⁻⁻	
K⁺	4		
Ca⁺⁺	5	Organic Acids	5
Mg⁺⁺	3	Protein	16

INTERSTITIAL FLUID — 153 mEq/l / 153 mEq/l

CATIONS		ANIONS	
Na⁺	144	Cl⁻	114
		HCO₃⁻	30
K⁺	4	SO₄⁻⁻	3
		PO₄⁻⁻⁻	
Ca⁺⁺	3	Organic Acids	5
Mg⁺⁺	2	Proteins	1

INTRACELLULAR FLUID — 200 mEq/l / 200 mEq/l

CATIONS		ANIONS	
K⁺	150	HPO₄⁼ / SO₄⁻⁻	150
		HCO₃⁻	10
Mg⁺⁺	40	Protein	40
Na⁺	10		

cular, extracellular fluid volume, obtained by subtracting the plasma volume from the measured total extracellular fluid volume, comprises approximately 15 percent of the body weight.

The interstitial fluid is further complicated by having, normally, a rapidly equilibrating, or functional, component, as well as several slower-equilibrating, or relatively nonfunctioning, components. The nonfunctioning components include connective tissue water as well as water that has been termed *transcellular,* which includes cerebrospinal and joint fluids. This nonfunctional component normally represents only 10 percent of the interstitial fluid volume (1 to 2 percent of body weight) and is not to be confused with the *relatively* nonfunctional extracellular fluid, often called a "third space," found in burns and soft tissue injuries.

The normal constituents of the extracellular fluid are shown in Fig. 2-2, with sodium the principal cation, and chloride and bicarbonate the principal anions. There are minor differences in ionic composition between the plasma and interstitial fluid occasioned by the difference in protein concentration. Because of the higher protein content (organic anions) of the plasma, the total concentration of cations is higher and the concentration of inorganic anions somewhat lower than in the interstitial fluid, as explained by the Gibbs-Donnan equilibrium equation.* For practical consideration, however, they may be considered equal. The total concentration of intracellular ions exceeds that of the extracellular compartment and would seem to violate the concept of osmolar equilibrium between the two compartments. This apparent discrepancy is due to the fact that the concentration of ions is expressed in milliequivalents (mEq) without regard to osmotic activity. In addition, some of the intracellular cations probably exist in undissociated form.

Osmotic Pressure

Relevant to a discussion of the complicated interactions between the various body fluid compartments is the definition of commonly used terms: The physiologic and chemical activity of electrolytes depend on (1) the *number of particles* present per unit volume [moles or millimoles (mM) per liter], (2) the *number of electric charges* per unit volume (equivalents or milliequivalents per liter), and (3) the *number of osmotically active particles,* or ions per unit volume [osmoles or milliosmoles (mO) per liter]. The use of the terms *grams* or *milligrams per 100 milliliters* expresses the weight of the electrolytes per unit volume but does not allow a physiologic comparison of the solutes in a solution.

A mole of a substance is the molecular weight of that substance in grams, and a millimole is that figure expressed in milligrams. For example, a mole of sodium chloride is 58 grams (Na—23, Cl—35), and a millimole is 58 milligrams. This expression, however, gives no direct informa-

---

*The product of the concentrations of any pair of diffusible cations and anions on one side of a semipermeable membrane will equal the product of the same pair of ions on the other side.

tion as to the number of osmotically active ions in solution or the electric charges that they carry.

The electrolytes of the body fluids then may be expressed in terms of chemical combining activity, or "equivalents." An equivalent of an ion is its atomic weight expressed in grams divided by the valence, whereas a milliequivalent of an ion is that figure expressed in milligrams. In the case of univalent ions, a milliequivalent is the same as a millimole. However, in the case of divalent ions, such as calcium or magnesium, one millimole equals two milliequivalents. The importance of this expression is that a milliequivalent of any substance will combine chemically with a milliequivalent of any other substance; in any given solution, the number of milliequivalents of cations present is balanced by precisely the same number of milliequivalents of anions.

When the osmotic pressure of a solution is considered, it is more descriptive to employ the terms osmole and milliosmole. These terms refer to the actual number of osmotically active particles present in solution, but are not dependent on the chemical combining capacities of the substances. Thus, a millimole of sodium chloride, which dissociates nearly completely into sodium and chloride, contributes two milliosmoles, and one millimole of sodium sulfate (Na_2SO_4), which dissociates into three particles, contributes three milliosmoles. One millimole of an un-ionized substance such as glucose is equal to one milliosmole of the substance.

The differences in ionic composition between intracellular and extracellular fluid are maintained by the cell wall, which functions as a semipermeable membrane. The total number of osmotically active particles is 290 to 310 mO in each compartment. Although the total osmotic pressure of a fluid is the sum of the partial pressures contributed by each of the solutes in that fluid, the *effective* osmotic pressure is dependent on those substances which fail to pass through the pores of the semipermeable membrane. The dissolved proteins in the plasma, therefore, are primarily responsible for effective osmotic pressure between the plasma and the interstitial fluid compartments. This is frequently referred to as the *colloid osmotic pressure.* The effective osmotic pressure between the extracellular and intracellular fluid compartments would be contributed to by any substance that does not traverse the cell membranes freely. Thus sodium, which is the principal cation of the extracellular fluid, contributes a major portion of the osmotic pressure, but substances that fail to penetrate the cell membrane freely, such as glucose, also increase the effective osmotic pressure.

Since the cell membranes are completely permeable to water, the effective osmotic pressures in the two compartments are considered to be equal. Any condition that alters the effective osmotic pressure in either compartment will result in redistribution of water between the compartments. Thus, an increase in effective osmotic pressure in the extracellular fluid, which would occur most frequently as a result of increased sodium concentration, would cause a net transfer of water from the intracellular to the extracellular fluid compartment. This transfer of water would continue until the effective osmotic pressures in the two compartments were equal. Conversely, a decrease in the sodium concentration in the extracellular fluid will cause a transfer of water from the extracellular to the intracellular fluid compartment. However, depletion of the extracellular fluid volume without a change in the concentration of ions will not result in transfer of free water from the intracellular space.

Thus, the intracellular fluid shares in losses that involve a change in concentration or composition of the extracellular fluid but shares slowly in changes involving loss of isotonic volume alone. For practical consideration, most losses and gains of body fluid are directly from the extracellular compartment.

CLASSIFICATION OF BODY FLUID CHANGES

The disorders in fluid balance may be classified in three general categories: disturbances of (1) volume, (2) concentration, and (3) composition. Of primary importance is the concept that although these disturbances are interrelated, each is a separate entity.

If an isotonic salt solution is added to or lost from the body fluids, only the *volume* of the extracellular fluid is changed. The acute loss of an isotonic extracellular solution, such as intestinal juice, is followed by a significant decrease in the extracellular fluid volume and little, if any, change in the intracellular fluid volume. Fluid will not be transferred from the intracellular space to refill the depleted extracellular space as long as the osmolarity remains the same in the two compartments.

If water alone is added to or lost from the extracellular fluid, the *concentration* of osmotically active particles will change. Sodium ions account for 90 percent of the osmotically active particles in the extracellular fluid and generally reflect the tonicity of body fluid compartments. If the extracellular fluid is depleted of sodium, water will pass into the intracellular space until osmolarity is again equal in the two compartments.

The concentration of most other ions within the extracellular fluid compartment can be altered without significant change in the total number of osmotically active particles, thus producing only a *compositional* change. For instance, a rise of the serum potassium concentration from 4 to 8 mEq/L would have a significant effect on the myocardium, but it would not significantly change the effective osmotic pressure of the extracellular fluid compartment. Normally functioning kidneys minimize these changes considerably, particularly if the addition or loss of solute or water is gradual.

An internal loss of extracellular fluid into a nonfunctional space, such as the sequestration of isotonic fluid in a burn, peritonitis, ascites, or muscle trauma, is termed a *distributional* change. This transfer or functional loss of extracellular fluid internally may be extracellular (e.g., as in peritonitis) or intracellular (e.g., as probably occurs in hemorrhagic shock). In any event, all distributional shifts or losses result in a contraction of the *functional* extracellular fluid space.

Volume Changes

Volume deficit or excess generally must be diagnosed by clinical examination of the patient. There are no readily available laboratory tests of benefit in the acute phase except measurement of the plasma volume. Changes secondary to long-standing derangements in volume, however, may be discernible by laboratory tests. For example, the blood urea nitrogen (BUN) level slowly rises with a long-standing extracellular fluid deficit of sufficient magnitude to reduce glomerular filtation. The concentration of serum sodium is *not* related to the volume status of extracellular fluid; a severe volume deficit may exist with a normal, low, or high serum sodium level.

VOLUME DEFICIT. Extracellular fluid volume deficit is by far the most common fluid disorder in the surgical patient. The loss of fluid is not water alone, but water and electrolytes in approximately the same proportion as that in which they exist in normal extracellular fluid. The most common disorders leading to an extracellular fluid volume deficit include losses of gastrointestinal fluids due to vomiting, nasogastric suction, diarrhea, and fistular drainage. Other common causes include sequestration of fluid in soft tissue injuries and infections, intraabdominal and retroperitoneal inflammatory processes, peritonitis, intestinal obstruction, and burns. The signs and symptoms of this state are easily recognized and are listed in Table 2-1. The central nervous system and cardiovascular signs occur early with acute rapid losses, whereas tissue signs may be absent until the deficit has existed for at least 24 hours. The central nervous system signs are similar to barbiturate intoxication and may be missed by the casual observer if the volume deficit is mild. The cardiovascular signs are secondary to a decrease in plasma volume and may be associated with varying degrees of hypotension in the patient with a severe extracellular fluid volume deficit. Skin turgor may be difficult to assess in the elderly patient or in the patient with recent weight loss and is not diagnostic in the absence of other confirmatory signs. The body temperature tends to vary with the environmental temperature. In a cool room, the patient may be slightly hypothermic, and the febrile response to injury may be suppressed.

VOLUME EXCESS. Extracellular fluid volume excess is generally iatrogenic or secondary to renal insufficiency. Both the plasma and interstitial fluid volumes are increased. In the healthy young adult, the signs are generally those of circulatory overload, manifested primarily in the pulmonary circulation, and of excessive fluid in other tissue (Table 2-1). In the elderly patient, congestive heart failure with pulmonary edema may develop rather quickly with a moderate volume excess.

Concentration Changes

Since the sodium ion is primarily responsible for the osmolarity of the extracellular fluid space, determination of the serum concentration of sodium generally indicates the tonicity of body fluids. Hyponatremia and hypernatremia may be diagnosed on clinical examination (Table

Table 2-1. EXTRACELLULAR FLUID VOLUME

Type of sign	Deficit		Excess	
	Moderate	*Severe*	*Moderate*	*Severe*
Central nervous system	Sleepiness Apathy Slow responses Anorexia Cessation of usual activity	Decreased tendon reflexes. Anesthesia distal extremities Stupor Coma	None	None
Gastrointestinal	Progressive decrease in food consumption	Nausea, vomiting Refusal to eat Silent ileus and distension	At surgery: Edema of stomach, colon, lesser and greater omenta and small bowel mesentary	
Cardiovascular	Orthostatic hypotension Tachycardia Collapsed veins Collapsing pulse	Cutaneous lividity Hypotension Distant heart sounds Cold extremities Absent peripheral pulses	Elevated venous pressure Distension of peripheral veins Increased cardiac output Loud heart sounds Functional murmurs Bounding pulse High pulse pressure Increased pulmonary 2d sound Gallop	Pulmonary edema
Tissue	Soft, small tongue with longitudial wrinkling Decreased skin turgor	Atonic muscles Sunken eyes	Subcutaneous pitting edema Basilar râles	Anasarca Moist râles Vomiting Diarrhea
Metabolic	Mild decrease temperature, 97–99°R	Marked decrease temperature, 95–98°R	None	None

2-2), but, in contrast to volume changes, they can be confirmed by laboratory tests.

HYPONATREMIA. Acute hyponatremia (sodium less than 130 mEq/L) clinically is characterized by central nervous system signs of increased intracranial pressure and tissue signs of excessive intracellular water. There are no cardiovascular signs per se. The hypertension is probably induced by the rise in intracranial pressure, since the blood pressure generally returns to normal with the administration of hypertonic solutions of sodium salts. Of importance with severe hyponatremia is the relatively rapid development of oliguric renal failure, which may not be reversible if therapy is delayed.

HYPERNATREMIA. Central nervous system and tissue signs, listed in Table 2-2, characterize acute symptomatic hypernatremia. This is the only state in which dry, sticky mucous membranes are characteristic. This sign does not occur with pure extracellular fluid volume deficit alone, and may be misleading in the patient who breathes through his mouth. Body temperature is generally elevated and may approach a lethal level, as in the patient with heatstroke.

While volume changes occur frequently without a change in serum sodium, the reverse is not true. The disease states that cause a significant acute alteration in the serum sodium frequently produce a concomitant change in the extracellular fluid volume.

Mixed Volume and Concentration Abnormalities

Mixed volume and concentration abnormalities may develop as a consequence of the disease state or occasionally may result from inappropriate parenteral fluid therapy. Moyer noted that the clinical picture associated with a combination of fluid abnormalities will tend to be an algebraic composite of the signs and symptoms of each state. Like signs produced by both abnormalities will be additive, and opposing signs will tend to nullify one another. For example, the tendency for the body temperature to fall with an extracellular volume deficit may be counteracted by the tendency for it to rise with severe hypernatremia.

One of the more common mixed abnormalities is an extracellular fluid deficit and hyponatremia. This state is readily produced in the patient who continues to drink water while losing large volumes of gastrointestinal fluids. It may also occur in the postoperative period when gastrointestinal losses are replaced with only water or a hypo-

Table 2-2. ACUTE CHANGES IN OSMOLAR CONCENTRATION

Type of signs	Hyponatremia (water intoxication)		Hypernatremia (water deficit)	
Central nervous system	Moderate: Muscle twitching Hyperactive tendon reflexes Increased intra-cranial pressure (compensated phase)	Severe: Convulsions Loss of reflexes Increased intra-cranial pressure (decompensated phase)	Moderate: Restlessness Weakness	Severe: Delirium Maniacal be-havior
Cardiovascular	Changes in blood pressure and pulse secondary to increased intracranial pressure		Tachycardia Hypotension (if severe)	
Tissue	Salivation, lacrimation, watery diarrhea "Fingerprinting" of skin (sign of intracellular volume excess)		Decrease saliva and tears Dry and sticky mucous membranes Red, swollen tongue Skin flushed	
Renal	Oliguria progressing to anuria		Oliguria	
Metabolic	None		Fever	

tonic sodium solution. An extracellular volume deficit accompanied by hypernatremia may be produced by the loss of a large amount of hypotonic salt solution, such as sweat, in the absence of fluid intake.

The prolonged administration of excessive quantities of sodium salts with restricted water intake may result in an extracellular volume excess and hypernatremia. This may also occur when pure water losses (such as insensible loss of water from the skin and lungs) are replaced with sodium-containing solutions only. Similarly, the excessive administration of water or hypotonic salt solutions to the patient with oliguric renal failure may rapidly produce an extracellular volume excess and hyponatremia.

Normally functioning kidneys may minimize these changes to some extent and compensate for many of the errors associated with parenteral fluid administration. In contrast, the patient in anuric or oliguric renal failure is particularly prone to develop these mixed volume and osmolar concentration abnormalities. Fluid and electrolyte management in these patients, therefore, must be precise. Unfortunately, the fact that a patient with normal kidneys who develops a significant volume deficit may be in a state of "functional" renal failure is often not appreciated. As the volume deficit progresses, the glomerular filtration rate falls precipitously, and the kidneys' unique functions for maintaining fluid homeostasis are lost. These changes may occur with only a mild volume deficit in the elderly patient with borderline renal function. In these elderly patients, the blood urea nitrogen level may rise higher than 100 mg/100 ml in response to the fluid deficit with a concomitant rise in the serum creatinine level. Fortunately, these changes are usually reversible with early and adequate correction of the extracellular fluid volume deficit.

Composition Changes

Compositional abnormalities of importance include changes in acid-base balance and concentration changes of potassium, calcium, and magnesium.

ACID-BASE BALANCE

The pH (the negative logarithm of the hydrogen ion concentration) of the body fluids is normally maintained within narrow limits in spite of the rather large load of acid produced endogenously as a by-product of body metabolism. The acids are neutralized efficiently by several buffer systems and subsequently excreted by the lungs and kidneys.

The important buffers include proteins and phosphates, which play a primary role in maintaining intracellular pH, and the bicarbonate–carbonic acid system, which operates principally in the extracellular fluid space. The proteins and hemoglobin have only minor influence in the extracellular fluid space, but the latter is of prime significance as a buffer in the red cell.

A buffer system consists of a weak acid or base and the salt of that acid or base. The buffering effect is the result of the formation of an amount of weak acid or base equivalent to the amount of strong acid or base added to the system. The resultant change in pH is considerably less than if the substance were added to water alone. Thus, inorganic acids (e.g., hydrochloric, sulfuric, phosphoric) and organic acids (e.g., lactic, pyruvic, keto acids) combine with base bicarbonate producing the sodium salt of the acid and carbonic acid:

$$HCL + NaHCO_3 \longrightarrow NaCl + H_2CO_3$$

The carbonic acid formed is then excreted via the lungs

as CO_2. The inorganic acid anions are excreted by the kidneys with hydrogen or as ammonium salts. The organic acid anions generally are metabolized as the underlying disorder is corrected, although some renal excretion may occur with high levels.

The functions of the buffer systems are expressed in the Henderson-Hasselbalch equation, which defines the pH in terms of the ratio of the salt and acid. The pH of the extracellular fluid is defined primarily by the ratio of the amount of base bicarbonate (majority as sodium bicarbonate) to the amount of carbonic acid (related to the CO_2 content of alveolar air) present in the blood:

$$pH = pK + \log \frac{BHCO_3}{H_2CO_3} = \frac{27 \text{ mEq/L}}{1.33 \text{ mEq/L}} = \frac{20}{1} = 7.4$$

pK represents the dissociation constant of carbonic acid in the presence of base bicarbonate and by measurement is 6.1. At a body pH of 7.4, the ratio must be 20:1, as depicted. From a chemical standpoint, this is an inefficient buffer system, but the unusual property of CO_2 to behave as an acid or change to a neutral gas subsequently excreted by the lungs makes it quite efficient biologically.

As long as the 20:1 ratio is maintained, regardless of the absolute values, the pH will remain at 7.4. When an acid is added to the system, the concentration of bicarbonate (the numerator in the Henderson-Hasselbalch equation) will decrease. Ventilation will immediately increase to eliminate larger quantities of CO_2 with a subse-

quent decrease in the carbonic acid (the denominator in the Henderson-Hasselbalch equation) until the 20:1 ratio is reestablished. Slower, more complete compensation is effected by the kidneys with increased excretion of acid salts and retention of bicarbonate. The reverse will occur if an alkali is added to the system. Respiratory acidosis and alkalosis are produced by disturbances of ventilation, with an increase or decrease in the denominator and a resultant change of the 20:1 ratio. Compensation is primarily renal, with a retention of bicarbonate and increased excretion of acid salts in respiratory acidosis and the reverse process in respiratory alkalosis.

The four types of acid-base disturbances are listed in Table 2-3. Use of the CO_2 combining power (approximates the plasma bicarbonate) or CO_2 content (includes bicarbonate, carbonic acid, and dissolved CO_2) and knowledge of the patient's disease may allow an accurate diagnosis in the uncomplicated case. However, use of the CO_2 content or CO_2 combining power alone is generally inadequate as an index of acid-base balance. Both these tests principally reflect the level of plasma bicarbonate, since dissolved CO_2 and carbonic acid contribute no more than a few millimoles under most circumstances. In the acute phase, therefore, respiratory acidosis or alkalosis may exist without any change in the CO_2 content; determinations of the pH and P_{CO_2} from a freshly drawn arterial blood sample are necessary for diagnosis. Thus, measurements of pH, bicarbonate concentration, and P_{CO_2} are required

Table 2-3. ACIDOSIS-ALKALOSIS

Type of acid-base disorder	Defect	Common causes	$\frac{BHCO_3}{H_2CO_3} = \frac{20}{1}$	Compensation
Respiratory acidosis	Retention of CO_2 (Decreased alveolar ventilation)	Depression of respiratory center—morphine, CNS injury Pulmonary disease—emphysema, pneumonia	↑ Denominator Ratio less than 20:1	Renal Retention of bicarbonate, excretion of acid salts, increased ammonia formation Chloride shift into red cells
Respiratory alkalosis	Excessive loss of CO_2 (Increased alveolar ventilation)	Hyperventilation: Emotional, severe pain, assisted ventilation, encephalitis	↓ Denominator Ratio greater than 20:1	Renal Excretion of bicarbonate, retention of acid salts, decreased ammonia formation
Metabolic acidosis	Retention of fixed acids or Loss of base bicarbonate	Diabetes, azotemia, lactic acid accumulation, starvation Diarrhea, small bowel fistulae	↓ Numerator Ratio less than 20:1	Pulmonary (rapid) Increase rate and depth of breathing Renal (slow) As in respiratory acidosis
Metabolic alkalosis	Loss of fixed acids Gain of base bicarbonate Potassium depletion	Vomiting or gastric suction with pyloric obstruction Excessive intake of bicarbonate Diuretics	↑ Numerator Ratio greater than 20:1	Pulmonary (rapid) Decrease rate and depth of breathing Renal (slow) As in respiratory alkalosis

Table 2-4. RESPIRATORY AND METABOLIC COMPONENTS
OF ACID-BASE DISORDERS

Type of acid-base disorder	Acute (uncompensated)			Chronic (partially compensated)		
	pH	P_{CO_2} (respiratory component)	Plasma HCO_3^-* (metabolic component)	pH	P_{CO_2} (respiratory component)	Plasma HCO_3^-* (metabolic component)
Respiratory acidosis...	↓↓	↑↑	N	↓	↑↑	↑
Respiratory alkalosis..	↑↑	↓↓	N	↑	↓↓	↓
Metabolic acidosis...	↓↓	N	↓↓	↓	↓	↓
Metabolic alkalosis..	↑↑	N	↑↑	↑	↑?	↑

*Measured as standard bicarbonate, whole blood buffer base, CO_2 content or CO_2 combining power. The *base excess value* is positive when the standard bicarbonate is above normal and negative when the standard bicarbonate is below normal.

for a more complete understanding of the acid-base status in most patients (Table 2-4).

Unfortunately, more complex acid-base disturbances are frequently encountered. Combinations of respiratory and metabolic changes occur and may represent compensation for the initial acid-base disturbance or may indicate two or more coexisting primary disorders (e.g., a *primary* respiratory acidosis complicated by a *primary* metabolic acidosis or alkalosis).

Usually primary acid-base disturbances are compensated to some extent. A primary metabolic disturbance is initially compensated by changes in pulmonary ventilation, while respiratory disturbances are compensated by renal mechanisms. For example, the initial compensation for an acute metabolic acidosis is an increase in the rate and depth of breathing to lower the arterial P_{CO_2}. As pointed out by Astrup et al., the actual state of the acid-base disorder may be characterized by the degree of compensation—*not compensated* (early or compensatory mechanisms not functioning), *partially compensated* (pH has not returned to a normal value), *compensated,* or *overcompensated.*

As previously noted, a knowledge of the pH, bicarbonate concentration, and P_{CO_2} will allow an accurate diagnosis of most acid-base disturbances. However, the clinical interpretation of these measurements is associated with some inherent problems. Although the arterial P_{CO_2} is considered an accurate index of primary respiratory disturbances, changes in the level may represent compensation for a primary metabolic alteration. Thus, a depressed P_{CO_2} (below 40 mm Hg) is characteristic of respiratory alkalosis but also represents the normal compensatory response to a metabolic acidosis. Similarly, the level of plasma bicarbonate cannot be regarded exclusively as an index of metabolic disturbances. An elevated plasma bicarbonate level may indicate a primary metabolic alkalosis or a compensatory response to chronic respiratory acidosis.

In an effort to separate the respiratory and metabolic components of acid-base disorders, two other approaches have been introduced: In 1948 Singer and Hastings introduced the concept of *whole blood buffer base,* and more recently Astrup and his colleagues proposed the use of the *standard bicarbonate* and *base excess* values. The approach advocated by Astrup has been the more popular of the two, although both are attempts to quantify the metabolic, or nonrespiratory, component in an acid-base disturbance and separate it from the respiratory component.

The standard bicarbonate is defined as the concentration of bicarbonate in plasma, when whole blood with fully oxygenated hemoglobin has been equilibrated with CO_2 at a P_{CO_2} of 40 mm Hg at a temperature of 38°C. This value may be rapidly and accurately determined using the Astrup technique by measuring pH values at two known levels of P_{CO_2} and reading the standard bicarbonate directly from a nomogram. The normal mean value for standard bicarbonate is 24.5 mEq/L of plasma. As a measure of bicarbonate concentration in plasma, the standard bicarbonate is probably superior to both the CO_2 content and CO_2 combining power values, since the latter two determinations vary with the actual P_{CO_2} and oxygen saturation. Unfortunately, the standard bicarbonate, unlike the whole blood buffer base, does not indicate the total amount of surplus acid or base present, since the bicarbonate–carbonic acid system does not account for the entire buffering capacity of the blood. This information can be obtained by expressing the base content of the blood as *base excess* or *base deficit.* Base excess (or deficit) directly expresses the amount, in milliequivalents, of fixed base (or fixed acid) added to each liter of blood. This value is obtained by multiplying the deviation of standard bicarbonate from the normal mean by a factor of 1.2. This factor corrects for the buffering capacity of the red cells and will vary slightly with changes in hemoglobin concentration. To avoid calculations, the base excess may be read directly from a nomogram. When the term *base excess* is used exclusively, the *positive* values represent the excess of base, and the *negative* values reflect the deficit of base (or excess of acid).*

In an excellent review of the Singer-Hastings and the Astrup systems, Schwartz and Relman state that neither system offers any advantage over the classic approach for the diagnosis of acid-base disorders. They question the validity of using an in vitro CO_2 titration curve as a measure of in vivo acid-base changes. Additionally, they note that the use of either of the two systems may be misleading in the analysis of chronic disorders. For example, a low pH with an elevated P_{CO_2}, a normal standard bicarbonate value, and a base excess value of zero are compatible with a diagnosis of primary uncompensated respiratory acidosis. After several hours or days, compensatory renal mechanisms would cause elevation of standard bicarbonate level above normal, resulting in a positive base excess value. This partially compensated respiratory acidosis, then, may be erroneously interpreted as a respiratory acidosis *plus* a metabolic alkalosis as indicated by a significant base excess.

Despite these shortcomings, either approach may be useful when properly interpreted as a single laboratory test. Other systems have been recommended, some with ingeniously devised nomograms, but all are subject to misinterpretation. Unfortunately, there are no shortcuts. Regardless of the methods used, the proper analysis of complex acid-base disorders requires a thorough knowledge of the clinical situation, good judgment, and a sound understanding of acid-base physiology.

RESPIRATORY ACIDOSIS. This condition is associated with retention of CO_2 secondary to decreased alveolar ventilation. The more common causes are listed in Table 2-3. Initially, the arterial P_{CO_2} is elevated (usually above 50 mm Hg), and the plasma bicarbonate concentration (measured as CO_2 combining power, CO_2 content, or standard bicarbonate) is normal. In the chronic form, the P_{CO_2} remains elevated, and the bicarbonate concentration rises as compensation occurs.

This problem may be particularly serious in the patient with chronic pulmonary disease in whom preexisting respiratory acidosis may be accentuated in the postoperative period. A number of conditions resulting in inadequate ventilation—airway obstruction, atelectasis, pneumonia, pleural effusion, hypoventilation due to the pain of upper abdominal incisions, or abdominal distension limiting diaphragmatic excursion—may exist singly or in combination to produce respiratory acidosis. Although restlessness, hypertension, and tachycardia in the immediate postoperative period may be due to pain, similar signs indicate inadequate ventilation with hypercapnia. The use of narcotics in this situation will compound the problem by further depressing respiration.

*The deficit or excess of base in the extracellular compartment can be estimated in milliequivalents by multiplying the negative or positive value for base excess, in milliequivalents per liter of blood, by 0.3 times the body weight in kilograms [Mellemgaard and Astrup].

Management involves prompt correction of the pulmonary defect, when feasible, and measures to ensure adequate ventilation. Endotracheal intubation and mechanical ventilation are occasionally necessary to achieve this objective. Strict attention to tracheobronchial hygiene during the postoperative period is an important preventive measure in all patients, particularly those with chronic pulmonary disease. Encouraging deep breathing and coughing, using humidified air to prevent inspissation of secretions, and avoiding oversedation are all indicated.

RESPIRATORY ALKALOSIS. Respiratory alkalosis is a more common problem in the surgical patient than previously recognized. Hyperventilation due to apprehension, pain, hypoxia, central nervous system injury, and assisted ventilation are all common causes. Any of these conditions may cause a rapid depression of the arterial P_{CO_2} and elevation of the pH. The plasma bicarbonate concentration is normal in the acute phase, but falls with compensation if the condition persists.

Mild respiratory alkalosis secondary to hyperventilation during the operative procedure frequently occurs. This is of little consequence in the majority of patients and generally requires no therapy. One important exception is the patient with impaired cerebral blood flow from obstructive arterial disease (or during performance of carotid endarterectomy), in whom modest hypocapnia with cerebral vasoconstriction may cause irreparable damage.

The majority of patients who require ventilatory support in the postoperative period will develop varying degrees of respiratory alkalosis. This may be inadvertent, due to improper use of the mechanical respirator, or it may occur during attempts to raise the P_{O_2} in an hypoxic patient. Proper management of the patient on a mechanical ventilator requires frequent measurements of blood gases and appropriate corrections of the ventilatory pattern when indicated. The arterial P_{CO_2} should not be allowed to fall below 30 mm Hg, as serious complications may occur, particularly in the presence of a complicating hypokalemia or metabolic alkalosis. Generally, the P_{CO_2} can be maintained at an acceptable level by proper adjustments of the ventilatory rate and volume. Increasing the pulmonary dead space is of doubtful benefit, while adding 5 percent CO_2 to the inspired air is potentially dangerous and poorly tolerated by most patients.

The dangers of a severe respiratory alkalosis are those related to potassium depletion and include the development of ventricular arrhythmias and fibrillation, particularly in patients who are digitalized or have preexisting hypokalemia. Other complications include a shift of the oxygen dissociation curve to the left, which limits the ability of hemoglobin to unload oxygen at the tissue level except at low intracellular P_{O_2}, and the development of tetany and convulsions if the level of ionized calcium is significantly depressed. The development of hypokalemia may be quite sudden and is related to entry of potassium ions into the cells in exchange for hydrogen and an excessive urinary potassium loss in exchange for sodium. Severe and persistent respiratory alkalosis is often difficult to correct and may be associated with a poor prognosis because of the underlying cause of hyperventilation. Treatment is primarily directed toward preventing the condition by the proper use of mechanical respirators and correcting any preexisting potassium deficits.

METABOLIC ACIDOSIS. Metabolic acidosis results from the retention or gain of fixed acids (diabetic acidosis, lactic acidosis, azotemia) or the loss of base bicarbonate (diarrhea, small bowel fistula, renal insufficiency with inability to resorb bicarbonate). The excess of hydrogen ion results in lower pH and plasma bicarbonate concentration. The initial compensation is pulmonary, with an increase of the rate and depth of breathing and depression of the arterial P_{CO_2}.

Renal damage may interfere with the important role of the kidneys in the regulation of acid-base balance. The kidneys serve a vital function in this regard through the excretion of nitrogenous waste products and acid metabolites and the resorption of bicarbonates. If renal damage occurs and these functions are lost, metabolic acidosis develops rapidly and may be difficult to control.

With normal kidneys, metabolic acidosis may develop when the capacity of the kidneys for handling chlorides is exceeded. This is particularly common in patients who have excessive losses of alkaline gastrointestinal fluids (biliary, pancreatic, small bowel secretions) and are maintained on parenteral fluids for an extended period of time. Continued replacement of these losses with fluids having an inappropriate chloride/bicarbonate ratio, such as isotonic sodium chloride solution, will not correct the pH change; the use of a balanced salt solution, such as lactated Ringer's, is indicated.

One of the most common causes of severe metabolic acidosis in surgical patients is acute circulatory failure with accumulation of lactic acid. This is a reflection of tissue hypoxia due to inadequate perfusion, although it is only one of the manifestations of cellular dysfunction. Acute hemorrhagic shock may result in a rapid and profound drop in the pH, and attempts to raise the blood pressure with vasopressors will simply compound the problem. Similarly, attempts to correct the acidosis by the infusion of large quantities of sodium bicarbonate without restoration of flow are futile. Following restoration of adequate tissue perfusion by proper volume replacement, the lactic acid is quickly metabolized and the pH returned to normal. The use of lactated Ringer's solution to replace the extracellular fluid deficit incurred with hemorrhagic shock concomitant with administration of whole blood does not accentuate the lactic acidosis. Instead, there is a rapid decrease in the lactate level and return of pH toward normal, as opposed to the results when whole blood alone is used.

The indiscriminate use of sodium bicarbonate during the resuscitation of patients in hypovolemic shock is discouraged for several reasons. A mild metabolic alkalosis is a common finding following resuscitation, in part due to the alkalinizing effects of blood transfusions and the administration of lactated Ringer's solution. After infusion (and partial restoration of hepatic blood flow), the citrate and lactate contained in the blood and the lactate in lactated Ringer's solution are metabolized, and bicarbonate is formed. If excessive quantities of sodium bicarbonate were administered simultaneously, severe metabolic alkalosis could result. An alkaline pH may be highly undesirable in this situation, particularly in patients with hypoxia or low fixed cardiac outputs, because it shifts the oxygen dissociation curve to the left. Other factors that tend to shift the oxygen dissociation curve to the left in this situation include the depressed level of erythrocyte 2,3-diphosphoglycerate in ACD-stored blood, and the development of hypothermia. If the curve shifts far enough to the left, significant interference with oxygen unloading at the cellular level may occur.

The treatment of metabolic acidosis, therefore, should be directed toward correction of the underlying disorder when possible. Bicarbonate therapy properly may be reserved for the treatment of severe metabolic acidosis, particularly following cardiac arrest, when *partial* correction of the pH is essential to restore myocardial function. Similarly, pH correction of more protracted states of metabolic acidosis may be indicated but should be accomplished slowly. Frequent measurements of serum electrolytes and blood pH are the best guides to therapy, since a satisfactory formula to estimate the amount of alkali needed has not been devised.

METABOLIC ALKALOSIS. Metabolic alkalosis results from the loss of fixed acids or the gain of base bicarbonate and is aggravated by any preexisting potassium depletion. Both the pH and plasma bicarbonate concentration are elevated. Compensation for metabolic alkalosis is primarily by renal mechanisms, since respiratory compensation is generally small and cannot be detected in most patients.

The majority of patients with metabolic alkalosis have some degree of hypokalemia. Depletion of cellular potassium results in entry of hydrogen and sodium ions into the cells with resultant lowering of intracellular pH and an extracellular alkalosis. Metabolic alkalosis, in turn, results in excessive urinary potassium loss in exchange for sodium, which further accentuates the alkalosis. The dangers of metabolic alkalosis are the same as discussed with respiratory alkalosis.

An interesting and not infrequent problem in the surgical patient is hypochloremic, hypokalemic metabolic alkalosis resulting from persistent vomiting or gastric suction in the patient with pyloric obstruction. Unlike vomiting with an open pylorus (involving a loss of gastric, pancreatic, biliary, and intestinal secretions), this entity results in loss of fluid with high chloride and hydrogen ion concentration in relation to sodium. The loss of chloride causes accelerated loss of sodium and bicarbonate in the urine and partial compensation of the alkalosis. In addition, the alkalosis itself causes increased renal excretion of potassium. As the volume deficit progresses, potassium and hydrogen ions are excreted into the urine in increasing quantities in an attempt to conserve sodium, resulting in an uncompensated alkalosis and hypokalemia. The initially alkaline urine becomes acid after a period of time due to the hydrogen ion excretion ("paradoxic aciduria"). Proper management includes replacement of the extracellular fluid volume deficit with isotonic sodium chloride solution in addition to replacement of potassium. A severe potassium depletion is invariably present but may be overlooked due to concentration of the serum potassium by a severe volume deficit. However, volume repletion should be started and a good urine output obtained before potassium is administered.

POTASSIUM ABNORMALITIES

The normal dietary intake of potassium is approximately 50 to 100 mEq daily, and in the absence of hypokalemia, the majority of this is excreted in the urine. Ninety-eight percent of the potassium in the body is located within the intracellular compartment at a concentration of approximately 150 mEq/L, and it is the major cation of intracellular water. Although the total extracellular potassium in a 70-kg male would approximate only 63 mEq (4.5 mEq/L × 14L), this small amount is critical to cardiac and neuromuscular function. In addition, the turnover rate in the extracellular fluid compartment may be extremely rapid.

The intracellular and extracellular distribution of potassium is influenced by many factors. Significant quantities of intracellular potassium are released into the extracellular space in response to severe injury or surgical stress, acidosis, and the catabolic state. A significant rise in serum potassium may occur in these states in the presence of oliguric or anuric renal failure, but dangerous hyperkalemia (greater than 6 mEq/L) is rarely encountered if renal function is normal. After severe trauma, however, normal or excessive urinary volumes may not reflect the ability of the kidney to clear solutes or to excrete potassium. (See the section High-Output Renal Failure.)

HYPERKALEMIA. The signs of a significant hyperkalemia are limited to the cardiovascular and gastrointestinal systems. The gastrointestinal symptoms include nausea, vomiting, intermittent intestinal colic, and diarrhea. The cardiovascular signs are apparent on the electrocardiogram initially, with high peaked T waves, widened QRS complex, and depressed ST segments. Disappearance of T waves, heart block, and diastolic cardiac arrest may develop with increasing levels of potassium.

Treatment of hyperkalemia consists of immediate measures to reduce the serum potassium level, withholding of exogenously administered potassium, and correction of the underlying cause if possible. Temporary suppression of the myocardial effects of a sudden rapid rise of potassium level can be accomplished by the intravenous administration of a solution containing 80 mEq of sodium lactate, 100 ml of calcium gluconate, and 100 ml of 50% dextrose in water. The administration of dextrose stimulates the synthesis of glycogen, resulting in an uptake of potassium. Insulin may also be given, but it should be limited to 1 unit per 5 Gm or more of glucose, since rebound hypoglycemia may be fatal. The sodium lactate raises the pH and shifts potassium intracellularly, and the calcium gluconate tends to counteract the myocardial effects of hyperkalemia. Administration of this solution over a 2-hour period allows time to prepare for definitive removal of the excess potassium by hemodialysis or peritoneal dialysis. A slow rise

of potassium level (less than 1 mEq/L/day) can be controlled by the use of cation-exchange resins, preferably in the sodium cycle,* administered by rectum in doses of 24 Gm every 12 hours. To prevent rapid absorption of water from the colon, 200 ml of 10% dextrose in water is used as the vehicle.

HYPOKALEMIA. The more common problem in the surgical patient is hypokalemia, which may occur as a result of (1) excessive renal excretion, (2) movement of potassium into cells, (3) prolonged administration of potassium-free parenteral fluids with continued obligatory renal loss of potassium (20 mEq/day or more), and (4) loss in gastrointestinal secretions.

Potassium plays an important role in the regulation of acid-base balance. Increased renal excretion occurs with both respiratory and metabolic alkalosis. Potassium is in competition with hydrogen ion for renal tubular excretion in exchange for sodium ion. Thus, in alkalosis, the increased potassium ion excretion in exchange for sodium ion permits hydrogen ion conservation. Hypokalemia itself may produce a metabolic alkalosis, since an increase in excretion of hydrogen ions occurs when the concentration of potassium in the tubular cell is low. In addition, movement of hydrogen ions into the cells as a consequence of potassium loss is partly responsible for the alkalosis. In metabolic acidosis the reverse process occurs, and the excess hydrogen ion exchanges for sodium with retention of greater amounts of potassium.

Renal tubular excretion of potassium ion is increased when large quantities of sodium are available for excretion. The more sodium ion available for resorption, the more potassium is exchanged for it in the lumen. Potassium requirements for prolonged or massive isotonic fluid volume replacement are increased, probably on this basis. The same mechanism may also explain the increased potassium ion excretion with steroid administration.

The renal excretion of potassium may be small when compared to the amount of potassium that may be lost in gastrointestinal secretions. The amount per liter in various types of gastrointestinal fluids is shown in Table 2-5. Although the average potassium concentration of some of these fluids is relatively low, significant hypokalemia will result if potassium-free fluids are used for replacement.

Hypokalemia also may be a serious problem in the patient maintained on intravenous hyperalimentation. Large quantities of supplemental potassium generally are necessary to restore depleted intracellular stores and to meet the requirements for tissue synthesis during the anabolic phase. (See the section Nutrition.)

In summary, most of the factors that tend to influence potassium metabolism result in excess excretion, and a tendency toward hypokalemia occurs frequently in the surgical patient except when shock or acidosis interferes with the normal renal handling of potassium.

The signs of potassium deficit are related to failure of normal contractility of skeletal, smooth, and cardiac muscle and include weakness that may progress to flaccid

*Kayexalate.

Table 2-5. COMPOSITION OF GASTROINTESTINAL SECRETIONS

Type of secretion	Volume (ml/24 hr)	Na (mEq/L)	K (mEq/L)	Cl (mEq/L)	HCO₃ (mEq/L)
Salivary	1,500 (500–2,000)	10 (2–10)	26 (20–30)	10 (8–18)	30
Stomach	1,500 (100–4,000)	60 (9–116)	10 (0–32)	130 (8–154)	
Duodenum	(100–2,000)	140	5	80	
Ileum	3,000 (100–9,000)	140 (80–150)	5 (2–8)	104 (43–137)	30
Colon	. . . .	60	30	40	
Pancreas	. . . . (100–800)	140 (113–185)	5 (3–7)	75 (54–95)	115
Bile	. . . . (50–800)	145 (131–164)	5 (3–12)	100 (89–180)	35

paralysis, diminished to absent tendon reflexes, and paralytic ileus. Sensitivity to digitalis with cardiac arrhythmias and electrocardiographic signs of low voltage, flattening of T waves, and depression of ST segments are characteristic. However, signs of potassium deficit may be masked by those of a severe extracellular fluid volume deficit. Repletion of the volume deficit may further aggravate the situation by lowering the serum potassium level secondary to dilution.

The treatment of hypokalemia involves, first, prevention of this state. In the replacement of gastrointestinal fluids, it is safe to replace the upper limits of loss, since an excess is readily handled by the patient with normal renal function. Potassium is available in 20-mEq and 40-mEq ampules for addition to intravenous fluids. No more than 40 mEq should be added to a liter of intravenous fluid, and the rate of administration should not exceed 40 mEq/hour unless the electrocardiogram is being monitored. In the absence of specific indications, potassium should not be given to the oliguric patient or during the first 24 hours following severe surgical stress or trauma.

CALCIUM ABNORMALITIES

The majority of the 1,000 to 1,200 Gm of body calcium in the average-sized adult is found in the bone in the form of phosphate and carbonate. Normal daily intake of calcium is between 1 and 3 Gm. Most of this is excreted via the gastrointestinal tract, and 200 mg or less is excreted in the urine daily. The normal serum level is between 9 and 11 mg/100 ml (depending on the individual laboratory's normal range), and approximately half of this is not ionized and is bound to plasma protein. An additional nonionized fraction (5 percent) is bound to other substances in the plasma and interstitial fluid, whereas the remaining 45 percent is the ionized portion that is responsible for neuromuscular stability. Determination of the plasma protein level, therefore, is essential for proper analysis of the serum calcium level. The ratio of ionized to nonionized calcium is also related to the pH; acidosis causes an increase in the ionized fraction, whereas alkalosis causes a decrease.

Disturbances of calcium metabolism generally are not a problem in the uncomplicated postoperative patient, with the exception of skeletal loss during prolonged immobilization. Routine administration of calcium to the surgical patient, therefore, is not needed in the absence of specific indications.

HYPOCALCEMIA. The symptoms of hypocalcemia (serum level less than 8 mg/100 ml) are numbness and tingling of the circumoral region and the tips of the fingers and toes. The signs are of neuromuscular origin and include hyperactive tendon reflexes, positive Chvostek's sign, muscle and abdominal cramps, tetany with carpopedal spasm, convulsions (with severe deficit), and prolongation of the Q-T interval on the electrocardiogram.

The common causes include acute pancreatitis, massive soft tissue infections (necrotizing fasciitis), acute and chronic renal failure, pancreatic and small intestinal fistulas, and hypoparathyroidism. Transient hypocalcemia is a frequent occurrence in the hyperparathyroid patient following removal of a parathyroid adenoma, owing to atrophy of the remaining glands. Asymptomatic hypocalcemia may occur with hypoproteinemia (normal ionized fraction), whereas symptoms may appear with a normal serum calcium level in a patient with severe alkalosis. The latter is due to a decrease in the physiologically active or ionized fraction of total serum calcium. Calcium levels also may fall with a severe depletion of magnesium.

Treatment is directed toward correction of the underlying cause with concomitant repletion of the deficit. Acute symptoms may be relieved by the intravenous administration of calcium gluconate or calcium chloride. Calcium lactate may be given orally, with or without supplemental vitamin D, in the patient requiring prolonged replacement. The routine administration of calcium during massive transfusions of blood in acid-citrate-dextrose solution is controversial. If the transfusions are administered slowly, the citrate binding of ionized calcium is generally compensated for by the mobilization of calcium from the bone. However, with rapid transfusion of blood, 1 Gm of calcium gluconate may be given with every 4 or 5 units of blood infused.

HYPERCALCEMIA. The symptoms of hypercalcemia are rather vague and of gastrointestinal, renal, musculoskeletal, and central nervous system origin. The early manifestations of hypercalcemia include easy fatigue, lassitude, weakness of varying degree, anorexia, nausea, vomiting, and weight loss. With higher serum calcium levels, lassitude gives way to somnambulism, stupor, and finally coma. Other symptoms include severe headaches, pains in the back and extremities, thirst, polydypsia, and polyuria. The critical level for serum calcium is between 16 and 20 mg/100 ml, and unless treatment is instituted promptly, the symptoms may rapidly progress to death. The two major causes of hypercalcemia are hyperparathyroidism and cancer with bony metastasis. The latter is most frequently seen in the patient with metastatic breast cancer who is receiving estrogen therapy.

The treatment of acute hypercalcemia crisis is an emergency. Measures to lower the serum calcium level are instituted immediately while preparations are being made for more definitive treatment. Of particular importance is the rapid repletion of the associated extracellular fluid volume deficit, which will immediately lower the calcium level by dilution. Other measures which have been used and may be of temporary benefit include the use of a chelating agent (EDTA), steroids, sodium sulfate solution, and hemodialysis. Recently, intravenous mithromycin has been shown to reduce the serum calcium level in normocalcemic and hypercalcemic patients. The definitive treatment of acute hypercalcemic crisis in patients with hyperparathyroidism is immediate surgery.

Treatment of hypercalcemia in the patient with metastatic cancer is primarily that of prevention. The serum calcium level is checked frequently; if it is elevated, the patient is placed on a low-calcium diet, and measures to ensure adequate hydration are instituted.

MAGNESIUM ABNORMALITIES

The infrequent occurrence of magnesium deficiency and the previous lack of a rapid, precise technique for measurement of magnesium ion concentration accounts for the late appreciation of this entity. The total body content of magnesium in the average adult is approximately 2,000 mEq, about half of which is incorporated in bone and only slowly exchangeable. The distribution of magnesium is similar to that of potassium, the major portion being intracellular. Plasma magnesium concentration normally ranges between 1.5 and 2.5 mEq/L. The normal dietary intake of magnesium is approximately 20 mEq (240 mg) daily. The larger part is excreted in the feces, and the remainder in the urine. The kidneys show a remarkable ability to conserve magnesium; on a magnesium-free diet, renal excretion of this ion may be less than 1 mEq/day.

MAGNESIUM DEFICIENCY. Magnesium deficiency is known to occur with starvation, malabsorption syndromes, protracted losses of gastrointestinal fluid, and prolonged parenteral fluid therapy with magnesium-free solutions. Other causes include acute pancreatitis, diabetic acidosis during treatment, primary aldosteronism, chronic alcoholism, and burns (late stage).

The magnesium ion is essential for proper function of most enzyme systems, and depletion is characterized by neuromuscular and central nervous system hyperactivity. The signs and symptoms are quite similar to those of calcium deficiency, including hyperactive tendon reflexes, muscle tremors, and tetany with a positive Chvostek sign. Progression to delirium and convulsions may occur with a severe deficit. A concomitant calcium deficiency occasionally is noted, particularly in those with clinical signs of tetany.

The diagnosis of magnesium deficiency depends on an awareness of the syndrome and clinical recognition of the symptoms. Laboratory confirmation is available but not reliable, as the syndrome may exist in the presence of a normal serum magnesium level. The possibility of magnesium deficiency should always be considered in the surgical patient who exhibits disturbed neuromuscular or cerebral activity in the postoperative period. This is particularly important in patients who have had protracted dysfunction of the gastrointestinal tract and require long-term maintenance on parenteral fluid therapy. Routine magnesium replacement should always be considered in the management of these patients.

Treatment of magnesium deficiency is by the parenteral administration of magnesium sulfate or magnesium chloride solution. As much as 2 mEq of magnesium/kg of body weight can be administered in a day in the face of a severe depletion. Magnesium sulfate (50% solution contains approximately 4 mEq of magnesium ion/ml) may be given intravenously or intramuscularly. The intravenous route is preferable for the initial treatment of a severe deficit. This can be accomplished by the addition of 80 mEq of magnesium sulfate (20 ml of 50% solution) to a liter of intravenous fluid which is administered over a 2- to 4-hour period. When large doses are given, the heart rate, blood pressure, respiration, and electrocardiogram should be monitored closely for signs of magnesium toxicity, which could lead to cardiac arrest. It is advisable to have calcium chloride or calcium gluconate available to counteract any adverse effects of a rapidly rising plasma magnesium level.

Partial or complete relief of symptoms may follow this infusion as a result of increased concentration of magnesium ion in the extracellular fluid compartment, although continued replacement over a 1- to 3-week period is necessary to replenish the intracellular compartment. For this purpose and for the asymptomatic patient who is likely to have significant magnesium depletion, 10 to 20 mEq of 50% magnesium sulfate solution is given daily by the intramuscular route or in infusion fluids. When magnesium sulfate is used, it should be given in divided doses or at multiple sites, since the intramuscular injection of this salt is painful. Following complete repletion of intracellular magnesium and in the absence of abnormal loss, balance may be maintained by the administration of as little as 4 mEq of magnesium ion daily.

Magnesium ion should not be given to the oliguric patient or in the presence of severe volume deficit unless actual magnesium depletion is demonstrated. If given to a patient with renal insufficiency, considerably smaller doses are used, and the patient is carefully observed for signs or symptoms of toxicity.

MAGNESIUM EXCESS. Symptomatic hypermagnesemia, although rare, is most commonly seen with severe renal insufficiency. Retention and accumulation of magnesium may occur in any patient with impaired glomerular or renal tubular function, and the presence of acidosis may rapidly compound the situation. Serum magnesium levels tend to parallel changes in potassium concentration in these cases. Therefore, magnesium levels should be carefully monitored in cases of acute and chronic renal failure and in selected patients with borderline renal function. Randall et al. have shown that in patients on ordinary dietary intakes of magnesium, increased serum concentrations of the ion do not occur until the glomerular filtration rate falls below 30 ml/minute. As noted by Henzel et al., however, magnesium-containing antacids and laxatives (milk of magnesia, epsom salts, Gelusil, Maalox) are commonly administered in quantities sufficient to produce toxic serum levels of magnesium where impaired renal function is present. Other conditions which may be associated with symptomatic hypermagnesemia include early-stage burns, massive trauma or surgical stress, severe extracellular volume deficit, and severe acidosis.

The early signs and symptoms include lethargy and weakness with progressive loss of deep tendon reflexes. Interference with cardiac conduction occurs with increasing levels of magnesium and changes in the electrocardiogram (increased P-R interval, widened QRS complex, and elevated T waves) resemble those seen with hyperkalemia. Somnolence leading to coma and muscular paralysis occur in the later stages, and death is usually caused by respiratory or cardiac arrest.

Treatment consists of immediate measures to lower the serum magnesium level by correcting any acidosis, replenishing any preexisting extracellular volume deficit, and withholding exogenously administered magnesium. Acute symptoms may be temporarily controlled by the slow intravenous administration of 5 to 10 mEq of calcium chloride or calcium gluconate. If elevated levels or symptoms persist, peritoneal dialysis or hemodialysis is indicated.

NORMAL EXCHANGE OF FLUID AND ELECTROLYTES

Knowledge of the basic principles governing both the internal and external exchanges of water and salt is mandatory for care of the patient undergoing major operative surgery. The stable internal fluid environment, which is maintained by the kidneys, brain, lungs, skin, and gastrointestinal tract, may be compromised by severe surgical stress or direct damage to any of these organs.

Water Exchange

The normal individual consumes an average of 2,000 to 2,500 ml water/day; approximately 1,500 ml water is taken by mouth, and the rest is extracted from solid food, either from the contents of the food or as the product of oxidation (Table 2-6). The daily water losses include 250

Table 2-6. WATER EXCHANGE (60–80 kg man)

Routes	Average daily volume, ml	Minimal, ml	Maximal, ml
H$_2$O gain:			
Sensible:			
Oral fluids	800–1,500	0	1,500/hr
Solid foods	500–700	0	1,500
Insensible:			
Water of oxidation . .	250	125	800
Water of solution . . .	0	0	500
H$_2$O loss:			
Sensible:			
Urine	800–1,500	300	1,400/hr (diabetes insipidus)
Intestinal	0–250	0	2,500/hr
Sweat	0	0	4,000/hr
Insensible:			
Lungs and skin	600–900	600–900	1,500

ml in stools, 800 to 1,500 ml as urine, and approximately 600 to 900 ml as insensible loss. A patient deprived of all external access to water must still excrete a minimum of 500 to 800 ml urine/day in order to excrete the products of catabolism, in addition to the mandatory insensible loss through the skin and lungs.

Insensible loss of water occurs through the skin (75 percent) and the lungs (25 percent) and is increased by hypermetabolism, hyperventilation, and fever. The insensible water loss through the skin is not from evaporation of water from sweat glands but from water vapor formed within the body and lost through the skin. With excessive heat production (or excessive environmental heat), the capacity for insensible loss through the skin is exceeded, and sweating occurs. These losses may, but seldom do, exceed 250 ml/day/degree of fever. An unhumidified tracheostomy with hyperventilation increases the loss through the lungs and results in a total insensible loss up to 1.5 liters/day.

A frequently overlooked source of gain is the water of solution, which is the water that holds carbohydrates and proteins in solution in the cell. Normally, gain of water from this source is zero, but after 4 to 5 days without food intake, the postoperative patient may begin to gain significant quantities of water (maximum 500 ml daily) from excessive cellular catabolism. The amount depends on the degree of trauma and the complications occurring postoperatively.

Salt Gain and Losses

In the normal individual, the salt intake per day varies between 50 and 90 mEq (3 to 5 Gm) as sodium chloride (Table 2-7). Balance is maintained primarily by the normal kidneys that excrete the excess salt. Under conditions of reduced intake or extrarenal losses, the normal kidney can reduce sodium excretion to less than 1 mEq/day within

Table 2-7. SODIUM (SALT) EXCHANGE
(60–80 kg man)

Sodium exchange	Average	Minimal	Maximal
Sodium gain:			
Diet	50–90 mEq/day	0	75–100 mEq/hr (oral)
Sodium loss:			
Skin (sweat) . .	10–60 mEq/day*	0	300 mEq/hr
Urine	10–80 mEq/day	<1 mEq/day†	110–200 mEq/L‡
Intestines	0–20 mEq/day	0	300 mEq/hr

* Depending on the degree of acclimatization of the individual.
† With normal renal function.
‡ With renal salt wasting.

24 hours after restriction. In the patient with salt-wasting kidneys, however, the loss may exceed 200 mEq/L of urine. Sweat represents a hypotonic loss of fluids with an average sodium concentration of 15 mEq/L in the acclimatized patient. In the unacclimatized individual, the sodium concentration in sweat may be 60 mEq/L or more. Insensible fluid lost from the skin and lungs, by definition, is pure water. For practical considerations then, normal losses may be relatively free of salt in the healthy individual with normal renal function.

The volume and composition of various types of gastrointestinal secretions are shown in Table 2-5. Gastrointestinal losses are usually isotonic or slightly hypotonic, although there is considerable variation in the composition. These should be replaced by an essentially isotonic salt solution. It is also important to reiterate that distributional or sequestration losses of extracellular fluid at any point in the operative or postoperative course also represent isotonic losses of salt and water.

FLUID AND ELECTROLYTE THERAPY

Parenteral Solutions

The composition of various parenteral fluids available for administration is shown in Table 2-8. There is sufficient variety to satisfy the majority of fluid requirements in the surgical patient. The proper choice of parenteral fluid in a given situation will correct the abnormalities but impose minimal demands on the kidneys.

A good available isotonic salt solution for replacing gastrointestinal losses and repairing preexisting volume deficits, in the absence of gross abnormalities of concentration and composition, is lactated Ringer's solution. This solution is "physiologic" and contains 130 mEq sodium balanced by 109 mEq chloride and 28 mEq lactate. This fluid has minimal effects on normal body fluid composition and pH even when infused in large quantities. The chief disadvantage of lactated Ringer's solution is the slight hypoosmolarity with respect to sodium. Each liter of lactated Ringer's solution furnishes approximately 100 to 150 ml free water. This rarely presents a clinical problem if

it is considered in calculating water replacement. The remainder of the solutions listed in Table 2-8 are used to correct specific defects. Choice of a particular fluid depends on the volume status of the patient and the type of concentration or compositional abnormality present.

Isotonic sodium chloride contains 154 mEq sodium and 154 mEq chloride/L. The high concentration of chloride above the normal serum concentration of 103 mEq/L imposes on the kidneys an appreciable load of excess chloride which cannot be rapidly excreted. Thus, a dilutional acidosis may develop.* This solution is ideal, however, for the initial correction of an extracellular fluid volume deficit in the presence of hyponatremia, hypochloremia, and metabolic alkalosis. In a similar situation with moderate metabolic acidosis, $M/6$ sodium lactate (167 mEq/L each of sodium and lactate) may be given. Another solution for this purpose can be made by adding one ampule of sodium bicarbonate (40 ml solution containing 40 mEq each of sodium and bicarbonate) to 1,000 ml lactated Ringer's solution.

Molar sodium lactate solution or 3 or 5% sodium chloride may be used to correct symptomatic hyponatremic states. The choice of anion (lactate or chloride) is determined by the accompanying acid-base derangement. The need for ammonium chloride solutions in the treatment of an uncompensated metabolic alkalosis is extremely rare. Indications for their use include very shallow or slow breathing with cyanosis or severe tetany. Following the correction of concentration or compositional abnormalities using specific repair solutions, a balanced salt solution is used to replenish the remaining volume deficit.

---

* Infusion of a large volume of isotonic sodium chloride solution may induce or aggravate a preexisting acidosis by reducing the amount of base bicarbonate in the body relative to the carbonic acid content.

Table 2-8. COMPOSITION OF PARENTERAL FLUIDS
Electrolyte content (mEq/L)

Solutions	Cations					Anions		
	Na	K	Ca	Mg	NH₄	Cl	HCO₃⁻	HPO₄⁻
Extracellular fluid.	142	4	5	3	.3	103	27	3
Lactated Ringer's	130	4	2.7			109	28*	
0.9% sodium chloride (saline)	154					154		
M/6 sodium lactate	167						167*	
M (molar) sodium lactate	1,000						1,000*	
3% sodium chloride	513					513		
5% sodium chloride	855					855		
0.9% ammonium chloride					168	168		

· * Present in solution as lactate which is converted to bicarbonate.

Preoperative Fluid Therapy

Preoperative evaluation and correction of existing fluid disorders is an integral part of surgical care. An orderly approach to these problems requires an understanding of the common fluid disturbances associated with surgical illness and adherence to a few simple guidelines. There are no shortcuts; close observation of the patient and frequent reevaluation of the clinical situation is the most rewarding approach.

The analysis of a fluid disorder may be facilitated by categorizing the abnormalities into *volume, concentration,* and *compositional* changes. Although some disease states produce characteristic changes in fluid balance, much confusion may be avoided by regarding each disturbance as a separate entity. For example, volume changes cannot be accurately predicted from a knowledge of the level of serum sodium, since an extracellular fluid volume deficit or excess may exist with a normal, low, or high sodium concentration. Similarly, any of the four primary acid-base disturbances may be associated with any combination of volume and concentration abnormalities.

CORRECTION OF VOLUME CHANGES

Changes in the volume of extracellular fluid are the most frequent and important abnormalities encountered in the surgical patient. Depletion of the extracellular fluid compartment without changes in concentration or composition is a common problem. The diagnosis of volume changes is made almost entirely on clinical grounds. The signs that will be present in an individual patient depend not only on the relative or absolute quantity of extracellular fluid which has been lost but also on the rapidity with which it is lost and the presence or absence of signs of associated disease.

Volume deficits in the surgical patient may result from external loss of fluids or from an internal redistribution of extracellular fluid into a nonfunctional compartment. Generally, it involves a combination of the two, but the internal redistribution is frequently overlooked.

The phenomenon of internal redistribution or translocation of extracellular fluid is peculiar to many surgical diseases; in the individual patient, the loss may be quite large. Although the concept of a "third space" is not new, it is generally considered only in relation to patients with massive ascites, burns, or crush injuries. Of more importance, however, is the "third space" loss into the peritoneum, the bowel wall, and other tissues with inflammatory lesions of the intraabdominal organs. The magnitude of these losses may not be fully appreciated without realization of the fact that the peritoneum alone has approximately 1 m² of surface area. A slight increase in thickness from sequestration of fluid, which would not be appreciated on casual observation, may result in a functional loss of several liters of fluid. Swelling of the bowel wall and mesentery and secretion of fluid into the lumen of the bowel will cause even larger losses. Similar deficits may occur with massive infection of the subcutaneous tissues (necrotizing fasciitis) or with severe crush injury.

These "parasitic" losses remain a part of the ex-

tracellular fluid space and may be measured as a slowly equilibrating volume. The term *nonfunctional* is used because the fluid is no longer able to participate in the normal functions of the extracellular fluid compartment and may just as well have been lost externally. Any transfer of intracellular fluid to the extracellular compartment for replenishment of the loss is insignificant in the acute phase. The patient with ascites may have an enormous total extracellular fluid volume although the functional component is severely depleted. The same is true of extensive inflammatory or obstructive lesions of the gastrointestinal tract, although the loss is not as obvious. These losses will evoke the signs and symptoms of an extracellular fluid volume deficit with or without the concomitant external loss of fluids.

Exact quantification of these deficits is impossible and, at the present time, probably unnecessary. The defect can be estimated on the basis of the severity of the clinical signs. A mild deficit represents a loss of approximately 4 percent of body weight, a moderate loss is 6 to 8 percent of body weight, and a severe deficit is approximately 10 percent of body weight. It is important to reemphasize the fact that cardiovascular signs predominate when there is acute rapid loss of fluid from the extracellular fluid compartment with few or no tissue signs. In addition to the estimated deficit, fluids lost during the period of treatment must be replaced.

Fluid replacement should be started and changed according to the response of the patient noted on frequent clinical observation. Reliance on a formula or single clinical sign to determine adequacy of resuscitation is fraught with danger. Rather, reversal of the signs of the volume deficit, combined with stabilization of the blood pressure and pulse, and an hourly urine volume of 30 to 50 ml are used as general guidelines. An adequate hourly urine output, although usually a reliable index of volume replacement, may be totally misleading. The excessive administration of glucose (over 50 Gm in a 2- to 3-hour period) may result in osmotic diuresis, while an osmotic agent such as mannitol tends to produce urine at the expense of the vascular volume. Patients with chronic renal disease or incipient acute renal damage from shock and injury also may have inappropriately high urinary volumes. In addition, the rapid administration of salt solutions may transiently expand the intravascular volume, increase the glomerular filtration rate, and result in an immediate outpouring of urine, although the total extracellular fluid space remains quite depleted.

The choice of the proper fluid for replacement depends on the existence of concomitant concentration or compositional abnormalities. With pure extracellular fluid volume loss or when only minimal concentration or compositional abnormalities are present, the use of a balanced salt solution, such as lactated Ringer's, is desirable.

CORRECTION OF CONCENTRATION CHANGES

If severe *symptomatic* hyponatremia or hypernatremia complicates the volume loss, prompt correction of the concentration abnormality to the extent that symptoms are relieved is necessary. Volume replenishment then should be accomplished with slower correction of the remaining concentration abnormality. For immediate correction of severe hyponatremia, 5% sodium chloride solution or molar sodium lactate solution is used, depending on the patient's acid-base status. In any case, the sodium deficit can be estimated by multiplying the decrease in serum sodium concentration below normal (in milliequivalents per liter) *times* the liters of total body water. Total body water averages 60 percent of the body weight in young adult males and 50 percent in young adult females. Initially, up to one-half of the calculated amount of sodium may be administered slowly, followed by clinical and chemical reevaluation of the patient before any additional infusion of sodium salts.

Example: A twenty-four-year-old female with symptomatic hyponatremia, weight = 60 kg, serum sodium = 120 mEq/L:

Total body water = 60 kg × 0.50 = 30 liters
Sodium deficit = (140 − 120 mEq/L) × 30 liters
= 600 mEq

Half of this amount (300 mEq) could be given by slowly infusing approximately 350 ml 5% sodium chloride solution.

Note that this estimate is based on total body water, since the effective osmotic pressure in the extracellular compartment cannot be increased without increasing this function proportionately in the intracellular compartment. Although absolute reliance on any formula is undesirable, proper use of this estimate will allow a safe quantitative approximation of the sodium deficit. Generally, only a portion of the total deficit is replaced initially to relieve acute symptoms. Further correction is facilitated when renal function is restored by correction of the volume deficit. If the total calculated deficit were given rapidly, severe hypervolemia might occur particularly in patients with limited cardiac reserve. In practice, the infusion of small, successive increments of hypertonic saline solution with frequent evaluation of the clinical response and serum sodium concentration is recommended.

In the treatment of moderate hyponatremia with an associated volume deficit, volume replacement can be started immediately with concomitant correction of the serum sodium deficit. Isotonic sodium chloride solution (normal saline) is used initially in the presence of metabolic alkalosis, whereas *M*/6 sodium lactate is used to correct an associated acidosis. Only a few liters of these solutions may be necessary to correct the serum sodium concentration; the remainder of the volume deficit may be repaired with lactated Ringer's solution.

Treatment of hyponatremia associated with volume excess is by restriction of water. In the presence of severe symptomatic hyponatremia, a small amount of hypertonic salt solution may be infused cautiously to alleviate symptoms. As this will cause additional volume expansion, it is contraindicated in patients with limited cardiac reserve; peritoneal dialysis or hemodialysis is preferred in this situation.

For the correction of severe, symptomatic hypernatremia with an associated volume deficit, 5% dextrose in water may be infused slowly until symptoms are relieved. If the extracellular osmolarity is reduced too rapidly, however, convulsions and coma may result. For this reason, correction of hypernatremia concomitant with repletion of the volume deficit by half-strength sodium chloride or half-strength lactated Ringer's solution is safer in most cases. In the absence of a significant volume deficit, water should be administered cautiously since dangerous hypervolemia may result; constant observation and frequent determinations of the serum sodium concentration are indicated. The problem is somewhat simplified once a sufficient quantity of fluid has been given to permit renal excretion of the solute load.

RATE OF FLUID ADMINISTRATION. This varies considerably, depending on the severity and type of fluid disturbance, the presence of continuing losses, and the cardiac status. In general, the most severe volume deficits may be safely replaced initially with isotonic solutions at a rate of 2,000 ml/hour, reducing the rate as the fluid status improves. Constant observation by a physician is mandatory when the administration exceeds 1,000 ml/hour. At these rates, a significant portion may be lost as urinary output owing to a transient overexpansion of the plasma volume.

In elderly patients, associated cardiovascular disorders do not preclude correction of existing volume deficits, but they do require slower, more careful correction with constant monitoring of all functions including the central venous pressure. Hypertonic salt solutions should be given under close supervision, and the rate of administration generally should not exceed 100 to 150 ml/hour.

COMPOSITION AND MISCELLANEOUS CONSIDERATIONS

Correction of existing potassium deficits should be started *after* an adequate urine output is obtained, particularly in the patient with metabolic alkalosis since this may be secondary to or aggravated by potassium depletion. Potassium chloride is available in 20-mEq and 40-mEq ampules for addition to intravenous fluids. A maximum of 40 mEq of potassium chloride per hour may be safely administered to the adult of average size who is not severely depleted of extracellular fluid volume, in frank hypovolemic shock, or in established oliguric or high-output renal failure. The concentration of potassium chloride should not exceed 40 mEq/L of intravenous fluids, with rare exception, such as the treatment of digitalis intoxication during which the electrocardiogram must be constantly monitored. Calcium and magnesium rarely are needed during preoperative resuscitation, but should be given if any doubt exists, particularly to patients with massive subcutaneous infections, those with acute pancreatitis, and those who have been chronically starved.

Fluid abnormalities also must be suspected in the patient for whom an elective procedure is planned. Chronic illnesses frequently are associated with extracellular fluid volume deficits, and concentration and compositional changes are not uncommon. Correction of anemia and recognition of the fact that a contracted blood volume may exist in the chronically debilitated patient is of obvious importance. The choice of whole blood versus packed cells for correction of anemia depends on the volume status. If there is any question, 1 unit of packed cells may be given and the hemoglobin and hematocrit determined subsequently. The hemoglobin generally increases approximately 1.5 following the infusion of 250 ml of packed cells into the adult of average size. The increase will be significantly greater than 1.5 Gm/100 ml in the patient with a contracted intravascular volume, indicating the probable need for whole blood transfusions. If available, measurement of the blood volume is obviously more accurate.

Of additional importance is the prevention of volume depletion during the preoperative period. Prolonged periods of fluid restriction in preparation for various diagnostic procedures, and the use of cathartics and enemas for preparation of the bowel may cause a significant acute loss of extracellular fluid. Prompt recognition and treatment of these losses is necessary to prevent complications during the operative period.

Intraoperative Management of Fluids

If preoperative replacement of extracellular fluid volume has been incomplete, hypotension may develop promptly with the induction of anesthesia. This can be quite insidious, as the ability of the awake patient to compensate for mild volume deficit is revealed only when the compensatory mechanisms are abolished with anesthesia. This problem is prevented by maintaining base-line requirements and replacing abnormal losses of fluids and electrolytes by intravenous infusions in the preoperative period.

Blood lost during the operative procedure should be replaced steadily. It is usually unnecessary to replace blood loss of less than 500 ml, but after the loss has exceeded this, replacement should begin. The warnings against the use of a single transfusion during operation have been somewhat confusing. There may be a very definite need for a single-unit transfusion in the patient who loses between 500 and 1,000 ml of blood during operation.

In addition to blood losses during operation, there appear to be extracellular fluid losses during major operative procedures. Some of these, including edema from extensive dissection, collections within the lumen and wall of the small bowel, and accumulations of fluid in the peritoneal cavity, are clinically discernible and well recognized. They generally are felt to represent distributional shifts, in that the functional volume of extracellular fluid is reduced but not externally lost from the body. These functional losses are often referred to as "a parasitic loss of extracellular fluid," "a third space edema," or "a sequestration" of extracellular fluid. Another source of extracellular fluid loss during major operative trauma is the wound itself. This is a relatively smaller loss and very difficult to quantify except in extensive and major operative procedures.

At the beginning of this century, surgeons became aware that many changes occurred in urinary output, blood volume, and fluid and electrolyte composition during and after surgery. Assessment of these changes, however, awaited the development of analytic techniques and their application to patient studies. In the following 25 years, saline solutions in varying combinations were given to patients undergoing operation, often in excessive amounts. Work in the late 1930s and early 1940s by Moyer and by many others indicated that during and after operative procedures, saline and water solutions should be withheld entirely, because most of the fluid administered was retained.

The possibility existed that the operative and postoperative retention of salt and water administered in relatively small amounts might simply be physiologic retention to replace a deficit of salt and water incurred by the operative procedure. Subsequent studies have revealed that functional extracellular fluid decreases with major abdominal operations, largely as sequestered loss into the operative site. This extracellular fluid volume deficit can be replaced during the operative procedure. These data have led to the conclusion that the need for an extracellular "mimic" in the form of balanced salt solution now can be clinically estimated. Intraoperative correction of the volume deficit with salt solution markedly reduces "postoperative salt intolerance," but is not intended to substitute for blood replacement. Rather, it is felt to be a physiologic supplement, or adjunct, to replace sequestered losses.

Thus, the pendulum has swung from indiscriminate use of salt solutions in the first quarter of this century to almost total withholding of fluid and electrolytes from surgical patients in the second quarter of the century; indications at present are that proper management lies somewhere between these two extremes. Some guidelines are necessary for the intraoperative administration of saline solutions as a "mimic" for the sequestered extracellular fluid. Since this varies from an almost imperceptible minimum to a high of approximately 3 liters during an uncomplicated procedure, quantification is extremely difficult with the presently available means of measuring functional extracellular fluid. Consequently, no accurate formula for intraoperative fluid administration can yet be derived. Some arbitrary but clinically useful guidelines are the following: (1) Blood should be replaced as lost, irrespective of any additional fluid and electrolyte therapy. (2) The replacement of extracellular fluid should begin during the operative procedure. Recent data reveal that if the operative replacement of extracellular fluid is delayed until the adrenal compensatory mechanisms have started to react to the operative trauma in the immediate postoperative period, dangerous overloads may be produced. (3) Balanced salt solution needed during operation is approximately $\frac{1}{2}$ to 1 liter/hour, but only to a maximum of 2 to 3 liters during a 4-hour major abdominal procedure, unless there are other measurable losses.

Postoperative Management of Fluids

IMMEDIATE POSTOPERATIVE PERIOD

Orders for postoperative fluids are not written until the patient is in the recovery room and the fluid status has been assessed. Evaluation at this point should include a review of preoperative fluid status, the amount of fluid loss and gain during operation, and clinical examination of the patient with assessment of the vital signs and urinary output. Initial fluid orders are written to correct any *existing* deficit, followed by maintenance fluids for the remainder of the day. For the patient with complications who has received or lost large amounts of fluid, it is frequently difficult to estimate the fluid requirements for the ensuing 24 hours. In this situation, intravenous fluids are ordered 1 liter at a time and the patient checked frequently until the situation is clarified. Proper replacement of fluids during this relatively short period will facilitate subsequent fluid management.

Immediately after operation, extracellular fluid volume depletion may occur as a result of continued losses of fluid at the site of injury or operative trauma—for example, into the wall or lumen of the small intestine. Several liters of extracellular fluid may be slowly deposited in such areas within a few hours or more during the first day or so from the time of the injury. Unrecognized deficits of extracellular fluid volume during the early postoperative period are manifest primarily as circulatory instability. The signs of volume deficiency in other organ systems may be delayed for several hours with this type of fluid loss. Postoperative hypotension and tachycardia require prompt investigation, followed by appropriate therapy. The generally accepted adequate blood pressure of 90/60 and a pulse of less than 120 in postoperative patients may not be sufficient to prevent renal ischemia unless, in addition to lack of signs of shock, urine flow is adequate. Evaluation of the level of consciousness, pupillary size, airway patency, breathing patterns, pulse rate and volume, skin warmth, color, body temperature, and a 30- to 50-ml hourly urine output, combined with critical review of the operative procedure and the operative fluid management, usually is rewarding. Since operative trauma frequently involves loss or transfer of significant quantities of whole blood, plasma, or extracellular fluid which can be only grossly estimated, circulatory instability is most commonly caused by underestimated initial losses or insidious, concealed continued losses. Operative blood loss is usually estimated by the operating surgeon to be 15 to 40 percent less than the isotopically measured blood loss from that patient. In addition, several liters of extravascular, extracellular fluid can be sequestered in areas of injury and manifested only by oliguria and mild depression of the blood pressure with a rapid pulse. For a patient with circulatory instability, further volume replacement of an additional 1,000 ml isotonic salt solution, while determining whether continuing losses or other causes are present, often resolves the problem. Contributing causes must be vigorously pursued with all diagnostic aids before excessive volumes of fluid have been administered.

It is unnecessary and probably unwise to administer potassium during the first 24 hours postoperatively, unless a definite potassium deficit exists. This is particularly important for the patient subjected to prolonged operative trauma involving one or more episodes of hypotension and for the posttraumatic patient with hemorrhagic hypotension. Oliguric renal failure or the more insidious high-output renal failure may develop, and the administration of even a small quantity of potassium may be quite detrimental.

LATER POSTOPERATIVE PERIOD

The problem of volume management during the postoperative convalescent phase is one of accurate measurement and replacement of all losses. In the otherwise healthy individual, this involves the replacement of measured sensible losses, which are generally of gastrointestinal origin, and the estimation and replacement of insensible losses.

The insensible loss is usually relatively constant and will average 600 to 900 ml daily. This may be increased by hypermetabolism, hyperventilation, and fever to a maximum of approximately 1,500 ml daily. The estimated insensible loss is replaced with 5% dextrose in water. This loss may be partially offset by an insensible gain of water from excessive tissue catabolism in the complicated postoperative patient, particularly if associated with oliguric renal failure.

Approximately 1 liter of fluid should be given to replace that volume of urine required to excrete the catabolic end products of metabolism (800 to 1,000 ml/day). In the individual with normal renal function, this may be given as 5% dextrose in water, since the kidneys are able to conserve sodium with excretion of less than 1 mEq daily. It is probably unnecessary to stress the kidneys to this degree, however, and a small amount of salt solution may be given in addition to water to cover urinary loss. In the elderly patient with salt-losing kidneys or in patients with head injuries, an insidious hyponatremia may develop if urinary losses are replaced with water. Urinary sodium in these circumstances may exceed 100 mEq/L and result in a daily loss of significant amounts of sodium. Measurement of urinary sodium will facilitate accurate replacement.

Urine volume is not replaced on a milliliter-for-milliliter basis. A urinary output of 2,000 to 3,000 ml on a given day may simply represent diuresis of fluids given during surgery or may represent excessive fluid administration. If these large losses are completely replaced, the urine output will progressively increase, and this may logically progress to a unique situation resembling diabetes insipidus with urinary outputs in excess of 10 liters daily.

Sensible losses, by definition, can be measured or, as in the case of sweating, the amount can be estimated. Gastrointestinal losses are usually isotonic or slightly hypotonic, and they are replaced with an essentially isotonic salt solution. When the estimated loss is slightly above or below isotonicity, appropriate corrections can be made in the daily water administration, while isotonic salt solutions are used to replace these losses volume for volume. Sweating is not usually a problem except with the febrile patient in whom losses may, but seldom do, exceed 250 ml/day/degree of fever. Excessive sweating may, in addition, represent a considerable loss of sodium in the unacclimatized individual.

Determination of serum electrolyte levels is generally unnecessary in the patient with an uncomplicated postoperative course maintained on parenteral fluids for 2 to 3 days. A more prolonged period of parenteral replacement or one complicated by excessive fluid losses requires frequent determinations of the serum sodium, potassium, and chloride levels, and carbon dioxide combining power. Adjustments then can be made with intravenous fluids of appropriate composition. For example, gastrointestinal losses should be replaced with isotonic sodium chloride solution in a patient with hyponatremia, hypochloremia, and mild metabolic alkalosis, and this should be continued until these abnormalities are corrected. In the hyponatremic patient with obvious overload, the amount of water given is restricted. In the presence of hyponatremia and mild metabolic acidosis, $M/6$ sodium lactate or lactated Ringer's solution with added sodium bicarbonate may be used. In this way, severe concentration and compositional changes can be avoided while an adequate extracellular fluid volume is maintained by appropriate maintenance fluids.

Maintenance fluids are administered at a steady rate over an 18- to 24-hour period as the losses are incurred. If given over a shorter period of time, renal excretion of the excess salt and water may occur while the normal losses continue over the full 24-hour period. For the same reason, fluids of different composition are alternated, and additives to intravenous fluids (e.g., potassium chloride and antibiotics) are evenly distributed in the total volume of fluid given.

In summary, daily fluid orders should begin with an assessment of the patient's volume status and a check for possible concentration or compositional disorders as reflected by proper laboratory determinations. All measured and insensible losses are replaced with fluids of appropriate composition, allowing for any preexisting deficit or excess. The amount of potassium replacement is 40 mEq daily for renal excretion of potassium in addition to approximately 20 mEq/L for replacement of gastrointestinal losses. Inadequate replacement may prolong the usual postoperative ileus and contribute to the insidious development of a resistant metabolic alkalosis. Calcium and magnesium are replaced when needed, as previously discussed.

SPECIAL CONSIDERATIONS IN THE POSTOPERATIVE PATIENT

VOLUME EXCESSES. The administration of isotonic salt solutions in excess of volume losses (external or internal) may result in overexpansion of the extracellular fluid space. The otherwise normal person in a postoperative state tolerates an acute overexpansion extremely well. Excesses administered over a period of several days, however, will soon exceed the kidneys' ability to excrete sodium; since water losses continue, hypernatremia will ensue. Therefore, it is important to determine as accurately as possible from intake and output records and serum sodium concentrations the actual needs of the patient managed over several postoperative days. Attention to the signs and symptoms of overload usually prevents this fluid abnormality. It arises most frequently with attempts to meet excessive volume losses that are not measurable, such as those occurring from incompletely controlled fistula drainage.

The earliest sign is a weight gain (when measurable) during the catabolic period, when the patient should be losing $\frac{1}{4}$ to $\frac{1}{2}$ lb/day. Heavy eyelids, hoarseness, or dyspnea on exertion may rapidly appear. Circulatory and pulmonary signs of overload appear late and represent a rather massive overload. Peripheral edema may be a sign, but it does not necessarily indicate volume excess. In the absence of additional evidence for volume overload, other causes for peripheral edema should be considered. Of particular importance is the fact that overexpansion of the *total* extracellular fluid may coexist with *depletion* of the functional extracellular fluid compartment. Central venous pressure measurements may be helpful during volume replacement but may be misleading, as a rapid rise may indicate an excessive rate of fluid administration or primary pump failure but it does not accurately establish volume status.

HYPONATREMIA. Significant postoperative alterations in serum sodium concentration are not frequently observed if the fluid resuscitation during operation has included adequate volumes of isotonic salt solutions. The kidneys retain the ability to excrete moderate excesses of salt water administered in the early postoperative period if functional extracellular fluid has been adequately replaced during the operative or immediate postoperative period. Previous studies of sodium balance have revealed that patients do excrete sodium after the functional deficit incurred by the shift of extracellular fluid has been replaced. Wright and Gann have demonstrated normal capacity to excrete water postoperatively when isotonic salt solutions are administered prior to a challenge with a water load. Thus, the commonly described hyponatremia associated with surgical procedures and traumatic injury is prevented by the replacement of extracellular fluid deficits. The daily maintenance of normal osmolarity is simplified by the replacement of observable losses of known sodium content.

Hyponatremia may easily occur when water is given to replace losses of sodium-containing fluids or when water administration consistently exceeds water losses. The latter may occur with oliguria or in association with decreased water loss through the skin and lungs, intracellular shifts of sodium, or the cellular release of excessive amounts of endogenous water. Severe or refractory hyponatremia, however, is difficult to produce if renal function remains normal.

Replacement of Sodium Losses with Water. A common error is replacement of gastrointestinal and other salt losses with only water or a hypotonic solution. Patients with head injury or with preexisting renal disease (loss of concentrating ability) may elaborate urine with a high salt concentration (50 to 200 mEq/L).

Progressive hyponatremia in the patient with head injury, despite adequate salt administration, is believed to be due to excessive secretion of antidiuretic hormone with consequent water retention. The loss of renal concentrating ability due to impairment of renal tubular function ("salt-wasting kidneys") is a common problem in elderly patients. This source of sodium loss is frequently not anticipated, since the blood urea nitrogen and creatinine levels usually fall within normal limits. Continued replacement of these urinary losses with water only eventually may result in symptomatic hyponatremia. The urine sodium concentration should be determined if the diagnosis is in doubt; with hyponatremia and normal renal function, the urine should be virtually free of sodium.

Decreased Urinary Volume. Oliguria, from whatever cause (prerenal or renal), reduces the daily water requirements if not corrected. Cellular catabolism and the metabolic acidosis produced by the retention of nitrogenous waste products increases the cellular release of water. Therefore, the gain of endogenous water decreases the total water requirement beyond that expected when the urinary volume is low.

Decreased Insensible Loss. Cutaneous vasoconstriction from any cause decreases both insensible and evaporative water loss by this route. This condition most commonly accompanies generalized hypothermia.

Endogenous Water Release. The patient maintained on intravenous fluids will, between the fifth and tenth days, gain significant quantities of water (maximum, 500 ml daily) from excessive cellular catabolism, thus decreasing the quantity of exogenous water required per day.

Intracellular Shifts. Systemic bacterial sepsis is often accompanied by a precipitous drop in serum sodium concentration. This sudden change is poorly understood, but usually accompanies loss of extracellular fluid as either interstitial or intracellular sequestrations. This can be treated by withholding free water, restoring extracellular fluid volume, and initiating treatment of the sepsis.

Many hyponatremic states are asymptomatic until the serum sodium level falls below 120 mEq/L. This moderate asymptomatic hyponatremia, however, signifies inappropriate therapy or indicates the basic underlying condition. Symptomatic hyponatremia, or water intoxication, is difficult to produce if renal function is normal. Convulsions and apnea from uncorrected water excesses occur most often in children and elderly adults. Within the limits imposed by the circulatory apparatus, these deficits should be corrected by the administration of hypertonic salt solution to a serum sodium level above 130 mEq/L. Mild or moderate degrees of hyponatremia may be simply corrected by temporary restriction of water intake.

In the presence of hyperglycemia, determination of the glucose concentration is necessary to evaluate the significance of a depressed serum sodium level. Since glucose does not enter cells by passive diffusion, it exerts an osmotic force in the extracellular compartment. This contribution to osmotic pressure is normally small, but with an elevated glucose concentration, the increased osmotic pressure causes the transfer of cellular water into the extracellular compartment, resulting in a dilutional hyponatremia. Hyponatremia therefore may be observed when the total effective osmotic pressure in the extracellular compartment is normal or even above normal. In terms of tonicity, each 100 mg/100 ml rise in the blood glucose *above normal* is roughly equivalent to a 3 mEq/L rise in the serum sodium concentration. Consider a patient with a serum sodium concentration of 125 mEq/L and a blood glucose level of 500 mg/100 ml. The glucose level is approximately 400 mg/100 ml above normal, which is equivalent to a 12 mEq/L rise in the serum sodium level. Thus, 125 + 12 = 137 mEq/L; the tonicity is normal despite the marked reduction in sodium concentration. In this instance, therapy is directed toward lowering the blood glucose level. The sodium concentration will return toward normal as the excess water leaves the extracellular compartment. In practice, a true sodium deficit may be secondary to the underlying disorder and must be corrected.

HYPERNATREMIA. Hypernatremia (serum sodium concentration above 150 mEq/L), although uncommon, is a dangerous abnormality. In contradistinction to decreased serum sodium concentration, hypernatremia is easily produced when renal function is normal. The extracellular fluid hyperosmolarity results in a shift of intracellular water from within the cell to the extracellular fluid compartment; in this situation, a high serum sodium level may indicate a significant deficit of total body water. In surgical patients hypernatremia arises most often from excessive or unexpected water losses, although it may result from use of salt-containing solutions to replace water losses. The following classification of water losses may be helpful in preventing and treating this abnormality.

Excessive Extrarenal Water Losses. With increased metabolism from any cause, but particularly associated with fever, the water loss through evaporation of sweat may reach several liters daily. Patients with tracheostomy in dry environments can (with excessive minute volume air exchange) lose as much as 1 to 1.5 liters of water/day by this route. Increased water evaporation from a granulating surface is of significant magnitude in the thermally injured patient, and losses may be as great as 3 to 5 liters/day.

Increased Renal Water Losses. Extremely large volumes of solute-poor urine may result from hypoxic damage to the distal tubules and collecting ducts or loss of antidiuretic hormone stimulation from damage to the central nervous system. In both instances, facultative water resorption is impaired. The former occurs in high-output renal failure; in our experience, this is the most common type of renal failure following severe injury or operative trauma. The latter occurs with extensive head injuries accompanied by temporary diabetes insipidus.

Solute Loading. High protein intake may produce an increased osmotic load of urea, which necessitates the excretion of large volumes of water. Hypernatremia, azotemia, and extracellular fluid volume deficits follow. In general, these can be prevented by an intake of 7 ml of water/Gm of dietary protein.

Excessive glucose administration results in the need for a large volume of water for excretion. Osmotic diuretics such as mannitol and urea also result in the obligatory excretion of a large volume of water as well as increasing urinary sodium losses. In addition, isotonic salt solutions, if used to replace pure water losses, rapidly produce hypernatremia.

HIGH-OUTPUT RENAL FAILURE. Acute renal insufficiency following trauma or surgical stress is a highly lethal complication. The diagnosis is classically based on persistent oliguria and chemical evidence of uremia after stabilization of the circulation. The clinical course is characterized by oliguria lasting from several days to several weeks, followed by a progressive rise in daily urine volume until both the excretory and concentrating functions of the kidney are gradually restored.

Uremia, occurring without a period of oliguria and accompanied by a daily urine volume greater than 1,000 to 1,500 ml/day, is a more frequent but less well recognized entity. Clinical experience and laboratory experiments suggest that high-output renal failure represents the renal response to a less severe or modified episode of renal injury than that required to produce classic oliguric renal failure. Its importance lies in the fact that it is a milder form of renal insufficiency and that realization of its presence, by serial measurement of blood urea nitrogen and serum electrolytes, permits intelligent chemical and fluid volume management with a much greater latitude because of the daily urine volume excretion. Normal extracellular fluid volume and normal serum sodium concentration, therefore, are quite easily maintained when accurate daily outputs of each are obtained and replaced accordingly. The sodium-containing fluids may be administered as lactate to control the mild metabolic acidosis that occurs. Severe acidosis may develop if isotonic losses from the gastrointestinal tract or renal excretion of sodium are replaced with sodium chloride.

The chief dangers of high-output renal failure are failure to recognize its existence because of normal output, and the intravenous administration of potassium salts. Good urinary output and gastrointestinal involvement requiring suction usually indicate the need for daily potassium replacement. With this type of renal failure, however, potassium intoxication may be produced. As little as 20 mEq of potassium chloride given intravenously may rapidly produce myocardial potassium intoxication requiring resin or hemodialysis treatment.

The typical course of high-output renal failure begins without a period of oliguria. The daily urine volumes are normal or greater than normal, often reaching levels of 3 to 5 liters/day while blood urea nitrogen is increasing. An attempt to decrease urine output by water restriction rapidly results in hypernatremia without a change in urine volume. On the average, urea nitrogen continues to increase for 8 to 12 days before a downward trend occurs. The blood/urine urea ratio is about 1:10 until a decrease occurs in the blood urea concentration.

Functionally, the lesion is characterized by a glomerular filtration rate of less than 20 percent of normal and complete resistance to vasopressin for 1 to 3 weeks after the blood urea nitrogen has declined. During the next 6 to 8 weeks, the glomerular filtration rate gradually rises, and the response to vasopressin becomes normal. The early recognition of high-output renal failure by serial blood determinations of blood urea nitrogen is important. Failure to recognize its presence may result in death from hyperkalemia, hypernatremia, or acidosis. As alluded to previously, it is unwise to administer potassium during the first 24 postoperative hours unless a definite potassium deficit exists. This is particularly important in the patient

subjected to prolonged operative trauma involving one or more episodes of hypotension and in the patient with posttraumatic hemorrhagic hypotension.

NUTRITION IN THE SURGICAL PATIENT

The majority of patients undergoing elective surgical operations withstand the brief period of catabolism and starvation without noticeable difficulty. However, maintaining an adequate nutritional regimen may be of critical importance in managing seriously ill surgical patients with preexisting weight loss and depleted energy reserves. Between these two extremes are patients for whom nutritional support is not essential for life but may serve to shorten the postoperative recovery phase and minimize the number of complications. Not infrequently a patient may become ill or even die from complications secondary to starvation rather than the underlying disorder. Therefore, it is essential that the surgeon have a sound grasp of the fundamental metabolic changes associated with surgery, trauma, and sepsis and an awareness of the methods available to reverse or ameliorate these events.

Body Fuel Reserves

The body must mobilize appropriate nutrients from fuel reserves in order to withstand the necessary periods of partial or complete starvation and to meet the additional requirements imposed by surgery, trauma, or sepsis. The extent and availability of these reserves may be of critical importance for successful recovery from an illness. Available information concerning body fuel composition and the rate of fuel consumption in man has recently been reviewed by Cahill and is summarized below.

Carbohydrates, proteins, and fats are the three sources of fuel in man. Their relative contributions both by weight and caloric potential are illustrated in Fig. 2-3. Carbohydrate stores, primarily in the form of liver and muscle glycogen, are relatively small and could supply basal caloric requirements for less than 1 day. However, this relatively small quantity is absolutely essential in the emergency situation for the production of high-energy phosphates during anaerobic metabolism. Although glucose yields approximately 4 kcal/Gm, its storage as glycogen requires the addition of 1 or 2 Gm of intracellular water and electrolytes. Therefore it yields only 1 or 2 kcal/Gm of wet weight.

Protein represents a considerably larger source of fuel, but, as emphasized by Cahill, every molecule of protein in the body has a specific purpose, such as an enzyme, a structural component, or a contractile protein in muscle. Thus, any protein loss represents loss of an essential function. Additionally, the amount of total body protein is relatively fixed in the normal healthy individual, and any additional protein is metabolized, the excess calories being stored as fat. Protein, like glycogen, represents an inefficient energy source relative to its wet weight, since it exists in an aqueous environment.

In contrast to glycogen and protein, fat is stored in a

relatively anhydrous state. By weight, then, it is a relatively rich source of energy, supplying approximately 9 kcal/Gm. Most of the fat in the body serves as a readily available energy source; the few areas where fat serves a specific function (e.g., mechanical fat pads) are the last to be mobilized during starvation.

In summary, protein and fat are the only major sources of fuel. Total protein mass is relatively fixed in amount, and caloric excess or deficiency is met by an increase or decrease in the body's fat mass. Fat depots serve as sources of energy, protein stores represent *potential* sources of energy but only through the loss of some important function, and the small stores of carbohydrates are generally protected except for emergency use during anaerobic glycolysis.

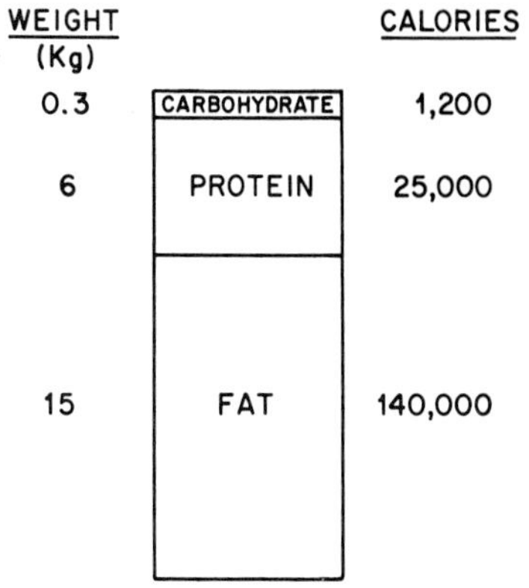

Starvation

During the first several days of complete starvation, caloric needs are supplied by body fat and proteins; the small glycogen reserve is largely spared. Previous studies have shown an obligatory loss of approximately 10 to 15 grams of nitrogen daily in the urine during this period, indicating the utilization of approximately 60 to 90 grams of protein (each gram of nitrogen represents approximately 6.25 grams of muscle protein). The majority of this protein, which is largely derived from skeletal muscle, is converted to glucose in the liver by the process of gluconeogenesis; most of this endogenously produced glucose is used by the brain. The remainder is used by certain tissues such as red blood cells and leukocytes which convert the glucose to lactate and pyruvate. These are returned to the liver and resynthesized into glucose (the Cori cycle). This obligatory nitrogen loss, then, reflects the use of amino acids derived from muscle protein for gluconeogenesis to supply glucose to the brain. No patient, however, should be allowed to starve completely. The administration of at least 100 Gm of glucose will obviate most of this gluconeogenesis and reduce the nitrogen loss by at least one-half—the well-known "protein-sparing effect" described by Gamble. Available evidence from Cahill indicates that this protein-sparing effect is regulated by insulin, which is released when exogenous glucose is infused for use by the brain. The slightly elevated insulin level reduces amino acid release from the muscle, amino acid extraction by the liver, and gluconeogenesis. In the diabetic with an absolute or relative lack of insulin, the infusion of glucose does not inhibit gluconeogenesis, and muscle breakdown to amino acids continues unabated. The liver derives its energy by oxidizing fatty acids to ketones, and the remainder of the body utilizes both fatty acids and ketones to meet caloric requirements. Generally a small quantity of the ketones is excreted into the urine.

If complete starvation continues for more than a few days, the obligatory nitrogen loss progressively decreases, as the brain begins to use fat as its fuel source. Unlike other body tissues, however, the brain cannot utilize free fatty acids, since they do not cross the blood-brain barrier. Instead, use of keto acids which are produced by the liver and readily cross the blood-brain barrier gradually dis-

Fig. 2-3. Body fuel composition in the normal individual. (*From G. F. Cahill, Jr., Bull Am Coll Surg, 55:12, 1970.*)

places the use of glucose by the brain. After prolonged starvation, the net effect of this adaptation to ketone utilization is a protein-sparing effect with reduction of urinary nitrogen excretion to approximately 4 Gm/day. This 4 Gm of nitrogen represents approximately 25 Gm of protein, or about 100 Gm of lean wet muscle. Thus, the normal individual with an average supply of fat and muscle may survive total starvation for several months. Insulin again may be the signal for the reduction in muscle catabolism and gluconeogenesis (coincident with the increased use of keto acids by the brain), according to Cahill. However, changes in the blood level of alanine, which is quantitatively one of the more important amino acids, may also play a role. A fall in the blood level of this amino acid appears to decrease gluconeogenesis and glucose production by the liver.

Surgery, Trauma, Sepsis

The sequence of metabolic and endocrine events occasioned by surgery, trauma, or sepsis may be divided into several phases. As pointed out by Moore (1960), the magnitude of the changes and the duration of each phase vary considerably and are directly related to the severity of the injury.

CATABOLIC PHASE. This phase has also been termed the *adrenergic-corticoid phase* since it corresponds to the period during which changes induced by adrenergic and adrenal corticoid hormones are most striking. Immediately following surgery or trauma, there is a sudden increase in metabolic demands and urinary excretion of nitrogen beyond the levels associated with simple starvation. The patient generally cannot eat, cannot lower his metabolic rate, and cannot effectively alter the source of endogenous fuels to spare protein utilization. This is in distinct contrast to events in the normal individual subjected to prolonged starvation, where most body tissues use fat as their main source of fuel, thereby sparing protein. Trauma apparently results in a continued and excessive mobilization of protein; unfortunately, the administration of moderate amounts of glucose to these individuals produces little or no change in the rate of protein catabolism. The exact

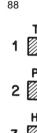

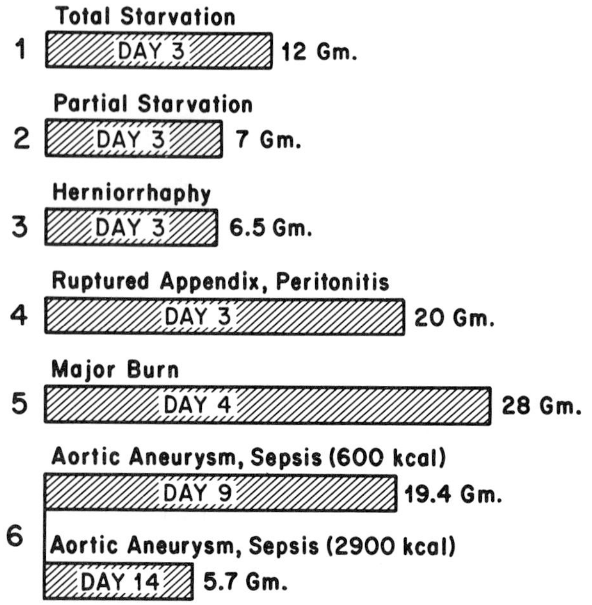

Total Starvation

1 DAY 3 12 Gm.

Partial Starvation

2 DAY 3 7 Gm.

Herniorrhaphy

3 DAY 3 6.5 Gm.

Ruptured Appendix, Peritonitis

4 DAY 3 20 Gm.

Major Burn

5 DAY 4 28 Gm.

Aortic Aneurysm, Sepsis (600 kcal)

DAY 9 19.4 Gm.

6 Aortic Aneurysm, Sepsis (2900 kcal)

DAY 14 5.7 Gm.

Fig. 2-4. The extent of negative nitrogen balance in adult patients during starvation alone and during various surgical illnesses associated with partial starvation. Note the difference in negative nitrogen balance in case 6 with low and high calorie parenteral supplementation. (*Cases 1 to 4 from W. D. Holden et al., Ann Surg, 146:563, 1957. Case 5 from J. M. Kinney, "Proceedings of a Conference on Energy Metabolism and Body Fuel Utilization," Harvard University Press, Cambridge, 1966. Case 6 from L. J. Lawson, Br J Surg, 52: 795, 1965.*)

stimulus for this continued protein utilization is not known at the present time, although it is not thought to be due to any of the presently known hormones such as adrenocortical steroids or insulin.

The reasons for this selective and extensive protein mobilization and use are also obscure. Kinney has shown that the modest increase in oxygen consumption cannot account for the extra energy requirements. It has been postulated that the reparative tissues themselves may be responsible, since it is known that polymorphonuclear leukocytes and immature fibroblasts use glucose as their main source of energy. Since the availability of oxygen in the area of injury may be limited due to inadequate perfusion, McMinn has suggested that these tissues may require glucose for anaerobic metabolism to lactate as the only energy source. Regardless of the cause, the stimulus for continued hypermetabolism remains and is not affected by the administration of exogenous glucose.

The extent of the negative nitrogen balance in these patients varies considerably and is largely related to the magnitude of the injury. In Fig. 2-4 daily net nitrogen losses during simple starvation with and without the administration of glucose are compared to losses sustained with moderate to severe surgical illness.

EARLY ANABOLIC PHASE. After several days or weeks, depending on the severity of injury, the body turns from a catabolic to an anabolic phase. This turning point, also known as the *corticoid-withdrawal phase*, is characterized by a sharp decline in nitrogen excretion and restoration

of a positive potassium balance. Generally, this transition period lasts no more than a day or two.

The prolonged anabolic phase may last from a few weeks to a few months and generally coincides with the resumption of oral intake. Nitrogen balance is positive, indicating synthesis of proteins, and there is a rapid and progressive gain in weight and muscular strength. The patient is usually active, has an excellent appetite, and generally is discharged from the hospital at this point. Positive nitrogen balance reaches a maximum of approximately 4 Gm/day, which represents the synthesis of approximately 25 Gm of protein and the gain of over 100 Gm of lean body mass/day. The total amount of nitrogen gain will ultimately equal the amount lost during the catabolic phase, although the rate of gain will be much slower than the rate of initial loss.

LATE ANABOLIC PHASE. The final period of convalescence or the late anabolic phase may last from several weeks to several months after a severe injury. This phase is associated with the gradual gain of fatty tissue as the previously positive nitrogen balance declines towards normal. Weight gain is much slower during this phase because of the higher caloric content of fat and can be realized only if intake is in excess of caloric expenditure. In most individuals, the phase ends with a gradual return to the previously normal body weight. The patient who is partially immobilized during this period of time, however, may exhibit a marked gain in weight due to decreased energy expenditure.

Base-Line Requirements

The normal caloric and protein requirements for individuals leading a sedentary life approximate 1 Gm of protein and 35 kcal/kg of body weight, or approximately 1400 kcal/m² of body surface area per day. These requirements, which have been recommended by the Food and Nutritional Board of the National Research Council, vary with age, sex, and the degree of daily activity.

These base-line requirements are totally inadequate for patients who have undergone surgery or who have suffered severe trauma or sepsis. The exact caloric and nitrogen requirements necessary to maintain an individual in balance after severe injury are unknown. However, guidelines for nutritional supplementation based on previous experimental data and clinical experience have been recommended. Moore has suggested that intakes in the region of 0.2 Gm of nitrogen/kg and 50 kcal/kg/day are necessary to maintain constant weight after moderate injury. Studies by Kinney suggest that a moderately positive caloric balance (1000 to 2000 kcal/day above resting expenditure) with a calorie-to-nitrogen ratio of approximately 150:200 may be appropriate for acutely ill surgical patients. Similarly, Dudrick et al. have noted that the average depleted or complicated major surgical patient requires between 2500 and 4000 kcal/day with approximately 12 to 24 Gm of nitrogen. These approximations are useful, although the quantity and composition of the nutrients must be tailored to meet individual needs.

The requirements for vitamins and essential trace minerals usually can be easily met in the average patient with an uncomplicated postoperative course, and vitamins usually are not given in the absence of preoperative deficiencies. The exception is vitamin C, essential for wound healing, which can be given orally or by subcutaneous or intravenous routes. The intravenous administration of vitamin C is associated with a large urinary loss, but since it is relatively nontoxic, large amounts (300 to 500 mg daily) can be given. Patients maintained on elemental diets or parenteral hyperalimentation require complete vitamin and mineral supplementation. Several commercial preparations are available for intravenous or intramuscular use, although most do not contain vitamin K and some do not contain vitamin B_{12} or folic acid. These, along with essential trace minerals, may be added to the mixture or given by other routes.

Indications and Methods for Nutritional Support

The selection of patients who require partial or complete nutritional support has become increasingly important. The ability to provide complete nutritional support in the starving patient and to counteract the nitrogen losses in catabolic states with elemental diets or parenteral hyperalimentation represents a substantial contribution. However, it should be emphasized that the majority of surgical patients do not require special nutritional regimens. The reasonably well-nourished and otherwise healthy individual who undergoes an uncomplicated major surgical procedure has sufficient body fuel reserves to withstand the catabolic insult and partial starvation for at least 1 week. Adequate quantities of parenteral fluids with appropriate electrolyte composition and a minimum of 100 Gm of glucose daily to minimize protein catabolism will be all that is necessary in most patients. Assuming that the patient has a relatively uncomplicated postoperative course and resumes normal oral intake at the end of this period, elemental diets or parenteral hyperalimentation are unnecessary and probably inadvisable because of the associated risks. During the early anabolic phase, the patient must be provided with an adequate caloric intake of proper composition to meet the energy needs of the body and allow protein synthesis. A high calorie-to-nitrogen ratio (optimal ratio approximately 200 kcal/Gm nitrogen) and an adequate supply of vitamins and minerals are necessary for maximum anabolism during this period.

In contrast to this group, there is a small but significant number of surgical patients for whom an adequate nutritional regimen may be of critical importance for a successful outcome. This category includes preoperative patients who are chronically debilitated from their diseases or malnutrition and patients who have suffered trauma, sepsis, or surgical complications and cannot maintain an adequate caloric intake for any number of reasons.

The methods for partial or complete nutritional supplementation in the surgical patient fall into three general categories: Nasopharyngeal, gastrostomy, and jejunostomy tube feedings are appropriate routes for alimentation in patients who have a relatively normal gastrointestinal tract but cannot or will not eat. Elemental diets may be administered by similar routes when bulk and fat-free nutrients requiring minimal digestion are indicated. Finally, parenteral hyperalimentation may be used for supplementation in the patient with limited oral intake or, more commonly, for complete nutritional management in the absence of oral intake.

NASOPHARYNGEAL TUBE FEEDING

Nasopharyngeal feedings, preferably through small, soft plastic tubes, should be used only in alert patients who are unable or unwilling to eat normally for various reasons; it is contraindicated in most other cases. The foremost contraindication for nasopharyngeal tube feeding is unconsciousness or lack of protective laryngeal reflexes, which may result in fatal pulmonary complications due to tracheal aspiration of regurgitated gastric content. Even with a tracheostomy, it is inadvisable to feed mentally obtunded patients via nasopharyngeal tubes, since such feedings often can be recovered from tracheostomy suction, indicating continued aspiration of gastric content even around a snugly fitting tracheostomy tube. An inflated tracheostomy tube cuff might prevent this, but the required constant inflation is inadvisable since it may cause pressure necrosis of the trachea. Furthermore, the prolonged use of a nasopharyngeal tube may cause severe discomfort, nasopharyngeal and laryngeal pressure necrosis, and esophagitis with stricture.

Pharyngeal tube feedings are often indicated for patients with oropharyngeal tumor; irritation may be prevented by inserting the tube into the pyriform sinus, as recommended by Graham and Royster. This technique also allows concealment of the feeding tube under the patient's clothing.

The nasopharyngeal tube may allow feeding beyond dysfunctional gastric stomas and high gastrointestinal fistulas. In such cases, it may be possible to maintain nutrition without a jejunostomy tube until stomal dysfunction relents or the fistula heals. This may be done by passing a Cantor tube or, preferably, a small polyethylene feeding tube weighted with a rubber finger cot filled with 1 ml of mercury distal to the faulty stoma or fistula, as recommended by Bachrach and Tecimer. The polyethylene feeding tube is prepared by passing a #1 silk thread through the tube with a wire. The mercury-filled finger cot is tied to the silk thread distad and the thread fixed to the tube proximally. The tube is then inserted through the nose into the stomach, and the patient is positioned so that the mercury weight tends to lead the small tube well into the jejunum. When the tube reaches the proper position (as noted on x-ray after the injection of a small amount of water-soluble opaque medium), the silk string is released proximally, and peristalsis carries the mercury-weighted finger cot and thread distad until they are passed per rectum. Feedings are started after a few hours when the string has cleared the tube. This small, flexible plastic tube and mercury weight may be more readily introduced into the intestine than the bulkier, more rigid, long intestinal tubes and is more conducive to patient comfort. More recently, Davis and Hofmann have described the use of a small, soft Penrose drain for a nasogastric feeding tube.

Experience indicates that this may minimize esophagitis and tracheal aspiration from gastric reflux.

GASTROSTOMY TUBE FEEDING

The administration of blended food through a gastrostomy tube is a good method for feeding patients with a variety of chronic gastrointestinal lesions arising at or above the cardioesophageal junction. However, gastrostomy tube feedings are contraindicated for mentally obtunded patients with inadequate laryngeal reflexes. This feeding method should be used only in alert patients or in patients with total obstruction of the distal esophagus.

Generally, gastrostomies of the Stamm (serosa-lined, temporary) or modified Glassman (mucosa-lined, permanent) type are constructed. The feeding mixture may be ordinarily prepared food converted by a blender into a semiliquid. Hyperosmolarity of the feeding formula is not generally a problem as long as the pylorus is intact. The jejunostomy formula outlined below also may be used.

JEJUNOSTOMY TUBE FEEDING

Jejunostomy tube feedings are generally required for patients in whom nasopharyngeal or gastrostomy tube feedings are contraindicated, e.g., comatose patients or patients with high gastrointestinal fistulas or obstructions. The jejunostomy may be of the Roux en Y (permanent) or the Witzel (temporary) type. The latter is constructed by inserting a #18 French rubber catheter into the proximal jejunum approximately 12 in. distal to the ligament of Treitz. The wall of the jejunum is inverted over the tube for about 3 cm as it emerges from the bowel to create a serosa-lined tunnel which allows rapid sealing of the jejunal opening when the tube is removed. The tube may then be brought out through a stab wound in the left upper quadrant of the abdomen. The jejunum is sutured to the anterior abdominal wall at the point of tube entry to seal it from the peritoneal cavity.

If the jejunostomy tube is inadvertently removed, blind attempts at reinsertion are contraindicated. If discovered within a few hours, the tube may be reinserted under fluoroscopic control to be sure it is in the bowel before feedings are resumed. The patient is observed for signs of peritonitis for 12 to 18 hours after feedings are restarted. If there is any doubt about the position of the tube, it should be replaced surgically. Feedings are safely begun 12 to 18 hours after jejunostomy construction, even though peristalsis is not audible. A progressive regimen of feeding modified from that recommended by Zollinger is preferable (Table 2-9). The full-strength formula suitable for most patients is simply a mixture of 1.5 cups of powdered milk, 1 qt of homogenized milk, and 1 ml of Tween 40 (an emulsifying agent allowing better fat absorption). This mixture contains about 1 kcal/ml, and, when given in the final volume recommended in Table 2-9, provides about 2500 kcal, 140 Gm of protein, and adequate carbohydrates. The fat content represents less than 4 percent of the total. Polyvisol and Fer-in-sol, 0.6 ml each, are added once daily to the formula. Many of the more complex jejunostomy feedings are difficult to prepare, likely to spoil before use,

Table 2-9. JEJUNOSTOMY FEEDING REGIMEN

1. 12–18 hours after jejunostomy—nothing.
2. First day—50 ml/hr × 20 of 5% dextrose/water.
3. Second day—100 ml/hr × 20 of 5% dextrose/water.
4. Third day—50 ml/hr × 20 of homogenized milk.
5. Fourth day—100 ml/2hr × 10 of homogenized milk.
6. Fifth day—180 ml/2hr × 10 of homogenized milk.
7. Sixth day—240 ml/2hr × 10 of homogenized milk.
8. Continue same regimen as on sixth day but add an additional half cup of powdered milk to each quart of homogenized milk daily until 1.5 cups per quart of homogenized milk is being used as feeding formula. Thereafter, give 240 ml of this mixture q. 2 h. × 10 daily. Feedings should begin at 6 A.M. and continue through 12 midnight. Additional water may be given between feedings when indicated.

too high in fat content, and excessively hyperosmolar, leading to a greater incidence of patient intolerance.

With proper care, about 85 percent of jejunostomy patients tolerate their feedings. Diarrhea is usually controlled if the concentration and volume of formula are temporarily reduced. Failing this, feeding is halted for a day, then resumed from the beginning of the feeding regimen, progressing somewhat more slowly than before. If mild diarrhea or cramping persists, a pulverized Lomotil tablet or 8 to 10 drops of tincture of belladonna may be given through the tube 30 minutes prior to formula infusion. At times it may be necessary to give 5 ml paregoric 15 to 30 minutes before the formula to control cramping and diarrhea, but this should be employed sparingly and for as short a period as possible. In many cases, symptoms are relieved if the rate and volume of infusion are reduced and cold formula avoided. Each feeding should be infused in about 20 minutes.

If the patient with a jejunostomy has a proximal bowel or biliary fistula draining more than 300 ml daily for prolonged periods, the fistular drainage may be collected by sump suction, cooled in an ice basin at bedside, and promptly refed in small increments throughout the day. To avoid jejunal overloading, the fistular fluid is refed between formula feedings. It is not advisable to refeed aspirated gastric juice, for this may cause jejunal irritation and profuse diarrhea. If the fistular drainage is profuse, it is usually not possible to refeed more than 2 liters/day, and fluid and electrolyte losses must be replaced by appropriate intravenous supplements. Additional water may be given with the feedings or administered between the feedings as indicated. Occasionally, an elemental diet, as discussed below, may be indicated when other jejunostomy formulas are not tolerated.

ELEMENTAL DIETS

Clinical experience with chemically formulated bulk-free elemental diets has been limited, but encouraging. These diets may be used for complete nutritional support or as dietary supplements for patients who are unable to eat or digest enough food to meet their energy requirements. They may be preferable to high-caloric parenteral feedings for patients who have at least part of the small bowel available for the absorption of simple sugars and amino acids. As outlined by Randall et al., elemental diets have been found useful for patients with depleted protein reserves secondary to gastrointestinal tract disease, such as ulcerative or granulomatous colitis and malabsorption syndrome; for patients with only partial function of the gastrointestinal tract, such as the short bowel syndrome, gastric or small bowel fistulas with feeding distal to the fistula; and for patients with accelerated metabolic states, such as multiple trauma or severe burns. The diets also have been used during preoperative bowel preparation and in place of ordinary jejunostomy feedings when the latter cannot be tolerated.

Elemental diets differ from conventional foods in that they are formulated synthetically out of known chemical nutrients, such as purified amino acids and simple carbohydrates. As commercially prepared, these diets also contain base-line electrolytes, water- and fat-soluble vitamins (except vitamin K), and trace minerals. They contain no bulk and therefore produce a minimum of residue. The compositions of three elemental diets which are currently available are shown in Table 2-10. The diets with lower protein content may be taken orally or by tube, while the diet with higher protein content is unpalatable and intended primarily for tube feeding. Unfortunately, patient acceptance of the flavored diets has been only fair, and they frequently must be given by tube.

The amount of elemental diet required to maintain weight and nitrogen balance varies with the individual

Table 2-10. ELEMENTAL DIETS*
Approximate composition per 1,800 ml†

	W-T low-residue Food	Vivonex-100	Vivonex-100 HN (high-nitrogen)
Kilocalories....	1800	1800	1800
Carbohydrates Gm......	408 (dextrin)	407 (glucose)	379
Protein, Gm ...	39	37	75
Nitrogen, Gm ..	5.4	5.9	12
Fat, Gm	1.3	1.3	0.8
Sodium, mEq ..	100	104	60
Potassium, mEq	54	54	32
Chloride, mEq..	151	128	94
Calcium, mEq ..	50	40	24
Magnesium mEq	33	13	17
Osmolality, mOsm/L....	650	1175	844

*All diets contain standard fat and water-soluble vitamins for normal daily requirements (based on 2000 kcal) and essential trace minerals. Contain only minimal quantities of vitamin K, which should be supplemented to the full therapeutic level. Additional quantities of B vitamins and vitamin C should also be added.

†Six 80-Gm packets diluted with water to a total of 1,800 ml.
SOURCE: VIVONEX-100, Eaton Laboratories, Norwich, N.Y.; W-I Low Residue Food, Warren-Teed Pharmaceuticals, Inc., Columbus, Ohio.

patient. In severe catabolic states the standard diet often fails to achieve positive nitrogen balance. The following guidelines are based on those recommended by Randall. For oral feedings, the diets are made up in standard dilution (25% weight/volume) and provide 1 kcal/ml of solution. The solution is cooled and ingested in small amounts of 100 to 150 ml at a time. Approximately 2,000 ml or more may be taken in a day, providing approximately 2000 kcal and 40 Gm of protein. Depending on patient tolerance, the volume of diet may be increased as indicated.

Either the high- or low-protein diets may be used for intragastric or jejunostomy tube feedings initially. The diet is mixed at half the standard dilution (12.5% weight/volume or less) and administered continuously by pump or gravity drip at a rate of 40 to 50 ml/hour. Once the individual has adjusted to the diet, the concentration may be gradually increased to the standard dilution and the volume increased in small increments until the desired caloric and protein intake is achieved. The development of nausea, vomiting, or diarrhea is an indication to slow or stop the infusion for a short period of time. The feeding may then be restarted at a slower rate or at a lower concentration. Lomotil tablets, tincture of belladonna, or paregoric may be indicated to control diarrhea as discussed previously. Using the high-protein diet, as much as 3000 ml/day may be administered, providing approximately 3000 kcal and 20 Gm of nitrogen.

Careful attention to water and electrolyte balance is mandatory, particularly when large quantities of fluid are being lost through fistulas or other routes. Additional sodium and potassium may be added to the mixture (not to exceed a total of 100 mEq), although they should be given in intravenous fluids when larger quantities are needed. Water may be added to the mixture in the face of excessive pure water losses.

Complications include nausea, vomiting, and diarrhea which develop because of the high osmolarity of the diets. This generally can be controlled by decreasing the rate and/or concentration of the mixture. Hypertonic nonketotic coma may occur in the presence of excessive water losses or if the diets are administered at concentrations above those recommended. Hyperglycemia and glycosuria may occur in any severely ill patient, particularly latent diabetics, and insulin may be indicated. Aspiration is a constant threat with intragastric feedings; for this reason, this route should not be used in the absence of laryngeal reflexes or in mentally obtunded patients.

PARENTERAL ALIMENTATION

The parenteral route for nutritional supplementation when oral or tube feedings into the gastrointestinal tract are not feasible has been tried for several decades but until recently has fallen short of expectations. Parenteral infusion of 5% dextrose solutions is totally inadequate to meet caloric requirements within the limits of fluid tolerance, while the use of hypertonic solutions of dextrose, fructose, or invert sugar has been limited by a high incidence of thrombophlebitis. The use of plasma and blood for nutritional supplementation is mentioned only to be condemned; they are very expensive and inefficient sources of calories, and their administration is associated with an unnecessary number of complications. High-caloric solutions, such as ethyl alcohol (7 kcal/Gm) and fat (9 kcal/Gm) have found limited use, although a satisfactory fat emulsion for clinical use is not presently available in this country.

Recently, Dudrick et al. have demonstrated the clinical practicality of providing complete nutritional needs for an extended period of time using high-caloric parenteral feedings. Parenteral hyperalimentation involves the continuous infusion of a highly concentrated solution containing carbohydrates, proteins, and other necessary nutrients through an indwelling catheter inserted into the superior vena cava. In order to obtain the maximum benefit, the ratio of calories to nitrogen must be adequate (at least 150 kcal/Gm nitrogen), and the two materials must be infused simultaneously. When the sources of calories and nitrogen are given at different times, there is a significant decrease in nitrogen utilization. These nutrients can be given in quantities considerably greater than the basic caloric and nitrogen requirements, and this method has proved to be highly successful in achieving growth and development, positive nitrogen balance, and weight gain in a variety of clinical situations. Unfortunately, intravenous hyperalimentation has not yet been shown to reverse the early catabolic response to surgery, trauma, or sepsis, although it has effectively minimized the level of negative nitrogen balance.

INDICATIONS FOR THE USE OF INTRAVENOUS HYPERALIMENTATION. The principal indications for parenteral hyperalimentation are found in seriously ill patients suffering from malnutrition, sepsis, or surgical or accidental trauma when use of the gastrointestinal tract for feedings is not possible. The safe and successful use of this regimen requires proper selection of patients with specific nutritional needs, experience with the technique, and an awareness of the associated complications. The number of reported complications has increased significantly since this technique has become more popular; it has been used in many instances either where it is not needed or where use of the gastrointestinal tract is more appropriate. For this reason, Dudrick et al. have recently outlined specific goals and indications for parenteral hyperalimentation, listed below:

1. Newborn infants with catastrophic gastrointestinal anomalies, such as tracheoesophageal fistula, gastroschisis, omphalocele, or massive intestinal atresia
2. Infants who fail to thrive nonspecifically or secondarily to gastrointestinal insufficiency associated with the short bowel syndrome, malabsorption, enzyme deficiency, meconium ileus, or idiopathic diarrhea
3. Adult patients with short-bowel syndrome secondary to massive small bowel resection or enteroenteric, enterocolic, enterovesical, or enterocutaneous fistulas
4. Patients with high alimentary tract obstructions without vascular compromise, secondary to achalasia, stricture, or neoplasia of the esophagus; gastric carcinoma; or pyloric obstruction
5. Surgical patients with prolonged paralytic ileus following major operations, multiple injuries, or blunt or open abdominal trauma, or patients with reflex ileus complicating various medical diseases

6. Patients with normal bowel length but with malabsorption secondary to sprue, hypoproteinemia, enzyme or pancreatic insufficiency, regional enteritis, or ulcerative colitis
7. Adult patients with functional gastrointestinal disorders such as esophageal dyskinesia following cerebral vascular accident, idiopathic diarrhea, psychogenic vomiting, anorexia nervosa, or hyperemesis gravidarum
8. Patients who cannot ingest food or who regurgitate and aspirate oral or tube feedings because of depressed or obtunded sensorium following severe metabolic derangements, neurologic disorders, intracranial surgery, or central nervous system trauma
9. Patients with excessive metabolic requirements secondary to severe trauma, such as extensive full-thickness burns, major fractures, or soft tissue injuries
10. Patients with granulomatous colitis, ulcerative colitis, and tuberculous enteritis, in which major portions of the absorptive mucosa are diseased
11. Paraplegics, quadriplegics, or debilitated patients with indolent decubitus ulcers in the pelvic areas, particularly when soilage and fecal contamination are a problem
12. Patients who will eventually require surgery but in whom prolonged progressive malnutrition has greatly increased the risk of operation
13. Patients in whom protein deficiency states are to be avoided, reduced, or corrected

Conditions *contraindicating* hyperalimentation include the following:

1. Lack of a specific goal for patient management, or where instead of extending a meaningful life, inevitable dying is prolonged.
2. Periods of cardiovascular instability or severe metabolic derangement requiring control or correction before attempting hypertonic intravenous feeding.
3. Feasible gastrointestinal tract feeding. In the vast majority of instances, this is the best route by which to provide nutrition.
4. Patients in good nutritional status, in whom only short-term parenteral nutrition support is required or anticipated.
5. Infants with less than 8 cm of small bowel, since virtually all have been unable to adapt sufficiently despite prolonged periods of parenteral nutrition. Intravenous hyperalimentation must be seriously questioned until bowel transplantation has been perfected for these neonates.
6. Patients who are irreversibly decerebrate or otherwise dehumanized.

INSERTION OF CENTRAL VENOUS INFUSION CATHETER. The successful use of intravenous hyperalimentation generally depends upon the proper placement and management of the central venous feeding catheter. A 16-gauge, 8- or 12-in. radiopaque catheter is introduced percutaneously through the subclavian or internal jugular vein and threaded into the superior vena cava. Although the technique for subclavian vein puncture advocated by Dudrick and others has been quite popular, the internal jugular approach as described by Jernigan et al. has been equally satisfactory (Figs. 2-5 and 2-6).

For insertion of the intravenous catheter through the subclavian vein, the patient is placed on his back in a 15° head-down position with a small pad placed between the shoulder blades to allow the shoulders to drop posteriorly. This allows expansion of the subclavian vein and easier penetration. The skin is scrubbed with ether or acetone to defat the surface and then with an iodophor compound. Drapes are carefully placed, and *scrupulous* aseptic precautions are observed. Local anesthetic is infiltrated into the skin, subcutaneous tissue, and periosteum at the inferior border of the midpoint of the clavicle. A 2-in.-long, 14-gauge needle attached to a small syringe is inserted, beveled down through the wheal, and advanced toward the tip of the operator's finger, which is pressed well into the patient's suprasternal notch. The needle should hug the inferior clavicular surface and go over the first rib into the subclavian vein. With slight negative pressure applied to the syringe, entrance into the vein will be noted by the appearance of blood. The needle is advanced a few millimeters further to be sure that it is entirely within the lumen of the vein. The patient is asked to perform a Valsalva maneuver, or the thumb is held over the needle hub as the syringe is removed. A 16-gauge, 8- or 12-in. radiopaque catheter is then introduced through the needle and threaded into the superior vena cava. The needle is then withdrawn from the patient, and a small plastic splint is fitted over the junction of the catheter and needle to prevent catheter severance by the needle. The catheter is connected to a sterile intravenous administration tubing, and a slow infusion is begun while the catheter is sewn to the skin with a small synthetic suture. Antibiotic ointment is applied around the entrance of the catheter into the skin, and an occlusive dressing is applied over it including the junction of the intravenous tubing with the catheter. A chest film is immediately obtained to confirm the position of the radiopaque catheter in the vena cava and to check for a possible pneumothorax.

Every 2 or 3 days, the intravenous tubing is changed, the catheter site is scrubbed as for an operative procedure, and antibiotic ointment and a new occlusive dressing are applied. In general, withdrawal or administration of blood through the catheter or the use of the catheter for central venous pressure measurements should be avoided, since the risk of contamination and catheter occlusion are significantly increased.

The use of the internal jugular approach has also been quite satisfactory and is probably the preferred technique for the pediatric age group. It is probably unwise, unless absolutely necessary, to place catheters into the inferior vena cava from the lower extremities because of the greater likelihood of sepsis and thromboembolic phenomena. Additionally, cut-down catheter insertions into the cephalic or basilic veins have not proved satisfactory.

PREPARATION AND ADMINISTRATION OF SOLUTIONS. The basic solution contains approximately 20% dextrose and 5% protein hydrolysate or crystalline amino acids in water. The solution may be prepared in bulk quantities by the pharmacist, or individual units can be prepared from available parenteral solutions under strict aseptic conditions. Commercially available kits containing the component solutions and transfer apparatus simplify the mixing procedure and reduce the possibility of contamination. Proper preparation and administration of these solutions are essential to avoid unnecessary complications. The following techniques and guidelines are based on those recommended by Dudrick and colleagues:

To prepare an individual unit, 750 ml of 5% protein hydrolysate (or crystalline amino acids) in 5% dextrose

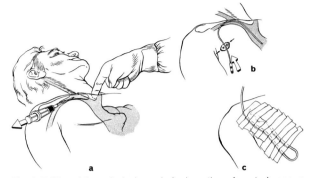

Fig. 2-5. Use of the subclavian vein for insertion of central venous catheter.

solution is mixed with 350 ml of 50% dextrose in water. This 1,100-ml mixture provides approximately 1000 kcal, 212 Gm of glucose, and 37 Gm of protein hydrolysates, equivalent to approximately 5.25 Gm of nitrogen (Table 2-11). Electrolytes, vitamins, and other micronutrients are added as required immediately prior to infusion.

For the average adult patient without significant cardiac, renal, or hepatic disease, approximately 40 mEq of potassium (as chloride and/or phosphate) and 50 mEq of sodium (as chloride and/or bicarbonate) are added to each liter of solution. The choice of sodium chloride or sodium bicarbonate depends on the acid-base status of the patient; in addition, part or all of the sodium should be added as bicarbonate when using base solutions of crystalline amino acids, since they already contain 35 to 50 mEq of chloride/L. These are only average recommended amounts of electrolytes to be added initially, and they will vary considerably in the individual patient. Daily serum electrolytes studies should be obtained in the first few days and frequently thereafter so that electrolyte content of the solutions can be altered appropriately. An intravenous preparation of fat- and water-soluble vitamins (e.g., MVI) should be added to any one bottle of the solution daily. This does not contain vitamin K, which should be given by subcutaneous injections—usually 10 mg three times a week. In addition, vitamin B_{12} and folic acid may be given weekly in required doses. Magnesium sulfate, 12 to 24

Fig. 2-6. Use of internal jugular vein for insertion of central venous catheter.

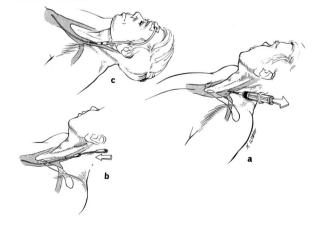

Table 2-11. PREPARATION OF HYPERALIMENTATION
SOLUTION, SINGLE-UNIT METHOD

350 ml 50% glucose *plus* 750 ml 5% glucose in 5% fibrin hydrolysate	Additions to only 1 unit daily (average adult):

Aseptic mixing technique under laminar-flow filtered-air hood:		Vitamin A . .	5,000–10,000 U.S.P. units
		Vitamin D . .	500–1,000 U.S.P. units
		Vitamin E . .	2.5–5.0 I.U.
Volume	1,100 ml	Vitamin C . .	250–500 mg
Calories	1,000 kcal	Thiamine . .	25–50 mg
Glucose	212 gm	Riboflavin . .	5–10 mg
Hydrolysates	37 gm	Pyroxidine . .	7.5–15 mg
Nitrogen	5.25 gm	Niacin	50–100 mg
Sodium	7 mEq	Pantothenic acid 12.5–25 mg	
Potassium	13 mEq		

ADDITIONS TO EACH UNIT OF BASE SOLUTION (Average Adult)	Optional additions to 1 unit (*Alternately May be Given in Daily or Weekly Dosages*)	
	Vitamin K	5–10 mg
	Vitamin B$_{12}$	10–30 μg
Sodium (chloride or	Folic acid	0.5–1.5 mg
bicarbonate) . . . . 40–50 mEq	Iron	2.0–3.0 mg
Potassium (chloride or	Calcium (gluconate)	4.5–9 mEq
phosphate) . . . . 30–40 mEq	Phosphate (potassium acid	
Magnesium (sulfate) . . . . . . 4–8 mEq	salt)	4–10 mEq

SOURCE: From S. J. Dudrick et al., General Principles and Techniques of Intravenous Hyperalimentation, in G. S. M. Cowan and W. L. Scheetz (eds.), "Intravenous Hyperalimentation,"
Chap. 1, Lea & Febiger, Philadelphia, 1972.

mEq/day, may be added to any one bottle of the solutions or divided equally in the total fluid allotment. Generally, 4 to 5 mEq of calcium and phosphorus may be added to each liter of fibrin hydrolysate or crystalline amino acid solution. The amounts vary in the individual patient, and serum levels of calcium and phosphorus should be determined at weekly intervals. If *casein* hydrolysate solutions are used, phosphorus should not be added, since these solutions already contain adequate phosphorus and severe hyperphosphatemia may occur. Iron may be given as indicated. After the patient has been on this regimen for over a month, replacement of essential trace minerals may be assured if 1 or 2 units of plasma are administered weekly.

The infusion is started at 1 to 2 liters/day in the average adult and gradually increased to tolerance (3 to 4 liters/day). Rarely, additional intravenous fluids and electrolytes may be necessary with continued abnormal large losses of fluids. Ideally, the patient should be in an intensive care unit for careful monitoring of both patient and infusion. Vital signs, central venous pressure, and urinary output are regularly observed, and the patient should be weighed daily. Frequent adjustments of the volume and composition of the solutions are necessary during the course of therapy. Electrolytes are drawn daily until stable and every 2 or 3 days thereafter, and the hemogram and blood urea nitrogen are determined weekly.

The urine sugar level is checked every 6 hours and blood sugar concentration at least once daily during the first few days of the infusion and at frequent intervals thereafter. Relative glucose intolerance may occur following initiation of parenteral hyperalimentation, and blood sugar levels may rise as high as 400 mg/100 ml or more. Subsequently, blood sugar levels usually fall toward normal, urine sugar

levels become negative to 2+, and insulin is not required in most cases. To avoid excessive glycosuria, the infusion is maintained at a rate which will not allow urinary glucose level to exceed a 3+ reaction. However, if blood sugar levels remain elevated or urine sugar levels again become 3 or 4+, insulin may be given subcutaneously as follows: 4+ urine sugar—10 units; 3+—5 units; 2+ to 0—no insulin; blood sugar 200 mg/100 ml—10 units; 150 mg/100 ml—5 units. Insulin should not be added routinely to the infusion fluid, since the initial rise in blood glucose level is generally temporary as the normal pancreas increases its output of insulin in response to the continuous carbohydrate infusion. In all patients with diabetes mellitus, crystalline insulin is given routinely by subcutaneous injection.

The administration of adequate amounts of potassium is essential to achieve positive nitrogen balance and replace depleted intracellular stores. In addition, a significant shift of potassium ion from the extracellular to the intracellular space may take place because of the large glucose infusion, with resultant hypokalemia, metabolic alkalosis, and poor glucose utilization. In some cases as much as 240 mEq of potassium ion daily may be required. Hypokalemia may cause glycosuria, which would be treated with potassium, not insulin. Thus, before giving insulin, the serum potassium level must be checked to avoid compounding the hypokalemia.

Often the blood urea nitrogen level rises, even in patients with a normal renal function, but this should not contraindicate giving the solution if the elevation is moderate, does not continue to rise sharply, and does not rise over approximately 80 mg/100 ml. Until greater experience is acquired, standard protein hydrolysate solutions should be used cautiously, if at all, for patients with more than moderate hepatic or renal dysfunction. The large amount of nitrogen may induce hepatic coma or increase uremic problems in these patients. More recently, however, Wilmore and Dudrick have demonstrated the safety and efficacy of parenteral hyperalimentation in patients with renal failure and some forms of hepatic disease. For this purpose, a special solution of essential L-amino acids is infused together with hypertonic dextrose in a volume within the daily fluid allowance of an oliguric patient.

There is usually a delay of about a week before weight gain and positive nitrogen balance become apparent; the patient then may gain as much as $\frac{1}{2}$ to 1 lb daily. After several days, one frequently notes marked improvement in the patient's general appearance and healing of previously indolent wounds and intestinal fistulas. Dramatic recovery often ensues, whereas formerly death from inanition inexorably occurred.

COMPLICATIONS. One of the more common and serious complications associated with long-term parenteral feeding is sepsis secondary to contamination of the solution, administration tubing, or the central venous catheter. This problem occurs more frequently in patients with systemic sepsis and in many cases is due to hematogenous seeding of the catheter with bacteria. More often, however, it is due to failure to observe strict aseptic precautions during preparation and administration of the solutions. One of the earliest signs of systemic sepsis may be the sudden development of glucose intolerance in a patient who previously has been maintained on parenteral hyperalimentation without difficulty. When this occurs or if fever develops without obvious cause, the solution and intravenous tubing are replaced. Other causes of fever should also be investigated; if fever persists, the infusion catheter should be removed and cultured. Antibiotics may be appropriate at this point in some cases. The catheter may be replaced in the opposite subclavian vein or into one of the internal jugular veins and the infusion restarted. In general, however, it is probably advisable to wait a short period of time before reinserting the catheter.

Other complications related to catheter placement include the development of pneumothorax, hemothorax, or hydrothorax; subclavian artery injury; cardiac arrhythmias if the catheter is placed into the atrium or the ventricle; air embolism or catheter embolism; and, rarely, cardiac perforation with tamponade. Thrombophlebitis or thrombosis of the superior vena cava has been an exceptionally rare complication. All these complications may be avoided by strict adherence to the techniques previously outlined.

Hyperosmolar nonketotic hyperglycemia may develop with normal rates of infusion in patients with impaired glucose tolerance or in any patient if the hypertonic solutions are administered too rapidly. This is a particularly common complication in latent diabetics and in patients following severe surgical stress or trauma. If blood and urine sugar concentrations are not monitored frequently, the blood sugar level may become markedly elevated with ensuing weakness, lethargy, and eventual coma. Treatment of the condition consists of volume replacement with correction of electrolyte abnormalities and the administration of insulin. This particularly serious complication can be avoided with careful attention to daily fluid balance and frequent determinations of urine and blood sugar levels and serum electrolyte content.

A number of volume, concentration, and compositional abnormalities may also develop, but these are largely avoided by careful attention to the details of patient management. This is particularly important for elderly patients and for patients with significant cardiovascular, renal, or hepatic disorders. Changes in the volume and composition of the administered solutions are often necessary to avoid complications. Additionally, the use of parenteral hyperalimentation in pediatric patients requires knowledge of the specific nutritional requirements of this age group and the special precautions that should be observed.

References

Fluid and Electrolyte Therapy

Andersen, O. S., and Engel, K.: A New Acid-Base Nomogram: An Improved Method for the Calculation of the Relevant Blood Acid-Base Data, *Scand J Clin Lab Invest,* **12:**177, 1960.

Astrup, P., Jorgensen, K., Andersen, O. S., and Engel, K.: The Acid-Base Metabolism: A New Approach, *Lancet,* **1:**1035, 1960.

Bartlett, W. C.: Acute Hyperparathyroid Crisis, *Am J Surg,* **114:**796, 1967.

Baxter, C. R., Zedlitz, W. H., and Shires, G. T.: High-Output Acute Renal Failure Complicating Traumatic Injury, *J Trauma,* **4:**567, 1964.

Berlinger, R. W., Kennedy, T. J., Jr., and Orloff, J.: Relationship between Acidification of the Urine and Potassium Metabolism, *Am J Med,* **11:**274, 1951.

Berry, R. E. L.: The Pathophysiology and Management of Complex Problems of Body Fluid Homeostasis Attending Surgical Disease States, *Surg Clin North Am,* **41:**1143, 1961.

Bunker, J. P.: Metabolic Effects of Blood Transfusion, *Anesthesiology,* **27:**446, 1966.

Canizaro, P. C., Prager, M. D., and Shires, G. T.: The Infusion of Ringer's Lactate Solution during Shock, *Am J Surg,* **122:**494, 1971.

Crandell, W. B.: Acid-Base Balance in Surgical Patients: I. A Survey of 62 Selected Cases, *Ann Surg,* **149:**342, 1952.

DeCosse, J. J., Randall, H. T., Habif, D. V., and Roberts, K. E.: The Mechanism of Hyponatremia and Hypotonicity after Surgical Trauma, *Surgery,* **40:**27, 1956.

Henzel, J. H., DeWeese, M. S., and Ridenhour, G.: Significance of Magnesium and Zinc Metabolism in the Surgical Patient: I. Magnesium, *Arch Surg,* **95:**974, 1967.

Hutchin, P.: Metabolic Response to Surgery in Relation to Caloric, Fluid and Electrolyte Intake, *Curr Probl Surg,* April, 1971.

Jenkins, M. T., and Beck, G. P.: Differential Diagnosis of Hypotension Occurring during Anesthesia and Surgery, *Clin Anesth,* **3:**106, 1963.

Kappagoda, C. T., Linden, R. J., and Snow, H. M.: An Approach to the Problems of Acid-Base Balance, *Clin Sci,* **39:**169, 1970.

McClelland, R. N., Shires, G. T., Baxter, C. R., Coln, C. D., and Carrico, C. J.: Balanced Salt Solution in the Treatment of Hemorrhagic Shock: Studies in Dogs, *JAMA,* **199:** 830, 1967.

Mellemgaard, K., and Astrup, P.: The Quantitative Determination of Surplus Amounts of Acid or Base in the Human Body, *Scand J Clin Lab Invest,* **12:**187, 1960.

Mengoli, L. R.: Excerpts from the History of Postoperative Fluid Therapy, *Am J Surg,* **121:**311, 1971.

Miller, R. D., Tong, M. J., and Robbins, T. O.: Effects of Massive Transfusion of Blood on Acid-Base Balance, *JAMA,* **216:**1762, 1971.

Moncrief, J. A., and Mason, A. D.: Water Vapor Loss in the Burned Patient, *Surg Forum,* **13:**38, 1962.

Moore, F. D., Olesen, K. H., McMurrey, J. D., Parker, H. V., Ball, M. R., and Boyden, C. M.: "Body Cell Mass and Its Supporting Environment: Body Composition in Health and Disease," W. B. Saunders Company, Philadelphia, 1963.

Moyer, C. A.: "Fluid Balance," The Year Book Medical Publishers, Inc., Chicago, 1954.

Pitts, R. F.: "Physiology of Kidney and Body Fluids," The Year Book Medical Publishers, Inc., Chicago, 1963.

Randall, H. T., and Roberts, K. E.: The Significance and Treatment of Acidosis and Alkalosis in Surgical Patients, *Surg Clin North Am,* **36:**315, 1956.

Randall, R. E., Jr., Cohen, M. D., Spray, C. C., Jr., and Rossmeisl, E. C.: Hypermagnesemia in Renal Failure: Etiology and Toxic Manifestations, *Ann Intern Med,* **61:**73, 1964.

Schwartz, W. B., and Relman, A. S.: A Critique of the Parameters Used in the Evaluation of Acid-Base Disorders, *N Engl J Med,* **268:**1382, 1963.

Shires, G. T., and Holman, V.: Dilutional Acidosis, *Ann Intern Med,* **28:**551, 1948.

Shires, T., Williams, J., and Brown, F.: Acute Changes in Extracellular Fluids Associated with Major Surgical Procedures, *Ann Surg,* **154:**803, 1961.

Shires, T., and Jackson, D. E.: Postoperative Salt Tolerance, *Arch Surg,* **84:**703, 1962.

Shires, T., Coln, D., Carrico, J., and Lightfoot, S.: Fluid Therapy in Hemorrhagic Shock, *Arch Surg,* **88:**688, 1964.

Shires, T., and Carrico, C. J.: Current Status of the Shock Problem, *Curr Probl Surg,* March, 1966.

Shires, G. T.: What's New in Surgery, Shock, and Metabolism, *Surg Gynecol Obstet,* **124:**284, 1967.

Singer, R. B., and Hastings, A. B.: An Improved Clinical Method for the Estimation of Disturbances of the Acid-Base Balance of Human Blood, *Medicine,* **27:**223, 1948.

Thompson, J. E., Vollman, R. W., Austin, D. J., and Kartchner, M. M.: Prevention of Hypotensive and Renal Complications of Aortic Surgery Using Balanced Salt Solution, *Ann Surg,* **167:**767, 1968.

Wacker, W. E. C., and Parisi, A. F.: Magnesium Metabolism: Parts I, II, and III, *N Engl J Med,* **278:**658, 712, 772, 1968.

Wright, H. K., and Gann, D. S.: Correction of Defect in Free Water Excretion in Postoperative Patients by Extracellular Fluid Volume Expansion, *Ann Surg,* **158:**70, 1963.

Nutrition

Bachrach, W. H., and Tecimer, L. B.: Use of a Feeding Tube in the Management of Gastric Retention following Gastroenteric Anastomosis, *Am Surg,* **30:**476, 1964.

Boles, T., and Zollinger, R. M.: Critical Evaluation of Jejunostomy, *Arch Surg,* **65:**358, 1952.

Bury, K. D., Stephens, R. V., and Randall, H. T.: Use of a Chemically Defined, Liquid, Elemental Diet for Nutritional Management of Fistulas of the Alimentary Tract, *Am J Surg,* **121:**174, 1971.

Cahill, G. F., Jr.: Body Fuels and Their Metabolism, *Bull Am Coll Surg,* **55:**12, 1970.

Cuthbertson, D. P.: The Disturbance of Metabolism Produce by Bony and Non-bony Injury, with Notes on Certain Abnormal Conditions of Bone, *Biochem J,* **24:**1244, 1930.

Davis, L. E., and Hofmann, W.: A Long-Term Nasogastric Feeding Tube Made from Modified Penrose Tubing, *JAMA,* **209:**685, 1969.

Dudrick, S. J., Groff, D. B., and Wilmore, D. W.: Long-Term Venous Catheterization in Infants, *Surg Gynecol Obstet,* **129:**805, 1969.

Dudrick, S. J., Ruberg, R. L., Long, J. M., Allen, T. R., and Steiger, E.: Uses, Non-Uses and Abuses of Intravenous Hyperalimentation, in G. S. M. Cowan, Jr., and W. L. Scheetz (eds.), "Intravenous Hyperalimentation," Lea & Febiger, Philadelphia, 1972.

Dudrick, S. J., Steiger, E., and Long, J. M.: Renal Failure in Surgical Patients: Treatment with Intravenous Essential Amino Acids and Hypertonic Glucose, *Surgery,* **68:**180, 1970.

Dudrick, S. J., Steiger, E., Long, J. M., Ruberg, R. L., Allen, T. R., Vars, H. M., and Rhoads, J. E.: General Principles and Techniques of Intravenous Hyperalimentation, in G. S. M. Cowan, Jr., and W. L. Scheetz (eds.), "Intravenous Hyperalimentation," Lea & Febiger, Philadelphia, 1972.

Dudrick, S. J., Wilmore, D. W., Vars, H. M., and Rhoads, J. E.: Long-Term Parenteral Nutrition with Growth, Development, and Positive Nitrogen Balance, *Surgery,* **64:**134, 1968.

Felig, P., Pozefsky, T., Marliss, E., and Cahill, G. F., Jr.: Alanine: Key Role in Gluconeogenesis, *Science,* **167:**1003, 1970.

Filler, R. M., Eraklis, A. J., Rubin, V. G., and Das, J. B.: Long-Term Total Parenteral Nutrition in Infants, *N Engl J Med,* **281:**589, 1969.

Graham, W. P., and Royster, H. P.: Simplified Cervical Esophagostomy for Long-Term Extraoral Feeding, *Surg Gynecol Obstet,* **125:**127, 1967.

Gump, F. E., Kinney, J. M., and Price, J. B., Jr.: Energy Metabolism in Surgical Patients: Oxygen Consumption and Blood Flow, *J Surg Res,* **10:**613, 1970.

Jernigan, W. R., Gardner, W. C., Mahr, M. M., and Milburn, J. L.: Use of the Internal Jugular Vein for Placement of Central Venous Catheter, *Surg Gynecol Obstet,* **130:**520, 1970.

Kinney, J. M.: A Consideration of Energy Exchange in Human Trauma, *Bull NY Acad Med,* **36:**617, 1960.

McMinn, R. M. H.: "Tissue Repair," Academic Press, Inc., New York, 1969.

Moore, F. D.: "Metabolic Care of the Surgical Patient," W. B. Saunders Company, Philadelphia, 1960.

————: Convalescence: The Metabolic Sequence After Injury, in The Committee on Pre and Postoperative Care, American College of Surgeons (eds.), "Manual of Preoperative and Postoperative Care," 2d ed., p. 19, W. B. Saunders Company, Philadelphia, 1971.

Randall, H. T., and Dudrick, S. J.: Surgical Nutrition: Parenteral and Oral, in The Committee on Pre and Postoperative Care, American College Of Surgeons (eds.), "Manual of Preoperative and Postoperative Care," 2d ed., p. 75, W. B. Saunders Company, Philadelphia, 1971.

Wilmore, D. W., and Dudrick, S. J.: Treatment of Acute Renal Failure with Intravenous Essential L-amino Acids, *Arch Surg,* **99:**669, 1969.

Chapter 3

Hemostasis, Surgical Bleeding, and Transfusion

by **Seymour I. Schwartz and Stanley B. Troup**

Biology of Normal Hemostasis

Tests of Hemostasis and Blood Coagulation

Evaluation of the Surgical Patient as a Hemostatic Risk
General Considerations
Evaluation of the Unsuspected Bleeder
Evaluation of the Suspected Potential Bleeder
Evaluation of the Patient Who Begins to Bleed During or
    After Surgical Procedures

Clinical Hemostatic Defects
Inheritance
Factor VIII Deficiency (Classical Hemophilia)
Von Willebrand's Disease (Pseudohemophilia)
Factor IX Deficiency (Christmas Disease)
Factor XI (PTA) Deficiency (Rosenthal's Syndrome)
Factor V (Proaccelerin) Deficiency (Parahemophilia)
Factor VII (Proconvertin) Deficiency
Factor X (Stuart-Prower) Deficiency
Inherited Hypoprothrombinemia (Factor II Deficiency)
Inherited Fibrinogen Abnormalities
Acquired Hypofibrinogenemia
    Defibrination Syndrome
    Fibrinolysis
Thrombocytopenia
Myeloproliferative Diseases
    Polycythemia Vera
    Myeloid Metaplasia
Other Diseases Associated with Increased Risk of Bleeding
Anticoagulation and Bleeding

Local Hemostasis
Mechanical Procedures
Thermal Agents
Chemical Agents

Transfusion
Background
Characteristics of Blood and Replacement Therapy
    Blood
    Replacement Therapy
Indications for Replacement of Blood or Its Elements
    Selective Therapy
    Specific Indications
Methods of Administering Blood
Complications

Few events in clinical medicine are so ominous as the failure of hemostasis. For the surgeon, few failures in normal physiology are potentially so catastrophic. Disruption in normal hemostasis often can be anticipated, just as the physiologic failure usually can be identified and corrected. In this chapter the reader will become acquainted with the events of normal hemostasis. Advances in understanding in this area have come largely from the laboratory, not the clinic. As a consequence of this and because of the complex nature of some of the events involved, disproportionate emphasis often is placed upon the laboratory in attempting to solve what, primarily, are clinical problems. We shall try to provide a background whereby the problems encountered can be solved by careful evaluation of the patient and judicious use of the laboratory. A desired by-product will be the evolution of logical therapeutic programs. These may include methods for local control of bleeding, replacement for the loss of circulating blood volume, and selective transfusion of physiologic products necessary to provide normal hemostasis.

BIOLOGY OF NORMAL HEMOSTASIS

Cessation of blood flow from an injured vessel, the cumulative phenomenon we call hemostasis, occurs as a result of many events. Blood coagulation frequently is equated with hemostasis. Coagulation is not, however, always the central or most important factor. Clinical testimony to this heresy is supplied by the patient with congenital afibrinogenemia. This illness, characterized in the laboratory by incoagulability of the blood, may present clinically as a relatively minor hemostatic problem. This paradox is explained by the important role of the platelets, which, in this setting, are able to function in a near-normal manner because of the trace amount of fibrinogen present on their surface.

The accomplishment of hemostasis depends, to a variable degree, on the clinical condition of the patient, the nature of insult to the blood vessel, the type of vessel or vessels injured, the anatomic site of injury, the coagulation mechanism, and fibrinolytic activity. A lateral incision in a small artery may remain open because of physical forces and can be associated with extensive and continued bleeding. In contrast, a complete transection of a similar-sized vessel, as Hunter demonstrated centuries ago, contracts to the extent that the bleeding may cease spontaneously. Illustrative of the importance of anatomic site of injury is the fact that bleeding from a small venule ruptured by trauma in the thigh of a healthy athlete may be negligible because of the support of surrounding muscle. Bleeding from a similar vessel due to trauma of the nasal mucosa may be extensive in the same individual. An elderly person with atrophy of the subcutaneous connective tissue or a patient who has received corticosteroid therapy for a long time may sustain a large ecchymosis from minor trauma to the dorsum of the hand, while a younger person might note no change secondary to comparable trauma at the same site. Normal hemostasis, then, results from the interplay of multiple factors. A gross defect in one function or a lesser defect involving multiple functions usually

HEMOSTASIS

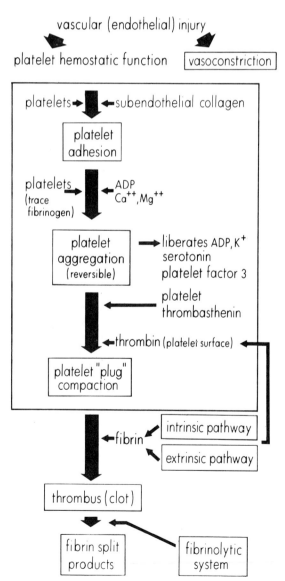

Fig. 3-1. Schematic representation of hemostasis.

proves necessary to effect significant bleeding. Description of the events of normal hemostasis will permit consideration of the points at which failure may occur and also provides an opportunity to correlate laboratory tests with their physiologic counterparts.

VASCULAR RESPONSE. The initial vascular response to injury, even at the capillary level, is that of vasoconstriction. Experimental observation has demonstrated that adherence of endothelial cell to endothelial cell, with obliteration of microdefects, may, in itself, be sufficient to effect hemostasis. Whether vasoconstriction of these small vessels is neurogenically or humorally mediated remains unsettled. Human platelets normally carry vasoactive amines, some of which are liberated at the site of injury. The initial vasoconstriction described, however, occurs prior to platelet adherence at the site of injury. Animal experiments demonstrate that when platelets have been depleted of serotonin in vivo and vascular injury has been produced, vasoconstriction still occurs.

Patients with a mild bleeding disorder have been described in whom the only laboratory abnormality is a prolonged bleeding time. Capillary microscopy in certain of these patients reveals that the capillary loops do not constrict following injury. A capillary structural defect has been postulated, and support for this concept is provided by the observation that, even in the absence of trauma, the capillary loops are dilated and tortuous.

PLATELET FUNCTION. In less than 15 seconds following vascular injury, platelets (Fig. 3-1) adhere to the injured margins of the vessels. For many years it was believed that the platelets adhered directly to the injured endothelial cells. More recently, phase microscopy and electron microscopic observations have revealed that this early platelet adherence is to subendothelial collagen fibrils. The mechanism of attraction between collagen fibrils and platelets has not been defined, nor has the physiologic significance clearly been established. Two types of observations suggest that the platelet-collagen interaction is important. Quick demonstrated that the bleeding time, fastidiously performed, may be lengthened in patients taking aspirin. Platelet-rich plasma derived from patients taking aspirin demonstrates an impairment of the platelet-collagen reaction in vitro. The second observation, related to the first, is that of Vigliano and Horowitz. These writers described a patient with multiple myeloma and hemorrhagic tendency in whom the principal laboratory abnormality was impairment of the collagen-platelet interaction.

Within seconds of the collagen-platelet response, platelets begin to adhere to one another at the site of injury. The initial aggregation is loose. The loose aggregates may be fragmented and dispersed by the pressure of blood issuing from tiny arteriols. This platelet aggregation is thought to occur as a result of a platelet-ADP (adenosinediphosphate) interaction. Gaarder et al. initially demonstrated that ADP, added in minute amounts, results in rapid platelet aggregate formation in whole blood or platelet-rich plasma. Trace amounts of calcium or magnesium are necessary for this reaction. Interestingly, and probably significantly, heparin does not interfere with this reaction. The maintenance of normal hemostasis in the heparinized patient may well be explained by the platelets' ability to aggregate loosely at sites of minimal trauma, even when the blood is relatively incoagulable.

A relatively rare clinical entity, thrombasthenia of the Glanzmann type, may represent a naturally occurring failure of hemostasis at this level. Platelets from such patients fail to aggregate in the presence of ADP. This is not their only abnormality of platelet function, for blood clots from these patients also display poor retraction. The platelets lack fibrinogen, and it is possible that all these abnormalities are related.

Following the formation of the loose platelet aggregate the mass of platelets begins to compact. When observed microscopically, the platelets lose their individual identity and begin to fuse with one another. The platelet granules concentrate toward the center of the platelet, and fibrin strands now can be identified scattered throughout the platelet mass. These changes are described as viscous metamorphosis and have a biochemical counterpart. During compaction the platelets, normally rich in adenosinetriphosphate (ATP), suffer a drop in content of this energy-rich compound and liberate ADP. Potassium and serotonin, normally present in platelets, also are liberated at this time. Platelet factor 3 (phospholipid) is made available for the clotting process, but a small amount probably becomes available earlier. Platelet factor 3 is a normal component within the platelet membrane as well as in certain of the platelet granules.

The events initiating these morphologic and biochemical processes have not been established with certainty. Probably trace amounts of the enzyme thrombin are formed at the surface of the platelet. All the necessary plasma factors are present in the immediate plasmatic environment of the platelet. All the observed platelet changes can be produced in vitro by the addition of trace amounts of thrombin. Indirect experimental data suggest that this also occurs in vivo.

The events culminating in the compaction of the loose platelet aggregate into a "platelet plug" seem to correspond to what we measure with the bleeding time. Failure of any of the early events described above can result in lengthening of the bleeding time.

Approximately 15 percent of human platelet protein is contractile. This material is called *thrombosthenin*. It is very similar to muscle actomyosin and is an ATPase. Compaction of the platelet plug is credited to the contractile protein, which participates in the biochemical events as well. The platelets' responses to thrombin end in destruction of the platelets as intact cells. The sequential changes in the platelets have been described as preaggregation, aggregation, thrombocytorrhexis, and thrombocytolysis.

The platelet is equipped to enhance its function in many ways. Laboratory studies have demonstrated that platelets are capable of liberating enough ADP during hydrolysis of the energy-rich ATP to supply their own stimulus for the ADP aggregation. Interestingly, ADP aggregation is facilitated by amines which also are liberated from the platelets early in their hemostatic function. The serotonin which is released may induce vascular constriction in the immediate area. While evidence for the importance of serotonin in normal hemostasis is lacking, its presence is provocative.

BLOOD COAGULATION. Until this point in the hemostatic process, the role of blood coagulation has been inferential and invoked only to explain the initiation of viscous metamorphosis by the platelets. Microscopic clotting, assumed to take place at the platelet surface, is thought to evolve through the effects of tissue thromboplastin on the plasma procoagulant substances at the platelet surface. Reliance on the concept of a *tissue* thromboplastin leading to microscopic clotting at the platelet surface, rather than an *intrinsic* thromboplastin, is explained by the normal platelet function and bleeding time with defects in intrinsic thromboplastin formation.

The complex series of reactions that ultimately leads to the transformation of the soluble protein fibrinogen to the insoluble fibrin clot constitutes the process of coagulation. Failure at any one of the stages may manifest itself as a potential bleeding disorder. The importance of blood coagulation has been appreciated since antiquity. Allowable exceptions to the covenant of circumcision demanded by the Old Testament are described in the Babylonian Talmud. While our understanding of blood clotting has become somewhat more precise since that time, a degree of faith remains requisite in the student of the hemostatic process. Nowhere is this better demonstrated than in the earliest step in the coagulation process, activation of factor XII.

Factor XII (Hageman factor) deficiency results in lengthening of the whole blood clotting time. Despite this gross laboratory abnormality, the deficiency is not associated with significant hemostatic problems. A patient named Hageman, the first patient demonstrated to have this deficiency, underwent gastrectomy without bleeding complication. Interestingly, the same patient succumbed to complications of thromboembolic disease many years later.

The concept of the blood coagulation mechanism representing a "waterfall," or "cascade," phenomenon was developed simultaneously and independently by Davie and Ratnoff and by Macfarlane (Fig. 3-2). These writers view the activation of factor XII as the initiation of the coagulation sequence. In vitro studies demonstrate that activation of factor XII is accomplished by virtually any nonendothelial surface. The activated factor XII, which differs from the inactive form in certain physicochemical features, has enzymatic properties. The substrate for activated factor XII is believed to be factor XI (plasma thromboplastin antecedent, PTA). Factor XI seemingly can be changed to its activated form without depending upon activated factor XII. This could explain the absence of hemostatic problems in patients with factor XII deficiency.

Deficiency of factor XI clinically is associated with a mild bleeding disorder known as *Rosenthal's syndrome.* This is inherited as an incompletely recessive autosomal trait. Factor XI behaves as an enzyme when activated either by factor XII or by some unexplained process. Factor IX (Christmas factor, plasma thromboplastin component, PTC) serves as the substrate for activated factor XI. This step requires the presence of ionized calcium. Deficiency of factor IX is characterized clinically by the disorder known as *Christmas disease, PTC deficiency,* or *hemophilia B.* This sex-linked recessive trait will be discussed later in the chapter.

Activated factor IX is believed to have enzymatic activity interacting with its specific substrate factor VIII (antihemophilic factor, AHF). The effect of factor IX upon factor VIII requires the presence of phospholipid (platelet factor 3) as well as ionized calcium. Although the phospholipid normally is contributed by the platelets, it is clear from in vitro studies that other tissues may serve as a source. Under pathologic circumstances, such as massive intravascular hemolysis, it is possible that the phospholipid can be derived from the red blood cell membrane. Inherited deficiency of factor VIII clinically is represented by classical hemophilia, or hemophilia A.

The events in blood coagulation described until this point are relatively time-consuming. The steps leading to the activation of factor VIII probably consume 90 percent of the time that is required for blood to clot grossly. Accordingly, defects within this portion of the clotting sequence are characterized by prolonged whole blood clotting time when severe or by abnormalities in other test systems which relate to this slower phase of blood coagulation.

Activated factor VIII is believed to use factor X (Stuart-Prower factor) as its substrate. Factor X deficiency is a rare but potentially serious disorder which may manifest laboratory abnormalities characteristic of both the earlier and later phases of blood coagulation. Thus, severe deficiency of factor X may result in a prolonged whole blood clotting time and impaired prothrombin consumption. Such a deficiency also invariably will prolong the one-stage *prothrombin time.* Activated factor X appears to act upon, or act with, factor V (proaccelerin). When this stage is completed, the activator *prothrombinase* has evolved. In the presence of ionized calcium, prothrombinase will split the prothrombin molecule (factor II) to form the smaller molecular species thrombin. Figure 3-2 schematically depicts the foregoing discussion. Examples of each of the clinical deficiencies will be discussed subsequently.

Normal hemostasis also requires the integrity of the extrinsic system of blood coagulation (Fig. 3-3). This pathway of blood coagulation takes origin with the interaction of tissue lipoprotein (tissue thromboplastin) and factor VII (proconvertin). Factor X then is activated, and the sequence continues as previously described for the intrinsic system. The formation of the platelet hemostatic plug, described earlier, is believed to be triggered by the effect of thrombin on the platelet surface. An explanation for this early appearance of a trace amount of thrombin, too soon to be explained by the more leisurely intrinsic pathway of blood coagulation, is the "shortcut" provided by tissue thromboplastin and factor VII as the extrinsic clotting system.

The in vitro equivalent of the extrinsic pathway is the one-stage prothrombin determination. In this test an extrinsic source of tissue lipoprotein and calcium is added

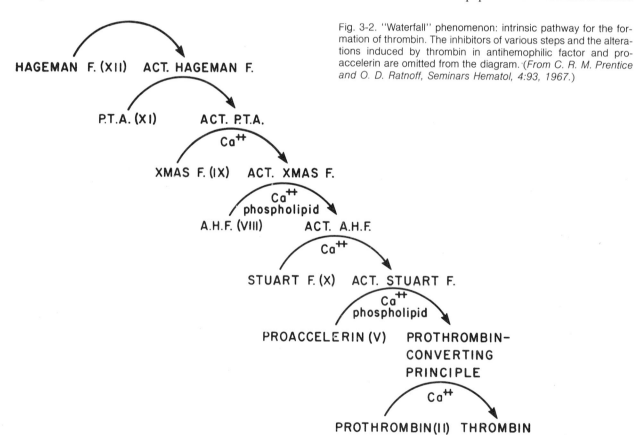

Fig. 3-2. "Waterfall" phenomenon: intrinsic pathway for the formation of thrombin. The inhibitors of various steps and the alterations induced by thrombin in antihemophilic factor and proaccelerin are omitted from the diagram. *(From C. R. M. Prentice and O. D. Ratnoff, Seminars Hematol, 4:93, 1967.)*

to plasma. Deficiencies in factor VII, factor X, factor V, or fibrinogen will lengthen the clotting time in this test. Since delays in clotting in this test are measured in seconds, it is clear that defects in this portion of the process will not noticeably lengthen the whole blood clotting time. The range of normal for the whole blood clotting time is appreciable, and even a substantial lengthening of the prothrombin time would be obscured within the variability of the whole blood clotting time.

The role of thrombin in the hemostatic mechanism has been the focus of much study. Thrombin probably serves as an initiator of the biochemical and functional platelet changes early in normal hemostasis. It has the ability to enhance strikingly the activation of certain of the blood clotting factors, e.g., factor V, factor VIII, and factor XIII (fibrin-stabilizing factor). The key position occupied by thrombin is emphasized further by our clinical approach to anticoagulation. On one hand the coumarin drugs are used to impair synthesis of those precursors that will lead to thrombin generation, while on the other hand the efficacy of heparin is its ability to impair or interfere with the effect of thrombin on fibrinogen.

The chemistry of the thrombin-fibrinogen reaction now is well characterized. Thrombin enzymatically cleaves two pairs of peptide chains from the fibrinogen molecule. The action of thrombin on fibrinogen ends at that point. Thereafter, the soluble fibrinogen monomers, which are the fibrinogen molecules minus the two pairs of peptide chains, unite by hydrogen bonding. This is a loose chemical bond that is easily separated. The weak formation is converted to a stable one through the enzymatic activity of factor XIII, fibrin-stabilizing factor. This enzyme probably works by facilitating conversion of sulfhydryl groups to disulfide bonds.

Inherited and acquired hemostatic abnormalities have been identified for these steps. Impaired organization of the fibrin monomers occurs in dysglobulinemic states, and the faulty clot structure has been blamed for the bleeding tendency. Congenital and acquired deficiencies of factor XIII have been described. Of interest to the surgeon is the repeated observation of impaired wound healing in patients with factor XIII deficiency. In vitro studies have suggested that fibroblasts grown on a medium lacking factor XIII show faulty organization, and it is possible that the biologic importance of factor XIII lies outside the immediate realm of hemostasis.

CLOT DISSOLUTION. Fibrinolysis (Fig. 3-4) is the mechanism by which dissolution of blood clots occurs. Although fibrinolysis is not necessarily part of the hemostatic mechanism, excessive fibrinolysis may cause failure of hemostasis. The process of clot dissolution is as complex as the clotting system itself but is not yet as thoroughly understood. The enzyme plasmin, which is derived from a precursor plasma protein (plasminogen), is essential to the mechanism of fibrinolysis. Under the influence of kinases, which may be blood activators, tissue activators, streptokinase, or urokinase, the precursor plasma protein (plasminogen) is converted into an enzyme with proteolytic activity (plasmin). There is some question as to whether the kinases act directly on plasminogen or transform a

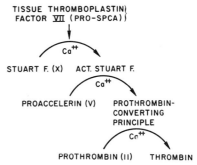

Fig. 3-3. Extrinsic pathway for the formation of thrombin. Inhibitors of the various steps and alterations induced by thrombin in proaccelerin are omitted from the diagram. (*From C. R. M. Prentice and O. D. Ratnoff, Semin Hematol, 4:93, 1967.*)

proactivator in the human plasma into an activator, which in turn converts plasminogen into plasmin. While fibrin is its preferred substrate, plasmin also can digest fibrinogen, factor V, and factor VIII. The fibrinolytic system can be activated in many ways, including by activated factor XII. It is likely that fibrinolysis progresses at the same time that the blood-clotting process itself is being activated. The initiation of fibrinolysis may arise from tissue sources, vascular endothelium representing a particularly likely possibility. Ischemia is a potent stimulator of the activation of the fibrinolytic system.

What Sherry has viewed as "physiologic proteolysis" results from the natural affinity of plasminogen for fibrin. The latter adsorbs the former during clot formation. The plasminogen then is in position to attack only the fibrin to which it is adsorbed, a locally controlled form of fibrinolysis resulting. On the other hand, pathologic proteolysis may occur when plasminogen free in the plasma is activated. The activated plasminogen may then attack other coagulant proteins as well.

The failure of hemostasis related to excessive activation or ineffective inactivation of the fibrinolytic system is due to several factors. The smaller fragments of fibrin liberated

FIBRINOLYTIC SYSTEM

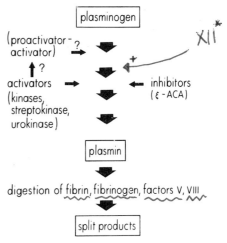

Fig. 3-4. Fibrinolytic system.

by proteolysis may interfere with normal platelet aggregation. The larger fibrin fragments are incorporated into the clot in lieu of normal fibrin monomers and create an unstable clot. When proteolysis is excessive, other plasma clotting factors also serve as substrates for protein digestion. Human blood normally has a high content of antiplasmin, which inhibits plasminogen activation, and platelets are also believed to possess an antifibrinolytic property.

TESTS OF HEMOSTASIS AND BLOOD COAGULATION

BLEEDING TIME. This is the time required for bleeding to cease after a standard skin incision has been made. The bleeding time probably corresponds to that time required for compaction of the platelet plug in the hemostatic process described above.

With the Duke technique, a clean 2- or 3-mm incision is made with a #11 Bard-Parker blade in the most dependent portion of the earlobe. A piece of filter paper is held below the wound, but not touching it, to catch each drop of blood as it forms and falls. The paper is held so that each drop strikes the margin of the filter paper serially. In this way, a permanent record of the bleeding time can be obtained and, if desired, entered in the patient's chart. The wound itself should not be disturbed, since this may prolong the bleeding time. When blood flow ceases, the time lapse following incision is recorded as the bleeding time. The upper limits of normal vary but probably should not exceed 5 minutes. The Ivy technique requires the placement of a blood pressure cuff above the elbow with inflation to 40 mm Hg pressure. A standard 5-mm incision is made to a depth of 2 mm on the volar surface of the forearm, taking care to avoid any obvious venules in the skin. Pressure within the cuff is maintained while a piece of filter paper is employed to touch the drops of blood carefully as they form. Once again, the wound must not be disturbed. With this method, a normal upper limit of 8 minutes is accepted.

In our experience, abnormalities of bleeding time usually are fairly clear-cut. In the case of an equivocal result, the test should be repeated using the opposite earlobe or forearm. The bleeding time usually is normal in patients with a platelet count greater than 75,000/mm³. Patients with a qualitative platelet abnormality (thrombocytopathia or thrombasthenia), patients with defective capillaries as described earlier in this chapter, or patients with von Willebrand's disease all may have prolonged bleeding time. The bleeding time can be of diagnostic value but in most hands should be considered a relatively gross test.

RUMPEL-LEEDE (TOURNIQUET) TEST. This test, to our view, has little clinical application today. It is designed to estimate capillary fragility. A blood pressure cuff is applied to the upper arm and inflated to a pressure midway between diastolic and systolic pressure. The pressure is maintained at that level for a maximum of 5 minutes—less if many petechiae appear on the forearm before that time. Semiquantification of capillary fragility is obtained by counting the number of petechiae seen within a predetermined area, which should be at some distance from the blood pressure cuff. The antecubital space is not used, for some normal individuals will show petechiae in this area. No more than 2 to 4 petechiae should be seen in a circle of 2.5 cm diameter.

The test need not be performed on patients known to have a low platelet count or prolonged bleeding time. The demonstration of capillary fragility will not contribute to the diagnosis in such circumstances. Rather, it results in some discomfort to the patient, and the petechiae merely serve as a frightening reminder that something is grossly abnormal. The test characteristically is abnormal when thrombocytopenia is present, but this may be determined readily by inspection of the blood smear or a direct platelet count. It also may be abnormal in the group of patients with prolonged bleeding time as well as in elderly patients with poor tissue turgor. Severe vitamin C deficiency also may result in a positive tourniquet test.

PLATELET ESTIMATION AND COUNT. Thrombocytopenia is the most common abnormality of hemostasis encountered in the surgical patient. Microscopic examination of a properly stained blood smear can provide much information about such patients. When an area where the red blood cells display their customary central pallor and where few of the red blood cells overlap one another is examined, 15 to 20 platelets per oil immersion field should be noted. If the blood is not anticoagulated before the smear is prepared, as many as half of these may be in clumps of three or four platelets. A well-stained blood smear that fails to display more than three or four platelets in at least every other oil immersion field can be considered significantly thrombocytopenic. In this situation, the patient's platelet count generally is less than 75,000/mm³. Blood smears which must be searched because platelets appear in only every four or five oil immersion fields usually represent platelet counts of fewer than 40,000/mm³. If cover slip smears have been prepared, the cover slips always should be mounted as matched pairs. Platelets occasionally stick to one of the cover slips, and examination of both will obviate a false impression of thrombocytopenia. Lightly stained blood smears may appear thrombocytopenic in that the platelets are not prominent enough to attract the examiner's attention.

Inspection of the blood smear has the other obvious advantage of permitting the examiner to identify additional pathologic features which may have meaning in the care of the patient. The presence of nucleated red blood cells or abnormal white cells can provide information important to the diagnosis. The presence of giant platelets or large fragments of megakaryocyte cytoplasm also will alert the examiner to possible pathologic platelet function.

Direct enumeration of blood platelets can be accomplished quite accurately. The most reliable microscopic method is that described by Brecher and Cronkite, employing the phase contrast microscope. With this method, normal values ranging from 160,000 to 350,000/mm³ are obtained. Electronic particle counters recently have been adapted for platelet counting. The degree of precision matches that obtained by phase contrast microscopy. *Spontaneous* bleeding only rarely can be related to thrombocytopenia with platelet counts greater than 50,000/mm³. Platelet counts of 60,000 to 70,000/mm³ usually are sufficient to provide adequate hemostasis following trauma or surgical procedures if other hemostatic factors are normal.

CLOT RETRACTION. Normal platelet function is responsible for retraction of the clot, but this gross phenomenon has no clear function in hemostasis. The macroscopic event, however, may well have its microscopic equivalent in the compaction of the platelet plug.

Semiquantification of this platelet function can be obtained. If an applicator stick, string, or partially straightened paper clip is suspended in 5 ml of freshly drawn blood and the blood permitted to clot undisturbed about this object, the clot can be removed 1 hour following coagulation and the serum that has been expressed from the clot measured. Clot retraction then can be expressed as a percentage of the serum related to the original volume of blood. With blood of normal hematocrit, the usual range is 40 percent or slightly higher. Normally, clot retraction in a test tube is complete within 3 or 4 hours at room temperature. A rough relationship exists between the platelet count and clot retraction. Significant thrombocytopenia can exist in the presence of normal clot retraction, since the clot will retract well if the platelet count is slightly less than 100,000/mm³.

OTHER TESTS OF PLATELET FUNCTION. The ability of the platelets to liberate platelet factor 3 (phospholipid), essential in tiny amounts at several stages of the blood-clotting process (Fig. 3-2), also can be measured. Impairment of platelet factor 3 release has been reported in conditions described as *thrombocytopathia*. This defect can represent a primary disease entity, but similar impairment has been described as a secondary phenomenon in uremia and liver disease. Whether the impairment plays a functional role, for example, in the bleeding associated with uremia, remains uncertain. The inability of the platelet to make platelet factor 3 available for the clotting process may be a part of a more fundamental surface membrane abnormality.

The role of ADP in platelet aggregation during hemostasis has been mentioned earlier. The ability of platelets to aggregate in plasma upon the addition of ADP serves as another test of platelet function. Failure of platelets to aggregate following the addition of ADP is seen in patients with the Glanzmann type of thrombasthenia and also, artifactually, when anticoagulants, such as EDTA, which tightly bind divalent cations, are used.

The ability of platelets to adhere to a standardized glass bead column also has been used as a measure of platelet function. This test, refined by Salzman, is reported to be grossly abnormal in patients with von Willebrand's disease. The test requires meticulous preparation of the glass bead column and, while of great interest, does not yet enjoy total acceptance.

WHOLE BLOOD COAGULATION TIME. This test is of historical interest as a diagnostic aid but is quite insensitive as a detector of coagulation defects. The most commonly employed method is a modification of the Lee-White method, in which venous blood is removed by clean venipuncture and 1-ml volumes are delivered into each of three tubes. The first tube is tilted every 30 seconds until no flow of blood is observed. A similar procedure is carried out sequentially on the second and third tubes. The clotting time is taken as the elapsed time from the drawing of blood until coagulation is observed in the third tube.

The coagulation time of blood so studied is influenced by many factors. Several of these relate to the amount of surface activation occurring during the procedure. The smaller the amount of blood relative to the size of the tube, the greater the surface contact and activation. If the tube is tilted more frequently than every 30 seconds, surface activation also is increased. If the venipuncture has not been made cleanly, even minute amounts of tissue juice (tissue thromboplastin) may accelerate the clotting time. To obviate the latter a two-syringe technique may be used. Following successful venipuncture, 1 or 2 ml of blood is drawn into the first syringe, which is carefully disconnected while the needle is held in place and the second syringe attached. Blood is then drawn into the second syringe and provides the sample for the determination. When 1 ml of blood is added, with care to avoid bubbling, to 3 to 10 mm inner diameter clean glass test tubes, the normal range for clotting in the third tube is between 9 and 14 minutes. For practical purposes, only severe deficiencies of factors VIII, IX, XI, XII, and rarely X will be detected by this method. The sensitivity of the test can be increased by employing silicone-coated syringes and clotting tubes or by using plastic syringes and plastic (Lusteroid) tubes. When the latter are employed, the normal clotting time is up to 40 minutes. The test performed with untreated glassware finds its principal use in the control of patients receiving anticoagulation treatment with heparin.

ONE-STAGE PROTHROMBIN TIME (QUICK TEST). This test measures the speed of the events described earlier as the extrinsic pathway of blood coagulation. A tissue source of procoagulant, ideally derived from acetone-dehydrated rabbit brain, as described by Quick, is added with calcium to an aliquot of citrated plasma and the clotting time determined. The laboratory should establish a normal dilution curve and normal values daily. The 100 percent value using the method of Quick should be 15 seconds. Using other sources of tissue thromboplastin, the 100 percent value may be as low as 11 seconds. The prothrombin time will be prolonged in the presence of even minute amounts of heparin. The presence of heparin, by its antithrombin action, will artificially prolong the clotting time of the mixture so that it appears that the prothrombin complex is low. Accordingly, an accurate prothrombin determination cannot be carried out in a patient receiving anticoagulation treatment with heparin until the heparin has disappeared from the plasma. This should be at least 5 hours following the last intravenous dose.

The use of tissue procoagulants in the test eliminates the roles of factors VIII, IX, XI, XII, and platelets. Properly done, the test will detect deficiencies of factors II, V, VII, X, and fibrinogen. The one-stage prothrombin time is the preferred method of controlling anticoagulation with the coumarin and indandione drugs.

PARTIAL THROMBOPLASTIN TIME (PTT). The partial thromboplastin time technically is a variant of the one-stage prothrombin time but provides broader information. The tissue source of procoagulant, commercially available, is extracted and refined so that the in vitro clotting system now is sensitive to factors VIII, IX, XI, XII, as well as the factors normally detected by the one-stage prothrombin time. The range of normal with this test varies with the product used, ranging from 45 to 85 seconds. Each laboratory should establish a normal dilution curve daily, and the patient's plasma must be compared with a normal control.

The partial thromboplastin time, when used in conjunction with the one-stage prothrombin time, can help to place a clotting defect in the first or second stage of the clotting process. If the partial thromboplastin time is prolonged and the one-stage prothrombin time is normal, factors VIII, IX, XI, or XII may be deficient. If the partial thromboplastin time is normal and the one-stage prothrombin time is prolonged, a single or multiple deficiency of factors II, V, VII, or X or of fibrinogen may be present. The partial thromboplastin time also is abnormal in the presence of circulating anticoagulants or during heparin administration. The sensitivity of the test is such that only extremely mild cases of factor VIII or IX deficiency may be missed. In one study of over 600 patients with clotting abnormalities, only two mild abnormalities failed to be detected with this test.

PROTHROMBIN CONSUMPTION TEST. The conversion of prothrombin to thrombin (prothrombin consumption) is a function of the speed of appearance and amount of prothrombin-converting activity generated during blood clotting. When the prothrombin-converting principle (prothrombinase) evolves slowly in clotting blood, the conversion of prothrombin to thrombin (the disappearance of prothrombin) is retarded. At the time of initial blood clotting in vitro, only small amounts of prothrombin have been converted to thrombin. If one examines the *serum* at that time, most of the prothrombin originally present in the plasma remains. When one examines the serum for its prothrombin content 1 hour following the clotting of normal blood, less than 25%, usually about 10%, of the prothrombin originally present in the plasma remains. These observations led to the development of the prothrombin consumption test.

The basis of the test is the comparison of the prothrombin content of the patient's serum 1 hour following clotting with the prothrombin content of the original plasma from which the serum has been derived. Abnormal results may be seen in those states characterized by deficiency of factors responsible for the evolution of the prothrombin-converting principle. These would include factors VIII, IX, X, XI, and XII and, to a lesser extent, platelets and factor V. The test also permits distinction between deficiency of factors VII and X, since factor VII is not necessary for the in vitro formation of prothrombin-converting principle in unassisted blood clotting. Accordingly, the patient with factor VII deficiency will have a prolonged one-stage prothrombin time but normal prothrombin consumption. In contrast, the patient with factor X deficiency will have a prolonged one-stage prothrombin time and an abnormal prothrombin consumption test.

THROMBIN TIME. The test is of value in detecting qualitative abnormalities in fibrinogen, in the detection of circulating anticoagulants and inhibitors of fibrin polymerization. The clotting time of the patient's plasma is measured following the addition of a standard amount of thrombin to a fixed volume of plasma. Controls of normal plasma must be run in parallel. Failure of the clot to form, in the absence of circulating inhibitors such as heparin, is consistent with severe diminution of fibrinogen, usually well below 100 mg/100 ml.

THROMBOPLASTIN GENERATION TEST (TGT). The development of this test permitted a distinction of deficiencies in the hemophilia family of diseases without requiring use of plasma from patients with known abnormalities. The thromboplastin generation test, or modification of it, has been used with success in performing assays of specific clotting factors of the first stage. In most laboratories in this country, the test has been replaced by the partial thromboplastin time test, or variations of it. The thromboplastin generation test has facilitated understanding of current concepts in blood coagulation and continues to be used with success in Great Britain, where it was developed. Preparation of the reagents can be time-consuming, and the test must be done with great precision in order to be reproducible.

TESTS OF FIBRINOLYSIS. The most gross and earliest determination of fibrinolysis was that of observing the whole blood clot for dissolution. Normally, this may not occur for 48 hours or more. When fibrinolysis is a significant factor in hemostatic failure, dissolution of the whole blood clot is observed in 2 hours or less. The test has the disadvantage of being time-consuming in a circumstance where time may be of the essence. In addition, a false impression of increased fibrinolytic activity may be gained from clots formed in patients with high hematocrits or in thrombocytopenia, where red cells may fall away from the clot. The euglobulin clot lysis time and dilute whole blood or plasma clot lysis time are more sensitive indices and permit more rapid evaluation of fibrinolysis.

OTHER TESTS OF HEMOSTASIS. Specific assays of all the known clotting factors now can be performed. The most popular of these assays are based upon modification of the partial thromboplastin time. The accuracy of these tests varies somewhat, but, on the average, the more accurate values are obtained when the factors are significantly reduced. Imprecision usually is found at the higher, clinically less important levels. These tests prove to be of significant clinical value but require an experienced laboratory staff.

Relatively simple tests permit identification of circulating anticoagulants. The simplest of these are based on the retardation of clotting of normal recalcified plasma by varying mixtures of the test plasma. The sensitivity of such tests usually can be increased by incubating the test plasma with the normal plasma for 30 minutes at body temperature prior to recalcification.

The *thrombotest*, devised by Owren, employs a refined tissue procoagulant which seems a little less sensitive than that used for the partial thromboplastin time but slightly more sensitive than that used for the standard one-stage prothrombin time. It has been credited with being more sensitive to factor X deficiency than the one-stage prothrombin time. While its developers have used it extensively, most laboratories will find the Quick one-stage prothrombin time test suitable.

The *thromboelastogram* is a graphic representation of clotting obtained by employing a special instrument, the thromboelastograph. The record obtained provides information about the clotting time, the speed of fibrin polymerization, and the strength and tendency toward dissolution of the clot. The instrument has provided information of research value but has not, in our experience, greatly aided the studies of clinical problems.

EVALUATION OF THE SURGICAL PATIENT AS A HEMOSTATIC RISK

General Considerations

Every patient viewed as a candidate for surgical treatment should be evaluated in terms of the risk of bleeding. The realities of time and economics dictate how exhaustive the approach to a given a patient will be. For the patient requiring surgical intervention on an elective basis several points can be emphasized. The nondirective, open-ended patient interview has proved of value in many diagnostic settings. Direct questioning, however, is required to elicit most hints of a bleeding tendency.

The history should determine if circumcision was accompanied by unusual bleeding, since such bleeding is a frequent occurrence in patients who have inherited hemostatic problems. Hemophilic infants have been circumcised, however, without bleeding when the circumcision was performed immediately following delivery. Sufficient factor VIII may be supplied by transplacental transfer. The dental history can be of great significance. Many patients with inherited bleeding disorders may have bleeding with eruption of the teeth or bleeding after extraction. In the case of the hemophiliac, bleeding may begin hours after extraction and continue to be a problem for several days. The patient with a bleeding disorder, either acquired or inherited, who does not bleed after tonsillectomy sufficiently to require reexploration or transfusion is rare. It also is unusual for the patient with a hemorrhagic diathesis to have hematemesis, epistaxis, or hemoptysis without some other hemorrhagic manifestation. The gastrointestinal tract has been regarded as an area of poor resistance in patients with hemostatic difficulties, but isolated gastrointestinal bleeding, *in the absence of bleeding or bruising tendency elsewhere,* usually is not associated with generalized hemostatic failure. More often, it may be related to local disease or associated with lesions such as hereditary hemorrhagic telangiectasia. Excessive menstrual flow, rather than intermenstrual bleeding, is a common complaint in patients with generalized hemostatic problems. It is not infrequent for such a patient, usually with thrombocytopenia, to be subjected to uterine curettage. Such an oversight can result in catastrophic complications. A detailed history of drug ingestion is essential, and it is wise to specify products by name. The patient may not regard aspirin, tranquilizers, and other pharmacologic agents which can affect the hemostatic process as drugs.

Special emphasis must be made of the family history. It is not enough to question the health of siblings and parents. Appreciation of simple genetic principles, such as the sex-linked recessive mode of transmission of some of the more serious clotting disorders, requires that we inquire into the health of grandparents, occasionally great grandparents, and certainly uncles and cousins. Patterns for the genetic transmission of hemorrhagic disorders are presented later in this chapter.

Certain findings on the physical examination should alert the examiner to the possibility of a hemostatic problem. The entire body should be inspected for ecchymoses or petechiae. These lesions are likely to appear at pressure points, where snug foundation garments are worn, or under belts or garters. Purpuric lesions are characteristically spontaneous in origin, often multiple, and frequently bilateral. The lesions of senile purpura are most common on forearms and hands, where tissue support is loose, while lesions of Henoch-Schönlein purpura generally are distributed over the buttocks, backs of the legs, elbows, and ankles. Spider angiomas are suggestive of liver disease. While not related, they may be associated with reduction in the prothrombin complex. Lesions characteristic of hereditary hemorrhagic telangiectasia are often found on the lips, under the fingernails, or around the anus. Examination of these areas is indicated in patients with gastrointestinal bleeding. When inspecting the skin, the site of a recent venipuncture should be evaluated for petechiae, ecchymoses, or hematoma.

Widespread lymph node enlargement, the presence of an enlarged liver or spleen, may suggest the possibility of reticuloendothelial disease. Jaundice, hepatomegaly, ascites, distended abdominal veins, and splenomegaly may be stigmata of liver disease. Again, these may be associated with a significant reduction in the level of the prothrombin complex.

Evaluation of the Unsuspected Bleeder

The surest method of identifying an unsuspected bleeder is to obtain a complete history and perform a thorough physical examination. The ideal laboratory test to detect these patients has yet to be described. The single most productive laboratory procedure, unquestionably, is the examination of the peripheral blood smear. Since thrombocytopenia is the most common abnormality resulting in failure of hemostasis and is so easily identified by simple inspection of a well-stained blood smear, the importance of this examination cannot be overemphasized. Other important information derived from examination of the blood smear has already been described.

Measurement of the bleeding time is an imperfect screening test. When abnormal, one must heed its warning. When normal, as it frequently is in a variety of serious hemostatic disorders, little confidence should be derived. Regrettably, this test historically has been coupled with the whole blood clotting time as a screening battery for the detection of hemostatic defects. The limitations of the whole blood clotting time as a diagnostic screening test also have been noted earlier. Fully one-third of patients affected by blood-clotting disorders that theoretically might be identified by this test will be missed. Observation of the clot retraction is another time-honored test which is not recommended for reliable screening. Platelet counts as low as 60,000 to 70,000/mm^3 can result in respectable clot retraction. Significant thrombocytopenia may go undetected if one relies too heavily on this test. Its one virtue is its simplicity.

Simple tests with reliability are available. The partial thromboplastin time, performed with care and with normal controls, is of sufficient sensitivity that abnormalities likely to result in life-endangering bleeding at operation are unlikely to be missed. The partial thromboplastin time will detect not only those abnormalities that would be identified by the whole blood clotting time but also those abnormalities characterized by defects in the prothrombin complex. The Quick one-stage prothrombin time also is a simple and accurate test which will identify abnormalities of factors V, VII, and X and prothrombin (factor II). When used in conjunction with the partial thromboplastin time, it can separate an abnormality into problems of the first stage (hemophilia group) and those of the second stage (prothrombin complex). For screening related to problems of fibrinolysis, as in patients with metastatic prostatic carcinoma or pancreatic disease, the dilute whole blood or plasma clot lysis tests are applicable.

Evaluation of the Suspected Potential Bleeder

The patient who is suspected of having hemostatic dysfunction requires a more comprehensive evaluation. This includes a particularly detailed history, a thorough physical examination, and more complete study in the laboratory. Accordingly, time must be set aside to permit these efforts. These can usually be done on an outpatient basis, or if the patient is already hospitalized and scheduled for operation, scheduling of the case should permit time for the

necessary evaluations. If suspicion of an abnormality is based on family history, every effort should be made to study other members of the family. If suspicion is based on previous bleeding following surgical treatment, every effort should be made to obtain the old hospital records, since they may provide important information. When the question of bleeding related to drug administration has been raised, identification of the drug through prescription files in pharmacies and obtaining the medications for inspection may be helpful.

If the history of drug exposure or the physical findings of petechiae or mucous membrane bleeding suggest the possibility of thrombocytopenia, in addition to the examination of the blood smear, direct platelet counting should be performed. Careful, and preferably multiple, bleeding times should be determined. Drug-related immunologic forms of thrombocytopenia can be evaluated with the clot retraction inhibition test. This takes advantage of the fact that antibody may remain in the patient's serum for 4 to 6 months. An aliquot of the patient's serum together with an aliquot of a saturated solution of the suspected drug are clotted together with an aliquot of the patient's blood. If the platelets are immunologically damaged in the presence of the drug, the clot retraction is inhibited. The use of appropriate normal controls is imperative. More detailed observations, such as the platelets' ability to aggregate in their native plasma following the addition of ADP, and measurements of platelet factor 3 release also can be performed.

If a blood coagulation defect is suspected, a combination of tests can help place the defect (Table 3-1). If the partial thromboplastin time is abnormal and the one-stage prothrombin time is normal, the defect is almost certainly in the first stage of clotting. One then has the option of performing mixing and matching studies or, more desirably, specific clotting factor assays. The former require samples of plasma from patients with proved abnormalities. One then tests the patient in question by determining if a small amount of the patient's plasma will correct the abnormality of the known deficient sample in vitro. Such

Table 3-1. DIAGNOSIS OF INHERITED DISORDERS OF COAGULATION

Deficient factor	Bleeding time	One-stage prothrombin time	Partial thromboplastin time	Thrombin time	Fibrinogen time	Platelet adhesiveness
I (fibrinogen)	Long or normal	Long	Long	Long	Low	Normal
II	Normal	Long	Long	Normal	Normal	Normal
V	Normal	Long	Long	Normal	Normal	Normal
VII	Normal	Long	Normal	Normal	Normal	Normal
VIII	Normal	Normal	Long	Normal	Normal	Normal
IX	Normal	Normal	Long	Normal	Normal	Normal
X	Normal	Long	Long	Normal	Normal	Normal
XI	Normal	Normal	Long	Normal	Normal	Normal
XII	Normal	Normal	Long	Normal	Normal	Normal
XIII	Normal	Normal	Normal	Normal	Normal	Normal
Von Willebrand's disease	Long	Normal	Long	Normal	Normal	Low

SOURCE: E. W. Salzman, Hemorrhagic disorders, in J. M. Kinney, R. H. Egdahl, and G. D. Zuidema (eds.), "Manual of Preoperative and Postoperative Care," p. 157, W. B. Saunders Company, Philadelphia, 1971.

tests can give reliable qualitative results in terms of establishing a specific diagnosis. Assays for individual blood-clotting factors can be performed by many laboratories. In addition to the specificity of the test, quantitative values are obtained, permitting estimation of the severity of the disease process. The specific assays are of particular value in controlling the transfusion program of affected patients undergoing surgical treatment.

Evaluation of the Patient Who Begins to Bleed During or After Surgical Procedures

The patient who bleeds excessively during or shortly following surgical procedures is an emergency problem. The approach to this difficult situation must be prompt and well organized. Generally, bleeding at the time of operation ultimately is identified as being due to, singly or in combination, (1) ineffective local hemostasis, (2) complications of blood transfusion, (3) a previously present but unsuspected hemostatic defect, (4) sepsis, (5) induced fibrinolysis or defibrination.

Bleeding from one site only, such as the surgical wound, usually is not due to a generalized hemostatic defect. The patient who manifests bleeding at the primary incisional site, for example, but not at the site of a stab wound where drains have been placed or the patient who is bleeding from a thoracotomy wound but not at all from his tracheostomy site is more likely to have a local problem that a generalized defect. One exception to this generalization should be noted: Occasionally following prostatic surgical treatment excessive bleeding from the prostatic bed is noted. The plasminogen activator present in prostatic tissue is activated by the urokinase normally present in the urine as it washes over the raw prostatic bed. Increased fibrinolysis occurs locally on the raw surface of the wound, and bleeding is aggravated. This is a failure of local hemostasis based, not on any mechanical problem, but rather on the increased activation of the local fibrinolytic process. A 24- to 48-hour period of interruption of this plasminogen activation by the administration of ϵ-aminocaproic acid (ϵ-ACA) usually suffices to still the blood loss.

Although one may be reasonably certain on clinical grounds that surgical bleeding is related to local problems, laboratory investigation must be confirmatory. Prompt examination of the blood smear to determine the number of platelets and an actual platelet count if the smear is not clear-cut should be done. A partial thromboplastin time, one-stage prothrombin time, and thrombin clotting time all can be determined within minutes. Correct interpretation of the results should confirm the clinical impression or identify the exceptional problem.

Complications of blood transfusion are an occasional cause of hemostatic failure. Massive blood transfusion with banked blood is a well-documented cause of thrombocytopenia. Most patients who receive 10 units or more of banked blood within a period of 24 hours will be measurably thrombocytopenic, but usually not sufficiently so to result in hemostatic failure. Patients who receive 14 units or more of banked blood in a period of 24 hours or less invariably will be significantly thrombocytopenic and may have frank bleeding as a result. *The patient in whom signs of hemostatic failure develop during or following operation when large quantities of banked blood have been used should be assumed to be thrombocytopenic until demonstrated otherwise.* The usual approach of examining the blood smear and determining the number of platelets should suffice to provide this answer. The therapeutic approach consists of supplying fresh platelets in the form of fresh blood if the patient requires volume or transfusion with fresh platelet-rich plasma or concentrated platelets if the red cells and blood volume are adequate. Preventive medicine can be practiced in relation to this complication. If the surgeon anticipates that a procedure may require massive transfusion, arrangement should be made in advance for fresh blood to be available. Prudent practice requires that with no patient should more than 10 units of banked blood be given without then using fresh blood. Following transfusion of 10 units of banked blood, at least equal volumes of fresh blood and banked blood should be employed as subsequent replacement.

Another cause of hemostatic failure involving transfusion is that of the hemolytic transfusion reaction. This complication, usually so readily detected in the conscious patient, can be difficult to recognize in the anesthetized patient. The characteristic chilly sensation, muscle ache, backache, headache, and ultimate hemoglobinuria will not be evident. The first hint to the experienced surgeon that the patient is undergoing hemolytic transfusion reaction may be progressive failure of hemostasis. Tissues in the operative field which have previously been dry begin to ooze.

The pathogenesis of this bleeding is not perfectly established, but several probable causes have been suggested. The release of ADP from the hemolyzed red cells may be sufficient to cause platelet aggregation, and the platelet clumps then are swept out of the circulation. Red blood cells also are a rich source of the procoagulant platelet factor 3 (phospholipid) necessary at several stages of blood coagulation. Release of these substances during hemolytic transfusion reaction may result in progression of the clotting mechanism and intravascular defibrination. In addition, the fibrinolytic mechanism may be triggered by the intravascular clotting. Both defibrination and fibrinolysis have been documented clinically and experimentally following hemolytic transfusion reaction. Their incidence is low but must be considered when the clinical events are consistent. The bleeding problem associated with hemolytic transfusion reaction should be considered due to thrombocytopenia until other laboratory measures suggest defibrination or fibrinolysis.

Transfusion purpura, which has been described in detail by Shulman and associates, is an uncommon but interesting cause of thrombocytopenia and associated bleeding following transfusion. In this circumstance, the donor platelets are of the uncommon Pl^{A1} group. These platelets sensitize the recipient, who makes antibody to the foreign platelet antigen. The foreign platelet antigen does not completely disappear from the recipient circulation but seems to attach to the recipient's own platelets. The antibody, which attains a sufficient titer within 6 or 7 days following the sensitizing transfusion, then destroys the recipient's own platelets. The resultant thrombocytopenia and bleeding may continue for several weeks. This uncommon cause of thrombocytopenia should be considered if bleeding follows transfusion by 5 or 6 days. Platelet transfusions are of little help in the management of this syndrome, since the new donor platelets usually are subject to the binding of antigen and damage from the antibody. Corticosteroids may be of some help in reducing the bleeding tendency. Posttransfusion purpura is self-limited, and the passage of several weeks inevitably leads to subsidence of the problem.

The patient with a hemostatic defect which manifests itself first during surgical treatment is likely to have other evidence of bleeding, such as ecchymoses at the sites of injection or venipunctures, and bloody drainage from nasogastric tubes or bladder catheters.

A hemostatic defect may be imposed iatrogenically during surgical treatment employing extracorporeal bypass. Many etiologic factors may be involved, but the most commonly implicated is the introduction of heparin into the circulation. Bleeding after discontinuation of extracorporeal bypass may be due to inadequate neutralization of heparin with protamine sulfate. Since both protamine sulfate and Polybrene are themselves anticoagulants when large doses are used, it is possible that bleeding was caused by these drugs. This is a rare occurrence. Rapid tests can be performed in vitro by adding small amounts of protamine sulfate to see if the clotting time is shortened. Other abnormalities attributed to extracorporeal circulation are defibrination and fibrinolysis. Fibrinolytic activity is often increased. These changes usually are related to the duration of pumping. We are impressed by the *lack* of clinical bleeding in the patients with laboratory evidence of fibrinolysis. Thrombocytopenia, hypofibrinogenemia, and reduction in factors V and VIII have been demonstrated. The thrombocytopenia usually is not severe, and the platelet count generally remains above 50,000/mm³. Evaluation of the patient with intraoperative or postoperative bleeding suspected of being due to hemostatic defect follows the same course previously outlined for preoperative evaluation of these patients.

At times, an operation performed in a patient with sepsis is attended by continued bleeding. Severe hemorrhagic disorders due to thrombocytopenia have occurred consequent to gram-negative sepsis. The pathogenesis of endotoxin-induced thrombocytopenia has been studied in detail, and it is suggested that a labile factor, possibly factor V, is necessary for this interaction. Defibrination and hemostatic failure also may occur with meningococcemia, *Clostridium welchii* sepsis and staphylococcal sepsis. Hemolysis appears to be one mechanism in sepsis leading to defibrination.

The appearance of pathologic fibrinolysis during surgical treatment is an uncommon but potentially serious event. It can occur subsequent to shock, following intravascular defibrination, and in association with operation on tissues rich in activators of the fibrinolytic mechanism. These include pancreas, prostate, and lung. Defibrination also can occur as a consequence of hemolytic transfusion reaction and sepsis.

The thrombin time can be of value in detecting abnormalities in fibrinogen. When fibrinolysis is a significant factor, dissolution of the whole blood clot is observed in 2 hours or less, but the euglobulin clot lysis and dilute whole blood clot lysis are more sensitive indices and permit more rapid evaluation.

CLINICAL HEMOSTATIC DEFECTS

Inheritance

The importance of a detailed family history in the evaluation of the patient with a possible hemostatic defect has been emphasized. The sensible use of this information requires an understanding of genetic principles and knowledge of the specific genetic features of the hemostatic disorders.

The modes of inheritance of hemostatic disorders, with few rare exceptions, are three in type: (1) autosomal dominant, (2) autosomal recessive, and (3) sex-linked recessive. The 46 chromosomes of man consist of 22 autosomal pairs, plus a pair of sex chromosomes, the X and Y. Since one chromosome of each of the 22 autosomal pairs normally is derived from each parent, any gene inherited as a part of an autosomal chromosome normally will occur with equal frequency among males and females. Each child of a parent carrying an autosomal dominant gene has one chance in two of inheriting that trait. The most common hemostatic disorder transmitted by the autosomal dominant mode is von Willebrand's disease. Hereditary hemorrhagic telangiectasia and factor XI deficiency also appear to be transmitted in this fashion.

A normal individual should transmit no disease to his progeny. Occasionally, in a pedigree with an autosomal dominant gene, an *apparently* normal person may transmit disease to his or her child. The parent clearly carried the gene, which clinically expressed no defect. Explanation of this phenomenon is not at hand. The gene activity in the parent is referred to as "incompletely penetrant."

In inherited hemostatic disorders, the difference in clinical expression between dominant and recessive genes is a graded one rather than an "all-or-none" phenomenon. The heterozygous individual with an autosomal recessive trait may have a measurable deficiency of the factor governed by that gene, but no clinical disease. In order to demonstrate clinical expression of disease, the individual must be homozygous. This appears to be the case, for example, in factor X deficiency. The homozygote with clinical disease, as described by Hougie, has less than 5% of factor X activity, while heterozygotes have levels ranging from 21 to 50%. Since the presumed heterozygotes within the same pedigree vary in factor X activity, it is convenient to suggest that the gene shows variable expression. Other hemostatic disorders probably inherited in this mode are factor V, factor VII, and factor I deficiencies. This mode of transmission could be regarded as incompletely dominant inheritance, rather than incompletely recessive, depending upon one's view. Since these traits are not very common, it is difficult to resolve this problem.

Sex-linked recessive inheritance governs true hemophilia (factor VIII deficiency) and factor IX deficiency (Christmas disease). The genes for these diseases are recessive in expression and are carried on the female (X) chromosome. When paired with the normal X chromosome (the female carrier state), clinical disease is not present. When the affected X chromosome is paired with the normal male (Y) chromosome, clinical disease is expressed.

Theoretically, with the "graded" expression, the female carrier should be detectable in the laboratory. In fact, since the range of factor VIII activity normally is so broad, most female carriers *appear* to fall in the low-normal range. Estimates vary, but possibly as many as 50 percent of female carriers can be identified. Although the sex-linked recessive mode of inheritance has been confirmed repeatedly in true hemophilia, it seems likely that an *autosomal* gene also may influence factor VIII activity. This probability is emphasized by the autosomal dominant mode of inheritance of von Willebrand's disease, characterized by low factor VIII activity, and also by the patterns of variation in factor VIII activity among individuals within the same normal family and among different normal families.

Despite the lack of complete understanding of genetic determinants in hemostatic disorders, detailed consideration of the family history facilitates accurate diagnosis.

Factor VIII Deficiency
(Classical Hemophilia)

Classical hemophilia (hemophilia A) is a disease of males. The failure to synthesize normal factor VIII activity is inherited as a sex-linked recessive trait. Incidence of the disease is approximately 1:25,000 population, and the clinical manifestations can be extremely variable.

CLINICAL MANIFESTATIONS. Characteristically, the severity of clinical manifestations is related to the degree of deficiency of factor VIII. Spontaneous bleeding and severe complications are the rule when virtually no factor VIII can be detected in the plasma. When plasma factor VIII concentrations are in the range of 25%, the patient may have no spontaneous bleeding yet may bleed severely with trauma or surgical treatment. Typically, members of the same pedigree with true hemophilia will have approximately the same degree of clinical manifestations.

While the severely affected patient may bleed during early infancy, significant bleeding typically is noted first when the child is a toddler. At that time, in addition to the classic bleeding into joints, bleeding may occur at other sites. Epistaxis and hematuria may be noted. Bleeding which is life-threatening may follow injury to the tongue or frenulum. We have seen tracheal compression following tonsillar infection and retropharyngeal bleeding. Vascular and neural compromise may occur in relation to pressure secondary to bleeding into a soft tissue closed space. Equinous contracture deformity may be seen in severely hemophilic patients secondary to bleeding into the calf.

Volkmann's contracture of the forearm and flexion contractures of the knees and elbows are also disabling sequelae of deep soft tissue bleeding.

Hemarthrosis is the most characteristic orthopedic problem. Bleeding into the joint may cause few symptoms until distension of the joint capsule occurs. Muscle spasm and pain around the joint arise from involvement of periarticular structures. A large hemarthrosis generally is manifested by a tender, swollen, warm, and painful joint. These signs may mimic infection. The same orthopedic problems are noted in association with severe factor IX deficiency (Christmas disease).

Retroperitoneal bleeding may follow lifting of a heavy object or strenuous exercise. Signs of posterior peritoneal irritation and spasm of the iliopsoas suggest the diagnosis. Hypovolemic shock may occur, since the amount of blood loss that can take place in this setting is enormous. The potential space in the retroperitoneal area readily accommodates several liters of blood in the adult. An intramural hematoma within the intestine also can pose problems of differential diagnosis. The clinical manifestations of nausea and vomiting, crampy abdominal pain, and signs of peritoneal irritation mimic those of appendicitis. Fever and leukocytosis may be noted. Roentgenograms of the abdomen may fail to reveal an abnormality or may display a modest amount of ileus. Upper gastrointestinal examination may demonstrate a uniform thickening of mucosal folds which has been described as a "picket fence" or "stack of coins" appearance (Fig. 3-5). Intramural hematomas of the intestine occur with other hemostatic disorders and, therefore, should be considered when any patient with a hemostatic problem presents with findings suggesting an acute intraabdominal process.

TREATMENT. This requires an appreciation of the transfusion therapy necessary to correct factor VIII deficiency as well as the application of specific surgical principles.

Replacement Therapy. The plasma concentration of factor VIII necessary for maintenance of hemostatic integrity is normally quite small. Patients with as little as 2 to 3% of factor VIII activity usually do not bleed spontaneously. Once serious bleeding begins, however, a much higher level of factor VIII activity, probably approaching 30%, is necessary to achieve hemostasis.

Following transfusion, the plasma level of factor VIII in vivo depends upon the potency of the administered preparation and the survival of the infused factor VIII. Many formulas have been developed as a guide to replacement. These should not be used in a cookbook fashion. We view laboratory control of the level of factor VIII as extremely important. This is particularly pertinent since the amount of factor VIII in individual aliquots of frozen plasma and cryoprecipitate varies considerably.

Following administration of a given dose of factor VIII, approximately one-half of the initial posttransfusion activity disappears from the plasma in 4 hours. This early disappearance is thought to be due, in large part, to diffusion from the intravascular space. The period of equilibration extends for as long as 8 hours, at which time only about one-quarter of the initial level remains in the circu-

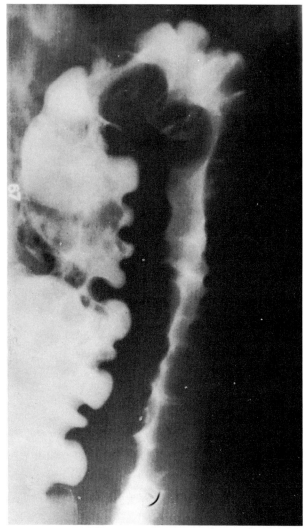

Fig. 3-5. Upper gastrointestinal roentgenogram of patient with "acquired hemophilia." Note thickening of mucosal folds indicative of an intramural hematoma. The spontaneous bleeding in this patient was ascribed to powerful circulating anticoagulant to factor VIII.

from which they are prepared. A hemophilic patient can be prepared for surgical treatment with a minimal initial dose of cryoprecipitate concentrated from an amount of plasma equal to one-half the patient's estimated blood volume. For a 70-kg patient undergoing major surgical treatment, the cryoprecipitate derived from 5 liters of plasma will be necessary to raise the factor VIII level to 60% of normal. Half that amount is subsequently administered every 12 hours to maintain a safe level. A promising factor VIII concentrate prepared as a glycine precipitate also is available. Concentrations as high as 70 or 80 units/ml are obtainable, simplifying the management of the hemophilic patient. Regardless of the preparation employed, continued laboratory assessment of circulating factor VIII level is an important element in the control of these patients.

Following major surgical treatment of the hemophiliac, transfusion replacement of factor VIII should be continued for at least 10 days. Wounds should be well healed and all drains removed prior to the termination of therapy. If sutures remain, transfusion should be reinstituted prior to their removal.

The virus of homologous serum hepatitis is transmitted by the various concentrates of plasma. Whether the new glycine precipitates are free of this virus remains to be demonstrated. Other complications of replacement therapy include the appearance of inhibitors of factor VIII, which may arise in the hemophiliacs who have had transfusion. These inhibitors have been characterized as antibodies of the γ G variety. They tend to diminish in several weeks if further transfusion is not employed. Laboratory search for these factors should be carried out in every hemophilic patient who is considered a candidate for elective surgical treatment, as their presence enormously complicates transfusion management.

Adjunctive Management. Treatment of soft tissue bleeding is directed at the prevention of airway obstruction and vascular and neural damage. These are accomplished best by the administration of sufficient factor VIII. Bed rest and cold packs can be of some assistance. In general, results of fasciotomy to relieve pressure have varied from disappointing to disastrous. The occasional development of large cysts has resulted in sufficient deformity and disability to require amputation.

The primary treatment of hemophilic hemarthrosis is directed at maintaining full range of motion and minimal destruction of the cartilage. Aspiration of blood from the hemophilic joint is not uniformly endorsed, and when regarded as necessary, it should be considered a major surgical event. Elevation of factor VIII level by transfusion is necessary. The procedure should be carried out in the operating room under strict sterile precautions. In most instances, aspiration is not required, and the combination of factor VIII replacement and local cold packing proves sufficient. Physiotherapy plays a critical role and should consist of *active* exercises, since the patient is unlikely to move the extremity to a point where bleeding will recur. Passive exercises often result in recurrence of bleeding. The reader is referred to the review by Curtiss for details of orthopedic management.

lating blood. From that time on, the slope of disappearance is less steep (Fig. 3-6). Twenty-four hours after a given dose, no more than 7 to 8% of administered factor VIII activity remains within the circulation.

One unit of factor VIII activity is considered that amount present in 1 ml of normal plasma. Theoretically, in a patient with 0% activity, to achieve an initial posttransfusion level of 60% of normal, using fresh plasma, a volume of plasma equal to 60% of the patient's estimated plasma volume would have to be administered. Remembering the loss from the circulation, one-half the initial dose would need to be supplied every 12 hours. The use of fresh plasma in such a circumstance would require a volume that is excessive. Factor VIII concentrates now available circumvent this problem. Cryoprecipitate concentrates of factor VIII can be regarded as containing one-half the amount of factor VIII present in the plasma

The management of intramural intestinal hematoma and retroperitoneal bleeding is predicated on appropriate transfusion therapy and avoidance of surgical treatment. It is to be emphasized that even when a relatively minor procedure, such as tracheostomy, is performed, the plasma level of factor VIII should be raised above 25 to 30%. Since dental hygiene usually is poor in hemophilic patients, dental and oral surgical treatment frequently are necessary. The same principles of transfusion therapy pertain, and the procedures should be delegated to well-trained personnel working where optimal care can be provided.

Recently, the question of transplantation of the spleen as therapy for hemophilia has been raised. Norman and associates have suggested that the spleen may be a site of factor VIII synthesis and/or storage. Also, it has been reported that the spleen is receptive to circulating factor VIII–trophic substance in the plasma of human hemophiliacs. In hemophilic dogs receiving heterotrophic splenic transplants, factor VIII levels were increased thirtyfold, to levels more than that required to prevent spontaneous bleeding. In an independent study, Webster and associates reported dissimilar results and an absence of significant effect on factor VIII. They warned against clinical applicability of this procedure. This concern has been reinforced by one subsequent clinical case of splenic transplantation in a human being, with continued postoperative bleeding and splenic infarction necessitating removal of the transplanted spleen. At this point, such imaginative but aggressive attempts cannot be recommended.

Von Willebrand's Disease (Pseudohemophilia)

Von Willebrand's disease occurs as commonly as true hemophilia. The increasing recognition is related to more reliable factor VIII assays. This hereditary disorder of hemostasis is transmitted as an autosomally dominant trait and, accordingly, appears in consecutive generations with males and females equally affected. The disease is characterized by a diminution of the level of factor VIII activity. The reduction of factor VIII activity usually is not as great as that seen in classical hemophilia. Also unlike classical hemophilia, where factor VIII activity remains constant, in the patient with von Willebrand's disease variation in the level of circulating factor VIII activity may be noted. Characteristically, these patients also have a prolonged bleeding time, but this is less constant than the factor VIII reduction. A given patient may have an abnormal bleeding time on one occasion and a normal bleeding time on another. Abnormalities of platelet adhesiveness in vitro, using Salzman's method, also have been described. Technical problems requiring exquisite standardization of the platelet adhesiveness test have limited its widespread use.

CLINICAL MANIFESTATIONS. The manifestations of bleeding usually are mild and often overlooked until trauma or the stress of surgical treatment makes them apparent. A careful clinical history is, therefore, of great importance in these patients. Spontaneous manifestations often are limited to bleeding into the skin or mild mucous membrane bleeding. Epistaxis and menorrhagia have been

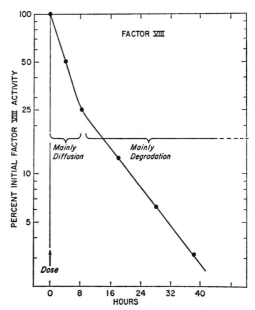

Fig. 3-6. Schematic representation of in vivo decay of a single dose of factor VIII. (*From N. R. Shulman, Mod Treat, 5:61, 1968.*)

relatively common in our personal experience. Serious bleeding following dental extractions and tonsillectomy also are not uncommon. Fatal bleeding from the gastrointestinal tract has been described.

TREATMENT. The typical patient with von Willebrand's disease will produce factor VIII activity in response to transfusion of modest amounts of plasma. This is unlike the classical hemophiliac in whom factor VIII concentration rises only in proportion to the amount of that substance actually transfused. In von Willebrand's disease, some 4 to 6 hours following transfusion an increase in circulating factor VIII activity to the range of five to eight times that which could be ascribed to transfusion alone is noted. This apparent synthesis continues for approximately 24 hours. Exceptions to this characteristic response recently have been described.

When a patient with von Willebrand's disease is scheduled to undergo surgical treatment, plasma transfusion should be instituted at least 48 hours prior to the operative procedure. In this manner, it can be determined whether the patient will respond to infusion with appearance of factor VIII activity. If factor VIII activity is not generated, a more ambitious program of transfusion is necessary to sustain the patient through the operative and postoperative period. In most patients, infusion of 10 ml of plasma/kg of body weight/24 hours will ensure hemostatically effective levels of factor VIII. Banked blood or plasma is effective as the stimulatory agent. Duration of treatment should be the same as that described for the patient with classical hemophilia.

Factor IX Deficiency (Christmas Disease)

Factor IX deficiency clinically is indistinguishable from factor VIII deficiency. These two entities were considered a single disease until 1952, when their unique deficiencies were documented. The incidence of factor IX deficiency is approximately 1:100,000 population.

TREATMENT. Factor IX, although not in the prothrombin complex, is dependent upon vitamin K for its synthesis in the liver. It is present in banked blood, plasma, and serum. Initially, the rate of disappearance of factor IX from the circulation is more rapid than that of factor VIII, but subsequently factor IX has a slower disappearance rate (Fig. 3-7). Half of the factor IX which is present 5 or 6 hours following transfusion remains after 24 hours. An infusion of plasma containing factor IX raises the recipient's factor IX level less than would be predicted. The extravascular space into which factor IX distributes itself may be larger than the distribution space for factor VIII. The longer survival of factor IX helps compensate for its more rapid initial disappearance following transfusion. Accordingly, a dose of 15 ml of plasma/kg of body weight administered over a 1- or 2-hour period 6 hours or more prior to operation usually serves to raise the plasma level to a suitable point. Half that volume then is administered every 12 hours as long as clinical indications require. An alternative method of treatment is that of administering 60 ml of plasma/kg over a 10- to 20-hour period 24 hours prior to anticipated surgical treatment and repeating doses of 7 ml/kg every 12 hours.

It should be emphasized that the patient with a mild factor IX deficiency, like the patient with a mild factor VIII deficiency, can bleed massively with surgical treatment and requires planned replacement therapy. At present, concentrated factor IX preparations are not widely available. Cryoprecipitates cannot be used in the treatment of factor IX deficiency. Cryoprecipitates which are rich in factor VIII contain only trace amounts of factor IX.

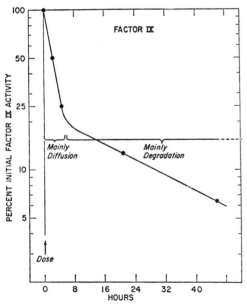

Fig. 3-7. Schematic representation of in vivo decay of a single dose of factor IX. (*From N. R. Shulman, Mod Treat, 5:61, 1968.*)

Factor XI (PTA) Deficiency (Rosenthal's Syndrome)

This uncommon and relatively mild disorder is inherited in an autosomally dominant fashion. Without careful laboratory testing, the affected males and females may be confused with von Willebrand's disease patients. A majority of patients are of Jewish ancestry.

Epistaxis is a common spontaneous clinical manifestation. The disease usually is recognized as a result of bleeding during and after operation. The bleeding usually is minor. Some patients have undergone major procedures without significant hemorrhage.

TREATMENT. Factor XI actually may gain in potency during storage, so that plasma is a suitable therapeutic medium. This factor disappears slowly from the circulation, and its biologic half-life may be as long as 48 hours. An initial dose of 10 ml of plasma/kg of body weight can be given 6 or 8 hours prior to anticipated surgical treatment, followed by a maintenance dose of 5 ml/kg administered every 24 hours. Therapy usually can be discontinued several days earlier than with patients with more serious hemostatic disorders.

Factor V (Proaccelerin) Deficiency (Parahemophilia)

This extremely rare deficiency usually is associated with mild bleeding, but serious bleeding may be encountered. The disease is transmitted as an autosomal recessive trait and is found in males and females alike. Only patients who presumably inherit the gene from both parents seem to be bleeders.

Factor V is synthesized in the liver but differs from prothrombin and factors VII, IX, and X in that factor V synthesis is not dependent upon vitamin K or inhibited by the administration of the coumarin drugs. Patients with severe parenchymal liver disease may be deficient in factor V.

TREATMENT. Excessive bleeding may occur at the time of operation, usually in patients who have levels of less than 1% of normal factor V concentration. No more than 25% of normal activity is necessary for hemostasis during operative procedures. This level can be achieved by administering 15 ml of fresh or freshly frozen plasma per kg of body weight 12 hours prior to operation. The administration of 7 to 10 ml/kg every 24 hours will suffice to maintain hemostasis until healing has occurred. Once again, it is wise to administer the factor at the time of suture removal. Factor V, also known as labile factor, loses its activity during storage. Only fresh plasma or plasma freshly frozen is applicable as therapy.

Factor VII (Proconvertin) Deficiency

Factor VII (stable factor) deficiency is an uncommon but not rare disease. Mild clinical manifestations are the rule. The deficiency is inherited as an autosomal gene of "intermediate penetrance." The homozygous state results in significant deficiency and may be associated with serious bleeding. In these patients, spontaneous epistaxis, genitourinary and gastrointestinal bleeding, and even hemarthroses, may be seen. The heterozygotes have minimal, if any, clinical manifestations.

Factor VII, like factors II, IX, and X, requires vitamin K for synthesis. The synthesis is blocked by coumarin administration. Coumarin inhibition of synthesis is reversed by vitamin K administration. The administration of vitamin K to patients *congenitally* deficient in these activities will *not* result in synthesis and increased plasma levels.

As is also true for factor V–deficient patients and in patients with deficiencies of factors II and X, the one-stage prothrombin time is prolonged in patients with factor VII deficiency. Since factor VII is active only in the "extrinsic" blood-clotting system, deficient patients have a normal prothrombin consumption test. In contrast, patients with factor X deficiency have abnormal prothrombin consumption, significant prothrombin remaining in the serum 1 hour after coagulation. Another laboratory distinction between factor VII and factor X deficiency can be made by the use of the Stypven time test. Factor X is necessary for the effect of this viper venom in blood coagulation, while factor VII is not. Accordingly, the factor VII–deficient patient has a normal Stypven time.

TREATMENT. The biologic half-life of factor VII probably is the briefest of any of the blood-clotting factors. The initial half-life, thought to be due to equilibration between the intravascular and extravascular compartments, probably is no more than 30 minutes. The remainder of the disappearance time presumably represents catabolism and is estimated at between 5 and 6 hours. Despite this relatively rapid disappearance, the transfusion management of patients with factor VII deficiency is not a great problem. Factor VII levels of less than 4 to 5% of normal are necessary before significant bleeding occurs. Even at these low levels of plasma activity, replacement transfusion is not always necessary for surgical procedures. Although the one-stage prothrombin time recognizes deficiency of factor VII, this test is not an effective guide to the treatment of factor VII–deficient patients. The test is markedly abnormal at factor VII levels at which the deficient patient may not bleed. Transfusion of banked plasma, 10 ml/kg of body weight, on the day of the operation, followed by half that amount daily for the next 5 or 6 days, provides adequate factor VII for hemostasis during major surgical treatment.

Factor X (Stuart-Prower) Deficiency

This relatively rare deficiency is inherited as an autosomal recessive trait and has been described in amyloidosis. Clinically, affected patients are homozygotes, while the heterozygotes are clinically well and only minimally affected. The latter may demonstrate mild abnormalities with the one-stage prothrombin test and the thromboplastin generation test.

TREATMENT. Little experience has been acquired in the surgical management of patients with factor X deficiency. Plasma levels of 15% of normal have proved sufficient to prevent significant bleeding following dental extractions.

Plasma transfusion experiments in patients with factor X deficiency have demonstrated an 8- to 10-hour first-phase disappearance time of half the administered activity, followed by a disappearance time estimated at 40 hours. Applying these data, plasma levels of 15% or greater could be achieved by infusing 15 to 20 ml of normal plasma per kg of body weight initially, followed by half that amount per 24 hours for 5 days. It is always prudent to give an additional infusion at the time of removal of the operative sutures.

Inherited Hypoprothrombinemia (Factor II Deficiency)

This deficiency, inherited as an autosomal recessive trait, is perhaps the most rare of the inherited disorders of hemostasis. The prothrombin levels reported in affected patients have averaged about 10% of normal. Although the level of prothrombin activity required for hemostatis following surgical treatment is not precisely established, it seems likely that a level of 15% of normal is effective.

TREATMENT. The disappearance time of prothrombin from the intravascular compartment approximates that of factor X. An initial equilibration time of 9 hours has been estimated, followed by a much slower disappearance of activity with another half-life of up to 3 days. Stored plasma contains factor II. Surgical treatment without faulty hemostasis should be possible in affected patients if an initial plasma infusion of 15 ml/kg of body weight is administered 12 to 24 hours prior to the scheduled operation. This can be followed by an infusion of half this amount once daily until healing has occurred.

When the transfusion programs outlined above for deficiency of the prothrombin group of factors (factors II, V, VII, and X) are employed, the one-stage prothrombin time does not return to normal. Rather, a one-stage prothrombin time slightly less than twice the control value is achieved. This is sufficient to result in normal hemostasis. Of the four "prothrombin" factors, only factor V must be provided as fresh or freshly frozen plasma. Stored plasma is equally effective as therapy for factors II, VII, and X.

Inherited Fibrinogen Abnormalities

For nearly 50 years following the first description of a patient with congenital afibrinogenemia, this rare abnormality was considered the only inherited defect involving fibrinogen. More recently, families with qualitatively abnormal fibrinogen have been identified. These latter patients have varied in their clinical manifestations as well as in laboratory features.

Congenital afibrinogenemia is ascribed to an autosomal recessive mode of inheritance. The parents of patients with this entity usually have normal concentrations of fibrinogen. The affected individuals presumably are homozygous for the trait. Plasma fibrinogen levels of less that 5 mg/100 ml are usual, and, occasionally, immunochemical methods have been necessary to identify even trace amounts of fibrinogen in the plasma of these patients. The deficiency, however, usually is less of a clinical problem than classical hemophilia. Severely affected infants have bled following sectioning of the umbilical cord. More often the clinical manifestations include bleeding following lacerations, purpura, epistaxis, and bleeding following loss of deciduous teeth. The characteristic laboratory defect is the failure of the blood to clot in vitro, even following the addition of thrombin.

Less profound inherited deficiencies of fibrinogen have been noted. The bleeding usually is more modest, and the treatment requires proportionately smaller amounts of fibrinogen concentrate or plasma. Patients with "dysfibrinogenemia" are uncommon. The characteristic abnormality is the retarded rate of clotting upon the addition of thrombin ("thrombin time"). Interestingly, thrombotic disease as well as bleeding disorders have been described in this heterogeneous group of patients. Although surgical experience with this type of patient has been negligible, the administration of normal fibrinogen should serve to diminish the hemorrhagic aspect of the problem.

TREATMENT. Approximately half the transfused fibrinogen given to a deficient patient disappears from the intravascular compartment in the first 24 hours. Following this, the biologic half-life is 3 days or more. The disappearance of fibrinogen is no more rapid in deficient patients than when fibrinogen is transfused into normal subjects, thus suggesting that accelerated fibrinogen catabolism is not a pathogenic mechanism. Although the hemostatically optimal level of fibrinogen is not known, a level of close to 100 mg/100 ml usually permits normal hemostasis. The fibrinogen level should be raised above this prior to major surgical treatment. The volume of normal plasma necessary to accomplish this could exceed 50 ml/kg of body weight initially. Fibrinogen replacement has been made easier by the use of concentrates. A dose of 1 Gm of fibrinogen/10 kg/day has proved adequate. Approximately one-fifth of this then is administered daily following the initial loading dose. A substantial risk of homologous serum hepatitis is incurred when fibrinogen fractions are used. These concentrates are prepared from pooled plasma. The hepatitis risk can be reduced by using the cryoprecipitate preparation described for the treatment of hemophilia. Approximately one-half of the fibrinogen in the initial plasma is available in the precipitate. A 60-kg patient requires the precipitate obtained from approximately 25 units of plasma as a loading dose.

Acquired Hypofibrinogenemia

DEFIBRINATION SYNDROME

The largest proportion of patients with fibrinogen-related problems of surgical concern are in this group. The fibrinogen deficiency rarely is an isolated defect, as thrombocytopenia and factor V and factor VIII deficiencies of variable severity usually accompany this state.

The majority of patients with acquired hypofibrinogenemia suffer from intravascular coagulation, more properly known as *defibrination syndrome* or *consumptive coagulopathy,* and it is to this group of patients that the term *disseminated intravascular coagulation* (DIC) has been applied. The syndrome, now recognized with increasing frequency, is caused by the introduction of thromboplastic materials into the circulation. Because this material is found in most tissues, many disease processes may activate the coagulation system. The hemorrhagic disasters of the perinatal period, e.g., retained dead fetus, premature separation of the placenta, and amniotic fluid embolus, primarily are due to this pathophysiologic mechanism. The hemorrhagic state following hemolytic transfusion reaction is also related to this process. Defibrination has been observed as a complication of extracorporeal circulation, disseminated carcinoma, lymphomas, thrombotic thrombocytopenia, rickettsial infection, snakebite, and shock. Release of thromboplastic material has long been a recognized complication of gram-negative sepsis and has been attributed to the effects of circulating endotoxin on platelets. More recently, it has been recognized that septicemia due to gram-positive organisms may also be associated with DIC.

The differentiation between DIC with secondary protective fibrinolysis from primary fibrinolytic states can be extremely difficult, as the thrombin time, which many consider to be the most useful single test in establishing the presence of significant DIC or fibrinolysis, is prolonged in both cases. The salient differentiating features are that DIC is more common and is associated with an increased amount of cold insoluble fibrinogen (cryofibrinogen) and, most important, thrombocytopenia.

TREATMENT. The most important facets of treatment are relieving the patient's primary medical or surgical problem and maintaining adequate capillary flow. The use of intravenous fluids to maintain volume and, at times, vasodilators to open the arterioles is indicated. If blood flow deficiency is related to inability of a damaged heart to pump, the use of drugs such as digitalis or Isuprel may be indicated. Viscosity may be affected by an increased hematocrit, and, therefore, a plasma expander may be beneficial.

In the past heparin has been regarded as the treatment of choice, since it provides the most direct interference with the coagulation process. The use of heparin is certainly indicated in some cases, but should follow procedures directed at maintaining capillary flow. Heparin may be completely inactivated in the presence of severe acidosis. The cautious administration of heparin can serve as a diagnostic aid in that a rise in the levels of platelets and fibrinogen can be noted within hours. Administration of fibrinogen should be limited, since it may result in further intravascular coagulation, and the use of ϵ-aminocaproic acid to inhibit secondary fibrinolysis is contraindicated, since uncontrolled disseminated intravascular coagulation may result.

FIBRINOLYSIS

The acquired hypofibrinogenemic state in the surgical patient also can be due to pathologic fibrinolysis. This may occur in patients with metastatic prostatic carcinoma, shock, sepsis, hypoxia, neoplasia, cirrhosis, and portal hypertension.

The pathogenesis of this bleeding disorder is complex.

Secondary to shock or hypoxia, a release of excessive plasminogen activator into the circulation occurs. This is thought to be endogenous kinases which can be released from vascular endothelium and other tissues. Pharmacologic activation of plasminogen also occurs with pyrogens, epinephrine, nicotinic acid, and acetylcholine. Electric shock and pneumoencephalopathy have also been reported to cause activation. Patients with cirrhosis and portal hypertension have a diminished ability to clear normal amounts of plasminogen activator from the blood.

In addition to the reduction in levels of plasma fibrinogen, diminution of factors V and VIII also occurs, since they also serve as substrates for the enzyme plasmin. Thrombocytopenia is not an accompaniment of the purely fibrinolytic state. Polymerization of fibrin monomers, a step in normal fibrin formation, is interfered with by the proteolytic residue of fibrinogen and fibrin. The fibrin and fibrinogen breakdown products usually disappear from the circulation in a matter of hours. The biologic half-life of the interfering products has been estimated at approximately 9 hours.

Streptokinase and urokinase have been used to induce therapeutic fibrinolysis, but enthusiasm for these drugs as treatment for venous thrombosis, pulmonary embolism, and carotid hemothorax is not widespread. As there is a limited endogenous supply of activator available, it is soon exhausted by the injections, and later injections fail to achieve the desired effect. Also, treatment with these drugs is frequently accompanied by chills and fever. Excessive bleeding has been noted in almost half the patients treated, and anemia has appeared beyond that anticipated by the amount of bleeding. At present, results of urokinase therapy for deep venous thrombosis should be regarded as encouraging but not conclusive.

TREATMENT. The successful treatment of the underlying disorder usually is followed by rapid spontaneous recovery, since the severity of fibrinolytic bleeding is dependent upon the concentration of breakdown products in the circulation. ε-Aminocaproic acid, a synthetic amino acid, interferes with fibrinolysis by inhibiting plasminogen activation. The drug may be administered intravenously or orally. An initial dose of 5 Gm for the average-sized adult is followed by another 5 Gm every 4 to 6 hours until the hemorrhagic state subsides. Treatment rarely is required for more than 2 or 3 days. Just as the administration of ε-aminocaproic acid to a patient with consumptive coagulopathy is potentially dangerous, the administration of heparin to the patient who has a primary pathologic fibrinolysis is fraught with danger. Thus, fine clinical judgment and reliable laboratories are needed to avoid therapeutic complications. Restraint in definitive treatment of both fibrinolysis and consumptive coagulopathy is recommended, while measures designed to reverse the shock and stabilize the patient are emphasized.

Thrombocytopenia

Thrombocytopenia, as stated earlier, is the most common abnormality of hemostasis resulting in bleeding in the surgical patient. A wide variety of diseases can lead to reduction in platelet count and purpuric bleeding. Thrombocytopenia may be primary and idiopathic (idiopathic thrombocytopenic purpura, or ITP) or secondary and symptomatic (lupus erythematosus, drug reaction, or portal hypertension). The lack of platelets may be associated with megakaryocytes in the bone marrow (ITP, congestive splenomegaly) or with absence of megakaryocytes (leukemia, following cytotoxic therapy).

Microscopic examination of a properly stained blood smear should suggest the diagnosis. The presence and extent of thrombocytopenia can be defined precisely by a quantitative platelet count. In general, 60,000 to 70,000 platelets per cubic millimeter are adequate for normal hemostasis, but often a poor correlation between bleeding and the platelet count is noted. The bleeding time may be prolonged with marked thrombocytopenia or, less commonly, with qualitative platelet abnormality. Clot retraction usually is abnormal when the platelet count is below 70,000. Thrombocytopenia obviously can exist in the presence of normal clot retraction. In patients with thrombocytopenia, the clotting time and one-stage prothrombin time are normal.

The numerous etiologic bases of thrombocytopenia create a therapeutic challenge for the surgeon. The problems can be reduced to manageable proportions by attempting to define the pathophysiology of the thrombocytopenic state. The patient whose bone marrow is replaced by leukemia, metastatic tumor, or fibrous tissue and is therefore not producing platelets will not benefit from splenectomy. If an immune mechanism is responsible for the thrombocytopenia, it is important to determine if this is related to an extrinsic stimulus, drug, or infection. If drug-related, the thrombocytopenia will correct itself within days to weeks of discontinuation of the medication. If thrombocytopenia is secondary to bacteremia, the repair usually occurs in a day or two. If thrombocytopenia is related to viral infection, the return of platelets may not take place for 3 weeks or longer. Occasionally, severe thrombocytopenia and bleeding are secondary to vitamin B_{12} or folic acid deficiency and are associated with a megaloblastic bone marrow. This may occur 2 or 3 years following total gastrectomy or in association with severe intestinal malabsorption. In either case, supplying the appropriate nutrient will correct the thrombocytopenia within 2 or 3 days. Thrombocytopenia has recently been reported in association with acute alcoholism in the noncirrhotic patient. The marrow megakaryocytes are normal, and the platelet count returns to normal 5 to 7 days after the alcohol intake ceases.

If the thrombocytopenia is associated with splenomegaly and megakaryocytes remain in the marrow, removal of the spleen offers a good chance for relief of thrombocytopenia.

TREATMENT. Treatment must be based upon consideration of the patient at hand. Management of the thrombocytopenic patient takes one of four forms, separately or in combination. These include (1) careful observation alone, (2) steroid therapy, (3) splenectomy, and (4) transfusion therapy.

Careful observation, a form of management, is neglected too often in our anxiety to do something for the patient.

This approach is applicable in the patient with chronic thrombocytopenia (75,000 to 85,000 platelets per cubic millimeter) and no bleeding symptoms or signs. The patient with drug-induced, immune-related thrombocytopenia or postinfectious thrombocytopenia also requires only careful observation if there is no significant bleeding.

Corticosteroid therapy is appropriate for the patient with thrombocytopenia who is having significant bleeding but is known to have a self-limited process. Although neither firm experimental data nor properly controlled clinical observations are available, a strong impression exists that corticosteroid administration to the thrombocytopenic patient reduces the bleeding tendency. This seems to be true even if there is no increase in the number of platelets in the peripheral blood. Corticosteroid administration to the patient with ITP can result in a partial or complete, temporary or permanent, remission. The incidence of success varies with the clinic. The most enthusiastic clinics do not report much more than 65 percent remission, either temporary or complete. Our experience suggests a figure of 50 percent or less, with fewer than 25 percent complete and permanent. The role of steroids in chronic ITP is to facilitate the management of acute bleeding episodes and to permit the scheduling of operations on a semielective basis.

Treatment of acute ITP is discussed in Chap. 33. Our approach is as follows: The patient is given 40 mg of prednisone daily in divided doses. If no return of platelets is noted after 4 weeks, the dose of prednisone is doubled. If no return of platelets occurs in 4 weeks with the higher dose, the patient then is considered a candidate for splenectomy. Should the platelets return during the course of prednisone treatment, the dose is decreased in a stepwise fashion over a 4- to 6-week period. If relapse occurs, the patient is considered a candidate for splenectomy rather than retreatment with steroids.

In certain patients, splenectomy may be considered because of relative contraindications to continued steroid therapy, e.g., an active peptic ulcer, serious psychologic changes, and diabetes in which difficulty of control is related to the steroid therapy.

Emergency splenectomy for ITP usually is limited to the patient who presents with central nervous system bleeding. If this is the case, the patient is given 200 mg of intravenous hydrocortisone immediately, and an intravenous infusion of 100 mg of hydrocortisone in 5% dextrose and water is administered over each 6-hour period. Platelet-rich plasma or platelet concentrates are administered preoperatively and during operation. Blood transfusions should consist of fresh whole blood. The platelet preparations and hydrocortisone are continued postoperatively until the platelets return. Remission occurs in 65 to 70 percent of patients, usually within 3 to 4 days. Occasionally, return of platelets occurs more slowly, over 10 to 14 days.

The use of platelet-rich plasma or platelet concentrate transfusions has definite limitations in the surgical patient. These preparations should be used shortly after collection and certainly within 6 hours, since the platelets lose their viability. If platelet preparations are not available, fresh blood may be used. In patients with normal hemo-

stasis, the life span of freshly infused platelets is about 8 to 10 days. When platelets are given to a patient with ITP or drug-related immune thrombocytopenia, the infused platelets circulate a relatively brief time, usually minutes to hours. Platelet-rich plasma or platelet concentrate transfusions are effective for longer periods of time in the patient with thrombocytopenia secondary to massive banked blood transfusion, marrow hypoplasia secondary to radiation injury, cytotoxic drugs, or other causes. Although a progressive decrease in platelet survival following multiple infusions has been noted, children being treated for acute leukemia have been given multiple platelet transfusions without this apparent decrease in survival of platelets.

Myeloproliferative Diseases

POLYCYTHEMIA VERA

Surgical treatment of the patient with polycythemia vera is complicated by distinctly increased morbidity and mortality. This is particularly true for the untreated patient but also applies, to some extent, to the patient who has been treated successfully. Spontaneous thrombosis is a complication of polycythemia vera and can be explained, in part, by increased blood viscosity, increased platelet count, and increased tendency toward stasis. Paradoxically, a significant tendency to spontaneous hemorrhage also is noted in these patients. Approximately one-third of patients with polycythemia vera have some form of hemorrhagic complaint at the time of initial diagnosis. The tendency to bleed usually is a function of an excessively high platelet count. Patients with spontaneous bleeding characteristically have a platelet count of 1.5 million per cubic millimeter or greater. The bleeding time may be prolonged. Evidence has been offered that the platelets in these patients may be qualitatively defective. Despite intensive study, the seeming paradox of hemorrhagic tendency accompanied by thrombocytosis is poorly understood.

The polycythemic patient with marked thrombocytosis is a major surgical risk. Operation should be considered only for the most grave surgical emergency. If possible, operation should be deferred until medical management has returned the blood volume, hematocrit, and hemostatic process to normal.

TREATMENT. Thrombocytosis can be reduced by the careful administration of alkylating agents such as busulfan or chlorambucil. These measures are time-consuming. Surgical procedure should be delayed weeks to months following institution of treatment. Ideally, the hematocrit should be kept below 48 percent and the platelet count less than 400,000 per cubic millimeter. The blood volume also can be reduced more rapidly by phlebotomy. Prior to operation, a thorough laboratory investigation of hemostatic function should be conducted. Any gross defect, such as deficiency of vitamin K–dependent factors or low plasma fibrinogen values, should be investigated and corrected when possible. When surgical treatment is judged imperative in these patients, the erythremic state should be reduced by phlebotomy. Operation, at all times, must be performed fastidiously. Postoperative fibrinolysis also has been known to occur, further complicating the postoperative course.

In one series reported from a clinic with considerable experience, 46 percent of polycythemic patients undergoing major procedures had complications at the time of operation or during the postoperative course, and a 16 percent mortality was associated with the surgical procedures. Significantly, 80 percent of the deaths were encountered in patients on whom operations were performed while the disease was not under control. In operations on patients in whom hemoglobin and hematocrit had been reduced prior to operation the mortality and incidence of complications decreased. Hemorrhage is the most common complication occurring during or following operation and accounts for greater than two-thirds of the deaths. Thrombosis, either venous or arterial, is the next most frequent complication. Infection also is surprisingly common, occurring in approximately 20 percent of patients.

MYELOID METAPLASIA

Myeloid metaplasia frequently represents part of the natural history of polycythemia vera. Approximately 50 percent of patients with myeloid metaplasia are postpolycythemic, while in the remainder the condition apparently occurs as a separate, possibly related, disease entity. Myeloid metaplasia is characterized by many of the features of polycythemia vera. Splenomegaly usually is more prominent and may be massive. Laboratory features include leukocytosis, which may be severe, or, at times, severe leukopenia. Young myeloid forms may be present. Platelets may be strikingly increased in number, but thrombocytopenia also may be present. The latter is usually characteristic of the patient who has myelofibrosis rather than a hyperplastic bone marrow. Examination of the peripheral blood smear may reveal large, bizarre platelets, fragments of megakaryocyte nuclei, occasional nucleated red cells, and bizarre variations in red cell shape. Evidence suggesting qualitative platelet abnormalities has been described. This is considered as a factor in bleeding in some myeloid metaplasia patients. Abnormalities of platelet factor 3 release have been demonstrated, as have abnormalities in platelet aggregation with ADP.

The morbidity rate following surgical treatment in patients with myeloid metaplasia has been reported as high as 68 percent in a small series. The mortality rate in the same experience was greater than 42 percent. Relatively innocuous surgical procedures have been accompanied by nearly uncontrollable bleeding. Spontaneous bleeding from esophageal varices in patients with myeloid metaplasia and massive splenomegaly also has been reported.

Other Diseases Associated with Increased Risk of Bleeding

A number of illnesses not primarily associated with hemostatic failure may be associated with increased risk of bleeding. These diseases frequently involve organs of formation or synthesis of products essential to hemostasis. Diseases such as leukemia, lymphoma, or multiple mye-

loma may lead to thrombocytopenia because of the replacement of the megakaryocytes in the bone marrow. Illnesses resulting in severe impairment of hepatic function may limit synthesis of plasma factors essential to normal coagulation. The patient with advanced cirrhosis may be lacking in factors of the prothrombin complex (II, V, VII, X), as well as factor XIII.

Illnesses increasing the removal of products essential to hemostasis also occur. Representative of this problem is the patient with splenomegaly in whom sequestration and removal of platelets proceeds at an abnormally rapid rate. Accelerated removal of plasma factors necessary for coagulation has been mentioned in the discussion of the consumptive coagulopathies. The reciprocal of the latter problem has been identified in the case of the patients with cirrhosis and portal hypertension who fail to clear the activators of fibrinolysis from the circulation. This results in a longer biologic survival of these activators and attendant increased fibrinolytic activity.

Some illnesses are characterized by the production of substances which interfere with the normal hemostatic mechanism. These diseases are associated with the production of abnormal proteins which may coat the platelets, as in macroglobulinemia, or bind with certain of the normal blood-clotting factors, as in multiple myeloma or in states associated with the production of cryoglobulin.

Certain diseases may be associated with multiple hemostatic defects. These may include qualitative and quantitative platelet problems, vascular abnormalities, and impaired metabolism and excretion of administered anticoagulant. Any combination of these problems may be noted in patients with renal failure and uremia. The most common problem in the group of patients is thrombocytopenia concurrent with qualitative platelet defects which parallel the degree of azotemia. The hemostatic problems of patients with severe liver disease may be multiple. Major hemorrhagic episodes in these patients usually are accompanied by significant thrombocytopenia, but this is rarely the sole cause. Deficiencies of the coagulation factors normally synthesized in the liver may be present, and increased fibrinolysis also may be evident.

Iatrogenic disorders may result from the administration of drugs which directly or indirectly influence the hemostatic process. Agents which may damage or inhibit the bone marrow include alkylating agents used in malignant disease, antibiotics, such as chloramphenicol, or antibiotics which occasionally result in immunologic removal of platelets, e.g., penicillin, ristocetin, streptomycin. In the idiosyncratic patient, a wide variety of agents may precipitate immune responses leading to platelet removal, e.g., quinidine, quinine, chlorothiazides. Vasculitis and purpura may follow the use of sulfonamides. Salicylates and phenylbutazone may interfere with the platelet-collagen reaction early in the hemostatic process.

TREATMENT. The management of the patient with liver disease is discussed in Chap. 30. Transfusion with freshly drawn whole blood or freshly prepared platelet-rich plasma may be necessary. When thrombocytopenia is significant, the administration of corticosteroids may diminish the bleeding tendency, even though the platelet count is not raised. Bleeding encountered in patients with bone marrow replacement or bone marrow destruction is thrombocytopenic in origin. The use of whole fresh blood, fresh platelet-rich plasma, or fresh platelet concentrates is indicated for control of acute bleeding episodes. Corticosteroids also have been helpful in this situation. Patients with dysproteinemia and attendant bleeding are particularly difficult to manage. Generally, surgical treatment should be deferred until the basic disease is ameliorated and the production of abnormal protein is diminished. In some instances, diminution of the hemorrhagic potential has been accomplished by intensive plasmapheresis with reduction in the level of the abnormal circulating protein.

Anticoagulation and Bleeding

Spontaneous bleeding may be a complication of anticoagulant therapy with either heparin or the coumarin and indandione derivatives. An exaggerated response to oral anticoagulants may occur if dietary vitamin K is inadequate. The anticoagulant effect of coumarin is consistently reduced in patients receiving barbiturates, and increased coumarin requirements have also been documented in patients receiving contraceptives, other estrogen-containing compounds, corticosteroids, and ACTH. Therefore, reduced anticoagulant dosage should be anticipated following discontinuance of any of these drugs. Medications known to increase the effect of oral anticoagulants include phenylbutazone, the cholesterol-lowering agent clofibrate, anabolic steroids (norethandrolone), D-thyroxine, glucagon, quinidine, and a variety of antibiotics.

The history is all-important in recognizing these patients. Questioning should be specific. The patient should be asked if he is presently taking drugs to "thin out" his blood or prevent clotting. Unexplained bleeding in medical and paramedical personnel occasionally is due to surreptitious anticoagulation. The onset of hematuria or melena in the patient receiving anticoagulants should be investigated, since it has been shown that anticoagulants may unmask underlying tumors. Patients with bleeding secondary to anticoagulation may present with only epistaxis, gastrointestinal hemorrhage, or hematuria. Physical examination, however, almost always reveals other signs of bleeding such as ecchymoses, petechiae, or hematoma. Bleeding secondary to anticoagulation is not an uncommon cause of rectus sheath hematoma, simulating appendicitis, and intramural intestinal or retroperitoneal hematoma.

Surgical intervention may prove necessary in patients receiving anticoagulant therapy. The typical example is the patient with rheumatic heart disease receiving long-term anticoagulation because of repeated arterial emboli, who then is seen subsequent to a critical embolic episode. Increasing experience suggests that surgical treatment can be undertaken without discontinuing the anticoagulant program. The risk of thrombotic complications reportedly is increased when anticoagulant therapy is discontinued suddenly. If so, this may not be related to what has been called the "rebound phenomena" but may represent an event in a patient who has an underlying thrombotic tendency.

When the clotting time is less than 25 minutes in the heparinized patient or when the prothrombin time is greater that 20% of normal in a patient on coumarin, reversal of anticoagulant therapy may not be necessary. Meticulous surgical technique is mandatory, and the patients must be observed closely.

Certain surgical procedures should not be performed in the face of anticoagulation. In sites where even minor bleeding can cause great morbidity, e.g., the central nervous system and the eye, anticoagulants should be discontinued and, if necessary, reversed. Because of the added problem of local fibrinolysis, prostatic surgical treatment should not be carried out in a patient on anticoagulants. Procedures requiring blind needle introduction should be avoided. Deaths have been reported following sympathetic block for peripheral vascular disease in patients receiving anticoagulation. Splenoportography has a markedly increased morbidity in patients in whom prothrombin times are less than 30% and who are thrombocytopenic.

Emergency operation occasionally is necessary in patients who have been heparinized as treatment for deep venous thrombosis. Reversal of heparinization may be desirable. The patient with repeated episodes of pulmonary embolization while fully heparinized is an example. Reversal of heparinization also can be a problem in cardiac surgical procedures employing extracorporeal circulation. The anticoagulant effect of heparin can be rapidly counteracted with protamine sulfate when the heparin has been given intravenously. Protamine sulfate also is administered intravenously. Theoretically, 1.28 mg should neutralize 1 mg of heparin. In fact, 1 milligram of protamine may be given for each milligram of heparin, provided the intravenous heparin was not given more than 2 hours previously. Protamine sulfate in large doses also has an anticoagulant activity. The formation of both extrinsic and intrinsic prothrombinase can be retarded, prolonging the one-stage prothrombin time test and the partial thromboplastin time test. Some patients exhibit the phenomenon of "heparin rebound" following apparently adequate heparin neutralization with protamine. Prolongation of the clotting time again recurs after adequate postoperative antagonism of the heparin. This can contribute to postoperative bleeding. In our experience, this is the major cause of "unexplained" postoperative bleeding following extracorporeal cardiac bypass surgical procedures. Activation of fibrinolysis and thrombocytopenia may also contribute to this problem.

Bleeding infrequently is related to hypoprothrombinemia if the prothrombin concentration is greater than 15%. We have successfully resected a ruptured aortic aneurysm and inserted a prosthetic graft in a patient with a prothrombin concentration at this level. Excessive bleeding was not encountered.

In the elective surgical patient receiving coumarin therapy adequately effecting anticoagulation, the drug can be discontinued several days prior to operation, and the prothrombin concentration then checked. A level greater than 50% is considered safe. If emergency surgical treatment is required, parenteral injection of vitamin K$_1$ can be used.

Since the reversal effect may take 6 hours, whole blood transfusion may be required. Parenteral administration of vitamin K also is indicated in elective surgical treatment of patients with biliary obstruction, malabsorption, and hypoprothrombinemia. The drug should result in a normal prothrombin time. In contrast, if the hypoprothrombinemia is related to hepatocellular dysfunction, vitamin K therapy is ineffective and should not be prolonged over a week if no response is noted. Vitamin K is an oxidant, and one must be aware that patients with red cell enzyme deficiencies may sustain hemolysis following its administration.

LOCAL HEMOSTASIS

Surgical bleeding, even when alarmingly excessive, is usually caused by ineffective local hemostasis. The goal of local hemostasis is to prevent the flow of blood from incised or transected blood vessels. This may be accomplished by interrupting the flow of blood to the involved area or by direct closure of the blood vessel wall defect. The techniques may be classified as mechanical, thermal, or chemical.

Mechanical Procedures

The oldest mechanical device to effect closure of a bleeding point or to prevent blood from entering the area of disruption is digital pressure. When pressure is applied to an artery proximal to an area of bleeding, profuse bleeding is reduced, permitting more definitive action. The Pringle maneuver of occluding the hepatic artery in the hepatoduodenal ligament as a method of controlling bleeding from a transected cystic artery or from the surface of the liver is a classic example. Direct digital pressure over a bleeding site, such as a lateral rent in the inferior vena cava, is also effective. The finger has the advantage of being the least traumatic vascular hemostat. All clamps, including the so-called atraumatic vascular clamps, do result in damage to the intimal wall of the blood vessel. The obvious disadvantage of digital pressure is that it cannot be used permanently.

The hemostat also represents a temporary mechanical device to stem bleeding. In smaller and noncritical vessels, the trauma and adjacent tissue necrosis associated with the application of a hemostat are of little consequence. These minor disadvantages are outweighed by the mechanical advantage that the instrument offers to subsequent ligation. When bleeding occurs from a vessel which should be preserved, relatively atraumatic hemostats should be employed to limit the extent of intimal damage and subsequent thrombosis.

In general, a ligature replaces the hemostat as a permanent method of effecting hemostasis in a single vessel. When a vessel is transected, a simple ligature usually is sufficient. For large arteries with pulsation and longitudinal motion, transfixion suture to prevent slipping is indicated. When the bleeding site is from a lateral defect in the blood vessel wall, suture ligatures are required. The adventitia and media constitute the major holding forces within the walls of large vessels, and therefore multiple fine sutures are preferable to fewer larger sutures.

Historically, Aulus Cornelius Celsus devised the use of ligatures in 100 A.D. Because of the strong influence of Galen, who was inclined to cautery, this method did not gain popularity. Paré, in 1552, rediscovered the principle of ligature. In 1800, Physick used absorbable sutures of buckskin and parchment. In 1858, Simpson introduced the wire suture, and in 1881 Lister employed chromic catgut. Halsted, in the early 1900s, emphasized the importance of incorporating as little tissue as possible in the suture and indicated the advantages of silk. In 1911, Cushing reported on the use of silver clips to effect hemostasis in delicate vessels in critical areas. Recently, a wide variety of staples made of different metals, which are relatively inert in tissue, have been employed. The advantages of stapling are speed, accuracy, minimal tissue trauma, and the ability to effect hemostasis in otherwise inaccessible areas. Staples have not replaced the ligature, since they are less reliable and harder to apply to larger vessels.

All sutures represent foreign material, and the selection is based on the characteristics of the material and the state of the wound. Nonabsorbable sutures, such as silk, nylon, and wire, evoke less tissue reaction than absorbable materials, such as catgut. The latter are preferable, however, in the face of overt infection. The presence of nonabsorbable material in an infected wound can lead to extrusion or sinus tract formation. Wire is the least reactive of the nonabsorbable sutures but the most difficult to handle. Monofilament wire and coated sutures have an advantage over multifilament sutures in the presence of infection. The latter tend to fragment and permit sinus formation due to the interstices.

Diffuse bleeding from multiple transected vessels may be controlled by mechanical techniques which employ pressure directly over the bleeding area, pressure at a distance, or generalized pressure. These techniques are based on the premise that as pressure and flow are decreased in the area of vascular disruption, a clot will occur. Pressure at a distance was effected by application of tourniquets and other pressure devices at pressure points proximal to bleeding sites as a standard procedure by military surgeons in the seventeenth century. Now it is generally felt that direct pressure is preferable and is not attended by the danger of tissue necrosis associated with prolonged use of tourniquets. In our present aerospace age, gravitational suits have been employed to create generalized pressure and to decrease temporarily bleeding from rupture of major intraabdominal vessels.

Direct pressure applied by means of packs affords the best method of controlling diffuse bleeding from large areas. At times, hemostatic chemical materials, such as oxidized cellulose, are incorporated in the packing. Rarely is it necessary to leave a pack at the bleeding site and remove it at a second sitting. If this is done, several days should elapse before removal, and the possibility of recurrent bleeding should be anticipated. The question as to whether hot wet packs or cold wet packs should be applied has been investigated. Unless the heat is so great as to denature protein, it may actually increase bleeding, whereas cold packs promote hemostasis by inducing vascular spasm and increasing endothelial adhesiveness. Bleeding from cut bone may be controlled by packing beeswax in the area. This material effects pressure and is relatively nonirritative to the body.

Thermal Agents

Galen's favoring of cautery influenced medicine for 1,500 years, until the teachings of Paré were appreciated. The use of cautery was revitalized in 1928, when Cushing and Bovie applied this technique for effecting hemostasis of delicate vessels in recessed areas, such as the brain. Heat achieves hemostasis by denaturation of protein, which results in coagulation of large areas of tissue. With actual cautery, heat is transmitted from the instrument by conduction directly to the tissue, whereas with electrocautery, heating occurs by induction from an alternating-current source.

When electrocautery is employed, the amplitude setting should be high enough to produce prompt coagulation but not so high as to set up an arc between the tissue and the cautery tip. This avoids burns outside the operative field and prevents exit of current through electrocardiographic leads or other monitoring devices. A negative plate should be placed beneath the patient whenever cautery is employed to avoid severe skin burns. The advantage of cautery is that it saves time, whereas the disadvantage is that more tissue is necrosed than with precise ligature. Certain anesthetic agents cannot be used with electrocautery because of the hazard of explosion.

A direct current can also result in electrical hemostasis. Since the protein moieties and cellular elements of blood have a negative surface charge, they are attracted to the positive pole, where a thrombus is formed. Direct currents in the 20- to 100-ma range have been applied to control diffuse bleeding from large serous surfaces.

At the other end of the thermal spectrum, cooling has been applied to control bleeding, particularly from the mucosa of the esophagus and stomach. Generalized hypothermia is of little avail, since, in order to reduce the blood flow to visceral organs, the systemic temperature must be brought down to the level of $35°C$. At this point shivering and ventricular fibrillation may be encountered. Thrombocytopenia may also be a consequence of generalized cooling. Direct cooling is effective and acts by increasing the local intravascular hematocrit and decreasing blood flow by vasoconstriction. A variety of gastric balloons and cooling devices have been employed locally to cool the stomach and distal esophagus as treatment for bleeding esophagogastric varices and gastritis.

Extreme cooling, i.e., cryogenic surgery, has been applicable particularly in neurosurgery. Temperature ranges of -20 to $-180°C$ are used, and freezing occurs around the tip of the cannula within 5 seconds. At temperatures of $-20°C$ or below, the tissue, capillaries, small arterioles, and venules undergo cryogenic necrosis. This is caused by dehydration and denaturation of lipid molecules. The muscular walls of large arteries are an exception. Although the major arteries and blood may be frozen solid, the blood contained in these vessels does not clot. When thawing occurs, normal circulation is resumed.

Chemical Agents

Chemical agents vary in their hemostatic action. Some are vasoconstrictive, while others have coagulant properties. Still others are relatively inert but possess hygroscopic properties which increase their bulk and aid in plugging disrupted blood vessels.

Epinephrine, applied topically, induces vasoconstriction, but extensive application can result in considerable absorption and systemic effects. The drug generally is used on oozing sites in mucosal areas, during tonsillectomy, for example.

Historically, skeletal muscle was one of the first materials with locally hemostatic properties to be employed, its use having been introduced by Cushing in 1911. Shortly thereafter, hemostatic fibrin was manufactured. The properties required for local hemostatic materials include handling ease, rapid absorption, nonirritation, and hemostatic action independent of the general clotting mechanism. The most widely used of the commercially available materials are gelatin foam (Gelfoam), oxidized cellulose (Oxycel), and oxidized regenerated cellulose (Surgicel). All these materials act, in part, by transmitting pressure against the wound surface, and the interstices provide a scaffold on which the clot can organize.

Gelfoam is made from animal skin gelatin which has been denatured. In itself, Gelfoam has no intrinsic hemostatic action, but it can be used in combination with topical thrombin, for which it serves as an absorbable carrier. Its main hemostatic activity is related to the contact between blood and the large surface area of the sponge and to the pressure exerted by the weight of the sponge and absorbed blood. Prior to application of Gelfoam, the sponge should be moistened in saline or thrombin solution, and all the air should be removed from the interstices.

Oxycel and Surgicel are altered cellulose materials capable of reacting chemically with blood and producing a sticky mass which functions as an artificial clot. These substances are relatively inert and are removed by liquefaction in 1 week to 1 month. They should be dry when they are applied. Like Gelfoam, these materials are nontoxic and relatively nonirritating but are somewhat detrimental to wound healing and require phagocytosis to be removed. Also, like Gelfoam, they serve as excellent culture media and potentiate infection.

Recently, adhesive chemicals have been developed literally to cement bleeding sites. One example is methyl-2-cyanoacrilate (Eastman 9-10), which is a rapidly polymerizing substance. These agents have little toxicity but do evoke a marked inflammatory response. Aneurysms have been reported subsequent to the application of cements to major blood vessels. Methyl-2-cyanoacrilate has been applied to the surface of the liver for hemostasis with reported success. Another local approach to the problem of bleeding from a large area is the application of tanned collagen sponge, which functions as a collagenous framework. This encourages the invasion and proliferation of fibroblasts while applying constant pressure against the wound to effect hemostatic action.

TRANSFUSION

Background

In 1967, the tercentenarial anniversary of the transfusion of blood into human beings was celebrated. In June of 1667, Jean Baptiste Denis and a surgeon, Emmerez, transfused blood from a sheep into a fifteen-year-old boy who had been bled many times as treatment for fever. The patient apparently improved, and a successful experience was reported simultaneously in another patient. Because of two subsequent deaths associated with transfusion from animals to man, criminal charges were brought against Denis. In April of 1668, further transfusions in man were forbidden unless approved by the Faculty of Medicine in Paris. It was not until the nineteenth century that human blood was recognized as the only appropriate replacement. In 1900, Landsteiner and his associates introduced the concept of blood grouping and identified the major A, B and O groups. In 1939, the Rh group was recognized. Numerous other groups have been uncovered since that time. Development of sensitive cross-matching procedures took place in the 1940s, and with the impetus of World War II blood transfusion became a common procedure. The introduction of various preservative solutions, such as acid citrate dextrose (ACD), contributed to the development of blood banking.

As the scope of surgery has expanded, the requirement for larger amounts of blood for transfusion has increased. Approximately 14 percent of all patients operated upon, exclusive of procedures performed in the outpatient department or emergency area, are transfused. Of 604 adults who received blood at a university medical center in association with surgical treatment, 125 required over 5,000 ml. The record administration in this hospital in a patient who survived was 100 units within a 36-hour period. The logistics of the problem have resulted in modernization of transfusion practices, including the use of plasma expanders and component therapy. Preservation of blood and its constituents has been achieved by freezing. Cadaver blood has been used in large amounts in the U.S.S.R.

Characteristics of Blood and Replacement Therapy

BLOOD

Blood has been described as a vehicular organ which perfuses all other organs. It provides transportation of oxygen to satisfy the metabolic demands and removes the by-product carbon dioxide. Blood also transports chemical nutriments for, and waste products from, metabolic activity. Homeostatic governors, including hormones, coagula-

tion factors, and antibodies, are carried to and from appropriate sites within the fluid portion of the blood. Red blood cells, with their oxygen-carrying capacity, white blood cells, which function in body defense processes, and platelets, which contribute to the hemostatic process, comprise the formed elements.

REPLACEMENT THERAPY

BANKED WHOLE BLOOD. Whole blood generally is collected in ACD solution and stored at 4°C. Such blood is considered suitable for administration any time up to 21 days of storage. Following this period, at least 70 percent of the transfused erythrocytes remain in the circulation 24 hours posttransfusion and are viable. Normal survival of red blood cells is 110 to 120 days. Sixty days after transfusion, approximately 52 percent of the cells will survive if the transfusion uses fresh blood. Fifty percent will survive if the transfusion is with ACD blood stored 14 days. In contrast, only 25 percent of erythrocytes survive at 60 days if the transfusion utilized blood stored for 28 days in ACD. The major loss occurs in the first 24 hours after transfusion, and subsequent to that time the survival slope for red cells from fresh blood and stored blood is identical.

Banked blood is a poor source of platelets, since they lose their ability to survive transfusion after 24 hours of storage. Among the clotting factors, factor II (prothrombin), factor VII, factor IX, and factor XI are stable in banked blood. Factor I (fibrinogen) is stable only in freshly banked blood, i.e., less than 24 hours after collection. Factor V is not stable in banked blood, while factor VIII also deteriorates during storage.

During the storage of whole blood, red cell metabolism and plasma protein degradation results in certain chemical changes in the plasma (Table 3-2). Lactic acid increases from 20 to 150 mg/100 ml, an amount which is insignificant in terms of transfusion at the end of 28 days. The pH decreases from 7 to 6.68 within 21 days. Little change in the sodium occurs, but the potassium concentration rises steadily to 32 mEq at the end of 21 days. This must be considered when transfusing patients with anuria, oliguria, or hyperkalemia. In these cases, fresh whole blood obviously is preferable. The ammonia concentration also rises steadily during storage from 50 to 680 μg at the end of 21 days. This may be of significance for the patient with hepatic disease. The hemolysis which occurs during storage for 21 days is insignificant, since lysis of only about 1 percent of the red cells occurs and the free hemoglobin is rapidly cleared from the circulation following transfusion.

Typing and Cross Matching. In selecting blood for transfusion, serologic compatibility is established routinely for the recipients' and donors' A, B, O, and Rh groups. Cross matching between the donors' red cells and recipients' sera (the "major" cross match) is performed. The donor sera and recipient cells ("minor" cross match) also are checked. As a rule, Rh-negative recipients should be transfused only with Rh-negative blood. Since this group represents 15 percent of the donor population, the supply may be limited. If the recipient is an elderly male who has not been transfused previously, the transfusion of Rh-positive blood

Table 3-2. CHARACTERISTICS OF PLASMA STORED IN
ACD SOLUTION AT $4 \pm 1°$C

Constituents	Unit value	Days stored				
		0	7	14	21	28
Dextrose	mg/100 ml	350	300	245	210	190
Lactic acid	mg/100 ml	20	70	120	140	150
Inorganic phosphate	mg/100 ml	1.8	4.5	6.6	9.0	9.5
pH*		7.0	6.85	6.77	6.68	6.65
Hemoglobin	mg/100 ml	0–10	25	50	100	150
Sodium	mEq/L	150	148	145	142	140
Potassium	mEq/L	3–4	12	24	32	40
Ammonia	μg/100 ml	50	260	470	680	

*Determined with glass electrode.
SOURCE: From M. M. Strumia, W. H. Crosby, J. G. Gibson II, T. J. Greenwalt, and J. R. Krevans, "General Principles of Blood Transfusion," J. B. Lippincott Company, Philadelphia, 1963.

is reasonable if Rh-negative blood is unavailable. Anti-Rh antibodies form in several weeks of transfusion. If further transfusions are needed within a few days, more Rh-positive blood can be used. Rh-positive blood should not be transfused to Rh-negative females who are capable of childbearing. Administration of hyperimmune anti-Rh globulin to Rh-negative women shortly after Rh sensitization largely eliminates Rh disease in subsequent offspring. This promising observation may serve as a model to facilitate transfusions. At present, however, type-specific transfusions remain the basis for therapy. Any Rh-negative woman who has borne children may have been sensitized during pregnancy.

A variety of cell-serum interactions may be detected by careful cross matching. Incompatibility may be due to the fact that either the donor or recipient has been wrongly grouped. An interaction may be caused by a difference in a subgroup, e.g., a donor who is A_1 and a recipient who is A_2 with anti-A_1 in the serum. Interactions may also be due to other naturally occurring antibodies such as anti-P_1 or anti-Le.

In the patient who is receiving repeated transfusions, serum drawn not more than 24 hours prior to cross matching should be utilized for matching with cells of the donor. The recipient cells used for the minor cross match also should be relatively fresh. Antigenic potency for certain blood groups is lost after several days of storage, and failure to detect minor incompatibility can result. Emergency blood transfusion can be performed with group O blood. If it is known that the prospective recipient is group AB, group A blood is preferable. The O donor blood should have low titers of anti-A and anti-B. Such emergency cases are extremely rare with the exception of battlefield casualties, and it should be possible to wait 45 minutes, during which time the patient's group can be determined and type-specific blood used. The use of plasma expanders in the meantime makes this particularly possible.

When the blood of multiple donors is to be transfused, such as in the case of extracorporeal circulatory procedures, the question arises as to whether all samples should be cross-matched with each other. In determining compatibility, screening is performed in the usual fashion. Major and minor cross matches are performed. Cold agglutinin titer of the recipient serum should be determined if hypothermia is to be employed. In patients with malignant lymphoma and leukemia cryoglobulins may be present, and the blood should be administered at room temperature. If these antibodies are present in high titer, hypothermia may be contraindicated.

In patients with thalassemia and, more particularly, with acquired hemolytic anemia, typing and cross matching may be difficult, and sufficient time should be allotted during the preoperative period to accumulate blood that may be required during the operation. Cross matching should always be carried out prior to the administration of dextran, since dextran interferes with the typing procedure.

FRESH WHOLE BLOOD. This refers to blood which is administered within 24 hours of its donation. In the patient who requires platelets, the blood must be transfused within 6 hours of donation. As noted earlier, such fresh blood also is a potential source of factors V and VIII.

PACKED RED CELLS AND FROZEN RED CELLS. Concentrated suspensions of red cells can be prepared by removing most of the supernatant plasma citrate from the blood following settling of the cells or centrifugation. A small amount of plasma citrate is left, so that the packed cell volume is approximately 70%.

The use of frozen red blood cells represents a recent addition to the transfusion armamentarium. The preparation is time-consuming and requires the addition of glycerol to assure uniform rate of intracellular crystal formation during freezing. At thawing, the cells are washed to remove the glycerol. An advantage of frozen red cells is that their use markedly reduces the risk of infusing hepatitis virus or antigens to which the patient has been previously sensitized. Either packed or frozen red cells are applicable in the treatment of anemia without hypovolemia. The use of packed red cells reduces the danger of circulatory overload. Reactions secondary to allergens in plasma to which the recipient is sensitive also can be minimized.

LEUKOCYTE AND PLATELET-POOR RED CELLS. These are prepared by aspirating the buffy coat and supernatant plasma, following slow centrifugation or settling. The red cells then are washed with sterile isotonic solution. The preparation is time-consuming and increases the possibility of bacterial contamination. This should be done only for patients with demonstrated hypersensitivity to either leukocytes or platelets (buffy coat reactions). Usually this syndrome is manifest by fever, chilly sensations, and urticaria in the absence of hemolysis.

PLATELET-RICH PLASMA AND PLATELET CONCENTRATES. The indications for platelet transfusion are as follows: thrombocytopenia due to massive blood loss and replacement with stored blood, thrombocytopenia due to inadequate platelet production, thrombocytopenia due to platelet destruction, and qualitative platelet disorders. The preparations should be used within 6 hours of blood donation. One unit of platelet-rich plasma has a volume of approximately 200 ml. The recovery of platelets in the recipient usually is no more than 60 percent of those present in the donor blood. The platelet concentrate consists of platelets prepared from a unit of platelet-rich plasma. These are resuspended in 30 ml of fluid and should be administered without a filter. The platelet concentrate has the advantage of obviating circulatory overload. Both preparations may harbor the hapatitis virus and account for allergic reactions similar to those due to whole blood. When treating thrombocytopenic bleeding or preparing thrombocytopenic patients for surgery, it is advisable to elevate the platelet levels to the range of 50,000 to 100,000/mm^3 in order to provide continued protection. The development of isoimmunity remains one of the most important factors limiting the usefulness of platelet transfusion. Isoantibodies are demonstrable in about 5 percent of patients after 1 to 10 transfusions, 20 percent after 10 to 20 transfusions, and 80 percent after more than 100 transfusions.

POOLED PLASMA. Plasma prepared from pooled blood is associated with a high incidence of hepatitis. Some investigators suggest that this may be reduced by storage at 31.6°C for 6 months. Banked plasma has been used to treat certain coagulation defects. Frozen plasma prepared from freshly donated blood or fresh plasma is necessary to provide factors V and VIII. The other plasma clotting factors are present in banked preparations. The use of plasma for therapy in patients with hypovolemia rarely is indicated. Ringer's lactate or buffered saline solution, administered in amounts two to three times the estimated blood loss, is effective in an emergency and is associated with fewer complications. Dextran or a combination of Ringer's lactate solution and normal human serum albumin are preferred for rapid plasma expansion. Commercially available dextran preparations probably should not be administered in amounts exceeding 1 liter/day, since prolongation of bleeding time and hemorrhage can occur. Low-molecular-weight dextran, i.e., molecular weight of 30,000 to 40,000, has achieved recent popularity because

it possesses a higher colloidal pressure than plasma and effects some reversal of erythrocyte agglutination.

CONCENTRATES. *Antihemophilic concentrates* are prepared from plasma and are available for the treatment of factor VIII deficiency. Some of these concentrates are twenty to thirty times as potent as an equal volume of fresh-frozen plasma. The simplest factor VIII concentrate, described initially by Pool and Shannon, is the plasma cryoprecipitate. Plasma is frozen rapidly by immersion of the plastic container in a dry ice–acetone mixture. The frozen plasma is thawed slowly (18 hours) at refrigerator temperature (4°C), and a sticky precipitate is found clinging to the bag. The thawed liquid plasma is expressed, and the precipitate, containing the bulk of the initial factor VIII activity, can be dissolved in 10 ml of sterile saline solution, pooled with other units if desired, and administered. *Desiccated human fibrinogen* is commercially available. The preparation is made from plasma pooled from many donors and carries a risk of transmitting the virus of hepatitis. *Albumin* also has been concentrated, so that 25 Gm may be administered and provide the osmotic equivalent of 500 ml of plasma. The advantage of albumin is that it is a hepatitis-free product. Salt-poor albumin is available for patients with sodium retention.

Indications for Replacement of Blood or Its Elements

VOLUME REPLACEMENT. The most common indication for blood transfusion in diseases of surgical interest is the replenishment of the circulating blood volume. It is difficult to evaluate the volume deficit accurately. Systolic blood pressure offers poor assessment of blood loss, particularly when the patient's base-line blood pressure is unknown. In a previously normotensive patient, a systolic pressure of 100 mm Hg may indicate a blood volume of at least 70% of normal.

A variety of techniques employing dyes or isotopically tagged colloids have been introduced to determine the blood volume more precisely. Values for "normal blood volume" are variable, and the techniques are relatively inaccurate when there is a rapidly changing situation, such as hemorrhage. Chronically ill and elderly patients may have a diminution of blood volume. In patients with cardiac decompensation, the blood volume may be greater than normal. Many patients with chronically reduced blood volume are well accommodated to that volume. Blood volume, in itself, does not serve as an absolute indication for transfusion. Measurement of hemoglobin or hematocrit also is used to interpret blood loss. This is misleading in the face of acute blood loss, since the hematocrit may be normal in spite of a severely contracted blood volume. Ebert et al. showed that after a healthy adult male lost approximately 1,000 ml of blood rapidly, the venous hematocrit fell only 3 percent during the first hour, 5 percent at 24 hours, 6 percent at 48 hours, and 8 percent at 72 hours, thus indicating the time required for the body to restore blood volume.

A healthy person can lose 430 ml in 20 minutes with only minor effects on the circulation and little change in blood pressure or pulse, as evidenced by the normal blood donor. The normal person may lose 1 liter of blood rapidly without a fall in blood pressure as long as he remains supine. About 40% of blood volume, or 2 liters of blood, usually is lost before significant hypotension develops. Loss of blood may be evaluated in the operating room by estimating the amount of blood in the wound and on the drapes and by weighing sponges. The loss determined by weighing sponges is only about 70% of true loss.

There is little justification for preparing the patient for operation by routine transfusion to meet an arbitrary level of hematocrit. Improvement of blood volume prior to operation should be reserved for patients with debilitating illnesses if reduction in blood volume has been demonstrated by accurate measurement. In these patients, transfusion should aim at increasing the red cell mass to about 70% of normal. The routine use of blood during operation cannot be justified. Evaluation of single unit transfusions given to 146 adults suggests that over 25 percent of such transfusions were of questionable indication and another 25 percent were definitely unnecessary.

IMPROVEMENT IN OXYGEN-CARRYING CAPACITY. This is primarily a function of the red cell. When anemia can be treated by specific therapy, transfusion should be withheld. Acute anemias, such as hemolytic anemia, are more disabling physiologically than chronic anemia, since most patients with chronic anemia have undergone an adjustment to the situation. In pregnancy, there is a moderate drop in hematocrit, and transfusions are not indicated to correct the physiologic anemia of pregnancy prior to surgical treatment. The correction of chronic anemia prior to surgical treatment, though often performed, is difficult to justify, and there is no indication that anemia predisposes to wound dehiscence. Peskin and associates have described a stroma-free hemoglobin solution which has the ability to carry and exchange oxygen and, in experimental animals, has demonstrated no toxicity. Blood volume may be replaced with dextran solution or Ringer's lactate solution with a reduction of the hemoglobin to levels below 10 Gm and little demonstrable change in the effects of a reduction in oxygen-carrying capacity or the capacity to remove metabolic gaseous by-products.

REPLACEMENT OF CLOTTING FACTORS. Transfusion of platelets and/or proteins contributing to coagulation may be indicated in specific patients either prior to or during operation. In the treatment of certain hemorrhagic conditions, it is to be appreciated that the clotting defects may be multiple and the injection of substitutes and extracts may be less effective than transfusion of fresh blood. Treatment with clotting factors requires an accurate diagnosis of the hemorrhagic disease with an appreciation of the changes which occur in the biologic properties of the factors during storage and the biologic effects and quantitative changes which occur after injection.

When transfusion with fibrinogen is deemed necessary, a plasma level greater than 100 mg/ml should be maintained. The hypofibrinogenemia encountered during surgical treatment is frequently related to excessive consumption. Adequate levels of fibrinogen frequently will return within hours without replacement therapy if the precipi-

tating cause is corrected. Deficiency of factor V, per se, is relatively rare; although transfusion will increase the level, there is suggestion that the biologic half-life is short and may not exceed 12 hours.

Hypoprothrombinemia and deficiency of factor VII in patients on anticoagulant therapy can be reversed with injection of vitamin K_1. In patients who are deficient in prothrombin, such as those with cirrhosis, and who require surgical treatment, transfusion with banked blood may effect immediate benefit.

Transfusion therapy for patients with hemophilia subjected to trauma or surgical procedures requires sufficient quantities to raise and maintain the level of factor VIII in the plasma to above 30% of normal. Transfusion of small amounts of factor VIII is not justified. If a life-threatening situation exists, large amounts must be used. The factor IX deficient patient subjected to surgery or trauma also requires levels of 20 to 30% for secure hemostasis. Such levels are difficult to attain with plasma infusions despite the stability of factor IX in stored plasma. Fortunately, factor IX concentrates now being tested offer considerable promise. The biologic half-life of factor IX is appreciably longer than that of factor VIII.

Usually, the hemostatic mechanism is not markedly altered with platelet counts greater than 50,000. If thrombocytopenia is more pronounced, however, the transfusion of fresh platelets may be indicated to prevent or treat active bleeding. The life span of freshly infused platelets is only about 10 days, and in some instances the recipient represents a hostile environment, and the survival is reduced to several hours.

SELECTIVE THERAPY

Johnson and Greenwalt recently pointed out that less than 50 years ago we were concerned with making blood transfusions easier to administer while presently we are searching for arguments with which to discourage the administration of unnecessary transfusions and methods to place transfusion on a more logical basis. If the patient has severe anemia and hypovolemia, which are usually associated with massive hemorrhage, whole blood represents the treatment of choice, and ordinary banked blood generally can be used. An alternative to this approach is a combination of packed red cells plus a plasma volume expander. Operative blood losses of 1,000 to 1,500 ml may be replaced without untoward difficulty using Ringer's lactate or buffered saline solution. When anemia exists without hypovolemia, packed red cells represent the treatment of choice. This can be accomplished with the standard packed cells or with frozen cells, which, although presently expensive, provide a method of storage for many years, avoid the complication of hepatitis, and reduce the incidence of fever, chills, and allergic reactions. The use of packed red cells is particularly applicable in patients with severe anemia who have diminished cardiac reserve or hypervolemia.

Thrombocytopenic bleeding is treated with platelet concentrates or platelet-rich plasma (Table 3-3). Deficiencies of factors VII, IX, X, or XI unaccompanied by anemia can be treated with stored plasma or any plasma prepara-

Table 3-3. REPLACEMENT OF CLOTTING FACTORS

Factors	Normal level	Life span in vivo ($\frac{1}{2}$ Life)	Fate during coagulation	Level required for safe hemostasis	Stability in ACD bank blood (4°)	Ideal agent for replacing deficit
I (fibrinogen)	200–400 mg/100 ml	72 hr	Consumed	60–100 mg/100 ml	Very stable	Bank blood; concentrated fibrinogen
II (prothrombin)	20 mg/100 ml (100%)	72 hr	Consumed	15–20%	Stable	Bank blood; concentrated preparation
V (proaccelerin, accelerator globulin labile factor)	100%	36 hr	Consumed	5–20%	Labile (40% at 1 week)	Frozen fresh plasma; blood under 7 days
VII (proconvertin, serum prothrombin conversion accelerator [SPCA] stable factor)	100%	5 hr	Survives	5–30%	Stable	Bank blood; concentrated preparation
VIII (antihemophilic factor [AHF], antihemophilic globulin, [AHG]	100% (50–150)	6–12 hr	Consumed	30%	Labile (20–40% at 1 week)	Fresh frozen plasma; concentrated AHF; cryoprecipitate
IX (Christmas factor, plasma thromboplastin component [PTC], hemophilia B factor	100%	24 hr	Survives	20–30%	Stable	Fresh frozen plasma, bank blood, concentrated preparation
X (Stuart-Prower factor)	100%	40 hr	Survives	15–20%	Stable	Bank blood; concentrated preparation
XI (plasma thromboplastin antecedent [PTA])	100%	Probably 40–80 hr	Survives	10%	Probably stable	Bank blood
XII (Hageman factor)	100%	Unknown	Survives	Deficit produces no bleeding tendency	Stable	Replacement not required
XIII (fibrinase, fibrin-stabilizing factor [FSF])	100%	4–7 days	Survives	Probably less than 1%	Stable	Bank blood
Platelets	150,000–400,000/mm^3	8–11 days	Consumed	60,000–100,000/mm^3	Very labile (40% at 20 hr; 0 at 48 hr)	Fresh blood or plasma; fresh platelet concentrate (not frozen plasma)

SOURCE: E. W. Salzman, Hemorrhagic disorders, in J. M. Kinney, R. H. Egdahl, and G. D. Zuidema (eds.), "Manual of Preoperative and Postoperative Care," p. 157, W. B. Saunders Company, Philadelphia, 1971.

tion. If patients with these defects are undergoing elective or emergency surgical treatment, stored blood may be preferable. Factor V deficiency requires fresh frozen plasma or fresh whole blood as therapy. Hemophilia without severe anemia should be treated with factor VIII concentrate or fresh frozen plasma as an alternative. If there is an accompanying severe anemia, the preferable treatment is packed red cells with either factor VIII concentrate or fresh frozen plasma, but fresh blood administered shortly after collection may be used. Congenital hypofibrinogenemia should be treated with whole blood or fibrinogen from small donor pools, while acute acquired hypofibrinogenemia requires, in addition to fibrinogen or whole blood, treatment of the underlying problem, i.e., heparin for defibrination and ε-aminocaproic acid for fibrinolysis.

SPECIFIC INDICATIONS

SINGLE-UNIT TRANSFUSION. There has been a general trend toward condemning all single-unit transfusion on surgical services. As has been previously mentioned, they are usually uncalled for. However, the Committee on Blood of the American Medical Association found it necessary to oppose this trend, pointing out that it is a poor practice to order 2 units of blood to escape criticism for using a single unit, and an appropriate volume of blood should be given whenever transfusion is required.

MASSIVE TRANSFUSION. The term *massive transfusion* implies a single transfusion greater than 2,500 ml or 5,000 ml transfused over a period of 24 hours. A variety of problems may attend the use of massive transfusion. Marked thrombocytopenia and deficiencies of several coagulation factors may occur. Although these are uncommon and usually responsive to the administration of platelet packs or fresh blood, they may be resistant to therapy and progress to the patient's death. The transfusion of large amounts of stored blood with a low pH theoretically may result in harmful effects, but the buffering reserve of the patient's body usually makes this a remote possibility. Howland et al. reported that the addition of 44 mEq of sodium bicarbonate significantly decreased the incidence of posttransfusion mortality in patients receiving large amounts of blood. When large volumes of citrated blood are transfused, particularly in young children and patients with severe liver disease, the citrate may cause primary skeletal conduction defects and cardiac conduction defects.

These are related to a depression of the ionized calcium level in the plasma and usually are corrected by spontaneous mobilization of calcium from extravascular sources. Since the citrate ion is rapidly metabolized, a markedly reduced serum calcium usually is associated with massive transfusions which are administered rapidly. When calcium reduction appears to be critical, it may be treated with calcium solution, which should not be added to the blood itself. It is generally felt that a high blood citrate level does not produce bleeding diathesis, and the administration of calcium may in itself lead to cardiac arrhythmias, especially ventricular fibrillation. The therapy of citrate excess generally is reserved for infants and patients in shock or with liver disease.

When large transfusions are administered, a heat exchanger may be used to warm the blood, since hypothermia may cause a decrease in cardiac rate and output and a reduction in the blood pH. Warming the blood significantly decreases the frequency of intraoperative cardiac arrest. The increased plasma potassium content of multiple units of stored blood generally does not produce clinical effects unless the patient has severe oliguria or anuria.

The use of blood from many donors increases the possibility of hemolytic transfusion reaction due to incompatibility. This can be reduced by screening each potential donor in the pool and eliminating those who show possible incompatibility. Paradoxically, patients who survive a massive transfusion do not have a high probability of developing isoantibodies subsequently, and the risk is no greater than that from a single transfusion. The risk of homologous serum hepatitis increases progressively with each succeeding unit.

EXTRACORPOREAL CIRCULATION. Fresh, heparinized blood generally has been used for open heart operations and other applications of extracorporeal circulation in order to decrease the danger of citrate effect. Subsequent to the procedure, the excess heparin is usually neutralized with protamine. Johnson and Greenwalt indicate that their experience with over 2,000 replacement transfusions demonstrates that this can be performed adequately with ACD blood which is less than 5 days old and modified by the addition of heparin and calcium. Prior to its use, the ACD blood is heparinized with 20 to 25 mg/unit and treated with 500 to 600 mg of calcium chloride/unit. When treated ACD blood is compared with heparinized blood, the pH of the former is lower during the first few minutes of perfusion, and the platelet counts are significantly lower 10 minutes after perfusion. By the end of perfusion there is no difference in the two series. A variety of physiologic compatible fluids, such as Ringer's lactate solution, buffered saline solution, and dextran, may be applied to prime the pump during extracorporeal circulation and reduce the need for blood.

Methods of Administering Blood

ROUTINE ADMINISTRATION. The rate of transfusion depends upon the patient's status. Usually, 5 ml/minute is administered for 1 minute, following which 10 to 20 ml/min may be administered to complete routine transfusion. When marked oligemia is being treated, the first 500 ml may be given within 10 minutes, and the second 500 ml may be given equally rapidly in most cases. Cold blood may be used for this amount, but when larger amounts are administered, warm blood is desirable.

The gauge of the needle is a critical factor in the rate of flow. Flow also is determined by the height at which the bottle is suspended. In patients with peripheral circulatory failure, the veins may be constricted with resultant increased resistance to flow, necessitating raising of the bottle. Positive pressure may be applied by some form of rotary pump or fingers which compress the tubing of the transfusion set and drive the blood onward. If plastic bags have been used as containers for the blood, they may be surrounded with a blood pressure cuff and pressure applied. Air pumped into the transfusion bottle has been used extensively as a method of increasing pressure, but this technique is associated with a definite danger of air embolism.

When large transfusions are administered, it is important not to overload the circulation, and the use of central venous pressure monitoring is particularly pertinent. There is no practical advantage in the use of intraarterial transfusion as compared with the intravenous route in the treatment of oligemia. It has been shown that coronary flow and systemic arterial pressure respond as rapidly and to the same extent whether the blood is administered intravenously or intraarterially. The theoretical advantage of intraarterial infusion for patients in whom the blood cannot pass from the venous to the arterial side of the circulation because of cardiac arrest or ineffective ventricular contraction is offset by the delay in setting up an intraarterial transfusion.

OTHER METHODS. Blood may be instilled intraperitoneally or into the medullary cavity of the sternum and long bones. Intrasternal and intramedullary transfusion may be painful, and the rate of administration is limited. Approximately 90 percent of red cells injected intraperitoneally enter the circulation, but uptake is not complete for at least a week, and therefore the method is not suitable when immediate transfusion is required.

In 1934, Tiber reported 123 autotransfusions using intraperitoneal blood in patients with ruptured ectopic gestation. There was only one death. This technique has also been applied to patients with ruptured livers and spleens. Blood is suctioned gently from the peritoneal cavity into a sterile container and then infused intravenously. Blood should not be reinfused if it has been within the peritoneal cavity for more than 24 hours.

Complications

HEMOLYTIC REACTIONS. Hemolytic reactions due to incompatibility of A, B, O, and Rh groups or many other independent systems may result from errors in the laboratory of a clerical or technical nature or the administration of the wrong blood at the time of transfusion. Hemolytic reactions are characterized by intravascular destruction of red blood cells and consequent hemoglobinemia and hemoglobinuria. Circulating haptoglobin is capable of binding 100 mg of hemoglobin/100 ml of plasma, and the complex is cleared by the reticuloendothelial system. When the binding capacity is exceeded, free hemoglobin circulates, and the heme is released and combines with albumin to form methemalbumin. When free hemoglobin exceeds 25 mg/100 ml of plasma, some is excreted in the urine, but in most subjects hemoglobinuria occurs when the total plasma level exceeds 150 mg/100 ml. The renal lesions which may occur consist of tubular necrosis and precipitation of hemoglobin within the tubules.

Clinical Manifestations. There is an increased hazard in patients with a previous transfusion reaction. If the patient is awake, the most common symptoms are the sensation of heat and pain along the vein into which the blood is being transfused, flushing of the face, pain in the lumbar region, and constricting pain in the chest. The patient may experience chills, fever, and respiratory distress, hypotension, and tachycardia from amounts as small as 50 ml. In patients who are anesthetized and undergoing operation, the two signs which may call attention are abnormal bleeding and continued hypotension despite adequate replacement. Abnormal bleeding may be related to the fact that thromboplastic substances are released as the cells are lysed. The mortality and morbidity resulting from hemolytic reactions is high if the patient receives a full unit of incompatible blood. Acute hemorrhagic diatheses occur in 8 to 30 percent of patients. There is a sudden fall in the platelet count, an increase in fibrinolytic activity, and consumption of coagulation factors, especially V and VIII, due to disseminated intravascular clotting.

Rudowski reported the following incidences of clinical manifestations in a large series with hemolytic posttransfusion reactions: oliguria, 58 percent; hemoglobinuria, 56 percent; arterial hypotension, 50 percent; jaundice, 40 percent; nausea and vomiting, 30 percent; flank pain, 25 percent; cyanosis and hypothermia, 22 percent; dyspnea, 20 percent; chills, 18 percent; diffuse bleeding, 16 percent; neurologic signs, 10 percent; and allergic reaction, 6 percent. The laboratory criteria are hemoglobinuria with a concentration of free hemoglobin over 5 mg/100 ml, a serum haptoglobin level below 50 mg/100 ml, and serologic criteria to show antigen incompatibility of the donor and recipient blood. The simplest clinical diagnostic test is insertion of a bladder catheter and evaluation of the color and volume of the excreted urine, since hemoglobinuria and oliguria are the most characteristic signs.

Treatment. If a transfusion reaction is suspected, the transfusion should be stopped immediately, and a sample of the recipient's blood should be drawn and sent along with the suspected unit to the blood bank for comparison with the pretransfusion samples. The residual blood from the transfusion should be cultured, and the serum bilirubin should be determined in the recipient. Each gram of hemoglobin is converted to about 40 mg of bilirubin. The hemolytic reaction is characterized by an increase in the indirect reacting fraction.

A Foley catheter should be inserted, and the hourly urine output recorded. Since renal toxicity is affected by the rate of urinary excretion and the pH and since alkalinizing the urine prevents precipitation of hemoglobin within the tubules, attempts are made to initiate diuresis and alkalinize the urine. This can be accomplished with 100 ml of 20% mannitol plus 45 mEq of bicarbonate. If marked oliguria or anuria occurs, the fluid intake and potassium intake are restricted, and the patient is treated as a case of renal shutdown. In some instances, dialysis is required. Following recovery from oliguria or anuria, diuresis is often copious and may be associated with significant losses of potassium and sodium which require replacement.

ALLERGIC REACTIONS. These are relatively frequent, occurring in about 1 percent of transfusions. Reactions are usually mild and are manifested by urticaria and fever. In rare instances, the reaction may be severe enough to cause anaphylactic shock. Allergic reactions are caused by transfusion of antibodies from hypersensitive donors or the transfusion of antigens to which the recipient is hypersensitive. Reactions may occur following the administration of whole blood, packed red cells, plasma, and antihemophilic factor. Treatment consists of antihistamines, epinephrine, and steroids, depending on the severity of the reaction.

BACTERIAL SEPSIS. Bacterial contamination of infused blood is rare and may be acquired either from the contents of the container or the skin of the donor. Gram-negative organisms, which are capable of growth at 4°C, are the most common cause. Clinical manifestations include fever, chills, abdominal cramps, vomiting, and diarrhea. There may be hemorrhagic manifestations and increased bleeding if the patient is undergoing surgical treatment. In some instances, bacterial toxins can produce profound shock. If the diagnosis is suspected, the transfusion should be discontinued and the blood cultured. Emergency treatment includes adrenergic blocking agents, oxygen, antibiotics, and, in some cases, judicious transfusion.

CITRATE TOXICITY. In the past, it was felt that the amount of citrate administered with massive transfusions resulted in hypocalcemia and a consequent bleeding diathesis. Citrate excess is, in fact, rarely encountered except in young children and in patients with marked impairment of liver function. Two liters of citrated blood can be given within 10 minutes, if liver function is not impaired, with no change in blood coagulation. In patients with liver disease, when citrated blood was infused at a rate of 500 ml/15 minutes, the plasma citrate concentration rose above 0.5 mM/liter, which approaches dangerous levels capable of producing asystole. The electrocardiographic changes associated with citrate toxicity include prolongation of the Q-T segments and depression of the P and T waves.

The injection of calcium reverses many of the toxic effects of citrates. Generally it is felt that if more than 2 liters of blood must be administered in a 20-minute period, it is reasonable to inject 10 ml of 10% calcium gluconate for every additional liter of citrated blood.

EMBOLISM. Although air embolism has been reported as a complication of intravenous transfusion, healthy animals tolerate large amounts of air injected intravenously at a rapid rate. In experimental animals, the minimal lethal dose averages 7.5 ml/kg, and the mortality rate accompanying this amount of air injection can be halved by placing the animal on the left side at the time of injection. This displaces the air away from the outflow tract in the right ventricle. It has been suggested that the normal adult generally will tolerate an embolism of 200 ml of air. Smaller amounts, however, can cause alarming signs and may be fatal. The most common method of producing air embolism during transfusion is by injecting air under pressure into the container in order to increase rate of flow. Manifestations of venous air embolism include a rise in venous pressure and cyanosis, a "mill wheel" murmur heard over the precordium, hypotension, tachycardia, and syncope. Death usually is related to primary respiratory failure. Treatment consists of placing the patient on the left side in a head-down position with the feet up. Arterial air embolism is manifested by dizziness and fainting, loss of consciousness, and convulsions. Air may be visible in the retinal arteries, and bubbles of air may flow from transected vessels.

Plastic tubes used for transfusion also have embolized after they have broken off within the vein. Plastic tubes have passed into the right atrium and the pulmonary artery, resulting in death. Embolized catheters have been removed successfully.

THROMBOPHLEBITIS. Prolonged infusions into peripheral veins using either needles, cannulae, or plastic tubes are associated with superficial venous thrombosis. Intravenous infusions which last more than 8 hours are more likely to be followed by thrombophlebitis. There is an increased incidence in the lower limb as compared to upper limb infusions. Treatment consists of discontinuation of the infusion and local compressing. Embolism from superficial thrombophlebitis of this nature is extremely rare.

OVERTRANSFUSION AND PULMONARY EDEMA. Overloading the circulation is a complication which is avoidable. It may occur with rapid infusion of blood, plasma expanders, and other fluids, particularly in patients with heart disease. The central venous pressure should be monitored in these patients and whenever large amounts of fluid are administered in order to prevent this complication.

Circulatory overloading is manifested by a rise in the venous pressure, dyspnea, and cough. Râles generally can be heard at the bases of the lung. Treatment consists of stopping the infusion, placing the patient in a sitting position, and, occasionally, venous section for removal of blood.

Although acute pulmonary edema occurs more frequently following large transfusions, it has been reported in patients receiving small transfusions. A syndrome which can be confused with pulmonary edema consists of postoperative hypoxia seen in patients who have undergone cardiac surgical treatment and extracorporeal bypass procedures. A damaging factor apparently is carried by the perfusing blood, and immature plasma cells are found in the interalveolar tissue. The lesion represents an immune response to homologous blood. The incidence is reduced by employing the hemodilution technique of pump priming.

TRANSMISSION OF DISEASE. Malaria and syphilis can be transmitted by blood transfusion. Positive serologic tests for syphilis may result 20 days after transfusion from donors with positive reactions.

Serum Hepatitis. Serum hepatitis is the most important disease transmitted by transfusion of blood components. The highest risks are associated with ultraviolet-exposed plasma pooled from many donors, platelet concentrates made from the blood of more than one donor, factor VIII concentrates, and commercial fibrinogen. The incidence of hepatitis transmission is thought to approximate 12 percent for pooled plasma. There is moderate risk with infusion of whole blood (approximately 1 percent), packed red blood cells, single-donor plasma, and single-unit platelet concentrates or factor VIII concentrates. Complement fixation tests for hepatitis-associated antigen (Australian) and antibody persist in 35 percent of those with serum hepatitis (SH; MS-2). Therefore, this test should be used to eliminate this proportion of dangerous donors. Currently there is no test for infectious hepatitis (IH; MS-1). A reduced incidence of hepatitis has been claimed for plasma stored for 6 months at 31.6°C, but the evidence is contradictory. The risk is definitely diminished by freezing the red cells and plasma. There is no risk from human serum albumin and other plasma protein fractions.

Intramuscular injection of 10 ml of γ-globulin within the first week of transfusion and again 1 month later to battle casualties reduced the incidence of icteric hepatitis from 8.9 to 1.3 percent. In patients undergoing cardiac surgical treatment, however, a similar dose of γ-globulin failed to reduce the incidence of hepatitis. Krugman et al. have reported that immune serum globulin is effective in preventing IH, or type A, hepatitis but inconsistent in effect for SH type. Using special γ-globulin having an anti-HAA titer 50,000 to 100,000 higher than the standard γ-globulin, several investigators have been able to confirm passive immunity against SH. Katz et al. added modified standard γ-globulin to blood before transfusion and reported encouraging results in reducing the incidence of hepatitis. However, the most effective prophylactic therapy has not yet been determined.

In recipients who are transfused with an average of 2 units of blood, an incidence of approximately 0.5 percent has been reported. The disease is caused by hepatitis virus B, which is present in the blood of a proportion of the population. There is a higher incidence of carriers among narcotic addicts and chronic alcoholics. Liver function tests have not proved valuable in detecting the carrier state. The incubation period is between 50 and 160 days, in contrast to infectious hepatitis, which has a shorter incubation period, 15 to 50 days, and also may be transmitted by transfusion. In a study using human volunteers who received injections of virus A and virus B, the "take rate" for the former was 20 percent and the latter 50 percent.

Clinical manifestations include lethargy, anorexia, and jaundice. The SGOT and SGPT levels are elevated. The mortality rate for serum hepatitis in the young age group is low but may be extremely high, up to 50 percent, in older patients. Some patients proceed to develop chronic hepatitis and cirrhosis.

References

General

Biggs, R. P., and Macfarlane, R. G.: "Human Blood Coagulation and Its Disorders," 3d ed., F. A. Davis Company, Philadelphia, 1962.

Hougie, C.: "Fundamentals of Blood Coagulation in Clinical Medicine," McGraw-Hill Book Company, New York, 1963.

Quick, A. J.: "Hemorrhagic Diseases and Thrombosis," Lea & Febiger, Philadelphia, 1966.

Ratnoff, O. D.: "Bleeding Syndromes," Charles C Thomas, Publisher, Springfield, Ill., 1960.

Ulin, A. W., and Gollub, S. S. (eds.): "Surgical Bleeding: Handbook for Medicine, Surgery, and Specialties," McGraw-Hill Book Company, New York, 1966.

Wintrobe, M. M.: "Clinical Hematology," Lea & Febiger, Philadelphia, 1967.

Biology of Normal Hemostasis

Astrup, T.: "Connective Tissue, Thrombosis, and Atherosclerosis," Academic Press, Inc., New York, 1959.

Davey, M. G., and Lüscher, E. F.: Biochemical Aspects of Platelet Function and Hemostasis, Semin Hematol, 5:5, 1968.

Davie, E. W., and Ratnoff, O. D.: Waterfall Sequence for Intrinsic Blood Clotting, Science, 145:1310, 1964.

Gaarder, A., Jonsen, J., Laland, S., Hellem, A., and Owren, P. A.: Adenosine Diphosphate in Red Cells as a Factor in the Adhesiveness of Human Blood Platelets, Nature (Lond), 192:531, 1961.

Macfarlane, R. G.: Enzyme Cascade in the Blood Clotting Mechanism and Its Function as a Biochemical Amplifier, Nature (Lond), 202:498, 1964.

Quick, A. J.: Effect of Aspirin on the Bleeding Time, Fed Proc, 25:498, 1966.

Rodman, N. F.: The Morphologic Basis of Platelet Function, in K. M. Brinkhous, R. W. Shermer, and F. K. Mostofi (eds.), "The Platelet," The Williams & Wilkins Company, Baltimore, 1971.

Sherry, S.: Present Concept of the Fibrinolytic System, Ser Haemat, 7:70, 1965.

Vigliano, E. M., and Horowitz, H. I.: Bleeding Syndrome in a Patient with IGA Myeloma: Interaction of Protein and Connective Tissue, Blood, 29:823, 1967.

Tests of Hemostasis and Blood Coagulation

Brecher, G., and Cronkite, E. P.: Morphology and Enumeration of Blood Platelets, J Appl Physiol, 3:365, 1950.

Budtz-Olsen, A. E.: "Clot Retraction," Charles C Thomas, Publisher, Springfield, Ill., 1951.

Bull, B. S.: A Semiautomatic Micro Sample Dilutor, Am J Clin Pathol, 47:549, 1967.

Cartwright, G. E.: "Diagnostic Laboratory Hematology," 4th ed., Grune & Stratton, Inc., New York, 1968.

DeNicola, P.: "Thromboelastography," Charles C Thomas, Publisher, Springfield, Ill., 1957.

Didisheim, P.: Screening Tests for Bleeding Disorders, Am J Clin Path, 47:622, 1967.

Duke, W. W.: The Relation of Blood Platelets to Hemorrhagic Disease: Description of a Method for Determining the Bleeding Time and Coagulation Time, and Report of Three Cases of Hemorrhagic Disease Relieved by Transfusion, JAMA, 55:1185, 1910.

Ivy, A. C., Shapiro, P. F., and Melnick, P.: The Bleeding Tendency in Jaundice, Surg Gynecol Obstet, 60:781, 1935.

Jim, R. T. S.: A Study of the Plasma Thrombin Time, J Lab Clin Med, 50:45, 1957.

Lee, R. I., and White, P. D.: A Clinical Study of the Coagulation Time of Blood, Am J Med Sci, 145:495, 1923.

Margolius, A., Jr., Jackson, D. P., and Ratnoff, O. D.: Circulating Anticoagulants: A Study of 40 Cases and a Review of the Literature, Medicine (Baltimore), 40:145, 1961.

Nye, S. W., Graham, J. B., and Brinkhous, K. M.: The Partial Thromboplastin Time as a Screening Test for the Detection of Latent Bleeders, Am J Med Sci, 243:279, 1962.

Owren, P. A.: Thrombotest: A New Method for Controlling Anticoagulant Therapy, Lancet, 2:754, 1959.

Quick, A. J.: Clinical Interpretation of the One-Stage Prothrombin Time, Circulation, 24:1422, 1961.

Salzman, E. W.: Measurement of Platelet Adhesiveness: A Sample In Vitro Technique Demonstrating an Abnormality in von Willebrand's Disease, J Lab Clin Med, 62:724, 1963.

Tocantins, L. M.: The Bleeding Time, Am J Clin Pathol, 6:160, 1936.

Evaluation of the Surgical Patient as a Hemostatic Risk

Biggs, R., and Macfarlane, R. G.: "Human Blood Coagulation and Its Disorders," 3d ed., F. A. Davis Company, Philadelphia, 1962.

Hougie, C.: "Fundamentals of Blood Coagulation in Clinical Medicine," McGraw-Hill Book Company, New York, 1963.

Shulman, N. R., Aster, R. H., Leitner, A., and Hiller, M. C.: Immunoreactions Involving Platelets. V. Posttransfusion Purpura Due to Complement-fixing Antibody against Genetically Controlled Platelet Antigen: Proposed Mechanism for Thrombocytopenia and Its Relevance, in "Autoimmunity," The Year Book Medical Publishers, Inc., Chicago, 1962–1963 ser.

Clinical Hemostatic Defects

Baldini, M.: Idiopathic Thrombocytopenic Purpura, N Engl J Med, 274:1245, 1966.

Biggs, R., and Macfarlane, R. G.: "Human Blood Coagulation and Its Disorders," 3d ed., F. A. Davis Company, Philadelphia, 1962.

Breckenridge, R. T., and Ratnoff, O. D.: Therapy of Hereditary Disorders of Blood Coagulation, Mod Treat, 5:39, 1968.

Curtiss, P. H., Jr.: Orthopedic Management of Patients with Hereditary Disorders of Blood Coagulation, Mod Treat, 5:84, 1968.

Griner, P. F.: Drug Effects on Oral Anticoagulants, in R. L. Weed (ed.), "Hematology for Internists," Little, Brown and Company, Boston, 1971.

Hardaway, R. M., III: Disseminated Intravascular Coagulation, Thromb Diath Haemorrh [Suppl], 56:207, 1971.

Hougie, C.: "Fundamentals of Blood Coagulation in Clinical Medicine," McGraw-Hill Book Company, New York, 1963.

Hoyer, L. W.: Disseminated Intravascular Coagulation, in R. L. Weed (ed.), "Hematology for Internists," Little, Brown and Company, Boston, 1971.

Klingensmith, W.: Surgical Implications of Hemorrhage during Anticoagulant Therapy, *Surg Gynecol Obstet,* **125:**1333, 1967.

Levine, B. B.: Induction of Immune Response and the Role of Antibody Specificity in Drug Hypersensitivity-Type Hemolytic Anemias and Thrombocytopenias, *Seminars Hematol,* **2:**338, 1965.

Norman, J. C., Covelli, V. H. and Sise, H. S.: Experimental Transplantation of the Spleen for Classical Hemophilia: A Rationale and Long-Term Results, *Bibl Haematol,* **34:**187, 1970.

Prentice, C. R. M., and Ratnoff, O. D.: Genetic Disorders of Blood Coagulation, *Semin Hematol,* **4:**93, 1967.

Ratnoff, O. D.: Hereditary Disorders of Hemostasis, in J. B. Stanbury, J. B. Wyngaarden, and D. S. Fredrickson, "The Metabolic Basis of Inherited Disease," 2d ed., McGraw-Hill Book Company, New York, 1966.

————: An approach to the Diagnosis of Disorders of Hemostasis, *Mod Treat,* **5:**11, 1968.

Sherry, S.: Urokinase, *Ann Intern Med,* **69:**415, 1968.

Shulman, N. R.: Surgical Care of Patients with Hereditary Disorders of Blood Coagulation, *Mod Treat,* **5:**61, 1968.

Smith, W. W.: Bleeding Disorders in Surgical Patients, *Monogr Surg Sci,* **1:**3, 1964.

Wasserman, L. R., and Gilbert, H. S.: Polycythemia Vera and Myeloid Metaplasia, in A. W. Ulin and S. S. Gollub (eds.), "Surgical Bleeding: Handbook for Medicine, Surgery, and Specialties," McGraw-Hill Book Company, New York, 1966.

Webster, W. P., Penick, G. D., Peacock, E. E., and Brinkhous, K. M.: Allotransplantation of Spleen in Hemophilia, *N Carolina Med J,* **28:**505, 1967.

Webster, W. P., Zukoski, C. F., Hutchin, P., Reddick, R. L., Mandel, S. R., and Penick, G. D.: Plasma Factor VIII Synthesis and Control as Revealed by Canine Organ Transplantation, *Amer J Physiol,* **220:**1147, 1971.

Local Hemostasis

Awe, W. C., Roberts, W., and Braunwald, N. S.: Rapidly Polymerizing Adhesive as a Hemostatic Agent: Study of Tissue Response and Bacteriological Properties, *Surgery,* **54:**322, 1963.

Cooper, P., and Christie, S. G.: Development of the Surgical Stapler, with Emphasis on Vascular Anastomosis, *Trans NY Acad Sci,* **25:**365, 1963.

Cushing, H.: The Control of Bleeding in Operations for Brain Tumor, *Ann Surg,* **54:**1, 1911.

Grey, E. G.: Fibrin as a Hemostatic in Cerebral Surgery, *Surg Gynecol Obstet,* **21:**452, 1915.

Halsted, W. S.: The Employment of Fine Silk in Preference to Catgut and the Advantages of Transfixing Tissues and Vessels in Controlling Hemorrhage, *JAMA,* **60:**1119, 1913.

Hinman, F., and Babcock, K. O.: Local Reaction to Oxidized Cellulose and Gelatin Hemostatic Agents in Experimentally Contaminated Renal Wounds, *Surgery,* **26:**633, 1949.

Jenkins, H. P., and Clarke, J. S.: Gelatin Sponge: A New Hemostatic Substance, *Arch Surg,* **51:**253, 1945.

Just-Viera, J. O., Puron-Del Aquila, R., and Yeager, G. H.: Control of Hemorrhage from the Liver without the Use of Sutures or Clamps: Preliminary Report, *Am Surg,* **28:**11, 1962.

Lindstrom, P. A.: Complications from the Use of Absorbable Sponges, *Arch Surg,* **73:**133, 1956.

Ravitch, M. M., Steichen, F. M., Fishbein, R. H., Knowles, P. W., and Weil, P.: Clinical Experiences with the Soviet Mechanical Bronchus Stapler (UKB-25), *J Thorac Cardiovasc Surg,* **47:**446, 1964.

Sawyer, P. N., and Wesolowski, S. A.: Electrical Hemostasis, in Conference on Bleeding in the Surgical Patient, *Ann NY Acad Sci,* **115:**455, 1964.

Schechter, D. S.: History of the Evolution of Methods of Hemostasis and the Study of Blood Coagulation, in A. W. Ulin and S. S. Gollub (eds.), "Surgical Bleeding: Handbook for Medicine, Surgery, and Specialties," McGraw-Hill Book Company, New York, 1966.

Schwartz, S. I., Muyshondt, E., and Penn, I.: Isotopic Evaluation of Bioelectric Factors Affecting Thrombogenesis, in Philip N. Sawyer (ed.), "Biophysical Mechanisms in Vascular Homeostasis and Intravascular Thrombosis," Appleton-Century Crofts, Inc., New York, 1965.

Waltz, J. M., and Cooper, I. S.: Cryogenic Surgery, in A. W. Ulin and S. S. Gollub (eds.), "Surgical Bleeding: Handbook for Medicine, Surgery, and Specialties," McGraw-Hill Book Company, New York, 1966.

Wangensteen, S. L., Orahood, R. C., Voorhees, A. B., Smith, R. B., III, and Healey, W. V.: Intragastric Cooling in the Management of Hemorrhage from the Upper Gastrointestinal Tract, *Am J Surg,* **105:**401, 1963.

Willman, V. L., and Hanlon, C. R.: The Influence of Temperature on Surface Bleeding: Favorable Effects of Local Hypothermia, *Ann Surg,* **143:**660, 1956.

Transfusion

Aggeler, P. M.: Physiological Basis for Transfusion Therapy in Hemorrhagic Disorders: A Critical Review, *Transfusion,* **1:**71, 1961.

Allen, J. G., Enerson, D. M., Barron, E. S. G., and Sykes, C.: Pooled Plasma with Little or No Risk of Homologous Serum Jaundice, *JAMA,* **154:**103, 1954.

American Medical Association Committee on Blood: Single Unit Transfusions, *JAMA,* **189:**955, 1964.

Barry, K. G., and Crosby, W. H.: The Prevention and Treatment of Renal Failure following Transfusion Reactions, *Transfusion,* **3:**34, 1963.

Bennett, P. J.: The Use of Intravenous Plastic Catheters, *Br Med J,* **2:**1252, 1963.

Blakeley, W. R., Bennett, L. R., and Maloney, J. V., Jr.: An Evaluation of Preoperative Blood Volume Determination in the Debilitated Surgical Patient, *Surg Gynecol Obstet,* **115:**257, 1962.

Braude, A. I.: Transfusion Reactions from Contaminated Blood: Their Recognition and Treatment, *N Engl J Med,* **258:**1289, 1958.

Bunker, J. P., Stetson, J. B., Coe, R. C., Grillo, H. C., and Murphy, A. J.: Citric Acid Intoxication, *JAMA,* **157:**1361, 1955.

Caceres, E., and Whittembury, G.: Evaluation of Blood Losses during Surgical Operations: Comparison of the Gravimetric Method with the Blood Volume Determination, *Surgery,* **45:**681, 1959.

Carter, J. F. B.: Reduction in Thrombophlebitis by Limiting Duration of Intravenous Infusions, *Lancet,* **2:**20, 1951.

Case, R. B., Sarnoff, S. J., Waithe, P. E., and Sarnoff, L. C.: Intra-arterial and Intravenous Blood Infusions in Hemorrhagic Shock: Comparison of Effects on Coronary Blood Flow and Arterial Pressure, *JAMA,* **152:**208, 1953.

Chaplin, H., Jr., Brittingham, T. E., and Cassell, M.: Methods for Preparation of Suspensions of Buffy Coat–poor Red Blood Cells for Transfusion, including a Report of 50 Transfusions of Suspensions of Buffy Coat–poor Red Blood Cells Prepared by a Dextran Sedimentation Method, *Am J Clin Pathol,* **31:**373, 1959.

Durant, T. M., Oppenheimer, M. J., Lynch, P. R., Ascanio, G., and Webber, D.: Body Position in Relation to Venous Air Embolism: A Roentgenologic Study, *Am J Med Sci,* **277:**509, 1954.

Ebert, R. V., Stead, E. A., and Gibson, J. G.: Response of Normal Subjects to Acute Blood Loss, with Special Reference to the Mechanism of Restoration of Blood Volume, *Arch Intern Med,* **68:**578, 1941.

Gollub, S., and Bailey, C. P.: Management of Major Surgical Blood Loss without Transfusion, *JAMA,* **198:**1171, 1966.

Grady, G. F., Chalmers, T. C., and the Boston Inter-Hospital Liver Group: Risk of Post-transfusion Viral Hepatitis, *N Engl J Med,* **271:**337, 1964.

Grossman, E. B., Stewart, S. G., and Stokes, J. S., Jr.: Post-transfusion Hepatitis in Battle Casualties: A Study of Its Prophylaxis by Means of Human Immune Serum Globulin, *JAMA,* **129:**991, 1945.

Harbrecht, P. J.: Abnormal Bleeding in Surgical Patients, *NY State J Med,* **66:**2428, 1966.

Hoff, H. E., and Guillemin, R.: The Tercentenary of Transfusion in Man, *Cardiovasc Res Cent Bull,* **6:**47, 1967.

Holland, P. V., Rubinson, R. M., Morrow, A. G., and Schmidt, P. J.: Gamma Globulin in the Prophylaxis of Post-transfusion Hepatitis, *JAMA,* **196:**471, 1966.

Howland, W. S., Schweizer, O., and Boyan, O. P.: Massive Blood Replacement without Calcium Administration, *Surg Gynecol Obstet,* **118:**814, 1964.

———, ———, and———.: The Effect of Buffering on the Mortality of Massive Blood Replacement, *Surg Gynecol Obstet,* **121:**777, 1965.

Huggins, C. E: Frozen Blood: Principles of Practical Preservation, *Monogr Surg Sci,* **3:**133, 1966.

———, and Grove-Rasmussen, M.: Advances in Blood Preservation, *Postgrad Med,* **37:**557, 1965.

Ingram, G. I. C.: The Bleeding Complications of Blood Transfusion, *Transfusion,* **5:**1, 1965.

Johnson, S. A., and Greenwalt, T. J.: "Coagulation and Transfusion in Clinical Medicine," Little, Brown and Company, Boston, 1965.

Katz, R., Rodriguez, J., and Ward, R.: Posttransfusion Hepatitis: Effect of Modified Gamma-Globulin Added to Blood In Vitro, *N Engl J Med,* **285:**925, 1971.

Kliman, A.: Complications of Massive Blood Replacement, *NY State J Med,* **65:**239, 1965.

Krevans, J. R., and Jackson, D. P.: Hemorrhagic Disorder following Massive Whole Blood Transfusions, *JAMA,* **159:**171, 1955.

Krugman, S., Giles, J. P., and Hammond, J.: Viral Hepatitis, Type B (MS-2 Strain): Prevention with Specific Hepatitis B Immune Serum Globulin, *JAMA,* **218:**1665, 1971.

Lalich, J. J., and Schwartz, S. I.: The Role of Aciduria in the Development of Hemoglobinuric Nephrosis in Dehydrated Rabbits, *J Exp Med,* **92:**11, 1950.

Langdell, R. D., Adelson, E., Furth, F. W., and Crosby, W. H.: Dextran and Prolonged Bleeding Time: Results of a Sixty-Gram, One-Liter Infusion Given to One Hundred and Sixty-three Normal Human Subjects, *JAMA,* **162:**346, 1958.

Lehane, D., Kwantes, C. M. S., Upward, M. G., and Thomson, D. R.: Homologous Serum Jaundice, *Br Med J,* **2:**572, 1949.

Luscher, E. F.: Biochemical Basis of Platelet Function, in K. M. Brinkhous, R. W. Shermer, and F. K. Mostofi (eds.), "The Platelet," The Williams & Wilkins Company, Baltimore, 1971.

MacCallum, F. O., McFarlan, A. M., Miles, J. A. R., Pollock, M. R., and Wilson, C.: Infective Hepatitis: Studies in E. Anglia during the Period 1943–7, *Med Res Counc Spec Rep Ser (Lond),* no. **273,** 1951

Macon, W. L., and Pories, W. J.: The Effect of Iron Deficiency Anemia on Wound Healing, *Surgery,* **69:**792, 1971.

Maloney, J. V., Jr., Smythe, C. McC., Gilmore, J. P., and Handford, S. W.: Intra-arterial and Intravenous Transfusion, *Surg Gynecol Obstet,* **97:**529, 1953.

McNair, T. J., and Dudley, H. A. F.: The Local Complications of Intravenous Therapy, *Lancet,* **2:**365, 1959.

Med Lett Drugs Ther, vol. 9, no. 22, issue 230, Nov. 3, 1967.

Mollison, P. L.: "Blood Transfusion in Clinical Medicine," 4th ed., F. A. Davis Company, Philadelphia, 1967.

Morton, J. H.: An Evaluation of Blood Transfusion Practices on a Surgical Service, *N Engl J Med,* **263:**1285, 1960.

———: Surgical Transfusion Practices, 1967, *Surgery,* **65:**407, 1969.

Moyer, C.: "Conference on Blood Groups and Blood Transfusion," Better Bellevue Association, New York, 1967.

Perrault, R., Jackson, J. R., Martin-Villar, J., and Smiley, R. K.: Experience with the Use of Frozen Blood, *Can Med Assoc J,* **96:**1504, 1967.

Peskin, G. W., O'Brien, K., and Rabiner, S. F.: Stroma-free Hemoglobin Solution: The "Ideal" Blood Substitute? *Surgery,* **66:**185, 1969.

Phillipps, E., and Fleischner, F. G.: Pulmonary Edema in the Course of a Blood Transfusion without Overloading the Circulation, *Dis Chest,* **50:**619, 1966.

Pool, J. G., and Shannon, A. E.: Production of High-Potency Concentrates of Antihemophilic Globulin in a Closed-Bag System, *N Engl J Med,* **273:**1443, 1965.

Pruitt, B. A., Jr., Moncrief, J. A., and Mason, A. D., Jr.: Efficacy of Buffered Saline as the Sole Replacement Fluid following Acute Measured Hemorrhage in Man, *J Trauma,* **7:**767, 1967.

Reece, R. L., and Beckett, R. S.: Epidemiology of Single-Unit Transfusion: A One-Year Experience in a Community Hospital, *JAMA,* **195:**801, 1966.

Rigor, B., Bosomworth, P., and Rush, B. F., Jr.: Replacement of Operative Blood Loss of More than One Liter with Hartmann's Solution, *JAMA,* **203:**399, 1968.

Rudowski, W. J.: Complications Associated with Blood Transfusion, in M. Allgower, S.-E. Bergentz, R. Y. Calne, and U. F. Gruber (eds.), "Progress in Surgery," S. Karger, New York, 1971.

Schwartz, S. I., Adams, J. T., and Bauman, A. W.: Splenectomy for Hematologic Disorders, *Curr Probl Surg,* The Year Book Medical Publishers, Inc., Chicago, May, 1971.

Shields, C. E., Dennis, L. H., Eichelberger, J. W., and Conrad, M. E.: The Rapid Infusion of Large Quantities of ACD Adenine Solution into Humans, *Transfusion,* **7:**133, 1967.

Shires, T., Coln, D., Carrico, J., and Lightfoot, S.: Fluid Therapy in Hemorrhagic Shock, *Arch Surg,* **88:**688, 1964.

Sneierson, H., Cunningham, J. R., and Artuso, D. A.: Autotransfusion for Massive Hemorrhage Due to Ruptured Spleen in Jehovah's Witness, *NY State J Med,* **67:**1769, 1967.

Strumia, M. M., Crosby, W. H., Gibson, J. G., II, Greenwalt, T. J., and Krevans, J. R.: "General Principles of Blood Transfusion," J. B. Lippincott Company, Philadelphia, 1963.

Tiber, L. J.: Ruptured Ectopic Pregnancy, *Calif Med,* **41:**16, 1934.

Tocantis, L. M., and O'Neill, J. F.: Infusion of Blood and Other Fluids into the General Circulation via the Bone Marrow: Technique and Results, *Surg Gynecol Obstet,* **73:**281, 1941.

Transfusion of Blood Components, *Med Lett Drugs Ther,* **9:**85, 1967.

Wallace, J. M., and Henry, J. B.: Isoimmunization after Massive Transfusion for Open Heart Surgery, *Transfusion,* **5:**153, 1965.

Walter, C. W.: Blood Donors, Blood and Transfusion, in J. M. Kinney, R. H. Egdahl, and G. D. Zuidema (eds.), "Manual of Preoperative and Postoperative Care," W. B. Saunders Company, Philadelphia, 1971.

Waterman, D. F., Birkhill, F. R., Pirani, C. L., and Levenson, S. M.: The Healing of Wounds in the Presence of Anemia, *Surgery,* **31:**821, 1952.

Wilson, R. F., Bassett, J. S., and Walt, A. J.: Five Years Experience with Massive Blood Transfusions, *JAMA,* **194:**851, 1965.

Young, L. E.: Complications of Blood Transfusion, *Ann Intern Med,* **61:**136, 1964.

Chapter 4

Circulatory Collapse and Shock

by **Richard C. Lillehei and Ronald H. Dietzman**

General Considerations

Traumatic Shock

Experimental Observations
    Hemodynamics
    Cell Metabolism
Traumatic Shock Other than External Bleeding

Gram-Negative Bacterial (Endotoxin) Shock

Experimental Observations
    The Bacterial Factor in Gram-Negative Septic
    Gram-Positive Infections
    Fungous Infections

Cardiogenic Shock

Experimental Observations

Specific Organ Involvement in Shock

Kidney
Lung
Pancreas

Tolerance to Shock

Treatment

Fluid Therapy
    Crystalloids
    Guides to the Administration of Fluids
Measures to Restore the Integrity of the Damaged
    Microcirculation and Reestablish Normal Cell
    Metabolism
        Vasopressor Therapy
        Vasodilators
        Isoproterenol
        Glucagon
        Beta-Blocking Agents
        Digitalis
        Clucocorticosteroids
Protocol
Buffers
Mechanical Support of the Circulation

GENERAL CONSIDERATIONS

Despite new knowledge, drugs, antibiotics, and blood substitutes, circulatory collapse and shock remain a major problem. While prompt use of blood, plasma, and other volume expanders have significantly reduced the incidence and mortality of traumatic shock, shock due to gram-negative bacteria and their endotoxins is increasing, and the mortality rate remains over 60 percent. This rate has not changed in the past half century despite antibiotic therapy. Indeed, there is good evidence that the increased incidence of gram-negative septicemia and shock may result from the promiscuous use of antibiotics, which have selectively eliminated gram-positive organisms, thus allowing unrestricted growth of gram-negatives.

The incidence of myocardial infarction and shock is also growing due to an increased incidence of coronary artery disease and a greater number of males over forty in the population. Over 1 million myocardial infarctions occur yearly in the United States; in 10 to 15 percent of these patients, cardiogenic shock occurs. The mortality of cardiogenic shock following infarction has remained over 80 percent for a generation. Cardiogenic shock also complicates the treatment of congestive heart failure from various causes and is a significant cause of mortality following cardiac surgical procedures, where it is often called the *low-output syndrome.*

In contrast to the continuing high mortality of septic and cardiogenic shock, we have made significant progress in reducing the mortality of traumatic shock, but this has been mainly in the handling of trauma secondary to wounds. The rapidly accumulated experience from World War II, the Korean war, and the war in Vietnam has greatly accelerated progress in this area, and rapid evacuation to centers superbly equipped and staffed now has reduced the mortality to less than 4 percent. Unfortunately, equivalent civilian facilities and personnel are only rarely available.

A principal problem in discussing shock is the lack of reliable statistics upon which to compare various methods of treatment. Despite this, all agree that we must improve our treatment of shock, principally preventing shock and correcting the hemodynamic and metabolic disturbances which result from shock. Clinical improvements must be based on solid experimental data.

Before discussing the physiology of shock, a suitable definition of shock is needed. Most would probably agree that shock results when tissue or organ blood flow is inadequate to sustain normal cell activities, and that this is usually accompanied by lowered arterial blood pressure (Fig. 4-1).

PATHOPHYSIOLOGY AND BIOCHEMISTRY. As early as 1879 Mapother called attention to the presence of intense peripheral vasoconstriction in shock. Malcolm in 1905

SHOCK

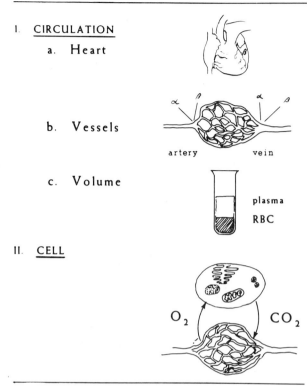

I. CIRCULATION

   a. Heart

   b. Vessels

artery   vein

   c. Volume

plasma

RBC

II. CELL

O_2 CO_2

Fig. 4-1. Shock occurs when nutritional blood flow is unable to support normal cell metabolism. Reduction of nutritional blood flow may be related to cardiac output, vascular response, or volume depletion. This results in altered cell metabolism and gaseous exchange. Shock is usually heralded by a systolic blood pressure below 90 mm Hg in a previously normotensive individual, a urine output of 25 ml/hour or less, and evidence of increased sympathetic activity causing cutaneous vasoconstriction.

confirmed these observations and in 1907 suggested heat, vasodilators, and saline solution as the treatment. Unfortunately, these observations did not attract much attention until the past decade. Rather, interest was directed toward elevating the lowered blood pressure which usually accompanies shock, using various natural and synthetic vasopressors. The major impetus toward improving tissue blood flow with vasodilating agents was stimulated by the independent work of Nickerson and of Lillehei and associates in the late 1950s and early 1960s, respectively. Now the pendulum began to swing back toward the concept that excessive vasoconstriction in shock is a factor in its continuing high mortality rate even though blood pressure is restored by vasopressors.

TRAUMATIC SHOCK

Experimental Observations

HEMODYNAMICS

Bleeding is the most common method of simulating the problems of traumatic shock in man. Hemorrhagic shock can be produced in a variety of animals, including the dog, rabbit, and rat, but most experience has been derived from the dog. In the dog, hemorrhagic shock is usually produced by bleeding the dog to a given, arbitrarily preset blood pressure or by bleeding to an arbitrarily preset percentage of the total blood volume. If the dog is bled to a mean arterial pressure of 35 mm Hg, maintained at this pressure for 2 hours, and then retransfused with all shed blood, survival is over 80 percent (Fig. 4-2). If this low mean pressure is maintained for 4 hours before pretransfusion, survival following retransfusion is less than 10 percent (Fig. 4-3).

The following chain of events is observed to occur in these experimental situations: With a reduction in the total blood volume, there is a reduction in the venous return to the heart and a reduction in the central venous or right atrial pressure. The reduced venous return is associated with a fall in both cardiac output and regional blood flow through splanchnic, renal, pulmonary, and cutaneous areas. Paralleling this is a rise in the total peripheral resistances. This rise represents a sum of the resistances of arterioles and venules throughout the circulatory system and is derived from the following formula: $(\bar{A}p - \bar{V}p)$ /C.O. $\times$ 80, where $\bar{A}p$ is the mean arterial pressure, $\bar{V}p$ is the mean central venous or right atrial pressure, and C.O. is the cardiac output; the factor 80 is a correction factor.

The increase in peripheral resistance in the various areas and organs results from the sympathoadrenal response triggered by the baroreceptors located in the aortic arch, carotid sinus, and probably many other locations including the hypothalamus–adrenal medulla axis. The baroreceptors respond to any event which lowers blood pressure, whether a fall in venous return due to bleeding, to peripheral pooling, or to a decrease in myocardial contractility as in cardiogenic shock, by a decrease in tone (Figs. 4-4, 4-5). This response activates the sympathetic nerve centers in the hypothalamus via afferent fibers in the glossopharyngeal and vagus nerves; the result is increased epinephrine secretion from the adrenal medulla and increased norepinephrine secretion from sympathetic postganglionic nerve endings. The adrenal cortex also takes part in this response by increasing cortisol production.

The sympathetic-induced vasoconstrictive response is selective; in the dog it occurs most noticeably in the adrenergically sensitive splanchnic, pulmonary, and cutaneous beds, where alpha receptors are highly concentrated. The alpha and beta receptors are conceptual structures proposed by Ahlquist in 1948 to explain changes occurring in the precapillary and postcapillary arterioles and venules. Stimulation of the alpha receptors by epinephrine and norepinephrine produces vasoconstriction of both arterioles and venules, and reduced capillary perfusion. Stimulation of the beta receptors, which are located primarily in the vasculature of the striated muscle, results in vasodilation. Beta receptors are also found in the myocardium; here stimulation causes an increase in the force and rate of heart contraction. It is interesting that the coronary and cerebral arterioles and venules probably have few if any alpha or beta receptors and generally react only to acid

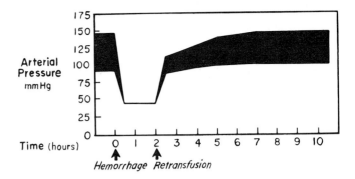

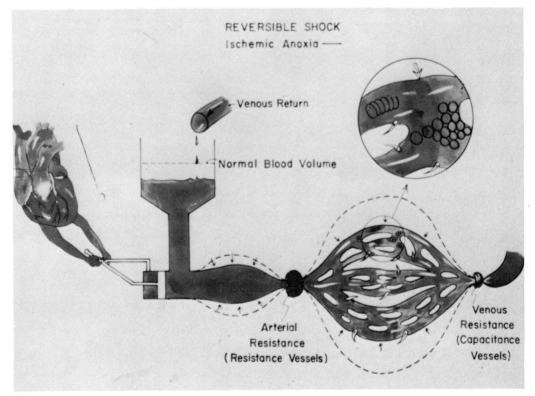

Fig. 4-2. Reversible shock; ischemic anoxia. Most dogs will survive mean arterial blood pressure reduced to 35 to 40 mm Hg by removal of about 50 percent of the total blood volume, if the shed blood is returned within 2 hours (see Fig. 4-6).

metabolites such as carbon dioxide, whose general effect is one of vasodilation.

Initially both the adrenergically sensitive (alpha receptors) precapillary and postcapillary arterioles and venules of the viscera and skin are constricted, producing ischemic anoxia and also reducing capillary hydrostatic pressure (Fig. 4-6). This results in a net inflow of extravascular fluid to replenish the diminished intravascular volume. This relation between hydrostatic forces tending to force fluid out of the capillaries and plasma osmotic pressure tending to pull fluid back into the capillaries is expressed in Starling's law of the capillaries: A volume loss of up to 1 liter, about 16 percent of the average adult blood volume,

usually can be tolerated because of viscerocutaneous vasoconstriction. Within 1 to 2 hours this volume deficit is eliminated by the passage of fluid into the vascular system, and the vasoconstriction relents. Even though the blood volume returns rather promptly to normal, the erythrocyte count will not reach normal for several weeks. This response to moderate volume losses is a very important factor in survival. Every donor giving 500 ml of blood in a blood bank manifests this same response; without it, blood donations would not be possible.

In contrast, if the blood volume loss is more than a liter and is not replaced, then reduced tissue perfusion and oxygen supply results in the accumulation of acid metabolites of anaerobic glycolysis such as lactic acid. The lowered pH incident to this accumulation apparently leads to a relaxation of the precapillary arteriolar vasoconstriction.

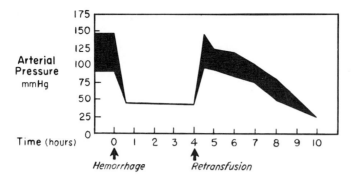

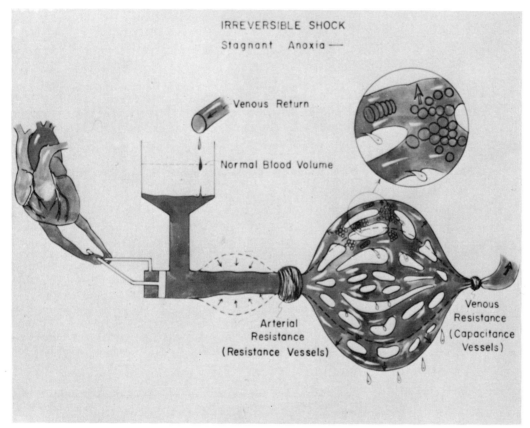

Fig. 4-3. Irreversible shock; stagnant anoxia. When the period of oligemic hypotension is extended to 4 hours before the shed blood is returned, most of the dogs die within 24 hours despite retransfusion (see Fig. 4-7).

The postcapillary venular vasoconstriction persists, however, and consequently there is an influx of blood into the microcirculation of the viscera and skin, and the hemodynamics of ischemic anoxia no longer pertain (Fig. 4-7). Hydrostatic pressures rise and begin to force fluid out of the vascular system. This fluid loss is abetted by the loss of albumin through the vascular membranes, whose integrity is breached as a result of anoxia, and a resultant decrease in plasma oncotic pressure. The stagnation in the viscerocutaneous microcirculation is intensified by aggregation of the formed elements of the blood. Red and white cells and platelets become more viscous as the velocity of flow through the microcirculation declines. In time, clumps of aggregated cells may form microthrombi, using up clotting factors of the blood in the process and giving rise to the dreaded, late phase of stagnant anoxia, disseminated intravascular coagulation (DIC).

Increasing intravascular stagnation and loss of fluid into the extravascular space further decreases the circulating blood volume. In the gastrointestinal tract plasma is initially found in the intestinal wall and finally in the intestinal lumen; in the lung plasma appears first in the interstitial spaces. Subsequently, cellular destruction and sloughing may occur, damaging the viscera and lung in such a manner that irreversible changes, or "irreversible shock," occur. In the dog this is heralded by bloody diar-

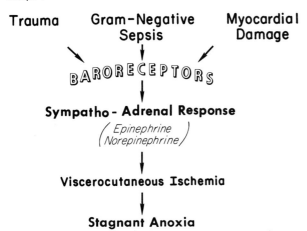

Fig. 4-4. The common, diverse insults causing shock: trauma, gram-negative bacteria and their endotoxins, or myocardial damage elicit a common response in the microcirculation of the viscera and skin because they affect the baroreceptors of the great vessels. Thus the body's response to these insults does not distinguish between them. However, the intensity of the response will certainly vary with the intensity of the insult as well as with the condition of the responding organism.

rhea and in man by hemorrhagic pneumonia and renal failure.

There is as yet no good explanation for the persistence of the venular tone and loss of arteriolar tone in severe or prolonged shock, but this has been observed by several investigators. Possibly, the venular sphincters are adapted to the lower pH and high lactic acid concentration which characterize severe stagnant anoxia, because the venous blood normally has a lower pH and contains higher concentrations of acid metabolites.

The role of the sympathetic nervous system in causing these changes is emphasized by studies of Fine, who noted that the vasoconstrictive response can be abolished by removing the sympathetic innervation to the involved area or organ prior to hemorrhage. When sympathectomies are done on segments of the intestine or spleen, vasoconstriction in response to bleeding does not occur in these areas. We have observed the same with total sympathectomies, spinal anesthesia, or high transection of the spinal cord. It appears that any method which blunts or ameliorates the sympathetic response to reduced intravascular volume usually increases survival.

The purpose of the selective vasoconstriction in response to bleeding is to divert the reduced blood volume to the brain, heart, and voluntary muscle. This response was labeled the "fight or flight" reflex by Cannon and is also part of the "alarm reaction" of Selye. It is probable that this response is evolutionary in origin and part of the "survival of the fittest" suggested by Darwin. Whatever its origin and original purpose, it can now be considered "Nature's first aid."

In most instances, the degree of vasoconstriction resulting from the sympathoadrenal response to blood loss is more than adequate. Further, if exogenous vasopressors such as levarterenol or metaraminol are added to maintain the blood pressure at near-normal levels, the microcircula-

tion deteriorates at an even more rapid rate, and the chance of survival is decreased.

Loss of blood is the initial insult leading to ischemic and ultimately stagnant anoxia. The effects of the anoxia on the cell require consideration since we originally defined shock in relation to cell function.

CELL METABOLISM

NORMAL CELL METABOLISM. In recent years, Schumer, Shires, Baue, Wilson, and others have contributed much to our understanding of shock by their studies of cell metabolism and/or correlation of function with ultrastructure using the electron microscope. To understand the aberrations of cell function occurring in shock, a review of normal cell structure and function is in order (Fig. 4-8).

The principal substrates of glucose, amino acids, fatty acids, and oxygen actively cross the cell membrane. Within the cytoplasm the glycolytic (anaerobic) cycle begins producing about 10 percent of the high-energy phosphate bonds, adenosine triphosphate (ATP), necessary for normal cell function. Pyruvate, the end product of the anaerobic cycle, then enters into the citric acid (anaerobic) or Krebs cycle (aerobic) within the mitochondria, where its further breakdown to carbon dioxide and water produces the other 90 percent of the high-energy ATP required for normal cell metabolism. While glucose is the principal substrate for producing the necessary energy, amino acids and fatty acids also are utilized for gluconeogenesis and may enter more or less directly into the anaerobic cycle.

The high-energy phosphate bonds of ATP are used by the cell to maintain the cell membrane potential which is responsible for the differential concentrations of sodium and potassium and other electrolytes within and without the cell. ATP is also used for energy to synthesize proteins, using ribosomes, in the endoplasmic reticulum.

The lysosomes of the cell contain potent hydrolysing enzymes which are used to destroy and dispose of bacteria and other foreign material after engulfment by the lysosome. These enzymes are prevented from damaging normal intracellular components by the protective lysosomal membrane which surrounds them.

CELL METABOLISM IN TRAUMATIC SHOCK. Minor blood loss, less than 1 liter, and even more significant blood loss if promptly replaced, cause little cellular dysfunction. When blood loss is large and the deficit not replaced, the effects of the anoxia can be assessed in many ways. Cell membrane integrity declines; this can be determined by isogravimetric techniques (Pappenheimer preparation), by measurement of cell membrane potential, and by assessment of intra- and extracellular concentrations of electrolytes, water, and ATP, as well as by measuring the various products of anaerobic and aerobic metabolism.

In the later phases of severe ischemic anoxia and by the time stagnant anoxia occurs, measurable shifts in sodium, potassium, and water take place; sodium and water move into the cell, while potassium moves out (Fig. 4-9). With a decrease in intracellular oxygen, pyruvate, the principal product of the anaerobic cycle, accumulates because of inability to enter the aerobic, or Krebs, cycle. Much of the pyruvate is converted to lactic acid. As lactic acid

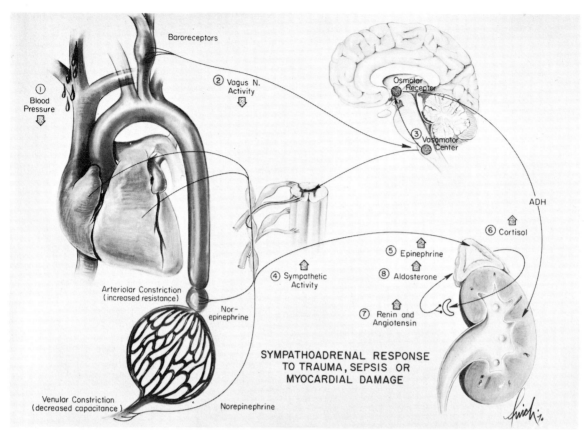

Fig. 4-5. The sympathoadrenal response results when blood pressure is lowered, which decreases the number of impulses in the nervous system connecting the baroreceptors of the great vessels and the sympathetic centers in the brainstem. These afferent nerve fibers are carried within the vagus nerves. The result is a sympathoadrenal stimulation, with outpouring of epinephrine from the adrenal medulla and norepinephrine from the postganglionic sympathetic nerve endings. The adrenal cortex also takes part in the sympathoadrenal response; there is an increase in cortisol production by the adrenal cortex and an increase in blood cortisol level.

accumulates, some finds its way back into the vascular system, where its measurement is used as an index of the degree of intracellular anoxia.

Within the cell, the decline in aerobic metabolism of pyruvate decreases the production of the high-energy ATP. Protein synthesis, which depends on ATP production, also declines.

It appears also that the lysosomal membranes surrounding the potent acid hydrolases lose their integrity, allowing these enzymes to indiscriminantly hydrolyze other intracellular structures. The resulting vasoactive peptides can cause further deterioration of the microcirculation. One such vasoactive peptide has been labeled myocardial depressant factor (MDF). Apparently it originates in the pancreas, but whether it is formed only in the pancreas and is a specific myocardial depressant is presently not clear.

Another aspect of abnormal metabolism important in shock is the entrance of increasing amounts of amino acids and fatty acids into the energy production cycle as available glucose and glycogen are used up. As a result, amino nitrogen increases at a time when the liver, the principal source of deamination, is unable to handle this increased load.

The mobilization of fatty acids theoretically should be of value because of the nearly double caloric value of fat compared with glucose or protein. Yet there are at least two problems associated with the increased fatty acid mobilization: The first is that considerable quantities of

ketone and acetone bodies, (acetoacetic acid, β-hydroxybutyric acid, and acetone) are formed. Usually these substances are produced in only small amounts and are easily metabolized by the liver and peripheral tissues. In shock, their production is increased, and the lack of oxygen for their aerobic breakdown adds further to the metabolic acidosis.

More recently, a second problem with increased fatty acid mobilization has been postulated. The fatty acid molecules may coalesce and form fat emboli which lodge in the lungs, leading to further oxygen deprivation. This has been supported by clinical observations indicating that fat embolism following trauma is lessened by providing high concentrations of exogenous glucose.

The result of these metabolic changes secondary to stagnant anoxia is that the organism reaches a state where correction of hemodynamic and metabolic aberrations will be of no avail because of extensive cell death. In the

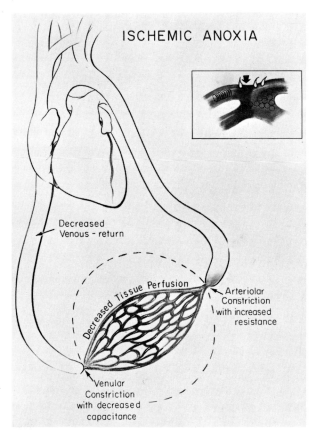

Fig. 4-6. Schema for ischemic anoxia. The initial response to a lowered arterial blood pressure includes constriction of arterioles and venules throughout the microcirculation of the viscera (including the lung) and skin. In this initial phase there is a decrease in intravascular hydrostatic pressure, whereas colloid osmotic pressure tends to remain unchanged. Thus, there is a net influx of fluids into the vascular system. This mechanism for autotransfusion can replace volume deficits up to 1 liter in the average adult if the loss has not been too rapid.

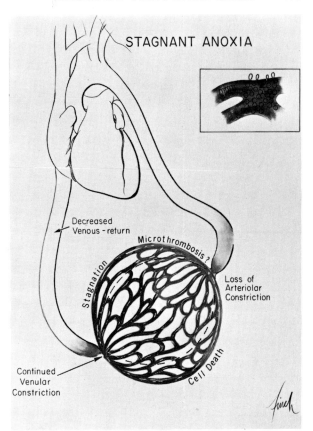

Fig. 4-7. With severe initial stress or insult, an unusually debilitated recipient, or combinations of insults of trauma, myocardial damage, or sepsis, ischemic anoxia gives way to stagnant anoxia. The period of time for this transition varies from minutes following overwhelming gram-negative bacterial sepsis to a period of years as in congestive heart failure. The appearance of the microcirculation now is quite different from that seen in Fig. 4-6. While there is continued venular constriction, arteriolar constriction is less intense and in some instances may even be absent. This allows blood to enter the microcirculation, but it cannot exit. As a result there is stagnation and pooling and an increase in hydrostatic pressure which tends to force fluid out of the vascular system. Edema, particularly in the lungs, characterizes this stage of the response. This edema is accentuated early in stagnant anoxia by the loss of plasma proteins through damaged anoxic endothelium and a decrease in colloid osmotic pressure. As the anoxia and acidosis continue, the anoxic endothelium of the microcirculation loses its integrity and allows blood cells to leave the vascular system, resulting in the typical hemorrhagic lesions of late shock seen in the abdominal viscera and in the lungs. Another common finding in stagnant anoxia is aggregation of the cellular components of the blood with the possibility that disseminated intravascular coagulation may occur with the using up of clotting elements of the blood. This is signaled by bleeding from mucous membranes or wounds and is more often a late consequence of septic shock than of traumatic or cardiogenic shock.

laboratory this state of "irreversible shock" can be defined with some precision because of the ability to control variables, but this is not the case clinically. Nonetheless, various investigators have described "patterns of shock" in man utilizing hemodynamic and metabolic measurements which often allow predictions of survival or death with a fair degree of accuracy.

Traumatic Shock Other than External Bleeding

In the preceding discussion, we have discussed a relatively "pure" type of traumatic shock in which the circulating blood volume is depleted by external loss in a controlled laboratory environment.

When dealing with traumatic shock in human beings, external blood loss often represents only a fraction of the total blood volume loss. Multiple fractures and/or soft tissue injuries often result in large volume losses in the tissues, the extent of which is often underestimated. Usually a single closed fracture of a long bone will result in

losses of 500 to 1,000 ml of blood into the surrounding tissue in a 70-kg adult. Moreover, chest trauma further compounds the anoxia of blood loss by interfering with normal gaseous exchange. These problems will be discussed in more detail in the section on treatment.

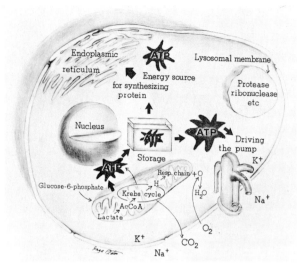

Fig. 4-8. The normal cell.

GRAM-NEGATIVE BACTERIAL (ENDOTOXIN) SHOCK

Until recently, the most common cause of septicemia and shock was the *Staphylococcus aureus*. This organism was also the one most frequently found in wound infections, but neither of these findings is still true. Gram-negative bacteria are now the most common organisms found in wound infections, abscesses, urinary tract infections, pneumonias, and septicemias. The reasons for this change are many, but probably the principal reason is that most of our antibiotics are far more effective against gram-positive bacteria than against gram-negative bacteria. Hence the gram-negative bacteria proliferate when competing gram-positive bacteria are reduced or eliminated. It appears also that many gram-negative bacteria are able to develop resistance to antibiotics.

Fig. 4-9. The abnormal cell.

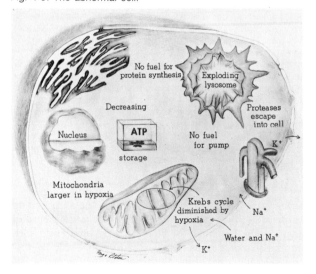

Presently the most common gram-negative bacteria isolated from skin, wounds, and blood of hospitalized patients is the *Escherichia coli* species. The *Klebsiella-Aerobacter* group follows closely in frequency. The bulk of the remaining gram-negatives are made up of members of the *Proteus, Pseudomonas,* and *Bacteroides* groups. *Herelea* species also are being reported with increasing frequency, especially in contaminated blood or plasma infusions.

The result of the change in flora of wound and other infections is that gram-negative bacteria have become initiators of shock nearly as frequently as trauma or myocardial infarction. The ability of gram-negative bacteria to cause shock is due principally to endotoxin, a complex lipopolysaccharide which is found in the cell walls of all gram-negative bacteria and is released following the death of the bacteria.

Endotoxin itself is an inert substance until it combines with one or more elements in the blood. Schumer has provided convincing evidence that activation of endotoxin occurs after combination with antibody and complement fixation. This combination leads to the formation of an anaphylotoxin, which in turn causes the release of vasoactive hormones such as epinephrine, norepinephrine, histamine, serotonin, and kinin (Fig. 4-10). The catecholamine and histamine release appears to cause most of the early cardiovascular effects of endotoxin. These effects have been studied extensively in the experimental animal and are summarized below.

Experimental Observations

Endotoxin shock can be induced in a variety of animals including the monkey, dog, rabbit, guinea pig, and mouse; endotoxins from any of the gram-negative bacteria can be used to produce shock. The most detailed hemodynamic and biochemical information is available from studies using the dog as a model and endotoxin from *E. coli* (Fig. 4-11). When this endotoxin is given intravenously to dogs, there is an almost immediate pooling of blood within the liver and intestine which is secondary to spasm of the hepatic veins and correlates with an increase in circulating histamine. The pooling reduces venous return to the right atrium and consequently reduces right atrial pressure. With the fall in venous return, there is a fall in cardiac output and in regional blood flow, particularly in the splanchnic and renal beds, and a subsequent fall in blood pressure. The hypotension affects the baroreceptors, and a sympathoadrenal response to restore blood pressure by viscerocutaneous vasoconstriction is mediated through the hypothalamus.

The hepatic venous vasoconstriction lasts only about 30 to 45 minutes and then gradually relents. Venous return to the right side of the heart is restored, and the sympathoadrenal response also relents for a time. The initial chain of events can be avoided by constructing a portacaval shunt to decompress the liver and intestine prior to administering the endotoxin. Yet elimination of this initial phase of hypotension in the dog due to portal congestion will not alter the subsequent lethality of the endotoxin.

The reestablishment of venous return to the right atrium

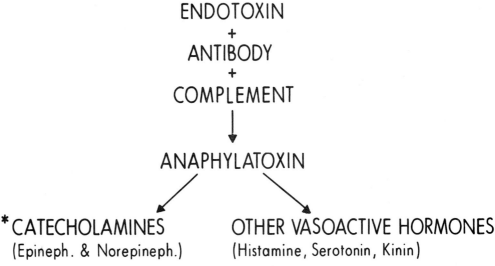

Fig. 4-10. Endotoxin is an inert substance until it combines with one or more elements in the blood. These elements are probably antibody and complement.

is short-lived. Approximately 1 hour after administration of the endotoxin, the venous return again falls and progressively decreases until the dog dies. This is secondary to intravascular pooling and also to an extravascular loss of plasma into the tissues. The blood volume falls and the hematocrit rises. Accompanying the falling venous return is a decrease in cardiac output; a decrease in regional blood flow to the splanchnic, pulmonary, and cutaneous beds; and a decrease in blood pressure, which initiates a new sympathoadrenal response. The pooling of blood in the viscerocutaneous beds as a result of stagnant anoxia is related both to the sympathomimetic effects of activated endotoxin and to the sympathoadrenal response triggered by the baroreceptors. The combination of increased circulating and tissue levels of the catecholamines (epinephrine and norepinephrine) and the direct effects of activated endotoxin causes intense vasospasm in the viscerocutaneous beds. Initially there are ischemic, then edematous, and finally hemorrhagic changes within the lung, liver, intestine, spleen, and kidneys, similar to those seen in prolonged hemorrhagic shock in dogs.

The chief difference in the visceral tissue changes between hemorrhagic and endotoxin shock is in the time it takes for the stagnant anoxia to occur. In hemorrhagic shock there is a slow progression from ischemic to stagnant anoxia in the microcirculation occurring over several hours. In endotoxin shock this same progression can occur in minutes depending on the dose of endotoxin injected and the susceptibility or sensitivity of the host animal. The result of the stagnation is a loss of plasma into the tissues due to increased hydrostatic pressure within the microcirculation; moreover, a fall in plasma oncotic pressure due to albumin loss accentuates the movement of fluid out of the vascular system. In addition to these extravascular losses, a significant portion of the blood volume is inactive within the stagnant microcirculation of the viscera. If the anoxia is prolonged, the endothelial cells of the microcirc-

ulation lose their integrity, and whole blood extravasates into the tissue, producing hemorrhagic congestion in the lungs, liver, intestine, and kidney. Additional evidence of reduced tissue perfusion and oxygen consumption is a fall in urine output and an increase in anaerobic metabolism manifested as an increase in blood lactic acid.

It is clear that the major problem in experimental endotoxin shock, as in hemorrhagic shock, is reduced nutri-

Fig. 4-11. The characteristic picture of endotoxic shock in the dog. Endotoxin from killed *Escherichia coli* was used here, but the effects are similar with all endotoxins.

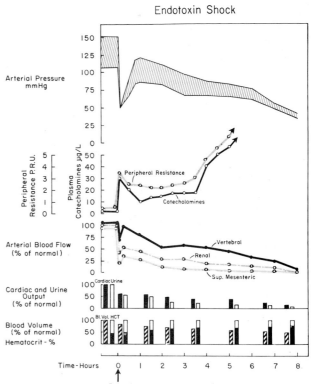

tional blood flow due to intense peripheral vasoconstriction and subsequent stagnation of the microcirculation. Again, these changes occur predominantly in the splanchnic, pulmonary, and cutaneous beds, while perfusion of the heart and brain is less affected.

The first suggestion of involvement of the sympathetic nervous system in endotoxin shock was made by Reilly et al. in 1936. They injected minute quantities of endotoxin directly into the splanchnic nerves and noted the development of intestinal hemorrhage, necrosis, and finally shock and death. This increased activity of the sympathetic nervous system after the administration of endotoxin has since been observed by several other investigators. Increased sympathetic activity can be correlated with increased tissue and plasma levels of the catecholamines and constriction of precapillary arterioles and postcapillary venules of the splanchnic, cutaneous, and pulmonary circulations, with increased resistance in these organs. Moreover, the sympathominetic effect of endotoxin further adds to tissue anoxia. With this knowledge of the changes wrought by activated endotoxin, it is clear why the addition of exogenous catecholamines such as levarterenol, metaraminol, or isoproterenol leads not to increased survival but to increased mortality.

In summary, experimental endotoxin shock is associated with intense arteriolar and venular vasospasm leading quickly to stagnant anoxia. These changes are initiated by endotoxin, which is itself a sympathomimetic agent when combined with antibody and complement and abetted by the sympathoadrenal response to lowered blood pressure initiated by the activated endotoxin.

Hemodynamically these changes are expressed as reductions in central venous pressure (CVP), cardiac output, and regional splanchnic, cutaneous, and pulmonary blood flows, as well as in reduced blood pressure and oxygen consumption. The metabolic effects of this process on the cell are similar to those discussed above for stagnant anoxia induced by trauma. Water and sodium pass into the cell, and potassium passes out. Aerobic metabolism decreases and lactic acid increases.

There are some differences between the hemodynamic and metabolic disturbances induced by endotoxin and those following blood loss, but they are more likely quantitative than qualitative. Some of the disturbances may have greater importance in septic shock. For example, the decrease in ATP formation results in decreased protein formation and decreased production of immune globulins. This in turn may reduce the ability of the organism to deal with the bacteria producing the endotoxin. Also, the aggregation of the formed elements of the blood in the stagnant microcirculation appears earlier following endo-

SHOCK

	Due to ENDOTOXINS	or to GRAM-NEGATIVE BACTERIA
Central Arterial Pressure	Low	Low
Central Venous Pressure	Low	Low
TPR	High	Low
C.I.	Low	High
Arterial O$_2$ Tension (Pa$_{O_2}$)	Normal	Low
Pulmonary A-V Admixture	Normal	High
Lactic Acidemia	High	High

Fig. 4-12. A comparison of the effects of endotoxin from killed bacteria and gram-negative bacterial sepsis.

toxin injection and is often associated with an earlier appearance of DIC (disseminated intravascular coagulation). With the depletion of fibrinogen, platelets, and factors II, V, and VIII, a bleeding diathesis occurs. Yet, while these effects on globulin synthesis and on clotting factors are more intense in endotoxin shock, in time they also occur in traumatic shock.

SPECIES DIFFERENCES. Much of the early work on endotoxin involved the use of mice, rats, rabbits, and dogs, all of which reacted to endotoxin in a similar fashion. More recently other investigators have used cats and subhuman primates, which show some differences in response to endotoxin, but these findings do not alter the basic concepts of the mechanisms by which endotoxin causes death. One fact that is clear from these comparative studies concerns the "shock organ" in each species, or the visceral organ showing the principal pathologic condition after endotoxin. These variations are shown in Table 4-1. There seems to be a hierarchy of sensitivity of the visceral organs to the stagnant anoxia induced by endotoxins. In man, the kidney and lung seem most sensitive. These species differences occur not only after endotoxin but after other insults such as trauma or myocardial damage, but they do not detract in any important way from the pathophysiology discussed above.

Table 4-1. TARGET ORGANS OF ACTIVATED ENDOTOXIN (ANAPHYLOTOXIN)

Rat	Rabbit	Cat	Dog	Monkey	Man
Intestine Liver Lung	Lung	Lung Liver	Intestine (early) Lung (late) Liver	Lung Liver	Kidney (early) Lung (late)

THE BACTERIAL FACTOR IN GRAM-NEGATIVE SEPTIC SHOCK. Until recently most investigators had assumed that most if not all the hemodynamic and metabolic changes in gram-negative septic shock were due to the endotoxins of the bacteria, ignoring the living bacterial factor. A rude awakening to the importance of the bacterial factor occurred when sufficient data on patients suffering gram-negative septic shock became available. Thus the human being suffering gram-negative septicemia seemed to present a hemodynamic picture which was at variance with the experimental observations noted above (Fig. 4-12). The most striking variation was the usually observed normal or high cardiac index coupled with low total peripheral resistance. Despite this apparent hyperdynamic circulation, the metabolic changes in man were similar to those in the animal with marked lactic acidosis indicative of severe cellular anoxia.

Some clinicians took these variations to mean that the experimental studies on endotoxin carried out over the past decade had no relevance to septic shock in man. Others such as Albrecht and Clowes, Thal, Siegel et al., Hinshaw, and Motsay et al. quickly realized that experimental endotoxin shock could not be equated with gram-negative septic shock in man until the living bacterial factor was introduced into the laboratory experiments. When a focus of infection and septicemia was induced in the dog along with endotoxin administration to more closely simulate the clinical situation, the hemodynamics in the dog were almost identical to those seen in man, i.e., a high cardiac index and low total peripheral resistance in the face of a severe metabolic acidosis. Hence, when conditions in the laboratory animal simulate those found in human septic shock, there are few if any major differences.

The paradox of high cardiac output, low total peripheral resistance, hypotension, stagnant anoxia, and lactic acidosis can be best explained by arteriovenous admixture, or shunting, in the area of infection and involvement of other organs such as the lung secondarily through blood-borne factors (Fig. 4-13).

Whether the shunting is due to opening anatomic or physiologic shunts, to uncoupling of oxidative enzyme systems, or to alterations in oxyhemoglobin dissociation cannot be determined at this time. All these mechanisms are likely involved to varying degrees, since there is at least some experimental evidence to support each.

At the turn of this century, Metchnikoff first noted the increased blood flow in areas of inflammation. He thought this was due to production of a local hormone. Now we are just beginning to appreciate the prescience of Metchnikoff's observations. There is increasing evidence that the interaction of bacteria and damaged tissue does activate a hormone. Kininogen is present in all tissues and in the blood and is easily converted to kinin. Kinin is found in high concentrations in inflamed areas and is a potent vasodilator. With increasing blood flow in inflamed areas oxygen consumption should increase, but this is usually not the case. Rather, arteriovenous oxygen difference decreases, indicating that the increased blood flow is not nutritional. This may be because it actually bypasses the

A.

ANATOMIC

Cirrhosis
Pleural surface of lung
Submucosa of intestine

PHYSIOLOGIC

Atelectasis
Local hormone production at site of bacterial infection,? Kinin?
Uncoupling of oxidative phosphorylation in mitochondria

Fig. 4-13. *A.* Sources of arteriovenous admixture, or shunting. *B.* Stagnant anoxia in septic shock. Living bacteria result in a shunting effect, while venular constriction causes stagnation within capillaries.

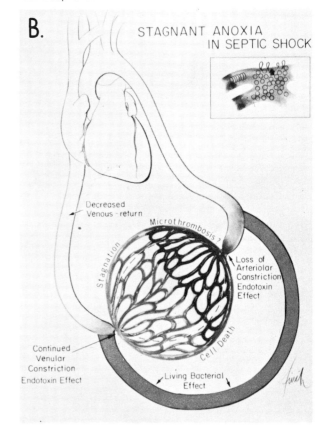

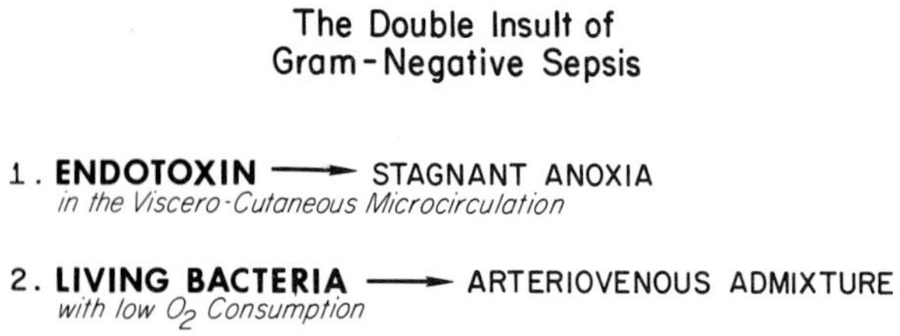

The Double Insult of Gram-Negative Sepsis

1. **ENDOTOXIN** ⟶ STAGNANT ANOXIA
   in the Viscero-Cutaneous Microcirculation

2. **LIVING BACTERIA** ⟶ ARTERIOVENOUS ADMIXTURE
   with low O$_2$ Consumption

Fig. 4-14. The double insult of gram-negative bacterial sepsis resulting from endotoxin-blood interaction and bacteria-tissue interaction.

cell or because there is a defect in oxygen transport or in oxidative phosphorylation. Evidence is available to suggest all these factors are involved. The result of this non-nutritional increased flow is a second anoxic insult in addition to that caused by the endotoxin (Fig. 4-14).

Almost all patients will show this hyperdynamic circulatory state if observed early in the course of septic shock. Later the cardiac output may fall as myocardial failure occurs, but many patients continue to show this hyperdynamic state almost until death occurs. It should be noted also that even though most patients suffering septic shock show a decreased arteriovenous oxygen difference and a decreased oxygen consumption despite the hyperdynamic

Fig. 4-15. Experimental cardiogenic shock induced in the dog with coronary artery embolization using microspheres. The hemodynamic and metabolic disturbances resulting from these diffuse myocardial infarctions closely resemble those seen in man.

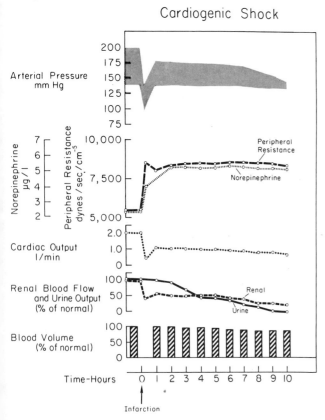

circulation, some patients have been observed with increased oxygen consumption; this finding does not alter the high mortality rate. It is clear that much remains to be learned about the metabolic response to the septic state. A major problem in assessing the problem in man is the lack of a reliable method to assay endotoxin in blood or tissues. Nevertheless, we may summarize our knowledge of gram-negative septic shock in man by indicting both the endotoxin which causes stagnant anoxia in the nutritional vasculature of the viscera and the living bacteria which cause blood to take a nonnutritional pathway, which further accentuates the stagnant anoxia caused by endotoxin.

GRAM-POSITIVE INFECTIONS

None of the gram-positive bacteria possess an endotoxin, and only a few such as the staphylococci produce an exotoxin. In contrast to an endotoxin, an exotoxin is produced by a living bacteria, and it does not need antibody or complement for its activation. Yet, in their effects on the circulation and metabolism exotoxins are very similar to activated endotoxins.

FUNGOUS INFECTIONS

In the 1970s we have witnessed an increase in fungous infections, principally those caused by *Candida albicans,* again probably due in part to the increasing effectiveness of the newer antibiotics against gram-negative organisms. The increasing use of immunosuppressive agents in transplantation, chemotherapy in cancer, and intravenous hyperalimentation also have contributed to the increasing frequency of *Candida* infections.

There is little experimental or clinical work available to characterize fungous infections according to their hemodynamic and metabolic disturbances, but our own observations suggest that the *C. albicans* infections have all the hyperdynamic and metabolic effects of the gram-negative bacteria. Cardiac indices of 6 to 10 liters/m^2/minute (two to three times normal) often have been measured in the face of striking decreases in arteriovenous oxygen differences, low oxygen consumption, and severe lactic acidosis.

CARDIOGENIC SHOCK

Experimental Observations

Numerous techniques have been tried to produce myocardial damage and cardiogenic shock which would resemble that seen in man. Practically, these techniques have been confined to the dog and have ranged from direct myocardial damage to coronary artery occlusions. The most reproducible technique is a closed-chest intracoronary artery plastic microsphere embolization model in the dog or subhuman primate.

Immediately after the production of myocardial damage with microspheres there is marked reduction in the cardiac output and blood pressure. The blood pressure then rises but stabilizes below the control level; however, the depressed cardiac output does not return toward normal in the same proportion. Hence increase in the blood pressure is secondary to an increase in total peripheral resistance resulting from the sympathoadrenal response to the fall in blood pressure mediated through the baroreceptors (Fig. 4-15). Experimental studies show that the baroreceptor-mediated peripheral vascular response to myocardial damage is similar to the responses to blood loss and endotoxins of gram-negative bacteria.

The catecholamines elaborated by the sympathetic nerve endings and the adrenal medulla stimulate the alpha receptors to cause vasoconstriction in the viscerocutaneous microcirculation. Pulmonary, hepatic, intestinal, and renal blood flows decline, and urine output decreases. This preserves blood flow to the brain and heart, the vasculature of which is not adrenergically sensitive. Yet a consequence of this increased total peripheral resistance is a greater work load (afterload) on the already damaged myocardium and a consequent greater oxygen demand at a time that such a demand cannot be met. As a result the size of the original infarct may expand, as has been shown experimentally by Braunwald and associates.

In the visceral microcirculation, the initial ischemic anoxia may progress to stagnant anoxia with all its disastrous hemodynamic and metabolic consequences, and these do not differ significantly from those described for traumatic or the endotoxic aspect of gram-negative septic shock.

In the experimental animal as in the human being the time sequence from myocardial infarction to cardiogenic shock may vary from a few minutes to a few hours, depending on the size of the initial infarct, the prior condition of the animal, and the nature of the treatment.

With the coronary embolization technique, about 40 to 50 percent of dogs will develop cardiogenic shock as defined by a 30 percent fall in systolic arterial pressure and a 50 percent fall in cardiac index. In patients suffering a myocardial infarction about 10 to 15 percent will develop shock as defined by a persisting systolic hypotension below 90 mm Hg, oliguria, and a decrease in cardiac index to below 2.5 liters/m^2/minute.

Chronic congestive heart failure can also lead to cardiogenic shock, but the process may extend over a period of many years. Nonetheless, the peripheral microcirculatory picture is one of stagnant anoxia with all its attendant hemodynamic and metabolic changes.

A third type of cardiogenic shock is that following surgery to repair congenital and acquired cardiac defects including septal defects, valve lesions and coronary artery obstructions. Although, as mentioned earlier, this type of cardiogenic shock is often called the low-output syndrome, it does not differ in its hemodynamic and metabolic findings from shock following myocardial infarction or chronic congestive heart failure. The cause of the low-output syndrome is threefold: First, there is the damage to the myocardium and lungs directly resulting from the cardiac defect, whether it be congenital, rheumatic, or secondary to coronary artery disease. Second, the response of the mammalian organism to cardiopulmonary bypass used during correction of the defect is similar to other types

of stress noted above. There is a sympathoadrenal activation, again via the baroreceptor mechanism, with catecholamine release. The initial effect on the visceral microcirculation is one of ischemic anoxia followed in time by stagnant anoxia characterized by a decrease in venous return to the pump-oxygenator. Hence cardiopulmonary bypass is a form of "controlled shock," and the longer the bypass, the more severe the resulting hemodynamic and metabolic disturbances.

The third aspect of the etiology of low-output syndrome concerns the damage to the heart which occurs in the repair of the defect. When right or left ventriculotomy is required, there is more interference with function than with atriotomy, aortotomy, or pulmonary arteriotomy. Also involved in the direct injury to the myocardium is the extent to which coronary artery perfusion can be maintained during the period of bypass.

SPECIFIC ORGAN INVOLVEMENT IN SHOCK

Kidney

We noted above that there are differences in organ susceptibility to anoxia among the mammalian species but that the same basic response of arterioles and venules occurs in all the visceral organs. The kidney and lung of man are especially sensitive to the anoxia of shock, and failure of either or both of these vital organs is a frequent cause of death, whatever the original insult causing the shock.

In the kidney, the cortex is more severely damaged than the medulla, with the result that acute tubular swelling or necrosis may occur. With tubular swelling, concentration is impaired and oliguria usually occurs early in shock. Subsequently the blood urea nitrogen level and creatinine and potassium levels may continue to rise for several days despite successful resuscitation of the patient and restoration of urine flow. In more severe anoxic damage to the cortex, anuria may occur and not relent even with resuscitation. This acute renal shutdown is usually thought to be caused by acute tubular necrosis (ATN); in reality, however, the tubule cells do not appear necrotic under the microscope but more often show only "cloudy swelling." In the situation of acute shutdown, peritoneal dialysis or hemodialysis may be required until tubular function is restored. Measures to prevent anuria from occurring during and following shock will be considered later. For the most part, renal failure as a cause of death from shock has greatly decreased with more prompt and physiologic resuscitation of the patient and the widespread use of peritoneal or hemodialysis.

The recent salutary advances in treating the renal complications of shock gave rise to overoptimism that the mortality of shock should greatly decrease. Mortality from this cause has decreased in some measure, but the lung has now replaced the kidney as a principal cause of death of shocked patients who are successfully resuscitated initially.

Lung

Until recently, little attention was given to the effects of shock on the lung, probably due to the concentration of efforts on resuscitating the patient from shock. More successful resuscitation and treatment of renal failure were largely overshadowed by the frequency of death from pulmonary insufficiency.

Prior to the acknowledgment of pulmonary insufficiency as a cause of death in clinical shock, only a few investigators had devoted their efforts to studying pulmonary physiology in this state. This was likely due to the fact that most experimental studies of shock are acute in nature, and the animal dies in less than 24 hours before pulmonary problems manifest themselves. The same was once true in the hospital; many patients could not be resuscitated from shock and did not live long enough to show pulmonary insufficiency.

Failure to recognize the problem was not the only reason for the paucity of knowledge. The study of pulmonary physiology has been neglected. Fortunately this is no longer the case; much new information is available to allow early treatment and even prevention of pulmonary insufficiency following shock.

We discussed earlier the effects of anoxia on membrane integrity. Passage of sodium and water into the cell and potassium out is just the beginning of the process of cell deterioration. Fluid passes from the circulation into the interstitial spaces of the lung, increasing the diffusion distance for oxygen. Albumin also is lost into these areas, accentuating the fluid loss and the interstitial edema. Within the stagnant pulmonary microcirculation, as elsewhere in the viscera, there is pooling of blood and aggregation of the formed elements of the blood. Using the electron microscope, leukocytes can be seen to plug capillaries as their outer cell membranes fuse with the endothelium of the capillary. Later the endothelial cells of the pulmonary microcirculation can be seen to "come apart" leaving larger gaps for red cells to escape into the interstitium and ultimately into the alveolus. The result of this process is that diffusion of oxygen from the alveolus to the pulmonary capillary is greatly decreased and in some areas of the lung may not occur at all even though blood is still passing by the alveolus. Circulation without oxygenation gives rise to the phenomenon of physiologic shunting.

With sepsis, these changes in the lung are even more pronounced than in traumatic or cardiogenic shock, and physiologic shunting, or admixture, may reach 40 to 50 percent of the cardiac output with a corresponding low oxygen uptake and consumption. The source of the sepsis does not have to be the lung but may be anywhere in the body. Blood-borne factors seem to be responsible for a picture of pulmonary insufficiency identical to that seen when the primary infection is in the lung. Moreover, most septic patients with nonpulmonary sources of infection soon develop a secondary septic process in the lungs.

We now see with increasing clarity that these changes within the pulmonary microcirculation set the stage for ensuing pulmonary insufficiency if resuscitation is successful. Moreover, overzealous use of fluids and inotropic agents during the resuscitation often compound the pulmonary damage. A similar problem arose a decade ago when renal failure was the most common cause of death following resuscitation. Our "tunnel vision" then focused only on blood pressure, with the result that the promiscuous use of vasopressors intensified the renal damage of shock, resulting in needless renal failure and death. It is clear that the first resuscitative efforts will determine the ultimate fate of the patients regardless of the initial or short-term success of these efforts.

Pancreas

Lysosomal membrane dissolution in the pancreas may release a specific MDF. Attention has been focused on the pancreatic reaction in shock because of reports that administration of glucose or glucose and insulin in late shock may improve the survival rate of experimental animals.

The typical finding in early experimental traumatic shock is an abrupt rise of insulin in the pancreatic venous blood at a time when blood glucose level is only gradually increasing. Later on, the blood glucose level continues to rise while the pancreatic release of insulin declines. These findings contrast with the pattern of blood glucose and insulin seen in the normal state, in which a rise in blood glucose precedes the insulin rise and the insulin then lowers the blood glucose.

The experimental pattern is postulated to arise from the sudden decrease in blood flow to the pancreas which may trigger the release of insulin stored within the beta cells. As the severity of shock deepens, the output of pancreatic insulin declines due to the inhibiting effects of the high levels of endogenous catecholamines and cortisol. The administration of exogenous insulin and glucose in late shock would then be expected to provide a needed source of energy. But the prompt disappearance of administered glucose from blood does not necessarily prove that oxidation to provide energy is the sole reason for the observed benefits.

In careful metabolic studies on dogs in hemorrhagic shock using ^{14}C-glucose, Gump et al. found that only 11 percent of the labeled glucose was oxidized, 5 percent was converted to lipid, and the remainder presumably was stored as glycogen in liver and muscle or converted to amino acids through gluconeogenesis, all being nonoxidative pathways of usage. These studies do not support a hypothesis that increased tolerance to shock following glucose administration is due principally to energy production.

Unexplained also is the effect of administered glucose and insulin of lowering the hyperkalemia which typically occurs in late shock whatever its origin. Such an effect is known to improve myocardial function by driving potassium into the cell.

Despite the conflicting data on the role of the pancreas in the pathophysiology of shock, the clinician should follow blood sugar levels in shock and probably give glucose and insulin intravenously to patients who do not respond promptly to standard resuscitative measures.

TOLERANCE TO SHOCK

Throughout the discussion of the pathophysiology of shock of any origin, there is a common theme of viscerocutaneous vasoconstriction with reduced tissue flow and anoxia in response to the sympathoadrenal response to stress. The purpose of this primitive reflex is to preserve flow to brain, heart, and voluntary muscles. However, this primitive survival response is also the beginning of the eventual destruction of the viscerocutaneous microcirculation if the response is perpetuated by delayed or inappropriate measures.

Some years ago we sought for means to blunt the sympathoadrenal response to shock. The induction of epinephrine tolerance in dogs proved to be one way to accomplish this. Epinephrine tolerance is induced by the thrice-weekly intravenous injection of increasing doses of epinephrine over a period of 6 weeks or more starting with a dose of <0.1 mg/kg of body weight and gradually increasing the dosage up to 2 mg/kg. Most dogs will die acutely if given 1 to 2 mg/kg of epinephrine intravenously initially, but if this dose is reached over a period of weeks, it is not lethal.

Epinephrine-tolerant dogs are then subjected to usually lethal hemorrhagic, endotoxic, or microsphere-induced cardiogenic shock. In contrast to controls, the experimental dogs have surprisingly high survival rates (Table 4-2). Subsequently we have assessed blood flow and arteriolar and venular resistance in the kidney, intestine, and lung of epinephrine-tolerant dogs subjected to each of these insults; we found that bood flow was significantly higher and arteriolar and venous resistance significantly lower than in normal dogs subjected to the same insults. These differences in hemodynamics apparently accounted for the increased survival of epinephrine-tolerant dogs. Moreover, using the Pappenheimer isogravimetric perfusion technique (Fig. 4-16) we found that the microcirculation of the forelimb, intestine, and lung of these dogs did not lose its integrity and leak fluid into the extravascular spaces of these organs.

Endotoxin can also be used to induce tolerance to vasoconstriction and confers increased survival on dogs subjected to usually lethal traumatic (drum shock), hemorrhagic, or cardiogenic shock. The interactions between different types of stresses causing shock are shown in more detail in Table 4-3.

These studies in cross tolerance to shock serve to emphasize similarity of responses of experimental animals subjected to a variety of insults. They also indicate the potential value of modifying the sympathoadrenal response of man in shock to increase survival, whatever the cause of the shock. We have called this approach the *unitarian concept.*

TREATMENT

In treating shock of any cause, there are two major problems to correct:

Table 4-2. EFFECT OF EPINEPHRINE TOLERANCE UPON SURVIVAL OF EXPERIMENTAL DOGS IN SHOCK

	Number of survivors*	
Type of shock	*Controls*	*Epinephrine tolerant*
Hemorrhagic	2/41 (5%)	8/10 (80%)
Endotoxin	6/37 (16%)	12/12 (100%)
Cardiogenic.	12/46 (26%)	18/18 (100%)

*Survived 72 hours or longer.

1. Deficiency in effective circulating blood volume
2. Disturbance in the peripheral circulation which leads to stagnant anoxia

Correcting these problems will restore normal blood pressure in a physiologic fashion. As blood pressure is the product of flow times resistance ($P = F \times R$), pressure also can be returned to normal by increasing resistance (R), but this approach will eventually decrease flow (F) and lead to further stagnant anoxia. With a background of the mechanisms of shock, we now can discuss in detail means to increase nutritional blood flow and decrease resistance in shock.

Fluid Therapy

The keystone of treatment of all shock is restoration of the effective circulatory blood volume. This usually means that intravenous volume should be administered. The need for volume is obvious in hemorrhagic shock, while in soft tissue and bony trauma the accurate assessment of volume loss is more difficult but no less necessary.

In septic shock there is also an urgent need for added volume, but here the assessment of the amount of loss is even more difficult. The volume deficit in septic shock is due to stagnation within the viscerocutaneous microcirculation and loss of volume into the extravascular spaces. With the use of ^{51}Cr or ^{131}I for measuring blood volume the stagnant volume along with more active circulating volume are measured together. Hence, blood volume is often found to be in the normal range in patients suffering septic shock.

In cardiogenic shock fluid administration must be even more cautious but may be equally lifesaving. Up to 20 percent of patients with myocardial infarction may be hypovolemic, and this is also frequently a problem after cardiopulmonary bypass.

While all agree on the need for added intravenous volume in most patients in shock, this agreement does not extend to the type of fluid to be used. As a rule blood is given when the hematocrit is below 35 percent or the hemoglobin level below 11 Gm; there is no benefit and some danger in going above these levels. Higher hematocrits are associated with increased viscosities, and viscosity is already high because of low velocity of flow. Some investigators believe that only 50 percent of estimated

Forelimb Isogravimetric Preparation

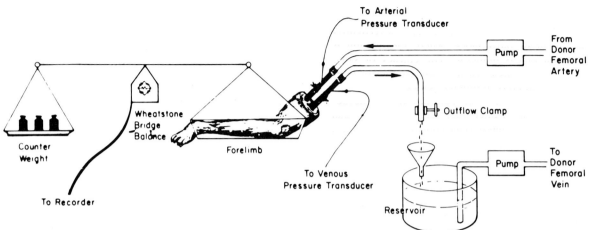

Fig. 4-16. The Pappenheimer isogravimetric perfusion technique of autologous organ is a precise method for measuring the integrity of the microcirculation. Epinephrine-tolerant dogs do not show a loss in the integrity of the microcirculation of the forelimb, intestine, or lung following usually lethal hemorrhagic, endotoxic, or cardiogenic shock.

blood losses should be replaced with blood and the other 50 percent with colloid and crystalloid. The lower viscosity of such a combination more than makes up for the lower oxygen-carrying capacity.

When the hematocrit is above 35 percent, the choice of fluid is colloid and crystalloid. The most frequently used colloid in the past was pooled plasma, but the relatively high incidence of serum hepatitis in recipients has resulted in the abandonment of this plasma preparation. Rather, single donor plasma or, more frequently, processed plasma protein fractions, which are mostly albumin with about 10 percent globulin, have virtually eliminated serum hepatitis in recipients. With the recognition that colloid osmotic pressure falls early in shock and contributes to the interstitial edema seen in the lung, concentrated, salt-poor albumin in 25 to 50 Gm doses is also often used. This preparation is also free from the risk of hepatitis.

Colloids made up of complex polysaccharides such as polyvinylpyrolidine, dextrans, and starch are also available. For practical purposes, only the dextrans are used to any extent. Here the physician may choose "clinical" dextran, with an average molecular weight of 70,000, or low-molecular-weight dextran, with an average molecular weight of 40,000. In the past the two dextrans have been

assigned quite different properties. Clinical dextran, which was introduced first, was thought to frequently cause aberrations in blood clotting leading to excessive bleeding, and also to cause allergic reactions. In contrast, low-molecular-weight dextran was said to be free of these problems and in addition more effective in lowering the viscosity of red and white cells, thus promoting increased flow in the microcirculation. In more recent studies, most investigators have minimized the differences between the two dextrans when the volume given is less than 1 liter/24 hours in the 70-kg adult. With this dosage there is a decrease of viscosity which will decrease the incidence of thromboembolism similar to the effect following Coumadin. Most of the dextran preparations are hypertonic, usually coming as 10% solutions in either 5% dextrose or 0.9% saline solution. By virtue of this hypertonicity, extravascular fluid is drawn into the vascular space in a volume equal to the administered dextran, and this also reduces viscosity.

Table 4-3. INTERRELATIONSHIP AND TOLERANCE BETWEEN VARIOUS
TYPES OF EXPERIMENTAL SHOCK

Tolerance and cross tolerance in shock	Experimental shock models						
Means of protection	Trauma (drum)	Bowel ischemia	Epinephrine	Endotoxin	Hemorrhage	Coronary embolism	Cardiac tamponade
Drum training	+ +	+	. . .	+	+		
Epinephrine tolerance.	+	. . .	+ +	+ +	+	+	
Endotoxin tolerance	+	+	+	+ +	+	+ +	
Adrenergic blockade	+	+	+ +	+ +	+ +	+ +	+ +
Synthetic corticoids	+	. . .	+	+ +	+	+	+ +

CRYSTALLOIDS

In the past 20 years there have been successive waves of enthusiasm for various crystalloid solutions. The need for large quantities of saline solution was first recognized in the treatment of burn shock, where the amount of interstitial fluid loss is immense. The efficacy of saline solution in burn treatment led to similar studies of other types of shock, notably traumatic shock. Here it was thought that large volumes of crystalloid were also needed due to the initial loss of interstitial fluid into the vascular space and later loss of fluid into the collagen matrix. Many of these investigations were stimulated by experience in the Korean conflict; many of these casualties exhibited the need for far more blood and crystalloid than could be accounted for by conventional calculations. Hence, when the Vietnam conflict began in the mid-1960s, there was great enthusiasm for treating casualties with vast amounts of crystalloid in addition to blood and plasma. The result of such treatment was a great increase in the success of initial resuscitation but an increase in pulmonary insufficiency as well. This condition, variously labeled in the past,* is now called "Vietnam lung." The great increase in postresuscitation pulmonary insufficiency probably represented the results of overzealous fluid replacement and an increase in salvage of the most severely wounded who now lived long enough for pulmonary complications to develop. The physiologic basis for these pulmonary problems is the loss of membrane integrity of the pulmonary microcirculation, as described above. The amount of crystalloid used was reduced in the later stages of the Vietnam conflict, and the number of instances of acute pulmonary insufficiency was similarly reduced.

Presently, the crystalloid used by most physicians is a balanced salt solution, usually Ringer's, to which sodium lactate is added as a buffer. The 5 mEq of potassium contained in Ringer's solution is certainly worthwhile, but more potassium than this is often needed. Moreover, laboratory and clinical studies fail to show that any of the balanced salt solutions are more effective than 0.9% saline solution in the initial resuscitation.

The addition of sodium lactate to crystalloid solution is based on the need for a buffer to counteract the metabolic acidosis of shock. However, the cardinal metabolic sign of shock is lactic acidosis resulting from the lack of oxygen to metabolize this product of anaerobic metabolism. Lactate given in crystalloid solutions, like the lactate accumulating from anoxia, needs oxygen in order to become a buffer. Hence, there appears to be little justification for the widespread popularity of lactated solutions for treating shock. Indeed, recent experiments by Schumer on subhuman primates in shock suggest that lactated solutions may damage the anoxic liver. If a buffer is given in shock, then it is wise to give bicarbonate, which is immediately available.

*World War I lung, blast injury lung, World War II lung, wet lung, congestive atelectasis, traumatic lung, postperfusion lung, respiratory lung, shock lung, septic lung.

GUIDES TO THE ADMINISTRATION OF FLUIDS

Whatever the various combinations of fluids administered in shock, they must be given in some proportion to the ability of the heart to handle the restored intravascular volume. The CVP (central venous pressure), measured via a catheter inserted into the superior or inferior vena cava or into the right atrium from a variety of access points, now is the standard guide for measuring this ability. The problem emerging from widespread use of the CVP is the tendency of some physicians to accord it all the virtues of the "philosophers' stone," said by the alchemists of old to change lead into gold.

Usually the right atrial or CVP changes in a more or less direct relation to the left atrial pressure, but the relationship is complex and variable. It is most accurate when there is no significant valvular disease or congestive failure, but it is in these very conditions where an accurate CVP is most needed. The CVP usually errs in not rising early enough in left ventricular failure. The pulmonary artery pressure or the pulmonary wedge pressure have been proposed as better guides than CVP, which they are, but it is not likely that the more complicated pulmonary artery cannulation will be widely used for some time, although the introduction of the Swan-Ganz catheter has greatly facilitated this cannulation (Fig. 4-17). CVP is still the most rapidly available guide to fluid therapy to be used in conjunction with other observations.

The access site to the central venous pool does not matter as long as the catheter tip is in the superior or inferior vena cava or in the right atrium; but it is best to avoid access sites in the legs or groin because of the higher incidence of thrombosis and thrombophlebitis in the inferior cava system. In practice, the most commonly used sites are the basilic vein, the infraclavicular subclavian vein, and the external or internal jugular vein. Once in place, the position of the catheter tip should be checked by x-ray; this will also rule out a pneumothorax if the subclavian approach has been used.

Fluids are best given in aliquots of 250 to 500 ml, and the CVP is checked frequently. Most patients tolerate a CVP of 10 cm of saline solution measured in the supine position at the midchest level and off the respirator, with little chance that pulmonary congestion will occur at this level. The chronic congestive failure of patients with preexisting heart disease may require a CVP pushed to 15 cm or more for optimal cardiac function, but some patients may also manifest pulmonary edema at this higher level. The simultaneous administration of diuretics can improve this situation, and a detailed treatment protocol is discussed below.

Measures to Restore the Integrity of the Damaged Microcirculation and Reestablish Normal Cell Metabolism

The disturbances in the microcirculation and in cell metabolism characterizing stagnant anoxia often cannot be corrected by fluid administration alone, as the adminis-

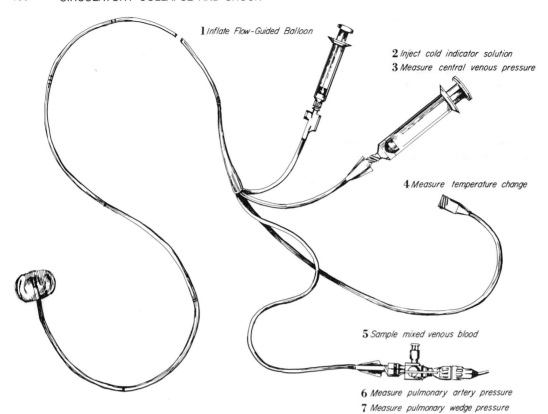

1 *Inflate Flow-Guided Balloon*

2 *Inject cold indicator solution*
3 *Measure central venous pressure*

4 *Measure temperature change*

5 *Sample mixed venous blood*

6 *Measure pulmonary artery pressure*
7 *Measure pulmonary wedge pressure*

Fig. 4-17. The Swan-Ganz catheter for cannulation of the pulmonary artery via a peripheral vein.

tered fluid may also pool within the stagnant microcirculation, increasing interstitial edema and contributing to further deterioration of the patient. This problem has long been recognized but corrective measures have been controversial. Proposed measures have been pharmacologic in nature and can be broadly divided into drugs which are vasopressor or vasodilatory in nature.

VASOPRESSOR THERAPY

Vasopressors are those agents which stimulate the alpha receptors in arterioles and venules to constrict, resulting in increased total peripheral resistance. The best example is levarterenol, synthetized by von Euler and introduced by Taintor for clinical use.

Levarterenol is the synthetic equivalent of the natural norepinephrine secreted by the postganglionic sympathetic nerve endings. Levarterenol also has beta-stimulating properties, so that myocardial contractility is increased and a chronotropic effect with increased heart rate could be expected. However, the increased total peripheral resistance secondary to the alpha effect and the rise in systolic blood pressure cause the baroreceptors to decrease the heart rate, so that the resulting rate usually is not changed or is slowed.

When introduced, levarterenol was believed to answer the need for a drug for use with fluids in treating shock. It does, indeed, raise arterial blood pressure but at the expense of further increases in resistance in the visceral microcirculation and decreased visceral blood flow. Hence its salutary results are usually short-lived. The high inci-

dence of postshock renal failure seen a decade ago was usually due to the overzealous use of levarterenol. More recently, most clinicians have found that levarterenol must be used in very low concentrations if at all so that the alpha effect is slight and the beta effect on the heart predominates, eliminating for the most part the increased visceral ischemia so characteristic of its use. Still, even the beta effect may not be as useful as once thought, because of the increased oxygen demand it imposes on the heart; this effect will be discussed below.

The adverse effect of levarterenol on the visceral circulation stimulated the search for less potent vasopressors. Metaraminol is one such drug which has been widely used. Like levarterenol it has both alpha- and beta-stimulating effects with the former predominating, but it appears to be less toxic. Interestingly, it acts by causing the release of norepinephrine from postganglionic nerve endings. It appears less likely to cause renal tubular damage, but most of the problems encountered with levarterenol develop with prolonged use. Some clinicians prefer epinephrine as a vasopressor because its alpha effect is less prominent than that of levarterenol. Yet, its beta effect often leads to an undesirable tachycardia unless it is used in very dilute solutions.

Drugs with a pure alpha effect such as mephentermine have also been tried, but they are even more toxic than the mixed alpha-beta drugs discussed above when used for any length of time. Angiotensin also enjoyed brief popularity for use in shock but was probably the most damaging drug of all on the visceral microcirculation. This drug is neither an alpha- nor a beta-receptor stimulant but acts directly on the arteriole to cause intense vasoconstriction.

Many other drugs similar to those discussed here have the adverse effects already mentioned without any redeeming features.

VASODILATORS

In the early 1950s Laborit introduced a "lytic" drug cocktail in combination with mild hypothermia, 33 to 35°C, for the treatment of the French casualties in Vietnam. The cocktail contained chlorpromazine, a moderately active alpha-blocking agent and a central nervous system depressant; phenothiazine, an antihistaminic and antiserotonin compound; and meperedine (Demerol) an analgesic. Laborit claimed a great increase in survival after treatment with this combination, and his publications stimulated worldwide experimental and clinical research. The various aspects of Laborit's regimen have been selected in order to assess their relative contributions to the total effect.

Apparently, reducing the metabolic rate by reducing the temperature below 37°C is offset by increased cardiac irritability and increased pooling of blood in the peripheral circulation. Thus, hypothermia does not contribute any significant increase in survival from traumatic shock in controlled experimental conditions, although there is some advantage in reducing an elevated temperature to normal.

Meperidine has some small value in shock by reducing pain and thereby reducing sympathetic nervous stimulation. Phenothiazine also provides some benefit under experimental shock conditions, probably related to its antagonism toward histamine and serotonin, which play a still uncertain roll in the genesis of the microcirculatory changes characteristic of stagnant anoxia.

Chlorpromazine was the most important agent in the "cocktail." The salutary effects of this drug seem to reside principally in its alpha-blocking potential. Unfortunately, the doses required often resulted in profound central nervous system depression. Nonetheless, Laborit's prescient observations stimulated others to search for more effective means to produce alpha blockade in shock.

Nickerson in 1955 published initial observations on the clinical use of phenoxybenzamine, a potent alpha-adrenergic blocking agent, in treating shock refractory to conventional treatment with fluids and vasopressors. Since then, a wealth of material has appeared on the experimental effects of phenoxybenzamine in a variety of types of traumatic, endotoxic, septic, and cardiogenic shock. Most investigators have shown improved microcirculation and metabolism when phenoxybenzamine is used just before shock or shortly after shock is induced. These improvements are usually associated with increased survival of a variety of experimental animals. Studies also have indicated that phenoxybenzamine is more than just an alpha-blocking agent and has membrane-sparing effects as well.

In the clinical area, the data supporting phenoxybenzamine are more sparse and more difficult to interpret because of the inability to control variables in an experimental fashion. The problem is compounded by the failure of this drug to win approval from the Federal Drug Administration for clinical trials in the United States.

Phenoxybenzamine is not the only alpha-blocking drug available, but it is the most potent and long-acting. Phentolamine (Regetine) is also an alpha blocker, but its effect is evanescent and requires continuous infusion closely supervised by a physician.

Recently, some clinicians have expressed renewed interest in the use of a reduced dose of chlorpromazine in treating human shock. Advocates say that a total dose of chlorpromazine of 5 to 10 mg given intravenously has an alpha-blocking effect which reduces the stagnant anoxia of shock, but hemodynamic and/or metabolic data supporting these impressions have not appeared.

Interest in alpha-blocking agents has led to studies with ganglionic blocking agents, such as hexamethonium, which block chemical transmission of nerve impulses at the ganglion through interference with the formation of the transmitter, actylcholine. The result is both parasympathetic and sympathetic blockade. While such agents are useful in controlling hypertension, their effects in shock states are variable and difficult to control and assess. They do not seem to have any advantage over alpha-adrenergic blocking agents and are even more difficult to use in the clinical setting.

ISOPROTERENOL

Isoproterenol was introduced for clinical use nearly a decade after levarterenol, a period of time sufficient for clinicians to realize that merely raising blood pressure at the expense of decreased flow did not correct the physiologic disturbances of shock. Isoproterenol appeared to be the ideal drug for treating the hypotension and low flow usually accompanying shock. Being a pure beta stimulator, it had none of the adverse effects on the visceral circulation which resulted from the alpha-stimulating action of levarterenol or similar agents. Moreover, there was usually an overall decrease in total peripheral resistance after its use in experimental or clinical shock. This effect is principally due to its ability to cause vasodilatation in the microcirculation of the voluntary muscle masses, whose vasculature is supplied predominantly with beta receptors. Finally its pure beta effect produces marked inotropic effects on the heart, with an increase in cardiac output and rate. The resulting tachycardia is often the factor limiting the use of isoproterenol because of possible arrthymias.

Isoproterenol is now most widely used in treating cardiogenic shock, but, while useful, is not the hoped for remedy. It is most helpful when used briefly for its inotropic effect, but this has made no impact on the continuing high mortality of cardiogenic shock, for several reasons: First, tachycardia often precludes continued use of the drug; second, its purely beta-stimulating effect does little to directly increase flow through the stagnant microcirculation of the viscera, although there may be some indirect benefit through the increase in cardiac output. Finally, there is increasing evidence that isoproterenol may actually extend the area of ischemia in myocardial infarction when used in the usual dose of 2 to 4 μg/minute. The basis for this is the creation of an increased oxygen demand in a myocardium with coronary circulation unable to respond with increased flow.

Some of the problems may be associated with the dosage usually used. When isoproterenol is given intravenously in doses of less than 1 μg/minute, the resulting increase in cardiac output is even higher than that obtained with the conventional doses of 2 to 4 μg/minute. Perhaps smaller doses will obviate at least some of the adverse effects.

Isoproterenol is probably most useful in treating patients with the low-cardiac-output syndrome associated with bradycardia in the early period following cardiopulmonary bypass and surgical correction of congenital or acquired defects. In this situation treatment with low concentrations of isoproterenol for brief periods is often lifesaving.

Although isoproterenol has not been used widely for traumatic shock, there are the same problems as with cardiogenic shock. The patient in traumatic shock often has a tachycardia, and isoproterenol merely accentuates this. In contrast, isoproterenol was widely used in septic shock in the past decade but again with no significant effect on the mortality rate. This failure is not surprising, because the basic hemodynamic pattern in this condition is high cardiac output and low total peripheral resistance due to the "shunting phenomenon" seen with gram-negative bacteria and tissue damage. Cardiac failure is usually not a factor in sepsis until near the time of death, but the cardiogram often shows ST-T–wave signs of myocardial ischemia. This is due more often to the low oxygen tension of the arterial blood in sepsis rather than to any intrinsic coronary or myocardial disease. In this situation isoproterenol may increase ischemia by creating a greater myocardial oxygen demand through its inotropism when the oxygen supply cannot be increased due to the "shunting" characteristic of sepsis. Tachycardia is also common in sepsis, further increasing the problems of using isoproterenol.

In summary, isoproterenol finds its best use in doses of less than 1 μg/minute in patients with bradycardia whose shock is not due to intrinsic coronary artery disease or to sepsis.

GLUCAGON

Glucagon is a poypeptide hormone produced exclusively by the alpha[2] cells of the islets of Langerhans of the pancreas. It appears that the biologic role of glucagon is to ensure, along with insulin, a steady supply of glucose, free fatty acids, and ketones. Normally the concentrations of glucagon and insulin are reciprocals of each other, and both are under the influence of the sympathetic nervous system. In shock, insulin secretion is usually suppressed, while glucagon concentrations increase and may be responsible for the "hyperglycemia" of shock.

Recently, some investigators have speculated that glucagon is also an inotropic agent. It is now well documented experimentally and clinically that glucagon will give a positive inotropic effect without the ventricular irritation often seen with beta stimulators. Its exact mode of action

on the myocardium is still largely unknown; further, we do not know if glucagon plays any role in regulating myocardial function in the normal state.

We have found glucagon to work best in relatively mild hypotensive states associated with transient myocardial insufficiency; in cardiogenic shock, it often is without effect. Nonetheless it should probably be used more often as the initial inotropic agent because of its safety. The usual adult dose is 3 to 5 mg by intravenous push followed by a micro drip of 3 to 5 mg in 100 ml of 5% dextrose in water.

BETA-BLOCKING AGENTS

Beta-blocking agents are most widely used to decrease myocardial contractility and oxygen demand in angina pectoris and thereby relieve pain. This depression of beta receptors is also useful in controlling tachycardia and arrthymias. Considering these effects, beta-blocking agents would not seem indicated in shock where all efforts are being made to improve myocardial function. Propranolol, the most frequently used drug of this type, is occasionally used in 1-mg doses intravenously to control arrthymias in shock, but more recently Berk and Holmagyi have advocated use of propranolol as part of the treatment protocol for traumatic or septic shock.

Holmagyi found that propranolol used in combination with phenoxybenzamine resulted in higher survival rates after experimental hemorrhagic shock than did the use of phenoxybenzamine alone. He attributed this to the ability of the propranolol to prevent the hyperthermia usually seen in the dog after retransfusion of the shed blood. Berk has presented clinical data to indicate that the hyperdynamic state characteristic of septic shock is converted to a normodynamic state when propranolol is given intravenously in doses of 0.5 to 1 mg/hour. He postulates the mode of action is through closing shunts in the visceral microcirculation. With this dose he found little evidence of myocardial depression, but he also advocated digitalization of patients so treated. Quantitative data are needed to support these observations. Furthermore, Berk's evaluation of the effects of propronolol is complicated by his use of large doses of glucocorticosteroids (see below).

DIGITALIS

Too often the physician is admonished to use digitalis only when obvious symptoms of failure appear, i.e., high venous pressure, congested lungs on x-ray, and bloody fluid in the tracheobronchial tree. By this time it is too late for the most effective use of digitalis. Most patients in shock show evidence of impaired myocardial function and may be greatly benefited by digitalis if no serious ventricular arrthymias are present and the serum potassium is above 4 mEq. Digitalis is the only drug with a direct inotropic effect on the myocardium which does not cause an increase in oxygen demand. This unique feature deserves wider appreciation.

Hinshaw and coworkers have recently contributed another reason for the early use of digitalis in septic shock. They have found in canine experiments that digitalis used early after the injection of endotoxin protected the myocardial ultrastructure from damage by the endotoxin and prevented early myocardial failure.

GLUCOCORTICOSTEROIDS

Almost 20 years ago we first noted that large intravenous doses of hydrocortisone, 50 mg/kg, would decrease the mortality of dogs receiving lethal intravenous dose of epinephrine. We did not relate these findings to our shock studies, which had begun a few years earlier, until we observed the common pattern of changes in the visceral microcirculation which followed experimental hemorrhagic, endotoxic, and cardiogenic shock. Subsequently, we used large doses of hydrocortisone to treat hemorrhagic, endotoxic, and cardiac shock in the dog. The results of this series of experiments were similar to those dealing with epinephrine shock—when the hydrocortisone was given early after the induction of shock, whatever its cause, mortality was significantly reduced. The common finding was a decrease in total peripheral resistance which resulted in increases in hepatic, gastrointestinal, renal, and pulmonary blood flows. The cardiac output also increased, but at that time we could not tell whether this was due to increased venous return, an improvement in *preload,* or venous, capacitance; to a decreased arterial resistance, the *afterload;* to a direct inotropic effect on the myocardium; or to a combination of these factors.

In our intensive care area, the effects of corticosteroids on central venous and intraarterial pressures, cardiac index, and the derived total peripheral resistance were next assessed along with measurements of lactic acid and oxygen consumption. Initially we used a bolus of hydrocortisone, 50 mg/kg, given intravenously over a 5-minute period. Soon we changed to an intravenous bolus of methylprednisolone sodium succinate, 30 mg/kg, which we had found to be more effective in the laboratory than the hydrocortisone. Moreover, the synthetic glucocorticoidlike compounds did not cause sodium retention and were less expensive.

Over the past decade more than 200 patients suffering shock from various causes have received one or more 30 mg/kg doses of methylprednisolone. It has not been possible to control all the variables clinically in the same manner as in the laboratory, but the data show that in patients suffering traumatic and cardiogenic shock total peripheral resistance is significantly lowered and cardiac index significantly raised after a single bolus of methylprednisolone (Fig. 4-18). In patients suffering shock due to gram-negative septicemia, there is an increase in oxygen consumption and a decrease in arteriovenous admixture in the lung following methylprednisolone (Fig. 4-19).

Compared with shocked patients similarly treated except for the use of one or more doses of methylprednisolone, those patients receiving the steroid have had a higher 30-day survival rate. Similar observations on the favorable effects of massive doses of hydrocortisone, methylprednisolone, or dexamethasone have now been reported by Shoemaker and by James for traumatic shock, by R. Wilson, Weil, Schumer, and James for gram-negative sep-

tic shock, and by Barzilai, James, and Wangensteen for cardiogenic shock.

Many clinicians fear that massive doses of glucocorticosteroids or their synthetic equivalents would result in gastrointestinal stress ulcerations, decreased wound healing, and increased susceptibility to infections. When massive doses of the corticosteroids are administered for less than 48 hours, these complications have not been noted any more frequently than in patients in shock not receiving corticosteroids. What is needed is a randomized, double-blind study using methylprednisolone in shock, and several such trials now are beginning.

The observed salutary effects of massive doses of synthetic glucocorticosteroids have redoubled the efforts of investigators to establish the physiologic basis of action. Most of the studies have utilized either methylprednisolone sodium succinate, 30 mg/kg, or dexamethasone sodium phosphate in an equivalent dose of 6 mg/kg, to treat experimental shock induced by bleeding, endotoxins, or myocardial damage. The results can be summarized as follows:

Decreases:

> in nerve impulse transmission in postganglionic sympathetic nerves
> in arteriolar and venular resistance of lung, intestine, kidney, forelimb
> in platelet adhesiveness
> in leukocyte adhesiveness
> in kinin production
> in extravascular lung water
> in myocardial infarct size
> in complement fixation by endotoxin-antibody complex

Increases:

> in visceral organ blood flow
> in cardiac index
> in coronary blood flow
> in oxygen consumption
> in lactic acid metabolism

Stabilization of lysosomal membranes:

> in lung
> in pancreas
> in liver and kidney

Restoration of vascular membrane integrity of lung, intestine, forelimb

Finally, Hinshaw has suggested from his studies controlling venous return (preload) and peripheral resistance (afterload) that methylprednisolone has a direct inotropic effect on the heart, although this is less prominent than the peripheral actions.

Although these investigations have largely dispelled the mystery shrouding the action of massive doses of glucosorticosteroids in shock, the proper place and timing for use in clinical shock requires more carefully documented studies. Glucocorticosteroids are indicated when standard regimens of treatment have failed. Glucocorticosteroids are not given to make up a deficiency in natural cortisol production by the adrenal cortex. Rarely does a patient in shock suffer from adrenal insufficiency; as in the sym-

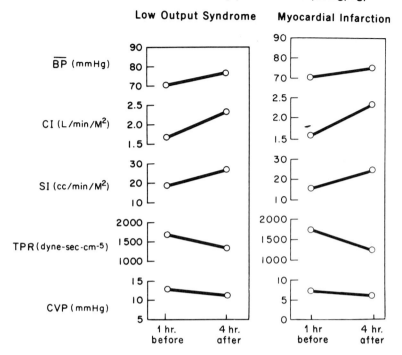

A

CARDIOGENIC SHOCK
Hemodynamic Changes
after Methylprednisolone (30mg/kg)

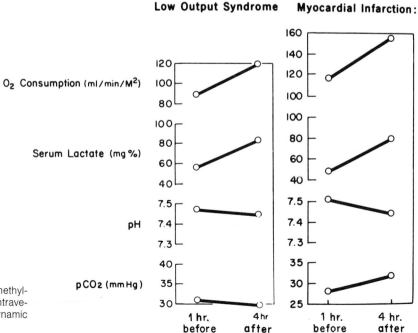

B

CARDIOGENIC SHOCK
Metabolic Changes
after Methylprednisolone (30 mg/kg)

Fig. 4-18. The effect of a single bolus of methyl-prednisolone, 30 mg/kg administered intravenously, in cardiogenic shock. A. Hemodynamic changes. B. Metabolic changes.

pathoadrenal response to stress, the adrenal cortex responds with increased production of cortisol so that blood cortisol levels are usually above normal. Hence the use of massive doses of glucocorticosteroids for brief periods is not related to their normal effects when present in the usual levels seen in the body but to their effect when given in massive doses. Failure to differentiate between physiologic and massive doses has led to needless confusion and controversy.

Protocol

We have discussed numerous disturbances in the normal hemodynamic and metabolic patterns which result from the insults of trauma, bacterial infection, and myocardial damage. Usually these result in all or most of the following problems: hypovolemia, aggregation of the formed elements of the blood, decrease in plasma osmotic pressure, decreased visceral organ blood flow with oliguria the most easily assessed result, hypoxemia, and lactic acidosis. Almost always these disturbances are associated with a decrease in systolic or mean arterial pressure. But we have seen that the hypotension results from the insult but does not cause shock. It is possible to raise blood pressure by increasing peripheral resistance, but the effects of this approach are usually of short duration, as is the patient's life, if the physician depends merely on blood pressure elevation. Arterial pressure is a product of flow times resistance (Fig. 4-20), and in most instances the hypotension is secondary to decreased flow and increased resistance. As the human organism has a great capacity for regaining hemostasis, most instances of traumatic shock can be treated by promptly administering fluids according to the volume and type lost and by stopping further losses. With large-volume losses, diffuse trauma, delayed treatment, and/or host resistance altered by other factors such as bacterial infection or myocardial failure, the treatment protocol becomes more complex (Fig. 4-21). A bolus of methylprednisolone, 30 mg/kg, or of dexamethasone, 6 mg/kg, will decrease venular outflow obstruction and restore toward normal cellular and intracellular membrane integrity. The decrease in osmotic pressure incident to loss of albumin through damaged endothelial membranes can be restored by giving 0.5 to 1 mg/kg of salt-poor albumin over the course of an hour or two.

Oliguria may continue despite blood volume restoration and progress to anuria with all its problems, notably further metabolic acidosis, hyperkalemia, and cardiac arrest. The prompt use of a diuretic such as furosemide will maintain urine flow despite tubular damage, even though

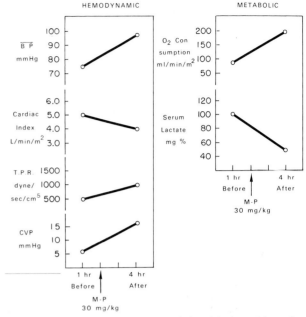

Fig. 4-19. The effect of a bolus of methylprednisolone, 30 mg/kg administered intravenously, in gram-negative septic shock.

the urine obtained is of the same osmotic pressure as the plasma. Intravenous doses of 10 or 20 mg of furosemide are usually given initially, but the dose can be increased to 100 mg or more. An effective, continuous stimulant to diuresis in the face of tubular damage is a solution of 500 ml of 5% dextrose to which is added mannitol to make a 20% solution and 500 mg of furosemide. This solution is then given intravenously at 15 to 25 ml/hour for the adult and in correspondingly smaller doses for the child. Furosemide is used in this situation because it has fewer toxic side effects than other potent diuretics such as ethacrynic acid, which can damage the eighth cranial nerve.

Of equal importance to restoration of the blood volume in traumatic shock is adequate oxygenation of the blood. Here it is better to provide respiratory support too early than too late. It is very difficult to make a "bedside" diagnosis of hypoxemia; even the experienced clinician is constantly surprised by the incongruities between the clinical assessment and the arterial oxygen and carbon dioxide measurements. The obtunded or comatose patient will usually tolerate an endotracheal or nasotracheal tube without problems; even the more alert patient tolerates a

Fig. 4-20. Goals in the treatment of shock related to pressure, flow, and resistance.

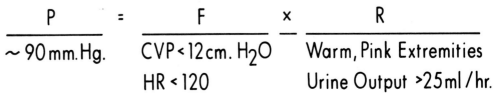

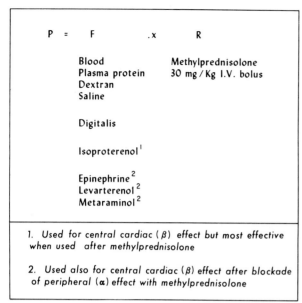

$$P = F \quad .x \quad R$$

Blood   Methylprednisolone
Plasma protein 30 mg / Kg I.V. bolus
Dextran
Saline

Digitalis

Isoproterenol[1]

Epinephrine[2]
Levarterenol[2]
Metaraminol[2]

1. Used for central cardiac (β) effect but most effective when used after methylprednisolone

2. Used also for central cardiac (β) effect after blockade of peripheral (α) effect with methylprednisolone

Fig. 4-21. Therapeutic regimen related to pressure, flow, and resistance.

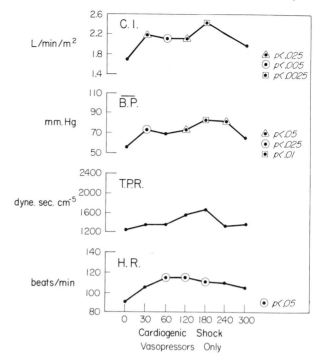

Fig. 4-22. The effect of levarterenol on cardiac index and total peripheral resistance in cardiogenic shock.

nasotracheal tube with little or no sedation. Tubes may be kept in place for several days under experienced care. Generally, tracheostomies now are done only when the patient still requires respiratory support after at least a 72-hour trial on an endotracheal tube and respirator.

The question of using positive end-expiratory pressure (PEEP) is still not completely settled. The rationale is to prevent complete collapse of the alveolus, but the amount of pressure needed is still controversial. Most advocate 3 to 5 cm H_2O positive pressure; others have advocated 25 cm or more when pulmonary congestion is severe, but these higher pressures can precipitate rupture of the lung and tension pneumothorax.

In traumatic shock uncomplicated by myocardial failure, there is little need for vasopressors in the treatment protocol. If the patient is brought to the emergency room without a discernible blood pressure, levarterenol or metaraminol may be used while fluids are being readied; but these agents are stopped promptly when fluids are started. Table 4-4 lists a suggested protocol for treating traumatic shock.

In cardiogenic shock the administration of fluids is often

Table 4-4. TREATMENT OF TRAUMATIC SHOCK DUE TO MULTISYSTEM INJURY

Condition to be corrected (restored)	Treatment
Hypovolemia	Blood, plasma fractions, dextran, crystalloids
Stagnant anoxia Membrane integrity	Synthetic glucocorticosteroids (methyl-prednisolone, dexamethasone)
Oncotic pressure	Albumin
Oliguria	Furosemide
Hypoxemia	Respirator (volume type; positive end-expiratory pressure)

as lifesaving as in traumatic shock, but it is far more difficult to gauge the amount needed. In obvious congestive heart failure, the central blood volume must be decreased, but in shock associated with myocardial infarction up to 20 percent of patients may be hypovolemic.

In the postcardiopulmonary bypass patient suffering shock, hypovolemia is also common even in the face of a normal or modestly elevated CVP (central venous pressure); a pulmonary wedge pressure or even a left atrial pressure determination will be more diagnostic.

When overt congestive heart failure with its characteristic pulmonary edema is present or suspected, digitalis may be administered as described earlier. If the potassium level is above 4 mEq/L, divided doses of 0.25 mg of digoxin can be given at 1- or two-hour intervals to a dose of 1 or 1.25 mg, and preceding each dose with an ECG strip.

In cardiogenic shock the inotropic agents such as levarterenol, metaraminol, or isoproterenol still have the widest usage but too often with disappointing results. All these agents increase myocardial oxygen demand as well as increasing myocardial contractility, and levarterenol and metaraminol further increase oxygen demand on the myocardium by increasing the peripheral resistance, or afterload (Fig. 4-22). A bolus of 30 mg/kg of methylprednisolone will increase cardiac index while at the same time decreasing total peripheral resistance (Fig. 4-18A); the mechanisms for this effect were discussed previously. Some patients still require an inotropic agent of the catecholamine type to maintain coronary perfusion; in this situation the combination of methylprednisolone with levarterenol, metaraminol, or isoproterenol is apparently effective (Fig.

4-23). The methylprednisolone prevents the peripheral constricting effects of the inotropic agent, thereby decreasing the afterload on the damaged myocardium. Also smaller concentrations of the inotropic agents can be used, thereby decreasing their adverse side effects. Other clinicians have used levarterenol in combination with the alpha-blocking agent, phentolamine, with similar results. Respiratory support, restoration of plasma osmotic pressure with albumin, and prevention of renal failure with furosemide are as important in cardiogenic shock as in traumatic shock. A suggested treatment protocol is outlined in Table 4-5.

The patient in septic shock presents all the problems of traumatic and cardiogenic shock as well as those due to the living bacterial factor. Activated endotoxin of gram-negative bacteria, or the exotoxin of gram-positive bacteria, has an effect on the visceral microcirculation related to the sympathomimetic effects of the activated endotoxin. Hence, intravenous volume, albumin, diuretics, synthetic glucocorticosteroids and respiratory support should be part of the treatment protocol. But, in addition to the favorable effects of synthetic glucocorticosteroids on arteriolar and venular resistance and membrane integrity, Schumer has found that complement fixation by endotoxin-antibody complex is decreased when massive doses of the synthetic corticosteroids are given early after endotoxin shock induced in experimental animals. Thus, clinical treatment of septic shock should include corticosteroids administered simultaneously with fluids (Fig. 4-24).

Eliminating the bacterial factor appears of equal importance to blocking the effects of endotoxin, as the interaction of bacteria and tissue leads to the arteriovenous admixture of shunting which characterizes septic shock in man. Eliminating the septic focus with drainage where possible and administering antibiotics will also eliminate the decreased oxygen consumption which characterizes septic shock in man. As most patients in septic shock have a gram-negative septicemia sensitive to gentamicin, this is the antibiotic of choice until culture and sensitivity results are available. While this antibiotic treatment may be initiated early, cultures of blood, urine, sputum, wounds, fistulas, and/or sinuses must be obtained first.

Usually a 1- to 2-mg/kg intravenous loading dose of gentamicin is given, and this dose is repeated at 8- to 12-hour intervals as long as urine output is adequate. If the creatinine or blood urea nitrogen concentration rises significantly, the gentamicin dose must be reduced accordingly. In septicemia of unknown origin, most clinicians will also add a synthetic penicillin to the antibiotic regimen to treat the occasional staphylococcal septicemia which might be resistant to gentamicin.

Gram-negative anaerobic organisms such as *Bacteroides* species are receiving more attention now that culture methods have improved. Many bacteriologists state that these culture methods show that this organism is associated with aerobic gram-negative infections in at least 25 percent of patients. Since not all *Bacteroides* are sensitive to gentamicin, the newest synthetic analog of penicillin, clindamycin, may be required when cultures and sensitivities so indicate.

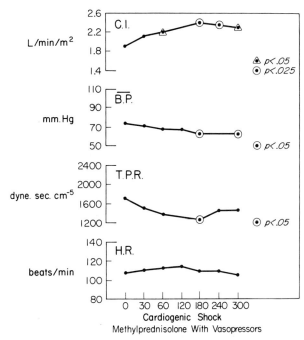

Fig. 4-23. The effect of a combination of methylprednisolone, 30 mg/kg administered intravenously, and levarterenol, 2 to 3 mg/kg/minute.

The *Pseudomonas* species are the one group of gram-negative bacteria which frequently cause shock but are often resistant to gentamicin. These bacteria are most often associated with chronic debilitated states and/or chronic infections in the respiratory or urinary tracts. As these patients often will have had previous cultures and sensitivities reported on their charts, the physician may have some forewarning of the likelihood of *Pseudomonas* involvement. In this situation, the combination of Colymicin and the new synthetic penicillin, carbenicillin, is probably the most effective treatment at this time.

A suggested protocol for the treatment of septic shock is listed in Table 4-6. This protocol is similar to those

Table 4-5. TREATMENT OF CARDIOGENIC SHOCK

Condition to be corrected (restored)	Treatment
Hypovolemia	Plasma fractions, dextran, crystalloids, blood (occasionally)
Stagnant anoxia	Synthetic glucocorticosteroids (methylprednisolone, dexamethasone)
Membrane integrity	
Infarct size	
Oncotic pressure	Albumin
Oliguria	Furosemide
Pulmonary edema	
Myocardial contractility	Digitalis
	Glucagon
	Beta stimulators
Hypoxemia	Respirator (volume type, positive end-expiratory pressure)

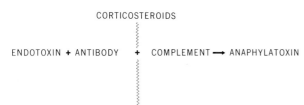

Fig. 4-24. The action of massive doses of glucocorticosteroids to decrease complement fixation by endotoxin will decrease the amount of activated endotoxin. This is an important basis for the early use of glucocorticosteroids to treat gram-negative septic shock.

presented earlier for traumatic and cardiogenic shock, but emphasis should be on early respiratory support, massive doses of corticosteroids, use of antibiotics, and determination of the source of the sepsis.

Buffers

Little was said about the use of buffers for the metabolic acidosis characteristic of shock. This omission was intentional so that the therapeutic emphasis would be on the restoration of nutritional blood flow. Provision of an adequate oxygen supply and restoration of normal cell metabolism will allow metabolism of the accumulated lactic acid and the production of adequate natural buffer. This does not mean that buffers such as sodium bicarbonate or THAM (tromethamine, or trishydroxymethylaminomethane) may not be needed in shock, but that their effects are short-lived if the hemodynamic and metabolic disturbances are not also corrected.

Buffers are indicated most often after a respiratory or cardiac arrest or when ventricular arrthymias occur. In these situations, bicarbonate in doses of 50 mEq or more is required. Some investigators have advocated the use of THAM rather than bicarbonate because the former has a higher pK value, enters cells more rapidly, and contains no sodium which may be harmful in patients with cardiac disease. Nonetheless, bicarbonate is still the buffer of

choice in most instances; it comes close to THAM in most of these effects, and THAM may have a negative inotropic effect in high doses and can cause respiratory arrest.

Mechanical Support of the Circulation

The continuing high mortality of cardiogenic shock secondary to massive and/or repeated infarction of the left ventricle despite all medical measures has stimulated the search for mechanical means to support circulation. Prolonged support was originally sought in order to allow recovery of the remaining viable myocardium, but more recently support for periods sufficient only to allow diagnostic coronary angiography and saphenous vein bypass of the obstructed arteries has been emphasized.

There are many devices designed to act as a pump-oxygenator. Intraaortic balloon assist has proved most promising because of its simplicity (Fig. 4-25). A catheter with a balloon designed to hold 20, 30, or 40 ml of helium is introduced into the femoral artery and advanced to the descending thoracic aorta. The balloon is rapidly inflated with helium during diastole and pumps blood both toward the coronaries and toward the periphery, increasing coronary and visceral organ flow and decreasing cardiac work. The correct timing is obtained from the ECG using the R wave. The device can be used for many days, but the best results have followed balloon support to gain time to obtain coronary angiography and to support the patient until the obstructed artery is bypassed under cardiopulmonary bypass. Survival rates up to 50 percent have been reported with balloon support used in this manner. In contrast, when balloon support is used as definitive treatment for the patient suffering cardiogenic shock unresponsive to medical treatment, the survival rate is less than 20 percent, or not significantly better than with medical treatment alone.

The balloon pump is also being used to support patients who cannot be weaned from cardiopulmonary bypass fol-

Fig. 4-25. Mechanical support of the circulation by intraaortic balloon assist.

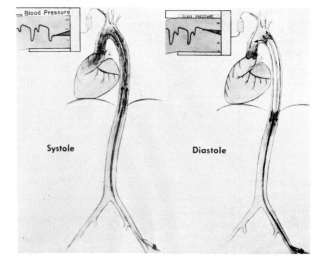

Table 4-6. TREATMENT OF SPETIC SHOCK

Condition to be corrected (restored)	Treatment
Hypovolemia	Plasma fractions, dextran, crystalloids, blood
Stagnant anoxia Membrane integrity Anaphylatoxin (activated endotoxin)	Synthetic glucocorticosteroids (methylprednisolone, dexamethasone)
Oncotic pressure	Albumin
Oliguria	Furosemide
Myocardial contractility (high-output failure)	Digitalis
Sepsis Arteriovenous admixture Hypoxemia	Antibiotics Eliminate source Respirator (volume type; positive end-expiratory pressure)

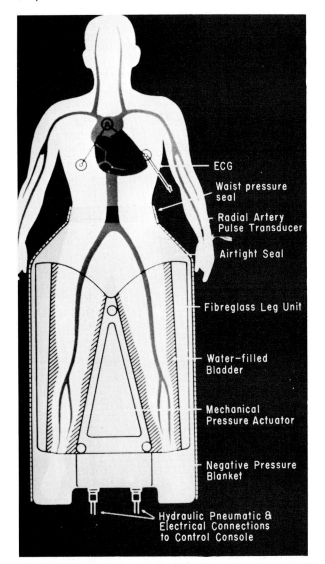

Fig. 4-26. Mechanical support of the circulation with external counterpulsation.

lowing correction of congenital or acquired heart defects, a variation of the low-output syndrome. Here the results are also promising.

A principal problem with all support devices which are "invasive" in nature is that they are not used early enough

in the shock syndrome. With this in mind, Soroff and colleagues have designed an external counterpulsation device also tuned with the R wave to give diastolic augmentation (Fig. 4-26). While somewhat less effective in diastolic augmentation than intraaortic balloon support, we have noted surprisingly similar results (Fig. 4-27). Moreover, the ease and rapidity with which the external device can be used means that it will be used earlier. Clinical studies so far are in the preliminary phases, but the device probably will enjoy widespread use in the near future.

SUMMARY

The hemodynamic and metabolic disturbances of shock, whatever the original insult, are largely determined by the sympathoadrenal response to the insult. Endogenous catecholamines and other released hormones such as histamine, catecholamine-like compounds such as activated endotoxin (anaphylatoxin), and administered synthetic catecholamines cause stagnant anoxia and cellular dysfunction in the viscerocutaneous microcirculation, and ultimate death. A significant increase in survival can be obtained by using fluids, drugs, and devices which modify the effects of the sympathoadrenal response to the shock-causing insult which result in a more equitable blood flow to all organs and restore normal cell metabolism.

References

Historical and General Consideration

Blalock, A.: Principles of Surgical Care: Shock and Other Problems, The C. V. Mosby Company, St. Louis, 1940.

Block, K. D. (ed.): "Shock: Pathogenesis and Therapy," Springer-Verlag OHG, Berlin, 1962.

Camron, W. B.: "Traumatic Shock," D. Appleton & Company, Inc., New York, 1923.

Forscher, B. K., Lillehei, R. C., and Stubbs, S. S. (eds.): "Shock in Low and High Flow States," Excerpta Medica, Amsterdam, 1972.

Gurd, F. N.: Fifty Years' Progress in Shock, *Bull Am Coll Surg,* **57:**27, 1972.

Hardaway, R. M., III: "Clinical Management of Shock," Charles C Thomas, Publisher, Springfield, Ill., 1968.

Hardy, J. D. (ed.): "Critical Surgical Illness," W. B. Saunders, Philadelphia, 1971.

Herman, C. M.: Advances and Newer Concepts in Shock—1972, in "Surgery Annual, 1972," Appleton Century Crofts, New York, 1972.

Hershey, S. G. (ed.): "Shock," Little, Brown and Company, Boston, 1964.

Johnson, P. C.: Renaissance in the Microcirculation, *Circ Res,* **31:**817, 1972.

Lefer, A. M.: Blood Borne Humoral Factors in the Pathophysiology of Circulatory Shock, *Circ Res,* **32:**129, 1973.

Lillehei, R. C., Longerbeam, J. K., Bloch, J. H., and Manax, W. G.: The Nature of Irreversible Shock: Experimental and Clinical Observations, *Ann Surg,* **160:**682, 1964.

Fig. 4-27. A comparison of the effects on diastolic augmentation of the arterial blood pressure of intraaortic balloon assist (IABP) and external counterpulsation (ECP).

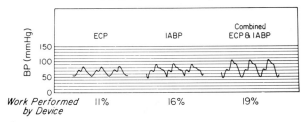

Malcolm, J. D.: The Condition of the Blood Vessels during Shock, *Lancet,* **2:**573, 1905.

Mapother, E. D.: Shock: Its Nature, Duration and Mode of Treatment, *Br Med J,* **2:**1023, 1879.

Nickerson, M.: Factors of Vasoconstriction and Vasodilation in Shock, *J Mich Med Soc,* **54:**45, 1955.

Scudder, J.: "Shock: Blood Studies as a Guide to Therapy," J. B. Lippincott Company, Philadelphia, 1940.

Selye, H.: The General Adaptation Syndrome and the Diseases of Adaptation, *J Clin Endocrinol Metab,* **6:**117, 1946.

Shepro, D., and Fulton, G. P. (eds.): "Microcirculation as Related to Shock," Academic Press, Inc., New York, 1968.

Shires, T., and Carreco, C. J.: Current Status of the Shock Problem, *Curr Probl Surg,* March 1966.

Shoemaker, W. C.: "Shock: Chemistry, Physiology and Therapy," Charles C Thomas, Springfield, Ill., 1967.

Starling, E. H.: On the Absorption of Fluids from Connective Tissue Spaces, *J Physiol* (*Lond*), **19:**312, 1896.

Thal, A. P.: "Shock: A Physiologic Basis for Treatment," Year Book Medical Publishers, Inc., Chicago, 1971.

——— and Wilson, R. F.: "Shock," *Curr Probl Surg,* September 1965.

Zweifach, B. W.: Functional Behavior of the Microcirculation, Charles C Thomas, Publisher, Springfield, Ill., 1961.

Hemorrhagic Shock

Ahlquist, R. P.: Study of the Adrenotropic Receptors, *Am J Physiol,* **153:**586, 1948.

Bane, A. E., Wurth, M. A., and Sayeed, M. M.: The Dynamics of Altered ATP-dependent and ATP-yielding Cell Processes in Shock, *Surgery,* **72:**94, 1972.

Cunningham, J. N., Shires, G. T., and Wagner, B. S.: Cellular Transport Defects in Hemorrhagic Shock, *Surgery,* **70:**215, 1971.

Fine, J.: "The Bacterial Factor in Traumatic Shock," Charles C Thomas, Publisher, Springfield, Ill., 1954.

Glenn, T. M. and Lefer, A. M.: Significance of Splanchnic Proteases in the Production of a Toxic Factor in Hemorrhagic Shock, *Circ Res,* **24:**338, 1971.

Lefer, A. M., Cowgill, R., Marshall, F. F., Hall, L. M., and Brand, E. D.: Characterization of a Myocardial Depressant Factor Present in Hemorrhagic Shock, *Am J Physiol,* **213:**492, 1967.

Lillehei, R. C.: Intestinal Factor in Irreversible Hemorrhagic Shock, *Surgery,* **42:**1043, 1957.

Pappenheimer, J. R., Renkin, E. M., and Borrero, L. M.: Filtration, Diffusion and Molecular Sieving through Peripheral Capillary Membranes: Contribution to the Pore Theory of Capillary Permeability, *Am J Physiol,* **157:**13, 1951.

Rosenberg, J. C., Lillehei, R. C., Longerbeam, J. K., and Zimmerman, B.: Studies on Hemorrhagic and Endotoxin Shock in Relationship to Vasomotor Changes and Endogenous Circulating Epinephrine, Norepinephrine and Serotonin, *Ann Surg,* **154:**611, 1961.

Schumer, W.: Metabolism of the Fat Cell in Low-Flow States, *J Surg Res,* **6:**254, 1966.

———: Localization of the Energy Pathway Block in Shock, *Surgery,* **64:**55, 1968.

——— and Kukeral: Metabolism of Shock, *Surgery,* **63:**630, 1968.

——— and Sperling, R.: Shock and Its Effect on the Cell, *JAMA,* **205:**215, 1968.

Shires, T., Cunningham, J. N., Baker, C. R. F., Reeder, S. F., Illner, H., Wagner, I. Y., and Maher, J.: Alterations in Cellular Membrane Function during Hemorrhagic Shock in Primates, *Ann Surg,* **176:**288, 1972.

Siegel, J. H., and Strom, B. L.: The Computer as a "Living Textbook" Applied to the Care of the Critically Injured Patient, *J Trauma,* **12:**739, 1972.

Wiggers, C. J.: "Physiology of Shock," The Commonwealth Fund, New York, 1950.

Wilson, J. W.: Pulmonary Morphological Changes Due to Extracorporeal Circulation: A Model for the 'Shock Lung' at Cellular Level in Humans, in "Shock in Low and High-Flow States," p. 160, Excerpta Medica Foundation, Amsterdam, 1972.

——— and Hackel, D. B.: A Unified Mechanism Producing a Microcirculatory Pulmonary Lesion in Response to Hemorrhagic Shock, Transfusion, and Pump-Oxygenator Procedures, *Anat Rec,* **160:**452, 1968.

———, Ratliff, N. B., and Hackel, D. B.: The Lung in Hemorrhagic Shock: I. In Vivo Observations of Pulmonary Microcirculation in Cats, *Am J Pathol,* **58:**337, 1970.

Septic Shock

Albrecht, M., and Clowes, G. H. Jr.: The Increase of Circulatory Requirements in the Presence of Inflammation, *Surgery,* **56:** 158, 1964.

Alho, A., Motsay, G. J., and Lillehei, R. C.: Effects of Therapy on Lysosomal Changes in Shock, in "Shock in Low and High-Flow States," p. 263, Excerpta Medica Foundation, Amsterdam, 1972.

Bacteroides in the Blood, Lancet, **1:**27, 1973. (Editorial.)

Bernhardt, H. E., Orlando, J. C., Benfield, J. R., Hirose, F. M., and Foos, R. Y.: Disseminated Candidiasis in Surgical Patients, *Surg Gynecol Obstet,* **134:**819, 1972.

Cann, M., Stevenson, T., Fiallos, E., and Thal, A. P.: Depressed Cardiac Performance in Sepsis, *Surg Gynecol Obstet,* **134:**759, 1972.

Caridis, D. T., Reinhold, R. B., Woodruff, P. W. H., and Fine, J.: Endotoxemia in Man, *Lancet,* **1:**1381, 1972.

Cavanaugh, D., and Rao, P. S.: Endotoxin Shock in the Subhuman Primate: I. Hemodynamic and Biochemical Changes, *Arch Surg,* **99:**107, 1969.

Clowes, G. H. Jr., Zuschneid, W., Dragacevic, S., and Turner, M.: The Non-specific Pulmonary Inflammatory Reactions Leading to Respiratory Failure after Shock, Gangrene, and Sepsis, *J Trauma,* **8:**899, 1968.

Fine, J., Frank, E. D., Ravin, H. A., Rutenberg, S. H., and Schweinburg, F. B.: The Bacterial Factor in Traumatic Shock, *N Engl J Med,* **260:**214, 1959.

Gaines, J. D., and Remington, J. S.: Disseminated Candidiasis in the Surgical Patient, *Surgery,* **72:**730, 1972.

Gilbert, R. P.: Mechanisms of the Hemodynamic Effect of Endotoxin, *Physiol Rev,* **40:**245, 1960.

Hardaway, R. M., and Johnson, D.: Clotting Mechanism in Endotoxin Shock, *Arch Intern Med,* **112:**775, 1963.

Hayasaka, H., and Howard, J. M.: Septic Shock: Experimental

and Clinical Studies, Charles C Thomas, Publisher, Springfield, Ill., 1964.

Hellebusch, A. A., Salama, F. and Eadie, E.: The Use of Mannitol to Reduce the Nephrotoxicity of Amphotericin B, *Surg Gynecol Obstet,* **134:**241, 1972.

Herman, C. M., McKie, A. E., Jr., Schilling, P. W., Dickson, L. G., Horwitz, D. L., Coran, A. G., Cryer, P. E., and Koprina, C. J.: The Baboon as a Subhuman Primate Shock Model, in "Shock in Low and High-Flow States,"p. 42, Excerpta Medica Foundation, Amsterdam, 1972.

Hermreck, A. S., and Thal, A. P.: Mechanisms for the High Circulatory Requirements in Sepsis and Septic Shock, *Ann Surg,* **170:**677, 1969.

Hinshaw, L. B.: Comparison of Responses of Canine and Primate Species to Bacteria and Bacterial Endotoxin, in "Shock in Low and High-Flow States," p. 245, Excerpta Medica Foundation, Amsterdam, 1972.

———, Archer, L. T., Block, W. B., Greenfield, L. J. and Guenter, C. A.: Prevention and Reversal of Myocardial Failure in Endotoxin Shock, *Surg Gynecol Obstet,* **136:**1, 1973.

———, Solomon, L. A., Holmes, D. D., and Greenfield, L. J.: Comparison of Canine Responses to *Escherica coli* Organisms and Endotoxin, *Surg Gynecol Obstet,* **127:**981, 1968.

Hirsch, E. F., Fletcher, J. R., and Lucas, S.: Hypotension and Lactic Acidemia in Sepsis following Combat Trauma, *J Trauma,* **12:**45, 1972.

Horwitz, D. C., Moquin, R. B., and Herman, C. M.: Coagulation Changes of Septic Shock in the Sub-human Primate and Their Relationship to Hemodynamic Changes, *Ann Surg,* **175:**417, 1972.

Kinney, J. M.: Energy Expenditure and Tissue Fuel in the Septic Patient, in "Shock in Low and High-Flow States," p. 145, Excerpta Medica Foundation, Amsterdam, 1972.

Kuida, H., Hinshaw, L. B., Gilbert, R. P. and Visscher, M. B.: Effect of Gram-negative Endotoxin on Pulmonary Circulation, *Am J Physiol,* **192:**335, 1958.

Kux, M., Coalson, J. J., Masson, W. H. and Guenter, C. A.: Pulmonary Effects of *E. coli* Endotoxin: Role of Leukocytes and Platelets, *Ann Surg,* **175:**26, 1972.

Lillehei, R. C., and MacLean, L. D.: The Intestinal Factor in Irreversible Endotoxin Shock, *Ann Surg,* **148:**513, 1955.

——— and ———: Physiological Approach to Successful Treatment of Endotoxin Shock in Experimental Animals, *Arch Surg,* **78:**464, 1959.

McCabe, W. R.: Serum Complement Levels in Bacteremia Due to Gram-negative Organisms, *N Engl J Med,* **288:**21, 1973.

Metchnikoff, E.: "Lectures on the Comparative Pathology of Inflammation," translated from the French by F. A. Starling and E. H. Starling, Kegan, Paul, Trensch, Truber & Co., Ltd., London, 1893.

Nicholas, G. G., Mela, L. M., and Miller, L. D.: Shock-Induced Alterations of Mitochondrial Membrane Transport: Effect of Endotoxin and Lysosomal Enzymes on Calcium Transport, *Ann Surg,* **176:**579, 1972.

Rangel, D. M., Byfield, J. E., Adomian, G. E., Stevens, G. H., and Fonkalsrud, E. W.: Hepatic Ultrastructural Response to Endotoxin Shock, *Surgery,* **68:**503, 1970.

Reichgott, M. J., and Melman, K. L.: Bradykinin and the Cardiovascular System, *Circulation,* **42:**563, 1970. (Editorial.)

——— and ———: Does Bradykinin Play a Pathogenetic Role in Endotoxemia? in "Shock in Low and High-Flow States," p. 59, Excerpta Medica Foundation, Amsterdam, 1972.

———, Forsyth, R. P., and Melmon, K. L.: Effects of Bradykinin and Autonomic Nervous System Intubation on Systemic and Regional Hemodynamics in the Unanesthetized Rhesus Monkey, *Circ Res,* **24:**367, 1971.

Reilly, J., Rivalier, E., Campagnon, A., Friedman, E. H. C., and DuBuit, H.: Le Râle du système neurovégétatif dans le réactions d'hypersensibilité, *Ann Med Interne (Paris),* **39:**165, 1936.

Siegel, J. H., Farrell, E. J., Goldwyn, R. M., and Friedman, H. P.: Myocardial Function in Human Septic Shock States, in "Shock in Low and High-Flow States," p. 250, Excerpta Medica Foundation, Amsterdam, 1972.

———, Goldwyn, R. M., and Friedman, H. P.: Pattern and Process in the Evaluation of Human Septic Shock, *Surgery,* **70:**232, 1971.

———, Greenspan, M., and DelGuercio, L. R. M.: Abnormal Vascular Tone, Defective Oxygen Transport, and Myocardial Failure in Human Septic Shock, *Ann Surg,* **165:**504, 1967.

Spink, W. W.: From Endotoxin to Snake Venom, *Yale J Biol Med,* **30:**355, 1958.

———: Endotoxin Shock, *Ann Intern Med,* **57:**538, 1962.

———: "The Role of Endotoxin Shock in Shock in Low and High-Flow States," p. 226, Excerpta Medica Foundation, Amsterdam, 1972.

——— and Anderson, D.: Experimental Studies on the Significance of Endotoxin in the Pathogenesis of Brucillosis, *J Clin Invest,* **33:**540, 1954.

Thal, A. P.: The Cardiovascular Response to Sepsis, in "Shock in Low and High-Flow States," p. 240, Excerpta Medica Foundation, Amsterdam, 1972.

Thomas, L.: The Physiological Disturbance Produced by Endotoxins, *Ann Rev Physiol,* **16:**467, 1954.

Weil, M. H., MacLean, L. D., Visscher, M. B., and Spink, W. W.: Studies on the Circulating Changes in the Dog Produced by Endotoxin from Gram-negative Microorganisms, *J Clin Invest,* **35:**1191, 1956.

Wilson, R. F., Thal, A. P., and Kindling, P. H.: Hemodynamic Measurements in Septic Shock, *Arch Surg,* **91:**121, 1965.

Wilson, W. R., Martin, W. J., Wilkowske, C. J., and Washington, J. A.: Anaerobic Bacteremia, *Mayo Clin Proc,* **47:**639, 1972.

Zimmerman, L. E.: Fatal Fungous Infections Complicating Other Diseases, *Am J Clin Pathol,* **25:**45, 1955.

Cardiogenic Shock

Agress, C. M., and Binder, M. J.: Cardiogenic Shock, *Am Heart J,* **54:**548, 1957.

———, Rosenburg, M. J., Jacobs, H. I., Binder, M. J., Schneiderman, A. and Clark, W. G.: Protracted Shock in Ten Closed Chest Dogs following Coronary Embolization with Graded Microspheres, *Am J Physiol,* **170:**536, 1951.

Bloch, J. H., Pierce, C. H., Manax, W. G., Lyons, G. W., and Lillehei, R. C.: Experimental Cardiogenic Shock, *Arch Surg,* **91:**77, 1965.

Braunwald, E., Corell, J. W., Marako, P. R., and Ross, J. Jr.: Effects of Drugs and of Counterpulsation on Myocardial Oxygen Consumption: Observation on the Ischemic Heart, *Circulation,* **40**(*Suppl* 4):220, 1969.

Dietzman, R. H., Lyons, G. W., Bloch, J. H., and Lillehei, R. C.:

Relation of Cardiac Work to Survival in Cardiogenic Shock in Dogs, *JAMA,* **199:**825, 1967.

Maroko, P. R., Kjekshus, J. K., Sobel, B. E., Watarabe, T., Covell, J. W., Ross, J. Jr., and Braunwald, E.: Factors Influencing Infarct Size following Experimental Coronary Artery Occlusions, *Circulation,* **43:**67, 1971.

Mueller, H., Ayres, S. M., Giannelli, S., Jr., Conklin, E. F., Mazzara, J. T., and Grace, W. J.: Effect of Isoproterenol, Norepinephrine, and Intraaortic Counterpulsation on Hemodynamics and Myocardial Metabolism in Shock following Myocardial Infarction, *Circulation,* **45:**335, 1972.

Replogle, R., Levy, M., DeWall, R. A., and Lillehei, R. C.: Catecholamine and Serotonin Response to Cardiopulmonary Bypass, *J Thorac Cardiovasc Surg,* **44:**638, 1962.

Rockley, C. E., and Russell, R. O., Jr.: Left Ventricular Function in Acute Myocardial Infarction and Its Clinical Significance, *Circulation,* **45:**231, 1972.

Swan, H. J. C., Ganz, W., Forrester, J., Marcus, H., Diamond, G., and Chonette, D.: Catheterization of the Heart in Man with Use of a Flow-directed Balloon-tipped Catheter, *N Engl J Med,* **283:**447, 1970.

Lung

Ashbaugh, D. G., and Petty, T. L.: Sepsis Complicating the Acute Respiratory Distress Syndrome, *Surg Gynecol Obstet,* **135:**865, 1972.

———— and ————: Positive End-expiratory Pressure: Physiology, Indications and Contraindications, *J Thorac Cardiovasc Surg,* **65:**165, 1973.

Berggren, P.: The Oxygen Deficit of Arterial Blood Caused by Non-ventilating Parts of the Lung, *Acta Physiol Scand,* **4**(*Suppl* 2):1, 1941.

Bert, P.: "Barometric Pressure Researches in Experimental Physiology," translated from the French by Mary and Fred A. Hitchcock, College Book Company, Columbus, Ohio, 1943.

Dietzman, R. H., Bloch, J. H., Feemster, J. A., Idezuki, Y., and Lillehei, R. C.: Mechanisms in the Production of Shock, *Surgery,* **62:**645, 1967.

Fleming, W. H., and Bowen, J. C.: The Use of Diuretics in the Treatment of Early Wet Lung Syndrome, *Ann Surg,* **175:**505, 1972.

Giordano, J. M., Joseph, W. L., Klingenmaier, C. H., and Adkiur, P. G.: The Management of Interstitial Pulmonary Edema, *J Thorac Cardiovasc Surg,* **64:**739, 1972.

Greenfield, L. J., Reif, M. E., Coalson, J. J., McCurdy, J. R., and Elkins, R. C.: Comparative Effects of Interstitial Pulmonary Edema Produced by Venous Hypertension or Hemodilution in Perfused Lungs, *Surgery,* **71:**857, 1972.

Hechtman, H. B., Reid, M. H., Dorn, B. C., Justice, R. E., and Weisel, R. D.: Shunting in the Lung: A Two-Compartment Model, *Surgery,* **72:**443, 1972.

Jenkins, M. T., Jones, R. F., Wilson, B., and Moyer, C. A.: Congestive Atelectasis: A Complication of the Intravenous Infusion of Fluids, *Ann Surg,* **132:**327, 1950.

Kellum, J. M., DeMeester, T. R., Elkins, R. C., and Zuidema, G. D.: Respiratory Insufficiency Secondary to Acute Pancreatitis, *Ann Surg,* **175:**657, 1972.

Lindsay, W. G., and Humphrey, E. W.: Measurement of Pulmonary Extravascular Water, *Surgery,* **71:**650, 1972.

Magilligan, D. J., Oleksyn, T. W., Schwartz, S. I., and Yu, P. N.: Pulmonary Intravascular and Extravascular Volumes in Hemorrhagic Shock and Fluid Replacement, *Surgery,* **72:**780, 1972.

Monaco, V., Burdge, R., Newell, J., Sardar, S., Leather, R., Powers, S. R., Jr., and Dutton, R.: Pulmonary Venous Admixture in Injured Patients, *J. Trauma,* **12:**15, 1972.

Moore, F. D.: Post-traumatic Pulmonary Insufficiency, in "Critical Surgical Illness," W. B. Saunders Company, Philadelphia, 1971.

————, Lyons, J. H., Jr., Pierce, E. C., Jr., Morgan, A. P., Jr., Drinker, P. A., MacArthur, J. D., and Dammin, G. J.: Post-traumatic Pulmonary Insufficiency, W. B. Saunders Company, Philadelphia, 1969.

Moss, G., Staunton, C., and Stein, A. A.: Cerebral Etiology of the "Shock Lung Syndrome," *J Trauma,* **12:**885, 1972.

Motsay, G. J., Alho, A. V., Schultz, L. S., Dietzman, R. H., and Lillehei, R. C.: Pulmonary Capillary Permeability in the Post-traumatic Pulmonary Insufficiency Syndrome, *Ann Surg,* **173:**244, 1971.

———— and Lillehei, R. C.: Acute Respiratory Distress Syndrome in Adults, *Int Surg,* **58:**304, 1973.

Peters, R. M., and Hilberman, M.: Respiratory Insufficiency: Diagnosis and Control of Therapy, *Surgery,* **70:**280, 1971.

Powers, S. R., Jr., Burdge, R., Leather, R., Monaco, V., Newell, J., Sardar, S., and Smith, E. J.: Studies of Pulmonary Insufficiency in Non-thoracic Trauma, *J Trauma,* **12:**1, 1972.

Shoemaker, W. C.: Cardiorespiratory Patterns of Surviving and Nonsurviving Postoperative Patients, *Surg Gynecol Obstet,* **134:**810, 1972.

Skillman, J. J.: Treatment of Acute Respiratory Distress Syndrome: Role of Albumen and Diuretics, in "Shock in Low and High-Flow States," p. 196, Excerpta Medica Foundation, Amsterdam, 1972.

Steer, M. I., Claeren, S. E., Bushnell, L. S., and Skillman, J. J.: Metabolic Alkalosis and Respiratory Failure in Critically Ill Patients, *Surgery,* **72:**408, 1972.

Szidon, J. P., Pietra, G. G., and Fishman, A. P.: The Alveolar-Capillary Membrane and Pulmonary Edema, *N Engl J Med,* **286:**1200, 1972.

Wilson, R. F., Christensen, C., and LeBlanc, L. P.: Oxygen Consumption in Critically-Ill Surgical Patients, *Ann Surg,* **176:**801, 1972.

Pancreas

Gump, F. E., Long, C. L., Wong, M., and Kinney, J. M.: Exogenous Glucose as an Energy Substrate in Experimental Hemorrhagic Shock, *Surg Gynecol Obstet,* **136:**611, 1973.

Jordan, G. L., Fischer, E. P., and Lefrak, E. A.: Glucose Metabolism in Traumatic Shock in the Human, *Ann Surg,* **175:**685, 1972.

Lan, T. S., Taubenfligel, W., Levene, R., Farago, G., Chan, H., Koven, I., and Drucker, W. R.: Pancreatic Blood Flow and Insulin Output in Severe Hemorrhage, *J Trauma,* **12:**880, 1972.

Lefer, A. M., and Barenholz, Y.: Pancreatic Hydrolases and the Formation of a Myocardial Depressant Factor in Shock, *Am J Physiol,* **223:**1103, 1972.

Majid, P. A., Sharma, B., Meeran, M. K. M., and Taylor, S. H.: Insulin and Glucose in the Treatment of Heart Failure, *Lancet,* **2:**937, 1972.

Moffat, J. G., King, J. A. C., and Drucker, W. R.: Tolerance to Prolonged Hypovolemic Shock: Effect of Infusion of an Energy Substrate, *Surg Forum,* **19:**5, 1968.

Spigelman, A., and Ozeran, R.: The Protective Effect of Insulin in Hemorrhagic Shock: *Surg Forum,* **21:**90, 1970.

Vegas, M., Hetenyi, G. J., and Haist, R. E.: Glucose Metabolism in Posthemorrhagic Shock in the Dog, *J Trauma,* **11:**615, 1971.

Tolerance to Shock

Dietzman, R. H., Feemster, J. A., Idezuki, Y., and Lillehei, R. C.: Tolerance to Lethal Vasoconstriction in Endotoxin Shock, *Surg Forum,* **18:**14, 1967.

———, Bloch, J. H., Lyons, G. W., and Lillehei, R. C.: Prevention of Lethal Cardiogenic Shock in Epinephrine Tolerant Dogs, *Surgery,* **65:**63, 1969.

———, Ersek, R. A., Idezuki, Y., and Lillehei, R. C.: Plasma Norepinephrine Levels during Cardiogenic Shock in Normal and Endotoxin Tolerant Dogs. *JAMA,* **204:**530, 1968.

Essex, H. E.: Further Observations of Certain Responses in Tolerant and Control Animals to Massive Doses of Epinephrine, *Am J Physiol,* **171:**78, 1952.

Hruza, Z.: Resistance to Trauma, Charles C Thomas, Publisher, Springfield, Ill., 1971.

Lillehei, R. C.: A Physiological Approach to the Treatment of Endotoxin Shock in the Experimental Animal, *Arch Surg,* **78:**464, 1959.

——— and MacLean, L. D.: Increased Resistance to Epinephrine Shock in Endotoxin Tolerant Dogs, *Physiologist,* **1:**48, 1958.

Motsay, G. J., Alho, A., Jaeger, T., Schultz, L. S., Dietzman, R. H., and Lillehei, R. C.: Effects of Methylprednisolone, Phenoxybenzamine and Epinephrine Tolerance in Canine Endotoxin Shock: Study of Isogravimetric Capillary Pressures in Forelimb and Intestine, *Surgery,* **70:**271, 1971.

Zweifach, B. W.: Relation of the Reticulo-endothelial System to Natural and Acquired Resistance in Shock, in "Shock," p. 113, Little, Brown and Company, Boston, 1964.

Vasoconstrictors and Vasodilators (including Cortico-steroids) in Shock

Beregovich, J., Reicher-Reiss, H., and Grishman, A.: Haemodynamic Effects of Isoprenaline in Acute Myocardial Infarction, *Br Heart J,* **34:**705, 1972.

Berk, J. L.: Use of Beta Blockers in Shock, in "Shock in Low and High-Flow States," p. 282, Excerpta Medica Foundation, Amsterdam, 1972.

Dietzman, R. H., and Lillehei, R. C.: The Treatment of Cardiogenic Shock: IV. The Use of Phenoxybenzamine and Chlorpromazine, *Am Heart J,* **75:**136, 1968.

Digitalis in Acute Myocardial Infarction, Editorial, *JAMA,* **223:**553, 1973.

Falicov, R. E., Lipp, H., Resnekov, L., and King, S.: Hemodynamic Effects of Low-Dose Isoproterenol and Aminophylline after Coronary Embolization in Dogs, *Cardiovasc Res,* **7:**63, 1973.

Holmagyi, D. F. J.: Combined Adrenergic Receptor Blockade in Experimental Post Hemorrhagic Shock, in "Shock in Low and High-Flow States," p. 49, Excerpta Medica Foundation, Amsterdam, 1972.

Koves, R. J., and Phillips, J. H.: Glucagon: Present Status in Cardiovascular Disease, *Clin Pharmacol Ther,* **12:**427, 1971.

Krassrow, N., Rolett, E. L., Yurchak, P. M., Hood, W. B., Jr., and Gorlin, R.: Isoproterenol and Cardiovascular Performance, *Am J Med,* **37:**514, 1964.

Laborit, H.: Le Choc traumatique, *Sem Hosp Paris,* **31:**1, 1955.

Majid, P. A., Sharma, B., Meeran, M. K. M., and Taylor, S. H.: Insulin and Glucose in the Treatment of Heart Failure, *Lancet,* **2:**937, 1972.

Nickerson, M.: Sympathetic Blockade in the Therapy of Shock, *Am J Cardiol,* **12:**619, 1967.

Skjoldborg, H.: Phenoxybenzamine in the Treatment of Septic Shock, *Acta Chir Scand,* **134:**85, 1968.

Tunnis, G. C., Lin, R., Ramos, R. G., and Gordon, S.: Prolonged Glucagon Infusion in Cardiac Failure, *JAMA,* **223:**293, 1973.

Von Euler, U. S.: A Specific Sympathomimetic Ergone in Adrenergic Nerve Fibers (Sympothin) and Its Relations to Adrenaline and Nor-Adrenaline, *Acta Physiol Scand,* **12:**73, 1946.

———: Twenty Years of Noradrenaline, *Pharmacol Rev,* **18:**29, 1966.

Wilson, R. E., Jablowski, D. V., and Thal, A. P.: The Usage of Dibenzyline in Clinical Shock, *Surgery,* **56:**172, 1964.

Glucocorticosteroids

Alho, A., Motsay, G. J., and Lillehei, R. C.: Effects of Therapy on Lysosomal Changes in Shock, in "Shock in Low and High-Flow States," p. 263, Excerpta Medica Foundation, Amsterdam, 1972.

Barzilai, D., Plavnick, J., Hazani, A., Einath, R., Kleinhaus, N., and Kanter, Y.: Use of Hydrocortisone in the Treatment of Acute Myocardial Infarction, *Chest,* **61:**488, 1972.

Bloch, J. H., Pierce, C. H., and Lillehei, R. C.: Adrenergic Blocking Agents in the Treatment of Shock, *Ann Rev Med,* **17:**483, 1966.

Christy, J. H.: Treatment of Gram-negative Shock, *Am J Med,* **50:**77, 1971.

Dietzman, R. H., and Lillehei, R. C.: The Treatment of Cardiogenic Shock: V. The Use of Steroids, *Am Heart J,* **75:**274, 1968.

———, Castaneda, A. R., Lillehei, C. W., Ersek, R. A., Motsay, G. J., and Lillehei, R. C.: Corticosteroids as Effective Vasodilators in the Treatment of the Low-Output Syndrome, *Chest,* **57:**440, 1970.

Knuth, O. E., Wagenknecht, L. V., and Madsen, P. O.: The Effect of Various Treatments on Renal Function during Endotoxin Shock, *Invest Urol,* **9:**304, 1972.

Lillehei, R. C., Dietzman, R. H., Motsay, G. J., Schultz, L. S., Romero, L. H., and Beckman, C. B.: The Pharmacologic Approach to the Treatment of Shock: I. Defining Traumatic, Septic and Cardiogenic Shock, *Geriatrics,* **27:**73, 1972.

———, ———, ———, ———, ———, ———: The Pharmacologic Approach to the Treatment of Shock: II. Diagnosis of Shock and the Plan of Treatment, *Geriatrics,* **27:**81, 1972.

———, Motsay, G. J., and Dietzman, R. H.: The Use of Corticosteroids in the Treatment of Shock, *Int J Clin Pharmacol,* **5:**423, 1972.

Motsay, G. J., Dietzman, R. H., Schultz, L. H., Romero, L. H., and Lillehei, R. C.: Effects of Massive Doses of Corticosteroids in Experimental and Clinical Gram-negative Septic Shock, in "Shock in Low and High-Flow States," p. 292, Excerpta Medica Foundation, Amsterdam, 1972.

Pierce, C. H.: Some Effects of Methylprednisolone in Controlled Hypoperfusion Induced Shock. (In press.)

——, Briggs, B. T., and Gutelius, J. R.: Methylprednisolone and Phenoxybenzamine in Experimental Shock: Cardiovascular Dynamics and Platelet Function, in "Shock in Low and High-Flow States," p. 183, Excerpta Medica Foundation, Amsterdam 1972.

Rao, P. S., and Cavanaugh, D.: Endotoxin Shock in the Subhuman Primate: II. Some Effects of Methylprednisolone Administration, *Arch Surg,* **102:**486, 1971.

Schumer, W., and Nyhus, L. W. (eds.): "Corticosteroids in the Treatment of Shock," The University of Illinois Press, Urbana, 1970.

——, Ervl, P. R., and Obernolte, R. P.: Mechanisms of Steroid Protection in Septic Shock, *Surgery,* **72:**119, 1972.

Schultz, L. S., Alho, A. V., Dietzman, R. H., Ersek, R. A., Motsay, G. J., Romero, L. H., Ruiz, J. O., and Lillehei, R. C.: Pharmacological Assistance in the Low Output Syndrome, in "Shock in Low and High-Flow States," p. 131, Excerpta Medica Foundation, Amsterdam, 1972.

Vyden, J. K., Corday, E., Parmley, W. W., and Swan, H. J. C.: Corticosteroids in the Management of Acute Myocardial Infarction and Cardiogenic Shock, *Clin Res.* (In press.)

Wilson, J. W.: Treatment or Prevention of Pulmonary Cellular Damage with Pharmacological Doses of Corticosteroid, *Surg Gynecol Obstet,* **134:**675, 1972.

Wilson, R. F., Ali, M., Anand, V., McCarthy, B., Pitt, J., Hayes, D., Perainel, A., and LeBlanc, L. P.: Effects of Vasoactive Agents in Clinical Septic Shock, in "Shock in Low and High-Flow States," p. 269, Excerpta Medica Foundation, Amsterdam, 1972.

Mechanical Support of the Circulation

Beckman, C. B., Romero, L. H., Shatney, C. H., Dietzman, R. H., Nicoloff, D. M., and Lillehei, R. C.: Clinical Comparison of Intraaortic Balloon Pump and External Counterpulsation for Cardiogenic Shock, *Trans Am Soc Artif Intern Organs,* vol. 19, 1973. (In press.)

Brickley, M. J., Sanders, C. A., and Austen, W. G.: Mechanical Circulatory Assistance for the Low Cardiac Output State, in "Shock in Low and High-Flow States," p. 140, Excerpta Medica Foundation, Amsterdam, 1972.

Intra-Aortic Balloon Pumping, *Lancet,* **2:**1238, 1972. (Editorial.)

Kantrowitz, A., Tjonneland, S., Freed, P. S., Phillips, S. J., Butner, A. N., and Sherman, J. L.: Initial Clinical Experience with Intraaortic Balloon Pumping in Cardiogenic Shock, *JAMA,* **203:**113, 1968.

Lande, A. J., Fillmore, S. J., Subramamon, V., Tiedemann, R. N., Carlson, R. G., Block, J. A., and Lillehei, C. W.: Twenty-four Hour Venous Arterial Perfusion of Awake Dogs with a Sample Membrane Oxygenator, *Trans Am Soc Artif Intern Organs,* **15:**181, 1969.

Sanders, C. A., Buckley, M. J., and Austen, W. G.: Mechanical Circulatory Assistance: Current Status, *N Engl J Med,* **285:**348, 1971.

Schultz, L. S., Koreski, W. R., Beckman, C. B., Romero, L. H., Dietzman, R. H., and Lillehei, R. C.: The Minnesota System for Cardiorespiratory Assistance: Test of a New System on Dogs, *Resuscitation,* **1:**183, 1972.

Soroff, H. S., Giron, F., Ruiz, O., Birtwell, W. C., Hirsch, L. J., and Deterling, R. A., Jr.: Physiologic Support of Heart Action, *N Engl J Med,* **280:**693, 1969.

Chapter 5

Infections

by Isidore Cohn, Jr. and George H. Bornside

Introduction

General Principles

Diagnosis
Surgical Therapy
Antibiotic Therapy
Hyperbaric Therapy

Some Common Surgical Infections

Principles of Antibiotic Therapy

Basic Considerations
Chemoprophylaxis
Intestinal Antisepsis
Intraperitoneal Antibiotic Therapy

Antimicrobial Agents

Antibiotics Active against Gram-positive Microorganisms
Antibiotics Active against Some Gram-positive or Some
    Gram-negative Microorganisms or Both
Antifungal Antibiotics
Sulfonamides

Streptococcal Infections

Erysipelas
Enysiperloid
Necrotizing Fasciitis
Streptococcal Myonecrosis
Progressive Synergistic Gangrene
Meleney's Ulcer

Staphylococcal Infections

Staphylococcal Enteritis
    Staphylococcal Enterocolitis (Pseudomembranous
        Enterocolitis)

Clostridial Infections

Clostridial Wound Infection
    Simple Contamination
    Clostridial Cellulitis
    Clostridial Myonecrosis (Gas Gangrene)
Infections of the Gastrointestinal Tract
Urogenital Infections
Tetanus

Infections Caused by Gram-negative Bacilli

Mycotic Infections

Actinomycosis

Blastomycosis
Other Fungal Infections
    Coccidiodomycosis
    Histoplasmosis
    Moniliasis

Surgical Asepsis

Sterilization
Degerming of Skin
Other Surgical Antiseptics

INTRODUCTION

Infection is a dynamic process involving invasion of the body by pathogenic microorganisms and reaction of the tissues to organisms and their toxins. Soon after birth, a variety of microorganisms colonize the external and internal surfaces of the human body. This indigenous microflora usually does no harm; it produces no detectable pathologic effects in tissues and may be beneficial. Indeed, current research indicates that the normal intestinal flora functions as a barrier providing natural resistance against enteric infections with pathogens such as *Salmonella* and *Shigella* species. Infection evolves into overt disease only when the equilibrium between host and parasite is upset. Of the thousands of species of microorganisms in nature, only a few hundred are known to be pathogenic for man.

Current thinking concerning clinical disease resulting from host and parasite interrelationships recognizes the role of the general health of the host, his previous contact with infectious microorganisms, his past clinical history, and various insults (toxic, traumatic, or therapeutic) of nonmicrobial origin. When the host's resistance is lowered, the indigenous microflora can become involved in infectious disease. This presents a dilemma to both the clinician and the microbiologist, as it must be decided which of the several microorganisms usually isolated from a clinical specimen are involved in the patient's disease. There are very few pathogenic species which cause disease at all times. Most organisms found in and on man often are harmless but are capable of causing disease in patients who are elderly, very young, or debilitated (Table 5-1).

Despite almost 80 years of aseptic surgery and 30 years of experience with antimicrobial agents, the surgeon finds that infections are as great a problem now as in the past. But the etiologic agents have changed. Streptococci and pneumococci are no longer the captains of death, because

Table 5-1. SOME INDIGENOUS MICROORGANISMS
AND SOME INFECTIONS WITH WHICH
THEY MAY BE INVOLVED

Microorganism	*Infection*
Aerobic or facultative:	
Achromobacter spp.	Bloodstream, burns, meningitis, urethritis
Alcaligenes fecalis	Bloodstream, conjunctivitis, meningitis, respiratory tract, urinary tract
Candida albicans	Bacterial endocarditis, pneumonitis, septicemia, thrush, vulvovaginitis
Enterobacteriaceae (*Escherichia, Klebsiella, Enterobacter, Proteus,* etc.)	Abscesses, bloodstream, meningitis, peritonitis, pneumonia, wounds, urinary tract
Hemophilus spp.	Bronchitis, conjunctivitis, meningitis, urinary tract
Moraxella spp.	Conjunctivitis
Nocardia spp.	Nocardiosis
Pseudomonas spp.	Bloodstream, burns, meningitis, urinary tract, wounds
Staphylococcus aureus	Abscesses, pneumonia, wounds
Staphylococcus epidermidis	Bacterial endocarditis, septicemia
Streptococcus fecalis	Bacterial endocarditis, bloodstream, urinary tract, wounds
Streptococcus viridans	Bacterial endocarditis
Anaerobic:	
Actinomyces spp.	Actinomycosis
Bacteroides spp.	Abscesses, bacterial endocarditis
Clostridium spp.	Cellulitis, myonecrosis
Fusobacterium spp.	Abscesses, myonecrosis
Lactobacillus spp.	Bacterial endocarditis
Peptostreptococcus spp.	Abscesses, myonecrosis
Veillonella spp.	Bacterial endocarditis

they can be controlled by antibiotics. Staphylococci continue to cause nosocomial (hospital-acquired) infections, and those gram-negative bacteria usually considered nonpathogens, opportunists, or secondary invaders have become a major problem. Nosocomial infection results from the transmission of pathogens to a previously uninfected patient from a source in the hospital environment (cross infection). Alternatively, the pathogens may come from the patient himself (autoinfection). He may be a carrier of the pathogen or become colonized with virulent hospital strains during hospitalization. Many nosocomial infections have a iatrogenic basis (i.e., result from treatment by the physician and his professional collaborators). Frequent or prolonged use of supportive procedures such as indwelling venous or urinary catheters, tracheostomies, and equipment for postoperative respiratory care are responsible for iatrogenic infections. Nosocomial infection causes morbidity, mortality, expense to the patient, and increasing malpractice liability for the surgeon and hospital.

A surgical infection is an infection which requires surgical treatment and has developed before, or as a complication of, surgical treatment. Thus, a postoperative wound infection is also a specific nosocomial infection. Surgical infections may be analyzed in relation to procedures in clean or contaminated fields, the anatomic site or system involved, and the pathophysiologic activities of the causative microorganisms (Table 5-2). The microorganisms commonly encountered in surgical infections are the staphylococci, streptococci, clostridia, bacteroides, and the enteric bacteria. Most surgical incisions are contaminated but not infected with normal skin flora (bacteria such as coagulase-negative staphylococci and anaerobic diphtheroids). However, traumatic wounds are usually contaminated if not yet infected, and operations on infected or "contaminated" tissue usually result in infection. Postoperative infections present a double hazard: First, the infection itself may result in toxemia or produce extensive tissue damage and perhaps septicemia. Second, the local effects of infection delay healing of the wound and may cause hemorrhage or disruption of the wound.

Table 5-2. CLASSIFICATION OF
SURGICAL INFECTIONS

I. Relative to final outcome
   A. Self-limiting infections: The patient recovers completely without medical or surgical treatment, or despite it (e.g., a boil).
   B. Serious infections requiring treatment: The outcome depends largely on the nature of treatment, the time after outset that it is administered, and clinical judgment (e.g., septicemia, pneumonia, empyema, primary peritonitis).
   C. Fulminating infections: These prove to be fatal or permanently disabling (e.g., retroperitoneal cellulitis).
II. Relative to time of onset
   A. Anteoperative surgical infections: These include all infections in which the microorganisms have gained entrance to the body before any operative procedure.
      1. Time and portal of entry are known—accidents.
      2. Time and portal of entry are not known—disease (infection) is established before the surgeon treats the patient.
   B. Operative surgical infections: These include all in which microorganisms gain entrance to the body during an operative procedure or as an immediate result of it (i.e., surgery may be considered either directly or indirectly responsible for the development of infection).
      1. Preventable operative surgical infections—failure of the surgeon or operating-room personnel to adhere to the principles of sterile procedure and all accepted and accredited practices
      2. Nonpreventable operative surgical infections
         a. Pathogenic microorganisms already resident within body tissues (e.g., incision seeded with *Staphylococcus aureus* resident in ducts and glands of normal skin)
         b. Microorganisms from a deep focus of infection (e.g., peritoneal abscess, lung abscess, etc.)
         c. Microorganisms resident on the surface of normal mucous membranes (e.g., intestinal tract, respiratory tract, genitourinary tract)
         d. Microorganisms on dust particles and borne by air currents
   C. Postoperative surgical infections: These are complications of the operation and may be manifested as
      1. Surgical wound infection
      2. Respiratory tract infection
      3. Urinary tract infection

SOURCE: From F. L. Meleney, "Treatise on Surgical Infections," Oxford University Press, New York, 1948.

GENERAL PRINCIPLES

Pathogenic species of bacteria have the capacity to invade and produce disease. However, disease is a biologic accident and represents a complex interaction between the microorganism and the host which occurs only under special circumstances. Healthy people may harbor pathogenic bacteria and yet be clinically unaffected. They are referred to as carriers of the particular pathogen. The healthy carrier of pathogenic microorganisms is the principal reservoir of most diseases. Although species such as *Staphylococcus aureus* and *Escherichia coli* are examples of pathogens, individual strains may be too feeble to cause infection. Feeble or noninvasive strains may cause infection if the resistance of the host is extremely low or if tremendous numbers of bacteria are introduced. Some bacteria which are nonpathogenic under ordinary conditions are opportunistic and may be pathogenic when the host-parasite equilibrium is upset, e.g., when normal flora is eliminated by antibiotics or when incision makes available a new area of the body. Antibiotic-resistant strains of *Staphylococcus aureus* of specific phage types, which cause nosocomial postoperative wound infections, may be endemic among carrier personnel of a particular hospital. The patient may become infected by direct contact with a carrier or may become infected with a hospital staphylococcus with which he has become colonized during hospitalization.

The term *virulence* refers to the tissue-invading powers of a specific strain of a pathogen and is used in two different ways: First, virulence describes quantitatively the smallest dose of a bacterial strain which will produce disease in a specified host. This assessment is usually conducted in experimental animals and may have no relation to human disease. Second, virulence describes an epidemiologic concept such as a given phage type of *Staphylococcus aureus* producing human disease more frequently than another. In this situation, virulence is based on ecologic advantage in the external environment but may not necessarily involve greater capacity to be virulent as measured by the critical dose of bacteria causing clinical infection.

A large infecting dose is favorable to the production of bacterial disease, because only a small number of bacteria may actually reach a favorable site in the host. A sudden change to a different environment or to a new site may injure most of the inoculum. Moreover, the defense mechanisms of the host often destroy a large proportion of the invading organisms before they can become established. The greater the number of bacteria introduced into the host, the greater the amount of preformed toxins that will be carried along. Preformed toxins may protect bacteria from destruction during the period when they are adapting to the new environment and are incapable of producing additional toxin. The resistance of the host is shown in his ability to keep bacteria out of the body initially and, failing in this, to localize and destroy them. A healthy, unbroken skin is the first line of resistance. Although mucous membranes are less resistant, even here minute breaks usually provide for bacterial entry. It is then that active defensive measures come into play. Primary defenses include the system of fixed phagocytic cells (i.e., the histiocytes of the reticuloendothelial system) and mobile phagocytes. These are aided by antibacterial substances in blood plasma, lymph, and interstitial fluid, by physical barriers to the spread of bacteria (i.e., ground substances, serous and fibrous membranes), and by local and systemic reactions such as hyperemia, fever, and leukocytosis. Secondary defenses are dependent upon the presence of specific antigenic stimuli (bacteria and bacterial products). The antibodies formed in response to these antigens inhibit or destroy bacteria, or neutralize their toxins. In the presence of sufficient antibodies, the primary defenses are greatly accelerated, bacteria are phagocytized and digested more quickly than before, and the ability of serum to neutralize bacterial toxins is increased many thousandfold. The presence of other disease may greatly reduce resistance to microbial infection. For example, diabetes predisposes to infection of the skin and the genitourinary tract. Influenza, measles, and other viral infections markedly predispose to secondary bacterial infections of the respiratory tract. Malignant disease, malnutrition, chronic alcoholism, etc., may interfere seriously with an individual's resistance to disease.

Bacteria cause disease by invading tissues and producing toxins. Bacterial invasion leads to demonstrable damage of host cells and tissues in the vicinity of the invasion, whereas bacterial toxins are transported by the blood and lymph to cause cytotoxic effects at sites removed from the initial lesion. Species such as *Streptococcus pyogenes* are both invasive and toxigenic. *Staphylococcus aureus* produces local damage but has little tendency to spread, although the local inflammatory response may be severe as in the case of carbuncles. *Clostridium tetani* is almost solely toxigenic. Generally, invasiveness and toxigenicity are not completely separable, since invasion involves some degree of toxin production and toxigenicity requires some degree of bacterial multiplication. Exotoxins are specific, soluble, diffusible, proteins produced by gram-positive bacteria as they multiply in a circumscribed area. Exotoxins lose their toxicity upon denaturation but retain much of their original antigenicity. Such modified exotoxins are called *toxoids*. Those prepared from *Clostridium tetani* are used to induce active immunity in man. The alpha toxin of *Clostridium perfringens* is a lecithinase which acts upon the membrane lipids of body cells and erythrocytes. Endotoxins are complex lipopolysaccharides of the bacterial cell wall produced by many gram-negative species. They are released only on partial or complete dissolution of the bacterial cell. Endotoxins are relatively heat-stable; many withstand temperatures of 60 to 100°C for 1 hour. They do not form toxoids. Their toxicity is associated with the phospholipid moiety of the molecule, whereas their antigenic determinants are associated with the polysaccharide moiety.

Diagnosis

The classic signs and symptoms of infection are redness, swelling, heat, and pain. Redness of the skin, due to intense hyperemia, is seen only in infections of the skin itself.

Swelling accompanies infection unless the infection is confined to bone which cannot swell. Heat results from hyperemia and may be detected in the absence of redness. Pain is the most universal sign of infection. Along with pain goes tenderness, or pain to the touch, which is greatest over the area of maximal involvement. Loss of function is another sign of infection. It is brought about by reflex and by voluntary immobilization. The patient immobilizes the painful part in the most comfortable position he can find. For example, a finger with an infected tendon sheath is kept flexed. In peritonitis, the abdominal muscles are maintained in a state of tonic contraction to keep the inflamed peritoneum beneath from moving. Fever and tachycardia are additional, albeit nonspecific, signs of infection. Fever and chills indicate septicemia, while an elevated pulse rate is a sign of a toxic state.

Leukocytosis accompanies an acute bacterial infection more often than a viral infection. The more severe the infection, the greater is the leukocytosis. In most surgical infections, the total leukocyte count is only slightly or moderately elevated. However, a high leukocyte count $(35,000/mm^3)$ occurs as a result of suppuration. The endotoxin released by gram-negative bacilli is thought to contribute to the production of high leukocyte counts. However, in the elderly, in the severely ill, and during therapy with antibiotic and immunosuppressive drugs, white cell counts may be normal or low. The leukopenia of overwhelming sepsis is probably due to exhaustion of the supply of leukocytes and to bone marrow depression. Although the total number of leukocytes is normal in some infections, there is a preponderance of immature granulocytes, which may be increased above 85 percent compared with the normal below 75 percent ("shift to the left"). A chronic infection may be evident only by fatigue, low-grade fever, and perhaps anemia. Moreover, massive pyogenic abscesses may occur without leukocytosis, fever, or tenderness.

Exudate from the area of infection should be examined for color, odor, and consistency. The microorganisms causing a surgical infection often may be seen microscopically on gram-stained smears. For each bacterial cell observed under the oil-immersion lens, there are approximately 10^5 similar organisms in each milliliter of exudate from which the smear was prepared. The staining and examination of slides are simple, rapid, inexpensive procedures which provide valuable and immediate information for the surgeon. Pus from deep-seated abscesses may be obtained by needle aspiration or at the time of definitive drainage. Exudate from surface infections may be examined directly. Specimens submitted to the bacteriologic laboratory should be collected before chemotherapy is begun and should be labeled adequately to identify the patient, the clinical diagnosis, and the nature and site of the specimen. The laboratory should be requested to do aerobic and anaerobic cultures and antibiotic-sensitivity tests. The surgeon must initiate treatment immediately upon clinical judgment, although the subsequent laboratory report will often enable him to make appropriate changes.

Biopsy is useful in establishing a diagnosis in granulomatous infections such as tuberculosis, syphilis, and my-coses. Additional sources of biopsy material are enlarged lymph nodes draining an area of infection or a sinus tract. Blood cultures are often helpful in identifying the microorganisms causing surgical infection. Transient bacteremias accompany the early phase of many infections and may result from manipulation of infected or contaminated tissues (surgical incision of furuncles or abscesses, instrumentation of the genitourinary tract, dental procedures, etc.). Bacteria usually enter the circulation via the lymphatic system. Consequently, when bacteria multiply at a site of local infection in tissues, the lymph drained from that area carries bacteria to the thoracic duct and eventually to the venous blood. However, a blood culture taken at the time of chill and fever may be negative for bacterias, as phagocytes promptly remove bacteria suddenly entering the bloodstream and chill and fever occur 30 to 90 minutes later. Thus, blood cultures should be taken at frequent intervals in a patient with febrile disease of unknown origin in an attempt to obtain blood before an expected chill and rise in temperature. A careful history and physical examination provide the basis for diagnosis and laboratory tests.

Surgical Therapy

It is necessary to distinguish between contamination and infection. Almost all wounds are contaminated with bacteria from the skin or from sources external to the patient. However, very few wounds become infected (i.e., exhibit disease manifested by inflammation, etc.). The major clinical responses to wound infection are suppuration and invasion. Bacteria grow in the wound on substrates consisting of blood clots, lymph, leukocytes, and necrotic debris. Extension of the local inflammatory response to adjacent tissues is associated with a systemic reaction. The hazard of generalized infection is associated with all traumatic wounds. These and preoperative surgical infections are treated to overcome existing infection and to prevent postoperative infection. Local treatment consists of debridement of all necrotic or injured tissue, drainage of abscesses, removal of foreign bodies, and therapy with antibiotics. Supportive measures governing the treatment of established surgical infections are bed rest, immobilization of the infected region, elevation to promote venous and lymphatic drainage, and relief of swelling and pain. Moist heat is applied to increase local blood supply, facilitate exudation, and hasten sloughing. The detailed management of wounds is discussed in Chap. 8 (Wound Healing and Wound Care).

Antibiotic Therapy

The adjunctive use of antibiotics in the treatment of infections is dependent upon an adequate blood supply and is most effective against acute infections such as cellulitis, septicemia, or peritonitis. Antibiotics have slight access to abscesses and penetrate by slow diffusion, if at all. In these situations, they should be used in conjunction with incision and drainage. Antibiotics are the primary treatment for acute spreading infections and should result in clinical improvement in 24 to 48 hours. Change to a more effective antibiotic may be based on the culture and sensitivity report.

Although clinical judgment frequently must be used to select an antibiotic and although the causative microorganism often is revealed on microscopic examination of a gram-stained smear of exudate or pus, the infecting microorganisms should be identified and antibiotic sensitivities determined by the laboratory. Accordingly, the specimen for culture (pus, exudate, blood, or urine) should be obtained before chemotherapy is begun. In severe infections, exudate can often be inoculated on a blood agar plate and antibiotic sensitivity discs positioned so that rapid, presumptive sensitivity information can be obtained after incubation overnight or for several hours. This crude procedure does not replace the official pure culture studies of all microorganisms isolated from the specimen.

Hyperbaric Therapy

Brummelkamp and associates in Amsterdam introduced the hyperbaric oxygen chamber for operative procedures. In 1963 they reported the first use of hyperbaric oxygen for gas-producing infections. Both the patient and medical personnel were placed in a room-sized chamber in which the air pressure was raised to three times that of the normal atmosphere (i.e., 2,200 mm Hg, or 3 atm absolute). For seven periods of $1\frac{1}{2}$ hours for 3 days, the patient inhaled 100% oxygen from a face mask, which increased the normal oxygen tension in plasma, lymph, and tissue fluids about fifteen to twenty times. Dramatic clinical improvement was described in most patients within the first day. The Amsterdam group advises that "operations be limited to opening the original wound and incising abscesses. Any further excision and removal of necrotic tissue can be done much later after clinical resolution. The advantage of postponement is that the operation can be performed in a dramatically improved patient who is no longer toxic." Large pressure chambers are expensive ($250,000 to $500,000) and available at only a few medical centers in the world. Much less expensive, single-patient isolators have been used to treat patients. Therapy with hyperbaric oxygen, antibiotics, and surgical debridement has been effective for clostridial infections. Hyperbaric oxygenation appeared to reduce toxemia and diminish the amount of tissue requiring excision. However, gas-producing infection due to anaerobic streptococci, *Escherichia coli,* and *Klebsiella* species showed no improvement after exposure to high-pressure oxygen. Although the use of hyperbaric oxygen is advocated by some as an adjunct to the surgical treatment of clostridial infections, the reliability of immediate surgical treatment and adjunctive antibiotic therapy remains unquestioned.

SOME COMMON SURGICAL INFECTIONS

Cellulitis is a nonsuppurative inflammation of the subcutaneous tissues extending along connective tissue planes and across intercellular spaces. There is widespread swelling, redness, and pain without definite localization. Central necrosis and suppuration may occur at a later stage. In severe infections, blebs and bullae form on the skin. Although a variety of aerobic and anaerobic bacteria produce cellulitis, the hemolytic streptococci are the classic etiologic agents. Treatment consists of antibiotic therapy and rest. Failure of the inflammatory swelling to subside after 48 to 72 hours of antibiotic therapy suggests that an abscess has developed, and that incision and drainage are needed.

Lymphangitis is an inflammation of lymphatic pathways which is usually visible as erythematous streaking of the skin. This is especially true in infections by hemolytic streptococci. Lymphangitis and the associated inflammatory swelling of lymph nodes (*lymphadenitis*) are a normal defense reaction against bacterial invasion and are frequently seen in the forearm of a patient with an infection of the hand or fingers. Most cases will respond to antibiotic therapy and rest.

Erysipelas is an acute spreading cellulitis and lymphangitis, usually caused by hemolytic streptococci which gain entrance through a break in the skin. There is a severe systemic as well as local reaction with abrupt onset, chills, fever, and prostration. The skin is red, swollen, and tender, and there is a distinct line of demarcation at the advancing margin of the infection. Erysipelas may develop on any cutaneous surface but commonly involves the face in a "butterfly lesion" over the nose and cheeks. Recurrent erysipelas in an extremity may lead to chronic lymphedema. Antibiotic therapy will usually halt the progress of the invasive infection, but the erythema disappears more slowly since it is a toxigenic consequence of bacterial invasion.

Infection in soft tissues is of paramount concern to the surgeon, and a variety of superficial infections will be discussed. An *abscess* is a localized collection of pus surrounded by an area of inflamed tissue in which hyperemia and infiltration of leukocytes is marked. A *furuncle,* or boil, is an abscess in a sweat gland or hair follicle. The inflammatory reaction is intense, leading to tissue necrosis and the formation of a central core. This is surrounded by a peripheral zone of cellulitis. An abscess beneath the corium of the skin is a *subepithelial abscess. Impetigo* is an acute contagious skin disease characterized by the formation of a series of intraepithelial abscesses. Gangrenous impetigo may occur as a complication in severe chronic debilitating diseases (e.g., chronic ulcerative colitis), and hemolytic streptococci and staphylococci can be cultured from the exudate. The lesions appear as multiple small pustules which extend and coalesce to form large areas of cutaneous gangrene and ulceration. Although management is similar to that of postoperative gangrene, favorable response is proportional to success in overcoming the primary disease. A *carbuncle* is a multilocular suppurative extension of a furuncle into the subcutaneous tissues. The nape of the neck, dorsum of trunk, hands and digits, and hirsute portions of the chest and abdomen are apt to be involved. Individual compartments in a carbuncle are maintained through persistence of fascial attachments to the skin. As these numerous component locules rupture separately, individual fistulas appear. Most abscesses are caused by pyogenic cocci, usually *Staphylococcus aureus.* However, gram-negative bacilli and streptococci may be found coincidentally.

The course of a furuncle is often self-limited and may require no specific therapy. However, a furuncle in the "dangerous" nasolabial area of the face bounded by the bridge of the nose and the angles of the mouth should not be disturbed by incision, squeezing, or other manipulation, since abscesses in this location may be complicated by septic phlebitis with intracranial extension along the nasal veins to the cavernous sinus. Treatment of facial furuncles consists of antibiotic therapy and warm compresses. Abscesses in regions other than the face should be incised and drained, and the patient treated with antibiotics.

Bacteremia is defined as bacteria in the circulating blood with no indication of toxemia or other clinical manifestations. Bacteremia is usually transient and may last only a few moments, as the reticuloendothelial system localizes and destroys these organisms under favorable conditions. The normal individual probably experiences bacteremia, unknowingly, many times each year. This state follows dental procedures, major traumatic wounds, or similar events, and may be the means by which apparently isolated infections arise in internal organs, e.g., osteomyelitis, pyelonephritis (descending type), or subacute bacterial endocarditis.

Septicemia is a diffuse infection in which infectious bacteria and their toxins are present in the bloodstream. Septicemia may arise directly from the introduction of infecting organisms into the circulation but, as a rule, is secondary to a focus of infection within the body. The major routes by which bacteria reach the blood are (1) by direct extension and entrance into an open vessel, (2) by release of infected emboli following thrombosis of a blood vessel in an area of inflammation, (3) by discharge of infected lymph into the bloodstream following lymphangitis. Many specific diseases, e.g., typhoid fever and brucellosis, include a septicemic phase. In the absence of systemic disease, beta-hemolytic streptococci (*Streptococcus pyogenes*) are most frequently responsible. Septicemia caused by alpha-hemolytic streptococci (*Streptococcus viridans*) is usually a consequence of subacute bacterial endocarditis. The majority of bacteria that produce suppurative lesions may give rise to secondary septicemia. *Pyemia* is septicemia in which pyogenic microorganisms, most notably *Staphylococcus aureus,* and their toxins are carried in the bloodstream and sequentially initiate multiple focal abscesses in many parts of the body. Before the advent of chemotherapy, staphylococcic pyemia was almost always fatal; the mortality is still high. In *toxemia,* toxins are circulating in the blood, though the microorganism producing the toxin need not be. Toxemia is usually associated with infection by toxin-producing bacteria (e.g., the clostridia of gas gangrene and the diphtheria bacillus), but this is not always so. For example, botulinum toxin and staphylococcal enterotoxin may be ingested directly to cause a profound toxemia without true infection.

PRINCIPLES OF ANTIBIOTIC THERAPY

Basic Considerations

Chemotherapeutic agents act primarily upon the parasite and not upon the host. They include antibiotics and metabolic antagonists such as the sulfonamides. An antibiotic is a chemical compound derived from, or produced by, living organisms and capable, at low concentrations, of inhibiting the life processes of microorganisms. *Bacteriostatic* agents prevent the growth of bacteria but do not destroy them. The defense mechanisms of the body then eliminate the bacteria which are unable to multiply. If the defenses are insufficient or if the bacteriostatic drug is withdrawn prematurely, then the bacterial population will resurge, and the patient will suffer a relapse. *Bactericidal* agents actively kill bacteria and must be employed in patients whose defense mechanisms are impaired or altered by disease or immunosuppressive therapy. The distinction between bactericidal and bacteriostatic effects is sometimes relative to duration of therapy and dosage. Some drugs are bacteriostatic at low concentrations and bactericidal at high concentrations. With most bactericidal drugs, the rate of killing increases with concentration. Antibiotic agents exert their effects in a variety of ways (Table 5-3). They may inhibit the synthesis of the bacterial cell wall and consequently interfere with the cell's osmotic defenses, or they may affect the barrier function of the cell membrane and cause loss of vital metabolites. An entirely different mode of action impairs the translation of genetic information and affects protein synthesis. Bacteriostatic drugs affect early stages of protein synthesis in the ribosome and result in an insufficiency, preventing growth and proliferation of bacteria without actually destroying them. However, bactericidal drugs cause the ribosome to miscode and consequently induce the manufacture of defective proteins or enzymes which poison the cell. Replication of deoxyribonucleic acid (DNA) in the chromosome at the level of the assembly of purine nucleotides may be affected by some antibiotics. Although their precise

Table 5-3. ANTIBIOTICS: MODES OF ACTION

Cellular site of action	Bactericidal	Bacteriostatic
Cell wall synthesis . . .	Penicillins Cephalosporins Vancomycin Bacitracin	
Barrier function of cell membrane. . . .	Polymyxin B Colistin Amphotericin B	Nystatin
Protein synthesis in ribosome	Streptomycin Kanamycin Neomycin	Tetracyclines Chloramphenicol Erythromycin Lincomycin
DNA replication in chromosome	Griseofulvin	

locus of action is not known, these drugs impede the replication of genetic information.

The addition of antibiotics to the armamentarium of the physician has revolutionized the practice of medicine, but has been a double-edged sword. It is pertinent to point out that the surgeon employs antibiotic drugs as adjunctive agents in the treatment of surgical infections, whereas the internist usually employs antibiotics as the primary treatment for medical infections. For the surgeon the aims of antibiotic therapy are much the same as those of surgical therapy, i.e., to control or eradicate bacterial infections acquired before or during hospitalization and to prevent infection from developing postoperatively. To obtain these goals, antibiotic agents are administered (1) systemically by either parenteral or oral routes, (2) preoperatively for preparation of the large intestine (intestinal antisepsis), or (3) locally by (a) topical irrigation, (b) topical application, (c) intraperitoneal, intrapleural, or intrathecal instillation or irrigation, and (d) intraluminal instillation into the large intestine. Antibacterial drugs may be administered preoperatively, intraoperatively, and postoperatively to prevent infection (prophylaxis) or to treat already established infection.

The fundamental principles governing the use of antibiotics are (1) administration of an agent active against the infecting microorganism, (2) adequate contact between the drug and the infecting microbe, (3) absence of (or minimal) toxic side effects or complications, and (4) utilization of host defenses to augment antibacterial effects of the antibiotic. The specificity of the antibiotic for the infecting microorganism is based upon laboratory identification and antibiotic-sensitivity studies. Clinical judgment is called upon in serious, rapidly developing infections, such as gram-negative shock, to administer antibiotics known to be effective. However, cultures should be taken, and the antibiotic changed, if necessary, when culture and antibiotic-sensitivity reports are available.

The antibiotic must come in contact with the infecting microorganism. In an acute, diffuse infection, blood flow into the area of infection will usually deliver adequate levels of systemic antibiotic. A spreading cellulitis with lymphangitis and lymphadenitis often responds within 24 hours to an appropriate antibiotic. However, since antibiotics cannot penetrate a thick-walled pyogenic abscess or an infected serous cavity, they should be used in conjunction with drainage of the abscess, debridement of necrotic tissue, and removal of any foreign bodies. These principles apply to every organ of the body. A spreading infection of the meninges responds to chemotherapy, but a brain abscess must be drained; a staphylococcal septicemia is treated by chemotherapy, but a pulp abscess of the fingertip must be drained.

The surgeon must be aware of toxic complications of antibiotics and should be prepared to treat them. Toxic effects range from minor skin rashes, drug fever, and gastrointestinal disturbances to renal tubular necrosis, loss of vision and hearing, irreversible blood dyscrasias, and anaphylactic shock. In addition, alterations in the normal flora of the body may occur in patients receiving antibiotic therapy. In most cases these changes produce no ill result, but in some the alterations of flora result in the rapid overgrowth of virulent, antibiotic-resistant bacteria which may have been present originally in small numbers (colonization). If the patient's general resistance to infection is depressed, a new infection may follow the antibiotic-induced alteration of flora (superinfection). The term *colonization* indicates an antibiotic-induced quantitative change in the resident microflora of the patient, a common consequence of antimicrobial therapy. There is no clinical evidence of secondary infection, and discontinuance of the antibiotic usually allows the normal flora to become reestablished. However, there is the risk that colonization will lead to superinfection, a clinical event which may be of great danger to the patient. The term *superinfection* usually refers to a new microbial disease induced by antibiotic therapy. Superinfection is often due to gram-negative bacilli and fungi which are more difficult to eradicate than are gram-positive streptococci and pneumococci. Superinfection may be fatal, usually occurs in elderly patients, and often follows therapy with aminoglycoside antibiotics (streptomycin, neomycin, and kanamycin) and other broad-spectrum drugs (either alone or in combination with penicillin). Clinical evidence of secondary infection (i.e., a rise in temperature, increased peripheral white blood cell count, and physical signs of a disease not present at the beginning of antibiotic therapy) indicates that colonization has progressed to superinfection.

Secondary or opportunistic infections may also occur in patients with noninfectious diseases. For example, mycotic infections may develop in patients with lymphoma or leukemia. Deficiencies in host resistance as a result of disease (e.g., diabetes mellitus, hematopoietic disorders, renal failure, liver disease) or as a consequence of therapy with radiation, antimetabolites, or corticosteroids confer the potential for pathogenicity on many ordinary nonpathogenic microorganisms. Indwelling venous or urinary catheters also contribute to lowered host resistance. It is suggested that the term *suprainfection* be retained for secondary infections unrelated to antibiotic therapy and that the term *antibiotic-induced suprainfection* be used to describe secondary infections arising during treatment with antimicrobial agents.

Chemoprophylaxis

Prophylactic antibiotics are administered to an uninfected patient who is in jeopardy of acquiring a bacterial infection. There is controversy regarding prophylactic antibiotic therapy because prophylaxis has not been as valuable as therapeutic use. In surgical patients, prophylactic antibiotics are administered to treat contaminated wounds before infection occurs. However, the administration of antibiotic drugs cannot be substituted for sound surgical judgment and good surgical technique. Prophylactic antibiotic therapy has no place in clean operative procedures or in those carrying a minimal risk of sepsis, but it should be considered for traumatic injuries and severe burns and for operations in infected tissues or those associated with heavy contamination (e.g., operations involving the large intestine). An equally beneficial role for chemoprophylaxis is prior to operations on patients especially prone to infection because of malnutrition, impoverished blood supply, or preexisting infection remote from the operative site. The patient undergoing immunosuppressive therapy and/or requiring insertion of a permanent prosthetic device is particularly prone to infection.

Surgical wounds have been designated as "clean," "contaminated," or "dirty" depending upon the presence or absence of prior infection and contact with the interior of the respiratory, urinary, or gastrointestinal tracts. Traumatic wounds are generally grossly contaminated, whereas elective clean surgical procedures may be slightly contaminated during the operative procedure. Infection does not necessarily follow contamination, since host factors as well as microbial factors are involved. However, the greater the contamination, the greater the possibility of consequent infection. Accordingly, in surgery of traumatic wounds or in elective "contaminated" or "dirty" surgery, prophylaxis should be started before the operation so that adequate levels of antibiotic may be obtained in tissue and body fluids during the operative procedure. Bernard and Cole (1964) investigated the use of antibiotics administered intramuscularly 1 to 2 hours prior to surgery, intravenously during the operation, and postoperatively when the patient was in the recovery room. They found a reduced incidence of postoperative infection (5 percent) with prophylactic treatment compared with administration of a placebo (25 percent). However, a prophylactic antibiotic regimen may not be successful if the drug is not effective against all potential pathogens or if the agent does not come in contact with susceptible pathogens at the site of infection. The antibiotic should be administered parenterally and in sufficient dosage to achieve high circulating blood levels. For treatment of patients with severe trauma, antibiotic therapy should be started prior to operation, as manipulation of wounds causes transient bacteremia.

Intestinal Antisepsis

The protocol for preoperative preparation of the large intestine includes the specific prophylactic use of antibiotics. Bacterial infection following elective colonic surgery results from unavoidable seeding of the wound with contents of the colon. This is manifested by intraabdominal abscesses and anastomotic disruption with resultant peritonitis and fistula formation. The ideal antibiotic agent for preoperative preparation of the colon has rapid bactericidal activity against pathogens in the gastrointestinal tract, minimal absorption, and the absence of undesirable or toxic side effects. The protocol we employ involves a 3-day period of hospitalization during which the patient is placed on a low-residue diet (some surgeons prefer a clear diet), given a cathartic and daily enemas, and administered a suitable chemotherapeutic agent for 72 hours. Although mechanical cleansing alone diminishes the volume of feces and, consequently, the total number of enteric bacteria, the remaining feces contain the usual large numbers of bacteria (on the order of 10^{11} bacteria per gram), and the

potential for postoperative infections remains a major hazard. Therefore, although there is no uniform agreement, we feel that antibiotic therapy along with mechanical cleansing is essential for an effective 3-day preoperative preparation of the large intestine. The antibiotics most frequently employed are kanamycin (1 Gm every hour for 4 hours, and then every 6 hours for a total of 72 hours) and Sulfathalidine-neomycin in combination (every hour for 4 hours, and then every 4 hours for a total of 72 hours). Intestinal antisepsis has been shown to reduce the incidence of postoperative complications related to bacteria but does not protect against errors of surgical skill or judgment.

Intraperitoneal Antibiotic Therapy

The most frequent indications for the intraperitoneal instillation of antibiotics are perforated and gangrenous appendicitis, perforated peptic ulcer, gangrenous intestinal obstruction, traumatic perforation of the gastrointestinal tract at any level, intraabdominal abscess, and excessive spillage associated with elective colonic, gastric, or small bowel surgery. Intraperitoneally administered antibiotics may be useful in pelvic inflammatory disease, acute pancreatitis, major intraabdominal vascular procedures, closure of evisceration, and repair of large abdominal incisional hernias. To be effective for routine intraperitoneal instillation, the antibiotic must provide adequate control of endogenous enteric bacteria that may be expected in the peritoneal cavity, with minimal accompanying pain and local or systemic reaction. Since intraperitoneal antibiotics are usually administered to anesthetized patients, the possible synergistic activity of the antibiotic and the anesthetic agent must be considered. This danger may be avoided if the catheter is placed in the peritoneal cavity after the operation, but before the incision is completely closed, and antibiotic instilled after the patient has recovered from anesthesia. Neomycin is safe for intraperitoneal administration only when the dosage is carefully controlled. Clinical success and safety have been achieved with kanamycin and also with cephalothin. Multiple postoperative instillations of kanamycin in patients with peritonitis reduce the incidence of wound infections and are more effective than a single instillation of the drug. The intraluminal administration of kanamycin into the colon to prevent perforation, slough, and leakage at the anastomosis has been recommended to support a colon anastomosis postoperatively.

ANTIMICROBIAL AGENTS

Antibiotics and chemotherapeutic agents which are currently useful in surgical practice are described briefly in this section. It is important to use an antibiotic agent for a sensitive microorganism and not to treat a particular disease. Precise antimicrobial therapy is based upon the laboratory culture and sensitivity report. Table 5-4 is a guide to the activities of antibiotics against microorganisms commonly involved in surgical infections. Table 5-5 sum-

Table 5-4. ANTIBIOTICS USEFUL AGAINST MICROORGANISMS COMMONLY INVOLVED
IN SURGICAL INFECTIONS

Microorganisms	First choice(s)	Second choice(s)	Third choice(s)
Streptococcus pyogenes	Penicillin G	Erythromycin	Cephalothin, lincomycin
Streptococcus viridans	Penicillin G ± streptomycin	Erythromycin	Cephalothin, lincomycin
Streptococcus fecalis	Penicillin G + streptomycin or kanamycin	Ampicillin ± streptomycin or kanamycin	
✱ Anaerobic streptococcus	Penicillin G		
Diplococcus pneumoniae.	Penicillin G	Erythromycin	Cephalothin, lincomycin, tetracycline
Neisseria gonorrhoeae	Penicillin G	Erythromycin, tetracycline	Cephaloridine, kanamycin
Staphylococcus (non-penicillinase-producing)	Penicillin G	Erythromycin	Cephalothin, lincomycin
Staphylococcus (penicillinase-producing)	Oxacillin, methicillin, cloxacillin	Cephalothin	Lincomycin
✱ Clostridium spp.	Penicillin G	Tetracycline	Erythromycin
Diphtheroids	Penicillin G	Cephalothin	Erythromycin, tetracycline
Pseudomonas aeruginosa	Colistin, polymyxin B	Carbenicillin	Gentamicin, kanamycin
Escherichia coli.	Kanamycin, gentamicin	Ampicillin, cephalothin	Tetracycline + streptomycin
Salmonella spp.	Chloramphenicol, ampicillin	Kanamycin	Tetracycline + streptomycin
Klebsiella-Enterobacter-Serratia group . . .	Kanamycin, gentamicin	Colistin	Tetracycline + streptomycin
Proteus mirabilis	Ampicillin, penicillin G	Kanamycin	Cephalothin
Other Proteus spp..	Kanamycin, gentamicin	Tetracycline + streptomycin	Cephalothin
Mima-Herellea group	Kanamycin + tetracycline		
✱ Bacteroides spp.	Tetracycline, penicillin G	Tetracycline, lincomycin	Chloramphenicol, clindamycin
Actinomyces israelii	Penicillin G	Cephalothin	Tetracycline
Candida albicans	Amphotericin B	Nystatin	

Table 5-5. ROUTES OF ADMINISTRATION AND DAILY DOSAGE OF
ANTIBIOTICS COMMONLY USED

Dose in grams per day

Drug	Oral	Intramuscular	Intravenous
Cephalosporins:			
Cephalexin.	1–4		
Cephalothin	. . . . . .	2–6	4–12
Cephaloridine	. . . . . .	1–2	1–2
Chloramphenicol	2–6	Not recommended	2–6
Erythromycin.	1–2	0.2–0.6	1–4
Gentamicin	. . . . . .	0.2–0.4	0.2–0.4
Kanamycin	4–7*	0.5–1	0.5–1
Lincomycin	1–2	1–2	1–2
Penicillins:			
Ampicillin	1–12	2–12	2–12
Carbenicillin.	. . . . . .	8–12	20–40
Cloxacillin	2–3		
Dicloxacillin	1–2		
Methicillin	. . . . . .	4–6	4–24
Nafcillin	2–6	2–6	3–24
Oxacillin	2–6	2–6	4–24
Penicillin G (crystalline)	0.5–1	2–12 million (units/day)	2–20 million (units/day)
Polymyxin B	. . . . . .	0.2–0.4	0.2–0.4
Colistin (Polymyxin E)	. . . . . .	0.2–0.4	0.2–0.4
Streptomycin	. . . . . .	1–2	
Tetracyclines:			
Oxytetracycline	1–2	0.2–0.8	1–2
Tetracycline	1–2	0.2–0.8	1–2

*Intestinal antisepsis only.

marizes the routes of administration and doses commonly employed. The selection of antibiotic and dosage for a specific infection depend upon clinical judgment, sensitivity tests, and toxicity of the drug. Individual agents are considered in terms of mechanism of antimicrobial action, absorption, distribution, metabolic fate, excretion, toxicity, and indications for use.

Antibiotics Active against Gram-positive Microorganisms

Penicillin G (benzyl penicillin) is active against almost all gram-positive pathogens. If necessary, very large doses can be given to combat infections by bacterial species which may be moderately resistant. Penicillin is bactericidal for susceptible bacteria; it blocks the synthesis of bacterial cell walls. Penicillin G is well absorbed but is not suitable for oral administration, because it is destroyed by gastric acidity. Therefore, it is injected intramuscularly or intravenously and becomes distributed throughout the body within a few minutes following injection. Excretion is mainly by the renal tubules. Hypersensitivity to penicillin is an important problem; it is usually manifested as urticaria, but almost any type of allergic response may develop. Anaphylactic reactions may occur in the highly sensitized patient within minutes after an injection and will require subcutaneous epinephrine. Penicillin G is recommended (provided hypersensitivity does not exist) for severe infections produced by beta-hemolytic streptococci, enterococci, pneumococci, gonococci, meningococci, clostridia, actinomycetes, and treponemata.

Penicillin V (phenoxymethyl penicillin) is a natural penicillin obtained when phenoxyacetic acid is the precursor during fermentation. It is acid-stable and may be administered orally. Penicillin V is more active than penicillin G against resistant staphylococci, because it is more slowly destroyed by penicillinase, and is slightly less active against streptococci. Penicillin V is not indicated for infections involving the respiratory tract or the urinary tract.

The natural penicillins have been superseded by several semisynthetic penicillins prepared by adding side chains to the 6-aminopenicillanic acid nucleus. The semisynthetic penicillins combine one or more of the following advantages: (1) they are acid-resistant and suitable for oral use; (2) they exert prolonged action in the body; (3) they are resistant to penicillinase produced by *Staphylococcus aureus* and some gram-negative bacilli; and (4) they are active against gram-negative bacteria.

Methicillin (Staphcillin) is sensitive to acid but resistant to staphylococcal penicillinase. It must be administered parenterally, and it is rapidly excreted by the renal tubules. Methicillin is inactivated by penicillinase 100 times more slowly than is penicillin G but has only one-tenth the potency of penicillin G. Methicillin is also the preferred parenteral semisynthetic penicillin against streptococci, pneumococci, and gram-negative bacteria.

Oxacillin, cloxacillin, and *dicloxacillin* are semisynthetic isoxazolyl penicillins combining resistance to penicillinase with resistance to acid. They can be administered orally and are effective against streptococcal infections compli-

cated by the presence of penicillinase-producing staphylococci. *Nafcillin* is also resistant to penicillinase and to acid. It may be used either orally or parenterally, but relatively low blood levels are obtained due to inactivation in the liver.

These penicillinase-resistant penicillins have been used to treat severe staphylococcal infections, such as pneumonia, septicemia, wound infection, and infections occurring as a consequence of malignant diseases or cardiac, hepatic, or renal disease. Although methicillin has the lowest activity against staphylococci, 60 percent of the dose is free in the blood. On the other hand, the acid-resistant penicillins have higher antibacterial activity, but only 5 percent is free. Accordingly, adequate doses of any one of these penicillins will achieve similar effects, and initial treatment of a severe staphylococcal infection should always be with one of these penicillins (unless the staphylococcus has been shown to be sensitive to penicillin G).

Cephalothin is one of a group of antibiotics known as the cephalosporins, which are structually similar to the penicillins. Cephalothin is effective against staphylococci, streptococci (except enterococci), and pneumococci. Most strains of *Escherichia coli, Proteus mirabilis,* and *Klebsiella* species are susceptible. *Enterobacter aerogenes* and *Pseudomonas aeruginosa* are resistant. Cephalosporin antibiotics, like the penicillins, are bactericidal and inhibit the synthesis of bacterial cell walls. Cephalothin must be administered parenterally, as it is not absorbed orally. Excretion is by the renal tubules. Intramuscular injections may be painful, and frequent injections are required if adequate levels of antibiotic are to be maintained. Phlebitis may occur with intravenous use; rashes are sometimes produced. Cephalothin may be administered to patients who are allergic to penicillin without danger of cross reaction, but sensitization to cephalothin itself may occur. The antibiotic is active against penicillin-resistant staphylococci. However, suprainfection with gram-negative bacilli or fungi can occur if indiscriminately large doses are used for 1 to 3 weeks. Cephalothin has a broader spectrum than ampicillin and is useful in treating urinary tract infections caused by sensitive enterobacteria.

Cephaloridine is a derivative similar to cephalothin both in its properties and indications for use. It is more stable in the body and is cleared more slowly. Renal toxicity has been encountered following large doses. Although it is not effective orally, there is little or no pain when it is injected intramuscularly. Cephaloridine is not a substitute for cephalothin since enterococci and staphylococci are not uniformly susceptible. Suprainfections have occurred.

Vancomycin is active against gram-positive organisms only, and it is of clinical importance against staphylococci and streptococci. Microorganisms sensitive to vancomycin do not acquire resistance. The antibiotic is bactericidal; it inhibits the incorporation of amino acids into the bacterial cell wall and suppresses the growth of protoplasts. Vancomycin is not absorbed from the alimentary tract and is administered intravenously; intramuscular injections cause pain and necrosis. The antibiotic is widely distributed, but little is found in bile or spinal fluid. Excretion is by glomerular filtration, but this is delayed in patients with impaired renal function, with deafness the most serious possible complication. Thrombophlebitis, fever, and rashes occur. Vancomycin is indicated for the treatment of severe staphylococcal or streptococcal disease in patients allergic or nonresponsive to other antibiotics (penicillin G, methicillin, cephalothin). Oral administration of vancomycin is recommended for the treatment of staphylococcal pseudomembranous enterocolitis.

Erythromycin is active against pneumococci, beta-hemolytic streptococci, enterococci, many staphylococci, gonococci (although less effective as an alternative agent than tetracycline), and clostridia. Erythromycin is bacteriostatic but may be bactericidal in high concentrations, inhibiting bacterial protein synthesis. Erythromycin may be administered orally or intravenously. The antibiotic is uniformly distributed throughout the body and is excreted in the urine and bile. However, the major portion of the drug is broken down in the body. Erythromycin base is generally well tolerated but may cause some gastrointestinal disturbance (nausea, vomiting, diarrhea, flatulence). Erythromycin estolate (the propionyl ester) can produce hepatic disease during prolonged administration. For this reason the plain erythromycin base is recommended. Erythromycin may be used as an alternative to penicillin for hemolytic streptococcal, staphylococcal, or pneumococcal infections in patients allergic to penicillin and for elimination of *Corynebacterium diphtheriae* from the pharynx of carriers. Bacterial resistance to erythromycin is common during long-term treatment.

Lincomycin resembles erythromycin in its antibacterial activity against staphylococci, hemolytic streptococci, and pneumococci. Bacteroides and anaerobic cocci are also sensitive. Enterobacteria and enterococci are resistant. Lincomycin is bacteriostatic; it inhibits protein synthesis. The antibiotic is absorbed from the gastrointestinal tract, but food delays absorption. The drug may also be administered intramuscularly; it becomes widely distributed, and significant levels occur in tissues and fluids. Therapeutic levels of lincomycin are found in bone. Excretion is primarily biliary; urine levels are low. Diarrhea has been the only toxic side effect reported. Lincomycin is recommended for the treatment of both acute and chronic osteomyelitis. Although the antibiotic is effective against severe staphylococcal and streptococcal infections, these diseases are readily treated with semisynthetic penicillins. Lincomycin resistance is easily induced, and the antibiotic has cross resistance with erythromycin.

Clindamycin is synthetically modified lincomycin (7-chloro-7-deoxylincomycin-HCl hydrate) which is more thoroughly absorbed and produces higher blood levels. Clindamycin is also more active against staphylococci and pneumococci and equally active against other species susceptible to lincomycin.

Bacitracin is a polypeptide active against gram-positive bacteria and pathogenic *Neisseria* species, but inactive against common gram-negative bacilli. It is bactericidal, and inhibits bacterial cell wall synthesis by binding to the cell membrane. Therefore, unlike penicillin, bacitracin is active against protoplasts. The antibiotic is not absorbed orally or by the skin. After intramuscular injection, which causes painful infiltrates at the site of injection, much of the antibiotic is bound by tissues so that systemic absorption is limited. Bacitracin does not cross the blood-brain barrier. It is excreted by the kidneys, and glomerular and tublar damage may occur. Bacitracin has no place in the systemic treatment of clinical infections, but it is useful for irrigating wounds, infected joints, or abscess cavities. It is used for topical application with neomycin and polymyxin.

Antibiotics Active against Some Gram-positive or Some Gram-negative Microorganisms or Both

Ampicillin is a semisynthetic penicillin which is slightly less active than benzyl penicillin against most gram-positive bacteria, is slightly more active against enterococci, and is destroyed by penicillinase. It is not indicated for staphylococcal infections, but it is effective against strains of gram-negative bacilli (e.g., *Escherichia coli, Proteus mirabilis,* and *Salmonella* and *Shigella* species). It is bactericidal and well absorbed when administered orally. Excretion is mainly renal, although some biliary excretion occurs. The toxicity of ampicillin is similar to that of penicillin G, but macular rashes are more frequent.

Carbenicillin is a semisynthetic, bactericidal penicillin. It is active against *Pseudomonas aeruginosa,* all species of *Proteus,* and some other enterobacteria, but it is inferior to benzyl penicillin against gram-positive bacteria. Synergism with gentamicin has been demonstrated, and combination therapy has been recommended because *Pseudomonas aeruginosa* may become resistant during treatment with carbenicillin alone.

Polymyxin B and *colistin* (polymyxin E) are basic polypeptide antibiotics having similar structure and antibacterial activity. Most species of gram-negative bacilli are sensitive to polymyxin. The exceptions are *Proteus* species, and *Neisseria* species. All species of gram-positive bacteria and fungi are resistant. Both these antibiotics are bactericidal and disrupt the cell membranes of susceptible bacteria. They are not absorbed from the alimentary tract but are well absorbed following intramuscular injection. Polymyxins lose about 50 percent of their activity in the presence of serum. They do not readily cross the blood-brain barrier. They are excreted in the urine. The polymyxins are nephrotoxic in the presence of renal disease and may be associated with respiratory arrest due to neuromuscular blockade, circumoral paresthesias, dizziness, and weakness. Polymyxin B is recommended for pseudomonal meningitis and pseudomonal endocarditis, and it may also be useful in treating infection by most strains of *Escherichia coli* and *Klebsiella-Enterobacter.* Colistin is recommended for treatment of systemic pseudomonal infections and may be useful for the same infections as those responsive to polymyxin. Both antibiotics must be injected intramuscularly. However, tablets may be used to treat diarrhea due to enteropathogenic *Escherichia coli.*

Chloramphenicol is a broad-spectrum antibiotic; it is bacteriostatic and inhibits protein synthesis by interfering with messenger ribonucleic acid (mRNA). It is well absorbed orally and parenterally. Excretion is mainly renal; about 90 percent can be detected in urine as an inactive conjugate with glucuronic acid; only about 10 percent appears as active antibiotic. Two different lethal toxic effects are known: First, total aplasia of the bone marrow with aplastic anemia may occur during treatment or as long as 4 months afterward. Second, because of deficiency in detoxifying enzymes, premature infants may accumulate sufficient free chloramphenicol to cause an acute and usually fatal circulatory collapse (gray syndrome). Minor toxic effects include soreness of the mouth from overgrowth of *Candida albicans* resulting from depression of normal flora due to antibiotic in the saliva, and optic neuritis in children with cystic fibrosis of the pancreas receiving treatment with chloramphenicol for pulmonary infection. Chloramphenicol should not be used for trivial infections or as a prophylactic agent to prevent bacterial infection. It is effective for typhoid fever and other severe *Salmonella* infections, but since most *Salmonella* infections will respond to ampicillin, chloramphenicol should be used only if the patient does not respond to ampicillin or is allergic to it. Chloramphenicol is recommended for patients who cannot tolerate tetracyclines and for those who have rickettsial disease, pssitacosis, or lymphopathia venereum. Most *Bacteroides* species are sensitive to chloramphenicol. The antibiotic should be restricted to specific indications.

The aminoglycosides include streptomycin and the neomycin group of antibiotics: neomycin, paromomycin, kanamycin, and gentamicin. They possess a wide range of bactericidal activity against gram-negative and gram-positive bacteria and mycobacteria. Bacteria acquire resistance to aminoglycosides slowly. There is little absorption from the alimentary tract and fairly slow renal excretion in unchanged form after intramuscular injection. This affords therapeutic levels for 6 to 8 hours. Aminoglycosides exhibit a high degree of mutual cross resistance, a strong tendency to damage the auditory branch of the eighth nerve, and some possibility of damage to the kidney.

Streptomycin is bactericidal and particularly active against *Mycobacterium tuberculosis,* gram-negative bacilli, and some strains of *Staphylococcus aureus.* Bactericidal effects usually occur during the phase of multiplication. There is damage to the cell membrane and interference with protein synthesis by disorganizing the proper attachments of mRNA to ribosomes. Streptomycin-resistant bacteria are frequently sensitive to neomycin and kanamycin, but strains which have developed resistance to neomycin and kanamycin usually also show resistance to streptomycin. Streptomycin usually is administered intramuscularly for systemic treatment. It is completely absorbed following parenteral injection, but it is absorbed poorly from the intestinal tract. Streptomycin levels in peritoneal fluid are high and in patients with peritonitis may be equal to those in serum. Streptomycin is rapidly excreted in the urine. Streptomycin combined with isoniazid and p-aminosalicylic acid is indicated for the treatment of tuberculosis. It also is important in the treatment of plague and tularemia, and sometimes is effective in treating infections due to *Pseudomonas aeruginosa, Proteus* species, and other coliform bacteria. However, it is not used without some

other antimicrobial agent, because bacterial resistance develops rapidly when it is given alone. Combined therapy with penicillin or cephalothin is synergistic against streptococcal infections. Streptomycin with tetracycline may be used to treat severe brucellosis and granuloma inguinale. Streptomycin with sulfadiazine is used to treat nocardiosis.

Neomycin is bactericidal; it is active against gram-negative enteric bacteria, some strains of staphylococci, and mycobacteria, but has limited usefulness because of its toxicity. Its major use is in ointments and solutions for topical application although skin sensitivity may occur. Following oral therapy, neomycin-resistant staphylococci are often found in the stool, and enteritis or even pseudomembranous enterocolitis may result. Neomycin inhibits absorption of oral penicillin V and has caused malabsorption of fat (with or without diarrhea). There is considerable risk of ototoxicity and nephrotoxicity when neomycin is given parenterally. Neomycin is used in treating patients with cirrhosis who have elevated levels of ammonia, and it is used in combination with other agents, such as sulfathalidine, bacitracin, or polymyxin B, for intestinal antisepsis prior to abdominal surgery. *Paromomycin* is similar to neomycin and kanamycin but generally administered orally. The main difference between paromomycin and other aminoglycosides is its activity against *Endameba histolytica.*

Kanamycin is bactericidal. It is rapidly absorbed after intramuscular injection, and behaves similarly to streptomycin with regard to blood levels, distribution, and excretion. It is necessary to limit the dose in accordance with renal function; the length of treatment should be limited to 7 to 10 days. Kanamycin is the drug of choice in the management of septicemias due to gram-negative bacilli and is recognized as a second-line drug for treatment of tuberculosis. Kanamycin is not absorbed and is used for preoperative intestinal antisepsis. Ototoxicity may occur; it is related to duration of therapy, blood level, and dosage greater than 15 mg/kg body weight/day.

Gentamicin is another bactericidal aminoglycoside. It is administered by intramuscular injection but is not absorbed orally. It is well-distributed in most highly vascular organs, and excretion is mainly renal. Gentamicin may exhibit nephrotoxicity and ototoxicity (affecting both vestibular and auditory branches of the eighth nerve), particularly in patients with any impairment of renal function. It should not be administered with streptomycin, kanamycin, colistin, polymyxin B, or vancomycin, as additional toxicity may result. Gentamicin is useful in treating bacteremia and severe soft tissue infections due to *Escherichia coli, Serratia marcescens,* and many *Proteus* species (but not *Proteus vulgaris*), and it is most effective in treatment of infections due to *Pseudomonas aeruginosa.* However, it is not recommended as an initial therapy of severe infections of unknown cause, because many gram-negative bacteria are resistant.

The tetracyclines are a family of closely related antibiotics. Those now widely used are *tetracycline, oxytetracycline,* and *doxycycline.* There is no good evidence that tetracycline has any advantage over oxytetracycline in the treatment of disease or in the production of fewer side effects in the adult. Doxycycline possesses the advantage, because of its slower excretion, of requiring only one dose daily. Members of this group are broad-spectrum and active against those gram-positive species which are also sensitive to penicillin, against many gram-negative species which are not sensitive to penicillin, against *Treponema pallidum* and other treponemata, and against *Mycobacterium tuberculosis*. The tetracyclines are bacteriostatic. They interfere with protein synthesis by inhibiting amino acid transfer from RNA to microsomal protein. Resistance may be due to decreased permeability to the antibiotic. A microorganism resistant to one tetracycline is equally resistant to the others. Tetracyclines are usually administered orally; they become distributed throughout the body and appear to have affinity for fast-growing tissues, such as liver, tumors, and new bone. They are slowly filtered by the renal glomeruli and are excreted in the urine unchanged. Some biliary excretion occurs. Tetracyclines are deposited in teeth during early stages of calcification, causing a yellow to brownish discoloration which is undesirable cosmetically. Therefore, tetracycline treatment should be avoided in early childhood except for imperative reasons or unless a short course will suffice. Liver damage has resulted from excessive doses. Replacement of suppressed normal flora by tetracycline-resistant microorganisms (suprainfection) causes gastrointestinal disturbance such as nausea, vomiting, diarrhea, and flatulence. Suprainfection with *Candida albicans* may produce soreness of the mouth and even thrush, which may spread to the pharynx and bronchi, or diarrhea and pruritus ani. Suprainfection with *Proteus* and *Pseudomonas* species resistant to tetracycline commonly produces diarrhea. Suprainfection with *Staphylococcus aureus* may produce a fatal staphylococcal enterocolitis. Tetracycline is effective against 50 percent of strains of *Bacteroides*. Tetracycline with penicillin is recommended for actinomycosis and, with sulfadiazine, for nocardiosis. If penicillin cannot be used, tetracycline is recommended for treatment of gonorrhea and syphilis.

Antifungal Antibiotics

Nystatin is effective in the treatment of candidiasis. It is fungistatic and damages the fungal cell membrane. The antibiotic is poorly absorbed from the gastrointestinal tract and skin. It is used to treat gastrointestinal candidiasis, which may result as a complication of therapy with broad-spectrum antibiotics. Nystatin is available in topical powders, creams, and ointments which may be useful in treating cutaneous and mucocutaneous candidiasis. Nystatin tablets may be sucked for candida stomatitis; vaginal tablets are available for treatment of vaginal candidiasis. Nystatin appears to be harmless by local application; no proved cases of human sensitivity have been reported. There have been occasional cases of diarrhea, nausea, and vomiting during oral therapy.

Griseofulvin has its greatest activity against dermatophytes and is useful in treating superficial dermatomycoses due to microspora, *Epidermophyton*, and *Trichophyton*. The antibiotic is fungistatic and administered orally. It is incorporated into liver, fat, keratin, and skeletal muscle. The antibiotic is well tolerated even during long courses of treatment, and toxic effects (skin reactions, gastric discomfort, and neurologic reactions) are uncommon and rarely severe. Griseofulvin has value in the systemic treatment of chronic fungal infection of the nails and hair.

Amphotericin B is the only antifungal antibiotic effective in the treatment of systemic mycotic infections. It is used in the treatment of systemic candidiasis, mucormycosis, disseminated active histoplasmosis, cryptococcosis, coccidioidomycosis, and pulmonary sporotrichosis. It is fungistatic and interferes with the permeability of the fungal cell wall. Amphotericin is not appreciably absorbed from the gastrointestinal tract or the skin; it is administered intravenously or intrathecally, or instilled directly into the site of infection. Initial toxic effects commonly include fever, chills, nausea, vomiting, and headache. Toxic effects brought on by continued usage may include anemia, thrombophlebitis at the site of injection, hypokalemia, rise of blood urea and serum creatinine levels, and permanent damage to the kidney.

Sulfonamides

Introduced in 1935, the sulfonamides initiated the modern antibacterial chemotherapeutic revolution in medicine. Their use antedates that of the antibiotics by several years, since penicillin did not become available until 1941. The sulfonamides are valuable agents in the management of some infections, particularly urinary tract infections due to *Escherichia coli,* and can be employed for the prophylaxis of recurrences of rheumatic fever. Although one of these compounds, mafenide acetate (Sulfamylon), has an important use in the topical therapy of severe burn wounds, the value of the sulfonamides in the treatment of surgical infections is severely limited by their inactivation by pus. The sulfonamides are bacteriostatic and active against both gram-positive and gram-negative bacteria. The drugs are strongly antagonized by p-aminobenzoic acid (PABA), an essential intermediate in the synthesis of folic acid by bacterial cells, and act as competitive inhibitors. Bacteria sensitive to the sulfonamides are unable to utilize preformed folic acid in the body and must synthesize it themselves. Folic acid acts as a coenzyme in the transfer of fragments containing one carbon atom, which are involved in the synthesis of amino acids (such as methionine and serine), purine, and thymine. These compounds also inhibit the activity of sulfonamides, but unlike PABA they are noncompetitive inhibitors, and their effect is not reversed by increasing the concentration of drugs. Accordingly, pus, which is rich in amino acids and purines made available by the breakdown of cellular protein and nucleic acids, inactivates the sulfonamides.

Some of the sulfonamides of use in surgical practice are sulfadiazine, which is the preparation of choice in treating nocardiosis; phthalylsulfathiazole (Sulfathalidine), which is poorly absorbed from the gastrointestinal tract and is used in combination with neomycin for preoperative preparation of the large intestine; sulfisoxazole (Gantrisin) and sulfamethoxazole (Gantanol), which are used for treating urinary tract infections; and mafenide (Sulfamylon), which is applied topically and used to treat burn wound infections. Mafenide is not inhibited by the products of tissue necrosis.

Except for nonabsorbable sulfonamides, orally administered sulfonamides are rapidly absorbed in the stomach and duodenum and become distributed in all tissues and fluids. The sulfonamides are bound to either serum albumin or to tissue proteins, and they are detoxified in the liver. Both the drug and its less active metabolites are excreted by glomerular filtration. Sensitivity to one sulfonamide frequently confers sensitivity to others. Toxic reactions limiting sulfonamide therapy range from nausea, vomiting, and dermatitis to crystalluria, renal injury, hepatic damage, and hematologic disorders.

STREPTOCOCCAL INFECTIONS

Streptococci form the dominant aerobic flora of the mouth and pharyngeal areas of man. They are gram-positive spherical or ovoid cells (rarely elongated into rods) arranged in pairs (short chains). Long chains are observed when the organism is cultured in fluid media. Although most species are aerobic or facultatively anaerobic, there are also species which are anaerobic or microaerophilic. They may be divided into those which produce a soluble hemolysin and those which do not. Aerobes producing a clear zone of hemolysis on blood agar (beta hemolysis) include most of the species associated with primary streptococcal infections in man and can be subdivided into 15 broad groups (Lancefield groups) which are identified by precipitin tests with group-specific antisera against specific carbohydrate haptens (C antigens) of the streptococci. Strains belonging to Lancefield group A (*Streptococcus pyogenes*) are responsible for over 90 percent of human streptococcal infections. These group A strains can be further subdivided for epidemiologic studies into Griffith types according to their surface protein antigens (M, T, and R) by capillary precipitin or slide agglutination tests.

Another group of streptococci produce an ill-defined zone of partial hemolysis having a green or brownish-green color (alpha hemolysis). These are strains of *Streptococcus viridans*. Streptococci which are without effect on blood agar (nonhemolytic) include the fecal enterococci (*Streptococcus fecalis*). Viridans and nonhemolytic streptococci are associated with chronic diseases or are nonpathogenic. *Streptococcus viridans* is part of the commensal flora of the mouth and throat and is dangerous in individuals with congenitally deformed or rheumatically damaged heart valves. It is the commonest cause of subacute bacterial endocarditis. *Streptococcus viridans* has been incriminated in apical tooth infections and is commonly found in carious teeth. Bacteremia frequently follows tooth extraction and even routine dental procedures. In otherwise healthy individuals the streptococci are rapidly removed from the circulation, but in those with heart lesions the organisms settle in or on the defective valves. Accordingly, patients with congenital or other valvular cardiac defects should be given penicillin prophylactically before and after any dental attention.

Nonhemolytic streptococci are always present in the colon and may be isolated from the terminal ileum and upper jejunum of 60 percent of surgical patients. In the laboratory, the enterococci (*Streptococcus fecalis*) withstand exposure to 60°C for 30 minutes, which kills other streptococci. These organisms can cause suppurative lesions and urinary tract infections. In our hospital, enterococci are isolated from 12 percent of surgical wound infections and from 8 percent of urinary tract infections. Some strains of *Streptococcus fecalis* produce a true beta hemolysis; they belong to Lancefield group D.

Group A beta-hemolytic streptococci (*Streptococcus pyogenes*) are the principal causes of streptococcal pharyngitis, scarlet fever, and rheumatic fever. They also cause bacteremias following surgical procedures in patients with malignant disease. Groups B, C, D, F, and G are usually less virulent. Although group B streptococci are often isolated from patients with puerperal sepsis, with meningitis of the newborn, with diabetes mellitus, and/or with peripheral vascular insufficiency, they are also involved in pneumonias and infections of the male genitourinary tract. Since group C streptococci are part of the skin flora, they may be isolated from wounds and exudates more often than group B strains. The group G streptococci involved in infections usually originate in the genitourinary tract or skin, but they may also originate in the upper respiratory tract or gastrointestinal tract. We find streptococci in 4 percent of surgical wound infections and in 6 percent of nosocomial respiratory tract infections.

Streptococcus pyogenes is an invasive microorganism; it secretes two distinct hemolysins (streptolysins O and S) and several other products which aid in invasion. Streptolysin O is cardiotoxic and leukocidic and may be identical with leukocidin. Streptolysin S is a pure hemolysin responsible for beta hemolysis on blood agar plates. Hyaluronidase hydrolyzes hyaluronic acid and allows increased permeability of tissues. Streptokinase reduces fibrinolysis by activating the plasmin system. Streptodornase depolymerizes DNA. Erythrogenic toxin produces erythema when injected intradermally and is responsible for the punctate erythema of scarlet fever. The hyaluronidase and streptokinase produced by most strains of *Streptococcus pyogenes* are responsible for the spreading cellulitis (erysipelas) which is the typical streptococcal lesion. When abscess occurs, the pus is watery and often blood-stained due to the action of streptodornase and streptokinase, since the viscosity of pus is due to DNA and fibrin.

Erysipelas

Erysipelas is a spreading streptococcal cellulitis and lymphangitis with raised, sharply defined, irregular, reddish borders. The classic lesion of erysipelas is a "butterfly" erythema centered around the nose and extending onto both cheeks. Since erythrogenic toxin is produced in variable amounts by hemolytic streptococci, the development of cutaneous erythema is an inconstant manifestation of streptococcal infection. Minor skin abrasions and fissures predispose to these infections of the skin. Erysipelas usually occurs in the elderly as a result of trophic changes in the skin. The cutis is edematous and reddened, with a palpably raised border; the lesion is hot, tender, and painful. The systemic manifestations of erisipelas may be severe and suggest invasion via the lymphatics or bloodstream. Penicillin is usually effective against the invasive infection, but the erythema disappears more slowly.

Erysipeloid

Erysipeloid, a nonstreptococcal disease distinct from erysipelas, is a type of cutaneous cellulitis. Erysipeloid often is contracted after contamination of a cutaneous abrasion of the hand, particularly the fingers. The typical lesion is a violaceous nodule, often having a curved shape, which differs from that of erysipelas by its tendency to central clearing and the absence of suppuration. Human cases of erysipeloid may also occur as either a severe, generalized cutaneous disease or as septicemia with or without cutaneous involvement and often associated with endocarditis. Penicillin therapy is specific for most cases. Erysipeloid is due to infection by *Erysipelothrix rhusopathiae,* a grampositive, nonsporulating, facultative anaerobe in the family Corynebacteriaceae. Erysipelothrix infection is considered an occupational disease of abattoir workers, fish handlers, and others exposed to meat, poultry, and fish products.

Necrotizing Fasciitis

This is a serious clinical infection which may occur in only one or two patients a year in large city-county hospitals. The most significant manifestation of the infection is extensive necrosis of the superficial fascia with resultant widespread undermining of surrounding tissue and extreme systemic toxicity. The bacteria involved in about 90 percent of cases have usually been beta-hemolytic streptococci, coagulase-positive staphylococci, or both. Gramnegative enteric pathogens alone have been associated with about 10 percent of cases of necrotizing fasciitis. The disease appears to be a clinical entity and not a specific bacterial infection. It has been described previously as hemolytic or acute streptococcal gangrene, gangrenous or necrotizing erysipelas, suppurative fasciitis, and hospital gangrene. Although necrotizing fasciitis may develop following surgical procedures such as appendectomy, the majority of cases have occurred outside the hospital following minor trauma such as abrasions, cuts, bruises, boils, and insect bites on the extremities. The chief diagnostic criterion for necrotizing fasciitis is superficial and widespread fascial necrosis. Cellulitis as well as edema (mild to massive) are present in most patients. The involved skin is pale red without distinct borders and with blisters or bullae. Pale red areas progress to a distinct purple. The diagnosis is confirmed by observation of (1) serosanguinous exudate, (2) swollen, stringy, dull gray, necrotic fascia with extensive undermining, and (3) a gram-stained smear of the pus or fluid.

TREATMENT. This consists of multiple linear incisions over the affected area. In an open wound, the extent of undermining can be ascertained by passing a sterile hemostat along the plane just superficial to the deep fascia. In simple cellulitis or erysipelas, the hemostat cannot be passed. Before operation, the patient should be given a full dose of systemic antibiotic(s) effective against both hemolytic streptococci and penicillinase-producing staphylococci. Therapy is continued postoperatively until the infection is controlled. Repeated debridement may be necessary if the patient continues to be febrile. With the appearance of clean granulation tissue after 5 to 10 days, the wound may be closed by skin graft or suture. Rea and Wyrick (1970) report a 30 percent mortality.

Anaerobic streptococci are also pathogenic. They are normal inhabitants of the mouth, intestine, and vagina. They are abundant in the presence of poor oral hygiene, and aspiration into the lungs and sinuses may lead to putrid lung abscess, empyema, and sinusitis. Brain abscesses often develop as complications of chronic or acute infections of the lungs, sinuses, or ears. Presently, *Peptostreptococcus putridus* is the only well-documented species of anaerobic streptococcus. It has been isolated from cases of puerperal sepsis, brain abscess, and infected wounds. *Nonclostridial crepitant anaerobic cellulitis* due to anaerobic streptococci was reported by Altemeier and Culbertson in 1948 as a consequence of operation or accidental contamination from the intestinal, respiratory, or urinary tract.

Streptococcal Myonecrosis

Anaerobic streptococci also can cause gas gangrene. *Streptococcal myonecrosis* resembles subacute clostridial gas gangrene and was not described until World War II. After an incubation period of 3 to 4 days, there is swelling, edema, and purulent wound exudate. These signs are followed by pain which rapidly becomes severe. Gas is present, and the infected muscle changes from pale and soft to bright red, striped with purple, and finally purple and gangrenous. The seropurulent discharge has a sour odor. In this disease, muscle is infected, in contrast to necrotizing fasciitis, in which the fascia is affected. Treatment consists of incision and drainage, antibiotic therapy, and supportive measures.

Progressive Synergistic Gangrene

The extensive studies of Meleney established the importance of microaerophilic and anaerobic streptococci in special wound infections known as progressive synergistic gangrene and chronic burrowing ulcer. *Meleney's progressive synergistic gangrene* characteristically develops in sutured, infected thoracic or abdominal incisions or around a colostomy, ileostomy, or simple abrasion. The initial lesion is a small, painful, superficial ulcer which gradually spreads. The central ulcerated area is surrounded by a rim of gangrenous skin, which is in turn encircled by a zone of purple erythema blending into a surrounding area of bright, painful erythema. There is seropurulent discharge. Cultures taken from the outer edematous part of the lesion yield microaerophilic or anaerobic nonhemolytic streptococci. Cultures taken from the central ulcerated area yield *Staphylococcus aureus* and sometimes gram-negative bacilli, such as *Proteus* species. However, clinical cases of progressive synergistic gangrene from which anaerobic or microaerophilic streptococci could not be isolated have been reported. Treatment involves wide excision and therapy with penicillin or chloramphenicol. Corticosteroids have been employed to aid healing.

Meleney's Ulcer

Chronic burrowing or undermining ulcer, often designated as *Meleney's ulcer,* is caused by a nonhemolytic anaerobic or microaerophilic streptococcus. The lesion begins as a small, superficial ulcer following trauma or surgery and may also originate from an infected lymph node or subcutaneous abscess. The ulcer is only mildly painful, and systemic reaction is minimal. Slow, progressive enlargement of the lesion occurs over months or years. Infection of subcutaneous tissue is associated with ulceration of the overlying skin. Cutaneous gangrene is absent, and the edges of the undermined skin roll inward. The periphery of the lesion is erythematous, and the advancing edge of the lesion is characterized by pain and tenderness. Meleney's ulcer occurs most frequently after incision of a lymph node in the neck, axilla, or groin and after operations on the genital and intestinal tracts. As the lesion spreads, multiple ulcers and sinuses develop, producing epithelial strands and undermined bridges of skin. Treatment consists of debridement, drainage of sinuses, penicillin therapy, and split-thickness skin grafts over denuded areas as soon as the wound appears clean.

Anaerobic streptococci, either in pure culture or mixed with bacteroides, are frequently involved in appendiceal abscesses, peritonitis, abdominal wall sepsis, perirectal abscesses, and superficial abscesses related to infections of pilonidal and sebaceous cysts. Most abscesses are treated successfully by incision and drainage, and penicillin therapy. Anaerobic streptococcal infections, including septicemias, commonly occur in the female pelvic area following septic abortion and postpartum sepsis.

STAPHYLOCOCCAL INFECTIONS

Staphylococci form part of the permanent bacterial flora of the normal skin and nasopharynx and may cause a variety of infections, often characterized by suppuration, ranging from mild, localized pustules to lethal septicemias. Surgical and traumatic wounds are particularly susceptible to purulent infection. In stained preparations of pus, staphylococci appear as spherical cells occurring singly, in pairs, or in small clusters. They are gram-positive and nonmotile, and produce no spores. Staphylococci are aerobic or facultatively anaerobic and grow on ordinary unenriched bacteriologic media. They may produce pigmentation varying from white, orange, or yellow to golden. Blood agar is often hemolyzed (beta hemolysis). Two species are of medical importance: *Staphylococcus aureus* and *Staphylococcus epidermidis* (formerly called *Staphylococcus albus*). *Staphylococcus aureus* is usually associated with disease, and will be discussed subsequently. On the other hand, *Staphylococcus epidermidis* usually has not been

considered a pathogen, but it has become recognized as an important cause of opportunistic infection following surgical procedures in which foreign materials and prostheses are placed in the patient. *Staphylococcus epidermidis* causes endocarditis following open heart surgery and occasionally produces septicemia.

The criteria identifying staphylococci are colonial appearance on blood agar, Gram-stain reaction, microscopic morphologic features, production of coagulase, and fermentation of mannitol. *Staphylococcus aureus* is coagulase-positive and produces acid from mannitol. *Staphylococcus epidermidis* produces neither coagulase nor acid from mannitol. Filtrates of cultures of *Staphylococcus aureus* contain hemolysins, dermonecrotic and lethal factors, leukocidins, and a number of enzymes. Strains of *Staphylococcus aureus* may be classified into groups on the basis of their susceptibility to various bacteriophages. Although phage typing of isolates is of value in epidemiologic investigations, it is an involved procedure and not employed by the diagnostic laboratory for routine identification of clinical isolates.

Staphylococci are readily phagocytized by polymorphonuclear leukocytes, which may then be killed by the bacteria, presumably by their leukocidins. Although leukocidins, hemolysins, and coagulase are antigenic, these antibodies provide little or no protection. Since the antigenic components of staphylococci responsible for virulence are unknown, it has not been possible to make effective vaccines.

Staphylococcal infections in man depend upon many factors, including the type and number of staphylococci, the route of introduction, and the toxic substances produced by the staphylococci. Of equal importance are the susceptibility of the host, his previous exposure to specific strains, his general health and nutritional state, and the amount of trauma he has sustained. Factors such as toxemia, allergic reactions, starvation, and diabetes influence the onset and course of staphylococcal infections. Foreign body reaction as a consequence of sutures is an important factor in staphylococcal infection.

The skin is the most common site of staphylococcal infections. Lesions range from furuncles (boils) and carbuncles to surgical wound infections. Hospital-acquired staphylococcal infection by antibiotic-resistant strains reached epidemic proportion during the 1950s. The development and use of semisynthetic penicillinase-resistant penicillins has controlled these infections. However, the antibiotic-resistant staphylococci are endemic in hospitals and pose a continual threat to the patient. A rapidly spreading cellulitis is sometimes seen with staphylococcal infections and should be treated vigorously with an appropriate antibiotic. Often there is pain, swelling, induration, patchy discoloration of the skin, and fever. Cellulitis may occur at the site of a venipuncture for intravenous cannulation. Staphylococcal abscesses characteristically begin in hair follicles or small sebaceous glands. An indurated area of cellulitis undergoes central necrosis and formation of an abscess having thick, odorless, and yellow or greenish pus. Staphylococci are a primary cause of acute wound sepsis and are involved in postoperative infections of "clean" incised wounds. The source of the infecting microorganisms is frequently exogenous. Virulent, antibiotic-resistant, hospital strains of *Staphylococcus aureus* may be carried in the nares and on the hands of physicians and hospital personnel, and these may be newly colonized on the skin of the patient. The air in the operating room may bear microorganisms from the nasopharynx, skin, hair, and clothing of the surgical staff and of the patient. Accordingly, it is essential to maintain strict, rigid rules for asepsis in the operating room. At our hospital, coagulase-positive staphylococci are isolated from 8 percent of postoperative surgical wound infections and account for 5 percent of nosocomial infections.

Infected incisions should be opened widely and allowed to drain. Therapy with antistaphylococcal antibiotics should be initiated. Fulminating septicemias may arise from severe wound infections. The patient is ill with high fever, leukocytosis, toxemia, and evidence of irritation of the central nervous system. The mortality rate in fulminating untreated infections may be as high as 90 percent. If the infection persists, metastatic abscesses form in lungs, heart, kidneys, gallbladder, appendix, liver, peritoneum, and bone. Meningitis and brain abscesses hasten death. Endocarditis is a frequent complication of staphylococcal septicemia. Staphylococcal pneumonia is another nosocomial postoperative infection. It may be severe and is often associated with a tracheostomy. In fatal cases, the major finding at autopsy is marked pulmonary edema with little destruction of tissue.

Staphylococcal Enteritis

Enteritis with a drug-resistant staphylococcus following oral administration of a broad-spectrum antibiotic was first described by Kramer in 1948. Generally, this disease is benign with mild to moderate symptoms including nausea, vomiting, diarrhea, abdominal distension, fever, and weakness, but may be fulminating and lead to septicemia and death. Discontinuance of the oral antibiotic usually leads to disappearance of symptoms. The prognosis is good so long as the intestinal mucosa remains intact.

STAPHYLOCOCCAL ENTEROCOLITIS (PSEUDOMEMBRANOUS ENTEROCOLITIS)

This is an acute inflammatory disease of the small and large intestine characterized by foci of epithelial necrosis and erosion of the mucosa. There is profuse, continuous diarrhea which soon becomes watery, contains desquamated, membranous patches, and often is greenish. The disease is a complication in debilitated surgical patients following therapy with broad-spectrum antibiotics. The use of neomycin in debilitated patients for preoperative intestinal antisepsis and for treatment of hepatic coma has resulted in staphylococcal enterocolitis. The major etiologic factors are suppression of normal gastrointestinal flora by a broad-spectrum antibiotic and acquisition of an enterotoxic strain of *Staphylococcus aureus* possessing multiple antibiotic-resistance. Secondary factors are debilitation and an empty small bowel (as a result of preoperative starvation). Although stool cultures from some patients yield a pure culture of *Staphylococcus aureus,* pseudo-

membranous enterocolitis may exist without culturable *Staphylococcus aureus.* Conversely, *Staphylococcus aureus may exist in pure culture in the intestine of a patient with the symptoms of enteritis but in the absence of a pseudomembrane.*

TREATMENT. Treatment consists of discontinuing previous antibiotics and employing a specific antistaphylococcal drug such as methicillin, hydration with intravenously administered fluids, replacement of electrolytes, intramuscular administration of corticosteroids, and attempts to reestablish a normal flora. The fulminating form of enterocolitis may be refractory to all forms of therapy and result in death.

CLOSTRIDIAL INFECTIONS

The clostridia are large, gram-positive, rod-shaped microorganisms. They are ubiquitous. *Clostridium perfringens* is more widespread than any other pathogen. Its principal habitats are the soil and the intestinal tract of man and animals. The most characteristic feature of clostridia is the presence of an oval, central, or subterminal spore. In the case of *Clostridium tetani,* the spore is spherical and terminally located and produces a characteristic drumstick appearance. The clostridia are obligate anaerobes and can be cultured only on media having a low oxidation-reduction potential. This may be achieved by employing fresh media incubated in an anaerobic atmosphere in specially designed jars or with liquid media exposed to the atmosphere, but containing added reducing agents (such as sodium thioglycolate, powdered iron, or chopped meat).

The lesions produced by the pathogenic clostridia are due to their exotoxins. Gas gangrene is a necrosis of tissue along with putrefaction and is usually caused by clostridia derived from the intestine or soil. The infection is localized but its systemic effects are far-reaching. Gas gangrene is rarely a pure culture infection. It usually involves *Clostridium perfringens* along with other clostridial species, such as *Clostridium novyi, Clostridium septicum, Clostridium bifermentans* (*sordelli*), sometimes *Clostridium tetani* and *Clostridium botulinum,* and often nonpathogenic but proteolytic *Clostridium sporogenes* and *Clostridium histolyticum.* In addition, gram-positive cocci and gram-negative enterobacteria are often present.

Clostridium perfringens is, nevertheless, the most important organism. Five types, A through F, have been described. They are differentiated on the basis of production of lethal toxins. All types produce alpha toxin, a lethal, necrotizing, hemolytic exotoxin, which is also a lecithinase. *Clostridium perfringens* type A produces the greatest amount of alpha toxin. In addition, some strains of type A produce variable amounts of hemolysin (theta toxin), collagenase (kappa toxin), hyaluronidase (mu toxin), and deoxyribonuclease (nu toxin).

Clostridial Wound Infection

MacLennan in 1962 described three types of anaerobic wound infection: simple contamination, clostridial cellulitis, and clostridial myonecrosis.

SIMPLE CONTAMINATION

Simple contamination of a wound by clostridia is common. It causes no discomfort to the patient and is of little concern to the surgeon. When anaerobes are digesting dead tissue, there may be a thin seropurulent exudate. If the necrotic material is removed, there will be no subsequent invasion of underlying tissues. The relatively common occurrence of clostridia in accidental wounds in the absence of anaerobic infection is probably due to the ubiquitous presence of these anaerobes and their spores. The absence of subsequent anaerobic infections is most likely due to unsuitable conditions for further multiplication of the contaminant and for toxin production. MacLennan estimated that between 10 and 30 percent of all severe civilian wounds were infected with spore-forming anaerobic bacilli. A high oxidation-reduction potential (Eh) due to the surrounding healthy tissues and possibly the presence of atmospheric oxygen prevent colonization of the tissues. In the absence of treatment, however, cellulitis or myonecrosis may develop from the simple contamination, and the three types of anaerobic wound infection may be considered as ascending grades of severity.

CLOSTRIDIAL CELLULITIS

This is a gassy, crepitant infection involving necrotic tissue (killed by ischemia or trauma, but not by bacterial activity). Intact, healthy muscle is not invaded. The cellulitis is characterized as a foul, seropurulent infection of the depths and crevices of a wound. There is often local extension along fascial planes, but involvement of healthy muscle and marked toxemia are absent. Although *Clostridium perfringens* may be present, the predominant organisms are proteolytic and nontoxigenic clostridia, such as *Clostridium sporogenes* and *Clostridium tertium*. Clostridial cellulitis generally has a gradual onset; the incubation period is from 3 to 5 days; systemic effects are usually mild; there is no toxemia; the skin is rarely discolored; and there is little or no edema. This distinguishes the infection from gas gangrene. The spread of the cellulitis in the tissue spaces often has been rapid and extensive, necessitating immediate radical surgical drainage.

CLOSTRIDIAL MYONECROSIS (GAS GANGRENE)

This infection is rapid-spreading. It may be crepitant, or noncrepitant and edematous, mixed, or toxemic. The lesion also has been described as a "myositis," which is not as precise a term as is *myonecrosis*. The infection occurs in association with severe wounds of large muscle masses that have become contaminated with pathogenic clostridia, especially *Clostridium perfringens*. Such wounds are most commonly caused by the high-velocity missiles of modern warfare and by accidental trauma. Sometimes clostridial myonecrosis follows clean elective surgical procedures. Many patients with clostridial myonecrosis harbor a variety of anaerobic as well as aerobic bacteria. In fatal cases it is rare for only a single species to be present. Clostridial myonecrosis is most likely to develop in wounds in which there has been extensive laceration or devitalization of thick muscle masses, such as the buttock, thigh, and shoulder. Associated with such trauma is impaired arterial supply to the limb or muscle group and gross contamination of the wound by soil, clothing, and other foreign bodies. These conditions provide an ideal substrate for the development of clostridia. In anoxic muscle glycolysis continues, and the oxidation-reduction potential (Eh) of the muscle falls. With the accumulation of lactate, alkaline reservoirs become depleted, and the pH also falls. As a consequence of lowered Eh and pH, the proteinases present and the amino acids produced not only lower the pH further but provide substrate for the growth of clostridia. Once bacterial growth is established and toxins and other products of bacterial metabolism accumulate, the invasion of uninjured tissue is promoted, and the anaerobic infection is established. The infection is further aided by the fact that neither phagocytes nor antibodies can enter the necrotic lesion. Gas gangrene is considered to have begun when the infecting pathogenic anaerobes have produced sufficient toxins to overcome local defenses. Gas gangrene is relatively infrequent in clinical practice. The overall incidence is less than 2 percent, although from 4 to 40 percent of wounds may be contaminated with clostridia.

TREATMENT. Early and adequate surgery is the most effective means of treating gas gangrene. Because of the rapid spread of the infection, a 24-hour delay in treatment may be fatal. The diagnosis of gas gangrene is based on clinical evidence. Multiple longitudinal incisions for decompression and drainage and surgical debridement usually arrest the disease. If not or if early diagnosis was not made, then amputation is necessary. Antibiotic therapy with penicillin G and tetracycline has been most effective as an adjunct to operative treatment. Antitoxin is of no value therapeutically or prophylactically and should not be used. Adjunctive hyperbaric oxygenation has been used with varied degrees of success.

Infections of the Gastrointestinal Tract

Clostridia are usually present among the mixed flora in peritonitis, appendicitis, and strangulation intestinal obstruction. Quantitatively, the most numerous flora in peritoneal and loop fluids of dogs with experimental strangulation intestinal obstruction are clostridia, coliforms, bacteriodes, and streptococci, in that order. Although it appears reasonable to assume that *Clostridium perfringens* actively participates in the pathophysiology of severe cases of appendicitis and acute cases of strangulated intestinal obstruction, direct clinical evidence is lacking. Experimental studies demonstrate that clostridial exotoxins contribute to the lethal activity of filter-sterilized strangulation fluids. However, this finding does not preclude a role for combinations of varying proportions of viable bacteria, bacterial endotoxins, and clostridial exotoxins. In biliary tract infections due to clostridia, acute emphysematous cholecystitis (gas gangrene of the gallbladder) and postcholecystectomy septicemia, it is generally believed that clostridia are transported to the liver from the gastrointestinal tract via the portal circulation and then excreted with the bile into the biliary tract. In postoperative gas gangrene of the abdominal wall, a rare complication of abdominal surgery, intestinal clostridia contaminate the abdominal wound at the time of operation. It occurs less often after operations on the stomach and duodenum than after those involving the lower intestinal tract. These infections are usually due to *Clostridium perfringens* and are fatal; they require awareness and early treatment. Gas gangrene of the abdominal wall must be distinguished from Meleney's progressive synergistic gangrene of the abdominal wall following drainage of appendiceal abscesses. Synergistic gangrene is a chronic, superficial progressive gangrene characterized by a slow, relentless progression, severe local symptoms, and absence of severe systemic symptoms. It is due to anaerobic cocci mixed with *Staphylococcus aureus, Streptococcus pyogenes, Pseudomonas aeruginosa,* or *Proteus* species.

Urogenital Infections

Postoperative infections due to *Clostridium perfringens* have occurred following procedures such as nephrectomy, lithotomy, and prostatectomy. Almost all uterine clostridial infections are due to *Clostridium perfringens.* They generally occur following criminal abortion and are rare following normal childbirth. Introduction of the organisms into the uterus is favored by instrumentation and manipulation. In modern obstetrics, the use of prophylactic antibiotic therapy and the wide use of cesarean section probably account for the decreasing frequency of this already rare form of uterine infection. In contrast, in cases of criminal abortion both endogenous and exogenous sources of contamination occur as the result of unskilled manipulations and the use of unsterile and unclean instruments and abortifacients. Once the interior of the puerperal or post-abortal uterus has been contaminated, fragments of blood clot and necrotic tissue provide conditions favorable for multiplication of clostridia. Early diagnosis depends upon clinical recognition of such signs as jaundice, hypotension, tachycardia, shock, hemoglobinuria, uterine or perianal tenderness, and offensive vaginal discharge. The simplest method for the rapid detection of *Clostridium perfringens* is the demonstration of gram-positive rods with rounded ends in direct smears from the cervical os or canal. The treatment of uterine gas gangrene involves immediate chemotherapy, hyperbaric oxygenation, treatment of shock, hysterectomy, and management of renal failure. Penicillin is the antibiotic of choice.

Tetanus

This disease is a toxemia resulting from the growth of contaminating *Clostridium tetani* at a traumatized site and consequent production of exotoxin. In contrast to the clostridia of gas gangrene, *Clostridium tetani* is noninvasive, and neurotoxin is responsible for the symptoms of tetanus. The conditions necessary for the development of tetanus are the presence of the organisms or spores in the wound and favorable anaerobic conditions for bacterial growth and the elaboration of exotoxin. The presence of *Clostridium tetani* in soil and in the intestine of man and

animals ensures that accidental wounds are exposed to the risk of contamination at the time of injury. However, as with other clostridial infections, the mere presence of *Clostridium tetani* or its spores in a wound is not followed by tetanus, and the organism may be isolated from wounds in individuals who never develop tetanus. A low oxygen tension is necessary if *Clostridium tetani* is to grow. Currently, tetanus commonly follows mild injuries because the routine protective measures employed in severe cases are frequently omitted. The type of lesions leading to the development of tetanus are penetrating wounds due to splinters, thorns, rusty nails, and even dirty abrasions. In about 50 percent of cases, it is presumed that the wound was slight and healed before evidence of intoxication developed. Such mild injuries may not induce significant local anoxia, but they may be accompanied by other infections which lower the oxidation-reduction potential of the tissues to a point at which the spores of *Clostridium tetani* can germinate. For example, chronic ulcers of the leg, measles rash, boils, paronychia, and dental extractions have been implicated as modes of entry. In the United States, tetanus has become a disease primarily of adults. The median age of patients with nonneonatal tetanus varies from fifty-five to fifty-seven years; the median age for those dying from tetanus is from fifty-five to sixty years.

Currently, tetanus is seen in urban centers of the United States as a complication of narcotic addiction; *urban tetanus* has a mortality of 90 percent. *Tetanus neonatorum* results from contamination of the cut surface of the umbilical cord and is an important cause of infant mortality in countries and areas where primitive unhygienic obstetric practices prevail. There is often continuous crying for hours followed by cessation of sucking and crying, convulsions, and fever. Severe spasm of the respiratory muscles is a common cause of death. *Postabortal tetanus* and *puerperal tetanus* result from unsterile manipulation or instrumentation of the genital tract. *Postoperative tetanus* sometimes follows elective surgical procedures, and is usually due to some breakdown in sterile technique, but it may also be caused by contamination from the patient's intestinal tract.

CLINICAL MANIFESTATIONS. The average incubation period for tetanus is from 7 to 10 days after injury, but it may range between 3 and 30 days. The incubation period is followed by the *period of onset,* that is, the time interval between the first symptom (usually trismus) and the onset of spasms. In severe cases reflex spasms may begin 12 hours after onset, in moderately severe cases after 2 to 3 days, and in milder cases after 5 or more days. In general, the shorter the periods of incubation and onset, the worse the prognosis. Even with modern treatment, the mortality rate is rarely less than 30 percent.

Trismus is the most common early symptom. It often is combined with pain and stiffness in the neck, back, and abdomen. Occasionally dysphagia appears first. These symptoms increase according to the severity of the attack. Twenty-four hours after the onset, a patient with a moderately severe attack has a characteristically anxious expression (*risus sardonicus*) in which the eyebrows and the corners of the mouth are drawn up. The muscles of the neck and trunk are rigid to varying degrees, and the back is usually slightly arched. The patient is usually comfortable except for occasional pain in the neck or back, which tends to be made worse by movement. Manipulation of a limb or palpation of any part of the body tends to increase muscular rigidity and may bring on cramplike pain. Initially, reflex spasms are brought on by external stimuli, such as moving the patient or knocking the bed, but later they occur spontaneously at regular and increasingly shorter intervals until the height of the disease is reached. Spasms often begin with a sudden jerk. Every muscle in the body is thrown into intense tonic contraction, the jaws are tightly clenched, the head is retracted, the back is arched, the chest and abdomen are fixed, and the limbs are usually extended. A severe spasm may stop respiration. Spasms may last a few seconds or several minutes. When spasms occur frequently, they lead to rapid exhaustion and sometimes to death from asphyxiation. Aspiration pneumonia is a common contributory cause of death.

Less common manifestations of the disease include local contracture of muscles in the neighborhood of the wound: *local tetanus.* This may precede the more generalized forms of involvement. *Cephalic tetanus* is a manifestation in which irritation or paralysis of cranial nerves appears early and dominates the picture. The facial nerve is affected most often, but ophthalmoplegia from involvement of the ocular nerves and spasm or paralysis of the tongue from involvement of the hypoglossal nerve may develop. Trismus and dysphagia may also be present. This condition, which is a type of local tetanus, follows wounds of the head and face, and the symptoms often appear first on the injured side.

Severe tetanus is terrible and often fatal, but those who recover do so completely. The patient who has survived tetanus is not immune and, unless immunized, is susceptible to a second attack. *Recurrent tetanus* in the same patient has been reported. Apparently a sublethal amount of tetanus toxin is not sufficient to provide an adequate antigenic stimulus for the production of active immunity.

The diagnosis of tetanus is a clinical one with bacteriologic confirmation sometimes possible. Frequently the presumed lesion has been so slight that it is not detectable at the time when clinical tetanus develops.

IMMUNIZATION. Prophylaxis with tetanus toxoid is the best means of preventing tetanus. For active immunization of individuals seven years old or over, the initial dose is 0.5 ml aluminum phosphate–adsorbed tetanus toxoid given intramuscularly, preferably in the left deltoid region, but it also may be given subcutaneously. This is repeated in 4 to 6 weeks, and a third injection is given in 6 to 12 months (or more). Only after this third injection is the basic series considered complete. For children six years old or under, diphtheria and tetanus toxoid combined with pertussis vaccine (DTP) is used. Delay in administering the second and third injections is not disadvantageous, and the series does not need to be restarted or repeated. Even after 25 years, a booster will rapidly recall complete active protection.

Following the initial dose of tetanus toxoid, nonimmun-

ized individuals require approximately 30 days to acquire a safe antibody level (at least 0.01 I.V. of serum antitoxin per milliliter of blood). Patients are passively immunized in the interim by intramuscular administration of human hyperimmune globulin containing 250 units of tetanus antitoxin simultaneously with the toxoid. This protects for about 4 weeks. Passive immunization is not recommended for individuals who have received previous active immunization.

TREATMENT. Surgical care of wounds should be immediate. The most important features of surgical wound care are thorough cleansing and debridement. Foreign bodies and necrotic tissue can be massively contaminated with *Clostridium tetani* and establish wound conditions promoting growth and exotoxin production by *Clostridium tetani.* The wound should be left open until the patient has recovered from the convulsive stage of the disease. Antibiotic therapy with penicillin is effective against vegetative cells of *Clostridium tetani.* Oxytetracycline or chloramphenicol may be used if an allergy to penicillin exists. Antibiotics also are important as prophylaxis against respiratory infections, which are common in tetanus. Treatment of the patient with severe tetanus involves the use of muscle relaxants, sedation with Pentothal sodium, balance of fluid and electrolytes, control of respiratory secretions, and elimination of visceral stimuli such as distension of the urinary bladder and fecal impaction. A tracheostomy is performed if needed or when the period of onset is 1 day or less. Constant nursing care is required.

COMPLICATIONS. Tetanus is a particularly lethal disease, and death is generally due to respiratory arrest. Some complications of tetanus and its treatment are drug intoxication, especially from barbituates; bronchopneumonia or other pulmonary infection; compression fracture of vertebrae, especially the thoracic vertebrae; anemia; and exhaustion, which may be so severe as a result of repeated convulsions that the patient lapses into coma and expires. Before human tetanus immune globulin was available, the risk of anaphylaxis complicated the use of bovine or equine tetanus antitoxin.

PROPHYLAXIS. The Committee on Trauma of the American College of Surgeons recommends the following guidelines in management of the tetanus-prone wound:

I. General principles
  A. For each patient the attending physician must determine the adequate prophylaxis against tetanus.
  B. Meticulous surgical care, including removal of all devitalized tissue and foreign bodies, should be provided immediately for all wounds regardless of the active immunization status of the patient. Such care is an essential part of the prophylaxis against tetanus.
  C. Each patient with a wound should receive adsorbed tetanus toxoid intramuscularly at the time of injury, either as an initial immunizing dose or as a booster for previous immunization, unless he has received a booster or has completed his initial immunization series within the past 12 months. As the antigen concentration varies in different products, specific information on the volume of a single dose is provided on the label of the package.
  D. Need for passive immunization with homologous (human) tetanus immune globulin must be considered in relation to the characteristics of the wound, the conditions under

which it was incurred, and the previous active immunization status of the patient.

E. Every wounded patient should be given a written record of the immunization provided, and instructed to carry the record at all times and, if indicated, to complete active immunization. For precise tetanus prophylaxis, an accurate and immediately available history regarding previous active immunization against tetanus is required.

F. Basic immunization with adsorbed toxoid requires three injections. A booster of adsorbed toxoid is indicated 10 years after the third injection or 10 years after an intervening wound booster.

II. Specific measures for patients with wounds
   A. For previously immunized individuals
      1. When the patient has been immunized within the past 10 years
         a. To the majority, give 0.5 ml of adsorbed tetanus toxoid as a booster unless it is certain that the patient has received a booster within the previous 12 months.
         b. To those with severe, neglected, and old (more than 24 hours) tetanus-prone wounds, give 0.5 ml of adsorbed toxoid unless it is certain that a booster was received within the previous 6 months.
      2. When the patient received active immunization more than 10 years previously and has not received a booster within the past 10 years
         a. To the majority, give 0.5 ml of adsorbed tetanus toxoid.
         b. To those with wounds which indicate an overwhelming possibility that tetanus might develop
            (1) Give 0.5 ml of adsorbed tetanus toxoid.
            (2) Give 250 units of tetanus immune globulin (human). Use different syringes, needles, and sites. For severe, neglected, or old wounds, 500 units of tetanus immune globulin (human) is advisable.
            (3) Consider administering oxytetracycline or penicillin prophylactically.
   B. For individuals not previously immunized
      1. With clean minor wounds in which tetanus is most likely, give 0.5 ml of adsorbed tetanus toxoid (initial immunizing dose).
      2. With all other wounds
         a. Give 0.5 ml of adsorbed tetanus toxoid (initial immunizing dose).
         b. Give 250 units of tetanus immune globulin (human). For severe, neglected, or old wounds, 500 units of tetanus immune globulin (human) is advisable.
         c. Consider administering oxytetracycline or penicillin prophylactically.

INFECTIONS CAUSED BY GRAM-NEGATIVE BACILLI

The gram-negative bacilli of importance to surgery are for the most part indigenous to man and often found in the intestinal tract. They are non-spore-forming rods, and they may be aerobes, facultative anaerobes, or obligate anaerobes. The role of some gram-negative bacilli as primary pathogens has long been known, e.g., *Pseudomonas aeruginosa* and *Salmonella typhi*. Others have been recognized only rarely as primary pathogens in human beings, e.g., *Serratia marcescens* and *Enterobacter aerogenes* (formerly *Aerobacter aerogenes*). However, since the development of modern chemotherapy after World War II, the gram-negative bacilli have become increasingly important

as causes of serious infection, particularly in hospitalized patients. Prior to the introduction of broad-spectrum antibiotics, the role of gram-negative bacilli as pathogens was usually overshadowed by the pneumococci, streptococci, and staphylococci. We now know that infection is most likely to occur when body defense mechanisms are either undeveloped or overtaxed, as in the case of infants and debilitated patients, and that therapeutic measures to combat one situation may provide an environment promoting the establishment of infection by almost any mixture of gram-negative bacilli. This situation prevails because of the great number of patients with impaired host defenses secondary to the use of multiple antibiotics, corticosteroids, immunosuppressive agents, antineoplastic drugs, and radiotherapy. Surgical procedures in which foreign bodies such as prosthetic valves or grafts are inserted appear to allow these less virulent species to become established and to produce infection. Indwelling venous and urethral catheters, endotracheal tubes and mechanical ventilators, peritoneal dialysis apparatus, and pump-oxygenators for extracorporeal circulation in cardiac surgery often serve as portals of entry for the gram-negative bacilli. The current taxonomic organization of gram-negative bacilli is outlined in Table 5-6.

Pseudomonas aeruginosa is widely distributed and frequently present in small numbers on healthy skin surfaces and in the normal intestinal flora. As a pathogen it is often associated with pyogenic cocci or with the Enterobacteriaceae. It is incriminated in primary infections such as meningitis resulting from lumbar puncture, traumatic injuries to the eye, and enteritis with associated bacteremia. Currently, pseudomonas infection is the cause of death in patients having large burns, and it is common in postoperative infections following the use of mechanical ventilators and indwelling urinary catheters. *Pseudomonas aeruginosa* is resistant to most antibiotics but is sensitive

Table 5-6. TAXONOMY OF GRAM-NEGATIVE BACILLI

Family	Tribe	Genus
Pseudomonaceae. . . .	. . . .	*Pseudomonas*
Enterobacteriaceae. . . .	Eschericheae	*Escherichia* (*E. coli*, including *Alkalescens-Dispar* group)
		Shigella
	Edwardsielliae	*Edwardsiella*
	Salmonelleae	*Salmonella*
		Arizona
		Citrobacter (including Bethesda-Ballerup group)
	Klebsielleae	*Klebsiella*
		Enterobacter (including *Hafnia*)
		Pectobacterium
		Serratia
	Proteae	*Proteus*
		Providencia
Bacteroidaceae.	. . . .	*Bacteroides*
		Fusobacterium

to polymyxin B, colistin, and mafenide. Although carbenicillin and gentamicin have been useful in the treatment of established infection, there is evidence that strains resistant to these agents are emerging. Currently, polyvalent *Pseudomonas* hyperimmune globulin and plasma for active protection and polyvalent *Pseudomonas* vaccines for passive immunization have been developed and are being evaluated as means of reducing mortality from *Pseudomonas* infection.

Escherichia coli is found in the intestinal tract of man and animals and is the predominant aerobic commensal in the normal intestinal flora. Although more than 145 different envelope capsular (K) antigens have been identified, the ability of a strain to be typed does not necessarily denote pathogenicity or virulence. Nevertheless, certain strains belonging to distinct antigenic types are enteropathogenic, and produce diarrheal disease, especially in infants. *Escherichia coli* may produce meningitis, septicemia, endocarditis, appendiceal abscess, peritonitis, septic wounds, and pyogenic infections, chiefly urinary tract infections (pyelitis, cystitis, etc.) in pure culture or in association with fecal streptococci. *Escherichia coli* also has the capacity to produce a potent endotoxin which enters the circulation and induces shock.

The *Salmonella* species are a large group of enteric bacteria causing enteric fevers (particularly typhoid fever), gastroenteritis, and septicemia. *Salmonella typhi* and *Salmonella enteritidis* invade the bloodstream and cause enteric fever. They may then be isolated from cerebrospinal fluid, bone marrow, etc. The primary sources of *Salmonella* infections are human and domestic animal reservoirs from which the microorganisms are transmitted to susceptible human beings via food or water. Infection of man with the *Salmonella* group is by ingestion, usually the result of transmission from sick individuals or healthy carriers to susceptible individuals. The organisms pass from the small intestine via the lymphatics to the mesenteric glands. After multiplication there, they invade the bloodstream via the thoracic duct. The onset of typhoid fever coincides with the entrance of *Salmonella typhi* into the bloodstream. During the bacteremia of the first 7 to 10 days, the liver, gallbladder, spleen, kidney, and bone marrow become infected. From the gallbladder a further invasion of the intestine results. The typhoid bacillus is found in other lesions occurring as suppurative periosteitis and osteitis, abscess of the kidney, acute cholecystitis, bronchopneumonia, empyema, and ulcerative endocarditis. Consequently, salmonellae may localize in joints, heart, lungs, or other organs, and produce local abscesses. Although postoperative wound infection due to *Salmonella typhi* is rare, recorded cases occur after gallbladder surgery in patients who are unsuspected typhoid carriers. Contaminated wound drainage and positive stools from such patients are distinct hazards to other hospitalized patients.

Before the introduction of modern chemotherapy, gram-negative bacilli of the tribe Klebsielleae were rarely noted as primary pathogens. However, along with other gram-negative bacilli, they have assumed increasing importance as causes of serious hospital-acquired infections.

Klebsiella pneumoniae (Friedlander's bacillus) in the past has been responsible for less than 1 percent of bacterial pneumonias but is important because more than 50 percent of these are fatal. *Enterobacter aerogenes* (formerly *Aerobacter aerogenes*) is a commensal in the intestinal tract of approximately 5 percent of healthy individuals. *Serratia marcescens* is another species formerly considered to be nonpathogenic for man. Although it too has low virulence for healthy individuals, it is now found primarily in hospitalized patients with some underlying disease. It may spread like other "hospital bacteria," and infection may not always produce clinical symptoms. Classically, *Serratia marcescens* has been recognized by its ability to produce a characteristic red pigment, and it has been thought to be an obligate pigment producer. However, the majority of strains of *Serratia marcescens* involved in hospital-acquired infections are nonpigmented and often have been mistaken for other enterobacteria. These nonchromogenic strains of *Serratia marcescens* now can be identified by appropriate biochemical tests. The *Klebsiella-Enterobacter-Serratia* species are often isolated in mixed culture from sputum, urine, blood, and wounds in which there are other potential pathogens such as streptococci, staphylococci, *Escherichia coli*, *Proteus* species, *Citrobacter* species, and *Pseudomonas aeruginosa*. Epidemiologic studies indicate that the particular strains and types of the gram-negative species producing infection are nosocomial and acquired in the intestinal tract of patients during hospitalization. They are often highly drug-resistant, and the overall mortality associated with bacteremia is approximately 50 percent. The risk of bacteremia appears to be related to the underlying disease of the patient and the nature of his infection (urinary tract, respiratory, wound infection, abscess, etc.).

Gram-negative bacilli in the genera *Proteus* and *Providencia* also compete for prominence with the other aerobic gram-negatives in infections. These organisms often occur in abscesses, in infected wounds, and also in burns as one component of a mixed infection. They are resistant to most antibiotics, and what was originally a mixed infection may be converted into a pure proteus infection as a result of antibiotic therapy. *Mima polymorpha* and *Herellea vaginicola* are two species of gram-negative pleomorphic aerobes capable of causing therapy-potentiated infection in hospitalized patients. There has been much confusion regarding the nomenclature of these two species in the tribe Mimeae, and as many as 15 different names have been applied to each species.

In addition to the enteric bacilli, the normal intestinal flora include enterococci, clostridia, and bacteroides. The bacteroides are obligately anaerobic, gram-negative, nonspore-forming bacilli. They are normal inhabitants of the oral cavity, gastrointestinal tract, and the external genitalia, but they may cause surgical infections as a complication of operations upon the gastrointestinal tract. Bacteroides are sometimes the only microorganisms found in clinical specimens but more often are found in association with other anaerobes and aerobes. Classification of the bacteroides is unresolved. Currently, human pathogens are assigned to the genus *Bacteroides* and the genus *Fusobacterium*. *Bacteroides* are rod-shaped cells with rounded ends and are sometimes coccobacillary; *Fusobacterium* may be bacilli with pointed ends or pleomorphic, filamentous forms with swellings and free, round bodies. Species causing infections in human beings are *Bacteroides fragilis, Bacteroides melaninogenicus, Fusobacterium fusiforme,* and *Fusobacterium necrophorus* (previously known as *Bacteroides fundiformis* and as *Sphaerophorus necrophorus*).

In circumstances such as chronic illness, malignant disease, surgical treatment, and cystoscopy, the bacteroides may invade the bloodstream to cause septicemia and penetrate tissue and organs to produce abscesses. The clinical spectrum of infections varies from superficial infections to deep abscesses with overwhelming bacteremia and shock. The gastrointestinal tract, especially the colon and appendix, appears to be the most frequent source of bacteroides infection. Gynecologic infections involve the vagina, uterus, and contiguous structures, and are related to malignancy of pelvic organs, septic abortions, and postpartum complications. Upper respiratory tract infections and those of the nasopharynx, mouth, and jaw (tonsillar and peritonsillar abscesses, chronic otitis media, and dentoalveolar abscesses) have become relatively uncommon since the widespread use of antibiotics (penicillin or tetracycline) for the treatment of undiagnosed pharyngitis. Brain abscesses are a well-known complication of these upper respiratory tract infections in which bacteroides are involved along with other microorganisms, such as anaerobic streptococci.

Bacteroides bacteremia is characterized by a spiking fever, jaundice, and leukocytosis. In the patient more than forty years old, it is associated with chronic debilitating disease, hypotension, and a high mortality. Bacteremias have followed primary infection in the gastrointestinal, pelvic, and pharyngeal areas, and may originate from thrombophlebitis in these sites of infection. An indication of *Bacteroides* infection is the presence of a foul-smelling exudate from wounds or abscesses which contain gram-negative forms but produce no growth on aerobic culture. There appears to be a disposition toward *Bacteroides* infection in patients with underlying malignant disease. Often these patients have undergone elective intestinal surgery after preoperative intestinal antisepsis. This suggests that changes in the normal intestinal flora may predispose to *Bacteroides* infection. Therefore, the surgeon should be alert to the possibility of *Bacteroides* infection. A changing pattern of pyogenic abscesses of the liver has been characterized by an increased incidence of *Bacteroides* as the pathogen.

Treatment of *Bacteroides* infections consists of surgical drainage of abscesses, and appropriate antibiotic therapy. This should be based upon the results of sensitivity tests, since most bacteroides are resistant to penicillin. About 50 percent of isolates are resistant to tetracycline and lincomycin, but almost 100 percent of bacteroides are sensitive to chloramphenicol and clindamycin (7-chloro-lincomycin). It is important to determine whether bacteremia is due to aerobic or anaerobic gram-negative organisms, since the antibiotics commonly used for aerobic gram-negative sepsis, such as kanamycin, colistin, and gentamicin, are not effective against *Bacteroides*.

MYCOTIC INFECTIONS

The relation of the surgeon to mycotic infection has changed in recent years. The need for surgical treatment has diminished because of more effective modern chemotherapy. However, the widespread use of cytotoxic agents, corticosteroids, and antibacterial drugs for patients with leukemia and neoplasms has increased the incidence of fungi in opportunistic infections. Fungal infection threatens severely burned patients and those with implanted prosthetic devices and transplanted organs. Some of the symptoms of mycotic disease are chronic skin or mucous membrane lesions, low-grade fever, weight loss, chronic pulmonary or meningeal involvement, hepatosplenomegaly, and lymphadenopathy. Mycotic disease should be suspected unless another cause is clearly established. A mycosis may coexist with a lymphomatous disease, e.g., the association of histoplasmosis and cryptococcosis with Hodgkin's disease. A presumptive clinical diagnosis of a mycosis must be confirmed in the laboratory. Serologic tests are useful in reaching a presumptive diagnosis. The morphologic features of the fungus in tissue and culture are significant in identification.

The majority of patients with fungal infections seen by the physician have serious illness and present with typical symptoms of infection. Symptoms of pulmonary involvement frequently are present. Hematogenous dissemination of the disease produces manifestations such as tender swollen joints, draining subcutaneous abscesses, ulcerative lesions of the oropharynx, and meningitis. Many patients with systemic mycoses, as well as those with dermatophytoses, have skin lesions which are painful, itching, weeping, crusting, malodorous, and disfiguring. Brain abscess is an ominous manifestation of cladosporiosis and nocardiosis, which is best treated with sulfonamides.

Actinomycosis

Actinomycosis, produced by *Actinomyces bovis,* is manifested by nodular granulomas which subsequently suppurate and form sinus tracts. The infection is locally progressive and spreads by burrowing into and through fascial planes as well as into more solid surrounding supportive structures. Actinomycosis is characterized by chronicity and gradual emaciation in the absence of systemic toxic manifestations. Microscopic examination of the pus may reveal lightly entwined mycelial filaments called *sulfur granules.*

There are three clinical types of actinomycosis: cervicofacial, thoracic, and abdominal. Cervicofacial lesions are characterized by moderately tender, firm, inflammatory nodules, which eventually suppurate. Progression of the infection follows the usual course of sinus tract formation and burrowing spread. The thoracic type is usually well advanced before it is recognized (see Chap. 17). The abdominal type is often confused with periappendiceal abscess or carcinoma of the cecum, as the firm, nodular, granulomatous process is frequently localized in and about the appendix. As the infection progresses, typical cutaneous fistulas with firm nodules form in the abdominal wall, followed by suppuration and sinus tract formation.

TREATMENT. Abscesses should be incised and drained as they appear, and it is sometimes possible to excise totally the extensive burrowing sinus tracts. The organism is best treated with penicillin for periods of several weeks.

Blastomycosis

Blastomycosis is caused by a yeastlike organism (*Blastomyces dermatitidis*) which produces a painless reddish papule that eventually ulcerates. The ulcer is characteristic in that it usually contains small intracutaneous abscesses within a violaceous indurated advancing margin and exhibits a tendency to central healing. Primary cutaneous blastomycosis, although a chronic disease, eventually heals. The cutaneous lesions of disseminated blastomycosis may resemble the lesions of the primary cutaneous type but more often present as papulopustules that slowly enlarge, with sanguinopurulent exudate. Firm subcutaneous nodules (particularly at sites of trauma) may develop; these eventually suppurate and progress into shaggy ulcerations with serpiginous margins. Primary pulmonary mycotic infection or involvement of bone may be noted (see Chap. 17).

TREATMENT. Therapy of primary cutaneous blastomycosis is early surgical excision of the lesion with the advancing margin. Cutaneous lesions of disseminated blastomycosis respond to systemic treatment by amphotericin B and local wound care. Untreated disseminated blastomycosis is frequently fatal, with mortality over 90 percent within 6 months of onset.

Other Fungal Infections

COCCIDIOIDOMYCOSIS

Coccidioidomycosis is caused by the fungus *Coccidioides immitis* and most frequently manifests itself as a pulmonary infection (see Chap. 17). It also is associated with skin lesions, subcutaneous nodules, and involvement of the bone and brain. It is diagnosed by demonstrating organisms in the smear, and skin tests also have been developed. Treatment is with amphotericin B.

HISTOPLASMOSIS

Histoplasmosis is caused by *Histoplasma capsulatum* and may be diagnosed by positive skin tests. There are many endemic areas in the Middle Western and some Eastern states. The clinical manifestations include granulomatous ulceration of the oropharynx and pulmonary involvement. There may be large regional lymph nodes, particularly in the cervical area. Diagnosis is obtained by demonstrating the organism by culture or biopsy. Treatment with amphotericin B in the acute and subacute stages has been successful.

MONILIASIS

Moniliasis is caused by the yeast *Candida albicans* and is of increasing importance in view of the widespread use of antibiotic therapy which reduces the normal bacterial flora. It causes mild vaginitis, particularly in diabetic or pregnant women, which is readily treated by topical application of gentian violet or nystatin. Systemic involvement is particularly common in debilitated patients and has been noted in mixed infections following transplantation. Amphotericin B is used as systemic treatment. *Candida* infections of the skin are best treated by local use of nystatin or amphotericin B in creams or ointments.

SURGICAL ASEPSIS

Surgical asepsis, the prevention of the access of microorganisms to an operative wound, is achieved by methods designed to destroy bacteria or remove them from all objects coming in contact with the wound. Modern surgery is aseptic in the use of sterile instruments, sutures, and dressings and in the wearing of sterile caps, gowns, masks, and rubber gloves by the operating personnel. Although this is presently the extent of routine sterility in surgical asepsis, the technology of germ-free research is able to provide sterile flexible plastic isolation chambers in which neonates or antibiotic-decontaminated patients may be maintained in a sterile environment. Operations may be performed in "surgical" isolators cemented to the operative site of the patient. The surgeon makes his incision through the site of attachment of the isolator, and the operation may be conducted in the absence of all microorganisms. There is currently considerable interest in unidirectional (laminar) airflow systems as a less absolute means of limiting the number of bacteria to which a patient is exposed. It is necessary to resort to the use of antiseptics to degerm the site of the operation on the patient's skin. The surgeon and operating-room personnel usually use soaps or detergents containing antiseptics for scrubbing their hands before donning gloves or else rinse in an antiseptic after the scrub. An *antiseptic* is a chemical agent which either kills pathogenic microorganisms or inhibits their growth so long as there is contact between agent and microbe. By custom as well as by federal law, the term "antiseptic" is reserved for agents applied to the body. The antiseptic may actually be a disinfectant used in dilute solutions to avoid damage to tissues. A *disinfectant* is a germicidal, chemical substance used on inanimate objects to kill pathogenic microorganisms but not necessarily all others. These germicidal agents are used to disinfect instruments and other equipment which cannot be exposed to heat. They are essential for good housekeeping practices in hospitals, where they are used to disinfect floors, fabrics, and excreta. The first step in any process of biologic decontamination is thorough mechanical cleansing with soap or detergent and water to remove all traces of blood, pus, proteins, and mucus before the antiseptic or disinfectant is employed.

Sterilization

Sterilization is the process of killing all microorganisms (bacteria, spores, viruses, mycotic agents, and parasites). It is the ultimate in disinfection. The practical criterion of sterility is the failure of microbial growth to appear on tests in suitable bacteriologic media. Sterilization can be achieved by either physical or chemical agents. *Steam under pressure* is the most reliable means of sterilizing surgical supplies because of its power of penetration, microbiologic efficiency, ease of control, and economy of operation. Application of steam under a pressure of 15 psi (pounds per square inch) for 15 to 45 minutes will destroy all forms of life. Free-flowing steam, like boiling water, has a temperature of 100°C, but the same steam under pressure of 15 psi exerts a temperature of 121°C. Steam gives up heat by condensing into water. Thus when a bundle containing surgical pads or sponges is sterilized, the steam contacts the outer layer. There a portion of it condenses into water and releases heat. The steam then penetrates to a second layer, where another portion condenses and gives up heat. The steam thus approaches the center of the package, layer after layer, until the whole package is sterilized. The time of exposure depends upon the size of the parcel and its wrappings. Sterilization by steam under pressure is carried out in an autoclave. A major caution to be recognized when operating an autoclave is that a mixture of air and steam has a lower temperature than does pure steam. Therefore, when air is present in the chamber, the killing power of the process is diminished in proportion to the amount of air present. Most autoclaves depend upon gravity displacement of air from the chamber and from within articles being sterilized. Thus, improperly packed and positioned articles in the autoclave may fail to become sterile even though all physical conditions of the run may be correct. A new development in autoclaves is the high-vacuum sterilizer. A vacuum pump is incorporated into the system, and a vacuum is pulled in the chamber at the beginning and end of the sterilizing cycle. There is a considerable shortening of the time needed for sterilization, as only 3 minutes are needed to achieve sterility rather than the 20 minutes on the regular systems. In addition, there appears to be less damage to rubber, fabrics, and sharp instruments because of reduced exposure to moisture. There is less danger of creating air pockets and less chance of the steam's failing to penetrate to the center of bundles. Materials emerge dry, and much greater tolerances in packing the chamber are afforded.

Dry-heat sterilization is commonly used for glassware, for items that are injured by moisture, and for materials that resist penetration by steam, such as talc, vaseline, fats, and oils. The process consists of baking the material to be sterilized in a hot-air oven. At a temperature of 121°C (250°F) it takes about 6 hours to sterilize glassware, but at 170°C (340°F) the time required is about 1 hour. *Gas sterilization* is practical with ethylene oxide, a gas employed as a sterilizing agent in specially designed chambers in which temperatures and humidity can be controlled and from which air can be evacuated. The killing action is slow, and an exposure period from 3 to 6 hours is needed. Sterilization employing ethylene oxide is used for delicate surgical instruments with optical lenses, for tubing and plastic parts of heart-lung machines and respirators, for prepacked commercial plastic products such as disposable syringes, and for blankets, pillows, and mattresses. Ethylene oxide is very soluble in water and easily permeates oils, organic solvents, rubber, and many plastics. *Radiation sterilization* refers to ionizing radiation by cobalt 60 sources (γ-radiation) and by electron accelerators (high-energy electrons). It is currently used commercially to sterilize disposable hospital supplies, such as plastic hyperdermic syringes and sutures. Radiation sterilization of heat-sensitive pharmaceuticals has been recommended.

Degerming of Skin

Antiseptics incorporated into soaps are used for preoperative preparation of the skin at the operative site and for surgical hand scrubs by operating personnel. The bacteriologic content of normal skin consists of a resident flora, composed of coagulase-negative *Staphylococcus epidermidis* and anaerobic diphtheroides (e.g., *Corynebacterium acnes*), which reside on the surface of the skin, in hair follicles and in the ducts of sebaceous glands. These bacteria can be diminished temporarily, although they cannot be permanently eradicated. They are not usually responsible for surgical infections. Superimposed upon the resident flora is a transient flora consisting of bacteria picked up as a result of temporary colonizing of the skin. In the hospital, this transient flora often consists of pathogens resistant to antibiotics and is likely to be composed of pathogenic strains of *Staphylococcus aureus* and gram-negative enterobacteria. Therefore, pathogenic bacteria on the hands of operating personnel at the time of operation must be removed by scrubbing and destroyed by an antiseptic agent. The patient's skin must be degermed in the area of operation prior to the incision. The most efficient method is a vigorous scrub with liquid soaps containing either hexachlorophene or an iodophor.

Hexachlorophene is a bisphenol which disinfects the skin slowly. Commercial preparations containing 3% hexachlorophene, a detergent, and liquid soap are used for surgical scrubbing. Over a period of days, regular use of these surgical soaps brings about a progressive decrease in the number of bacteria on and in the skin. The hexachlorophene leaves an active film, which is renewed with each scrubbing. Consequently, its antibacterial activity persists so long as one continues to wash with soap containing hexachlorophene. A single washing with ordinary soap removes the antibacterial film. Hexachlorophene is effective against gram-positive pathogens such as *Staphylococcus aureus,* but it is without activity against gram-negative bacteria, such as the pseudomonas and the enterobacteria. This fact should be seriously considered by anyone using hexachlorophene, since gram-negative bacteria are currently responsible for the majority of nosocomial infections.

Iodophors are organic complexes of iodine and a synthetic detergent. About 1% iodine is available in the formula, whose germicidal action results from the liberation of free iodine when the compound is diluted with water. The detergent in the complex enhances the bactericidal activity of the iodine. Advantages of iodophors are that they destroy both gram-positive and gram-negative bacterial cells, but not spores; they do not stain skin and clothing; and they do not produce allergic reactions. Iodophors have been incorporated into surgical scrub soaps for hands and for the operative site.

Other Surgical Antiseptics

Isopropyl alcohol is slightly more effective than ethyl alcohol when used as 70% solutions and is less expensive. It may be obtained readily because it is not a potable beverage. As a group, alcohols possess many desirable features. They are bactericidal, have a cleansing action, and evaporate readily. They do not kill bacterial spores, however, and the skin should be thoroughly washed before the antiseptic solution is applied. The best one can hope to accomplish is to reduce the number of viable bacteria and to destroy pathogens which may be on the skin as transients. Isopropyl alcohol may also be used for the chemical sterilization of instruments if they are cleansed of all blood, pus, and body fluids. In the absence of spores, alcohol is an effective sterilizing agent.

Quaternary ammonium compounds, such as benzalkonium chloride (Zephiran chloride), are cationic surfactants. They are potent bactericides in vitro and because of their positive charge have an affinity for bacterial cells, which are negatively charged at physiologic pH. They are incompatible with anionic detergents, such as soap and phospholipids, since oppositely charged surfactants precipitate each other. They may be used together, however, if there has been a very thorough interim rinsing. Quaternary ammonium compounds may be used to preserve the sterility of heat-sterilized surgical instruments and sometimes are applied to minor lacerations and abrasions. They should be used for preoperative antisepsis of intact skin and mucous membranes with the knowledge that they are deposited on the skin as a sterile, invisible film beneath which bacteria remain viable.

References

Introduction; General Principles

Brachman, P. S., and Eickhoff, T. C., (eds.): "Proceedings of the International Conference on Nosocomial Infections," American Hospital Association, Chicago, 1971.

Brummelkamp, W. H., Boerema, I., and Hoogendyk, L.: Treatment of Clostridial Infections with Hyperbaric Oxygen Drenching: A Report of 26 Cases, Lancet, 1:235, 1963.

Dubos, R. J.: "Biochemical Determinants of Microbial Diseases," Harvard University Press, Cambridge, Mass., 1954.

Hentges, D. J.: Enteric Pathogen–Normal Flora Interactions, Am J Clin Nutr, 23:1451, 1970.

Jacobson, J. H., II, Morsch, J. H. C., and Rendell-Baker, L.: The Historical Perspective of Hyperbaric Therapy, Ann NY Acad Sci, 117:651, 1965.

Maibach, H. I., and Hildick-Smith, G., (eds.): "Skin Bacteria and Their Role in Infection," McGraw-Hill Book Company, New York, 1965.

Meleney, F. L.: "Treatise on Surgical Infections," Oxford University Press, New York, 1948.

Meleney, F. L.: "Clinical Aspects and Treatment of Surgical Infections," W. B. Saunders Company, Philadelphia, 1949.

Pulaski, E. J.: Common Bacterial Infections: Pathophysiology and Clinical Management," W. B. Saunders Company, Philadelphia, 1964.

Roding, B., Groeneveld, P. H. A., and Boerema, I.: Ten Years of Experience in The Treatment of Gas Gangrene with Hyperbaric Oxygen, Surg Gynecol Obstet, 134:579, 1972.

Rosebury, T.: "Microorganisms Indigenous to Man," McGraw-Hill Book Company, New York, 1962.

Slack, W. K., Hanson, G. C., and Chew, H. E. R.: Hyperbaric Oxygen in the Treatment of Gas Gangrene and Clostridial Infection: A Report of 40 Patients Treated in a Single-Person Hyperbaric Oxygen Chamber, Br J Surg, 56:505, 1969.

Wangensteen, O. H., Wangensteen, S. D., and Klinger, C. F.: Surgical Cleanliness, Hospital Salubrity, and Surgical Statistics, Historically Considered, Surgery, 71:477, 1972.

Williams, R. E. O., Blowers, R., Garrod, L. P., and Shooter, R. A.: "Hospital Infection: Causes and Prevention," 2d ed., Lloyd-Luke (Medical Books) Ltd., London, 1966.

Basic Considerations of Antibiotic Therapy

Crofton, J.: Some Principles in the Chemotherapy of Bacterial Infections, Br Med J, 2:137, 209, 1969.

Ellis, H.: The Place of Antibiotics in Surgical Practice To-day, Ann R Coll Surg Eng, 45:162, 1969.

Kabins, S.: Interactions among Antibiotics and Other Drugs, JAMA, 219:206, 1972.

Kantor, H. S., and Shaw, W. V.: Microbial Suprainfection. Recognition and Management, Med Clin North Am, 55:471, 1971.

Klainer, A. S., and Beisel, W. R.: Opportunistic Infection: A Review, Am J Med Sci, 258:431, 1969.

Weinstein, L., and Musher, D. M.: Antibiotic-induced Suprainfection, J Infect Dis, 119:662, 1969. (Editorial.)

Yale, C. E., and Peet, W. J.: Antibiotics in Colon Surgery, Am J Surg, 122:787, 1971.

Chemoprophylaxis; Intestinal Antisepsis; Intraperitoneal Antibiotics

Bernard, H. R., and Cole, W. R.: The Prophylaxis of Surgical Infection: The Effect of Prophylactic Antimicrobial Drugs on the Incidence of Infection following Potentially Contaminated Operations, Surgery, 56:151, 1964.

Cohn, I., Jr.: Intraperitoneal Antibiotic Administration, Surg Gynecol Obstet, 114:309, 1962.

Cohn, I., Jr.: "Intestinal Antisepsis," Charles C Thomas, Publisher, Springfield, Ill., 1968.

Cohn, I., Jr.: Intestinal Antisepsis, Surg Gynec Obstet, 130:1006, 1970.

Cohn, I., Jr., Langford, D., and Rives, J. D.: Antibiotic Support of Colon Anastomoses, Surg Gynecol Obstet, 104:1, 1957.

Cohn, I., Jr., and Rives, J. D.: Antibiotic Protection of Colon Anastomoses, Ann Surg, 141:707, 1955.

Cotlar, A. M., and Cohn, I., Jr.: Antimicrobial Therapy for Surgical Gastrointestinal Disease, in B. M. Kagan (ed.), "Antimicrobial Therapy," chap. 22, W. B. Saunders Company, Philadelphia, 1970.

DiVincenti, F. C., and Cohn, I., Jr.: Prolonged Administration of Intraperitoneal Kanamycin in the Treatment of Peritonitis, *Amer Surg,* **37:**177, 1971.

Laufman, H.: Surgical Judgment, in L. Davis (ed.), "Christopher's Textbook of Surgery," 9th ed., chap. 40, W. B. Saunders Company, Philadelphia, 1968.

McMullan, M. H., and Barnett, W. O.: The Clinical Use of Intraperitoneal Cephalothin, *Surgery,* **67:**432, 1970.

Mortimer, E. A., Jr.: Rational Use of Prophylactic Antibiotics, in B. M. Kagan (ed.), "Antimicrobial Therapy," chap. 31, W. B. Saunders Company, Philadelphia, 1970.

Nichols, R. L., and Condon, R. E.: Preoperative Preparation of the Colon, *Surg Gynecol Obstet,* **132:**323, 1971.

Antimicrobial Agents

Garrod, L. P., and O'Grady, F.: "Antibiotic and Chemotherapy," The Williams & Wilkins Company, Baltimore, 3d ed., 1971.

Kagan, B. M., (ed.): "Antimicrobial Therapy," W. B. Saunders Company, Philadelphia, 1970.

McCracken, G. H., Jr., Eichenwald, H. F., and Nelson, J. D.: Antimicrobial Therapy in Theory and Practice: I. Clinical Pharmacology: II. Clinical Approach to Antimicrobial Therapy, *J Pediatr,* **75:**742, 923, 1969.

Pankey, G. A.: "A Manual of Antimicrobial Therapy," Charles C Thomas, Publisher, Springfield, Ill., 1969.

Rutenberg, A. M.: Observations on Current Antibiotic Usage in the Surgical Patient, *Surg Clin North Am,* **49:**603, 1969.

Sandusky, W. R.: Infection and Antimicrobial Agents, in J. M. Kinney, R. H. Egdahl, and G. D. Zuidema (eds.), "Manual of Preoperative and Postoperative Care," chap. 5, W. B. Saunders Company, Philadelphia, 2d ed., 1971.

Streptococcal Infections

Abrams, J. S.: Role of Steroids in the Management of Phagedenic Ulcer, *Surgery,* **66:**297, 1969.

Altemeier, W. A., and Culbertson, W. R.: Acute Non-clostridial Crepitant Cellulitis, *Surg Gynecol Obstet,* **87:**206, 1948.

Armstrong, D., Blevins, A., Louria, D. B., Henkel, J. S., Moody, M. D., and Sukany, M.: Groups B, C, and G Streptococcal Infections in a Cancer Hospital, *Ann NY Acad Sci,* **174:**511, 1970.

Bornside, G. H., Welsh, J. S., and Cohn, I., Jr.: Bacterial Flora of the Human Small Intestine, *JAMA,* **196:**1125, 1966.

Brewer, G. E., and Meleney, F. L.: Progressive Gangrenous Infection of the Skin and Subcutaneous Tissues, following Operation for Acute Perforative Appendicitis: A Study in Symbiosis, *Ann Surg,* **84:**438, 1926.

Eickhoff, T. C., Klein, J. O., Daly, A. K., Ingall, D., and Finland, M.: Neonatal Sepsis and Other Infections Due to Group B Beta-hemolytic Streptococci, *N Engl J Med,* **271:**1221, 1964.

Grieco, M. H., and Sheldon, C.: *Erysipelothrix rhusopathiae, Ann NY Acad Sci,* **174:**523, 1970.

MacLennan, J. D.: Streptococcal Infection of Muscle, *Lancet,* **1:**582, 1943.

Meleney, F. L., Friedman, S. T., and Harvey, H. D.: The Treatment of Progressive Bacterial Synergistic Gangrene with Penicillin, *Surgery,* **18:**423, 1945.

Meleney, F. L., and Johnson, B. A.: Further Laboratory and Clinical Experiences in the Treatment of Chronic, Undermining, Burrowing Ulcers with Zinc Peroxide, *Surgery,* **1:**169, 1937.

Rea, W. J., and Wyrick, W. J., Jr.: Necrotizing Fasciitis, *Ann Surg,* **172:**957, 1970.

Strasberg, S. M., and Silver, M. S.: Hemolytic Streptococcus Gangrene: An Uncommon but Frequently Fatal Infection in the Antibiotic Era, *Am J Surg,* **115:**763, 1968.

Staphylococcal Infections

Altemeier, W. A., Hummel, R. P., and Hill, E. O.: Staphylococcal Enterocolitis following Antibiotic Therapy, *Ann Surg,* **157:**847, 1963.

Andriole, V. T., and Lyons, R. W.: Coagulase-negative Staphylococcus, *Ann NY Acad Sci,* **174:**533, 1970.

Dearing, W. H.: Micrococcic Enteritis and Pseudomembranous Enterocolitis as Complications of Antibiotic Therapy, *Ann NY Acad Sci,* **65:**235, 1956.

Elek, S. D.: "Staphylococcus Pyogenes and Its Relation to Disease," Livingstone Ltd., London, 1959.

Gresham, G. A., and Gleeson-White, M. H.: Staphylococcal Bronchopneumonia in Debilitated Hospital Patients: A Report of Fourteen Fatal Cases, *Lancet,* **1:**651, 1957.

Hardaway, R. M., III, and McKay, D. G.: Pseudomembranous Enterocolitis: Are Antibiotics Wholly Responsible? *Arch Surg,* **78:**446, 1959.

Kramer, I. R. H.: Fatal Staphylococcal Enteritis Developing during Streptomycin Therapy by Mouth, *Lancet,* **2:**646, 1948.

Wilson, T. S., and Stuart, R. D.: *Staphylococcus albus* in Wound Infection and in Septicemia, *Can Med Assoc J,* **93:**8, 1965.

Clostridial Infections

Altemeier, W. A., and Fullen, W. D.: Prevention and Treatment of Gas Gangrene, *JAMA,* **217:**806, 1971.

Altemeier, W. A., and Hummel, R. P.: Treatment of Tetanus, *Surgery,* **60:**495, 1966.

Athavale, V. B., and Pai, P. N.: Tetanus—Clinical Manifestations in Children, *J Pediatr,* **65:**590, 1964.

Bornside, G. H., and Cohn, I., Jr.: Clostridial Toxins in Strangulation Intestinal Obstruction in the Rabbit, *Ann Surg,* **152:**330, 1960.

Bornside, G. H., and Cohn, I., Jr.: Intestinal Bacteriology of Closed Loop, Strangulated Obstruction in Dogs, *Gastroenterology,* **41:**245, 1961.

Bornside, G. H., Floyd, C. E., and Cohn, I., Jr.: Clostridium sordelli Toxin in Strangulation Obstruction: Further Studies of Serial Changes of Intestinal Contents, *J Surg Res,* **4:**233, 1964.

Brooks, G. F., Buchanan, T. M., and Bennett, J. V.: Tetanus Toxoid Immunization of Adults: A Continuing Need, *Ann Intern Med,* **73:**603, 1970.

Cherubin, C. E.: Clinical Severity of Tetanus in Narcotic Addicts in New York City, *Arch Intern Med,* **121:**156, 1968.

Clay, R. C., and Bolton, J. W.: Tetanus Arising from Gangrenous Unperforated Small Intestine, *JAMA,* **187:**856, 1964.

DeJongh, D. S.: Postoperative Synergistic Gangrene, *JAMA,* **200:**227, 1967.

Dickinson, K. M., and Edgar, W. M.: Anaerobic Cellulitis of the Abdominal Wall after Prostatectomy and Orchidectomy, *Lancet,* **1**:1139, 1963.

Grainger, R. W., MacKenzie, D. A., and McLachlin, A. D.: Progressive Bacterial Synergistic Gangrene: Chronic Undermining Ulcer of Meleney, *Can J Surg,* **10**:439, 1967.

Heyningen, W. E. van: General Characteristics, in S. J. Ajl, S. Kadis and T. C. Montie (eds.), "Microbial Toxins," vol. 1, chap. 1, Academic Press, Inc., New York, 1970.

Isenberg, A. N.: *Clostridium welchii* Infection, *Arch Surg,* **92**:727, 1966.

Lowbury, E. J. L., and Lilly, H. A.: Contamination of Operating-Theatre Air with *Cl. tetani, Br Med J,* **2**:1334, 1958.

MacLennan, J. D.: The Histotoxic Clostridial Infections of Man, *Bacteriol Rev,* **26**:177, 1962.

McNally, M. J., and Crile, G., Jr.: Diagnosis and Treatment of Gas Gangrene of the Abdominal Wall, *Surg Gynecol Obstet,* **118**:1046, 1964.

Meleney, F. L.: Bacterial Synergism in Disease Processes: With a Confirmation of the Synergistic Bacterial Etiology of a Certain Type of Progressive Gangrene of the Abdominal Wall, *Ann Surg,* **94**:961, 1931.

Oakley, C. L.: Gas Gangrene, *Br Med Bull,* **10**:52, 1954.

Shapiro, B., Rohman, M., and Cooper, P.: Clostridial Infection following Abdominal Surgery, *Ann Surg,* **158**:27, 1963.

Treadway, C. R., and Prange, A. J., Jr.: Tetanus Mimicking Psychophysiologic Reaction: Occurrence after Dental Extraction, *JAMA,* **200**:891, 1967.

Willis, A. T.: "Clostridia of Wound Infection," Butterworth Scientific Publications, London, 1969.

Pseudomonal Infections

Alexander, J. W.: Pseudomonas Infections in Man, in P. S. Brachman and T. C. Eickhoff (eds.), "Proceedings of the International Conference on Nosocomial Infections," p. 103, American Hospital Association, Chicago, 1971.

Forkner, C. E., Jr.: "Pseudomonas Aeruginosa Infections," Grune & Stratton, Inc., New York, 1960.

Sandusky, W. R.: Pseudomonas Infections: Sources and Cultural Data in a General Hospital with Particular Reference to Surgical Infections, *Ann Surg,* **153**:996, 1961.

Enterobacterial Infections

Alami, S. Y., and Riley, H. D., Jr.: Infections Caused by Mimiae, with Special Reference to *Mima polymorpha:* A Review, *Am J Med Sci,* **252**:537, 1966.

Clayton, E., and Von Graevenitz, A.: Nonpigmented *Serratia marcescens, JAMA,* **197**:1059, 1966.

Eickhoff, T. C., Steinhauer, B. W., and Finland, M.: The *Klebsiella-Enterobacter-Serratia* Division: Biochemical and Serologic Characteristics and Susceptibility to Antibiotics, *Ann Intern Med,* **65**:1163, 1966.

Graber, C. D., Rabin, E. R., Mason, A. D., Jr., and Vogel, E. H., Jr.: Increasing Incidence of Nosocomial Herellea vaginicola Infections in Burned Patients, *Surg Gynecol Obstet,* **114**:109, 1962.

Reisig, G., and Schaffner, W.: Postoperative Detection of *Salmonella typhi, Arch Surg,* **104**:349, 1972.

Steinhauer, B. W., Eickhoff, T. C., Kislak, J. W., and Finland, M.: The *Klebsiella-Enterobacter-Serratia* Division: Chemical

and Epidemiologic Characteristics, *Ann Intern Med,* **65**:1180, 1966.

Wilkowske, C. J., Washington, J. A., II, Martin, W. J., and Ritts, R. E., Jr.: *Serratia marcescens:* Biochemical Characteristics, Antibiotic Susceptibility Patterns, and Clinical Significance, *JAMA,* **214**:2157, 1970.

Bacteroides Infections

Altemeier, W. A., Schowengerdt, C. G., and Whiteley, D. H.: Abscesses of the Liver: Surgical Considerations, *Arch Surg,* **101**:258, 1970.

Bartlett, J. G., and Finegold, S. M.: Clinical Features and Diagnosis of Anaerobic Pleuropulmonary Infections, *Antimicrob Agents Chemother 1970,* 1971, p. 78.

Bodner, S. J., Koenig, M. G., and Goodman, J. S.: Bacteremic Bacteroides Infections, *Ann Intern Med,* **73**:537, 1970.

Bornstein, D. L., Weinberg, A. N., Swartz, M. N., and Kunz, L. J.: Anaerobic Infections: Review of Current Experience, *Medicine,* **43**:207, 1964.

Brodine, W. N., and Schwartz, S. I.: Pyogenic Hepatic Abscesses: Review of Representative Literature and Presentation of Ten Cases, *NY State J Med.* (In press.).

Finegold, S. M., Marsh, V. H., and Bartlett, J. G.: Anaerobic Infections in the Compromised Host, in P. S. Brachman and T. C. Eickhoff (eds.), "Proceedings of the International Conference on Nosocomial Infections," p. 123, American Hospital Association, Chicago, 1971.

Gelb, A. F., and Seligman, S. J.: Bacteroidaceae Bacteremia: Effect of Age and Focus of Infection upon Clinical Course, *JAMA,* **212**:1038, 1970.

Heineman, H. S., and Braude, A. I.: Anaerobic Infection of the Brain, *Am J Med,* **35**:682, 1963.

Saksena, D. S., Block, M. A., McHenry, M. C., and Truant, J. P.: Bacterioidaceae: Anaerobic Organisms Encountered in Surgical Infections, *Surgery,* **63**:261, 1968.

Sinkovics, J. G., and Smith, J. P.: Septicemia with Bacteroides in Patients with Malignant Disease, *Cancer,* **25**:663, 1970.

Mycotic Infections

Bernhardt, H. E., Orlando, J. C., Benfield, J. R., Hirose, F. M., and Foos, R. Y.: Disseminated Candidiasis in Surgical Patients, *Surg Gynecol Obstet.,* **134**:819, 1972.

Conant, N. F., Smith, D. T., Baker, R. D., and Callaway, J. L.: "Manual of Clinical Mycology," 3d ed., W. B. Saunders Company, Philadelphia, 1971.

Emmons, C. W., Binford, C. H., and Utz, J. P.: "Medical Mycology," 2d ed., Lea & Febiger, Philadelphia, 1970.

MacMillan, B. G., Law, E. J., and Holder, I. A.: Experience with *Candida* Infections in the Burn Patient, *Arch Surg,* **104**:509, 1972.

Nash, G., Foley, F. D., Goodwin, M. N., Jr., Bruck, H. M., Greenwald, K. A., and Pruitt, B. A., Jr.: Fungal Burn Wound Infection, *JAMA,* **215**:1664, 1971.

Surgical Asepsis

Bornside, G. H., Crowder, V. H., Jr., and Cohn, I., Jr.: A Bacteriological Evaluation of Surgical Scrubbing with Disposable Iodophor-Soap Impregnated Polyurethane Scrub Sponges, *Surgery,* **64**:743, 1968.

Crowder, V. H., Jr., Bornside, G. H., and Cohn, I., Jr.: Bacteri-
    ological Comparison of Hexachlorophene and Polyvinyl-
    pyrrolidine-Iodine Surgical Scrub Soaps, *Am Surg,* **33:**906,
    1967.
Lawrence, C. A., and Block, S. S., (eds.): "Disinfection, Sterili-
    zation, and Preservation," Lea & Febiger, Philadelphia, 1968.

Levenson, S. M., Trexler, P. C., Malm, O. J., LaConte, M. L.,
    Horowitz, R. E., and Moncrief, W. H.: A Plastic Isolator for
    Operating in a Sterile Environment, *Am J Surg,* **104:**891, 1962.
Rubbo, S. D., and Gardner, J. F.: "A Review of Sterilization and
    Disinfection," Lloyd-Luke (Medical Books) Ltd., London,
    1965.

Chapter 6

Trauma

by G. Tom Shires

General Considerations

Initial Resuscitation of the Severely Injured Patient
    Priority by Injury
Immediate Nonoperative Surgical Care
Diagnosis and Management of Unapparent Injury

Metabolic Response to Trauma

Endocrine Response
Catabolic Response
Metabolic Requirements
Management

Anesthesia

Complicating Problems
Assessment of the Patient's Status
Premedication
Choice of Anesthetic
Postoperative Management

Principles in the Management of Wounds

Primary Wound Management
    Local Care of Wounds
Emergency Laparotomy
Antibiotics

Bites and Stings of Animals and Insects

Rabies
Snakebites
Stinging Insects and Animals
    Hymenoptera
    Stingrays
    Portuguese Man-of-War
Spider Bites
    Black Widow Spider
    North American Loxoscelism

Penetrating Wounds of the Neck and Thoracic Inlet

Specific Injuries

Abdominal Trauma

Evaluation of Blunt Trauma
Penetrating Trauma
    Stab Wounds
    Gunshot Wounds
Stomach
Duodenum
    Intramural Hematoma
Small Bowel
Colon Injuries

Liver
Extrahepatic Biliary Tree
    Penetrating Injuries
    Blunt Trauma
Pancreas
Spleen
Retroperitoneal Hematoma
Inferior Vena Cava
Female Reproductive Organs
Abdominal Wall

GENERAL CONSIDERATIONS

(*By G. Tom Shires and Ronald C. Jones*)

The magnitude of the problem of trauma in the United States is probably not adequately appreciated. In this country trauma is the leading cause of death in the first three decades of life. It ranks overall as the fourth leading cause of death in the United States today; if arteriosclerosis is considered as a single entity, trauma is the third leading cause of death. Fifty million injuries occur annually in the United States, over ten million of them being disabling. Over 100,000 deaths occur each year from accidents. Automobile accidents alone kill more Americans each year than were lost during the entire Korean conflict. Unlike many serious disease entities in the United States, the incidence of and mortality from injuries is increasing each year.

Accident patients take up to 22 million hospital bed days a year in the United States—more than are needed to take care of the delivery of all the babies in a given year, more than are needed by all the heart patients, and four times more than are needed by all cancer patients. Even during wartime, deaths from accidents always exceed battle deaths. In World War II, United States battle deaths were 292,000; accidental civilian deaths during the same period in the United States alone were 450,000. And more military personnel die from accidents than from combat during a period of national involvement.

An attempt will be made in this chapter to cover certain principles related to injuries, as well as selected areas of bodily injury. The following discussions of certain specifics of the patient who has sustained trauma will, of necessity, omit several critical areas concerned with care of the traumatized patient. These related problems are being discussed elsewhere in the text and include related principles such as those of shock, cardiac arrest, transfusion problems, pulmonary ventilation, and surgical infections initiated by trauma. Other organ system injuries covered elsewhere include burns, injuries to central nervous system, thoracic trauma, and genitourinary trauma. Similarly, complications including renal failure and embolism are covered in detail in separate chapters.

Initial Resuscitation of the Severely Injured Patient

The patient with multiple injuries is best managed by one physician. When the responsibility is divided, evaluation of the patient's overall problems may be lacking, and complications may not be recognized for several hours.

PRIORITY BY INJURY

There are three categories of patients, according to immediacy of injury. The first group includes injuries which interfere with vital physiologic function and therefore immediately threaten life, such as obstruction of an airway or bleeding from a gunshot wound. The primary treatment is to establish an airway and control the bleeding. This type of patient may require surgical treatment for massive internal bleeding within 5 to 10 minutes following arrival in the emergency room. The operating room should be alerted when the patient is admitted to the emergency room, and no time is wasted in getting the patient into "operative" condition. Often the control of hemorrhage is dependent on a rapid thoracotomy or laparotomy to occlude injured major vessels.

A second group of patients are those with injuries which offer no immediate threat to life. These include patients who have received gunshot wounds, stab wounds, or blunt trauma to the chest and abdomen but whose vital signs are stable. The majority of injured patients are in this category. Although they will require surgical procedures within 1 to 2 hours, there is time for additional information to be obtained. Blood for typing and cross matching is drawn, and blood is made available if there is any possibility that the patient will require surgical intervention. If vital signs are stable, x-rays may be obtained to determine the course of the missile and the extent of possible associated injuries, such as fractures. Cystography and pyelography may be done to assess hematuria. Since patients with penetrating and blunt abdominal injuries may develop shock at any moment, a physician must be in constant attendance during all evaluations. Patients who suddenly go into shock are immediately taken to the operating room without additional diagnostic procedures.

The third group of patients are those whose injuries produce occult damage. This group is composed primarily of patients who have sustained blunt trauma to the abdomen which may or may not require surgical intervention and in whom the exact nature of the injury is not apparent. These patients usually have time for extensive laboratory studies, x-rays, and more complete physical examination. Surgical intervention in this group may be delayed hours or days, as with delayed rupture of the spleen.

Patients who are severely injured should be admitted to the emergency room in a trauma area equipped for emergency resuscitation. This room should contain such items as intravenous fluids, overhead operating-room light, oxygen, cardiac monitor and defibrillator, and a portable carriage which is suitable for an operating-room table in an emergency situation. A cabinet should be in the room containing a tracheostomy tray, closed chest drainage tray, venous section tray, closed-chest drainage bottle, intravenous fluids with tubing and needles, and syringes for four-quadrant abdominal paracentesis and pericardiocentesis. The cabinet shelf should have clearly visible labels under each tray or set of instruments. These trays and instruments should be kept in this trauma room and not in central supply, as a waiting period of even 5 minutes may prove fatal.

ADEQUATE AIRWAY. The first and most important emergency measure in the management of the severely injured patient is to establish an effective airway. A cabinet should be available at the head of the emergency room carriage in which a laryngoscope and cuffed endotracheal tubes of various sizes are available. Endotracheal intubation is a most rapid method of obtaining an adequate airway. Once an airway is established, a means of positive-pressure breathing should be available, such as an Ambu bag or an intermittent positive-pressure breathing machine. A cuffed endotracheal tube is desirable, so that positive-pressure breathing may be accomplished if needed in the resuscitation or in the administration of anesthesia. Either wall suction or a portable suction machine must be available in the trauma room to remove pulmonary secretions, foreign bodies, and, frequently, blood from the upper respiratory tract. When an endotracheal tube cannot readily be inserted, a tracheostomy may be done.

SHOCK AND HEMORRHAGE. Shock is usually controlled while the patient's airway is being cleared by another person. Internal hemorrhage will require immediate surgical intervention. Hypovolemic shock is best prevented or controlled by starting intravenous infusions in at least two extremities, using 18-gauge needles or cutdown catheters of comparable size. At least one upper extremity should be chosen for the intravenous infusion in the presence of abdominal wounds. If the inferior vena cava or one of its major tributaries is partially severed, the intravenous fluid may pour from the lower extremity into the retroperitoneal space, depriving the heart of any infusion from the lower extremities. A balanced salt solution such as Ringer's lactate solution is usually started until blood is available. Blood for typing and cross matching is drawn at the time the intravenous fluid is started, and the balanced salt solution is given in addition to the blood. Shock resulting from a blood loss of 500 to 750 ml can usually be corrected by rapid administration of 2 liters of Ringer's lactate solution over a 15- to 20-minute period. Blood loss in excess of 750 ml usually requires the administration of whole blood in addition to balanced salt solution. Often, 2 liters of balanced salt solution will replace the volume and correct hypotension so that no blood is necessary, reducing the possibility of blood transfusion reaction. When a patient initially responds to 1 to 2 liters of balanced salt solution, as evidenced by a normal blood pressure and decrease in pulse rate, but subsequently becomes hypotensive, whole blood usually is indicated. However, by this time, type-specific blood usually is available and often cross-matched, which reduces the chances for a transfusion reaction. Should a patient not respond to the rapid administration of 2 liters of balanced salt solution, un-cross-matched, type O, Rh-negative blood is administered without hesitation. The administration of blood from plastic bags markedly decreases the possibility of an air embolus when blood is being pumped.

External bleeding is best controlled by direct finger pressure on the bleeding wound or vessel. Tourniquets are of little benefit in the control of major arterial bleeding and often injurious if they occlude collateral circulation. A frequent mistake is the placement of a tourniquet on an extremity tight enough to obstruct venous return but loose enough not to inhibit arterial flow; this only increases the blood loss and edema. The danger of tissue loss from tourniquet use is always present.

Superficial vessels may be ligated if they are readily seen; however, wounds are not probed in a blind attempt to place a hemostat on a vessel. As soon as bleeding is controlled, the wound is covered with a sterile dressing, and the patient is taken to the operating room, where the wound is more adequately visualized and proper instruments are available. The needless probing of wounds in the emergency room may lead to severe infection, which can be avoided by proper exploration including adequate irrigation and sterile surgical technique in the operating room.

NEUROLOGIC EVALUATION. After an adequate airway has been obtained and hemorrhage has been controlled, a gross neurologic evaluation of the patient is undertaken. Motor function in the four extremities should be verified. A progressing neurologic deficit following injury to the spinal cord may indicate an emergency laminectomy. Decompression of a hematoma may result in return of function. Thoracoabdominal injuries usually take precedence over orthopedic or neurologic injury.

CHEST INJURIES. Airway obstruction may be due to mucus, fragments of bone from facial fractures, dirt and debris, and, commonly, broken teeth or dentures. If the patient does not ventilate normally after an endotracheal tube is inserted or a tracheostomy has been performed, several injuries should be considered. These include pneumothorax, hemothorax, cardiac tamponade, flail chest, and a ruptured bronchus.

Pneumothorax. If a pneumothorax is questionable, an 18-gauge needle may be inserted into the chest in the anterior axillary line and aspiration done to reveal the presence of air. A chest x-ray is preferable, but often severe respiratory distress precludes time for x-ray confirmation. Tension pneumothorax with mediastinal shift is suggested by displacement of the trachea to the opposite side. Auscultation of the chest may reveal decreased breath sounds. The patient with a pneumothorax is treated with closed-chest drainage. As there is little danger from the insertion of a chest tube in the absence of a pneumothorax, an anterior chest tube should be inserted if there is doubt.

Hemothorax. Diagnosis of hemothorax is similar to that of pneumothorax. If the patient on the emergency-room cart is in distress, a needle may be inserted in the eighth interspace in the posterior axillary line and aspiration done to reveal a hemothorax. This is best drained with both anterior and posterior chest tubes. The anterior chest tube is placed in the second interspace in the midclavicular line, and the posterior chest tube is placed in the eighth interspace in the posterior axillary line in the region between the midaxillary and posterior axillary line. Chest tubes are of large caliber and soft rubber so that adequate drainage may be maintained. Thoracotomy may be indicated, depending on the rate of bleeding or the presence of intrathoracic clots.

Cardiac Tamponade. During initial observation, an unsuspected cardiac tamponade may develop secondary to blunt or penetrating trauma. This is often not present on arrival in the emergency room but may develop after 1 to 2 hours of observation. The clinical signs pathognomonic for cardiac tamponade are increased venous pressure, decreased pulse pressure, particularly with a paradoxical pulse and with or without cyanosis, and subsequent development of hypotension and decreased heart sounds. Emergency treatment includes aspiration of the pericardial sac with an 18-gauge needle through the xyphocostal angle. As little as 20 ml of aspirated blood may make a remarkable difference in the patient's vital signs. Depending on the cause of cardiac tamponade, immediate thoracotomy may be required to repair the cardiac wound, or the patient may be observed until a second aspiration is necessary. Following the development of the second cardiac tamponade, almost all patients will require an emergency thoracotomy. When a patient arrives at the emergency room in shock without evidence of blood loss, this diagnosis should be suspected.

Flail Chest. Unless patients sustaining blunt trauma to the thorax and abdomen are fully disrobed in the emergency room, a flail chest may not be recognized. Patients sustaining flail chest are best treated immediately with tracheostomy and intermittent positive-pressure breathing (IPPB). This promptly expands the lungs and provides adequate ventilation, often preventing the development of atelectasis and pneumonia. Some type of stabilizing apparatus such as towel clips may be beneficial. However, towel clips alone may not be effective, since the patient may not ventilate as well without intermittent positive-pressure breathing. Sandbags are of little value and may lead to the development of pulmonary complications such as atelectasis.

Ruptured Bronchus. After rupture of a bronchus, respiratory distress, hemoptysis, cyanosis, and a massive air leak with both mediastinal and subcutaneous emphysema and/or tension pneumothorax may be observed. Often the diagnosis is not obvious. There is a close relationship between fractures of the first and second ribs and rupture of a bronchus. If extrapleural hematoma is noted, special views of the first ribs are indicated. A ruptured bronchus is treated initially with closed-chest drainage. If this does not effectively keep the lung expanded, open thoracotomy with repair of the bronchus is indicated.

Open Chest Wounds. The patient with a chest injury resulting in a sucking chest wound is best managed by immediately covering the open wound with whatever material is available, such as a large gauze bandage. This prevents further shifting of the mediastinum and allows ventilation of the opposite lung. Chest tubes are usually inserted prior to operation, and immediate surgical intervention is indicated.

Ruptured Thoracic Aorta. The diagnosis may be suspected from chest x-ray showing a widened mediastinum and confirmed by arteriography. Immediate operation usually is indicated.

PENETRATING WOUNDS OF THE ABDOMINAL WALL. All penetrating injuries to the abdominal wall are explored locally in the emergency room to determine if the peritoneal cavity is penetrated. Exploration is usually accomplished by extending the stab wound and determining its depth. In the event that the extent of penetration cannot be determined or if the stab wound violates the posterior rectus abdominis sheath, the abdominal cavity is explored. The use of radiopaque material to determine abdominal cavity penetration has been reported, but until the accuracy of this method is better confirmed, questionable penetrating injuries of the abdominal cavity should be explored. The mortality and morbidity from a negative abdominal exploration is negligible, but failure to discover such injuries as colon or liver injury for several hours may allow peritonitis and other complications to develop. All gunshot wounds of the abdomen should be explored whether penetration is evident or not. Shock waves from nonpenetrating gunshot wounds of the abdominal wall often easily transect bowel or lacerate the liver or spleen without entering the abdominal cavity.

THE UNCONSCIOUS PATIENT. Patients with closed head injuries who are unconscious must have an airway established immediately. Hypotension rarely results from a closed head injury but is almost always caused by blood loss, usually in the thorax or abdomen. The cause of the blood loss is most rapidly determined by using an 18-gauge needle for immediate abdominal and chest taps, which may reveal nonclotting blood. The absence of blood does not rule out an intraabdominal or thoracic injury. Extreme care should be used in moving unconscious patients until injuries of the spine have been ruled out, as repositioning the head may result in transection of the spinal cord.

Immediate Nonoperative Surgical Care

HEMATURIA. A Foley catheter is routinely inserted, particularly following blunt trauma to the abdomen, to determine the presence of hematuria as well as to follow the urinary output during and immediately following the surgical procedure. Gross hematuria is evidence of urinary tract injury resulting from contusion, laceration, or rupture. If the patient's vital signs are stable and hematuria is present, a combined cystogram and intravenous pyelogram should be done. A single 15-minute film is usually adequate to determine kidney function as well as indicate extravasation from the bladder, ureter, or kidneys. Failure to demonstrate extravasation does not rule out the possibility of a ruptured bladder or kidney. Should a nephrectomy be required during a laparotomy, functioning of the kidney on the opposite side should be proved. It is useless to attempt to visualize the kidneys by intravenous pyelogram when the patient is hypotensive. X-rays are delayed until the patient has been resuscitated and bleeding has been controlled in the operating room. If time is not available preoperatively for an intravenous pyelogram, a cassette may be placed under the patient prior to the start of surgical procedures and a pyelogram obtained intraoperatively.

FRACTURES. Fractures of the extremities are best managed immediately with splints, such as a Thomas splint for the lower extremities and an arm board for the upper extremities. Immobilization may prevent additional nerve and blood vessel injury and conversion of a closed fracture to an open one. The presence or absence of pulses in the fractured extremities should be noted on initial examination. Intravenous infusions should not be started in an injured extremity. Massive thoracoabdominal bleeding takes precedence over fractures, unless there is an accompanying arterial injury of such magnitude that there is danger of loss of limb. In such instances, it is often necessary to have two surgical teams working simultaneously.

Pelvic fractures usually are managed conservatively with a pelvic binder, traction, or only bed rest. Inability to insert a Foley catheter into the urethra following a pelvic fracture may indicate a fractured urethra.

ARTERIAL INJURIES. Any penetrating injury in the region of a major blood vessel or nerve requires surgical exploration. On initial examination, 18 percent of subsequently proved arterial injuries are noted to have a normal pulse distal to the arterial injury, and one-third of the patients have a palpable but diminished distal pulse. Arteriography is time-consuming and often will not demonstrate extravasation if the vessel injury is covered by a clot. If the platysma muscle in the neck has been violated, the neck is explored, and carotid and/or subclavian vessels also are explored. Vessel exploration in the region of the neck should be done under endotracheal anesthesia and may require resection of a portion of the clavicle for adequate visualization. Early recognition of an arterial injury is the most important factor in preserving a viable extremity or functioning distal organ.

Diagnosis and Management of Unapparent Injury

Blunt trauma to the abdomen may produce severe intraperitoneal or retroperitoneal injury with minimal physical findings. Bowel sounds may not be lost for several hours, and evidence of retroperitoneal or intraabdominal injury may not become apparent for as long as 18 hours.

An abdominal paracentesis may be performed early in the observation period in patients with injuries from blunt trauma to the abdomen. A 95 percent diagnostic accuracy is associated with the positive abdominal tap, and even a tap which yields only a few drops of nonclotting blood is indication for abdominal exploration. A negative abdominal tap does not rule out intraabdominal injury; if injury is still suspected, peritoneal lavage is indicated. Strong suspicion of intraabdominal injury in the female with a negative abdominal tap calls for culdocentesis.

Patients with signs of peritoneal irritation require exploratory laparotomy even in the absence of a positive abdominal tap.

ROENTGENOGRAMS. These are taken when a patient's vital signs remain stable but are omitted for patients in severe shock. X-rays of the chest and abdomen are routinely performed to rule out foreign bodies such as knife blades within the depths of the wound. Patients sustaining gunshot wounds should have x-rays when possible in an attempt to trace the course of the missile. Patients sustaining blunt trauma often require multiple x-rays to rule out obscure fractures of the vertebral spine and retroperitoneal injuries. X-rays of extremities will be of value in determining whether or not the missile struck bone, fractured bone, or passed near vital structures.

NASOGASTRIC INTUBATION. A Levin tube is routinely inserted in the severely injured patient. Passage of the tube may provoke vomiting and empty the stomach of large particles, preventing subsequent aspiration during anesthesia. Stomach injury from penetrating or blunt trauma may be diagnosed by finding bright red blood in the Levin tube drainage. Gastric intubation prevents gastric dilatation during tracheal intubation and aids in the prevention of postoperative distension of the small bowel.

PROPHYLACTIC ANTIBIOTICS. Antibiotics are administered preoperatively to all patients sustaining penetrating wounds of the abdomen, beginning as soon as possible after the injured patient arrives in the emergency room. They may be discontinued if exploratory laparotomy is negative. Considerable experimental evidence indicates that prophylactic antibiotics in trauma are of benefit if administered within the first 3 hours following injury. A recent review of a group of patients at Parkland Memorial Hospital, Dallas, Texas, who sustained penetrating abdominal injuries showed that there was a statistically significant decrease in the incidence of wound infection in those patients who received antibiotics preoperatively or intraoperatively as opposed to those who received antibiotics in the immediate postoperative period or therapeutically. Following injury, immunized patients are administered a tetanus toxoid booster. In unimmunized patients the wound is debrided, and 250 units of tetanus human immune globulin is administered. Patients who were previously immunized but are now taking steroids, immunosuppressive therapy, or chemotherapy or who have had extensive irradiation should receive human immune globulin, since they may not have normal antibody response. Contaminated wounds should be left open or converted to open wounds when feasible.

METABOLIC RESPONSE TO TRAUMA

(By Malcolm O. Perry)

Trauma acutely and extensively alters the delicate integration of endocrine and metabolic systems in man (see Chap. 1). The wide range of response correlates with the magnitude of injury and the metabolic adjustments of which the patient is capable. Moore has divided the metabolic response into four phases: (1) the initial injury reaction, lasting 2 to 4 days; (2) the turning point, requiring 1 to 2 days; (3) an anabolic period, characterized by protein synthesis and lasting 2 to 5 weeks; (4) a period of several months of final adjustment in which "fat gain" is preponderant. These metabolic responses can be conveniently grouped into two categories: endocrine and catabolic.

Endocrine Response

Following injury, there is increased urinary excretion of epinephrine, norepinephrine, and their metabolic products. Although the measurement of blood levels of catecholamines does not always correlate well with the clinical findings, sympathicoadrenal activity is present. During the early stages the patient frequently exhibits tachycardia, sweating, and vasoconstriction, and is pale and apprehensive. Although the clinical signs may disappear relatively rapidly, elevated urinary levels of catecholamines and their metabolic products may persist for 1 or 2 days. If no complications follow the initial traumatic episode, the primary effects of sympathicoadrenal action are noted only during the early stages of the injury and pass rather rapidly.

Many of the metabolic changes noted following injury are similar to those induced by the administration of excessive amounts of cortisone or hydrocortisone. Urinary excretion of conjugated steroids is increased in the posttraumatic period. The normal excretion of 10 to 20 mg of 17-hydroxycorticosteroids may be tripled during the first 3 to 4 days following an injury of moderate severity. If shock or liver injury has not occurred, peak blood levels of 17-hydroxycorticosteroids are obtained about 6 hours after trauma. This reaction appears to be nonspecific and more closely related to the severity of the injury than to the specific type of injury. There is a less exact correlation between the negative nitrogen balance and the increasing levels of corticosteroid production. It has been observed that even in adrenalectomized rats urinary nitrogen excretion increases after injury if the animals are maintained on constant amounts of adrenocortical extracts, suggesting that the metabolic changes which follow injury are not directly related to the absolute level of corticosteroid production. This observation accords with the concept of the corticosteroids exerting a "permissive" or "conditioning" action.

The exact relationship between injury and the function of other endocrine glands remains unclear. The increase in oxygen consumption and carbon dioxide production following injury suggests that the thyroid gland may play an essential role, but similar effects can be produced by a variety of influences in the absence of trauma. Various measurements of thyroid function fail to correlate well with energy changes in the traumatized patient. The increased calcium excretion following injury can be related quite well to immobilization, and parathyroid function need not be invoked to explain calcium loss. Somatotropin, or growth hormone, has a profound effect on body metabolism, particularly skeletal growth and the synthesis of protein. Normal growth and development seem to be directly related to its presence, but there is no evidence that this hormone is necessary for normal convalescence. At the present time, the exact reaction of these other endocrine glands to injury is unclear.

Catabolic Response

Catabolism is increased following injury. Dissolution of body protein is reflected by increased urinary nitrogen excretion; after extensive trauma or with infection, levels of 15 to 20 Gm/day may be reached. The increased rate of excretion may persist for 3 to 5 days in the uncomplicated case. This can be reduced by the administration of exogenous protein and other compounds which supply calories, thus decreasing the effect of starvation. The inability to prevent these nitrogen losses completely indicates a definite catabolic effect in excess of that produced by starvation.

If water gain and loss are kept at minimal rates, careful weight measurements will reveal a loss of body tissue. A urinary loss of approximately 10 Gm of nitrogen represents about 62 Gm of protein loss, or about 300 Gm of wet lean muscle. The protein in bone and connective tissue and in plasma less readily reflect these changes. There can be, in fact, large losses or gains in protein without detectable changes in the concentrations of plasma proteins.

As initial responses to injury dissipate, a relatively abrupt change toward normal occurs in urinary nitrogen excretion. With sufficient caloric intake, protein balance is restored. If subsequent complications do not occur, net protein gain is prominent, and recovery proceeds rapidly. This gain, however, is usually much slower than the initial loss. It will often require three to six times as long to repair the protein deficit as it took to create it. If protein and caloric intake are satisfactory, the level eventually obtained is quite close to that prior to the loss.

Metabolic Requirements

ENERGY. The normal person at rest may require 2000 kcal/day, but a febrile, severely injured patient may use 4000 kcal in a single day. Variable periods of starvation almost inevitably follow severe trauma, and weight loss in excess of water loss may reach as high as 100 Gm daily as the energy demands are met by the consumption of body tissue.

Initial energy needs are supplied by the body stores of carbohydrate, 300 to 500 Gm being present as liver and muscle glycogen. The supply is exhausted within 14 to 18 hours after severe trauma, and subsequent energy requirements must be supplied by body tissues. In the postinjury period, 200 to 500 Gm of fat may be oxidized daily to yield 1800 to 4500 kcal. This is greatly in excess of the 1000 to 1300 kcal liberated by the oxidation of 100 to 150 Gm of fat/day in starvation.

Although the major contribution to energy needs comes from the oxidation of fat, protein catabolism yields a significant number of calories. Normal daily intake of 70 Gm of protein results in the urinary excretion of some 10 Gm of nitrogen daily. Following extensive injury, urinary nitrogen may reach levels as high as 20 Gm/day, representing the liberation of more than 500 kcal.

The production of energy is dependent upon the oxidation of metabolites via the tricarboxylic cycle. The two carbon fragments, active acetate or coenzyme A (CoA), assume a pivotal position in this important process. Acetyl CoA combines with oxyloacetic acid to form citric acid, which is subsequently degraded stepwise to yield eight hydrogen atoms, two molecules of carbon dioxide, and oxyloacetic acid. The eight electrons liberated by specific dehydrogenases then are introduced into the electron transport charge for transfer to oxygen. By oxidative phosphorylation the energy of foodstuffs is thus converted to adenosinetriphosphate (ATP), which is the ultimate driving force for most of the energy reactions within the cells (Fig. 6-1).

Intravenously administered carbohydrate solutions may supply a significant portion of the caloric needs for these energy processes. These solutions also may exert a protein-sparing effect, thus reducing the dissolution of lean body tissue. Approximately 100 Gm of carbohydrate appears to be adequate to obtain maximal protein sparing. As the first phase of injury passes, parenteral feeding is replaced by oral intake, and anabolic processes approach normal although the need for increased caloric supply often continues. Moore indicates that approximately 1 Gm of nitrogen and 20 kcal/kg of body weight/day are necessary to ensure restoration of body tissues during early convalescence.

CARBOHYDRATES. Although present in relatively small amounts, the monosaccharide glucose occupies a very important position because of its ready availability for energy. The two carbon fragments are intermediates in fatty acid metabolism and energy production. Via transamination reactions, glucose eventually may be converted to amino acids and proteins. Thus, glucose is an important precursor to fat and protein, as well as a supplier of oxidative energy.

Approximately 55 percent of absorbed carbohydrate is rapidly introduced into the Krebs cycle and converted into energy, carbon dioxide, and water. A portion of the remaining carbohydrate is converted to fat or protein, and about 5 percent is stored as liver and muscle glycogen. The carbohydrate in muscle is not readily available for use except by the muscle, but liver glycogen can easily be broken down and used elsewhere in the body. This glycogen is rapidly depleted in periods of starvation and in less than 5 hours may be exhausted if gluconeogenesis is interdicted. Without supplemental carbohydrate body tissues must be used to meet energy requirements.

FAT. Fat is rapidly oxidized to yield energy during starvation. From 75 to 100 Gm daily is mobilized under these conditions, but after extensive injury, as much as 500 Gm/day may be used. In addition to energy, free water is obtained. Although neutral fat contains little free water, the oxidation of 1 kg of fat liberates more than 1,000 ml of water.

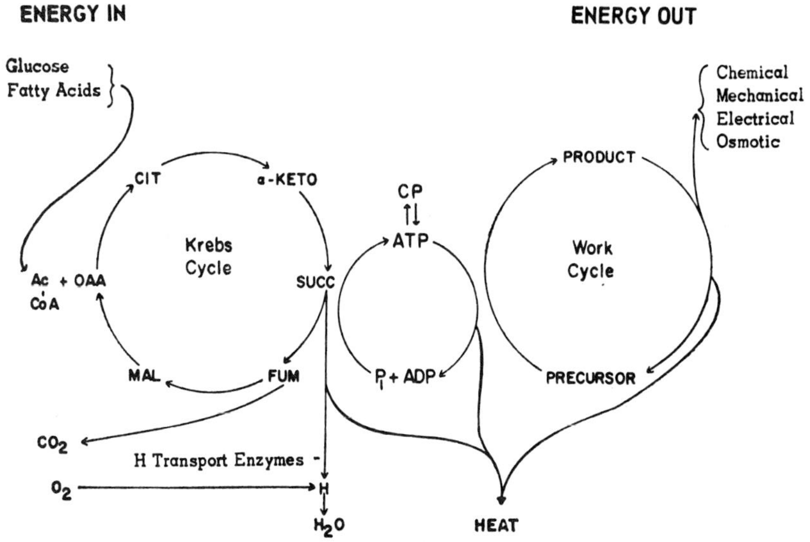

ENERGY IN   **ENERGY OUT**

Fig. 6-1. Schema of the mechanism of energy produced within the cell. OAA, oxalacetic acid; CIT, citric acid; α-KETO, α-ketoglutaric acid; SUCC, succinic acid; FUM, fumaric acid; MAL, malic acid; ADP, adenosinediphosphate; P_1, inorganic phosphate; ATP, adenosinetriphosphate; CP, creatine phosphate. (*From R. E. Olson, JAMA, 183:471, 1963.*)

VITAMINS. The suggested daily requirements of vitamins have been outlined by the National Research Council Committee on Nutrition. The exact vitamin requirements of the injured patient are not known, but it is probable that the vitamin C requirement is increased out of proportion to those of the other vitamins. There is a great individual variability in requirement for ascorbic acid in healthy adults, and it has been observed that blood level or buffy coat determinations for vitamin C do not necessarily reflect the magnitude of the deficit. It is widely held that the failure of wound healing and subsequent dehiscence is related more to the lack of vitamin C than to actual caloric starvation or protein depletion. It appears reasonable that the intake of vitamin C required to maintain normal body function in the posttraumatic patient is considerably higher than that customarily given for daily maintenance. If vitamin C is given intravenously in high levels, the renal threshold is soon exceeded, and a large portion of the administered dose is lost in the urine.

Most patients on parenteral therapy for short periods following surgical procedures for trauma will not require supplemental vitamins A and D. However, in addition to C, thiamine is certainly needed, as body stores of thiamine are rapidly depleted after the administration of large amounts of glucose. One of the important coenzymes in the tricarboxylic acid cycle necessary for oxidative decarboxylation of pyruvate to acetyl CoA is cocarboxylase, or thiamine pyrophosphate. The defect in oxidation of pyruvate therefore may be related to a preexisting thiamine deficiency in some patients.

Management

Most patients will reach the operating room in satisfactory nutritional status, but this desirable goal is not easily attained after extensive trauma. Preexisting nutritional and vitamin deficits may further complicate the severe metabolic response following trauma. Patients with hypoproteinemia may exhibit diminished tolerance to blood loss and reduced antibody production. There may be impaired wound healing and delayed union of fractures, and perhaps fatty infiltration of the liver in patients who are severely hypoproteinemic.

Although the normal patient at bed rest can be maintained easily on approximately 1 Gm of protein and 30 kcal/kg of body weight, after extensive trauma these requirements may be doubled or tripled. In the past it has been quite difficult to supply sufficient calories by the intravenous route.

Although protein may be supplied via administered blood plasma or albumin, these solutions are expensive, they require considerable metabolic work for their assimilation and caloric equilibrium for maximal use, and their caloric values are quite low. At one time there was widespread interest in the use of intravenous solutions containing protein hydrolysates and fat emulsions, which theoretically appeared to be more useful. However, this nutritional technique was not extensively employed because of doubtful effectiveness in preventing nitrogen losses and because of certain hazards attending their use. In 1968, Dudrick and associates reported that large quantities of protein hydrolysates and dextrose could be administered through a catheter inserted in the superior vena cava to consistently and safely achieve a positive nitrogen balance and weight gain. In over 300 patients, Dudrick and his colleagues induced weight gain and promoted healing of fistulas and wounds by this technique of *parenteral hyperalimentation*. Intravenous solutions containing adequate protein, essential amino acids, fat, carbohydrate, and vitamins to meet chronic nutritional requirements are now available. This important development in the pre- and postoperative care of patients is particularly useful when protein and caloric requirements are quite high and convalescence is prolonged.

Improvements in infusion technique are primarily responsible for the success of parenteral hyperalimentation, particularly the technique of catheterizing the subclavian vein to approach the superior vena cava for instillation of the concentrated solutions. As the subclavian vein is large, the catheter does not usually produce irritation of the vein wall and subsequent thrombosis, and the rapid blood flow prevents clotting and reduces bacterial growth. Placement of the catheter tip in the superior vena cava permits rapid dilution of the hypertonic solutions, thus decreasing the incidence of chemical phlebitis. Rigid sterile technique in placement and care of these catheters has allowed an acceptably low infection rate.

It is clear that with careful attention to strict asepsis and antisepsis in preparing and infusing these solutions (see Chap. 2) parenteral hyperalimentation may be considered a primary mode of both acute and long-term therapy, rather than a modified method of intravenous treatment, and can provide all essential nutrients without exceeding the daily fluid requirements. Initially, the solutions were prepared just prior to administration, but commercial products with a wide range of constituents now are available. Minor adjustments of essential amino acids, vitamins, and ion supplementation facilitate the preparation of individualized solutions.

ANESTHESIA

(By A. H. Giesecke, Jr. and E. R. Johnson)

Complicating Problems

Distinct problems differentiate the injured patient requiring emergency operation from the patient well prepared for elective operation (see Chap. 11). The major problems are possible airway difficulties, lack of comprehensive preoperative evaluation, multiple injuries, the full or nonemptied stomach, intoxication with alcohol or drugs, and shock.

AIRWAY OBSTRUCTION. Establishment and maintenance of the patient's airway may be the most important step in successful resuscitation. Some form of artificial airway is indicated for any patient with respiratory obstruction, inability to clear secretions, need for artificial ventilation, or unconsciousness. The type of airway must be individualized, but oropharyngeal or nasopharyngeal airways, orotracheal tubes, nasotracheal tubes, or tracheostomy should be considered.

Endotracheal intubation, if technically possible, is an effective method of rapidly clearing an airway obstruction to allow a more orderly, unhurried tracheostomy. Intubation should be performed under direct vision with a laryngoscope so that loose fragments of bone, teeth, or tissue will not be carried into the trachea by the advancing tube. The tube may be left in place for 48 hours or longer, if necessary, to support ventilation or maintain the airway until the patient can satisfactorily perform these functions. Meticulous care is as important for the indwelling endotracheal tube as for the tracheostomy. Inspired gases should be completely humidified. Periodic saline solution instillation followed by suctioning with a sterile catheter and hyperinflation of the lungs every other hour are prerequisites for proper management. Chest physiotherapy consisting of postural drainage, percussion, and vibration are beneficial in preventing and treating atelectasis.

For desperate asphyxia with supraglottic obstruction, a rapid flow of oxygen can be administered via a 15-gauge needle inserted through the cricothyroid membrane into the tracheal lumen. This will provide sufficient oxygenation for establishing an adequate airway by tracheal intubation or tracheostomy.

LACK OF COMPREHENSIVE PREOPERATIVE EVALUATION. Morbidity and mortality of trauma are inversely related to the preinjury state of health, but no patient should be assumed to have been healthy before injury. Evidence of prior diseases, allergies, or chronic drug therapy should be sought from the patient or an available informant. The main categories of drugs which create hazardous interactions with anesthetics are hormones (corticosteroids, insulin), psychopharmacologics, antihypertensives (including diuretics), cardiac drugs (including digitalis), and anticoagulants.

MULTIPLE INJURIES. When injuries involve many areas, problems arise in establishing priorities for operative intervention. In patients with head injuries, associated injuries may compel initial consideration. However, one must be alert to change in the patient's neurologic status during the anesthesia. Usually the pupils are the best indicators, and reduced requirement for anesthesia may indicate progression of the neurologic deterioration. Conversely, if the head injury is the primary surgical target, the anesthesiologist should be alert for progression of associated trauma, such as tension pneumothorax, hemoperitoneum, and cardiac tamponade. As shock rarely is directly caused by head injuries, its occurrence in the presence of head injury should engender suspicion of other injury. Unusual diagnostic skill may be needed to assess associated injuries with effects that become apparent only after an operation is progressing in another area. For example, hemorrhage from a torn spleen or liver may be minimal at the beginning of operation to correct extremity trauma but will require careful consideration if hypotension occurs. The diagnosis may be masked and delayed by the empiric administration of vasopressors for hypotension of uncertain cause.

THE FULL OR NONEMPTIED STOMACH. The chief hazard of the unprepared stomach is vomiting and aspiration of the vomitus. Peristalsis may cease at the time of the accident because of shock, anxiety, or abdominal or central nervous system trauma. For this reason all traumatized patients should be managed as if the stomach were full regardless of the interval since the last oral intake. Where appropriate, regional anesthesia should be selected for these patients, although aspiration remains a hazard. Regional analgesia is technically contraindicated for agitated, intoxicated patients and for those with significant hypovolemia.

Awake intubation with or without topical anesthesia has been shown to be safe for the emergency patient with a full stomach. An alternative choice for a vigorous patient is rapid induction with an intravenous thiobarbiturate followed by a paralyzing dose of succinylcholine to facilitate tracheal intubation. The hazard of anesthetic over-dosage exists if, following intubation, volatile inhalation agents are pumped into the lungs by controlled ventilation. The stomach should be previously decompressed with a nasogastric tube. Following administration of the thio-barbiturate, an assistant should exert continuous pressure on the cricoid cartilage to occlude the esophagus. This should not be released until the tube is securely in the trachea and the cuff inflated. The endotracheal tube should not be removed until the patient is conscious postopera-tively and has protective laryngeal reflexes to prevent aspi-ration during extubation.

Two clinical pictures of aspiration have been described: First is the aspiration of undigested food resulting in respi-ratory obstruction and distress. Depending on the amount of material aspirated, patients may have acute respiratory distress with cyanosis and cardiac arrest or may exhibit a milder, chronic course leading to lobar pneumonitis and lung abscess. A second form, Mendelson's syndrome, is caused by aspiration of liquid acid gastric secretions. This is equally hazardous in terms of morbidity and mortality and is manifest by generalized bronchospasm, dyspnea, tachypnea, and cyanosis. In severe cases cardiac arrest may develop. Immediate therapy includes oxygen, endotracheal suctioning, methylprednisolone given intravenously, and broad-spectrum antibiotics. Bronchoscopy is indicated if particulate material is found in the vomitus or if signs of obstructive atelectasis develop. Tracheobronchial lavage with large volumes of saline solution is no longer recom-mended.

ALCOHOL AND DRUG INTOXICATION. Based largely on animal studies, the statement has been repeatedly made that the manifestations of shock are more severe in the drunk patient than in the sober patient. However, mild to moderate intoxication (blood alcohol less than 250 mg/100 ml) is reported to have no effect on the incidence of hypotension, morbidity, or mortality of surgical treat-ment for trauma. Higher levels of blood alcohol are ex-pected to increase intraoperative anesthetic complications. Regional anesthesia is not technically feasible for the agi-tated and intoxicated patient; intravenous induction is preferred. The airway should be protected by rapid endo-tracheal intubation.

Patients intoxicated with cannabis, LSD, and/or am-phetamines may exhibit altered responses to anesthetics. Intoxication with barbiturates and methyl alcohol may result in delayed emergence from anesthesia.

SHOCK. The severely hypovolemic patient, unrespon-sive to pain or verbal stimulus, should receive no anesthetic drugs which may depress the cardiovascular system. Such a patient needs endotracheal intubation, ventilation with oxygen, and restoration of circulating volume. Satisfactory operating conditions should be provided, with muscle re-laxants and analgesic concentrations of nitrous oxide.

Other aspects of care for the severely hypotensive, hypo-volemic patient include (1) simultaneous infusion of large quantities of blood and electrolyte solutions, warmed to avoid myocardial hypothermia and irreversible cardiac arrhythmias; (2) administration of calcium as an antagonist

to hyperkalemia, to prevent citrate intoxication and to strengthen myocardial force; (3) administration of sodium bicarbonate to correct the acidosis produced by anaerobic metabolism and infusion of acidotic blood; and (4) admin-istration of large doses of steroids, although their efficacy is not firmly established.

Assessment of the Patient's Status

Blood pressure, pulse, skin color, capillary filling time, and pupil size should be monitored during all anesthetia. In addition, the central venous pressure of the severely traumatized patient should be monitored to detect early failure of the myocardium and overload with colloid solu-tions. The hourly urine output should be monitored to determine the efficacy of fluid therapy. Output should be at least 50 ml/hour if the extracellular fluid volume is being sufficiently replaced with a balanced salt solution.

Premedication

The emphasis in anesthesia for trauma is on resusci-tation. An obligation exists to relieve suffering of a patient whose physical condition will tolerate the effects of anal-gesic drugs. However, hypoxic agitation must be differenti-ated from suffering. Barbiturates should not be used if the patient is in pain, as in this circumstance they tend to produce the paradoxic response of excitement or depressed agitation rather than sedation. Narcotics are contraindi-cated for patients with closed head injuries, because they deepen the depression, produce miosis, and mask the progression of intracranial injuries. For its drying effects and vagal depressant characteristics, an anticholinergic drug should be used for nearly all patients.

Choice of Anesthetic

The choice of agent varies from oxygen alone for the patient in hypovolemic shock to the full range of anesthetic agents for the patient with intact homeostatic mechanisms. Those agents and techniques should be chosen which tend to facilitate successful resuscitation. The patient who is hypoxic preoperatively should be managed with an anes-thetic which can be given with the highest concentration of oxygen. Nitrous oxide is acceptable for obtunded or inebriated patients. Spinal anesthesia is useful for patients with injuries of the lower extremities if the central nervous system is not involved, if the blood volume has been replaced, and if the patient is not otherwise unmanageable.

A guiding principle in the choice of anesthetic agents and techniques is that complete supression of sensation is not necessary and may be harmful if achieved by deep anesthesia. Extensive surgical procedures can be per-formed in analgesic planes of nitrous oxide, ether, cyclo-propane, or halothane, or by combining light general and local anesthesia. Severely traumatized and unconscious patients will require oxygen only and perhaps a muscle relaxant.

Postoperative Management

Not all the effects of massive trauma may be apparent at the same time. Following definitive correction of damage in one area, the patient must be closely observed for evidences of injury in other areas. The usual principles of recovery-room care must be applied. These include oxygen by mask, at least until the patient is awake and oriented; periodic use of intermittent positive-pressure breathing; frequent turning from side to side; and monitoring of the blood pressure, pulse rate, adequacy of ventilation, urine output, fluid infusion, gastric suction, emergence from anesthesia, and evidences of continued or recurring blood loss.

Delayed emergence from anesthesia may be caused by many factors, including possible head injury from the initial trauma or brain damage from prolonged shock or hypoxia. Progression of nervous system lesions should be watched for even if head injury was not suspected prior to operation. If the patient remains motionless except for breathing, anesthetic overdosage may be the cause, but the differential diagnosis should include spinal cord injury, brain damage, persistent partial curarization, overdosage with curare antagonists, hypothermia, and alcohol or drug intoxication. Bizarre causes for failure to awaken include myasthenia gravis, hypothyroidism, hypoglycemia, sickle cell crisis, intermittent porphyria, and nonketotic hyperosmotic coma.

Hypoventilation is a difficult problem to assess clinically in the postoperative patient. It can be caused by one condition or by a combination of several perplexing conditions. The list of reasons for hypoventilation includes most of those considered in delayed emergence from anesthesia, i.e., anesthetic overdosage or idiosyncrasy, relaxant overdosage or idiosyncrasy, overdosage with narcotics given for postoperative pain, endocrinopathies including myasthenia gravis and hypothyroidism, fluid overload, shock, neomycin or streptomycin administered intraperitoneally, upper and/or lower airway obstruction, respiratory restriction by dressings or casts, pneumothorax or hemothorax, abdominal distension, and pain.

An informed suspicion is required for the early diagnosis of hypoventilation, since the classic syndrome appears late and may be masked. Signs include restlessness, stridor or retractions, air hunger, disorientation or stupor, diminution of respiration (volume and/or frequency), hypertension which progresses to hypotension, tachycardia changing to bradycardia, and pallor or cyanosis. Chest roentgenograms may show atelectasis, pneumonitis, pneumothorax, or hemothorax. Spirometer measurements will confirm diminished tidal ventilation. Arterial blood-gas analysis will show hypercapnia, acidosis, and arterial unsaturation.

The proper treatment for hypoventilation is directed primarily at respiratory assistance or control with a breathing apparatus. Other measures may be indicated for specific causes: atropine and neostigmine to reverse residual paresis from curare; levallorphan or naloxone to antagonize narcotics; and analeptics. All are useful but are secondary to good ventilatory support.

PRINCIPLES IN THE MANAGEMENT OF WOUNDS

(By Ronald C. Jones and G. Tom Shires)

Primary Wound Management

The most important single factor in the management of contaminated wounds is adequate debridement. This old surgical principle frequently has been forgotten since the advent of antibiotics. All tissue which is dead, has a poor blood supply, or is heavily contaminated should be removed if at all possible. This is particularly true of subcutaneous fat and muscle. Skin with impaired blood supply should be removed initially because of its tendency to suppurate and become infected. Granulation tissue formation and later grafting procedures are preferable. Following sharp debridement and hemostasis, the wound is irrigated with copious quantities of saline solution, depending on the area and degree of soft tissue injury and contamination. That the incidence of wound infection is inversely proportional to the amount of irrigation and debridement at the time of injury has been demonstrated by Singleton et al. and by Peterson and confirmed clinically many times.

LOCAL CARE OF WOUNDS

Glass or sharp instruments usually carry a minimal amount of foreign material into a wound and cause a minimal amount of tissue trauma. X-rays should be taken of any area in which the depth of the wound cannot clearly be seen. It is not uncommon for the deep portion of a stab wound to contain the tip of a knife blade or other foreign body. Stab wounds of soft tissues are explored in the emergency room with the gloved finger or under local anesthesia by extending the length of the laceration to determine the direction and extent of the wound and to rule out any major vessel, nerve, or organ injury. The wound is then irrigated with copious amounts of saline solution. If the solution is found not to penetrate the peritoneal cavity, a small, soft-rubber Penrose drain is inserted, and the wound is left open for drainage. The drain is removed in 24 hours. Gunshot wounds are debrided externally and left open for drainage. Suturing these wounds leaves a closed contaminated space, and the infection can easily spread to surrounding soft tissue structures. Deep lacerations involving the extremity with damage to major vessels and tendons and massive muscle injury are managed by controlling major vessel bleeding and immediately wrapping the wound in sterile dressings. An x-ray is taken, if indicated, but a severe laceration is not explored until the patient is in the operating room. This procedure prevents undue contamination of the wound in the emergency room before the patient is adequately prepared. Minor lacerations can be managed in the emergency room.

Muscles usually can be approximated and, depending on the type of wound, the skin and subcutaneous tissue may or may not be closed initially. These wounds are often left open and have delayed primary closure in 3 to 5 days. Damaged muscle due to gunshot wounds is debrided, hemostasis is obtained, and the wound is irrigated as outlined above. The wounds are packed open and closed with delayed closure. All patients with such wounds receive antibiotics and tetanus toxoid.

Antibacterial soaps or detergent materials are not used to irrigate wounds when muscle, tendon, or blood vessels are visible. Severe chemical irritation to these structures may occur, with resultant structure impairment and delayed wound healing.

Cosmetic appearance is a secondary consideration; the primary aim is to avoid infection and cover vital structures. No attempt at plastic repair is made at the initial closure of a potentially contaminated wound. Jagged edges of skin with poor blood supply are trimmed, and any resulting unpleasant scar can be cared for at a later date when no infection is present. Most lacerations, regardless of location, will never need revision if they meet the criteria previously outlined for the primary closure.

PUNCTURE WOUNDS. The most frequent puncture injury is that caused by a rusty nail in the foot. Initial treatment consists of ellipsing a small area of skin and subcutaneous tissue around the puncture site. A simple method of excising a portion of skin uses cuticle nippers. The wound is then irrigated with copious amounts of saline solution and left open for drainage. The patient is started on antibiotics both to prevent secondary infection and to aid in the prevention of tetanus, since this wound is not completely open to the air.

Puncture wounds elsewhere in the body are debrided more conservatively if they involve only the skin and subcutaneous tissue. Human tetanus immune globulin is reserved for the more massively contaminated tetanus-prone wound; otherwise, the routine is debridement with conversion to an open wound and the administration of antibiotics and tetanus toxoid, whether or not the patient has been previously immunized.

POWER MOWER INJURIES. Injuries resulting from the use of power mowers have increased in recent years. These include injuries from flying objects thrown from the power mower and from the mower itself to the hands and feet, particularly the fingers and toes. Treatment has consisted of covering exposed bones with muscle and leaving the entire wound open. These injuries almost uniformly become infected if an attempt is made to close the wound primarily. Patients are treated with systemic antibiotics and tetanus toxoid, and the wounds are packed with fine-mesh gauze. Skin grafting and reconstructive procedures should be delayed.

Emergency Laparotomy

INCISIONS. A longitudinal midline incision is regularly used for exploratory laparotomy in patients with abdominal trauma and does not endanger the abdominal muscle blood supply or nerve supply, or damage aponeuroses. Skin towels are routinely sewn into place, if time permits, to prevent skin contamination and drying of subcutaneous tissues. Minimal ligatures are used on bleeders which are contained in small bits of tissue, as each extra ligature is

a foreign body and enhances the chance of a wound infection. Tissues should be kept moistened and gently handled. Surgical technique governs the development of wound infection as significantly as any single factor.

SUTURE. Number 30 stainless steel wire is the suture material of choice for closing the uncomplicated midline abdominal incision, particularly in operations for traumatic lesions. This has been shown to cause the least reaction and is of sufficient strength. It has not been the cause of draining sinuses following postoperative wound infections. Suture placement is probably the most important factor in the prevention of wound dehiscence. There is no longer need to overlap fascia, since new tissue comes from surrounding tissue, and if fascia is freed to allow overlapping, this surrounding tissue is damaged. Sutures should not be placed at equal distances from the edge of the fascia, as they will fall in the same group of fibers; should one suture tear the fascia longitudinally, the tear may extend from suture to suture until dehiscence occurs. Sutures should be staggered or placed at varying intervals from the edge of the fascia. With such a closure, there should be no fear in having a patient cough vigorously for adequate postoperative pulmonary care. No problem has occurred with wire sutures protruding through the skin. An occasional patient with minimal subcutaneous tissue will complain of pain in the incision when the wire is under a pressure point such as a belt. These sutures are easily removed under local anesthesia.

Simple interrupted suture is used to close the fascia and peritoneum in a single layer. This is felt to be superior to the figure-of-eight suture, because less tissue is gathered and the suture can be placed faster, thus reducing anesthesia time. Interrupted sutures are used instead of running sutures, because a break in the suture material will not loosen the entire incision. Regardless of the type of suture or method of placement, the fascia should be loosely approximated and not strangulated. Tightening fascial sutures may lead to necrosis with the suture subsequently cutting through the tissue. Retention sutures have not been regularly used. Routine antibiotic irrigation of the wound for the prevention of infection has not been necessary. Fragmentation of wire sutures has been described as a complication, but this must be quite rare; we have seen no patients with fragmentation with erosion into a viscus such as the small bowel.

Through-and-Through Closure. Several local and systemic factors noted at the time of the original operation may make through-and-through closure the procedure of choice (Fig. 6-2). This uses plastic bridges and #4 stainless steel wire swaged on a large cutting needle. The bridges prevent cutting of skin by the wire and allow for swelling which occurs in the first 24 to 48 hours postoperatively. These sutures usually do not require postoperative adjustment. Wounds massively contaminated from shotgun wadding and fecal material, in patients on steroids, or associated with massive infection and peritonitis are best handled with through-and-through closure. Often a single patient may have several indications for this type of closure such as chronic pulmonary disease, obesity, and/or chronic

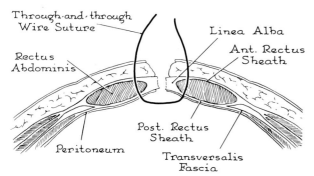

Fig. 6-2. Through-and-through wire closure. (From G. T. Shires, "Care of the Trauma Patient," p. 37, McGraw-Hill Book Company, New York, 1966.)

debilitating disease. Occasionally through-and-through closure is used at the end of a lengthy operation with a long incision to shorten anesthesia time if the patient is not tolerating the procedure well. This type of closure is routinely used in the patient requiring reoperation in the early postoperative period because of gastrointestinal bleeding or intestinal obstruction. The wires are left in place for 3 weeks. This measure has proved to be sure, safe, timesaving, and often lifesaving.

INFECTION. Infection and severe abdominal distension are frequently mentioned as causative factors in dehiscence. Routine use of the Levin tube may prevent the latter. A severe wound infection may be prevented in the markedly contaminated abdomen by leaving the skin and subcutaneous tissue open down to the fascia for delayed primary closure. This method is frequently used in long operations or with excessive contamination such as from feces. Staphylococcus remains the number one organism causing wound infections in trauma patients. Abdominal wounds freqently harbor coliform organisms if bowel injury has been sustained. These wounds are packed open with fine-mesh gauze, changed daily for debridement, and either closed at 5 days or allowed to granulate until closure. This procedure will usually result in an excellent scar. Reoperation in the same area of a previous wound infection, even months later, will frequently result in a second wound infection.

DRAINS. Subcutaneous drains will not substitute for good hemostasis. Failure to obtain hemostasis will give rise to a hematoma which is an excellent culture medium for an already contaminated wound. Drains from the abdominal cavity are usually brought out through a separate stab wound which will easily admit two fingers and by the most direct route, which occasionally may be through the midline incision. This is especially true for some liver and pancreatic injuries. Drainage of the free peritoneal cavity is not attempted unless drainage of a particular organ or a well-localized abscess is specifically indicated.

Antibiotics

Sepsis is related to the length of time which elapses between bacterial contamination of the traumatic wound or surgical incision and the start of treatment designed to prevent sepsis. The "golden period" for wound infection has been stated to be 6 hours, but the effectiveness of preventive antibiotics in surgical wounds has been shown to be no more than 3 hours. In fact, the shorter the time between contamination or surgical incision and the administration of antibiotics, the more effective are the antibiotics in preventing a bacterial infection.

Burke has demonstrated in animals injected with staphylococci that the steps which determine the size of a bacterial lesion take place very shortly after the bacteria reach the tissue. As the time interval between the injection of bacteria and the administration of an antibiotic increases, the antibiotic effect on the size of the lesion produced is decreased. Most of the antibiotic effect is over in 1 to 2 hours. As antibiotics injected more than 3 hours after staphylococci have been introduced have no effect on the size of the 24-hour lesion, it appears that there is little benefit from antibiotics administered 3 hours following the injection of staphylococci. This indicates that the antibiotic should be given early, so that it is in the tissue when the bacteria arrive. If given postoperatively, the antibiotic may reach the local dead tissue after the time period considered safe for traumatic injuries, and bacteria already may be beginning to multiply.

Viable bacteria can be demonstrated in many surgical wounds at the time of closure; however, only a minimal number later become infected. Therefore, the number of bacteria encountered in clean operations is not alone sufficient to produce sepsis. There is considerable evidence that other factors produce decreased host resistance.

Various regions of the body respond differently to wound contamination. Clinical experience has long shown an inverse relationship between the vascularity of an area and its susceptibility to infection. This probably is reflected in the low incidence of infection in head and neck operations, compared with the higher incidence with abdominal operations. Normal tissues have remarkable resistance to microorganisms, but devitalized tissues have limited resistance. Thus, the development of local wound infection depends greatly on the altered physiologic state of the wound. In addition, Ollodart and Mansberger have demonstrated in both animals and man that bacterial resistance is decreased following hypovolemic shock.

Surgical materials and technique are also important. Suture material enhances the virulence of staphylococci several-fold. Altemeier and Wulsin have shown that this occurs less with monofilament suture than with twisted or braided material. However, Condie and Ferguson have shown that dead space is more important in the production of wound infection than is increased amount of suture material.

Since the advent of the sulfa drugs, the administration of antibiotics intraperitoneally has been advocated. Artz et al. demonstrated that following the intraperitoneal injection of a fecal suspension into the dog, bacteremia was not detected in the bloodstream during the first 2 hours after injection, but bacteria began invading at the third hour and increased in number until the dog's death. They also demonstrated that antibiotics administered intravenously 2 hours after the fecal suspension had been injected intraperitoneally gave the same degree of protection as did intraperitoneal administration, without its complications. Because of the degrees of respiratory depression following intraperitoneal administration of neomycin and kanamycin, the concentration should be no greater than $\frac{1}{2}$%. Cohn and Kotler have shown that kanamycin has a greater margin of safety than does any other antibiotic currently available for intraperitoneal administration. Altemeier and Wulsin recommend the early preoperative institution of intravenously administered antibiotics to obtain in the peritoneal fluid an antibacterial concentration of antibiotics prior to the operative procedure. Probably antibiotics should not routinely be given intraperitoneally in the abdominal cavity unless massive fecal contamination has occurred.

A recent review at Parkland Memorial Hospital of a series of patients sustaining gunshot and stab wounds to the abdomen indicated that the incidence of infection in patients sustaining abdominal injuries who received prophylactic antibiotics in the emergency room or intraoperatively was much lower than that in patients who did not receive antibiotics until the immediate postoperative period or therapeutically. Patients are often in shock, and this complication may affect the method chosen for the administration of antibacterial agents. If shock is present, absorption of the antibiotic agents by the intramuscular route may be decreased or inadequate. For this reason, the intravenous route is recommended until shock has been adequately controlled. If no significant injury is present at the time of laparotomy, antibiotics may be discontinued in the recovery room or during the first 24 hours postoperatively. In the event of severe contamination, the antibiotics are administered for 5 days.

BITES AND STINGS OF ANIMALS AND INSECTS

(By Ronald C. Jones and G. Tom Shires)

Rabies

INCIDENCE. In the United States an estimated 2 million human beings are bitten by animals yearly, and $\frac{1}{2}$ million are bitten by dogs. Any mammalian animal may carry rabies. In 1971 there were 4,392 laboratory confirmed cases of rabies. This increase of more than 14 percent over the previous 5-year average resulted from substantially more cases of skunk and bat rabies. For the first time rabies cases were reported from all the contiguous states and from Alaska. The animals most frequently reported infected and the percentage of the cases they accounted for were skunks (46 percent), foxes (15 percent), bats (11 percent), cattle (9 percent), dogs (5 percent), cats (5 percent), and raccoons (4 percent). In 1971, 80 percent of the rabies in this country was in wildlife species. For the eleventh consecutive year, skunks were the animals most frequently infected with rabies. More states reported bat rabies than in any previous year. Wildlife rabies was also reported in coyotes, opossum, otter, bobcats, bear, squirrel, deer, mink, woodchucks, coatis, and a badger. Domestic rabies was reported in

cattle, dogs, cats, horses, mules, sheep, goats, swine, and guinea pigs in 1971. The Communicable Disease Center estimates that this represents less than 10 percent of the cases that actually exist. In the past 5 years, there has been an average of two cases of human rabies per year. Table 6-1 shows the incidence and frequency of reported rabies in the United States in various animals and in human beings by states or territory in 1971. Many of the few cases of human rabies reported in the past 10 years have resulted from exposure abroad.

EPIDEMIOLOGY. Saliva from a rabid animal contains large numbers of the rabies virus and is inoculated through a bite, any laceration, or break in the skin. Animal experiments and at least two human infections indicate that animals and man can become infected by bats, without being bitten, by inhalation of rabies virus. Girard examined bats and demonstrated rabies virus in the brain, kidney, urine, salivary gland, adrenal gland, and liver using the fluorescent antibody test. Most cases of racoon rabies are reported from Florida and Georgia, the only part of the United States where a cycle of transmission in raccoons has been established.

The maintenance of wild and exotic animals such as skunks, raccoons, ocelots, and bobcats as household pets is discouraged since many of these animals are infected with rabies. If people insist on maintaining wild and exotic animals as household pets, these animals should be quarantined for a minimum of 90 days after capture and vaccinated at least 30 days prior to being released to an owner. Annual vaccination is recommended.

Dogs and cats bitten by a known rabid animal should be destroyed immediately. If the animal has been vaccinated within the previous 3 years, it should be revaccinated immediately and confined for 90 days.

DIAGNOSIS. Circumstances of the Bite. Circumstances surrounding the attack frequently furnish vital information as to whether or not vaccine is indicated. Most domestic animal bites are provoked attacks; if this history is obtained, rabies vaccine can usually be withheld if the animal appears healthy. Children are frequently bitten while attempting to separate fighting animals or while teasing or accidentally hurting the animal. Bites during attempts to feed or handle an apparently healthy animal should generally be regarded as provoked. Frequently the patient has attempted to handle a sick animal.

Although vaccination of the animal does not totally rule out the possibility of transmitting rabies, it is over 90 percent effective. A small number of dog rabies have apparently involved vaccine failure.

Bites from rodents, including squirrels, chipmunks, rats, and mice, seldom require specific rabies prophylaxis. Each case of possible exposure must be studied individually before a conclusion can be reached as to whether antirabies therapy is indicated.

Extent and Location of Bite Wound. The likelihood that rabies will result from a bite varies with its extent and location. For convenience in approaching management, two categories of exposure are widely accepted:

Severe: Multiple or deep puncture wounds, or any bites on the head, face, neck, hands, or fingers.

Table 6-1. CONFIRMED RABIES CASES IN THE UNITED STATES, BY STATE AND ANIMAL, 1971

State	Dogs	Cats	Cattle	Horses and mules	Sheep and goats	Domestic animal totals	Skunks — Striped	Skunks — Spotted	Skunks — Not specified	Bobcats	Coyotes	Foxes — Gray	Foxes — Red	Foxes — Not specified	Raccoons	Bats	Other animals	Wild animal totals	Human beings	Total
Totals	235	222	398	48	30	941	1,773	10	235	10	15	282	159	230	190	465	88	3,449	2	4,392
Alabama	2		4		1	7			1					47	2	4		54		61
Alaska	4					4							32				6 Arctic fox, 1 land otter	39		43
Arizona	2		2	1		5			10	4	4			4		10	1 bear, 2 coatis	35		40
Arkansas	5	8	8	1	2	24	65					6	4			8	1 swine	84		108
California	1	2	4	1	2	10	197					6				106	1 deer, 1 squirrel	311	1	322
Colorado	1	2	1			4	10									18		29		33
Connecticut																17		17		17
Delaware																4		4		4
Dist. of Columbia																				0
Florida	1	3				4	1		2					4	48	17		72		76
Georgia	2		1			3						10	5	1	118	9		143		146
Hawaii																				0
Idaho																3	1 swine	4		4
Illinois	13	9	20	1	2	45	247					7	9			8	2 wood chucks	273		318
Indiana	2	1	1	1	1	6	66					2	1			7	2 guinea pigs	76		82
Iowa	11	22	52	1	1	88	133	2				2			3	8	1 wood chuck, 1 badger, 1 mink, 1 swine	152		240
Kansas	26	4	4			8			101		1					2		104		112
Kentucky	26	8	27	3		64			23			58	11	27	1	2	1 mink	123		187
Louisiana	10	1				11	5		1		2	42				1		51		62
Maine	13	21	30	4	17	85			6					93	8	4	3 swine, 2 deer	113		198
Maryland																3		3		3
Massachusetts																6		6		6
Michigan	1	3	5	4		13	10						14		1	9	1 weasel	35		48
Minnesota	13	18	36	4		71	178		2						1	9		194		265
Mississippi																5		5		5
Missouri	11	8	14	1		34	44		55			2	6	2		5		114		148
Montana	1		1			2	2									2		4		6
Nebraska									12									12		12
Nevada											1			2		2		5		5
New Hampshire																3		4		4
New Jersey																19		19		20
New Mexico											1					1		9		9
New York		4	20	3		27	20		7		1	1	45	13		29		109		136
North Carolina																5		5		5
North Dakota	5	22	23			50	133		3		6		1		1	2		143		193
Ohio	16	1	9	1		27	70					4	1	14	1	6		96		123
Oklahoma	5	11	33	1		50	221	2				1	1		2	6		233		283
Oregon							1						3			5		9		9
Pennsylvania	3		2			5						1				10		18		23
Rhode Island																1		1		1
South Carolina								1					4	2	2		1 opossum	20		20
South Dakota	6	17	28			51	66	3	4	1		25	3	9	1	4		116		167
Tennessee	9	10	9	4		32	28					21		2	1	9		76		108
Texas	18	21	24	6	2	71	158					56				38		252		323
Utah							2									7		9		9
Vermont		1	2	1		4							3			4		12		16
Virginia	2	4	2	2		10	47		3				7	4		7		67		79
Washington																1		5		5
West Virginia	34	15	14	2	2	67						37	5	6		5	1 opossum	54		121
Wisconsin	15	2	14	2		33	47					1	1			11		60		93
Wyoming				1		1	7		2							4		13		14
Guam																				0
Puerto Rico	5	5	8	4	1	23											57 mongooses	57		80
Virgin Islands																				0

Mild: Scratches, lacerations, or single bites on areas of the body other than the head, face, neck, hands, or fingers. Open wounds, such as abrasions, suspected of being contaminated with saliva also belong in this category.

Laboratory Diagnosis. The fluorescent antibody test described by Goldwasser and his associates appears to be a more accurate test than the stain for Negri bodies. The intracerebral inoculation of mice combined with the microscopic examination of brain tissue for Negri bodies is still one of the most useful tests in the laboratory diagnosis of rabies and should be used whenever human beings have been bitten by suspect animals and the fluorescent antibody test is negative.

MANAGEMENT OF BITING ANIMALS. Most animal bites of human beings are caused by dogs and cats, and in most instances it is possible to observe the biting animal for the development of rabies. Domestic animals that bite a person should be captured and observed for symptoms of rabies for 10 days. If none develop, the animal may be assumed to be nonrabid. If the animal dies or is killed, the head should not be damaged but should be sent promptly to a public health laboratory for examination. The tissue requires refrigeration but not freezing, and transportation to the laboratory following death of the animal should be rapid. Clinical signs of rabies in wild animals cannot be interpreted reliably; therefore, any wild animal that bites or scratches a person should be killed at once (without unnecessary damage to the head) and the brain examined for evidence of rabies.

Information from the county health department regarding which animals, both domestic and wild, have been reported to be rabid within the past 10 years in the particular area may indicate a possible specific animal transmitting rabies.

EXPOSURE OF PERSONS PREVIOUSLY IMMUNIZED. For mild exposure of a person who has demonstrated an antibody response to antirabies vaccination received in the past, a single booster dose of vaccine is recommended. In the case of severe exposure, five daily doses of vaccine should be given followed by a booster dose 20 days later.

If it is not known whether an exposed person has had antibody, the complete postexposure antirabies treatment should be given. Because of variation in vaccine potency and individual response, immunization should not be considered complete until antibody is demonstrated in the serum. Farrar et al. have demonstrated that most persons receiving three or more injections of any rabies vaccine within 4 years will show antibody in the blood 30 days after a single booster injection of duck embryo vaccine (DEV), a killed virus.

PREEXPOSURE PROPHYLAXIS. The relatively low frequency of reactions to DEV has made it more practical to offer preexposure immunization to persons in high-risk groups, e.g., veterinarians, animal handlers, certain laboratory workers, and individuals, especially children, living in areas where rabies is a constant threat. Others whose vocations or avocations result in frequent contact with dogs, cats, foxes, skunks, or bats should also be considered for preexposure prophylaxis.

A significant number of citizens of the United States have been and, with increasing frequency, will continue to be exposed to rabies in other countries where rabies in dogs is a major problem. Because rabies in animals is widespread in large areas of Asia, Africa, and Latin America, the Foreign Quarantine Program of the United States Public Health Service has recently advised that preexposure immunization against rabies with DEV be suggested for Americans traveling in these areas.

Two 1-ml injections of DEV given subcutaneously in the deltoid area 1 month apart should be followed by a third dose 6 to 7 months after the second dose. This series of three injections can be expected to have produced neutralizing antibody in 80 to 90 percent of vaccinees by 1 month after the third dose. For more rapid immunization, three 1-ml injections of DEV should be given at weekly intervals with a fourth dose 3 months later. This schedule elicits an antibody response in about 80 percent of those vaccinated. All who receive the preexposure vaccination should have their serum tested for neutralizing antibody 3 to 4 weeks after the last injection. Tests for rabies antibody can be arranged with or through state health department laboratories. If no antibody is detected, booster doses should be given until a response is demonstrated. Persons with continuing exposure should receive 1-ml boosters every 2 to 3 years.

ACCIDENTAL INOCULATION WITH LIVE RABIES VIRUS VACCINE. Persons inadvertently inoculated with attenuated rabies vaccines for use in animals, such as the Flury strain vaccine, are not considered at risk, and antirabies prophylaxis is not indicated.

POSTEXPOSURE PROPHYLAXIS. Incubation Period. It is generally accepted that the incubation period for rabies in human beings ranges from 10 days to 1 year, most cases occurring within 4 months of the time of exposure. In cases of exposure of the head, neck, or upper extremities, the incubation period is potentially less than 30 days.

Immediate Local Care. Not all persons bitten by rabid animals contract the disease. Vigorous local treatment to remove possible rabies virus may be as important as specific antirabies therapy. Free bleeding from the wound is encouraged. Local care of an animal bite should consist of:

1. Thorough irrigation with copious amounts of saline solution.
2. Cleansing with a 20% soap solution.
3. Swabbing with a 1 or 2% solution of benzalkonium chloride (all soap should be removed before application of quaternary ammonium compounds, because soap neutralizes the activity of such compounds).
4. Debridement.
5. Administration of antibiotic when indicated to prevent bacterial infection.
6. Administration of tetanus toxoid.
7. Immediate suturing of the wound generally is not advised, since it may contribute to the development of rabies, but a severe laceration secondary to a dog bite may be sutured if exposure to rabies is unlikely.

Passive Immunization. This in combination with vaccine is considered the best postexposure prophylaxis. The only preparation of antirabies serum now available in the United States is of equine origin; therefore skin testing is necessary prior to administration.

Hyperimmune serum is recommended for most exposures classified as severe, and for all bites by rabid animals and unprovoked bites by wild carnivores and bats. When indicated, antirabies serum should be used regardless of the interval between exposure and treatment.

The dose recommended is 1,000 units (one vial) per 40 lb of body weight. A portion of the antiserum should be used to infiltrate the wound, and the rest administered intramuscularly. If the wound is particularly extensive or on the head, a larger dose of 50 to 100 I.U./kg should be given. In the United States, rabies hyperimmune serum is obtainable in 1,000-unit vials. It is presently recommended that serum be given on one occasion only and as early as possible following exposure. The use of serum should be accompanied by a 14-day course of vaccine (Table 6-2).

Active Immunization. *Primary Immunization.* At least 14 daily injections of DEV are recommended by the manufacturer. These should be given subcutaneously in the abdomen, lower back, or lateral aspect of thighs; rotation of sites is recommended. For severe exposure, 21 doses of vaccine are recommended. These may be given as 21 daily doses or 14 doses in the first 7 days (either as two separate injections or a double dose), and then 7 daily doses. A shorter course of vaccine is not recommended, since passive immunity induced by serum may limit response to vaccine. The vaccine may be stopped if the animal is proved not to be rabid. Previous experience indicates that the rabies vaccine is most effective in preventing rabies when given immediately after exposure and when the incubation period exceeds 30 days.

Booster Doses. Two booster doses are recommended, one 10 days and the other at least 20 days after completing the primary course. The two booster doses are particularly important if antirabies serum was used in the initial therapy (Table 6-2).

Side Reaction to Vaccine and Antiserum. Rabies vaccine should not be given unless there is a definite indication for its use. Local reactions to DEV are frequent. These consist of erythema, pruritus, pain, and tenderness at the site of inoculation. Generalized reactions occasionally are observed, usually after five to eight doses.

Neurologic reactions following DEV are rare. Perhaps one death has been attributed to its use. Neurologic reactions to nerve tissue vaccine constitute the principal hazard to its use. They occur in three main types: peripheral neuritis, the spinal form, and the cerebral form with acute encephalitis. Dorsolumbar paralysis may be either flaccid or spastic. Peripheral neuritis may involve facial, oculomotor, glossopharyngeal, or vagal nerves.

Immediate reactions may occur in an individual sensitive to avian tissue. Epinephrine is helpful in anaphylactic reactions. Should a complication develop and if, in view of the severity of the exposure, the amount of immunization already obtained is considered adequate, the vaccine may be discontinued. If further immunization is indicated, steroids and antihistamines should be administered.

Antirabies serum is obtained from immunized horses and may be expected to produce side reactions in approxi-

Table 6-2. POSTEXPOSURE ANTIRABIES PROPHYLAXIS GUIDE*

The following recommendations are intended only as a guide. They may be modified according to knowledge of the species of biting animal and circumstances surrounding the biting incident. Each case of possible exposure to rabies from species of animals other than those listed here must be studied individually.

Animal bite		Exposure and treatment		
Species	Status at time of attack	No lesion	Mild*	Severe*
Dog or cat	Healthy	None	None[1]†	S[1]
	Signs suggestive of rabies	None	V[2]†	S + V[2]
	Escaped or unknown	None	V	S + V
	Rabid	None	S + V	S + V
Skunk Fox Raccoon Coyote Bat	Regard as rabid in unprovoked attack.	None	S + V	S + V

*See definitions in text.
Code: V = rabies vaccine.
     S = antirabies serum.
[1] = Begin vaccine at first sign of rabies in biting dog or cat during holding period (preferably 7–10 days).
[2] = Discontinue vaccine if biting dog or cat is healthy 5 days after exposure or if acceptable laboratory negativity has been demonstrated in animal killed at time of attack. If observed animal dies after 5 days and brain is positive, resume treatment.
SOURCE: Recommendations on rabies prophylaxis for the United States by Public Health Advisory Committee on Immunization Practices, October, 1969.

mately 20 percent of persons. Serum sickness occurs in approximately 5 percent of persons.

Effectiveness of Vaccines in Human Beings. Over 30,000 people receive antirabies vaccine yearly. Comparative effectiveness of vaccines can be judged only by reported failures. During the years 1957 through 1968 when both nerve tissue vaccine and DEV were available, there were six rabies deaths among 125,000 individuals receiving the nerve tissue vaccine, or 1:20,800, and eight among the 225,000 treated with DEV, or 1:28,100. It is the opinion of the National Communicable Disease Center that the clinical effectiveness of the two vaccines has not been significantly different. Therefore, the lower frequency of central nervous system reactions with DEV makes it preferable to nerve tissue vaccine. Antibody tends to develop somewhat earlier following DEV than following nerve tissue vaccine, but the titers tend to be lower. Human beings may contract rabies even after 14 doses of DEV, particularly when the incubation period has been less than 30 days.

MANIFESTATIONS AND TREATMENT OF DISEASE. Rabid dogs are noted to have purposeless movements with snapping, drooling, and vocal cord paralysis. Death usually occurs in 2 to 5 days. Man dies essentially the same way. There are 2 to 4 days of prodromal symptoms before the patient reaches the excited stage. Paresthesia in the region of the bite is an important early symptom. Symptoms noted with the onset of clinical rabies include headaches, vertigo, stiff neck, malaise, lethargy, and severe pulmonary symptoms including wheezing, hyperventilation, and dyspnea. The patient may have spasm of the throat muscles with dysphagia. The outstanding clinical symptom of rabies is related to swallowing. Drooling, maniacal behavior, and convulsions ensue and are followed by coma, paralysis, and death.

Instead of sedation and symptomatic treatment only, it is now recognized that intensive respiratory supportive care may be beneficial, in view of a case of human rabies in which the patient survived. Strict attention was given to the management of airway, pulmonary care, cardiac arrhythmias, and seizures. This included tracheostomy, vigorous suctioning, Dilantin for seizures, close monitoring of blood gases, electrocardiograms, electroencephalograms, and a ventricular shunt. Nursing care is extremely important. Probably many organs are involved, including brain, heart, and lungs.

Snakebites

INCIDENCE. In North America all the poisonous snakes of medical importance are members of the family Crotalidae, or pit vipers, with exception of the coral snake. Coral snakes are scattered from Florida to southern Arizona, are biologically related to the Indian cobra, and produce a different envenomation syndrome than the crotalids. The pit vipers include the rattlesnake, cottonmouth moccasin, and copperhead.

Approximately 6,000 to 7,000 persons are bitten each year by poisonous snakes. Over 98 percent of snakebites occur on the extremities. Thirty-five percent of snakebites occur in children less than ten years of age, usually in an area around their homes. Since 1960, an average of 14 victims have died annually as a result of snakebites. Seventy percent of all such deaths occur in five states: Texas, Georgia, Florida, Alabama, and Southern California. Rattlesnakes are responsible for approximately 70 percent of all deaths due to snakebite. Death from the bite of a copperhead snake is extremely rare, probably not exceeding an incidence of 0.01 percent.

POISONOUS VERSUS NONPOISONOUS SNAKES. Pit vipers are named for the characteristic pit, a heat-sensitive organ, that is located between the eye and the nostril on each side of the head. As a rule, these snakes may be identified by their elliptical pupils, as opposed to the round pupil of harmless snakes. Nonpoisonous snakes do not have pits. However, the coral snake does have a round pupil and lacks the facial pit. Pit vipers have two well-developed fangs that protrude from the maxillae, whereas nonpoisonous snakes have rows of teeth without fangs. Pit vipers also may be identified by turning the snake's belly upward and noting the single row of subcaudal plates. Nonpoisonous snakes have a double row of subcaudal plates (Fig. 6-3). The coral snake is a brightly colored small snake with red, yellow, and black rings. This color combination occurs also in nonpoisonous snakes, but the alternating colors are different. Only the coral snake has a red ring next to a yellow ring; when red touches yellow, it is a coral snake. The nose of the coral snake is black.

The venoms of poisonous snakes consist of enzymatic, complex proteins which affect all soft tissues. Venoms have been shown to have neurotoxic, hemorrhagic, thrombogenic, hemolytic, cytotoxic, antifibrin, and anticoagulant effects. Phospholipase A is probably responsible for hemolysis. Most venoms contain hyaluronidase, which enhances the rapid spread of venom by way of the superficial

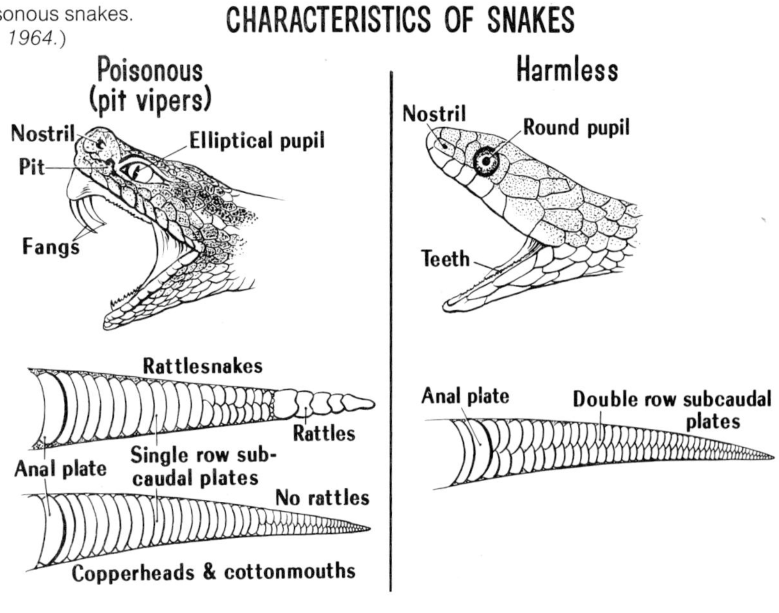

Fig. 6-3. Characteristics of poisonous and nonpoisonous snakes. (*From H. M. Parrish, Texas State J Med, 60:592, 1964.*)

CHARACTERISTICS OF SNAKES

lymphatics. There may be considerable variation in the venom effect. Either neurotoxic features such as muscle cramping, fasciculation, weakness, and respiratory paralysis or hemolytic characteristics may predominate depending on the snake and the patient.

CLINICAL MANIFESTATIONS OF POISONOUS SNAKEBITES. Pain from the bite of a poisonous snake is excruciating and probably the symptom that most easily differentiates poisonous from nonpoisonous snakebites. Poisonous snakes characteristically produce one or two fang marks, whereas nonpoisonous snakes may produce rows of punctures. Swelling, tenderness, pain, and ecchymosis appear within minutes at the site of the venom injection. If no edema is present within 30 minutes following the injury, the pit viper probably did not inject any venom.

Rattlesnake. Most rattlesnakes probably eject less than 50 percent of their venom during a single biting act. Following a rattlesnake bite ecchymosis, hemorrhagic vesiculations, swelling of the regional lymph nodes, weakness, fainting, and sweating commonly are reported. The venom produces deleterious changes in the blood cells, defects in blood coagulation, injuries to the intimal linings of vessels, damage to the heart muscles, alterations in respiration, and, to a lesser extent, changes in neuromuscular conduction.

Coral Snakes. The coral snake contributes only 1.5 percent of all deaths from poisonous snakes. Bites by the coral snake occasionally provoke blurred vision, ptosis, drowsiness, increased salivation, and sweating. The patient may notice paresthesia about the mouth and throat, sometimes slurring of speech, and nausea and vomiting. Pain is not a constant complaint, nor is edema a constant finding.

LOCAL TREATMENT OF SNAKEBITES. The treatment of the bite of a poisonous snake varies considerably but is related to the length of time from the bite until treatment is instituted. The tourniquet, and incision and suction as well, are appropriate if employed within 1 hour from the time of the bite.

Immobilization. Patients are kept quiet, and the extremity is immobilized. Splinting the limb may inhibit the local diffusion of venom by stopping the movement of muscle bellies within their sheaths. Snyder and Knowles have shown in animals that exercise greatly enhances the absorption of venom, and as much as 30 percent may be absorbed within 30 minutes following vigorous exercise.

Tourniquet. The snake injects venom into the subcutaneous tissue, and this is absorbed by the lymphatics. As almost none of the venom is absorbed through the bloodstream, the tourniquet is applied loosely to obstruct only venous and lymphatic flow. The index finger should be easily inserted beneath the tourniquet after its application. The tourniquet is not released once applied and may be left in place during the 30 minutes that suction is being applied. Snyder and Knowles have injected ^{131}I-tagged venom into dogs and have demonstrated that if the tourniquet is applied promptly, less than 10 percent of the venom leaves the leg of the dog in 2 hours.

Incision and Suction. Incision and suction should be accomplished as soon as possible after snakebite. Approximately 50 percent of subcutaneously injected venom can be removed when the suction is started within 3 minutes. Treatment in the first 5 minutes is important, since half the value of suction is lost after 15 minutes and almost all after 30 minutes. A 30-minute period of suction extracts about 90 percent of the venom which can be removed by this procedure. The incision should be $\frac{1}{4}$ in. long and $\frac{1}{8}$ to $\frac{1}{4}$ in. deep, longitudinal and not cruciate. When two fang marks are seen, the depth of the venom injection is generally considered to be three-quarters of the distance between the fang marks. A good rule of thumb has been to incise the skin and subcutaneous tissue the same distance between the fang marks to ensure adequate drainage. A superficial incision may be easily accomplished by raising the skin with a pinch between two fingers. This procedure rarely results in penetration of fascia or muscle. Incisions made proximal to the bite will usually recover venom insufficient to make the procedure worthwhile.

When a suction cup is not available after incisions have been made, mouth suction may be used if the mucosa of the mouth is intact. Snake venom is not absorbed through an intact oral mucosa but may be absorbed when there is any denuded area or minor laceration of the mucosa. The digestive juices neutralize poisonous snake venom if it is swallowed.

Russell has demonstrated that the serosanguinous fluid removed during suction contains substances which when injected into animals produced a fall in systemic blood pressure and changes in respiratory rates, and alterations in the electrocardiogram and electroencephalogram similar to those observed following injection of crude *Crotalus* venom. If exudate removed during suction contains venom, its removal should increase the chances of survival.

Excision. Snyder and Knowles showed that wide excision of the entire area around the snakebite within 1 hour from the time of injection can remove most of the venom. Excision of the fang marks including skin and subcutaneous tissue should be considered in severe bites and in patients known to be allergic to horse serum who are seen within 1 hour following the bite.

Most fatalities from snakebites do not occur for 6 to 48 hours following the bite, giving time to institute these first-aid measures.

Cryotherapy. This form of therapy has been used but is not recommended, as it probably only increases the local area of necrosis. McCollough and Gennard analyzed cryotherapy in relation to amputation and noted that 75 percent of children requiring amputation following snakebite had received cryotherapy. In seven of nine snakebite cases requiring amputations in California, cryotherapy had been used. Cooling or refrigeration experimentally produces intense vasoconstriction and thus decreases the amount of antivenin getting into the area of the bite. Gill found that dogs developed edema and ecchymosis just as rapidly and extensively with cryotherapy as without it. There was no evidence to suggest inactivation of venom by tissue temperature of 15°C and below.

SYSTEMIC TREATMENT. The most important treatment for a snakebite is antivenin. Most snakebite fatalities in the United States during the past 20 years have involved either delay in obtaining treatment, no antivenin treatment, or inadequate dosage. Because antivenin contains horse serum, its administration requires prior skin testing.

Information concerning identification of a snake or proper antivenin frequently can be obtained from the nearest zoo herpetarium. A major problem with bites by exotic poisonous snakes is the choice and availability of suitable antiserum. Physicians confronted with this situation may obtain advice from the local poison control center or from the Antivenin Index Center of the American Association of Zoological Parks and Aquariums in Oklahoma City, Oklahoma.

Because the rattlesnake, cottonmouth moccasin, and copperhead belong to the same biologic family, their bites can be treated by the same antivenin (antivenin Crotalidae polyvalent).

The coral snakebite is rare, and the antivenin is different from that for the pit vipers. A North American coral snake (*Micrurus fulvius*) antivenin has recently been developed and released. It effectively treats *Micrurus* coral snake bites but is not effective in treating bites of *Micruroides,* the genus native to Arizona and New Mexico. Coral snake antivenin can be obtained from many state public health departments. Also, a large supply has been stocked at the United States Public Health Service National Communicable Disease Center in Atlanta, Georgia.

The time of antivenin administration depends upon the snake involved. If the bite is from a snake with quick-acting venom, such as a king cobra or mamba, an initial dose of antivenin may be required as part of the first-aid treatment. However, for bites by most snakes, such as rattlesnakes and others with less virulent venom, antivenin should be withheld until a physician can determine if it is indicated. Approximately 30 percent of all poisonous snakebites in the United States result in no venenation.

The indication for antivenin is governed by the degree of venenation, as outlined by Wood et al. and modified by Parrish and by McCollough and Gennard:

Grade 0—no venenation: One or more fang marks; minimal pain; less than 1 in. of surrounding edema and erythema at 12 hours; no systemic involvement.
Grade I—minimal venenation: Fang marks; moderate to severe pain; 1 to 5 in. of surrounding edema and erythema in the first 12 hours after bite; systemic involvement usually not present.
Grade II—moderate venenation: Fang marks; severe pain; 6 to 12 in. of surrounding edema and erythema in the first 12 hours after bite; possible systemic involvement including nausea, vomiting giddiness, shock, or neurotoxic symptoms.
Grade III—severe venenation: Fang marks; severe pain; more than 12 in. of surrounding edema and erythema in first 12 hours after bite; grade II symptoms of systemic involvement usually present and may include generalized petechiae and ecchymoses.
Grade IV—very severe venenation: Systemic involvement is always present, and symptoms may include renal failure, blood-tinged secretions, coma, and death; local edema may extend beyond the involved extremity to the ipsilateral trunk.

Antivenin usually is not required for grades 0 or I venenation. Grade II may require three or four ampules, and grade III usually requires five ampules or more. If symptoms increase, several vials may be required during the first 2 hours. Because children are smaller, they receive relatively larger doses of venom, which places them in a higher-risk group. Thus, the smaller the patient, the relatively larger the required dose of antivenin. Proper dosage can be estimated by observing the clinical signs and symptoms.

The injection of antivenin locally around the bite is not advised, as massive edema usually occurs in that area. Therefore, absorption from this area is poor, and additional antivenin fluid will further decrease perfusion and perhaps increase tissue anoxia.

Antivenin is given by intravenous drip in 250 ml of normal saline solution or 5% glucose solution. McCollough and Gennard have demonstrated in studies with radioisotopes that antivenin accumulates at the site of the bite more rapidly after *intravenous* than after *intramuscular* administration. The dose of intravenously administered antivenin can be more easily titrated with response to treatment. When it is obvious that antivenin therapy will be instituted, the tourniquet should be left in place until antivenin is started intravenously.

Complications of Antivenin. If too much time has elapsed for excision to be effective and the patient is allergic to horse serum, a slow infusion of one vial of antivenin in 250 ml of 5% glucose solution may be given over a 90-minute period with constant monitoring of the blood pressure and electrocardiogram depending on the seriousness of the bite. If an immediate reaction occurs, the antivenin is stopped, and a vasopressor, epinephrine, and perhaps an antihistamine may be required, depending on the severity of the reaction.

The incidence of serum sickness is directly related to the volume of horse serum injected. Of patients receiving 100 to 200 ml of horse serum, 85 percent will have some degree of sensitivity in 8 to 12 days following injection. This complication will have to be dealt with at a later time since some patients may require from one to five vials of antiserum every 4 to 6 hours.

Steroids have been used but are of questionable benefit. Russell experimentally used doses of methylprednisone up to 100 mg/kg in mice and noted that steroids neither affected survival nor prevented tissue damage and inflammation. When used in association with the antivenin, there is a decreased incidence of serum sickness. According to Parrish, cortisone and ACTH do not affect the survival rate of animals poisoned with pit viper venom.

Intravenous fluids are frequently required to replace the decreased extracellular fluid volume resulting from edema formation. Fascial planes may become very tense, with obstruction of venous and later arterial flow, requiring fasciotomy.

Blood should be immediately drawn for typing and cross matching, since hemolysis may later make this difficult. Since hemolysis and injury to kidneys and liver may occur, it is important to follow alterations in clotting mechanism and renal and liver function as well as electrolyte status. Bleeding and clotting time, platelet count, prothrombin time, fibrinogen level, and partial thromboplastin times are included in the base-line studies. These patients may need blood, since anemia can develop from the hematologic effects. As afibrinogenemia has been reported, fibrinogen may be required. Vitamin K may also be required, according to Stahnke. The patient is started on antibiotics immediately to prevent secondary infection, and tetanus toxoid is administered on arrival at the emergency ward. Prolonged artificial ventilation may be required for respiratory failure.

Stinging Insects and Animals

HYMENOPTERA

The most important insects that produce serious and possibly fatal anaphylactic reactions are the arthropods of the order Hymenoptera. This group includes the honeybee, bumblebee, wasp, yellow and black hornet, and fire ant. The venom of these stinging insects is just as potent as that of snakes and causes more deaths in the United States yearly than are caused by snakebites. Davidson states that, drop for drop, the venom of the bee is just as potent as that of the rattlesnake. Parrish noted that, of 460 deaths between 1950 and 1959, 50 percent were due to Hymenoptera, 30 percent due to poisonous snakes, and 14 percent due to spiders. Scorpions accounted for eight deaths. No other poisonous creature killed more than five persons.

Insects of the Hymenoptera group, except the bee, retain their sting and are in a position to sting repeatedly, each time injecting some portion of the venom sac contents. The worker honeybee sinks its barbed sting into the skin, and it cannot be withdrawn. As the bee attempts to escape, it is disemboweled. The stinger with the bowel, muscles, and venom sac attached are left behind. The muscles controlling the venom sac, although separated from the bee, rhythmically contract for as long as 20 minutes, driving the sting deeper and deeper into the skin, and continuing to inject venom.

Bee venoms contain histamine, serotonin, acelytcholine, formic acid, phospholipase A, hyaluronidase, and other proteins. Once the proteins of these insects are injected, the patient may become sensitized and be a candidate for anaphylactic response with the next sting.

CLINICAL MANIFESTATIONS. Symptoms consist of one or more of the following: localized pain, swelling, generalized erythema, a feeling of intense heat throughout the body, headache, blurred vision, injected conjunctiva, swollen and tender joints, itching, apprehension, urticaria, petechial hemorrhages of skin and mucous membranes, dizziness, weakness, sweating, severe nausea, abdominal cramps, dyspnea, constriction of the chest, asthma, angioneurotic edema, vascular collapse, and possible death from anaphylaxis. Fatal cases may manifest glottal and laryngeal edema, pulmonary and cerebral edema, visceral congestion, meningeal hyperemia, and interventricular hemorrhage. Death apparently results from a combination of shock, respiratory failure, and central nervous system changes.

The acute, allergic phase of the simple reaction is thought to be due to protein allergens rather than to toxicity of venom. These allergens may be found in dust from the wings, bodies, venom, saliva, or feces of the insect. Most deaths from insect stings occur within 15 to 30 minutes following the bite or sting.

TREATMENT. Early application of a tourniquet may prevent rapid spread of the venom. Affected persons should be taught to remove the venom sacs if present, being careful not to squeeze the sac. It may be necessary for some patients to carry an emergency kit, which is commercially available, supplied with a tourniquet, sublingual isoproterenol in 10-mg tablets, epinephrine hydrochloride aerosol for inhalation to reduce bronchospasm and laryngeal edema, and tweezers to remove the sting and venom sac until a physician is available. The patient should be taught to give himself an epinephrine injection. Patients having severe reactions should first receive 0.3 to 0.5 ml of a 1:1,000 solution of epinephrine intravenously. Antihistamines also may be intravenously administered, and oxygen may be given. If wheezing continues, aminophylline may be given slowly intravenously. Occasionally the patient may require a tracheostomy.

DESENSITIZATION. The Insect Allergy Committee of the American Academy of Allergy noted that 50 percent of people who had a severe generalized reaction to stings had no previous history of a severe reaction. A sharp rise was noted in the proportion of serious reactions after the age of thirty, suggesting increasing sensitivity as the total number of stings increase. Patients with a history of severe local or systemic involvement following insect stings should be desensitized.

The efficacy of desensitization to insect stings has been demonstrated. Of persons desensitized and stung again, 88 percent experienced milder reactions than they had previously, and only 3 percent suffered more severe reactions. By comparison, 63 percent of those patients stung again but not desensitized suffered more severe reactions. It has been suspected that a refractory period of 10 to 14 days persists following an insect sting during which skin tests may be negative. Therefore, skin tests should be delayed several weeks after stinging and be performed with extreme caution. Cross reactions to the wasp, bee, and yellow jacket may occur.

Because the antigens eliciting hypersensitive reactions are present in the insect's body as well as its venom, whole insect extract should be used for skin testing before hyposensitization therapy is begun. The initial dilution should be weak, since shocklike reactions have been reported after intradermal testing with a 1:1 million dilution. Immunotherapy consists of weekly subcutaneous injections of whole body extract, containing equal parts of bee, hornet, wasp, and yellow jacket whole body extracts, administered for at least 3 years, perhaps indefinitely.

STINGRAYS

Approximately 750 persons each year are stung by stingrays. However, during the past 60 years, only two deaths in this country have been attributed to the venom of the stingray.

As the spine, which is curved and has serrated edges, enters the flesh, the sheath surrounding the spine ruptures, and venom is released. As the spine is withdrawn, fragments of the sheath may remain in the wound. The wound edges are often jagged and bleed freely. Pain is usually immediate and severe, increasing to maximum intensity in 1 to 2 hours and lasting for 12 to 48 hours.

TREATMENT. This consists of copious irrigation with water to wash out any toxin and fragments of the spine's integumentary sheath. Russell noted that the venom is inactivated when exposed to heat. Therefore, the area of the bite should be placed in water as hot as the patient can stand without injury for 30 minutes to 1 hour. After soaking, the wound may be further debrided and treated appropriately. Patients treated in this manner were shown to have rapid and uncomplicated healing of the wound. Patients not treated with heat had tissue necrosis with prolonged drainage and chronically infected wounds.

PORTUGUESE MAN-OF-WAR

This coelenterate is commonly found along our southern Atlantic coast. Its tentacles are covered with thousands of stinging cells, the nematocytes, capable of emitting microscopic organelles, the nematocysts, each of which consists of a small sphere containing a coiled hollow thread. When activated by touch, the thread is uncoiled with such force that it can penetrate skin and even rubber gloves. On contact, venom in the cyst is injected into the victim through the thread. This sting produces extreme pain and often signs of clinical shock; however, no deaths have been reported due to this sting alone.

Following a severe sting there may be almost immediate severe nausea, gastric cramping, and constriction and tightness of throat and chest with severe muscle spasm. There is intense burning pain with weakness and perhaps cyanosis with respiratory distress.

TREATMENT. Demerol and Benadryl may dramatically relieve the pain and symptoms. Covering the area with alcohol inactivates undischarged nematocysts. Lathering the area and shaving it with a razor relieves the pain probably by removing tentacular material. Application of baking powder or dry sand and rubbing may remove some of the material. Aerosol corticosteroid-analgesic balm may be helpful.

Spider Bites

BLACK WIDOW SPIDER

The most common biting spider in the United States is the black widow (*Latrodectus mactans*) (Fig. 6-4). This spider is black and globular, with a red hourglass mark on the abdomen. The bite of this species in the 10-year period 1950–1959 accounted for 63 deaths. *Latrodectus* venom is primarily neurotoxic in action and appears to center on the spinal cord. Following a bite by the black widow spider, the patient usually experiences sudden pain, and in a few minutes a small wheal with an area of erythema appears. The most prominent physical finding is generalized muscle spasm. Even if bitten on an extremity, the spasm may involve the abdomen and chest. Although the abdomen is rigid, it is nontender. The severe symptoms last from 24 to 48 hours.

TREATMENT. Treatment has consisted of narcotics for the relief of pain and a muscle relaxant for relief of spasm.

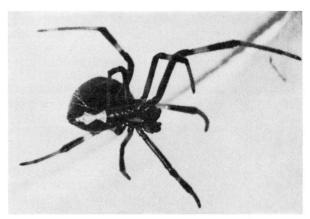

Fig. 6-4. Abdominal view of a female black widow spider showing the hourglass marking. (*From B. C. Paton, Surg Clin North Am, 43:537, 1963.*)

Either methocarbamol (Robaxin) or 10 ml of a 10% solution of calcium gluconate relieves symptoms. Methocarbamol can be administered intravenously, 10 ml over a 5-minute period, with a second ampule started in a saline solution drip. Specific treatment involves the use of antivenin. This is administered intramuscularly, after appropriate skin tests, since it contains horse serum.

NORTH AMERICAN LOXOSCELISM

The distinguishing mark of the *Loxosceles reclusa* is the darker violin-shaped band over the dorsal cephalothorax (Fig. 6-5). The spider is native to the South Central United States and is found both indoors and outdoors and under cliffs and overhanging rocks. The first recognized and documented case in the United States of a bite by *Loxosceles reclusa* was not published until 1957.

CLINICAL MANIFESTATIONS. The bite may go unnoticed because pain may not occur until 6 to 8 hours afterward. A generalized macular and erythematous rash may appear in 12 to 24 hours. Erythema develops, with bleb or blister formation surrounded by an irregular area of ischemia. A zone of hemorrhage with induration and a surrounding halo of erythema may develop peripherally. The central ischemia turns dark, an eschar forms by the seventh day, and by the fourteenth day the area sloughs, leaving an open ulcer. Approximately 3 weeks is required for the lesion to heal. Severe systemic manifestations may occur in 24 to 48 hours in small children, with fever, chills, malaise, weakness, nausea, vomiting, joint pain, and even petechial eruption. The two principal systemic effects, hemolysis and thrombocytopenia, have been responsible for two deaths. Hemoglobinemia, hemoglobinuria, leukocytosis, and proteinuria may also occur. *Loxosceles* venom is chiefly cytotoxic in action.

TREATMENT. Immediate excision with primary closure has been advocated as the treatment of choice. This usually is not possible since the patient rarely can be certain of what bit him or has failed to recognize the type of spider. Several writers immediately administered steroids. The dose has varied from 30 to 80 mg of methylprednisolone daily, tapered over a period of several days. This seems

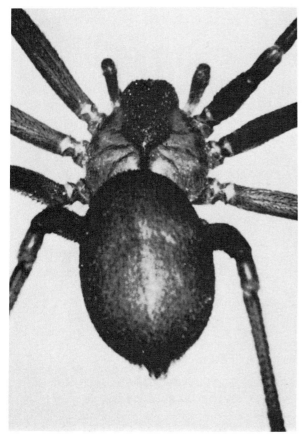

Fig. 6-5. The distinguishing mark of the *Loxosceles reclus* is the darker violin-shaped band over the dorsal cephalothorax. *(From C. J. Dillaha, G. T. Jansen, W. M. Honeycutt, and C. R. Hayden, JAMA, 188:33, 1964.)*

to be the preferred treatment. Excision of the necrotic area with skin grafting may be required at a later date.

PENETRATING WOUNDS OF THE NECK AND THORACIC INLET

(By Robert F. Jones, G. Tom Shires, and William H. Snyder III)

INCIDENCE. Although major wounds of the soft tissues of the neck are relatively uncommon in civilian surgical practice, the number of vital structures in the small volume of the neck makes it imperative that every penetrating neck wound be considered a serious surgical problem.

Prior to World War II, the treatment of penetrating wounds of the neck was largely nonsurgical unless major bleeding or deep injuries were obvious. Reported mortality rates were 18 percent of 188 cases in the Spanish-American War and 11 percent of 594 cases in World War I. During World War II the mortality rate fell to 7 percent, probably because of a variety of factors, including earlier tracheostomy, earlier and more frequent surgical exploration, antibiotics, and improvements in surgical and anesthetic techniques.

Since 1960, several civilian series have been reported with no further reduction in mortality rate, which seems to have leveled off at about 10 percent. In the three previous series, the total number of deaths was 57. Of these, 43 were a direct result of blood vessel injuries. The other 14 deaths were due principally to complications from wounds of the larynx, trachea, and esophagus. In the study of Shirkey et al. 6 of the 22 deaths occurred in the group in which exploration was delayed beyond 6 hours or omitted entirely. Fogelman and Stewart pointed out that the mortality rate for their cases which were promptly explored was 6 percent, whereas for those in which surgical intervention was omitted or postponed the mortality rate was 35 percent. Their overall mortality was 11 percent. Since the initial phase of the Fogelman and Stewart series, it has been the policy at Parkland Memorial Hospital to "treat the platysma like the peritoneum" and explore virtually all neck wounds that penetrate the platysma in the operating room under general endotracheal anesthesia, regardless of preoperative opinion as to the extent and severity of the damage.

Recently, 274 penetrating wounds of the neck treated at Parkland Memorial Hospital have been reviewed. There were 11 deaths, for a mortality rate of 3.6 percent. Of the fatalities, four were due to complications from spinal cord injuries, three from massive hemorrhage, one from extensive aspiration of blood from a bleeding tracheal wound, one from blast injury to the brainstem, one from a cerebral embolus following repair of a common carotid artery injury, and one from blast injury to the trachea unrecognized at the original exploration and leading to laryngeal edema and obstruction in the absence of a tracheostomy.

Of the 274 cases, 103 explorations were negative, i.e., with no hematoma, no significant bleeding, and no damage to any named structure in the neck, although the tract of injury frequently was within millimeters of vital structures. Of these negative cases, there were no deaths and no complications except one superficial wound infection which cleared promptly with drainage. These patients usually were discharged within 72 hours to clinic follow-up if there were no associated injuries.

Table 6-3 summarizes the injuries found in 15 patients with clinically "negative" neck wounds, i.e., with no visible bleeding, no visible hematoma, no evidence of hemorrhagic shock. At some hospitals these wounds would not have been explored, and many probably would have

Table 6-3. INJURIES IN 15 CLINICALLY "NEGATIVE"* NECK WOUNDS

Total series = 274 patients

Innominate vein	2
Subclavian vein	1
Internal jugular vein	5
Thyrocervical artery	3
Thoracic duct	2
Esophagus (blast injury)	2
Ascending pharyngeal artery	1

*No visible bleeding, no visible hematoma, no shock.

healed uneventfully without surgical exploration. However, unexplored patients, apparently free of significant injury on examination in the emergency room, may bleed massively later when a blood clot is shaken loose, or a deep abscess may develop from a small perforation of the esophagus, or other complications may develop from unrecognized injuries. Even those less serious injuries associated only with damage to subcutaneous tissues and muscles will heal faster with less chance of infection if hemostasis, debridement, and adequate drainage are accomplished. It is a fundamental fact that bacteria thrive on extravasated blood and damaged tissue, and every penetrating wound is contaminated.

TREATMENT. The safest treatment for penetrating neck wounds appears to be prompt and thorough surgical exploration under local or general anesthesia.

Initial Treatment. On admission to the emergency room, all patients with neck injuries are immediately evaluated regarding their systemic condition, i.e., airway and adequacy of ventilation, blood pressure, pulse, mental state, and peripheral signs of shock such as sweating, cold skin, and collapsed veins. If there is external bleeding, some type of pressure is applied for temporary hemostasis. If there is upper airway obstruction, an endotracheal tube is passed immediately, or if there is sufficient time, a tracheostomy is performed. Meanwhile, one or two large-bore intravenous cannulas or needles are inserted in peripheral veins and Ringer's lactate solution is started while blood is drawn for typing and cross matching. If shock is present, the fluid is given rapidly, and if there is no evidence of significant blood loss, the intravenous infusions are kept going by slow drip. When indicated, whole blood is administered as soon as it is available. Usually the salt solution will temporarily reverse the shock state until cross-matched blood is available. If shock is severe and is not improved promptly by the Ringer's lactate solution, type O, Rh-negative low-titer unmatched blood is infused rapidly until the matched blood is available. Plasma has also been used, but there is little advantage over salt solutions; i.e., both are quite helpful temporarily, although neither is a substitute for whole blood.

If it is apparent that blood or air is free in a pleural cavity, closed-chest drainage is immediately instituted. If there is no clinical evidence or a pneumothorax or hemothorax and the missile or blade could have possibly reached the pleura, and if the patient's systemic condition is stable, an upright chest film is obtained with a physician in constant attendance. Special x-ray studies such as arteriograms have rarely been worthwhile.

If the depth of the injury is not apparent, the wound is very gently probed with a small hemostat only to the depth of the platysma muscle. If the platysma has been penetrated, the probing is discontinued. Nonbleeding neck wounds should not be deeply probed in an emergency room. The patient is then transferred to the operating room. No attempt is made to pass a nasogastric tube in the emergency room because of the danger of hemorrhage with coughing or gagging.

Anesthesia. Virtually all neck wounds are explored under general anesthesia, using an orotracheal airway with an inflatable cuff. The anesthetic agent varies considerably according to the specific problem, necessity for rapid induction, circulatory status, preexisting disease, etc. There are no specific contraindications in neck injuries per se to any of the commonly used anesthetic agents or relaxants.

The chest is again examined just prior to induction, since pneumothorax or hemothorax may develop slowly following a neck wound, appearing an hour or longer after an initially negative chest x-ray. Wounds at the root of the neck following a downward path may barely penetrate the pleura so that a pneumothorax is not apparent initially and may not be manifest until after the patient is intubated. This should be kept in mind as a cause for hypotension or hypoxia during anesthesia, especially if closed thoracotomy drainage has not been instituted.

Technique of Exploration. With adequate control of the ventilatory and cardiovascular systems, the surgeon can now safely and adequately explore the structures that are apparently or potentially injured. The incision is planned to allow full exposure of the tract of injury. Proximal and distal control of the major vessels must also be considered in the length and position of the incision. The sternocleidomastoid muscle and/or any other neck muscles are transected whenever necessary to provide adequate exposure. An oblique incision along the anterior border of the sternocleidomastoid muscle is often useful, or any transverse incision may be used if it gives adequate exposure. The tract of injury is followed to its depth, with systematic examination of each structure in or near the tract. It should also be pointed out that blast injury from gunshot wounds may not be immediately apparent in the tissues adjacent to the tract.

Specific Injuries

CERVICAL BLOOD VESSELS. If injuries to the major vessels are suspected, umbilical tapes are passed around the vessels proximal and distal to the point of suspected injury before local clots are removed if bleeding has previously occurred and stopped. This happens frequently with venous and occasionally with arterial injury. The vessels are then carefully inspected, all clots are removed, and repair is carried out.

When the injury involves the low anterior neck, it may be necessary to resect a portion of the clavicle or to split the sternum to obtain proximal control and prevent uncontrollable hemorrhage. The medial one-third or one-half of the clavicle is resected whenever necessary, disarticulating the sternoclavicular joint. There is no significant disability following this procedure, and if the periosteum is preserved, bony regeneration will usually occur. When this does not adequately expose the great vessels for repair or for proximal control, the entire clavicle is removed, or the sternum may be split with a Lebsche knife. The sternal incision may be carried off laterally into the second or third intercostal space to avoid opening the full mediastinum unnecessarily.

The internal carotid, common carotid, subclavian, and innominate arteries should be repaired if at all possible. An internal or external shunt may be utilized during carotid repair, as with carotid grafting or endarterectomy, or the vessel may be partially occluded with a curved vascular clamp to allow partial flow during repair. The vertebral artery is usually very difficult to repair in the bony canal but may be controlled by prolonged pressure, suture ligatures, and bone wax. The external carotid artery and/or its branches may be ligated except in patients with carotid arteriosclerosis with an occluded common or internal carotid vessel. In these cases, the external carotid may be a major source of collateral flow.

When the carotid arteries are to be handled or pressed upon in the region of the bifurcation, the adventitia of the carotid bulb is infiltrated with a local anesthetic to prevent hypotension from reflexes originating in pressor receptors of the carotid sinus. Atropine may be given at intervals during the procedure when hypotension results from such stimuli.

The internal jugular vein is repaired if feasible but may be ligated unilaterally if necessary without adverse sequelae. All other neck veins are routinely ligated if injured. Prompt pressure on an open vein and a slight head-down tilt to the table will prevent the occurrence of air embolism.

BLOOD VESSELS OF THORACIC INLET. Injuries to the major vascular structures in the base of the neck or thoracic inlet are a significant challenge in management. Rapid resuscitation, liberal surgical exploration, and a thorough knowledge of the operative approach are the necessary ingredients of success. The vascular structures involved are the common carotid, subclavian, and innominate arteries and their corresponding veins. A penetrating wound due to an act of violence is the usual cause. Indications for early surgical exploration are listed in Table 6-4. Diagnostic errors and subsequent inappropriately conservative management rarely occur with overt signs of major vascular injury. Unfortunately, a significant number of these injuries appear innocuous at the time of presentation, and a high index of suspicion is necessary. It is in this context that platysmal penetration and proximity of the wound to a major vascular structure must be regarded as absolute indications for surgical exploration. This concept is emphasized by data from a recent Parkland Memorial Hospital series, to be presented later. Arteriog-

Table 6-4. FINDINGS SUGGESTING MAJOR VASCULAR INJURY

Obvious or direct evidence of injury:
1. Circulatory instability
2. Excessive external bleeding
3. A large or progressing hematoma
4. Distal pulse deficit
5. Neurologic deficit involving nerves anatomically adjacent to major vascular structures
6. Massive or continued intrathoracic bleeding

Indirect evidence indicating exploration:
1. A wound above the clavicle or manubrium that penetrates the platysma muscle
2. Thoracic wounds whose trajectory traverses the superior mediastinum or thoracic inlet
3. Mediastinal widening demonstrated roentgenographically

raphy to modify the principle of proximity and penetration exploration remains controversial. It may prove useful if always immediately available. However, valuable time should not be wasted obtaining studies if objective evidence of major vascular injury exists.

Immediate formal exploration in the operating room generally is recommended. Massive bleeding progressing to exsanguination can occur rapidly from a wound that initially appears innocent if increased intrathoracic pressure dislodges a tamponading clot. For this reason, every effort is made to avoid vomiting, coughing, or agitation. Smooth anesthetic induction is most important. Endotracheal intubation of patients with wounds in the base of the neck is most safely accomplished following infusion of muscle relaxants, thus minimizing the danger of "bucking the endotracheal tube" with a sudden increase in intravascular pressure.

As preoperative prediction of the specific vessels injured often is inaccurate, a flexible operative approach is necessary. The entire neck, thorax, and proximal arms are included in the surgical field. The supine position with slight cervical extension provides the greatest flexibility for performing the primary incision and any necessary extensions. The major technical problem is to provide adequate exposure for establishing proximal and distal vascular control prior to dissecting the area of injury. Familiarity with several basic incisions and their extensions is necessary. These are demonstrated in Fig. 6-6. They include the oblique neck incision, the horizontal clavicular incision with resection of the medial portion of the clavicle, the median sternotomy, and the bilateral fourth intercostal space anterolateral thoracotomies.

The right oblique incision generally is adequate to expose the entire right common carotid artery. The horizontal clavicular incision with subperiostial resection of the medial half of the clavicle adequately exposes the right subclavian vessels. Extension to a median sternotomy generally is necessary to expose the innominate artery; the distal left common carotid artery is easily exposed through a left oblique neck incision. The proximal left common carotid and the distal left subclavian can be reached through a horizontal clavicular incision; further exposure can be gained by extension to a median sternotomy. However, the proximal portion of the left subclavian artery is best approached through a left anterolateral thoracotomy. The entire left subclavian artery is adequately exposed through a combined left clavicular and left anterolateral thoracotomy incision. The construction of a musculoskeletal flap, or "trapdoor," has been used by some to expose the innominate and subclavian vessels. This is formed by combining horizontal clavicular, superior median sternotomy, and anterolateral thoracotomy incisions. As a general rule, the majority of these injuries are exposed through the oblique neck or horizontal clavicular incisions. Major extensions should be made without hesitation when these incisions provide inadequate exposure. The vascular repair seldom is difficult and most often can be accomplished by lateral arteriorrhaphy or end-to-end anastomosis. When graft interposition is required, autogenous material is preferred.

INCISIONS AND EXTENSIONS
FOR
BASE OF THE NECK VASCULAR INJURIES

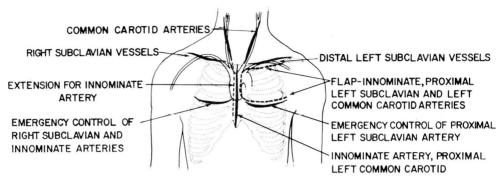

Fig. 6-6. Incisions and extensions for base-of-the-neck vascular injuries.

Important factors in the management of these injuries are emphasized by a recent series from Parkland Memorial Hospital. During a 10-year period, 99 patients with 122 injuries of the major vascular structures at the base of the neck were seen. Arterial injuries accounted for 40 percent, including 23 injuries to the subclavian artery, 21 to the common carotid, and 3 to the innominate artery. Of 74 venous injuries, there were 35 to the subclavian vein, 31 to the internal jugular, and 8 to the innominate vein. Signs and symptoms of significant vascular injury were equivocal in many patients and totally absent in 32 patients. These patients were explored on the basis of platysmal penetration and the proximity of the wound to a major vascular structure. The overall mortality was 5.1 percent, generally related to the magnitude of associated injuries or the extent of blood loss prior to operation. Eleven percent of the patients with arterial trauma died, compared with 1.3 percent of those with venous injuries. Postoperative complications were related to vascular injury or repair in only 20 percent of patients. Essentially all injuries of the common carotid arteries or internal jugular veins were exposed through oblique neck incisions. Extension into a median sternotomy or horizontal clavicular incision was required only with associated vertebral or subclavian vessel injuries or when the proximal left common carotid artery was involved. Horizontal clavicular incisions with resection of the medial portion of the clavicle adequately exposed injuries of the subclavian vessels in most instances. An anterolateral thoracotomy was necessary only for immediate control of bleeding or when the proximal portion of the left subclavian artery was involved. The majority of the innominate vein injuries could be managed through horizontal clavicular incisions. However, median sternotomy was necessary to adequately expose innominate artery injuries. Early and liberal surgical exploration with emphasis on adequate exposure has resulted in the low mortality and morbidity rates in this large series.

LARYNX AND TRACHEA. Whenever laryngeal or tracheal injury is apparent in the emergency room, tracheostomy is performed promptly, prior to transfer of the patient to the main operating suite. If the injury is not apparent until the time of exploration, a tracheostomy is done during exploration. When the patient is hoarse or the wound is near the thyroid or larynx, indirect laryngoscopy is performed preoperatively when feasible to determine the integrity of the recurrent laryngeal nerve. Laryngeal blast injury may result from a bullet tract near the larynx; in such a case, a tracheostomy is also performed.

Subcutaneous air may be present with such injuries and may increase rapidly under observation. However, air may spread subcutaneously from outside via the entrance wound in the absence of tracheal, pharyngeal, or esophageal penetration. Cervical extension of mediastinal air from an injured bronchus or lung may also occur.

Clean lacerations of the trachea or larynx are closed using a nonabsorbable suture, usually cotton or silk. If the defect cannot be closed primarily, a fascial flap may be used as a patch. Synthetic patch grafts such as Marlex have been successful. The tracheostomy is maintained until healing is complete and laryngeal or tracheal edema has subsided, usually 4 to 8 days.

PHARYNX AND ESOPHAGUS. If a small esophageal injury is suspected but cannot be demonstrated during exploration, an anesthetic mask may be applied to the nose and mouth and positive pressure exerted while the wound is filled with saline solution. Bubbles may disclose the point of injury. The pharynx and esophagus may be repaired primarily using chromic catgut suture, following debridement as necessary. It is vital to drain all such wounds, since infection and/or a salivary leak is not an infrequent complication. If there is massive loss of tissue, as with a close-range shotgun blast, it may be necessary to perform a cutaneous esophagostomy for feeding purposes and cutaneous pharyngostomy for salivary drainage. A secondary plastic reconstruction will be required after initial healing is complete. A small plastic nasogastric tube is used for feeding for 8 to 10 days following all esophageal injuries, unless for some reason a gastrostomy is deemed preferable.

NERVES. A preoperative neurologic examination is performed whenever possible to identify an injured nerve. The brachial plexus, the deep cervical plexus, the phrenic nerve, and the cranial nerves are systematically tested. The vagus and recurrent laryngeal nerves can be checked by examination of the vocal cords. A hypoglossal or spinal accessory nerve injury is particularly easy to miss unless a preoperative neurologic examination is performed. An associated head injury or alcoholic intoxication will frequently complicate the neurologic evaluation.

Whenever possible, all severed or lacerated nerves are debrided and repaired primarily, using interrupted fine silk sutures on the perineurium. If a motor nerve deficit is apparent, an expendable sensory nerve such as the great auricular nerve may be interposed as a nerve autograft to allow anastomosis without tension.

THYROID. After debridement of devitalized tissue, hemostasis may be secured by suture ligature. Adequate drainage is particularly important.

THORACIC DUCT. Wounds near the inferior segment of the left internal jugular vein may sever the thoracic duct at or below the point of entry; the location is quite variable. Repair of the duct is not feasible because of its friability, but simple ligation is adequate. Since the duct may divide just before entering the vein or there may be tributaries for the head and arm, multiple ligatures may be required for lymphostasis. The area should be thoroughly dried and inspected before closing, since a large collection of lymph may occur postoperatively from even a small leak. If lymph does accumulate, incision and drainage with the application of a bulky pressure dressing will usually allow closure of the lymph fistula within a few days. Occasionally, an injured right lymphatic duct is encountered on the opposite side in the same location and is treated in like manner.

SALIVARY GLANDS. A sialogram may be used preoperatively to establish the diagnosis, or it may be determined during exploration. Injuries to the gland may be handled by debridement, hemostasis, and simple drainage. In the absence of ductal obstruction, a salivary fistula will rarely occur following injury to the gland substance. When the major duct is injured, it may be repaired with fine silk over a ureteral catheter stent. The catheter should be removed after repair is effected. When repair is not feasible because of the patient's condition or for some other compelling reason, the duct may be ligated and the gland allowed to atrophy, or the duct may be reimplanted in the mucosa at a later time.

When the parotid gland is involved, the major facial nerve branches should be identified and repaired if injured. Primary repair has a better prognosis for nerve function than does delayed repair, unless there is gross bacterial contamination or massive loss of tissue.

If a salivary fistula does occur postoperatively and fails to close spontaneously, irradiation is usually effective in arresting salivary flow but is not used for this purpose in children or young adults.

CLOSURE. Almost all soft tissue neck wounds are drained for 24 to 48 hours using soft Penrose drains to prevent the accumulation of blood and serum. If the pharynx or esophagus is injured, drainage is continued for 4 to 8 days. All muscles are repaired. In the case of massive gunshot wounds, such as a close-range shotgun injury, the wound is left open initially and a delayed primary closure performed 3 to 4 days later, if possible.

ABDOMINAL TRAUMA

(*By Robert N. McClelland, Ronald C. Jones, Malcolm O. Perry, G. Tom Shires and Erwin R. Thal*)

The incidence of abdominal trauma increases each year. About 5 million persons in the United States are injured yearly in automobile accidents, and many of these injuries are abdominal. Blunt abdominal trauma generally leads to higher mortality rates than penetrating wounds and presents greater problems in diagnosis. The spleen, liver, kidneys, and bowel are the most frequently injured abdominal viscera. In a review of several series of abdominal trauma by Griswold and Collier, the frequency of injury was determined (see Table 6-5).

Evaluation of Blunt Trauma

The greatest difficulty in the management of blunt abdominal trauma is in the diagnosis. This is largely due to masking of abdominal injury by associated injuries. The most frequently associated injuries are head trauma, chest trauma, and fractures. Often the patient is unconscious because of alcoholism, shock, or associated head injury. Another misleading factor in diagnosis, often not recognized, is that relatively trivial injuries may rupture abdominal viscera. The index of suspicion of abdominal trauma must be high, even in cases of supposedly minor abdominal trauma, if diagnostic errors are to be avoided.

CLINICAL MANIFESTATIONS. The evaluation of the patient with blunt abdominal trauma begins with a careful history and physical examination. The entire patient must be examined as well as the abdomen because of the high incidence of associated trauma. Fitzgerald et al. have reported extraabdominal injuries in 97 percent of patients with abdominal injuries who were dead on arrival at the hospital and in 70 percent of those admitted alive. When the diagnosis is doubtful, one must often depend on repeated physical examinations alone, done at frequent intervals by the same examiner to decide whether the patient requires laparotomy.

Abdominal pain and tenderness are the most frequent findings. Abdominal rigidity, or involuntary guarding, is

Table 6-5. FREQUENCY OF INJURY
IN ABDOMINAL TRAUMA

Viscera injured	Frequency, %
Spleen	26.2
Kidneys	24.2
Intestines	16.2
Liver	15.6
Abdominal wall	3.6
Retroperitoneal hematoma	2.7
Mesentery	2.5
Pancreas	1.4
Diaphragm	1.1

the most helpful sign and even when present alone warrants exploratory laparotomy. Hinton, in 1929, recommended a period of watchful waiting before exploration because of fear of uncontrollable hemorrhage and infection, as well as the difficulty of performing the necessary surgical procedures under adverse conditions. There is no excuse for this course today, and a policy of watchful waiting frequently may be disastrous. Fitzgerald et al. reported no deaths of patients who had exploratory laparotomy without a finding of intraabdominal injury. However, three deaths in their series occurred from intraabdominal hemorrhage because abdominal injury was masked by associated head injuries. The absence of any mortality for negative abdominal exploration in Parkland Memorial Hospital cases of suspected abdominal trauma is similar to that quoted above.

In patients with blunt abdominal trauma, determinations of alterations in blood pressure are often useful. In a series of patients with blunt trauma reviewed recently from this institution, approximately 65 percent had systolic blood pressures below 80 mm Hg on admission to the emergency room. It was found that a valuable sign of continuing intraabdominal hemorrhage was transient elevation of the blood pressure to normal levels for a few minutes followed by return to hypotensive levels with rapid infusion of 500 to 1,000 ml of Ringer's lactate solution. Patients who are hypotensive from minimal blood loss or from neurogenic shock usually do not behave in this manner. The Ringer's lactate solution generally is infused over a period of 15 to 20 minutes while other measures, such as blood typing and cross matching, are being carried out. Postural hypotension, when the patient assumes the erect position, is another useful sign of continuing intraabdominal bleeding.

DIAGNOSTIC PROCEDURES. Berman et al. state that if the leukocyte count is greater than 15,000 following abdominal trauma, a ruptured solid viscus is likely, especially if other findings are compatible with that diagnosis. Knopp and Harkins and Williams and Zollinger, however, have not found the leukocyte count to be so helpful. Several studies of the hemoglobin and hematocrit done at intervals of 30 minutes to 1 hour in suspicious cases may be helpful, but they may be misleading if the findings are overinterpreted. Naffziger and McCorkle note that the serum amylase level is valuable in recognizing acute pancreatic trauma. Elevated amylase levels may also indicate injury to the upper small bowel and duodenum with leakage of amylase-containing fluid from the injured bowel into the peritoneal cavity, where the amylase is freely absorbed into the blood. Studies of urinary sediment are useful, since hematuria may indicate injury to the genitourinary tract. If the patient with abdominal injury cannot void, catheterization should be done to obtain urine for examination. Examination of vomitus or insertion of a nasogastric tube to obtain gastric contents to be checked for evidence of upper gastrointestinal tract bleeding is helpful.

Roentgenographic Findings. For patients who have sustained severe abdominal injury and in whom other clinical signs obviously point to such injury, roentgenography for diagnosis may dangerously delay surgical intervention.

However, for about one-third of patients with stable vital signs and questionable diagnoses of intraabdominal injury, x-ray studies may be helpful. Roentgenography is of least aid in injury to solid viscera, notably the liver, spleen, and pancreas.

King has outlined a pattern to be followed by the roentgenologist in diagnosing injuries to the abdominal viscera by indirect and direct evidence. X-ray films of the abdomen should be made in the erect, supine, prone, lateral, and left lateral decubitus positions to check for the following points: (1) Skeletal parts are checked for fractures or dislocations. (2) Examination of the soft tissues may give information concerning alterations of size, shape, or position of many viscera. (3) Pneumoperitoneum may be diagnosed with the patient in the erect or lateral decubitus positions. (4) Indirect evidence of solid viscera rupture with secondary hemorrhage may be presumed by an increase in density in the region, by displacement of neighboring viscera, or by accumulation of fluid between the gas shadows of bowel loops. Also, if a gastric, duodenal, or upper jejunal rupture is possible, the frequency of pneumoperitoneum may be increased by injecting 750 to 1,000 ml of air into a nasogastric tube, after which the patient sits in a semierect position for 10 minutes before an upright chest film or left lateral decubitus film of the abdomen is made. Films should also be made prior to the air injection for purposes of comparison if the patient's condition permits.

Another study which may be useful is examination of the upper gastrointestinal tract by x-ray after ingestion of a water-soluble opaque medium, which may indicate injury of the stomach, duodenum, or upper small bowel. The use of barium mixtures for this is dangerous, since a severe peritoneal reaction is caused by barium if it leaks through a perforation in the gastrointestinal tract. This is especially true if there is fecal contamination in the peritoneal cavity from concomitant colon injury.

Intravenous or retrograde pyelograms should be done if feasible for patients with hematuria or other evidence of genitourinary injury, not only to establish the nature of the injury, but also to determine if both kidneys are functioning prior to surgical intervention in case an injured kidney must be removed. If necessary, intravenous pyelograms may be done during the surgical procedure to determine the presence of a functional kidney on one side before removing the other kidney.

Cystograms may also be useful for diagnosing bladder injury or perforation from blunt abdominal trauma, but normal cystograms do not rule out bladder injury.

Intravenous cholangiography has also been helpful at times in suspected trauma to the hepatobiliary system.

Levin Tubes. Levin tubes are inserted in all patients sustaining blunt abdominal trauma. The stomach contents are aspirated, and the aspirate is examined for the presence of blood. In addition, a Levin tube provides for decompression of the stomach, prevents gastric dilatation, and prevents aspiration with the induction of anesthesia.

Paracentesis. Needle abdominal paracentesis is a useful diagnostic aid only for those cases of abdominal trauma in which, after physical examination, the examiner continues to suspect intraabdominal hemorrhage. The abdominal tap has been particularly useful as a diagnostic adjunct for comatose patients with head injury in whom adequate physical examination of the abdomen is not possible. A recent review of Parkland Memorial Hospital experience with this procedure shows a diagnostic accuracy of 95 percent with positive paracentesis. A negative tap is not definitive, particularly if other elements of the physical examination indicate other reasons for exploring the abdomen. In female patients with suspected intraabdominal hemorrhage, culdocentesis may be positive for blood when abdominal taps are negative.

The technique is well described by Drapanas and McDonald and illustrated in Fig. 6-7. The abdomen is surgically cleansed with pHisoHex or an iodophor compound. An 18-gauge short-bevel spinal needle is attached to a syringe and inserted through the abdominal wall after prior infiltration of the site of tap with a local anesthetic agent. Suction is applied to the syringe as the needle is slowly advanced into the abdomen at the sites illustrated. Return of a minimum of 0.1 ml of nonclotting blood constitutes a positive tap. Occasionally, an intraabdominal blood vessel may be entered, but this blood will clot and differentiate it from blood obtained from the free peritoneal cavity. If the tap is negative in one quadrant, it is repeated at the other sites. Bilateral flank taps are as reliable as four quadrant taps and may be more reliable if only small amounts of blood are present. Puncture of the rectus abdominis sheath anteriorly should be avoided to prevent a rectus abdominis sheath hematoma from injury to the epigastric vessels and to diminish the chance of the needle's penetrating the bowel, since gas-filled loops of bowel tend to float anteriorly in the abdomen containing fluid or blood. Actually, the danger of penetrating the intestine is slight; several studies have shown that penetration with an 18-gauge needle is harmless, as a hole in the bowel seals off quite rapidly with no leakage. Other technical considerations include the following:

1. Areas of abdominal scars or other points of possible bowel fixation to the abdominal wall should be avoided.
2. The direction of the needle inside the abdominal cavity should be changed only by withdrawing the point of the needle just superficially to the peritoneum, redirecting the needle, and reintroducing it into the peritoneal cavity.
3. Peritoneal taps should be avoided in the presence of markedly distended bowel, because abnormally elevated intraluminal pressure may cause continued leakage.

Paracentesis is simple and quick with relatively few complications. The major drawback is the high percentage of false-negative results.

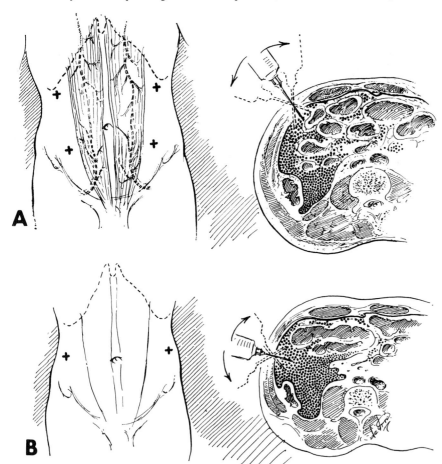

Fig. 6-7. *A.* Technique for four-quadrant peritoneal taps. Preferred location for aspiration of each quadrant is shown. Note that puncture through the rectus abdominis sheath is avoided. *B.* Technique for bilateral flank taps. Aspiration is performed in each flank midway between the costal margin and iliac spine. In our experience, bilateral flank taps are equally reliable as, and more easily performed than, four-quadrant taps in cases of abdominal trauma. (*From T. Drapanas and J. McDonald, Surgery, 50:742, 1961.*)

Peritoneal Lavage. Because of the poor reliability of paracentesis, other procedures have been developed to detect intraabdominal injury. Canizaro et al. described in 1964 the use of intraperitoneal saline infusions in animals. Root et al. described in 1965 the technique of peritoneal lavage in human beings and subsequently reported a series of 304 patients with a 96 percent accuracy. A recent review of this procedure at Parkland Memorial Hospital has proved peritoneal lavage to be a safe and reliable adjunctive procedure for evaluating patients with blunt abdominal trauma. The indications for this technique are closed head injuries, altered consciousness, spinal cord injuries, equivocal abdominal findings, and negative needle paracentesis. It is not recommended for patients with either gunshot or stab wounds to the abdomen, multiple abdominal procedures, dilated bowel, pregnancy, or positive needle paracentesis.

The technique used is similar to that described by Perry et al. A point is selected in the lower midline below the umbilicus approximately one-third of the distance between that and the pubic symphysis. After decompression of the urinary bladder, the skin is cleansed and prepared with an iodinated antiseptic solution. A wheal is raised with 1% lidocaine and the skin incised with a # 11 scalpel. A standard peritoneal dialysis catheter (McGaw V-4900) is inserted, and the trocar is advanced carefully until it just penetrates the peritoneum (Fig. 6-8). Once the peritoneum is penetrated, the trocar is removed and the dialysis catheter advanced toward the pelvis. A syringe is then attached to the catheter and the peritoneal cavity aspirated.

Nonclotting blood often will be aspirated through the larger catheter even with a negative needle paracentesis. If no blood or fluid is aspirated, a liter of balanced saline solution (Ringer's lactate) is rapidly infused into the peritoneal cavity over 5 to 10 minutes, using 10 ml/kg for small adults and children. The patient is then turned from side to side in order to further mix the blood and fluid. If other injuries such as pelvic or long bone fractures are present, this step is eliminated.

The empty intravenous-fluid bottle is lowered and the fluid siphoned out of the peritoneal cavity. A sample is sent to the laboratory for quantitative analysis. In addition to obtaining red cell and white cell counts, it is important to determine the presence or absence of amylase, bile, or bacteria. Some have recommended colorimetric methods, but these do not appear to be as accurate as quantitative analysis of the fluid. The criteria for positive peritoneal lavage include the following determinations: gross blood in lavage fluid; greater than 100,000 RBC/mm³; greater than 500 WBC/mm³; elevated amylase level; bacteria or bile.

It must be emphasized that the lavage is very inaccurate in indicating retroperitoneal injuries. Unless the posterior peritoneum has been torn or considerable time has elapsed between the injury and lavage, most pancreatic injuries are not detected. The same is true for duodenal, urologic, and major vessel injuries which are retroperitoneal. Complications occur frequently enough that lavage is not recommended for every patient suspected of abdominal injury.

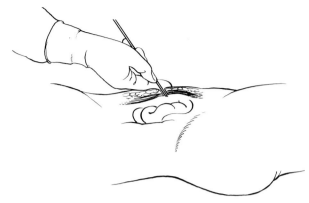

Fig. 6-8. Insertion of catheter for peritoneal lavage in the lower midline below the umbilicus.

However, a negative lavage may spare the patient exploratory laparotomy.

Arteriography. Selective arteriography is another available aid to the diagnosis of blunt abdominal trauma. This procedure, advocated by Freeark, employs percutaneous retrograde arteriography by the Seldinger method. Depending upon the skill of the technician, selective catheterization of celiac, mesenteric, or renal vessels may be performed. The arteriogram provides visualization of the arteries supplying the abdominal viscera and pelvis. A film taken several minutes after injection can be used as an excretory urogram.

The benefits of arteriography are directly related to the capabilities of the radiology department. Again, it must be emphasized that time should not be wasted on adjunctive procedures when surgical intervention is indicated.

Scintiscanning. Both liver and splenic scanning have been described in conjunction with blunt abdominal trauma. This technique primarily is limited to those patients whose diagnoses are uncertain and whose conditions remain stable. The radionuclide most frequently used is ^{99m}Tc sulfur colloid. Most series reporting results of this technique are small and emphasize the relative inaccuracy of the examination.

A filling defect representing a parenc.hymal hematoma frequently is seen with damage to the spleen or liver. In addition, displacement, increased size, and mottled appearance of the spleen may increase the suspicion of splenic trauma. Filling defects also may indicate cysts, abscesses, infarcts, or tumors secondary to trauma.

Penetrating Trauma

STAB WOUNDS

The diagnosis of penetrating injuries of the abdomen does not usually present the difficult problem often posed by blunt abdominal trauma. Three methods of managing stab wounds of the abdomen have evolved: (1) routine exploration of all abdominal stab wounds, (2) selective management, and (3) laparotomy following demonstration of peritoneal cavity penetration.

Abdominal stab wounds frequently were managed by routine exploration. Since the incidence of negative laparotomy results was as high as 60 percent in some series, a more conservative approach recommending selective management for those patients with abdominal stab wounds and no clinical evidence of intraabdominal injury has been advocated. The vital signs should be stable, with no evidence of upper or lower gastrointestinal bleeding, pneumoperitoneum, or signs and symptoms of peritoneal irritation if the patient is to be selectively managed. These patients are admitted to the hospital and reevaluated frequently, preferably by the same observer. If the patient's condition deteriorates or changes significantly, exploratory laparotomy is performed. Objections to selective management are that (1) minimal physical findings may be common in spite of significant visceral injury, (2) peritonitis may develop prior to laparotomy, and (3) the incidence of negative laparotomies may still run as high as 30 percent.

Instead of subjecting the patient to general anesthesia and exploratory laparotomy, it is often possible to determine by other means whether the wound has penetrated the peritoneal cavity. Cornell et al. have described the diagnostic injection of radiopaque contrast material. Following aseptic preparation of the wound site, a small catheter is inserted into the wound and held tightly by a purse-string suture. Fifty to one hundred milliliters of contrast media is injected, and anteroposterior, lateral, and oblique films of the abdomen are obtained. Contrast media seen within the peritoneal cavity is an indication for surgery. Objections to this technique are the following: (1) Some patients are hypersensitive to the radiopaque material. (2) Injection of this material may be quite painful, thereby masking further evaluation. (3) The incidence of false-positive and false-negative results may be as high as 15 to 25 percent in some series. (4) The technique is impractical for multiple stab wounds.

Local exploration may provide useful information. The abdominal wall is prepared with an antiseptic agent, and, with local anesthesia, the abdominal wound is opened sufficiently to visualize the complete course and depth of the wound. Often with adequate light, instruments, assistance, and exposure it is obvious that a wound thought to have penetrated the peritoneal cavity is actually superficial and not damaging to viscera. These patients are managed by simple drainage and outpatient follow-up if other injuries do not require hospitalization. Usually, local wound exploration involves more than simple instrument probing to determine penetration. This blind probing may be misleading since a tortuous wound tract may allow passage of the probe for only a short distance, creating a false impression of nonpenetration. In this case, the course of penetration must be directly visualized. If the end of the tract cannot be visualized or if the peritoneum is penetrated, the patient is taken to surgery. This technique is equally useful for stab wounds of the back, although the thickness of the paraspinous muscles may prevent visualization of the end of the wound tract and exploration in the operating room may be necessary. Frequently, innocuous small stab wounds of the back significantly damage such retroperitoneal structures as the inferior vena cava, ureter, pancreas, or duodenum.

Many wounds which appear to penetrate only the thorax also penetrate the abdomen, injuring abdominal viscera as well as intrathoracic organs. Figure 6-9 indicates the diaphragmatic excursion on maximal expiration and maximal inspiration; it is apparent that certain penetrating wounds of the lower thoracic region often involve the diaphragm and adjacent abdominal viscera. Consequently, an exploratory laparotomy is performed when penetrating injuries involve the lower thoracic region.

Prior to abdominal exploration of these thoracic wounds, anterior and posterior chest tubes are inserted to drain air and blood from the thorax and to prevent pulmonary complications during the operative procedure from concurrent thoracic injuries. Although a pneumothorax or hemothorax may not be indicated by x-ray or physical examination, prophylactic insertion of an anterior chest tube will decrease the danger of a tension pneumothorax developing during induction of anesthesia and subsequent abdominal exploration.

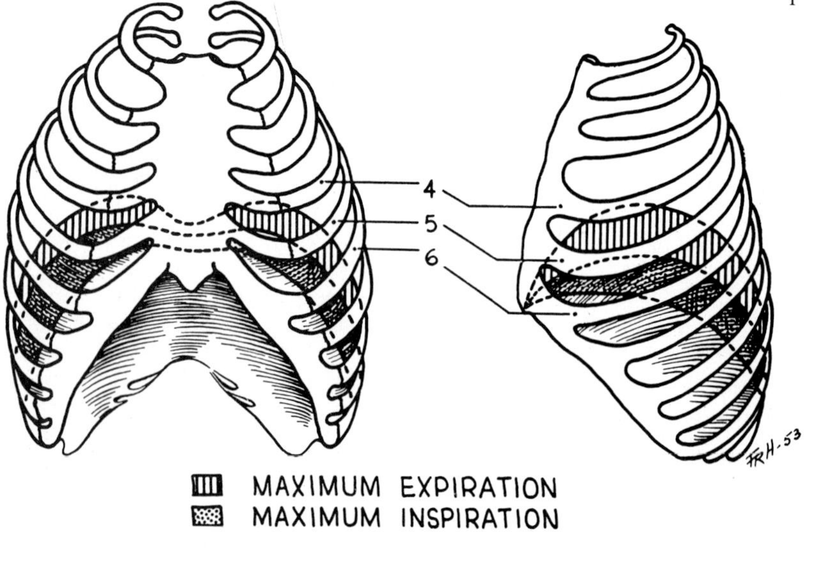

Fig. 6-9. Maximum diaphragmatic respiratory excursion. (*From L. M. Shefts, Surg Clin North Am, 38:1577, 1958.*)

4
5
6

▥ MAXIMUM EXPIRATION
▨ MAXIMUM INSPIRATION

GUNSHOT WOUNDS

Any bullet passing in proximity to the peritoneal cavity requires laparotomy, since visceral injury from "blast effect" may occur whether or not the cavity is entered. If the patient's condition permits, anteroposterior and lateral films of the abdomen should be made to locate the missile and determine its probable trajectory. Selective management, the use of radiopaque material, or local exploration are not recommended.

Once the diagnosis of intraabdominal injury is established and resuscitation instituted, the abdomen is explored. A long midline incision is preferred for the following reasons: (1) It may be made much more rapidly than other incisions—a matter of vital importance when attempting rapid control of exsanguinating hemorrhage; (2) it gives wide access to all parts of the abdomen, which transverse incisions do not; (3) it may be readily extended into either side of the thorax in case of combined thoracoabdominal injury or when better abdominal exposure is required; and (4) it may be rapidly closed, which is of great importance in decreasing the anesthesia and operative time for gravely injured patients.

Stomach

Injuries to the stomach from blunt trauma are not frequent, perhaps because of the relative lack of fixation of the stomach and its protected position. However, penetrating injuries of the stomach from gunshot wounds occur frequently.

DIAGNOSIS. The diagnosis is generally suspected from the course of the penetrating object, and, at times, additional suspicion of gastric injury arises from the presence of bloody fluid aspirated from the Levin tube. Generally, wounds of the anterior stomach wall are easily seen at laparotomy. Because of the possibility of missing posterior stomach wall wounds, it is important in all cases of proved or possible gastric injury to open the lesser sac through the gastrocolic omentum. This allows the entire posterior aspect of the stomach to be searched for injury. The points of insertion of the greater and lesser omentum into the greater and lesser curvature of the stomach, respectively, should also be carefully inspected. If a hematoma is noted at the mesenteric attachment, it should be evacuated and the stomach wall at that site carefully inspected for injury of that part of the wall located between the leaves of the greater or lesser omentum.

TREATMENT. Gastric wounds are repaired by first placing a continuous locked 2-0 chromic catgut suture through all the layers of the gastric wall; a purse-string suture does not give adequate hemostasis. This hemostatic stitch is very important to control extensive bleeding which may occur from the rich submucosal network of blood vessels in the stomach. Following the first layer closure, an outer inverting row of interrupted nonabsorbable mattress sutures of the Lembert or Halsted type is placed. The outer row of sutures provides adequate serosal approximation of the stomach wall, seals off readily, and prevents leaks. These sutures in the outer layer should not be through-and-through, as is the first row of sutures, but should extend through the seromuscular coat and the submucosal layer of the stomach. Wounds of the stomach are not drained, since they are unlikely to break down and leak, as duodenal wounds sometimes do. However, it is very important to suction the peritoneal cavity, with particular attention to the subhepatic and subphrenic spaces and the lesser sac, so that all food particles and gastric juice spilled into these areas are removed.

After operation for a gastric wound, Levin tube suction should be maintained for several days until active peristalsis has resumed and the danger of postoperative gastric dilatation has passed. The gastric aspirate should be observed for inordinate bleeding, which may occur if the hemostatic suture line is inadequate. If bleeding is brisk or persists, the patient should be immediately reexplored for control of the gastric bleeding point. After peristalsis resumes, gastric aspiration is discontinued, and the patient is started on clear liquids in the usual fashion and advanced to a normal diet over the next few days.

COMPLICATIONS. Complications which may develop following stomach wounds are hemorrhage from, or leakage of, the suture line and development of subhepatic, subphrenic, or lesser sac abscesses secondary to spilling of contaminated gastric contents. The development of such abscesses is suspected following gastric wounds in patients who fail to do well postoperatively and who persist with unexplainable fever for more than a few days. If contamination seems heavy, the skin should be left open until the wound appears clean.

Duodenum

Injuries to the duodenum and small bowel comprise about 24 percent of blunt and penetrating abdominal trauma. Lauritzen reported the mortality rate for retroperitoneal duodenal perforation as approximately 60 percent and related it to the difficulty in establishing an early diagnosis. A mortality of 55.9 percent has been reported for abdominal wounds with all types of duodenal injury. Burrus et al. have reported a series of 86 duodenal injuries with a total mortality of 26 percent.

DIAGNOSIS. The diagnosis of blunt trauma to the duodenum and small bowel is considerably more difficult than that of penetrating trauma to these organs. With duodenal or small bowel trauma, all the characteristic signs of trauma to abdominal viscera may be minimal or absent, particularly in the early period following injury for several reasons: (1) The injury of the duodenum following blunt trauma is frequently retroperitoneal, so that duodenal contents leak into the retroperitoneal area, rather than into the free peritoneal cavity. (2) Duodenal and small bowel fluid is generally sterile and does not lead to early signs of bacterial peritonitis, as occurs following colon injury. (3) The pH of the small bowel contents if frequently nearly neutral and, thus, produces only slight chemical irritation of the peritoneum. This is not true of injuries to the duodenum, in which duodenal fluid freely flows into the peritoneal cavity. The highly alkaline pH of this fluid causes immediate chemical irritation of the peritoneum and physical signs of such irritation.

One should be suspicious of injuries to the duodenum or upper small bowel in any patients who have received a blow to the upper abdomen or lower chest, such as from a steering wheel. Testicular pain should raise suspicion of a retroperitoneal duodenal rupture. Also, pain referred to the shoulders, chest, and back is associated with perforation of the duodenum and small intestine.

Several diagnostic aids may be helpful in determining rupture of the duodenum or small bowel. First, needle paracentesis of the abdomen, particularly in the right gutter region or in the upper quadrants, may be helpful if blood, bile, or abnormal amounts of small bowel content are aspirated. Roentgenograms are helpful and may be diagnostic, but the absence of free intraperitoneal air does not rule out bowel perforation. Retroperitoneal rupture of the duodenum is not often diagnosed by x-ray. The diagnosis may be based on finding a large accumulation of air about the right kidney. It is also important to inspect the psoas muscle margins on the plain film of the abdomen for the presence of air, indicating retroperitoneal rupture of a viscus. After x-ray films of the abdomen and upright chest films are made to search for free air collections, it is valuable to inject air through the Levin tube in order to produce or enlarge these air collections. Such a maneuver frequently increases the diagnostic accuracy of x-ray films for free air. An additional aid is to give the patient a water-soluble radiopaque dye orally and then to make abdominal x-ray films to detect any dye leak from the duodenum or small bowel. Such diagnostic procedures are unnecessary if other clinical signs indicate the need for exploratory laparotomy.

When laparotomy is done for suspected intraabdominal injury, duodenal lesions are often missed, especially retroperitoneal lesions of the third and fourth portions of the duodenum. This is due to superficial observation, inadequate exposure, and lack of persistence on the part of the surgeon. Hinton has reported that duodenal perforations have been missed initially in 33 to 50 percent of the various reported series of retroperitoneal duodenal injuries. To avoid overlooking duodenal trauma and contributing to the high mortality from duodenal wounds, it is important to inspect the entire duodenum during abdominal exploration for trauma. This is particularly true if a retroperitoneal hematoma is noted near the duodenum or if there is crepitation or bile-stained fluid along the lateral margins of the duodenum retroperitoneally. If these signs are noted or if the duodenum is contused, it should be widely mobilized by the Kocher maneuver, incising the peritoneum along its lateral margins, so that it is completely mobilized along with the head of the pancreas. Thus, small areas of perforation in the retroperitoneal aspect of the duodenum may be seen. Often retroperitoneal wounds of the duodenum which have been missed are not recognized until several days later, when bile-stained fluid drains from the abdominal wound of a patient who has continued to do poorly postoperatively. As Cohn et al. state, the following signs, in addition to those mentioned previously, indicate careful exploration of the duodenum and the retroduodenal area: elevation of the posterior peritoneum with a glassy edema; petechiae or fat necrosis over the ascending and transverse

colon or mesocolon; retroperitoneal phlegmon; hematoma over the head of the pancreas extending into the base of the mesocolon; fat necrosis of the retroperitoneal tissues; and/or discoloration of retroperitoneal tissues—dark from hemorrhage, grayish from suppuration, or yellowish from bile.

TREATMENT. The local treatment of the duodenal perforation itself will depend more on the size of the perforation than any other single factor. Generally, an attempt is made to close the duodenal perforation if this can be done without decreasing the lumen of the duodenum. This closure is done with a continuous locking 3-0 chromic catgut suture through all layers of the duodenal wall, followed by an outer layer of nonabsorbable interrupted mattress sutures in the seromuscular layer of the duodenum. After this, the duodenum should be carefully palpated to exclude stenosis. If the perforation is so large that closure will cause a stricture of the duodenum, consideration should be given to (1) complete division of the duodenum and an end-to-end anastomosis or (2) division of the duodenum, closure of both ends, and gastroenterostomy.

Kobold and Thal have reported another method of handling large duodenal defects, which previously might have necessitated one of the above techniques of duodenal division. This consists of using a retrocolic loop of proximal jejunum with suture over the large defect in the duodenum, with an inner row of absorbable catgut sutures taken between the torn edge of the duodenum and the seromuscular layer of the jejunum and an outer layer of nonabsorbable mattress sutures taken between the seromuscular coats of the duodenum and the jejunum. Animal studies, as well as clinical usage, have demonstrated the feasibility of this "patching" technique in managing large duodenal defects (Fig. 6-10).

Large duodenal wounds and duodenal wounds which have dehisced also have been managed by anastomosing the open end of a defunctionalized Roux en Y loop of proximal jejunum over the duodenal defect.

The common bile duct should be identified with insertion of a T tube if the region of the ampulla is involved in a duodenal injury, since reimplantation of the common bile duct sometimes may be necessary. Approximately 75 to 80 percent of all duodenal injuries may be closed by debridement of the wound edges and simple suture. For the other 20 to 25 percent, however, one of the reparative procedures described above or recommended by Cleveland and Waddell is used. Rarely, even a pancreatoduodenectomy may be necessary to manage large defects of the duodenum with extensive trauma to the duodenum and periampullary region (Fig. 6-11).

A recent report from the Lahey Clinic describes a technique for wide exposure of the third and fourth portions of the duodenum. This involves mobilizing the cecum, right colon, hepatic flexure of the colon, and mesenteries of these organs up to and including the ligament of Treitz, carrying the dissection of the mesocolon along the attachment at the root of the small bowel mesentery, as shown in Fig. 6-12.

It is also frequently important after duodenal injuries

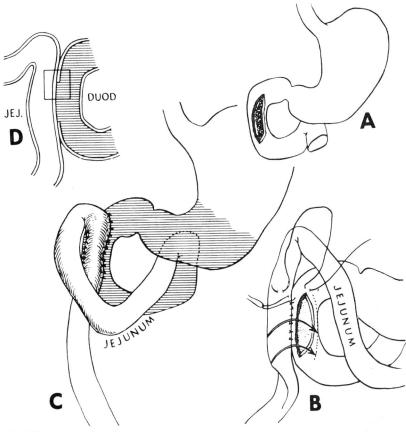

Fig. 6-10. *A.* Area of excision of duodenal wall. *B.* Technique of placement of intact jejunum over the wound to form a patch. *C.* The completed closure. *D.* Cross section of the completed closure showing the relationship of the intact jejunum to the duodenal perforation. The boxed area is the site from which tissue was subsequently removed for study. (*From E. E. Kobold and A. P. Thal, Surg Gynecol Obstet, 116:340, 1963.*)

to establish adequate drainage. This is done by placing two or three Penrose drains near the injury, bringing them out of the abdomen by the most direct route possible. This reduced markedly the mortality from duodenal wounds in the several series in which drainage was evaluated. It is even more important to institute drainage if there appears to be associated pancreatic injury, as often occurs.

Fistulas. Fistula formation following duodenal injury occurs frequently because of poor blood supply, infection, excessive tension on suture lines, distal obstruction, etc., and leads to approximately a 50 percent mortality. The occurrence of a fistula may be related to the lack of a serosal surface in which to sew the retroperitoneal portion of the duodenum, so that an insecure closure is obtained. Fistulas may be prevented by prolonged decompression of the duodenum following closure of the wound. This is especially indicated in more severe injuries of the duodenum and is accomplished by several means:

1. A Levin tube may be threaded through the entire course of the duodenum with sufficient holes in the tube to allow simultaneous decompression of the duodenum and stomach. The tube may be brought through the an-

terior wall as a gastrostomy tube and placed on suction or may be inserted through the nasopharynx.

2. A #10 Foley catheter may be placed through a small stab wound in the duodenum, adjacent to the area of duodenal injury, to serve as a vent. The tube is maintained on gentle suction until active bowel sounds return. At this time, suction is discontinued, and the tube is attached to a glass Y tube fixed to a stand at the level of the duodenum. This arrangement does not allow siphonage of duodenal contents, as does gravity drainage, but does provide a decompressive vent if the pressure rises in the duodenum. After 9 or 10 days, at which time a fibrinous tract has formed about the small Foley catheter, the bag, which contains only 2 ml of water, is deflated. The Foley tube is again placed on gentle suction and is pulled just outside the duodenum, where it remains on suction for an additional 24 hours. At the end of the 24-hour period, the Foley catheter is removed if drainage is minimal. This small tube has been used for duodenal trauma at Parkland Memorial Hospital and also has been used to decompress the duodenum following gastric resection in which closure of the duodenal stump is insecure. In none of the approximately 75 cases in which the Foley tube was used following gastric resection and duodenal trauma has there been a significant complication, and no fistulas have occurred.

Postoperative Care. Postoperative care of these patients may be extremely difficult. Extracellular fluid volume deficits may be large, particularly if fistulas, retroperitoneal

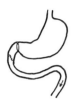
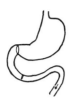
I   II

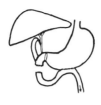
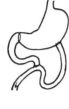
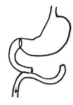
III   IV

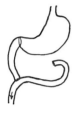
V   VI   VII

inflammation, or pancreatitis occur. It is very important to maintain the extracellular fluid volume with adequate infusions of balanced salt solution. In addition, these patients should be maintained on adequate doses of broad-spectrum intravenously administered antibiotics. Gastric and duodenal decompression should be continued for long periods of time in order to protect the suture lines. The average period of gastroduodenal decompression for duodenal wounds is about 5 to 7 days following exploration. If fistulas form, gastroduodenal decompression should be continued for longer periods, and a sump drain should be inserted into the drain site for continuous active suction of the fistular tract. This is instituted to prevent the collection of duodenal fluid with possible spread throughout the peritoneal cavity, to promote collapse and healing of the fistular tract, to prevent digestion of the skin by duodenal fluid draining onto the skin, and to aid calculation and replacement of fluid and electrolyte losses. Although several types of sump drains are now available

Fig. 6-11. Diagrammatic representation of various operative procedures in a series of cases. I, Simple closure; II, end-to-end duodenoduodenostomy; III and IV, closure of both ends of duodenum and gastroenterostomy; V, closure of distal duodenum and duodenojejunostomy; VI, duodenojejunostomy and gastroduodenostomy; VII, resection of fourth part of duodenum and duodenojejunostomy (*From H. C. Cleveland and W. R. Waddell, Surg Clin North Am, 43:413, 1963.*)

Fig. 6-12. A technique for the exposure of the third and fourth portions of the duodenum. *A and B.* Initial dissection for mobilization of the right side of the colon, small intestine, and mesentery. *C.* Exposure obtained of the third and fourth portions of the duodenum. (*From R. B. Cattell and J. W. Braasch, Surg Gynecol Obstet, 111:379, 1960.*)

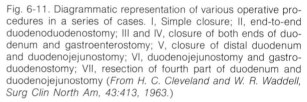

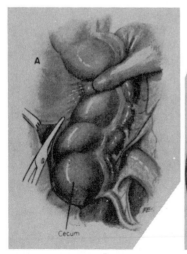
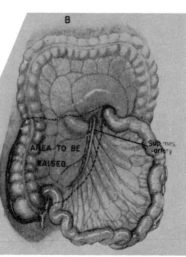
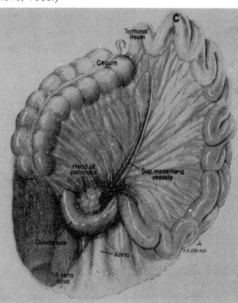

commercially, recent experience with a simple sump drain made from two red rubber catheters has shown it to be more effective. A #18 French and a #14 French red rubber catheter are sewn together with nonabsorbable suture material at two or three points along the distal one-third of the catheters. Extra holes are cut in the sides of both tubes in their distal thirds. This sump drain is placed among several large Penrose drains through the abdominal drainage site. Postoperatively, suction is applied to the #18 catheter, and the smaller tube parallel to it serves as an effective air vent. This sump device was adapted from Waterman et al., although we have found it to be more effective when placed among several Penrose drains rather than through a single Penrose drain.

When a duodenal fistula develops, the patient should be placed on central intravenous hyperalimentation according to the principles of Dudrick and associates, which are discussed in Chap. 2. This regimen maintains excellent nutrition and may reduce the volume of gastrointestinal secretions.

With central intravenous hyperalimentation, it is now frequently unnecessary to perform feeding jejunostomies to provide nutritional support for patients with duodenal fistulas. If for some reason central intravenous feeding is not possible or if copious fistular drainage persists, a jejunostomy may become necessary. Two tubes are inserted through separate Witzel (serosal-lined) tunnels in the proximal jejunum and brought out through separate sites in the left upper quadrant of the abdomen. One jejunostomy tube is inserted in a retrograde direction so that its tip lies within the duodenum just below the duodenal fistula, and the other tube is inserted in an antegrade direction into the upper jejunum. Suction is applied to the retrograde tube lying within the duodenum; this usually greatly reduces the volume of drainage and promotes closure. Standard jejunostomy feedings are given through the antegrade tube in the proximal jejunum. Also, the duodenal fluid is slowly refed through this tube as it is removed by suction from the sump drain in the fistula and from the retrograde jejunostomy tube. This feeding is ideally done with constant slow infusions through a Barron pump.

If, after 5 to 7 days of Levin tube or gastrostomy decompression of the duodenum, the patient is doing well, shows no evidence of duodenal leak, and has adequate bowel activity, he is given 1 oz of water orally every hour for approximately 12 hours, after the Levin tube is removed or the gastrostomy tube clamped. If water is tolerated, the diet is increased in the usual fashion. Also, after feeding has been instituted for 1 to 2 days and there has been little or no drainage, the Penrose drains are advanced and removed over 3 days unless further drainage ensues. In the face of continued drainage, the drains should be left for at least 2 or 3 weeks, or as long as any significant drainage continues. After about 3 weeks, if drainage persists, the Penrose drains may be removed; the only drainage tube which should remain is the previously described sump drain, which is removed when drainage has dropped to a minimum.

Occasionally, the duodenal fistula does not close despite adequate nonoperative treatment described above. In such cases, when a reasonable trial of conservative treatment has been made and the patient is in optimal condition for reoperation, the abdomen is opened and completely explored to rule out distal bowel obstruction which may be causing the fistula to persist. The fistula is exposed at its origin from the duodenum, and a Roux en Y defunctionalized limb of proximal jejunum is brought up to the fistula and anastomosed to it. This anastomosis may use either the end or the side (after closing the end of the jejunal limb) of the defunctionalized jejunum. This procedure permanently diverts the fistular drainage internally and has been very effective in treating persistent duodenal fistulas.

INTRAMURAL HEMATOMA

Another interesting but infrequently reported lesion of the duodenum secondary to trauma is intramural hematoma of the duodenum. Up to 1963 only 33 cases had been reported, according to Moore and Erlandson.

This lesion is generally caused by blunt abdominal trauma which causes rupture of intramural duodenal blood vessels with formation of a dark, sausage-shaped mass in the submucosal layer of the duodenal wall. This hematoma causes partial or complete duodenal obstruction, usually partial. The patient shows signs of a high small bowel obstruction, with nausea and vomiting associated with upper abdominal pain and tenderness, and sometimes a suggestion of a right upper quandrant mass. Flat films of the abdomen may show an ill-defined right upper quadrant mass and obliteration of the right psoas shadow. An upper gastrointestinal tract series is almost diagnostic, showing dilatation of the duodenal lumen with the appearance of a "coiled spring" in the second and third portions of the duodenum due to the crowding of the valvulae conniventes by the hematoma, according to Felson and Levin. The serum amylase level may be elevated. The lesion has occurred spontaneously in patients on anticoagulants.

Treatment ideally consists of laparotomy, evacuation of the duodenal hematoma, and closure of the defect in the seromuscular coat of the duodenum with interrupted nonabsorbable sutures after control of any bleeding points. The prognosis is excellent.

Small Bowel

Injuries to the small bowel are more frequent than injuries to the duodenum or colon. Counseller and McCormack, in a review of 1,313 cases of intestinal trauma, found that 80 percent of bowel injuries occur between the duodenojejunal junction and the terminal ileum, with approximately 10 percent each in the duodenum and large intestine. The usual mechanism of small bowel injury from blunt trauma is the crushing of the small bowel against the vertebral column. Rupture of the small bowel is also caused by shearing and tearing forces applied to the abdomen, and rarely by sudden elevation of the intraluminal pressure of the bowel with bursting from such sudden high pressure. Work by Williams and Sargent has shown that rupture due to sudden elevation of pressure is quite unusual.

In exploring the abdomen for injuries to the small bowel, it is important to inspect minutely the entire circumference of the small bowel and its attached mesentery from the ligament of Treitz to the ileocecal valve. The bowel may be completely transected in one or more places by blunt trauma with or without severe injury to the mesentery and its blood supply; at times, the mesentery may be torn from a segment of bowel, thus depriving the bowel of its blood supply. Penetrating trauma to the small bowel from a gunshot wound or stab wound is frequent, although, surprisingly, it has been noted at times that in patients with a stab wound of the abdomen the small bowel has been spared. This is probably because the great mobility of the small bowel allows it to slide away from the knife, a much less likely occurrence with gunshot wounds than with stab wounds.

TREATMENT. Small, single perforations of the small bowel may be closed safely with a single layer of interrupted nonabsorbable mattress sutures which include and invert the seromuscular and submucosal coats of the bowel. A hemostatic stitch, as required for stomach wounds, is not necessary for small bowel wounds, because the small bowel does not tend to continue bleeding from the submucosal plexus, as does the stomach. Individual bleeders, however, should be ligated with fine suture material. An advantage of a single-layer closure is its rapidity of performance, which is important in patients in precarious condition following multiple trauma.

Two small perforations of the bowel which are very close together may often be repaired by converting the wounds into one and closing the resulting defect as a single linear wound. This type of repair does not constrict the lumen of the bowel as much as two separate lines of suture placed close together and is more secure. Multiple perforations of the small bowel may occur following injury from shotgun pellets. Each one of these injuries should be carefully sought out and closed with interrupted rows of nonabsorbable mattress sutures.

Long linear lacerations of the lumen also should be closed with a single row of nonabsorbable sutures after ligating any persistent bleeders with small nonabsorbable suture. Longitudinal lacerations may be closed in a longitudinal direction or transversely according to the Heineke-Mikulicz principle.

Small bowel injuries produced by high-velocity missiles cause severe contusions of tissue surrounding the actual perforation. Because the contusion is a site of potential tissue necrosis and bowel leakage caused by thrombosis of vessels in the area of blast injury, it should be debrided. The debridement should extend into viable bowel where active bleeding is obtained.

If the wound is too large or is long and longitudinal, the bowel may not be adequately closed without loss of lumen, and the damaged segment should be resected. Also, if there are multiple wounds in a short segment of bowel, it is much safer and easier to resect the injured segment than to attempt to suture each of the closely spaced wounds, with resulting impairment of the bowel lumen and blood supply and subsequent obstruction and/or necrosis and leakage. Perforations or lacerations to the mesenteric border, unless they are quite small, are difficult to repair and frequently are associated with vascular impairment. They also should be managed by resection of the involved bowel if an adequate closure cannot be obtained without interference with blood supply. Bowel transections should be reanastomosed after debriding contused and damaged bowel on either side of the wound back to normal bowel with good blood supply. Careful attention should be given to leaving uninjured mesentery adjacent to the suture line of the reanastomosis. Extensive segments of bowel may be avulsed from the mesentery, so that the bowel loses its blood supply. All the necrotic or potentially necrotic bowel and injured mesentery must be resected and an end-to-end anastomosis made between uninjured bowel attached to uninjured mesentery.

Contusions of the small bowel should be assumed to be larger than is apparent. Such injuries are dangerous, since they may lead to necrosis and perforation. Contusions up to 1 cm in diameter may be turned in with a row of fine, nonabsorbable mattress sutures. Larger contusions should be resected.

Postoperative care of patients with wounds of the small bowel includes maintenance on nasogastric suction and no oral intake until adequate bowel activity has returned. Also, these patients are usually maintained on antibiotics, most frequently penicillin and tetracycline, which are given preoperatively and postoperatively. Usually, the antibiotic is discontinued at about the time that the nasogastric tube is removed, unless there is some other indication to continue antibiotic treatment. Leakage from suture lines and intestinal obstruction are rarely seen if the wounds are properly managed. In the report of Giddings and McDaniel concerning wounds of the jejunum and ileum during World War II, leakage from suture lines occurred in only 1 percent and intestinal obstruction in 1.7 percent, in a series of 1,168 patients with small bowel injuries, most of whom had multiple visceral injury. Again, extracellular fluid volume deficits should be replaced in patients with small bowel injury, with adequate amounts of balanced salt solution given during the surgical procedure and in the postoperative period to maintain sufficient urine volume and prevent extracellular fluid volume deficit.

Colon Injuries

The morbidity and mortality from acute injuries to the colon and rectum have been significantly reduced by an aggressive surgical approach. This has been largely influenced by the experiences of military surgeons during World War II and the Korean conflict. In the American Civil War, wounds of the abdomen carried a mortality rate of approximately 90 percent; it was not until the Boer War that the mortality rate of 80 percent of cases treated conservatively was thought to be excessive and active intervention was viewed more favorably. During this time, the fatalities from wounds of the colon eventually dropped to less than 60 percent. In World War II, an impressive improvement in the mortality from wounds of the colon was noted. This was due to several factors including improved methods of triage and transportation, effective replacement of blood and fluid, and early surgical intervention combined with ancillary use of antibiotics.

The mortality rate for wounds of the colon of 37 percent in World War II was reduced to approximately 15 percent during the action in Korea. The majority of military surgeons treating acute injuries of the colon tended to exteriorize the wound as an artificial anus to prevent further soilage of the peritoneal cavity. This approach to these particular wounds was duly carried over into civilian practice and reflected in the subsequent reduction in mortality and morbidity. In the later phase of the Korean conflict, however, some modification of the aggressive technique was noted in that small, primary wounds treated early were handled by primary closure without exteriorization.

Acute wounds of the colon which occur in a civilian environment exhibit features that may modify the indications for exteriorization of the wound. The types of injury usually noted in a military situation resulted from either high-velocity missiles or fragmentation missiles in which there was massive destruction of tissue and usually gross soilage of the peritoneal cavity. In the civilian environment, the wounds more often are caused by low-velocity missiles and usually are unassociated with massive destruction of surrounding organs and tissue. The time from wounding to initial treatment in the civilian situation is generally somewhat less than that noted during military conflict. Similarly, associated injuries occurring in civilian accidents do not tend to be so numerous nor so massive as those in a military environment, and this has a definite influence on morbidity and mortality.

ETIOLOGY. Acute injuries of the colon and rectum may be divided into penetrating wounds and wounds resulting from blunt trauma. In the former group, accidental colon injuries may be the result of industrial accidents involving explosions resulting in impalement, penetrating injuries from flying objects, or blast injuries. These injuries may be either the direct result of explosives or the result of accidents involving sources of greatly compressed air. External acts of violence constitute an important source of injuries to the colon, and these are generally penetrating injuries caused by guns or knives or, on rarer occasions, blunt abdominal trauma. Wounds of the rectum, particularly, may be the result of instrumentation during the process of sigmoidoscopy or the administration of enemas. There may also be perforations of the colorectum by foreign bodies which pass through the alimentary canal into the colon. Inadvertent penetration of the colon or rectum may occur during difficult operations; this is especially true of operations in the pelvis for severe neoplastic or inflammatory disease. Falls resulting in impalement upon sharp objects may produce wounds of the rectum. Automobile accidents and other forms of blunt trauma may produce acute injuries to the colon and rectum.

DIAGNOSIS. A systematic diagnostic approach to problems of abdominal trauma is necessary, but specific examinations of the colon and rectum may be necessary to delineate an injury. This is particularly pertinent in those instances in which instrumentation is the cause of suspected perforation of the rectum or colon. Rectal examination and sigmoidoscopy should occupy a prominent place in the examination of these patients. Diagnostic abdominal x-ray studies should be employed to determine if there is a perforated colon with leakage of air into the free peritoneal cavity. Anteroposterior and lateral decubitus views are particularly helpful in these instances. Contrast studies of the colon should be employed rarely and cautiously in view of the high morbidity and mortality associated with leakage of barium and feces into the free peritoneal cavity. Aqueous opaque media, such as Gastrografin, are preferable when penetration of the colon is suspected.

TREATMENT. The general principles of management of patients with abdominal trauma apply to those patients who have acute injuries of the colon. It is important that the time from wounding to definitive operation be as short as possible, and aggressive replacement of fluid and blood losses should be undertaken at once. Preoperatively, penicillin and tetracycline should be started in all patients suspected of having penetrating injuries of the colorectum. Two million units of aqueous penicillin and 0.5 Gm of tetracycline are added to the intravenous solution.

These patients are explored through a midline incision in order to allow access to all parts of the abdominal cavity. A thorough and complete exploration of all abdominal viscera is made, for the morbidity and mortality vary directly with the number of associated injuries. Bleeding should be controlled as rapidly as possible and immediate efforts made to reduce peritoneal soilage from any penetrating wound of an abdominal viscus. The specific care of the wound of the colon should be approached by noting the anatomic differences between the intraperitoneal and extraperitoneal large intestine. Particular attention must be paid to the type of wound, its location, the amount of tissue destruction, the presence of associated injuries, and the time from wounding to definitive care.

Wounds of the intraperitoneal colon may be divided into two groups: First, small, primary wounds located on the antimesenteric border which are seen quite early, in which there is minimal tissue destruction, and minimal or no peritoneal soiling. These wounds, especially of the left colon and in the absence of associated injuries of other abdominal viscera, may often be adequately managed by a primary two-layer closure. The mucosa is approximated with a running lock suture of 3-0 chromic catgut, and the seromuscular layers are closed with interrupted #50 cotton sutures, the Lembert technique. Second, wounds of the right colon, containing liquid feces, are less amenable to this type of primary closure, for often gross and extensive peritoneal soiling follows the colon penetration. High-velocity missile wounds should rarely, if ever, be closed primarily, for tissue destruction is often excessive and may not be readily apparent. The injured area should be extensively debrided.

Acute injuries of the intraperitoneal colon resulting from high-velocity missiles which are associated with extensive destruction of tissues or which are large and ragged in nature and are located near or involve the mesenteric border should not be closed primarily. If located in the ascending, transverse, or descending colon, the wound may be exteriorized as a colostomy. Similarly, if the time from wounding to definitive care is relatively long, allowing seeding of the peritoneal cavity with a large number of bacteria, some type of colostomy should be performed either as a wound exteriorization or as a proximal diverting colostomy. Primary closure of the distal wounds is then permissible. Although a loop colostomy may be done for expediency, a completely diverting double-barrel colostomy is favored. It is preferable to open the loop colostomy immediately, usually with the cautery, and secure early, complete fecal diversion. This is performed in the operating room after all the wounds are closed and dressed. When there are associated massive injuries to other viscera, although the colon wound itself might fulfill the indications for primary closure, a colostomy is indicated. In some instances, there may be massive injury of the cecum or of the ileocecal area, in which case it will be necessary to resect the injured bowel and do an ileotransverse colostomy. This is preferable to an ileostomy and, with suitable antibiotic coverage and intraluminal antibiotics, is an adequate procedure.

Localized minor wounds of the right colon and cecum which do not produce extensive destruction of the large bowel and are not associated with massive soilage or serious injuries to other viscera may often be managed by primary closure and appendicostomy. In these instances, after debridement and careful closure of the laceration of the cecum, tube appendicostomy is performed to decompress this segment. Seromuscular sutures are placed about the base of the appendix and secured to the lateral parietal peritoneum in order to prevent intraperitoneal leakage about the area of tube insertion. By this technique, suitable decompression of the cecum and right colon may be obtained, and removal of the tube appendicostomy permits the vent to close spontaneously. This route may also be used for intraluminal installation of neomycin or kanamycin solutions, which may offer some protection from bacterial invasion of the suture line.

The extraperitoneal perforations of the rectum must be evaluated under the same principles employed for colon injuries within the peritoneal cavity. If clean lacerations with minimal spillage are seen early, primary bowel repair may be indicated if the wound is accessible. Presacral drains should then be inserted. Associated perineal wounds should be debrided and, if grossly contaminated, left open. If debridement is adequate and these wounds are clean, they may be closed with drainage. Any damage to the anal sphincter may be repaired at this time. When a perineal wound is present but not penetrating the colon, it should be debrided widely and if not grossly contaminated then may be closed with drainage. Where there is no perineal wound but there is significant tissue destruction about the extraperitoneal rectum, presacral drainage should be instituted.

For all injuries of the rectum, complete diversion of the fecal stream is mandatory and can be accomplished by constructing a proximal double-barrel colostomy. Even in those instances where the rectal wound has been closed and diverting colostomy performed, presacral drainage is often helpful; it always should be employed when there are significant posterior wounds of the rectum.

Early closure of the colostomy is indicated in patients who have completely recovered and have no distal colon injury. It is desirable to close the simple colostomy in 2 or 3 weeks. Prior to closure, both limbs of the colon should be visualized radiographically to assure that no lesion persists. Mechanical and bacterial cleansing of the colon is effected preoperatively. First, 8 to 12 Gm of Sulfasuxidine is given daily for 5 days. Then 24 hours preoperatively, oral neomycin is begun: 1 Gm is administered every hour for four doses, and then every 4 hours until the surgical procedure starts. Cleansing saline solution enemas are given the night before operation, and then 200 ml of 1% neomycin solution is instilled into the rectum. Intramuscular penicillin and oral tetracycline are begun the night before the surgical procedure. In most instances, the skin and subcutaneous tissues are not approximated at this time. Delayed closure is then effected in 3 to 4 days when it is apparent that the wound is not infected.

Adjunctive Measures. Aggressive replacement of fluid and blood loss should be undertaken immediately and general supportive measures instituted. Attention to possible injuries elsewhere is mandatory. The systemic antibiotics begun in the preoperative period are continued for 5 to 7 days postoperatively. The use of peritoneal and intraluminal instillation of antibiotics has been advocated by many. Certainly, removing all gross fecal material from the peritoneal cavity is indicated, but instillation of intraperitoneal antibiotics has been followed by some complications, notably respiratory depression. These have been most frequently seen in anesthetized patients who received intraperitoneal neomycin. Extensive lavage of the peritoneal cavity with saline solution may actually result in dissemination of fecal material and is not recommended. The use of an intraluminal catheter for postoperative instillation of antibiotics as advocated by Cohn may add further protection from late wound disruption. The antibiotics may be instilled through a small polyethylene catheter, which is inserted into the bowel proximal to the areas of injury. It is desirable to place the catheter through a taenia and secure it with a purse-string suture. The bowel is then sutured to the parietal peritoneum at the point of entrance of the catheter. A 1% solution of neomycin or 15 ml of sterile saline solution with 1 Gm of kanamycin may be instilled at 6-hour intervals for the first three or four postoperative days. The small polyethylene catheter may then be removed without difficulty. The use of antibiotics systemically and locally may reduce the incidence of septic complications, particularly septic shock.

Liver

Several factors improve survival figures for hepatic injuries:

1. Early exploration aided by diagnostic peritoneal tap or peritoneal lavage saves many patients before fatal hemorrhage develops.
2. Optimal amounts of blood and balanced electrolyte solution are used. In addition to massive loss of blood in many of these patients, there is a large loss of extracellular fluid, both externally and by an internal shift into a nonfunctional space, which must be replaced.

3. The use of adequate drainage in every case of hepatic injury and elimination of gauze packs to control hemorrhage greatly decrease the mortality and morbidity from liver injuries. Madding et al. noted that the decrease in mortality from liver wounds from 60 percent in World War I to approximately 27 percent in World War II was due largely to these two factors.

4. Antibiotics are used in all cases of hepatic trauma to prevent or decrease the high incidence of infectious complications occurring with this injury, particularly when associated with other lesions of the gastrointestinal tract.

5. Finally, liver resection for massive liver trauma has reduced the mortality and morbidity from massive liver trauma for the following reasons: (a) The incidences of hemorrhage and hematobilia, which occur frequently with other forms of treatment for massive liver trauma, are reduced. (b) Purulent complications are more adequately prevented by the removal of necrotic hepatic tissue, better drainage, and reduced foreign material in the wounds, such as packs or Gelfoam, which tend to prevent drainage and sequester infected necrotic material with the liver. (c) The incidence of biliary fistulas, often high following suture repair or gauze-pack tamponade, is much lower following resection. This is due to the ligation of separate bile ducts during resection, more effective wound drainage, and reduced retention of necrotic tissue and foreign bodies in the wound.

TREATMENT. Treatment may be accomplished by drainage alone, suture and drainage, or varying extents of hepatic resection.

Drainage Alone. Approximately 30 percent of liver wounds may be treated by drainage alone without the use of sutures. The wounds so managed should be simple lacerations or perforations of the liver which are not bleeding at the time of surgical intervention. In the experience at Parkland Memorial Hospital, about 55 percent of patients with hepatic injuries had continuing hemorrhage during the surgical procedure, which is more than other reports have indicated. It is possible that suturing small nonbleeding lacerations of the liver may lead to tissue strangulation and necrosis more serious than any slight rebleeding or drainage which might occur if the small wound were not sutured. Also, difficult rebleeding may occur when sutures are placed in a small, nonbleeding laceration which could be adequately treated by drainage alone. None of the 100 patients treated at Parkland Memorial Hospital without suture experienced any episodes of rebleeding, biliary fistula, bile peritonitis, or excessive drainage of bile from the drain site. Crosthwait and associates have also reported no difficulties with the treatment of certain hepatic lacerations by the nonsuture method with adequate drainage.

Suture and Drainage. About 60 percent of patients with hepatic trauma should be treated by suture and drainage. As indicated above, the wounds which are treated in this manner are generally larger than those treated by the nonsuture technique, and they continue to bleed at the time of the surgical procedure, thus requiring suture for control of bleeding as well as reestablishment of anatomic continuity. The preferred suture is #1 chromic catgut swaged on a long curved needle with a tapered point. It is placed as a broad interlocking horizontal mattress suture, approximately 2 to 3 cm from the edge of the laceration on each side, and deeply into the liver. Some reports state that these sutures should be tied over a bolster, using a

material such as Ivalon or Gelfoam, to prevent cutting through the liver, but generally this is not necessary if the sutures are placed properly and tied without excessive tension. Occasionally, when a bolster beneath the suture is indicated because of the friability of hepatic tissue, the insertion of an omental tag beneath the suture and over the laceration provides a more physiologic substance than synthetic materials. However, this usually is not necessary.

Another advisable departure from common therapeutic practice is less frequent use of hemostatic agents, such as Gelfoam and Oxycel, which are often wedged into lacerations in an attempt to control hemorrhage. Whitcomb and Ponka point out that such Gelfoam wedges may extend the depth of the laceration, causing more bleeding deep to the Gelfoam. Thus, infected and necrotic tissue and blood may be trapped within the depths of the laceration and may lead to secondary hemorrhage, bile drainage, hepatic abscess, or hematobilia. In one case in our experience, a large piece of Gelfoam was pressed deeply into a hepatic laceration; that case is the only one in which there was prolonged and copious bile drainage in the entire experience with hepatic injury at Parkland Memorial Hospital. Foreign materials thrust into lacerations to control hemorrhage also prevent close coaptation of the wound surfaces and slow healing even though none of the other complications occurs. Occasionally, it may be absolutely necessary to use such agents for hemostasis when this cannot be obtained by suture alone, by individual ligation of bleeding vessels within the laceration, or by hepatic resection and debridement. However, these materials generally are not required and certainly should not be used routinely.

In addition to suturing large wounds which continue to bleed, it is very important, as pointed out by Madding et al. in their review of World War II liver injuries, to establish extensive drainage of all liver injuries, no matter how slight. Crosthwait et al. noted the occurrence of fatal bile peritonitis in two of their patients in whom drainage was not used following hepatic injuries; this has been the experience at Parkland Memorial Hospital with a few liver wounds which were not drained or were inadequately drained. Adequate drainage consists of several 1-in. Penrose drains placed in the subphrenic space, down to the laceration directly, and in the subhepatic space in Morison's pouch. The drains should be placed through the shortest and most direct route. They are left in until there is no further drainage, with the exception of minimal tissue fluid, and then they are removed over a period of 2 or 3 days. However, when drainage of bile or other material continues, the drains remain in place until drainage ceases or until a permanent tract has formed about the drains, which requires about 3 weeks.

Resection. Approximately 10 percent of hepatic injuries should be treated by hepatic resection or debridement of varying extent. Nearly half of the cases of blunt trauma to the liver may be managed by a lobar or sublobar resection. However, a third of our hepatic resections have been done for shotgun or high-velocity bullet wounds. Wounds of the liver which produce extensive stellate lacerations and destroy great portions of hepatic tissue should be

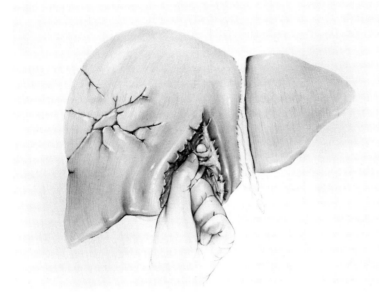

Fig. 6-13. Typical liver injury requiring hepatic resection.

treated by resection (Fig. 6-13). In the past, these wounds were treated by gauze tamponade, which was very ineffective and usually led to death from recurrent hemorrhage and infection. Because as little normal hepatic tissue as possible is removed, these resections might more accurately be termed *debridement resections.*

The techniques for controlling bleeding in hepatic resection are described in detail in Chap. 30. However, it might be noted here that a recent report by Miller indicates that extending a midline abdominal incision into a median sternotomy incision, as in open heart surgery, may give superior exposure of the suprahepatic vena cava and the hepatic veins and permit more rapid and better control of bleeding from these vessels than is possible through the usual right thoracoabdominal incision. The median sternotomy also gives good exposure of the heart for insertion of an intracaval shunt into the inferior vena cava through the right atrial appendage, as described by Schrock et al. This shunt allows complete vascular isolation of the liver while maintaining venous return to the right atrium and permits repairs of hepatic venous and/or vena cava injuries associated with liver injuries which otherwise would not be possible. The authors have described and used such an intracaval shunt, which can be inserted into the infrahepatic inferior vena cava for vascular isolation of the liver before the chest is opened. The median sternotomy approach may make the shunt which is inserted through the right atrial appendage preferable to the shunt inserted through the abdominal vena cava.

Although Merendino et al., Longmire and Marable, and Perry and LaFave suggested that T-tube drainage of the common bile duct should be carried out after hepatic resections, recent reports by Lucas and by Pinkerton et al. suggest that septic complications and bleeding from gastroduodenal stress ulcers are significantly increased by this. However, Lane et al. and Wasowski, in separate recent reports, do not concur that T-tube drainage is harmful and

state that it should continue to be used after liver resection. Although T-tube drainage may not lower pressures in the common bile duct and therefore probably does not prevent bile leakage from the liver and bile collections in the operative site, the T tube does help identify the right and left hepatic ducts with certainty during liver resections and thus aids in preventing operative injury to the remaining major bile duct. Also, the T tube does provide a useful port through which such postoperative complications as hematobilia and biliary fistula formation can be recognized and the type of drainage observed. Cholangiography may also be done through the tube postoperatively, and this may be very useful in determining the cause of prolonged jaundice after hepatic resections. Currently, the authors are continuing to insert T tubes into the common bile duct during hepatic resections unless the duct is so small that a #10 or #12 tube cannot be easily inserted. If a T tube is forced into a small common bile duct, acute biliary obstruction and later bile duct stricture caused by the T tube have been observed. The increased likelihood of bleeding from gastroduodenal stress ulcers caused by T-tube drainage of the common bile duct after hepatic resection may be offset by frequently lavaging the stomach with antacid solutions through the Levin tube to maintain a high intragastric pH for several days postoperatively, as recently suggested by Silen.

Four or five large Penrose drains are brought out through a separate stab wound placed subcostally and anterolaterally in the abdominal wall. After right lobar resections, when the abdomen is closed and the anterior drains are in place, the patient is turned to a lateral position, a separate incision is made over the twelfth rib for resection of this rib, the peritoneal cavity is entered from behind through the bed of the twelfth rib, and four or five more 1-in. Penrose drains are inserted to establish through-and-through drainage of the resected liver bed.

The incision over the twelfth rib is made as in the Ochsner-Nather approach to draining subhepatic abscesses (see Chap. 34).

COMPLICATIONS. Major nonfatal complications occur after approximately 20 percent of liver injuries. Major complications occur in about one-third of the resected cases, which does not seem inordinately excessive in view of the extensiveness of the hepatic injuries which are treated by resection. The thorax is involved in approximately 40 percent of hepatic injuries; so there is a high incidence of pulmonary complications. Next in incidence are purulent intraabdominal or intrathoracic collections which require subsequent drainage. Approximately 50 percent of such purulent complications are associated with colon injuries, and these are among the worst injuries which can be associated with hepatic injuries. With an adequate index of suspicion and early recognition, however, few with hepatic injury who develop such complications should die. Other significant complications have been the development of renal failure in only slightly more than 1 percent and bleeding phenomena in only 1.5 percent of all the patients with hepatic injury in the Parkland Memorial Hospital experience. The low incidence of these two latter complications is felt to be due to the adequate replacement of extracellular fluid volume deficit and judicious, but not excessive, use of whole blood in these patients.

All the patients with major lobar resections may be expected to have some degree of postoperative bilirubin elevation, secondary probably to transient biliary obstruction by blood clots and temporary hepatic insufficiency (due to shock, loss of hepatic mass, and operative trauma, and, on occasion, perhaps secondary to postoperative sepsis). Such hyperbilirubinemia usually disappears in about 3 weeks with no further surgical treatment for the relief of jaundice required. Liver function studies generally demonstrate hepatic impairment, such as a lowered serum albumin level, elevated alkaline phosphatase level, and positive flocculation tests, which usually return to normal after several weeks. Studies indicate that survival is possible with only 20 percent of the normal hepatic mass and that within 1 to 2 years most of the resected hepatic tissue is replaced as the result of hepatic regeneration.

Hematobilia, which develops when a hematoma or abscess within the substance of the liver erodes into one of the bile ducts, may become manifest 1 to 3 weeks following initial hepatic trauma or much later. It is probable that the wider use of hepatic resection for extensive hepatic trauma will lead to better control of injured blood vessels deep within the substance of the liver and less hematobilia. The presence of hepatic subcapsular hematomas at the time of initial exploration should be noted, and if they seem to be growing, they should be opened and the offending vessels ligated to prevent hematobilia. Once hematobilia is recognized, operation is indicated. The intrahepatic cavity may be detected during the surgical procedure by inspection and needle aspiration or using hepatic angiography. It is best treated by resection of the offending lobe of the liver, but if the cavity is near the surface, it may be more practical to unroof the cavity and

ligate the bleeding vessel. Cholecystostomy and T-tube drainage, which have previously been employed, are unsatisfactory therapy.

Half of the deaths from hepatic trauma occur as the result of massive uncontrollable hemorrhage during the surgical procedure. With a single, small penetrating injury, involving only the liver, the death rate should be 1 percent or less. The overall mortality rate for hepatic trauma at Parkland Memorial Hospital was 11 percent in a series of 259 hepatic injuries. The mortality rate is directly related to the number of intraabdominal viscera injured other than the liver. The mortality rises to approximately 60 percent when the liver and five or more other intraabdominal viscera are injured. In our series of 25 patients in whom the severe hepatic injury was treated by resection, the mortality rate was only 20 percent. The mortality rate from blunt trauma to the liver which was managed either by resection or by suture has been only 26 percent, whereas a summary of the literature concerning blunt hepatic trauma shows a mortality rate of approximately 65 percent.

Extrahepatic Biliary Tree

PENETRATING INJURIES

The diagnosis of penetrating injuries of the extrahepatic biliary tree generally presents no problem as compared with the diagnosis of blunt trauma of the biliary tree, which may be difficult unless intraabdominal hemorrhage occurs. When the hepatic artery and portal vein are involved, the mortality rate is inordinately high because of massive hemorrhage which may be virtually impossible to control before irreversible hypoxic damage occurs to the brain and myocardium. Probably most patients with injuries to the extrahepatic biliary tree and one of the major vessels in the hepatoduodenal ligament do not survive to come to surgical exploration. This is particularly true when the wounding agent is a large-caliber, high-velocity missile. In contrast, wounds of the gallbladder which are seen frequently following penetrating abdominal trauma have a low mortality rate and are not so frequently associated with injuries to the major vessels in the hepatoduodenal ligament.

On opening the abdomen, blood and bile seen issuing from the subhepatic region indicate possible injury to the biliary tree. At times, the amount of bile, blood, or contusion may be minimal, and the gallbladder, cystic duct, and hepatoduodenal structures must be carefully inspected to evaluate the significance of any subserosal hematoma or bile staining. If the patient has survived to be surgically explored, generally no massive bleeding from the subhepatic region will be noted initially. However, many times in obtaining exposure of the hepatoduodenal ligament structures, clots which have formed and caused tamponade of major bleeding sites may be dislodged, with recurrence of vigorous bleeding from the portal vein, hepatic artery, or their branches, which are so frequently injured when the bile ducts are injured.

Generally, the hemorrhage may be immediately arrested by placing the fingers in the foramen of Winslow and compressing the hepatoduodenal ligament. Following this, after removing the free blood and obtaining good exposure while maintaining finger tamponade as above, more definitive control of the hemorrhage may be obtained by placing vascular clamps or rubber-shod clamps across all structures in the hepatoduodenal ligament. One clamp should be placed as far distad as possible on the hepatoduodenal ligament, and this maneuver is aided by dividing the lateral serosal reflection of the duodenum and reflecting the duodenum and the head of the pancreas mediad. Another clamp is then placed on the hepatoduodenal ligament through the foramen of Winslow as near the liver hilus as possible.

After hemorrhage is controlled, the serosa of the hepatoduodenal ligament at the point of the hematoma formation is incised, and the disruption of the portal vein or hepatic artery is visualized by rapidly dissecting out these structures. When the defects in the major vessels are located, repair is done with 5-0 silk arterial sutures using the general principles and techniques of vascular surgery. The vascular repair should be done only after careful exposure of the defect but also with dispatch, since the safe occlusion period of hepatic vascular inflow is only 15 to 20 minutes unless the patient is under hypothermia.

After repair of any vascular injuries, the biliary tract is carefully dissected out along the course of the penetrating missile. Knife wounds of the bile ducts may be closed with interrupted 4-0 silk suture. The common duct should be decompressed with a T tube inserted through a separate incision in the ductal system a short distance above or below the injury, so that one arm of the T tube serves as a stent for the wounded portion of the bile duct. For injuries caused by bullets or other large penetrating objects which may produce destruction or avulsion of a segment of the biliary ductal system, the wound should be carefully debrided and all devitalized ductal tissue removed. This may require completing a partial transection of the bile ducts, so that an end-to-end anastomosis may be made between viable portions of the common duct. This anastomosis is again made with interrupted simple sutures of 4-0 silk, and the repair is stented with a rubber T tube placed through a separate incision in the duct, above or below the injury. Medial reflection of the duodenum relaxes tension and allows the ends of the divided ducts to come together more readily, particularly when duct tissue has been destroyed and the ducts are shortened.

If the loss of biliary ductal structure is extensive, end-to-end repair of the duct may not be possible, and a bypass procedure is necessary. Generally, the Roux en Y bypass is effective. This is done by bringing up a 30-cm Roux en Y limb of jejunum made by transecting the jejunum about 30 cm below the ligament of Treitz. The end of the defunctionalized limb of jejunum is closed with two layers of suture. Following this, the distal end of the common duct is doubly ligated with heavy nonabsorbable suture material, and the choledochojejunostomy is performed in the following manner: a small incision is made in the side of the defunctionalized limb of jejunum about 2 cm from the closed end, at a site where the free limb of jejunum comfortably opposes the divided proximal bile duct. The anastomosis is performed by placing a posterior row of 4-0 silk arterial sutures between the seromuscular coat of the jejunum and the common duct. Usually, it is possible to place only two or three silk sutures in the posterior layer of the anastomosis.

After this, the inner row of the anastomosis is made with 4-0 chromic gastrointestinal catgut sutures, placing the sutures so that the knots are tied within the lumen of the anastomosis. These catgut sutures are continued around from the posterior to the anterior row, and, again, it is usually possible with a small duct to place only about four of these catgut sutures. Following this, the anterior row of silk sutures is placed in the same manner as described above for the posterior row. It is best to perform this anastomosis over a T-tube stent to help prevent stenosis of the anastomosis and to reduce bile leakage from the anastomosis in the immediate postoperative period. The T tube should be placed in the bile duct, just above the anastomosis to the jejunum, so that one limb of the tube goes across the anastomosis. If the anastomosis is made so high in the hilus of the liver that it is impossible to place a T tube above it, then the T tube may be placed through a stab wound in the wall of the jejunal limb and one limb led through the anastomosis into the biliary ductal system. A purse-string suture should be placed in the jejunum about the T tube to secure it in position.

The abdomen should be closed with extensive drainage of the biliary-jejunal anastomosis. The T tube should be left in place for 3 or 4 weeks, following which cholangiography is performed to ensure adequate healing and patent anastomosis, and the T tube is removed. The drains are left in until all biliary drainage has ceased, or until a firm drainage tract has formed, which occurs about 3 weeks postoperatively.

If the gallbladder and cystic duct are intact, the bypass also may be done between the gallbladder and jejunum with ligation of the distal and proximal limbs of the damaged common duct. Also, it may be more expedient at times to use a simple loop of jejunum instead of a Roux en Y limb to perform the bypass procedure.

If the patient is in poor condition and cannot tolerate a prolonged procedure for definitive repair, then the defects of the biliary ductal structures may be repaired by simple bridging with a T tube fixed in place with a suture at either end of the ductal defect; secondary repair may be done later as soon as the patient can tolerate it. If possible, however, definitive repair should be done, since recurrent strictures are more likely to occur following the more difficult secondary repairs of the bile ducts.

Injuries to the gallbladder generally may be handled in one of two ways: (1) If the patient has other extensive injuries or is in poor condition from hemorrhagic shock and other complications, the most rapid means of dealing with the gallbladder injury is to suture the wound with a one-layer row of interrupted nonabsorbable mattress sutures and to decompress the gallbladder with a #28 to 30 French mushroom catheter, placed in the fundus of the gallbladder through a purse-string suture. The catheter is brought out through a separate stab wound in the right upper quadrant of the abdomen. This catheter remains for approximately 3 weeks, or until a good tract has formed around it in order to prevent bile leakage into the peritoneal cavity following removal of the tube. Before removing the tube, cholangiography should be done through it to demonstrate patent cystic and common ducts. (2) If the patient is in good condition, however, it is preferable to remove the gallbladder when it has been injured.

BLUNT TRAUMA

Blunt trauma to the biliary tree deserves separate discussion, not because the surgical management differs, but because of its relative rarity and difficulty of diagnosis. Barnes and Diamonon reported in 1963 that only 48 cases of traumatic rupture of the gallbladder due to blunt trauma to the abdomen had been reported up to that time. According to Rydell, complete division of the common duct by blunt trauma was reported in 25 cases up to 1970. The usual means of closed injury to the extrahepatic biliary tree is a shearing force applied to the common duct or impingement of the bile duct between the vertebral column and a crushing force applied to the abdominal wall.

When blunt trauma to the biliary tree is severe enough to result in a free flow of bile, the characteristic picture of bile peritonitis occurs. According to Sturmer and Wilt, the usual history reveals a crushing injury to the right upper quadrant, the epigastrium, or the lower part of the chest, which results in severe pain and is followed by shock. The shock usually is of relatively short duration, seldom more than a few hours. Generally during this period, the diagnosis of probable intraabdominal injury may be established by signs of peritoneal irritation, such as abdominal rigidity and guarding. Bile or nonclotting blood may be found on peritoneal tap done in the flanks or in the right upper quadrant of the abdomen, but the tap may be negative. Shock is usually secondary to the marked outpouring of extracellular fluid into the peritoneal cavity due to the chemical irritation of the peritoneum by bile. The initial chemical peritonitis caused by bile may be followed shortly by a bacterial peritonitis. If biliary leakage is minimal, shock may be of relatively short duration or absent, and abdominal signs initially may be slight. This may be followed by the recovery and well-being of the patient, which lasts for periods up to 5 or 10 days. However, the onset of jaundice on about the third day is a fairly constant sign. The appearance of clay-colored stools and the presence of bile in the urine may be noticed from about the second to the fifth day after injury.

A considerable gradual increase in abdominal size occurs during the first 10 days that may be unattended by the usual signs of peritonitis. This condition is accompanied by progressive signs of extracellular fluid volume deficit and by evidence of infection, such as rising temperature and elevated white cell count. In the reported cases of complete transection of the common duct, the site of transection was uniformly in the retroduodenal area, thus again indicating the importance of extensive medial reflection of the duodenum to explore the retroperitoneal duodenum as well as the distal common duct and pancreas.

When blunt trauma to the extrahepatic biliary tract is diagnosed, the repair is generally the same as in the previous discussion of penetrating trauma. End-to-end repair of the ducts over a T tube should be done, if possible, or a bypass procedure between the ducts and the jejunum should be done by bringing up a Roux en Y limb or loop of jejunum to perform an anastomosis between the biliary tract and the jejunum as described in the discussion of penetrating trauma. The ducts should not be implanted in the duodenum, since anastomotic leaks occur more often with this than with the anastomosis to a defunctionalized limb of jejunum. Leak of a choledochoduodenal anastomosis produces not only a biliary fistula but a duodenal fistula as well, with all the grave consequences of such a fistula. If a biliary-jejunal anastomosis leaks, only a bile leak occurs, which is easier to manage generally and has a better prognosis than a biliary duodenal fistula.

The postoperative therapy of biliary tract injuries, in which bile peritonitis is an important complicating feature, should include adequate replacement of extracellular fluid volume deficits, which may require several liters of balanced salt solutions in 24 hours. These solutions should be given as soon as possible preoperatively and continued throughout the surgical procedure and postoperatively to avoid extracellular fluid volume deficit. Broad-spectrum antibiotics should be given prior to the surgical procedure and continued throughout the procedure and for several days after, until the chances of sepsis and infection have diminished.

Mortality from biliary tract injuries should be below 5 to 10 percent if they are discovered early and treated by adequate reconstruction, adequate drainage and decompression of the biliary tree, adequate coverage with antibiotics, and proper fluid replacement. Patients with more severe injuries probably do not survive to be diagnosed and treated.

Pancreas

(By Ronald C. Jones and G. Tom Shires)

The first pancreatic injury was reported by Travers in England in 1827. Due to the increasing number of high-speed automobile accidents and other acts of violence, more pancreatic trauma has been observed in the past 5 years than was treated in the previous 15 years. During the past 20 years, 175 patients have received initial management and surgical therapy for pancreatic trauma at Parkland Memorial Hospital.

DIAGNOSIS Diagnosis includes physical examination, serum amylase level determination, and adequate visualization of the pancreas at surgical exploration. The clinical signs and symptoms depend not only upon the type and extent of injury to the gland but also to a great extent upon the associated injuries. There are no early signs pathognomonic for pancreatic trauma. Injuries to retroperitoneal organs such as the pancreas may not produce clinical findings of loss of bowel sounds, tenderness, and guarding or spasm for 12 to 24 hours afterward. The possibility of pancreatic injury should be considered in all abdominal injuries, and frequent determinations of serum amylase in the initial studies, particularly following blunt trauma, are essential. Serum amylase level elevation may be the only early evidence of pancreatic injury. If retroperitoneal duodenal perforation is suspected, Gastrografin is injected into the stomach and films obtained to determine extravasation or obstruction.

Serum Amylase Determination. Over 20 years ago Matthewson and Halter advocated routine serum amylase level determinations in patients sustaining blunt trauma and emphasized that pancreatic injury was more common than had been previously appreciated. Serum amylase elevation alone has not been considered an indication for exploratory laparotomy. If signs of peritonitis are present, such as spasm, tenderness, and absent bowel sounds, then a laparotomy is performed. Unrecognized severe pancreatic injury can be a fatal lesion, particularly when it is accompanied by disruption of pancreatic tissue and leakage of pancreatic juice.

Many patients have been found to have an elevated serum amylase level but negative abdominal findings. These patients are closely observed for evidence of peritonitis or until the amylase returned to normal. An amylase determination is performed on peritoneal lavage, but the elevation is more often due to small bowel injury than to pancreatic injury.

The preoperative serum amylase has been very useful in detecting injuries to the pancreas secondary to blunt trauma, since 91 percent of these patients have an elevated serum amylase level. In contrast, only one-fourth of the patients sustaining penetrating pancreatic trauma have a preoperative serum amylase elevation. Although an elevated serum amylase following blunt trauma indicates pancreatic injury, it does not relate to the severity of the injury. A prolonged elevation of the serum amylase may be an indication that a pseudocyst is developing.

Surgical Exploration. It is helpful to know the serum amylase level at the time of laparotomy. When it is elevated, the pancreaticoduodenal area must be carefully examined for any pancreatic injury. During abdominal exploration, if there is any evidence of trauma to the periampullary region, such as retroperitoneal hematoma, crepitation, or bile-stained fluid, then complete medial mobilization of the duodenum and pancreatic head is performed. The lesser sac is opened through the gastrocolic ligament, and the pancreas is examined throughout its length.

In the past, untreated disruption of the pancreatic ductal system has been the main source of the morbidity associated with pancreatic injuries. If there is question concerning the integrity of the pancreatic duct, it may be necessary to obtain a pancreatogram to confirm continuity before deciding to leave the injured portion of the gland in place.

ASSOCIATED INJURIES. Isolated pancreatic injury is rare. Associated injuries are usually more obvious indications for surgical exploration than suspected pancreatic injury. Death and serious complications are frequent in pancreatic trauma but are only rarely caused by the pancreatic injury. Massive hemorrhage from associated vascular, hepatic, or splenic injury is the main cause of death.

Although the pancreas is a vascular organ, it is not often responsible for uncontrollable hemorrhage. When profuse bleeding occurs from the pancreatic area, the pancreas is mobilized and the superior mesenteric, splenic vessels, aorta, and vena cava inspected, since they are often the source of severe hemorrhage. Because of the location of the pancreas, injuries to the liver and stomach are frequent.

Of the 175 pancreatic injuries in the Parkland Memorial Hospital series, 58 percent had an associated retroperitoneal injury in addition to the pancreatic injury; therefore, all retroperitoneal hematomas are explored.

MANAGEMENT OF PANCREATIC INJURIES. The surgical procedure used to repair a pancreatic injury is determined by the extent of the injury, associated organ injury, and the overall condition of the patient. The treatment of pancreatic injuries has consisted primarily of suture and drainage techniques. In the last decade more aggressive treatment has included radical resection and Roux en Y drainage procedures.

For simple contusion and lacerations in which there is no loss of pancreatic tissue and no major ductal involvement, Penrose drainage in association with sump drainage has been adequate. Only if there is bleeding is suture repair of the lacerated capsule required. Fragmentation of pancreatic tissue requires debridement and adequate drainage. Ductal injury should be determined depending on proximity to major pancreatic ducts. If this cannot be accomplished by direct visualization, then a pancreatogram is indicated.

Drainage. Since it has been shown that pancreatic injuries may normally drain for 2 to 4 weeks, it is essential to have adequate and effective drainage. The sump drain has been used in association with the Penrose drain. A properly functioning sump drain allows air to enter the tract, preventing the occurrence of a vacuum. It also allows measurement of the amount of pancreatic juice being lost and helps prevent skin digestion. The Penrose drains are brought out through the bed or at the tip of the twelfth rib for direct drainage. The drains are left in place for 10 days to 2 weeks since moderate drainage may not occur during the first week following injury.

Distal Pancreatectomy. Adequate exposure and complete exploration of the retroperitoneal area are mandatory following blunt trauma. Any hematoma present in the region of the pancreas is opened, but complete transection of the pancreas may occur without extensive hematoma formation. Distal pancreatectomy is an effective method for treating extensive damage of the body and tail of the organ; traumatized and devitalized tissue are removed and the occurrence of postoperative pancreatic complications are decreased.

When performing a distal pancreatectomy, suture stick ties are placed in the superior and inferior borders of the pancreas approximately $1\frac{1}{2}$ to 2 cm from the edge. This, along with isolation of the splenic vessels during distal pancreatectomy, prevents unnecessary blood loss and provides better visualization. A splenectomy is almost always necessary. In resecting the distal pancreas the cut edge is beveled in a fish mouth fashion. This enables a better closure of the proximal end of the pancreas. Following penetrating trauma, the proximal pancreas is oversewn with permanent suture material, and when possible, the pancreatic duct is ligated.

Distal Pancreatectomy with Roux en Y Anastomosis. This has been utilized in patients receiving blunt trauma to the pancreas when the extent of damage to the proximal pancreatic duct is uncertain and when partial duct obstruction secondary to edema could give rise to a pancreatic fistula. In the critical patient with multiple organ involvement oversewing of the distal pancreas is a satisfactory method of treatment.

Complete Transection of Pancreas

The mechanism of pancreatic transection secondary to blunt trauma appears to be a sudden severe compression of the upper abdominal viscera between the object, such as a steering wheel, and the spinal column at the time of impact. For the transected pancreas, drainage alone is inadequate. Transection requires identification of the pancreatic duct which may be quite difficult.

The mortality for 18 patients in the Parkland Memorial Hospital series who sustained complete transection of the pancreas was 39 percent. Blunt trauma accounted for 13 of the complete transections, with a mortality of 31 percent. No patient in the Parkland Memorial Hospital series who has undergone a distal pancreatectomy is known to have subsequently developed pancreatic insufficiency or diabetes in the PMH series although resected specimens have measured up to 14 cm in length. (The average normal pancreas has a length of 15 cm, is 3 cm thick, and weighs 65 to 125 Gm.) Freeark et al have reported patients who have developed diabetes, one of whom also had diarrhea, following extensive distal pancreatectomy.

Roux en Y Pancreaticojejunostomy. Several methods of treating pancreatic transection have been described. For the completely transected pancreas over the superior mesenteric vessels and to the right of these vessels, a Roux en Y anastomosis suturing both ends of the pancreas into this limb has proved satisfactory (Fig. 6-14). This has been the preferred treatment for injuries which require removal of 75 percent or more of the pancreas. Variations of this method described by Letton and Wilson are also applicable. A Roux-en-Y anastomosis to both ends of the severed pancreas has eliminated the need to find a severed duct or to reanastomose it. This method leaves all functioning pancreatic tissue, thereby avoiding the possibility of pancreatic insufficiency or diabetes. The risk of injury to the underlying superior mesenteric vessels seems less with this mode of treatment than with resection. The possibility of fistula, and pseudocyst formation is also minimized.

The easiest method of accomplishing the Roux en Y anastomosis to both ends of the severed pancreas is an end-to-end anastomosis of pancreas to jejunum and end of pancreas to side of jejunum. This is accomplished using permanent sutures placed approximately 1 cm apart in a single layer anastomosis. Once this anastomosis is accomplished, drainage with Penrose and sump drains is placed to the pancreatic injury.

Jordan and associates advocate complete transection of the pancreas and a Roux en Y anastomosis to the distal pancreatic fragment with oversewing of the proximal pancreas.

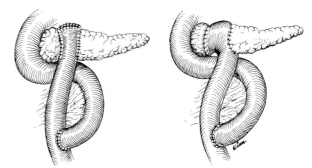

Fig. 6-14. Technique of Roux en Y anastomosis of both ends of transected pancreas.

creas. The Roux en Y limb should be at least 30 cm in length and is usually passed through the transverse mesocolon to the site of injury. As long as the duodenum is intact and viable there is little justification for a pancreaticoduodenectomy for this type of injury.

Unless the completely severed pancreatic duct is managed with definitive surgery, a pseudocyst or fistula will almost always result. A Roux en Y anastomosis to one fragment of the severed pancreas is little more time-consuming than resection of the distal fragment, which requires a splenectomy.

If the location of the pancreatic injury suggests the possibility of injury to the intrapancreatic portion of the common bile duct, the common bile duct is opened in its supraduodenal position and a cholangiogram obtained. If a partial tear of the distal common duct has occurred but some ductal continuity remains, a T-tube is inserted for decompression.

Repair and Stent of Pancreatic Duct. It is difficult to locate the pancreatic duct in this case, with bleeding and hematoma, and even more difficult to suture it after it is found. Nevertheless, several reports have appeared in which the pancreatic duct has been identified, found to be completely transected in the region of the neck of the pancreas, and successfully repaired by stenting and suture repair. The stent may be inserted into the duct at the area of injury and threaded through the ampulla into the duodenum. The second method by which this has been accomplished is by duodenotomy and catheter cannulation of the pancreatic duct through the ampulla, with or without a sphincterotomy, with passage into the distal pancreatic duct past the point of transection. The pancreatic duct is then reapproximated with #6 or #7 nonabsorbable suture material. This is not a preferred but an alternate method, which might be of some benefit in selected cases in which the injury would require radical resection of the pancreas in the critically ill patient. Although either fistula, late stricture formation at the site of injury, or recurrent pancreatitis secondary to partial obstruction of the pancreatic duct is possible, these complications have not been reported.

Anterior Roux en Y Pancreaticojejunostomy. A Roux en Y pancreaticojejunostomy. may be placed to the anterior surface of the pancreas over the injury in selected cases. This method of treatment has been satisfactory only if the posterior pancreatic capsule is intact. If the posterior pancreatic capsule is broken, drainage will continue into the retroperitoneal space rather than into the Roux en Y limb and result in abscess, pseudocyst, or fistula formation.

Combined Pancreaticoduodenal Injuries

Kerry and Glass reported a mortality of 73 percent in 11 cases of combined pancreaticoduodenal injuries. Cleveland et al reported deaths in five of six patients with combined duodenal and pancreatic injury. However, Sheldon, et al. have found that combined pancreaticoduodenal injuries were not by themselves especially lethal. Of seven patients who had pancreaticoduodenal injuries, only one died. These findings correlate well with the observations in the Parkland Memorial Hospital series.

Combined pancreaticoduodenal injuries in the region of the head of the pancreas and duodenal "C" loop occurred in 30 patients in the PMH series, who therefore could be considered possible candidates for a pancreaticoduodenectomy depending on the severity of the injury. The overall mortality for these 30 pancreaticoduodenal injuries was 27 percent. Due to the severity of the injury, three patients did undergo pancreaticoduodenectomy with survival. Of the remaining 27 patients, eight expired; six of these expired on the operating table from massive injuries to retroperitoneal vessels. Of the two remaining patients, one died of renal failure, and the other died of multiple injuries including a combined pancreaticoduodenal injury. Therefore, only one of 27 patients with combined pancreaticoduodenal injury not treated by pancreaticoduodenectomy died as a result of the injury. Most of the high mortality associated with pancreaticoduodenal trauma appears to be secondary to major vessels located in this area.

Pancreaticoduodenectomy. When a pancreaticoduodenectomy is considered for penetrating pancreatic trauma, pancreatic ductal injuries should be verified. This may be accomplished by duodenotomy, cannulation of the pancreatic duct, and pancreatogram. The common duct is identified and proved to be intact by cholangiogram. An alternate method of determining ductal injury is by mobilizing the tail of the pancreas and performing a pancreatogram through the distal pancreatic duct. Hemostatic sutures are placed 1.5 to 2 cm into the superior and inferior portion of the pancreas prior to incising the tail of the pancreas, since large vessels are often in this area. If the common bile duct and major pancreatic duct system are intact and the duodenal injury can be closed, then a pancreaticoduodenectomy is usually not indicated. Reports of high mortality secondary to combined pancreaticoduodenal injuries do not always take into account the major vessel injury which is often responsible for the death of the patient on the operating table, as occurred in this series. If these patients are excluded, the mortality secondary to combined injuries would be less.

Some feel that pancreaticoduodenectomy, with its high mortality under circumstances of multiple organ injury, is unwarranted if the duodenum is viable despite extensive damage to the pancreatic head. Over 30 patients have been reported to have undergone pancreaticoduodenectomy for trauma; the mortality following this procedure is approximately 30 percent. None of the cases reported were obviously intraoperative deaths, which makes this a relative higher mortality, since the high mortality associated with other series of combined pancreaticoduodenal injuries in which a lesser procedure was performed includes the intraoperative deaths. The most common cause of death associated with pancreatic injury is hemorrhage. It becomes quite obvious that pancreaticoduodenectomy be performed only for strict indications.

Indications for pancreaticoduodenectomy include rupture of the duodenum and head of the pancreas, avulsion of the common duct from the duodenum with avascular duodenal wall, and stellate fracture with bleeding from crushing injury of the head of the pancreas. This procedure also is indicated for combined injuries to the head of the pancreas and duodenum with destruction of both to control hemorrhage, remove devitalized tissue, and restore ductal continuity. Perhaps the only indication for a pancreaticoduodenectomy when the duodenum is viable and intact is uncontrolled hemorrhage from sheering of branches from major vessels beneath the head of the pancreas, or severe hemorrhage from the head of the pancreas including severe stellate fractures of the head of the pancreas. The overall condition of the patient and associated injuries must be considered prior to submitting the patient to several more hours of surgery. There are times when this procedure is necessary but they are rare, particularly if the duodenum is intact. Complications following pancreaticoduodenectomy are common. Thus, mortality of pancreaticoduodenectomy must be low to justify its use if any other form of management can be employed.

In addition to fistula formation and abscesses, marginal ulceration with upper gastrointestinal bleeding has occurred following pancreaticoduodenectomy in which a vagotomy or an extensive subtotal gastric resection was not performed. Symptoms of dumping, diabetes, and weight loss with diarrhea and semi-formed bowel movements have occurred following pancreaticoduodenectomy for trauma. Foley and associates have reported a postoperative complication following pancreaticoduodenectomy of bleeding into the intestinal tract from the site of the pancreaticojejunostomy which was demonstrated by arteriographic studies and required operation to suture the bleeding point. Warren, Poulantzas, and Kune have noted that patients with limited gastric resection developed jejunal ulcers 6 months to 2 years after surgery, whereas none of the patients who had subtotal gastrectomy and vagotomy developed jejunal ulcer. Complications following total pancreatectomy are diabetes and steatorrhea.

For combined pancreaticoduodenal injuries, Donovan and Hagen have advocated closure of the duodenal perforation with accompanying vagotomy and antrectomy with gastrojejunostomy, gastrostomy, duodenostomy, and choledochostomy when indicated. This is performed in an attempt to defunctionalize the duodenal perforation and decrease pancreatic stimulation following the vagotomy and antrectomy. The mortality for nine patients with combined duodenal and pancreatic injuries was 33 percent. Further improvements in mortality can be expected as pancreaticoduodenectomy is used in carefully selected patients for severe injuries to the duodenum and head of the pancreas.

Avulsion of the Common Duct

Upper abdominal visceral injuries should be suspected in all patients with upper abdominal or lower thoracic injuries, especially following steering wheel injuries. A pattern of injury involving great force is applied directly to the right upper quadrant of the abdomen which may produce compound injuries of the duodenum, pancreas, and the bile duct has been described by Thal and Wilson. The pancreatic head and second portion of the duodenum are crushed postero-inferiorially against the vertebrae, and the liver and bile ducts are abruptly displaced upward with consequent disruption of the periampullary duct structures from the duodenum. If the duodenum is viable, this injury may often be treated with closure of the duodenum and a Roux en Y anastomosis to the avulsed ampulla of Vater but may occasionally require a pancreaticoduodenectomy.

Duodenostomy. In combined pancreaticoduodenal injury a duodenostomy is usually performed using a #10 Foley catheter placed through a small stab wound in the anterior duodenal wall adjacent to the injury.

COMPLICATIONS. Complications following pancreatic trauma include fistula, pancreatic abscess, vascular necrosis with hemorrhage from the drain site, pseudocyst formation, and duodenal fistula secondary to suture line breakdown from pancreatic juice activation.

Pancreatic enzymes liberated in the inactive form do not digest living tissue. In extensive injuries, duodenal and biliary enzymes are often released and the proteolytic pancreatic enzymes activated. Trypsinogen activated by enterokinase and hydrolyzed to trypsin breaks down protein. Mixtures of bile, gastric, and pancreatic juice are capable of digesting soft tissues with which they come in contact. As a result of digestion of surrounding tissues, any attempt at delayed definitive operation in this area becomes hazardous.

Fistula. Jordan et al. have reported the occurrence of pancreatic fistula as the most common complication following operative therapy, occurring in 35 percent of the cases and usually following blunt trauma. Most pancreatic fistulas are minor and close within a period of less than 1 month. Major pancreatic fistulas have been arbitrarily defined as those which drained for longer than 1 month. The serum amylase is frequently elevated while the fistula is present, probably due to transperitoneal absorption of amylase.

Almost all pancreatic fistulas will eventually close spontaneously; therefore treatment is mainly conservative. Attention must be given to preventing autodigestion of the surrounding skin. Vigorous fluid replacement with balanced salt solution to prevent volume deficit is indicated; the volume may be equal to that lost through the fistula. Baker, Strohl, and associates advocate continuous suction with sump drainage to prevent skin maceration as well as to obtain accurate estimates of fluid loss. They have shown a decrease in volume of pancreatic secretion of greater than 50 percent with the administration of 1 mg of atropine intramuscularly every 4 hours.

Pseudocyst. A pancreatic pseudocyst is a cyst whose wall of inflammatory fibrous tissue does not contain epithelium but is made up of structures surrounding the region of the pancreas in the retroperitoneum. The most frequent symptoms associated with a pancreatic pseudocyst are an abdominal mass, pain, nausea, and vomiting. The serum amylase level is usually elevated for a prolonged period of time during this illness. The pseudocyst rarely resolves spontaneously. Pancreatic pseudocyst is now a rare complication following pancreatic trauma if the pancreas has been explored. The preferred method of draining pancreatic pseudocysts is internally by either cyst gastrostomy or Roux en Y cyst jejunostomy.

Sepsis. Intraabdominal abscess is a common complication following multiple abdominal trauma. Although pancreatic fistulas rarely cause death, they occasionally give rise to pseudocyst formation and lesser sac abscess requiring reoperation for drainage. Lesser sac abscess may contribute to either sepsis or to retroperitoneal bleeding and death. Cultures of the abscess and fistula grow a predominance of mixed gram negative organisms; however, staphylococcus and enterococcus may often be present. The serum amylase is not consistently elevated in patients with a pancreatic or lesser sac abscess.

The method of management of a pancreatic abscess consists of adequate debridement and drainage and insertion of gastrostomy and feeding jejunostomy tubes. Complications are often associated with a duodenal fistula. If this is present, a Roux en Y jejunostomy is placed over the duodenal fistula when possible. Antibiotics are instituted early in all cases.

Although several methods of management have been advocated for pancreatic trauma, identification or strong suspicion of pancreatic ductal injury at the initial operation and the institution of appropriate definitive treatment are most important.

MORTALITY. The mortality for penetrating injuries to the pancreas is approximately 20 percent and is related to the type and severity of the injury (Table 6-6). Blunt trauma to the pancreas yields a mortality of 16 percent which was very close to the overall mortality of 18 percent.

The mortality correlates with the location of the injury, with injuries to the head having the highest mortality. Early surgical intervention in both blunt and penetrating abdominal trauma, meticulous intraabdominal examina-

Table 6-6. MORTALITY AND TYPE OF TRAUMA

	No. of patients	Died	Mortality
Penetrating	143	27	19%
Stab	30	2	6%
Gunshot	95	14	15%
Shotgun	18	11	61%
Blunt	32	5	16%
Total	175	32	18%

Table 6-7. MORTALITY FROM ISOLATED TRAUMA TO PANCREAS

Author	Review period	Patients operated	Penetrating	Deaths	Blunt	Deaths	Overall mortality
Walters . . .	1939–1963	131	73	15	58	9	18%
Jordan. . . .	1940–1967	140	117	23	23	2	18%
Stone	1948–1961	62	56	12	6	1	21%
Thompson .	1948–1963	73	39	10	34	4	17%
PMH*	1950–1970	175	143	27	32	5	18%
Freeark . . .	1952–1961	82	59	10	23	5	17%
Blaisdell. . .	1952–1968	56	33	10	23	6	29%
Walt	1956–1965	84	45	12	39	15	32%
Total . . .		803	565	119(21%)	238	47(20%)	21%

*Parkland Memorial Hospital.

tion of all organs, and an aggressive surgical approach to pancreatic injuries, including resection when indicated, are essential if mortality is to be lowered. Due to more aggressive management of pancreatic injuries, the mortality for blunt trauma of the pancreas has decreased to 8 percent during the past 5 years. Mortality for the pancreatic injury is less than 5 percent. Approximately 45 percent of the deaths in the Parkland Memorial Hospital series were patients who expired on the operating table of uncontrolled hemorrhage or brain injury. Of all pancreatic injuries approximately 70 percent are the result of penetrating trauma, and 30 percent follow blunt trauma. In a review of 800 cases of pancreatic trauma reported in the literature within the past 10 years, a mortality of 21 percent has occurred following penetrating pancreatic trauma and 20 percent following blunt trauma, with an overall mortality of 21 percent (Table 6-7).

Spleen

The spleen is the abdominal organ most frequently injured by blunt trauma, representing approximately one-quarter of all blunt injuries of abdominal viscera. The spleen also is often injured by penetrating abdominal injuries and is frequently associated with blunt and penetrating thoracoabdominal injuries (see Chap. 33).

TREATMENT. The only acceptable treatment of any type of splenic injury is splenectomy. Even a slight nonbleeding tear of the splenic capsule may lead to recurrent fatal bleeding. Also, it is likely that a splenic hematoma will increase in size secondarily to increasing osmotic pressure of the hematoma and imbibition of fluid, even though no further hemorrhage occurs. The splenic hematoma eventually reaches such size that the spleen ruptures, either spontaneously or following slight trauma, causing massive bleeding from the spleen which may be rapidly fatal.

Nonoperative treatment was recognized very early to carry a high mortality rate; when no operation is performed, the mortality rate is 90 to 95 percent. If an attempt is made to suture the spleen to stop bleeding or to tamponade with omentum or Gelfoam tacked over the injured site, the estimated mortality rate ranges from 25 to 50 percent because of the high incidence of rebleeding. The

average mortality for several series with splenectomy is about 20 percent, but if the spleen alone is injured, the operative mortality should be 5 percent or less according to Griswold and Collier. The technique is presented in Chap. 33.

Retroperitoneal Hematoma

The management of traumatic retroperitoneal hematoma is a controversial problem. The most common cause of retroperitoneal hemorrhage, according to Baylis et al. and according to the experience at Parkland Memorial Hospital, is pelvic fracture, which accounts for about 60 percent of all traumatic retroperitoneal hematomas. The diagnosis of retroperitoneal hematoma is most difficult following blunt, nonpenetrating trauma to the abdomen and should be suspected in any patient following trauma who has signs and symptoms of hemorrhagic shock but no obvious source of hemorrhage. The hemorrhage within the retroperitoneal area may be massive and may exceed 2,000 ml of blood. Experimental data have shown that as much as 4,000 ml of fluid can extravasate into the retroperitoneal space under pressure equal to that in the pelvic vessels.

DIAGNOSIS. Abdominal pain occurs in approximately 60 percent of the patients, and back pain in about 25 percent. The abdominal pain is usually vague and generalized, but is occasionally is localized over the hematoma. Local or generalized tenderness is present in about two-thirds of the patients, and shock occurs in approximately 40 percent. Occasionally, a tender mass is palpable through the abdomen or in the flanks, and in some cases, rectal examination will reveal a boggy mass anterior or posterior to the rectum. Dullness to percussion over the flanks or the abdomen which does not vary with changing positions of the patient has been recorded in some instances. At times, discoloration of the flanks from retroperitoneal hemorrhage has been noted after the lapse of a few hours (Grey Turner's sign). Progressive decrease in the hemoglobin and hematocrit is a consistent finding, and hematuria is found in 80 percent of patients—hematuria may represent the first clue to the development of retroperitoneal hematoma.

Somewhat more than half of the patients produce free

nonclotting blood on diagnostic paracentesis of the abdomen, which generally is related to the presence of both retroperitoneal and intraabdominal hemorrhage. However, if the retroperitoneal hematoma which occurs without intraperitoneal hemorrhage is large enough to yield a so-called "false-positive" peritoneal tap from retroperitoneal hemorrhage alone, then the hematoma itself may require abdominal exploration to search for the persistent source of retroperitoneal bleeding.

Roentgenography, according to Baylis et al., has been valuable in several respects: Approximately two-thirds of the patients with retroperitoneal hematoma have had fractures of the pelvis, and other x-ray findings have included obliteration of the psoas shadows in 30 percent, abdominal mass in 5 percent, and paralytic ileus in 8 percent. Also, displaced bowel gas shadows and fractured vertebrae have been noted. Baylis et al. also noted that in one patient a pelvic phlebolith was displaced by an expanding retroperitoneal hematoma. Intravenous pyelograms and/or retrograde cystograms are routinely obtained in all patients with suspected retroperitoneal hematomas, if the patient's condition is stable enough to have these studies performed. In the deteriorating patient, however, immediate exploration is performed without obtaining such studies, in order to attempt rapid control of progressive bleeding. Most retroperitoneal hematomas from pelvic fractures will tampon themselves within a short time, and the patient's condition will remain stable and the hematocrit normal, perhaps after transfusion of several units of blood.

TREATMENT. It has been recommended by some that retroperitoneal hematomas not be explored at the time of operation. This nonexploration is considered poor practice, an opinion based on experience which indicates that nonoperative treatment of retroperitoneal hematomas, with the exception of retroperitoneal hematomas secondary to pelvic fracture, has led to an excessive mortality from continued or recurrent hemorrhage from injured retroperitoneal vessels such as the vena cava, aorta, lumbar veins, or renal veins. In addition, it is felt that nonexploration of retroperitoneal hematomas adjacent to partially extraperitoneal bowel is dangerous because of the possibility of missing a perforation in the bowel's extraperitoneal portion (e.g., duodenum). Consequently, it has been our practice to explore all retroperitoneal hematomas discovered during laparotomy for the source of bleeding, as well as for associated injuries to the bowel, kidney, ureter, bladder, etc. This is done regardless of the size of the hematoma or whether it is increasing in size or not at the time of exploration. This policy has not been associated with any complications arising solely from such exploration.

Warnings have been made that if a small hematoma which is not enlarging is disturbed, uncontrollable bleeding may occur. However, it is felt that if such bleeding is to occur, it is best for it to take place at the time of the surgical procedure rather than postoperatively. If major vessels are not explored when hematomas occur near them, major and sometimes fatal postoperative bleeding may occur. Present-day vascular surgical techniques obviate the fear of incurring massive hemorrhage as a contraindication

to exploring retroperitoneal hematomas. This is with the sole exception to the treatment of large retroperitoneal hematomas due to pelvic fracture.

In massive pelvic retroperitoneal hematomas following pelvic fractures, it is often impossible adequately to control multiple small bleeding points. Consequently, it is advisable not to explore this type of massive pelvic hematoma for fear of causing bleeding which may be very difficult to control unless the hemorrhage from the fracture sites fails spontaneously to tampon itself and exsanguination threatens. However, spontaneous tamponade usually occurs.

Seavers et al. advise that ligation in continuity of one or both hypogastric arteries may, at times, control persistent bleeding in the pelvic retroperitoneal space from pelvic fracture sites which cannot be controlled by any other means This will often control venous bleeding from this source, also. Certainly, it is preferable to locate a single vessel which is bleeding and either ligate or repair it, rather than blindly ligate the hypogastric arteries. However, because of the multiple bleeding points from the fracture sites and the large amount of edema which may be associated with pelvic retroperitoneal hematoma, hypogastric artery ligation may be the only feasible procedure and may be lifesaving.

Inferior Vena Cava

By Ronald C. Jones and G. Tom Shires

Over a 10-year period ending in 1968, 84 patients with injuries of the inferior vena cava were surgically treated at Parkland Memorial Hospital. Of this group, 51 survived, yielding a survival rate of 61 percent. There were 14 injuries of the suprarenal vena cava, 18 injuries at the level of the renal veins, and 51 injuries of the infrarenal vena cava (Table 6-8).

Associated retroperitoneal injuries of such organs as the pancreas, duodenum, kidney, and aorta were present in 79 percent of the patients. These accompanying injuries strongly support exploration of retroperitoneal hematomas.

Approximately 70 percent of the patients with injuries of the inferior vena cava were in shock upon admission to the emergency room. Immediate correction of hypovolemic shock was initially accomplished by the administration of balanced salt solution via intravenous catheters placed in the upper extremities. Type-specific blood was then administered if required.

OPERATIVE MANAGEMENT. At the time of exploration,

Table 6-8. LOCATION OF INJURY

	Total	Lived	Died	Mortality
Above renals	14	6	8	57%
At renals	19	8	11	58%
Below renals	39	28	11	28%
Bifurcation	12	9	3	25%

Simple Anterior Repair

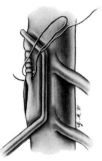

Fig. 6-15. Repair of anterior laceration of the inferior vena cava. Note the use of a partially occlusive clamp.

a midline incision is employed. When the abdomen is explored and brisk bleeding encountered, finger pressure is used to control hemorrhage. Sponge stick tamponade of the major vessels against the vertebral column or digital pressure above and below the injury may be utilized to control bleeding. Injuries of the upper portion of the inferior vena cava are approached by reflecting the duodenum. The lower vena cava is exposed either through the small bowel mesentery or by medial reflection of the right colon. Injuries involving the hepatic veins are approached by rotating the right lobe of the liver medially. Those injuries immediately below the diaphragm are exposed by freeing the attachments of the left lobe of the liver from the diaphragm and reflecting the left lobe laterally. Once the

Fig. 6-16. Repair of through-and-through injury to the inferior vena cava. *A.* Anterior laceration is enlarged to permit closure of the posterior wall from within the lumen. *B.* Rotation of the posteroinferior vena cava.

Anterior and Posterior Rotation Repair Repair

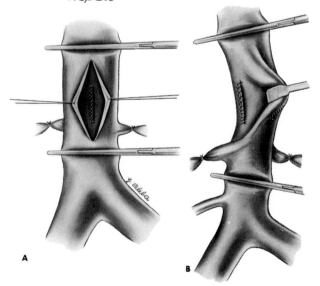

A   B

bleeding is controlled, definitive repair should be deferred until adequate restoration of volume and perfusion is attained.

TECHNIQUE OF REPAIR. Wounds of the anterior wall or tangential injury of the infrarenal vena cava are controlled with a partial occlusion clamp and repaired with vascular suture (Fig. 6-15). Heparin is not administered.

Through-and-through injuries of the inferior vena cava present a more difficult technical problem, but after proximal and distal control is obtained, repair may be accomplished by one of two procedures. The anterior hole may be enlarged and the posterior wound repaired through this opening; the anterior defect is then sutured (Fig. 16-16A). An alternate method of repairing the posterior inferior vena cava injury is by rotation of the vessel. This often required ligation and division of one or more lumbar veins (Fig. 16-16B).

SUPRARENAL CAVAL INJURIES. In the management of suprarenal caval injuries, only two surviving cases have been reported following ligation at this level. Other investigators have reported successful ligation of the suprarenal cava following urologic procedures with nephrectomy for nephrosis or tumor. Ligation of the cava above and below the renal veins was reported by Fitzsimmons and Garvey, but an adjunctive left spleno-renal shunt was performed.

Caplan et al. reported removal of a segment of suprarenal inferior vena cava in a patient undergoing tumor resection. He measured pressure in the distal segment of the inferior vena cava and found it to be 14 cm of saline. A cavagram performed 7 weeks postoperative demonstrated collateral circulation and large ascending lumbar veins. This is consistent with cavagrams performed following ligation of the infrarenal vena cava.

This extensive collateral circulation has been experimentally demonstrated by Wear and by Ripstein et al., and consists of channels through the vertebral, lumbar, azygous, and hemiazygous veins. Some connections with ovarian, adrenal, and splanchnic circulation also occur. Because of collateral circulation through the spermatic and ovarian veins, the left kidney perhaps has a better chance for survival than does the right following suprarenal caval ligation.

Experimental studies by Lespinasse suggest that survival in animals can be increased by ligation of the infrarenal cava whenever suprarenal caval ligation is indicated. He believes that the high survival rate is due to a reduction in the degree of passive congestion of the kidney.

Despite the fact that adequate collaterals are potentially available, ligation of the suprarenal cava is rarely indicated. If a major segment of vein is destroyed, a patch graft may prevent narrowing of the lumen (Fig. 6-17). Autogenous graft interposition is favored in those cases in which extensive venous damage is present and primary repair is impossible. Venous interposition grafts may be obtained from the infrarenal cava or, in some cases, the common iliac vein (Fig. 6-18). These techniques are considered preferable to ligation of the suprarenal cava. In patients with infrarenal caval injury, when primary repair cannot be accomplished or associated injuries are so severe as to require limiting the surgical procedure, ligation is justified. Synthetic prostheses are of limited value because of the high incidence of thrombosis in this low pressure system.

Schrock et al. have advocated the use of an internal shunt for injuries of the intrahepatic vena cava. The shunt may be inserted from either above or below the diaphragm and allow flow through the vena cava while the repair is accomplished. McClelland and Canizaro have employed a similar technique to manage suprarenal caval injuries. The portal triad may be occluded to further reduce bleeding (Fig. 6-19).

MORTALITY. If the inferior vena cava is found to be actively bleeding at laparotomy, the mortality usually exceeds 80 percent. This finding correlates more closely with survival than any other single factor.

When the suprarenal vena cava is injured, or there is an injury at the level of the renal veins, the mortality is twice that of an injury of the infrarenal cava. This high mortality occurs because of the difficulty of exposure and control of hemorrhage. In contrast, injuries of the infrarenal cava are more accessible and produce the lowest mortality rate.

Mortality has been directly related to the incidence of injuries to major vessels and associated wounds of other organs. Twenty percent of the patients in Parkland experience had an associated injury to the renal vessels and of this group, 70 percent died. Of the 33 patients who succumbed of their wounds, 75 percent had from one to four associated major vessel injuries. Death of 23 patients was from hemorrhage. Of patients who had one or more major vessel injuries, 67 percent died; only 13 percent with no associated major vessel injury died.

In managing patients with abdominal trauma, one frequently encounters retroperitoneal hematomas. It is difficult to know the extent of the retroperitoneal trauma until this area is adequately explored. There is no correlation of the severity of the injury with the size of the hematoma or whether or not it is expanding at the time of laparotomy. If there is suspicion of major vessel injury, proximal and distal control is obtained when possible prior to exploring major vessels. An exception to retroperitoneal exploration is the pelvic fracture with hematoma formation and without evidence of other retroperitoneal injury. Release of a large hematoma secondary to a pelvic fracture may cause uncontrollable bleeding from numerous veins and bone fragments.

Quast and associates reported that tamponade of the retroperitoneal wound occurred; if exploration was not performed, there was a tendency for bleeding to recur in the postoperative period after restoration of blood pressure and blood volume to normal. They reported increased late mortality from this cause.

COMPLICATIONS. Transient leg edema may occasionally appear following ligation of the infrarenal cava. Rarely an ileofemoral thrombosis following suture repair may occur, requiring a thrombectomy.

The principle factors determining survival have been: associated major vessel injury, the level of vena cava injury, and most important, whether or not the vessel was actively bleeding at the time of laparotomy.

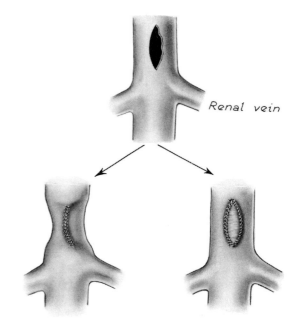

Fig. 6-17. Repair of the inferior vena cava using a patch graft to prevent stenosis.

Female Reproductive Organs

Injuries of the female reproductive organs are infrequently seen following either blunt or penetrating trauma of the abdomen. A series reported by Quast and Jordan revealed only 27 patients with gynecologic injuries in a 16-year period at their hospital. Two of those injuries resulted from blunt trauma with rupture of the uterus in patients who were in the immediate postpartum period.

Fig. 6-18. Construction of an inferior vena caval conduit from the saphenous vein.

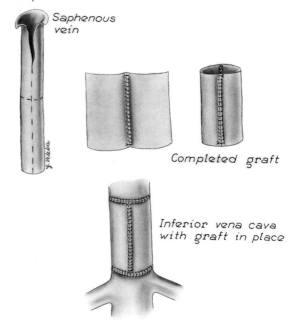

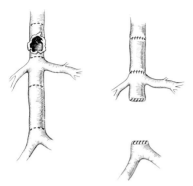

Fig. 6-19. Interposition of an excised segment of the infrarenal inferior vena cava to establish continuity of the suprarenal inferior vena cava.

These are apparently the only cases recorded of rupture of the nonpregnant uterus. The remaining injuries were penetrating wounds. An enlarged uterus was present in 10 of their patients. Six patients were pregnant, two had large uterine myomas, and two were in the postpartum period. No cases of rupture of the unenlarged uterus by blunt trauma have been recorded, however. Rupture of the pregnant uterus due to blunt trauma is rare but has occurred in a number of instances. Of blunt and penetrating wound to the female reproductive tract, 90 percent involve the uterine corpus, and 10 percent involve the remaining adnexa.

TREATMENT. According to Griswold and Collier, the signs and symptoms from a ruptured pregnant uterus are those of abrupt and massive intraperitoneal hemorrhage. Shock is immediate. Associated with these findings are generalized abdominal pain and tenderness, abdominal distension, ileus, and absence of fetal heart sounds and movements. If the patient arrives at the hospital alive (which is not often the case), immediate blood volume and extracellular fluid replacement must be instituted through several large-bore intravenous catheters, preferably placed in the upper extremities, since there may be an interference with venous return from the lower extremities of these patients. The use of type-specific or O, Rh-negative un-cross-matched blood is usually necessary, because massive hemorrhage does not allow time for the usual typing and cross-matching procedures. Urgent laparotomy is necessary to control hemorrhage, even though the patient is still in shock at the time of laparotomy, since the only means of controlling the shock is to stop the hemorrhage. Probably the only anesthesia which will be required is assisted respiration with 100% oxygen administered through an endotracheal tube. Other agents may be added if and when shock abates. The treatment of choice is evacuation of the uterus, closure of the disruption with large chromic catgut sutures, and thorough peritoneal toilet with removal of all blood and foreign tissue.

Wounds of the uterus and adnexa are repaired by figure-of-eight chromic catgut sutures without drainage in most instances, although in occasional patients hysterectomy is indicated, as in injury of the lower uterine segment

and major uterine vessels caused by high-velocity missiles. In these instances, hysterectomy is preferable to an attempted suture repair, since repair could cause stenosis of the cervical canal with resultant hematometra and dystocia. Also, hysterectomy for lower uterine segment injuries is indicated to obtain proper control of bleeding vessels and to help rule out and prevent ureteral injury at the point where the ureter and uterine artery are in juxtaposition.

It is wise to leave the vaginal cuff partially open following hysterectomy for trauma, because of the likelihood of vaginal cuff or cul-de-sac abscess formation, especially if there is appreciable blast injury or concomitant colon injury. If abscesses occur and the vaginal cuff has been left open, it is usually a relatively simple matter to drain the abscess with a finger inserted through the vagina into the open cuff. If gross fecal contamination is present from colon injury, the cuff should be left open and a Penrose drain led out of the vagina from the cul-de-sac. This drain may be secured to the vaginal cuff by a single small chromic catgut suture.

If massive uncontrollable or recurrent bleeding occurs following trauma to the female pelvic organs, it may be rapidly and adequately controlled in most instances by bilateral in-continuity ligations of the hypogastric arteries with nonabsorbable suture material, as recommended by Reich and Nechtow. This will not often be required but should be borne in mind as a very helpful and possibly lifesaving procedure.

Following injury to the pregnant uterus, the loss of pregnancies is quite high. Quast and Jordan reported a salvage of only 1 of 10 pregnancies. The one patient, who was pregnant at the time of a tangential knife injury of the uterus, had a uterine repair for penetrating trauma and subsequently delivered the child uneventfully *per vaginam.* Other instances have been reported in which penetrating uterine injury during pregnancy has been repaired with ensuing normal delivery. Quast and Jordan found that 81 percent of their patients with uterine injuries during pregnancies delivered subsequently *per vaginam* with no difficulty. The cesarean section rate was 19 percent. Of the patients they followed after uterine injury, all who were in the childbearing age subsequently were able to conceive children. In this group, the abortion rate for these later pregnancies was 16 percent, with no apparent cause found.

By far the majority of pregnant patients with uterine injuries will abort shortly after the injury, frequently requiring curettage to control bleeding after spontaneous abortion. Others will require elective emptying of the uterine contents at the time of laparotomy in order to secure adequate hemostasis and uterine repair. Intravenous oxytocin should be given in such instances to aid in uterine contraction and hemostasis after hysterotomy.

Abdominal Wall

Injury to the abdominal wall without intraperitoneal injury is often difficult to diagnose. Muscular guarding and rigidity are frequently present, and it may be impossible to rule out intraabdominal injury until laparotomy is done and no injury is found in the peritoneal cavity. Instead, a hematoma of the abdominal wall causing muscular guarding and rigidity is found. Such hematomas are usually due to rupture of the rectus abdominis muscle or the epigastric artery by direct trauma or severe muscular exertion. The epigastric artery may be injured also by penetrating trauma, so that a hemoperitoneum results, and the patient may go into shock from such an injury because of the severe intraperitoneal bleeding which sometimes occurs. If any doubt exists whether abdominal muscle spasm is due to local trauma to the abdominal wall or to intraperitoneal trauma, the safest course to pursue is to perform a laparotomy, since only in this manner will no significant lesions be overlooked.

The mass from the rectus abdominis hematoma is below the umbilicus in over 80 percent of the cases. To distinguish this mass from intraperitoneal masses, the patient should be requested to raise his head against resistance; the mass should disappear if it is intraperitoneal and remain the same if it is in the abdominal wall. This sign is not completely reliable, and, again, if in doubt, abdominal exploration should be done.

References

General Considerations

Patman, R. D., Poulos, E., and Shires, G. T.: The Management of Civilian Arterial Injuries, *Surg Gynecol Obstet,* **118:**725, 1964.

Shires, G. T.: "Care of the Trauma Patient," McGraw-Hill Book Company, New York, 1966.

Metabolic Response to Trauma

Abbott, W. E., Krieger, H., Holden, W. D., Bradshaw, J., and Levey, S.: Effect of I.V. Administered Fat on Body Weight and Nitrogen Balance in Surgical Patients, *Metabolism,* **6:**691, 1957.

Artz, C. P.: Newer Concepts of Nutrition by the I. V. Route, *Ann Surg,* **149:**841, 1959.

Cohn, I., Singleton, S., Harterj, Q. L., and Atile, M.: New I.V. Fat Emulsion, *JAMA,* **183:**755, 1963.

Coon, W. W.: Ascorbic Acid Metabolism in Postoperative Patients, *Surg Gynecol Obstet,* **114:**522, 1962.

Doolas, A.: Planning Intravenous Alimentation of Surgical Patients, *Surg Clin North Am,* **50:**103, 1970.

Dudrick, S. J., Wilmore, D. W., Vars, H. M., and Rhoads, J. E.: Long-Term Total Parenteral Nutrition with Growth, Development, and Positive Nitrogen Balance, *Surgery,* **64:**134, 1968.

———, ———, ———, and ———: Can Intravenous Feeding as the Sole Means of Nutrition Support Growth in the Child and Restore Weight Loss in an Adult?, *Ann Surg,* **169:**974, 1969.

Elman, R.: Acute Starvation following Operation or Injury with Special Reference to Caloric and Protein Needs, *Ann Surg,* **120:**350, 1944.

Hardy, J. D.: "Surgery and the Endocrine System: Physiologic

Response to Surgical Trauma—Operative Management of Endocrine Dysfunction," W. B. Saunders Company, Philadelphia, 1952.

Krebs, H. A., and Lowenstein, J. M: "Tricarboxylic Acid Cycle: Metabolic Pathways," vol. 1, Academic Press, Inc., New York, 1960.

Lehr, H. B., Rhoads, J. E., Rosenthal, O., and Blakemore, W. S.: The Use of I.V. Fat Emulsion in Surgical Patients, *JAMA,* **181:**745, 1962.

Moore, F. D.: Hormones and Stress-Endocrine Changes after Anesthesia, Surgery, and Unanesthetized Trauma in Man, *Recent Prog Horm Res,* **13:**511, 1957.

———: Systemic Mediators of Surgical Injury, *Can Med Assoc J,* **78:**85, 1958.

———: "Metabolic Care of the Surgical Patient," W. B. Saunders Company, Philadelphia, 1959.

Olson, R. E.: The Two-Carbon Chain in Metabolism, *JAMA,* **183:**471, 1963.

Peden, J. C., Olin, A., Williams, P. T., and Weathers, H.: I.V. Protein Hydrolysates, *Arch Surg,* **87:**59, 1963.

Rea, W. J., Wyrick, W. J., Jr., McClelland, R. N., and Webb, W. R.: Intravenous Hyperosmolar Alimentation, *Arch Surg,* **100:**393, 1970.

Selye, H.: "Conditioning" vs. "Permissive" Actions of Hormones, *J Clin Endocrinol Metab,* **13:**122, 1954.

Shires, G. T., Williams, J., and Brown, F.: Acute Changes in Extracellular Fluids Associated with Major Surgical Procedures, *Ann Surg,* **154:**803, 1961.

Zimmerman, M. M., and Levine, R.: "Physiologic Principles of Surgery," W. B. Saunders Company, Philadelphia, 1957.

Anesthesia

Bastron, R. D., and Hamilton, W. K.: Perils of Rapid Induction Techniques, *JAMA,* **201:**875, 1967.

Beck, G. P., and Neill, L. W.: Anesthesia for Associated Trauma in Patients with Head Injuries, *Anesth Anal (Cleve),* **42:**687, 1963.

Bowers, W. F.: Priority of Treatment in Multiple Injuries and Summation of Surgery for Acute Trauma, *Arch Surg,* **75:**743, 1957.

Clark, K.: The Incidence and Mechanisms of Shock in Head Injury, *South Med J,* **55:**513, 1962.

Crighton, H. C., and Giesecke, A. H.: One Year's Experience in the Anesthetic Management of Trauma—1964, *Anesth Anal (Cleve),* **45:**835, 1966.

Greene, N. M.: General Considerations in Anesthesia for Emergency Surgery, *Clin Anesth,* vol. 2, 1963.

Hamilton, W. K.: Atelectasis, Pneumothorax and Aspiration as Postoperative Complications, *Anesthesiology,* **22:**708, 1961.

Jacoby, J. J., Hamelberg, W., Ziegler, C., Flory, F. A., and Jones, J. R.: Transtracheal Resuscitation, *JAMA,* **162:**625, 1956.

Lee, J. F., Jenkins, M. D., and Giesecke, A. H.: The Anesthetic Management of Trauma: Influence of Alcohol Ingestion, *South Med J,* **60:**1240, 1967.

Nicholas, T. H., and Rumer, G. F.: Emergency Airway: A Plan of Action, *JAMA,* **174:**1930, 1960.

Sellick, B. A.: Cricoid Pressure to Control Regurgitation of Stomach Contents during Induction of Anesthesia, *Lancet,* **2:**404, 1961.

Walts, L. F.: Anesthesia of the Larynx in the Patient with a Full Stomach, *JAMA*, **192:**705, 1965.

Principles in the Management of Wounds

Alexander, J. W., Kaplan, J. Z., and Altemeier, W. A.: Role of Suture Materials in the Development of Wound Infection, *Ann Surg*, **165:**192, 1967.

Allen, K. G., Harkins, H. N., Moyer, C. A., and Rhoads, J. E.: "Surgery Principles and Practice," J. B. Lippincott Company, Philadelphia, 1961.

Altemeier, W. A., and Wulsin, J. H.: Antimicrobial Therapy in Injured Patients, *JAMA*, **173:**527, 1960.

Artz, C. B., Barnett, W. O., and Grogan, J. B.: Further Studies concerning the Pathogenesis and Diagnosis of Peritonitis, *Ann Surg*, **155:**756, 1962.

Burke, J. F.: The Effective Period of Preventive Antibiotic Action in Experimental Incisions and Dermal Lesions, *Surgery*, **50:**161, 1961.

Cohn, I., Jr., and Kotler, A. N.: Intraperitoneal Kanamycin, *Ann Surg*, **155:**532, 1962.

Condie, J. P., and Ferguson, D. J.: Experimental Wound Infections: Contamination versus Surgical Technique, *Surgery*, **50:**367, 1961.

Crawford, D. T., and Ketcham, A. S.: Late Complications of Wire Sutures and Some Causative Factors, *Am J Surg*, **106:**898, 1963.

Douglas, D. M.: The Healing of Aponeurotic Incisions, *Br J Surg*, **40:**79, 1952.

Dunphy, J. E., and Jackson, D. S.: Practical Applications of Experimental Studies in the Care of the Primarily Closed Wounds, *Am J Surg*, **104:**273, 1962.

Houston, A. N., Roy, W. A., Faust, R. A., and Ewin, D. M.: Tetanus Prophylaxis in the Treatment of Puncture Wounds of Patients in the Deep South, *J Trauma*, **2:**439, 1962.

Localio, S. A., Lowman, E. W., and Gibson, J.: Wound Healing in the Paraplegic Patient, *Surgery*, **44:**625, 1958.

Mann, L. S., and Levin, M. J.: Respiratory Depression with Intraperitoneal Neomycin, *Arch Surg*, **81:**690, 1960.

———, Spinazzola, A. J., Lindesmith, G. G., Levine, M. J., and Kuzerepa, W.: Disruption of Abdominal Wounds, *JAMA*, **180:**99, 1962.

Ollodart, R., and Mansberger, A. R.: The Effect of Hypovolemic Shock and Bacterial Defense, *Am J Surg*, **110:**302, 1965.

Peterson, L. W.: Prophylaxis of Wound Infection, *Arch Surg*, **50:**177, 1945.

Robertson, W. H.: Postoperative Wound Disruption, *Am Practitioner Dig Treat*, **9:**1615, 1958.

Rosen, R. G., and Enquist, I. F.: The Healing Wound in Experimental Diabetes, *Surgery*, **50:**525, 1961.

Singleton, A. O., Jr., David, D., and Julian, J.: The Prevention of Wound Infection following Contamination with Colon Organisms, *Surg Gynecol Obstet*, **108:**389, 1959.

Sisson, R., Lang, S., Serkes, K., and Parevia, M. D.: Comparison of Wound Healing in Various Nutritional Deficiency States, *Surgery*, **44:**613, 1958.

Smith, P. S.: Management of Abdominal Incision: A Survey of Current Practices, *Arch Surg*, **88:**515, 1964.

Spencer, F. C., Sharp, E. H., and Jude, J. R.: Experiences with Wire Closure of Abdominal Incisions in 293 Selected Patients, *Surg Gynecol Obstet*, **117:**235, 1963.

Thorngate, S., and Ferguson, D. J.: Effect of Tension on Healing of Aponeurotic Wounds, *Surgery*, **44:**619, 1958.

Wagner, D. H.: Errors in the Choice of Abdominal Wall Incisions and in Their Closure, *Surg Clin North Am*, **38:**175, 1958.

Bites and Stings of Animals and Insects

Bitseff, E. L., Garoni, W. J., Hardison, C. D., and Thompson, J. M.: The Management of Stingray Injuries of the Extremities, *South Med J*, **63:**417, 1970.

Constantine, D. G.: Rabies Transmission by Nonbite Toute, *Public Health Rept (US)*, **77:**287, 1962.

Davidson, T.: Inside World of the Honeybee, *Natl Geograph*, **154:**188, 1959.

Dillaha, C. J., Jansen, G. T., Honeycutt, W. M., and Hayden, C. R.: North American Loxocelism, *JAMA*, **188:**33, 1964.

Fardon, D. W., Wingo, C. W., Robinson, D. W., and Masters, F. W.: The Treatment of Brown Spider Bites, *Plast Reconstr Surg*, **40:**482, 1967.

Farrar, W. E., Warner, A. R., and Vivona, S.: Pre-exposure Immunization against Rabies Using Duck-Embryo Vaccine, *Milit Med*, **129:**960, 1964.

Gill, K. A.: The Evaluation of Cryotherapy in the Treatment of Snake Envenomization, *South Med J*, **63:**552, 1970.

Girard, K. F., Hitchcock, H. B., Edsall, G., and MacCready, R. A.: Rabies in Bats in Sourthern New England, *N Engl J Med*, **272:**75, 1965.

Goldwasser, R. A., and Kissling, R. E.: Fluorescent Antibody. Staining of Street and Fixed Rabies Virus Antigens, *Proc Soc Exp Biol Med*, **98:**219, 1958.

———, ———, and Carski, T. R.: Fluorescent Antibody Staining of Rabies Virus Antigens in the Salivary Glands of Rabid Animals, *Bull WHO*, **20:**579, 1959.

Hattwick, M. A. W., Weis, T. T., Stechschulte, C. J., Baer, G. M., and Gregg, M. B.: Recovery from Rabies: A Case Report, *Ann Intern Med*, **76:**931, 1972.

Hershey, F. B., and Aulenbacher, C. E.: Surgical Treatment of Brown Spider Bites, *Ann Surg*, **170:**300, 1969.

Hildreth, E. A.: Review: Prevention of Rabies, *Ann Intern Med*, **58:**833, 1963.

Insect Allergy Committee of the American Academy of Allergy: Insect-Sting Allergy, *JAMA*, **193:**109, 1965.

Langlois, C.: Allergic Reaction to Insect Stings, *Postgrad Med*, **45:**190, May, 1969.

Levine, M. I.: Insect Stings, *JAMA*, **217:**964, 1971.

McCollough, N. C., and Gennard, J. F., Jr.: Evaluation of Venomous Snake Bite in Southern United States, *J Fla Med Assoc*, **49:**959, 1963.

McQueen, J. L., Lewis, A. L., and Schneider, N. J.: Rabies Diagnosis by Fluorescent Antibody, *Am J Public Health*, **50:**1743, 1960.

Marr, J. J.: Portuguese Man-of-War Envenomization, *JAMA*, **199:**115, 1967.

Owen, C.: Poisoning by Venomous Animals, *Am J Med*, **42:**107, 1967.

Parrish, H. M.: Fatalities from Venomous Animals, *Am J Med Sci*, **245:**129, 1963.

———: Intravenous Antivenin in Clinical Snake Venom Poisoning, *Mo Med*, **60:**240, 1963.

———: Texas Snakebite Statistics, *Tex State J Med*, **60:**592, 1964.

————: Incidence of Treated Snakebites in the United States, *Public Health Rept (US),* **81:**269, 1966.

———— and Carr, C. A.: Bites by Copperheads in the United States, *JAMA,* **201:**927, 1967.

———— and Schwichtenberg, A. E.: Treatment of Venomous Snakebites: Fiction versus Fact, *Med Times,* **97:**153, 1969.

Paton, B. C.: Bites: Human, Dog, Spider and Snake, *Surg Clin North Am,* **43:**537, 1963.

Portuguese Man-of-War, *JAMA,* **192:**994, 1965. (Editorial.)

Recommendations of the Public Health Service Advisory Committee on Immunization Practices, October, 1969.

Russell, F. E.: Injuries by Venomous Animals in the United States, *JAMA,* **177:**903, 1961.

————: Portuguese Man-of-War Sting, *Mod Med,* **34:**121, 1966.

———— and Emery, J. A.: Effects of Corticosteroids on Lethality of *Ancistrodon Contortrix* Venom, *Am J Med Sci,* **241:**135/507, 1961.

———— and ————: Incision and Suction following Injection of Rattlesnake Venom, *Am J Med Sci,* **241:**66, 1961.

———— and Lewis, R. D.: Evaluation of the Current Status of Therapy for Stingray Injuries, in E. E. Buckley and N. Porges (eds.), "Venoms," p. 43, American Association for the Advancement of Science, Washington, 1956.

————, Quilligan, J. J., Jr., and Rao, S. J.: Snake Bite, *JAMA,* **195:**596, 1966.

Schnaper, H. W.: The Emergency Therapy of Poisonous Snakebite, *Med Clin North Am,* **46:**575, 1962.

Shaffer, J. H.: Stinging Insects: A Threat to Life, *JAMA,* **177:**473, 1961.

Sikes, R. K.: Guidelines for the Control of Rabies, *Am J Public Health,* **60:**1133, 1970.

Snakebite Symposium, *J Fla Med Assoc,* **55:**307, 1968.

Snyder, C. C., and Knowles, R. P.: Snake Bite! *Consultant (SKF),* **3:**44, 1963.

Sparger, C. F.: Problems in the Management of Rattlesnake Bites, *Arch Surg,* **98:**13, 1969.

Stahnke, H. L., and McBride, A.: Snake Bite and Cryotherapy, *J Occup Med,* **8:**72, 1966.

Steele, J. H.: Rabies in Man and Animals, *J La State Med Soc,* **114:**427, 1962.

U.S. Department of Health, Education, and Welfare, Public Health Service, unpublished vital statistics.

————, Center for Disease Control Zoonoses Surveillance: Annual Summary Rabies, 1971.

Wood, J. T., Hoback, W. W., and Gran, T. W.: Treatment of Snake Venom Poisoning with ACTH and Cortisone, *Va Med Mon,* **82:**130, 1955.

Penetrating Wounds of the Neck and Thoracic Inlet

Ashworth, C., Williams, L. F., and Byrne, J. J.: Penetrating Wounds of the Neck, *Am J Surg,* **121:**387, 1971.

Brawley, R. K., Murray, G. F., Crisler, C., and Cameron, J. L.: Management of Wounds of the Innominate, Subclavian and Axillary Blood Vessels, *Surg Gynecol Obstet,* **130:**1130, 1970.

Bricker, D. L., Noon, G. P., Beall, A. C., Jr., and DeBakey, M. E.: Vascular Injuries of the Thoracic Outlet, *J Trauma,* **10:**1, 1970.

Fitchett, V. H., Pomerantz, M., Butsch, D. W., Simon, R., and Eiseman, B.: Penetrating Wounds of the Neck, *Arch Surg,* **99:**307, 1969.

Fogelman, M. J., and Stewart, R. D.: Penetrating Wounds of the Neck, *Am J Surg,* **91:**581, 1956.

Hubay, C. A.: Soft Tissue Injuries of the Cervical Region, *Surg Gynecol Obstet,* **111:**511, 1960.

Hunt, T. K., Blaisdell, F. W., and Okimoto, J.: Vascular Injuries of the Base of the Neck, *Arch Surg,* **98:**586, 1969.

Imamoglu, K., Read, R. C., and Huebl, H. C.: Cervicomediastinal Vascular Injury, *Surgery,* **61:**274, 1967.

Jones, R. F., Terrell, J. C., and Salyer, K. E.: Penetrating Wounds of the Neck: An Analysis of 274 Cases, *J Trauma,* **7:**228, 1967.

Shirkey, A. L., Beall, A. C., and DeBakey, M. E.: Surgical Management of Penetrating Wounds of the Neck, *Arch Surg,* **86:**955, 1963.

Steenburg, R. W., and Ravitch, M. M.: Cervico-thoracic Approach for Subclavian Vessel Injury from Compound Fracture of the Clavicle: Considerations of Subclavian-Axillary Exposures, *Ann Surg,* **157:**839, 1963.

Stone, H. H., and Callahan, G. S.: Soft Tissue Injuries of the Neck, *Surg Gynecol Obstet,* **117:**745, 1963.

Abdominal Trauma

Backwinkel, K.: Rupture of the Rectus Abdominis Muscle, *Arch Surg,* **90:**35, 1965.

Baker, R. J., Bass, R. T., Zajtchuk, R., and Strohl, E. L.: External Pancreatic Fistula following Abdominal Injury, *Arch Surg,* **95:**556, 1967.

————, Dippel, W. F., Freeark, R. J., and Strohl, E. L.: The Surgical Significance of Trauma to the Pancreas, *Arch Surg,* **86:**180, 1963.

Barnes, J. P., and Diamonon, J. S.: Traumatic Rupture of the Gallbladder Due to Nonpenetrating Injury, *Tex State J Med,* **59:**785, 1963.

Baylis, S. M., Lansing, E. H., and Glas, W. W.: Traumatic Retroperitoneal Hematoma, *Am J Surg,* **103:**477, 1962.

Biggs, T. M., Beall, A. C., Jr., Gordon, W. B., Morris, G. C., and DeBakey, M. E.: Surgical Management of Civilian Colon Injuries, *J Trauma,* **3:**484, 1963.

Bolot, F., Germain, J., Ponson, R., and Masotte, J.: Blessure par balle de la veine cave inferieure au-dessus des pedicules renaux. Ligature de la veine cave inferieure, guerison, *Mem Acad chir,* **81:**396, 1955.

Bracey, D. W.: Complete Rupture of the Pancreas, *Br J Surg,* **48:**575, 1961.

Brawley, R. K., Cameron, J. L., and Zuidema, G. D.: Severe Upper Abdominal Injuries Treated by Pancreaticoduodenectomy, *Surg Gynecol Obstet,* **126:**516, 1968.

Bull, J. C., Jr., and Mathewson, C., Jr.: Exploratory Laparotomy in Patients with Penetrating Wounds of the Abdomen, *Am J Surg,* **116:**223, 1968.

Burrus, G. R., Howell, J. F., and Jordan, G. L.: Traumatic Duodenal Injuries: An Analysis of 86 Cases, *J Trauma,* **1:**96, 1961.

Buscaglia, L. C., Blaisdell, W., and Lim, R. C.: Penetrating Abdominal Vascular Injuries, *Arch Surg* **99:**764, 1969.

Butler, E., and Carlson, E.: Pain in Testicle, Symptoms of Retroperitoneal Traumatic Rupture of Duodenum, *Am J Surg,* **11:**118, 1931.

Canizaro, P. C., Fitts, C. T., and Sawyer, R. B.: Diagnostic Abdominal Paracentesis: A Proposed Adjunctive Measure, *U.S. Army Surg Res Unit Annl Rept,* June, 1964.

Caplan, B. B., Halasz, N. A., and Bloomer, W. E.: Resection and

Ligation of the Suprarenal Inferior Vena Cava, *J Urol,* **92:**25, 1964.

Cassebaum, W. H., Bukanz, S. L., Baum, V., and Azzi, E.: Ligation of the Inferior Vena Cava above the Renal Vein of a Sole Kidney with Recovery, *Am J Surg,* **113:**667, 1967.

Cattell, R. B., and Braasch, J. W.: A Technique for the Exposure of the Third and Fourth Portions of the Duodenum, *Surg Gynecol Obstet,* **111:**379, 1960.

Chunn, C. F.: Wounds of the Rectum, *Surg Clin,* 1960, p. 1649.

Clark, K.: The Incidence and Mechanisms of Shock in Head Injury, *South Med J,* **55:**513, 1962.

Cleveland, H. C., and Waddell, W. R.: Retroperitoneal Rupture of the Duodenum Due to Nonpenetrating Trauma, *Surg Clin North Am,* **43:**413, 1963.

———, Reinschmidt, J. S., and Waddell, W. R.: A Study of Traumatic Pancreatitis; An Increasing Problem, *Surg Clin North Am,* **43:**401, 1963.

Cohn, I., Jr.: Intraluminal Antibiotic Administration following Surgery of the Colon, *Am J Surg,* **103:**18, 1962.

———, Hawthorne, H. R., and Frabese, A. S.: Retroperitoneal Rupture of the Duodenum in Nonpenetrating Abdominal Trauma, *Am J Surg,* **84:**293, 1952.

Cornell, W. P., Ebert, P. A., Greenfield, L. J., and Zuidema, G. D.: A New Nonoperative Technique for the Diagnosis of Penetrating Injuries to the Abdomen, *J Trauma,* **7:**307, 1967.

Counseller, V. S. and McCormack, C. J.: Subcutaneous Perforation of Jejunum, *Ann Surg,* **102:**365, 1935.

Crosthwait, R. W., Allen, J. E., Murga, F., Beall, A., and DeBakey, M. E.: The Surgical Management of 640 Consecutive Liver Injuries in Civilian Practice, *Surg Gynecol Obstet,* **114:**640, 1962.

Donovan, A. J., and Hagen, W. E.: Traumatic Perforation of the Duodenum, *Am J Surg,* **111:**341, 1966.

Doubilet, H., and Mulholland, H. F.: Some Observations of the Treatment of Trauma to the Pancreas, *Am J Surg,* **105:**741, 1963.

Drapanas, T., and McDonald, J.: Peritoneal Tap in Abdominal Trauma, *Surgery,* **100:**22, 1960.

Feldman, E. A.: Injury to the Hepatic Vein, *Am J Surg,* **11:**244, 1966.

Felson, B., and Levin, E. J.: Intramural Hematoma of the Duodenum: Diagnostic Roentgen Sign, *Radiology,* **63:**828, 1954.

Fitzgerald, J. B., Crawford, E., and DeBakey, M. E.: Surgical Considerations of Abdominal Injuries: Analysis of 200 Cases, *Am J Surg,* **100:**22, 1960.

Fitzsimons, L. E., and Garvey, F. K.; Inferior Vena Caval Injury: Case Report, *J Urol,* **82:**285, 1959.

Fogelman, M. F., and Robison, L. J.: Wounds of the Pancreas, *Am J Surg,* **101:**698, 1961.

Foley, W. J., Gaines, R. D., and Fry, W. J.: Pancreaticoduodenectomy for Severe Trauma to the Head of the Pancreas and the Associated Structures: Report of Three Cases, *Ann Surg,* **170:**759, 1969.

Freeark, R. J.: Role of Angiography in the Management of Multiple Injuries, *Surg Gynecol Obstet,* **128:**761, 1969.

———, Kane, J. M., Folk, F. A., and Baker, R. J.: Traumatic Disruption of the Head of the Pancreas, *Arch Surg,* **91:**5, 1965.

Giddings, W. P., and McDaniel, J. R.: Wounds of the Jejunum and Ileum, in "Surgery of World War II," chap. 19, Office of the Surgeon General, Washington, 1955.

——— and Wolff, L. H.: Penetrating Wounds of the Stomach, Duodenum, and Small Intestine, *Surg Clin North Am,* **38:**1605, 1958.

Gonzalez, E., Leiter, E., Jemerin, E. E., and Brendler, H.: Renal Survival after Renal Vein Ligation, *JAMA,* **200:**171, 1967.

Graham, A. S.: Penetrating Wounds of the Colon, *Surg Clin,* 1960, p. 1639.

Griswold, R. A., and Collier, H. S.: Blunt Abdominal Trauma, *Surg Gynecol Obstet,* **112:**309, 1961.

Haddad, G. H., Pizzi, W. F., Fleishmann, E. P., and Moynahan, J. M.: Abdominal Signs and Sinograms as Dependable Criteria for the Selective Management of Stabwounds of the Abdomen, *Ann Surg,* **172:**61, 1970.

Hannon, D. W., and Sprafka, J.: Resection for Traumatic Pancreatitis, *Ann Surg,* **146:**136, 1957.

Hinshaw, D. B., Turner, G. R., and Carter, R.: Transection of the Common Bile Duct Caused by Nonpenetrating Trauma, *Am J Surg,* **104:**104, 1962.

Hinton, J. W.: Injuries to Abdominal Viscera: Their Relative Frequency and Their Management, *Ann Surg,* **90:**351, 1929.

Jones, R. C., and Shires, G. T.: The Management of Pancreatic Injuries, *Arch Surg,* **90:**502, 1965.

———, McClelland, R. N., Zedlitz, W. H., and Shires, G. T.: Difficult Closures of the Duodenal Stump, *Arch Surg,* **94:**696, 1967.

——— and Shires, G. T.: Pancreatic Trauma, *Arch Surg,* **102:**424, 1971.

Jordan, G. L., Burns, G. R., and Howell, J. F.: Surgical Management of Pancreatic Injuries, *Am J Trauma,* **1:**32, 1940.

Kerry, R. L., and Glas, W. W.: Traumatic Injuries of the Pancreas and Duodenum, *Arch Surg,* **85:**133, 1962.

King, J. C.: Trauma to the Abdominal and Retroperitoneal Viscera As It Concerns the Radiologist, *Southern Med J,* **49:**109, 1956.

Knopp, L. M., and Harkins, H. N.: Traumatic Rupture of the Normal Spleen, *Surgery,* **35:**493, 1954.

Kobold, E. E., and Thal, A. P.: A Simple Method for the Management of Experimental Wounds of the Duodenum, *Surg Gynecol Obstet,* **116:**340, 1963.

Lane, T. C., Johnson, H. C., and Walker, H. S. J., Jr.: Extrahepatic Biliary Decompression in Traumatized Canine Livers, *Surgery,* **62:**1039, 1967.

Lauritzen, G. K.: Subcutaneous Retroperitoneal Duodenal Rupture, *Acta Chir Scand,* **96:**97, 1947.

Lespinasse, V.: Ligation of the Vena Cava above the Renal Veins with or without Nephrectomy, *Q Bull Northwestern Med School,* **21:**312, 1947.

Letton, A. H., and Wilson, J. P.: Traumatic Severance of Pancreas Treated by Roux-y Anastomosis, *Surg Gynecol Obstet,* **109:**473, 1959.

Longmire, W. P., and Marable, S. A.: Clinical Experiences with Major Hepatic Resections, *Ann Surg,* **154:**460, 1961.

Lucas, C. E.: What Is the Role of Biliary Drainage in Liver Trauma? *Am J Surg,* **120:**509, 1970.

——— and Walt, A. J.: Critical Decisions in Liver Trauma, *Arch Surg,* **101:**277, 1970.

McClelland, R. N., and Shires, T.: Management of Liver Trauma in 259 Consecutive Patients, *Ann Surg,* **161:**248, 1965.

———, ——— and Poulos, E.: Hepatic Resection for Massive Trauma, *J Trauma,* **4:**282, 1964.

————, Jones, R. C., Shires, G. T., and Perry, M. O.: Trauma to the Abdomen, in G. T. Shires (ed.), "Care of the Trauma Patient," McGraw-Hill, New York, 1966, chap. 18.

————, Canizaro, P. C., and Shires, G. T.: Repair of Hepatic Venous Intrahepatic Vena Caval and Portal Venous Injuries, in Madding, G. F. and Kennedy, P. A., "Trauma to the Liver," 2d ed., Saunders, Philadelphia, 1971, chap. 10, pp. 146–153.

Madding, G. F., Lawrence, K. B., and Kennedy, P. A.: War Wounds of the Liver, *Tex J Med,* **42:**267, 1946.

———— and Kennedy, P. A.: "Trauma to the Liver," W. B. Saunders Company, Philadelphia, 1971.

Martin, L. W., Henderson, B. M., and Welsh, N.: Disruption of the Head of the Pancreas Caused by Blunt Trauma in Children: A Report of Two Cases Treated with Primary Repair of the Pancreatic Duct, *Surgery,* **63:**697, 1968.

Matthewson, C., Jr., and Halter, B. L.: Traumatic Pancreatitis With and Without Associated Injuries, *Am J Surg,* **83:**409, 1952.

Maynard, A. L., and Oropeza, G.: Mandatory Operation for Penetrating Wounds of the Abdomen, *Am J Surg,* **115:**307, 1968.

Mehta, A. R., Rajpal, R. M., and Jussawalla, D. J.: Suprarenal Ligation of the Inferior Vena Cava with a Solitary Horseshoe Kidney, *Am J Surg,* **116:**925, 1968.

Merendino, K. A., Dillard, D. H., and Cammock, E. E.: The Concept of Surgical Biliary Decompression in the Management of Liver Trauma, *Surg Gynecol Obstet,* **117:**285, 1963.

Miller, D. R.: Median Sternotomy Extension of Abdominal Incision for Hapatic Lobectomy, *Ann Surg,* **175:**193, 1972.

Moore, S. W., and Erlandson, M. E.: Intramural Hematoma of the Duodenum, *Ann Surg,* **157:**798, 1963.

Naffziger, H. C., and McCorkle, H. J.: Recognition and Management of Acute Trauma to Pancreas with Particular Reference to Use of Serum Amylase Test, *Ann Surg,* **118:**594, 1943.

Nance, F. C., and Cohn, I., Jr.: Surgical Judgment in the Management of Stab Wounds of the Abdomen: A Retrospective and Prospective Analysis Based on a Study of 600 Stabbed Patients, *Ann Surg,* **170:**569, 1969.

Nesbit, R. M., and Wear, J. B.: Ligation of the Inferior Vena Cava above the Renal Veins, *Ann Surg,* **154:**332, 1961.

O'Mara, R. E., Hall, R. C., and Dombroski, D. L.: Scintiscanning in the Diagnosis of Rupture of the Spleen, *Surg Gynecol Obstet,* **131:**1077, 1970.

Oschner, J. L.: Discussion of Buscaglia, L. C., Blaisdell, W., and Lim, R. C.: Penetrating Abdominal Vascular Injuries, *Arch Surg,* **99:**764, 1969.

Pantazelos, H. H., Kerhulas, A. A., and Byrne, J. J.: Total Pancreaticoduodenectomy for Trauma, *Ann Surg,* **170:**1916, 1969.

Pellegrini, J. N., and Stein, I. J.: Complete Severance of the Pancreas and Its Treatment with Repair of the Main Pancreatic Duct of Wirsung, *Am J Surg,* **101:**707, 1961.

Penberthy, G. C., and Reiners, C. R.: Visceral Injury Resulting from Nonpenetrating Abdominal Trauma, *J Mich State Med Soc,* **54:**1057, 1955.

Perry, J. F., Jr., DeMeules, J. E., and Root, H. D.: Diagnostic Peritoneal Lavage in Blunt Abdominal Trauma, *Surg Gynecol Obstet,* **131:**742–743, 1970.

———— and LaFave, J. W.: Biliary Decompression without Other External Drainage in Treatment of Liver Injuries, *Surgery,* **55:**351, 1964.

Pinkerton, J. A., Sawyers, J. L., and Foster, J. H.: A Study of the Postoperative Course after Hepatic Lobectomy, *Ann Surg,* **173:**800, 1971.

Pringle, J. H.: Notes on the Arrest of Hepatic Hemorrhage Due to Trauma, *Ann Surg,* **48:**541, 1908.

Quast, D. C., and Jordan, G. L.: Traumatic Wounds of the Female Reproductive Organs, *J Trauma,* **4:**839, 1964.

————, Shirkey, A. L., Fitzgerald, J. B., Beall, A. C., and DeBakey, M. E.: Surgical Correction of Injuries of the Vena Cava: An Analysis of Sixty-one Cases, *J Trauma,* **5:**3, 1965.

Quattlebaum, J. K., and Quattlebaum, J. K., Jr.: Technique of Hepatic Lobectomy, *Ann Surg,* **149:**648, 1959.

Ramnath, R., Walden, E. C., and Caguin, F.: Ligation of the Suprarenal Vena Cava and Right Nephrectomy with Complete Recovery, *Am J Surg,* **113:**667, 1967.

Reich, W. J., and Nechtow, M. J.: Ligation of the Internal Iliac (Hypogastric Arteries): A Life-saving Procedure for Uncontrollable Gynecologic and Obstetric Hemorrhage, *J Intern Coll Surg,* **36:**167, 1961.

Richie, J. P., and Fonkalsrud, E. W.: Subcapsular Hematoma of the Liver, *Arch Surg,* **104:**781, 1972.

Ripstein, C. B., Seropian, D., Schor, G., and Levine, A.: Obstruction of the Inferior Vena Cava above the Renal Veins, *Surg Forum,* p. 292, 1952.

Resnicoff, S. A., Morton, J. H., and Bloch, A. L.: Retroperitoneal Rupture of the Duodenum Due to Blunt Trauma, *Surg Gynecol Obstet,* **125:**77, 1967.

Roof, W. R., Morris, G. C., and DeBakey, M. E.: Management of Perforating Injuries to the Colon in Civilian Practice, *Am J Surg,* **99:**641, 1960.

Rydell, W. B., Jr.: Complete Transection of the Common Bile Duct Due to Blunt Abdominal Trauma, *Arch Surg,* **100:**724, 1970.

Ryzoff, R. I., Shaftan, G. W., and Herbsman, H.: Selective Conservatism in Abdominal Trauma, *Surgery,* **59:**650, 1966.

Salyer, K., and McClelland, R. N.: Pancreaticoduodenectomy for Trauma, *Arch Surg,* **95:**636, 1967.

Sawyers, J. L., Carlisle, B. B., and Sawyers, J. E.: Management of Pancreatic Injuries, *South Med J,* **60:**385, 1967.

Schrock, T., Blaisdell, F. W., and Mathewson, C.: Management of Blunt Trauma to the Liver and Hepatic Veins, *Arch Surg,* **96:**698, 1968.

Schwartz, S. I., Adams, J. T., Cockett, A. T. K., and Morton, J. H.: Blunt Trauma to the Upper Abdomen, *Surg Annu,* **3:**273, 1971.

Seavers, R., Lynch, J., Ballard, R., Jernigan, S., and Johnson, J.: Hypogastric Artery Ligation for Uncontrollable Hemorrhage in Acute Pelvic Trauma, *Surgery,* **55:**516, 1964.

Shefts, L. M.: The Management of Thoraco-abdominal Wounds, *Surg Clin North Am,* **38:**1577, 1958.

Sheldon, G. F., Cohn, L., and Blaisdell, W.: Surgical Treatment of Pancreatic Trauma, *J Trauma,* **10:**795, 1970.

Shires, G. T., Jackson, D., and Williams, J.: Temporary Duodenal Decompression as an Adjunct to Gastric Resection for Duodenal Ulcer, *Am Surg,* **28:**709, 1962.

Silen, W.: Personal Communication, 1971.

Smith, A. D., Jr., Woolverton, W. C., Weichert, R. F., and Drapanas, T.: Operative Management of Pancreatic and Duodenal Injuries, *J Trauma,* **11:**570, 1971.

Smithwick, W., III, Gertner, H. R., Jr., and Zuidema, G. D.:

Injection of Hypaque (Sodium Diatrizoate) in the Management of Abdominal Stab Wounds, *Surg Gynecol Obstet,* **127:**1215, 1968.

Sparkman, R. S.: Massive Hemobilia following Traumatic Rupture of the Liver, *Ann Surg,* **138:**899, 1953.

Sperling, L., and Rigler, L. G.: Traumatic Retroperitoneal Rupture of Duodenum: Description of Valuable Roentgen Observation in Its Recognition, *Radiology,* **29:**521, 1937.

Starzl, T. E., Kaupp, H. A., Beheler, E. M., and Freeark, R. J.: Penetrating Injuries of the Inferior Vena Cava, *Surg Clin North Am,* **43:**387, 1963.

Stone, H., Stowers, K. B., and Shippy, S. H.: Injuries to the Pancreas, *Arch Surg,* **85:**187, 1962.

Sturim, H. S.: The Surgical Management of Pancreatic Injuries, *Surg Gynecol Obstet,* **122:**133, 1966.

Sturmer, F. C., and Wilt, K. E.: Complete Division of the Common Duct from External Blunt Trauma, *Am J Surg,* **105:**781, 1963.

Thal, A. P., and Wilson, R. F.: A Pattern of Severe Blunt Trauma to the Region of the Pancreas, *Surg Gynecol Obstet,* **119:**773, 1964.

Thal, E. R., and Shires, G. T.: Peritoneal Lavage in Blunt Abdominal Trauma, *Am J Surg,* **125:**64, 1973.

Thomoret, G., et al.: Traumatic Ruptured Liver: Severe Secondary Digestive Hemorrhages Caused by Arterio-biliary Fistula; Controlled Right Hepatectomy; Recovery, *Nouv Acad Chir (France),* **83:**16, 1957.

Thompson, R. J., and Hinshaw, D. B.: Pancreatic Trauma, *Ann Surg,* **163:**153, 1966.

Travers, B.: Rupture of Pancreas, *Lancet,* **12:**384, 1827.

Trunkey, D., Hays, R., and Shires, G. T.: Rectal Trauma, *J Trauma.* (In press.)

Vannix, R. S., Carter, R., Hinshaw, D. B., and Joergensen, E. J.: Surgical Management of Colon Trauma in Civilian Practice, *Am J Surg,* **106:**364, 1963.

Walters, R. L., Gaspard, D. J., and Germann, T. D.: Traumatic Pancreatitis, *Am J Surg,* **111:**364, 1966.

Warren, K. W., Poulantzas, J. K., and Kune, G. A.: Life after Total Pancreatectomy for Chronic Pancreatitis, *Ann Surg,* **164:**830, 1966.

Wasowski, J. R.: Drainage of the Common Bile Duct in Experimental Injury to the Liver, *Am J Surg,* **115:**787, 1968.

Waterman, N. G., Walsky, R., Kasdan, M. L., and Abrams, B. L.: The Treatment of Acute Hemorrhagic Pancreatitis by Sump Drainage, *Surg Gynecol Obstet,* **126:**963, 1968.

Wear, J. B.: Ligation of the Inferior Vena Cava above the Renal Veins, *J Urol,* **86:**301, 1961.

Weckerson, E. C., and Putman, T. C.: Perforating Injuries of the Rectum and Sigmoid Colon, *J Trauma,* **2:**474, 1962.

Werschky, L. R., and Jordan, G. L.: Surgical Management of Traumatic Injuries to the Pancreas, *Am J Surg,* **116:**768, 1968.

Whitcomb, J. G., and Ponka, J. L.: A Revised Suture Method for Repair of Hepatic Lacerations: An Experimental Study with an Illustrative Clinical Case, *Henry Ford Hosp Med Bull,* **8:**116, 1960.

Williams, R. D., and Sargent, F. T.: The Mechanism of Intestinal Injury in Trauma, *J Trauma,* **3:**288, 1963.

—— and Zollinger, R. M.: Diagnostic and Prognostic Factors in Abdominal Trauma, *Am J Surg,* **97:**575, 1959.

Wilson, R. F., Tagett, J. P., Pucelik, J. P., and Walt, A. J.: Pancreatic Trauma, *J Trauma,* **7:**643, 1967.

Chapter 7

Burns

by **John A. Moncrief**

Heat Transfer and Thermal Injury

Depth of Skin Destruction

Local Results of Thermal Injury

Alterations in Host Defense

Systemic Changes
Cardiovascular
Renal
Pulmonary
Gastrointestinal

Therapy
Sedation
Maintenance of Airway
Intravenous Resuscitation
Tetanus Prophylaxis
Antibacterial Therapy
Care of the Burn Wound

Complications
Pneumonia
Gastrointestinal Lesions
Hypertension in Children

Burns of the Head

Burns of the Hands

The victim of thermal injury presents to the surgeon a picture of altered anatomy which is immediately apparent and which requires skill, patience, and devotion to reconstruct. Of even greater importance, although less often appreciated, are the tremendous physiologic alterations occurring during the postburn period. These are of a magnitude surpassing that of other types of trauma, and the duration of these changes far exceeds that known to occur in injuries of other types. Without an understanding of these physiologic mechanisms to use as the basis for intelligent treatment, little can be anticipated in terms of survival or improvement in morbidity.

HEAT TRANSFER AND THERMAL INJURY

Burns are caused by the application of heat to the body, by direct contact or indirectly by radiant heat. The resulting burns vary only in degree, which depends upon (1) intensity and duration of application of heat, in turn dependent upon the heat source, and (2) the conductivity of the tissues involved, which varies with density, water content, and other factors.

Direct contact with the heat source, such as a hot piece of metal or a flame, leads to thermal conduction. This is the transfer of heat from one object to another, the thermal gradient, or heat transfer, being from the higher temperature to the lower temperature. Should the environmental temperature be higher than the body in question, heat is transferred to the body and under appropriate circumstances can destroy tissue. Conversely, if the ambient temperature is less than that of the body in question, thermal energy is transferred from the body to its environment. If the gradient is large enough, tissue destruction can result from the rapid loss of temperature from the tissues to the ambient environment, as in cold thermal injury. This is seen clinically in patients with frostbite. Only thermal injury due to heat is considered in this chapter.

Inanimate objects, particularly those composed of materials of uniform density and conductivity, respond to the laws of thermodynamics in a predictable manner. Biologic systems, such as the human body, do not respond in a rigidly predictable manner under a given set of circumstances. However, the direction in which the responses progress and the processes by which the body can alter these progressions are rather well understood.

The specific heat conductivity of specific local tissue determines the rate and amount of thermal transfer and thus the speed and degree with which thermal injury may be forced upon the local cells. Water content, local natural oils or secretions of such organs as the skin, amount and distribution of local pigmentation, and the presence of efficient insulating materials such as the cornified keratin layer of the skin are the most significant factors in determining specific tissue conductivity. In addition, alterations of the local circulation have a profound effect upon heat transfer and distribution, not only in local areas but in the body in general. Total heat transferred to the body is of little importance, but the speed with which the heat transfer takes place is critical. If this is significantly greater than the body's rate of heat dissipation, local tissue damage occurs. The speed of heat transfer depends upon the intensity of the heat source and the local conductivity of the tissues.

Inability to conduct the heat away efficiently will result in varying degrees of tissue death. If inefficient conduction is localized, only local tissue destruction or individual cell death may occur, while generalized failure to conduct heat adequately may result in rapid death of the organism. The amount of heat to which the body can be exposed therefore varies considerably according to the circumstances of exposure. In addition, cellular structures of different functional capacities have varying resistances to heat. Damage as a result of heat rarely occurs below 45°C, and between 45 and 50° varying degrees of cell injury may occur. Above 50°, denaturation of protein elements of the cell becomes apparent, and variable degrees of cellular destruction occur. Ultimate recovery under these circumstances is dependent upon the duration of exposure. Above 60°C some denaturation of protein occurs, and above 65°C cell death routinely results as protein coagulation takes place.

While it is difficult to quantify precisely the amount and intensity of heat required to result in a predictable degree of tissue damage, this has been rather well documented for burns due to a radiant heat source. Under such circumstances the amount of heat to which the local tissue is exposed is characteristically expressed as calories per square centimeter per second. Investigations utilizing a radiant heat source reveal that a 0.54-second exposure of human skin to 3.9 cal/cm²/second results in a definite second-degree burn, and increasing heat to 4.8 cal/cm²/second produces full-thickness skin destruction.

The principles previously elucidated can be appreciated clinically if one considers the mechanism by which the thermal injury has occurred in a specific patient, the area of tissue involved, and the duration of heat application to the body surface. Flame burns and immersion scalds are the result of more prolonged contact of the body with the heat source than are flash burns and spill scalds. As a result, the latter have a more superficial area of skin destruction, and the former are characteristically deep burns. The immersion scald, since it exposes tissue to a uniform intensity of heat for the same duration, results in a homogeneous degree of tissue destruction, whereas the flame burn more characteristically varies in the intensity of exposure of different segments of the body and thus results in a mixture of full-thickness and partial-thickness skin destruction.

DEPTH OF SKIN DESTRUCTION

In any consideration of thermal injury, it is imperative that the terms used to describe depth of tissue destruction be strictly defined. Burns are classified as of first, second, or third degree (Table 7-1). First-degree burns are characterized by simple erythema of the skin with only microscopic destruction of superficial layers of the epidermis. This is typical of mild sunburn and is of little clinical significance. Second-degree burns demonstrate greater tissue destruction located primarily in the epidermis but involving areas of dermis and superficial layers of adjacent tissue to varying degrees. While the depth of cellular death

Table 7-1. CLASSIFICATION OF BURNS

Classification	Morphology	Clinical appearance	Cause
First degree	Only superficial layers of epidermis devitalized; dilatation and congestion of intradermal vessels.	Erythema only— blanches on pressure.	Ultraviolet exposure (ultraviolet light, sunburn), very short flash
Second degree	Destruction of varying depths of epidermis with coagulation necrosis; clefting of epidermis with fluid collection (blister formation); congestion and coagulation in subdermal plexus.	Erythematous, weeping, painful. Blisters and bullae often present. Superficial layers of skin can be readily wiped away.	Short flash, spill scald
	Some skin elements remain viable (often only skin appendages), from which epithelial regeneration can occur.*	Remaining skin elements waxy white, soft, dry, insensitive.	
Third degree	Destruction of all skin elements; coagulation of subdermal plexus.	Dry, hard, inelastic, translucent, with thrombosed veins visible.	Flame, immersion scald, chemical contact, electrical

*Initial injury is partial-thickness, with only dermal appendages (hair follicles and glands) remaining, but these skin elements are readily destroyed by infection, with resulting conversion to full-thickness (third-degree) burn.

in the skin itself may vary in second-degree burns, if any epithelial elements remain from which regeneration can occur, the burn by definition is of no greater severity than second degree. Since regeneration can occur from remaining epithelial elements, second-degree burns are described as "partial-thickness." Third-degree burns, by definition, are characterized by total, irreversible destruction of all the skin, dermal appendages, and epithelial elements. Thus, in third-degree burns, spontaneous regeneration of epithelium is not possible. The terms "partial-thickness" and "full-thickness" more accurately describe the depth of burn.

Since skin varies in thickness in different parts of the body and is itself a poor conductor of heat, application of the same intensity of heat for a given period of time will result in a burn the depth of which is dependent upon (1) the thickness of the skin itself in the local area and (2) the existence and degree of development of the dermal appendages (sweat glands and hair follicles) and dermal papillae. Thus in the very old, in whom dermal papillae and appendages are atrophic, and in the very young, in whom they have yet to develop fully, deeper burns result from the same heat intensity that produces a moderate second-degree burn in the average adult. The skin of the back is the thickest and that of the inner arm the thinnest. Dermal appendages penetrate to varying depths in different areas, those in the scalp and male beard being notably deep. Skin from the thickest areas regenerates more readily.

LOCAL RESULTS OF THERMAL INJURY

While it is often overlooked in the consideration of the various organs of the body, the skin is the largest organ of the body, and destruction of large areas of the integument results in impairment of its functional integrity. The homeothermic nature of man demands that his internal environment be regulated within a relatively narrow range. This regulation is one of the prime functions of the skin, and the destruction of significant areas of this elastic envelope within which man lives greatly impairs the homeostatic mechanism, exposing the body to damaging effects of elements of the ambient environment. Were it not for the protective and relatively impervious skin, the water contained within the body would readily evaporate from the tissues, and death by dehydration and inspissation would result. The keratin layers and the lipid content of the skin as well as other as yet unknown factors prevent the passage of water vapor from the saturated tissues to the relatively dry environment. In thermal injury the protective layers are removed in proportion to the depth of injury, and the normal vapor barrier of 35 mm Hg is totally eliminated in the full-thickness burn. As a result, body water evaporates through the area of injury at the same rate that it would from an open pan of water under the same conditions of ambient temperature and humidity. In the second-degree burn there is only a partial loss of the vapor barrier, but evaporation of water still proceeds at an accelerated rate. Thus the insensible water loss occurring in the burned patient is far in excess of that seen in the person with a normal integument. The normal unburned individual evaporates by the insensible route (primarily from the respiratory tree) 15 to 21 ml/hour/m² of body surface. The average adult with a flame burn covering 40 percent of the body surface will lose by the insensible route (primarily from the burn wound) 100 ml/hour/m² of body surface.

This excessive loss of water by evaporation has several important results. Unless it is recognized and replaced by equal volumes of salt-free water, an insidious but inexorable dehydration of the body results. Also, the body is cooled both locally and systemically by this evaporation, since 560 kcal of heat is lost from the body with evaporation of each liter of water. Since these kilocalories cannot be produced from an external source, the metabolic demand upon the patient may be greatly increased under such circumstances. These factors are very important in the consideration of the fluid therapy and caloric intake of severely injured patients.

The skin also protects from assault by the host of microorganisms present in the daily environment. The precise mechanism by which this protective barrier is maintained is unknown, but the results of thermal destruction of the skin and its effects upon this barrier are quite clear. As the result of thermal injury the skin undergoes coagulation necrosis. Varying degrees of thrombosis in the blood vessels within the skin and in immediately adjacent subcutaneous tissue occur. This is most marked in full-thickness destruction. In the second-degree burn, in the absence of significant infection, recanalization of the underlying vascular tree begins at about 48 hours postburn and is complete by the end of the first week. With full-thickness thermal injury to the skin, the vascular-destructive nature of the lesion persists, and the vascular tree does not become functional again in the affected area. At the interface between normal and thermally denatured tissue, however, a granulation tissue barrier, rich in fibroblasts and new capillaries, begins to appear near the end of the second week and is well established at 3 weeks. Infection may severely alter the course of these events.

Subsequent to the thermal injury, microorganisms contaminating the surface of the wound and persisting in the depth of the hair follicles and sweat glands begin a rapid proliferation, which by 48 hours postburn has reached 100 million (10^8) organisms per gram of tissue in the superficial areas of the burn wound. This initial proliferation and colonization of the superficial layers of the burn wound is most characteristically accomplished by the gram-positive organisms, primarily the staphylococci. Gradually proliferation progresses, being most marked in the area of the hair follicles, where the bacterial growth rapidly penetrates through the perifollicular capsule into the adjacent tissue. By the fifth day following thermal injury the gram-negative bacilli are found in significant numbers and by the end of the first week postburn are the predominant organisms noted. At this time rapid proliferation and active invasion of the adjacent subcutaneous tissue is occurring in the uncontrolled burn wound. Qualitative bacteriologic study reveals *Pseudomonas aeruginosa* to be the

Table 7-2. BURN WOUND SEPSIS

Definition

The proliferation and active invasion of the burn wound by microorganisms in the quantity of 100,000 or more per gram of tissue.

Clinical picture

Onset of sepsis rare before third or after fourteenth postburn day. Deterioration of local wound, with red-brown discoid or serpiginous lesions of second-degree wounds and black punctate coalescing lesions of granulations or areas of full-thickness loss with formation of pseudoeschar. Abdominal distension and ileus, disorientation, and terminal hypotension and oliguria.

Microscopic picture

Initial colonization by gram-positive cocci, supplanted by active invasion of burn wound by gram-negative bacilli at 5–7 days. *Pseudomonas* predominant. Invasion primarily via lymphatics, with perivascular and perineural involvement. Visceral metastases late, and death often occurs with infection localized to wound.

primary pathogen, and quantitative counts show the microorganisms to be actively invading the adjacent subcutaneous tissue in numbers exceeding 100,000 organisms (10^5) per gram of tissue; in most instances there are more than 10 million (10^7) bacteria per gram of tissue (Table 7-2).

It should be noted that the mere presence of a positive blood culture is not evidence of burn wound sepsis, nor does the absence of a positive culture militate against it. The gram-negative bacilli, invading primarily by way of the lymphatics, are cultured from the blood only late in the disease, and death often occurs from wound sepsis without bloodstream invasion. A common reason for positive blood cultures (and primarily causing growth of gram-positive organisms) is septic phlebitis resulting from use of intravenous catheters.

The lack of an effective blood supply in the local area precludes any active blood-borne host resistance. Thus the third-degree burn characteristically shows extensive vascular thrombosis and an almost complete lack of cellular inflammatory reaction. In contrast, the second-degree burn shows, by the third postburn day, a patent vascular tree and an active cellular inflammatory response. If infection by virulent microorganisms goes unchallenged, however, a progressive thrombosis occurs even in the second-degree burn with resultant devitalization of tissue. Thus avascular necrosis is added to the progressive tissue necrosis resulting from the proliferation of large numbers of organisms, and the original partial-thickness burn wound is converted to full-thickness skin destruction.

The local circulatory changes in the burn wound are important in the consideration of local or systemic therapy of the burn wound itself.

ALTERATIONS IN HOST DEFENSE

The immediate postburn period is characterized by increased susceptibility to infection related to diffuse trapping of neutrophils throughout the capillary bed. Gradually this defensive weakness fades, and granulation tissue forming at the site of injury establishes a barrier to invasive bacterial growth. Owing to the ability of granulation tissue to promptly provide many phagocytic cells, healthy granulations can withstand bacteria in numbers exceeding 10^7/Gm of tissue.

The capability of the neutrophils to kill ingested bacteria normally waxes and wanes in cyclic fashion. In the burn victim this is often exaggerated, and it is during the periods of depressed ability that burn sepsis develops. Humoral defenses manifest alterations of a different nature. Complement is depressed but not to levels affecting function. Immunoglobulin levels drop rapidly, in part due to loss in tissues. λ-G-globulin (IgG) and λ-M-globulin (IgM) return to normal levels by the second or third week except in cases of sepsis, when the IgG often is quite low. For this reason supplemental γ-globulin is advocated by some. Antibody formation in response to injected antigen varies. An anamnestic response is promptly and markedly elicited by such humoral antigens as tetanus toxoid, but cellular antigens may evoke no response. Prolonged but temporary skin homograft survival may result. The immunologic picture is far from clear, but the persisting antibody-producing capability has been used in limited clinical trials to stimulate active immunity to the major bacterial pathogen in the early postburn period, *P. aeruginosa*.

SYSTEMIC CHANGES

Systemic changes occurring subsequent to thermal injury are rapid in onset, prolonged in duration, dramatic in intensity, and fatal in outcome if not treated or corrected.

Cardiovascular

Major physiologic alterations involve the cardiovascular system, and while the precise relationships are poorly understood, the changes which occur have been fairly well documented. The blood vessels themselves, particularly the capillaries, undergo an immediate functional if not physical alteration, and the substances normally contained within the vascular tree not only demonstrate physical alterations but take part in massive shifts through the various body tissues. In general, these changes are directly proportional to extent and depth of burn. Reversion to normal ordinarily begins between 24 and 36 hours postburn, although it may not be complete until the fifth or sixth postburn day. There is a rapid and massive loss of red blood cells as the result of the direct hemolysis attendant upon the exposure of red cells to extremes of heat. This hemolysis occurs in two phases: Immediate hemolysis occurs in the first 1 to 2 hours postburn and may involve as much as 60 percent of the total red cell mass. In some patients hemolysis has been estimated as being 0.5 percent of the red blood cell mass for each 1 percent of full-thickness burn. Delayed hemolysis occurs 2 to 7 days postburn and results from increased fragility of the spherocytic red cells commonly seen in the immediate postburn period. The magnitude of this loss may be as great as 10 percent of the total red blood cell mass.

Protein denaturation and coagulation occur as the result of exposure to heat, but unless the temperature is extreme (and thus immediately fatal) or persists for long periods of time, the amount of denaturation is not of clinical significance. There does occur, however, some polymerization of the large protein molecules such as fibrinogen as the result of a general response to stress. The marked increase in capillary permeability results in loss of large amounts of protein from the vascular compartment into the extracellular space, with an increase of lymph protein from 1 Gm/100 ml to 4 Gm/100 ml. In contrast, the total protein of the vascular compartment may drop precipitously to 3 Gm with reversal of the albumin/globulin ratio, which persists for several weeks. The rapid loss of protein in the 4 days immediately following burning equals twice the total plasma pool. Half of this is lost from the body through the wound, and the remainder lies sequestered in the extravascular space for 3 weeks or more before being returned to the blood. There is an additional increase in the catabolism of all proteins at a rate twice normal. This also contributes to the low total protein level and the reversal of the albumin/globulin ratio (Table 7-3).

The most significant loss from the vascular compartment in terms of volume is that of the salt water component. While the precise rate is unknown, the loss from the vascular compartment is extremely rapid, and within 3 hours following major thermal injury 50 percent of the total plasma volume can be lost. In the first 8 hours as much as an 80 percent deficit in plasma volume has been measured. With moderate thermal injury (e.g., 40 percent), the plasma volume deficit is in the range of 25 percent, and the functional extracellular fluid volume shrinks between 40 and 50 percent within the first 18 hours postburn. In clinical practice it is more practical to consider that, except for the very large thermal burn, the greatest losses in extracellular fluid and plasma are complete by 12 hours postburn, although some additional loss at a much slower rate may continue for another 6 to 12 hours. Loss into the extravascular space is due to the marked increase in capillary permeability, which is confined to the burned area in burns of 30 percent or less but is generalized in the larger burns. Some substances have been inferentially implicated as etiologic agents, but no precise cause has yet been found. The increased protein concentration in the extravascular space removes water from the vascular compartment simply by reversing the osmotic gradient.

Table 7-3. LOSS OF BODY FLUIDS SUBSEQUENT TO BURN

Component and time postburn	Amount lost	Cause	Result
Red cells: 1–2 hr	Proportional to depth of burn; can be as much as 60%; rough estimate is 0.5% of red blood cell mass for each percent third-degree burn.	Direct effect of heat on red blood cells causing immediate hemolysis.	Loss of red blood cell mass not evident until intravascular volume replenished.
2–7 days	Much less than immediate loss but may be 10% of red blood cell mass.	Delayed hemolysis due to spherocytosis with increased fragility.	Hemoglobinemia and hemoglobinuria prominent in deep extensive burns
Protein: 0–24 hr	Extremely rapid beginning within 30 min postburn; as much as 50% of original protein mass can be lost in first 5 hr postburn.	Increased capillary permeability due to unknown factors (in burn area in 30% burn, in all areas in larger burn).	Decrease in total protein with reversed albumin globulin ratio; increased protein content of extracellular fibrinogen; lymph protein rises to 4 Gm/100 ml.
0–21 days	20 Gm albumin utilized daily (normal 8 Gm/day).	Rate of catabolism of albumin and globulin twice normal; peak at 3–6 days postburn.	Hypoproteinemia.
Salt water: 0–24 hr	Extremely rapid; plasma volume loss can be 50% in first 2 hr postburn and 80% in first 5 hr.	Increased capillary permeability; loss of protein increases extravascular pressure to as much as 200 mm Hg with resulting loss into tissues by diffusion.	Sharp drop in intravascular volume, decreased cardiac output, increased blood viscosity, and decreased glomerular filtration rate.
Salt-free water: 0–10 days	Minimal first 48 hr, then increases to peak at 10 days; loss proportional to area, with loss in children greater than adults; average adult loss 100 ml/m²/hr, in children may be 2–3 times as much.	Loss of vapor barrier of normal skin due to loss of keratin layer and lipids (third-degree has total barrier loss, second-degree and donor sites have vapor barrier of 10 mm Hg).	Dehydration; evaporative loss requires 560 kcal/L, resulting in increased metabolic rate and relative or absolute decrease in core temperature.
10+ days	Gradual decline as wound heals or is grafted; until healed wound is mature may still lose 2–3 times normal.	Normal barrier 32–35 mm Hg.	

In addition to the peripheral changes, alterations in central hemodynamics also are noted. There is a sudden and marked decrease in cardiac output concomitant with increased pulse rate, decreased stroke volume, and a precipitous and marked rise in peripheral vascular resistance. These hemodynamic changes are due primarily to constriction of the peripheral arteriolar tree but also in part to increased viscosity secondary to protein polymerization and loss of noncellular blood components in excess of red cell mass. There is an immediate and profound impairment of myocardial fuction which in major thermal injury can be attributed to a myocardial depressor. This humoral substance, which circulates freely in the bloodstream, is of unknown cause, but it is readily demonstrable both experimentally and clinically. Capable of immediately arresting myocardial contraction, either in the intact animal or in the isolated muscle preparation, the substance is dialyzable, has a molecular weight less than 1,000, produces fluorescence at 420 to 435 mμ, is no known kinin or amine, and is probably identical to a substance demonstrable in the blood of experimental animals subjected to profound hypovolemic shock secondary to blood loss. Prolonged impairment of the peripheral circulation, decreased vascular volume, and pumping against severe and protracted increases in peripheral resistance gradually lead to failure of the unassisted heart. Thus restoration of vascular volume, decrease in peripheral vascular resistance, and support of the myocardium represent the logical therapy for alterations of cardiocirculatory dynamics.

Renal

Acute tubular necrosis following thermal injury has been regarded as a natural consequence but should not be, since there is no major impairment of renal function as a primary result of thermal injury. Renal function tests designed for steady-state situations are difficult to interpret in the presence of the marked dynamic changes occurring in the immediate postburn period. An increase in permeability of the glomerulus in the burned patient is reflected by the appearance of large amounts of protein in the urine. A gradual and progressive increase in capillary permeability permits the loss of increasingly larger molecular components from the glomerulus. By the third postburn day, substances of a molecular weight of 150,000 are found in the urine, but after this period the lesion gradually heals. Although glomerular filtration rate may fall in the first few postburn hours, it rapidly returns to normal levels with adequate resuscitation. Tubular integrity, as reflected in the ability to resorb sodium and chloride, excrete potassium, and differentially handle water, creatinine, urea, etc., remains unimpaired. Thus, with adequate resuscitation therapy, renal function, although temporarily deranged in some aspects, can remain adequate and rapidly return to normal.

Pulmonary

Changes in pulmonary function dependent upon thermal injury are poorly understood, although they are among the most significant changes in the immediate postburn period. Most studies have been morphologic. The few functional studies do demonstrate that in the larger burns an increase in minute ventilation is readily demonstrable by the third postburn day. This rapidly rises to a peak at the fifth postburn day and then gradually declines. The increase in ventilation appears related to the size of burn injury, occurring regularly with burns of more than 40 percent but independently of lung clearance index, forced vital capacity, or changes in static compliance. Airway resistance does not appear to be significantly increased except in cases of inhalation injury. As with other types of major injury, oxygen consumption rises in the immediate postburn period and then gradually declines, but it shows no consistent relationship to ventilatory levels. Arterial blood-gas studies reflect changes identical to those accompanying other types of major injury, with an initial depression of the P_{O_2} to levels below 80 mm Hg and spontaneous return to normal levels by the end of the first week unless significant complications supervene.

It is frequently stated that a "pulmonary burn" has occurred. This misnomer should be deleted from the surgical literature because it implies actual thermal injury to the respiratory tree at some point below the larynx. The fallacy of this is readily apparent from examination of postmortem tissues and an understanding of thermal dynamics. It is impossible to produce actual thermal damage to the respiratory tree below the larynx by inhalation of superheated air: the heat-carrying capacity of air is so poor that the normal moisture residing in the mouth and posterior pharynx cools it rapidly. Studies clearly show that air expired through the larynx is hotter than that which was inspired and subsequently cooled before reaching the larynx. However, if steam, with a heat-carrying capacity 4,000 times that of air, is inhaled, an actual thermal burn of the pulmonary tree can result. Such burns are unusual.

Most patients who have been classified as manifesting "pulmonary burns" were forced to inhale combustion products which are extremely irritating to the tracheobronchial mucosa. This results in an intense inflammatory reaction in the mucosa and submucosa of the pulmonary tree, which is characterized by a heavy inflammatory infiltrate, congestion of the submucosal veins and bronchial arteries, and marked edema of the mucosa with outpouring of secretions and sloughing of extensive areas of the tracheobronchial mucosa. While these changes can be detected histologically in the first few hours following the inhalation of the combustion products, they do not ordinarily appear clinically until the second 24-hour postburn period. The production of carbonaceous sputum in the immediate postburn period, however, should be considered a strong indication that such complication will ensue.

Gastrointestinal

Gastrointestinal changes following thermal injury are readily perceived, but the basis for the anatomic lesions is not clear, nor are many of the functional alterations delineated. An intestinal ileus of varying degrees is frequently seen in larger burns, and it is unusual for a patient with burns of more than 30 percent of total body surface to tolerate oral fluids. The regurgitation of coffee-grounds material is very common in these patients, but it is not necessarily a cause for anxiety. The most significant alteration in the gastrointestinal physiology is that manifested by massive melena or hematemesis of bright blood, characteristically resulting from Curling's ulcer. This lesion, first described in 1842 and until recently considered to occur in only 4 percent of burned patients, can actually be demonstrated in 8 to 50 percent of burn deaths and in 25 percent of the hospitalized burn population.

The precise mechanism of its inception is unknown, but there appears to be neither dependence upon gastric secretory hyperactivity nor preexistent peptic ulcer. The lesions appear to be associated with a marked congestion of mucosal capillaries in the gastroduodenal region. These delicate vessels rupture into the gastric or duodenal lumen, accounting for the early coffee-grounds emesis. The congestion often becomes intense and localized to discrete areas of the gastric or duodenal mucosa, and sloughing of the tissue results. It is possible that this local plethora, along with changes in the character of gastric mucus, could result in local mucosal susceptibility to digestion by normal quantities of gastric acid. Should such a focal area overlie a major branch of the arterial blood supply, exsanguinating hemorrhage can occur. While these local lesions have been demonstrated, alterations in gastric mucus production are yet to be clarified.

THERAPY

Physiologic responses to thermal injury form the basis for intelligent therapy. The response to the injury is rapid, frequently of tremendous magnitude, and often complicated by preexistent disease. Variations in response to injury and to therapy demand close observation of the patient throughout the postburn course. The multitude of problems simultaneously affecting the burned patient preclude a therapeutic regimen which can be followed in a rigid fashion. Each case presents certain aspects of therapy which take priority over others, and this priority may change from time to time, particularly in the first 48 to 72 hours. This does not preclude an orderly approach to each patient based upon sound understanding of physiologic mechanisms involved in both injury and reparative therapy.

Sedation

Sedation is probably one of the most grossly misused aspects of the care of the burned patient. An insignificant burn of a minute area incurred during a common household mishap may be quite painful. Projecting this experience has resulted in an overevaluation of the pain associated with a major burn. If there is full-thickness skin destruction, the intrinsic sensory nerve endings have also been destroyed, and the wound itself is painless. In contrast, the second-degree burn may be quite painful initially. The requirement for sedation is thus inversely proportional to the depth of the initial thermal injury.

Sedation should be kept at an absolute minimum to prevent clouding of the clinical picture, and it is rarely required beyond 48 hours.

Topical analgesia can be quite effective in the burn wound but should be avoided in all but small burns. Applied to extensive burn areas, whether full- or partial-thickness, these analgesic compounds, which are systemically toxic, are rapidly and extensively absorbed.

Because of the massive and rapid shifts of fluid to the burned area from the unburned area, with concomitant impairment of peripheral circulation, any substances administered intramuscularly or subcutaneously are subject to erratic uptake. Such routes should be avoided during the first 4 or 5 days. Analgesics or sedatives must be administered by the intravenous route to assure predictable action and to prevent overloading when capillary integrity returns and edema resolves. Once this resolution is complete, an intramuscular or subcutaneous route is preferred. Barbiturates are frequently ineffective and may result in excitation rather than sedation.

Maintenance of Airway

In thermal injury, as in other types of trauma, maintenance of an adequate airway demands high priority, for without it all other therapy is of no avail. Although actual thermal damage to the tracheobronchial tree is a physical impossibility except after inhalation of live steam, the majority of patients who have sustained burns of 30 percent or more will have some type of airway or pulmonary problem. The reason for this high percentage is only partially understood. Inhalation of irritating combustion products and poor ventilation due to associated injuries, restriction of the thoracic cage by burn and immobilization, and thickened secretions which also may be increased in volume are the more obvious factors. Decrease in pulmonary compliance is known to occur, but gas-exchange problems are initially those of distribution rather than diffusion.

In the past, tracheostomy for all patients who have sustained burns of the face and neck has been advocated. Careful studies indicate not only that this is not necessary in all such patients but that severe and sometimes fatal complications can result. The tracheostomy made through a burn wound frequently results in constant inoculation not only of the tracheobronchial tree but of the peritracheal tissues as well. Well-documented cases have been reported of fatal sepsis originating in the peritracheal tissues and mediastinum, as well as from pneumonia; these fatalities occurred in the absence of significant sepsis elsewhere in the body. Autopsy studies have indicated that in every case in which a tracheostomy tube was in place for 5 days or more, the tip of the tracheostomy tube had eroded the anterior tracheal wall. In virtually every case in which the tube was present for more than 7 days, local invasive submucosal infection was well established. Thus it is imperative that a tracheostomy be done only when necessary and be cared for in a meticulous manner, and that the tube be removed as soon as possible, preferably prior to the fifth postburn day.

There are circumstances, of course, in which a tracheostomy is mandatory. For patients who have obvious difficulty in clearing the tracheobronchial tree of thick or copious secretions, nasotracheal suction should first be tried. The object of such suction, as well as suction through a tracheostomy, is not to insert the catheter tip as far as possible into the lower bronchi and aspirate vigorously, but rather to stimulate the patient to cough vigorously. This accomplishes two purposes: (1) It expands areas of the peripheral pulmonary parenchyma, and (2) it delivers the secretions to the upper tracheobronchial tree from which they can be more gently aspirated. The only thing accomplished by too vigorous suction is further traumatization of the already inflamed, edematous, sloughing tracheobronchial mucosa.

If the secretions cannot be adequately cleared, by the more conservative means, tracheostomy should be done. Also, the individual who has a deep burn of the face and neck may require such a procedure prophylactically. The inelastic deep eschar of full-thickness skin destruction prevents the edema fluid from expanding outward, with the result that the soft tissues of the neck and posterior pharynx swell markedly and can impinge upon the posterior airway. Of even greater importance is the fact that many such patients are nauseated and regurgitate stomach contents. The inelastic eschar, holding the mouth in a closed position, prevents the egress of vomitus, and aspiration may occur.

The tracheostomy should be done under optimal conditions, with good lighting and adequate assistance and in an unhurried manner. Care should be taken to enter the trachea between the second and third tracheal rings. At this level the thyroid isthmus is rarely encountered; it is not high enough to result in any laryngeal stenosis, and it is high enough to prevent the standard tracheostomy tube from riding on the tracheal carina or slipping down one of the main stem bronchi. It is necessary to remove a block of the anterior tracheal wall so that the tracheostomy tube will fit without difficulty and the stoma will not immediately close if the tube is dislodged.

Bypass of the oral pharynx, while circumventing some immediate problems, poses others. During the actual operative procedure, either or both of the apical pleura may be inadvertently opened. The resulting pneumothorax can be fatal if unrecognized. This happens most frequently in struggling children or infants with the incision placed low in the hyperextended neck. Following the completion of the operative procedure, careful ausculation of the chest should be carried out to detect any possible pneumothorax and to determine whether both lung fields are being adequately aerated. A tube projecting down one main stem bronchus and occluding the other will result in aeration of only one-half the pulmonary tree; this frequently can be detected by the coughing or bronchospasm which the patient experiences.

Endotracheal suction through the tracheostomy opening should be done as often as necessary to maintain an adequate airway. Such suctioning should be as atraumatic as possible and aimed primarily at stimulating coughing. It is not unusual for simple catheter suctioning to be inadequate. Under such circumstances, bronchoscopy through the tracheostomy opening should be performed without hesitation. This usually accomplishes more efficient tracheobronchial toilet and more effective stimulation of coughing than the routine catheter suction.

The tracheostomy stoma must not be left exposed to dry room air. Every effort must be made to provide humidified air or oxygen by ultrasonic nebulization or heated mist. Mechanical apparatus providing such moisture requires close attention. The common practice of delivering oxygen to a tracheostomy by way of a bubble water trap is erroneously thought to provide an oxygen source of high humidity; actually, as the oxygen under pressure in the container expands rapidly when it emerges, the gas is cooled to a point at which its water-carrying capability (in spite of the bubble trap) is less than that of ambient room air.

A tracheostomy opening facilitates anesthesia, but this is not a primary indication for its establishment or maintenance. While orotracheal or nasotracheal intubation may be much more difficult in a patient with a face burn, it is much safer. Particularly among younger children and infants, it may be necessary to gradually wean the patient away from the tracheostomy by temporarily occluding the tube for several days prior to its removal. This is rarely seen when the tracheostomy tube has been in place less than 7 days.

Intravenous Resuscitation

Much has been written concerning fluid resuscitation therapy for thermal injury. Most of this has been directed toward modification of the constituent quantities of the resuscitation fluids, both in quantity and in rate of administration, but the basic principles of fluid resuscitation have remained unchanged. Formulas are merely guidelines for initiating resuscitation; therapy must be modified in both type of fluid and rate of administration according to the individual patient's response.

If we consider the extent and depth of burn to indicate the magnitude of thermal injury, the volume of resuscitive fluid should vary in direct proportion to the magnitude of injury. This has been demonstrated in the experimental animal and is readily verified clinically. Therefore, it is necessary to begin therapy with some indication of the magnitude of injury from which to determine the necessary volume of fluids.

The extent of the body surface involved is most commonly estimated by the "Rule of Nines" (Table 7-4). This is arrived at by dividing major anatomic portions of the body into multiples of 9 percent of the body surface area. This is not a precisely accurate measure of body surface area, but more exact measurements involve odd numbers and fractions of percentages which are much more difficult to remember and use and are of little value except for statistical purposes. Variations in response to resuscitation therapy far exceed the variations in surface area measurements by the simple Rule of Nines. However, in estimating

Table 7-4. "RULE OF NINES" FOR ESTIMATING PERCENTAGE OF BODY SURFACE INVOLVED IN BURNS

Anatomic area	Percent of body surface
Head	9
Right upper extremity	9
Left upper extremity	9
Right lower extremity	18
Left lower extremity	18
Anterior trunk	18
Posterior trunk	18
Neck	1

the extent of burn, individual anatomic areas such as the arm or leg must be calculated separately and the total derived from simple summation of the different areas.

Simultaneously with estimating the extent of burn, one must estimate depth. For practical purposes, first-degree burns can be ignored; simple division into second- and third-degree burn is all that is necessary. While specific percentages of full-thickness skin destruction as opposed to partial-thickness are of no exact significance in determining fluid requirements, the deeper burn wound generally requires greater total fluid volume replacement. Also, in the later stages of resuscitation beyond the first 24 hours, the response to colloid replacement therapy may be more significant than with lesser injuries. Hemolysis of red cells will have been more extensive, which will be reflected by a more significant depression of the hematocrit when the plasma volume reexpands.

While much is yet to be learned about the cardiocirculatory response to thermal injury, present knowledge does allow a rational approach. Thus, the intravascular volume must be reconstituted with fluids approximating as closely as possible both the magnitude of fluid deficit and the constituent quantities lost. The loss of plasma into the burn wound can be qualitatively corrected by available colloid in the form of plasma or by artificial colloids (dextran) and salt solutions resembling extracellular fluid such as Ringer's lactate. The quantitative correction of the fluid volume deficit is titrated only by the individual patient's response to the resuscitation therapy.

It is customary to initiate fluid resuscitation therapy on the basis of one of several formulas which are available for this purpose. *It is of no consequence which formula is utilized to begin such therapy as long as this is modified according to the patient's needs.* The formula shown in Table 7-5 was developed at the U.S. Army Surgical Research Unit, Brooke Army Medical Center, and is merely a modification of earlier formulas. The formula shown in Table 7-6 has been popularized by Baxter. He emphasizes that the salt and fluid volumes are almost identical in the Parkland and Brooke formulas but that the rates of administration vary. In the Parkland formula, *all the salt is given in the first 24 hours.*

Until recently, most resuscitation therapy combined colloid and salt-containing solutions such as Ringer's lactate in ratios depicted in the formulas. However, recent experi-

Table 7-5. BROOKE FORMULA FOR FLUID RESUSCITATION THERAPY*

First 24 hours:

Colloid (plasma, dextran)† . . . . . 0.5 ml/kg body wt/% burn
Electrolyte (Ringer's lactate) . . . . 1.5 ml/kg body wt/% burn
Dextrose/water‡ . . . . 2,000 ml

Second 24 hours:

One-half the amount calculated for colloid and electrolyte during the first 24 hr, but the same amount of electrolyte-free water (2,000 ml dextrose/water)

*For calculating fluids, 50% burn is upper limit in adults, 30% in children.
†Unless concomitant injuries demand it, blood is not given until hematocrit level has fallen and need is demonstrated.
‡This requirement is relatively greater in children, being 160 ml/kg up to 2 years of age, 100 ml/kg at 2–5 years, and 80 ml/kg at 6–8 years.

ments have clearly demonstrated that plasma volume expansion in the immediate postburn period, when capillary integrity as a semipermeable membrane no longer exists, depends upon the *rate* of fluid administration rather than the composition of fluids. With significant thermal injury, obligatory loss of plasma volume continues until the rate of infusion *exceeds* 4.4 ml/kg/hour, at which time plasma volume expansion begins. These studies form a rational basis for the use of Ringer's lactate solution as the sole means of resuscitation in the immediate postburn period, and this is the heart of the Parkland Formula. It is important to realize that with this type of resuscitation therapy *only Ringer's lactate solution is given in the first 24 hours postburn.* Since it is mildly hypotonic, no additional electrolyte-free water is required, and serum sodium concentrations characteristically will remain in the range of 135 mEq/L. *In the second 24 hours no electrolyte solutions are administered,* and the patient is maintained on glucose and water. If this therapy does not maintain adequate urinary output, colloid is administered. During this period the capillary integrity has been restored, and the administration of colloid during the second 24 hours results in rapid expansion of plasma volume and a sustained increase in cardiac output which cannot be realized with continued administration of salt water.

While red cell hemolysis may be extensive, particularly

Table 7-6. PARKLAND FORMULA

First 24 hours:

Colloid . . . . None
Electrolyte (Ringer's lactate) . . . . . 4 ml/kg body wt/% burn
Dextrose/water . . . . None

Second 24 hours:

No further electrolyte is administered. Hydration and urine flow are maintained by dextrose/water, and colloid is administered only if it is required to maintain urine output.

with the larger burn, the loss of the noncellular components of the intravascular volume, protein and salt water, so far exceeds it that a rising hematocrit level is characteristic. Under these circumstances, the administration of whole blood is contraindicated. The main problem at this time is not increasing the unit oxygen-carrying capacity of the blood but rather improving peripheral flow. Whole blood would merely increase viscosity and impair peripheral flow, while expansion of intravascular volume by the use of protein and salt water results in a more adequate tissue perfusion. Rapid infusion of solutions free of red blood cells in the immediate postburn period rarely results in any rapid lowering of hematocrit level, indicating the speed with which such substances are leaving the vascular compartment (Table 7-3).

Response to resuscitation therapy is measured by several criteria. In the absence of extensive burns of the extremities, the capillary flow in the digits may indicate the effectiveness of therapy. In addition, the patient's sensorium in the absence of respiratory hypoxia is used as an indication of cerebral circulation. However, the most readily available and most commonly used index of adequacy of resuscitation is the hourly urinary output. This will vary with the type of resuscitation and with the vigor of application. Generally it is recommended that fluids be administered at a rate sufficient to maintain a urinary output of 30 to 50 ml/hour. With the Parkland type of resuscitation the urinary output is closer to 100 ml/hour in the adult and 30 to 50 ml/hour in children in the first 24 hours after burn. As colloid is administered in the second 24 hours or later, the rate of urinary output may rise markedly as a result of mobilization of edema fluid. Under some circumstances this may result in a rather precipitous overexpansion of plasma volume and occasionally pulmonary edema. This is treated in the customary fashion with diuretics, rotating tourniquets, positive pressure ventilation, and phlebotomy if necessary.

While salt and colloid replacement are obviously needed, the requirement for salt-free water gradually increases in the early postburn period. A minimum of 2,000 ml/day is necessary for basal adult requirements, and in the larger burns 100 to 150 ml/m² body surface/hour is average in the adult. Because of the greater surface area in proportion to weight of infants and children, the salt-free water requirement is often as much as 300 ml/m²/hour. Variations in individual rates of evaporative water loss can be readily monitored by following the serum sodium concentration, which is an accurate guide to the state of hydration. Though the normal kidney is capable of correcting many mistakes in fluid therapy, it is wise to consider a serum sodium value above 140 mEq/L indicative of dehydration and one below 130 mEq/L indicative of dilutional hyponatremia.

There are important aspects of burn therapy for children determined by the following facts: (1) the body area is much greater in respect to body weight than in adults; (2) requirements for electrolyte-free water are relatively greater; (3) evaporative water loss is much greater than in adults (often doubled per unit area); (4) renal ability to handle water and salt does not fully develop until the child is one year of age; (5) overhydration and dehydration are constant dangers in the very young. Therefore, infant fluid resuscitation should be accomplished with solutions containing 40 to 70 mEq of sodium. This avoids the dilutional hyponatremia secondary to diffusion of dextrose/water and the hypernatremia resulting from the excess sodium which accompanies normal saline or Ringer's lactate solution resuscitation and heavy evaporative water loss.

Often overlooked in fluid therapy is the need for potassium replacement. Thermal injury impairs the functional capacity of tissue at the periphery of the wound, with loss of intracellular potassium. Of even greater magnitude is the loss by renal mechanisms as a result of the aldosterone response to volume deficit, which initiates sodium retention by the renal tubule and reciprocal potassium loss. When, during resuscitation, large volumes of salt solutions are administered, the kidney is subjected to a heavy salt load. The sodium presented to the renal tubule is increased markedly, and more sodium is retained by the tubule to repair the volume deficit. As the reciprocal relation continues, a greater loss of the potassium occurs. Thus potassium requirements are 80 to 120 mEq/L/day for the thermal injury itself. This is given intravenously as potassium chloride or potassium phosphate by drip bottle, not syringe.

Intravenous administration of fluids to the burned patient must be carefully attended and frequently inspected to ensure against complications. The incidence of phlebitis in the lower extremities is much greater than in the upper extremities, which therefore should be used whenever possible. While it is common practice to introduce small-bore plastic tubes within the veins, these should be removed, or at least the site changed, after 3 days to minimize the likelihood of septic phlebitis, which can be a major problem. In addition, the Foley catheter which provides a means of monitoring urinary output should be removed as soon as possible. Studies have shown that local bladder irritation always occurs when the catheter has been in place more than 5 days. It is rarely necessary to maintain such drainage for that period of time, but if it is required, the Foley catheter should be removed and controlled drainage established by means of an external condom catheter.

An almost universally avoidable but relatively common occurrence in the postburn period is acute renal failure. The exact cause is unknown, but it is probably primarily due to tubular obstruction by protein precipitate, with shock per se a contributing factor. This lesion may be prevented, even after shock, by maintenance of a grossly clear urine output. Conversely, acute tubular necrosis occurs in individuals with normal blood pressure but with large quantities of hemoglobin in the urine. It is imperative, therefore, to maintain not only an adequate volume of urine output but to provide for the gross clearance of the pigment. This can be accomplished most readily by using sufficient volumes of intravenous fluids (water load) to result in a urinary volume in excess of 30 to 50 ml/hour. Once the urine has cleared grossly, the volume of fluid administered can be decreased. On occasion it is necessary to utilize an osmotic diuretic such as mannitol in order to assure initial clearing of urine. The mannitol is administered by syringe intravenously in a single 25-Gm dose in a fluid load of 300 to 500 ml over 30 minutes. If a good urinary response does not occur in the presence of an adequate fluid load, the further administration of mannitol will be of no value, since acute tubular necrosis has probably been established. If a good response does occur, diuresis should be maintained by fluid load alone rather than mannitol to permit monitoring of the rate of urine output. Alkalinization of the urine with sodium bicarbonate or tromethamine buffer is indicated to prevent precipitation of heme pigment.

Tetanus Prophylaxis

Whenever dead tissue is present, clostridial infections, particularly tetanus, may appear. Prior to active immunization against tetanus, the incidence of this disease among the thermally injured was as high as 20 percent. With almost routine use of active immunization in early childhood or infancy, this incidence has been markedly reduced. However, there are still some patients, particularly older females, who have not received active immunization. Under such circumstances, protection against anaerobic infection must be given. The method of choice today is the administration of 250 units of hyperimmune human antitetanus γ-globulin. This will provide protection for a period of at least 6 weeks and can be repeated at that time if the danger of tetanus still exists. If the hyperimmune γ-globulin is not available, one must combine active and passive immunization, administering the tetanus antiserum for passive immunization and alum-precipitated toxoid as the initial dose of the active immunization program.

Antibacterial Therapy

Recently it has been recognized that the primary cause of death following thermal injury is burn-wound sepsis. This entity, which in the past has accounted for 86 percent of burn deaths in a well-studied series, is characterized by the active invasion of microorganisms, primarily the gram-negative bacilli, in numbers exceeding 100,000 per gram of tissue. The avascular nature of the burn wound precludes bloodstream delivery of systemically administered drugs to the local area. Even the natural body defense mechanisms, the leukocytes, are not transported to the areas, as evidenced by their singular lack of appearance in the third-degree burn wound. Also, clinical experience shows that even large doses of multiple antibiotics effective in vitro against the primary pathogens fail to influence the mortality rate in the burn population. Complete withholding of systemic antibody therapy fails to demonstrate any increase in mortality, thus indicating that systemic therapy is of no benefit.

In order for any antibacterial therapy to be effective against the organisms proliferating in the burn wound, the agent must be not only effective against the major pathogens but also nontoxic both systemically and locally, read-

ily available, easy to apply, and rapidly excreted or easily metabolized and should not interfere with wound healing. Since early 1964, two substances have been found to meet these general criteria, although some problems have been encountered in their use. They are 0.5% aqueous silver nitrate solution and 10% mafenide (para-aminomethylbenzene sulfonamide, Sulfamylon*) (Table 7-7).

The 0.5% aqueous silver nitrate solution is applied directly to the burn wound by means of wet compresses composed of 40 layers of coarse-mesh gauze thoroughly soaked with the aqueous solution every 4 hours and changed entirely every 12 hours. Applications are begun as soon as evaluation of the patient is complete and resuscitation therapy has been instituted. Each day, as the dressings are changed, the wound is debrided, and as a clean tissue bed is prepared, the area is covered with grafted skin. A light cotton blanket placed over the patient is sufficient to inhibit evaporative water loss and maintain an ambient temperature which will greatly reduce the metabolic requirements of the patient, compared with those from the exposed burn wound.

As silver nitrate is applied in aqueous solution, the biochemical composition of local and systemic tissues alters. The magnitude of these changes is proportional to the extent and depth of burn and is most serious in children and infants. The changes consist of precipitation of silver chloride, absorption of significant quantities of distilled water, and leaching of body sodium into the wet dressings. They result in hypochloremic, hyponatremic alkalosis which requires monitoring by means of blood pH and blood electrolyte determinations at least daily in adults in the first several postburn days. In small children and infants monitoring can be required as often as every 3 to 4 hours. Loss of sodium and chloride requires replacement by either the oral or the intravenous route, depending on which is feasible. Large quantities of these solutions may be necessary. Also, silver nitrate solution causes a relatively permanent discoloration of the linens, mattress, sick-room furniture, and the patient. Experience is required to distinguish burned from unburned tissue after one week's application of silver nitrate.

Mafenide was initially utilized as a hydrochloride salt but presently is applied as an acetate salt. A mixture of 10% powder in a water-soluble base is applied topically with the gloved hand to the local burn wound. Application is made at least twice a day over the entire burn wound. Areas in which the medication has been removed by bed linens or changes of position are subject to reapplication as necessary. Because of the hygroscopic nature of the drug, a burning sensation of varying intensity lasting from 15 to 60 minutes is experienced for the first 5 to 7 days of application. This can ordinarily be controlled by simple analgesics but sometimes requires morphine or meperidine. There is a 5 percent incidence of sensitivity to this sulfonamide-like drug, ordinarily manifested by maculopapular rash; this usually occurs in the second week of

---

*It is common practice to use the terms mafenide, para-aminomethylbenzene, and Sulfamylon interchangeably; in this chapter the term mafenide is used for this preparation.

Table 7-7. COMPARISON OF TOPICAL ANTIBACTERIAL BURN THERAPIES

	10% mafenide	*0.5% silver nitrate*
Chemistry............	Methylated sulfonamide $H_2N{-}CH_2{-}\bigcirc{-}SO_2{-}NH_2$	Inorganic silver salt $AgNO_3$
Antibacterial activity.......	Bacteriostatic, with inhibition of growth allowing phagocytosis; bactericidal only in extremely high concentrations; precise mechanism unknown	Primarily bacteriostatic with weak bactericidal activity but active in very minute quantities; activity dependent upon liberation of silver ions but specific mechanism unknown—may be associated with protein fixation
Local and systemic effects	Penetrates burn tissue in high concentration of active form Immediately broken down by amine oxidases to inactive *p*-carboxy salt Rapidly absorbed and excreted as highly soluble salt in urine Strong carbonic anhydrase inhibition	Penetrates burn tissue well and ionizes rapidly Rapidly precipitated as silver chloride in local tissues Very scant absorption from tissues; argyria no problem Leaching of tissue sodium and absorption of large quantities of distilled water
Biochemical changes	Acid-salt breakdown product results in heavy $H+$ load Renal buffering blocked by carbonic anhydrase inhibition with high HCO_3 and negligible NH_4 excretion in urine Metabolic acidosis compensated by hyperventilation and low P_{CO_2}	Hypochloremia from AgCl precipitation Hyponatremia due to leaching of sodium and absorption of large quantities of distilled water Hypochloremic alkalosis corrected by intravenous saline solutions
Method of use..........	Applied topically twice daily as 10% of drug in water-soluble base Medication washed off daily and wound debrided	Dressings of 40 thicknesses of gauze changed twice daily and saturated every 4 hours Wound debrided with dressing changes
Advantages............	Wide spectrum of activity Not inactivated by PABA, blood, or tissue fluids as are other sulfonamides Nontoxic Clean and simple to use	Wide spectrum of activity Not inactivated by specific antagonists Nontoxic in this concentration Sensitivity nil Comfortable to patient
Disadvantages..........	Painful to second-degree burn for a short time Sensitivity in 5% of cases Biochemical alterations significant if pulmonary problems supervene	Messy and difficult to use Discolors tissues making recognition difficult Biochemical alterations of serious import in infants and children Requires precise methods for use
Results	Both substances essentially nontoxic to tissues and allow progressive and simultaneous debridement and grafting; with proper use, both result in effective suppression of bacterial growth and elimination of burn-wound sepsis	

therapy and is rarely severe enough to require discontinuation of therapy.

Topical mafenide therapy is begun immediately after evaluation of the patient and institution of resuscitation therapy. As soon as the patient's condition is stable, which even in patients with large burns is about 48 hours postburn, he is taken to the hydrotherapy room. The topical medication is washed from the burn surface and thorough but gentle debridement carried out to the point of active bleeding and discomfort to the patient. The patient is then removed from the hydrotherapy tank, returned to his bed, and topical medication reapplied. As a clean, viable wound surface becomes available, it is gradually covered with the appropriate type of wound-closure material, which is described later in this chapter.

Biochemical alterations occur also with use of this topical sulfonamide-like preparation. The drug itself retains at best only slight traces of activity in the systemic circulation, since it is immediately broken down by monoamine oxidase. Thus systemic toxicity is no problem, nor is systemic activity any asset. Active diffusion of the drug through the burn wound results in large quantities being absorbed into the systemic circulation, and after its breakdown the resulting acid salt imposes a heavy hydrogen ion load upon the buffer system. In addition, the drug is a strong carbonic anhydrase inhibitor, thus preventing active participation by the renal buffering mechanism. This is reflected by a high urinary bicarbonate level, an extremely low urinary ammonia level, and a urinary pH which is on the alkaline side. Under these circumstances, the drug itself and the breakdown product are quite soluble, and there is no danger of crystalluria as there is with the true sulfonamides. An additional manifestation of this acid load and renal buffer block is the hyperventilation which is characteristic of this state of compensated acidosis. Most patients receiving such topical therapy hyperventilate but adequately can compensate for this moderate acidosis by means of pulmonary ventilation. Only when some pulmonary complication develops is the patient in danger of decompensating. Under these circumstances the drug must be removed from the burn surface, systemic buffering by means of intravenous sodium bicarbonate accomplished, and the pulmonary problem vigorously corrected. If ventilatory compensation can be reestablished within 3 to 4 days, the topical therapy can be reinstituted with little danger of losing ground in the battle against burn-wound sepsis.

Biochemical monitoring of blood gases, pH, and electrolytes is necessary in patients who have sustained large burns and are being treated by the topical sulfonamide therapy. It is rarely necessary to obtain such values more than once daily, and after the first week postburn, unless a pulmonary problem supervenes, twice a week is adequate. In contrast to silver nitrate therapy, children and infants appear to tolerate topical sulfonamide better than adults. The precise reason is unknown, but it may be related to lack of preexistent pulmonary disease among younger patients.

Recently another substance attacking the burn wound flora has come upon the scene. Combining the known effectiveness of sulfonamides and the antibacterial properties of the silver ion, this silver sulfadiazine complex presently is being used experimentally. It appears that some binding of the silver ion to the deoxyribonucleic acid (DNA) of the bacteria occurs. As silver sulfadiazine supposedly reacts very slowly with tissue fluids, its release is slow enough to preclude any significant systemic toxicity, and blood levels usually range from 3 to 5 mg/100 ml. Sulfonamide sensitivity occurs in a small percentage of patients, as with mafenide, and absorption is greatest in areas of second-degree burn. Although effectively controlling the burn wound flora in most instances, silver sulfadiazine has been of limited effectiveness with deep and extensive burns, as have the other substances. Usually it has been applied topically, like mafenide. In general, the results have been equivalent to those from silver nitrate or mafenide except with established infections, where mafenide appears to be the most effective of the substances presently available.

Another effective technique which has recently gained popularity is the direct instillation into the subeschar space of large volumes of solution containing antibiotics. The technique is identical to that of a hypodermoclysis. To preclude salt or water overload, one-half- or one-quarter-strength normal saline solution is preferred. Ringer's lactate solution is avoided because its calcium is incompatible with many of the antibiotics. The major principles of the technique include determination of the appropriate antibiotic by tissue culture and sensitivity and the administration of the maximum recommended daily dose to aliquots of 200 to 250 ml placed in the subeschar space by multiple long spinal needles which deliver each aliquot to an area

of approximately 8 to 10 cm^2. Of the antibiotic agents available, erythromycin is not used because subcutaneous administration is very painful, and Coli-mycin, novobiocin, and cephaloridine are not effective.

All types of topical therapy have had rather significant effects upon the overall metabolic response in the early postburn period. Since silver nitrate is applied in aqueous solution and the sulfonamide-like drug is applied in a base which is 63 percent water, evaporative water loss through the burn wound is markedly reduced and thus the caloric demands upon the patients are lessened. As frequent operating-room sessions with general anesthesia and the occasionally consequent anorexia or vomiting are obviated, a more adequate caloric intake can be maintained. Reduced bacterial activity in the burn wound also reduces caloric demand. As a result, weight loss in these patients, rather than being the 20 to 30 percent routinely seen in the extensive burn with prior therapy, presently runs 10 to 15 percent. This is coupled with good appetite, clear sensorium, maintenance of muscular activity and joint motion, and remarkable absence of the odor of acute and chronic infection so prevalent in burn wards in the past.

Systemic antibiotic therapy has not been relegated to the past, since there are specific indications for its proper use in the burned patient. In young children and infants who frequently have preexisting or concomitant upper respiratory tract or middle ear infection, penicillin is almost routinely administered for the first 5 to 7 postburn days. Most patients, children and adults, receive this type of therapy during the first postburn week. Preexisting disease or concomitant injury, such as an open fracture of the extremities or the skull or an abdominal or chest wound, receive systemic antibiotic therapy.

Antibiotic therapy also is directed toward complications of thermal injury such as pneumonia. One of the most common and most significant uses of systemic antibacterial therapy is in the treatment of cellulitis, which may develop to a striking degree about the margins of the burn wound. This is not considered significant unless it extends 2 cm beyond the wound margin, becomes indurated, is associated with lymphangitis, or is quite intense in its appearance. Under these circumstances, systemic antibiotic therapy is directed toward the organisms most frequently involved in the inflammatory reaction, the streptococcus and/or staphylococcus. While gram-negative organisms most frequently predominate in the burn wound itself, peripheral cellulitis is most frequently due to gram-positive cocci. Under these circumstances, initial empiric therapy is penicillin, given intramuscularly or intravenously as feasible, in a dose of 1 to 2 million units/day. If cellulitis is streptococcal in origin, a good clinical response should be apparent within 48 to 72 hours. If this does not occur, the patient is given one of the semisynthetic penicillins effective against staphylococcus. The vast majority of patients respond quite promptly and adequately to this empiric therapy.

Care of the Burn Wound

The burn wound itself usually should be considered last during the immediate postburn period, although a circumferential third-degree burn of the extremity may demand immediate attention. The inelastic, constricting eschar beneath which the obligatory edema continues to form results in venous stasis initially, but as the pressure increases, total obliteration of the arterial circulation results. As a consequence, ischemic necrosis of the distal tissues may develop, requiring amputation of the distal, perhaps unburned, portion of the extremity.

It is often difficult clinically to determine precisely how much embarrassment of peripheral circulation has occurred. The Doppler flowmeter has been of considerable aid in this situation. If flow in the palm or digits can be demonstrated, adequate circulation must exist. However, if no signal is detectable distal to the constricting eschar, circulatory embarrassment may be due entirely to the accumulation of edema fluid beneath the constricting eschar. Elevation of the extremity and active exercise of the muscles to augment the return of fluid from the limb frequently will reestablish the Doppler signal. If this is successful, no surgical intervention is required. However, if there is no palpable or audible distal pulse, surgical intervention is necessary in order to preclude ischemic necrosis of the distal tissues.

Simple splitting of the eschar with the scalpel is sufficient. This can be accomplished in the bed without topical, local, or general anesthesia, as the third-degree eschar is insensitive. Ordinarily, little bleeding is encountered, and rarely does the incision require extension into the fascia investing the underlying muscle. Some have objected to this procedure on the ground of the appearance of clostridial myositis in wounds thus treated. However, the clostridial organisms will not grow and produce clinical infection in the absence of dead tissue. Thus, in those cases in which clostridial myositis has occurred subsequent to escharotomy, this surgical procedure had been delayed for so long that ischemic necrosis of the muscle had already occurred. The object is to relieve the circulatory embarrassment before it has progressed to such a degree. In several hundred escharotomies at the Surgical Research Unit, Brooke Army Medical Center, not a single instance of clostridial myositis or cellulitis has been detected.

If the constricting eschar is located about the trunk, particularly overlying the thoracic cage, marked restriction of excursion of the ribs may occur and cause severe respiratory embarrassment. Under these circumstances also, escharotomy should be performed immediately in a manner identical to that described for the extremities. The incision should extend across the chest below the clavicle and along the costal margins inferiorly, and these incisions should be joined by similar ones extending vertically over the sternum and at both anterior axillary lines. If necessary, another incision can be carried transversely just below the nipple line to allow for further rib excursion. This situation is unusual, but when this type of escharotomy is required, the effect is quite dramatic.

In general, the wound may be treated by the exposure method or by the occlusive dressing method. It may be excised in toto in the early postburn period, with early or immediate graft coverage. Most commonly the necrotic tissue is gradually removed by repeated debridement, with closure accomplished in stages.

Except during transportation, when patients are more comfortable when covered with an occlusive dressing, burned victims are more readily cared for and the burn wound better attended when treated by the exposure method. Any occlusive dressing utilized in the immediate postburn period should be bulky and provide even, resilient, compressive force to the burn surface.

Such a dressing cannot be properly placed about the head and neck without impairing respiratory exchange or encouraging aspiration of vomitus, and the perineum does not lend itself well to any type of dressing. An occlusive dressing placed about the chest restricts respiratory excursion to a deleterious degree and impairs auscultation not only of the chest but of the abdomen as well. Extremities lend themselves fairly well to the application of an adequate compressive dressing, but improper application frequently results in a multiple tourniquet effect, and complete coverage of the tips of the digits impairs evaluation of the peripheral circulation. This method is still used by many in the immediate postburn period.

Occlusive dressings must be bulky in order to provide even compression and absorptive capacity at the same time. The material immediately next to the wound is fine-mesh gauze lightly impregnated with carbowax or petroleum jelly. The bulky dressing is then applied and consists of cotton sheets and fluff gauze. The preconstructed one-piece dressings are by far the best. With the occlusive dressing method, the patient is taken to the hydrotherapy tank every 2 to 3 days, the dressings are removed, and debridement is performed.

The exposure method, sometimes referred to as "open treatment," is so frequently synonymous with "open neglect" that it is in danger of falling into disrepute in some areas. Unfortunately, those who utilize this method merely place the patient in bed carefully surrounded by sterile sheets, totally ignore the victim, and expect him to get well spontaneously. Such a result rarely ensues; the exposure method requires more active supervision of the burn than does the occlusive dressing method.

The burn wound is open, and advantage must be taken of the opportunity to inspect the wound several times each day and care for it as necessary in order to obtain optimal results. Soft areas in the third-degree eschar and crust beneath which purulence exists must be unroofed and the areas cleansed thoroughly with soap and water and allowed to dry. The patient is taken to the hydrotherapy tank daily, the entire wound cleansed gently with soap and water, and debridement of the burn wound carried out to the point of tolerance and active bleeding. As the eschar begins to separate, the exposure method is converted to a partial occlusive dressing method in which wet saline compresses are placed over the burn area and changed every 4 to 8 hours depending upon the nursing facilities available. The dressings are initially wet with saline solution, which is then allowed to evaporate slowly. Gentle but active debridement results from removal of the dressings, and the wound can be rapidly cleansed.

In large burns, one trip to the operating room is necessary for active surgical debridement of the burn wound to remove eschar, which may be densely adherent in many areas. The entire burn wound is subsequently covered with relatively light occlusive dressings. With small wounds, the entire debriding process can be completed by wet dressings.

HOMOGRAFTING

As the burn wound gradually is cleared of its necrotic tissue, some type of closure must be accomplished. None of the synthetic skin coverings are of value. To date there is still no substitute for skin, but it is not necessary to use the patient's own skin initially, particularly when only small patches can be covered at a time and the risk of graft loss is great. Under these circumstances, homograft obtained from cadaver donors is placed over the areas from which necrotic tissue has been removed. Debridement continues each day, with more and more of the eschar being removed and replaced by homograft. None of the homograft is allowed to remain in place more than 3 to 4 days, and frequently it must be removed sooner because of graft failure or purulent collections beneath it.

The homograft can be placed over a freshly debrided wound in the absence of any significant granulation tissue if the majority of necrotic eschar has been removed. Small amounts of eschar remaining behind, however, can result in rapid purulent collections beneath a graft; the graft must then be removed and replaced, frequently on a daily basis. Once the burn wound has been completely covered with patches of homograft in different stages, the patient can be debrided more thoroughly in the operating room and the entire burn area again covered with a fresh homograft. Two to three days later, upon return to the operating room, the homograft is stripped mechanically from the recipient site and the entire area covered with autograft. If the autograft donor area is limited, a portion of the homograft may be allowed to remain in place and progress to homograft rejection, at which time the area can be covered with autograft taken again from the original donor site.

Porcine heterograft can be used in a manner similar to homograft. The porcine heterograft used within 24 hours of harvesting ranks in effectiveness just below the fresh homograft and above the lyophilized homograft. The commercially available lyophilized, or frozen, porcine heterograft is not as satisfactory as the fresh heterograft, nor is it as effective as the lyophilized homograft. However, its superior performance compared to other artificial skin dressings presently available has stimulated a large commercial undertaking. The only significant problem so far encountered has been occasional bacterial contamination of the porcine heterograft, most commonly by enterococcus (*Streptococcus fecalis*). For this reason the skin is often prepared with neomycin solution, and if large areas are covered, systemic neomycin toxicity may occur.

While homografts can be obtained from living donors, this poses great sociologic and economic problems which should be avoided. A good educational program is necessary to obtain an adequate supply of homograft for a large burn service, and there is little reason why the occasional burned patient requiring homograft cannot be supplied with this tissue on demand. The body of any recently deceased person, provided that he has not died with cutaneous malignant metastases, hematogenous malignant disease such as leukemia, hepatitis, syphilis, or other contagious disease, is a suitable source.

Ideally, the skin should be obtained within 4 to 6 hours of the death of the donor and applied to the recipient within 8 hours. However, if the need for homograft is a continuing one or if the need is great in a specific patient, skin obtained at almost any period after the death of the donor and prior to embalming can be used. The skin is obtained in the operating room under aseptic conditions. The donor sites are thoroughly shaved and the dermatome set at 0.012 to 0.014 in. The upper layers of skin are removed from clavicles to ankles and wrists. Removal of the skin is greatly facilitated by the infiltration of saline solution subcutaneously over the thoracic cage and the bony prominences.

If the skin is to be used immediately, the only safeguard needed is to prevent it from drying out. If storage for later use is anticipated, a thin strip of gauze impregnated with petroleum jelly is spread on the epidermal side of the skin. An opened 4- by 8-in. sponge dampened with saline solution is then placed over the dermal side, which is exposed, and several strips of the skin are placed in a large Petri dish with $\frac{1}{4}$ Gm of streptomycin and 500,000 units of aqueous penicillin. The Petri dish is sealed and deposited in the general refrigerator area. Care must be taken not to place the Petri dish in the freezing compartment, since the skin will rapidly deteriorate. Skin viability diminishes rapidly, so that 5 days of storage at 4°C results in a 50 percent deficit in oxygen consumption. However, clinical use clearly shows that functional viability rather sharply diminishes after 12 hours of storage, is unpredictable after 24 hours, and except for very clean wounds is not an effective protective covering after it has been stored more than 3 or 4 days.

Homografts can be utilized not only to cover temporarily areas of obvious full-thickness skin loss but also to test the acceptability of a recipient site of autograft. In many instances early autograft coverage is desirable, but because of limited donor area, failure of any initial autografting cannot be tolerated. Under such circumstances, homografts can be placed over the recipient area, and if a good pink, viable take occurs, the homograft can be stripped from the recipient bed within 48 to 72 hours of application and immediate autografting accomplished with the assurance of an excellent take. In addition, reepithelization of deep dermal burns can be hastened by the application of homograft to the surface. Under these circumstances, changing of the homograft every 24 to 48 hours is necessary to prevent the destruction of the new epithelium by the purulence which may collect between the deep dermal burn and the homograft. Use of homograft for this purpose is reserved for those instances in which homograft is available in plentiful quantities.

The greatest value of homograft is as a temporary but

extremely effective method of closing the burn wound prior to the availability of autograft. The homograft is as effective as the autografting in preventing evaporative water loss, reducing caloric demand, returning the patient to a feeling of comfort and high spirits, and, most importantly, preventing invasive burn-wound infection. While the precise mechanism is unknown, it has been well documented that either homograft or autograft applied to a burn wound in the absence of necrotic tissue will sterilize the wound within 48 hours.

AUTOGRAFTING

Autogenous skin can be obtained by various methods, including the presently popular use of the Brown electric dermatome. It is of little consequence how the skin is obtained if suitable skin coverage is provided and the donor site is handled properly.

The choice of donor site is dictated by two factors: The distribution of the initial thermal injury itself determines not only what must be ultimately covered by autograft but also the sources of the autograft. One must choose donor skin which will provide the optimal cosmetic and functional coverage for the recipient site. At the same time, one must anticipate which areas will be required for future reconstruction. In general, the skin of the back is the thickest, and skin taken at an intermediate thickness from this source (0.012 to 0.014 in.) will be relatively inelastic, since it is composed entirely of epidermis with little dermis and none of the dermal papillae. Skin obtained from the anterior surface of the trunk and the medial aspect of the upper extremities or the thigh will be the most elastic if taken at the same thickness, because it will contain most of the dermal papillae which provide the skin's elasticity. Skin from the lateral aspect of the thigh and upper extremities will be intermediate between the preceding sites. If one wishes to cover the dorsum of the hand, for example, the desideratum would be an elastic piece of skin which would allow for a full range of hand motion. Conversely, to cover areas of the trunk, the thigh, or other areas of the extremity exclusive of major joints, the relatively inelastic skin of the back would suffice.

The skin of those at the extremes of age must be taken as a relatively thin sheet, since the dermal papillae and appendages are atrophic in the older age group and less well developed in the younger.

It is best to apply autograft to a surface which has been previously homografted, because one is then applying it to a sterile and receptive wound. It is not necessary that granulation tissues be present or that the wound be sterile. However, necrotic tissue must be absent, and a viable bed must exist. The main organism of significance in relation to graft survival is the beta-hemolytic streptococcus. This causes extensive graft loss, which can be prevented by administering 600,000 units procaine penicillin for 24 hours before and after grafting.

Sutures are to be avoided in the grafting procedure, since they more than double the operating period, cause bleeding beneath the graft, and by 2 to 3 days after grafting are the site of microabscesses. Should some type of graft immobilization be necessary or desirable, a simple expedi-

ent is to anchor the grafts to the adjacent grafts or surrounding healed areas with Steri-strips. This rapid technique avoids the problems encountered with sutures. However, sutures are usually required in the hand, where motion would adversely affect the take. Dressings may be placed over the grafted area but are better omitted, to allow for daily or twice daily inspection of the burn wound and the early evacuation of seromas, hematomas, or purulent collections which may develop beneath the graft or destroy adjacent viable skin. Absence of dressings also permits the meticulous trimming of the graft at points where it may overlap the margins of the wound or adjacent graft. In circumferential burns of the trunk or extremities, either the anterior or the posterior surface can be grafted initially, the opposite side being covered 7 to 10 days later when the initial graft site can withstand the weight.

COMPLICATIONS

The victim of thermal injury often is beset by various complications, singly or in combination. While most of these occur in the early postburn period (the first 2 weeks), they also frequently occur several weeks after the initial injury.

Pneumonia

Pneumonia, already referred to, is discussed again here to emphasize its importance and frequency. In the years before effective topical antibacterial therapy, the most common type of pneumonia was hematogenous pneumonia due primarily to gram-negative organisms. It was part of the generalized picture of burn-wound sepsis. With the successful control of burn-wound sepsis the picture has changed considerably, and the process is commonly a rapidly advancing, confluent bronchopneumonia associated frequently with the inhalation of irritating combustion products. It can be anticipated that the patient will have some pulmonary difficulty if within the first 24 to 48 hours coughing produces a carbonaceous sputum. Careful auscultation of the chest at this time will reveal only some heavy rales and rhonchi which clear fairly well on coughing. Within the next few hours these findings become more pronounced, and a wheezing expiratory grunt characteristic of bronchospasm appears. A chest x-ray at this time is ordinarily clear but may occasionally show some early pneumonic process in addition to increased bronchovascular markings. These findings should arouse suspicion of an impending fulminant bronchopneumonia.

While it may require 5 to 7 days to develop, the full-blown clinical picture is ordinarily apparent within 48 to 72 hours after the burn, and vigorous steps must be directed toward its resolution. Sputum smears and cultures are utilized to determine the appropriate antibiotic therapy, which must be supplemented by vigorous physical measures to support the respiration and clear the tracheobronchial tree. Bronchoscopy must be used, sometimes twice daily, in order to clear the tracheobronchial tree thoroughly, stimulate coughing, and provide lavage of the distal segments of the bronchi if necessary. Assisted respiration or intermittent positive-pressure breathing or a combination of the two can be accomplished through a tracheostomy, which may be required in order to decrease the amount of functional dead space.

If bronchospasm is severe, it may interfere with ventilation and cause death. A bronchodilator, such as aminophylline, should be tried initially but ordinarily is of little benefit. Large, single-shot doses of steroids given intravenously will occasionally relax the bronchospasm. Heavy sedation with meperidine may permit use of a respirator to provide assisted respiration. Controlled respiration of a patient paralyzed with curare is occasionally necessary but requires close attention. Unfortunately, patients who require controlled respiration seldom survive. Whether it is a reflection of the basic disease process or a complication of the respirator and/or oxygen therapy is unknown, but many at postmortem examination demonstrate hyaline membrane changes in the pulmonary alveoli. A rapidly fatal pneumonia frequently occurs secondarily to aspiration, often during transportation; this can be obviated by using a nasogastric tube.

Gastrointestinal Lesions

One of the most dramatic and rapidly fatal complications which befall the thermally injured is acute ulceration of the gastrointestinal tract. These ulcers, first described by Curling in 1842 and bearing his name, occur in 20 percent of hospitalized burn cases. While originally described as being limited to the duodenum, these lesions occur most commonly on the gastric side of the pylorus, may be multiple, and may occur in the stomach and duodenum simultaneously. Those in the duodenum are more characteristically associated with massive hemorrhage. Fatal bleeding often results from those located in the stomach. Although the cause is unknown, the manifestations should be recognized. The most startling symptom is the sudden passage of a large, tarry stool or the vomiting of large amounts of bright red blood. This occurs in over 40 percent of the cases without prodomal symptoms; in others it may be preceded by mild upper abdominal distension or discomfort.

Bleeding characteristically occurs near the end of the first postburn week, and while it is seen occasionally with the very small burn, it is noted most often with burns exceeding 30 percent of total body surface. Initial therapy is conservative, with replacement of the blood loss. If adequate blood volume replacement cannot be provided or if the patient bleeds anew, operative intervention is mandatory. The abdominal cavity can be and often must be opened through the burn wound; if this is done, the subcutaneous tissue and skin are left open at the time of closure. The bleeding source is identified by gastrotomy or duodenotomy and blood volume replacement continued until the patient's condition is stable. At this time a gastric resection encompassing the actual bleeding point is performed. A hemigastrectomy and vagotomy have usually proved to be adequate, but occasionally a more extensive resection is necessary in order to include the bleeding site.

A gastrojejunostomy reconstitutes the continuity of the alimentary tract, and the abdominal wall is closed with figure-of-eight buried stainless-steel sutures.

Although initial experience with this procedure indicated that there might be some impairment of healing of the gastrointestinal anastomosis, this has not been confirmed. In the last 42 cases reported from the U.S. Army Institute of Surgical Research, Brooke Army Medical Center, there has been no impairment of anastomotic healing, although in three instances there has been disruption of the anterior abdominal wall incision. While many patients continue in their postoperative recovery only to die later of complications unrelated to the surgery, they nevertheless are able to reestablish oral alimentation in most instances, thus demonstrating the benefit of surgical intervention.

Hypertension in Children

For a number of years there have been British and European reports of hypertension and convulsive disorders occasionally accompanying thermal injury of children. Until recently this received little attention in this country. However, recent investigations now clearly show that of children sustaining thermal injury approximately 30 percent will be hypertensive as defined by a diastolic pressure exceeding 90 mm Hg. Approximately 10 percent of these will have convulsive seizures. Although associated with prolonged elevation of catecholamine levels, also seen in those not hypertensive, the precise cause is unknown. Marked elevation in renin levels to as high as 6,000 $m\mu g/100$ ml have been measured, but correlation with the hypertension and the convulsive episodes is uncertain. The elevated blood pressure characteristically occurs within the first 2 weeks postburn but may be present at any time during the first 8 to 10 weeks. All pediatric age groups have been involved, and symptoms range from simple irritability or somnolence to severe grand mal seizures. Duration usually is brief, but the hypertension and symptoms have been reported to persist for several weeks to 2 months. Treatment has been essentially symptomatic with reserpine or hydralazine, and the therapy is withdrawn as the symptoms subside with healing of the wound.

BURNS OF THE HEAD

Because of its exposed position, the head with its appendages and orifices is the anatomic area most frequently burned. The protective action of the lids and the constant moisture which surrounds the ocular structures prevent the eyes from being directly involved by thermal injury except in cases of contact, chemical, or electrical burns. Injury due to these agents results in total destruction of the globe, perforation of the cornea with resultant delayed destruction, or opacification of the cornea, which frequently precludes graft correction. However, even though the eye may escape immediate initial thermal damage, the infection present in the burned skin of the lids, the malar area, the brow, and the nose subject the conjunctival sac to constant bacterial insult. This, coupled with the drying effect of chronically retracted lids, sets the stage for a very erosive and destructive ocular infection. To obviate this, extreme care must be directed toward protecting all the structures of the eye, and particularly the cornea. If the cornea cannot be covered by the lids because of burn retraction, the lids must be sutured together, either by a tarsorrhaphy or a blepharorrhaphy. Repeated daily irrigations with sterile saline solution must be performed, and bland ointment should be instilled into the conjunctival sac. As soon as possible, skin should be grafted over the lids and other periocular structures in order to protect the eye.

Burns of the ears result in unpredictable amounts of disability due to secondary involvement of the supporting cartilaginous structures of the pinna. While seen most often in cases of full-thickness skin destruction of the ear, purulent necrosis of the cartilage may also occur in individuals who have sustained only partial-thickness skin damage in this area. Characteristically, the ear becomes painful and swollen, with most of the enlargement initially manifested at the base of the ear. Treatment is directed toward evacuation of the necrotic infected cartilage and results in almost immediate relief of the extreme pain. The cartilage may be removed surgically either through an elliptic incision at the margin of the helix or by removal of a window of skin in the anterior surface of the ear in the midportion of the antihelix. This latter method, if successful in arresting the necrosis, is cosmetically preferable.

BURNS OF THE HANDS

The most common functional disability which occurs as the result of thermal injury is loss of coordinated movements of the hand. Disability may not be due to the burn per se. If edema of the hand is allowed to persist for several days and subsequently becomes organized, a frozen hand results in spite of spontaneous healing of a second-degree burn or excellent graft coverage in the case of full-thickness loss. To prevent this it is imperative that the hand be elevated as early as possible and to as extreme a degree as possible during the first several postburn days, until the edema has completely subsided. In addition, in spite of the pain and discomfort which the patient experiences, he should be made to use his hands for all simple tasks whenever possible and should exercise in the hydrotherapy tank at least once and preferably twice a day. This is not possible on so frequent a schedule for the patient with an extensive major burn, but active use of the hands still must be encouraged.

When partial-thickness skin destruction has occurred, the necrotic superficial tissue may be removed by progressive debridement in the whirlpool. More rapid epithelization can be accomplished and a less painful hand results if the hand is completely covered with homograft or porcine heterograft. It is not necessary to enclose the hand in dressings, since the skin will adhere firmly within a few minutes. If the graft is placed in sections which meet over the knuckles, a full range of motion can be provided.

Full-thickness skin loss to the palm or the proximal flexor surface of the digits is rare in the absence of contact, chemical, or electrical burns. However, full-thickness destruction of the flexor surface of the tips of the digits and the entire dorsum of the hands frequently occurs because the skin in this area is so thin. In addition, the delicate middle slip of the extensor tendon is readily destroyed by thermal denaturation or bacterial proteolytic digestion. Every effort must be made to save this extensor network. This can be realized only by bacterial suppression and early coverage of the hand. If the initial thermal injury has resulted in tendon destruction, the joint must be fused in a more appropriate position of function than it would naturally assume because of the flexion contracture of the unopposed flexor muscles. Fusion is carried out by pinning across the joint with a Kirschner wire and leaving the wire in place until bony ankylosis has occurred.

Major joints may be involved by soft tissue contractures or periarticular calcification. The former are difficult to avoid in the extensively burned patient with limited donor area, but in the patient with a smaller burn, in which earlier coverage can be obtained, they can be avoided by early and active motion. The same process must be encouraged in order to prevent periarticular calcification, which is so prone to occur about the elbow joints. This process can severely restrict motion of the elbow in either extension or flexion, and although adequate range of motion may ultimately be acquired, marked disability is a frequent permanent concomitant.

Nothing can be done to reverse tissue destruction resulting from thermal injury, but every effort must be expended to prevent progressive tissue loss, functional disability, and death. The treatment period is a long one beset with many complications, but much can be accomplished through an intelligent approach based on available knowledge and sound surgical principles.

References

General

Artz, C. P., and Moncrief, J. A.: "The Treatment of Burns," W. B. Saunders Company, Philadelphia, 1969.

Blocker, T. G., Jr., Washburn, W. W., Lewis, S. R., and Blocker, V.: A Statistical Study of 1,000 Burn Patients Admitted to the Plastic Surgery Service of the University of Texas Medical Branch, 1950–1959, *J Trauma*, **1**:409, 1961.

Bull, J. P., and Squire, J. R.: A Study of Mortality in a Burns Unit, *Ann Surg*, **130**:160, 1949.

Hockmuth, R. E., and Ziffren, S. E.: Results of the Treatment of Severe Burns, *Surg Gynecol Obstet*, **117**:540, 1963.

Monafo, W. W.: "The Treatment of Burns: Principles and Practice," W. A. Green, Inc., St. Louis, 1971.

Polk, H. S., and Stone, H. H.: "Contemporary Burn Management," Little, Brown and Company, Boston, 1971.

Pruitt, B. A., Jr., Tumbusch, W. T., Mason, A. D., Jr., and Pearson, E.: Mortality in 1,100 Consecutive Burns Treated at a Burns Unit, *Ann Surg*, **159**:396, 1964.

Shuck, J. M., and Moncrief, J. A.: The Management of Burns, *Curr Probl Surg*, Year Book Medical Publishers, Inc., Chicago, 1969.

Heat Transfer and Thermal Injury

DuBois, E. F.: Heat Loss from the Human Body, *Bull NY Acad Med,* **15**:43, 1939.

James, G. W., III, Purnell, O. J., and Evans, E. I.: The Anemia of Thermal Injury: I. Studies of Pigment Excretion, *J Clin Invest,* **30**:181, 1951.

Moritz, A. R., and Henriques, F. C.: Studies of Thermal Injury: II. The Relative Importance of Time and Surface Temperature in the Causation of Cutaneous Burns, *Am J Pathol,* **23**:695, 1947.

Pearse, H. E., and Kingsley, H. D.: Thermal Burns from the Atomic Bomb, *Surg Gynecol Obstet,* **98**:385, 1954.

———, Payne, J. T., and Hogg, L.: Experimental Study of Flash Burns, *Ann Surg,* **130**:774, 1949.

Ponder, E.: The Coefficient of Thermal Conductivity of Blood and of Various Tissues, *J Gen Physiol,* **45**:545, 1962.

Price, P. B., Call, D. E., Hansen, F. L., and Zerwick, C. J.: Penetration of Heat in Thermal Burns, *Surg Forum,* **5**:443, 1954.

———, ———, and Zerwick, C. J.: Histopathologic Changes in Experimental Thermal Wounds, *Surgery,* **36**:664, 1954.

Depth of Skin Destruction

Hinshaw, J. R.: Progressive Changes in the Depth of Burns, *Arch Surg,* **87**:993, 1963.

Jackson, D. Mac G.: Diagnosis in the Management of Burns, *Br Med J,* **1**:1263, 1959.

Local Results of Thermal Injury

Caldwell, F. T., Jr., and Lavitsky, K.: Nitrogen Balance after Thermal Burns, *Arch Surg,* **86**:500, 1963.

Foley, F. D.: The Burn Autopsy, *Am J Clin Pathol,* **52**:1, 1969.

Hardy, J. D., Neely, W. A., and Wilson, F. C., Jr.: Thermal Burns in Man: "Insensible Fluid Loss," *Surgery,* **38**:692, 1955.

Harrison, H. N., Moncrief, J. A., Duckett, J. W., Jr., and Mason, A. D., Jr.: The Relationship between Energy Metabolism and Water Loss from Vaporization in Severely Burned Patients, *Surgery,* **56**:203, 1964.

Jelenko, C., and Ginsburg, J.: Water-holding Lipid and Water Transmission Through Homeothermic and Poikilothermic Skins, *Proc Soc Exp Biol Med,* **136**:1059, 1971.

Lamke, L. O.: "Evaporative Water Loss from Normal and Burnt Skin: A Methodological and Clinical Study," Linkoping, 1971.

McClure, G. S.: Evaporation of Water from Superficial Burns, *Arch Surg,* **32**:747, 1936.

Moncrief, J. A.: Changing Concepts in Burn Sepsis, *J Trauma,* **4**:233, 1964.

——— and Mason, A. D., Jr.: Evaporative Water Loss in the Burned Patient, *J Trauma,* **4**:180, 1964.

Order, S. E., Mason, A. D., Jr., Switzer, W. E., and Moncrief, J. A.: Arterial Vascular Occlusion and Devitalization of Burn Wounds, *Ann Surg,* **161**:502, 1965.

———, ———, Walker, H. L., Lindberg, R. B., Switzer, W. E., and Moncrief, J. A.: Vascular Destructive Effects of Thermal Injury and Its Relationship to Burn Wound Sepsis, *J Trauma,* **5**:62, 1965.

——— and Moncrief, J. A.: Vascular Destruction and Revascularization in Severe Thermal Injuries, *Surg Forum,* **15**:38, 1964.

Teplitz, C., Davis, D., Mason, A. D., Jr., and Moncrief, J. A.: *Pseudomonas* Burn Wound Sepsis: I. Pathogenesis of Experimental Pseudomonas Burn Wound Sepsis. *J Surg Res,* **4**:217, 1964.

———, ———, Walker, H. L., Raulston, G. L., Mason, A. D., Jr., and Moncrief, J. A.: *Pseudomonas* Burn Wound Sepsis: II. Hematogenous Infection at the Junction of the Burn and the Unburned Hypodermis, *J Surg Res,* **4**:217, 1964.

Walker, H. L., Mason, A. D., Jr., and Raulston, G. L.: Surface Infection with *Pseudomonas aeruginosa, Ann Surg,* **160**:297, 1964.

Wilson, J. S., and Moncrief, J. A.: Vapor Pressure of Normal and Unburned Skin, *Ann Surg,* **162**:130, 1965.

Zwacki, B. E., Spitzer, K. W., Mason, A. D., and Johns, L. A.: Does Increased Evaporative Water Loss Cause Hypermetabolism in Burned Patients?, *Ann Surg,* **171**:236, 1970.

Systemic Changes

Alexander, J. W., Diongi, R., and Meakins, J. L.: Periodic Variations in the Antibacterial Function of Human Neutrophils and Its Relation to Sepsis, *Ann Surg,* **173**:206, 1971.

Allison, S. P., Hinton, P., and Chamberlain, M. J.: Intravenous Glucose Tolerance, Insulin and Free Fatty Acid Levels in Burned Patients, *Lancet,* **2**:1113, 1968.

Arturson, G.: Experimental and Clinical Studies of Capillary Permeability in Burns, in "Bahama International Conference on Burns," Dorrance & Co., Inc., Philadelphia, 1964.

———, Johansson, S. G. O., Hogman, C. F., and Killander, J.: Changes in Immunoglobulin Levels in Severely Burned Patients, *Lancet,* **1**:546, 1969.

Beer, S.: Serum and Plasma Proteins in Thermally Injured Patients Treated with Plasma, Its Admixture with Albumin or Serum Alone, *Ann Surg,* **161**:112, 1965.

Birke, G., Liljedahl, S. D., and Linderholm, H.: Studies on Burns: IV. On the Possibility of Prolonged Use of an Indwelling Catheter in the Pulmonary Artery for Studies of Circulation and for Intravenous Infusion, *Acta Chir Scand,* **116**:362, 1958–1959.

———, ———, and ———: Studies on Burns: V. Clinical and Pathophysiological Aspects of Circulation and Respiration, *Acta Chir Scand,* **116**:370, 1958–1959.

———, ———, Plantin, L. O., and Reizenstein, P.: Studies on Burns: IX. The Distribution and Losses Through the Wound of ^{131}I-Albumin Measured by Whole Body Counting, *Acta Chir Scand,* **134**:27, 1968.

Brown, A.: Studies of Burns and Scalds: IV. Blood Changes and Blood Pressure in Burned Patients, *Med Res Counc Spec Rep Ser (London),* no. 249, p. 114, 1942–1943.

———: Morphological Changes in the Red Cells in Relation to Severe Burns, *J Pathol,* **58**:367, 1946.

Caldwell, F. T., Jr., Casali, R. E., Boswer, B., Smith, V., Enloe, J., and Rose, D.: On the Failure of Heat Production in the Immediate Postburn Period, *J Trauma,* **11**:936, 1971.

Cameron, J. A., and Miller-Jones, C. M. H.: Renal Function and Renal Failure in Badly Burned Children, *Br J Surg,* **54**:132, 1967.

Cook, W. A., Baxter, C. R., and Ferrell, J. M., Jr.: Pulmonary Circulation after Dermal Burns, *Vasc Surg,* **2**:1, 1968.

Davies, J. W. L., and Liljedahl, S. E.: Protein Catabolism and Energy Utilization in Burned Patients Treated at Different

Environmental Temperatures, in R. Proter and J. Knight (eds.), *Ciba Found Symp Energy Metabolism Trauma,* p. 59, 1970.

Eklund, J.: Renal Regulation of Body Osmolal Balance in Burns, *Acta Chir Scand [Suppl],* vol. 410, 1970.

Epstein, B. S., Hardy, D. L., Harrison, H. N., Teplitz, C., Villarreal, Y., and Mason, A. D., Jr.: Hypoxemia in the Burned Patient: A Clinical-Pathologic Study, *Ann Surg,* **158:**924, 1963.

Graber, I. G., and Sevitt, S.: Renal Function in Burned Patients and Its Relationship to Morphological Changes, *J Clin Pathol,* **12:**25, 1959.

Ham, T. H., Shen, S. C., Fleming, E. M., and Castle, W. B.: Studies on the Destruction of Red Blood Cells: IV. Thermal Injury: Action of Heat in Causing Increased Spheroidicity, Osmotic and Mechanical Fragilities and Hemolysis of Erythrocytes; Observations on the Mechanisms of Destruction of Such Erythrocytes in Dogs and in a Patient with Fatal Thermal Burn, *Hematology,* **3:**373, 1948.

James, G. W., III, Purnell, O. J., and Evans, E. I.: The Anemia of Thermal Injury: I. Studies of Pigment Excretion, *J Clin Invest,* **30:**181, 1951.

Michie, D. D., Goldsmith, R. S., and Mason, A. D., Jr.: Effects of Hydralazine and High Molecular Weight Dextran upon the Circulatory Responses to Severe Thermal Burns, *Circ Res,* **13:**468, 1963.

——, ——, ——, and Moncrief, J. A.: Hemodynamics of the Immediate Postburn Period: I. Hemodynamic Alterations Produced by Thermal Burns, *J Trauma,* **3:**111, 1963.

Moncrief, J. A.: The Effect of Various Fluid Regimens and Pharmacologic Agents on the Circulatory Hemodynamics of Immediate Postburn Period, *Ann Surg,* **164:**723, 1966.

——, Switzer, W. E., and Teplitz, C.: Curling's Ulcer, *J Trauma,* **4:**481, 1964.

Morris, A. H., and Spitzer, K. W.: Pulmonary Pathophysiologic Changes following Thermal Injury, in "U.S. Army Institute of Surgical Research Annual Research Progress Report, FY 1971," sec. 52, Brooke Army Medical Center, Fort Sam Houston, Texas, 1971.

Muir, I. F. K.: Red-cell Destruction in Burns, *Br J Plast Surg,* **14:**273, 1961.

O'Neill, J. A., Pruitt, B. A., Jr., and Moncrief, J. A.: Studies of Renal Function During the Early Postburn Period, in "Research in Burns: Transactions of Third International Congress on Research in Burns, Prague," p. 95, Hans Huber Verlag, Bern, 1970.

Pruitt, B. A., Jr., Mason, A. D., Jr., and Moncrief, J. A.: Hemodynamic Changes in the Early Postburn Patients: The Influence of Fluid Administration and of a Vasodilator, *J Trauma,* **11:**36, 1971.

Shen, S. C., and Ham, T. H.: Studies on the Destruction of Red Blood Cells: III. Mechanism and Complications of Hemoglobinuria in Patients with Thermal Burns: Spherocytosis and Increased Osmotic Fragility of Red Blood Cells, *N Engl J Med,* **229:**704, 1943.

Taylor, F. W., and Gumbert, J. L.: Cause of Death from Burns: Role of Respiratory Damage, *Ann Surg,* **161:**497, 1965.

Topley, E., Jackson, D. M., Cason, J. S., and Davies, J. W. L.: Assessment of Red Cell Loss in the First Two Days after Severe Burns, *Ann Surg,* **155:**581, 1962.

Wilmore, D. W., Curreri, R. W., Spitzer, K. W., Spitzer, M. E.,

and Pruitt, B. A., Jr.: Supranormal Dietary Intake in Thermally Injured Hypermetabolic Patients, *Surg Gynecol Obstet,* **132:**881, 1971.

Therapy

Alexander, J. W.: Immunologic Considerations and the Role of Vaccination in Burn Injury, in H. C. Polk and H. H. Stone (eds.), "Contemporary Burn Management," p. 265, Little, Brown and Company, Boston, 1971.

Baxter, C. R.: Topical Use of 1.0 Percent Silver Sulfadiazine, in H. C. Polk and H. H. Stone (eds.), "Contemporary Burn Management," p. 203, Little, Brown and Company, Boston, 1971.

Bruck, H. M., Asch, M. J., and Pruitt, B. A., Jr.: Burns in Children: A 10 Year Experience with 412 Patients, *J Trauma,* **10:**658, 1970.

Canizaro, P. C., Sawyer, R. B., and Switzer, W. E.: Blood Loss during Excision of Third-Degree Burns, *Arch Surg,* **88:**800, 1964.

Curreri, P. W., Wilmore, D. W., Mason, A. D., Newsome, T. W., Asch, M. J., and Pruitt, B. A., Jr.: Intracellular Cation Alterations following Major Thermal Trauma: Effect of Supranormal Caloric Intake, *J Trauma,* **11:**390, 1971.

Dennis, D. L., and Peterson, C. G.: Candida and Other Fungi, in H. C. Polk and H. H. Stone (eds.), "Contemporary Burn Management," p. 329, Little, Brown and Company, Boston, 1971.

Epstein, B. S., Hardy, D. L., Harrison, H. N., Teplitz, C., Villarreal, Y., and Mason, A. D., Jr.: Hypoxemia in the Burned Patient: A Clinical-Pathologic Study, *Ann Surg,* **158:**924, 1963.

——, Rose, L. R., Teplitz, C., and Moncrief, J. A.: Experiences with Low Tracheostomy in the Burn Patient, *JAMA,* **183:**1966, 1963.

Fox, C. L., Jr.: Silver Sulfadiazine: A New Topical Therapy for *Pseudomonas* in Burns, *Arch Surg,* **96:**184, 1968.

——: Evaluation of Various Salt Solutions, in "Research in Burns, Transactions of Third International Congress on Research in Burns, Prague," p. 67, Hans Huber Verlag, Bern, 1970.

Harrison, H. N., Bales, H., and Jacoby, F.: The Behavior of Mafenide Acetate as a Basis for Its Clinical Use, *Arch Surg,* **103:**449, 1971.

Henry, C. L., and Amspacher, W. H.: Potassium Migration in Experimental Burns, *Surgery,* **36:**740, 1954.

Janzekovic, Z.: A New Concept in the Early Excision and Immediate Grafting of Burns, *J Trauma,* **10:**1103, 1970.

Larson, D. L., Abston, S., Evans, E. B., Dobrokovsky, M., and Linares, H. A.: Techniques for Decreasing Scar Formation and Contractures in the Burned Patient, *J Trauma,* **11:**807, 1971.

——, Evans, E. B., and Abston, S.: Skeletal Suspension and Traction in the Treatment of Burns, *Ann Surg,* **168:**981, 1968.

Lindberg, R. B., Moncrief, J. A., Switzer, W. E., Order, S. E., and Mills, W., Jr.: The Successful Control of Burn Wound Sepsis, *J Trauma,* **5:**601, 1965.

MacMillan, B. G.: Comparison of Topical Antimicrobial Agents, in H. C. Polk and H. H. Stone (eds.), "Contemporary Burn Management," p. 227, Little, Brown and Company, Boston, 1971.

Metcoff, J., Buchman, H., Jacobson, M., Richter, H., Jr., Bloomenthal, E. D., and Zacharias, M.: Losses of Physiologic Requirements for Water and Electrolytes after Extensive Burns in Children, *N Engl J Med,* **265:**101, 1961.

Miller, T. A., Switzer, W. E., Foley, F. D., and Moncrief, J. A.: Early Homografting of Second-Degree Burns, *Plast Reconstr Surg,* **40:**117, 1967.

Monafo, W. W., Jr., and Moyer, C. A.: Effectiveness of Dilute Silver Nitrate in the Treatment of Major Burns, *Arch Surg,* **91:**200, 1965.

———: The Treatment of Burn Shock by the Intravenous and Oral Administration of Hypertonic Lactated Saline Solution, *J Trauma,* **10:**575, 1970.

Moncrief, J. A.: Changing Concepts in Burn Sepsis, *J Trauma,* **4:**233, 1964.

———: Burns of Specific Areas, *J Trauma,* **5:**278, 1965.

———: The Effect of Various Fluid Regimens and Pharmacologic Agents on the Circulatory Hemodynamics of the Immediate Postburn Period, *Ann Surg,* **164:**723, 1966.

———: Topical Therapy of the Burn Wound: Present Status, *Clin Pharmacol Ther,* **10:**439, 1969.

———, Lindberg, R. B., Switzer, W. E., and Pruitt, B. A., Jr.: The Use of Topical Antibacterial Therapy in the Treatment of the Burn Wound, *Arch Surg,* **92:**558, 1966.

———, Switzer, W. E., and Rose, L. R.: Primary Excision and Grafting in the Treatment of Third-Degree Burns of the Dorsum of the Hand, *Plast Reconstr Surg,* **33:**305, 1964.

Moyer, C. A., Brentano, L., Gravens, D. L., Margraf, H. W., and Monafo, W. W., Jr.: Treatment of Large Human Burns with 0.5% Silver Nitrate, *Arch Surg,* **90:**812, 1965.

———, Margraf, H. W., and Monafo, W. W., Jr.: Burn Shock and Extravascular Sodium Deficiency Treatment with Ringer's Solution with Lactate, *Arch Surg,* **90:**799, 1965.

Moylan, J. A., Jr., Reckler, J. M., and Mason, A. D., Jr.: Hypertonic Lactated Saline Resuscitation in Thermal Injury, in "U.S. Army Institute of Surgical Research Annual Progress Report, FY 1971," Brooke Army Medical Center, Fort Sam Houston, Texas, 1971.

Olson, R. E.: "Excess Lactate" and Anaerobiosis, *Ann Intern Med,* **59:**960, 1963.

Order, S. E., Mason, A. D., Jr., Switzer, W. E., and Moncrief, J. A.: Arterial Vascular Occlusion and Devitalization of Burn Wounds, *Ann Surg,* **161:**502, 1965.

———, ———, Walker, H. L., Lindberg, R. B., Switzer, W. E., and Moncrief, J. A.: The Pathogenesis of Second and Third-degree Burns and Conversion to Full Thickness Injury, *Surg Gynecol Obstet,* **120:**893, 1965.

——— and Moncrief, J. A.: Vascular Destruction and Revascularization in Severe Thermal Injuries, *Surg Forum,* **15:**38, 1964.

Pruitt, B. A., Jr., Lotke, P., Sell, K., O'Neill, J. A., Jr., Lindberg, R. B., Moncrief, J. A., and Switzer, W. E.: Clinical Evaluation of Freeze Dried and Fresh-frozen Homograft in Burned Patients, in "U.S. Army Surgical Research Unit Annual Report, FY 1966," sec. 10, Brooke Army Medical Center, Fort Sam Houston, Texas, 1966.

Reiss, E., Stirman, J. A., Artz, C. P., Davis, J. H., and Amspacher, W. H.: Fluid and Electrolyte Balance in Burns, *JAMA,* **152:**1309, 1953.

Shuck, J. M., Pruitt, B. A., Jr., and Moncrief, J. A.: Homograft Skin for Wound Coverage, *Arch Surg,* **98:**472, 1969.

Soroff, H. S., Pearson, E., Arney, G. K., and Artz, C. P.: Metabolism of Burned Patients: An Estimation of the Nitrogen Potassium Requirements for Equilibrium, in "Research in Burns," p. 126, *Am Inst Biol Sci Publ 9,* 1962.

Stone, H. H., and Kolb, L. D.: The Evolution and Spread of Gentamycin-resistant *Pseudomonas, J Trauma,* **11:**586, 1971.

Switzer, W. E., Jones, J. W., and Moncrief, J. A.: Evaluation of Early Excision of Burns in Children, *J Trauma,* **5:**540, 1965.

Taylor, P. H., Moncrief, J. A., Pugsley, L. Q., Rose, L. R., and Switzer, W. E.: The Management of Extensively Burned Patients by Staged Excision, *Surg Gynecol Obstet,* **115:**1, 1962.

Teplitz, C., Davis, D., Mason, A. D., Jr., and Moncrief, J. A.: *Pseudomonas* Burn Wound Sepsis. I. Pathogenesis of Experimental *Pseudomonas* Burn Wound Sepsis, *J Surg Res,* **4:**217, 1964.

———, ———, Walker, H. L., Raulston, G. L., Mason, A. D., Jr., and Moncrief, J. A.: *Pseudomonas* Burn Wound Sepsis: II. Hematogenous Infection at the Junction of the Burn Wound and the Unburned Hypodermis, *J Surg Res,* **4:**217, 1964.

———, Epstein, B. S., Rose, L. R., and Moncrief, J. A.: Necrotizing Tracheitis Induced by Tracheostomy Tube, *Arch Pathol,* **77:**14, 1964.

———, ———, ———, Switzer, W. E., and Moncrief, J. A.: Pathology of Low Tracheostomy in Children, *Am J Clin Path,* **42:**58, 1964.

Zaroff, L. I., Mills, W., Jr., Duckett, J. W., Jr., Switzer, W. E., and Moncrief, J. A.: Multiple Uses of Viable Cutaneous Homografts in the Burned Patient, *Surgery,* **59:**368, 1966.

Complications

Lowrey, G. H.: Hypertension in Children with Burns, *J Trauma,* **7:**140, 1967.

Moncrief, J. A., Switzer, W. E., and Teplitz, C.: Curling's Ulcer, *J Trauma,* **4:**481, 1964.

Pruitt, B. A., Jr., Divencenti, F. C., Mason, A. D., Foley, F. D., and Flemma, R. J.: The Occurrence and Significance of Pneumonia and Other Pulmonary Complications in Burned Patients: Comparison of Conventional and Topical Treatments, *J Trauma,* **10:**519, 1970.

———, Foley, F. D., and Moncrief, J. A.: Curling's Ulcer: A Clinical Pathologic Study of 323 Cases, *Ann Surg,* **172:**523, 1970.

Sevitt, S.: Duodenal and Gastric Ulceration after Burning, *Br J Surg,* **54:**32, 1967.

Burns of the Head

Georgiade, N. G., Matton, G. E., and Von Kessel, F.: Facial Burns, *Plast Reconstr Surg,* **29:**68, 1962.

Moncrief, J. A.: Burns of Specific Areas, *J Trauma,* **5:**278, 1965.

Robinson, D. W.: Electrical Burns: A Review and Analysis of 33 Cases, *Surgery,* **57:**385, 1965.

Burns of the Hands

Foley, F. D., and Shuck, J. M.: Burn Wound Infection with *Phycomycetes* Requiring Amputation of the Hand, *JAMA,* **203:**596, 1968.

Griswold, M. L., Jr.: Extra-articular Bone Formation as a Burn Complication, *Plast Reconstr Surg,* **32:**544, 1963.

Gronley, J. K., Yeakel, M. H., and Grant, A. E.: Rehabilitation of the Burned Hand, *Arch Phys Med Rehabil,* **43:**508, 1962.

Miscellaneous

Arturson, G.: Pathophysiological Aspects of the Burn Syndrome, *Acta Chir Scand* [*Suppl*], vol. 274, 1961.

Cope, O., Graham, J. B., Mixter, G., Jr., and Ball, M. R.: Threshold of Thermal Trauma and Influence of Adrenal Cortical and Posterior Pituitary Extracts on the Capillary and Chemical Changes, *Arch Surg,* **59:**1015, 1949.

Evans, E. I., Purnell, O. J., Robinett, P. W., Batchelor, A., and Martin, M.: Fluid and Electrolyte Requirements in Severe Burns, *Ann Surg,* **135:**804, 1952.

Goodpastor, W. E., Levenson, S. M., Tagnon, H. J., Lund, C. C., and Taylor, F. H. L.: A Clinical and Pathologic Study of the Kidney in Patients with Thermal Burns, *Surg Gynecol Obstet,* **82:**652, 1945.

Schlegel, J. W., and Jorgensen, H.: Studies in Metabolism of Trauma: II. Treatment of Burns, *Ann Surg,* **149:**252, 1959.

Chapter 8

Wound Healing and Wound Care

by **Erle E. Peacock, Jr.**

Introduction

Wound Contraction

Epithelization

Ground Substance

Collagen

Sequence of Events: Summary

Wound Care

Skin Grafts

INTRODUCTION

During the course of man's evolution he lost a valuable defense mechanism—the ability to regenerate compound tissues—and accepted in its place a much less complicated and far less valuable process—the phenomenon of healing. Although the ability to heal has been of enormous importance in natural selection, restoration of physical integrity by synthesis of scar tissue can be regarded, at best, as only a method of preserving homeostasis and cannot be compared to the more pristine function of multi-germ-layer regeneration. Moreover, the fibrous tissue synthesis stage of healing can itself be detrimental even to the extent of destroying the organism which it sought to preserve. Examples are the potentially fatal deformity of valve leaflets incurred during healing of rheumatic fever valvulitis and the development of posthepatic cirrhosis. In both cases the patient may survive the initial disease only to succumb months or years later from complications of fibrous tissue synthesis during healing.

Posthepatitis cirrhosis is of special interest to students of the healing phenomenon because the liver is probably the only human example of a compound organ in which almost embryonic propensity for secondary regeneration appears to be retained. Under most circumstances, the liver can be counted upon to regenerate about four-fifths of its preinjury mass; in fact, the failure of regeneration to occur in severe nodular cirrhosis gives the distinct impression that only the overgrowth of fibrous tissue may have prevented hepatic regeneration. The significance of this hypothesis is based on the possibility that fibrous protein synthesis anywhere in the body chokes or overpowers cellular regeneration; from an evolutionary standpoint, such a hypothesis has some factual basis. The hydrozoan *Tubularia* will sometimes regenerate an amputated hydranth without formation of a connective tissue scar; at other times the organism will merely heal the wound by formation of typical scar tissue, and when scar tissue is found, only an abortive attempt at regeneration can be identified. There is a very critical time in the development of newts when the ability to regenerate is disappearing. If during this time connective tissue synthesis is blocked by pharmacologic methods, the power to regenerate a new limb will be slightly prolonged, and a poor but definite new extremity will be formed.

With the exception of the liver, regeneration in man is essentially limited to simple tissue such as epithelium; compound structures such as skin, deep organs, and nervous system can heal only by sealing the wound in a manner to be described. The sealing process varies, depending upon whether structural integrity is merely interrupted or tissue substance is removed. In both types of wounds, epithelization is the fundamental process which seals the wound, and fibrous tissue synthesis is the process which provides structural strength. When tissue is missing, an additional process—contraction—moves viable margins of tissue into closer approximation so that epithelization and fibrous protein synthesis can accomplish their objectives. Simple as this description may sound, most of the mistakes made by physicians in treating wounds are attributable to failure to realize and understand the limitations and end results of each of these fundamental processes and how they differ from pristine regeneration. Thus the best wound management demands a detailed knowledge of epithelization, fibrous protein synthesis, and the biology of wound contraction. Study of these processes requires, in addition, some knowledge of the milieu in which they operate—the ground substance.

WOUND CONTRACTION

In 1793 John Hunter wrote, "In the amputation of the thick thigh (which is naturally 7, 8, or more inches in diameter) . . . the cicatrix shall be no broader than a crown piece." The essence of this quotation is that full-thickness wounds of organs (including skin) do not heal by synthesis of a fibrous scar with the exact dimensions of the original defect. A crown piece in Hunter's time was $1\frac{1}{2}$ in. in diameter, thus over 90 percent of the amputation wound was closed by centripetal movement of the skin edges. This process is called *contraction*—a term denoting the action, which should not be used interchangeably with "contrac-

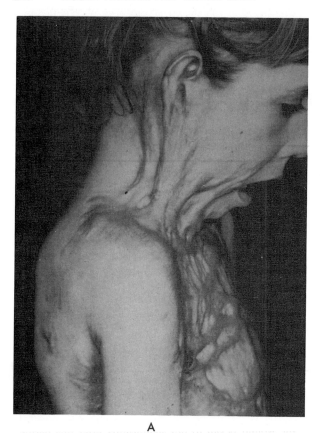

A

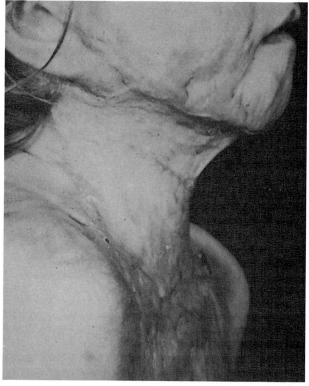

B

Fig. 8-1. *A*. Severe contracture produced by full-thickness skin loss in burn wound of neck and face. Note ectropion of lower lip. *B*. Release of contracture in same patient shown in Fig. 8-1*A*. Contracture was released by excising scar tissue and resurfacing the defect with several split-thickness skin grafts. Note absence of wrinkling of graft and restoration of cervical profile. Facial scars ultimately will be excised and resurfaced.

ture," the term for the end result (Fig. 8-1*A* and *B*). Just as loss of brain or stomach produces a permanent defect in man, loss of skin also is permanent, and when a defect in the integument occurs, restoration of integrity is largely dependent upon stretching the surrounding skin to cover the exposed subcutaneous tissue. Obviously, stretching skin will distort movable features such as the lips, eyelids, breasts, or digits. The fundamental process in contraction can be illustrated perfectly and the end result predicted positively by simply grasping the edges of a gaping wound and manually coapting them. This replication of the contraction process produces the exact deformity that will result from natural wound contraction over a longer period of time. If it is not physically possible to coapt the edges of a wound by reasonable external force, one can be certain that natural processes also will not be effective, as the amount of skin present is all that will be available to be stretched over the wound. The area which remains uncovered will either remain as an open granulating wound or, if it is small enough, be covered by epithelium, which is a poor substitute for normal skin and establishes a potentially dangerous area for the development of epidermoid carcinoma.

Thus the effectiveness of the contraction process in producing complete wound closure and the cosmetic and functional deformity which closure by contraction will produce are related to the amount of skin available in a given area of the body. Because the hands and face of a young person do not contain any excess skin, closure of a defect by contraction will cause distortion of facial features and restriction of joint motion. In areas where there is a redundancy of skin, such as the cervical region or face of old people, wound contraction can be extremely effective in closing defects without producing cosmetic or functional abnormalities. Where an excess of skin is not present but flexion or extension of a joint will move wound edges together, wound contraction inexorably results in movement of the joint into an extreme position. After healing has occurred, the joint will be fixed because of lack of a satisfactory envelope. Last, when loss of skin occurs over an area such as the malleolar area of the lower leg and ankle, wound contraction simply cannot occur because there is not enough skin to stretch over the defect. In this instance the wound either becomes covered by a thin, almost gelatinous film of epithelium or remains open for an indefinite length of time.

Three questions immediately arise about the contraction process: What starts it? What stops it? What is the mechanism by which it occurs? At first glance the answer to the first question appears obvious, in that interruption of the integrity of skin always seems to be the initiating stimulus. Close examination of the series of events which occur following removal of a piece of full-thickness skin, however, reveals that wound contraction does not begin immediately and that about 4 days elapse before movement of the edges is measurable. The so-called "lag phase" of healing seems to include the contraction phenomenon, and it can only be surmised that a set of conditions must be established or an assembly of cells or energy source completed before the actual work of mobilizing the skin edges begins. One might surmise also that reestablishment of physical integrity is the stimulus which stops contraction; but again, measurement of the timing of other events reveals that contraction of a wound does not stop immediately with closure; indeed, wounds which were not caused by a loss of tissue and which have their edges approximated immediately will sometimes undergo considerable contraction. Even closure of a wound by the application of a free split-thickness skin graft or pedicle graft does not stop the contracting process once movement of the wound edges has begun (Fig. 8-2). An interesting observation is that the rate of wound contraction is not the same for all points on the circumference of a wound unless the wound is a perfect circle. The ultimate configuration of the scar produced by a contracting wound is the result of variations in the rate of movement of different segments as well as the firmness of attachment of different areas of the skin to both movable and immovable structures.

The first step in studying the mechanism of wound contraction is to try to define precisely where the fundamental process is located. In the crudest analysis it must be determined whether centripetal movement occurs because an energy or power source located outside the defect is pushing the skin edges in or whether a centrally located power source is pulling the skin edges inward. Curiously, even after 15 years of intensive study, the answer is not entirely clear. There is good evidence that energy is being expended in both areas, and the question becomes whether both processes are effective or whether only one is effective and the other is either reacting to wound contraction or is insufficient to produce effective tissue movement.

Over the years most people have assumed that either central granulation tissue in a contracting wound was retracting and pulling the normal skin over the granulating base or contents of the wound were being absorbed as the skin edges moved toward the center. In 1958, Grillo et al. awakened interest in this question by reporting some experiments designed to determine whether changes in the central mass of wound tissue were pulling the skin edges together or whether central wound tissue was merely adjusting to movement of wound edges propelled by peripheral force. The commonly held opinion that dehydration of wound tissue was responsible for contraction was destroyed by their measurements, which showed that water content of central wound tissue at the beginning of wound contraction had not changed significantly at the end of contraction. The assumption that collagen synthesis and contraction might be responsible for drawing wound edges together also was disproved by direct measurements of the collagen content of wound tissue during the process of contraction. Although collagen content increased markedly

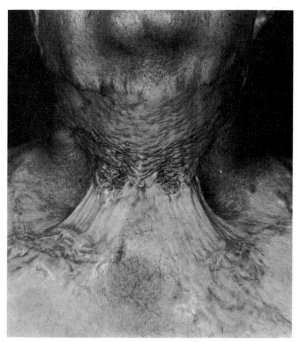

Fig. 8-2. Appearance of split-thickness skin graft applied to granulating wound while it was undergoing contraction. Note wrinkled appearance of graft and effect of continued contraction on surrounding skin.

between the fifth and eighth day of healing, total collagen in the wound began to fall significantly after this period and could not be correlated with rate of wound contraction.

The result of these studies was that attention was focused upon living cells as the motor units in the contraction process. Wound contraction occurs only in living organisms, and the force producing migration of the edges is generated by living cells. As might be expected, cytochrome poisons, such as potassium cyanide, can be shown to impair wound contraction although they do not abolish it completely. Migration of mesodermal cells in tissue culture also have been shown to be sharply restricted by cytochrome poisons. These observations are readily reversible, which suggests an inverse relationship between inhibition of aerobic respiration and cell migration.

In an attempt to see if the cells responsible for wound contraction were located in granulation tissue, Grillo excised all the central wound tissue from wounds in guinea pigs every day during the contracting process. Curiously, excision of the central tissue did not affect the rate of wound contraction. These data are not conclusive in localizing the mechanism of wound contracture, however, because they cannot be correlated with the results produced by other manipulations of the central mass of wound tissue. For instance, if a square of granulation tissue in the center of a healing wound is outlined by tattoo marks and then separated from the rest of the wound tissue by circumferential incision during wound contraction, two interesting observations can be made: The centrally migrating wound edge will retract peripherally, and the centrally circumcised area of granulation tissue will contract centrally. This finding leads one to the inescapable conclusion that the granulation tissue between the two wound edges was not being compressed by peripheral skin moving inward but was under considerable tension between the wound edges. Moreover, in other experiments, wounds which were splinted for several days and then released did not show marked acceleration of wound contraction following removal of the splint if any of the central granulation tissue was incised. Additional evidence that tension in the granulation tissue is causally related to wound contraction is found in the ingenious experiments of James and Newcombe, who measured the contraction force of granulation tissue and plotted it against the length of tissue elements and the cross-sectional area of the granulation tissue. No significant correlation between wound tension and overall wound area could be shown, but a highly significant correlation was found between cross-sectional area of granulation tissue and the tension which was developed during wound contraction. These studies suggest that granulation tissue under tension resembles stretched elastic tissue, in that the amount of tension produced is related to cross-sectional area and not to overall length or surface area. These data, plus the demonstration that granulation tissue contains cells of a type which can exert migratory force of a magnitude necessary to mobilize skin edges, strongly suggests that the machinery for wound contraction is located in the central granulating mass. A recent discovery by Majno et al. of highly specialized cells (which he termed *myofibroblasts*) with smooth muscle-like contracting powers lends additional support to this concept.

In subsequent experiments Grillo found that although wound contraction was not inhibited by excising the entire central mass of granulation tissue, it could be stopped decisively by excising a very limited zone of tissue just beneath the advancing dermal edge. He coined the term "picture frame area" to describe the strategic location of cells which appeared to constitute the machinery for wound contraction. Histologic examination of the "picture frame area" reveals a collection of large, stellate, pale-staining cells which have been thought to be the cells responsible for moving the overlying dermis.

Presently it can be said only that recent investigations have eliminated changes in nonliving materials as the cause of wound contraction and have established that the movement of wound edges requires a high order of energy transfer which is performed by living cells. No unifying hypothesis exists by which all the available data can be explained or the exact site or mechanism of action of wound contraction identified. The apparently incompatible findings of Grillo and of Abercrombie and James concerning the importance of the central granulation tissue can be explained in one of three ways. The first involves the contribution of the panniculus carnosus muscle, which is well developed in some animals and not as well developed in others. The excision of central or peripheral tissue could have vastly different effects on wound contraction depending upon the presence or absence of this structure and whether it was cut in either the primary wound or the

secondary excision. The second explanation is that although central granulation tissue can and obviously does contract to some extent during wound contraction it may be contracting as the result of peripheral wound-edge movement and not actually producing it. The third, and in the opinion of the author the most likely, explanation for the seemingly incompatible data of Grillo and Abercrombie is that the wound margin makes its way over the surface of the movable granulation tissue, and as it does so, it forces it by counteraction in a centrifugal direction, thus putting it under enough tension to cause retraction when it is excised or divided. Whatever the mechanism may be, however, the phenomenon of wound contraction is one of the most predictable and powerful of all biologic reactions and must be positively reckoned with in the management of all types of wounds.

EPITHELIZATION

An attempt to cover by regenerating epidermis any area of the body denuded of skin is the first irrefutable sign of wound repair and occurs long before any evidence of connective tissue synthesis can be detected. Factors which control the movement of epidermal cells and the mechanism by which they cover a denuded area are important to students of wound healing for two reasons. The first is that epithelization is necessary in the repair of all types of wounds if a watertight seal is to be developed. Protection from fluid and particulate-matter contamination and maintenance of an internal milieu are dependent upon the physical characteristics of keratin. It should be pointed out, however, that just as the plastic liner of a home swimming pool contributes only a watertight seal while structural stability is maintained by concrete blocks, the epidermis provides very little structural strength for the wound. It is the surrounding fibrous protein framework which gives strength to the scar (Fig. 8-3). Actually, no cellular structure or globular protein can impart much strength in the repair of a wound. When structural strength is needed, fibrous protein must be synthesized. Thus highly cellular organs, such as liver, spleen, kidney, or brain, have almost no structural strength and cannot be sutured as effectively as fibrous tissue organs, such as dura, dermis, fascia, or peritoneum. A wound healed only by epithelium will stop "weeping" and be safe from bacterial invasion as long as the epithelium is intact, but the slightest trauma will literally wipe off what is hardly more than a gelatinous film; thus no degree of permanent safety has been achieved.

Second, epithelization is of great importance in the study of wound healing because when certain variations in the control of cell division and cell movement occur, normal epithelization becomes uncontrolled growth, with awesome invasive potential. The recognized propensity to development of cancer in certain types of wound scars (radiant-energy-induced wounds particularly) and in all wounds which are prevented from healing emphasizes the close similarity between cancer and the healing process (Fig. 8-4A and 4B). Actually, a histologic section from a 5-day-old healing wound can be interpreted easily as fibrosarcoma if none of the historical details are available. Healing is dependent upon what may be thought of as a return to embryonic status; at certain times in the healing process the overall picture—characterized by mitosis, pleomorphism, disorganization, and loss of polarity—strongly resembles the uncontrolled growth of a malignant neoplasm. One major difference exists, however: the factor of control. In a healing wound, the embryonic state is temporary and some controlling influence brings order out of disorder, a resting state to rapidly multiplying cells, and a remodeling of recently synthesized fibrous tissue to produce purposeful structural patterns. In the neoplasm, however, one may consider the situation as a healing wound in which the factor of control never reappears, so that healing continues without purpose or control until the entire organism is consumed by direct extension or metastasis of the products of regeneration. Considered in this way, there may be only a very fine distinction between healing and malignant growth; it may be that when we understand all the factors which influence cells to return to embryonic activity during healing, and even more important, the factors which control their growth and movement after healing has been accomplished, an important step will have been taken in solving the riddle of cancer. For now, however, it is important to remember only that the stimulus to return to an embryonic state is one of the most powerful and predictable phenomena in biology.

Apparently cell division and ameboid movement cease only when cells are surrounded by other cells of their own type, and this characteristic behavior of individual cells has something to do with determining the direction in which a mass of cells will move. Weiss observed that when epithelial and mesenchymal cells are mixed and suspended in a proper medium, random movement of the cells will occur, causing numerous collisions. Collisions of dissimilar cells (i.e., epidermal and mesenchymal) results in repulsion, whereas collision of similar cells results in the two cells sticking together and later developing protoplasmic bridges and protofibrils. Thus random movements and collisions over a sufficient period of time invariably result in all the cells of one type becoming agglutinated on one side of the medium and the remainder of the cells becoming agglutinated in a similar manner on the other side. As increasing portions of the circumference of a cell membrane become satisfied by attaching to cells of similar lineage, the remaining unsatisfied sides become the exploring or searching surface; thus some degree of polarity for the whole mass may be established. Failure to achieve complete surface contact with other cells results in a continued state of embryonic activity. One does not have to use much imagination to predict that as the cells continue to be driven by an insatiable desire to contact cells of their own types, the risk of loss of control over replication and locomotion increases with time. Until more is known about the factors involved in the control of cell growth and movement, however, one can only take cognizance of the fact that any wound which is prevented from healing is potentially a malignant neoplasm.

Wounds caused by certain agents such as radiant energy or specific chemicals have an unusual propensity for de-

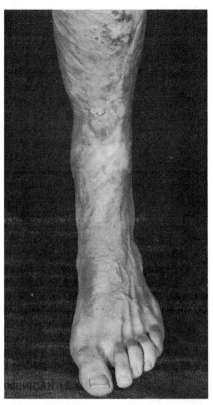

Fig. 8-3. Third-degree burn of lower leg following healing by epithelization. Absence of dermis accounts for shiny appearance and relative fragility of the surface.

veloping cancer in healed scars or unhealed wounds. In wounds induced by radiant energy, the length of time before cancer develops appears to be directly proportional to the wavelength of the damaging ray. Thus thermal burn wounds and scars may require 20 years for invasive cancer to develop, while in gamma- or x-ray wounds cancer may develop in a matter of a few months. Solar and cosmic radiation, a causative agent in most human skin cancer, is short-wavelength radiation, but because it is filtered by atmosphere and melanin, human development of epidermoid cancer from this source usually does not occur until late in life.

The development of cancer is more rare in surgical or traumatic wounds than in radiant-energy or chemical-induced wounds. No type of wound is exempt, however, when healing has been prevented by constant reinjury or inadequate skin replacement. Even in postphlebitic leg ulcer (a common chronic ulcer) cancer may develop over a long period of time.

The mechanism by which epithelium attempts to close a wound has caused considerable speculation. Previous descriptions of the process, based on the assumption that mitosis was not a prominent occurrence, are not correct. Although it is difficult to find mitotic figures in the advancing margin of epithelium, the works of Bullough and of Gillman and Penn have shown conclusively that mitosis does occur in several layers of epithelium and that it is an important part of epithelization. Theoretically, it should

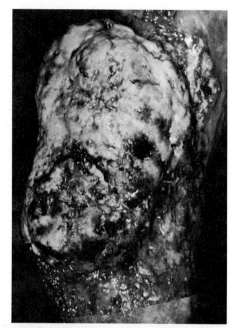

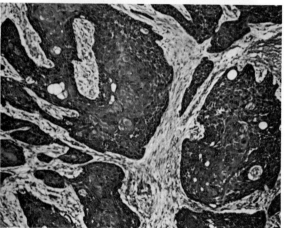

Fig. 8-4. *A.* Epidermoid carcinoma in open third-degree burn wound of thigh. Burn is 15 years old. *B.* Microscopic appearance of carcinoma shown in Fig. 8-5. Carcinoma developing in burn wounds metastasizes by vascular routes more frequently than other carcinomas.

be possible for a wound of any size to be epithelized, although there is a practical limit to the size of the area which can be covered. Mitosis is not an unlimited operation which assures that enough cells will always be present to cover any area.

One of the important gross and histologic differences between normal epithelization in a healing wound and abnormal epithelial growth in epidermoid cancer is the size and shape of the peripheral cell mass. A striking feature in a normally healing wound is the diminishing thickness to monolayer proportions of the advancing cell front (Fig. 8-5*A* and *B*). In carcinoma, cells pile up and tumble over one another to produce a grossly umbilicated appearance (Fig. 8-6*A* and *B*). Thus in normal epithelial regeneration,

even though mitosis does occur, the most fundamental process is dedifferentiation and cell movement by development of ruffled membranes and pseudopods. The process begins very early (within hours) and results in flat, thin, resting cells at the margin of the wound, that develop ruffled membranes and move across fat or granulation tissue in the center of the wound. When this occurs, the cell seems to adopt the characteristics of a typical basal cell; if it comes to rest in a more superficial position, it becomes a typical prickle cell.

In incised and sutured wounds, epithelization produces a watertight seal in 24 hours even though there is a dip where the cells have migrated into the crevice. Although the area of regeneration thickens with the addition of more cells, the center of the wound remains somewhat inverted until underlying connective tissue synthesis pushes the epithelium into an everted position. Gillman and Penn have pointed out that the cutaneous tract of a skin suture on either side of the scar is also a wound of the epithelium, and that the inverted contour of the epithelium over the main wound also occurs along the path of a suture to the extent that a completely epithelized tract may be produced or a small cyst formed after a suture is removed. These observations are important in the selection of materials and methods for closing wounds.

Epithelization of a surface wound (whether partial thickness of skin such as an abrasion, or split-thickness skin-graft donor site, or full-thickness wound such as postphlebitic ulcer of the ankle) involves similar movement of epithelial cells but over a much more hazardous terrain and greater distance than incised and sutured wounds. The early escape of blood and serum in open wounds produces a scab, and the regenerating epithelium moves beneath the scab, literally detaching it from the underlying surface as it seals the wound. Actually, epithelium does not move along the interface between dermis or fat and the scab but seems to prefer to infiltrate or actually cut through the fibrous tissue substrate by elaborating an enzyme which renders collagen soluble. This mysterious behavior has been somewhat clarified recently by identification of a collagenolytic enzyme found at the interface between epithelium and mesenchymal tissue. Confirmation of the observation that epithelium literally cuts its own path through fibrous tissue may be extremely important in understanding the remodeling of deep fibrous tissue to produce a new dermis.

The protective influence of a scab or some other cover (eschar, surgical dressing, etc.) to prevent physical trauma, drying, hemorrhage, contact with caustic materials, and the like is the basis for medical care of secondarily healing wounds. In the final analysis, successful epithelization occurs only if the cumulative effect of physical manipulation, drying, bacterial enzymes, wound area, etc., does not exceed the finite capacity of the available cells to divide, dedifferentiate, and move across the surface. Considered in the simplest analysis, it may be that interruption of epidermis merely allows the epidermis to do what it normally would do if it had room, since cell movement and cell division are to a large extent prevented in the intact epidermis by the compression effect of surrounding cells; to interrupt the integrity of an epithelium-lined surface may merely allow the cells to do what they would naturally do if they were not orderly and compactly arranged.

GROUND SUBSTANCE

Even as late as 1952, some treatises on wound healing made no mention of the role of ground substance. The mystery surrounding ground substance is nowhere better exemplified than in the name itself, a mistranslation of the German *grundsubstance,* which referred to a mysterious matrix from which all the formed elements of connective tissue were believed to originate. A similar connotation was expressed by the French *substance fondamentale.* Modern definitions have done little to clarify the true nature of this amorphous material, and the best that can be said even now is that the term "ground substance" usually refers to a continuous nonfibrillar matrix including water and electrolytes through which metabolites diffuse between blood vessels and cells. Histologically, ground substance is identified by a remarkable propensity to absorb certain dyes such as toluidine blue and to undergo characteristic reactions with periodic acid. By such staining reactions it can be seen that ground substance is relatively organized in some areas, such as basement membrane, and undergoes, during inflammation and healing, characteristic changes in staining reaction called *metachromasia.* Such histochemical reactions seem to be due to reactions with mucopolysaccharides, many of which contain hexosamine. Because of the characteristic staining reactions which they produce, attention has been focused on the acid mucopolysaccharides, even though it must be remembered that they account for only a small portion of the ground substance. As a result, errors have been made by measuring hexosamine in connective tissues and drawing conclusions about the relative amount and importance of the ground substance on the basis of change in one small sugar moiety.

Meyer's division of the acid mucopolysaccharides into two major groups has been useful in the study of wound healing. These groups are nonsulfated mucopolysaccharides, of which hyaluronic acid and chondroitin can be easily identified, and sulfated mucopolysaccharides, of which chondroitin sulfate A, chondroitin sulfate B, chondroitin sulfate C, hepartin sulfate and keratosulfate have been identified. Presently it seems that the nonsulfated group is the main component of the structureless gel fraction of ground substance and that the sulfated group is most closely associated with the fibrillar elements of connective tissue. Thus changes in the sulfated acid mucopolysaccharides are most likely to be of significance during the healing process, and, indeed, these substances are found to be increased during the early stages of wound healing. Determination of actual amounts of any of the components of ground substance may be misleading, however, as we are dealing with a very complex substance which involves polymerizing reactions and the formation

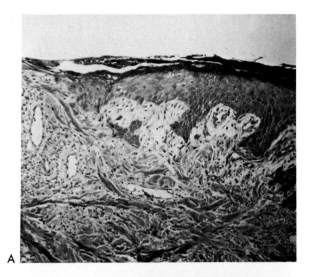

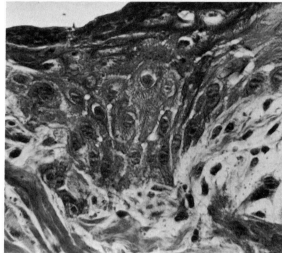

Fig. 8-5. *A.* Low-power view of epithelium advancing over granulating surface in a human wound. Note decreased thickness of advancing margin. *B.* High-power view of advancing epithelium in granulating human wound. Note dedifferentiation of cells, deep migratory activity suggesting subsurface enzyme activity at epithelial-mesenchymal tissue interface, and absence of mitotic activity.

of giant molecules with molecular weight varying between 10,000 and 10,000,000.

Because the healing process is characterized by polymerizing, cementing reactions, it is interesting to speculate upon the role of these complex substances. Discovery that acid-sulfated mucopolysaccharides accumulate during healing raises the question of whether linkages between fibrillar proteins and ground substance occur. The same question has been raised about normal tissues such as tendons, where chondroitin C is a prominent portion of the ground substance; stabilization of tendon by cross linkages between collagen fibrils and chondroitin C has not been demonstrated conclusively. Chondroitin A protein complex seems important in stabilization of cartilage,

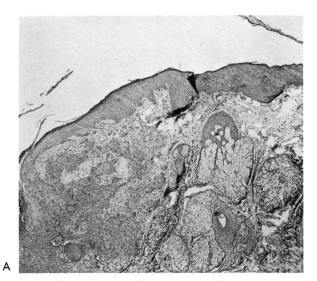

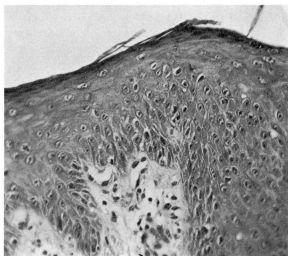

Fig. 8-6. *A.* Low-power view of epidermoid carcinoma of skin. Note accumulation of cells producing increased thickness of epithelium without purposeful migratory activity. *B.* High-power view of epidermoid carcinoma. Note numerous mitotic figures.

and destruction of this complex by local injection of papain in a rabbit's ear will produce a lop-ear deformity which will return to normal as soon as the complex is reconstituted. It seems likely that ground substance is most important in the phenomenon of healing because of its relation to collagen synthesis and remodeling. Although chemical linkages between mucopolysaccharides and collagen have been extremely difficult to identify, chemical bonds are present which may be important in the development of strength or orientation of collagen fibers and fibrils. Certainly the assembly of collagen subunits into fibrils and fibers is dependent upon many environmental conditions, which ground substance provides. Variations in the relative amounts of sulfated fractions are believed by many to be instrumental in determining the configurations of collagen fibrils, but how much this complicated sub-

stance actually participates in other aspects of the healing process awaits further investigation.

COLLAGEN

As far as the questions which patients ask their physicians following repair of wounds are concerned, fibrous protein synthesis is the essence of healing. Accurate answers to such questions as "When do the stitches come out?" "When can I go back to work?" "How bad will the scar be?" and others are dependent upon a thorough knowledge of collagen synthesis, collagen degradation, and the factors which influence the equilibrium between the two. Unfortunately, there are gaps in our knowledge about collagen metabolism; but enough is known so that the care of wounds does not have to be a mixture of craft and religion, as Paré expressed it, but can be, in most instances, a scientific exercise with a predictable outcome. Even such seeming trivia as the selection of a suture or dressing material can be the result of logical reasoning based upon factual knowledge.

Collagen is an extracellular secretion from specialized fibroblasts, and the monomeric particles or basic molecules which fibroblasts synthesize are frequently called *tropocollagen.* The tropocollagen molecule is one of the largest biologic macromolecules, with a molecular weight of about 300,000 and dimensions of 15 Å in width and 2800 Å in length. It is a stiff, elongated rod which can be visualized by an electron microscope and is soluble in cold salt solution. Thus tropocollagen is sometimes referred to as saline-extractable, or salt-soluble, collagen.

The amino acids found only in collagen, and used to identify it in analytical procedures, are hydroxyproline and hydroxylysine. The amount of collagen in a specimen of tissue is determined by measuring the amount of hydroxyproline and multiplying the result by a factor of 7.8. Other fibrous tissues such as elastin do not contain significant amounts of hydroxyproline. Formerly it was believed that hydroxyproline in collagen had much to do with the formation of various intra- and intermolecular cross links which give collagen molecules, fibers, and fibrils their characteristic rigidity. The three-plane fixation of the triple helix structure results, teleologically speaking, in our being able to rely on collagen to transmit energy accurately in tendons or to support nonfibrous structures such as muscle. The supporting nonelastic properties of collagen can be destroyed by rupturing cross links within and between molecules, but fortunately, the destruction of cross links to this extent requires rather harsh treatment for mature collagen, such as temperatures over 70°C or exposure to strong acids or alkalies. Under these circumstances, what is produced is gelatin, which, of course, has no structural strength even though the essential amino acids are present. It seems evident now that hydroxylation of proline and lysine is more important in transport of the molecule across cell membranes than in controlling physical strength.

Synthesis of collagen is an intracellular phenomenon which occurs on polysomes; a critical stage in construction of the molecule is the hydroxylation of proline to produce hydroxyproline. Externally administered hydroxyproline is rapidly excreted in the urine and apparently cannot be utilized by fibroblasts to synthesize collagen. Among other things, one of the metabolic defects which can be identified in collagen-deficiency diseases such as scurvy is the accumulation of proline-rich precursors and deficiency of hydroxyproline containing polypeptides. During active collagen synthesis the ergastoplasm of fibroblasts forms characteristic parallel lines, or canaliculi, and it appears that monomeric molecules are excreted into the extracellular milieu through these canaliculi. In ascorbic acid deficiency, the microsomes do not form parallel lines of canaliculi but are arranged, instead, in large cystic spaces. It is from these areas that proline-rich and hydroxyproline-poor amorphous material is found.

Monomeric collagen particles exposed to proper pH, temperature, osmotic conditions, etc., in the intercellular milieu aggregate or polymerize rapidly by the formation of cross links of various types. The most important such cross links are covalent ester bonds such as a Schiff's base between an amino group of one molecule and an aldehyde group of another. Oxidative deamination of lysine by an important enzyme, lysyl oxidase, is a necessary first step to formation of covalent ester cross links. In addition, other types of cross links, such as oppositely charged electrostatic groups and Van der Waals interactions, are involved in assembling monomeric particles into polymerized aggregates.

The rodlike collagen molecules appear to lie in staggered, overlapping, parallel formation, with one-quarter-length overlap. It is this staggered one-quarter-overlap arrangement of tightly packed units which gives collagen its typical repeating axial periodicity of 640 Å. Whenever collagen molecules are assembled under physiologic conditions such as those provided by the extracellular ground substance, typical fibrils with 640 Å repeating periods are produced. In certain laboratory preparations, however, it is possible to alter the characteristic 640 Å periodicity by forcing the monomeric particles to line up exactly parallel or end-on. This can be accomplished by adding glycoprotein to the milieu or by charging the preparation with a high-energy system such as adenosine triphosphate. Under these conditions, fibrils with band widths of 2000 Å can be produced; such atypical fibers are called *segment long-spacing fibers,* or *fibrous long-spacing fibrils.* These preparations have been extremely valuable in the laboratory, as they have revealed much about the size and method of polymerization of collagen molecules; they are not of any physiologic importance, however, as far as is known.

The formation of various cross links in the assembly of collagen molecules, like all polymerizing processes, is subject to acceleration and retardation by alteration of the external environment. For example, in addition to the ionic strength, temperature, and pH influences previously mentioned, various amino acids and inorganic substances have been shown by in vitro measurements of the rate of gelation of soluble collagen to have an extraordinary regulating effect. Thiocyanate, iodine, and lysine have marked accelerating influences, and urea, histamine, and creatine inhibit gelatinization. Some of the more powerful in vitro gelation accelerators have been tested for possible effect on rate of gain of tensile strength in the wounds of laboratory animals. Negative results obtained in each case strongly suggest that conditions imparted by the normal ground substance (and its changes during the healing process) are about ideal for the gelation process; none of the in vitro accelerators exerts a measurable beneficial effect on gain of tensile strength in a healing wound. Apparently monomeric collagen is, for all practical purposes, virtually nonexistent under physiologic conditions. Although it is possible to extract a tiny amount of collagen from most tissues with cold 0.45 *M* saline solution, the temperature and salt are imparting abnormal conditions which merely destroy new cross links, making very recently polymerized collagen soluble. Collagen which is soluble under these circumstances is so flimsily cross-linked that it does give some idea as to the rate of collagen synthesis and breakdown in a specimen of tissue.

Although the collagen molecule is basically a triple-helix molecule with a spiral configuration, heat-sensitive intramolecular cross links prevent it from having elastic or recoil properties. However, if a collagen fiber or fibril is placed in a water bath with a small weight suspended from one end and the temperature of the bath is elevated, a point will be reached when the heat-sensitive intramolecular cross links will be destroyed and recoil of the spiral polypeptide chain will occur. The temperature at which this phenomenon occurs is called the *thermal shrinkage temperature,* and the magnitude of this reaction is such that a fiber or fibril will shrink to one-third of its physiologic length. The thermal shrinkage temperature of collagen, therefore, is an excellent indicator of the strength and degree of inter- and intramolecular bonding. By measuring the thermal shrinkage temperature of various types of collagen, it has been possible to learn something about variations in bonding under physiologic conditions and, in some instances, to correlate the development of physical properties of collagen with the extent of cross linking. From such studies it has become clear that cross linking, among other factors, is a function of aging; the older a specimen of collagen becomes, the firmer and more numerous the cross links are. Thus, collagen gel which is only a few minutes old has relatively few cross links and a low thermal shrinkage temperature and is so flimsy that cold salt solution solubilizes it. If the gel is allowed to mature for 24 hours, the number and strength of the cross links increase to the extent that a weak acid may be needed to depolymerize even a portion of it and a higher temperature will be required to cause it to undergo thermal shrinkage. If the aggregate is allowed to polymerize for several weeks, the maximum number and firmness of cross links will be realized, with the result that a strong acid may be needed to get even a portion of the collagen into monomeric units and the thermal shrinkage temperature will be the highest yet. In summary, therefore, both solubility and thermal shrinkage temperatures can be used to measure the age of collagen as represented by the effectiveness of the cross-linking process.

In addition to naturally occurring cross links such as ester bonds, artificial cross links can be added to change the physical properties of collagen. Just as adding an agent which shares electrons easily, such as a sulfur molecule, will increase the stength of rubber (vulcanization) sevenfold, addition of a similar agent such as the methyl group in formaldehyde will increase the number and kinds of cross links in collagen. Just how much the addition and destruction of cross links has to do with the physical properties of wound-repair collagen in scar tissue is not known. It has been shown, however, that addition of methyl or amide cross links will increase the tensile strength of scar tissue in incised and sutured wounds in rats as much as threefold on the eighth postwound day. That variations in cross linking are partially responsible, however, for the final appearance, texture, or elasticity of human scars is becoming more certain for many investigators. Comparison of thermal shrinkage temperatures of collagen from primary and secondary wounds of the same age revealed a higher thermal shrinkage temperature in secondary-wound collagen than in primary-wound collagen of the same age. This finding raised the question of whether some of the markedly increased tensile strength of secondary wounds could be due to a different type or number of cross links, since the amount of collagen in the wounds is approximately equal. However, recent data strongly suggest that the phenomenon of secondary healing really is nothing more than briefly interrupted primary healing. Apparently brief physical disruption of coapted skin edges has little or no effect upon the fundamental biology and biochemistry involved in tensile strength gain of a healing wound.

At this point, other factors involved in tensile strength must be considered, for cross linking may have very little to do with tensile strength after fibrils and fibers have been formed. It is highly unlikely, in the opinion of the author, that fibrils and fibers are cross-linked very efficiently, because the average distance between fibrils is of the order of 1 μ. Chemical cross links are approximately 2.8 Å, which means that the distance is roughly 500 times too great for the usual types of cross links to span the distance between fibrils. However, because addition of cross links such as methyl or amide bonds definitely increases tensile strength in wet scar tissue, the inescapable conclusion seems to be that rupture of scar tissue must occur, to some extent, along inter- and intramolecular planes. There is not uniform agreement on this point, and the question of the importance of cross linking in the development of strength in scar tissue must be investigated further.

After a certain amount of collagen has been synthesized, the most important factor in gain of strength may be the physical weave of fibrils and fibers. Certainly it is possible to vary the physical properties of other fibrous materials by varying the weave of the small components exclusive of any chemical bonds. A good example of this principle is to be found in the physical weave of a nylon stocking. Nylon thread is nonelastic, yet a nylon stocking can be made elastic by properly weaving the fibers. Transposed to a biologic system, nonelastic tendon or fascia shows physical characteristics similar to nylon thread, while elasticity of the wall of the aorta is similar to that of a nylon stocking.

The old concept of collagen as a static, adynamic substance—the excelsior of the body—is erroneous. Actually, as will be shown later, collagen in wound scar is a relatively dynamic structure which, like other tissues, is undergoing constant remodeling and replacement. After the forty-second day of wound healing there is no measurable increase in the amount of collagen in a healing wound, yet the scar continues to gain strength for at least 2 years. Thus changes in collagen, such as increased cross linking and rearrangement of fibers and fibrils, must be occurring.

Before leaving the subject of remodeling, it is important to mention a disease, lathyrism, which has been useful in the study of collagen metabolism and which may have far-reaching implications for control of human scar tissue. The disease, recognized by Hippocrates, is caused by excessive ingestion of certain peas of the genus Lathyrus. Considerable differences exist between the human form of the disease, which is manifested by spastic paralysis, and the disease in laboratory animals, which is characterized by skeletal and cardiovascular abnormalities secondary to altered collagen metabolism. Curiously, attempts to produce neurolathyrism in rats have been unsuccessful; the Lathyrus species toxic to man and domestic animals are not toxic to rats, which thrive on them. The active and highly potent fraction which produces altered collagen metabolism is beta-aminopropionitrile. Considerable data are available on the effect of this substance on both developing and mature tissues. Most of these data support the hypothesis that the primary effect of beta-aminopropionitrile is to block the formation of inter- and intramolecular cross links during all stages of collagen aggregation. Thus beta-aminopropionitrile affects growing tissue more than adult tissue. Characteristically, beta-aminopropionitrile produces an enormous increase in the saline-extractable collagen, as it seems to block the assembly of monomeric collagen units into stable fibrils and fibers. There is some evidence to indicate that fibril formation is not stopped during lathyrism but that cross linking in fibrils is so unstable that cold saline will solubilize most of the collagen which was assembled during beta-aminopropionitrile poisoning. Growing embryos literally become saline-soluble under the effect of beta-aminopropionitrile, and mature animals will develop hernias or die suddenly of dissecting aneurysms. Wound healing, as might be predicted, is affected by beta-aminopropionitrile; there is a cessation of gain in tensile strength within hours after the agent is administered, while saline-extractable collagen increases approximately ten times. Clinical implications of the beta-aminopropionitrile effect are exciting, for it is a clear-cut demonstration that it is possible to alter the physical properties of collagen in dramatic fashion. Because some of the effects of fibrous tissue healing in specialized organs, such as the liver or heart, can be more ruinous to the health of the individual than the disease or injury which preceded healing, the demonstration that some control over deep scar formation is possible is an exciting one. If, in addition, mature recently synthesized collagen also could be solubilized selectively, a major breakthrough in many disease processes could evolve.

Several times in this chapter the term "remodeling" of scar tissue has been used. The thoughtful student is likely to be concerned over such a term, as it connotes not just synthesis of collagen but collagen breakdown as well. Because no enzyme able to lyse collagen had been identified in human beings until recently, collagen turnover in either normal tissue or wound scar was suspect. Even though no such mechanism could be demonstrated, however, indirect evidence has been abundant that some enzyme or mechanism for solubilizing collagen must exist. There is always some extractable collagen in the skin of even the oldest and most depleted individuals. Obviously, if all this tropocollagen were going into the skin, the dermis would soon be as thick as elephant hide. Some collagen must be coming out of the dermis, and the relatively constant thickness of skin only attests to an equilibrium which exists between collagen synthesis and degradation. Surface scars are always raised above the surface 2 to 4 weeks after injury; yet they usually soften, become pliable, and decrease considerably in size with the passage of more time. The loss of 50 percent of collagen from the gravid uterus 36 hours after parturition and the rapid disappearance of dermis when tetraplegic patients are allowed to lie unattended attest that man possesses an extremely effective enzyme capable of degrading mature collagen. Search for such an enzyme previously has been unsuccessful because it was assumed that the enzyme could be extracted from tissues. In 1963, Gross, Lapiere, and Tanzer hypothesized that collagenolytic enzyme was the product of living cells and that contact with a living cell was necessary in order for collagenolysis to occur. In one of the most important experiments performed in the wound-healing field during the last decade, they tested their hypothesis by preparing culture plates of reconstituted collagen and amphibian Tyrode culture medium. Specimens of tissue from the rapidly absorbing tail of a metamorphosing tadpole (a structure containing mostly collagen which is absorbed and not broken off during metamorphosis) were placed on the collagen–Tyrode substrate, and the culture plates were incubated under suitable tissue culture conditions. After several days a clear zone appeared around each implant, and if the tissues were kept alive long enough, the entire substrate became lysed by collagenolytic activity. Failure of the cells to survive stops collagenolytic activity immediately; even after lysis has begun, it can be stopped by killing the cells. Thus Gross and Lapiere demonstrated that collagenolytic enzyme is a product of living cells and that cells which produce enzyme need to be in close contact with collagen fibers for lysis to occur. Grillo, using the same tissue-culture technique, cultured wound tissues from actively healing wounds in guinea pigs and found extremely active enzyme activity at the wound edge. Moreover, the most active lysis in a secondary healing wound appeared to be at the epidermis-dermis interface of an advancing wound margin. Riley and Peacock cultured a variety of normal and pathologic human tissues and found collagenolytic enzyme to be widely distributed, particularly in epithelium-containing structures.

The most uniformly positive tissue for collagenolytic enzyme in human beings is cutaneous scar. Scar tissue reveals positive lytic activity approximately 10 days after closure of a cutaneous laceration, and a high level of activity has been found in dermal scars as long as 30 years after injury. Granulation tissue is only slightly active; burn eschar does not show any activity for about 2 weeks. Between 2 and 3 weeks after a third-degree burn, however, cultures of separating dermal eschar are strongly positive for collagenolytic activity. These findings suggest that invasion of dead eschar by underlying connective tissue cells or undermining epidermal cells is necessary for contact between cells and heat-tanned collagen.

By measuring both collagen synthesis and collagen breakdown, it is now possible to study healing from the standpoint of variations in metabolic equilibrium. Considered as such, scar tissue becomes a product of opposing forces of collagen synthesis and collagen destruction, and the result of these forces will vary according to the relative rate and effectiveness of each. The maximum amount of total collagen in a healing wound is found by the forty-second day. Although increased amounts of saline-extractable collagen (compared with nonwounded resting dermis) can be extracted from the scar for as long as 18 months, there is no further gain in insoluble (or mature) collagen. The conclusion would seem to be that, even though remodeling of the collagen continues, equilibrium has been established between collagen synthesis and collagen destruction. Recent demonstration by Cohen of accelerated collagen synthesis and deposition and collagenolytic activity in human keloids probably represents an abnormality of such an equilibrium.

The concept that all collagen to some extent, and healing wound collagen particularly, is undergoing simultaneous construction and destruction can serve as a basis for speculation concerning some of the previously unexplainable findings in the healing process. One such enigma is the behavior of wounds during ascorbic acid depletion. In the classic descriptions of scurvy it is important to remember that sailors' wounds did not just fail to heal; they actually disrupted months after they had healed perfectly. This observation has been verified in animals and raises the question of whether collagen is dependent upon ascorbic acid for structural integrity. It is known that collagen can be repeatedly depolymerized and reconstituted in the laboratory without contact with ascorbic acid, and artificially reconstituted collagen does not lose tensile strength. Therefore, the notion that vitamin C has anything to do with strength of mature scar tissue is untenable. Because synthesis of new collagen is blocked during ascorbic acid deficiency, and because collagenolytic activity probably proceeds normally, a possible explanation for old scar dehiscence would seem to be that tissue previously in equilibrium becomes unbalanced by having synthesis knocked out and lysis continue. Inexorably, the scar will become weaker until a point is reached where normal tissue tension produces complete disruption.

Although to some extent hypothetical (actual quantitative measurements of lysis and synthesis are not sensitive enough now to prove or disprove the equilibrium hypothesis), the theory is important as it relates to the whole field of conditions erroneously referred to in the past as "collagen diseases." The collagen in these diseases is precipitated under physiologic conditions and, as might be predicted, is normal as far as can be determined by electron or light microscopy, x-ray defraction, or amino acid analysis. Thus all the evidence supports the idea that so-called "collagen diseases" represent abnormal amounts of collagen in abnormal places but are not specific diseases of the collagen molecule or fibril. Such an explanation is entirely logical, as one cannot have a disease of a nonliving structure. Collagen is a long-chain polymer in which the nearest thing that could be classified as a disease process is the abnormal construction of collagen during lathyrism. The collagen in such diseases as rheumatic fever, dermatomyositis, and scleroderma is probably much more accurately considered as the ash or scar from a burnt-out primary wound or inflammatory process. The concept of the collagen system as a dynamic, constantly remodeling one, however, opens the door for investigation of a large number of diseases of unknown cause which are characterized by deficient or excessive collagen formation.

SEQUENCE OF EVENTS: SUMMARY

Once the basic processes in the healing phenomenon have been mastered, the student has only to relate them to one another in proper sequence to be ready to start the study of what physicians can do to aid healing. The most important concept in this regard is the understanding that healing is not a series of events but is a concert of simultaneously occurring processes, some of which continue for many years after physical integrity of wounded tissue has been reestablished. The most dramatic events, such as sealing the wound, regaining tensile strength sufficient to permit normal stress, and acquiring a scar which is cosmetically acceptable, occur in a relatively short period of time. Long-term processes, such as remodeling of collagen and development of cancer in scar tissue, fortunately are not processes which cause patients much concern. Although the basic processes are much the same in an incised and sutured wound properly coapted (healing by primary intention) and a wound in which tissue has been lost so that healing must occur by contraction and epithelization (secondary healing, or healing by secondary intention), the time required for secondary healing is so much longer and the area involved usually so much greater that it is convenient to study the secondary healing process to see how the basic steps in wound healing relate to one another.

The first thing which happens after full-thickness skin loss is that normal elasticity of the skin and external tension produced in some areas by muscle pull enlarges the defect according to the amount of force exerted and the direction over which it acts. Thus the shape of a skin defect may have little relation to the size or shape of the fragment of tissue which was removed. If hemorrhage is not too severe, a clot forms quickly, then contracts and dehydrates to form a scab. Because a scab is essentially a dehydrated, fully contracted blood clot, it is less durable and effective in closing the wound than collagenous eschar. Nevertheless, a scab serves an extremely useful purpose in providing limited protection from external contamination, satisfactory maintenance of internal hemostasis, and a surface beneath which cell migration and movement of the wound edges can occur. Classically, the beginning of wound healing is described as the "lag" phase—an inaccurate term which carries the connotation that there is a period when nothing of importance is happening. Actually, a great number of extremely important things are happening even though they usually are not considered part of the healing process. One soon recognizes, however, that almost instantly following infliction of an injury the stage for healing is set, and the props and background for the events which are to follow are essentially those of controlled inflammation. Study of the biology of repair has emphasized that the most successful reparative processes occur against a background of inflammation and that, up to the point of necrosis, how well the wound heals is directly related to the amount of inflammation present. Specifically, the release of various amines from connective tissue mast cells, perfusion of capillaries surrounding the defect, change in permeability of capillary walls, release of enzymes, fluid, and protein into extracellular spaces, accumulation of white blood cells and connective tissue cells, and formation of thrombi in peripheral lymphatic channels are all well-known changes in general inflammation which are extremely important in providing the best milieu for repair to proceed. It is only when bacteria, foreign bodies, medications, or accumulation of destructive enzymes cause necrosis of tissue that inflammation becomes a deterrent to healing. Therefore the author prefers to see the term "lag" phase replaced by strong emphasis on inflammation as an active part of the reparative process.

Approximately 12 hours after injury has occurred, and at a time when inflammation is definite, epithelial migration—the first clear-cut sign of rebuilding—occurs. In a primary wound, epithelization is complete in a few hours; in a secondary healing wound, migration of cells is rapid at first, but as the line of cells from the wound margin becomes extended and the epithelial probe dwindles to a monolayer, progress becomes slower, so that days or even weeks elapse before epithelization is complete. After 4 or 5 days, however, epithelization is greatly assisted as the machinery of wound contraction begins, and the wound margins begin centripetal movement.

A great amount of activity takes place in the center of the wound after a scar or eschar has been removed and before epithelium has covered the surface. Grossly, the surface which was once gray or yellow-brown and perfectly smooth becomes bright red and granular. The reason for this is an extravagant proliferation of richly perfused capillary loops. The knuckles or loops of blood vessels impart a granular appearance to the surface, and it is because of them that the wound is often described as granulating or showing granulation tissue. Granulation tissue provides a good defense against invasion by surface contaminants, but it is fragile and produces a difficult terrain for advancing epithelial cells to negotiate. This is particularly true if surface infection, edema, or deep fibrous tissue interferes with return circulation. When this happens, the fiery red granular dots will change to a purple, soggy, gray-black cluster which may fill the entire wound cavity and spill over the wound edge, thus eliminating the possibility of epithelization.

Although no visible signs of collagen synthesis can be found until the fourth to sixth day, biochemical evidence of collagen synthesis can be found between the second and fourth days. The level of hydroxyproline in wound tissue rises rapidly, and the saline-extractable-collagen level becomes elevated shortly thereafter. Before these signs of collagen synthesis occur, the ground substance changes, as evidenced by the accumulation of sulfated mucopolysaccharides and the development of metachromasia. On or about the seventh day wounds will show a delicate fine reticulum of young collagen fibrils. Actually, the gelation process which is occurring at this time is so random that polymerization of new collagen fibrils is much like that of a new gel in a laboratory beaker—without purposeful orientation or polarity. There is a short period during this time when young fibrils and fibers will take silver stains selectively, and it is thought that this property reflects the presence of large numbers of unsatisfied bonding sites which will be used later; mature collagen fibers do not stain selectively with silver. As fibrogenesis proceeds, purposefully oriented fibers seem to become thicker, presumably because they are accruing more collagen particles; nonpurposefully oriented fibers seem to disappear. The overall effect appears to be one of lacing the wound edges together by a three-dimensional weave. In secondary wounds the mass of scar tissue becomes dense, compact, and smaller in circumference but shows little in the way of purposeful organization. The overall direction is one of replacing granulation tissue, allowing the surface to become covered with epithelium, and filling in the remaining skin defect with scar tissue after contraction is complete. As far as filling the defect is concerned, contraction is the major influence; it exerts full potential before scar-tissue synthesis is complete. The central scar seems to remodel itself to fill the defect after contraction is over. Thus wounds surrounded by mobile and redundant skin will have a small central scar, while wounds surrounded with tight nonmovable skin will have relatively large central scars regardless of the size of the defect.

Development of tensile strength (strength per unit of scar tissue) and burst strength (strength of the entire wound) are the results initially of blood vessels growing across the wound, epithelization, and coagulation of globular protein. Later, collagen synthesis is important. The effect of vascularization and epithelization, although relatively small, is usually adequate on the fifth day to hold wound edges, if not under excessive tension, coapted without sutures. The really significant gain in tensile strength begins about the fifth day, however, when collagen synthesis becomes apparent; tensile strength measurements in laboratory animals usually are recorded from that day. Increase in strength is rapid for 17 days and slow for an additional 10 days; there is an almost imperceptible gain

in tensile strength for at least 2 years. In spite of the measurable increase in tensile strength for such a long period, the strength of the scar in rat skin never quite reaches that of unwounded skin.

Collagen content of the wound tissue rises rapidly between the sixth and the seventeenth days but increases very little after the seventeenth day and none at all after the forty-second day. Gain in strength after the seventeenth day, therefore, is due primarily to remodeling of collagen and, hence, is not correlated with total collagen content except for a very short portion of the healing curve.

When a normally healing wound is mechanically disrupted after the fifth day and immediately resutured, the return of tensile strength is so rapid that within 2 days the burst strength is nearly what it would have been had the secondary wound not occurred. This phenomenon, commonly called the *secondary healing effect,* has been studied intensely to determine the exact mechanism of rapid gain of tensile strength following a secondary wound. Curiously, it is neither more rapid collagen synthesis nor more rapid assembly of collagen subunits; secondary wounds contain slightly less collagen than primary wounds of the same age. Because the thermal shrinkage temperature of secondary wound collagen is significantly higher than that of primary wounds of the same age, it has been suggested that more effective cross linking or better physical weave of collagen subunits is responsible for the rapid gain in strength of secondary wounds. The recent demonstration by Madden and Smith that secondary healing is really nothing more than continued primary healing (without a lag phase) invalidates previous cross-linking theories of secondary wound healing. Whatever the explanation, however, the machinery for producing rapid gain in tensile strength in secondary wounds is limited to an area of 7 mm around the first wound. Excision of skin edges more than 7 mm circumferential to the primary wound results in secondary wound healing at the same rate as in a primary wound.

WOUND CARE

From a treatment standpoint, there are essentially two types of wounds: those which are characterized by loss of tissue and those in which no tissue has been lost. Lacerations are an example of wounds without tissue loss, and avulsions or burns are examples of wounds which, in addition to interruption of surface continuity, result in destruction of tissue. A question which must be answered for both is whether immediate closure can be done safely. Whether the wound can be closed by suturing the edges together or a graft of some sort is required, a decision must be reached about whether closure can be immediate or should be delayed until the danger of infection is past.

The history of wound surgery is, in large measure, the history of military surgery, and the decision of many surgeons about whether to close a wound primarily or to delay closure is based on principles and practices developed in military hospitals. The tendency of many surgeons to set a certain number of hours after a wound is sustained as the time during which primary closure can be performed safely probably dates back to World War I and a study of wound bacteriology made in French military hospitals. In an attempt to determine the number of hours within which immediate wound closure would be safe and beyond which closure should be delayed, many wounds were cultured and the growth of bacteria measured. It was determined that about 12 hours after wounding, the number of colonies on the wound surface doubled; this was interpreted as meaning that debridement and wound closure were safe before 12 hours had elapsed but likely to be dangerous after that time. It is interesting to follow the effect of this study through subsequent years and to note the difficulties that surgeons have encountered in performing primary wound closure in any predetermined length of time. As troubles have been encountered in following a set time for closure, the time has been shortened to the point where it is sometimes recommended that wounds not be closed more than 2 hours after injury. Obviously, there is no fixed length of time within which primary closure is always safe and beyond which secondary closure must be done. The key to deciding when a wound should be closed is an understanding of the difference between contamination and infection; the trick to determining when one has become the other is the ability to recognize and interpret signs of inflammation. A contaminated wound can be converted by skillfully performed surgery into a clean wound which can then be closed safely; an infected wound cannot be surgically debrided without high risk of failure, including the potentially lethal complications of interfering with natural localizing processes. The history and physical examination contribute valuable information, because the length of time needed for contamination to become infection reflects, among other things, the strength of the bacterial inoculum and the ability of the substrate to combat invasion. A clean razor slice of highly vascular skin of the face might be closed safely 48 hours after injury, whereas a stable-floor-nail penetration of the foot of an elderly person might not be closed safely 1 minute after injury.

Once the decision has been made to close a laceration, the surrounding skin should be prepared with a suitable antiseptic and a local anesthetic injected. A good guide to the application of antiseptic is never to put anything in the wound that could not be tolerated comfortably in the conjunctival sac. Any caustic solution which is capable of sterilizing the surface of the skin will also destroy delicate cells on the surface of the wound. Therefore, harsh antiseptics should be applied only up to the edges of the wound, never within it. Debridement of a wound can be done either hydrodynamically or mechanically. When the wound contains only surface contaminants not attached to wound tissues, a copious stream of saline solution will flush foreign bodies and undesirable organisms out of the wound cavity. When devitalized or contused tissue fragments are still attached to the wound tissues and external contaminants are partially driven into the tissues, however, surgical excision of affected tissues must be performed. When there is a redundancy of tissue and there are no important structures in the depth of the wound, such as

nerve or tendon, the best type of debridement is excision of the entire wound to produce under optimal conditions a new wound which is surgically clean. When there is a shortage of tissue or when a wound involves important structures which cannot be sacrificed without producing disability, damaged tissue must be carefully dissected out of the wound until all dead tissue and extraneous material have been meticulously removed. In a wound of the hand involving numerous tendons and nerves, this type of debridement may be extremely tedious and require several hours to perform.

After the wound has been debrided, proper suture materials must be selected for closure. There are two main types of sutures, absorbable and nonabsorbable, and selection of the proper one should be based on what has been learned about the biology of the healing process. For the most part, absorbable sutures, which are made of sheep intestines, are used when infection is known to be present or when debridement has been difficult and thoroughness is in doubt.

Plain gut sutures will be solubilized by tissue collagenase in less than 10 days, while gut which has been tanned lightly with chromium salts will remain structurally intact for approximately 3 weeks. Absorbable sutures are usually not used when they can be avoided, because the reaction to a foreign animal protein is considerably greater than to such substances as cotton, silk, and nylon. Synthetic absorbable sutures, recently available, may not be as locally irritating as animal proteins. Because the collagen-synthesis stage of wound healing is barely under way at 10 days and the scar tissue is far from mature even at 3 weeks, a more permanent material is needed if widening of the scar is to be prevented. Chromic gut sutures produce less soft tissue reaction than plain gut sutures, possibly because more available cross-linking sites have been satisfied by the tanning agent.

Nonabsorbable sutures are usually preferable because they produce less tissue reaction and can remain permanently below the surface of the integument. The major disadvantage of permanent sutures is that if they are placed in areas where infection develops, the suture material can harbor organisms; hence infection will not subside until the sutures are removed. A nonabsorbable suture of steel or some alloy may be mechanically irritating, and sometimes an inflammatory reaction develops around nonabsorbable sutures which resembles a local allergic phenomenon. Sutures are placed in different types of tissue for different reasons; before selecting and placing a suture in a wound, one should ask these questions: What is the suture being asked to do? and How long does it need to do it? Sutures which are placed in tissues to hold wound edges together under tension need to be placed in fibrous tissue. Moreover, if the final appearance of the surface scar is important and tension on the suture line is unavoidable, permanent sutures should be used. Even a suture which lasts 15 days would not be acceptable under these circumstances, as collagen synthesis and, more important, remodeling of recently synthesized scar have barely gotten under way at this time. Sutures placed in cellular tissues such as fat, epidermis, liver, or kidney provide little structural strength, as they tend to cut through such tissues, which have no appreciable strength of their own. Sutures in these tissues usually are used to obliterate a potential cavity (dead space), provide hemostasis, or act as a fine-adjustment leveling device on the surface of the skin. Objectives for these sutures are met in a few hours, thus absorbable sutures can be used satisfactorily if they are desirable.

A typical facial wound involving skin, subcutaneous fat, fascia, and superficial muscle might be repaired in the following way: After local anesthesia has been administered, the skin prepared, contaminants flushed out with saline solution, and any dead fragments of tissue excised, closure is performed. The muscle, being primarily cellular, would not support the pull of a suture, so the fibrous tissue surrounding it is closed with a permanent suture of silk or cotton. If hemorrhage has been significant in the muscle, a separate suture or ligature may be used to control it. If the skin is closed in a single layer, the retracted subcutaneous fat might not come together completely, thus producing a cavity which would become filled with blood and possibly infected. Another loosely tied stitch, which has no strength because it does not pass through fibrous tissue, is frequently used to obliterate a cavity in the subcutaneous area and discourage hemorrhage of a capillary type. After the subcutaneous tissue has been closed, a decision should be made about the desired final appearance of the surface scar. The width of the wound following closure of the subcutaneous tissue will be a good indicator of how wide the final cutaneous scar will be if the next sutures merely approximate the skin edges and are tied on the outside. The reason is that, if suture marks are to be avoided, silk sutures should be removed in 6 to 8 days because of development of inflammatory reaction, epithelial lined tracts, or small stitch abscesses. Although the wound edges may be accurately coapted with only a hairline scar at the time that such sutures are removed, the wound is held together only by epithelium, blood vessels, and globular protein. Even though it usually will not dehisce before collagen production takes over, the scar will stretch and widen during the ensuing 21 days while collagen formation and remodeling are occurring. The result usually is that a 7-day-old 1-mm-wide scar may become a 1-cm-wide scar 3 weeks after the sutures have been removed. The best way to prevent widening of a scar after skin sutures are removed is to place permanent sutures in the fibrous protein layers of the skin to bring the edges together. This is accomplished by a subcuticular or intradermal suture of fine silk or cotton. The overlying epidermis is gently retracted, and the sutures are placed in the lower part of the dermis. The knot is sometimes placed deep in the subcutaneous tissue, but it can be tied superficially provided that the ends of the suture are cut close and the knot and suture ends are covered by overlying epithelium. It is important to use a very fine suture that will not be palpable beneath the epithelium and a clear or light-colored suture material that will not show through the translucent epithelium.

After subcuticular sutures have been placed, the skin edges will be as close together as it is possible to bring

them, yet the overlying epithelial edges may be vertically uneven. A final row of sutures of very fine silk or nylon which serve as a fine adjustment or leveler of the epithelial edges is frequently used to produce an even surface. Because these sutures are in cellular tissue, they contribute little to the strength of the wound and should not be placed more than 1 mm away from the wound edge. They should be tied loosely and removed before any epithelial reaction develops. Actually, external sutures in a wound closed in this manner could probably be removed in a few hours or as soon as the plasma clot seals the epithelial edges. For practical purposes, however, they are not removed until the first dressing, whenever that may be. In recent years the use of external cutaneous sutures has been partially eliminated by the development of various types of adhesive tapes which can be used to hold the skin edges together without producing epithelial sinuses or reaction.

When do you remove the stitches? is a question frequently asked of surgeons. The answer is simple: when they have done the job they were put in to do, namely, hold the wound edges together until adequate tensile strength has developed. To set a finite period of time for removal of sutures is to imply that wounds heal at a standard rate; but the rate of healing is extremely variable even in different parts of the body and under different conditions in a single individual. Instead of counting days until sutures can be removed, the wound must be examined; sometimes one or two sutures must be removed to see if the skin edges are sufficiently adherent to permit removal of all sutures. In wounds where a narrow scar is important and where some tension is unavoidable, it is advisable to splint the immature scar with adhesive strips for 2 or 3 weeks or until new collagen has attained sufficient strength and reliability.

The appearance of a linear scar is always worse between the third and fifth weeks after wound closure than it is at the time that sutures are removed. The irregular, raised, purplish appearance of immature scar tissue at this time can be a cause of great concern to young patients. Resorption of excess collagen, development of pliability, and the fading of undesirable color are called *maturation* of the scar, and maturation occurs more rapidly in older people than in the young. Children and teen-age patients, particularly, may have a distressing amount of red in their scars for several years. This condition is always a temporary one, however, and redness should never be an indication for secondary surgical revision.

Scars should be revised secondarily only after they have undergone maximum maturation. Beefy, red, hypertrophic, immature scars usually recur after excision, and it is often amazing how much natural improvement will occur if sufficient time is allowed. It is seldom wise to attempt surgical improvement of a scar in less than 6 months; often natural improvement will continue for as long as 12 months.

Secondary revision should never be performed with the idea of changing the color of a scar or with the idea that a scar can be eliminated completely. All that secondary revision can accomplish is to take out a scar which resulted from unskilled closure or closure under unsatisfactory conditions and to close the defect as skillfully as possible under the best conditions. Leveling uneven edges, changing direction of the scar so that it does not cross lines of changing dimensions, and narrowing a wide scar by the use of meticulously placed subcuticular sutures are the main improvements which can be accomplished. If scar tissue is elevated slightly above the level of surrounding skin, abrasion of that area by sandpaper or rotating brush will produce a smooth denuded surface over which new epithelium will spread in a more even sheet.

Wounds characterized by a loss of skin can be allowed to heal by contraction and epithelization if there is sufficient skin to be stretched across the defect. This is usually permitted only when infection prevents primary closure and when contraction does not produce a contracture which would interfere with function or produce a cosmetically unacceptable scar. In all other wounds, a skin graft should be performed to replace the skin which has been lost.

At the moment, there is no known catalyst to speed up wound healing; about all that a physician can do to aid normal healing is to protect the wound from physical, chemical, or bacteriologic complications which retard or prevent healing. Protection usually means the use of an artificial dressing unless a good natural dressing material, such as an eschar or scab, can serve the same purpose. Once the scar or eschar deteriorates, however, it, like any other dressing material, must be changed (debrided), and either definitive coverage provided or an artificial dressing applied. As in the selection of suture materials, choosing dressing materials involves a clear understanding of the objectives of each component of the dressing and the fundamental biologic processes that the dressing is supposed to protect. The first layer of a dressing is usually made of fine-mesh gauze, so that granulation tissue will not penetrate the interstices and cause hemorrhage when the dressing is removed. A long search for a pharmacologic substance to incorporate in the gauze to stimulate epithelial growth has been unsuccessful so far. Because certain by-products of the azo dye industry are carcinogenic, it was hoped that related dyes such as scarlet red might offer epithelial stimulation without being carcinogenic. All such substances have been disappointing, however, although most surgeons do use a gauze impregnated with some bland substance such as petroleum jelly or topical antibiotic in a water-soluble base. The main value of such medicated dressings is that there is less adherence of epithelium and vascular tissue to the dressing, hence less interference with wound healing when the dressing is changed. Dry gauze is a perfectly satisfactory dressing for most wound surfaces, however, and when carefully applied and removed, it can be as atraumatic as any other material. The usual coarse 4×4 hospital gauze sponge with its cotton-filled center is not a good material to place against open wounds; the interstices permit permeation by vascular tissue, and the cotton lint which is included becomes embedded in the wound. Sponges, mechanics' waste, bulk cotton, and the like are used to give bulk to a dressing after the fine-mesh gauze has been applied to make the dressing conform to a desired shape and immobilize the wounded part. Nonstretchable, firm, roller gauze bandage and adhesive tape are used to complete the dressing in a typical occlusive (erroneously called "pressure") type of dressing. The nonstretchable gauze and adhesive tape provide a compact and stable immobilizing influence. A clean wound has very little drainage and no odor, and does not have to be dressed very often.

Infected wounds have considerable drainage and odor and, therefore, must be dressed often to provide suitable drainage and tolerable appearance. It is common practice to use a wet dressing on infected wounds, which means that the inside layers of the dressing are intentionally moistened with saline solution or some other substance. The realization that there is no catalytic effect upon healing or any control of infection from water and that maceration of skin or eschar produces favorable conditions for bacterial or fungus growth throws doubt upon the beneficial effects to be obtained by applying a wet dressing. The usual answer is that drainage is increased by capillary action or that debridement is accomplished as detritus sticks to the dressing. Such reasoning has never seemed logical to the author; a dry dressing will absorb more wound drainage than a saturated one, and debridement can usually be accomplished more efficiently by mechanical means. It often appears that wounds become cleaner more quickly with the use of wet dressings, but in the author's experience this is partly because wet dressings are changed more often. Of course, less pain may be associated with wet-dressing changes than with dry-dressing changes. However, when dry dressings are changed frequently and skillfully, surface detritus may be removed more effectively by dry dressings than by wet ones. One sound reason for using a wet dressing, however, is that wet heat is more penetrating than dry heat, and when additional warmth is desirable to increase the local inflammatory response, a warm moist dressing is very effective. Failure to keep a moist dressing warm by the addition of external heat, however, results in a cold soggy dressing which has no particular virtue and which is definitely inferior to a frequently changed dry one.

SKIN GRAFTS

Skin grafts are classified as free grafts (meaning that they are separated completely from their donor sites before being transferred to recipient areas) and pedicle grafts (which maintain a vascular connection with the general circulation). Free grafts are full-thickness (which means that the entire thickness of the skin, including epidermis and dermis, is transferred) and split-thickness (which means that the entire epidermis and only a portion of the dermis are transferred). The remainder of the dermis after split-thickness skin grafting remains at the donor site.

The "take" of a free graft refers to the pink appearance of a graft which occurs between the third and fifth days after transfer, signifying that vascular connections have developed between the recipient bed and the transplant. Before this time, free grafts are white and do not show any change in color when pressed upon and released. It is a matter of considerable conjecture whether there is any diffusion of gases and nutrients between the cells of the graft and the underlying capillaries prior to the development of actual vascular connections, and it has been assumed in the past that diffusion was necessary to keep cells nourished during the first few days. When grafts which include more than full thickness of the skin do not survive as free transplants, or when split-thickness grafts with pus or blood interposed between the graft and the capillary bed do not survive, it has been considered that diffusion could not occur through fat, pus, blood, etc. It seems more likely now, however, that diffusion is not important in the take of a graft and that mechanical barriers such as pus, blood, or fat prevent the take of a free graft by preventing vascular connections from occurring. Whatever the reason, the thicker the graft, the more likely will be the failure of take if mechanical or inflammatory conditions at the graft-wound interface are less than optimal. For this reason, thin grafts are used to cover less than ideally prepared wounds; full-thickness grafts are reserved for surgically produced wounds under optimal conditions.

In taking a full-thickness skin graft the surgeon will produce a wound which will have to be closed by suturing the edges together or by applying a split-thickness skin graft from another donor site. If this is not done, closing of the wound in one area with the graft will leave a wound of the same size and shape at the donor site. Full-thickness grafts are usually small grafts which can be taken from a place where there is an excess of thin skin, such as the inframammary fold or the groin, where the donor site can be closed by suturing the skin edges together.

It was once thought that split-thickness skin grafts must be taken through the level of the dermal-epidermal undulating interface so that small islands of stratum germinativum cells would remain to reepithelize the denuded surface. Because of this notion, surgeons were careful to take grafts as thin as possible, and the taking of a split-thickness skin graft was relegated to only a few highly skilled individuals (Fig. 8-7). It seems obvious now that if it were possible to take a graft through only the epithelium, a satisfactory take would be unlikely. Most of the cells would be dead, and the covered wound would be resurfaced by cells which would provide no better coverage than that which would have occurred from normal epithelization. The qualities of skin other than waterproofing (strength, flexibility, appearance, etc.) which are desired in a graft are qualities provided by the dermis. The final appearance of both the recipient and donor sites, therefore, reflects the amount of dermis which has been transferred and the amount of dermis which is left behind. Epithelial cells migrate out of deeply located glands and hair follicles, and donor sites which do not extend through the entire depth of the dermis will be reepithelized from these sources. Dermis, being a complex organ and not a simple tissue, does not regenerate, however, and if all the properties of normal dermis are desired in the recipient area, full-thickness dermis must be transferred; if less than the full thickness is transferred, the resulting graft will be abnormal in appearance and function.

In choosing the thickness of a free skin graft, the qualities which are desired in the recipient area must be balanced against the cost incurred in the donor site. How these factors influence selection of graft thickness can be

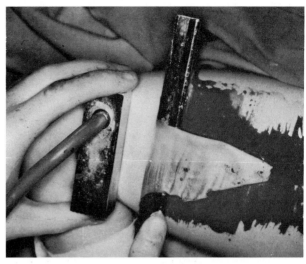

Fig. 8-7. Removal of thick split-thickness skin graft with a free-hand knife. The largest possible grafts can be taken by this method.

illustrated by comparing two extremes in wound and donor-site conditions. In a large thermal burn, the recipient area is far from optimal in that it is usually infected and edematous and involves a large area. The take of a graft is therefore uncertain, and revascularization is problematic. From the standpoint of the donor site, it may be necessary to procure several grafts from the same area to obtain enough skin for the entire wound; thus rapid healing, with a remaining dermis thick enough for subsequent grafts to be taken, is mandatory. In this case, both donor-site and recipient conditions require thin grafts. In contrast, a 2-cm-diameter wound caused by loss of skin from the cheek of a young person presents an entirely different set of requirements for an optimal graft. The recipient bed should be optimal if excised immediately or prepared later in the operating room. The need for full-thickness dermis is mandatory so that normal texture, color, and thickness will produce the most cosmetically acceptable result. The graft is small, so a variety of areas with a 2-cm redundancy of skin can be found for a donor site. Thus all factors point to the selection of a full-thickness graft. In other wounds the choice may not be quite so clear, but the principles involved in these two cases are the factors which must be considered in selection of any free graft (Fig. 8-8*A* and *B*).

Split-thickness skin grafts have a tendency to develop deep pigmentation after transfer. The thinner the graft, the more pronounced is postoperative pigmentation for 6 to 9 months following transfer. It is important to warn patients who have recently had split-thickness skin grafts placed on exposed areas of the body that protection from solar radiation is mandatory for at least 6 months. Thick grafts have less tendency to develop undesirable pigment, and they will usually blend into their new surroundings more quickly than thin ones.

Finally, a word should be said about the concept of the "dressing graft." Split-thickness skin is the best possible dressing material for an open wound, and failure of many surgeons to take advantage of this fact in treating compli-

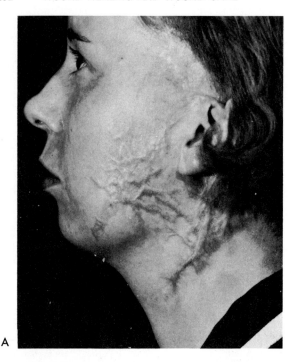

A

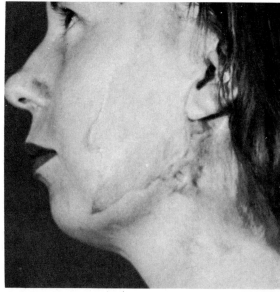

B

Fig. 8-8. *A.* Hypertrophic scar produced by deep second-degree burn. Although a significant amount of full-thickness skin has not been lost, overproduction of collagen has produced an unsightly scar. *B.* Patient shown in Fig. 8-8*A* following excision of facial portion of scar and application of a thick split-thickness skin graft. Cervical portion of scar will be resurfaced later. A single graft covering facial and cervical areas would obliterate submandibular groove. Note that scar at junction of graft and skin is most prominent near angle of mouth where motion and tension are unavoidable. Although different in texture, hue, and thickness from normal skin, the graft provides a smooth surface over which cosmetics can be applied more effectively than over previous scar.

cated wounds is usually based on the mistaken notion that placing a split-thickness skin graft on a wound is tantamount to closing the wound. Although the possibility that some portion or all of the graft may take and thus close the wound is the main advantage in using split-thickness skin grafts as a dressing material, placing the graft on a wound of questionable suitability for closure does not in itself produce a closed wound in the same manner as suturing two full-thickness skin edges together. Actually, a skin dressing does not close the wound any more than a petroleum jelly gauze dressing. If the wound has been inadequately debrided or infection is not yet controlled, the graft will slough in a few days and may completely disappear by the time of the first dressing. By dressing wounds of questionable suitability for closure with a split-thickness skin graft, however, the surgeon provides a definite biologic cover. If the wound is not ready for closure, the graft will not take, and nothing will have been lost except a few square centimeters of split-thickness skin from the donor area. Dressing a questionable wound of relatively small size with split-thickness skin, therefore, is a sort of biologic test to determine suitability for closure, as well as providing some benefit if even a part of the graft survives. Xenografts of porcine skin and human allografts of split-thickness skin are useful also as biologic dressings and seem to improve various aspects of the healing process. Such grafts should be removed before take occurs and often are changed several times before optimum conditions for autograft application are obtained.

When more than the skin has been lost, and the skin plus some other tissue such as fat, tendon, muscle, or nerve must be replaced to restore function and appearance, transfer of skin by pedicle flap is required (Fig. 8-9). As the name implies, pedicle transfers maintain vascular connection with the host, so that interruption of the capillary circulation never occurs. The vessels which are most important during transfer of tissue are the vessels in the subdermal plexus. These vessels are relatively large, frequently longitudinally oriented, and found on the undersurface of the dermis between it and the subcutaneous fat. One frequently hears that a predicle flap has been made thicker than actually needed for cosmetic or functional purposes in order to provide a safe blood supply. Fat on the undersurface of a flap does not add any appreciable blood supply, and it may be removed safely to produce as thin a pedicle as needed, provided that surgical manipulation does not injure the important vessels lying on the undersurface of the dermis. The problem in transplanting tissue by the pedicle method is to design a pedicle so that the base is as narrow as possible in relation to the length needed to cover the deficient area. It becomes a matter of considerable judgment, therefore, to gauge the shape and dimensions of a flap so that blood supply through the intact pedicle will be adequate to nourish the distal end of the flap. A great deal depends upon the natural profuseness of vascular beds; thus it is possible to move a pedicle flap on the face or cervical region which is three times as long as it is wide, while it may not be possible (without performing preliminary procedures to increase the blood supply) to transfer a flap on the leg which is no longer than it is wide. The blood supply in the base of a contemplated flap can be improved by performing a procedure commonly referred to as delay of the flap. The principle of delay is gradually to reduce blood supply to small segments of the circumference of the flap and thus improve the remaining blood supply to the point where a pedicle which was of insufficient width before the flap was delayed becomes adequately vascularized to nourish the flap. The mechanism by which delay (gradual interruption of a portion of the blood supply to a flap) improves the circulation in the base is not completely clear. It seems doubtful that new blood vessels actually grow into the area, although casual observation of changes in the vessels at the base suggests that this is what may happen. The rapidity with which delay improves the circulation strongly suggests, however, that the release of various amines, probably in response to changes in pH secondary to increased anaerobic metabolism, causes a closure of normally open shunts that prevent perfusion of the entire capillary network. The effect is a substantial hyperemia at the base of the flap; over a period of several weeks and after several delaying procedures, the vessels in the pedicle base become racemose in appearance, and the amount of blood flow is increased to the extent that a relatively long flap can be transferred on a narrow pedicle. Following transfer of the flap, circulation must be observed carefully for the first 48 hours, as signs of impending circulatory embarrassment occur before irreversible thrombosis and cell death occur. It is not unusual for the distal end of a flap to be a little dusky following transfer; venous spasm secondary to the trauma of rotation may be all that is involved. Improvement usually occurs in a few hours, but during this time the danger of a venous thrombosis is increased; if there is any progression of cyanosis and edema, the possibility that tension on veins is interfering with return circulation must be investigated by removing a few sutures. Perhaps the most serious, but still reversible, sign of impending venous thrombosis is the development of a sharp line of color differentiation. A gradual change from normal pink to slight cyanosis is not so significant as a clear-cut line demarcating the area of circulatory deficiency from normal circulation. Even if all the sutures have to be removed and the flap returned to its original bed, the sign must be attended to, or an irreversible demarcation will soon develop, signifying complete thrombosis and certain distal necrosis. In sensibly planned and adequately prepared flaps, one does not have to be particularly concerned about arterial insufficiency; venous drainage is the function in which complications develop. Complications usually are the result of too much tension, poor dressing, hematoma, or infection. The use of heparin and low-molecular-weight dextran have seemed to be beneficial in dangerously compromised circulation. Hyperbaric oxygenation has been reported instrumental in saving flaps of laboratory animals, but is not practical for managing human flaps.

Advancement flaps and rotation flaps are the simplest pedicle transfers. These are dependent upon a redundancy of soft tissue adjacent to a defect so that the donor defect can be closed by approximating the skin edges or applying

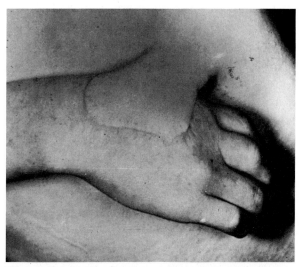

Fig. 8-9. Abdominal pedicle flap applied to dorsum of hand. Scar on hand has been turned back to resurface the raw side of pedicle and a portion of the donor site. Flap will be separated from the abdominal wall in 18 days.

split-thickness skin grafts. More complicated flaps require the use of an arm as a carrier to provide circulation during the period that skin is detached from the original donor site, such as abdominal wall, and transferred to a distant site, such as the lower leg. Because of similarity of tissue characteristics, safety in transfer, and expense and time involved, it is desirable to design flaps as close to the point where they are needed as possible.

Perhaps the most sophisticated flap is the island pedicle flap (Fig. 8-10), which combines the pedicle principle of intact blood and nerve supply with some of the advantages of a free graft. The principle of the island pedicle is that careful dissection of the artery and vein (and sometimes the nerve) to a piece of skin can be performed so that the skin is detached from all surrounding skin and remains attached to the body only by the barest essentials for survival—an artery, a vein, and sometimes a nerve. Depending on the length of these structures, it is possible to move a full-thickness skin and fat graft, or an intact finger, or a portion of a finger or toe, a surprising distance. Transfer of hair-bearing portions of the scalp on a temporal artery-and-vein supported flap to the supraorbital region for eyebrow reconstruction and transfer of a finger to replace a missing thumb are examples of island pedicle transfers which are useful. Complete freedom in transferring composite-tissue grafts, however, awaits further developments in microsurgical technique for anastomosing small vessels. A few skilled investigators in this area have become reasonably proficient in anastomosing animal blood vessels of the order of 1 mm in diameter, but such technical feats are not yet a standard part of the restorative surgeon's technique.

Finally, it should be pointed out that, in the opinion of many, maturity in restorative surgery can be measured, in part, by how often one thinks of a pedicle flap as the only means of rebuilding a damaged area and then devises a way to make a free graft do as well. Pedicles are dra-

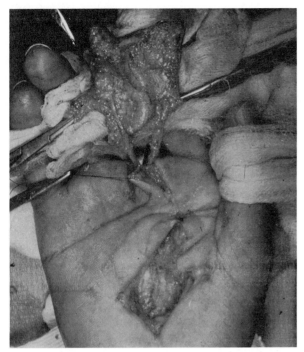

Fig. 8-10. Island pedicle flap developed during amputation of long finger. The flap is nourished by a single digital artery and nerve. Sensation is preserved by including a digital nerve in the vascular pedicle.

matic, particularly as used by military surgeons to rebuild enormous tissue defects caused by high-explosive wounds; fortunately, however, civilian injuries are not often so devastating, and the practical points of expense, length of time away from work, shortage of hospital facilities, and the like have to be considered in each case where a pedicle could be used. In addition, although areas such as the face may appear in photographs to have been superbly restored by massive flaps, yet it must be remembered that flaps have no dynamic function; they are expressionless, and often look better in photographs than they do as part of the constantly moving facial features. When a pedicle flap is needed, nothing else will suffice, and pedicles are an extremely valuable part of restorative surgery. The high cost of donor-site mutilation, length of time required for transfer, and adynamic features, however, make the pedicle flap definitely second choice to a free graft if a free graft can be used as well.

References

General

Douglas, D. M.: "Wound Healing and Management: A Monograph for Surgeons," The Williams & Wilkins Company, Baltimore, 1963.

Hartwell, S. W.: "The Mechanism of Healing in Human Wounds," Charles C Thomas, Publisher, Springfield, Ill., 1955.

McDowell, F., and Brown, J. B.: "Skin Grafting," J. B. Lippincott Company, Philadelphia, 1958.

Montagna, W., and Billingham, R. E.: Advances in Biology of Skin, vol. V, "Wound Healing," *Proc Brown Univ Symp Biol Skin, 1963,* The Macmillan Company, New York, and Pergamon Press, New York, 1964.

Patterson, W. B.: Wound Healing and Tissue Repair, *Dev Biol Conf Ser Rept, 1956,* The University of Chicago Press, Chicago, 1959.

Williamson, M. B., (ed.): "The Healing of Wounds: A Symposium on Recent Trends and Studies," McGraw-Hill Book Company, New York, 1957.

Wound Contraction

Abercrombie, M., Flint, M. H., and James, D. W.: Wound Contraction in Relation to Collagen Formation in Scorbutic Guinea-Pigs, *J Embryol Exp Morphol,* **4:**167, 1956.

———, James, D. W., and Newcombe, J. F.: Wound Contraction in Rabbit Skin, Studied by Splinting the Wound Margins, *J Anat,* **94:**170, 1960.

Billingham, R. E., and Russel, P. S.: Studies on Wound Healing with Special Reference to the Phenomenon of Contracture in Experimental Wounds in Rabbit's Skin, *Ann Surg,* **144:**961, 1956.

Danes, B., and Leinfelder, P. J.: Cytological and Respiratory Effects of Cyanide on Tissue Cultures, *J Cell Comp Physiol,* **37:**427, 1951.

Grillo, H. C., and Gross, J.: Studies in Wound Healing: III. Contraction in Vitamin C Deficiency, *Proc Soc Exp Biol Med,* **101:**268, 1959.

———, Watts, G. T., and Gross, J.: Studies in Wound Healing. I. Contraction and Wound Contents, *Ann Surg,* **148:**145, 1958.

James, D. W.: Intussusceptive Growth of Skin Islands within Wounds, *J Anat,* **93:**161, 1959.

———, and Newcombe, J. F.: Granulation Tissue Resorption during Free and Limited Contraction of Skin Wounds, *J Anat,* **95:**247, 1961.

Majno, G., Babbiani, G., Hirschel, B. J., Ryan, G. B., and Statkov, P. R.: Contraction of Granulation Tissue *in vitro:* Similarity with Smooth Muscle, *Science,* **173:**548, 1971.

Paul, H. E., Paul, M. F., Taylor, J. D., and Masters, R. W.: Biochemistry of Wound Healing: II. Water and Protein Content of Healing Tissue of Skin Wounds, *Arch Biochem,* **17:**269, 1948.

Phillips, J. L., and Peacock, E. E.: Importance of Horizontal Plane Cell Mass Integrity in Wound Contraction, *Proc Soc Exp Biol Med,* **117:**539, 1964.

Van den Brenk, H. A. S.: Studies in Restorative Growth Process in Mammalian Wound Healing, *Brit Surg,* **43:**525, 1956.

Watts, G. T., Grillo, H. C., and Gross, J.: Studies in Wound Healing: II. The Role of Granulation Tissue in Contraction, *Ann Surg,* **148:**153, 1958.

Epithelization

Abercrombie, M.: The Control of Growth and the Cell Surface, *Lect Sci Basis Med,* **8**(1958–1959):19, 1960.

Arey, L. B., and Covode, W. M.: The Method of Repair in Epithelial Wounds of the Cornea, *Anat Rec* **86:**75, 1943.

Brophy, D., and Lobitz, W. C.: Injury and Reinjury to Human Epidermis: II. Epidermal Basal Cell Response, *J Invest Dermatol,* **32:**495, 1959.

Bullough, W. S.: Mitotic and Functional Homeostasis, *Cancer Res,* **25:**1683, 1965.

———. and Lawrence, E. B.: The Control of Epidermal Mitotic Activity in the Mouse, *Proc R Soc Land [Biol]*, **B151**:517, 1960.

Coman, D. R.: Decreased Mutual Adhesiveness: A Property of Cells from Squamous Cell Carcinomas, *Cancer Res*, **4**:625, 1944.

Gelfant, S.: Initiation of Mitosis in Relation to the Cell Division Cycle, *Exp Cell Res*, **26**:395, 1959.

Gillman, T., and Penn, J.: Studies on the Repair of Cutaneous Wounds, *Med Proc*, **2**(*Suppl.* 3):121, 1956.

Hartwell, H. F.: Surgical Wounds in Human Beings, *Arch Surg*, **19**:835, 1929.

Howes, E. L.: The Rate and Nature of Epithelialization in Wounds with Loss of Substance, *Surg Gynecol Obstet*, **76**:738, 1943.

Lobitz, W. C.: The Histochemical Response to Controlled Injury, *J Invest Dermatol*, **22**:189, 1954.

Medawar, P. B.: Biological Aspects of the Repair Process, *Br Med Bull*, **3**:70, 1945.

Meyer, K., Hoffman, P., and Linker, A.: Chemistry of Ground Substances, in I. Page (ed.), "Connective Tissue, Thrombosis and Atherosclerosis," p. 181, Academic Press, New York, 1959.

Needham, A. E.: "Regeneration and Wound Healing," Methuen & Co., Ltd, London, 1952.

Pace, D. M., and Layon, M. E.: Effect of Cell Density on Growth in HeLa Cells, *Growth*, **24**:355, 1960.

Pinkus, H.: Examination of the Epidermis by the Strip Method of Removing Horny Layers: I. Observation on the Thickness of the Horny Layer and on Mitotic Activity After Stripping. *J Invest Dermatol*, **16**:383, 1951.

Sullivan, D. J., and Epstein, W. S.: Mitotic Activity of Wounded Human Epidermis, *J Invest Dermatol*, **41**:39, 1963.

Weiss, P.: The Biological Foundations of Wound Repair, *Harvey Lect*, **(55)**(1959–1960):**13**, 1961.

Winter, G. D.: Formation of the Scab and the Rate of Epithelialization of Superficial Wounds in the Skin of the Young Domestic Pig, *Nature (Lond)*, **193**:293, 1962.

Collagen

Allgower, M., and Hulliger, L.: Origin of Fibroblasts from Mononuclear Blood Cells: A Study of *in vitro* Formation of the Collagen Precursor, Hydroxyproline, in Buffy Coat Cultures, *Surgery*, **47**:603, 1960.

Cohen, I. K., Keiser, H. R., and Sjoersma, A.: Collagen Synthesis in Human Keloid and Hypertrophic Scar, *Surg Forum*, **22**:488, 1971.

Dunphy, J. E., and Udopa, K. N.: Chemical and Histochemical Sequences in Normal Healing of Wounds, *N Engl J Med*, **253**:847, 1955.

Gould, B. S.: Ascorbic Acid and Collagen Fiber Formation, *Vitam Horm*, **8**:89, 1960.

Grillo, H. C.: Origin of Fibroblasts in Wound Healing: An Autoradiographic Study of Inhibition of Cellular Proliferation by Local X-irradiation, *Ann Surg*, **157**:453, 1963.

Gross, J.: On the Significance of the Soluble Collagens, in I. H. Page (ed.), "Connective Tissue, Thrombosis and Atherosclerosis," pp. 77–95, Academic Press, Inc., New York, 1959.

———, Highberger, J. H., and Schmitt, F. O.: Extraction of Collagen from Connective Tissue by Neutral Salt Solutions, *Proc Natl Acad Sci USA*, **41**:1, 1955.

——— and Kirk, D.: The Heat Precipitation of Collagen from Neutral Salt Solutions: Some Rate-regulating Factors, *J Biol Chem*, **233**:355, 1958.

——— and Lapiere, C. M.: Collagenolytic Activity in Amphibian Tissues: A Tissue Culture Assay, *Proc Natl Acad Sci USA*, **48**:1014, 1962.

———, ———, and Tanzer, M. L.: Organization and Disorganization of Extracellular Substances: The Collagen System, in "22nd Growth Symposium," p. 175, Waverly Press, Baltimore, 1963.

Jackson, D. S.: Some Biochemical Aspects of Fibrogenesis and Wound Healing, *N Engl J Med*, **259**:814, 1958.

Leven, C. I., and Gross, J.: Alterations in State of Molecular Aggregation of Collagen Induced in Chick Embryos by Aminopropionitrile (lathyrus factor), *J Exp Med*, **110**:771, 1959.

Madden, J. W., and Peacock, E. E.: Studies on the Biology of Collagen during Wound Healing: III. Dynamic Metabolism of Scar Collagen and Remodeling of Dermal Wounds, *Ann Surg*, **174**:511,1971.

———, and Smith, H. C.: Studies on the Biology of Collagen during Wound Healing: II. Rate of Collagen Synthesis and Deposition in Dehisced and Resutured Wounds, *Surg Gynecol Obstet*, **130**:487, 1970.

Orekovitch, V. N., and Shipikiter, V. O.: Procollagens, *Science*, **127**:1371, 1958.

Peacock, E. E.: Production and Polymerization of Collagen in Healing Wounds of Rats: Some Rate Regulating Factors, *Ann Surg*, **155**:251, 1962.

———: Some Aspects of Fibrogenesis during the Healing of Primary and Secondary Wounds, *Surg Gynecol Obstet*, **115**:408, 1962.

——— and Biggers, P. W.: Measurement and Significance of Heat-labile and Urea-sensitive Cross Linking Mechanisms in Collagen of Healing Wounds, *Surgery*, **54**:144, 1963.

Porter, K. R., and Pappas, J. G.: Collagen Formation by Fibroblasts of the Chick Embryo Dermis, *J Biophys Biochem Cytol*, **5**:153, 1959.

Prockop, D. J., Peterkofsky, B., and Udenfriend, S.: Studies on the Intracellular Localization of Collagen Synthesis in the Intact Chick Embryo, *J Biol Chem*, **237**:1581, 1962.

Randall, J. T., and Jackson, S. F.: "Nature and Structure of Collagen," Butterworth Scientific Publications, London, 1953.

Riley, W. B., Jr., and Peacock, E. E., Jr.: Identification, Distribution, and Significance of a Collagenolytic Enzyme in Human Tissue, *Proc Soc Biol Med*, **214**:207, 1967.

Ross, R., and Benditt, E. P.: Wound Healing and Collagen Formation: I. Sequential Changes in Components of Guinea Pig Wounds Observed in the Electron Microscope, *J Biophys Biochem Cytol*, **11**:677, 1961.

——— and ———: Wound Healing and Collagen Formation: III. A Quantitative Autoradiographic Study of the Utilization of Proline H^3 in Wounds from Normal and Scorbutic Guinea Pigs, *J Cell Biol*, **15**:99, 1962.

Schiffman, E., and Martin, G. R.: Spontaneous Generation of Cross-Links in Aldehyde Containing Collagen, *Arch Biochem*, **138**:226, 1970.

Woessner, J. F.: Catabolism of Collagen and Non-collagen Protein in the Rat Uterus during Post-partum Involution, *Biochem J*, **83**:304, 1962.

Chapter 9

Oncology

by **Donald L. Morton, Frank C. Sparks, and Charles M. Haskell**

Introduction

Epidemiology

Etiology

Biology
Immunobiology
    Clinical Evidence for Tumor-specific Antigens in Human Neoplasms

Pathology

Clinical Manifestations of Cancer

Cancer Diagnosis and Staging Extent of Cancer
Diagnosis
Staging Extent of Cancer

Therapy
General Considerations
Surgical Therapy
    Cancer Surgery
Radiation Therapy
Chemotherapy
Immunotherapy
    Active Immunotherapy
    Passive and Adoptive Immunotherapy
    Nonspecific Immunotherapy

Prognosis

Psychologic Management of the Cancer Patient

INTRODUCTION

Oncology (from the Greek *onkos,* mass, or tumor, and *logos,* study) is the study of neoplastic diseases. Neoplasms are an altered cell population characterized by an excessive, nonuseful proliferation of cells that have become unresponsive to normal control mechanisms and to the organizing influences of adjacent tissues. Malignant neoplasms are composed of cancer cells that exhibit uncontrolled proliferation and impair the function of normal organs by local tissue invasion and metastatic spread to distant anatomic sites. Benign neoplasms are composed of normal-appearing cells that are not locally invasive, or characterized by metastatic spread.

Cancer has plagued man since antiquity, and many of its clinical manifestations were described by Hippocrates (460–375 B.C.) Neoplasms have been identified in all species of animals including the lower vertebrates, such as amphibia and fish. The wide distribution of neoplasia in natural and human history suggests that cancer may be common to all multicellular organisms.

Neoplastic disease is the second most frequent cause of death in the United States. The magnitude of the cancer problem is exemplified by the fact that one of every four persons living today has or will develop cancer. An estimated 50 million of the 200 million people presently alive in the United States will develop cancer, and 34 million will die of the disease. Thus, only one of every three cancer patients can be cured by present methods of therapy. Until recently those facts caused many physicians and surgeons to approach the cancer patient with feelings of pessimism and despair that frequently interfered with adequate therapy. This aversion to the problems of cancer was reflected by the paucity of physicians willing to devote full time to its clinical studies. Furthermore, basic scientists were somewhat hesitant to investigate fundamental problems posed by the malignant state.

Fortunately, recent exciting developments in tumor immunology, viral oncology, and molecular biology, and advances in the therapy of some neoplasms have led to a rebirth of interest in the basic biologic and clinical problems posed by cancer. The United States government has launched a massive Conquest of Cancer Program which should expend $1 billion each year by 1976 for cancer research. Specialty boards have been established in medical oncology and gynecologic oncology. A wide variety of scientists from many disciplines have been attracted to its study. As a result, it is probable that more advances will be made in cancer therapy during the next few years than in all previous times. This chapter is designed to introduce the student to general principles that can be used as the basis for acquiring further knowledge in this rapidly growing field.

EPIDEMIOLOGY

The changes in death rates caused by cancer by body site for males and females in the United States during the past 40 years are summarized in Fig. 9-1 and 9-2. Although there has been a decrease in mortality from certain neoplasms, the overall cancer death rates continue to show a slow, steady increase.

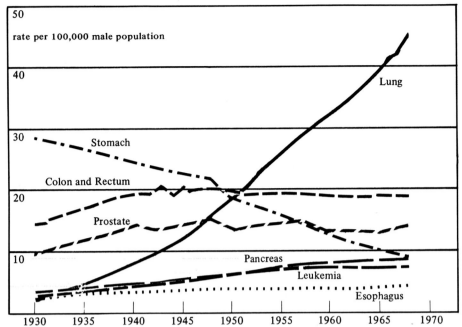

Fig. 9-1. Male cancer death rates by site, United States, 1930–1968 (standardized for age on the 1940 United States population). (*From National Vital Statistics Division and Bureau of the Census, United States.*)

The mortality rates from lung cancer have increased steadily and probably represent the most dramatic change for any cancer site. Compared with 40 years ago, the mortality is now eighteen times greater for men and six times greater for women. Lung cancer represents the leading cause of cancer death when both sexes are considered.

Pancreatic cancer death rates also have steadily increased through the years. Today, the rates are twice what they were in women and three times that in men when compared to 1930.

There has been a striking reduction during the past 40 years in death rates caused by cancers of the stomach and uterus. The stomach cancer death rate is now less than one-third the 1930 rate in men and less than one-fourth the 1930 rate in women, although there has been little

Fig. 9-2. Female cancer death rates by site, United States, 1930–1968 (standardized for age on the 1940 United States population). (*From National Vital Statistics Division and Bureau of the Census, United States.*)

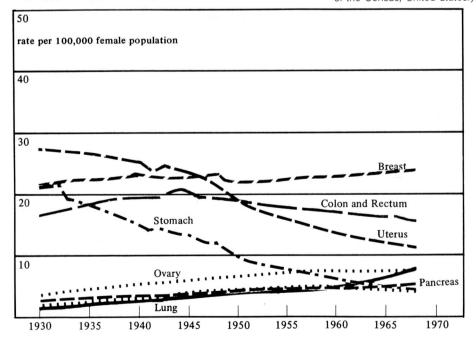

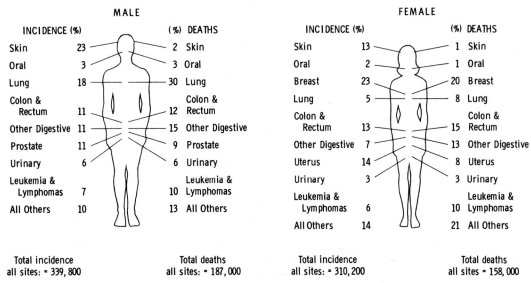

MALE

INCIDENCE (%)		(%)	DEATHS
Skin	23	2	Skin
Oral	3	3	Oral
Lung	18	30	Lung
Colon & Rectum	11	12	Colon & Rectum
Other Digestive	11	15	Other Digestive
Prostate	11	9	Prostate
Urinary	6	6	Urinary
Leukemia & Lymphomas	7	10	Leukemia & Lymphomas
All Others	10	13	All Others

FEMALE

INCIDENCE (%)		(%)	DEATHS
Skin	13	1	Skin
Oral	2	1	Oral
Breast	23	20	Breast
Lung	5	8	Lung
Colon & Rectum	13	15	Colon & Rectum
Other Digestive	7	13	Other Digestive
Uterus	14	8	Uterus
Urinary	3	3	Urinary
Leukemia & Lymphomas	6	10	Leukemia & Lymphomas
All Others	14	21	All Others

Total incidence
all sites: = 339,800

Total deaths
all sites: = 187,000

Total incidence
all sites: = 310,200

Total deaths
all sites = 158,000

Fig. 9-3. Estimated cancer incidence and resultant deaths by site and sex.

improvement in the survival rates of stomach cancer. The decreasing mortality is due to a decreased incidence of stomach cancer in both sexes. The reason for this declining incidence is unknown.

There has been a similar striking decline in death rates due to uterine cancer with mortality rates today only one-third what they were 40 years ago. In this case, the causes of the reduction are known to be earlier detection and improved treatment for cancer of the uterine cervix and corpus.

The incidences of cancer in different sites and the mortality rate in each sex are compared in Fig. 9-3. The sites most frequently causing cancer death in males, in order of decreasing frequency, are (1) lung, (2) colon and rectum, (3) prostate, (4) pancreas, and (5) stomach. The sites, in order of decreasing frequency in females, are (1) breast, (2) colon and rectum, (3) uterus, (4) lung, and (5) ovary. It is obvious that there are differing incidences of kinds of cancer occurring in the male and female.

The incidence of various types of neoplasms differs from the death rates for the same neoplasms (Fig. 9-4) because different forms of cancer are not equally lethal. The most significant 5-year survival rates are achieved in patients with cancer of the skin (94 percent) and uterus (70 percent); the lowest survival occurs in patients with lung cancer (9 percent). Lung cancer is the leading cause of cancer death even though skin cancer occurs more commonly.

Females tend to have a greater number of 5-year survivals with cancers of any given primary site than males, although the reasons are unknown at this time. The overall

Fig. 9-4. A. Cancer death rates by sex, United States, 1900–1968 (standardized for age on the 1940 United States population). B. Forecast of cancer deaths based on present trends. (From National Vital Statistics Division and Bureau of the Census, United States.)

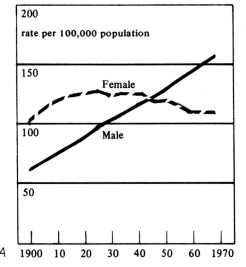

A   1900   10   20   30   40   50   60   1970

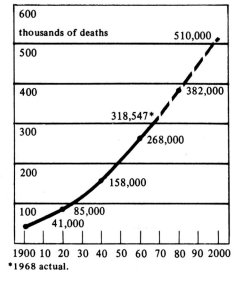

B   1900 10 20 30 40 50 60 70 80 90 2000
*1968 actual.

5-year survival for women with cancer is 50 percent, compared with only 31 percent for men.

ETIOLOGY

The primary etiologic factors responsible for most neoplasms in man are still unknown. In experimental animals, a wide variety of causative agents have been identified. These agents may be classified as chemical and physical, viral and genetic. There is no reason to doubt that a similar variety of factors is responsible for causing human cancer. Although the primary mechanisms by which these agents cause neoplastic transformation is unknown, it seems relatively certain that the inciting agents represent but one link in the chain of factors that leads to the development of cancer. Therefore, the identification of carcinogenic agents, although their mechanisms of action are unknown, can be extremely important in cancer prevention.

CHEMICAL CARCINOGENS. The first cause-and-effect relation between a carcinogenic stimulus and the development of cancer in man was described by Percival Pott, an English surgeon, in 1775, when he described a cancer of the scrotum frequently occurring in the chimney sweeps. However, Yamagiwa and Ichikawa, working from 1915 to 1918, identified the carcinogen when they experimentally produced cancers by painting the ears of rabbits with coal tar. Kennaway and Cook in studies from 1924 to 1932, demonstrated that pure hydrocarbons, such as 1, 2-dibenzanthracene and similar compounds isolated from coal tar, were carcinogenic agents. Subsequently, a variety of chemical agents have been found that are capable of inducing neoplasms in experimental animals and in man. These chemicals are called *carcinogens.* There may be many years separating the time of exposure to a carcinogen and subsequent development of a neoplasm. Consequently, the present-day evaluation of the safety of food additives or other products for human consumption that are chronically ingested over long periods of time is a most difficult task.

A variety of chemicals which have been associated with different types of human neoplasms are summarized in Table 9-1. Aromatic amines are known to cause tumors of the urinary tract; workers in the dye industry have a higher incidence of this type of cancer. Benzene has been associated with acute leukemia, in shoe repairmen in Italy, solvent manufacturers, painters, and printers who use it as a solvent. Coal tar, pitch, creosote, and anthracene have been associated with cancer of the skin, larynx, and bronchus. A variety of paraffin oils, waxes, and tars are associated with cancer of the skin. Isopropyl oil has been associ-

Table 9-1. CHEMICAL AND PHYSICAL CARCINOGENS IN HUMAN BEINGS

Carcinogen	Site of neoplasm	Site exposed	Persons at risk
Chemical agents:			
Aromatic amines, especially β-naphthylamine	Urinary tract	Cutaneous and respiratory	Chemical workers producing dye stuffs, rodenticides, laboratory reagents
Benzol or benzene	Blood, lymphatic organs	Cutaneous and respiratory	Coal tar refiners, solvent manufacturers, painters, printers, mechanics
Coal tar, pitch, creosote, anthracene, tobacco	Skin, larynx, bronchus	Cutaneous and respiratory	Coke oven workers, coal tar distillers, lumber industry workers, chemical workers, smokers
Petroleum, shale and paraffin oils, waxes, tars	Skin	Cutaneous	Workers in oil refineries, wax and asphalt producers, mechanics
Isopropyl oils	Sinus, larynx, bronchus	Respiratory	Producers of isopropyl alcohol
Asbestos	Bronchus, mesothelioma of pleura	Respiratory, generally > 2 years	Abestos miners, shippers, millers
Chromium	Bronchus	Respiratory and cutaneous	Workers engaged in chromate ore reduction
Nickel	Nasal cavity, sinus, bronchus	Respiratory	Nickel miners, shippers, and refiners
Arsenic	Skin, bronchus, bladder	Respiratory	Smelters, pesticide manufacturers
Physical agents:			
Ionizing radiation	Skin, thyroid, tongue, tonsil, sinus, bone, blood	Local or systemic, therapeutic (e.g., treatment of spondylitic polycythemia)	Radium dial workers
	Bronchus	Respiratory	Pitchblend miners
Ultraviolet radiation	Skin	Cutaneous	Farmers, other outdoor workers, sailors, fishermen, and fair-skinned people in tropical climates

ated with cancer of the sinuses, larynx, and bronchus in workers exposed to it. Mesotheliomas occur very frequently in miners and ship workers who have been exposed to asbestos. Certain metals have been associated with tumors, including chromium, nickel, and arsenic.

PHYSICAL CARCINOGENS. Ionizing radiation was found in the 1920s to be carcinogenic when subcutaneous sarcomas were induced by radium implants in experimental animals. The carcinogenic effects of radiation in man was recognized when radium dial painters who commonly licked brushes containing radioactive materials developed bone cancers. Since then, many examples of the carcinogenic effects of radiation in man have been recognized. In physicians and dentists who experience multiple x-ray exposures recurrent skin cancer has developed. Cancer of the thyroid in adults is frequently associated with neck irradiation in early childhood. The survivors of the atomic bomb detonations show an increased incidence of leukemia. Ultraviolet light on exposed areas may foster the development of skin cancer. Farmers and sailors have an increased incidence of skin cancers from excessive exposure to sunlight, as do fair-skinned people living in tropical regions.

Mechanical Irritation. Chronic mechanical irritation may be associated with the development of cancer, although the exact mechanisms are unknown. Examples include the malignant degeneration in old burn scars (the chronic ulcer of Marjolin), and cancer of the liver and bladder subsequent to parasitic infestation by schistosomes.

VIRUSES. These are carcinogenic in several animal species, and it is likely that some cancers in man are caused by viruses. Many animal-oncogenic viruses have been described since 1911 when Rous discovered a filterable agent which caused sarcoma in chickens. At least two distinct classes of viruses can cause tumors. Ribonucleic acid (RNA) viruses have been associated with sarcomas, lymphomas, leukemias, and mammary cancer in chickens, mice, rats, cats, monkeys, and gibbons. Deoxyribonucleic acid (DNA) viruses also are oncogenic. The polyoma virus can cause multiple tumors in mice, rats, and hamsters. Simian virus (SV-40) can cause a sarcoma in hamsters; papilloma virus causes papillomas in a variety of animals; adenoviruses have caused sarcomas in rodents. Pox viruses have been associated with fibromas in the rabbit and squirrel, and a tumor in the monkey. Herpes viruses cause neoplasms in frogs, chickens, and monkeys.

Despite clear-cut evidence for a viral cause of a variety of animal tumors, there has been no proof that viruses can cause human neoplasms. Yet, it would be surprising if man were not susceptible to some form of viral carcinogenesis because it is so common in all other animal species, and basic biologic phenomena are generally quite similar throughout nature. In fact, there is increasing evidence linking viruses with certain types of human neoplasms and suggesting a prominent role in etiology. The Epstein-Barr (EB) virus, probably the cause of infectious mononucleosis in man, is linked to the occurrences of Burkitt's lymphoma in Africa and to nasopharyngeal cancer in the Orient. RNA viruses of a characteristic type (type C) similar to those agents known to cause leukemias, and sarcomas in mice,

have been associated with leukemias, sarcomas, and papillary urinary neoplasms in man. RNA viruses resembling the mammary tumor virus of mice have been found in the breast cancers and milk from women with this malignant disease.

Two modes of oncogenic viral transmission, vertical and horizontal, have been described. Vertical transmission involves passage of virus from parent to offspring. For example, the mouse mammary tumor virus is transmitted to progeny in the mother's milk, and the Gross leukemia virus is transmitted in the gametes of the parents to the offspring. Horizontal transmission is passage of virus to close contacts in excreta and airborne particles, as with the polyoma virus.

Experimental animals must be infected as newborn offspring with almost all oncogenic viruses to produce neoplastic change in adulthood. The immunologic immaturity of the neonate allows viral infection and induction of neoplastic transformation. Adult animals are resistant to infection with oncogenic viruses unless they are immunosuppressed.

Studies of viral oncogenesis can become quite complex in situations where multiple factors may interact to produce a situation which ultimately causes cancer. The development of mouse mammary cancer depends upon the cooperation of (1) genetic susceptibility, (2) proper hormonal stimuli, and (3) infection with the virus in the first 6 weeks of life. When all these conditions have been met, the breast cancer still requires 1 to 2 years to develop.

HEREDITARY FACTORS. Genetic factors have been demonstrated to be of major importance in determining the effectiveness of chemical, physical and viral carcinogens in animals.

Clear-cut examples of genetic factors playing a role in human cancer development are demonstrated when the same type of cancer occurs in identical twins, when colon cancer develops in persons with familial polyposis, and with the familial patterns associated with breast cancer. Cancer of the breast is about three times more common in the daughters of women with breast cancer and in women whose blood relatives have had at least two incidences of breast cancer. Furthermore, the daughters develop breast cancers at a younger age than did their mothers.

A more indirect genetic role was noted in certain families who seemed to have an increased incidence of neoplastic diseases. A clearly defined pattern of inheritance has been established for some of these tumors. It is often difficult to assess the importance of environmental factors in these cases. Substantiated examples include a pattern of dominant inheritance in some families for diseases such as retinoblastoma, lipomatosis, and colonic polyposis. In other families, there may be an association of multiple diseases that may include one or more neoplasms. An example of this is the association of pheochromocytoma with medullary (amyloid-producing) carcinoma of the thyroid, cerebellocortical hemangioblastoma, or neurofibromatosis. Other examples where tumors appear to be inherited in families as a dominant trait include some cases of polyendocrine adenomas (pituitary, parathyroid, pancreas), including the Zollinger-Ellison syndrome and hereditary adenocarcinomatosis (adenocarcinoma of the colon, stomach, uterus, and ovary occurring in different members of the same family). There are also several relatively rare heritable nonneoplastic diseases which have been associated with malignant tumors with great frequency. An example of this is the high incidence of skin cancer in patients with xeroderma pigmentosa. There also is an association between dermal inclusion cysts and multiple carcinomas of the colon, polyposis, multiple bony exostoses, and benign connective tissue tumors (Gardner's syndrome).

There are marked differences in the frequency of certain neoplastic diseases with respect to age, sex, and other constitutional factors suggesting that additional host determinants may be important. Acute lymphocytic leukemia is essentially a disease of childhood, whereas malignant melanoma is essentially a postpubertal disease. Testicular tumors and Hodgkin's disease are more frequent in young adults, and breast cancer is far more common in women than in men. In many other tumors, the frequency in both sexes increases markedly with increasing age.

GEOGRAPHIC FACTORS. Neoplasms may be found in all human populations, but there are some striking racial and regional differences in the occurrence of specific types of cancer. Although it is difficult to separate the genetic from the environmental factors, such as diet or habits, it is important to be aware of certain particularly strong differences. In a comparison study with the Caucasian population of the United States, Shimkin noted the following differences in cancer incidence:

1. High incidence of cancer of the stomach in Scandinavia, Iceland, and Japan
2. High incidence of primary cancer of the liver in South and West Africa
3. High incidence of cancer of the nasopharynx in China
4. High incidence of cancer of the urinary bladder in Egypt
5. Low incidence of cancer of the breast in Japan
6. Low incidence of cancer of the uterine cervix in Israel and in Jewish women in general
7. Low incidence of cancer of the skin in Negroes
8. Low incidence of cancer of the prostate in Japan and China

Custom and environment obviously play an important role in the development of cancer. It is almost certain that some of the geographic factors noted above are due more to environmental factors than to genetic ones. Migration of populations usually causes a shift toward the patterns of cancer incidence of the host country. For example, in Japan there is a very high incidence of stomach cancer and a relatively low incidence of lung cancer. However, a second generation Japanese-American has a low risk of stomach cancer, and if a heavy smoker, he has as high a risk of lung cancer as his smoking American counterpart.

For unknown reasons, socioeconomic factors may also influence cancer incidence. Cancer of the stomach and of the cervix are three to four times more frequent in lower economic groups than in middle and higher economic groups. On the other hand, cancer of the breast, leukemia,

and multiple myeloma are more frequent in higher socioeconomic groups.

PRECANCEROUS CONDITIONS. Some clinical disorders are described as precancerous because they are so frequently followed by the development of cancer. It is particularly important that the physician be aware of these conditions in order to conduct careful follow-up of these patients. Some precancerous conditions are leukoplakia, actinic keratoses, polyps of the colon or rectum, neurofibromas, dysplasia of the cervix or bronchial mucosa, and chronic ulcerative colitis.

MULTIFACTORIAL ETIOLOGY. It is likely that in any given individual cancer is the result not of just one but of multiple factors. There may be an interaction of an oncogenic virus with a chemical or physical carcinogen. It is also possible that two chemical carcinogens may act synergistically to increase the incidence of cancer. A chemical may be a carcinogen only in those with a hereditary susceptibility. When condensations of smog or cigarette smoke are applied separately to the cheek pouch of the golden hamster, there is a low but definite incidence of tumor. However, a synergistic interaction is observed when they are applied together, with a markedly increased incidence of tumors. Similarly, viruses have enhanced the oncogenic effects of smog and cigarette smoke in tissue culture. It is very possible that such synergistic interactions also occur in man.

The possibility that multiple factors may be involved in the etiology of human neoplasia, although it makes the proof of any one factor as a causative agent more complex, may in itself increase the chances of ultimate cancer prevention by providing a larger number of factors to be manipulated. For example, in carcinoma of the lung, it may be that in addition to heavy cigarette smoking (perhaps only chronic irritation), one requires a specific genetic background (since not all heavy smokers develop cancer of the lung), suitable male hormonal factors (since males are more frequently affected), and a virus. In addition, the latent period between start of smoking and high incidence of lung cancer is roughly 35 years. Although cigarette smoking may not be the only cause of lung cancer, it is the only factor which is known at the present time that can be controlled. On the basis of present knowledge, lung cancer could be prevented by eliminating cigarette smoking altogether or by limiting cigarette smoking to a shorter period of time.

Custom and environment obviously play an important part in the etiology of cancer. Although cigarette smoking has been strongly implicated as a cause of squamous cell carcinoma of the lung, the habit is sufficiently ingrained in people in the United States to make its total elimination extremely difficult. Habits and customs in other parts of the world may be equally difficult to eliminate. The inhalation of snuff and the mastication of betel nuts have been associated with nasal and oral pharynx tumors, but the use of such materials continues despite their known carcinogenic effects. Nevertheless, efforts to identify the causative factors and to educate people regarding these factors must be continued.

BIOLOGY

Regardless of the etiologic agent, the cancer cell is a progeny of a normal cell that has lost its cellular mechanisms for controlling proliferation. The cancer cell differs from a normal cell in a variety of ways, but none of its new characteristics are absolutely indicative of malignancy. Cytogenetic studies of some cancer cells have revealed various abnormalities in chromosome number and appearance. However, these changes have not been shared by all cancer cells, and many cancer cells have normal chromosomal profiles.

Almost all malignant neoplasms seem to arise from a single cell that has undergone malignant transformation to form a malignant clone (group of cells); however, other human neoplasms such as the neurofibromas occurring in von Recklinghausen's disease may develop from multiple clones of cells. Simultaneously multifocal origins of carcinoma of the breast, oral pharynx, colon, and other organs also have been observed. Studies of breast carcinoma have demonstrated that at least 30 percent have other areas involved with in situ carcinoma. Nevertheless, the primary tumor mass which was the cause for clinical presentation arises from a single cell alone.

Although the proliferative rate of cancer cells is generally greater than the overall average of normal cells, the former do not divide more rapidly than some normal cells, such as leukocytes or cells of the intestinal mucosa. The proliferative rate of cancer cells generally decreases as the tumor mass grows. It has been shown that the proportion of cells undergoing mitosis is much greater when there are only a few cancer cells present than when there are many cells present in a large tumor mass. There are many rapid changes in the mitotic fraction of neoplasms during the initial growth phase, but after the tumor mass is 1 cm in diameter, the rate of division usually follows a predictable pattern.

After neoplastic transformation has occurred, the cancer cell differs from the normal cell not only in proliferative index but also in morphology, biochemistry, antigenetic expression, and many other aspects.

MORPHOLOGIC CHANGES. Malignant cells tend to revert to more primitive cell types, that is, to dedifferentiate. The normal orderly tissue patterns are lost or replaced by the random piling up of malignant cells without definite pattern. Other histologic changes may include cellular pleomorphism, a high index of mitoses, and hyperchromatism in the nucleus and nucleoli. Invasion of adjacent normal structures also may be seen microscopically. These morphologic changes are the basis for histopathologic or cytologic diagnoses of cancer and usually allow very accurate diagnosis of neoplastic diseases.

BIOCHEMICAL CHANGES. The biochemical activity of cancer cells is similar, though not identical, to that of normal cells. A great diversity exists in the biochemical characteristics of different tumor cells, usually correlating with rate of proliferation. Changes in DNA, RNA, and the chemical architecture of the cellular membrane of malignant cells are associated with the loss of contact inhibition to proliferation and intercellular adhesiveness. However, no single biochemical alteration has yet been defined that is absolutely characteristic of malignant transformation.

Reversion of the normal cellular biochemistry to that of the embryonal cells produces distinctive embryonal substances whose presence in the adult may be used to diagnose cancer. The carcinoembryonic antigen associated with gastrointestinal cancers, and α-fetoglobulin associated with hepatoma and embryonal cancers are thought to be examples of this type. The synthesis of these substances may be due to depression of fetal gene function that occurs during oncogenesis.

Malignant cells may also produce biologically active substances that are normally produced by the cells from which the neoplasm originated. The release of these substances may cause symptoms similar to hyperfunction of that particular organ, for example, hyperparathyroidism produced by parathyroid carcinomas. Neoplasms may also produce biologically active substances that are not normally produced by the cells of origin. Some bronchogenic carcinomas may produce parathyroidlike hormones, ACTH, antidiuretic hormones, and other hormones.

The mechanism of this ectopic hormone secretion is based upon the hypothesis of variable genetic activity or *selective derepression* of a specific gene. All cells contain the same genes; however, only about 10 percent of these genes are expressed in any one cell type; the remainder are repressed. Cancer cells are primitive cells; with the dedifferentiation, they acquire the ability to express some of these previously repressed genes. This new genetic expression is responsible for the production of a new specific-messenger RNA and the production of new polypeptides and hormones.

GROWTH RATES OF NEOPLASMS. Approximately two-thirds of the growth of human neoplasms occurs before they are clinically detectable. If one assumes that a cancer begins from a single cell, then it takes about 30 exponential divisions to produce a 1-cm nodule (1 billion cells). At 45 exponential divisions the patient is apt to be dead from the sheer bulk of the malignant tumor.

The growth rate of tumors can be expressed by the *tumor doubling time,* i.e., the time it takes for a tumor to double in volume. Tumor doubling times appear to be an accurate and precise method for comparing the biologic aggressiveness of neoplasms in different patients. This measurement is particularly applicable to metastatic pulmonary lesions, since these are usually peripheral in location and are discretely delineated on chest roentgenograms, so that accurate serial measurements are easily obtainable.

The method used in the measurement of the tumor doubling time is illustrated in Fig. 9-5. Briefly, the average of the greater and the lesser diameters of each metastatic nodule is determined from successive chest roentgenograms. The averages are plotted on semilogarithmic paper against the time in days between these points; the slope of this line represents the rate of tumor growth. Where this line crosses any two doubling lines, the horizontal distance between them represents the tumor doubling time

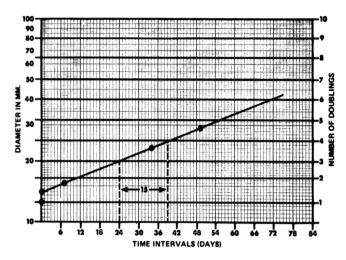

Fig. 9-5. Method of plotting tumor doubling time, based upon the direct measurement of the changing diameters of metastatic pulmonary nodules. (*From W. L. Joseph et al., J Thorac Cardiovasc Surg, 61:23, 1971.*)

in days. This measurement has been shown to be an accurate and reproducible method for the quantitation of the rate and pattern of tumor growth in individual patients.

The tumor doubling time of neoplasms varies from 8 to 600 days, most tumors doubling in 20 to 100 days. The measurement of tumor doubling times can be extremely helpful in determining prognosis, in evaluating response to chemotherapeutic agents, and in comparing responses to different therapeutic regimens.

In a recent study the tumor doubling times of a large series of patients with pulmonary metastases from tumors of different histologic types were measured. Wide variations within particular types of neoplasms were found. The tumor doubling time correlated closely with the length of survival in three distinct groups of patients. This is illustrated in Fig. 9-6. This correlation might be expected, because the tumor doubling time represents the balance between the intrinsic proliferative rate of the tumor cell and the patient's inhibiting defense mechanisms.

Based on growth dynamics, most human tumors have been present in the body for at least 1 year and many for as long as 10 to 15 years prior to their clinical detection. Thus, it appears that there is a long period of time between the inception of neoplastic transformation and the development of clinical cancer. During this time, detection may be possible and surgical treatment might result in cure. Tests must be perfected to detect cancer earlier, thus

shorten this preclinical interval, and make surgical treatment more successful.

Immunobiology

The concept that cancer patients may develop an immune response against their neoplasms is not new. This view became very popular at the turn of the century when it was found that strong immunity could be induced against transplantable neoplasms in randomly bred laboratory rodents. A period of intense laboratory and clinical investigation followed, in anticipation that tumor immunity might lead to control of malignant disease. However, it soon became evident that the immunity was not directed against tumor-specific antigens (TSA), but instead against normal tissue antigens in the neoplasm due to genetic differences between tumor donor and recipient. Thereafter, interest in tumor immunology declined because no antigens other than the transplantation antigens could be demonstrated in neoplasms.

Interest in the immunology of neoplastic diseases was reawakened in the 1950s when tumor-specific antigens were conclusively demonstrated in methylcholanthrene-induced sarcomas of mice. In order to eliminate any histocompatibility factors the investigators used inbred strains of rodents that, after many years of inbreeding, had the genetic homogeneity of monozygotic twins. Specific tumor

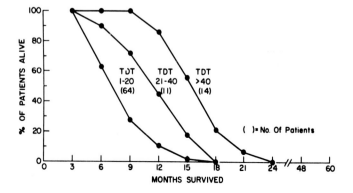

Fig. 9-6. Survival curves in 89 untreated patients following the onset of pulmonary metastases, showing three groups based upon tumor doubling time. (*From W. L. Joseph et al., J Thorac Cardiovasc Surg, 61:23, 1971.*)

transplantation resistance was induced by presensitization with a transplant of tumor tissue which was allowed to grow for a time and then was excised. The immunized rodents were then resistant to challenge with further transplants of the same neoplasm (Fig. 9-7). However, the limitations of tumor immunity were evident by the fact that the immunity induced in these animals was relative, not absolute. Whereas a challenge with 100,000 tumor cells produced a growing tumor in control mice, it did not in the immune mice. Challenge with larger numbers of cells (1 to 10 million), however, usually overwhelmed the immunologic defense, and progressive tumor growth was observed.

During the past 15 years there has been tremendous progress in tumor immunology. Tumor-specific antigens have been demonstrated in most viral, chemical, and physical-carcinogen-induced neoplasms, as well as in many spontaneous tumors. These tumor-specific antigens can elicit tumor-specific immunity against tumor transplantation in syngeneic animals; thus, they are known as *tumor-specific transplantation antigens* (TSTA).

ANTIGENIC SPECIFICITY OF ANIMAL NEOPLASMS. The wide variety of viral, chemical, and physical-carcinogen-induced neoplasms for which tumor-specific transplantation antigens have been demonstrated are summarized in Table 9-2. The antigenic specificity of these major types of carcinogenic agents have been found to be quite different.

Tumor-specific Antigens of Neoplasms Induced by Chemical and Physical Carcinogens. These are individually distinct for each tumor, even if induced by the same carcinogen, in the same strain, and of the identical histologic type (Fig. 9-8). For example, injection of a chemical carcinogen such as benzpyrene in two inbred mice of the same strain will result in two antigenically different tumors, t_1 and t_2. If mouse *A* is immunized with irradiated tumor cells from t_1, it will subsequently reject tumor cells from the same tumor transplanted into an intermediate host. However, the same animal, immune to t_1, will develop a tumor when injected with the same number of tumor cells from t_2.

Tumor-specific Antigens of Neoplasms Induced by Viral Carcinogens. In contrast to the unique tumor-specific antigens of chemical-carcinogen-induced tumors, the tumor-specific antigens of viral-induced neoplasms are common to all neoplasms induced by the same virus, but differ from those induced by other viruses (Fig. 9-9). For example, with inbred mice of the same strain, mouse *A* is immunized with SV-40 virus alone, mouse *B* is immunized with *irradiated* tumor cells from a SV-40 virus–induced mouse tumor, and mouse *C* is immunized with tumor cells from a SV-40 virus–induced rat tumor. All will reject challenge of tumor cells from SV-40 virus–induced tumor t. However, challenge with the same tumor cells in mice *D* and *E*, immunized with either polyoma virus alone or polyoma virus–induced tumor cells, leads to progressive tumor growth and death.

Although the generalization that virus-induced neoplasms contain common antigens and chemical-carcinogen-induced neoplasms contain individually distinct antigens is usually correct, more recent studies have

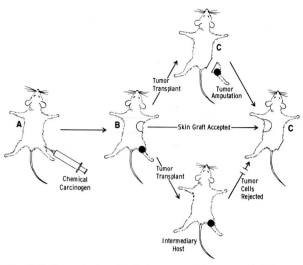

Fig. 9-7. Tumor induced with benzpyrene in mouse A is transplanted into mouse B. Mouse C, immunized by amputation of a tumor-bearing extremity, demonstrates tumor-specific immunity by rejecting tumor cells while accepting a normal skin graft from the same mouse.

Table 9-2. TUMOR-SPECIFIC ANTIGENS CAPABLE OF INDUCING REJECTION RESPONSES IN SYNGENEIC HOSTS

Inducing agent	*Antigenic specificity*
Chemical carcinogens:	
3-Methylcholanthrene	
1,2,5,6-Dibenzanthracene	
9,10-Dimethylbenzathracene	
3,4,9,10-Dibenzpyrene	
3,4-Benzpyrene-dimethylam-	
inoazobenzene	Antigens distinct for
Physical agents	each individual
Films	neoplasm
Millipore filter	
Cellophane film	
Radiation:	
Ultraviolet	
^{90}Sr	
Virus:	
DNA:	
Polyoma	
SV-40	
Adenovirus 12,18	
Shope papilloma	
RNA:	
Mammary tumor agent	Common antigens in
Leukemia	each neoplasm in-
Gross	duced by the same
Moloney	virus
Rauscher } Shared common	
Friend } antigens	
Graffi	
Rich	
Rous (Schmidt-Ruppin)	

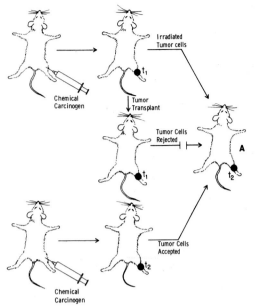

Fig. 9-8. Mouse A, immunized with benzpyrene-induced tumor t, resists subsequent challenge with t tumor cells. Challenge with cells from another benzpyrene induced tumor, t_2, leads to progressive tumor growth and death of the mouse.

demonstrated that this distinction is not as absolute as originally believed. Common antigens related to leukemia viral antigens have been found in chemical-carcinogen-induced sarcomas, and some carcinogen-induced neoplasms arising in the bladder have contained common antigens. Furthermore, spontaneous mouse mammary carcinomas induced by the mammary tumor virus contain individually distinct antigens in addition to the common antigens of the mammary tumor virus.

MECHANISMS OF TUMOR-SPECIFIC IMMUNE REJECTION. The immune response against tumor-specific antigens on tumor cells is similar to the immune response against the histocompatibility antigens of tissue or organ allografts. Two types of immune response are elicited against the tumor-specific antigens of growing neoplasms—humoral antibodies and cell-mediated immune responses.

The cellular immune response is thought to be more important in controlling tumor rejection than the response of the humoral antibodies for several reasons: (1) tumor-specific immunity can be adoptively transferred by lymphoid cells (Fig. 9-10) much more readily than with humoral antibody, and (2) immune lymphocytes or macrophages that kill tumor cells both in vitro and in vivo can be easily demonstrated at all phases of tumor growth.

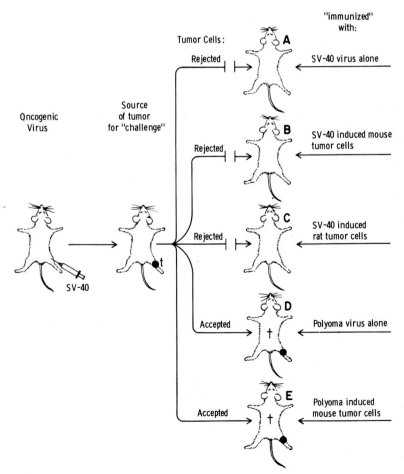

Fig. 9-9. Mice A, B, and C, immunized with SV-40 virus or SV-40 virus–induced tumor cells, reject challenge of tumor cells from SV-40 virus–induced tumor t. Challenge with the same tumor cells in mice D and E, immunized with polyoma virus or polyoma virus–induced tumor cells, leads to progressive tumor growth and death of the mouse.

Although the mechanism by which lymphocytes and macrophages kill tumor cells is unknown, close contact between the tumor cell and the immune lymphocyte is essential for the cytolytic effect. After attachment to the antigenic site on the tumor cell surface, a lytic effect on the cell membrane resulting in cell death may follow. It is evident that lymphocytes unsensitized to tumor cells are increased to sufficiently high numbers.

Macrophages probably play an important role in the tumor-host relationship. Specifically, sensitized macrophages are able to destroy tumor cells in tissue culture or in vivo. In addition, recent studies have shown that nonspecific activation of macrophages by a number of agents will cause them to destroy tumor cells both in vivo and in vitro.

Humoral antibodies also have inhibited tumor growth in vivo and destroy tumor cells in vitro in the presence of complement. Usually, antibody must be given prior to or immediately after tumor transplantation in order to be effective. The sensitivity of various types of neoplasms to cytotoxic antibodies varies considerably. Leukemias and lymphomas are most sensitive, whereas sarcomas and carcinomas are more resistant. There appears to be a correlation between sensitivity of the tumor to cytoxic antibodies in vitro and its response to antibodies in vivo. It is clear that there are considerable differences in the ability of different classes of antibodies to reduce tumor cell viability in vitro and tumor growth inhibition in vivo. IgM classes of antibodies are generally more effective in inducing immunity by passive transfer.

IMMUNE SURVEILLANCE. The concept of immunologic surveillance is based upon the premise that carcinogenesis occurs frequently as a spontaneous mutation, from chemical carcinogens or from oncogenic viruses. Burnet postulated the teleologic explanation for the immune system was to recognize the foreignness of tumor-specific antigens on the neoplastic cells and to mount an immune response capable of eliminating them. In this context, clinical cancer would represent a failure of the mechanisms for immunologic destruction, although it may be the exception rather than the rule.

Mechanisms for Evasion of Immune Surveillance. If neoplastic cells are capable of eliciting a host immune response that leads to their specific destruction, it is pertinent to ask why or how cancer develops. A variety of possible ways by which cancer cells evade the immune surveillance mechanisms have been described:

Insufficient antigenicity to evoke an immune response may account for the growth of some neoplasms. Tumor-specific antigens are usually weaker immunogens than transplantation antigens. Some neoplastic cells may have either an extremely weak tumor-specific antigen or an extremely low density of tumor-specific antigens on the cell surface. Thus, the tumor cell with the stronger tumor-specific antigen may be recognized and eliminated, whereas those cells with weak tumor-specific antigens may escape detection and destruction.

Antigenic modulation of a thymus leukemia (TL) antigen has been observed on a murine lymphoma cell. The TL antigen disappears when the cell is transplanted in im-

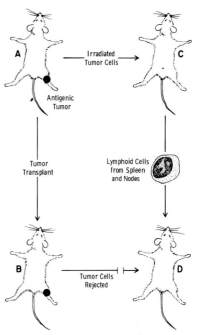

Fig. 9-10. Tumor induced in mouse A with benzpyrene is serially passed into another mouse, B, of the same strain. Mouse C is immunized with irradiated tumor cells of the same tumor. Immune lymphocytes transferred from mouse C to mouse D confer tumor-specific immunity to subsequent tumor challenge.

munized hosts or carried in tissue culture containing specific antibody, but it will reappear when the tumor cells are passed in tissue culture without antibody or transplanted in unimmunized hosts. Furthermore, antigenic shift may be another form of antigenic modulation whereby tumor cells escape control of immunologic surveillance. This phenomenon has been described with certain animal neoplasms in which the lung metastases are antigenically different from the primary tumor.

Immunologic indifference may explain the observation by Old and associates that small numbers of tumor cells having tumor-specific antigens develop into progressively growing tumors although larger numbers of cells are rejected. In this instance the small number of cells may not be immunogenic enough and can "sneak through" the host immune response.

Immunosuppression by irradiation, neonatal thymectomy, chemotherapy, or steroid or antilymphocyte globulin administration usually increases the frequency and growth rate, and shortens the latency period, for both virus- and carcinogen-induced neoplasms in experimental animals. The incidence of cancer in man increases significantly with advancing years as his immune response to a variety of antigens decreases. Furthermore, in human beings with congenital immunodeficiency diseases, the incidence of spontaneous cancer is 10,000 times that of the general age-matched population. In human organ transplant recipients on immunosuppressive drugs, the incidence of spontaneous cancer is more than seventy times that of the general age-matched population.

Immunologic tolerance that develops during the fetal or

neonatal periods due to exposure to tumor-specific antigens or an oncogenic virus may account for tumor growth in some animals when the immunologic surveillance system would otherwise afford protection. Bittner discovered in 1936 that C3H female mice transmitted mammary tumor virus (MTV) through the milk to their nursing young which later induced mammary tumors in a high percentage of their adult female progeny. Morton demonstrated that mice infected as neonates subsequently became tolerant to the tumor-specific antigens of the MTV-induced neoplasms and consequently could not be immunized against them as adults. Newborn mice foster-nursed on non-MTV-carrying mothers from another strain were not tolerant to the virus and, when adult, could be effectively immunized against the MTV-induced mammary tumors. The incidence of mammary tumors in these foster-nursed mice was much lower than in those nursed on MTV infected mothers.

Low-dose immunologic tolerance similar to that seen with transplantation systems, but secondary to prolonged exposure to small amounts of weak tumor-specific antigens may account for the growth of some tumors. Low-dose tolerance may explain the development of metastases from breast cancer in immunocompetent patients many years after radical mastectomy.

Immunologic enhancement refers to the facilitated growth of some tumors in the presence of specific antibody against the tumor-specific antigen. The antibody may work on the afferent limb, the efferent limb, or the central portion of the immune response.

Afferent enhancement occurs when the antibody coats the antigen on the tumor cell and prevents processing of the tumor-specific antigen, either at the regional node or by a macrophage at the tumor cell. *Central enhancement* occurs when the antibody directly inhibits the reactivity of the immunocompetent cells. *Efferent enhancement* occurs when the antibody coats the antigenic site and prevents intimate contact between the immune cell and the tumor cell.

An important point to stress concerning the enhancement of tumor growth by specific antibody concerns the temporal relation between the transfer of antibody and tumor or organ allotransplantation. The antibody must be administered shortly before, at the same time as, or shortly after tumor or organ transplantation in order for enhancement to occur. If administration of the antibody is delayed for a week, the host cellular immune response has already been stimulated, and tumor rejection occurs in a normal fashion. Most animal and human neoplasms have a long latency period prior to clinical detection, and the host immune response is already sensitized to the tumor-specific antigens. Therefore, it is unlikely that immunologic enhancement by antibody is responsible for tumor enhancement or plays an important role in evasion of immunologic surveillance in naturally occurring neoplasms.

CLINICAL EVIDENCE FOR TUMOR IMMUNITY IN MAN

Until recently there was little evidence for the existence of tumor-specific antigens on human neoplasms. For obvious reasons the tumor transplantation techniques used to demonstrate these tumor-specific antigens of animal neoplasms were not applicable to the study of human tumors. Nevertheless, there are a number of well-documented clinical observations which suggest human host immune defenses against cancer. Although other physiologic, endocrinologic, and biologic explanations can be given for these observations, they are most easily explained on an immunologic basis:

1. Spontaneous regression of established tumors is a rare but well-documented phenomenon. Sometimes these regressions have followed a minor viral or bacterial infection. Although spontaneous regression has been observed in many different tumor types, it is most frequently seen in neuroblastomas of children, malignant melanoma, choriocarcinoma, adenocarcinoma of the kidney, and soft tissue sarcomas. However, spontaneous regression occurs less frequently than 0.5 percent in all types, except for neuroblastomas.

   Spontaneous regression of small pulmonary metastases following the surgical removal of the primary tumor has been observed and occurs most frequently in hypernephromas. Spontaneous regression also may account for the prolonged survival or cure of patients after incomplete surgical excision of the cancer.

2. Recurrence of tumor 10 years after successful treatment of the primary is often manifested by rapid tumor growth and death. Although endocrinologic changes may account for some of these observations in breast cancer, in other tumors this course suggests a host defense which inhibits the tumor growth during the disease-free interval.

3. Microscopic evidence of the histiocytic, plasmocytic, lymphocytic, and esosinophilic infiltration, which resembles that seen in an organ transplant or tumor transplant that is undergoing rejection in man, is associated with an improved prognosis. For example, in stomach cancer, these findings correlate better with survival than does adequate surgical removal of the tumor.

4. The presence of many tumor cells in the peripheral blood, lymphatics, pleural cavity, and operative wounds of patients who subsequently never develop metastases suggests host immune defense.

5. There is a low incidence of successful growth of tumor tissue, or autotransplants in patients with advanced disease. The resistance against tumor growth was relative rather than absolute, since challenge with greater numbers of cancer cells usually resulted in tumor growth. The immune nature of this resistance was suggested when autologous leukocytes or plasma was mixed with these tumor cells, and cancer growth decreased in approximately half the patients studied.

IMMUNOLOGIC EVIDENCE FOR TUMOR-SPECIFIC ANTIGENS IN HUMAN NEOPLASMS. During the past decade, a variety of sensitive serologic techniques have demonstrated that every human neoplasm adequately studied contained specific antigens which elicited both cellular and humoral responses in cancer patients.

Humoral antibodies have been shown by the immunofluorescence, complement fixation, immunocytolosis, and immunodiffusion techniques. Cellular immunity has been demonstrated by lymphocyte-mediated cytotoxicity (the ability of lymphocytes to kill tumor cells in tissue culture), lymphocyte blastogenesis tests (the ability of lymphocytes to be stimulated to proliferate by tumor-specific antigens), and migration inhibition tests (macrophages or other blood leukocytes inhibited in their migration by tumor-specific antigens). Finally, it has been found that cancer patients develop delayed cutaneous hypersensitivity reactions to tumor-specific antigens. Thus, it has become increasingly apparent that tumor-specific antigens are capable of eliciting an immune response which can be monitored by the immunologic techniques used to study other types of immune reactions. The wide variety of human neoplasms in which tumor-specific antigens have been detected are listed in Table 9-3.

The antigenic pattern of most human neoplasms is similar. Neoplasms of the same histologic type contain common tumor-specific antigens which differ from tumor-specific antigens of other types of neoplasms. Thus, human sarcomas share a common antigen which is different from the antigens shared by bladder cancer.

In addition, some neoplasms such as malignant melanoma have additional antigens with a pattern of more limited specificity, as well as the common melanoma-specific antigen. This pattern of both individually distinct and common antigens may be characteristic of other types of human neoplasms as well, although studies undertaken thus far have not demonstrated it. The discovery of the common antigen in neoplasms of the same histologic type may allow precise immunotherapeutic and immunoprophylactic maneuvers based upon vaccines prepared for this common tumor antigen rather than from each patient's own tumor-specific antigens.

Carcinoembryonic, or Fetal, Antigens. Most of the tumor-associated antigens described above are located on the cell surface, where they are susceptible to immune attack by antibodies or lymphocytes. Thus, they are probably of considerable importance in the tumor-host relationship. However, there are other types of antigens which may not be located at the cell surface, although they are more or less specific for the neoplastic state. One such group is composed of the fetal, or carcinoembryonic, antigens.

Fetal antigens are produced by normal fetal organs during embryonic development. Their production is repressed shortly after birth, and they are not produced in significant quantities in normal adult organs. However, during neoplastic transformation, reversion of the cell to the embryonic state is accompanied by a renewed production of these fetal antigens. The fetal antigens are thought to represent the phenotypic expression of genes active during fetal life but not expressed during normal adult life. Their occurrence in tumors is thought to be secondary to alterations in the pattern of gene regulation as the result of the dedifferentiation and reversion of the cell to a primitive embryonic state.

The carcinoembryonic, or fetal, antigens may be a useful means of detecting malignant disease before other clinical evidence of disease is apparent or as a detector of recurrence following therapy to provide a basis for further treatment. Fetal antigens that are common to many different histologic types of human neoplasms have been described, as have those that are restricted to the organ of origin.

α-Fetoglobulin. The α-fetoglobulin circulating in approximately 70 percent of patients with primary hepatomas is found in normal human fetal serum up to 1 year after birth. The fetal antigen also has been found occasionally

Table 9-3. HUMAN NEOPLASMS WITH DEMONSTRATED TUMOR-SPECIFIC ANTIGENS

Burkitt's lymphoma
Malignant melanoma
Neuroblastoma
Osteosarcoma
Soft tissue sarcomas
Colon carcinoma
Breast carcinoma
Leukemia
Lung carcinoma
Bladder carcinoma
Renal carcinoma

in patients with gastric cancer, prostatic cancer, and primitive testicular tumors such as teratomas, although it appears to be relatively specific for hepatomas. The specificity of the test was demonstrated when adult monkeys were given hepatic carcinogens; α-fetoglobulin appeared in the serum of a high percentage of these monkeys prior to any histologic evidence of neoplastic change.

The α-fetoglobulin test has been clinically evaluated and found to be useful in the diagnosis of hepatomas. It is not positive in patients with rapidly dividing cells due to hepatic regeneration following liver resection or in those with cirrhosis.

Carcinoembryonic Antigen. The carcinoembryonic antigen (CEA) reported in 1965 by Gold and Friedman is another tumor-associated antigen occurring in fetal gut, liver, and pancreas during the first two trimesters of gestation. This antigen was originally thought to be specific for adenocarcinomas arising in the gastrointestinal tract and pancreas, but more recently it has been found in a variety of carcinomas, sarcomas, and lymphomas of many different histologic types.

Since the CEA appears in the bloodstream, it was initially thought to be of great importance as a diagnostic tool for malignant disease prior to other clinical evidence of cancer. A radioimmunoassay capable of detecting nanogram quantities of CEA in the blood was developed. However, elevated CEA levels were found in patients with a variety of nonmalignant conditions including alcoholic cirrhosis, pancreatitis, cholecystitis, colonic diverticulitis, and ulcerative colitis. As a result, the incidence of elevated CEA levels in mass screening of normal or hospitalized populations has been over 10 percent in some series. Therefore, it would appear that this test will not become useful as a serologic method for the diagnosis of malignant tumor.

The serum levels of CEA do appear to correlate with the extent of known carcinomas of the colon. Less than 20 percent of patients with early lesions (Dukes Stage A or B) have elevated CEA levels, whereas one-half of patients with Dukes C lesions and almost all patients with Dukes D lesions have elevated levels of CEA. Metastasis to the liver is frequently associated with the highest levels. These statistics suggest that CEA may have limited use in detecting early carcinoma of the bowel. It has been shown that the CEA level drops during the postoperative period in those patients who have successful resection of the tumor. Patients who develop tumor recurrence often show a rise in CEA titer to the preoperative levels. Thus, CEA may be extremely useful in following the clinical course of patients with known malignant disease in order to detect evidence of recurrence prior to its becoming clinically detectable.

γ-Fetoprotein. Edynak and associates have recently described a new type of fetal antigen occurring in a wide variety of human neoplasms of different histologic types, in human fetal tissues and serum, in benign neoplasms, and in normal breast tissue adjacent to breast carcinomas, but not in the serum of normal individuals. This antigen was also found in the serum of 10 percent of cancer patients; unfortunately, in only 23 of 210 patients with a variety of cancers was this antigen detectable in the serum. Furthermore, in only 8 of 1,518 patients with cancer was there antibody to this antigen in the serum. This test can become useful as a screening procedure for primary or recurrent cancer when it is more sensitive to both the γ-fetoprotein antigen and the antibody.

GENERAL IMMUNE COMPETENCE OF CANCER PATIENTS. A number of studies have tested the general functional capacity of the cancer patient's immunologic system. Such studies can be grouped into two categories—those concerned with humoral antibody production and those dealing with cell-mediated immune reactions.

Formation of humoral antibody to known antigenic substances has been studied by many investigators, who have found most cancer patients have the ability to form humoral antibodies against a variety of antigenic substances, even in the presence of advanced disease. There is no evidence to implicate a defect in humoral antibody production in most cancer patients.

The cell-mediated immune reactions have been measured by the cancer patient's ability to manifest delayed cutaneous hypersensitivity to a variety of common skin test antigens to which most normal persons are reactive by virtue of previous exposure such as to mumps, tuberculin, streptokinase, or streptodornase. In addition, a primary immune response was tested against a new antigen by

studying the survival of skin allografts and by sensitizing patients to an antigen, such as the contact sensitizer dinitrochlorobenzene (DNCB). DNCB reacts with proteins in the skin and forms a hapten which sensitizes the immunocompetent patient (Fig. 9-11). Cell-mediated immunity can be studied with an in vitro test which requires lymphocyte recognition and proliferation in response to foreign tissue antigens or mitogens such as phytohemagglutinin.

These immunologic studies revealed that cell-mediated immune reactions are significantly impaired in patients with lymphoreticular neoplasia. Since these diseases usually diffusely involve the immune effector system, this might be expected. However, a similar impediment in cell-mediated immune reactions was found in patients with localized or advanced solid neoplasms that did not involve the immune system. The explanation for this immunologic defect in cancer patients is unknown, but there does appear to be a strong correlation between an impaired cell-mediated response and the clinical course of the malignant disease.

This correlation becomes particularly evident when the postoperative course of cancer patients is compared with their ability to become sensitized to DNCB (Fig. 9-12). More than 95 percent of normal control volunteers, patients with benign neoplasms, patients free of disease 5 years or more following cancer surgery, and patients with a history of spontaneous regression of cancer could be sensitized to DNCB. On the other hand, only 65 percent of patients who presented for definitive cancer surgery could be sensitized to this chemical. Seventy-two percent of these immunocompetent patients had localized neoplasms that could be resected, and they subsequently remained free of disease for at least 6 months after surgery. However, those patients who were anergic had a uniformly poor prognosis following operation. Ninety-nine percent were inoperable because of local or metastatic spread of the disease or, when resected, had recurrence of disease within 6 months after surgery. Regardless of the histologic type of neoplasm, patients who had severe impairment of their cell-mediated immune reactions apparent from cutaneous anergy to DNCB had a uniformly poor prognosis after operation.

There were considerable differences, however, in the pattern of DNCB reactivity in patients with different histologic types of solid neoplasms. Patients with epidermoid carcinoma of the cervix, mouth, pharynx, or larynx showed a very strong correlation between the positive DNCB response and a good prognosis after cancer surgery. Most of these patients who could be sensitized were operable and free of disease for at least 6 months, whereas those who were anergic had a uniformly poor prognosis. There was little correlation between a positive DNCB test and recurrence after surgery with the skeletal or soft tissue sarcomas and melanomas; many of these patients developed a recurrence even though they were immunologically competent. The explanation for the differences in cutaneous reactivity with various tumor types is unknown at the present time. It is possible that these patterns are indicative of some important variations in either the causes of or the response to the different types of human neo-

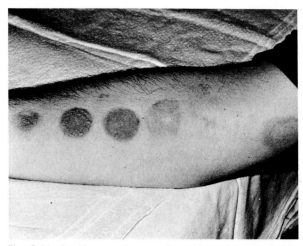

Fig. 9-11. Positive reaction to dintrochlorobenzene (DNCB), showing initial exposure and subsequent challenges.

Patients	DNCB Positive	DNCB Negative
Control	19/20 = 95%	1/20 = 5%
Benign	10/10 = 100%	0/0 = 0%
Longterm survival (>5 yrs) .	16/16 = 100%	0/16 = 0%
Spontaneous regression . . .	8/8 = 100%	0/8 = 0%
All cancer patients	152/237 = 64%	85/237 = 35%
Free of disease (6 mo) . . .	110/152 = 72%	1/85 = 1%
Inoperable or early recurrence	42/152 = 28%	84/85 = 99%

Fig. 9-12. Correlation between delayed cutaneous hypersensitivity to DNCB and prognosis.

plasms. In some instances, it appears that the presence of a neoplasm is clearly related to the immunosuppression, because resection of the neoplasm results in return of immunologic competence. This is particularly true in patients with large, bulky skeletal and soft tissue sarcomas. However, in all cases, the preoperatively anergic patients developed recurrence of the neoplasm even though their general immune competence returned following surgery.

It is apparent that cutaneous anergy indicates a poor prognosis even in patients otherwise considered curable by definitive cancer surgery. Therefore, it is possible that this may become a useful prognostic test in the preoperative evaluation of the patient with cancer.

CORRELATIONS BETWEEN IMMUNE RESPONSE TO TUMOR-SPECIFIC ANTIGENS AND CLINICAL COURSE OF HUMAN CANCER. More sophisticated immunologic studies demonstrated a correlation between the cell-mediated and humoral immune responses and the clinical course of malignant disease. Such studies show that patients with a normal immune response to DNCB may have instead abnormalities in their response to the tumor-specific antigens of their neoplasms that can be detected by other immunologic techniques.

While the antibody role in controlling tumor growth is controversial at the present time, there is a marked correlation between the antibody titer detectable by immunofluorescence and complement fixation and the clinical course in patients with melanomas and sarcomas. This correlation was especially striking when sera from sarcoma patients was tested by complement fixation.

Analyses of sera from patients who enjoyed long-term survival from previous sarcomas showed a persistently elevated antisarcoma antibody titer (Fig. 9-13). Little variation was noted, and persistence of antibody was evident 3 to 4 years after removal of the primary tumor. When sequential antisera samples were obtained before and after surgery for primary sarcomas, it was found that all those patients who had primary surgery and continued to be free of disease had at least a fourfold rise in tumor antibody following removal of the tumor. These antibody titers remained elevated as long as those patients remained free of disease (Fig. 9-14). In contrast, most patients who had no antisarcoma antibody preoperatively with no increase in antibody titer following surgery developed recurrence within 6 months. Furthermore, of the several patients with

low antibody titers preoperatively who had a transient rise in antibody titer following tumor removal, all who developed subsequent pulmonary metastases showed a progressive decline in antisarcoma antibody titers to nondetectable levels as the metastatic disease progressed (Fig. 9-15). In careful, frequent sampling of a few sarcoma patients, it appeared that the antibody titer fell 2 to 3 months prior to development of detectable pulmonary metastatic disease. Thus, careful monitoring of the sarcoma patient's complement fixing antibody titer in the postoperative period may be helpful in early detection of recurrence of disease.

The observation of Hellstrom and associates regarding the presence of blocking factors in the sera of sarcoma patients who have growing neoplasms or who subsequently will develop recurrent disease is probably of considerable importance in the tumor-host relationship. They found that lymphocytes specifically cytotoxic for tumor cells can be demonstrated throughout the course of malignant disease regardless of whether patients have been cured of

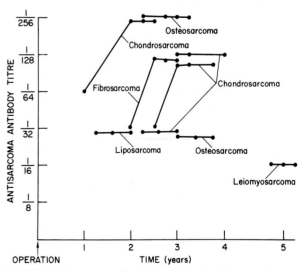

Fig. 9-13. Antisarcoma antibody titers determined by complement fixation against the HuSA-I liposarcoma antigen. Serial serum samples obtained from patients who remained free of disease up to 5 years after resection of the primary sarcoma. (From D. L. Morton et al., Ann Intern Med, 74:587, 1971.)

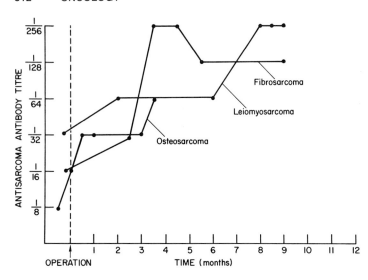

Fig. 9-14. Antisarcoma antibody titers determined by complement fixation against the HuSA-I liposarcoma antigen. Serial serum samples obtained following resection of the primary sarcoma in patients who remained free of disease. (*From D. L. Morton et al., Ann Surg, 172:740, 1970.*)

their tumors or have growing neoplasms. However, the sera of those patients with growing tumors contained blocking factors that inhibited the cytotoxic action of the killer lymphocytes upon tumor cells in vitro. Further studies suggested that the blocking factors were probably circulating tumor antigen-antibody complexes or tumor antigen alone rather than simple enhancing antibodies. This blocking factor could be completely neutralized by admixture with serum that had the cytotoxic or deblocking antibodies from patients free of malignant disease. A most significant correlation to clinical course was found when these in vitro studies demonstrated the deblocking antibodies in patients free of disease but found the blocking serum factors in patients who had recurrence of the disease. Obviously such techniques can be useful in predicting in which patients the disease will recur. The day may come when the balance between antibody and cellular immunity may be manipulated to the patient's benefit through such studies as this.

In addition to the correlations of clinical course to specific humoral immunity, it does appear that delayed cutaneous hypersensitivity reactions to tumor-specific antigens extracted from various types of human neoplasms also correlate in a general way with clinical course. Patients with arrested melanomas, Burkitt's lymphoma, and leukemia exhibit delayed skin reactions to antigens extracted from their tumor cells. These skin reactions become negative with relapse.

POSSIBLE APPLICATIONS OF IMMUNOBIOLOGY TO CANCER THERAPY. There are many possible applications of cancer immunobiology to cancer therapy besides those of the immunotherapy. Immunoprevention by vaccine prepared from the common tumor antigens or tumor viral antigens is theoretically possible. However, because of the long latency period of most human neoplasms, it would require several decades to evaluate such a vaccine even if it were already in hand.

Immunobiology has great potential as a guide to standard cancer therapy. Immunologic monitoring of cancer patients undergoing therapy for malignant disease could be extremely useful in determining choice of therapy, as well as determining the patient's response to the therapy.

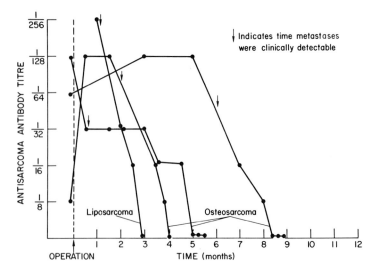

Fig. 9-15. Antisarcoma antibody titers determined by complement fixation against the HuSA-I liposarcoma antigen. Serial serum samples obtained following resection of primary sarcoma in patients who developed recurrent disease with pulmonary metastases. The time at which pulmonary metastases were detected on the chest roentgenogram is indicated by an arrow. (*From D. L. Morton et al., Ann Intern Med, 74:587, 1971.*)

Immunologic testing also may be useful in following the patient's response to certain therapeutic modalities that are known to be immunosuppressive, such as chemotherapy or radiation therapy, so that therapeutic regimens that are nonimmunosuppressive may be devised. Furthermore, with multiphasic immune monitoring, it may become possible to carry out immunologic engineering in patients with defective immune responses. The deficiencies then might be corrected by appropriate adjunctive therapy once the site of the defect has been diagnosed.

PATHOLOGY

When confronted with a tumor mass, the clinician must first determine whether it is a neoplastic or inflammatory process and, if neoplastic, whether it is benign or malignant. This is usually accomplished by biopsy of the mass.

In general, biopsy of a neoplasm should always be obtained before therapy is instituted. The pathologist's interpretation of materials submitted for microscopic examination depends not only upon his experience and the quality of the material submitted but also upon the clinical history and findings on the patient and a review of any previous biopsy material. The features to which the pathologist must direct his attention are partly histologic, that is, the arrangement of the tumor cells and their relation to the surrounding tissue, and partly cytologic, namely, the nature of the tumor cells and, in particular, the appearance of the nucleus and nucleoli.

The characteristics of benign and malignant neoplasms are listed in Table 9-4. *Anaplasia* means lack of differentiation. *Polarity* is the normal orderly alignment of epithelial cells, which are arranged in sheets. One of the early signs of malignant change is the loss of this normal polarity, so that the cells may present as a disorderly arrangement in relation to the surface and to each other. *Nuclear changes* of the malignant cells are often seen as enlarged and hyperchromic nuclei. These three features may all be seen before invasion of the deeper tissues has occurred. This is known as *preinvasive carcinoma*, or *carcinoma in situ.*

One of the most characteristic features of malignant disease is *local infiltration of adjacent tissues,* i.e., malignant colonic epithelial cells invading the muscular or serosal layers of the colon. In contrast, a benign tumor grows by expansion, compressing the surrounding tissues to form a capsule.

Based upon these microscopic criteria, the pathologist usually has no difficulty in determining whether the neoplasm is malignant or benign. Sometimes the microscopic diagnosis is difficult and opinions are divided among the different pathologists examining the tissue. When this happens, several paths are open to the clinician: If the biopsy is not adequate, more material should be obtained. Special stains are sometimes helpful, such as oil red O, to show fat globules as in liposarcoma. Outside expert opinion may be useful, such as from the Armed Forces Institute of Pathology or the National Cancer Institute, which act as referral centers for patients with unusual malignant neoplasms.

The electron microscope has been helpful in diagnosing some undifferentiated tumors, such as malignant melanoma and soft tissue sarcomas. Tissue culture characteristics also may be useful in identifying some malignant neoplasms. Hormonal assay may be helpful, as in diagnosing a glucagon-producing alpha cell cancer of the pancreas. However, it is well to remember that sometimes tumors produce biologic substances that are not normally produced by the tissue from which they originated.

It may not be possible, in certain situations, to differentiate histologically between a benign and a malignant neoplasm, as with the parathyroid carcinomas, giant cell sarcomas of bone, and thymomas. In these cases, clinical characteristics of the lesions in terms of the development of recurrence, metastases, and progressive growth may be the only differentiating criteria available to the clinician.

CLASSIFICATION OF NEOPLASMS. Many different classifications of tumors exist, but the most useful one is based upon the cell type of tissue of origin. When the neoplasm is undifferentiated, the special methods discussed above may help to classify it.

Neoplasms arising from epithelial cells regardless of whether in the ectoderm or the entoderm are known as

Table 9-4. GENERAL CHARACTERISTICS OF BENIGN AND MALIGNANT NEOPLASMS

Characteristic	Benign neoplasms	Malignant neoplasms
Nuclear structure	Normal size, staining and shape	Large, hyperchromatic with variation in size and shape
Mitotic figures	Usually rare	Frequent and perhaps atypical
Anaplasia.	Absent	Varying degree
Polarity	Orderly arrangement	Disorderly arrangement
Local invasion or infiltration	Absent (except angioma	Usually present
Capsule	Present	Absent or a pseudocapsule
Recurrence	Absent or rare	Frequent
Metastases	Absent	Frequent
Growth	Slow, self-limited	Often rapid
Systemic effects	Rare, except for neoplasms	Frequent

carcinomas. Sarcomas arise from connective tissue and include tumors of fibrous, muscular, fatty, vascular, and skeletal origin. Teratoma signifies a neoplasm in which anaplastic, immature somatic cells, comparable to blastoderm, are usually dominant; it exhibits varying degrees of differentiation into mature somatic cells of ectodermal, mesodermal, and entodermal types. Teratomas occur in the testis, ovary, and mediastinum. A simplified classification of benign and malignant neoplasms arising from different sites is given in Table 9-5.

GRADING OF MALIGNANCY. Broders classified carcinomas into four grades according to their degree of differentiation, the appearance of cells, their nuclei, and the number of mitotic figures. On this basis, the least malignant are classified as grade 1, and the most malignant are grade 4. In general, the lower-grade, more differentiated neoplasms are less malignant and tend to metastasize less frequently than the higher-grade, more anaplastic ones. Although the grading of neoplasms is sometimes useful, growth rate and presence of metastasis may be more important in determining prognosis.

CARCINOMA IN SITU AND OTHER PREMALIGNANT LESIONS. Carcinoma in situ is a lesion with the cytologic characteristics of malignant tumors but with no detectable invasion into the surrounding tissue. It seems to develop into invasive cancer after variable delay periods. The interval between the detection of carcinoma in situ of the cervix and invasive carcinoma may be 10 to 15 years. Carcinoma in situ also occurs in the skin, bronchus, stomach, and pharynx. When these lesions are adequately treated, a complete cure is assured.

ROUTES FOR SPREAD OF NEOPLASMS. There are few subjects of greater importance to the oncologist than the spread of cancer. Much is known about the routes of spread but little about the conditions which determine that spread. Some cancers are metastatic at the time of their clinical discovery, while others of the same type and in the same organ tissue may remain localized for years.

Metastases may entirely dominate the clinical picture, while the primary tumor remains latent and asymptomatic. For example, neoplasms of the brain secondary to silent cancers in the bronchus or the gastrointestinal tract are often mistaken for primary brain tumors.

Knowledge of the particular manner in which different types of cancer spread is important in planning therapy. In general, a malignant tumor may spread by four routes: directly by infiltrating surrounding tissue; via lymphatics; by vascular invasion; or by implantation in serous cavities (Fig. 9-16). Knowledge of the patterns of neoplastic spread in different types of cancer is important in planning definitive therapy. Metastatic patterns of various types of human tumors are summarized in Table 9-6.

Direct Extension. Cancer cells may spread by direct extension through tissue spaces. Some neoplasms, such as soft tissue sarcomas and adenocarcinomas of the stomach or esophagus, may extend for considerable distances (10 to 15 cm) along tissue planes beyond the palpable tumor mass. Other neoplasms, such as basal cell carcinoma of skin, rarely extend for more than a few millimeters beyond the visible margin.

Lymphatic Spread. Tumor cells can readily enter lymphatics and extend along these channels by permeation or embolism through the regional lymphatics to lymph nodes. Permeation is the growth of a colony of tumor cells along the course of the lymph vessel. This occurs commonly in the skin lymphatics in carcinoma of the breast and in the perineural lymphatics in carcinoma of the prostate.

Spread along the lymphatics by embolism to the regional nodes or distant lymph nodes is of much greater importance. Lymph node metastases are first confined to the subcapsular space; at this stage the node is not enlarged and may appear normal to the naked eye. Gradually the tumor cells permeate the sinusoids and replace the parenchyma. There is little direct spread from node to node, because the capsule is not penetrated until a late stage. The tumor cells travel by anastomosing lymphatics, and

Table 9-5. SIMPLE CLASSIFICATION OF NEOPLASMS

Tissue of origin	Site of origin	Benign	Malignant
Epithelial origin (ectoderm or entoderm)	Skin, mouth, larynx, lung, esophagus, urinary tract, cervix	Papilloma	Squamous cell carcinoma
	Breast, stomach, colon pancreas, liver	Adenoma	Adenocarcinoma
Mesodermal origin	Fibrous tissue	Fibroma	Fibrosarcoma
	Muscular tissue	Leiomyoma, rhabdomyoma	Leiomyosarcoma, rhabdomyosarcoma
	Fatty tissue	Lipoma	Liposarcoma
	Vascular tissue	Angioma	Angiosarcoma
	Hemopoietic tissue		Leukemia, multiple myeloma, lymphoma
	Bone	Osteoma, chondroma	Osteogenic sarcoma, chondrosarcoma
Special types:			
Melanocytes	Skin, eye	Nevus	Malignant melanoma
Neural tissue	Brain, spinal cord nerve	Astrocytoma	Glioblastoma multiforme
		Ganglioneuroma	Neuroblastoma
Trophoblast	Placenta testis	Chorioepithelioma	Choriocarcinoma
Notochord	Spine	Chordoma	Chordoma
Blastoderm	Mediastinum, ovary, testis	Teratoma	Teratoma

the spread occurs in other nodes by way of collateral lymph channels.

The lymph from the abdominal organs and lower extremities drains into the cisterna chyli and then into the thoracic duct, which finally opens into the left jugular vein. Tumor cells pass from the lymph to the bloodstream by this route. Spread along the thoracic duct explains those cases in which cancer of the gastrointestinal tract is associated with pulmonary metastasis while the liver remains clear. Involvement of the supraclavicular lymph nodes is usually related to entrapment of tumor emboli from the thoracic duct behind the valves near the termination of the duct, followed by extension of these cells along the lymphatics to the node. Thus, lymphatic spread may eventually become vascular dissemination.

Lymphatic spread is extremely common in epithelial neoplasms of all types, except basal cell carcinoma of the skin, which does not metastasize to regional lymphatics. Sarcomas metastasize to lymph nodes in only a minority of cases, usually less than 10 percent.

VASCULAR SPREAD. Cancer cells may reach the bloodstream either by the thoracic duct, as just described, or by invasion of blood vessels. The veins are invaded frequently, the arteries rarely. The chief reason for the striking differences in invasion characteristics between arteries and veins appears to be that lymphatics frequently penetrate the walls of the large veins from without and form a plexus reaching to the subendothelial region, thus providing a portal of entry for tumor cells through the vein wall. When the vascular endothelium is destroyed, a thrombus forms that is quickly invaded by tumor. It is this combination of thrombus and tumor which detaches to form the emboli that result in metastases. Vascular invasion is commonly seen in both carcinomas and sarcomas and is frequently associated with a poor prognosis. Some

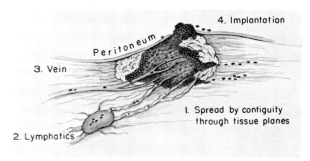

Fig. 9-16. Four mechanisms of the dissemination of cancer cells. This is a diagramatic illustration; the original tumor could be one of many organs with cells disseminating by the four mechanisms. (*From W. H. Cole, et al., "Dissemination of Cancer," Appleton-Century-Crofts, Inc., New York, 1961.*)

types of neoplasms have a remarkable tendency to grow as a solid column along the course of veins, for example, renal carcinomas and sarcomas. Renal carcinomas have been known to grow out of the renal vein into the inferior vena cava and up the inferior vena cava to the right atrium.

Spread through Serous Cavities. Tumor cells occasionally gain entrance to serous cavities via direct growth of tumor through the wall of certain organs, or by growth on the surface of such potential spaces. Many tumor cells are capable of growth in suspension without a supporting matrix. In either case, it is common for tumor cells to spread widely when they encounter a space lined with a serous surface. Thus, widespread peritoneal seeding is commonly seen with gastrointestinal neoplasms and tumors of ovarian origin. A similar mechanism appears to operate in the case of malignant gliomas, which may spread widely within the central nervous system via cerebral spinal fluid.

Table 9-6. ESTIMATED FREQUENCY* OF PATTERNS OF NEOPLASTIC SPREAD FOR COMMON HUMAN NEOPLASMS

Neoplasm	Hematogenous	Lymphatic	Local infiltration (expressed as local recurrence)
Adenocarcinoma			
Breast	3	3	2
Colon	3	3	1
Stomach	4	4	3
Pancreas	4	4	3
Epidermoid carcinoma			
Lung	4	3	2
Oral pharynx	1	3	3
Larynx	1	3	2
Cutaneous neoplasm			
Squamous cell carcinoma	1	2	1
Melanomas	3	3	2
Basal cell carcinomas	0	0	1
Sarcomas			
Bones	4	1	1
Soft tissue	4	1	3
Brain neoplasms	0	0	4

*0—Does not occur, 1—1 to 15 percent, 2—15 to 30 percent, 3—>30 percent, and 4—>50 percent.

CLINICAL MANIFESTATIONS OF CANCER

The manner in which neoplastic disease presents itself clinically is varied and inconstant. Current ability to define, detect, and quantify the neoplastic state is limited. Cancer may present as an asymptomatic lesion too small to be seen without magnification, as an asymptomatic lump, or as symptomatic disease. Often, symptoms are nonspecific and resemble those of nonmalignant diseases. The clinical abnormalities produced by advancing neoplastic diseases may be grouped into two categories—those abnormalities which stem directly from the presence of a tumor mass and those physiologic derangements which are produced indirectly. By including the possibility of neoplastic disease in every differential diagnosis and by teaching patients those key symptoms which require medical evaluation, one may be able to achieve earlier diagnosis and treatment, thereby improving the survival of cancer patients.

The onset of the neoplastic state is difficult to date in human beings. As previously discussed, a prolonged latent or induction period is likely before clinically detectable disease evolves. Therefore, the use of the word "early" in describing a cancer may lead to confusion. To avoid this, we will use the terms "early" and "late" in relation to the clinical stage of a neoplasm rather than to indicate its duration in the body. When viewed in this manner, the curable cancer may have been present a long time prior to its diagnosis and therapy. The term *early* usually means a neoplasm that can be effectively treated. These neoplasms are small rather than large, do not extend into essential organs, and have not metastasized. Some lesions that have been present for years still may be early, whereas other lesions with more rapid growth rates may be *late* even if present for only a few months.

The "Seven Danger Signals of Cancer," as formulated by the American Cancer Society, are listed in Table 9-7. These may be helpful in the ongoing effort to educate people and increase the frequency of early diagnosis for certain major tumors. The more common patterns of clinical presentation, and some of the more common syndromes related to cancer will be discussed in detail in the paragraphs which follow.

Carcinoma in situ and other premalignant lesions were discussed earlier under pathology and will not be discussed further here.

SIGNS OF EXPANSILE GROWTH. The signs attributable to the expansile growth of a tumor depend upon its location. When the neoplasm is either on or near the surface of the body, it may present simply as a visible or palpable mass. In the gastrointestinal, biliary, respiratory, and uri-

Table 9-7. CANCER'S SEVEN WARNING SIGNALS

Change in bowel or bladder habits
A sore that does not heal
Unusual bleeding or discharge
Thickening or lump in breast or elsewhere
Indigestion or difficulty in swallowing
Obvious change in wart or mole
Nagging cough or hoarseness

nary tracts, signs are frequently related to obstruction. Examples are vomiting, jaundice, cough, or urinary retention. Within the central nervous system, expansile growth may cause pain and paralysis.

Expansile growth of a tumor may also result in destruction of host tissues. Examples are pathologic fractures, hepatic insufficiency, and Addison's disease.

SIGNS OF INFILTRATIVE GROWTH. Pain and paralysis may result when tumor infiltrates nerves. Frequently, signs of nerve invasion are also signs of incurability. Examples are lumbosacral plexus pain in cancer of the cervix and rectum, dorsal and lumbar spine pain in cancer of the pancreas, and the shoulder and arm pain and palsy when carcinoma of the lung infiltrates the brachial plexus. Other signs of infiltration generally denoting incurability are thickening of the uterine ligaments in cancer of the cervix and fixation to the chest wall in breast cancer.

SIGNS OF TUMOR NECROSIS: BLEEDING AND INFECTION. Tumors may become necrotic, ulcerate, and bleed. Fatigue and weakness may be the only symptoms or signs in cancer of the stomach or right colon, because the tumor ulceration and bleeding has resulted in anemia. If gastric or colonic cancer becomes ulcerated and infected, the signs of inflammation include edema, pain, tenderness, and fever. The inflammation caused by cecal cancer can mimic the clinical symptoms of acute appendicitis or cholecystitis. Therefore, response of such inflammation to antibiotics or the healing of an ulcer does *not* necessarily indicate a nonneoplastic lesion.

Tumor necrosis at any site may produce fever, leukocytosis, elevation of sedimentation rate, anorexia, and malaise. Such necrosis constitutes one of the causes of the "fever of unknown origin." Keller and Williams, in studies of 46 patients with unexplained fever, found that in 19 who underwent exploratory laparotomy the cause of the fever was intraabdominal malignant disease.

UNKNOWN PRIMARY TUMORS PRESENTING AS METASTASES. Although the primary neoplasm often grows to considerable size before metastatic lesions are seen, in other cases the primary neoplasms may be so small as to be undetectable. The initial presentation of a tumor may be at a distance from its origin. In fact, the primary neoplasm giving rise to the metastases may have regressed completely and may never be detected in some neoplasms, such as malignant melanoma and carcinomas of the oral pharynx.

The most frequent sites of presentation of metastatic neoplasms are the cervical and supraclavicular lymph nodes, lungs, liver, bones, and brain. The most common metastatic sites for unknown primary neoplasms are listed in Table 9-8.

SYSTEMIC MANIFESTATION OF MALIGNANT DISEASE. Tumors may have a variety of remote and systemic effects that contribute to morbidity. Cancer patients frequently develop unusual symptoms and physiologic derangements which cannot be attributed to the mechanical presence of primary or metastatic disease, or to physiologic changes resulting from hormones normally secreted by the tissue of origin.

Some symptoms, such as the cachexia of carcinomatosis,

may result from competition between the tumor and the host for basic components of the same metabolic pool. However, the pathogenesis of many of these disorders is unknown. Some of these nonmetastatic, systemic manifestations of malignant tumors are thought to result from (1) the ectopic production of known hormones, (2) the secretion of unidentified, physiologically active substances which do not resemble known hormones, (3) autoimmune phenomena in which the host is sensitized to an antigen from the tumor, and/or (4) toxic substances secreted from the tumor.

The nonmetastatic clinical manifestations of malignant disease and the neoplasms with which they are associated are presented in Table 9-9. Sometimes palliative surgery is indicated to treat these systemic manifestations, for example, resection of metastases which are producing hormones that induce hypercalcemia, or of a pulmonary osteoarthropathy.

CANCER DIAGNOSIS AND STAGING EXTENT OF CANCER

Diagnosis

Diagnosis of cancer should proceed in an orderly fashion: careful history, thorough physical examination with examination of the blood and urine, and investigation of suspicious findings by appropriate radiologic examinations and radioisotope scans.

A history of any of the following is suspicious and should prompt a search for cancer: weight loss; loss of appetite; bleeding or a discharge from any body orifice or nipple; a sore that has not healed in 3 weeks; changing color or size of a mole; persistent cough or wheeze; change in voice; difficulty in swallowing; growing lump either in or under the skin, in the breast, in the abdomen, or in the muscles; and/or change of bowel habits.

Physical examination includes a thorough search of the entire skin surface for squamous cell and basal cell carcinomas, indurated lesions, ulcers, suspicious or irritated nevi, nodules, and other signs of malignant disease. Lymph nodes should be palpated for enlargement. Breasts should be palpated with the patient rotated to take the tension off the suspensory ligaments. All body orifices should be examined. A Papanicolaou smear from the cervix should be examined prior to a bimanual pelvic examination. Rectal examination should include proctoscopic examination of patients who have hemorrhoids or rectal symptoms. The oral pharynx should be examined with special attention to the floor of the mouth. Indirect laryngoscopy should be performed if the patient is hoarse or is suspected of having an intrathoracic neoplasm in cancer of the thyroid gland.

Laboratory examination should include complete blood cell count, urinalysis, examination of stool for occult blood, and chest roentgenogram. Other tests should be ordered where indicated by symptoms. Before operating on a patient for cure or palliation, a metastatic work-up should be done, directed by symptoms and the most likely site

Table 9-8. UNKNOWN PRIMARY TUMORS PRESENTING AS METASTASES

Site of metastasis	Primary neoplasm
Lymph nodes:	
Cervical nodes	Nasopharynx, pharynx, oral cavity, thyroid, larynx, lymphomas
Supraclavicular nodes	Bronchus, breast, stomach, esophagus, pancreas, colon, testis, ovary, cervix
Axillary nodes	Breast, melanoma, lymphoma
Inguinal nodes	Genitalia, anus, melanoma
Skin and subcutaneous tissues	Melanoma, breast, bronchus, stomach, kidney
Lung	Breast, colon, kidney, stomach, testis, melanoma, thyroid, sarcomas
Liver	Stomach, colon, breast, pancreas, bronchus
Ovary	Stomach, colon
Bones	Breast, bronchus, prostate, thyroid
Central nervous system	Breast, bronchus, kidney, colon
Serous cavities	Bronchus, breast, ovary, lymphoma

of metastases. Prior to extensive disfiguring or disabling procedures, tomograms of the lungs, bone marrow biopsy, scalene node biopsy, isotope scans, or arteriography may be useful in determining whether the neoplasm is still localized. Cytologic examination should be performed if a pleural effusion or ascites is present.

Diagnosis of solid tumors rests upon locating a space-occupying lesion and taking a portion of it for histologic examination. This goal is most easily fulfilled when the tumor is near the body surface or involves one of the orifices of the body that can be examined with appropriate visual instruments, such as a bronchoscope, proctoscope, or cystoscope. Carcinomas of the breast, tongue, or rectum can be seen or palpated, and a portion can be excised for definitive diagnosis.

The most difficult cancers to diagnose, and unfortunately the most lethal ones, occur in the internal organs. Space-occupying lesions in the internal organs may grow quite large before causing symptoms. Techniques which may be useful in localizing such lesions include barium examinations of the stomach and colon, examination of the bronchial tree with soluble contrast media, selective arteriography of major vessels supplying internal organs, and the use of radioisotopes and radiopaque dyes that concentrate in various organs such as the liver, gallbladder, kidney, and lymph nodes. Despite the use of such indirect means of examination, major surgery is often required to confirm the diagnosis.

CANCER DETECTION EXAMINATION. Both physicians and patients have been rather slow to adopt the habit of regular examinations to detect asymptomatic neoplasms. The lack of popularity of cancer detection examinations is in direct relation to the low yield of cancers diagnosed.

Table 9-9. SYSTEMIC MANIFESTATIONS OF MALIGNANT DISEASE

Clinical manifestations	*Associated neoplasms*
Cutaneous	
Acanthosis nigricans	Cancer of stomach, lung, and breast
Dermatomyositis	Cancer of stomach, breast, lung, and ovary
Erythema multiforme, exfoliative dermatitis, bullous phemphigoid	Allergic response to a variety of neoplasms, lymphoma, myeloma
Peutz-Jeghers syndrome	Intestinal polyposis
Hematologic	
Abnormal red cell mass	
Erythrocytosis (increased erythropoietin)	Renal cell carcinoma, hepatoma, uterine myoma, cerebellar tumors, pheochromocytoma
Anemia:	
Myelophthisic	All tumors
Hypoproliferative	Thymoma, renal cell carcinoma
Hemolytic	Hematopoietic neoplasm
Miscellaneous causes (infection, bleeding, radiation effects, uremia, etc.)	
Abnormal leukocyte or platelet mass	
Leukemoid reactions	Miscellaneous neoplasms
Leukopenia	Hemopoietic neoplasms, lung, pancreas
Thrombocytosis	
Coagulation and bleeding disorder	
Disseminated intravascular coagulation (DIC)	Mucin-secreting adenocarcinoma
Vascular	
Thrombophlebitis	Cancer of lung, reproductive tract, pancreas, and breast
Fibrinogen deficiency (increased fibrinolysin)	Cancer of prostate and lung
Flushing, vasodilatation, violaceous skin, asthma	Carcinoid tumor
Hormonal and metabolic effects of nonendocrine tumors	
Hypoglycemia (mechanism unknown)	Retroperitoneal or mediastinal mesenchymal tumors, hepatic tumors
Cushing's syndrome (increased ACTH)	Cancer of the lung, malignant thymoma, pancreatic cancer
Hypercalcemia (increased PTH, vitamin D–like substances or bone destruction)	Cancer of lung, kidney, breast, uterus, sarcomas, hemopoietic neoplasms
Hyponatremia (increased ADH)	Cancer of lung, intracranial tumors
Hyperthyroidism (increased TSH)	Choriocarcinoma, testicular embryonal carcinoma
Precocious puberty and/or gynecomastia (increased gonadotropin)	Hepatoma, lung, adrenal cancer, testicular tumors
Zollinger-Ellison syndrome (increased gastrin) or secretion	Pancreatic nonbeta islet cell adenomas
Elevated liver enzymes	Renal cell carcinoma
Anorexia and weight loss	Most neoplasms

Clinical manifestations	*Associated neoplasms*
Hyperuricemia	Hemopoietic neoplasms
Atypical carcinoid syndrome	Pancreatic duct, islet cell, gastric, thyroid, and oat cell cancer of lung
Nonmetastatic neuromuscular	
Multifocal leukoencephalopathy	Hemopoietic neoplasms
Subacute cerebellar degeneration	Multiple neoplasms, especially of lung, ovary, and breast
Polyneuropathy and/or myopathy	Multiple neoplasms, especially of lung, ovary, and breast
Myasthenia gravis	Thymoma

SOURCE: Modified from A. H. Owens, Jr., Neoplastic Diseases, in A. M. Harvey, et al., "The Principles and Practice of Medicine." Appleton-Century-Crofts, New York, 1972.

Any given individual stands approximately 1 chance in 4 of developing cancer during his lifetime. Therefore, in screening 1,000 persons for an entire life span, we will find cancer in 250 of them. Since a person can harbor more than one primary cancer and a second lesion will develop with increasing frequency as the number of people who have survived the first one increases, we might count on a very crude estimate of 350 cancers in our population of 1,000. Since we expect people to live an average of 72 years, we must carry out 72,000 annual examinations to discover 350 cancers, or less than 5 cancers per 1,000 examinations. By directing our search to the middle and late adult years when the incidence is highest, we might conceivably double the yield to 10 per 1,000. Thus, the chances of detecting cancer in a given annual examination are no more than 1 in 100 even under the most optimal circumstances.

The problem of cancer detection is further complicated by the relative insensitivity of our methods for clinical cancer detection. The earliest neoplasms must be at least 1 cm in size before they are detectable by physical examination, and often tumor masses up to 10 cm in diameter will go undetected if in the liver, retroperitoneum, or other "silent" areas.

Therefore, the best chance for early diagnosis will depend upon the development of biochemical or serologic methods for cancer diagnosis rather than on routine cancer examinations in asymptomatic patients.

BIOPSY. It is imperative that microscopic proof of malignant disease be obtained prior to institution of treatment, since significant morbidity and mortality may result from all forms of cancer therapy. Significant errors have been made when biopsies were not obtained; examples are radical mastectomies for fat necrosis and radiation therapy for renal cysts.

Even when biopsy reports from another hospital are available, the slides of the previous biopsy must be obtained and reviewed prior to the institution of therapy. This is essential because, not infrequently and particularly in rare neoplasms, an erroneous interpretation may have been made. *Definitive therapy cannot be planned rationally without knowing the nature of the neoplastic lesion.*

Three methods for biopsy of suspicious tissue are commonly used. They are the *needle,* the *incisional,* and the *excisional,* or open, biopsy; each has its advantages and disadvantages. Regardless of method used, the pathologic interpretation of the tumor mass can be valid only if a representative section of tumor is obtained. A problem of "sampling error" can occur with the needle and the incisional biopsies when only a small portion of the total tumor mass is submitted for pathologic examination.

Needle biopsy is the simplest method and may be used for biopsy of subcutaneous masses, muscular masses, and some internal organs, such as liver and kidney. Further, this method is inexpensive and causes minimal disturbance of the surrounding tissue. There is less chance of disrupting lymphatics and spreading cancer cells along tissue planes. The danger of implanting tumor cells in a needle tract during aspiration biopsy is extremely small and can be avoided if the location of the needle tract is such that it can be excised easily at the time of the definitive surgical procedure. Needle biopsy may be disadvantageous when the specimen is quite small and not representative of the total tumor, or the needle may miss the space-occupying lesion within the liver or kidney. Hence, a needle or aspiration biopsy does require experience to interpret. A negative report for malignant disease is always viewed with skepticism and should be followed by incisional or excisional biopsy if there is any doubt.

Incisional biopsy involves removal of only a portion of a tumor mass for pathologic examination. It is best performed under circumstances where, if tumor cells are spilled at the time of biopsy, the incisional wound can be encompassed and totally excised at the time of the definitive surgical procedure. Incisional biopsy includes removal of portions of tumor with forceps during endoscopic examination of the bronchus, esophagus, rectum, and bladder. Incisional biopsy is indicated for deeper subcutaneous or muscular tumor masses when needle biopsy fails to establish a diagnosis.

The incisional biopsy is also used when a tumor is so large that total local excision would prejudice any subsequent adequate, wide, locally curative resection because of the wide tissue planes that are necessarily exposed by biopsy. Such biopsy should take a deep section of tumor, as well as a margin of normal tissue, if possible. Incisional biopsy does suffer from the same hazard as the needle biopsy in that the removed portion may not be representative of all the involved tissue; hence, a negative biopsy does not preclude the presence of cancer in the remaining mass. Another theoretic objection to the incisional method is the possibility that the surgeon may seed cancer cells into the operative wound or that exposed open lymphatics may transport the cells to distant sites. Despite these dangers, one must keep in mind that definitive surgical procedures cannot be planned rationally without knowing the nature of the neoplastic lesion.

Excisional biopsy is total local removal of the tumor mass. This is used for small, discrete masses, 2 to 3 cm in diameter, when local removal will not interfere with the wider excision required for permanent local control. A major advantage of an excisional biopsy is that it gives the entire lesion to the pathologist. However, this method is contraindicated in large tumor masses because, again, the biopsy procedure often scatters tumor cells throughout a large biopsy incision that must be widely and totally encompassed by subsequent definitive surgical procedures. Therefore, excisional biopsy is usually contraindicated for skeletal and soft tissue sarcomas, although it is ideally suitable for superficial squamous or basal cell carcinomas and malignant melanomas. The surgeon should always mark the excisional biopsy margins with sutures so that if removal is incomplete, he will know where tumor margin was positive should further excision be indicated.

Biopsy incisions should be closed with meticulous hemostasis, since it may be possible for a collecting hematoma to extend tumor cell contamination by widespread infiltration of tissue planes. Contaminated instruments, gloves, gowns, and drapes should be discarded and replaced with noncontaminated substitutes when the definitive procedure is to follow immediately after the biopsy procedure.

The excisional method is principally used for polypoid lesions of the colon, for thyroid and breast nodules, for small skin lesions, and for equivocal partial biopsies. An unbiopsied lump is surgically removed when the suspicious character of the lesion, the need for its removal whatever the diagnosis, and the nonmutilating nature of the operation make such an approach reasonably definitive. Examples of such procedures include hemithyroidectomy for thyroid nodules, partial colectomy for lesions at any point beyond the reach of the sigmoidoscope, or a right colectomy for a cecal mass that might be inflammatory or neoplastic.

Lymph nodes should be carefully selected for biopsy. Cervical lymph nodes should not be biopsied until a careful search for a primary tumor has been made. Indirect laryngoscopy, pharyngoscopy, esophagoscopy, and bronchoscopy are included in the work-up. Enlargement of the upper cervical nodes is usually due to metastases from laryngeal, oropharyngeal, and nasopharyngeal neoplasms. Supraclavicular nodes are more frequently enlarged from metastases originating in the thoracic or abdominal cavity.

The specimen may be prepared for pathologic examination by either frozen or permanent sections. Frozen sections are made immediately, and pathologic diagnosis can be obtained within 10 to 20 minutes. Although frozen sections may be as adequate as permanent sections for diagnosis of some neoplasms, most pathologists would prefer to make a definitive diagnosis in questionable cases on permanent sections. Unfortunately, such sections require 1 to 2 days for processing. Therefore, frozen sections are used when the diagnosis is required at the time of major surgery and when it is in the patient's best interests to have the definitive resectional surgery carried out at that time. Examples in which the therapeutic decision will be based upon the results of frozen section examination include (1) deciding between a local or radical operation in carcinoma of the breast, (2) limiting the extent of excision in carcinomas of the lip or face, (3) determining the adequacy of surgical margins, and (4) identifying small structures such as parathyroid glands.

Occasionally, an exploratory thoracotomy or laparotomy will be necessary to obtain tissue for microscopic examination and confirmation of diagnosis. As a general rule, regardless of the clinical picture, the neoplastic nature of the disease process must be confirmed by frozen section examination prior to closure of the wound. This is critical because the permanent sections may fail to confirm the neoplastic nature of the pathologic process.

Exfoliative cytology constitutes one possible method for the early diagnosis of certain types of neoplasms. This technique is based upon the fact that cancer cells are shed from the surfaces of neoplasms arising in epithelial-lined body cavities and orifices, such as the vagina, bronchus, and stomach. These cells can be collected, stained, and recognized as malignant because of their individual morphologic changes.

Staging Extent of Cancer

The extent of the patient's tumor at a given point in time is expressed as its *clinical stage.* In addition to making an exact histologic diagnosis of cancer, it is essential that the clinical stage of the disease be determined prior to making a decision regarding therapy. This is especially important when the patient initially presents for treatment, but also it is often desirable to repeat some of the diagnostic procedures periodically during the patient's course in order to assess his true status. The recognized importance of this staging has led to a variety of international and national attempts to standardize the staging of the patient with cancer. To date, no single system has been universally accepted. However, Stage I usually indicates a neoplasm confined to its primary site of origin, Stage II indicates metastases to the regional lymph nodes, and Stages III and IV indicate distant metastatic spread.

The Union Internationaux Contra Cancer (UICC) has attempted to standardize one system for all nations. This has been called the TNM system because it relies on a statement of tumor extent in terms of the primary tumor (T), presence or absence of node metastases (N), and the presence or absence of distant metastases (M). The system was developed following careful analysis of the results of treatment in patients with various constellations of clinical findings. It was found that patients with larger tumors did less well than those with smaller tumors; hence, the separation of various stages on the basis of tumor size. For different tumors size criteria vary, but in this system decreasing prognosis is indicated by increasing numbers after the T, such as T1, T2, T3, or T4 for lesions of increasing sizes. The presence or absence of regional spread is usually indicated by variations in the secondary category, under N for nodes. The absence of nodal metastasis is designated as N_0; the presence of nodal metastasis is N_1; for more extensive nodal involvement, additional numbers may be used. Finally, distant metastases are indicated by adding a subscript 1 following M for metastases, or a subscript

0 for their absence. Thus, a small lesion that has neither spread to regional nodes nor metastasized would be designated as a $T_1N_0M_0$ lesion. A lesion which was larger and involved regional nodes but without distant metastases might be identified as a $T_2N_1M_0$ lesion. A larger neoplasm with both regional and distant metastases would be designated a $T_3N_1M_1$ lesion.

Specific staging systems have been developed for Hodgkin's disease and other lymphomas. A distinction is made between the clinical stage, as defined by clinical tests, and the pathologic stage, as defined by biopsy or major operation. Stage I relates to diseases localized to one lymph node–bearing area. Stage II would be disease into adjacent regional areas, but on one side of the diaphragm and restricted to lymph node–bearing areas including the spleen and Waldeyer's ring (tonsilar area). Stage IV represents widespread metastases in organs, such as bone, bone marrow, liver, or lung.

Hodgkin's disease, which spreads from a localized region directly into an organ, in this classification scheme is identified as the respective stage plus the subscript E, for extension. Thus, a patient with disease in the mediastinum and neck, with extension into the pulmonary parenchyma adjacent to the mediastinal lesion, would have Stage II_E disease. For lymphomas, the importance of symptoms in prognosis is further identified by adding a designation for the absence or presence of symptoms. Patients with symptoms of night sweats, weight loss, or fever are identified as having Stage B disease, whereas patients lacking these symptoms are identified as having Stage A disease (for example, Stage II_EA). The tremendous importance of accurate staging is underlined by the fact that for many lymphomas an accurate decision regarding therapy may require pathologic staging of the presence or absence of disease below the diaphragm. Thus, patients with disease clinically limited to extensive areas above the diaphragm are commonly subjected to an abdominal exploratory operation in order to remove the spleen, examine the liver, and biopsy lymph nodes. This allows a much more precise designation of the extent of disease, and the findings frequently lead to a change in decision regarding a choice of therapy. Specifically, Hodgkin's disease in Stages I and II is curable by radiation therapy, while Stages IIIB and IV are generally treated with chemotherapy.

The importance of accurate staging when designating a therapeutic program for a patient with cancer cannot be overemphasized. It is an important consideration when comparing the results of therapy in different centers, and as therapeutic methods for cancer improve, it is only by careful staging that new forms of therapy can be appropriately evaluated.

Unfortunately, one of the great difficulties in the present staging methods is their inability to detect subclinical microscopic metastatic lesions. Many patients who are treated for apparently localized cancers already have disseminated metastases. For example, about one-half of those patients who have cancer of the breast and who undergo mastectomy have subclinical distant metastasis at the time of operation.

THERAPY

General Considerations

At present, 55 percent of all cancer patients are treated by surgical resection (40 percent by surgery alone); 34 percent by radiation therapy (16 percent by radiation therapy alone); and 22 percent by chemotherapy alone or in combination with the other modalities. Fifteen percent of cancer patients receive no treatment.

Surgery and radiation therapy today represent the most successful means of dealing with cancer as long as it remains localized to the primary site and regional lymph nodes. Neither can be considered curative once the disease has metastasized beyond the local region, although both methods of therapy may be useful as palliative treatment. Chemotherapy and immunotherapy, unlike surgery and radiation therapy, represent systemic forms of treatment effective against tumor cells already metastatic to distant organ sites. These systemic therapeutic modalities have a greater chance of curing patients with a minimum number of tumor cells than those with clinically evident disease. Thus, though surgery and radiation therapy cannot be curative unless the tumor is confined locally or regionally, they can decrease the patient's tumor burden so that chemotherapy or immunotherapy may become more effective. During the past several years, enough evidence has accumulated to suggest that treatment combining surgery, radiation therapy, chemotherapy, and, possibly, immunotherapy will significantly improve cure rates above those achieved with any single therapeutic modality.

Future cancer treatment, therefore, will be approached in an interdisciplinary manner. Just as oncology should be approached as a unique field of study, so cancer should be regarded as a single but complex disease requiring a multidisciplinary approach. The practice of assigning certain types of neoplasms to surgery, radiation therapy, or medicine with a further division into various anatomically oriented specialties should be discontinued.

GOALS OF THERAPY—CURE OR PALLIATION. Once the diagnosis of malignant disease has been made and the extent of disease determined, a decision must be made about the specific therapy. *Is the patient curable?* This is the foremost question that must be answered before the physician recommends aggressive therapy with its attendant complications. The goals of therapy vary with the extent of the cancer. If the cancer is localized without evidence of spread, the goal is to irradicate the cancer and cure the patient. However, when the cancer is spread beyond local cure, the goal is to control the patient's symptoms and to maintain his maximum activity for the longest possible period of time. Palliation should be measured in terms of useful life. Diabetes is not cured, but the manifestations of the disease are controlled so that a patient has many years of activity and useful life. Goals for the palliation of patients living with cancer are similar.

Patients are generally judged as incurable if they have distant metastases or evidence of extensive local infiltration of adjacent organs or structures. The most common criterion for incurability is distant metastases. However, some patients are potentially curable even if they have distant metastases. For example, patients with solitary pulmonary metastases may be curable by resection, and even those with widespread metastases who have choriocarcinoma may be curable with chemotherapy. Histologic proof of distant metastases should be obtained before the patient is assessed as incurable. Occasionally, an exploratory celiotomy or thoracotomy may be necessary to determine the nature of equivocal lesions in the lungs or liver. In some situations, e.g., multiple pulmonary metastases, the clinical situation may point so overwhelmingly to distant metastases that the patient may safely be considered incurable without biopsy.

Local extension may be a criterion of incurability. For each anatomic site, there are certain local criteria which place the patient unequivocally in an incurable status, while others imply a poor prognosis but are not absolutely indicative of incurability. In equivocal situations after extensive studies have failed to demonstrate metastatic or incurable local extension, the patient deserves the benefit of doubt and should be treated for cure.

CHOICE OF THERAPY. Surgery, radiation therapy, and chemotherapy are the most frequently used therapeutic modalities in the fight against cancer. Each may play a role in both curative and palliative therapy. Immunotherapy is a new modality that has a limited role in cancer therapy at the present time, but one which should become increasingly useful in the future. In choosing therapy, a variety of factors must be considered regardless of whether the aim is cure or palliation. The natural history of the disease and the results obtained from each type of therapy must be known prior to choosing a modality or combination of modalities.

The patient's general medical condition and the presence of any coexisting disease must be considered in planning therapy. Surgery may be contraindicated in a patient who has recently experienced a myocardial infarction. A patient with preexisting diabetes will be much more susceptible to the toxic effects of hormonal therapy with corticosteroids. Renal disease may increase the toxicity of some of the chemotherapeutic drugs, such as methotrexate. In addition, any evidence of infection or bleeding in a patient may make any form of cancer therapy dangerous, requiring vigorous treatment prior to the initiation of definitive therapy.

The psychologic makeup of the patient and the patient's life situation must be considered. A patient who is unable to accept the realities of a given treatment should be offered an alternative approach when possible. This is particularly true of any surgical procedures that significantly alter appearance or that involve change of organ function requiring the patient's daily care, such as colostomy. Experimental forms of therapy, such as intraarterial infusion of drugs, should also be avoided by some patients. Obviously, a patient who is going to be unwilling to tolerate the inconvenience of an intraarterial catheter and who might remove it without medical approval should not undergo such treatment.

Surgical Therapy

Surgical treatment represents the most frequently used and the most successful single method of cancer therapy currently available. More patients are cured of cancer by surgery than by any other therapeutic modality. However, only about one-third of cancer patients are cured by surgery alone, since surgical therapy, with few exceptions, is curative only in those patients in whom the disease is localized in the primary site and regional nodes.

Cancer surgery is based upon the concept that cancer begins as a local disease and spreads in an orderly fashion from the primary site to adjacent tissues by direct extension, to the regional lymph nodes by lymphatics, and through the blood vessels. The surgical procedure is designed to remove the primary neoplasms and the usual contiguous routes of spread with the aim of removing *every* cancer cell from the body.

Advances in surgical techniques, anesthesia, and supportive care (blood transfusion, antibiotics, and fluid and electrolyte management) have permitted the development of more radical and extensive operative procedures. This has resulted in significant improvements in the cure rates for certain human neoplasms. Ultraradical cancer surgery has extended operations to their anatomic limits, permitting the surgical removal of nearly all organs. Unfortunately, these more radical procedures have often failed to significantly increase cure rates.

There have been few significant improvements in the management of most human neoplasms by surgery alone during the past two decades. Furthermore, advances in cancer surgery techniques beyond those presently practiced are unlikely to significantly change the cure rates of most human neoplasms. It would appear, then, that any therapeutic advances must come from the combination of other modalities with cancer surgery.

PREOPERATIVE PREPARATION. Often, the physical condition of cancer patients is relatively poor. Many malignant tumors seem to have a toxic effect on the host disproportionate to the size of the lesion. Patients may have a poor nutritional status because of interference with normal alimentary function as with cancers of the oral pharynx, esophagus, and intestinal tract. Pain may contribute to anorexia and severe electrolyte disorder. Anemia, vitamin deficiencies, and defects in the coagulation mechanisms must be corrected before an operation can be safely performed.

Every effort should be made to correct nutritional deficiencies, restore depleted blood volumes, and correct hypoproteinemia prior to extensive surgical procedures. Otherwise the operative morbidity and mortality following extensive cancer operations will be excessive.

CANCER SURGERY

Once the decision has been made to proceed with surgical therapy, the operative procedure should be planned carefully. It is essential to realize that the best, and often the only, opportunity for cure is at the time of the first operation. If the neoplasm is incompletely excised at that time, tissue planes, lymphatics, and blood vessels are violated and tumor cells seeded throughout the wound. Any recurrence that follows may be difficult to separate from the inflammatory reaction and scarring that can distort tissue planes to a point where tumor margins are indistinct. Therefore, enucleation or incomplete excision of tumor masses is *never* indicated as a therapeutic measure.

PREVENTION OF CANCER CELL IMPLANTATION DURING SURGERY. Local recurrence of cancer following surgery may be due to incomplete removal or spillage of cancer cells into the operative area (Fig. 9-17). The cancer surgeon constantly must be aware of the possible danger of transferring cancer cells by inoculation into the surrounding tissues during the course of an operation. As soon as the incision is made, all edges of the wound must be protected with a plastic drape to prevent tumor cell contamination. This precaution is exemplified best when laparotomy or thoracotomy is performed for malignant disease within the abdomen or thorax.

Tumor cells may be inadvertently transplanted from the primary site to other sites during the surgical procedure. When preliminary biopsy has been done, the entire operative field should be reprepared after the biopsy incision is closed. The instruments and gloves used during the biopsy are not used again, because they may have been contaminated. Even the basin of saline solution in which the surgeon dips his gloved hand may be contaminated with cancer cells. The importance of this is illustrated by a patient with breast cancer who had a skin graft taken from the thigh to close a skin defect after a mastectomy. Later, tumor nodules having the same histologic characteristics as the primary neoplasm developed on the thigh at the skin graft donor site.

If the tumor is entered during the operative procedure, the risk of implanting cancer cells into the wound is greatly increased. Should this happen, the operative field must be isolated; the cut surface of the tumor must be cauterized with the electrocautery and isolated from the remainder of the wound; and the contaminated knife, instruments, and gloves must be discarded. Then, and then only, can the operation continue through a new plane of dissection allowing a much wider margin around the tumor.

Many different cytotoxic solutions have been used to irrigate the wound following cancer surgery in an effort to sterilize the operative site. None have been very effective in decreasing the local recurrence rate, with the exception of 0.5% formaldehyde used to prevent local recurrence from carcinoma of the cervix. Sodium hypochlorite solution, nitrogen mustard, and thiotepa have all been tried, with little success.

The rate of local recurrence in the suture line following resection for carcinoma of the colon is about 10 percent. There has been some success with various techniques to prevent this local recurrence. Ligation of the bowel with umbilical tape proximal and distal to the tumor, or anastomosis, or irrigation of the cut ends of the colon with bichloride of mercury solution and then excision of the edge of each end of the bowel have been used and have decreased the recurrence rate to less than 2 percent. The use of closed anastomosis and iodized sutures has decreased the anastomotic recurrence rate in the laboratory.

PREVENTION OF VASCULAR DISSEMINATION AT SURGERY. Blood-borne metastases are a major factor in the death of patients with most tumors. Although cancer cells have been identified in the blood of many cancer patients, only a small number of these circulating cancer cells survive because of host resistance and other factors. Thus, tumor embolism and metastases are not synonymous. In fact, there appears to be little difference in the prognosis of patients with or without tumor cells in their blood preoperatively. However, there is a correlation between the tumor cells seen during surgery and the prognosis. Furthermore, manipulation of the tumor at surgery can greatly increase the number of cancer cells recovered from the blood.

Definite measures should be taken to prevent the dissemination of tumor cells during surgery. These can include (1) avoiding manipulation of the tumor ("no-touch" technique), (2) early ligation of the vascular pedicle, (3) the use of tourniquets on all extremity tumors.

Since any manipulation of the tumor mass results in exfoliation of tumor cells into the lymphatics and blood, such manipulation must be kept to a minimum prior to surgery, during preparation of the skin with antiseptic agents, as well as during the operative procedure. Furthermore, it is imperative to use incision of proper size to minimize unnecessary manipulation of the tumor. One that is too small will not permit the necessary wide excision without excessive handling. Turnbull and associates have reported a significant higher survival in left colon cancer using the no-touch technique which combines minimal manipulation, early ligation of the vascular pedicle, and wide excision.

TYPES OF CANCER OPERATIONS. Local Resection. Wide local resection in which an adequate margin of normal tissue is removed with the tumor mass may be adequate treatment for certain low-grade neoplasms that do not metastasize to regional nodes or widely infiltrate adjacent tissues. Basal cell carcinomas and the mixed tumors of the parotid gland are examples of such neoplasms.

Radical Local Resection. Some neoplasms may spread widely by infiltration into adjacent tissues. This is especially true for soft tissue sarcomas and esophageal and gastric carcinomas. For this reason, it is necessary to remove a wide margin of normal tissue with the neoplasm in these cases. The wide normal-tissue margin between the line of excision and the tumor mass also acts as a protective barrier against tumor cell spill into the severed lymphatics and vessels. The greater the thickness of normal tissue between the plane of dissection and the tumor, the greater likelihood of a complete local excision.

If the tumor was previously explored but not removed or if an incisional biopsy was performed, it is extremely important that a wide segment of skin and the underlying muscles, fat, and fascia be removed far beyond the limits of the original incision.

It must be constantly emphasized that malignant neoplasms are not well encapsulated. A pseudocapsule composed of a compression zone of neoplastic cells usually covers the tumor. This apparent encapsulation offers a great temptation for simple enucleation, because the tumor

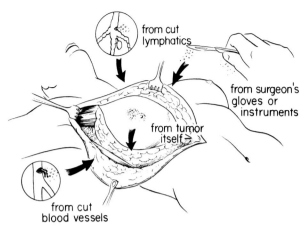

Fig. 9-17. During the operative procedure, cancer cells may be seeded in the wound by direct contact with the primary tumor, with lymph nodes containing metastatic tumor, or with contaminated gloves and instruments. Cancer cells may also enter the wound via cut lymphatics and divided blood vessels. (*From W. H. Cole et al., "Dissemination of Cancer," Appleton-Century-Crofts, Inc., New York, 1961.*)

may be dislodged from its bed so easily. However, this temptation must be resisted. The surgeon must cut through normal tissue at all times and should never encounter the neoplasm during its removal. Dissection should proceed with meticulous care to avoid tumor cell spill. Retraction always should be away from, rather than toward, the tumor. It is important for the surgeon to remember that he must be as far as possible from the gross extent of the tumor on all sides including the deep aspect. He must be prepared to sacrifice important nerves, muscles, and blood vessels if necessary in order to encompass the tumor. Skin, subcutaneous fat and muscle usually can be sacrificed with impunity and little functional loss. However, involvement of major vessels, nerves, joints, or bones may require sacrifice of these structures and even amputation in order to obtain a curative result. During the surgical procedure, the extent of operation should be determined only by the concern for cure.

All deeply situated sarcomas lying between or within muscle groups require the removal of all muscle bundles from their origin to insertion within that particular fascial compartment; all surrounding or adjacent fascia, periosteum, vessels, nerves, and connective tissues; and all skin adjacent to the lesions. These procedures are imperative because sarcomas of the soft somatic tissues tend to infiltrate along fascial and muscle planes far beyond the palpable limits of the tumor. As the surgeon proceeds with the operation, he may be forced to alter his initial operative plan as he visualizes the extent of tumor and as the pathology reports of frozen section examinations of surgical margins are made available. These decisions as to extent of resection are difficult and require experienced judgment. In borderline situations, it is usually better to proceed with a potentially curative resection of the tumor mass unless there is histologic confirmation that the lesion has extended beyond the boundaries of possible surgical resection.

Radical Resection with En Bloc Excision of Lymphatics. Since many neoplasms commonly metastasize by way of the lymphatics, operations have been designed to remove the primary neoplasms and the regional lymph nodes draining that area in continuity with all the tissues intervening between the primary neoplasm and regional nodes. Conditions are best for this type of operation when the collecting nodes of the lymphatic channels draining the neoplasm lie adjacent to the primary site or if there is a single avenue of lymphatic drainage which can be removed without sacrificing vital structures. The regional nodes farthest from the tumor should be dissected first, with dissection proceeding toward the tumor mass in order to prevent any exfoliation of tumor cells from the primary tumor into the regional lymphatics of the venous system.

This principle was applied to breast cancer by Meyer and by Halsted at the turn of the century and has formed the foundation of cancer surgery for many years. At the present time, it is generally agreed that such en bloc regional lymph node dissections should be performed in patients having clinical involvement of nodes by metastatic tumor. However, in many such cases, the tumor has already spread beyond the regional nodes, and the cure rates following such procedures may be quite low.

The high rate of cancer recurrence following surgical removal when lymph nodes are grossly involved and the high error rate when trying to ascertain by palpation those nodes involved by tumor have led to routine dissection of regional nodes close to the primary tumor even though they are not clinically involved. Microscopic examination of the excised lymph nodes in these patients who have no clinical evidence of palpable enlargement reveals evidence of tumor spread in 20 to 40 percent of carcinomas. This concept is supported by comparison of the higher 5-year survival rate of patients showing microscopic involvement of lymph nodes with that of patients in whom lymph node involvement was clinically recognizable.

Recently, some surgeons have challenged the concept of elective or prophylactic resection in cases where the regional nodes are not obviously involved, because of the possibility that such removal may interfere with the patient's immune response to the tumor. This concept originated from experiments in laboratory animals in which removal of the regional nodes within 1 to 2 weeks after implantation of tumor transplants in an extremity interfered with the development of tumor immunity. The validity of these experiments must be challenged, however, because it has been demonstrated with other animal tumors that regional lymphadenectomy has little influence upon host immunity if the removal of the regional nodes is delayed 4 to 6 weeks until the immune response is already underway. The differences between these two sets of experiments depends upon the well-established observation that early excision of regional nodes will interfere with a primary immune response.

It is possible that the immune response against cancer in man is similar. Most human neoplasms have been present in the body for many months or years prior to clinical detection. Hence, cancer patients already have an active systemic immune response to their malignant condition, best demonstrated by the presence of killer lymphocytes in the blood and circulating antitumor antibodies. Thus, the importance of the regional lymph nodes as an immune barrier controlling tumor dissemination in man probably should not be considered an adequate argument against regional lymphadenectomy. In addition, when metastatic cancer cells are found in 20 to 40 percent of operative specimens, it seems likely that the regional nodes obviously are not doing an effective job of controlling the dissemination of cancer.

Nevertheless, this is a very controversial issue at the present time, with sufficiently numerous conflicting reports concerning the effectiveness of elective regional lymphadenectomy that a definite conclusion regarding its use cannot be made. We advocate regional lymphadenectomy in selected patients with clinically negative nodes who have neoplasms which frequently metastasize to lymph nodes because of data supporting higher 5-year survival rates with this technique. Furthermore, most studies comparing identical stages of primary disease have shown slightly improved survival when lymphadenectomy was done. There has been little evidence that removal of the regional nodes adversely affects the survival figures.

This controversy can be settled by a controlled clinical trial to demonstrate the effectiveness of elective or prophylactic lymph node dissections. Such studies are currently underway for several different types of neoplasms. Until more data are available, en bloc resection of regional nodes should continue as standard therapy for carcinoma of the mouth, pharynx and larynx, colon and rectum, breast, uterus and cervix, malignant melanoma, and testicular neoplasms.

Extensive Surgical Procedures. Some slow-growing primary tumors may reach enormous size and may locally infiltrate widely without developing distant metastasis. Supraradical operative procedures can be undertaken in these extensive, nearly inoperable tumors, with cure of occasional patients. Although surgical care, anesthesia, blood replacement, and physiologic monitoring are much improved over the past, these procedures should not be undertaken except by experienced surgeons who can select those patients most likely to benefit from such procedures. Since these extensive surgical procedures sometimes offer a chance for a cure that is not possible by other means, they are justified in selected situations when extensive laboratory work-up shows no evidence of distant metastases. However, the surgeon must be willing to accept the responsibility for the postoperative emotional rehabilitation of the patient before undertaking such extensive procedures as the pelvic exenteration, hemipelvectomy, forequarter amputation, or mutilating operations for head and neck carcinomas.

Pelvic exenteration is a well-conceived operation capable of curing patients with radiation-treated recurrent cancer of the cervix and certain well-differentiated and locally extensive adenocarcinomas of the rectum. This operation removes the pelvic organs (bladder, uterus, and rectum) and all soft tissues within the pelvis. Bowel function is restored with colostomy. Urinary tract drainage is established by anastomosis of ureters into a segment of bowel (ileum or sigmoid colon). The 5-year survival cure rate from pelvic exenteration is 25 percent in this situation.

Hemipelvectomy (resection of the lower extremity and iliac bone) can sometimes be curative for skeletal sarcomas limited to the head of the femur or acetabulum or to one-half of the pelvic structures, and in some slowly growing soft tissue sarcomas of the upper thigh and buttock which recur locally but metastasize slowly. Forequarter amputation (resection of the upper extremity and scapula) can offer similar cure when the neoplasm is limited to the bones of the scapula and upper humerus or to the soft tissues of the shoulder girdle.

SURGERY OF RECURRENT CANCER. There is a definite role for surgical resection of localized recurrent neoplasms of low-grade malignancy and slow growth where further resection may produce a long period of remission. Additional surgical procedures are frequently successful in controlling recurrent soft tissue sarcomas, anastomotic recurrences of colon cancer, and certain basal and squamous carcinomas of skin.

Gilbertsen and Wangensteen advocate routine "second look" operations over a scheduled period, perhaps 6 months after the original procedure, whether or not symptomatic or objective evidence of recurrence is evident. An extensive re-resection of tissue at the operative site is performed at the time of this reexploration. The results of these operations have not been impressive, although a few patients experienced an unexpected long-term control of their disease. However, many of these patients might have been salvaged anyway if reoperation and excision had been delayed until a symptomatic recurrence developed, since this is not uncommon. Thus, it is difficult to prove the second-look theory; for this reason, second-look operations have not become common practice.

RESECTION OF METASTASES. Although logic would suggest that once a neoplasm has metastasized to a distant site it should no longer be curable by surgical resection, removal of metastatic lesions in the lung, liver, or brain has occasionally resulted in a clinical cure. Therefore, in selected patients with slowly growing neoplasms, resections of the metastatic lesions may be indicated especially if the metastasis is solitary. Prior to undertaking resection, an extensive laboratory work-up should rule out metastatic spread to other body areas.

The results of resection of pulmonary metastatic lesions have been much more satisfactory than those of resection of liver or brain metastases. In fact, resection of solitary pulmonary metastases has given a higher rate of 5-year survival than has resection of primary bronchogenic carcinoma of the lung. Resection of pulmonary metastases may be indicated even when more than one metastatic lesion is present. Many patients die with pulmonary metastases and no other evidence of tumor at autopsy; resection of the pulmonary metastases could have resulted in cure. Our experience has shown measurement of the tumor doubling time to be useful in selecting those patients who will benefit most from resection of pulmonary metastases. Patients with tumor doubling times greater than 40 days received significant palliation from their pulmonary resections and remained free of disease for as long as 5 years. In contrast, patients with tumor doubling times of less than 20 days have not significantly benefited from resection of their metastatic lesions (Fig. 9-18).

Hepatic Dearterialization. Hepatic dearterialization has been advocated for the treatment of liver metastases, based upon the observation that metastases derive their blood supply predominately from the hepatic artery whereas normal liver tissue receives blood from both the arterial and portal systems. In the absence of hypotension and sepsis, hepatic artery ligation is surprisingly well tolerated and results in selective necrosis of liver tumors. Because some tumor cells remain viable, postoperative chemotherapy is necessary to help control tumor growth. This procedure is not without risk and needs further evaluation to determine its role in managing patients with either primary hepatic carcinoma or hepatic metastases.

ADMINISTRATION OF CHEMOTHERAPY BY ARTERIAL INFUSION OR ISOLATED PERFUSION. The concentration of chemotherapeutic drugs can be greatly increased when the drug is administered directly into the artery supplying the neoplastic lesion. Continuous infusion of chemotherapeutic drugs over a period of weeks can be carried out with portable infusion pumps attached to a catheter placed in the artery. Some striking remissions using this technique have been observed, although they usually have been of short duration. It appears logical to assume that this manner of administering chemotherapeutic agents would increase their effectiveness because of the greater concen-

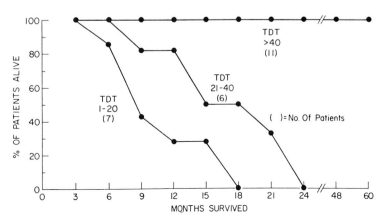

Fig. 9-18. Survival curves of 24 untreated patients following onset of pulmonary metastases. (*From W. L. Joseph et al., J Thorac Cardiovasc Surg, 61:23, 1971.*)

trations obtainable. However, it is not known at the present time whether intraarterial infusion produces significantly greater response than the usual intravenous administration.

One ingenious method of administering increased concentrations of chemotherapeutic drugs involves the isolated perfusion technique. The artery and veins supplying the tumor-bearing extremity are cannulated and isolated from the systemic circulation by connection to a pump-oxygenator. The tumor is then perfused for up to 90 minutes with oxygenated blood containing cancerocidal drugs in amounts that would be prohibitively poisonous if perfused through the general circulation.

Recently it has been found that heating the blood with a heat exchanger similar to that used for cardiopulmonary bypass appears to increase the effectiveness of the chemotherapeutic drugs. Hyperthermic perfusion with chemotherapeutic agents may be worthwhile in treating satellite or intransient metastasis from malignant melanoma and primary or recurrent sarcomas of the extremities. Some long-term survivors with malignant melanoma treated by this technique have been reported. Furthermore, Stehlin reports that hyperthermic perfusion of chemotherapeutic drugs, when combined with radiation therapy, may decrease the necessity of amputation in some primary or recurrent sarcomas which are bordering on vital structures of the extremity.

Despite a long experience with intraarterial infusion and regional perfusion for the administration of chemotherapeutic drugs, there is still no general agreement about their usefulness. Many chemotherapists believe systemic administration of drugs would be equally effective.

PALLIATIVE SURGERY. Surgical procedures are sometimes indicated to relieve symptoms, to reduce the severity of the patient's illness, or to prolong a useful comfortable life without attempting to cure the patient. Such surgery is justified to relieve pain, hemorrhage, obstruction, or infection when it can be done without great risk to the patient, and when it improves the quality of life even if it does not prolong it. Surgery that only prolongs a miserable existence certainly does not benefit the patient.

Some examples of palliative surgical procedures are (1) colostomy, enteroenterostomy, or gastrojejunostomy to relieve obstruction; (2) chordotomy to control pain; (3) cystectomy for infected, bleeding tumors of the bladder; (4) amputations for painful infected tumors in the extremities; (5) simple mastectomy for carcinoma of the breast, even in the presence of distant metastases, when the primary tumor is infected, large, ulcerated, and locally resectable; and (6) colon resection in the presence of hepatic metastases.

Radiation Therapy

Radiation therapy, like surgery, can cure only localized cancer. The palliative effects of radiation therapy in treating symptoms of metastatic or recurrent cancer are well recognized. In fact, 40 percent of all cancer patients will receive radiation therapy at some time in the course of their disease. Irradiation can destroy neoplastic tissue with a minimum of damage to normal tissues surrounding the tumor and thus, when successful, leads to good functional and cosmetic results. Some neoplasms are best treated by this method, whereas other neoplasms can be managed equally well with surgery. Radiation therapy and surgery need not be competitive if specialists in each of the two areas understand the indications and limitations of each form of treatment. Often the two modalities can be used in combination to increase the cure rates for certain types of neoplasms.

MECHANISM OF ACTION. Regardless of the primary source of radiation energy, radiation penetrates and collides with the atoms in tissue, releasing energy that causes the ionization of water in cells. The hydroxy and peroxide radicals thus formed cause DNA and chromosome breaks in both tumor cells and normal cells. Thus, the mechanism of radiation damage relates to a direct effect on certain vital substrates within living cells. Although such effects occur in both normal and neoplastic cells, there are quantitative differences in toxicity, apparently related primarily to a more adequate mechanism for cellular repair in the normal cells, which can be translated into a useful therapeutic effect.

The cellular effects of radiation are both immediate and delayed. Changes in the appearance and behavior of individual cells are observed within a few minutes of exposure, whereas gross changes in irradiated tissue may not appear until weeks, months, or even years after exposure. Microscopic changes occur in both the cytoplasm and nucleus of the cell. Vacuoles often appear in the cytoplasm of the cell, which then becomes swollen. Nuclear chromatin may clump and shrink. The chromosomes may appear abnormal in the cell undergoing mitosis at the time of radiation exposure. Although the radiation may not cause immediate cell death, the cell may be unable to divide again.

The *rad* is the unit of measurement used to express the amount of radiation absorbed. With unidirectional radiation therapy, the dose varies throughout the depth of the radiation field and is dependent upon the energy of the radiation source (Fig. 9-19). Since a tumor is three dimensional, the dose varies across the tumor volume. There is a maximum and a minimum tumor dose. Without further qualification, a dose of 4,500 rads refers to the average tumor dose within the whole field.

By using various techniques such as multiple ports, rotational fields, lead shielding, and others, it is often possible to deliver larger doses of radiation to the tumor-bearing area than to the surrounding tissue.

Usually, patients tolerate radiation therapy much better when the total dose is fractionated over a number of days or when it is split into two treatment courses, allowing for a rest period between. The margin of safety between destruction of tumor and damage to surrounding tissue also is increased by these techniques.

Rets express the relation between the total dose delivered, the number of fractions, and the time it took to deliver the dose. The ret concept is a method of comparing dissimilar treatment schedules by reducing them to a similar unit of measurement.

There are three basic types of radiation: *alpha particles, beta, or electron, particles,* and *electromagnetic rays,* such

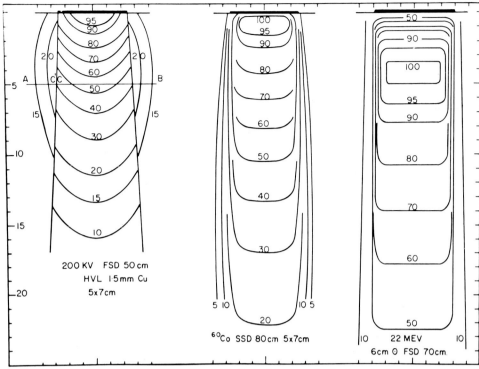

Fig. 9-19. Typical isodose distributions for low-energy (200 kv), high-energy (⁶⁰Co), and very high energy (22 Mev) radiation. The average patient is 20 cm thick. When treating a tumor situated midway through the patient, or at 10 cm, each of the three sources would deliver a different percentage of the maximum dose at that point—25 percent with 200 kv, 52 percent with ⁶⁰Co, and 83 percent with 22 Mev.

as gamma rays and x-rays. Their qualitative effects upon tissue are similar. However, there is great variation in the distance to which these rays can penetrate tissues. Alpha particles penetrate only a few microns and are stopped by the epidermis. Beta particles penetrate tissue in proportion to their energy and in inverse proportion to the density of the tissue, but they do not usually penetrate tissues for more than a few millimeters. Gamma rays can penetrate several centimeters of metal, depending upon the energy and the distance from the target source. The penetration of x-rays depends upon the voltage of the machine used to produce the radiation and the distance from the source. Supervoltage machines producing 1,000 to 50,000 kv of energy are available. Such radiation can penetrate to greater depth and will cause less ionization, hence less skin damage, as it passes through the skin than the 250-kv machines used routinely in the past.

The relative biologic effectiveness of x-rays, gamma rays, and beta rays are approximately equal, although neutrons and alpha rays are ten to twenty times as effective, respectively. Therefore, it is possible that new types of neutron radiation may eventually prove very useful in reaching those deep-seated tumors which are relatively insensitive to the present forms of radiation treatment.

RADIOSENSITIVITY VERSUS RADIOCURABILITY OF TU- MORS. Radiosensitivity and radiocurability are *not* synonymous terms. A tumor may be radiosensitive but not radiocurable, because of recurrence developing either locally or at a distant site. For instance, very few patients with Ewing's sarcoma, a very radiosensitive tumor, can be cured with radiation therapy, because they develop distant metastases. Some tumors, such as undifferentiated soft

tissue sarcomas, initially may respond very rapidly, only to recur locally several months later. Other tumors, such as epidermoid carcinoma of the cervix or adenocarcinoma of the uterus, do not disappear immediately, but hysterectomy several months later may reveal no evidence of tumor, and the patient may be cured.

Radiocurability depends upon radiosensitivity; however, tumors differ in their response to radiation therapy, as shown in Table 9-10. In general, tumor cells which are undifferentiated or in active mitosis are more sensitive to radiation. Furthermore, radiosensitivity of malignant tumors usually parallels the radiosensitivity of their cell of origin. Hemopoietic cells, epidermoid cells, lymphocytes, germ cells of the gonads, and the lining epithelium of the alimentary tract are most sensitive to radiation. Usually tumors derived from these cells are also radiosensitive. However, there are exceptions, such as adenocarcinoma of the stomach and gonads. Tumor volume, tumor oxygenation, and the histology of the tumor are of equal importance in determining radiosensitivity and radiocurability.

COMPLICATIONS OF RADIATION THERAPY. Although usually associated with no immediate mortality, the morbidity, complications, and long-term effects of radiation therapy may be considerable. The complications of radiation therapy, itself, may limit the dose and the rate of

Table 9-10. RELATIVE RADIOSENSITIVITY OF
MALIGNANT TUMORS

(Listed in order of decreasing radiosensitivity)

Malignant tumors arising from hemopoietic organs (lympho-
    sarcoma, myeloma)
Hodgkin's disease
Seminomas and dysgerminomas
Ewing's sarcoma of the bone
Basal cell carcinomas of the skin
Epidermoid carcinomas arising by metaplasia from columnar
    epithelium
Epidermoid carcinomas of the mucous membranes, mucocutaneous
    junctions, and skin
Adenocarcinomas of the endometrium, breast, gastrointestinal
    system, and endocrine glands.
Soft tissue sarcomas
Chondrosarcomas
Neurogenic sarcomas
Osteosarcomas
Malignant melanomas

SOURCE: From L. V. Ackerman and J. A. del Regato, "Cancer:
Diagnosis, Treatment, and Prognosis," 4th ed., The C. V. Mosby
Company, St. Louis, 1970.

delivery. Both systemic and local complications of radiation therapy may be seen, as well as the less frequent
genetic and carcinogenic effects. The acute and chronic
local effects of radiation on different organs are outlined
in Table 9-11. The acute changes are caused by edema and
inflammation, while the chronic changes are caused by
scarring and fibrosis. Megavoltage radiation has largely
obviated the skin changes seen in the past with lower-
voltage radiation.

Many patients undergoing radiation therapy temporarily
develop systemic symptoms associated with malaise, nausea, vomiting, weakness, and weight loss. These symptoms
are directly related to dose, volume, and rate of delivery,
and to type of tissue treated. Radiation sickness usually
can be prevented, and the nausea and vomiting can be
successfully treated with antiemetics such as Compazine.

The genetic and carcinogenic effects of radiation therapy

are seen less frequently as these problems have become
better understood. The genetic effects of radiation expressed as mutations and congenital abnormalities have
been demonstrated in lower animals, but not conclusively
in human beings. The late carcinogenic effects of radiation
are manifested by lung tumors in uranium miners, skin
cancer in radiologists, bone tumors in clock dial painters,
leukemia in radiologists and atomic bomb survivors, and
thyroid cancer in patients who have had radiation in childhood for an enlarged thymus.

INDICATIONS FOR RADIATION THERAPY. A variety of
localized neoplasms can be cured with radiation therapy.
Curative radiation therapy usually requires doses of 4,500
to 6,000 rads, delivered over 4 to 6 weeks. As most patients
are unable to work during this time, the total time the
patient is incapacitated is similar for both radiation therapy and surgery. The doses and complications for curative
radiation therapy are significantly higher than those for
palliative radiation therapy. To avoid unnecessary complications, it is vital that the stage of the tumor be carefully
established in order to assure that the disease is still localized and therefore curable by radiation therapy. The best
example of this is Hodgkin's disease, which is treated by
aggressive and curative radiation therapy for Stages I, II,
and possibly III without organ involvement other than the
spleen. If other organs are involved, then systemic chemotherapy is indicated.

When the cure rate for a particular tumor appears equal
by either radiation therapy or surgery, a variety of other
factors must be considered by the surgical oncologist before making a decision on treatment. These include age,
operative risk, cosmetic and functional deformity, and
logistical problems such as distance and time. Squamous
cell and basal cell carcinomas of the skin are good examples. Many of these tumors can be cured with a simple
and quick diagnostic biopsy as an outpatient procedure.
However, if these tumors are located in areas where surgery would lead to extensive cosmetic deformity, such as
the nose or eyelid, then radiation therapy is usually the
treatment of choice.

Some useful generalizations regarding choice between
radiation therapy and surgery can be made. Usually sur-

Table 9-11. LOCAL EFFECTS OF RADIATION

Organ	Acute changes	Chronic changes
Skin	Wet or dry epidermitis	Running
	Radiodermatitis	Ulceration
	Epilation	
Gastrointestinal tract	Edema, ulceration, infection, diar-rhea, hepatitis	Stricture, ulceration, and per-foration
Kidney		Nephritis, renal insufficiency
Bladder	Dysuria	Ulceration
Gonads	Sterility	Atrophy, menopause
Hemopoietic tissue	Lymphopenia	Pancytopenia
Bone	Cessation of epiphyseal growth	Necrosis
Lung	Pneumonitis	Pulmonary fibrosis
Heart	Acute pericarditis, myocarditis	Chronic pericarditis, myocarditis
Eye	Conjunctivitis	Cataracts
Nervous system	Cerebral edema	Radiation myelitis

gery, rather than radiation therapy, should be used to treat radiation-induced (actinic) skin cancer in people with prolonged exposure to the sun. Radiation therapy may be the preferred treatment for recurrent carcinomas when the primary therapy was surgery, and vice versa. However, surgery is more likely to salvage a cure after a radiation failure, especially in the head and neck area.

Neoplasms in which radiation therapy is preferred to surgical therapy are lymphomas, Ewing's sarcoma, some malignant thymomas, locally unresectable carcinoma of the breast, oat cell carcinoma of the lung, locally advanced carcinoma of the prostate, and carcinomas of the skin (basal or epidermoid) where surgery would lead to extensive cosmetic deformity. Table 9-12 compares the effectiveness of radiation therapy to surgery in the treatment of various types of neoplasms.

Palliative Radiation Therapy. Radiation therapy can relieve symptoms such as pain, hemorrhage, intractable cough, inability to swallow, intestinal obstruction from tumor, edema such as that produced by lung carcinomas with an associated superior vena cava syndrome, pathologic fractures, spinal cord compression, and varying degrees of paralysis secondary to brain metastases from a number of different tumors. In the presence of diffuse metastases, aggressive radiation therapy should not be given except for specific indications, because patients may be made more uncomfortable by the side effects of the radiation itself. An exception would be palliative radiation of metastases in weight-bearing bones such as the neck of the femur; this can prevent pathologic fractures and unnecessary hospitalization.

Even when a tumor is considered to be radioresistant, a trial of radiation therapy will sometimes result in unexpected palliation with regression or stabilization of the tumor. For instance, soft tissue sarcomas are not considered by many to be very radiosensitive or radiocurable. Yet, radiation therapy for palliation of soft tissue sarcomas often produces an objective response and relief of symptoms. However, radiation therapy should not be used for radioresistant tumors such as melanoma and osteogenic sarcoma unless it is clearly the best form of therapy or other methods of therapy are no longer available.

Combined Radiation Therapy and Surgery. Radiation therapy is a logical adjunct to surgery for treating many *locally advanced neoplasms.* Table 9-13 lists the tumors for which preoperative or postoperative radiation therapy has improved the cure rate or decreased the local recurrence rate.

Preoperative Radiation Therapy. Radiation therapy can sometimes convert an inoperable tumor into an operable one by decreasing both the size of the tumor and its fixation to surrounding tissues. In this manner, radiation therapy is a logical adjunct to surgery, because it is known that the cells at the periphery of a tumor are more radiosensitive because of their more rapid rate of growth and the availability of adequate oxygen. In contrast, tumor cells in the center of the tumor are often hypoxic and more slowly dividing, which makes them less sensitive to radiation therapy.

Preoperative radiation therapy may increase the cure

Table 9-12. COMPARISON OF RADIATION THERAPY AND SURGERY IN TREATMENT OF MALIGNANT TUMORS

A. Cure rate higher with radiation therapy
  1. Lymphomas and Hodgkin's disease
  2. Ewing's sarcoma
  3. Certain malignant thymomas
  4. Carcinoma of the breast (locally unresectable)
  5. Certain basal and epidermoid carcinoma of the skin where surgery would lead to extensive cosmetic deformity
  6. Oat cell carcinoma of the lung
  7. Carcinoma of prostate (locally advanced)
B. Cure rate higher with surgery
  1. Carcinoma
    a. Gastrointestinal tract [esophagus (distal one-third), stomach, pancreas, liver and biliary ducts, colon and rectum]
    b. Lung
    c. Breast (localized to breast and axilla)
    d. Urinary tract [kidney, renal pelvis, ureter, bladder, and prostate (early)]
    e. Genital tract (ovary, testis, penis, vulva, vagina, uterus, in situ cervix)
    f. Thyroid and parathyroid glands
    g. Salivary glands
    h. Adrenal gland
    i. Carcinoma from any site with lymph node metastases (not bulky or mixed)
  2. Neuroblastoma
  3. Sarcomas (skeletal and soft tissue)
  4. Melanoma
  5. Cancer of the brain and spinal cord
C. Cure rate of radiation therapy and surgery approximately equal (choice depends on stage, size of tumor, and other factors—see text).
  1. Epidermoid carcinoma
    a. Skin
    b. Cervix
    c. Anus
    d. Lip
    e. Oral pharynx (tongue, floor of mouth, tonsil, gingiva)
    f. Nasopharynx and paranasal sinuses
    g. Hypopharynx
    h. Larynx
    i. Esophagus, upper two-thirds (low cure rate)

rate or decrease the rate of local recurrence from tumor cells disseminated into the wound, lymphatics, or body cavities during surgery, either by killing the cells or by destroying their ability to multiply. In experienced hands, preoperative radiation therapy usually can be given with little increased morbidity or mortality. Its usefulness needs to be further evaluated for a number of neoplasms, such as carcinomas of the breast, pancreas, stomach, and rectum.

Preoperative radiation is not justified when a cancer is small and freely movable, and can be removed with a wide margin of normal tissue. With these tumors there is both a high cure rate and a very small chance of local recurrence.

Postoperative Radiation Therapy. When the "tumor margin" of normal tissue surrounding the tumor is inadequate or when further surgery is either impossible or unacceptably deforming, postoperative radiation therapy is indicated. However, it should not be given in place of proper

Table 9-13. RADIATION THERAPY AS AN ADJUNCT TO SURGERY (LOCALLY ADVANCED CANCERS)

Preoperative radiation therapy
Cure rate increased with these locally advanced carcinomas:
    Larynx
    Laryngopharynx
    Esophagus
    Bladder
    Uterus
    Retinoblastoma
    Paranasal sinuses
    Superior pulmonary sulcus
    Soft tissue sarcomas (liposarcomas)
    Bulky cervical node metastases from epidermoid carcinoma of the head and neck
Local recurrence decreased with these locally advanced carcinomas:
    Rectum
    Endometrium
    Head and neck (epidermoid) with clinically positive lymph nodes
Postoperative radiation therapy
Carcinoma of the lung for mediastinal node metastases
Seminoma (periaortic and iliac node areas)
Medulloblastoma (after biopsy)
Wilms' tumor
Bladder
Ovary (dysgerminoma, granulosa cell, and cystadenocarcinoma)

(adequate) surgery or when further "curative" surgery can be performed.

Postoperative radiation therapy is given routinely for Wilms' tumor, medulloblastoma, seminoma (to treat periaortic and iliac node-bearing areas), and in Stage II cancer of the ovary. For carcinoma of the bladder, both preoperative and postoperative radiation therapy appears to have some benefit in selected cases, though the data are not totally convincing.

Recent evidence suggests that postoperative radiation therapy may be useful in carcinoma of the lung for treating residual mediastinal node metastases. For breast cancer, radiation therapy can be effective in treating local recurrences and bone metastases. However, the routine use of postoperative radiation therapy, even in patients with positive nodes, has not been found to be of value in increasing the cure rate.

Combined Radiation Therapy, Chemotherapy, and Surgery. Combined modality therapy, utilizing radiation therapy and surgery in combination with chemotherapy, appears to be exceedingly effective for childhood neoplasms.

The effectiveness of similar multimodality therapy has not as yet been demonstrated for adult neoplasms. The cure rate for localized retinoblastoma and other sarcomas in children has been increased with radiation therapy and chemotherapy with cyclophosphamide. The cure rate for Wilms' tumor approaches 75 percent if surgery is followed by radiation therapy and chemotherapy with actinomycin, compared to 40 percent with surgery alone. Similarly, embryonal rhabdomyosarcoma responds best to combined radiation therapy, chemotherapy, and surgery.

Chemotherapy

The treatment of cancer with drugs was initiated in 1941 by Huggins and Hodges, with the discovery that estrogens palliated prostatic cancer. Polyfunctional alkylating agents were developed in the later 1940s, as a result of experimental work performed during World War II. Since then there has been a tremendous increase in the number of chemotherapeutic drugs available; at present at least five major classes of drugs, plus an additional group of miscellaneous drugs, are available (Table 9-14). Although full elucidation of this complex field is beyond the scope of this chapter, certain general principles will be described regarding the use of chemotherapy. This section will consider the mechanisms of action of the major classes of chemotherapeutic drugs, the biologic and pharmacologic factors which are important in understanding drug therapy, and guidelines for the use of chemotherapy in patients with nonhematologic malignant conditions.

MECHANISMS OF ACTION. The majority of antineoplastic drugs appear to affect either enzymes, directly, or substrates of enzyme systems. In most cases the effects on enzymes or substrates relate to DNA synthesis or function, apparently by inhibiting cells which are undergoing DNA synthesis. Drugs which act by inhibiting the enzymes of nucleic acid synthesis are called *antimetabolites*, or *structural analogs*. Methotrexate, a structural analog of folinic acid, appears to act as an irreversible inhibitor of the active site of the enzyme dihydrofolate reductase, which is necessary for DNA synthesis. Another commonly used antimetabolite is 5-fluorouracil, which appears to act as a reversible inhibitor of the enzyme thymidylate synthetase necessary for incorporation of thymidine into DNA. This class of compounds acts directly on enzymes as either reversible or irreversible inhibitors, leading to the synthesis of abnormal DNA due to the incorporation of an abnormal building block or to disruption of DNA synthesis due to the lack of an essential building block.

Other major drugs appear to work primarily by affecting substrates. The usual substrate affected is the DNA macromolecule, although some of these agents will interfere with other substrates, such as proteins, and may have other diverse effects. Three major chemical classes of drugs appear to act by affecting specific substrates. The alkylating agents are extremely reactive compounds which can substitute an alkyl group (for example, $R—CH_2—CH_2^+$) for the hydrogen atoms of many organic compounds. The primary compounds affected appear to be the nucleic acids, especially DNA. Such alkylation produces breaks in the DNA molecule and cross linking of the twin strands of DNA, thus interfering with DNA replication and the transcription of RNA. Since these effects are somewhat similar to that seen with ionizing radiation, alkylating agents are sometimes called "radiomimetic." Another group of compounds which appear to work primarily on substrates are the *antibiotics*. These are natural products derived from certain soil fungi. They produce their antineoplastic effect by forming relatively stable complexes with DNA, thereby inhibiting the synthesis of DNA and RNA. The final class of drugs acting primarily on sub-

Table 9-14. DRUGS USED IN TREATMENT OF NONHEMATOLOGIC NEOPLASMS

Drugs	Route of administration	Cell cycle phase specificity*	Acute toxicity†	Principle delayed or cumulative toxicity†
Alkylating agents:		Nonspecific	N & V§	BM§; cyclophosphamide may cause alopecia, hemorrhagic cystitis, jaundice.
Nitrogen mustard	I.V.		N & V	
Chlorambucil	P.O.§		None	
Phenylalanine mustard	P.O., I.V.‡, I.A.‡		None	
Cyclophosphamide	P.O., I.V.		N & V	
Thiotepa	I.V.		None	
Antimetabolites:				
Methotrexate	P.O., I.M., I.V.	Specific	None	BM, stomatitis, hepatitis.
5-Fluorouracil	P.O.‡, I.V.	Nonspecific	N & V	BM, stomatitis, diarrhea, nausea, alopecia.
Hydroxyurea	P.O., I.V.‡	Specific	None	BM.
Cytosine arabinoside*	I.V.	Specific	N & V	BM.
Antibiotics:				
Actinomycin D	I.V.		N & V	BM, alopecia, stomatitis.
Mithramycin	I.V.		None	BM & hemorrhagic diathesis.
Adriamycin‡	I.V.		N & V, fever	BM, cardiac toxicity, stomatitis, alopecia.
Bleomycin	I.V., S.C.		Fever	Skin changes, pulmonary fibrosis.
Vinca alkaloids:				
Vincristine	I.V.	Specific	N & V, rare	Constipation, BM, peripheral neuropathy, alopecia.
Vinblastine				
Steriod hormones				
Adrenal corticoids	P.O., I.V., I.M.	(?) Nonspecific	None	Hypertension, peptic ulcer, diabetes, increased susceptibility to infection.
Androgens	P.O., I.M.	Unknown	None	Fluid retention, masculinization; may cause hypercalcemia in breast cancer.
Estrogens	P.O.	Unknown	N & V, occasional	Fluid retention, uterine bleeding; may cause hypercalcemia in breast cancer.
Progestins	P.O., I.M.	Unknown	None	May cause hypercalcemia in breast cancer.
Miscellaneous				
Nitrosoureas‡	I.V., P.O	Nonspecific	N & V	BM (may be delayed 4–6 weeks), liver dysfunction.
BCNU				
CCNU				
Imidazole	I.V., IA‡	Nonspecific	N & V	BM, hepatotoxicity, fever.
Mitotane (o, p-DDD)	P.O.	Unknown	N & V	Skin eruptions, mental depression, muscle tremors.

*The distinction between a phase-specific and non-phase-specific drug may not be absolute. Some authorities distinguish additional categories or use different names for these categories, but these are not considered in this chapter since their clinical relevance remains to be defined.

†See manufacturer's package inserts for usual doses and for additional toxicity data.

‡Experimental drug or route of administration; not yet approved by the Federal Drug Administration or Division of Biological Standards; it may be available from the Cancer Chemotherapy National Service Center, Bethesda, Maryland.

§N & V = nausea and vomiting; BM = bone marrow depression; P.O. = orally (per os); I.A. = intraarterial.

strates is the *vinca alkaloids*. Although their total mechanism of action may not be completely defined, it is apparent that they can bind to microtubular proteins necessary for cell division. These proteins form the spindle apparatus which allows the chromosomes to separate to either end of the dividing cell; the vinca alkaloids appear to be able to dissolve this protein, leading to death of the cell during mitosis.

Other than these two known major mechanisms of drug action, the mechanisms of action for many drugs useful in the treatment of cancer are unknown. In some cases there may be combinations of activities, particularly for those steroid hormones which are active in treating cancer.

Table 9-14 lists representative examples of each group

along with selected characteristics of their clinical importance.

BIOLOGIC AND PHARMACOLOGIC FACTORS IN CANCER THERAPY. A major theme in pharmacology has been the study of variations in drug absorption, distribution, metabolism, and excretion as related to a stable, invariant biologic receptor. In cancer chemotherapy, however, the biologic receptor, the cancer cell, is a variable and fluctuating target. Thus, the kinetics of tumor growth must be given as much attention as the kinetics of drug absorption or metabolism when considering cancer chemotherapy. Specifically, four general principles of tumor biology relevant to treatment appear to be extremely important. These include an understanding of (1) antineoplastic drug action as a function of the cell cycle, (2) tumor cell population growth, (3) the log–cell kill hypothesis, and (4) the critical role of drug scheduling in optimizing therapy.

Drug Action and the Cell Cycle. The life cycle of all cells, both normal and neoplastic, starts with mitosis, or cell division. This is followed by either differentiation or a series of biochemically distinct phases known, in sequence, as G_1 (the first "gap" phase), S phase (DNA synthesis), G_2 (second "gap" phase), and mitosis (Fig. 9-20). Although these events are similar in neoplastic and normal cells, there appear to be some quantitative differences in the duration of the cycle and the sensitivity of cells to drugs during various phases of the cell cycle. Because of these differences, it has become apparent that one must differentiate between drugs which kill cells only during specific phases of the cycle (*phase-specific*), and drugs which kill cells during all or most phases of the cell cycle (*phase-nonspecific*). The distinction between a phase-specific and phase-nonspecific drug may not be absolute. Some authorities distinguish additional categories or use different names for these categories. In particular, some workers separate the phase-nonspecific drugs into an additional two categories: *cycle-specific* and *non-cycle-specific*. For this discussion, drugs which can affect multiple phases of the cell or which appear to be effective against nondividing cells are grouped together under the term *phase-nonspecific*, since the clinical usefulness of this group appears to be correlated with their lack of phase specificity.

Gompertz and Cell Population Growth. The human organism consists of communities of cells, many of which are capable of self-renewal through cell division. Generally these renewable populations grow rapidly when they are small in number and slowly when they are large. Thus, the fetus grows rapidly, but the adult organism remains constant in size, thanks to a balance between cell production and cell loss. This relation between size and growth rate may be expressed quantitatively in either of two ways: (1) as a function of volume doubling times (time for any given number of cells to double in number) or (2) as a function of the growth fraction (that fraction of cells un-

dergoing division at any one time). Figure 9-21 presents a logarithmic plot of human fetal and childhood growth against time and includes specific data on the volume doubling times during growth. Growth in the early years is clearly exponential with a high growth fraction and very short volume doubling times. As time passes, the doubling time lengthens and the growth fraction decreases. The general slope of this curve can be expressed mathematically as an exponentially decreasing function. The specific equation describing this relationship was originally derived by the eighteenth-century mathematician Gompertz; therefore, biologic growth that conforms to this pattern is referred to as *Gompertzian growth*. Interestingly, evidence that not only normal cell growth but neoplastic cell growth follows a Gompertzian pattern is increasing. At least 18 different animal tumors conform to a Gompertzian growth curve, and Sullivan and Salmon have recent, preliminary evidence suggesting that human myeloma follows a Gompertzian growth pattern.

The Log–Cell Kill Hypothesis. Antineoplastic drugs are incapable of killing all cancer cells at any given exposure; rather, they will kill a variable fraction of cells from a very few up to a maximum of 99.99 percent. The fractional cell kill observed can usually be graphed as a line with a negative exponential slope, and so experimental chemotherapeutic data is usually expressed in logarithmic terms. Since the body burden of tumor cells in man with an advanced malignant tumor may be greater than 10^{12} cells, and since the best one can hope for with a single maximal exposure of tumor cells to a drug is 2 log cell kill, it is apparent that treatment must be repeated many times in order to achieve even partial control. Theoretically, this hypothesis also suggests that chemotherapeutic drugs may not be capable of totally eradicating any given population of tumor cells. There is good evidence that immunotherapy does not face this restriction, since it can completely eradicate small numbers of tumor cells; however, it may be totally ineffective against larger tumor cell masses (greater than 0.1 mg of tumor in most model systems).

DRUG SCHEDULING AND COMBINATION THERAPY. Studies with experimental animal tumors have conclusively demonstrated the critical importance of drug scheduling in therapy. Cytosine arabinoside, an antimetabolite which kills only cells in S phase, must be given frequently in order to assure contact with cancer cells during this critical period. When this drug is so employed, it is possible to "cure" some forms of murine leukemia, whereas maximally tolerated doses of the drug given at less frequent intervals fail to prolong survival. On the other hand, cyclophosphamide (Cytoxan), which is phase-nonspecific, achieves optimal suppression of most experimental neoplasms when given on an intermittent schedule.

A second factor related to drug scheduling is the growth status of any given tumor. In general, solid tumors with a large tumor mass will be growing slowly, and will have a small growth fraction (less than 10 percent) and a prolonged tumor volume doubling time. Since relatively few of these cells are dividing, these tumors are generally resistant to phase-specific drugs. Thus, the usual treatment for advanced nonhematologic tumors has been with

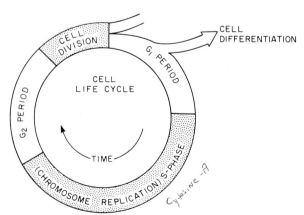

Fig. 9-20. Schematic diagram of the cell life cycle. G_1 is the first "gap" period, and G_2 is the second "gap" period. (*From R. Baserga (ed.), "The Cell Cycle and Cancer," Marcel Dekker, Inc., New York, 1971.*)

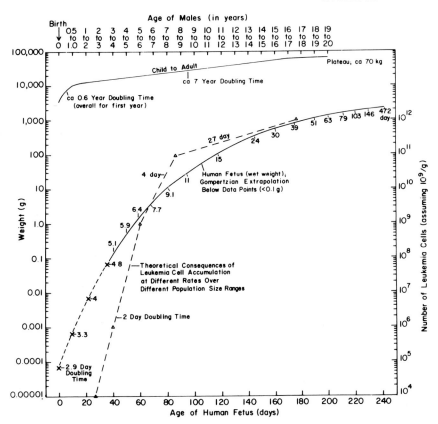

Fig. 9-21. Human fetal and childhood growth as a Gompertzian process, and the theoretic consequences of accumulation of leukemic cells at different rates over varying population ranges. (*From H. E. Skipper and S. Perry, Cancer Res, 30:1883, 1970.*)

phase-nonspecific drugs, such as the alkylating agents or 5-fluorouracil. However, successful treatment with such phase-nonspecific drugs may render the tumor more susceptible to phase-specific drugs, by converting the tumor from one with a low growth fraction with few of the cells in S phase to one with a higher growth fraction with many cells in S phase. Good experimental data exist supporting this concept. Schabel has shown that a hamster plasmacytoma, which grows with Gompertzian kinetics, can be "cured" with cyclophosphamide therapy when followed by cytosine arabinoside therapy. When either drug is used alone or in the reverse sequence, "cures" were not seen. These results are consistent with tumor conversion, i.e., by changing an insensitive tumor with a low growth fraction and few cells in S phase to one with a higher growth fraction and many cells in S phase and therefore sensitive to the phase-specific drug cytosine arabinoside.

Theoretic Model for Combination Chemotherapy. The practical application of these concepts in man remains to be accomplished, but studies are in progress. One approach (Fig. 9-22) is proposed by Schabel. The vertical axis gives the number of viable tumor cells in a patient, on a log scale, versus arbitrary time units on the horizontal axis. At the initial tumor mass of 100 Gm, a likely growth fraction of less than 10 percent can be predicted. The class of drug to be used initially will be phase-nonspecific because of the low growth fraction. A 2 log cell kill with such drugs is possible in many types of tumors. During the recovery time only those viable tumor cells that are

in the cell division cycle will repopulate the tumor. A phase-specific drug might be capable of suppressing this process by a selective effect on dividing cells, although doses and scheduling would have to be carefully chosen to minimize toxicity to the vital normal cells of the patient. Alternating courses of the phase-nonspecific and phase-specific agents, provided cellular resistance or excessive host toxicity does not intervene, would be expected to result in progressively more successful killing of tumor cells. This prediction (Fig. 9-22*E* and *G*) relates to the decreasing tumor cell mass and the associated increase in tumor cell growth fraction. Specifically, as the tumor cell mass becomes smaller, the percentage of cells in S phase or mitosis will be greater, leading to increased cell killing by drugs specific for such phases. Finally, "cure" may be possible with continued chemotherapy, or possibly by appropriate immunotherapy.

CHEMOTHERAPY AS AN ADJUVANT TO CANCER SURGERY. The proved ineffectiveness of surgical resection alone for many types of neoplasms has led many investigators to the use of cancer chemotherapeutic agents as adjunctive treatment. It was postulated that these agents might control microscopic foci of cancer already disseminated in the body. Controlled clinical trials have been carried out to determine the effectiveness of single chemotherapeutic agents when combined with surgical resection for carcinomas of the breast, lung, stomach, and colon. No significant benefits have been demonstrated thus far. However, the chemotherapeutic agents chosen for these

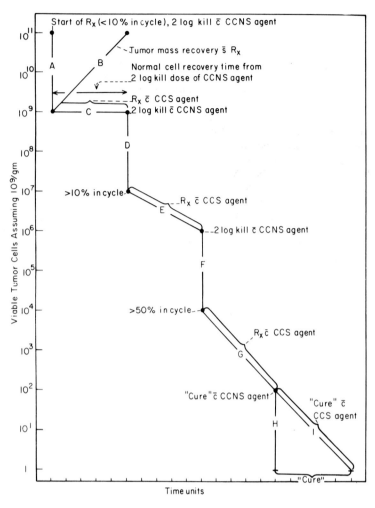

Fig. 9-22. Idealized approach to "curative" therapy of advanced tumors using a phase-nonspecific (CCNS) agent (for example, an alkylating agent) followed by a phase-specific (CCS) agent (for example, certain antimetabolites) in repeated courses. (*From F. M. Schabel, Jr., Cancer Res, 29:2384, 1969.*)

studies, their dosage, and the duration of administration may not have been optimal for the desired result. It is likely that future applications of this concept using newer chemotherapeutic agents in combination for prolonged periods of time may well result in improved survival for these patients. This approach may be further enhanced by advances in immunotherapy and radiation therapy.

CLINICAL PHARMACOLOGY. In addition to the principles relating to tumor biology described above, numerous pharmacologic principles must be considered in cancer chemotherapy. The first such consideration relates to the route of administration of a drug or a combination of drugs. A variety of routes can be chosen, such as oral, intravenous, intramuscular, intraarterial, or local application. By using a carefully selected parenteral route of administration, difficulties related to absorption of drug are avoided. It also may be possible to improve the antitumor effect of a given drug. Particularly promising in this regard has been the use of intraarterial administrative drugs, such as when the primary tumor is in the liver or on an extremity. Using a portable infusion pump, drugs can be continuously infused over weeks or months. An extension of this approach has been with isolation-perfusion of an extremity

with high doses of chemotherapy. As newer drugs are developed, particularly drugs with very short half-life periods, it is likely that the choice of the route of administration will become increasingly important.

A second consideration relates to transport mechanisms for the drug in question. If the drug is transported on serum proteins, it is possible that other drugs may alter significantly the proportion of the bound and free anticancer drug. An example of this is the ability of salicylates to displace methotrexate from its binding site on albumin. In this setting, high doses of salicylates may result in augmented host toxicity from methotrexate.

Another consideration is the possible effect of drug interactions when drugs are given in combinations. One well-established drug interaction involves allopurinol, a xanthine oxidase inhibitor, when it is used with 6-mercaptopurine (6-MP). Since degradation of 6-MP is catalyzed by xanthine oxidase, the use of allopurinol along with full doses of 6-MP has been shown in the past to be deleterious. Normal function of organs important in drug metabolism or degradation may be critical to the biologic fate of a drug. For example, serious liver disease may increase the toxicity of drugs which are cleared by that route, such as vincristine. Severe neurotoxicity has been observed in patients with concomitant liver disease when given otherwise clinically well-tolerated doses of vincristine.

The route of excretion of a drug may be critical. Methotrexate is primarily excreted by the kidney, and even modest elevation of the BUN (blood urea nitrogen) may be associated with major hematologic toxicity from the use of relatively low doses of methotrexate. For this reason the status of the kidneys must be observed very closely in all patients receiving methotrexate therapy. In fact, it is wise to observe renal function in all patients receiving cancer chemotherapeutic drugs, since nearly all of them have some extent of excretion by the renal route. In addition, it is not unusual for a brisk response to chemotherapy to result in elaboration of large amounts of uric acid, from the breakdown of the nucleic acids of the destroyed cancer cells. Uric acid nephropathy may result. Pretreatment with allopurinol may prevent this complication.

A final factor relates to the ability of a given drug to enter the cancer cell: many drugs require direct access to a specific biochemical pathway within the cell, and failure to gain entry will be associated with drug resistance. To some extent this effect may be overcome by giving very large doses of the drug, but the inability of the drug to gain access to the cell generally precludes any cytotoxicity. In some cases this mechanism has been studied carefully. In the case of some alkylating agents, particularly nitrogen mustard and chlorambucil, it appears that drug uptake is coupled with choline transport into the cell. It is possible that future work relating to these factors may be capable of improving the therapeutic/toxic ratio for such drugs by influencing factors of drug uptake.

Ultimately, all factors which might alter either the concentration of the critical drug at its primary site of action or the duration of time available for such activity should be considered in the use of drugs. This may be expressed as a function of concentration times time, and because of its importance it is commonly referred to as the $C \times T$ function.

GUIDELINES FOR THE USE OF CHEMOTHERAPY IN PATIENTS WITH NONHEMATOLOGIC MALIGNANT TUMORS. The initial major question a physician must ask himself when considering chemotherapy for any patient with a neoplasm is whether benefit will result with tolerable toxicity. The physician must have all the facts regarding the patient, including the type, extent, and grade of the malignant tumor, its expected natural history, the results of current therapy, and the psychologic makeup of the patient. In addition, he must consider the following three principles:

1. The patient should have a histologic diagnosis of a malignant disease that is known to respond in a reasonable percentage of cases in a manner beneficial to the patient. Table 9-15 outlines the current status of cancer chemotherapy for a variety

Table 9-15. CURRENT STATUS OF CANCER CHEMOTHERAPY FOR NONHEMATOLOGIC NEOPLASMS

Disease	Agent	Benefit
Highly responsive neoplasms:		
Trophoblastic tumors	Methotrexate, actinomycin L, alkylating agents, vinca alkaloids	80% response with permanent regression
Carcinoma of prostate	Estrogens	80% response; prolonged survival
Wilms' tumor	Actinomycin D,	80% 2-year survival with combined
Neuroblastoma	Vincristine	surgery, radiation therapy, and chemotherapy
Carcinoma of breast	Estrogens, androgens, 5-fluorouracil, alkylating agents, combination chemotherapy	25–50% response; prolonged survival for responders
Moderately responsive neoplasms:		
Carcinoma of bowel and stomach	5-Fluorouracil	Clinical improvement in 15–25%
Carcinoma of ovary	Alkylating agents	Clinical improvement in 30–50%
Testicular carcinoma, germinal cell tumors	Actinomycin D, vinca alkaloids, methotrexate, alkylating agents, mithramycin	Clinical improvement in approximately 30%
Adrenal carcinoma	o, p′-DDD	Occasional clinical improvement, sometimes prolonged
Carcinoma of endometrium	Progestins	Clinical improvement in 25%
Minimally responsive neoplasms:		
Hepatic, pancreatic tumors	5-Fluorouracil	10% objective response
Carcinoma of cervix	Alkylating agents	5% objective response
Sarcomas of bone and soft tissue	Actinomycin D, vinca alkaloids, alkylating agents	5% objective response
Lung cancer	Alkylating agents	10% objective response
Melanoma	Imidazole carboxamide (experimental drug	20% objective response but duration of response usually short

SOURCE: Modified and updated from M. J. Cline, "Cancer Chemotherapy," pp. 8, 9, W. B. Saunders Company, Philadelphia, 1971.

of nonhematologic neoplasms. Brief comments on specific drug-sensitive neoplasms will be presented subsequently. In general, patients in whom disease usually or often responds to chemotherapy should receive drug treatment, unless these is a specific contraindication. Such therapy would be questionable for those patients with a tumor known to be minimally inhibited by commercially available drugs. Experimental therapy may be warranted for these patients.

2. It is absolutely essential that there be adequate facilities to monitor the potential toxicity outlined in Table 9-14, and a physician should not initiate therapy unless he is adequately trained in the use of drugs and committed to monitoring the patient. Chemotherapy is generally contraindicated for patients with nonhematologic malignant conditions if they have major bleeding or infection, although patients with leukemia and, in some cases, lymphomas may require treatment even during such episodes in order to control life-threatening bleeding or infection. Patients with major dysfunction of an organ system particularly susceptible to the toxicity of a cancer chemotherapeutic drug must be followed carefully and may be more suitably treated with an alternative drug. An example of this latter situation would be a patient with a severe neuromyopathy, who might be better treated with drugs other than vinca alkaloids, as these may exacerbate the condition. Patients in whom a rapid response to therapy is possible or who have preexisting renal disease should be treated with allopurinol to prevent the complication of uric acid nephropathy. Finally, patients who are under active chemotherapy and develop severe toxicity may require aggressive support with platelets, red blood cells, or in some cases, white blood cells for control of infection.

3. Cancer chemotherapeutic drugs are toxic. In order to minimize unwarranted toxicity it is essential that patients have at least one major parameter which can be closely followed to assess the response to therapy. Ideally, several parameters of tumor response should be followed; some factors which can be considered are described in more detail in Table 9-16.

Table 9-16. CRITERIA FOR RESPONSES IN PATIENTS WITH SOLID TUMORS

Tumor size	Palpation and measurement with calipers. Radiologic measurement. Radioisotope scans. Ultrasound.*
Tumor products	Quantitative level of chorionic gonadotropin (choriocarcinoma and certain testicular tumors). Quantitative level of carcinoembryonic antigen (CEA) in bowel cancer.* Quantitative level of α-fetoprotein in hepatoma.* Serum or urine paraproteins in myeloma Urinary adrenal hormone (adrenal carcinoma treated with o,p'-DDD).
Improvement in symptoms or sign of tumor	Improvement in hypercalcemia (particularly with carcinoma involving bone). Improvement in obstruction due to tumor (such as bowel obstruction or obstructed ureter). Disappearance of effusions from tumors involving pleura, peritoneum, or obstructing lymphatics. Subjective symptoms are important to patient but are generally poor indicators of antitumor response.

*Under experimental study to define usefulness as indicator response.

Some suggestions for chemotherapy, based on current therapeutic research, can be found in Table 9-15 and in the following section illustrating selected neoplasms. Sometimes the package inserts included with each drug can be a useful source of information especially in regard to questions of toxicity. However, they may not give up-to-date information regarding optimal treatment schedules and combinations. Other useful sources of ongoing information include the *Medical Letter on Drugs and Therapeutics,* which periodically publishes information on the choice of therapy in the treatment of cancer (February 2, 1973); the *Washington University Manual of Medical Therapeutics* (revised every 2 years); and the specialty journals of cancer (*Cancer; Cancer Chemotherapy Reports; Cancer Research*).

ILLUSTRATIVE NEOPLASMS HIGHLY RESPONSIVE TO CHEMOTHERAPY. Trophoblastic Tumors of the Uterus.

Metastatic gestational choriocarcinoma is curable in 80 to 90 percent of women using chemotherapeutic drugs alone. The discovery by Li et al. in 1956 that methotrexate could control metastatic disease in women with choriocarcinoma represents a landmark in the history of cancer chemotherapy. Subsequent systematic study of this disease has markedly increased our understanding about cancer and its treatment. Certain points are worthy of special mention.

1. Methotrexate must be started as soon as possible after the diagnosis has been made. This relates to the finding that the best prognosis, with cure rates of 95 to 100 percent, is seen in patients whose disease is treated within 4 months of onset, in whom metastases are limited to the lungs or pelvis, and in whom 24-hour urine quantities of human chorionic gonadotropins are less than 100,000 I.U.

2. Sequential use of other drugs, or combination chemotherapy, should be used if the initial response to chemotherapy is suboptimal. Second-line drugs for this disease include actinomycin D, vincristine, and alkylating agents.

3. Therapy should be continued for 6 months after the chorionic gonadotropin titer has returned to normal. This is even more important than eliminating radiographic evidence of disease, since residual pulmonary lesions may be present despite cure of clinical growths. This is analogous to the residual changes of many nonneoplastic diseases, such as tuberculosis.

Carcinoma of the Prostate. The mainstays of therapy for disseminated cancer of the prostate are orchiectomy and estrogen therapy. These modalities have increased survival of these patients two- to threefold. Many different doses of the most commonly used estrogenic hormone have been employed. However, data from the Veterans Administration Cooperative Research Group have shown up to a 25 percent increased mortality from cardiovascular diseases in a group of patients treated with moderately high doses (5 mg daily) of diethylstilbestrol. A prospective study has since proved that a low dose of 1 mg daily results in good antitumor effects without significant cardiovascular toxicity.

Wilms' Tumor. Improvements in survival for patients with Wilms' tumor have developed steadily in recent years. Whereas this was once considered a hopeless tumor to treat, it is now possible to control the disease for substantial periods of time in 80 percent of children with the disease. This improvement involves the sequential use of optimal surgery, radiation therapy, and chemotherapy with actinomycin D and/or vincristine. A rationale study group is currently trying to resolve the optimal combination of these modalities; however, it is clear that the addition of effective chemotherapy has substantially improved the care of these patients.

Carcinoma of the Breast. Although considerable controversy exists over the optimal therapy for disseminated breast cancer, it is very clear that some patients may receive major benefit from a wide variety of hormonal and nonhormonal chemotherapeutic drugs. Discussions of surgical ablative and hormonal treatment in both pre- and postmenopausal patients appear elsewhere in this textbook, and so the present comments will be restricted to the use of single-agent and combination chemotherapy.

The first nonhormonal drugs proved to be useful in treating advanced breast cancer were the alkylating agents. Of this group, cyclophosphamide has been the most extensively studied and is generally acknowledged at present to be the alkylator of choice for this disease. It can be given in a variety of doses and schedules. Prolonged administration on a daily basis has resulted in a reported overall response rate of 35 percent (from 10 percent to 62 percent). The response rate with intermittent schedules has not been clarified.

The most commonly employed antimetabolite for breast cancer has been 5-fluorouracil. It has been administered in a variety of doses and schedules. The two most commonly employed programs are initial therapy with a 5-day loading course followed by weekly maintenance, or weekly treatment from the very beginning with a dose of 15 mg/kg given as a rapid intravenous injection. Although the optimal program has yet to be defined, preliminary data suggest that the latter program is less toxic. From a review of 1,263 patients with breast cancer treated with 5-fluorouracil, 324 responses were noted, for an overall response rate of 25.7 percent.

A variety of other drugs have been employed for advanced breast cancer including the vinca alkaloids, methotrexate, corticosteroids, and antibiotics. All these are capable of killing breast cancer cells, although response rates are difficult to define because the number of patients reported has been small.

Much recent interest has centered on the use of combined therapy for breast cancer. Following the initial lead of Cooper, many physicians are currently treating advanced breast cancer with combinations of drugs. One combination includes 5-fluorouracil, cyclophosphamide, vincristine, methotrexate, and, sometimes, prednisone. Response rates have varied between 56 and 90 percent; the duration of response may be substantial, although data are presently inadequate to give precise figures for this important parameter.

Immunotherapy

One of the basic problems associated with all forms of cancer therapy is caused by the similarities in the biochemical and subcellular constituents of the cancer and normal cells. Although some cancer cells may have a rapid rate of cell division when compared to normal cells of the same organ, there are other normal cells in the body (e.g., those in the bone marrow and intestinal epithelium) that may grow even more rapidly. Hence, any therapy designed to inhibit the proliferation rate of cancer cells may also inhibit the function of these normal cells. Herein lies the fundamental deficiency of both radiation and chemotherapy. Similarly, cancer surgery often requires the sacrifice of normal tissues and organs to ensure an adequate margin around the cancer cells. In contrast, immunotherapy depends upon basic antigenic differences between neoplastic and normal cells for its therapeutic effect. Because the immune attack is directed only at those cells possessing tumor-specific antigens, while sparing normal cells from damage, this treatment method can achieve a specific tumor cell kill greater than any other known therapeutic modality. At the present time, however, immunotherapy has limited potency.

Immunity against cancer is relative rather than absolute. Host defenses are quite capable of destroying small numbers of tumor cells, 1 to 10 million, but 100 million tumor cells almost always result in progressive tumor growth. Since a neoplasm only 1 cm in diameter contains approximately 1 billion tumor cells, by the time most tumors are clinically detectable, they have already outgrown the patient's immune defenses. Therefore, it is unlikely that immunotherapy alone will ever bolster host offenses sufficiently to reverse tumor growth in patients with advanced disease.

In contrast, immunotherapy is a logical adjunct for the treatment of subclinical microscopic disease following definitive cancer surgery, radiation therapy, or chemotherapy, for the following reasons: (1) Patients who have only small foci of cancer cells remaining after destruction of the major tumor bulk are the most likely to benefit from immunotherapy, because the tumor mass that must be destroyed is smallest at that time. (2) The specificity of the immune response provides a possible therapeutic tool that has selectivity for small numbers of cancer cells not possible with any other therapeutic modality. (3) Patients with disease in earlier stages are more likely to respond to immunotherapeutic maneuvers, since the cancer patient's general immune competence is greatest when the disease is localized and is often impaired after metastasis. (4) Immunotherapy should complement rather than interfere with currently available methods of cancer therapy. However, since both irradiation and chemotherapy are immunosuppressive, the use of immunotherapy in combination with these therapeutic modalities must be carefully controlled. Because these treatment modalities can stimulate immune response when immunization is carried out under special conditions, the results of cancer therapy may improve when the influence of radiation therapy and chemotherapy upon the immune response is better understood.

Numerous attempts at immunotherapy of cancer have been undertaken since the turn of the century. Although an occasional striking regression was obtained, in most cases the results were neither impressive nor consistent, and interest in this treatment modality declined until recently. A rational basis for cancer immunotherapy was provided only during the past 7 years as compelling evidence accumulated indicating the participation of immune responses in human cancer. It was found that cancer patients develop two types of immune response to the antigens of their neoplasms, *humoral antibodies* and *cell-mediated immune reactions.*

The relative importance of these two types of immune responses and their influence upon the host's defense against cancer is somewhat controversial at the present time. Most approaches to immunotherapy do, in fact, stimulate both types of immune response. Three possible approaches to immunotherapy in man will be discussed—active; passive, or adoptive; and nonspecific.

ACTIVE IMMUNOTHERAPY

The greater effectiveness of active immunization over passive immunization in infectious diseases provided a strong stimulus for studies of active immunotherapy against cancer. The rationale for this approach is based upon animal studies demonstrating that a growing tumor does not induce a maximum immune response in the host (Fig. 9-23). In this method of treatment, efforts are made to increase the patient's tumor immunity by altering the tumor-specific antigen in such a way that it becomes more antigenic, or by stimulating the patient's lymphoreticular system with immunologic adjuvants.

Most attempts at immunotherapy in man have involved vaccines composed of whole tumor cells inactivated by a variety of different methods to render the cells incapable of proliferation. These methods have included radiation, mitomycin C treatment, freezing and thawing, or heat treatment. Although such techniques have prevented pro-

gressive tumor growth, they may have inactivated the tumor-specific antigens as well. For example, the same freezing and thawing technique frequently used to prepare human tumor vaccines has often inactivated tumor-specific antigens of carcinogen-induced animal neoplasms.

Studies with animal neoplasms demonstrate that living tumor cells administered intradermally in numbers insufficient for progressive tumor growth generally are the most effective immunogens. The possibility that living tumor cells might result in tumor growth at the inoculation site has inhibited the use of such vaccines in man. However, it would seem that with certain tumors that share common tumor-specific antigens, such as skeletal and soft tissue sarcomas, one patient could be immunized with an allogenic vaccine of living tumor cells from another patient. An immune response could be induced against the foreign HLA transplantation antigens on the tumor cells, causing their rejection. Theoretically this immunization should induce a strong immune response against a common cross-reacting tumor-specific antigen as well.

Repeated attempts have been made to increase the antigenicity of tumor vaccines by modifying the tumor cells in a variety of ways. These have included coupling highly antigenic carrier proteins such as rabbit γ-globulin to the tumor cells, and chemical treatment by agents such as iodoacetate and, more recently, with neuraminidase and concanavalin A. Regression of established tumors has been observed in animals following active immunotherapy with such vaccines.

Many of these experiments have used immunological adjuvants as well, such as bacillus Calmette-Guérin (BCG) vaccine, *Corynebacterium parvum,* and Freund's adjuvant, in an attempt to enhance the host's immune response to the native or modified tumor antigens.

The ideal tumor vaccine in many respects, however, would be one composed of the isolated and purified tumor-specific transplantation antigens from the cell surface. Such vaccines would have the advantages of safety, stability, and ease of administration. Previous experience gained with guinea pig sarcomas from which isolated and partially purified tumor-specific antigen preparations induced good immunity to tumor challenge suggests that success can be anticipated for this approach. However, to date, there has been little progress along these lines with the human tumor-specific transplantation antigen.

In summary, active immunotherapy using vaccines prepared in a variety of ways combined with many different types of immunoadjuvants has been used in clinical trials. It can be demonstrated clearly that such autoimmunization procedures do enhance the patient's immune response to his own tumor (Fig. 9-24). Results to date, however, have not been impressive in patients with advanced disease where active immunization is used alone. Active immunotherapy has great potential when used in combination with other types of cancer therapy, such as surgery, chemotherapy, or radiation therapy. Preliminary experiences by Mathe with leukemia and Morton with melanomas and sarcomas would suggest that this potential will become increasingly evident in the future.

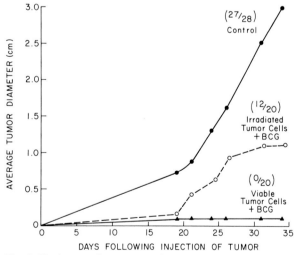

Fig. 9-23. Immunotherapy experiments with a transplantable liposarcoma in syngeneic strain 2 guinea pigs: 1×10^5 liposarcoma tumor cells were inoculated intramuscularly into the leg, and immunotherapy was initiated intradermally in four sites on the back with 1×10^6 living or 1×10^7 irradiated tumor cells mixed with bacillus Calmette-Guérin (BCG). (*From D. L. Morton et al., Ann Surg, 172:740, 1970.*)

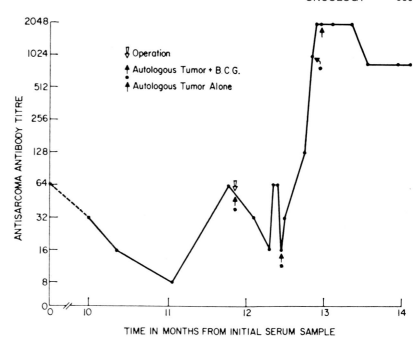

Fig. 9-24. Antisarcoma antibody titers determined by complement fixation against the HuSA-I liposarcoma antigen on serial serum samples from a sixteen-year-old boy with a primary osteosarcoma of the right femur in whom pulmonary metastases developed 10 months after resection of the primary, for which a left pneumonectomy was performed and immunotherapy initiated. (*From D. L. Morton et al., Ann Surg, 172:740, 1970.*)

PASSIVE AND ADOPTIVE IMMUNOTHERAPY

Since patients with cancer develop two types of immune responses to their neoplasms—humoral antibodies and cell-mediated immune responses—passive immunotherapy is logically based upon the administration of either antitumor sera or lymphoid cells.

PASSIVE IMMUNOTHERAPY WITH ANTITUMOR SERA. In the past, antitumor sera produced in a foreign species proved to be very toxic to the recipient, because it contained antibodies against normal tissue antigens of the host. However, this problem may be resolved soon when successful isolation and purification of the tumor-specific transplantation antigens are achieved so that the antisera can be directed specifically against the tumor-specific transplantation antigens of the tumor cells. Another source of potential antisera may be from those patients cured of their malignant condition who demonstrate high titers of cytotoxic or deblocking antibodies.

An important new concept of antisera therapy concerns the discovery of certain blocking factors that appear to inhibit the effectiveness of the lymphocytes. Thought to be circulating antigen or antibody-antigen complexes, these blocking factors may contribute to tumor growth by interfering with cellular immunity. In experiments using mouse and guinea pig sarcomas, as well as leukemias, tumor regression can be induced with antisera containing high titers of antitumor antibody. The mechanism for antitumor effectiveness is unclear. It could be due to a direct cytotoxic effect on tumor cells acting as cytophilic antibody that induces macrophages or lymphocytes to kill tumor cells or by neutralizing blocking factors. Nevertheless, these observations clearly indicate that antitumor sera can induce regression of established neoplasms and as such should receive serious consideration for immunotherapy of cancer.

IMMUNOTHERAPY WITH LYMPHOID CELLS. Adoptive immunotherapy with lymphoid cells from an immunized donor was accomplished with ease between inbred laboratory animals of the same strain and suggested that antitumor immunity was primarily cell-mediated. However, these animal experiments indicated that the transferred lymphocytes must persist in the host to have a significant immunotherapeutic effect. As studies were done in human cancer, the primary difficulty was with rejection of the transferred lymphocytes due to HLA differences between host and donor. This problem was overcome when the lymphoid cells were obtained from family members who were identical by HLA matching or by bulk growth of the patient's own lymphocytes in tissue culture. The lymphocytes of the family members may be already sensitized to the tumor-specific antigens in certain neoplasms, such as human sarcomas, where our investigations have shown a high incidence of antibodies in close family members.

As with antisera, another source of lymphocytes may be those cancer patients who have been cured of their malignant disease. Sumner and Foraker reported one of the earliest successes by this means when they transfused a melanoma patient with whole blood from a second melanoma patient who had undergone complete remission.

Moore and Gerner attempted to increase the lymphocyte ratio to tumor cells by growing a patient's lymphocytes in tissue culture and reinfusing them back to the patient. They reported significant regressions in two of three patients. However, the logistic problems of growing such large numbers of lymphocytes are considerable.

IMMUNOTHERAPY FOLLOWING IN VITRO ACTIVATION OF LYMPHOCYTES. Further studies of adoptive immunotherapy have concerned in vitro, nonspecific stimulation of lymphocytes with agents such as phytohemagglutinin. Some success has been reported when these treated autologous lymphocytes were reinfused into the patient or injected directly into tumor deposits. Another approach has involved specific sensitization of lymphocytes with tumor cells in vitro by incubation with mitomycin C-treated tissue culture tumor cells. The mitomycin C prevented replication of the tumor cells by eliminating their potential to form metastases. Though the results were not impressive in these human investigations, recent animal experiments suggest this means as a very effective way to induce an effective antitumor immunity. The ability to obtain large numbers of lymphocytes from any donor by continuous lymphophoresis using the NCI-IBM blood cell separator has considerably increased the feasibility of this approach.

IMMUNOTHERAPY WITH LYMPHOCYTES SENSITIZED BY TRANSPLANTATION OF TUMORS. Several investigators have attempted passive immunotherapy with cross immunization with tumor tissue followed by cross transfusions of lymphocytes or lymphocytes and serum. These studies have been undertaken in the following manner: Patients with incurable cancer were paired according to blood type and tumor types. Tumors from patients in group A were transplanted subcutaneously to patients in group B, and vice versa. Following sensitization to each other's tumors, the transfusions of lymphocytes from patients in group B to patients in group A, or vice versa, were begun and continued daily for variable periods of time. The response rate reported following this type of immunotherapy is from 15 to 20 percent. However, the criteria for therapeutic response have varied between investigators and in many cases have not met rigid specifications acceptable to many oncologists.

IMMUNOTHERAPY WITH EXTRACTS OF SENSITIZED LYMPHOID CELLS. One particularly appealing method of immunotherapy concerns the transfer of informational molecules. These molecules can arouse a specific immune response from the recipient's own immune system. The two reported substances that have this remarkable ability are Lawrence's transfer factor and immune RNA described by Deckers and Pilch.

Lawrence's transfer factor is capable of transferring immunity to skin grafts, tuberculosis, and a variety of other antigens. It has not been used extensively for immunotherapy of cancer, but preliminary reports appear encouraging.

Deckers and Pilch found that immune RNA, extracted from the lymphoid tissues of a xenogenic host following immunization with tumors, could induce immunity in syngeneic recipients of tumor transplants. This model is most advantageous because the immune RNA can be produced in a host other than man.

Both these methods of immunology have considerable promise, because each bypasses many of the problems associated with passive and adoptive immunotherapy, such as HLA incompatibility, serum sickness, and anaphylaxis.

NONSPECIFIC IMMUNOTHERAPY

The theoretic basis for nonspecific immunotherapy depends upon the observation that certain substances, such as mixed bacterial toxins and fractions of the tubercle bacillus, have the ability to nonspecifically enhance host resistance to most viral, fungal, and bacterial agents. Although the exact mechanism is unknown, these agents do appear to stimulate immune response to a wide variety of antigens, including tumor-specific antigens.

Historically, a type of nonspecific immunotherapy was described by Bradford Coley at the turn of the century in one of the first reports of a tumor regression possibly induced by immunologic means. Coley's interest in the possible value of such therapy was stimulated when he observed a recurrent inoperable sarcoma of the neck regress completely for 7 years after the patient had had attacks of erysipelas. This observation led to the development of Coley's toxins, a mixture of killed bacterial vaccines. Coley injected this admixture directly into tumor lesions or gave it intravenously. Some impressive regressions of tumors and long-term cures resulted from these agents. Because the responses were inconsistent, Coley's toxins never received widespread use, and interest in them died out. Recently a nonspecific immunotherapy of a similar type has been revived using attenuated bovine tuberculosis bacillus (BCG) to treat patients with malignant melanoma. More than a decade ago BCG was discovered by Old and his associates to have significant antitumor activity against a wide variety of animal neoplasms.

Our own work with this agent in man began more than 5 years ago when patients with malignant melanoma who had metastatic nodules in the skin and subcutaneous tissues were treated by direct intralesional injection of BCG vaccine. Approximately 90 percent of the melanoma nodules directly injected with BCG were observed to regress in patients who were immunologically competent, as judged by their ability to be sensitized to DNCB as well as to react positively to tuberculin following BCG therapy. In addition, nodules of malignant melanoma at sites different from the BCG inoculation also regressed in approximately 20 percent of these immunologically competent patients. These patients remained free of disease for periods of 2 to 5 years. Similar instances of tumor regression have been seen in breast cancer and other neoplasms when the lesions were confined to the skin.

There are several possible mechanisms to explain tumor regression in these patients following BCG injections; both specific and nonspecific immune reactions were probably involved. BCG is known to be a potent immunologic adjuvant capable of increasing host immune responses to a wide variety of tumor-specific antigens. Nevertheless, the fact that the observed regression of melanoma nodules occurred only in tuberculin-positive patients following direct injection of nodules suggests that a large part of the antitumor effect was nonspecific and resulted from the induction of a delayed hypersensitivity reaction within the melanoma nodule. It is obvious that BCG had no direct antitumor effect, since it did not cause tumor regression in tuberculin-negative patients.

In addition to the nonspecific effect, a specific immune response to the melanoma tumor-specific antigens also occurred in some patients because an associated rising titer of antimelanoma antibody was observed following BCG immunotherapy. Sequential biopsies of tumor nodules following BCG inoculation revealed that the regression of these nodules was associated with a granulomatous infiltration of lymphocytes, monocytes, and fibroblasts surrounding and infiltrating the melanoma cells. Furthermore, the regression of melanoma nodules not given injection with BCG was accompanied by the appearance of lymphocyte infiltrates within the regressing melanoma tumor nodules (Fig. 9-25). The specific antitumor effect may result from more lymphocytes and macrophages coming into contact with the tumor cells so that the afferent limb of the immune response is increased. Conversely, it may work via the effector limb of the immune response by bringing greater numbers of both stimulated and unstimulated lymphocytes to the tumor.

Since our original report, these observations have been confirmed by many investigators. The response to immunotherapy in melanoma patients occurs primarily in those whose diseases are limited to the skin, subcutaneous tissue, and regional lymph nodes. Patients who have large amounts of tumor metastatic to the parenchymal organs such as the lung, liver, and brain generally have shown little response to BCG immunotherapy. However, from the natural history of malignant melanoma in man, we know that many of the patients in whom malignant melanoma appears to be limited to the skin and subcutaneous tissues when initially seen also have subclinical disease at metastatic sites in other organs. Since 20 percent of these patients remain disease-free for long periods of time following BCG immunotherapy, we must conclude that the immunotherapy was successful in eliminating these smaller metastatic sites of melanoma in the parenchymal organs, and that it has both a systemic and local effect.

Of major significance is the fact that BCG immunotherapy of malignant melanoma demonstrates that a human cancer, even when disseminated, can be made to regress for long periods of time by immunologic means provided the tumor burden is small. This alone proves the feasibility of cancer immunotherapy in man for subclinical microscopic disease.

Further impressive observations demonstrating that local immunotherapy results in tumor regression (by induction of delayed hypersensitivity reactions) come from the studies of Klein in patients with basal and squamous cell carcinomas of the skin. Here the induction of delayed hypersensitivity reactions to DNCB results in the resolution of more than 90 percent of superficial basal or squamous cell carcinomas. Klein observed that multiple antigens increased the delayed hypersensitivity and effectiveness of this form of immunotherapy.

Another example of nonspecific immunotherapy is acute leukemia. Mathé and associates have reported a significant improvement in the survival of patients with acute leukemia when, after the induction of complete remission by standard chemotherapeutic agents, they were placed on BCG immunotherapy for prolonged periods of time. Al-

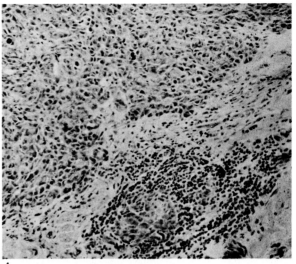

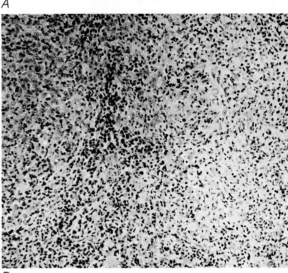

Fig. 9-25. *A.* Subcutaneous metastasis of malignant melanoma prior to immunotherapy with BCG. Note the absence of lymphocytic and monocytic infiltration among the tumor cells. *B.* Subcutaneous metastasis which had decreased in size from 10 to 5 mm during the 6-week period following immunotherapy with BCG injections into other melanoma nodules. BCG was *not* injected into this nodule. Note the marked lymphocytic and monocytic infiltration among the melanoma cells. (*From D. L. Morton, et al., Ann Surg, 172:740, 1970.*)

though some investigators have been unable to confirm Mathé's early observations, differences in methods of applying BCG are the most likely explanation for these discrepancies.

At the present time, nonspecific immunotherapy with BCG for malignant melanoma or with DNCB for squamous cell carcinomas of the skin are the only two methods of immunotherapy that have been consistently useful in the treatment of human cancer. BCG is only one of a wide variety of agents that can nonspecifically stimulate the immune system's response to a variety of different types of antigens. Examples of other agents would include *Corynebacterium parvum,* MER (methanol extractable residue of BCG), bacterial endotoxins, and polynucleotides. We can anticipate that in the future this approach will be applied to a wider variety of neoplasms and that new immunologic adjuvants will be developed.

Obviously, the rational application of immunotherapy to human cancer will depend, to a large extent, upon a better knowledge of the nature of tumor-specific antigens in human neoplasms and methods for increasing the immune response against these antigens. Specificity for cancer cells cannot be achieved by any other known therapeutic means, but at the present time its potency is limited.

The observation that organ transplant patients with disseminated neoplasms, inadvertently transplanted at the time of kidney transplantation, have regressions of their tumors after cessation of immunosuppressive drugs suggests that the immune response can cause regression of disseminated cancer if the tumor-specific antigens are sufficiently strong. The recent exciting experiments with animal neoplasms in which established sarcomas and mammary carcinomas regressed following the treatment with neuraminidase and BCG suggest that the strength of the tumor-specific antigens and the host immune response to these antigens can be sufficiently enhanced to cause tumor regression in selected situations.

At the present time, the tumor immunologist is faced with a paradox in the clinical application of immunotherapy. Ideally, the patients who are most likely to respond to this therapeutic modality are those who are in the early stages of the disease and have minimal residual tumor burden following treatment with other therapeutic modalities. However, many of these patients may have been cured of the cancer by the primary treatment, so the results of such therapy can be evaluated only by controlled clinical trials containing large numbers of patients. It should be emphasized, however, that the toxicity, dosage, indications, and therapeutic results of immunotherapy are largely unknown at the present time.

PROGNOSIS

Predicting the future course of a patient's malignant disease is one of the most difficult problems an oncologist faces. At the present time, it is impossible to predict the future course of a given patient except in general terms. However, a number of known factors are important in determining prognosis.

The *site of origin* of the primary tumor is one of the most important factors influencing prognosis. The propensity of a neoplasm to metastasize to distant sites varies according to its tissue of origin. Over 90 percent of carcinomas of the lung, pancreas, and esophagus spread beyond their primary site and cause death, whereas carcinomas of the skin, breast, and thyroid glands are frequently localized and curable, even when metastatic in some patients.

The *stage of disease* at the time of initial treatment is of considerable importance in determining survival for all types of neoplasms. The chance for cure is best when the neoplasm is confined to the organ of origin. The smaller the primary neoplasm, the better the prognosis, as well. Thus, in situ carcinoma of the cervix, carcinomas of the breast less than 1 cm in diameter, and small polypoid carcinomas of the colon are generally curable; larger neoplasms may not be curable. Direct extension into adjacent organs or metastases to regional nodes suggest a more guarded prognosis, although many patients are still curable at this stage of the disease. The spread of cancer by the bloodstream with metastases to distant sites portends a grave prognosis, and few patients are curable at this stage. As a general rule, lymph node involvement sharply reduces survival probability by about one-half that of patients without involved nodes. If only one node is involved, the prognosis is better than if the majority of lymph nodes are involved.

The *histopathologic features* of the neoplasm correlate in a general way to prognosis. The more undifferentiated, highly malignant-appearing neoplasms with frequent mitosis are more likely to develop early distant spread and local recurrence. However, some very malignant neoplasms still can be cured with adequate treatment. Venous invasion is a grave prognostic factor in all types of neoplasia.

Host immune factors, as previously discussed, may be the most important single factor in determining prognosis. Immunologic methods for monitoring immune responses are currently under development. It is already apparent that those patients who have spontaneous depression of their immune responses have a uniformly poor prognosis following therapy.

The *age of the patient* may be an important factor affecting prognosis. Some oncologists believe that neoplasms in younger patients carry a poorer prognosis than the same tumors in middle-aged or elderly patients, although elderly patients may have associated medical problems that do not permit adequate treatment of the cancer. While there may be some validity in this concept, it should not be overemphasized, because many young patients have a good prognosis. In fact, some have a much better prognosis than adults with the same neoplasms. Those neoplasms which occur prior to one year of age generally have a better prognosis than those which occur later in childhood. This can be determined in the following manner: The child is usually cured of the neoplasm if he is free of disease for 9 months after treatment, plus double the age at the time treatment was begun. This concept is based upon the supposition that if the earliest cancer cell started with conception and if the cancer grew at a constant rate, then it would reach a certain size at the time treatment was initiated. If treatment was successful in eliminating all cancer cells except one, then in a period equal to 9 months plus double the age of the child, the cancer size would again be equivalent to the original tumor mass. Therefore, if there is no recurrence after this time span, it can be assumed that the patient is cured.

The *adequacy of treatment* is most relevant to prognosis for certain types of neoplasms. The cure rate for some neoplasms, such as soft tissue sarcomas and certain child-hood neoplasms, may be twice as high in sophisticated cancer centers when compared to cure rates in small community hospitals. Furthermore, some patients with seemingly hopeless prognoses may be cured with aggressive therapy by an experienced oncologist, whereas they might not be by the physician who only occasionally treats cancer patients and might be unwilling to undertake the aggressive therapy.

PSYCHOLOGIC MANAGEMENT OF THE CANCER PATIENT

The cancer patient's great fear of his disease usually can be decreased by understanding derived from free and open communication with the physician. Psychologic support and education to deal with any disability that may result from therapy are important. Examples include training in the care of a stoma following curative surgery for colonic and rectal cancer or referral to lay groups associated with the American Cancer Society for counseling the anxious patient with an altered body image resulting from mastectomy.

Despite the prognostic factors discussed previously, it is still impossible to predict the exact course of any malignant tumor. Patients with the most grim prognoses are occasionally cured by aggressive therapy, and spontaneous regressions are sometimes observed even in patients with metastases. In contrast, some patients with apparently localized disease may be dead of disseminated cancer in a few months. This uncertainty about the future is one of the most difficult adjustments faced by the cancer patient and his family. Most reassuring in this regard is to emphasize that for each month that passes following successful treatment of the primary neoplasm, the chances for cure improve. This is particularly correct for tumors such as squamous cell carcinoma of the lung or oral pharynx. Although other, more slowly growing neoplasms, such as carcinoma of the breast and malignant melanoma, may recur after disease-free intervals of 10 or 20 years, the chances of recurrence also decrease with time. Recognition that cancer is a chronic disease is an important aspect of management. Long-term, consistent follow-up provides opportunities for reassurance and usually can ensure detection of recurrence at an early stage.

Some patients do not want to know about their illness for fear of having their suspicions verified. Never lie to a patient, if possible, even if requested by the family. In general, gentle and optimistic truth is best. Untruths often create barriers between the patient and his family which can lead to psychologic isolation of the patient who is unable to discuss his fears and anxieties with those he needs most.

With the patient for whom primary cancer therapy has failed, one of the most difficult problems faced by the physician is "What should the patient be told?" Most oncologists who deal exclusively with cancer patients agree that the incurable patient also must be told the truth as gently and optimistically as possible. Hope and reassurance as to the physician's continuing concern are best sustained by continuing active treatment until it is certain that the patient can no longer benefit. Realistic and consistent support is actually more important to the patient and the family at this stage of the disease than earlier. There is increasing evidence that patients tolerate the process of dying much better when cared for in this manner.

Some incurable patients are unable to accept the realities of the situation. In this case, it is essential that a responsible family member be informed. The life duration of the incurable patient is so uncertain that predictions should be avoided. If, as frequently happens, the relatives insist upon some estimate, a combined minimum-maximum prognosis, such as from 6 months to 2 years, will help the family accept this uncertainty.

The basic aim in caring for the patient with advanced cancer is to prolong useful life, but not useless suffering. The patient should be permitted to die with dignity when active therapy can no longer benefit him.

References

Etiology

Barratt, R. W., and Tatum, E. L.: Carcinogenic Mutagens, *Ann NY Acad Sci,* **71:**1072, 1958.

Blum, H. F.: Sunlight as a Causal Factor in Cancer of the Skin, *Cancer Res,* **5:**592, 1945; **9:**247, 1948.

Buell, P., and Dunn, J. E., Jr.: Cancer Mortality among Japanese Issei and Nisei of California, *Cancer,* **18:**656, 1965.

Burdett, W. J.: "Viruses Inducing Cancer," University of Utah Press, Salt Lake City, 1966.

Cutler, S. J.: A Review of the Statistical Evidence on Association between Smoking and Lung Cancer, *J Am Statis Assoc,* **50:**267, 1955.

Haenszel, W.: Cancer Mortality among the Foreign Born in the United States, *J Natl Cancer Inst,* **26:**37, 1961.

Hammond, E. C., and Horn, D.: The Relationship between Human Smoking Habits and Death Rates, *JAMA,* **155:**1316, 1954.

Heuper, W. C.: Environmental Cancer, in F. Homburger (ed.), "The Physiopathology of Cancer," p. 919, Harper & Row, Publishers, Incorporated, New York, 1959.

Kennaway, E. C.: The Formation of a Cancer Producing Substance from Isoprene (2-Methyl-Butadiene), *J Pathol Bacteriol,* **27:**233, 1924.

Khanolkar, V. R.: Oral Cancer in Bombay, India: A Review of 1,000 Consecutive Cases, *Cancer Res,* **4:**313, 1944.

Lorenz, E.: Radioactivity and Lung Cancer: A Critical Review of Lung Cancer in the Miners of Schneeburg and Joachimstall, *Cancer Res,* **5:**1, 1944.

Martland, H. S.: Occupational Poisoning in Manufacture of Luminous Watch Dials: General Review of Hazard Caused by Ingestion of Luminous Paint with Special Reference to the New Jersey Cases, *JAMA,* **92:**466, 1929.

Mayo, C. W., DeWeerd, J. H., and Jackman, R. J.: Diffuse Familial Polyposes of the Colon, *Surg Gynecol Obstet,* **93:**87, 1951.

Pifer, J. W., Toyooka, E. T., Murray, R. W., Ames, W. R., Hempelmann, L. H., Crump, S. L., and Dutton, A. M.: Neoplasms in Children Treated with X-rays for Thymic Enlargement: I. Neoplasms and Mortality; II. Tumor Incidence as a Function of Radiation Factors; III. Clinical Description of Cases, *J Natl Cancer Inst,* **31:**1333, 1357, 1379, 1963.

Porter, C. D., and White, C. J.: Multiple Carcinomata following Chronic X-ray Dermatitis, *Ann Surg,* **46:**649, 1970.

Prehn, R. T.: Specific Isoantigenicities among Chemically Induced Tumors, *Ann NY Acad Sci,* **101:**107, 1962.

Rous, P.: Transmission of a Malignant New Growth by Means of a Cell-free Filtrate, *JAMA,* **56:**198, 1911.

Shimkin, M. B.: Cancer Research, in L. V. Ackerman and J. A. Del Regato (eds.), "Cancer," pp. 35–57, The C. V. Mosby Company, St. Louis, 1962.

Biology and Immunobiology

Black, M. M., Opler, S. R., and Speer, F. D.: Structural Representations of Tumor-Host Relationships in Gastric Carcinoma, *Surg Gynecol Obstet,* **102:**599, 1956.

Burnet, F. M.: "Immunological Surveillance," Pergamon Press, New York, 1970.

Edynak, E. M., Old, L. J., Vrana, M., and Lardis, M.: A Fetal Antigen in Human Tumors Detected by an Antibody in the Serum of Cancer Patients, *Proc Am Assoc Cancer Res,* **11:**22, 1970.

Eilber, F. R., and Morton, D. L.: Impaired Immunologic Reactivity and Recurrence following Cancer Surgery, *Cancer,* **25:**362, 1970.

Everson, T. C., and Cole, W. H.: "Spontaneous Regression of Cancer," W. B. Saunders Company, Philadelphia, 1966.

Fass, L., Ziegler, J. L., Herberman, R. B., and Kiryabwire, J. W. M.: Cutaneous Hypersensitivity Reactions to Autologous Extracts of Malignant Melanoma Cells, *Lancet,* **1:**116, 1970.

Fenyö, E. M., Klein, E., Klein, G., and Swiech, K.: Selection of an Immunoresistant Moloney Lymphoma Subline with Decreased Concentration of Tumor-specific Surface Antigens, *J Natl Cancer Inst,* **40:**69, 1968.

Foley, E. J.: Antigenic Properties of Methylcholanthrene-induced Tumors in Mice of the Strain or Origin, *Cancer Res,* **13:**835, 1953.

Gatti, R. A., and Good, R. A.: Occurrence of Malignancy in Immunodeficiency Diseases: A Literature Review, *Cancer,* **28:**89, 1971.

Gold, P., and Freedman, S. O.: Specific Carcinoembryonic Antigens of the Human Digestive System, *J Exp Med,* **122:**467, 1965.

Goodwin, W. E.: Regression of Hypernephromas, *JAMA,* **20:**609, 1968.

Griffiths, J. D., McKinna, J. A., Rawbotham, H. D., Tsolakidis, P., and Salsbury, A. J.: Carcinoma of the Colon and Rectum: Circulating Malignant Cells and 5-Year Survival, *Cancer,* **31:**226, 1973.

Hammond, W. G., Fisher, J. C., and Rolley, R. T.: Tumor Specific Transplantation Immunity to Spontaneous Mouse Tumors, *Surgery,* **62:**124, 1967.

Hellstrom, I., Sjogren, H. O., Warner, G., and Hellstrom, K. E.: Blocking of Cell-mediated Tumor Immunity by Sera from Patients with Growing Neoplasms, *Int J Cancer,* **7:**226, 1971.

Klein, G.: Tumor Antigens, *Annu Rev Microbiol,* **20:**223, 1966.

Morton, D. L.: Acquired Immunological Tolerance and Carcinogenesis by the Mammary Tumor Virus: I. Influence of Neonatal Infection with the Mammary Tumor Virus on the Growth of Spontaneous Mammary Adencarcinomas, *J Natl Cancer Inst,* **42:**311, 1969.

———, Eilber, F. R., Joseph, W. L., Wood, W. C., Trahan, E., and Ketcham, A. S.: Immunological Factors in Human Sarcomas and Melanomas: A Rational Basis for Immunotherapy, *Ann Surg,* **172:**740, 1970.

———, Holmes, E. C., Eilber, F. R., and Wood, W. C.: Immunological Aspects of Neoplasia: A Rational Basis for Immunotherapy, *Ann Intern Med,* **74:**587, 1971.

Old, L. J., and Boyse, E. A.: Antigens of Tumors and Leukemias Induced by Virus, *Fed Proc,* **24:**1009, 1965.

———, ———, and Stockert, E.: Antigenic Properties of Experimental Leukemias: I. Serological Studies In Vitro with Spontaneous and Radiation-induced Leukemias, *J Natl Cancer Inst,* **31:**977, 1963.

———, Stockert, E., Boyse, E. A., and Kin, J. H.: Antigenic Modulation: Loss of TL Antigen from Cells Exposed to TL Antibody: Study of the Phenomenon In Vitro, *J Exp Med,* **127:**523, 1968.

Piessens, W. F.: Evidence of Human Cancer Immunity, *Cancer,* **26:**1212, 1970.

Prehn, R. T., and Main, J. M.: Immunity to Methylcholanthrene-induced Sarcomas, *J Natl Cancer Inst,* **18:**769, 1957.

Sjogren, H. O.: Transplantation Methods as a Tool for Detection of Tumor-specific Antigens, *Prog Exp Tumor Res,* **6:**289, 1965.

Smith, R. T.: Tumor-specific Immune Mechanisms, *N Engl J Med,* **278:**1207, 1968.

Sophocles, A. M., and Nadler, S. H.: Immunologic Aspects of Cancer, *Surg Gynecol Obstet,* **133:**321, 1971.

Southam, C. M., Brunschwig, W., Levin, A. G., and Dixon, Q. S.: The Effect of Leukocytes on Transplantability of Human Cancer, *Cancer,* **19:**1743, 1966.

Sugarbaker, E. V., and Cohen A. M.: Altered Antigenicity in Spontaneous Pulmonary Metastases from an Antigenic Murine Sarcoma, *Surgery,* **72:**155, 1972.

Zamcheck, N., Moore, T. L., Dhar, P., and Kupchic, H.: Immunologic Diagnosis and Prognosis of Human Digestive Tract Cancer: Carcinoembryonic Antigens, *N Engl J Med,* **286:**83, 1972.

Pathology

Anderson, W.: The General Pathology of Tumors, in "Boyd's Pathology for the Surgeon," p. 92, W. B. Saunders Co., Philadelphia, 1967.

Bloom, H. J. G., Richardson, W. W., and Harries, E. J.: Natural History of Untreated Breast Cancer (1805–1933): Comparison of Untreated and Treated Cases according to Histological Grade of Malignancy, *Br Med J,* **2:**213, 1962.

Boyd, W.: "An Introduction to the Study of Disease," p. 210, Lea & Febiger, Philadelphia, 1971.

Cole, W H., McDonald, G. O., Roberts, S. S., and Southwich, H. W.: "Dissemination of Cancer," Appleton-Century-Crofts, Inc., New York, 1961.

Collins, V. P., Leoffler, R. K., and Tivey, H.: Observations on Growth Rates of Human Tumors, *Am J Roentgenol Radium Ther Nucl Med,* **76:**988, 1956.

Cowan, D. R.: Mechanisms Responsible for the Origin and Distribution of Blood-borne Tumor Metastases, *Cancer Res,* **13:**397, 1953.

Everson, T. C.: Spontaneous Regression of Cancer, *Ann NY Acad Sci,* **114:**721, 1964.

Garland, L. H., Coulson, W., and Wollin, E.: The Rate of Growth and Apparent Duration of Untreated Primary Bronchial Carcinoma, *Cancer,* **16:**694, 1963.

Knox, L. C.: The Relationship of Massage to Metastases in Malignant Tumors, *Ann Surg,* **75:**129, 1922.

MacMahon, B., and Feng, M. A.: Prenatal Origin of Childhood Leukemia: Evidence from Twins, *N Engl J Med,* **270:**1082, 1964.

Moertel, C. G.: Incidence and Significance of Multiple Primary Malignant Neoplasms, *Ann NY Acad Sci,* **114:**886, 1964.

Pearson, H. A., Grello, F. W., and Cane, E. C., Jr.: Leukemia in Identical Twins, *N Engl J Med,* **268:**1151, 1963.

Pund, E. R., Nettles, T. B., Caldwell, T. D., and Nieburgs, H. E.: Preinvasive and Invasive Carcinoma of the Cervix Uteri: Pathogenesis, Detection, Differential Diagnosis, and Pathologic Basis for Management, *Am J Obstet Gynecol,* **55:**831, 1948.

Rigler, L. B.: Natural History of Untreated Lung Cancer, *Ann NY Acad Sci.* **114:**755, 1964.

Russell, W. O., Ibanex, M. L., Clark, R. L., and White, E. C.: Thyroid Carcinoma: Classification, Intraglandular Dissemination, and Clinicopathologic Study Based upon Whole Organ Sections of 80 Glands, *Cancer,* **16:**1425, 1963.

Slaughter, D. P.: Multicentric Origin of Intraoral Carcinoma, *Surgery,* **20:**133, 1946.

Clinical Manifestations

Barrie, J. G., Knapper, W. H., and Strong, E. W.: Cervical Nodal Metastases of Unknown Origin, *Am J Surg,* **120:**466, 1970.

Bhattacharya, S. K., and Sealy, W. C.: Paraneoplastic Syndromes Resulting from Elaboration of Ectopic Hormones, Antigens, and Bizarre Toxins, *Curr Probl Surg,* May, 1972.

Greenberg, B. E.: Cervical Lymph Node Metastases from Unknown Primary Sites, *Cancer,* **19:**1091, 1966.

Jesse, R. H., and Neff, L. F.: Metastatic Carcinoma in Cervical Nodes with an Unknown Primary Lesion, *Am J Surg,* **112:**547, 1966.

Keller, J. W., and Williams R. D.: Laparotomy for Unexplained Fever, *Arch Surg,* **90:**494, 1965.

Myers, W. P. L., Tashima, C. K., and Rothschild, E. O.: Endocrine Syndromes Associated with Non-endocrine Neoplasms, *Med Clin North Am,* **50:**763, 1966.

Owens, A. H., Jr.: Neoplastic Diseases, in A. M. Harvey, R. J. Johns, A. H. Owens, and R. S. Ross (eds.), "The Principles and Practice of Medicine," p. 641, Appleton-Century-Crofts, Inc., New York, 1972.

Smith, P. E., Krementz, E. T., and Chapman, W.: Metastatic Cancer without a Detectable Primary Site, *Am J Surg,* **113:** 633, 1967.

Diagnosis and Staging

Commission on Clinical Oncology of the Union Internationale Contre Cancrum: "TNM Classification of Malignant Tumors," International Clinics against Cancer, Geneva, 1968.

Copeland, M. M.: American Joint Committee on Cancer Staging and End Results Reporting: Objectives and Progress, *Cancer,* **18:**1637, 1965.

Glatstein, E., Guernsey, J. M., Rosenberg, S. A., and Kaplan, H. S.: The Value of Laparotomy and Splenectomy in the Staging of Hodgkin's Disease, *Cancer,* **24:**709, 1969.

Goldman, J. M.: Laparotomy for Staging of Hodgkin's Disease, *Lancet,* **1:**125, 1971.

Kennedy, W. B.: History and Physical Examination in the Diagnosis of Cancer, in T. F. Nealon, Jr. (ed.), "Management of the Patient with Cancer," p. 62, W. B. Saunders Co., Philadelphia, 1966.

Surgery

Ansfield, F. J., Ramirez, G., Skibba, J. L., Bryan, G. T., Davis, H. L. Jr., and Wirtanen, G. W.: Intrahepatic Arterial Infusion with 5-Fluorourocil, *Cancer,* **28:**1147, 1971.

Aune, S., and Schistad, G.: Carcinoid Liver Metastases Treated with Hepatic Dearterialization, *Am J Surg,* **123:**715, 1972.

Barnes, J. P.: Physiologic Resection of the Right Colon, *Surg Gynecol Obstet,* **94:**722, 1952.

Cole, W. H., Packard, D., and Southwich, H. W.: Carcinoma of the Colon with Special Reference to Prevention of Recurrence, *JAMA,* **155:**1549, 1954.

Deckers, P. J., Ketcham, A. S., Sugarbaker, E. V., Hoye, R. C., and Thomas, L. B.: Pelvic Exenteration for Primary Carcinoma of the Uterine Cervix, *Obstet Gynecol,* **37:**647, 1971.

Flanagan, L., and Foster, J. H.: Hepatic Resection for Metastatic Cancer, *Am J Surg,* **113:**551, 1967.

Gilbertsen, V. A., and Wangensteen, O. H.: A Summary of Thirteen Years' Experience with the Second Look Program, *Surg Gynecol Obstet,* **114:**438, 1962.

Gulesserian, H. P., Lawton, R. L., and Condon, R. E.: Hepatic Artery Ligation and Cytotoxic Infusion in Treatment of Liver Metastases, *Arch Surg,* **105:**280, 1972.

Halsted, W. S.: The Results of Operations for the Cure of Cancer of the Breast Performed at the Johns Hopkins Hospital from June 1889 to January 1894, *Ann Surg,* **20:**297, 1894.

Huggins, C., and Bergenstal, D. M.: Inhibition of Human Mammary and Prostatic Cancer by Adrenalectomy, *Cancer Res,* **12:**134, 1952.

Kiselow, M., Butcher, H. R., and Bricker, E. M.: Results of the Radical Surgical Treatment of Advanced Pelvic Cancer: A Fifteen-Year Study, *Ann Surg,* **166:**436, 1967.

Krementz, E. T., Creech, O. J., Ryan, R. F., and Reemstma, K.: Appraisal of Cancer Chemotherapy by Regional Perfusion, *Ann Surg,* **156:**417, 1962.

————, and Ryan, R. E.: Chemotherapy of Melanoma of the Extremities by Perfusion: Fourteen Years Clinical Experience, *Ann Surg,* **175:**900, 1972.

Miles, W. E.: A Method of Performing Abdomino-perineal Excision for Carcinoma of the Rectum and the Terminal Portion of the Pelvic Colon, *Lancet,* **2:**1812, 1908.

Miller, D. R., and Albritten, F. F., Jr.: Principles of Surgery for Cancer, in T. F. Nealon Jr. (ed.), "Management of the Patient with Cancer," p. 154, W. B. Saunders Company, Philadelphia, 1966.

Mockman, S., Curreri, A. R., and Ansfield, F. J.: Second-Look Operation for Colon Carcinoma after Fluorouracil Therapy, *Arch Surg,* **100:**527, 1970.

Pierce, E. H., Clagett, O. T., McDonald, J. R., and Gage, R. P.: Biopsy of the Breast Followed by Delayed Radical Mastectomy, *Surg Gynecol Obstet,* **103:**559, 1956.

Roberts, S. S., Hengesh, J. W., McGrath, R. G., Valaitis, J., McGrew, E. A., and Cole, W. H.: Prognostic Significance of Cancer Cells in the Circulating Blood: A Ten Year Evaluation, *Am J Surg,* **113:**757, 1967.

Stearns, M. W., and Schottenfeld, D.: Techniques for the Surgical Management of Colon Cancer, *Cancer,* **28:**165, 1971.

Stehlin, J. S.: Hyperthermic Perfusion with Chemotherapy for Cancer of the Extremities, *Surg Gynecol Obstet,* **129:**305, 1969.

Turnbull, R. B., Kyle, K., Watson, F. R., and Spratt, J.: Cancer of the Colon: The Influence of the No-Touch Isolation Technic on Survival Rates, *Ann Surg,* **166:**420, 1967.

Watkins, E., Khazei, A. M., and Nabra, K. S.: Surgical Basis for Arterial Infusion Chemotherapy of Disseminated Carcinoma of the Liver, *Surg Gynecol Obstet,* **130:**581, 1970.

Watkins, E. W., Jr., and Sullivan, R. D.: Cancer Chemotherapy by Prolonged Arterial Infusion, *Surg Gynecol Obstet,* **118:**3, 1964.

Wilkens, E. W., Jr.: The Surgical Management of Metastatic Neoplasms of the Lung, *J Thorac Cardiovasc Surg,* **42:**298, 1961.

Woodington, G. F., and Waugh, J. M.: Results of Resection of Metastatic Tumors of the Liver, *Am J Surg,* **105:**24, 1963.

Radiation Therapy

Johns, H. E., and Cunningham, J. R.: in "The Physics of Radiology," p. 345, Charles C Thomas, Publisher, Springfield, Ill., 1971.

Moss, W. T., and Brand, W. N.: "Therapeutic Radiology; Rationale, Technique, Results," 3d ed., The C. V. Mosby Company, St. Louis, 1969.

Paulson, D. L., Shaw, R. R., Kee, J. L., Mallams, J. T., and Collier, R. E.: Combined Preoperative Irradiation and Resection for Bronchogenic Carcinoma, *J Thorac Cardiovasc Surg,* **44:**281, 1962.

Powers, W. E., and Tolmach, L. J.: Preoperative Radiation Therapy: Biologic Bases and Experimental Investigation, *Nature (Lond),* **201:**272, 1964.

Chemotherapy

Bailor, J. C., and Byar, D. P.: Estrogen Treatment for Cancer of the Prostate, *Cancer,* **26:**257, 1970.

Baserga, R.: "The Cell Cycle and Cancer," Marcel Dekker, Inc., New York, 1971.

Bertino, J. R., and Hyrniuk, W. M.: Disorders of Cell Growth, in K. L. Melmon, and H. F. Morrelli (eds.), "Clinical Pharmacology," p. 511, The Macmillan Company, New York, 1972.

Bruce, W. R.: The Action of Chemotherapeutic Agents at the Cellular Level and the Effects of These Agents on Hematopoietic and Lymphomatous Tissue, *Can Cancer Conf,* **7:**53, 1966.

Calabresi, P., and Welch, A. D.: Cytotoxic Drugs, Hormones and Radioactive Isotopes, in L. S. Goodman and A. Gilman (eds.), "The Pharmocological Basis of Therapeutics," The Macmillan Company, New York, 1970.

Carter, S. K.: Single and Combination Nonhormonal Chemotherapy in Breast Cancer, *Cancer,* **30:**1543, 1972.

Cline, M. J.: "Cancer Chemotherapy," W. B. Saunders Company, Philadelphia, 1971.

D'Angio, G. J.: Management of Children with Wilms' Tumor, *Cancer,* **30:**1528, 1972.

Frei, E., and Zubrod, C. G.: Principles of Chemotherapy for Hematologic Neoplasms: in C. Mengel et al. (eds.), "Hematology, Principles and Practice," Year Book Medical Publishers, Inc., Chicago, 1972.

Gilman, A.: The Initial Clinical Trial of Nitrogen Mustard, *Am J Surg,* **105:**574, 1963.

Huggins, C., and Hodges, C. V.: Studies on Prostatic Cancer: I. The Effect of Castration, of Estrogen and of Androgen Injection on Serum Phosphatases in Metastatic Carcinoma of the Prostate, *Cancer Res,* **1:**293, 1941.

Laird, A. K.: Dynamics of Growth in Tumors and in Normal Organisms, *Natl Cancer Inst Monogr,* **30:**15, 1969.

Lewis, J. L.: Chemotherapy of Gestational Choriocarcinoma. *Cancer,* **30:**1517, 1972.

Li, M. C., Hertz, R., and Spencer, D. B.: Effect of Methotrexate Therapy upon Choriocarcinoma and Chorioadenoma, *Proc Soc Exp Biol Med,* **93:**361, 1956.

Mathé, G.: Scientific Basis of Cancer Chemotherapy, *Recent Results Cancer Res,* **21:**1, 1969.

————: Immunotherapy in the Treatment of Acute Lymphoic Leukemia, *Hosp Prac,* **6:**43, 1971.

Morton, D. L., Haskell, C. M., Pilch, Y. H., Sparks, F. C., and Winters, W. D.: Recent Advances in Oncology, *Ann Intern Med,* **77:**431, 1972.

Salmon, S. E., and Apple, M.: Cancer Chemotherapy, in F. H. Meyers, E. Jawetz, and A. Goldfien (eds.), "Review of Medical Pharmacology," Lange Medical Publications, Los Altos, Calif., 1972.

Schabel, F. M., Jr.: The Use of Tumor Growth Kinetics in Planning "Curative" Chemotherapy of Advanced Solid Tumors, *Cancer Res,* **29:**2384, 1969.

Skipper, H. E.: Cancer Chemotherapy is Many Things: G.H.A. Clowes Memorial Lecture, *Cancer Res,* **31:**1173, 1971.

————, and Perry, S.: Kinetics of Normal and Leukemic Leukocyte Populations and Relevance to Chemotherapy, *Cancer Res,* **30:**1883, 1970.

————, Schabel, F. M., Jr., and Wilcox, W. S.: Experimental Evaluation of Potential Anticancer Agents: XIII. On the Criteria and Kinetics Associated with "Curability" of Experimental Leukemia, *Cancer Chemother Rep,* **35:**1, 1964.

Strawitz, J. G.: Cancer Chemotherapy Using Isolation Perfusion, in I. Brodsky, S. B. Kahn, and J. H. Moyer (eds.), "Cancer Chemotherapy," vol. II, p. 443, Grune & Stratton, Inc., New York, 1972.

Sullivan, P. W., and Salmon, S. E.: Kinetics of Tumor Growth and Regression in IgG Multiple Myeloma, *J Clin Invest,* **51:**1697, 1972.

Sullivan, R. D., and Semel, C. J.: Arterial Infusion Cancer Chemotherapy for Solid Tumors. in I. Brodsky, S. B. Kahn, and J. H. Moyer (eds.), "Cancer Chemotherapy," vol. II, p. 453, Grune & Stratton, Inc., New York, 1972.

Immunotherapy

Deckers, P. J., and Pilch, Y. H.: RNA-mediated Transfer of Tumor Immunity: A New Model for Immunotherapy of Cancer, *Cancer,* **28:**1219, 1971.

Halpern, B. N., Biozzi, G., Stiffel, C., and Mouton, D.: Corrélation entre l'activité phagocytaire du système reticulo-endothelial et la proction d'anticorps antibacteriens, *Compt Rend Soc Biol,* **152:**758, 1958.

Klein, E.: Hypersensitivity Reactions at Tumor Site, *Cancer Res,* **29:**2351, 1969.

Lawrence, H. S.: Transfer Factor, *Adv Immuno,* **11:**195, 1969.

McKhann, C. F.: Immunobiology of Cancer, in J. S. Najarian and R. L. Simmons (eds.), "Transplantation" p. 297, Lea & Febiger, Philadelphia, 1972.

Mathé, G., Schwarzenberg, L., and Amiel, J. L.: Bone Marrow, in J. S. Najarian and R. L. Simmons (eds.), "Transplantation," p. 588, Lea & Febiger, Philadelphia, 1972.

Moore, G. E., and Gerner, R. E.: Cancer Immunity: Hypothesis and Clinical Trial of Lymphocytotherapy for Malignant Diseases, *Ann Surg,* **172:**733, 1970.

Morton, D. L.: Immunotherapy of Cancer: Present Status and Future Potential, **30:**1647, 1972.

———, Eilber, F. R., Joseph, W. L., Wood, W. C., Trahan, E., and Ketcham, A. S.: Immunological Factors in Human Sarcomas and Melanomas; A Rational Basis for Immunotherapy, *Ann Surg,* **172:**740, 1970.

———, Haskell, C. M., Pilch, Y. H., Sparks, F. C., and Winter, W. D.: Recent Advances in Oncology, *Ann Intern Med,* **77:**431, 1972.

Old, L. J., Benacerraf, B., Clark, D. A., Carswell, E. A., and

Stockert, E.: The Role of the Reticuloendothelial System in the Host Reaction to Neoplasia, *Cancer Res,* **21:**1281, 1961.

Sumner, W. C., and Foraker, A. C.: Spontaneous Regression of Human Melanoma: Clinical and Experimental Study. *Cancer,* **13:**79, 1960.

Prognosis

Berkson, J., and Gage, R. P.: Specific Methods of Calculating Survival Rates of Patients with Cancer, in G. T. Pack and I. M. Ariel (eds.), "Treatment of Cancer and Allied Diseases," Harper & Row, Publishers, Incorporated, New York, 1958.

Kelly, W. D., and Friesen, S. R.: Do Cancer Patients Want to be Told? *Surgery,* **27:**822, 1950.

Wangensteen, O. H.: Should Patients Be Told They Have Cancer? *Surgery,* **27:**944, 1950.

Psychologic Management

Sherman, C. D., Jr., and Feasel, W. P.: "General Aspects of Cancer," University of Rochester School of Medicine and Dentistry, Rochester, N.Y., 1969–1970. (Syllabus.)

Silverberg, E., and Holleb, A. I.: "Cancer Statistics 1972," American Cancer Society, Inc., New York, (Reprinted from *CA,* **22:**2, 1972.)

Chapter 10
Transplantation

by **Richard L. Simmons, John E. Foker, Richard R. Lower, and John S. Najarian**

Immunobiology of the Allograft

Transplantation (Histocompatibility) Antigens
  The Nature of Histocompatibility Antigens
  The Immunogenetics of Histocompatibility
The Immune Apparatus
Immunologic Events in Allograft Rejection
  Induction of Immunity
    Immunogen Release from the Graft
    Processing of the Immunogens
    Role of the Macrophage in the Induction of Allograft Immunity
    Recognition of the Immunogen by Lymphocytes
    Cellular Interactions during the Induction of Immunity
    Morphological Changes of the Small Lymphocyte in Response to Immunological Challenge
    Proliferation and Differentiation of Stimulated Lymphocytes
  Expression of Immunity
    Role of Specifically Immunized Lymphocytes in Allograft Rejection
    Role of Antibody in Allograft Rejection
Complement
The Clotting System
Interrelationships of the Molecular Cascade Systems
  An Integrated View of the Rejection of Organ Allografts

Circumventing Rejection

Immunosuppression
  Methods Involving the Destruction of Immunocompetent Cells
    Extirpation of Lymphoid Tissue
    Thymectomy
    Thoracic Duct Drainage
    Extracorporeal Irradiation
    Antilymphocyte Globulin
  Methods Preventing the Proliferation of Immunocompetent Cells
    Radiation
    Immunosuppresive Drugs
  Methods Designed to Inhibit the Expression of Immunity
Immunological Tolerance
Immunological Enhancement
Privileged Sites for Allografts
Histocompatibility Matching
  Leukocyte Typing
  Mixed Lymphocyte Culture (MLC)

Clinical Tissue and Organ Transplantation

Skin
Vascular Grafts
  Autograft
  Allograft
Fascia
Tendon
Nerve
Cornea
Bone
Cartilage
  Composite Grafts of Bone and Cartilage
    Epiphyseal Growth Plates
    Osteochondral Grafts
    Transplants of Hemijoints or Whole Joints
Extremity Replantation
Hemopoetic and Lymphoid Tissues
  Bone Marrow
  Thymus
  Spleen and Lymph Node
Endocrine Grafts (Other than the Pancreas)
Pancreas
Gastrointestinal Transplants

Liver
  Experimental Transplantation in Animals
    Orthotopic Transplantation
    Heterotopic Transplantation
  Clinical Liver Transplantation
    Indications
    Precautions
    Technique of Orthotopic Hepatic Transplantation
    Technique of Auxiliary Liver Transplantation
    Operative Complications
    Postoperative Care
    Results
Heart
  Historical Background
  Selection of Patients
  Technique
  Postoperative Care
  Results
Lung
  Autotransplantation
    Experimental Studies
    Clinical Experience
  Allotransplantation
    Experimental Studies
    Clinical Experience
Kidney
  Recipient Selection and Indications for Trans-
    plantation
    Criteria for Selection
    Workup of Potential Recipients and Timing of
      Dialysis
    Preparation for Hemodialysis and Trans-
      plantation
      Principles of Hemodialysis

Selection and Evaluation of Living Donors
  Ethical Problems
Selection of a Cadaver Donor
  Criteria of Brain Death
Organ Harvest
  Related Living Donor
  Cadaver Donor
Preparation of the Recipient for Transplantation
  Nephrectomy
Technique of Renal Transplantation
  Operative Management
  Anesthesia in Anephric Patients
Routine Posttransplant Care
  Routine Posttransplant Laboratory Determi-
    nations
  Prophylactic Immunosuppression
Complications of Renal Transplantation
  Renal Failure
    Early Anuria and Oiliguria
    Rejection
Renal Failure due to Recurrent Disease
  Complications of Immunosuppressive Therapy
Results of Renal Transplantation
  Transplant Registry Results
  Transplantation in Children
  Multiple Transplants
  Rehabilitation

Xenografts

Organ Preservation

Methods on Viable Organ Preservation
  Organ Freezing
Storage of Nonviable Tissues by Freeze-Drying

Man does not burst like a balloon—he falls apart, piece by piece. Clinical organ transplantation is designed to replace the exhausted parts as they fall. Because the immunologic barrier of allograft rejection stands in the way of attaining chimerism between host and graft, immunologists and the surgeons have been working in conjunction since World War II to circumvent the rejection reaction and achieve a real reconstructive surgery. Unfortunately, the problems remain unsolved. Despite the establishment of kidney transplantation as a true therapeutic modality organs are still rejected, and attempts to prevent rejection can be fatal. The field of clinical transplantation, though no longer totally experimental, remains in flux, and apparently well-founded principles are soon washed away. Much of the material presented in this chapter will not survive the decade.

The first part of this chapter discusses the immunobiology of the allograft, its rejection, and the means for retaining the graft. The current and incipient clinical applications of these biologic principles and techniques to the human patient are discussed in the second section.

IMMUNOBIOLOGY OF THE ALLOGRAFT

Tissue or organ grafts between individuals of the same species (allografts, or homografts) are rejected with a vigor proportional to the degree of the genetic disparity between them. Grafts between individuals of different species (xenografts, or heterografts) are rejected even more rapidly. Grafts between identical twins (isografts, isogeneic grafts, or syngeneic grafts), or from an individual to himself (autografts, or autogenous grafts) survive indefinitely once vascular supply has been reestablished to the host.

Allografts normally survive surgical manipulation as well as isografts. If the recipient has not previously encountered the antigens present on the donor graft, the allograft is not morphologically or physiologically distinguishable from the isograft in the early posttransplant period—the rejection process normally takes several days. Medawar, in his classic demonstration of the immunologic nature of the allograft response, noted that skin grafts between randomly selected adult rabbits appeared normal until the fourth or fifth day. At that time inflammation appeared within the graft bed in the form of a dense leukocyte infiltrate which led to necrosis of the entire graft by about the tenth day. Medawar further demonstrated that the rejection process, whatever its complexities, is the result of immunologic mechanisms. Whereas the "first-set rejection" takes place in 10 or 11 days, a second graft from the same rabbit resulted in an accelerated "second-set rejection." This process of first-set and second-set rejection of allogeneic graft takes place whether or not the graft is orthotopic (a graft placed in the anatomic position normally occupied by such tissue) or heterotopic (those grafts placed in abnormal recipient locations). The reaction is immunologically specific for the antigens involved, and the second-set rejections occur only when the recipient has previously encountered the antigens of the first graft.

Transplantation (Histocompatibility) Antigens

Tissue transplanted from one individual to another will be rejected if the new host can recognize that tissue as foreign. Foreignness is equated with the presence of antigens on the donor cells which the host does not possess and thereby recognizes as nonself. Foreign antigens on a tissue or organ graft are considered histocompatibility antigens if they can be related to graft rejection. Any histocompatibility antigen will lead to graft rejection if the antigen is present on donor tissue but absent from the host. In fact, some histocompatibility differences are probably present in all donor-recipient combinations, with the exception of identical twins in man, and inbred strains in other animal species. However, the "strength" of different antigenic incompatibilities can lead to graft rejection within 8 days, and others can permit graft survival of well over 100 days. The strongest antigens are xenogeneic antigens, i.e., those which elicit the rejection of grafts from animals of a different species. One of the weakest histocompatibility antigens is linked to the Y chromosome of male mice, so that female mice will gradually reject grafts from male mice of the same inbred strain.

THE NATURE OF HISTOCOMPATIBILITY ANTIGENS

Histocompatibility alloantigens are products of histocompatibility genes. They are probably present in all tissues, but tissues vary with respect to the relative amount of alloantigen present, and the products of different genetic loci often have different distributions. For example, in the mouse the strong alloantigens governed by the H-2 locus (see Immunogenetics of Histocompatibility, below) are found in high concentration in the spleen and liver and in lymphoid tissue. The kidney, lung, adrenal gland, and gastrointestinal tract contain intermediate amounts of the H-2 alloantigen, and the heart, skeleton, muscles, and brain contain very little. Furthermore, while the mouse H-2 alloantigens are relatively poorly represented on red blood cells, the antigenic products of the weaker H-5 and H-6 histocompatibility loci have a very large quantity of the antigen on the red cells, and a variable to small amount on the cells of liver and spleen. Alloantigens appear early in the course of development—Simmons and Russell found histocompatibility antigenicity expressed at as early a stage as the fertilized egg.

It is generally conceded that histocompatibility antigens are found on the cell surface; however, a certain amount of antigenic activity is also thought to be present on microsomal membranes. Since the plasma membrane is itself a multimolecular complex of lipid, protein, glycoprotein, and carbohydrate, even "purified" membranes are too complex (without further processing) to yield precise information on the specific chemical structure of such components as histocompatibility determinants. The membrane has been disrupted by various methods to release these antigens in biologically reactive forms, so that they might be purified and chemically characterized. In general, several different approaches to membrane extraction have been employed, including treatment with detergents and organic solvents, low-intensity sound, proteolytic enzymes, and solutions of high ionic strength.

The results of these investigations are compatible with the fluid mosaic model for cell membrane structure (Fig. 10-1). This model suggests that the separate histocompatibility antigens are expressed on separate globulin proteins which move freely in the fluid lipid bilayer of the cell membrane. Extensive ultracentrifugal analyses have revealed that the antigens, themselves, are homogenous molecular entities. Determination of sedimentation velocity and molecular weight have shown that the strong human histocompatibility (HL-A) antigens have a sedimentation coefficient ($S_{20'_w}$) of 2.3 and a molecular weight of 31,000 dalton, assuming a partial specific volume of 0.72. The purified antigenic moiety resolves as a single sharp peak upon acrylamide gel electrophoresis under a variety of conditions. Cryptic peptide maps of highly purified antigens and amino acid analyses also suggest their purity. There is additional evidence suggesting that the HL-A determinants are essentially polypeptide in nature and that there are probably less than two residues of lipid on carbohydrate per mole of 31,000. It is difficult, however, to rule out any role of the carbohydrates in the expression of histocompatibility determinants. The differences in amino acid composition of electrophoretically homogenous transplantation antigens suggest that the polypeptide chains possess regions of amino acid sequence variability and constancy. The evidence strongly supports the idea that each antigenic specificity is contained on a separate protein molecule.

THE IMMUNOGENETICS OF HISTOCOMPATIBILITY

The strongest (but not all) transplantation antigens on cell surfaces appear to be the expression of a single complex genetic locus called HL-A in man, H-2 in mice, AGB in rats, etc. Until recently it was generally accepted that the major histocompatibility locus consisted of a series of regions (genes) which coded for antigens detectable both by serologic and transplantation methods. Most recently, this view has been replaced by the so-called two-gene model, which postulates that all serologic and transplantation effects can be explained by assuming the existence of two histocompatibility genes or gene clusters within the larger major histocompatibility region (Fig. 10-2). Thus, the HL-A histocompatibility antigens can be arranged into two series, in which members of the same series show mutual exclusiveness. One region codes for the "first" series of antigens and the other for the "second" series of antigens. Biochemical analysis has shown that antigens coded by the first locus and antigens coded by the second locus are present on separate molecules and they never occur on the same molecule. The two genes on each chromosome are usually inherited together, and each pair is called a *haplotype*. The inheritance of HL-A antigens is illustrated in Fig. 10-2. Nevertheless the two regions (there may be more than two) are separated by a considerable amount of genetic material, which in the mouse has been estimated to include some 500 genes. The two genes are far enough apart for recombination to occur within the major histocompatibility complex in approximately 1 of 200 animals (Fig. 10-2).

The antigens coded by these genes are commonly detected by antisera directed against these antigens. Whether these antigens, which are detected by serologic techniques, truly code for the antigenic determinants that control graft rejection has recently been questioned. It is possible that a locus closely linked to the HL-A complex could actually control the foreignness of a graft. Evidence for this hypothesis lies in the finding that immune stimulation of lymphocytes in culture can occur even between siblings who share all four HL-A antigens.

This hypothetic locus governing all immune stimulation in vitro has been called the *mixed lymphocyte culture* (MLC) locus, but its importance has not yet been determined. Other loci within this same histocompatibility region apparently code for the ability of a person to respond to certain types of antigens (Ir locus). This type of ongoing genetic analysis is particularly important in view of the failure to correlate clinical transplantation results with detectable serologic differences in HL-A antigens (see discussion of tissue typing under Histocompatibility Matching later in this chapter).

The Immune Apparatus

It is now agreed that there is a single hemopoietic stem cell, which is first found in the extraembryonic yolk sac and migrates to various centers for further differentiation. Within these centers progenitor cells for erythrocytes, eosinophils, basophils, neutrophils, and lymphoid cells arise, depending on the local microchemical environment.

Fig. 10-1. Schematic three-dimensional and cross-sectional views of the lipid-globular protein mosaic model with a lipid matrix (the fluid mosaic model). The solid bodies with stippled surfaces represent the globular integral proteins, which at long range are randomly distributed in the plane of the membrane. At short range, some may form specific aggregates, as shown. (*From S. J. Singer and G. L. Nicolson, The Fluid Mosaic Model of the Structure of Cell Membranes, Science, 175:720, 1972.*)

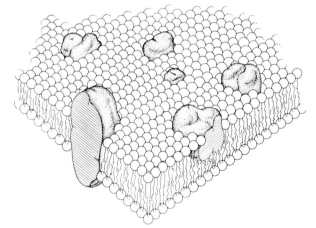

It is likely that the further proliferation of these progenitor stem cells depends on the action of "poietins" which tend to expand the populations of specialized cells in the way that erythropoietin acts on the erythrocyte line (Fig. 10-3).

The lymphoid cell line first appears within two primary (or central) lymphoid tissues. The thymus governs the development of cellular immunity. In birds, the bursa of Fabricius governs the development of humoral immunity. The bursa exists as a clearly defined central lymphoid structure only in birds. The equivalent of the bursa of Fabricius has not been clearly defined in mammals, but there is evidence that a functional bursal equivalent does exist. In man the characteristics of sex-linked agammaglobulinemia of the Bruton type—very low levels of immunoglobulins, levels of circulating lymphocytes within normal limits, and delayed cellular reactivity—suggest that the bursa equivalent has failed to develop.

Both the thymus and the bursa (or its equivalent) are responsible for the further development of the peripheral lymphoid tissues, i.e., spleen, lymph nodes, Peyer's patches. Certain areas of the lymph node can be shown to be dependent on the functional presence of the thymus and bursa. The paracortical regions between the cortical germinal centers and the medulla are dependent on the thymus, while the germinal centers themselves and the medullary cord lymphoid tissue are under the developmental control of the bursal equivalent. Therefore, thymectomy early in the neonatal period or congenital thymic deficiency results in failure of development of the paracortical regions of the lymph nodes. In chickens, bursectomy leads to failure of development of germinal centers and medullary cord lymphoid tissues.

During ontogeny, the thymus is the site of a vigorous cell proliferation. Many of these cells migrate to the paracortical areas of lymph nodes. All such cells which were once dependent on the thymus for their development are

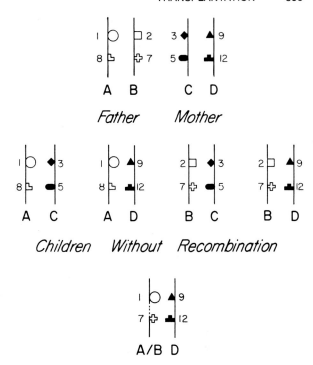

Fig. 10-2. Hypothetic examples of inheritance of HL-A antigens. Four offspring of mating between parents, with chromosomes labeled AB and CD, and one possible result of recombination within the HL-A region are shown. Genes coded for "first series" antigens are indicated at the top of each chromosome, and the genes coded for the "second series" antigens are indicated at the bottom of each chromosome. The antigens determined by the gene are labeled with arabic numbers.

Fig. 10-3. Schematic representation of developmental relations in the lymphoid system. Note that the lymphoid stem cell, which exists in fetal liver and bone marrow, has the capacity to come under the differentiative influence of either of two central lymphoid organs, to develop into either a T cell system or a B cell system. The two separate systems of lymphoid cells subserve separate functions. T cells are responsible for the cellular immunities (cell-mediated immune responses), whereas B cells represent the immunoglobulin-producing and secreting lymphoid cells and plasma cells. (*From R. A. Good and J. Finstad, Structure and Development of the Immune System, in J. S. Najarian and R. L. Simmons (eds.), "Transplantation," p. 26, Lea & Febiger, Philadelphia, 1972.*)

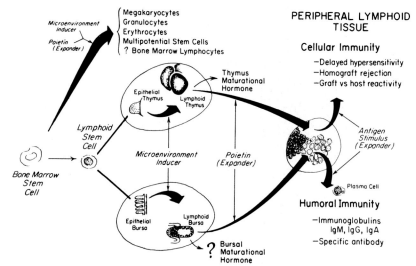

called *T cells*. The T cells represent the immunocompetent cell population responsible for the development of cellular immunity, rather than humoral immunity. These reactions include delayed hypersensitivity reactions as well as many of the early reactions responsible for allograft rejection.

Once these cells have migrated from the thymus, they seldom return. There is some evidence that the thymus produces a "hormone" (thymosin), perhaps a poietin, that is necessary for the maintenance of the full functional capacity of the T cell system. The thymus increases in size until puberty, at which time it begins to atrophy. This atrophy progresses throughout adult life, but the function of the T cell system is maintained by the bone marrow and peripheral lymphoid tissue.

The lymphoid populations in the medullary and far cortical areas of the lymph node are under the developmental influence of the bursa of Fabricius in birds or its equivalent in mammals (Fig. 10-4). A humoral factor similar to that secreted by the thymus may also be at work here in maturing and maintaining the population of immunocompetent cells known as *B cells*. The B cells descend from stem cells in the bone marrow and become responsible for the manufacture of circulating immunoglobulins and thus for humoral immunity (Fig. 10-3).

Although the bursal and thymic developmental systems appear to be independent, they frequently interact. For example, the presence of T cells seems to be necessary for development of immunity against many antigens that primarily elicit a humoral response. They perhaps contribute by recognizing the antigen and enlisting B cells. Thus, thymectomy early in embryonic development, prior to the maturation of the peripheral lymphoid tissues, or thymectomy followed by sublethal irradiation leads to deficiencies not only in the cellular immunity system but also in humoral immunity.

A number of subclassifications of lymphoid cells have developed, and it is likely that new lymphoid cell types and subtypes with differing functions will soon emerge. At present, however, it appears certain that the lymphoid system is the seat of the body's immunologic response and the small mature lymphocytes and the plasma cells are the immunocompetent cells. Once the lymphocytes (T or B cells) have migrated to the peripheral lymphoid tissue, they are fully immunocompetent. It is likely that Burnet's clonal selection theory holds true—a state of preparedness for a certain antigen or group of related antigens exists within a lymphoid cell so that it is capable of responding to only a narrow range of antigenic specificities. Whether this degree of specificity is "built in" or acquired during embryonic or early postnatal life is unknown. Nevertheless, only a small percentage of the lymphocytes in the body will respond to a specific antigen. Conversely, each cell can respond to only a narrow spectrum of antigens.

The B cells appear to be relatively sessile within the germinal centers and the medullary cord lymphoid tissues of lymph nodes and spleen. Their end products, immunoglobulins and antibodies, can interact with foreign antigens at distant sites. The T cells responsible for cell-mediated immunity are of necessity more peripatetic and must migrate to the periphery in order to neutralize foreign antigens. Such T cells, which appear to be "small lymphocytes," have a patterned migration pathway. They migrate from the peripheral blood (from which they enter the lymph nodes or spleen via highly specialized regions in the postcapillary venules), percolate through the lymphoid organs, enter the lymph, pass into the thoracic duct, and return to the bloodstream to begin circulating again.

Immunologic Events in Allograft Rejection

Mature lymphocytes appear to sit in a state of immunologic readiness. Whatever role other cells play in the development of immunity, there is little doubt that the small lymphocyte is the seat, and perhaps the only specific site, of immunologic recognition. The small lymphocyte has the capacity to recognize whether or not a molecule is foreign. Once having reacted to an immunogen, the small lymphocyte, or its descendants, produces the molecules (antibodies

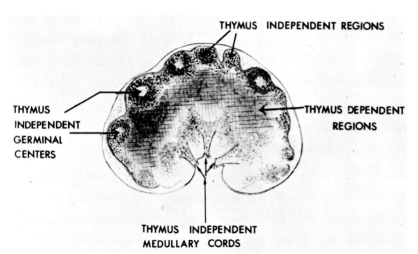

THYMUS INDEPENDENT REGIONS

THYMUS INDEPENDENT GERMINAL CENTERS

THYMUS DEPENDENT REGIONS

THYMUS INDEPENDENT MEDULLARY CORDS

Fig. 10-4. The thymus-dependent and thymus-independent areas are illustrated in this schematic representation of a lymph node. (*From R. A. Good and J. Finstad, Structure and Development of the Immune System, in J. S. Najarian and R. L. Simmons (eds.), "Transplantation," p. 26, Lea & Febiger, Philadelphia, 1972.*)

or cellular receptor sites) that recognize and react with the antigenic determinants of the immunogen.

One of the major proofs in immunology was the demonstration of the ability of a virtually pure suspension of small lymphocytes from the thoracic duct of parental-strain rats to cause a graft-versus-host (GVH) immune reaction in F_1 hybrid animals. Large lymphocytes, in comparison, were considerably less effective in producing a GVH reaction. Similarly transfused small lymphocytes can bring about the adoptive destruction of long-tolerated skin allografts in rats.

Gowans and associates observed that the small lymphocyte did not divide and did not take up tritiated thymidine into deoxyribonucleic acid (DNA) until an appropriate immunogenic stimulus was encountered. When stimulated, the small lymphocyte transformed in the lymphoid tissue to large activated cells. The large lymphocyte population is less effective in producing the GVH reaction, presumably because many of these cells have been recently activated by prior antigenic exposure and are "committed" to these antigens.

Small lymphocytes also carry immunologic memory. Gowans and Uhr showed that thoracic duct lymphocytes taken from rats immunized with phage particles would respond with high antibody titers after transfer to syngeneic irradiated recipients. These cells, or a portion thereof, have a life-span of many months in rats and many years in human beings. It is tempting to conclude that the small lymphocyte can carry out primary, secondary, and memory functions of the lymphoid system for allograft response, if not for all immunologic situations.

INDUCTION OF IMMUNITY

As stated above, the small lymphocyte recognizes the immunogenic determinants and translates that recognition into an immunologic response. The mechanisms of immunogen release and recognition and the mode of translation into antibody formation is unknown although they have been the subject of considerable investigation.

The first phase of the immunologic response has been called the *afferent arc*. It involves the grafting process itself, the release of the immunogenic histocompatibility antigens from the graft, the processing of the immunogens, and the stimulation of the responsive lymphoid cell population.

IMMUNOGEN RELEASE FROM THE GRAFT. The immunogens of a grafted organ, being surface components of the cell membrane, are readily available to the recipient's immune system. They might be shed into either veins or lymphatics and thereby reach the immunocompetent centers, or the immunogens might be recognized by circulating cells of the host immune system. Both mechanisms may be operative. The route of administration of the immunogen is important in determining the onset of immunity, as well as its strength. The intravenous route will evoke the earliest response, but it is also the poorest immunogenic route and results in a less profound and less persistent state of immunity. The subcutaneous and the intraperitoneal avenues are more effective, and an intradermal route is the most efficient immunizing route. Thus permanent strong immunity follows intradermal injection of allogeneic cells, and only weak immunity results from the intravenous infusion of dissociated cells. These findings may well account for the capacity of vascularized allografts (i.e., kidney, liver, heart) to withstand graft rejection better than nonvascularized grafts (i.e., skin), which must develop a blood supply as they heal. Skin grafts appear to immunize primarily via the lymphatic system, whereas vascularized organ grafts immunize by the bloodstream, a far less immunogenic route.

PROCESSING OF THE IMMUNOGENS. There is some evidence that lymphocytes may migrate to a graft and become immunized there. Most sensitization to allografts, however, probably takes place within the peripheral lymphoid tissue of the host to which the immunogens migrate. Nossal and associates studied the travels of microgram quantities of ^{125}I-labeled *Salmonella adelaide* flagella after injection into rats. By combined electron micrograph and radioautography, it was found to be taken up by both the medullary and cortical areas of lymph node follicles, but no studies using labeled transplantation antigens have been performed. Flagellar immunogen trapped in the medullary sinuses was overwhelmingly located in macrophages. Uptake of the immunogen by medullary macrophages may be an important part of sensitization and is compatible with the hypothesis that macrophages process the immunogen as the first step toward immunity. There appeared, however, to be no unique spatial relationship between the immunogen macrophages and the plasma cells within the medulla and no evidence for the intracellular location of immunogen in plasma cells. Therefore, by the admittedly restricted morphologic criteria, Nossal et al. could find no proof of the importance of medullary uptake of immunogen in the development of immunity.

The remainder of the injected flagellar immunogen lodged in the cortical folliculllar areas of the lymph node. In contrast to the immunogen taken up by the medullary macrophages, the immunogen in the follicular area was retained in an extracellular location for as long as 3 weeks. It was most frequently found at or near the surface of fine cellular processes, usually in the branches of dendritic reticular cells. An important finding would seem to be that the antigen-containing processes of the reticular cells often interdigitate with the equally fine processes of lymphoctyes (Fig. 10-5). The long residence of immunogens on these exposed positions could allow the development of immunity among the neighboring lymphocytes. Evidence of this development is the finding of *transformed lymphocytes* in the area. These transformed cells are identical morphologically to lymphocytes responding to antigens in vitro. When the rats had been previously sensitized to the flagellar antigen the number of these responding cells in the cortical area was greatly increased.

Admittedly, these morphologic events are the response of an "experimental animal" to a bacterial flagellar immunogen, but nonetheless the events should be applicable to histocompatibility immunogens arriving at a lymph node.

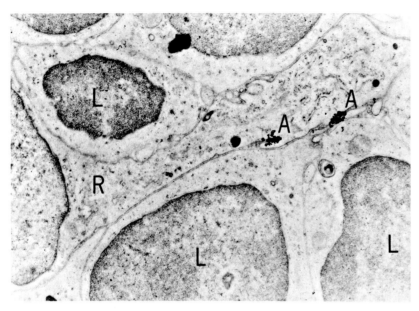

Fig. 10-5. An electron microscope radio-autograph of a primary lymph node follicle which includes a reticular cell (*R*) and several lymphocytes (*L*). The labeled antigen (*A*) is located within or near surface invaginations of the reticular cell membrane and in close proximity to the lymphocytes. This relationship of lymphocytes, reticular cells, and antigens is appealing as a site of immunization. (*From G. J. V. Nossal, A. Abbot, J. Mitchell, and Z. Lummus, Antigens in Immunity: XV. Ultrastructural Features of Antigen Capture in Primary and Secondary Lymphoid Follicles, J Exp Med, 127:277, 1968.*)

It is not clear, however, whether the lymph node represents a mere way station for the antigen which happens to be structurally advantageous for the development of immunity or whether it possesses unique conditions for essential cell-to-cell contact. The ensnarement of the immunogen on the surface of the dendritic reticular cell may only enhance the chance of contact with a receptive lymphocyte. Alternatively, the role of this cell may be more complex and may include either the physical preparation of the immunogen or a function as an inducer cell to the differentiation of the lymphocytes.

ROLE OF THE MACROPHAGE IN THE INDUCTION OF ALLOGRAFT IMMUNITY. Certain data indicate that the macrophage may participate early in the afferent arc and function as processor of antigen. Macrophages gathered from the peritoneum of normal mice are required to induce antibody formation in vivo, after exposure to *Shigella* antigen in vitro. Other studies have shown that following a 24-hour incubation of antigen and macrophages with lymphoid cells, the macrophages could be removed without diminution of the subsequent antibody response. The macrophage response, including ingestion and processing of antigen, is therefore necessary, but its job is complete and the information is transferred to lymphoid cells within a single day.

Considerable investigation has been carried out to determine the precise role of the macrophage. Fishman incubated either bacteriophage or hemocyanin antigens with peritoneal macrophages, and a hemogenate from the cells. Incubation of this subcellular fraction with a suspension of lymph node cells led to an antibody response 5 days later. Thus a substance recovered from an intracellular location in macrophages can stimulate the induction of antibody production by lymphocytes in vitro. Control experiments, in which bacteriophages were incubated with lymph node cells, produced no significant phage-neutralizing antibody.

Other investigations have minimized the role of intra-cellular processes during interaction of the antigen with the macrophage. Three possible mechanisms of macrophage-immunogen interaction are indicated in Fig. 10-6.

RECOGNITION OF THE IMMUNOGEN BY LYMPHOCYTES. The center of the immune response lies in the reaction of the lymphocyte to the immunogen. This most certainly requires direct interaction of the lymphocyte with the antigen or its products, since the most striking aspect of the immune response is its specificity. For each unique stimulus a distinctive population of antibodies or immune cells are elicited which show a greater complementarity for the specific inciting determinants than for structures resembling these antigens. The specificity of the immune response provides an important clue regarding the nature of the antigen receptors on the antigen recognition cells. The receptor sites must be at least as discriminatory as the antibody-combining sites or the cellular recognition sites on hypersensitive cells. It is probable that the receptors on B lymphocytes are antibodies themselves. This evidence has been based on (1) the ability of antisera to immunoglobulins to transform the cells, (2) the ability of radioactive antigens to interfere with the immune responsiveness of the cells, (3) inhibition of the response of hapten-sensitive cells by the haptens themselves, (4) the removal of these cells by passage through antigen-coated columns, and (5) the direct demonstration of immunoglobulin on lymphoid cell membranes.

The demonstration of immunoglobulin on cells which are thought to be responsible for delayed hypersensitivity reactions (including allograft rejection) has been difficult to demonstrate. Only Greeves et al. have shown inhibition of purified protein derivative (PPD) stimulation of tuberculin-sensitive cells by antisera to the light-chain component of the immunoglobulin, and most investigators cannot demonstrate that T cells possess immunoglobulins on their surfaces. It is possible, however, that not enough immunoglobulins are present on the surfaces of T cells to be detectable by immunofluorescent techniques or that

Fig. 10-6. Schematic presentation of the possible ways reticular cells and mobile macrophages could participate in the afferent limb of immunity. The first possibility (A) is that the reticular cell–lymphocyte interaction is a surface phenomenon in which the reticular cell retains the immunogen in an exposed position facilitating recognition by the lymphocyte. The second (B) and third (C) mechanisms are similar in that the immunogen is ingested and processed by macrophages. In both, the result of this digestion is the production of RNA, which apparently has the ability to transfer specific sensitivity to lymphocytes. The question is whether a portion of the immunogen is linked to the RNA molecule (B) or not (C) and thus whether the immunogen or the RNA conveys the specificity. (From J. E. Foker, R. L. Simmons, and J. S. Najarian, Allograft Rejection: I. The Induction of Immunity: The Afferent Arc, in J. S. Najarian and R. L. Simmons (eds.), "Transplantation," p. 63, Lea & Febiger, Philadelphia, 1972.)

THEORETICAL MODES OF IMMUNOGEN PROCESSING AND PRESENTATION TO LYMPHOID CELLS

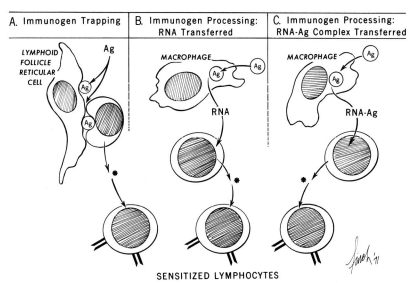

the immunoglobulins on T cells are of a different type. Mitchison has suggested that there is a unique, nonsecretable immunoglobulin class, "IgX," bound on the surface of T cells.

It must be remembered that most of the data discussed and theories presented relate to cells immune to an immunogen. For these cells the recognition molecules (antibody or IgX) may be the product of prior exposure to the immunogen. The nature of the recognition molecule on a true immunologically virgin cell is less clear. The recognition molecule may prove to be the same. Burnet's clonal selection theory would suggest this possibility. This theory proposes that clones of cells reactive to a specific antigen arise, probably by somatic mutation, prior to antigen exposure. The cells are precommitted to the immunogen before encountering it and are not potentially reactive to all immunogens. The molecule these cells use to recognize their complementary immunogen might be immunoglobulin or a form of cell-associated immunoglobulin among T cells.

CELLULAR INTERACTIONS DURING THE INDUCTION OF IMMUNITY. The reaction of an immunogen with an antigen receptor will trigger the cellular response necessary either for antibody production or cell-mediated immunity. Although the specific combination of immunogen and receptor activates the lymphocyte, interactions with other cells are necessary to the development of immunity. One example, involving the macrophage and its role in antigen processing, has previously been discussed. The relation between macrophage and lymphocyte is only one of a number of cellular interactions which may be necessary to transform an uncommitted lymphocyte into a specifically immune cell.

Most studies seem to indicate that there is a cooperative effect between T cells and B cells which results in specifically immune cells. When adult thymus and bone mar-

row cells were injected together with sheep red blood cells into an irradiated recipient, hemolysin-producing colonies formed in the normal way. These two cell types, acting synergistically, were able to form functional (antibody-producing) units. Together their competence was similar to the mixed T and B cell population of spleen, lymph nodes, or thoracic duct. Alone neither the bone marrow nor thymocytes had such competence. Thus, the bone marrow must contain immunocompetent cells which will produce antibody only under the influence of the thymus. The relevance of this hemolysin-producing system to allograft rejection was experimentally established by Globerson and Auerbach. Thymus tissue restored the competence of spleen slices from irradiated animals to evoke a rejection reaction in vitro. Presumably the more immature radioresistant cells within the spleen became immunocompetent under the influence of thymic factors.

All studies of the cooperativeness of T cells and B cells have shown that the B cells, not the T cells, are the specific effector cells. Nossal et al. studied antibody-forming cells arising in the irradiated mouse reconstituted with thymus and bone marrow cells. Using chromosomal markers they found a preponderance of the antibody-forming cells were of bone marrow origin. Therefore, in either combination, the bulk of observed immunologic responses is produced by cells newly enlisted from the bone marrow. In experiments with the GVH reaction the cells derived from the bone marrow also proved to be the effector cells. The thymus cells did not themselves mediate the reaction and acted only in recruitment.

One function of the thymus-derived cells in these experiments seems to be recognition of the immunogen. These cells must have contact with immunogen in some systems prior to interacting with bone marrow cells. When thymocytes were injected into an irradiated thymectomized animal, the spleen cells removed from that animal would not respond to an immunogen in a second thymectomized host unless the first host was also injected with that immunogen. Thus, the helper effect of the thymus results from a specific interaction with the immunogen. The recognition function of the thymocytes is important in the allograft situation. When C3H mouse thymus and CBA mouse bone marrow cells were used to reconstitute thymectomized irradiated CBA mice, skin grafts of the C3H strain were not rejected by the reconstituted animal.

Some data indicate that part of the thymus effect is mediated by a humoral factor. Thymosin, apparently an endocrine product of the thymus, will at least partially restore both antibody production and the ability to produce the GVH reaction in neonatally thymectomized mice. In contrast thymosin was not able to return adult, thymectomized, lethally irradiated mice, given syngeneic bone marrow, to antibody production against sheep cells. But even in adult animals a humoral factor is of importance in delayed reaction. Thymocytes that were encased in a cell-impermeable filter reconstituted the ability of bone marrow cells to produce a rejection reaction in vitro.

In summary, the cell-to-cell relations in allograft rejection are still hazy, but the preceding evidence suggests the following sequence (Fig. 10-7): An allograft is first recognized by long-lived memory cells if the immunogens are familiar to the host. If not, recognition takes place in the regional lymphoid tissue or by circulating uncommitted lymphocytes. The cells accomplishing the recognition are T cells, but thereafter the bulk of the specifically sensitized cells are drawn from the bone marrow. The B cells thus serve as a source of uncommitted cells which can be matured and sensitized, and T cells seem capable not only of responding to a given antigen but also of recruiting B cells. The details of the journey of the recruited effector cells remain obscure, but residence in lymphoid tissue may be necessary to the final induction of competence before migration to the graft. Even in the adult animal, a thymic influence is required at some stage of the developmental sequence of the infiltrating cells.

MORPHOLOGIC CHANGES OF THE SMALL LYMPHOCYTE IN RESPONSE TO IMMUNOLOGIC CHALLENGE. Scothorne and McGregor first described the cellular changes which occurred in the regional lymph nodes and spleen following the placement of skin allografts in the rabbit. In these nodes, large lymphoid cells appeared which stained with methyl green pyronine, indicating ribonucleic acid (RNA) synthesis. Hall and Doty studied the lymph draining the skin allograft sites in sheep and found many large basophilic cells; lymph from autograft sites contained few of these cells. Again the supposition was that lymphoid cells had enlarged, or had transformed in response to allograft stimulation, and that the transformation involved RNA synthesis. Cells of this morphologic description are also found as a major component of the diverse invading population of cells in kidney allografts.

The development of cell culture techniques allows a more detailed study of the morphologic and molecular responses of the lymphocyte than is possible in the intact animal (Fig. 10-8). When lymphocytes from the peripheral blood are cultured in serum and a simple culture medium, little morphologic change is seen over a period of several days. The lymphocytes remain small and presumably still correspond to the resting state of the cruising peripheral lymphocytes. If the lymphocytes are taken from previously sensitized animals and cultured in the presence of the antigen, many are transformed after several days from small cells with dense nuclei and scanty cytoplasm into cells with larger, more open nuclei, prominent nucleoli, and considerably more capacious, polysome-filled cyto-

SCHEMATIC PRESENTATION OF T-CELL AND B-CELL INTERACTIONS

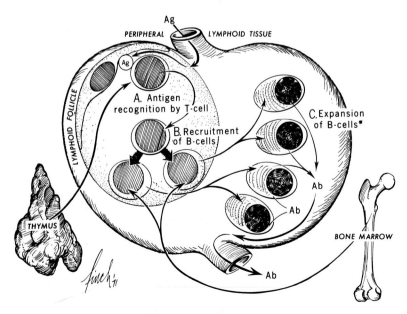

Fig. 10-7. The postulated relation between T cells and B cells is schematically presented within a lymph node. Antigen (*Ag*) in the lymph draining the site of an allograft enters the regional lymph node and is entrapped on the surface of a reticular cell within the lymphoid follicle. Recognition of the antigen is made by a T cell (*A*). The antigen stimulates the T cell to enlist, by an unknown mechanism, B cells from the bone marrow (*B*). The B cells, in turn, divide and differentiate into mature immunocompetent cells (*C*). The terminal cells here are plasma cells and produce antibody (*Ab*), but cells capable of producing delayed hypersensitivity may also result. (*From J. E. Foker, R. L. Simmons, and J. S. Najarian, Allograft Rejection: I. The Induction of Immunity: The Afferent Arc, in J. S. Najarian and R. L. Simmons (eds.), "Transplantation," p. 63, Lea & Febiger, Philadelphia, 1972.*)

plasm. The lessened density of the nucleus by electron micrography is correlated with the presence of more euchromatin, which in turn is the form of chromatin active in RNA production. The cells with predominantly dense heterochromatin in the nuclei are relatively quiescent. The cytoplasm also increases, and the expansion of the polysome population in the transformed cells presumably greatly increases the protein-synthesizing capability.

Allogenic stimulation between two populations in cell cultures has become the basis of one clinical test of histocompatibility. The amount of immunogenic stimulation and hence blast transformation is measured by the uptake of tritiated thymidine. The ability of histocompatibility antigens on intact cells to stimulate lymphocyte transformation is compelling evidence that similar cell activation occurs in vivo when an organ is allografted. Furthermore, this suggests the applicability of the in vitro work on transformation to the allograft situation.

The teleologic conclusion is that the circulating small lymphocyte is a peripatetic nucleus conserving energy and synthetic tasks while awaiting immunologic stimulation. After antigenic challenge, it converts to a form which is able to synthesize effector molecules in larger numbers.

PROLIFERATION AND DIFFERENTIATIONS OF STIMU-LATED LYMPHOCYTES. Stimulation of lymphocytes by histocompatibility antigens results in DNA synthesis and cell replication after gene activation takes place. The initial bursts of protein and RNA synthesis are followed by DNA synthesis which is apparent within 48 hours and is maximal approximately at 96 hours. As expected, numerous mitoses appear at about the same time. Dutton and Mishell have provided evidence that lymphoid differentiation to antibody-producing cells is accompanied by cellular proliferation. By combining uptake of tritiated thymidine with a cellular assay of antibody production (Jerne plaque assay) they found virtually all the antibody-forming cells had taken up large amounts of label, presumably synthesizing DNA. In addition, they discovered a lag period of 24 to 36 hours before DNA synthesis began. These results argue that production of antibodies involves cellular differentiation and requires proliferation. Not all results have agreed with this interpretation, however, and some experiments have indicated that antibody production is possible in the absence of cell proliferation.

DNA synthesis and cell division seem to be an important part of producing a population of immunologically competent cells. The descendants of this proliferation, however, are not uniform, and a progression of cell types results from the original immunogenic stimulus. Sercarz and Coons postulated at least three distinct stages (X, Y, and Z) in the development of immunologically competent cells (Fig. 10-9). The first level is inhabited by the uncommitted but potentially responsive X cell. Following activation by an antigen, X cell development (and presumably differentiation and division) leads to the Y cell, which, in addition to acquiring some immunologic capability, continues to multiply. The immunologic memory cell which accounts for the anamnestic response is postulated to be one consequence of these cell divisions. The Z cell, the antibody-producing cell (or immune B cell), is the result

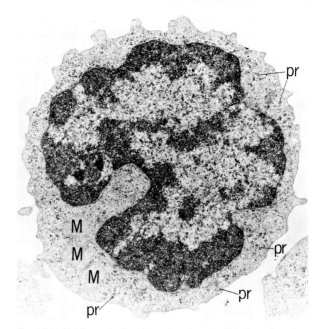

Fig. 10-8. Rat thoracic duct large lymphocyte. This large lymphocyte has a larger, more open nucleus than that of the small lymphocyte. In addition, many polyribosomes (*pr*) and several mitochondria (*M*) are visible. (*Courtesy of Joseph D. Feldman, M.D. From J. E. Foker, R. L. Simmons, and J. S. Najarian, Allograft Rejection: I. The Induction of Immunity: The Afferent Arc, in J. S. Najarian and R. L. Simmons (eds.), "Transplantation," p. 63, Lea & Febiger, Philadelphia, 1972.*)

of continued differentiation. Progression from the Y to the Z cell may require a second contact with the antigen.

For the immunoglobulin-producing cell line, the presumed Z cell is the plasma cell which has an abundance of rough endoplasmic reticulum engaged in the specialized production of antibody. Conversion from a transformed cell to a plasma cell is seen within a few days of grafting, in both organ allografts and the lymphoid tissues stimulated by these transplants. Although an equivalent level of morphologic differentiation has not been identified with certainty within the T cell line, a similar progression probably takes place.

EXPRESSION OF IMMUNITY

The efferent arc of immunity begins with the recognition of the antigen by presensitized cells or antibodies. Recognition in the efferent limb requires previously committed cells, whereas afferent recognition is restricted to immunologically uncommitted cells. The mechanisms of recognition in both the afferent and efferent arcs may, however, prove to be similar.

The recognition of antigens by sensitized cells or antibodies marks the beginning of the active effort of disposal of the foreign graft, but the reaction of an antibody or an immune cell with a graft antigen will not by itself destroy the graft. The recognition phase merely triggers the activation of several cascading enzyme systems which include the complement, clotting, and probably the kinin pathways. In addition, a number of cellular mediators

POSTULATED STAGES OF LYMPHOCYTE DIFFERENTIATION AND ANTIBODY PRODUCTION

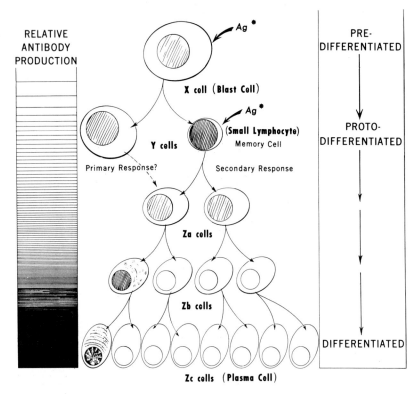

Fig. 10-9. Stages of lymphocyte differentiation. The development of antibody-producing cells is schematically represented here using the X, Y, and Z nomenclature of Sercarz and Coons. Antigenic stimulation (* perhaps requiring prior macrophage processing) of an immunoblast (X cell) leads to cell division and production of a Y cell able to produce a primary immune response. This cell might produce the IgM immunoglobulin characteristic of the primary response. Subsequent division and differentiation by this cell may occur, and the more mature Z cells may be produced later in the primary response. Small lymphocyte memory cells may also result from this initial encounter with antigen. Subsequent antigenic stimulation or the continued presence of antigen would produce a secondary response. Progressive differentiation of the Z cells in association with cell division would occur. The plasma cell (Zc) is the final stage of differentiation. In the secondary response IgG antibody is the major immunoglobulin produced. As the cellular differentiation passes through the predifferentiated, proto-differentiated, and differentiated stages shown, the corresponding ability to produce antibody increases from none to low levels to high levels of synthesis. (*From J. S. Foker, R. L. Simmons, and J. S. Najarian, Allograft Rejection: I. The Induction of Immunity: The Afferent Arc, in J. S. Najarian and R. L. Simmons (eds.), "Transplantation," p. 63, Lea & Febiger, Philadelphia, 1972.)*

(lymphocytes, macrophages, platelets, and polymorphonuclear leukocytes) are recruited both as a consequence of the specific immunologic reaction itself and as a result of the subsequent enzymatic events. All play an active role in disposing of the allograft. Thus, the efferent limb of the allograft reaction has both an immunologically specific (recognition) phase and an immunologically nonspecific (effector or amplification) phase.

ROLE OF SPECIFICALLY IMMUNIZED LYMPHOCYTES IN ALLOGRAFT REJECTION. Until a dozen years ago the specifically sensitized lymphocyte was believed to affect rejection primarily by direct contact with the grafted cells. Murphy first suggested this function in a series of experiments reported in 1926. He observed the appearance of lymphoid cells at the junction of a skin allograft and the host. Nevertheless, polymorphonuclear leukocytes (PMNs) and eosinophils may be present, and plasma cells may be visible during the later stages of the rejection process. Electron micrographs have shown the "rejection cells" to be composed of a variety of mononuclear forms, usually with ample mitochondria and a small complement of endoplasmic reticulum.

The presence of inflammatory cells at the time and site of graft rejection has always had a strong influence on immunobiologic thinking. The earliest and simplest explanation was that sensitized lymphocytes both recognized and destroyed the graft, but debate has long raged on the relative importance of sensitized cells and antibody in recognition of an allograft. Recognition in both cases is

probably provided by antibodylike molecules which for the sensitized cell are attached to the cell surface. The question now centers on the relative importance of antibody from B cells and sensitized cells from the T cell line in initiating allograft rejection. Immune cells and antibody can both recruit immunologically nonspecific cells and molecules to produce damage of the target cells.

The question of whether allografts were rejected by cells or antibody was investigated in the classic experiments of Mitchison and Dube. They showed that specific sensitivity to grafts could be transferred by means of lymphoid cells from one individual to another, but not by means of serum even when high titers of antibody could be demonstrated in the donor. Although the conclusions have been challenged in more recent years, the basic findings were frequently confirmed, and passive transference of transplantation immunity of skin grafts with immune serum has always been difficult.

Further substantiation of cellular participation in allograft immunity was provided by Brent et al. They showed that skin allograft immunity in guinea pigs could be made to express itself as a typical delayed-type hypersensitivity reaction. When living cells or "cell-free antigenic material" from a skin graft donor were injected intradermally into a guinea pig who had rejected the skin of that donor, a tuberculinlike reaction was seen at the rejection site. Furthermore, when lymphoid cells from the sensitized recipient were injected intradermally into the original allograft donor, a similar reaction was seen. The "transfer reaction"

ACTIVITIES OF LYMPHOCYTES IN ALLOGRAFT REJECTION

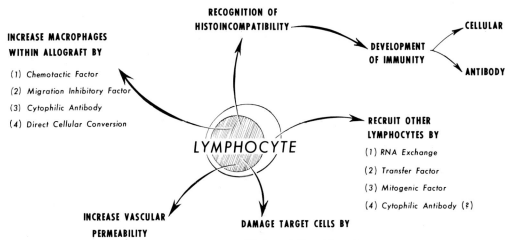

INCREASE MACROPHAGES WITHIN ALLOGRAFT BY

(1) *Chemotactic Factor*

(2) *Migration Inhibitory Factor*

(3) *Cytophilic Antibody*

(4) *Direct Cellular Conversion*

RECOGNITION OF HISTOINCOMPATIBILITY

DEVELOPMENT OF IMMUNITY

CELLULAR

ANTIBODY

LYMPHOCYTE

RECRUIT OTHER LYMPHOCYTES BY

(1) *RNA Exchange*

(2) *Transfer Factor*

(3) *Mitogenic Factor*

(4) *Cytophilic Antibody (?)*

INCREASE VASCULAR PERMEABILITY

DAMAGE TARGET CELLS BY

(1) *Cytotoxic Factor(s)*

(2) *Antibody Triggered Systems*

Fig. 10-10. Complex of activities carried out by lymphocytes in allograft rejection. Lymphocytes are responsible for the original recognition of tissue incompatibility and for the subsequent development of cellular and humoral (antibody) immunity. In addition, sensitized lymphocytes would seem able to injure target cells directly or at least release antibodies that can initiate damage. They may expand the population of specifically immune cells by exchanging RNA, transfer factor, mitogenic factor, or cytophilic antibody. In an analogous way they can recruit immunologically nonspecific macrophages by releasing chemotactic and migration inhibition factors, releasing cytophilic antibody, or by directly converting to macrophages. Finally, the release of a factor that increases vascular permeability causes induration and edema. Most of the recruitment factors, whether for macrophages or lymphocytes, have been studied only in vitro, and the functional importance for allograft rejection is unknown. (*From J. S. Najarian and J. E. Foker, Allograft Rejection: II. The Expression of Immunity: The Efferent Arc, in J. S. Najarian and R. L. Simmons (eds.), "Transplantation," p. 94, Lea & Febiger, Philadelphia, 1972.*)

is mediated by leukocytes or peritoneal exudate cells, but not by serum.

Another demonstration of the importance of cells in transplantation was obtained from the studies of Weaver et al., who showed sustained survival of allogenic cells enclosed in cell-impermeable millipore chambers. These cells survived not only in unsensitized recipients but also in recipients who had previously been sensitized by the donor tissue. It was believed at that time that antibodies and complement diffused freely into such chambers, but Amos and Wakefield later showed that these molecules diffuse poorly into millipore chambers of that type.

Najarian and Feldman were among the first to raise doubts that virtually unaided sensitized cells both recognized and rejected allografts. They showed that the cellular infiltrate seen at the sites of delayed hypersensitivity reactions (including first-set skin allograft rejection) contained few specifically sensitized cells. Tritium-labeled lymphoid cells from specifically sensitized animals were transferred to isogenic recipients at the time the antigenic stimulus was given. Yet these cells comprised less than 1 percent

of the infiltrating cellular population at the site of the graft toward which their specific sensitivity was directed. These results were independently confirmed by the team of McClusky, Benacerrof, and McClusky, and also by Prendergast. Thus, it became apparent that a small number of specifically sensitized lymphoid cells could initiate the rejection reaction but that the completion of the reaction appeared to require many nonsensitized mononuclear cells, as well as PMNs, eosinophils, and plasma cells. Furthermore, it raised the question of whether or not the immune cells were operating at a distance from the graft and had sent antibody as their mediator (Fig. 10-10).

In Vitro Lysis of Target Cells by Lymphocytes. The specifically sensitized lymphoid cells which collect at the site of an allograft have long been thought to damage the donor tissues directly. Recent in vitro studies support such a role for the specifically sensitized lymphocyte.

Govaerts first demonstrated the apparent ability of a sensitized lymphocyte to kill an antigen-bearing target cell in vitro. He incubated lymphocytes from dogs, sensitized by kidney transplantation, with cultured cells from the remaining kidney of the transplant donor. Maximal destruction of the kidney target cells reached 50 percent after 48 hours. No detectable antibody was found. Similar experiments, in which the source of the sensitizing or target cells were varied, produced the same result; immune lymphoid cells will damage a majority of the target cells they encounter within about 48 hours.

In these experiments direct contact between the sensitized lymphocyte and the target cell appeared to be important. Appendages from the lymphocytes have been described which touch target cells, but such projections have also been found in mixed lymphocyte culture (MLC) extending to both macrophages and lymphoblasts. The ameboid lymphocyte contacts the target cells with its uropod and remains attached for 10 minutes. The lymphocyte then moves off, and 10 to 20 minutes later the target cells lyse. Although this contact may be important, it does not identify the mechanism of cell membrane damage, and a variety of cytotoxic agents have been found which may be released by the lymphocytes. Such cytotoxic factors may well be the effector agent of cell-mediated immunity.

Effector Molecules Released by Activated Lymphocytes. The release of cytotoxic factors by lymphocytes infiltrating an allograft would be the most direct way these cells could damage foreign tissue, but it may not be the most efficient. Several other kinds of molecules have been found to be released by stimulated immune cells. In general these factors work by initiating immunologically nonspecific mechanisms. These pathways may prove to be the most effective means whereby an allograft is rejected.

Two factors released by immune lymphoid cells in the presence of the target antigen have similar properties and may be the same. Under the individual experimental circumstances, one is *migration inhibitory factor* (MIF), and the other is *chemotactic factor* (CF). The principal consequence of the release of MIF and CF is to increase the number of activated macrophages in the area of the stimulated lymphocytes. This mechanism for the amplification of the nonspecific cells infiltrating an allograft will be discussed later in the section.

A *mitogenic factor* has also been found that will stimulate blast cell transformation in normal lymphocyte cultures. It can be found in the supernatants of MLCs and after the addition of specific antigen to human being or guinea pig sensitized lymphocytes. There may be more than one mitogenic factor present. The substance which stimulates cell division among lymphocytes is probably immunologically nonspecific and may more properly belong in the discussion of the afferent arc of immunity. Its relevance to allograft rejection is unknown.

Transformed lymphocytes appear to produce a *vascular permeability factor* in addition to cytotoxic agents. On injection to an experimental animal it will produce the induration characteristic of a delayed hypersensitivity reaction. At this time, little else is known about the permeability factor(s), and no description of the effect, if any, in allograft rejection has been made. A prominent feature, however, of the rejecting organ allograft is edema.

The list of factors given off by specifically stimulated lymphocytes will almost certainly continue to grow. Further investigation should elucidate the role played by these molecules in allograft immunity. To date most have been investigated only in in vitro model systems.

Two other factors should not be forgotten. They differ from the preceding in that they are immunologically specific. *Transfer factor* is released on the interaction of the sensitized cells with antigen and confers specific immunity on nonsensitized lymphocytes. Lastly, *antibodies* themselves can be produced by the interaction of sensitized lymphocytes with specific antigen. Such antibodies could have a variety of roles, and though initially considered to be of little importance in classic allograft immunity, they have been shown subsequently to be of great importance.

Recruitment of Specifically Sensitized Cells. It is apparent that the few specifically sensitized cells which migrate to the site of the allograft cannot be totally responsible for graft death. A number of mechanisms have now been uncovered which allow the specifically sensitized cells to amplify their graft-destructive potential at the graft site. These can be broadly classified into two groups: (1) those which increase the number of specifically sensitized cells and (2) those which are nonspecific in nature.

It is likely that the specifically immune cell, upon encountering the antigen which elicited its maturation, can recruit specifically sensitized cells from unsensitized lymphocytes in their environment. Among the antibody-producing population there is evidence that the number of active cells is expanded in this way. When the kinetics of plaque-forming (antibody-producing) cells were looked at in one experiment, more cells arose than could be accounted for by cell division. Recruitment of lymphocytes producing cellular hypersensitivity may be accomplished in several ways: A recognition molecule manufactured and released by the specifically sensitized cell could be attached to the cell surfaces of adjacent cells. Such factors would quickly convert lymphoid cells into specific cells which on encountering the antigen could transform and become metabolically active. The impressment of the cells in this manner would allow quick amplification of the number of sensitized cells.

One recognition molecule that could be transferred from lymphocyte to lymphocyte is specific antibody. Clark and Weiss showed that immunoglobulin synthesis of cultured and stimulated lymphocytes appeared simultaneously with their ability to inflict cellular damage. Cell-bound or cytophilic antibody released in the presence of unsensitized lymphocytes does adhere to those lymphocytes. It has not yet been established, however, that cytophilic antibody can enlarge the lymphocyte population specifically sensitized to an allograft.

A second recognition molecule which may expand the sensitized cell population is the transfer factor described by Lawrence. Transfer factor is dialyzable material of less than 10,000 molecular weight which can be extracted from specifically sensitized lymphocytes, and will convert previously unsensitized lymphocytes to a specific antigen-responsive state both in vitro and in vivo. When the converted lymphocytes are subsequently exposed to the specific antigen, they will transform and proliferate. Transfer factor itself appears not to be an immunoglobulin but has a polypeptide-polynucleotide composition, although it is resistant to pancreatic ribonuclease (RNase). Transfer factor may act as a transmitter of immunologic information. Much controversy revolves around its presence and nature, however, and some writers regard it as transferred antigen or question its importance in allograft rejection.

Another potential mechanism for recruitment of specifically sensitized cells would be by transfer of the information needed to produce recognition molecules. In addition to the possible role of RNA in the transfer of processed antigenic information from macrophage to lymphocyte, RNA from sensitized cells may enlist other lymphocytes into specific immunity. Mannick and Egdahl were the first to extract RNA from the nodes of rabbits immunized to skin allografts. This RNA fraction conferred the capacity to produce transfer reactions on normal lymphoid cells when they were injected into the skin of the graft donor. In later experiments, they demonstrated that rabbit spleen cells exposed in vitro to RNA extracted from the lymph nodes of immune rabbits would sensitize isogenic rabbits to subsequent grafts from the skin donor. These RNA extracts would confer sensitivity to the immunizing antigen on lymph node cells as measured by the ability to inhibit the migration of macrophages or the production of delayed skin hypersensitivity.

The obvious conclusion has been that the transfer and incorporation of a messenger RNA (mRNA) will establish immunity in lymphoid cells. Although these experiments suggest such a conclusion, more understanding of the development of immunity at the molecular level will be needed before it can be established. In addition, it has not been shown that the RNA comes from lymphocytes. The RNA could be from macrophages.

This discussion has assumed that lymphocytes, if stimulated to differentiate, will become increasingly immunologically specific. Other pathways of differentiation, however, may be opened to a lymphocyte. Several studies indicate that lymphoid cells can convert to macrophages. Macrophages in turn may or may not be specifically directed against the graft. Macrophages have acquired increased resistance against certain bacterial species. This capability has considerably less precision and retention than the immune system, but could be effective against an allograft. The recruitment, or horizontal expansion, of sensitized cells is an appealing concept, and certain evidence suggests it may be true; however, it has not been established for immunity in general, and its role in the allograft reaction is unknown.

ROLE OF ANTIBODY IN ALLOGRAFT REJECTION. Any discussion of the role of humoral antibody in the rejection of allografted tissues should take into consideration two recognized facts: First, circulating antibody is not an obligatory participant in the rejection of solid tissue allografts. In fact, the inability to make an immunoglobulin of any recognizable type does not preclude graft rejection. Animals incapable of making antibody (neonatally bursectomized chickens or bursectomized irradiated chickens) can still reject allografts. Agammaglobulinemic fetal sheep were also found to be capable of rejecting skin allografts even in the presence of heterologous antisheep immunoglobulins.

Second, humoral antibody provides only the recognition portion of graft rejection and tends to be obscured by the effector mechanisms it activates. Unlike cell-mediated immunity, where the recognition system is intimately associated with the destruction of the target, humoral antibody must activate other systems in order to effect cell death.

Even during the early days of organ transplantation it was known that antibodies are formed in concert with allograft rejection. It was initially concluded, however, that antibodies were formed in association with rejection but were not of great functional significance. Experimental work with tumor allografts provided some of the earliest

evidence that antibodies were truly involved in the rejection process. Gorer and later Gorer and Kaliss showed both the in vitro cytotoxic effects of antibody to tumor cells and the ability to retard tumor growth by passive transfer. Boyse et al. found that all tumors could show damage initiated by cytotoxic antibodies if the techniques were sufficiently sensitive.

Despite this evidence, most early investigators believed that rejection occurred as the result of cellular immunity only. Experiments that supported such a view were derived primarily from the failure of transferred antibody to destroy solid tissue allografts: (1) allogenic cells survived in millipore chambers even in hosts sensitized against them, (2) attempts to passively transfer allograft sensitivity to unaltered hosts by an immune serum were frequently unsuccessful, and (3) all attempts to passively transfer serologic immunity to tolerant hosts failed.

These three observations have all been challenged. Antibody and complement penetrate millipore chambers with difficulty, but, even so, humoral factors can destroy tissue enclosed within them, and sensitized lymphoid cells enclosed in a millipore chamber could accelerate the rejection of skin grafts. More recently even tolerance has been abolished by humoral antibody, and an increasing number of investigators have shown that immune serum can accelerate skin graft rejection. There are several reasons why the skin graft model was not the best model to demonstrate this effect: (1) the skin graft is isolated from the circulation prior to revascularization; (2) the endothelium which revascularizes the graft is of host origin; and (3) the antibody may not reach the graft or may be eluted from the graft before effector mechanisms can be mobilized.

The destruction of vascularized allografts with immune serum is made easier by the vasculature's being composed of donor cells, but it is made more difficult by the size of the organ. Clark et al. first demonstrated the effect of antibody even in an isogenic host. A kidney was grafted to a dog, after 4 days it was removed, and the dog was lethally irradiated. The second kidney from the same donor was then transplanted to the leukopenic sensitized host for 4 hours and then returned to the donor. This provided efficient perfusion of the kidney with humoral immune factors in the absence of sensitized cells. On return to the donor the kidney was promptly infiltrated with autologous cells, and the urine output ceased. The functional effectiveness of antibodies has also been convincingly demonstrated in clinical transplantation when preformed antibodies were present. Kidney allografts can reject within hours of transplantation. Such "hyperacute" rejections are usually due to antibodies directed against donor histocompatibility antigens.

Effector Pathways and Their Amplification: Antibody-induced Molecular Cascade Systems. Although antibodies bind to allografts, such binding is of no consequence by itself, and the antibody would probably be cleared during the course of normal cell membrane repair. The combination of antibody with the antigen produces an active complex, which triggers a number of nonspecific effector pathways (Fig. 10-11). Each effector pathway typically consists

ANTIBODY STRUCTURE

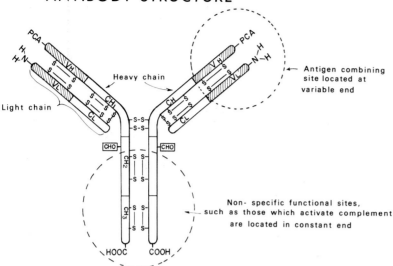

Fig. 10-11. Structure of the IgG antibody molecule. V_H and V_L are the variable portions of the heavy and light chains, respectively, and together they form the antigen-combining site. C_L is the constant portion of the light chain. CH_1, CH_2, and CH_3 are the subunits forming the invariable area of the heavy chain. The approximate positions of the inter- and intrachain disulfide bridges are shown. (*From J. E. Foker, R. L. Simmons, and J. S. Najarian, Allograft Rejection: I. The Induction of Immunity: The Afferent Arc, in J. S. Najarian and R. L. Simmons (eds.), "Transplantation," p. 63, Lea & Febiger, Philadelphia, 1972.*)

of a sequential activation of enzymes which attract and hold active cells, produce vascular permeability, release enzymes capable of degrading cell surfaces and other proteins, release factors causing smooth muscle contraction, and precipitate the formation of fibrin clots.

The immunologic response can be therefore both efficient and discriminatory. Relatively few specifically differentiated cells can produce molecules that will perform the recognition function. Since few cells are committed to each antigen, many more antigens can be discriminated. The antibodies in turn initiate a relatively general effector mechanism which can destroy the graft.

Complement

The combination of antibody with antigen changes the conformation of the antibody molecule. The constant (Fc) end of the antibody molecule is then responsible for the activation of the complement system (Fig. 10-11). The complement system consists of circulating protein molecules which, when activated, react in a sequential fashion.

At present, the system is known to be made up of at least nine major components, at least one of which (C_1) includes three subcomponents: C_{1q}, C_{1r}, C_{1s} (Fig. 10-12). For the most part the molecules seem to have enzymatic activity with the next molecule as the substrate.

The first component of complement is activated by certain antibodies when they are in combination with their respective antigens. The first participant, C_{1q} binds with the antigen-antibody complex; then, with the addition of C_{1r} and C_{1s}, esterase activity is produced. This enzyme activates C_4 and C_2, triggering the cascade of complement component interaction (Fig. 10-12).

An important biologic characteristic of the complement system, as well as the other cascade systems discussed in this section, is that they are capable of self-amplification. Thus, in one study, while 450 C_4 molecules were found fixed to sensitized sheep red blood cells, each erythrocyte had approximately 100,000 C_3 components on its surface. In addition, the C_3 components were distributed over the cell membrane surface rather than confined to the site of antigen-antibody combination, thus enlarging the area of

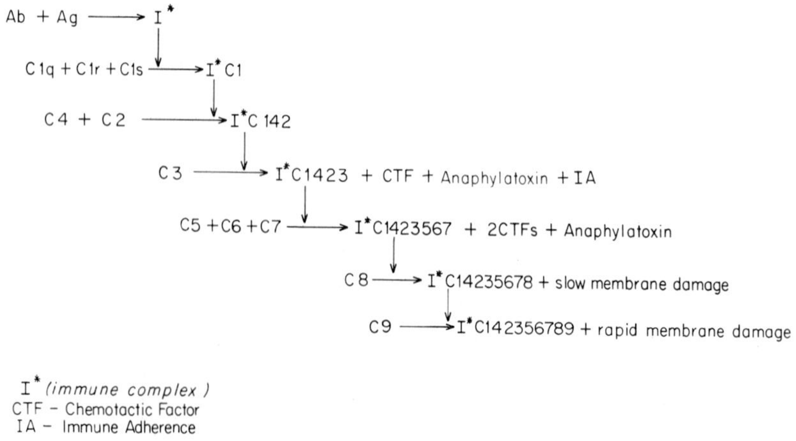

Ab + Ag ⟶ I*

C1q + C1r + C1s ⟶ I*C1

C4 + C2 ⟶ I*C 142

C3 ⟶ I*C1423 + CTF + Anaphylatoxin + IA

C5 + C6 + C7 ⟶ I*C1423567 + 2CTFs + Anaphylatoxin

C8 ⟶ I*C14235678 + slow membrane damage

C9 ⟶ I*C142356789 + rapid membrane damage

I* (immune complex)
CTF – Chemotactic Factor
IA – Immune Adherence

Fig. 10-12. The complement cascade system. Immune complexes (I*) trigger the cascade. The many steps in the cascade, most of them enzymatic, considerably amplify the effect on allografted tissue. Chemotactic factors (CTF) cause infiltration by polymorphonuclear leukocytes (PMNs). The anaphylatoxins increase vascular permeability and probably aid the cellular infiltration, as well as produce edema. Immune adherence leads to platelet and PMN clogging of the vessels. Finally, the last two steps can lead to direct damage of cell membranes and possibly basement membranes. (*From J. S. Najarian and J. E. Foker, Allograft Rejection: II. The Expression of Immunity: The Efferent Arc, in J. S. Najarian and R. L. Simmons (eds.), "Transplantation," p. 94, Lea & Febiger, Philadelphia, 1972.*)

effect. Although this step produces the greatest numerical amplification, other steps in the complement system also sequentially enlarge the number of active molecules.

The activation of C_3 is the first step in which other biologic activities are produced. The partial degradation of the C_3 molecule cleaves off at least two low-molecular-weight proteins which have biologic activity. One of these molecules, with a molecular weight of approximately 6,000, has the ability to attract PMNs. Anaphylatoxin, a second and presumably separate molecule produces increased capillary permeability, smooth muscle contraction, and the release of histamine from mast cells. Histamine thus is an effector molecule of the anaphylatoxins and contributes to their action.

In addition, the presence of C_3 molecules fixed to the cell surface will lead to the adherence of PMNs and platelets, and C_3 activation is sufficient to stimulate release of histamine by the platelets. Consequently, these cells are also activated by this step of the complement sequence. More anaphylatoxic factors and CFs (chemotactic factors) are produced as the cascade progresses through the C_5, C_6, and C_7 steps. Continued activation through C_7, C_8, and C_9, when tripped by soluble antigen-antibody complexes, produces histamine release from platelets. More importantly, however, the activation of the terminal C_8 and C_9 steps produces the ability to damage cell membranes. Fluorescent-labeled tagging techniques can detect complement within the rejecting organ itself. In the inbred-rat allograft model, complement was found on capillary basement membranes in concert with IgG deposition 2 or 3 days after grafting.

The Clotting System (Fig. 10-13)

Theoretically the deposition of fibrin in the allografted organ may arise in two ways: The first, the so-called *extrinsic pathway* of thrombin formation, requires tissue thromboplastin to initiate the sequence of events. The release of this cellular substance may follow damage to the endothelial cell membranes either by antibody and complement or through the direct cytotoxic effect of lymphocytes. The activation of complement through C_3 would also promote the adherence of platelets which, in turn, would stimulate platelet retraction and release of platelet phospholipids. These phospholipids have been shown to promote clotting.

The second method of inducing clot formation, the *intrinsic pathway,* has the potential to be activated directly by immunologic reaction. In the intrinsic pathway, Hageman factor (factor XII) begins a sequence which proceeds through factors XI, IX, VII, and V to the activation of prothrombin factor to form thrombin with the eventual polymerization of fibrin. Antigen-antibody complexes will activate Hageman factor to trigger this cascade and produce clotting in vitro in the absence of platelets. Thus, an entry into the intrinsic pathway is present within the interactions of antigens and antibodies (Fig. 10-13).

As the reaction proceeds and tissue damage is produced, tissue thromboplastin is released, collagen fibers are exposed, and clotting is facilitated. It is now generally hypothesized that the progressive obliterative vascular reaction of a chronically rejecting allograft is a by-product of fibrin laid down along endothelium that has been damaged by immune mechanisms.

Interrelation of the Molecular Cascade Systems (Fig. 10-14)

Antigen-antibody complexes activate complement and Hageman factor. Hageman factor in turn produces clotting, activates plasmin, and perhaps directly activates complement. Plasmin in turn can activate C_3 to produce, among

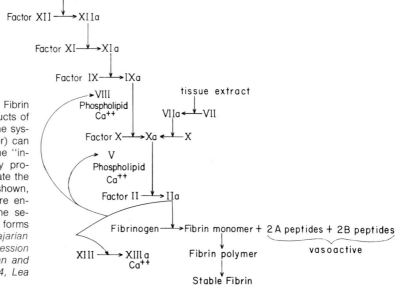

Fig. 10-13. The coagulation cascade system. Fibrin and two vasoactive peptides are the final products of the cascade. The two modes of activation of the system are diagrammed. Factor XII (Hageman factor) can be activated by immune complexes initiating the "intrinsic pathway." Tissue damage (presumably produced by immunologic damage) could precipitate the extrinsic system. In both systems, the factors shown, with the probable exceptions of V and VIII, are enzymes. Activation of the pathways involves the sequential conversions of these enzymes to active forms (represented by XIIa, XIa, etc). (*From J. S. Najarian and J. E. Foker, Allograft Rejection: II. The Expression of Immunity: The Efferent Arc, in J. S. Najarian and R. L. Simmons (eds.), "Transplantation," p. 94, Lea & Febiger, Philadelphia, 1972.*)

RECOGNITION

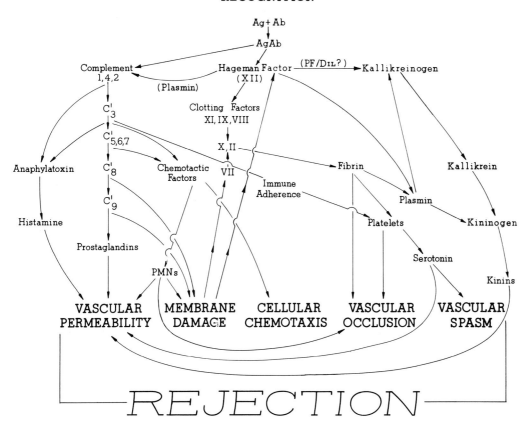

Fig. 10-14. Integration of the humoral amplification system in graft rejection. This diagram suggests the complexity of allograft rejection. The three main cascade pathways—complement, clotting, and kinin—generate many active molecules, including the kinins, chemotactic factors, anaphylatoxins, histamine, and serotonin. These molecules, together with platelets and polymorphonuclear leukocytes (PMNs), produce the destructive effects on the graft. The most prominent consequences include increased vascular permeability (edema), spasm, and occlusion as well as cell and basement membrane damage and cellular chemotaxis (infiltration). It is clear that these systems do not operate singly but tend to activate each other. Not shown are the many interlocking inhibitory factors that keep these systems in check once they are activated. (*From J. S. Najarian and J. E. Foker, Allograft Rejection: II. The Expression of Immunity: The Efferent Arc, in J. S. Najarian and R. L. Simmons (eds.), "Transplantation," p. 94, Lea & Febiger, Philadelphia, 1972.*)

other effects, CFs. Activation of Hageman factor also leads to kinin production; kinins are small polypeptides that increase vascular permeability. Activation of the complement system produces aggregation of platelets and, consequently, initiation of the clotting mechanism. Thrombin formation, in turn, stimulates the production of plasmin from plasminogen. Prostaglandin activity is released following complement activation, and may contribute to vascular permeability, although the significance of this in allograft rejection remains unclear.

Not only are the activators of these systems interrelated, but also the inhibitors are intertwined. The C_1 esterase inhibitor also decreases the activity of the kinin and plasmin systems. Neither activation nor inhibition of one system can occur without affecting the other pathways.

Efferent Pathways and Their Amplification: Cellular Mechanisms. The property of amplification does not seem to be confined to the molecular cascade system; analogous mechanisms are available to increase the numbers of cellular participants at the site of immunologic reactions. Following immunologic recognition many nonspecific cells, including mononuclear cells, PMNs, and platelets, can be enlisted.

We have already discussed the evidence that indicates that the mononuclear cells infiltrating an allograft are not all specifically sensitized to it. A few specifically sensitized cells seem able to recruit many uncommitted mononuclear cells. The mechanisms involve the release of certain factors from the specifically sensitized cell which attracts or holds the uncommitted cell in the region of the graft.

Migration Inhibitory Factor (MIF). Rich and Lewis made the curious observation that mononuclear cells from either the buffy coat or the spleen of an animal sensitized to tuberculin did not migrate in the presence of the antigen. George and Vaughn designed a simple but elegant and quantifiable system based on the predictable migration of leukocytes placed in a capillary tube. When antigens were present with the sensitized cells in the capillary tube, migration out of the end of the tube did not occur. Inhibition of migration occurs only when the cells are from an animal that would show delayed hypersensitivity to the antigen when challenged in vivo.

Bloom showed the amplification potential of MIF and demonstrated much of its significance to the allograft rejection reaction. Among a large preponderance of macrophages only 2 percent of the cells need to be lymphocytes to inhibit migration. Thus, specifically sensitized lymphocytes can amplify their destructive ability by enlisting macrophages. Because of the design of the in vitro experiments the active substance was called MIF. In a transplanted organ a specifically sensitized lymphocyte activated by histocompatibility antigen would presumably release MIF and induce wandering macrophages to stay.

Complement. Additional factors may also contribute to the accumulation of mononuclear cells at an allograft site. For example, complement receptors are apparently present on macrophages and will cause them to adhere to erythrocytes in the presence of complement. This may be akin to the phenomenon of immune adherence and provides another mechanism for the concentration of macrophages in an allograft.

Chemotactic Factor (CF). Ward has produced evidence that mononuclear cells will respond to CF. When immune complexes were added to serum, a substance was produced that caused mononuclear cells to migrate within millipore chambers. Thus, it would seem that mononuclear cells can respond to a concentration gradient of attracting molecules and migrate toward their source.

Cytophilic Antibody. Cytophilic antibodies would seem to be another mechanism by which macrophages are concentrated at a site of immunologic activity. Large numbers of macrophages accumulate at skin or kidney allograft sites, although their contributions to immunologic damage has not been established. Some have proposed that they act only as scavengers and possible processors of antigen. There is evidence that the macrophage has a more active role, however, and for those cells carrying cytophilic antibodies the participation would be immunologically specific.

Cytophilic antibody has been found predominately in the 7S globulin fraction. The fact that digestion by papain destroys the cytophilic properties of these antibodies indicates that the Fc fragment of the molecule contains the macrophage binding site. Macrophages carrying cytophilic antibody seem to cause damage by phagocytizing the cellular membrane of the target cells.

Volkman and Gowans first demonstrated that the macrophage population which rapidly infiltrates a site of injury arises in the bone marrow. Thus, it would appear that there is a large actively proliferating population of cells arising in the bone marrow which can be attracted to the site of immune reaction and greatly amplify the effect of the specifically sensitized cells (Fig. 10-15). There are other indications that small lymphocytes can also transform into macrophage-like cells. Boak et al. observed that thoracic duct cells, comprised almost entirely of small lymphocytes, were able to transform into phagocytic cells dwelling in the liver reticuloendothelial network. Their work suggested

that under normal conditions the bone marrow is the principal source for these cells.

The majority of round cells infiltrating an allograft are probably not specifically sensitized to it, and many are drawn from the rapidly replicating pool of macrophages originating in the bone marrow. Other round cells, such as fibroblasts, might have a strictly reparative function. Most of the macrophage enlistment probably results from release of CF and MIF at the site of immune reaction, but immunologic specificity acquired by cytophilic antibody or lymphocyte-to-macrophage transformation may contribute to the influx of macrophages (Fig. 10-15).

Similar mechanisms have also been postulated to explain the presence of PMNs at the site of rejection. Antigen-antibody complexes which activate complement produce at least two factors which are attractive to PMNs: The gradient of CF molecules will allow PMNs to actively migrate to the source. The PMNs may also be retained by immune adherence, another function of activated complement. Neutrophils as well as platelets will adhere to a site of antigen-antibody reaction when complement is present and activated.

PMNs have frequently been found in allografts, especially during an active rejection reaction. The greater frequency of their numbers correlates best with an increasing vigor of the reaction. Because the cell is active, its life span is rather short when stimulated by an immunologic reaction in the presence of material to be phagocytized. Consequently, a significantly larger percentage of PMNs probably contributes to an allograft rejection reaction than is apparent from any single biopsy.

Functional assessments for the potency of PMNs has shown PMNs to be much more effective and more rapidly active in producing allogenic target cell death than are lymphoid cells. The basis for the potency of PMNs in the allograft rejection reaction is easily demonstrated. The neutrophil is a highly differentiated cell, packed full of lysosomes—cytoplasmic bodies filled with digestive enzymes. The cell fraction containing the cytoplasmic granules has been found to contain acid phosphatase, alkaline phosphatase, lysozyme, collagenase, lipase, RNase, deoxyribonuclease (DNase), and β-glucuronidase. In addition, proteolytic enzymes have been found of which cathepsins D and E may play an important part in producing immunologic damage. At least four basic proteins from rabbit neutrophil granules, which can induce both vascular and glomerular basement membrane permeability, have been isolated. Finally, slow-reacting substances or anaphylatoxins and a kinin-generating factor seem to be associated with neutrophils (Fig. 10-14).

Large immune complexes, greater than 19S in density, seem prone to lodge in arterial and arteriolar wall. PMNs are attracted to these sites, wedge past the intimal cells, and begin phagocytizing the complexes. This in turn apparently activates the PMN, causing lysosome degranulation and release of active enzymes. Damage to the internal elastic membrane and medial necrosis result.

Platelets, as with PMNs, have only recently been conceded to be of any significance in allograft rejection reac-

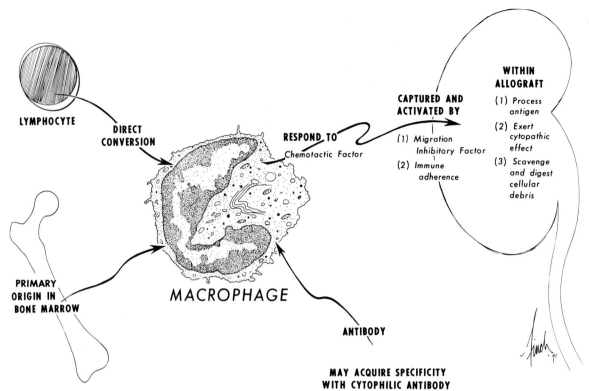

LYMPHOCYTE

DIRECT CONVERSION

RESPOND TO Chemotactic Factor

CAPTURED AND ACTIVATED BY
(1) Migration Inhibitory Factor
(2) Immune adherence

WITHIN ALLOGRAFT
(1) Process antigen
(2) Exert cytopathic effect
(3) Scavenge and digest cellular debris

PRIMARY ORIGIN IN BONE MARROW

MACROPHAGE

ANTIBODY

MAY ACQUIRE SPECIFICITY WITH CYTOPHILIC ANTIBODY

Fig. 10-15. Complex of activities carried out by macrophages in allograft rejection. Evidence for each of these activities exists. In most instances, however, it comes from model systems, and the functional importance to rejection has not been established. As depicted in the illustration, the macrophages arise primarily from a stem cell source in the bone marrow, although direct conversion of lymphocytes does take place. More than one mechanism for the arrival of macrophages at the allograft has been suggested by experimental evidence. If the macrophage takes up cytophilic antibody, it would acquire immunologic specificity for the target antigens. The macrophage has a receptor site on its surface for the constant portion (*Fc* fragment) of the immunoglobulin molecule. It is also possible that antibody, complexed with antigen within the allograft, could arrest passing macrophages. In addition, there are other means for recruiting macrophages. Chemotactic factor, migration inhibitory factor, or a type of immune adherence would concentrate macrophages at sites of immunologic activity. Once within the allograft, the macrophage may contribute to the development of immunity by processing antigen and presenting it on its surface to lymphocytes. The macrophage may also process the antigen to a smaller component complexed in some way with RNA and transfer this to lymphocytes. It should be noted, however, that no evidence yet exists that the development of immunocompetence occurs within an allograft. More certain activities of the macrophage include the scavenging and digesting of cellular debris within the allograft. Finally, these cells may exert a direct cytopathic effect on the allograft, perhaps on those cells already damaged or in some way sensitized. (*From J. S. Najarian and J. E. Foker, Allograft Rejection: II. The Expression of Immunity: The Efferent Arc, in J. S. Najarian and R. L. Simmons (eds.), "Transplantation," p. 94, Lea & Febiger, Philadelphia, 1972.*)

tions. Identification of platelets in a histologic section requires electron microscopy; thus the number of studies are fewer than those which implicate other cells. Platelets are now thought to be important components of the rejection reaction and contribute to allograft damage by several mechanisms. Platelets contain many cytoplasmic granules, at least some of which have been found to contain acid phosphatase and glucuronidase. This finding implies that at least some of these granules are lysosomes and contain various other enzymes capable of tissue degradation.

The phospholipids found in cell membrane fractions as well as in isolates of platelet granules are important in both the extrinsic system of blood coagulation, initiated by tissue factors (including those of platelets), and the intrinsic system, which occurs in the absence of cellular damage. Activation and damage of platelets would release these factors and engage the clotting pathways.

Another important consequence of platelet function is the release of vasoactive amines. Serotonin is released by human platelets, and both histamine and serotonin are released by rabbit platelets. It is not known whether these vasoactive amines are synthesized or merely stored in the platelets.

Platelet activity, which seems to begin with aggregation of these cells, can be initiated by exposed collagen fibers as well as cells coated with immune complexes. Consequently, immunologic damage may precipitate thrombosis by the uncovering of collagen fibers in basement membrane structures beneath the endothelial cells of capillaries and larger vessels. Platelet aggregation may also be initiated by damage to endothelial cells which exposes adenosine triphosphatase (ATPase) beneath the cellular membranes. The formation of adenosine diphosphate (ADP) by these enzymes would then promote platelet thrombosis. Such aggregation could effectively clog small vessels.

In the allograft rejection reaction they may well congregate secondary to the association of antibody with antigen and the activation of complement. The presence of C_3 products on cell surfaces might be expected to retain the platelets by immune adherence, although this phenomenon did not occur in vitro with sensitized sheep erythrocytes as the target cells. In addition, platelets may accumulate by adhering to collagen fibers exposed by other mechanisms, such as PMN-released digestive enzymes or macrophage-induced damage.

The complexity of the allograft reaction is just beginning to be understood. It involves a variety of recognition molecules (antibodies) and presumably a similar variety of specifically sensitized cells. In addition, the main force of the reaction is produced by a bewildering array of amplifying chain reactions which include both molecular amplification schemes and cellular amplifiers. The activation of complement, the clotting system, kinin formation and the stimulation of PMN, macrophages, and platelet assault produce a variety of damage to the transplanted organ. Included are occlusive phenomena within the graft vessels, induced permeability of these same vessels with interstitial edema accumulation, disruption of cellular basement membranes, and the infiltration of the graft with a profusion of cell types (Fig. 10-14).

AN INTEGRATED VIEW OF THE REJECTION OF ORGAN ALLOGRAFTS

Rejection morphology has two main components: The first component is the host response, and it is composed of effector cells and molecules, both immunologically specific and nonspecific. In rapid rejections these comprise most, if not all, of the pathologic picture so that the speed of the reaction virtually precludes response by the organ cells. The second component becomes prominent only with longer survival of the transplanted organ and encompasses the various morphologic alterations of the organs. In fact, the responses of these cells can form an important part of the pathologic picture.

A predictable series of events ensues when an unsensitized patient is allografted. The first visible change is a perivascular infiltration of round cells accomplished by migration through the cytoplasm of the endothelial cells (Fig. 10-16). The accumulation of cells is not significant for several hours after transplantation but can reach considerable numbers within 24 hours. This delay suggests that although the immunogenicity of the graft may be a sufficient stimulus to transmigration by the lymphoid cells, the host cells may first need to synthesize a recognition molecule or have other cellular events transpire before migration occurs. The confrontation between graft and host immunocompetent cells may be important in the development of this infiltrate.

The temporal aspects have been best worked out for the kidney, but the sequence appears to be the same for most organs. During the first 48 hours following grafting the number of infiltrating cells continues to increase. The original enclaves around small vessels spread, and the interstitial space is further infiltrated. A potpourri of cells accumulates: cells resembling small lymphocytes are seen, as well as large transformed lymphocytes with basophilic cytoplasm. Large histiocytes or macrophages are just beginning to arrive in numbers. Plasma cells are still relatively scarce: as a terminal product of cellular differentiation, they may require several cell divisions before they appear in the organ (Fig. 10-17).

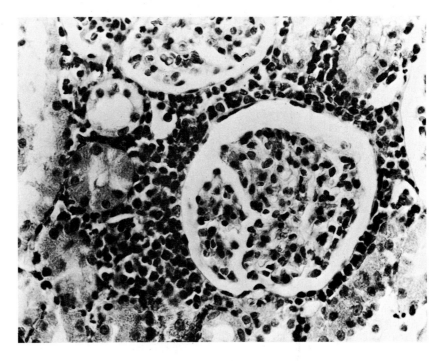

Fig. 10-16. Canine renal allograft 48 hours after transplantation into unmodified recipient. Round cell infiltration, usually the first overt sign of host activity against the allograft, is apparent within 6 to 12 hours after transplantation. By 48 hours the number of invading cells is substantial. The original perivascular infiltrate has surrounded a glomerulus and adjacent tubules. (*From J. E. Foker and J. S. Najarian, Allograft Rejection: III. The Pathobiology of Organ Rejection, in J. S. Najarian and R. L. Simmons (eds.), "Transplantation," p. 122, Lea & Febiger, Philadelphia, 1972.*)

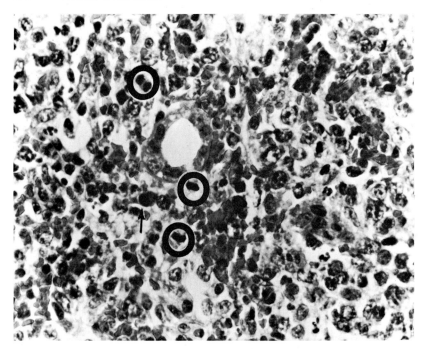

Fig. 10-17. Canine renal allograft 4 days after transplantation into an unmodified recipient. Invading cells all but obscure the architecture of the kidney. Numerous mitoses (circles) can be found, and this cellular proliferation may be producing immunologically competent cells within the graft. A plasma cell (arrow) is present, but most of the cells resemble lymphocytes and macrophages. (*From J. E. Foker and J. S. Najarian, Allograft Rejection: III. The Pathobiology of Organ Rejection, in J. S. Najarian and R. L. Simmons (eds.), "Transplantation," p. 122, Lea & Febiger, Philadelphia, 1972.*)

Antibody and complement are deposited in the area of the capillaries, and some of the infiltrating lymphoid cells are producing immunoglobulins by the third day. Recognition molecules (antibody) as well as sensitized cells are therefore present early in the allograft reaction.

Sensitized lymphoid cells, upon recognizing the foreign tissue, release several mediators of inflammation and cell damage. The release of cytotoxic factors directly injures membranes of adjacent cells. Mitogenic products stimulate division of lymphoid cells, perhaps expanding the immunocompetent population. Activated, phagocytic macrophages are effectively concentrated in the area by MIF (migration inhibitory factor) and other CFs. In addition vascular permeability agents are released.

Meanwhile, complement is fixed, thereby producing CFs, anaphylatoxins, and finally cellular damage when the terminal components (C_8 and C_9) are activated. Capillary permeability is increased by anaphylatoxins from the complement chain and probably by kinins. Interstitial edema becomes prominent. At the same time there are several additional inducements to cellular infiltration. The complement cascade generates molecules which produce immune adherence and others which have chemotactic activity. Damaged cells release additional compounds which contribute to infiltration by PMNs as well as other cells. PMNs in turn release vasoactive amines (including histamine or serotonin, depending on the species) and additional vascular permeability–promoting factors. The PMNs squeeze through the enlarged endothelial cell junctions and release proteolytic cathepsins D and E, causing basement membrane damage.

Fibrin, and α-macroglubulins, whose contribution is not understood, are deposited by 7 days. During this time, lymphoid cells have continued to accumulate and, joined by significant numbers of plasma cells and PMNs, obscure

the normal architecture. The round cell population presumably contains many macrophages and other immunologic nonspecific cells at this point. Increasingly frequent mitoses may indicate the production of immunocompetent cells within the graft.

The small vessels become plugged with fibrin and platelets, diminishing the perfusion and preventing function. In this relatively rapid sequence of events the organ has little chance to respond, and the pathologic process is dominated by the host effector pathways.

Obviously, rejection modified by immunosuppressive agents is not a distinct morphologic classification but is only a continuation of the events comprising the rejection reaction. The morphologic features associated with this more chronic rejection become dominated by the response of the organ tissue itself. Here the normal response of tissue to injury predominates in the pathologic picture. A good deal of endothelial cell damage occurs in the allograft, and the responses of cellular repair, hypertrophy and hyperplasia, follow.

Endothelial cell damage also elicits repair processes. Aggregations of platelets within the intimal layer are resolved, and the dissolution of the thrombi is accompanied by the infiltration of macrophages and foam cells. The result is a thickened intimal layer with the loss of smooth endothelial lining and the presence of vacuolated cells. The lumen narrows as a result. Narrowing of the vessel lumen is also a consequence of the medial thickening. Studies using nonimmunologic disease models have shown that most of the cells proliferating in response to the stimulus of injury are smooth muscle cells. A reasonable extrapolation is that hyperplasia of these cells produces much of the lumenal narrowing in the allograft (Fig. 10-18).

Although the exposed position of the endothelial cells and the striking proliferation of the smooth muscle cells

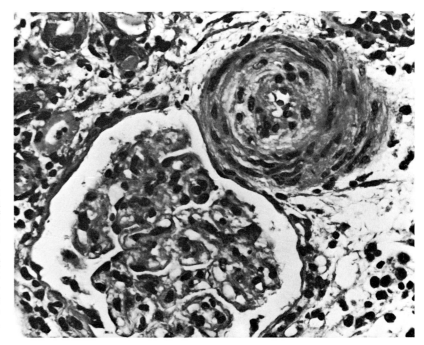

Fig. 10-18. A rejected human allograft removed 18 months posttransplant. The lumen of the arteriole has all but disappeared as a consequence of hyperplasia of the cells of the vessel. Most of the thickening of the wall is probably due to proliferation of smooth muscle cells, with spindle-shaped nuclei. Endothelial cells, with rounder nuclei, almost fill the lumen. (*From J. E. Foker and J. S. Najarian, Allograft Rejection: III. The Pathobiology of Organ Rejection, in J. S. Najarian and R. L. Simmons (eds.), "Transplantation," p. 122, Lea & Febiger, Philadelphia, 1972.*)

argue for their being an important target of the immune reaction, there is evidence that the basement and elastic membranes of the vessel absorb a major portion of immune-mediated damage. Either immune complexes or antibodies to the vascular basement membrane activate complement and attract polymorphonuclear cells. These nonspecific effector cells release at least four protein factors which increase the permeability of the vessel and in addition produce cathepsins D and E, which digest basement membranes. The PMNs are active in reaching the basement membrane and will lift the endothelial cells to gain this access.

Platelets may be of greater significance than PMNs in mediating damage. Immune complexes (which activate complement) will result in platelet adherence and the release of vasoactive substances. Platelet aggregation leads to the release of histamine, serotonin, and other capillary permeability factors which expose more basement membrane; the exposed collagen fibers of the basement membrane further enhance platelet aggregation. Platelets and PMNs drawn to these sites release cathepsins, elastases, and phosphatases which increase destruction and attract other nonspecific cellular effectors including macrophages (Fig. 10-19).

The myocardial cell is the characteristic cell of the heart, the tubular cell of the kidney, the acinar and islet cell of the pancreas, etc. The differentiation and function of this cell demand an ample oxygen supply and do not permit further cellular division. Therefore, compromise of respiration by vascular endothelial and medial hypertrophy, intravascular aggregations of platelets, and interstitial accumulations of edema and mononuclear cells will have predictable consequences for these cells. They will atrophy, and because some have poor regenerative ability, cell death may be followed by replacement fibrosis (Fig. 10-19).

The interstitial area concomitantly increases in size. The interstitial area, however, has much activity in its own right. Repair of immunologic damage stimulates many fibroblastic cells to proliferate, and it attracts macrophages. The persisting immunogenic capacity of the allograft is indicated by the inevitable presence of infiltrating plasma cells and lymphoid cells.

It is impossible to determine what proportions of these effects result from ischemia produced by vascular occlusion, interstitial edema, or cellular infiltrates. Similarly, the contribution made by the direct cytotoxic action of specific and nonspecific effector cells and molecules is unknown.

CIRCUMVENTING REJECTION

Immunosuppression

Theoretically, there are seven methods by which the immune response can be suppressed: (1) by destroying or eliminating the immunocompetent cells and their progeny, (2) by interfering with the ability of these cells to react with antigen, (3) by blocking the interaction of immunocompetent cells with the macrophages that process the antigen, (4) by inhibiting the differentiation and proliferation of these cells, (5) by neutralizing the ability of these cells to synthesize or secrete immunoglobulins, (6) by interfering with the action of immunoglobulins on the target antigen, or (7) by interfering with the cellular and noncellular mediators of tissue damage activated by the antigen-antibody complex. In fact, the methods of immunosuppression of clinical usefulness depend for the most

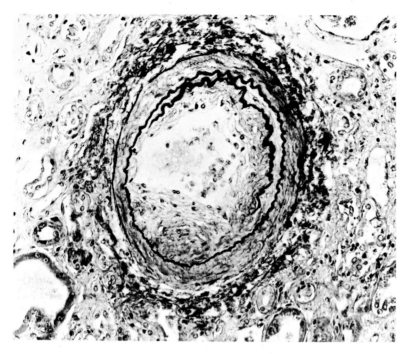

Fig. 10-19. Extensive damage to this small artery in a human renal allograft removed 14 months posttransplant is apparent. The elastic membranes are badly frayed, and the elastica interna has been destroyed entirely along half the circumference of the vessel. The intimal layer shows extensive disruption and loss of cells. The cells remaining are often vacuolated. The lumen is narrowed by tissue from several origins: proliferation of smooth muscle cells in the media, endothelial cell swelling and hyperplasia, and the presence of an organized thrombus. The adventitial area shows damage and edema formation. Note also that severe tubular atrophy and interstitial fibrosis are present. (*From J. E. Foker and J. S. Najarian, Allograft Rejection: III. The Pathobiology of Organ Rejection, in J. S. Najarian and R. L. Simmons (eds.), "Transplantation," p. 122, Lea & Febiger, Philadelphia, 1972.*)

part on the destruction or elimination of the immunocompetent cells or on inhibiting the differentiation and proliferation of these cells. Methods that depend on neutralizing preformed immunoglobulins or interfering with the mediators of tissue damage activated by immune complexes have been almost totally ineffective.

METHODS INVOLVING THE DESTRUCTION OF IMMUNOCOMPETENT CELLS

It is obvious that destruction of the small lymphocyte, which is the resting immunocompetent cell, would be of major potential value for immunosuppression. One subpopulation of thymic-derived lymphocytes has a very long life span, perhaps on the order of 10 years, and it repeatedly circulates in the blood and in the lymphatic system. These cells are probably the source of immunologic memory. The shorter-lived B lymphocytes are more sessile and reside in the spleen and lymph nodes.

EXTIRPATION OF LYMPHOID TISSUE. Immunity becomes rapidly systemic and is not confined to the regional lymph nodes or to a single major lymphoid organ like the spleen for prolonged periods. In experimental situations, interruption of lymphatic channels, the placement of grafts in sites with poor lymphatic drainage, or the excision of local lymphoid tissue will delay the acquisition of immunity for only brief periods. Vascularized organ grafts do not require lymphatic drainage, and the excision of locally draining lymph nodes or spleen is ineffective as an immunosuppressive technique.

THYMECTOMY. The adult mammalian thymus continues to be important in maintaining the immunologic responsiveness of the animal. Its extirpation, especially when combined with administration of immunosuppressive agents or irradiation, results in a failure of normal immunologic capacity. Thymectomy might be expected to be an immunosuppressive treatment of some potential usefulness. Unfortunately, although thymectomy can be performed rather simply through a cervical incision as well as by the classic transsternal route, it has not proved to be of great use in clinical immunosuppression in man. Starzl utilized thymectomy in a number of patients in the early development of renal transplantation and found little improvement in results. It is possible that the thymus in an adult man has completed its inductive functions and removal has no consequences; it is also possible that thymectomy has not received an adequate trial. Even if successful, it may not be desirable to produce general immunologic incompetency in transplant recipients. Bursectomy in man, of course, is not yet possible, since the mammalian equivalent of the avian bursa of Fabricius has not been found.

THORACIC DUCT DRAINAGE. Cannulation and drainage of the thoracic duct will successfully deplete the body of a large proportion of its circulating small lymphocytes. Such depletion will lead to marked prolongation of allograft survival as well as lesser, but real, decrease in the capacity for antibody synthesis. Thoracic duct cannulation and drainage have been used for clinical immunosuppression. Although they seem to produce prolongation of allografts, they are cumbersome; the indwelling cannula can become plugged or infected, and protein depletion can result. A modification that permits the irradiation of thoracic duct lymphocytes and reinfusion of them has also been used in animals.

EXTRACORPOREAL IRRADIATION. Blood can be circulated through an extracorporeal source of radiation and returned to the patient without great risk of infection or protein depletion. Continuous or intermittent irradiation of the circulating lymphocytes will deplete them and re-

duce the immunocompetence of the patient. The ineffi-
ciencies of the system and the need for nearly continuous
irradiation make this technique impractical for clinical use.

ANTILYMPHOCYTE GLOBULIN. The use of heterologous
antisera directed against human lymphocytes has been
a major advance in clinical immunosuppression.
Metchnikoff first described the destruction of white cells
by heterologous antiserum in 1889. He noted that guinea
pig antisera prepared against rabbit or rat lymph node or
spleen cells agglutinated and killed PMNs of the donor
species. Flexner noted lymphoid cell hypoplasia in animals
treated with rabbit anti-guinea pig lymph node serum;
Chew and Lawrence showed that daily administration of
similar serum produced a fall in the total lymphocyte
counts of the recipient guinea pigs. In the early 1960s
Interbitzen, Waksman, and Woodruff and Anderson noted
that heterologous sera made against lymphoid tissues depressed certain immunologic reactions, i.e., tuberculin sensitivity and allograft rejection, but the sera were of low
potency and appeared unpromising. The work of Monaco
et al., however, demonstrated that potent antisera were
profoundly effective in prolonging mouse skin grafts across
strong histocompatibility barriers and even across xenogenic barriers. Monaco et al. further demonstrated that such
sera could prolong canine renal allografts and skin grafts
in man. Starzl was the first to use antilymphocyte serum
in clinical kidney transplantation, and subsequently the use
of these preparations has become widespread.

Antilymphocyte globulins (ALG) are produced when
lymphocytes (thoracic duct, peripheral blood, or lymph
node cells, thymocytes, or spleen cells) are injected into
animals of a different species. Cell membranes or cultured
lymphocytes can also provide the stimulation so that a
standard reproducible lymphocyte immunogen can be
given. In general, the addition of adjuvants to the stimulating heterologous lymphocytes produces sera that are
consistently more immunosuppressive than those prepared
without adjuvants. The rabbit, goat, and horse are most
commonly utilized to produce antisera for human use.

Most of the antibody that is relatively specific for human
lymphocytes rests in the IgG fraction, and the serum can
be purified in a number of ways—Cohn fractionation,
column chromatography, and forced-flow electrophoresis.
The resulting antibody is not totally specific for lymphocytes, however, and there are usually cross reactions with
platelets, red cells, and other tissues. If a purer lymphocyte
antigen, i.e., cultured human lymphocyte or thoracic duct
lymphocytes, is used, these cross-reacting antibodies can
be minimized but not totally avoided. Antibodies against
erythrocytes and platelets can be absorbed out without
complete loss of immunosuppressive potency. The purified
material can be administered intravenously, intramuscularly, or subcutaneously.

Most evidence now points toward a direct effect of the
ALG on the circulating small lymphocyte. The antibody-
coated lymphocyte is either lysed or opsonized, and removed by the reticuloendothelial system. More prolonged
administration depletes the paracortical regions of the
lymph nodes where T cells reside, and high doses will even
affect the B cells in the medullary regions and follicles of
the nodes.

If the long-lived peripheral circulating small T cell lymphocytes are depleted, there will be marked inhibition of
cellular immunity. ALG can even abolish preexisting, delayed hypersensitivity reactions (i.e., tuberculin) and will
prolong skin or renal allograft survival. Larger doses will
produce marked prolongation of some xenografts. ALG
has a definite but lesser effect on humoral antibody production. The immunosuppression that does appear may be
attributable to a direct action either on B lymphocytes or
on those T cells which recognize an antigen prior to stimulation of the B cell system.

The effectiveness of ALG in clinical renal transplantation can easily be demonstrated (Fig. 10-20). A series
of cadaver kidney recipients were treated with increasing
doses of ALG without change in other aspects of the
immunosuppressive regimen. The results were remarkably
improved in all patient categories. Rapid rejection of almost all kidneys took place in 3 or 4 months when ALG was
not used. ALG thus appears to be a major adjunct in
clinical immunosuppression. Figure 10-21*A* and *B* illustrates the effect of ALG dose on the survival of both
ideal-risk and high-risk recipients of cadaver renal transplants.

The toxicity of any heterologous serum prepared against
human tissue depends on two factors: its cross reactivity
with other tissue antigens and the ability of the patient
to make antibodies against the protein itself. When administered intramuscularly, ALG produces an area of striking
erythematous induration accompanied by considerable
fever. This probably represents the action of the antibodies
with cross-reacting antigens in the injected tissues. Similarly, anemia and thrombocytopenia have been reported
after injection of ALG and presumably represent the result
of a reaction between ALG and erythrocytes and platelets.
Some investigators have also found that ALG binds to
renal glomerular basement membranes, thereby initiating
a nephrotoxic serum nephritis. When the ALG is manufactured from either cultured or thoracic duct lymphocytes
(rather than lymphoid tissues), these cross reactions can
be minimized or eliminated.

The allergic reactions to the antiserum are the most
common problem associated with the clinical use of ALG.
Urticaria, serum sickness, and anaphylactoid reactions
have all resulted when the patient became immune to the
heterologous globulin. To prevent these reactions, one can
induce immunologic unresponsiveness to the foreign proteins in ALG. The development of immunologic unresponsiveness to the heterologous globulin is of value because the ALG can be administered for more prolonged
periods and may actually be more potent in equivalent
dose than if there were antibodies directed against it.

One of the great advantages of ALG is that it can be
used with other immunosuppressive agents which will
potentiate or prolong its activity. Almost all the chemical
immunosuppressants are useful in augmenting the immunosuppressive effect of ALG. This allows one to use large
doses of ALG as a priming agent and follow with smaller

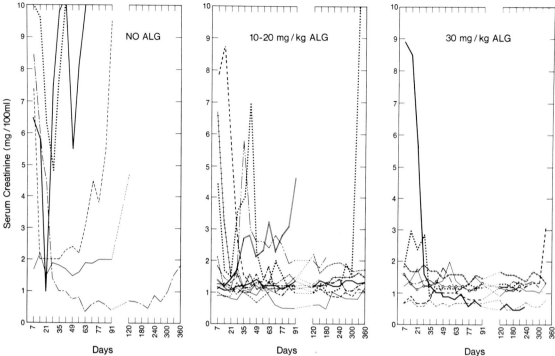

Fig. 10-20. Effect of increasing doses of ALG on functional survival of kidney allografts from unrelated (cadaver) donors. All patients received ALG for a course of only 2 to 3 weeks. Azathioprine and prednisone in identical doses were used in each group. When ALG was not used, kidney rejection usually took place in the first 3 to 4 months. As the doses of ALG were increased, functional survival dramatically improved. Rejection episodes could not be detected in the majority of the recipients of the high-dose ALG therapy. (*From J. S. Najarian and R. L. Simmons, The Clinical Use of Antilymphocyte Globulin, New Engl J Med, 285:158, 1971.*)

doses of the more toxic chemical immunosuppressants. Thymectomy and thoracic duct drainage will likewise potentiate the lymphocytic depletion and immunosuppressive effects of rather small doses of ALG.

The major problem in the production of a standardized antihuman ALG has been the inability to develop a mode of assaying its immunosuppressive potency. Most immunosuppressive drugs are available in measurable quantities, and reproducibility of response can be expected. Unfortunately, ALG preparations are made in different ways by different investigators, and a standard method of assay has not yet been developed. Cytotoxic assays, the formation of cellular rosettes, and animal assays for immunosuppressive potency have all been attempted, but their correlation with graft prolongation is uncertain. This is of importance since batches of ALG prepared by the same method will have variable immunosuppressive potency; it would be desirable to be able to discard the inferior lots.

METHODS PREVENTING THE PROLIFERATION OF IMMUNOCOMPETENT CELLS

Aside from ALG, conventional immunosuppressive agents (x-rays, antimetabolites, alkylating agents, and toxic antibiotics) have all been borrowed from cancer chemotherapy, where they were devised or chosen for their antiproliferative activity. Being antiproliferative, they inhibit the full expression of the immune response by preventing the differentiation and division of the immunocompetent lymphocyte after it encounters the antigen.

RADIATION. Radiation was probably the first agent utilized as an immunosuppressive agent. Ionizing radiation (x-rays, beta rays, alpha rays) affects both the protein and the nucleic acids of the cell. Although relatively small

doses of irradiation will disrupt the secondary structure formed by hydrogen bonding and consequently will also affect the tertiary structure of proteins, biologically effective and persistent alterations of protein functions seem to require rather high doses. Most of the immunosuppressive effects of x-radiation are due to changes produced in nucleic acids, particularly DNA, thereby interfering with cellular replication. Although several modes of damage to nucleic acids are inflicted by x-radiation, the most important is the production of scattered breaks in the sugar-phosphate backbone of DNA (Fig. 10-22). Disruption of the carbon-carbon bonds of the deoxyribotides or of bonds involving the phosphate groups interrupts one of the DNA strands to form single breaks. Less commonly, both strands are broken at the same point (double breaks). Other sites of damage, e.g., the bases themselves, are even more infrequent.

Repair mechanisms exist to mend the breaks, although in the dividing cell insufficient time may be available for this. Consequently, the effectiveness of radiation is highly dependent upon the phase of the cell cycle in which the cell is found. The cell cycle is illustrated in Fig. 10-23 and is generally divided into four distinct phases: (1) G_1, which consists of the gap between the completion of the previous

A

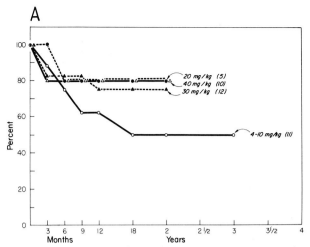

B

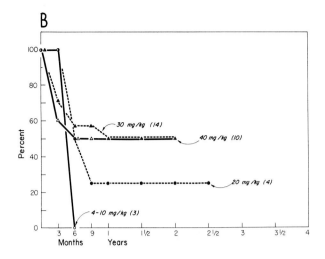

Fig. 10-21. *A.* Effect of ALG dose on the function of cadaver kidney transplants (ideal risk). Ideal-risk patients were all children one to sixteen years old and all adults aged sixteen to forty-five who had primary renal disease, normal lower urinary tracts, and no evidence of infection and/or malignant disease. *B.* Function of cadaver kidney transplants (high risk). High-risk patients were considered to be those aged forty-five or more with diabetes (Kimmelstiel-Wilson disease), previous malignant disease (Wilms' tumor), previous tuberculosis, evidence of gastrointestinal bleeding due to peptic ulceration, lupus erythematosis, or polyarteritis nodosa, or those with abnormal lower urinary tracts requiring the construction of an ideal bladder. (*From R. L. Simmons, R. Condie, and J. S. Najarian, Antilymphoblast Globulin for Renal Allograft Prolongation, Transplant Proc, 4:487, 1972.*)

mitosis and the next DNA synthesis, the phase of the resting nonproliferating cell; (2) DNA synthesis (S phase); (3) the second gap, G_2, the relatively short interval between the end of the S phase and the beginning of mitosis; and (4) the mitosis, or M, phase. Cells in the M or G_2 phase are most sensitive to irradiation. Presumably DNA breaks would not be repaired quickly enough, and the proteins needed for mitosis and cell division would often be nonfunctional. The early G_1 phase and the latter part of the S phase are the most resistant portions of the cell cycle. Therefore, irradiation must take place just prior to or during mitosis for its effect to be maximal.

The effect of irradiation on the immune response, consequently, depends greatly on its timing with relation to antigen exposure. If the antigen is presented soon after the irradiation, the immune response will be inhibited, since there is insufficient time for recovery of the immunocompetent cell population before the antigen is encountered. On the other hand, if antigenic stimulation is delayed long enough to allow recovery of the precursor cells, there will be slight stimulation of the response. Similarly, if radiation is given during the time of maximal proliferation of the immunocompetent population to an antigen (soon after antigen administration), marked inhibition of the response will be seen. Radiation is ineffective, however, if given somewhat later when there is a mature population of antibody-synthesizing cells. Mature plasma cells and presumably mature effector lymphocytes are radioresistant. Irradiation is, therefore, relatively ineffective in blocking

secondary response in a preimmunized animal. Paradoxically, an augmented antibody response takes place under certain circumstances, and the timing of irradiation must be carefully planned for immunosuppressive effect.

Local Irradiation of the Graft. Local irradiation of the graft has been found both to be an effective prophylactic method of immunosuppression and to interfere with ongoing rejection episodes within the graft. However, the mechanism of action is unclear. Irradiation of the graft

Fig. 10-22. X-ray-induced damage of DNA molecule. Irradiation frequently induces single breaks in the deoxyribotide backbone of the DNA double helix. More rarely, irradiation induces double breaks within the backbone. (*From R. L. Simmons, J. E. Foker, and J. S. Najarian, Principles of Immunosuppression, in D. C. Sabiston, Jr. (ed.), "Davis-Christopher Textbook of Surgery," p. 471, W. B. Saunders Company, Philadelphia, 1972.*)

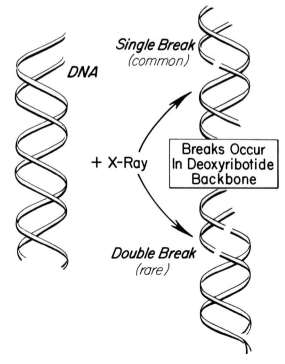

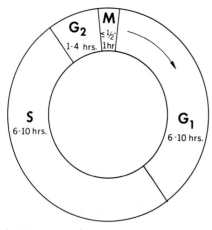

Fig. 10-23. Cell cycle showing phases, with their approximate duration, of most somatic cells of higher plants and animals. Cells are most sensitive to irradiation in the M or G₂ phase. Cells are most resistant to irradiation in the G_1 phase and the late S phase. (*From T. Makinodan and G. B. Price, Circumventing Graft Rejection: V. Radiation, in J. S. Najarian and R. L. Simmons (eds.), "Transplantation," p. 251, Lea & Febiger, Philadelphia, 1972.*)

may well damage immunocompetent cells invading the graft which will ultimately become immune or which are damaging the graft itself. There may also be nonspecific anti-inflammatory effects of local irradiation that are not clearly understood.

IMMUNOSUPPRESSIVE DRUGS. The plethora of investigational drugs used for immunosuppression has been reduced to a few for clinical use. All these drugs, however, fall into one of two broad mechanistic categories: either they are structural analogs of needed metabolites, or they combine with components of the immunocompetent cells, such as DNA, and thereby interfere with function. The former group, the antimetabolites, because of their structural similarity, either competitively inhibit enzyme systems or are incorporated by these enzymes to produce faulty synthesis. The antimetabolites comprise purine, pyrimidine, and folic acid antagonists, and include azathioprine, the most useful suppressant of clinical transplantation rejection reactions. The antimetabolites are most effective against proliferating and differentiating cells, and hence are given at the time of transplantation when the immunocompetent cells have been stimulated. Because the stimulus to the immune system is continuous, these agents are given for the life of the graft. It is hoped that the ability to produce tolerance to transplantation antigens will some day allow earlier discontinuance.

Those compounds which combine with DNA and other cellular components include the alkylating agents and certain antibiotics. Although these agents may theoretically be useful in the pretransplant period to reduce the number of effective immunocompetent cells in the recipients, and thereafter to prevent proliferation, their use in practice has been limited because of toxicity.

Purine Analogs. The purine analog azathioprine (Imuran) is the most widely used immunosuppressive drug in clinical organ transplantation. Azathioprine is 6-mercaptopurine (6-MP) with the addition of a side chain to protect the labile sulfhydryl group. In the liver this side chain is split off, and the 6-MP is converted to the metabolically active 5′-phosphotide. The structural resemblance of this molecule to inosine monophosphate is obvious, and it inhibits the enzymes that begin the conversion of this molecule to adenosine and guanosine monophosphate (Fig. 10-24). In addition the antimetabolite slows the entire purine biosynthetic pathway by feedback inhibition of an early step. Consequently, the synthesis of cellular RNA, DNA, and certain cofactors and active nucleotides is affected.

The biologic activity of azathioprine is therefore essentially that of 6-MP, inhibition of the development of both humoral and cellular immunity by interference with the proliferative response of the lymphocyte. It is on these rapidly replicating cells that the inhibition of nucleic acid synthesis by azathioprine is most effective. Once the proliferation and differentiation of the immunocompetent cells have been accomplished, as in the case of the secondary response, nucleic acid synthesis is less important and azathioprine is less effective. The effectiveness of azathioprine in transplantation may be due not only to its effect on lymphoid cells but also to its effect on neutrophils and macrophages and hence inflammation in general.

The primary toxic effect of azathioprine is on the bone marrow, and leukopenia is occasionally a problem in clinical transplantation. This is particularly true during rejection episodes when deterioration of renal function appears

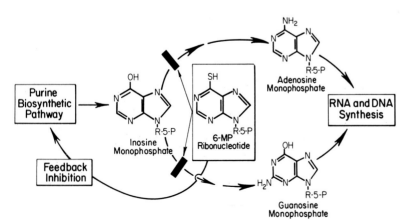

Fig. 10-24. Mechanism of antimetabolite action. 6-Mercaptopurine (6-MP) ribonucleotide resembles inosine monophosphate in its steric configuration. It thereby competes with inosine in its transformation into adenosine monophosphate and guanosine monophosphate and their subsequent incorporation into RNA and DNA. In addition, 6-MP inhibits the purine biosynthetic pathway, since it resembles a product of that biosynthetic pathway (feedback inhibition). (*From R. L. Simmons, J. E. Foker, and J. S. Najarian, Principles of Immunosuppression, in D. C. Sabiston, Jr. (ed.), "Davis-Christopher Textbook of Surgery," p. 471, W. B. Saunders Company, Philadelphia, 1972.*)

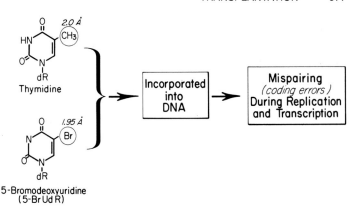

Fig. 10-25. Mechanism of antimetabolite action. 5-Bromodeoxyuridine (5BrUdR) strongly resembles thymidine in its steric configuration. Even the bromine molecule is similar in size to the methyl. 5-BrUdR thereby competes with thymidine incorporation into DNA. (*From R. L. Simmons, J. E. Foker, and J. S. Najarian, Principles of Immunosuppression, in D. C. Sabiston, Jr. (ed.), "Davis-Christopher Textbook of Surgery," p. 471, W. B. Saunders Company, Philadelphia, 1972.*)

to interfere with azathioprine clearance. Less frequently liver toxicity is seen.

Pyrimidine Analogs. Pyrimidine analogs have not been as extensively studied as immunosuppressants as have the purine analogs, and none are yet used clinically. The structure of 5-bromodeoxyuridine resembles that of thymidine, and it is incorporated into DNA (Fig. 10-25). Once incorporated, it does not have the precision in base pairing that thymidine has, and subsequent DNA synthesis is faulty, leading to ineffective progeny. Although 5-bromodeoxyuridine will prolong skin grafts and act in synergy with antilymphocyte globulin, its use is only experimental. Another pyrimidine analog, cytosine arabinoside, also inhibits effective DNA synthesis and hence affects the proliferative phase of immune response. Experimentally its immunosuppressive effect has been more easily seen by a decrease in humoral antibody response than by a decreased cellular response.

Folic Acid Antagonists. The immunosuppressive effect of a diet deficient in pteroylglutamic acid was originally noted by Little, thereby setting the stage for the use of the folic acid antagonists Aminopterin and methotrexate. Both drugs inhibit the enzyme dihydrofolate reductase, thus preventing the conversion of folic acid to tetrahydrofolic acid. This step is necessary for the synthesis of DNA, RNA, and certain coenzymes. Again proliferating cell systems would be most affected. Although some of the toxicity of these drugs can be abrogated by the administration of folic acid some hours after the use of the antagonist, the ratio of immunosuppression to toxicity has not justified their clinical use.

Alkylating Agents. The alkylating agents combine with nucleophilic centers of other molecules, i.e., molecules possessing $-NH_2$, $-COOH$, $-SH$, $-PO_3H_2$, and tertiary nitrogen compounds in heterocyclic systems. Obviously many of the components of these cells have such groups including DNA, RNA, and the enzyme and structural proteins. The high-energy ring of the alkylating agents breaks and combines with these constituents to form stable covalent bonds (Fig. 10-26). Combination with the DNA molecules is most detrimental to the cell, presumably because fewer copies of this molecule are present and if they are not repaired replication of the cell will be faulty.

Consequently, the administration of alkylating agents just before stimulation by the antigen would most interfere with the ability of the immunocompetent cells to respond to that antigen. Continued use of the alkylating agents would also muffle the proliferative responses of these cells in the face of a persistent stimulus. In general, the usefulness of these agents, which include nitrogen mustard, L-phenylalanine mustard, busulfan, and so forth, is limited by their toxicity, and they are not clinically useful for immunosuppression although they are used in the treatment of various malignant diseases.

Cyclophosphamide (Fig. 10-26), however, is an alkylating agent that has been used extensively in experimental immunosuppression and now more frequently in clinical bone marrow transplantation, where tolerance of both host to the graft and graft to the host is desired. Part of its usefulness in bone marrow transplantation is related to its ability to potentiate radiation effects, presumably through a cumulative action of the alkylating agent and radiation on DNA. Leukemia is one indication for bone marrow transplantation, and preparation of the recipient includes elimination of the leukemic cells. With cyclophosphamide, lower doses of radiation are required. More recently cyclophosphamide has been used in renal transplantation when liver toxicity has prevented the use of azathioprine; it has performed satisfactorily.

Antibiotics. Included in this category are mitomycin C and actinomycin D, which affect cellular DNA, and chloramphenicol and puromycin, which interfere with cellular protein synthesis. Actinomycin D has been extensively studied, and it has been found to bind to the guanine residue of DNA, thereby sterically inhibiting RNA polymerase and consequently inhibiting DNA-directed RNA synthesis. Despite this potentially effective means of suppressing the induction of immunity, the toxicity of this compound has limited its usefulness; it has been less and less frequently utilized clinically.

Mitomycin C combines with the DNA of the cell and interferes with cellular replication. Again, this would be useful in preventing the development of allograft immunity. As with actinomycin D, however, the general toxicity of this compound has precluded its clinical utilization. Mitomycin C is useful, however, in the mixed lymphocyte

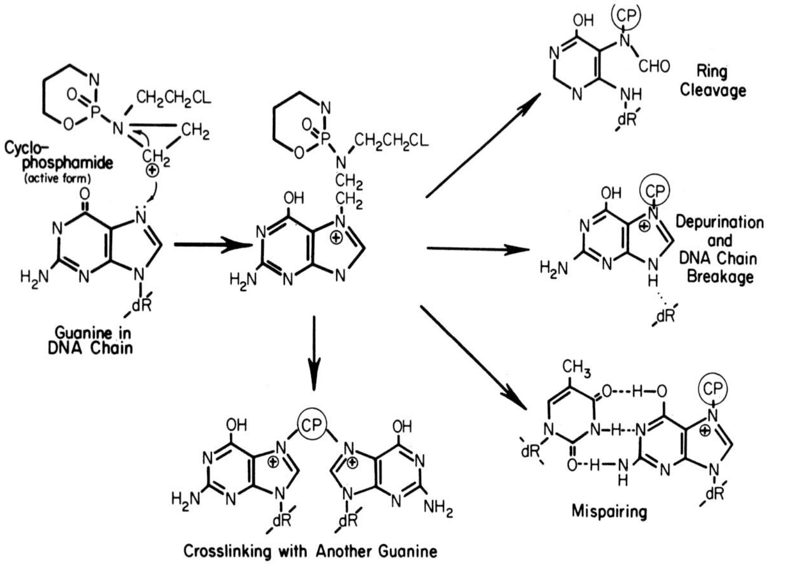

Fig. 10-26. Mechanism of the action of the alkylating agent cyclophosphamide (CP). CP binds to the guanine molecule within the DNA chain. The guanine-CP complex leads to further damage to the DNA molecule. Four examples of the damage to DNA are shown. (*From R. L. Simmons, J. E. Foker, and J. S. Najarian, Principles of Immunosuppression, in D. C. Sabiston, Jr. (ed.), "Davis-Christopher Textbook of Surgery," p. 471, W. B. Saunders Company, Philadelphia, 1972.*)

reaction in vitro. This reaction of lymphocytes toward foreign cells will probably become increasingly important in the assessment of tissue matches between prospective donors and recipients. Mitomycin C is used to block replication by the target or donor cells and hence allows assessment of recipient cell response as measured by DNA synthesis and uptake of tritiated thymidine.

Chloramphenicol and puromycin both inhibit protein synthesis and can be immunosuppressive. Chloramphenicol is most potent in prokaryotic (e.g., bacterial) cell systems and presumably exerts its effect on mammalian cells by inhibiting the mitochondria, which seem to be derived from prokaryotic cells. Puromycin resembles an amino acid-charged transfer RNA (tRNA) molecule and is accepted into the ribosome, resulting in premature termination of the peptide chain. Although protein synthesis is obviously central to immunologic expression, it is too general a requirement for other cells of the body to allow an effective inhibitory concentration to be reached without toxicity. Therefore, these agents are not used clinically. In general, only agents that primarily affect DNA synthesis are successful in treading the thin line between inhibition of the rapidly proliferating immune system and inhibition of other dividing cell systems such as the bone marrow and intestinal epithelium.

Adrenal Steroids. Adrenal steroids are the most commonly used immunosuppressants in clinical practice and are effective in a wide variety of immunologically based situations from transplantation to the treatment of lupus erythematosus, childhood nephrotic syndrome, and asthma. Their action, however, cannot be attributed solely to their lympholytic or antiproliferative activity. Corticosteroids interfere with both the acquisition of immunity by immunocompetent cells and the expression of immunity by the various effectors of the immune response. The wide variety of immunologic systems that steroids will suppress indicates that their effectiveness against the rejec-

tion reaction is probably the sum of many activities. There may well prove to be a common discrete point of inhibition for all these effects, however, when they are understood at the molecular level.

The effectiveness of cortisone in suppressing the allograft reaction was first observed in rabbits, where it was found to prolong the survival of skin grafts. Subsequently it was shown to increase skin graft survival in mice and guinea pigs, although it is ineffective by itself in pigs, dogs, monkeys, and man. Similarly, antibody production has often, but inconsistently, been found to be suppressed by the presence of steroids. Steroids are catabolic to lymphoid cells but not to liver cells, where they are anabolic. Protein and RNA synthesis are diminished by these compounds, and in sufficient concentration they cause the death of lymphoid cells. Results indicate that steroids may affect T cells more profoundly than B cells. Effector pathways are also inhibited, and one of the important effects of steroids seems to be their ability to stabilize lysosomal and cellular membranes. Steroids prevent the increased formation of lysosomes and lysosomal enzymes seen in normal stimulated lymphocytes and macrophages. They also inhibit the degranulation and release of enzymes by polymorphonuclear leukocytes, as well as phagocytosis. Steroids probably interfere with both the processing of antigens by macrophages and the digestion of allograft tissues by these active cells. Also the full expression of the complement system with its several active products is impaired by the presence of steroids.

The beneficial effect of steroids in prolonging clinical allograft survival is therefore probably the sum of several actions. They are not sufficiently active alone to prevent allograft rejection; together with azathioprine, they are potent in both preventing and reversing rejection reactions. Steroids, azathioprine, and antilymphocyte serum now compose the backbone of immunosuppression in clinical transplantation.

METHODS DESIGNED TO INHIBIT THE EXPRESSION OF IMMUNITY

When the lymphocyte has been exposed to the antigen and undergoes gene activation, proliferation, and differentiation, the product is either the sensitized T cell or humoral antibody in the form of immunoglobulin. The recognition of antigens by sensitized cells or antibodies marks the beginning of the active effort of disposal of the foreign antigen. The combination of the antigen with the sensitized cell or antibody sets off the second phase, which consists of the recruitment of a multitude of effector systems by which the antigen is removed or the graft destroyed. The reaction of antibody and immune cell with an antigen will not, by itself, eliminate the antigen or destroy the graft. The recognition phase triggers the activation of several cascading enzyme systems which include the complement, clotting, and probably the kinin pathways (Fig. 10-14). In addition, a number of cellular mediators (lymphocytes, macrophages, platelets, and PMNs) are recruited both as a consequence of the specific immunologic reaction itself (Fig. 10-10) and as a result of the subsequent enzymatic events (Fig. 10-14). All play an active role in disposing of the allograft. Thus, the efferent limb of the allograft reaction has both an immunologically specific (recognition) phase and the immunologically nonspecific (effector or amplification) phase.

It is conceivable that one could reduce the effect of an immune response by (1) promoting faster elimination of antibody, (2) interference with the complement, clotting, and kinin cascades that are activated by antigen-antibody complexes, (3) destruction of factors secreted by activated cells that recruit other activated cells (MIF, CF, cytophilic antibody, RNA, transfer factor, mitogenic factor), or (4) the neutralization of the vascular permeability factors, lysosomal enzymes, lymphotoxins. To this end a number of agents or combinations of agents that interfere with the expression of immunity have been tried. For example, anticoagulants (heparin), agents that interfere with platelet aggregation (dipyridamole, aspirin), and fibrinolytic agents have been employed to interfere with the thrombosis of graft vessels. These agents are ineffective in themselves although they may be useful adjuncts. Anticomplementary drugs (vitamin A, cobra venom factor) are not clinically useful. Antimacrophage globulin (AMG), carrageenin, and silica all destroy macrophages, but are rather weak immunosuppressants. Antibodies to lymphotoxins or MIFs and other effector molecules are in the early experimental phase. Antihistamines and antiserotonin agents have also been found to be relatively weak immunosuppressant drugs. Steroids that interfere with both the afferent and efferent limbs of the allograft reaction and with the efferent limb at multiple sites are the only immunosuppressants currently in use that may be effective after the development of immunity.

In short, it is extremely difficult to interfere with the immune response after antibody has been synthesized and after large numbers of immunologically committed effector cells have been mobilized. It is, in fact, difficult to inhibit the secondary, or anamnestic, response of any im-mune reaction. Successful interference with the effector mechanism of graft rejection is prohibited by both the complexity and the interdependence of the reaction. Many pathways and cellular participants, such as the complement, coagulation, and kinin systems, as well as lymphocytes, platelets, PMNs, and macrophages, need to be blocked. In addition, there are points of cross activation between these which make it difficult to effectively inhibit any or all of them. If true immunosuppression is to be achieved with respect to a certain antigen, one must interfere with the early phases of the primary immune response, and most accepted immunosuppressive agents act either to prevent perception of the antigen or to prevent the proliferation and synthetic response of the immunocompetent cell to the antigen.

The immunosuppressive drugs and antilymphocyte globulin all act by suppressing the capacity of the immunocompetent cell to respond to any antigen. Thus, even ALG, with its predilection for cellular immunity, cannot select between T cells destined to reject an allograft and T cells necessary for immunity against viruses and tumors. The complications of immunosuppression constantly reinforce the importance of developing modes of immunosuppression that will be specific for the histocompatibility antigens present on the graft. Experimentally, two general approaches have been tried to induce nonreactivity to a given antigen: The injection of the antigen itself, leading to a specific negative adaptation to the antigen (called immunologic tolerance) and the infusion of specific antibody (called the induction of immunologic enhancement). Both have shown promise.

Immunologic Tolerance

Immunologic tolerance refers to an immunologic nonreactivity to a specific antigen.

An animal injected with an antigen may either be stimulated to produce an immune response or, alternatively, develop a state unresponsive to subsequent exposure to the same antigen. This immunologically unresponsive state has been called *immunologic tolerance*. It is specific for the antigen and differs from chemical immunosuppression in that is is antigen directed. The best example of antigen-directed immunologic unresponsiveness is the unresponsive state enjoyed by animals to their own body constituents. During early life, before maturation of the immune mechanisms, animals apparently develop a state immunologically unresponsive to their own body constituents which is usually maintained throughout life. This unresponsive state appears to result from direct contact between the "self" components and the antigen-reactive cells. Following Burnet's prediction that specific unresponsiveness could be induced to antigenic material by injection during early life, Billingham et al. demonstrated the induction of immunologic unresponsiveness in mice to histocompatibility antigens by the neonatal injection of replicating allogenic cells. Numerous investigators have since shown that immunologic unresponsiveness can be induced to a variety of nonliving substances, as well as living cells, by injecting these substances into neonatal animals or, under selected conditions, into adult animals.

The conditions for producing immunologic unresponsiveness directed against foreign antigens are complex; the dose of antigen given must be carefully chosen. It appears that the maintenance of a critical concentration of antigen throughout all the tissue fluids is more important than the amount initially injected. The age of the recipient or the status of his immunologic competence is also important. In neonatal animals immunologic unresponsiveness to an antigen is more likely to develop than in adult animals.

Certain antigens (like serum proteins) are endowed with properties that are particularly favorable for the induction of immunologic unresponsiveness, i.e., the ability to persist in the circulation and equilibrate within the extravascular spaces, thereby coming in contact with antigen-reactive cells in effective concentration. Viral and bacterial antigens and transplantation antigens do not have these properties and, in addition, may possess multiple antigenic specificities. The conditions for the induction of tolerance to one specificity may not be conducive to the induction of tolerence to others on the same macromolecule.

The degree of tolerance produced by a mixture of histocompatibility antigens is inversely proportional to the "strength" of the antigen; i.e., it is difficult to induce immunologic tolerance to the stronger H-2 antigens but relatively simple to induce unresponsiveness to H-1 and H-3 antigens of the mouse.

Total immunologic unresponsiveness cannot be induced by tissue grafts except against the "weakest" histocompatibility antigens. Prolonged tolerance to strong antigens still requires the injection of replicating hemopoietic or lymphoid cells in the immunologically incompetent host. Chimeras with living cells of both donor and host result. If the genetic disparity between donor and host is great enough, the immunocompetent grafted cells may actually react against the host, producing a GVH reaction. GVH reaction can be circumvented in inbred animals by using donor hybrid cells injected into parental strain recipients. In these cases, permanent cellular chimerism can be established because of the inability of the grafted cells to react against the host. Surviving donor cells can be identified by a number of techniques, but the most common test of chimerism and immunologic unresponsiveness involves the persistence of an orthotopic skin graft from the donor strain. A further common test for chimerism involves the injection of lymphoid cells of the presumed chimera into an immunologically competent recipient of the host strain. Persistence of the donor cells may then be recognized by sensitization of the second recipient to those donor cells.

The proper choice of closely histocompatible donor-recipient pairs will result in immunologic unresponsiveness to histocompatibility antigens in mice without GVH disease. Tissue typing techniques have permitted a similar selection of donors for bone marrow transplantation.

It is likely that a state unresponsive to organ allografts in man will have to be induced by the use of relatively pure histocompatibility antigens. Although a state unresponsive to allografts can be induced by neonatal injections of replicating cells, such an unresponsive state does not lend itself to organ transplantation because of both GVH reaction and the necessity of predicting the need of an organ transplant at birth. An unresponsive state could undoubtedly be induced in adults to allografts if the histocompatibility antigens were injected in the proper form and if conditions were selected so that an immune response temporarily did not occur.

In order for the histocompatibility antigens to induce an unresponsive state following injection, they would probably have to equilibrate throughout the body fluid and persist at the antigen reactive cells in a critical concentration and for a critical period of time. Histocompatibility antigens have been solubilized by detergents, organic solvents, enzymatic degradation, and sonic energy. However, the yield of active material is very low. Furthermore, the chemical nature of these antigens and the small molecular size of the more purified peptides suggest that, following injection of even large amounts of the antigens, they would neither persist in the body fluid nor equilibrate into extravascular fluid space in sufficient amount to maintain critical concentrations at the antigen-sensitive cells. Despite the above obstacles, the chances of inducing lasting immunologic unresponsiveness in the future are quite good. In fact, even crude preparations of soluble transplantation antigens injected intravenously tend to induce prolonged graft survival. The induction of immunologic unresponsiveness to histocompatibility antigens depends first on isolation of these antigens in relatively pure form and in reasonable amounts and, second, on the injection of these antigens under selective conditions which do not result in an immune response.

Irradiation, chemical immunosuppression, and ALG have been used to inhibit the immune response and permit development of a state relatively unresponsive to an antigen administered while immunocompetence is depressed. The major barrier to an attempt at induction of immunologic tolerance in adult transplant patients is the fear that immunity, rather than tolerance, will be induced.

It is likely that, even now, clinical transplantation depends on the establishment of a degree of immunologic unresponsiveness to the antigens implanted in the form of the transplanted organ.

Immunologic Enhancement

It is possible that total immunologic unresponsiveness represents a specific negative response to an antigen. The state of relative unresponsiveness is more likely due to the presence of an antibody that itself interferes with the further development of immunity.

The amount of antibody formed in response to any antigen appears to be restricted over a wide range of antigen dosages and a variety of immunization regimens. As a rule, antibody reaches predictable maximal levels despite continued immunization. The mechanisms that regulate these events so precisely are still largely unknown, but the apparent presence of a feedbacklike regulation has long suggested that antibody might prove to be a specific immunosuppressant. The immune response to many antigens can be totally abrogated by the passive transfer of specific antibodies prior to or shortly after the administration of antigen. Even antibody fragments (Fab fragments) will suppress the immune response. Two general mechanisms of antibody action have been proposed. Originally, investigators termed the antibody blockade of immunologic response the *enhancement phenomenon* from results obtained with tumors. In these experiments animals were immunized with allogenic tumor extracts, provoking humoral antibody response. When the animal was subsequently grafted with tumor, the graft grew more readily than normal. It has now been shown that, under certain conditions of sensitization, blocking antibodies will be produced. These antibodies do not seem to have the same functional capabilities as do the usual antibodies and hence do not trigger the effector mechanisms of graft rejection. Instead they bind to the antigen and block the action of more cytotoxic antibodies.

The second general way in which antibodies could act as immunosuppressants would be by feedback inhibition. One can inhibit the response to any antigen by passively immunizing the animal with antiserum. The most striking practical use of this phenomenon is seen in the prevention of erythroblastosis fetalis by the administration of anti-Rh antiserum to the pregnant mother. Here, the administration of the antibody inhibits the immune response to the fetal Rh antigen.

Whatever the mechanism, immunologic "enhancement" has been so named because its realization requires the presence of antigraft antibody in the prospective host. The token of enhancement is "permanent" survival of the allograft (for cancer grafts this means premature death of the host) or a delay in rejection.

Enhancement can be induced by prior exposure of the graft recipient to the histocompatibility antigens of the donor, i.e., active enhancement. The state of the antigen and the timing of first exposure with relation to the test graft are crucial. In addition, the conditions for each antigen differ, and each strain and species of animal appear to react in a different way.

The induction of enhancement by passively transferred antiserum, in particular by γ-globulin (passive enhancement), is more effective. Experience has shown that late hyperimmune sera are more efficient than early ones, although enhancing serum can be recovered from mice 4 days after they have been sensitized with live tumor. Assays of serum fractions place enhancing activity in the 7S immunoglobulins. More specifically, enhancement has been ascribed to IgG-γ_2. Even microliter (and smaller) quantities of passive antibody may be effective.

Impressive results have been obtained with kidney allografts in rats and dogs. In rats, Stuart et al. obtained uncurtailed survivals for $(L \times BN)F_1$ kidneys implanted in Lewis rats that had received injections of viable F_1 spleen cells 18 to 24 hours before grafting, with treatment continued on alternate days after grafting up to 62 days. The best results followed combined intravenous injection of spleen cells and specific alloantiserum, the antibody being given 2 hours before and 1 hour after grafting. Survival

was equally good with antibody administration continued for either 6 or 62 days after grafting. Either antigen or antibody alone was not as effective. The grafts were not affected adversely by antibody. The donor-host combination differed at the strong Ag-B histocompatibility locus. Similar results have been achieved in immunosuppressed dogs, and the line differentiating immunologic tolerance and enhancement have become blurred.

Immunosuppression by antibody enhancement, and immunosuppression by antigen tolerance may, therefore, be essentially identical mechanisms of specific immunosuppression. The presence of such antibodies cannot always be detected in "tolerant" individuals, but antibodies can be detected in patients with excellent long-term functioning human renal allografts.

Privileged Sites for Allografts

First-set grafts require either a vascular or a lymphatic conduit for sensitization, although the presensitized recipient can reject a second-set allograft before vascular connection develops. Certain sites within the recipient, therefore, permit extended graft survival of first-set grafts.

The anterior chamber of the eye has been the most frequently used privileged space for allografts and xenografts of both normal and malignant tissues. Grafts at this site were originally thought to survive because of their inability to sensitize the host, and not because they are protected from immunologic mediators of rejection. Tissues in the anterior chamber are rejected if the host is sensitized by conventional means. Therefore, the anterior chamber of the eye has been considered an excellent site for the study of the afferent arc of immunity. It is one of the rare locations in which lymphatic vessels are completely lacking, and the prolonged survival of grafts provides further evidence for the importance of lymphatic connections in host sensitization.

Absence of lymphatic connections may not be the only explanation. Raju and Grogan have presented evidence that grafts within the anterior chamber become vascularized rapidly and sensitize the recipient only slightly less rapidly than other grafts. Despite such sensitization, however, the grafts continue to survive unless sensitization is induced by more conventional techniques. Implants in unsensitized recipients become infiltrated by small round cells which somehow are *not* associated with graft destruction. The extended survival of grafts in the anterior chamber may represent a combination of both afferent arc delay and efferent arc blockade.

Other sites provide a special environment for allografts. It has been known for almost 50 years that the meninges of the brain shelter grafts. The implants must be within the meninges and without encroachment on the ventricles. The extended survival is dependent on a lack of vascular connections to the host, which in turn prevents sensitization. The immunologic insulation of the testis may relate to its circuitous lymphatic supply. Presentation of the antigens may be inefficient.

The cheek pouch of the hamster has been used as a

location for a variety of foreign grafts. Once again, graft survival is due to reduced ability to sensitize the host, since grafts will not survive in the cheek pouches of hamsters previously sensitized to donor antigens. Even well-established grafts will be rejected promptly if the host is sensitized through conventional means. The immunologic arc seems to be interrupted on the afferent side because the mucopolysaccharide-containing connective tissue of the pouch acts as an immunologic insulator.

Histocompatibility Matching

It is obvious that, other things being equal, the less antigenic the graft, the less the host will react against the graft. In human transplantation, when the donor and recipient are identical twins, there is no antigenic difference of any significance, and the tissues will be readily accepted. When the donor and recipient are siblings or when a parent donor is used for offspring, there is a greater statistical likelihood of antigen sharing between donor and recipient than when a cadaver or other unrelated donor is used.

Several methods have been developed for the purpose of demonstrating antigenic similarities between donor and recipient prior to transplantation, so that donor and recipient pairs may be selected which are relatively histocompatible. This should lessen the need for large doses of immunosuppressive drugs and increase the likelihood of an ultimately successful outcome. Although many methods have been tried, the currently most promising are leukocyte typing and MLC (mixed lymphocyte culture).

LEUKOCYTE TYPING

The rationale for leukocyte typing is based upon two observations: The first is that leukocytes are capable of immunizing animals to a subsequent skin or kidney graft and thus must share many important antigens with these and other tissues of the body. The second rationale is that antisera from certain patients who have received multiple transfusions will react with cells from some patients but not from others. Investigators observed that antisera of this type were also found in certain multiparous women. Subsequently, many antisera obtained from multiply transfused patients or from women with multiple pregnancies (and occasionally from other sources) have been assembled and tested for their ability to detect leukocyte antigens. Some of the antisera seem to recognize groups of antigens, and others recognize single antigens (monospecific antisera). Using the patient's leukocytes and a group of standard antisera it is thus possible to characterize many, if not all, of the strong (HL-A) histocompatibility antigens on the human lymphocyte membrane. This is done for both donor and recipient, and the two patterns are then compared to determine whether the donor is likely to be compatible with the recipient or not (Table 10-1).

Antigens found less frequently have been identified which appear not to be at this locus; it is likely that other antigenic loci may be defined in the future. The inheritance of HL-A antigens was discussed above. Weaker histocompatibility antigens at other loci have not been detected by serologic techniques in man.

Currently antigens are detected by isolating lymphocytes from the peripheral blood of potential donors or recipients. The cells are incubated with antisera of various specificities and rabbit serum as a source of complement. Cells which react with antibodies in the serum die in the presence of complement and can be stained with vital dyes. Typing sera is becoming increasingly standardized. A typical set of results from the University of Minnesota typing laboratories is illustrated in Table 10-1.

Histocompatibility typing is useful in determining the best match between donor and recipient when family donors are utilized. Siblings who share all four HL-A antigens in common and who have inherited identical

Table 10-1. LYMPHOCYTE ANTIGEN TYPING REPORT OF THEORETIC FAMILY*

Family member	ABO	Genotype	HL-A locus (LA)								HL-A 2d locus (four)														
			HL-A1	HL-A2	HL-A3	HL-A9	HL-A10	HL-A11	W19	W28	HL-A5	HL-A7	HL-A8	HL-A12	HL-A13	W5	W10	W14	W15	W16	W17	W18	W21	W22	W27
Father AB	A	AO	+	+	−	−	−	−	−	−	−	+	+	−	−	−	−	−	−	−	−	−	−	−	−
Mother CD	A	AO	−	−	+	+	+	−	−	−	+	−	··	+	−	−	−	−	−	−	−	−	−	−	−
Son AC (patient)	O	OO	+	−	+	−	−	−	−	−	+	−	+	−	−	−	−	−	−	−	−	−	−	−	−
Son AD	A	?	+	−	−	+	+	−	−	−	−	−	+	+	−	−	−	−	−	−	−	−	−	−	−
Daughter BC	O	OO	−	+	+	−	−	−	−	−	+	+	−	−	−	−	−	−	−	−	−	−	−	−	−
Daughter BD	A	?	−	+	−	+	+	−	−	−	−	+	−	+	−	−	−	−	−	−	−	−	−	−	−
Daughter AC	O	OO	+	−	+	−	−	−	−	−	+	−	+	−	−	−	−	−	−	−	−	−	−	−	−

*The specificities for the first and second loci are those currently used at the University of Minnesota.

Son AC is the prospective transplant recipient. Daughter AC is a perfect match for all four antigens; she shares the inheritance of both HL-A haplotypes and is the ideal donor. Both parents, son AD, and daughter BC share only one haplotype with the potential recipient and are theoretically not as good donors. Daughter BD shares no HL-A haplotypes with the recipient and is the poorest donor in the family.

More important than the HL-A type are the ABO blood types. The father, mother, son AD, and daughter BD *cannot* donate, because they are all blood group A and the recipient is blood group O and possesses anti-A antibodies in his serum.

HL-A haplotypes from their parents are the best possible donor-recipient pair. But there are several points about histocompatibility matching which deserve emphasis: (1) Recipients receiving grafts even from donors who are "perfect" matches with them will still reject the graft (although more slowly) unless immunosuppressive drugs are utilized. Only an identical twin is truly a perfect match. In the context used here "perfect" simply means that there are no detectable antigenic differences between donor and host with the antisera employed and that the degree of compatibility is sufficiently high so that, with the judicial use of immunosuppressive drugs, the outcome is likely to be good. (2) Even with poor histocompatibility matches between relatives the results are frequently good. Those results probably indicate that, with the current immunosuppressive drugs, it is sometimes possible to suppress even great degrees of antigenic incompatibility. (3) Even in the presence of a good histocompatibility match the graft may fail if the host happens to have preformed antibodies against a donor's tissues. These antibodies can be recognized if recipient serum is allowed to react with donor lymphocytes in a cytotoxicity test. This test is called *cross matching* and should be performed with fresh serum as a final test of compatibility prior to transplant. Preformed cytotoxic antibodies to donor tissue cannot be detected by the usual typing procedure itself. (4) The presence of anti-A (or anti-B) antibodies will lead to the prompt rejection of tissue bearing A (or B) blood group substances. Transplants in the face of such barriers should not be performed. (5) Despite the results of tissue typing, a related donor will generally yield better transplant results than an unrelated (cadaver) donor. This statement is controversial, but the results of kidney transplantation strongly support it. (6) Tissue typing for unrelated cadaver donors is not as successful as typing for related donors. Most American kidney transplant centers cannot make good correlations between closeness of typing and satisfactory results of kidney transplantation.

MIXED LYMPHOCYTE CULTURE (MLC)

The other method of detecting degrees of histocompatibility between donor and recipient is the MLC test, which is still being explored to some extent. Lymphocytes of the recipient are mixed with lymphocytes of the donor in tissue culture. If significant antigenic differences exist between the two, they will respond by transformation into blasts, DNA synthesis, and mitosis. The incorporation of tritiated thymidine into DNA can be quantitated to assess the degree of stimulation. As the test was originally devised, it was a two-way test—cells of the donor were capable of reacting against cells of the recipient and vice versa. In order to isolate and quantitate the response of the recipient cells to the donor antigens, the donor lymphocytes can be inactivated by irradiation or exposure to mitomycin C.

The MLC test is very sensitive and does not distinguish between subtle shadings of incompatibility. It may, however, be useful in demonstrating degrees of incompatibility which are not detectible in tissue typing. For example, one of every four sibling pairs will have inherited identical HL-A antigens. Occasionally the lymphocytes of such siblings will stimulate each other in MLC. Whether the MLC test is useful in predicting transplant success or failure in that circumstance is still under study.

CLINICAL TISSUE AND ORGAN TRANSPLANTATION

Clinical allotransplants may be of several types: (1) temporary free grafts, such as skin allografts, and blood transfusions; (2) partially inert struts which provide a framework for the ingrowth of host tissue, such as bone, cartilage, nerve, tendon, and fascial grafts; (3) permanent, partially privileged, structural free grafts, such as cornea, blood vessels, and heart valves; (4) partially privileged functional free grafts such as parathyroid, ovary, and testes; (5) whole organ grafts, such as pancreas, kidney, liver, lung, and heart. Immunosuppression has been given only to patients with grafts in the last category. Because of the danger of immunosuppressive therapy it is seldom warranted for grafts not essential for life. Lymph nodes and spleen grafts, which are highly antigenic have the immunologic potential to react against the host and have not proved useful in man. Tooth bud and thyroid grafts, which would require immunosuppression for any success, are trivial grafts and are easily replaced by prostheses or medication.

Clinical autotransplants have been carried out with hair, skin, teeth, kidney, legs, arms, veins, arteries, pericardium, valves, bone, cartilage, fascia, fat, tendons, nerves, stomach, bowel, parathyroid, thyroid, ovary, testis, adrenal, and hemopoietic tissue. Allotransplants have been carried out employing cornea, teeth, thyroid, parathyroid, adrenal, ovary, testis, pituitary, spleen, lymph node, skin, bone, cartilage, fascia, tendons, nerves, arteries, valves, veins, hemopoietic tissue, pancreas, duodenum, kidney, liver, lung, and heart. Xenografts of skin, valves, heart, kidney, testis, bone, and cartilage have been tried in recent years.

Skin

Autotransplants of skin containing hair are used to reconstruct eyebrows or to replace the scalp after traumatic avulsion. Autotransplants of individual hair roots are sometimes used as a treatment for baldness. Skin autotransplants have been used to reconstruct the esophagus, urinary tract, vagina, and hernial weaknesses as well as the usual surface defects. The main use of skin autographs is to cover and replace areas destroyed by trauma, burn, or operation.

Skin allotransplants are also used quite extensively in burned patients. They are used in three different ways: In the first they are applied as a dressing to the burned area and are removed after 3 or 4 days. At this time additional allografts are reapplied if the area does not appear to be clean enough to accept autografts. If the area does appear to be clean, autografts are applied. The theory behind this is that the skin allograft provides a better coverage than any other material, and during the period of time when it is taking, it prevents the continued spread of sepsis. In the second method the allograft is applied and allowed to take. When it begins to be rejected, it is removed, and autografts are applied. The third method is to place alternate thin strips of autografted and allografted skin side by side to cover large defects. As the allografted skin is gradually rejected, it is replaced by epithelial cells which grow in from the autografts.

The burned patient appears to have some depression of his immunologic defenses and will tolerate skin allografts for somewhat longer periods of time than the normal patient. Nevertheless the grafts are ultimately rejected, but by this time the patient's general condition has improved to the point where autografts can be carried out. If the burned patient happened to have an identical twin, of course, this would be an ideal circumstance, since the skin, being antigenically identical to his own, would take indefinitely. In fact, an exchange of skin grafts between two individuals thought to be identical twins used to be the method by which this relationship was definitely established. Despite earlier reports that fetal skin might have some advantage over adult skin, none of these grafts have survived permanently.

Vascular Grafts

AUTOGRAFT

Vein autografts have been used for over 50 years to replace segments of damaged arteries. This is still by far the best bypass graft for occluded vessels in the lower extremity below the level of the inguinal ligament. It is also possible to carry out successful autologous vein grafts to bridge defects in veins, although veins are less likely to stay open than arteries. After a period of time in the arterial circuit the vein wall thickens, and the vein becomes somewhat arterialized. Although there are occasional instances in which vein grafts weaken and rupture, by and large they make very satisfactory arterial substitutes. The two most common usages at the present time are in femoropopliteal artery–saphenous vein bypass grafts and aortorenal artery–saphenous vein bypass grafts. Pieces of autologous vein are also used as patch grafts either for small stenotic areas, such as the renal artery, or over long segments of endarterectomized artery. Autologous vein grafts have also been used as tendon sheath and bile duct replacement without success.

Autografted arteries are sometimes used as vascular replacements. An occluded superficial femoral artery may be excised, opened, endarterectomized, and resutured over a stent for use as a bypass graft or for replacing another arterial segment.

Pieces of pericardium are sometimes used to form vessels or as a patch graft on some partially occluded vessel or intracardiac defects. An autologous pulmonary valve is sometimes removed and used to replace a defective aortic valve. The pulmonary valve is then replaced with a prosthesis or a homografted valve. However, this procedure has very little clinical applicability.

ALLOGRAFT

The use of allografted arteries had a considerable vogue a few years ago, but they are seldom used now. There are three reasons for this: The first is that when allografts were used to replace the abdominal aorta, aneurysms sometimes occurred, with rupture and a fatal outcome. Secondly, the advent of Dacron and other plastic prostheses have proved so suitable for the larger blood vessels that they are far superior to allografts in convenience and results. Finally, for smaller blood vessels the use of the autologous saphenous vein has proved to be better than either prostheses or homografts. Arterial allografts, even if viable, do not survive but in part are replaced by host tissue and in part persist as semi-inert material. These changes occur whether the graft is fresh, frozen, or freeze-dried. When allografts have been used to repair coarctation of the aorta in small children, it has been observed that as the child grows, the graft is capable of some increase in diameter, as well as in length. This is perhaps the one advantage which an allograph has over a plastic graft.

When organs are transplanted, the artery supplying the organ becomes an arterial allograft. It has been shown that the epithelium of smaller blood vessels is highly antigenic. Although this is less so in the larger vessels, some degree of allograft rejection occurs in vascular grafts, which probably accounts for the difference in the results between experimental arterial autografts and allografts, the latter being distinctly inferior to the former.

Allografted valves have been used quite extensively. They appear to elicit a very minimal antigenic response when compared even to arterial homografts.

Vein allografts have been used for a number of years in a sporadic fashion. It was shown some years ago that apart from vein autografts the only type of graft which would remain patent in small veins was a vein allograft. The results with the allograft were inferior to the results of the autograft but were superior to every other material tried. Vein allografts have been used to perform femoropopliteal arterial bypass grafts but have been found by most workers to become occluded with the passage of time. There is, of course, no reason whatsoever for the inferiority of arterial and venous grafts to autografts of the same type *except* for the antigenicity of the homograft and the mild rejection reaction which these grafts elicit. For some reason there has been a great reluctance among surgeons and others to accept the fact that arterial and venous allografts are antigenic. It is true that the antigenicity is relatively mild and that the graft can provide a structural function even in the face of the immunologic response. Some changes occur in allografted arteries, however, even in the immunosuppressed individual.

The use of allografted veins is being reinvestigated with an assessment of the relative histocompatibility of the donor and host to see whether appropriate matching might lead to results with vein allografts which are comparable to those obtained with autografts. The situation occasionally arises in which either autografts are unobtainable or the diameter of the distal vein is too small to permit an adequate flow. The matched vein allograft may provide an answer for some of these cases.

Fascia

Fascial autografts, either free or attached at one end, are used as living sutures to repair inguinal hernias; for the repair of chest wall defects, torn ligaments and tendons, abdominal wall hernias, and defects in the pleura, dura, diaphragm, trachea, and esophagus; for wrapping aneurysms; in arthroplasty; for fascial slings to correct paralysis of the facial muscles; in the stabilization of fractures and joints; in the construction of flexor sheaths; and to correct urinary incontinence. Fascial autografts have been used almost exclusively because of their convenience and ready availability. Some preserved fascial xenografts have been used, however, and these dead grafts have united with muscle nearly as quickly as living fascia but evoke a much more marked inflammatory response and fail to retain their elasticity as well as autologous fascia.

Tendon

Free tendon autografts are used every day in standard surgical procedures. By far the most common use is that of repairing severed flexor tendons to the fingers. Usually the palmaris longus or extensor tendons of the toes are used, and the graft is inserted from the level of the mid-palm of the hand to the distal phalanx.

Until lately very little success had been obtained with allografts, and these were almost never used. Peacock and Madden have reported the results of 11 homografts in 10 patients. The technique they used is to remove both flexor tendons and all surrounding tissue from the hand and finger of a cadaver and to maintain the integrity of this entire block of tissue when inserting the graft into the recipient. Under these circumstances adhesions form only to the outer layer of the tissue, and the graft continues to glide against the inner surfaces which are normally against it. Experiments in animals have shown that there is very little antigenicity of these grafts, since they are composed largely of collagen, which is nonantigenic. They do not immunize the animal for subsequent skin grafts, for example. The results of these grafts have been extremely good, with a 70 percent functional success rate. At the present time the use of allografts is indicated in patients who have already experienced failure of an autograft or in a situation where the trauma to the extremity has been so great that there is little likelihood that an autograft would succeed. This technique is an ingenious one, and the results have been extremely good. It seems likely that it will acquire wider application.

Nerve

Nerve autotransplants are used to bridge defects in important motor nerves or sometimes to transfer the function of one nerve into the distal end of another, to repair a severed facial or recurrent laryngeal nerve, for instance. It has been nearly 100 years since it was demonstrated that a nerve autograft was capable of conducting impulses across a nerve defect. The autografts undergo wallerian degeneration with proliferation of Schwann cells and are penetrated by regenerating fibers of the host's nerve after a few weeks. When the nerve graft is thick, the center of the graft may develop a zone of avascular necrosis in which regeneration fails to occur, whereas this does not happen with thin grafts. As a consequence of this some investigators have advocated the use of cable grafts consisting of several strands of smaller nerves to bridge defects in nerves of large caliber. Sensory recovery can occur as well as motor recovery.

When allografts are used, wallerian degeneration also takes place but occurs a little more slowly than in autografts. The proliferation of Schwann cells is not as vigorous as in autografts, and after a few days the cells appear to become necrotic. Despite this fact allografts are capable of penetration by the nerve fibers and have permitted return of nerve function across the defect. The rate and intensity of nerve fiber penetration is less in allografts than in autografts. The ultimate outcome of allografts is clearly far inferior to that obtained with autografts, and in general they should probably be used only when autografts cannot be obtained. Xenografts have been tried but appear to be of no value to man. It is likely that the inflammatory rejection response interferes with the passage of autologous nerve endings down the transplanted nerve sheath.

Cornea

Perhaps the most common clinical allotransplant is that of the cornea. The eye should be harvested from cadavers within at least 1 hour after death, although intervals up to 5 hours are permissible. Eyes removed more than 15 hours after death are unsuitable for corneal transplantation. The whole eye is generally preserved in sterile liquid paraffin at a temperature of 3 to 5°C, and the graft is cut from it at the time of use. The eye is suspended from a suture passed through the severed optic nerve to keep it from coming in contact with the sides of the vessel. Frozen corneas are not as good as those preserved this way, and freeze-dried corneas are completely unsatisfactory. Xenografts are useless.

Two types of corneal transplants are utilized: the full-thickness graft and the lamellar, or partial-thickness, graft. The full-thickness graft should give the best results, but complications such as secondary glaucoma, anterior synechiae, and a partial lifting off of the graft, causing astigmatism or opacification, are frequent. These complications are avoided in lamellar keratoplasty, which is the operation of choice when the corneal opacity does not involve the full thickness of the cornea. In order to achieve a successful graft there must be good apposition between the graft and the host, the graft must be in contact with healthy cornea at some point in the circumference if it is to remain transparent, and blood vessels must not invade the graft to any appreciable extent.

The best patients for grafting are those with central corneal scars and healthy surrounding cornea with no vascularization; keratoconus, especially if the apex of the cone is beginning to break down; corneal dystrophy; indolent corneal abscesses; and perforating ulcers of the cornea which have resulted in a descemetocele. The results are somewhat less good in acne rosacea and herpetic keratitis because of the danger of recurrence of the disease.

Corneal grafts are apparently so successful because they remain effectively isolated from the host's cells so long as the graft itself, and the cornea directly around it, remain avascular. Many corneal grafts remain clear indefinitely, although occasionally a graft which has remained clear for several weeks becomes opaque. Apparently the fibrous barrier which is formed at the junction between the host and the graft is almost impervious to blood vessels and helps to maintain the isolation of the graft even when vessels have entered the host's cornea. The clouding over of a previously clear graft is due to the allograft reaction, usually because of vascularization. It has been demonstrated experimentally that if a graft of skin from the donor of the cornea is put on 2 to 6 weeks after corneal transplantation, the graft becomes opaque, whereas if a skin homograft from another donor is applied, nothing happens. Skin from the original donor transplanted 6 weeks or more after the corneal transplantation is no longer capable of causing it to become opaque. This is presumably due to adaptation, the development of the scar tissue barrier between the host and the graft, or replacement of the cells of the graft by host's cells.

Bone

Bone implants are used for the following indications: (1) to hasten the healing of defects and cavities, e.g., the use of cancellous bone chips in the residual defect after curettage of a unicameral bone cyst; (2) to supplement the arthrodesis of joints, e.g., extraarticular arthrodesis of the tuberculous hip; (3) to achieve bony union in cases of delayed healing or pseudarthrosis arising after fracture, e.g., sliding or barrel stave grafts for nonunion of tibial shaft fractures; (4) to supplement the healing of certain fresh fractures for which open reduction and internal fixation are required, e.g., cancellous implants for fractures of both bones of the forearm in an adult; (5) for reconstruction of major skeletal defects arising as a result of trauma, disease, or congenital malformation; (6) for reconstruction of contour, e.g., replacement of calvarial defects after surgery for trauma by compact bone implants.

A variety of grafting techniques has been devised to meet the differing clinical requirements. The most frequent types of bone grafts are inlay grafts, onlay grafts and/or internal fixation, barrel stave grafts, sliding grafts, and application of cancellous chips. In addition, there are pedicled grafts of two types, those with a bony base and muscle pedicle grafts. The pedicle technique applies strictly to autografts and was devised to circumvent devitalization, thereby hastening healing.

Autografts are preferred for clinical use, since the cellular elements of bone allografts usually elicit a rejection response. Bone allografts do elicit new bone formation (osteoinduction) and serve as struts for the ingrowth of autologous bone (osteoconduction). As such, allografts are

of great clinical use although they are always somewhat inferior to autografts.

For the most part stored or processed bone allografts are used in human beings. Preservation methods include (1) refrigeration, (2) freezing, (3) freeze-drying, (4) boiling or autoclaving, (5) deproteinization, (6) decalcification, (7) any one of the above plus irradiation for sterilization, and (8) removal of marrow elements and replacement by autologous marrow. Such nonviable grafts mainly serve to stimulate and conduct new autologous bone formation.

Cartilage

It has been long known that cartilage can be successfully transferred between individuals of different genetic backgrounds without the need for immunosuppression therapy. This immunologic privilege is attributable to the presence of the mucoprotein matrix, which acts as an insulation to prevent host lymphocytes from reaching the graft chondrocytes. Cartilage cells can elicit allograft responses, but cartilage grafts will survive even in highly immunized hosts.

Free autografts of cartilage have been used most extensively in plastic reconstructive surgery (1) to rebuild the contours of the nose after congenital or posttraumatic deformity, (2) to reconstruct the pinna, and (3) to fill out defects in the facial bones and the skull.

The fresh cartilage autograft comes closest to fulfilling the description of an ideal cartilage graft: it should maintain its structure, have the potential for growth and repair, provoke no untoward reaction, and form a firm union with host tissues, persisting without loss of viability or absorption.

The fresh cartilage allograft, however, has been a reasonable substitute for the autograft, particularly because of its greater ease of procurement. The major drawback of such grafts is that despite the immunologic privilege of cartilage, the bulk of experimental and clinical evidence suggests that the tendency for late deterioration and absorption is somewhat greater than that of autografts.

The preserved cartilaginous allograft has been used as a substitute for the fresh implant primarily for the convenience that storage of such implants in cartilage banks provides. Boiled, refrigerated, frozen, and chemically pressured cartilage have all been used with success.

The cartilage xenograft should be mentioned since it enjoys a prolonged survival and relative exemption from transplantation rejection unrivaled by any other tissue. Even so, the exemption is not complete, and some xenografts elicit strong inflammatory responses and are absorbed.

COMPOSITE GRAFTS OF BONE AND CARTILAGE

Composite grafts involve the surgical transfer of entire functional units rather than the implantation of bits and pieces of cartilage or bone.

EPIPHYSEAL GROWTH PLATES. The object of the transplantation of epiphyseal growth plates is to restore longitudinal growth in hypoplastic limbs, whether congenital or acquired. This type of procedure has been used in efforts to improve the function of children with congenital deficiency of the radius. In these cases, autotransplantation of the proximal fibula has been used as a substitute for the radial deficiency. Although, in some cases, enlargement of the transplant could be demonstrated, this was always inferior to the natural growth potential and has not been sufficient to justify incorporation of this procedure into the surgical armamentarium.

OSTEOCHONDRAL GRAFTS. The diseases that destroy the articular cartilage are common. The osteochondral or osteoarticular graft might be a useful substitute. Transplants of articular cartilage, in conjunction with a very thin shell of subchondral supporting bone, are still in the experimental stage. Such operations will require allografting.

TRANSPLANT OF HEMIJOINTS OR WHOLE JOINTS. The experimental transplantation of joints was initiated by Judet in 1908. Autografts tend to heal their osteosynthesis sites, revascularize the bony component, and in general maintain the articular surfaces in a fair state of preservation. On the other hand, both fresh and preserved allogeneic transplants begin to deteriorate progressively about 6 months after surgery. These changes in the allogeneic groups are associated with delayed revascularization of the bony component, subchondral fracture and collapse, and the late development of degenerative arthritic change. Clinical joint transplantation has been sporadically performed for half a century. In general, joint function is satisfactory at first, but degenerative changes occur.

Extremity Replantation

Autotransplants or replantation of extremities have been carried out. This has usually involved the upper extremity, because the chances for nerve regeneration are far greater in the arm than in the leg. Satisfactory prostheses exist for the lower extremity, but they are much more complex and unsatisfactory for the upper. Shortening of the severed extremity usually is necessary, and this produces much more incapacity in the leg than in the arm. Replantation of the leg might be considered when the opposite leg has been extensively damaged or lost or when the amputation has been so high that good prostheses are not available.

The technique of limb replantation initially requires a general evaluation of the patient to assess other associated injuries. This should include an x-ray of the proximal stump as well as the amputated extremity itself, and particularly the spine to be certain that the spinal roots to the extremity have not been avulsed. After securing hemostasis and being certain that no serious injury has been overlooked, the replantation can begin. During this initial phase the severed limb should be packed in ice. If the facilities are available, the artery of the limb should be perfused with cold Ringer's lactate solution to which albumin and heparin have been added. The limb may be replanted even though several hours have elapsed between its severance and the start of replantation. The exact critical period has not definitely been established, but it appears that at least 6 hours and sometimes even more can elapse with successful results after replantation. Satisfactory hypothermia of the extremity increases this period.

The more distal the amputation, the better the preservation of the extremity, and the more prolonged is the tolerance to ischemia.

When perfusion is completed and replantation is about to begin, a limited debridement of grossly devitalized tissue is carried out. Questionably viable tissue is not removed. Then the bone is fixed so that the limb will be stabilized before beginning the repairs of the vessels and nerve supply. The bone is usually shortened about 2 in. to freshen up the ends and to gain additional length for relaxation of the arteries and nerves. Intramedullary fixation is used whenever possible.

After proper fixation of the bones the blood vessels are joined. The largest vein is joined first, so that there will be an outflow tract at the moment when the blood is ready to flow through the artery. A triangulation technique is used for the veins, to prevent constricting them and for ease of anastomosis. An autologous saphenous vein graft can be used to bridge any defect.

If the nerve injury has been a crushing one, nerve repair is delayed until healing is complete. If the nerve has been cleanly severed with a sharp instrument, particularly if the injury has been at the level of the wrist, immediate primary repair is carried out. With either primary or secondary nerve repair sections are sliced from the ends of the nerve until a fresh end of pure, scar-free nerve is encountered. After each end is prepared in this fashion, the two are apposed very carefully, and the epineurium is sutured with interrupted fine nonabsorbable sutures. It is probably important to avoid tension on the nerve ending, and this usually is accomplished by the previous shortening of the bone carried out as the first step in replantation. While the results of nerve allografts are still highly problematic, an autograft or allograft should be used to bridge any large defect in the nerve. A better result is obtained in distal nerve transections than in proximal ones, and in young people as compared with older ones. Motor recovery in the median nerve is much more common than in the ulnar nerve.

After completing the arterial and venous anastomoses and after either joining the ends of the nerves or deciding to perform nerve suture as a secondary procedure, attention is turned to the soft tissues. With the blood supply restored viability of tissues is easier to ascertain, and debridement can be completed. The shortening of the bone makes it possible to join several muscles together with a particular view to covering the blood vessels with living tissues. If soft tissue loss is minimal, the covering can be achieved with the skin of the extremity, and other defects can be covered with split-thickness skin grafts. If the soft tissue defect is great and no covering is available, the defect must be covered by a pedicle flap.

In the postoperative period the patient's arm must be kept in an elevated position to avoid the swelling which is almost inevitable. It is important to do a fasciotomy at the end of the replantation to avoid severe ischemia from swelling if damage to the arm was severe. Heparin and dextran are not generally used postoperatively. Some degree of hypotension may occur as a consequence of leakage of plasma into the replanted extremity. This is particularly true of a lower extremity. The hypotension is counteracted by the administration of plasma. There may be an acute period of acidosis as a consequence of absorption of metabolic products from the ischemic extremity, and this is counteracted by the administration of bicarbonate. Both bicarbonate and mannitol are administered to protect against renal damage, and prophylactic antibiotics are also administered. If early severe sepsis supervenes, the extremity may have to be amputated. Low-grade late infection, usually consisting of osteomyelitis, is treated by drainage and irrigation, and the fixation materials are left in place until the bone heals even in the face of sepsis— because fixation must be achieved if possible.

Passive movement of all joints is begun immediately and continued throughout the course of treatment. Galvanic stimulation of the intrinsic muscles of the hand is utilized to maintain the tone of the muscles. Extensive physical therapy is instituted. If primary nerve suture has not been carried out, the nerves are reexplored 6 weeks or more after the injury, and repair is carried out then.

Surprisingly, some good results of limb replantation have been achieved. Malt replanted the arm of a twelve-year-old boy $3\frac{1}{2}$ hours after it was severed just below the shoulder. A secondary repair of the nerves was carried out using end-to-end suture and autografts. Two years later the boy had good strength in the flexor muscles of the forearm, some opposition of thumb, and excellent sensation in all fingers. A transposition of the pectoralis major muscle to the reversed detached end of the extensor carpi radialis longus muscle produced good flexion of the elbow to aid a weak biceps. Wrist fusion and tendon transfers were subsequently performed, and the patient was able to use this arm fairly successfully some 3 years after the injury. Several replantations of the hand and distal forearm have been carried out with even better results.

Hemopoietic and Lymphoid Tissues

BONE MARROW

Bone marrow is easily destroyed by whole-body ionizing irradiation by many drugs and chemicals. The stem cell compartment of red bone marrow is the major sensitive site. Its final products, the mature peripheral blood cells, are in most instances not sensitive to injury by irradiation by chemical substances, but these cells have relatively short life spans in the normal steady state. Peripheral blood cells are essential for life, and they will disappear unless there is a regular supply of new cells coming into the blood from the marrow. In leukemia the bone marrow is crowded out by tumor cells, a situation effectively the same as that existing when marrow is destroyed by other means.

Experimental bone marrow transplantation has a long history. If an animal is exposed to lethal radiation, the marrow can be repopulated and the animal saved by an infusion of normal marrow from a genetically identical donor.

Injury to bone marrow by drugs and chemicals is a major problem in human medicine. Bone marrow trans-

plants between identical twins have been successfully carried out on many occasions. In one case the recipient was a worker who had been exposed to an apparently lethal dose of radiation from an accelerator. He survived with the aid of the transplant from his identical twin. Bortin cites recovery in five of seven individuals who received marrow from an identical twin as treatment for aplastic anemia. Autologous marrow transplantation has also been found useful in a few patients after planned treatment with toxic levels of alkylating agents.

Marrow allotransplants are far less successful, but intensive investigations are being carried out. Marrow is highly immunogenic and will be readily rejected by the immunologically normal host. If, however, the marrow is allotransplanted into an immunologically crippled (irradiated, immunosuppressed) host, a chimera is produced; the donor marrow, which contains potentially competent stem cells, will induce a GVH immunologic reaction.

The idea that a graft of foreign cells can attack the host came to the attention of transplantation investigators in the early 1950s. This phenomenon is not seen with skin, kidney, heart, liver, and many other organ allografts, but it is a major, still unsolved, problem in the transplantation of foreign bone marrow, white blood cells, and lymphatic tissues.

Not long after the first bone marrow and spleen transplants had been performed in mice exposed to lethal doses of radiation, prompt recovery from bone marrow failure took place, but during the next few weeks death occurred from a secondary wasting disease. The secondary disease did not occur when blood-forming tissue genetically identical to the host material was grafted. Theory predicts, and practice shows, that secondary disease does not occur in bone marrow transplants between identical twins in man, and in marrow grafts within an inbred strain of mice, rats, or guinea pigs (that is, when the relation between donor and host is syngeneic). An important additional point is the finding of reduced severity of the GVH reaction when the donor and host, even though not genetically identical, have been closely matched by histocompatibility testing.

The major sites of injury in GVH reactions are the lymphatic tissues, the skin, the intestine, and possibly the liver of the host. The failure of lymphatic tissues to regenerate as they do in syngeneic grafts means that the recipient animal or man cannot adequately control the microorganisms present in the flora of the skin, intestine, and other tissue. Dermatitis of an extremely serious kind, diarrhea, loss of weight, and sometimes poor liver function are additional manifestations of a GVH reaction.

The GVH reactions in bone marrow transplantation in human beings have been of overwhelming importance and are the major problem in these experiments.

Congdon has summarized some of the experimental and clinical approaches to the problem of the control of GVH disease (Table 10-2). A combination of tissue typing and immunologic suppression are the most common attempts to control the GVH reaction in man.

A long-range goal in marrow transplantation is to use marrow grafts as a means of promoting acceptance of other

Table 10-2. SOME APPROACHES TO THE CONTROL
OF GRAFT-VERSUS-HOST DISEASE

A. Immunologic compatibility: histocompatibility typing and
   matching of donor and recipient
B. Immunologic suppression
   1. Treatment of marrow recipient
      a. Methotrexate
      b. Cyclophosphamide
      c. Antilymphocyte serum
   2. Treatment of marrow donor: antilymphocyte serum
C. Removal of immunologically active cells
   1. Manipulation of the marrow in vitro
   2. Cell separation
D. Innate absence of immunocompetent cells: use of fetal and
   newborn blood-forming tissue from the donor

organs, such as liver, heart, and kidney. Investigations in
the mouse have shown that once the foreign marrow is
established, a state of immunologic tolerance (or enhancement) is conferred. Then skin taken from the same donor
as the marrow can be successfully transplanted without
further immunosuppression. The transplantation of foreign
bone marrow in laboratory animals constitutes the important feasibility experiment for many of the goals in organ
transplantation, in particular that of achieving immunosuppression with only a single-pulsed injury to the host.

In practice, human bone marrow allotransplantation has
enjoyed some limited success. HL-A identical marrow
transplants (from identical twins and other siblings) have
been used to treat aplastic anemias. HL-A matched but
nontwin transplants produce a milder (but occasionally
lethal) GVH reaction. Dramatic success has been achieved
in the treatment of certain congenitally immunodeficiency
diseases, in some of which no GVH reaction is possible,
so that host immunosuppression is not required. In all
other patients, known allotransplantation requires doses of
immunosuppressive cytotoxic drugs much larger than those
used to gain acceptance of kidney grafts. Combination of
chemotherapy for leukemia followed by marrow transplantation accomplished two aims: (1) rendering the host
immunosuppressed and (2) killing the leukemia cells.
Though a few patients with leukemia have been helped
by this treatment, most die of GVH disease, recurrent
leukemia, or infection.

THYMUS

The congenital absence of thymic tissue presents the
maturation of the entire T cell system. Such patients are
deficient in cell-mediated immune responses and, to a
lesser extent, in those which require T cell and B cell
interaction. Transplantation of an embryonic thymus into
such patients has resulted in considerable improvement in
these normal defense mechanisms. The exact indications
and success rate have not been fully defined, but this is
a promising field of investigation.

SPLEEN AND LYMPH NODE

Patients with agammaglobulinemia have been treated by
free transplantation of lymph nodes or by transplantation
of the spleen with vascular anastomoses. No success has
been achieved, but, surprisingly, neither have any serious

difficulties eventuated. If a patient with agammaglobulinemia were indeed able to accept allotransplants readily, it
might be expected that the spleen or lymph node would
react against the immunologically inadequate host.

Several splenic allografts have been carried out in man
for a variety of indications. These include attempts (1) to
transplant immunoglobulin-producing tissue for agammaglobulinemia, (2) to transplant enzyme-producing tissues
to treat congenital enzymatic deficiencies (e.g., Gaucher's
disease), and (3) to treat cancer with spleen immune to
tumor antigens. None of these transplants were successful.
Spleen transplants have also been proposed to treat hemophilia, since splenic tissue may be one source of antihemophilic globulin. Since the spleen and lymph nodes
are highly antigenic tissues, their successful transplantation
must require one of two circumstances: (1) either that the
host have a severe type of congenital immunologic deficiency, thus permitting a successful allotransplant but subjecting the patient to the GVH disease, or (2) if the host
has a somewhat greater degree of immunologic competence, that immunosuppressive drugs be administered, thus
rendering the host even more vulnerable than before to
serious infection. These transplants do not, therefore, hold
out much hope of clinical success, and bone marrow transplantation may be a better solution which does not entail
an operating procedure.

Most of the clinical experience with endocrine allografts
has had only historical significance, because little scientific
information has been acquired and there has been only
doubtful benefit to the patient. At best such clinical attempts provided temporary indirect evidence of function.
Claims of long-term success were never supported by
histologic proof.

Endocrine Grafts (Other than the Pancreas)

The placement of endocrine fragments as autografts into
intramuscular pockets has proved successful in several
clinical situations.

The requirements of fragment size and delicate handling
which have been emphasized in experimental transplants
must be observed. When it appears possible that the patient may be rendered deficient of thyroid or parathyroid
tissue because of the amount of normal tissue removed
at surgery, the implantation of 1- to 2-mm-thick slices into
the exposed neck or chest wall muscles has repeatedly been
proved worthwhile. Thus in a child with lingual thyroid,
the implanted tissue derived from the lingual mass may
be the only functional thyroid. While margins should not
be compromised in thyroid cancer therapy, parathyroid
glands inadvertently removed with surgery in the patient
with a benign thyroid should be sliced and implanted into
an intramuscular pocket of the sternocleidomastoid muscle
or other accessible site.

Woodruff has made a similar plea for the autotransplantation of ovarian fragments into the rectus muscle in
selected cases. Testicular slices have been successfully autotransplanted (albeit without histologic documentation) to
prevent the need for replacement therapy in a case of

accidental castration. Such a procedure should always be attempted when uncontaminated tissue is available with placement of the implants in a readily accessible muscle in the thigh or abdominal wall.

In adrenal hyperplasia with Cushing's syndrome the accepted surgical therapy has changed from subtotal adrenalectomy to total adrenalectomy with indefinite steroid replacement therapy, due to the high incidence of recurrent hyperfunction and the difficulty in secondary removal of residual tissue. Yet autotransplantation of hyperplastic slices with functional and histologic success has been reported, with placement of the grafts at a site accessible for secondary removal. It may represent a reasonable surgical alternative in selected cases of Cushing's syndrome.

Similarly, subtotal excisional surgery for parathyroid hyperplasia secondary to chronic renal failure has clearly proved its value. But neck reexploration for recurrent hyperactivity of the remnant has been necessary and has led some to the prescription of total parathyroidectomy. In view of the possibility of spontaneous disappearance of the hyperactivity after renal transplantation, and especially in children in whom normal skeletal molding requires some parathyroid hormone, autotransplantation of hyperplastic parathyroid glands should be tried. Fragments equivalent to two of the hyperplastic glands can be placed in several individual muscle pockets in the axilla or thigh, from which they later may be removed in stages if indicated by continued hyperactivity.

The prognosis of clinical parathyroid allotransplants, however, has been insistent and recurrently hopeful. It is true that parathyroid deficiency is not treated with specific hormone replacement but rather with calcium and vitamin D, which often give only inadequate results. The early reports of successes with human parathyroid fragments implanted along the axillary sheath (after passage through culture medium containing serum from the prospective host) encouraged other attempts. Treatment of parathyroid deficiency with en bloc thyroparathyroid allografts with vascular anastomoses was reported by several surgeons with claims of prolonged beneficial effect. But all such "successes" have been based on indirect evidence of decreased replacement therapy, and none have been substantiated by histologic evidence. There has been no documentation that parathyroid tissue is immunologically privileged in human beings despite good evidence that this is true in rats. The associated complications of immunosuppressive therapy have not been considered worth the risk, except in a single patient already under immunosuppressive treatment.

Although endocrine allografts are of little current clinical usefulness, endocrine transplantation has been important in the progress of endocrinology. Harris and Jacobsohn first illustrated the control of the pituitary secretion by the releasing factors from the hypothalamus, which reach the gland through the portal vessels descending from the median eminence. They used pituitary transplants which functioned normally in that location but did not function when vascularized by the temporal lobe vessels. Barnicot's observation of the histologic evidence of bone resorption to parathyroid glands transplanted onto the surface of parietal bone was the cornerstone of the accepted hypothesis that parathyroid hormone acts directly on bone to raise the calcium in the blood. The previous concept stated that the parathyroid hormone acted only indirectly by its phosphaturic effect on the kidney.

Pancreas

Even with insulin replacement diabetics have shortened life spans, because the unremitting and progressive vascular changes continue. The solution of this problem would be successful transplantation of the pancreas. The pancreas, however, does not seem to have been blessed with any significant degree of antigenic privilege, and furthermore its cells are likely to be self-digested by pancreatic enzymes.

Free transplants of cultured canine pancreatic fragments taken from duct-ligated glands and placed in pancreatectomized animals are rapidly rejected. Neonatal pancreatic tissue has been transplanted experimentally in the cheek pouch of the hamster made diabetic by alloxan, and improvement has been noted. The hamster cheek pouch is a privileged site, however, permitting prolonged survival of allografts. Fetal rat pancreatic fragments have been injected into the testis, also a privileged site, of recipient rats made diabetic by alloxan. The hyperglycemia of the recipients disappeared within 48 hours. Pancreatic tissue taken from rats with duct ligation and placed in the anterior chamber of the eye has survived histologically.

Most recently pancreatic islets have been isolated from minced pancreatic tissue by treatment with collagenase. These can be allotransplanted into diabetic animals, where they are rejected in the usual fashion. Isografts of pancreatic islets will reverse the renal disease of diabetic rats, suggesting an important ultimate clinical role for this type of transplant.

Clinically, slices of embryonic pancreas have been placed beneath the rectus abdominis sheath in juvenile diabetics without any demonstrable benefit. Temporary success has been claimed in one human diabetic in whom tissue-cultured insulinoma was implanted along the axillary artery. It seems unlikely, however, that an allograft take was achieved. Attempts have also been made in human beings to transplant pancreatic fragments in millipore chambers, but these also failed. Two patients had short-lived reduction of insulin requirements for 6 weeks after subcutaneous implantation of insulinoma fragments.

Experimentally, many workers have transplanted the whole pancreas in the dog. No long-term success was achieved in one series of cases in which the duct had not been ligated previously. In another series pancreatic allotransplants were carried out in one group of animals without previous duct ligation and in a second group with ligation. The functional survival of the second group was much better, the longest survival of the group being 21 days. These animals were given immunosuppressive drugs. In several other series it was demonstrated that poor results were obtained when the pancreatic duct had not been ligated previously. This led workers to do transplants of the total pancreas and the duodenum so that the exocrine secretion of the pancreas could drain to the outside. Here the results have been better, and several workers have achieved somewhat prolonged graft survival.

Pancreatic transplants have been carried out in a number of diabetic patients—sometimes in conjunction with renal transplants and sometimes alone. The major technical problem has been to deal with the pancreatic exocrine secretions. Pancreaticoduodenal transplantations have been tried the most often. The graft is placed in the iliac fossa, and the vein is anastomosed to the systemic circulation. The duodenum is brought out to the skin (Fig. 10-27). A standard immunosuppressive regimen is azathioprine and prednisone. There is good evidence for normal exocrine and endocrine function, but no patient has survived for more than a year.

Later the duodenum is anastomosed to the intestine (Fig. 10-28), but the rejection of the duodenum has too frequently been a fatal complication. Pancreatic islet transplantation appears to be a better future alternative.

Gastrointestinal Transplants

Although various segments of intestine have been experimentally autotransplanted in the animal by removal from the body and reimplantation, most clinical transplants into man involve only the transfer of the structure from place to place. Stomach, small bowel, and colon can all be used to replace esophagus with reimplantation of the vascular supply. Some true autotransplants of bowel are occasionally carried out when the bowel is completely resected together with its blood supply and moved up in the neck to reconstruct the cervical esophagus; the blood supply is then reanastomosed to vessels in the neck, which then continue to nourish it. Allotransplantation of the small bowel and stomach have been carried out experimentally (Fig. 10-29). These grafts are rejected in the usual fashion, and within the same general time period as for kidneys and other organs. Although there is no real clinical use for a gastric transplant, there is a definite clinical need for transplantation of the small bowel. Infarction of the bowel sometimes requires excision of the entire small bowel, and this leads to a nutritional deficiency which is fatal. If small bowel transplants could be carried out successfully, they would unquestionably find a useful place in the surgeon's armamentarium. A few attempts in man have been successful for several months, but no long-term survival has been achieved.

Liver

EXPERIMENTAL TRANSPLANTATION IN ANIMALS

Two major surgical approaches to the transplantation of the liver are presently employed. The graft may be positioned in the normal anatomic location (orthotopic transplantation) following a recipient hepatectomy. Alternatively, the donor organ is placed in an ectopic site (heterotopic transplantation), generally with retention of the host's liver (auxiliary transplantation). Each of these

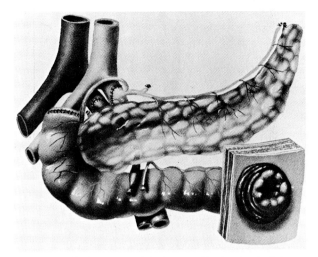

Fig. 10-27. Technique used for pancreaticoduodenal allotransplantation in the first four patients. The distal end of the duodenum was brought out as a cutaneous duodenostomy. (*From R. C. Lillehei and J. O. Ruiz, Pancreas, in J. S. Najarian and R. L. Simmons (eds.), "Transplantation," p. 627, Lea & Febiger, Philadelphia, 1972.*)

Fig. 10-28. Present technique of grafting donor duodenum to recipient small intestine. Both renal and pancreaticoduodenal allografts are illustrated. (*From R. C. Lillehei and J. O. Ruiz, Pancreas, in J. S. Najarian and R. L. Simmons (eds.), "Transplantation," p. 626, Lea & Febiger, Philadelphia, 1972.*)

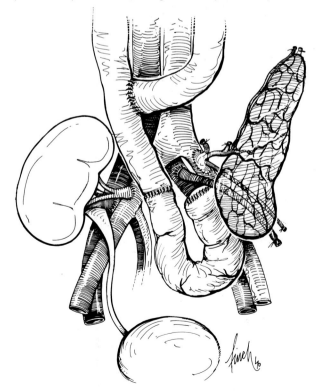

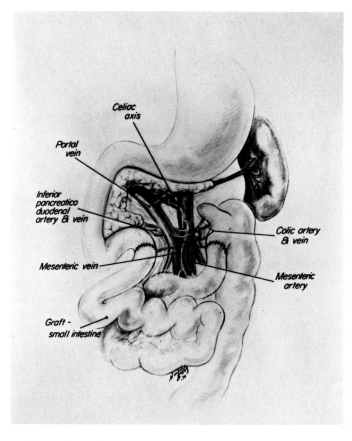

Fig. 10-29. Diagram showing the operative technique of orthotopic transplantation of the entire small intestine in a dog. (*From J. O. Ruiz, H. Uchida, and R. C. Lillehei, Intestine, in J. S. Najarian and R. L. Simmons (eds.), "Transplantation," p. 646, Lea & Febiger, Philadelphia, 1972.*)

techniques has unique inherent advantages, disadvantages, and requirements. The greatest success has been obtained with orthotopic transplantation, even though it is more technically difficult.

ORTHOTOPIC TRANSPLANTATION. The earliest studies evaluating orthotopic liver transplantation in the dog had an extremely high operative mortality. The technical and biologic prerequisites for transplantation of this intricate organ were soon elucidated. Initially, the inferior vena cava and portal vein of the anhepatic dog recipient were cross-clamped during total extirpation of the host's liver prior to receipt of the graft. Dogs subjected to this insult, without an adequate pathway for return of blood from the intestines and lower extremities, often died. To circumvent this dilemma, two decompressing external shunts from the inferior vena cava and portal vein into both external jugular veins were used. Alternatively, an internal side-to-side portacaval shunt would permit a single external vena cava–jugular bypass for decompression of both the systemic and splanchnic venous systems (Fig. 10-30). These precautions are not necessary in pigs. In man collateral venous networks usually develop as a consequence of existing liver disease, thereby eliminating the clinical need for shunts.

Experimentally, the donor organ is removed in continuity with the hepatic artery and a segment of aorta. The graft is transplanted in its normal anatomical position by performing vena cava–to–vena cava and portal vein–to–portal vein anastomoses. An arterial anastomosis is

created between the aorta of the graft and the aorta of the recipient. Biliary drainage is provided through construction of a cholecystoenterostomy (Fig. 10-31), after ligating the transected end of the graft's common duct. The vascular shunt can then be removed.

With good surgical techniques and adequate short-term preservation, an operative survival rate of 85 to 95 percent can be obtained following orthotopic allotransplantation in the dog. There is little or no evidence of coagulation defects, severe acidosis, hypoglycemia, or biochemical derangements indicative of a significant hepatic injury pattern.

In the nonimmunosuppressed dog recipient, a pattern of rejection is almost invariably present by the fifth day. Elevations in the alkaline phosphatase, serum glutamic oxaloacetic transaminase (SGOT), and serum glutamic pyruvic transaminase (SGPT) develop at the same time as, or shortly prior to, the onset of jaundice. By the seventh day there is usually a progression of hyperbilirubinemia and other biochemical parameters reminiscent of biliary obstruction, as well as hepatic parenchymal cellular injury. A periportal mononuclear cell infiltrate, centrilobular necrosis, and intracanalicular bile stasis are present on microscopic examination. The recipient usually dies by the tenth postoperative day.

The pig appears to have inherent advantages as an experimental animal compared to the dog. In the pig there is infrequent presence of naturally occurring indigenous bacteria within the liver parenchyma, resistance to devel-

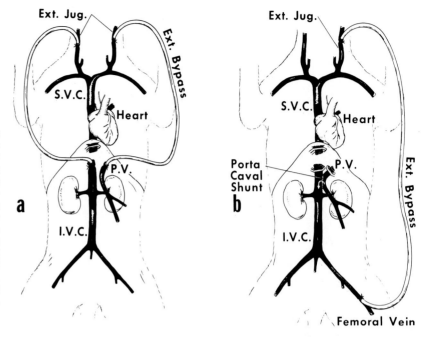

Fig. 10-30. Various splanchnic and systemic venous decompression techniques are employed during removal of the recipient liver in the healthy dog prior to revascularization of a hepatic graft. *A.* Two external shunts may provide for venous return from the inferior vena cava and portal vein into the jugular veins. *B.* Alternatively, a temporary side-to-side portacaval anastomosis establishing continuity between both venous systems permits the use of a single external bypass between the femoral and external jugular veins. (*From L. Brettschneider, Liver: I. Experimental (Transplantation), in J. S. Najarian and R. L. Simmons (eds.), "Transplantation," p. 497, Lea & Febiger, Philadelphia, 1972.*)

opment of the "outflow block" syndrome, and the requirement for a single (rather than double) decompressing bypass system during the recipient operation. Most remarkably, a number of liver transplant recipients have lived beyond several weeks, and occasionally for many months, without any evidence of rejection or with a uniquely weak and highly reversible immune response. The cause of the absent or mild rejection pattern following transplantation of the pig liver is speculative. Most evidence supports the idea that the pig's reactions to vascularized organ grafts are less strong and more easily attenuated. The pig rejects skin and renal allografts in the usual fashion, which argues against a generalized immune incompetence of the species. In experiments where both the liver and a kidney from the same donor were concomitantly transplanted following a bilateral nephrectomy, the magnitude of rejection of the transplanted kidney and liver was reduced.

HETEROTOPIC TRANSPLANTATION. The theoretic advantages of auxiliary liver homotransplantation are great. The procedure is technically less arduous than orthotopic transplantation, retains the residual function of the host's liver, and avoids the necessity of removing the diseased organ from a critically ill recipient. These theoretic advantages have proved to be less useful in practice, however, because of complicating mechanical and physiologic factors.

The original technique (Fig. 10-32) placed the allograft outflow into the transected vena cava of the host below the renal vessels, with the arterial supply originating from the aorta or iliac artery. Portal venous inflow was provided by the distal transected vena cava or iliac vein. A cholecystoenterostomy affords biliary drainage. Deviations from the original preparation relating to the donor portal circulation have comprised exclusion of a portal blood supply to the graft, arterialization of the portal vein, establishing

Fig. 10-31. Orthotopic transplantation involves total substitution of the host's own liver with the donor organ placed in its normal location. The vena cava and portal vein are generally reestablished anatomically. In the earlier experiences, a segment of donor aorta in continuity with the celiac artery was sutured to the recipient's aorta. A cholecystoduodenostomy afforded biliary drainage. (*From L. Brettschneider, Liver: I. Experimental (Transplantation), in J. S. Najarian and R. L. Simmons (eds.), "Transplantation," p. 496, Lea & Febiger, Philadelphia, 1972.*)

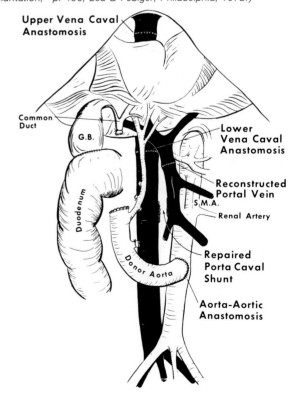

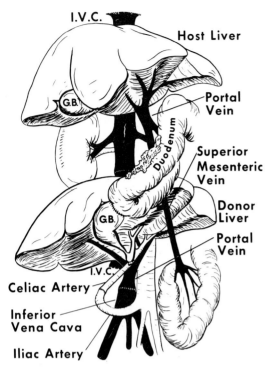

Fig. 10-32. Canine heterotopic transplantation as described by Welch. Anastomosis of the host's vena cava with the portal vein of the donor organ provides a systemic venous inflow. The hepatic artery is anastomosed to the transected iliac artery. Biliary drainage is afforded through a cholecystoduodenostomy. Graft atrophy is almost invariably noted following this procedure. (*From L. Brettschneider, Liver: I. Experimental (Transplantation), in J. S. Najarian and R. L. Simmons (eds.), "Transplantation," p. 496, Lea & Febiger, Philadelphia, 1972.*)

splanchnic venous flow to the transplant, or creation of a host portacaval shunt.

The failure rate following auxiliary transplantation is extremely high. The "outflow block" syndrome is common in the dog following revascularization of the allograft. This complication may be due in part to torsion of the graft around its vascular pedicles. In addition, mechanical compression by the surrounding organs may further contribute to the development of this syndrome, since the abdomen cannot easily contain two livers. Thus, a 25 to 50 percent incidence of vascular thrombosis is associated with the operative procedure.

Survival can be obtained for several weeks in canine recipients of auxiliary homografts with the employment of immunosuppression (azathioprine), but the transplanted organ atrophies after 2 to 3 weeks, while the host's own liver is not affected. Following removal of the recipient's own liver, the graft is incapable of sustaining life.

The lack of splanchnic venous blood flow to the auxiliary transplant probably contributes to hepatic allograft atrophy.

If splanchnic blood flow to the allograft is maintained, atrophy can be prevented. Marchioro et al. provided a visceral venous inflow to the canine allograft (Fig. 10-33). An anastomosis between the donor portal vein and recipi-

ent superior mesenteric view was followed by ligation of the host's portal vein. This provided for retrograde flow of portal blood through the allograft, rather than the host's own liver. In the immunosuppressed dog, the recipient's liver underwent atrophy. The allograft was favorably affected and did not demonstrate shrinkage. Obviously, the organ receiving a splanchnic venous blood flow has a definite physiologic advantage.

The recipient's liver will have already been severely compromised when this procedure is applied to man. A splanchnic blood supply may not be essential in the clinical setting with extensive preexisting liver damage, since competition from the host liver will be negligible. Thus far, however, neither the acute nor the long-term survival data following canine heterotopic liver transplantation have compared favorably with those results obtained after orthotopic allotransplantation in the dog.

CLINICAL LIVER TRANSPLANTATION

Clinical hepatic transplantation is still in its infancy, as was renal transplantation only 10 years ago. Even so, definite progress is being made.

INDICATIONS. In the United States, approximately 15,000 persons, between the ages of five and sixty years, died in 1963 as a result of primary hepatic disease (45,000 persons were thought to die as a result of primary renal disease). Some of these patients will never be good candidates for liver transplantation, but certain indications are clear.

Intrahepatic or extrahepatic congenital biliary atresia, if not surgically correctable, will generally lead to death before the age of two; few patients survive up to five years. Such a child is the ideal candidate for a liver transplant.

Patients with either *primary hepatomas* or *cholangiocarcinomas* are far less ideal candidates. If, however, it can be ascertained that the malignant condition is entirely confined to the liver, these patients should be considered for liver transplantation. Often the final diagnosis of disease confined to the liver may not be made until the operation.

The patient with *cirrhosis* raises additional problems. The inevitability of rapid death is not as certain in these patients as in those with biliary atresia or primary malignant disease. On the other hand, the terminal stages of the cirrhosis make these patients extremely poor candidates for any operative procedure. Patients with postnecrotic cirrhosis without a history of alcoholism may be better risks, as will be the patient with primary biliary cirrhosis, Wilson's hepatolenticular degeneration, and hemachromatosis.

Acute liver failure may represent one of the best indications for liver transplantation, especially in those patients who have been exposed to hepatotoxins. Viral hepatitis, on the other hand, may or may not recur in the transplanted liver.

Each indication may require a different type of transplant. For example, acute liver failure may respond well to the temporary support of an auxiliary liver that allows the host liver to recover. The child with biliary atresia will almost certainly require an orthotopic transplant with total hepatectomy, since the small child also has no abdominal space for an auxiliary liver. Patients with hepatic malignant disease will also require total hepatectomy and orthotopic transplantation.

Choosing a hepatic donor should follow the same guidelines as choosing a donor for cadaver renal transplantation. Size is a more important criterion in liver transplantation than it is in renal transplantation, particularly when children with congenital biliary atresia are the potential recipients. Usually these children (3 to 15 kg) cannot tolerate a liver larger than that from a child weighing 30 kg. Severe postoperative respiratory distress has occurred when donor livers from larger children were used.

PRECAUTIONS. The hepatic transplantation candidate is usually in severe preterminal hepatic failure. In addition, anemia, pulmonary insufficiency, myocardial fibrosis, inanition and protein depletion, and ascites may be present singly or in combination. The anemia should be corrected with packed red blood cells and protein-containing solutions as soon as transplantation is contemplated.

Pulmonary insufficiency in hepatic failure can be traced to several causes: First, chronic abdominal ascites restricts the diaphragm and fosters compression atelectasis of the lower portions of the lungs. Also, extensive collateral circulation consequent to portal vein hypertension shunts blood from the portal system to the pulmonary veins via enlarged paraesophageal, mediastinal, and bronchial veins, resulting in venous admixture of systemic blood. Intrapulmonary shunts may also develop in cirrhotic patients so that arterial hypoxemia is frequently encountered. These conditions make it more difficult for the anesthesiologist to provide adequate ventilation and oxygenation during surgery and require that he avoid techniques employing borderline oxygen concentration.

In cirrhotic patients diffuse myocardial fibrosis frequently develops that reduces ventricular contractility, stroke volume, and work capacity.

The bedridden patient with hepatic failure invariably suffers from debilitation and poor nutrition, which make him vulnerable to hypotension following anesthesia, moderate hemorrhage, or positional change. Drugs which ordinarily produce mild vasodilation often evoke unusually severe and prolonged effects in the cirrhotic patient that are out of proportion to the dose administered. Most anesthetic drugs provoke such responses and must therefore be administered slowly in small increments. Sudden removal of ascitic fluid may also precipitate or exaggerate hypotension, but the mechanism of this response is obscure.

It is apparent from these considerations that, in undertaking to provide anesthesia for the transplant patient, the anesthesiologist faces several difficult challenges. He must, on the one hand, provide conditions adequate for a massive intraperitoneal procedure; at the same time, he must keep in mind that his patient will probably not tolerate deep anesthesia and that the implanted liver may be slow to metabolize and detoxify anesthetic drugs. Most of all, intraoperative and postoperative respiratory distress must be anticipated and minimized. In addition, there is almost no time for proper patient preparation. Once a donor is

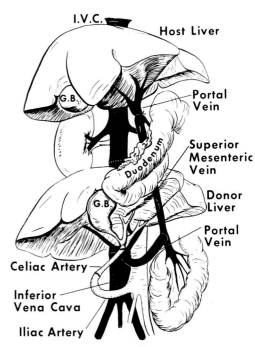

Fig. 10-33. Marchioro et al. modified the technique described in Fig. 10-32. By ligating the portal blood supply to the host's own liver and diverting the splanchnic blood to the homograft by creating an anastomosis between the graft's portal vein and the in situ superior mesenteric vein, homograft atrophy was prevented. (*From L. Brettschneider, Liver: I. Experimental (Transplantation), in J. S. Najarian and R. L. Simmons (eds.), "Transplantation," p. 496, Lea & Febiger, Philadelphia, 1972.*)

available, the operation must commence promptly so that agonal ischemia of the donor organ be as brief as possible. The recipient frequently comes to surgery unexpectedly, perhaps an hour or two after a meal. A full stomach is added to the already imposing list of preoperative problems.

The following preparatory procedures are carried out either before anesthesia is induced or immediately after: (1) A central venous pressure catheter is positioned in the right atrium or superior vena cava. (2) A second large-bore plastic needle is placed in an upper extremity vein for fluid and blood replacement; it is important to remember that intravenous input via the lower extremities is not adequate during the actual transplantation phase, since the inferior vena cava is clamped. (3) Another needle is placed in either the brachial or radial artery for direct blood pressure monitoring and arterial blood sampling. (4) ECG electrodes are applied to each extremity. (5) A rubber warming blanket is placed under the patient and kept between 100 and 105°F. (6) An esophageal temperature probe is positioned so that its sensor lies directly behind the heart. (7) A catheter is placed in the urinary bladder and connected to a graduated collecting flask.

TECHNIQUE OF ORTHOTOPIC HEPATIC TRANSPLANTATION. A transverse abdominal incision with an extension into the thorax, if necessary, is the most common incision.

Recipient hepatectomy must be preceded by careful

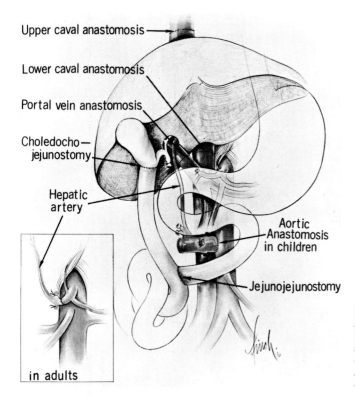

Upper caval anastomosis

Lower caval anastomosis

Portal vein anastomosis

Choledocho—jejunostomy

Hepatic artery

Aortic Anastomosis in children

Jejunojejunostomy

in adults

Fig. 10-34. Orthotopic liver transplantation in children and adults. In children an aortic cuff can be used for anastomosis; in adults (inset) a direct anastomosis of the hepatic artery and celiac axis can be used. (*From J. S. Najarian, Liver: III. Clinical (Transplantation), in J. S. Najarian and R. L. Simmons (eds.), "Transplantation," p. 522, Lea & Febiger, Philadelphia, 1972.*)

inspection to determine the feasibility of the procedure. This is particularly true of patients with primary hepatic neoplasms to ensure that no extrahepatic spread of the tumor has occurred.

The allograft anastomoses are shown in Fig. 10-34. The suprahepatic caval anastomosis is the most difficult to perform. The second anastomosis is usually the hepatic artery, but if visceral congestion is great, the portal vein anastomosis should be performed before the hepatic artery to relieve the venous congestion of the intestine. After the hepatic artery or portal vein anastomosis is completed, the inferior hepatic caval clamps should be briefly removed, leaving the suprahepatic vena cava clamped. The arterial or portal vein inflow should be opened to allow the liver to be perfused with warm blood. This sequence is useful to remove the cold perfusate from the liver and prevent systemic hypothermia and heparinization. As soon as the perfusate is washed from the liver and it becomes firm and pink, the intrahepatic vena cava is clamped, and the suprahepatic vena cava clamp is removed. The remaining vascular anastomoses can then be accomplished.

Following anastomoses biliary drainage must be obtained. A Roux en Y cholecystojejunostomy is most often used, but occasionally a cholecystoduodenostomy is employed. Because bile leakage may be a fatal complication and since the cystic artery is an end artery, the anastomosis is best made from the proximal gallbladder to a defunctionalized intestinal loop.

Finally, the liver is fixed in position by suturing the donor and recipient falciform ligaments together. If possible, the triangular ligaments can also be attached for further support of the liver.

TECHNIQUE OF AUXILIARY LIVER TRANSPLANTATION. Auxiliary, or heterotopic, transplantation is the second alternative for patients with benign liver disease. The major disadvantage of this procedure is its requirement for abdominal volume in which to accommodate the second large organ. When auxiliary transplants are performed, the recipient's own liver is retained to offer some metabolic support during and after the operation. Thus, with the auxiliary liver transplant there is no urgent need for immediate function of the graft, and the operation is shorter and less traumatic.

As noted above, splanchnic blood should be supplied to the graft. This technique is illustrated in Fig. 10-35. The portal vein may be anastomosed to the side of the superior mesenteric vein or to the end of the splenic vein. The advantage of this technique is twofold. It provides for the decompression of the hypertensive recipient portal system, and it provides splanchnic blood flow through the auxiliary liver transplant.

OPERATIVE COMPLICATIONS. *Technical Complications.* Bleeding is the major technical problem during hepatic transplantation. Portal hypertension predisposes to an extensive collateral venous circulation, and laceration of any smaller vein precipitates extensive bleeding, especially during recipient hepatectomy. The failure of the diseased liver to produce a normal quota of coagulation factors compounds this problem.

Other operative complications are far less common. It is important to remember that the cystic duct may not enter the common duct except in its terminal course. Therefore, during the donor operation one must be sure that the common duct is ligated distal to its anastomosis with the cystic duct, if bile is to be expected to flow down the common duct and into the gallbladder. Similarly, it is important to remember that 30 to 40 percent of patients have double hepatic arteries, and one of them arises from the superior mesenteric artery. Care must be taken during the donor operation to preserve this arterial supply.

A common complication is paralysis of the right side of the diaphragm, which apparently results from crushing of the right phrenic nerve by the vascular clamp applied to the suprahepatic inferior vena cava. Enough length must be preserved during total hepatectomy for the clamp to be applied without impinging on the diaphragm.

Metabolic Complications. Because pulmonary insufficiency is common following hepatic transplantation, a nasotracheal tube should be placed at the outset of anesthesia, with the intention of maintaining intubation and mechanical ventilation until respiratory competence is reestablished. A sterile tube is used to obviate nosocomial infection, which is a significant hazard in patients receiving immunosuppressive drugs.

Because of increased tissue uptake of glucose and reduced glycogen conversion, hypoglycemia develops insidiously in response to hepatic ischemia, hypotension, and acidosis. Hyperglycemia is a hazard of hypertonic glucose infusion. The blood sugar should be regularly measured, and glucose infusion should be modified according to the values obtained.

Since precise measurement of blood loss and fluid sequestration is not possible, evaluation and correlation of suction loss, weight loss, arterial blood pressure, cardiac rate, venous pressure, acid-base status, and urine volume must be made frequently by the anesthetist. At this point of the operative procedure central venous pressure measurement is useful as a guide to the adequacy of the filling pressure of the right side of the heart, but manipulation of the liver and its great vein attachments may produce high-pressure artifacts.

Hypotension is a particular danger during the anhepatic period, its severity depending upon the adequacy with which collateral venous circulation maintains venous return to the heart. If blood pressure is seriously depressed, the transfusion rate is increased, but often the hypotension cannot be fully overcome until the caval clamps are removed. This disturbance of cardiac output is the major cause of the progressive metabolic acidosis that characterizes this portion of the transplant operation.

When the anastomoses are completed, further dangerous metabolic and hemodynamic changes occur. The great veins draining the intestines and lower half of the body now discharge blood containing a heavy load of acid metabolites. At the same time, the vascular space within the liver takes up a considerable volume of blood and discharges additional products of ischemia as it again becomes an integral part of the circulation. Thus the metabolic acidosis suddenly worsens and is accompanied by hypovolemia. Severe hypotension, cardiac arrhythmias, bradycardia, and other bizarre configurations of the ECG pattern appear abruptly at this point. Blood loss from leaks in the vascular anastomoses frequently compounds the hemodynamic problems. Whole blood must be rapidly

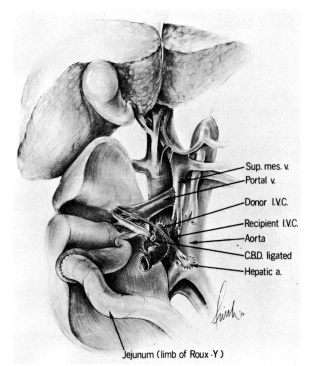

Fig. 10-35. The method of auxiliary liver transplantation utilizing splanchnic blood flow. The hepatic arterial supply comes directly from the aorta, and the portal vein supply to the liver is derived from the splanchnic circulation. The portal vein can be anastomosed either to the superior mesenteric vein, as shown, or to the portal vein, whichever is most convenient. The donor's inferior vena cava is anastomosed end to end to the inferior vena cava. In this method portal decompression is provided, as well as splanchnic circulation to the transplanted liver. (*From J. S. Najarian, Liver: III. Clinical (Transplantation), in J. S. Najarian, and R. L. Simmons (eds.), "Transplantation," p. 522, Lea & Febiger, Philadelphia, 1972.*)

administered at this phase of the operation until the systolic arterial blood pressure stabilizes at 100 mm Hg or better. Simultaneously, blood-gas analyses are made every 5 minutes to provide guidance in adjustment of acid-base balance at this critical juncture.

Hypothermia is a concomitant hazard as the donor liver is revascularized. The whole transplantation procedure with its extensive visceral exposure and heavy blood loss fosters hypothermia. Furthermore the donor liver is flushed with iced saline solution prior to transplantation into the host's circulation to increase its tolerance of ischemia. The *coup de grâce* therefore is the sudden inclusion of this ice-cold organ directly upstream of the heart. Consequently the core temperature usually falls 3 to 4°C within 2 minutes of release of the clamps. Such abrupt cardiac cooling fosters arrhythmias and poor myocardial function. Perfusion of the liver through the infrahepatic vena cava prior to opening the suprahepatic vena cava will warm the liver and work out the cold perfusate. In addition, irrigation of the abdominal cavity with warm saline solution (40°C) and transfusion with warm blood can also compensate.

Potassium disturbances impose an additional hazard during revascularization. Several factors (hepatocellular ischemia, massive blood replacement, and metabolic acidosis) favor hyperkalemia when hepatic circulation is restored. There may be a concomitant decrease in serum calcium due to the heavy citrate load imposed by the multiple transfusions and the impaired capacity of the new liver to metabolize that load. These cation shifts have not been systematically quantitated, but the abrupt appearance of peaked T waves and conduction disturbances have been observed on the ECG as liver circulation is reestablished. Disturbance of the potassium/calcium ratio is known to depress myocardial function and cardiac output; when acidosis, hypothermia, and a sudden increase in the vascular bed add their own special depressant effects, severe hypotension and arrhythmias result. Prompt correction of hypovolemia and acidosis are the keys to success in negotiating this critical period. Then, if myocardial weakness still persists one can assume that a potassium/calcium ratio disturbance is present and slowly inject 0.5 to 1.0 Gm of calcium chloride. The serum electrolyte determinations made every 15 minutes until the circulation stabilizes provide guidance in adjusting ionic balance. Hypokalemia is the most prominent electrolyte problem in the early postoperative period.

POSTOPERATIVE CARE. There is a high potential for postoperative respiratory insufficiency in most hepatic transplant patients, because pulmonary dysfunction is always present in some degree. The extensive upper abdominal incision causes abdominal muscle splinting and reduces vital capacity. Often the transplanted liver is significantly larger than the organ it replaces, so that breathing is further compromised until abdominal wall accommodation takes place. The nasotracheal tube is therefore usually left in place after surgery. Mechanical ventilation is applied for at least 12 hours or until the patient's own respiratory competence is proved by normal blood gases. Strict adherence to sterile technique in respiratory care is essential because of the patient's immunosuppressed state. Sterile distilled water should be used to provide humidification of respiratory gases.

After operation, the transplant recipient is nursed in a 30°-angle head-up position to reduce the pressure of the abdominal contents on the diaphragm. He is also turned from side to side each hour, and vibratory chest percussion is applied each time a positional change is made. Chest roentgenograms are made daily to detect atelectasis, which is dealt with by postural pummeling, directional tracheobronchial suction, and hyperinflation with a self-inflating bag.

Most of the remaining problems are related to metabolic changes that may be minimal if the quality of the new liver is good. If, however, the liver quality is impaired by prolonged ischemia or agonal changes in the donor, the liver is unable to regulate blood sugar, and both hypoglycemia and hyperglycemic nonketotic coma will have occurred.

The coagulation changes that accompany the transplantation of the liver have been thoroughly discussed by the Denver group. Since most of the coagulation factors are hepatic in origin and the liver is involved in the clearing of substances active in coagulation and fibrinolysis, a damaged liver frequently fails to produce sufficient coagulation factors to prevent hemorrhage. The problem is compounded by the probability that intravascular coagulation accompanies the trauma and shock of the procedure, thereby consuming whatever factors are present. A rapid return of coagulation tests to normal in the early posttransplant period is a good indicator of satisfactory hepatic function.

Hepatic transplant recipients receive the same immunosuppressive drugs used in renal transplant recipients (azathioprine, prednisone, and ALG). The hepatotoxicity of azathioprine, however, requires that a reduced level be utilized (1 mg/kg), although the levels of prednisone and ALG remain the same. Cyclophosphamide has recently been used in place of azathioprine by Starzl and his colleagues.

Diagnosis of Rejection. Mild rejection episodes may occur at any time posttransplantation. This diagnosis can usually be made by laboratory determinations of modest rises in the levels of serum bilirubin, transaminase, and alkaline phosphatase.

While the milder rejection episodes may not be clinically apparent, severe rejection crises are accompanied by systemic signs that may mimic toxic hepatitis. Fever, malaise, anorexia, and hepatomegaly are present, and the patient generally appears quite ill. The laboratory findings reveal elevated serum bilirubin, alkaline phosphatase, and serum transaminase levels. The 99m technetium liver scan will reveal either a patchy or diffuse decrease in hepatic uptake and an increased uptake in the bone marrow and lungs. The serum bilirubin level is such a reliable indication that it should be performed two or three times weekly in the posttransplant period.

Septic infarcts within the liver are among the most severe problems encountered after liver transplants; they are usually fatal. This syndrome appears as a distinct clinical triad: (1) gram-negative septicemia, (2) evidence of massive liver necrosis with increased serum levels of liver enzymes, and (3) liver scans showing persistent absence of isotope concentrations in the liver allograft. Hepatic septic infarcts are associated with severe rejection involving the vascular supply to the liver. Ischemic infarction then follows, and the liver can no longer deal with the enteric organisms normally traversing through the portal venous system or possible from the cholecystojejunostomy anastomosis. The ischemic segment soon becomes abscessed. An increase in serum transaminase, a positive blood culture, and an area that fails to concentrate the isotope on liver scan are all positive indications of an abscessed ischemic segment.

Increased immunosuppressive therapy and antibiotics should be instituted. Drainage or a formal hepatic resection may even be necessary in an attempt to save the recipient.

RESULTS. The ACS/NIH (American College of Surgeons/National Institutes of Health) Organ Transplant Registry collects the results of hepatic transplantation. Between March of 1963 and January 1, 1973, 145 orthotopic and 37 heterotopic (auxiliary) hepatic transplants had been performed on 178 patients (4 patients received 2 transplants). Of these patients, 67 had biliary atresia, 57 had other benign disease (41 had types of cirrhosis; 9, hepatitis; 2, hepatic necrosis; 2, Wilson's disease; 1, α_1-trypsinase deficiency; 1, lupoid hepatitis; and 1, galactosemia), and 54 patients had hepatic malignant tumors (48 with primary malignant tumors and 6 with metastatic malignant tumors).

There are 16 liver recipients still living (15 orthotopic, 1 heterotopic). Fourteen of these patients survived more than 1 year, and six lived more than 2 years after their transplants. The longest survivor is in excellent health over 4 years after liver replacement. Most recipients died during the first month after the operation from complications directly related to the graft or from hepatic insufficiency not relieved by transplantation. Other patients died from sepsis or circulatory and respiratory failure. The results for heterotopic transplantation are obviously poorer than those of orthotopic transplantation. Problems peculiar to heterotopic grafts are technical difficulties in construction of nonanatomic vascular anastomosis and overfilling of the abdomen with consequent respiratory distress.

Despite the numerous difficulties associated with liver transplantation, the number of patients with extended postoperative survival is significant. An appreciably better rate than that of the total series has been achieved by the group with the greatest experience in the field. Selection of recipients, greater experience with the technical procedure, and improved methods of immunosuppression (ALG) can be expected to improve the results in the future.

Heart

Cardiac transplantation is emerging as a truly therapeutic intervention for some patients with terminal or intractable heart disease for whom no alternative therapy is currently available. By June 1973, over 200 cardiac transplants were performed in human beings by 61 teams in 34 countries of the world. While the overall survival rate has been disappointingly low, the potential for long-term survival has been established by six patients who are currently alive between 4 and 5 years after transplantation. Equally gratifying is their high degree of rehabilitation.

HISTORICAL BACKGROUND

Prior to the initiation of human trials, a number of fundamental areas required extensive laboratory investigation—development of a surgical technique, demonstration of adequate postoperative function of the acutely denervated heart, early detection and prevention of homograft rejection, and resuscitation and preservation of the cadaver heart. An encouraging degree of progress was made in each of these areas during the 10 years preceding the first clinical transplant in Cape Town, South Africa, in December of 1967.

Before the development of modern methods for cardiopulmonary bypass, studies of cardiac transplantation, of necessity, were confined to placement of the heart in an ectopic position, usually in the neck of a larger dog. As early as 1905, Carrel and Guthrie, using previously un-

known suturing techniques, carried out heterotopic transplantation of the heart and of the heart and lungs and demonstrated the capacity of the transplanted heart to continue beating despite severance from its nerve supply. Subsequent studies by other investigators using various modifications of the original preparation added considerably to our knowledge of the transplanted heart. Much was learned about the susceptibility of the heart to the process of rejection; its vulnerability to hypoxia, thrombosis, and air embolism; and the protective effect of hypothermia against the metabolic abnormalities which occur with transplantation. In addition to these studies, the heterotopically transplanted heart has been investigated as a means of assisting circulation. In contrast to the recently developed mechanical assist pumps, the asynchronously beating transplant can be expected only to support an isolated segment of the circulation, rather than to augment the general circulation. Synchronized artificial pacing of the transplant could possibly overcome this disadvantage.

Subsequent to the development of techniques for generalized hypothermia and extracorporeal circulation, the possibility of complete cardiac replacement was investigated by several groups. Survival in the initial dog studies was limited to a few hours, but much was learned about the technical problems. In December of 1959, Lower et al. demonstrated that a dog could recover fully after orthotopic replacement of the heart with a homograft. In an initial series of 10 animals, 6 survived from 6 to 21 days without immunosuppression. Five days of survival was also achieved after orthotopic homotransplantation of the heart and both lungs as a unit.

Subsequent animal studies demonstrated that the ECG voltage was a useful means of monitoring the transplant in order to detect impending rejection episodes and that prolonged survival could be achieved in some animals by appropriate use of azathioprine and high doses of steroid to combat rejection crises. The feasibility of using cadaver hearts was also established, as was the successful hypothermic storage of the donor heart for several hours prior to transplantation.

Extensive physiologic studies of autotransplanted dog hearts confirmed the capacity of the denervated heart to function normally for several years under a variety of physiologic stresses and demonstrated that signs of autonomic reinnervation would frequently reappear within months to a year after transplantation. These laboratory investigations established the technical and physiologic feasibility of cardiac transplantation in man and set the stage for the clinical trials which were initiated in December of 1967 and carried out most extensively in 1968 in several centers. In subsequent years, because of the high rate of immunologic failure of the grafts, cardiac transplantation has been performed less frequently and only in a few centers as carefully studied clinical investigations.

SELECTION OF PATIENTS

Because of the relatively high risk of allograft failure from rejection or of death from complications of immunosuppression, patient selection for cardiac transplantation generally has been reserved for those under age fifty with terminal or intractable heart failure for whom no alternative therapy is available. The majority have had severe coronary disease with multiple infarctions and extensive or diffuse loss of left ventricular myocardium. Many of these patients have been failures of prior revascularization attempts, but these have proved to be an especially favorable group (see below). Another group for consideration includes patients with cardiomyopathy who do not respond satisfactorily to medical therapy. It has now been established in some long-term survivors that the cardiomyopathy is not likely to recur in the transplanted heart, and one such patient is alive after 4 years with normal cardiac function. Another group is composed of infants with the hypoplastic left-heart syndrome for whom transplantation from anencephalic donors might prove successful. Of particular interest is the high success rate reported by the Stanford University Medical Center group for patients who had prior cardiopulmonary bypass procedures, which suggest that, rather than the anticipated high rate of sensitization to donor antigens, some measure of graft enhancement may have occurred.

Up to the present time histocompatibility typing has provided no predictive value in matching donor and recip-

ient, but to avoid the problem of accelerated rejection a lymphocyte cross match must establish that the recipient harbors no preformed antibodies against the potential donor. Otherwise, successful transplantation has required only the geographic and temporal proximity of recipient and donor with appropriate ABO compatibility. Cardiac donors have sustained brain death usually from trauma or from spontaneous intracerebral hemorrhage, and complete cessation of brain function has been certified by an independent team of neurologists and neurosurgeons.

TECHNIQUE

The operative approach (Fig. 10-36) for cardiac transplantation used by most groups follows with a few modifications the procedure which proved successful in the animal model. The recipient is prepared for cardiopulmonary bypass using a median sternotomy incision. Venous drainage catheters are placed through the right atrial wall in a posterior position, or they may be inserted through peripheral veins. Arterial cannulation is via the femoral artery or ascending aorta. The recipient's diseased heart is excised by appropriate incisions in the right and left atrial walls and atrial septum, retaining in the recipient the posterior portions of both atria. This residual atrial tissue not only facilitates anastomosis of the donor heart but preserves some of the afferent innervation to the atria which may play a significant role in maintaining homeostatic fluid balance in the postoperative period. Blood supply to the retained atrial tissue is adequately provided by the bronchial circulation, but retention of excessive amounts, particularly the appendages, is avoided to minimize the risk of ischemia, stasis, and thrombosis. The aorta and pulmonary artery are transected at a convenient point distal to the semilunar valves.

Simultaneously, the donor is heparinized and the heart exposed by a second team. Removal of the donor heart is carried out by division of the venae cavae, the pulmonary veins, and the great arteries. The excised heart is then immersed in saline solution at 5 to 10°C to provide protective cooling of the myocardium during transport to the recipient, as well as during the remainder of the transplantation procedure. Further preparation of the donor heart includes suture ligation of the superior vena cava, incision of the lateral right atrial wall from the inferior vena cava to the atrial appendage avoiding the major internodal pathways, and preparation of the left atrium by incision between the pulmonary venous openings.

Implantation of the donor heart consists of suturing the left atrial wall, atrial septum, and right atrial wall in succession by continuous suture, followed by anastomosis of the pulmonary artery and ascending aorta. Prior to completing the final anastomosis, care is taken to evacuate all residual air from the cardiac chambers. With release of the aortic clamp and rewarming of the heart, cardiac rhythm often returns spontaneously, or ventricular fibrillation may require electrical cardioversion. In each of our cases, the transplanted heart has resumed vigorous contractions once coronary circulation has been restored, and cardiopulmonary bypass has been discontinued.

Fig. 10-36. *A*. The recipient has been prepared for cardiopulmonary bypass with insertion of caval catheters through the posterior portion of the right atrium. *B*. The recipient's heart has been excised leaving in place the posterior remnants of right and left atria. *C*. Suturing of the donor heart is begun with the left atrial wall, followed in sequence by the atrial septum, right atrium, pulmonary artery, and aorta. *D*. Suturing is complete, and coronary circulation is restored by removal of the aortic clamp. (*From R. R. Lower, Cardiac Transplantation, in J. C. Norman (ed.), "Cardiac Surgery," 2d ed., p. 599, Appleton Century Crofts, New York, 1972.*)

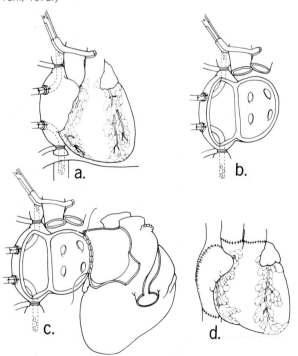

POSTOPERATIVE CARE

The most immediate problem in the postoperative period is the capacity of the transplanted right ventricle to cope with the preexisting pulmonary hypertension which usually results from long-standing failure of the left side of the heart. Under these circumstances, the heart may temporarily require inotropic support for 1 or 2 days. The precise level of pulmonary hypertension which precludes a successful transplant has not yet been defined, but adequate cardiac function without prolonged pharmacologic support has been recovered in most instances despite the additional theoretic problems of acute denervation and interrupted cardiac lymphatics.

Once the posttransplant circulatory status is stable, the major emphasis in management shifts to the immunologic problem. The heart transplant recipient appears to be less immunologically depressed than a kidney transplant recipient with prolonged uremia and thus requires higher levels of immunosuppression in the early posttransplant weeks. Azathioprine is given in the maximally tolerated daily dose of 3 to 4 mg/kg, with careful observation for signs of hematologic toxicity. Prednisone is begun at a dose of 200 mg/day and tapered gradually to 60 mg/day by the end of 2 weeks. Further tapering of the dose is more gradual, reaching a level of 30 mg/day at 3 months, if the clinical condition permits. Antithymocyte globulin is administered over a 10-day period, although its importance and dosage are incompletely known at this time. To minimize the emergence of resistant microorganisms, antibiotics are administered only at the time of operation and for specific indications thereafter.

Monitoring for episodes of impending rejection depends almost entirely on daily or twice daily observation of the ECG. The majority of patients will have a rejection episode during the first 2 postoperative weeks, and the most significant ECG changes will include a stepwise decrease in voltage, rightward shift in the frontal plane axis, and the occasional occurrence of atrial arrhythmias or right bundle branch block (Fig. 10-37). An epicardial electrode implanted at operation serves to enhance the accuracy of voltage changes in the first few postoperative weeks.

Clinical signs of rejection may include the development of a protodiastolic gallop sound and the murmur of tricuspid insufficiency. Other signs and symptoms, such as pericardial friction rub, fever, and malaise, are rather nonspecific in the early postoperative period and therefore of little diagnostic value. Other confirmatory diagnostic maneuvers include fluoroscopy or ultrasound to demonstrate cardiac chamber enlargement, decreased amplitude of ventricular wall pulsations, and diminished ventricular compliance. A suspected rejection crisis may be further confirmed by transvenous endocardial muscle biopsy as described by the Stanford University Medical Center group (Fig. 10-38).

The treatment of a rejection episode requires a large intravenous dose of steroid, usually 1 Gm of methylprednisolone on the first day and 0.5 Gm on the second day, with subsequent return to maintenance levels if the clinical condition permits. The adjunctive value of graft irradiation

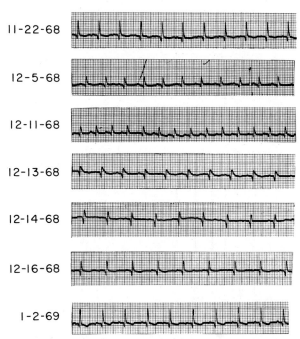

CARDIAC TRANSPLANT L.R. ECG LEAD III

11-22-68

12-5-68

12-11-68

12-13-68

12-14-68

12-16-68

1-2-69

Fig. 10-37. ECG evidence of an acute rejection episode 3½ months after cardiac transplantation. The significant changes include a decrease in voltage and the development of right bundle branch block; these changes were reversed with a temporary increase in the steroid dose, and the patient remains the longest surviving transplant 5 years after operation. (*From R. R. Lower, Cardiac Transplantation, in J. C. Norman (ed.), "Cardiac Surgery," 2d ed., p. 599, Appleton Century Crofts, New York, 1972.*)

and anticoagulant therapy is incompletely settled at the present time. Late postoperative management includes a vigorous exercise program to minimize the catabolic effects of steroid therapy. The likelihood of acute rejection diminishes after 4 months, and ECG studies are reduced to twice weekly.

The major late problem, aside from infectious complications, has been the development of vascular lesions characteristic of chronic rejection. Even small lesions may produce ischemic damage to the conduction system, and the occurrence of conduction defects may require transvenous pacing. The value of prolonged therapy with warfarin and dipyridamole is under investigation in the hope of minimizing the vascular complications. Control of hyperlipidemia is also carefully managed in the appropriate patients.

RESULTS

Survival data have been periodically compiled and published by the ACS/NIH Organ Transplant Registry. The majority of cardiac transplants from 1971 to 1973 were performed at the Stanford University Medical Center, and this group has also published several detailed analyses of their steadily improving results which currently indicate a 48 percent 1-year and 38 percent 2-year survival rate.

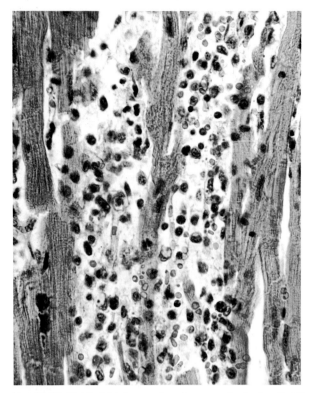

Fig. 10-38. Right atrial myocardium from a patient who died 7 days after cardiac transplantation from acute rejection. There are marked interstitial edema, hemorrhage, and an extensive mononuclear cell infiltration. (*From R. R. Lower, Cardiac Transplantation, in J. C. Norman (ed.), "Cardiac Surgery," 2d ed., p. 599, Appleton Century Crofts, New York, 1972.*)

Twenty-six patients are currently alive in the world experience, of which ten have survived more than 3 years and six more than 4 years after operation. A total of 22 patients have lived 2 years or more, attesting to the therapeutic potential of this procedure. Late deaths occurring more than 3 months after operation have usually resulted from infectious complications or from the graft arteriosclerosis associated with chronic rejection (Fig. 10-39). Four patients have died of disseminated malignant disease.

The majority of patients surviving beyond 6 months have returned to an active and productive existence and have enjoyed an excellent exercise tolerance. Postoperative cardiac catheterization studies reported by the Stanford group on seven patients 12 to 14 months after operation revealed normal resting pressures in the right and left sides of the heart and a fall in pulmonary vascular resistance from a preoperative average of 5.8 units to an average of 2.4 units in the postoperative study. There was no evidence in any patient of autonomic reinnervation, but the cardiac index increased from 2.5 liters/min/m^2 at rest to 4.8 liters/min/m^2 during moderate exercise with a concomitant increase in left ventricular end-diastolic pressure to an average of 21 mm Hg. It is thus concluded from the patient and animal studies that the denervated transplanted heart increases cardiac output during exercise by two sequential mechanisms: in the initial phase of 2 to

3 minutes there is predominantly an increase in stroke volume due to the Starling mechanism with little change in rate, followed later by a gradual increase in heart rate in response to peripherally produced catecholamines.

Lung

Transplantation of the lung presents three rather unique problems: First is that for a long time it appeared that technical factors related to denervation of the transplanted lung would make it impossible to achieve normal or even adequate function of the transplant. This, however, no longer seems to be the case. Second is that with the currently employed immunosuppressive agents the lung is by far the most common site of infection, even in patients with kidney homotransplants. Most patients with kidney transplants who die do so because of the complications of pulmonary infection, because the lung is normally exposed to the outside air, with its microorganisms and viruses. As an allotransplant, with the added hazard of the immunologic onslaught of the host, it is even more likely that the lung will become involved in bacterial, fungal, or viral infections which lead to its destruction and to the death of the host. Despite these formidable barriers to successful transplantation of the lung, some progress has been made in this field.

AUTOTRANSPLANTATION

EXPERIMENTAL STUDIES. Autotransplantation of the lung involves division of pulmonary and bronchial arteries, the pulmonary veins, the nerves, and the lymphatics. Each of these structures has a relation to pulmonary physiology. Permanent division of the pulmonary artery results in fibrosis, but no necrosis, of the lung. Simple ligation of the bronchial arteries is without adverse effect upon the function of the lung but probably contributes to the high incidence of disruption, leakage, and sterosis at the bronchial anastomosis after lung transplantation. Unilateral denervation of the lung by hilar stripping has sometimes been said to produce a decrease in ventilation, oxygen consumption, and compliance, while in other instances no alteration of pulmonary function has been observed. Bilateral denervation by hilar stripping reduces lung function but permits survival of the animal.

The chief technical advance in transplantation of the lung has been the technique described by Metras and later by Neptune et al. in which a portion of the left atrium is removed along with the pulmonary veins, so that the anastomosis can be made through the wall of the left atrium instead of through each individual pulmonary vein (Fig. 10-40). When the lung has been completely removed and replaced by division and anastomosis of the pulmonary artery, left atrium, and bronchus, usually a transient depression of ventilation and oxygen consumption with a return toward normal a few days later is seen. On occasion a severe loss of function and pulmonary hypertension is noted. This could easily be demonstrated by ligation of the contralateral pulmonary artery, which is followed by a sharp rise in the pulmonary artery pressure and edema of the transplant.

It has been shown that isolated division and reanastomosis of the left atrium just proximal to the insertion of the pulmonary veins produces no physiologic or morphologic change, provided the anastomosis remains adequately patent. If partial obstruction to the venous outflow occurs, there is decreased ventilation and decreased oxygen consumption similar to that seen in transplants. Pulmonary hypertension does not develop when the contralateral artery is clamped unless there is partial obstruction to the venous anastomosis. It would appear, therefore, that most of the abnormalities observed in the early experiments with lung autotransplants were related to technical problems with the venous anastomosis. If this procedure is carefully carried out, unilateral autotransplantation of the lung does not significantly alter function or structure. While temporary alterations of pulmonary alveolar surfactant have been described in lung autotransplants, other investigators have found no alteration in this parameter.

Bilateral autotransplantation of the lung in dogs has been accomplished by many investigators. Initially attempts were often made to carry out simultaneous bilateral autotransplantation, but death always resulted. It was discovered, however, that after autotransplantation of one lung the second lung could be removed and reimplanted after an interval of 3 to 12 months. It was felt that during this period of time some type of adaptation had occurred which permitted the successful removal and reimplantation of the second lung. It was thought that this might be due to nerve regeneration, but the Hering-Breuer reflex did not return after reimplantation.

Haglin and Arnar in 1964 carried out staged bilateral reimplantations at intervals of 7 to 10 days in baboons. This seemed to demonstrate for the first time that bilateral pulmonary transplantation could be successfully accomplished without nerve regeneration. It also showed that lung autotransplantation could be done more easily and with a greater degree of success in the baboon than in the dog. However, several dogs have now survived bilateral reimplantation of the lung. More recently it has been possible to carry out reimplantation of the contralateral lung in the dog 7 days after autotransplantation, with long-term survival. Division of the vagal nerve fibers does appear to have a more deleterious effect upon pulmonary function than division of the lymphatics or the bronchial arteries. Regeneration of the lymphatics appears to take place in 7 to 12 days.

In comparing the effect of contralateral pneumonectomy at various intervals after reimplantation of one lung, Haglin and Arnar performed contralateral pneumonectomy in 34 surviving dogs from 1 week to 2 years following reimplantation. Thirty-one dogs died. These investigators carried out the same procedure in the baboon, in which, by contrast, 8 of 11 animals tolerated contralateral pneumonectomy 2 years after unilateral reimplantation.

CLINICAL EXPERIENCE. Autotransplantation has been used in the treatment of severe bronchial asthma in man. A single lung was replaced in six patients, and in one additional patient bilateral staged autotransplantations were carried out. Two patients died ultimately of pulmonary hemorrhage from bronchovascular fistulae, while the

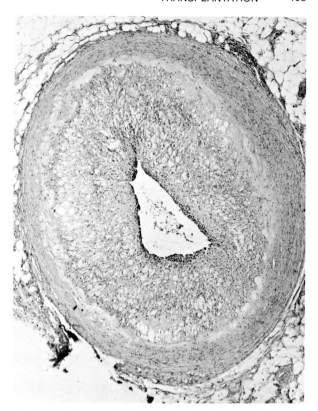

Fig. 10-39. An epicardial coronary artery from a patient dying 8 months after cardiac transplantation showing marked arteriosclerosis characteristic of chronic rejection. (*From R. R. Lower, Cardiac Transplantation, in J. C. Norman (ed.), "Cardiac Surgery," 2d ed., p. 599, Appleton Century Crofts, New York, 1972.*)

other five patients, including the one with bilateral reimplantation, survived. The asthma was said to be improved. The procedure is not recommended.

ALLOTRANSPLANTATION

EXPERIMENTAL STUDIES. As with renal and hepatic transplantation the function of the allotransplanted lung in the untreated recipient lasts for 6 to 8 days. Death of the recipient usually occurs within 2 weeks. A variety of drugs have been used in attempts to obtain prolonged survival of lung allotransplants. The function of the transplanted lung is often severely diminished even in those animals which survive for long periods of time. If the contralateral lung is removed or the contralateral pulmonary artery ligated in animals living for a long time with a lung homograft, only a few animals survive.

CLINICAL EXPERIENCE. More than 30 lung transplants have been performed in patients with end-stage pulmonary disease. Although there has been some significant survival (one patient survived as long as 10 months), all efforts have ultimately failed. These failures have provided important knowledge and have served to indicate areas for further evaluation and study.

Certain technical considerations should be kept in mind. The transplanted lung must be capable of immediate function: there are no adequate artificial lungs available with

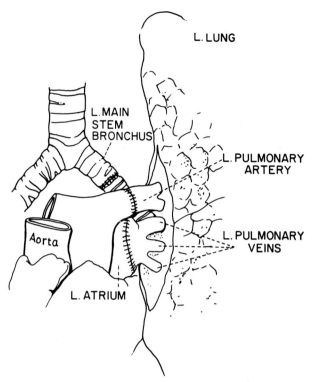

L. LUNG

L. MAIN
STEM
BRONCHUS

L. PULMONARY
ARTERY

Aorta

L. PULMONARY
VEINS

L. ATRIUM

Fig. 10-40. Technique for lung transplantation (described by Metras). A portion of the left atrium is removed along with the pulmonary veins, so that the anastomosis can be made through the wall of the left atrium instead of through each individual pulmonary vein.

which life can be maintained while waiting for the transplanted lung to function. Therefore, it is particularly important to perform a perfect venous anastomosis between the pulmonary veins and the left atrium. If this anastomosis is defective, thrombosis will occur in most cases, and even those patients with patency will demonstrate an increased vascular resistance and poor function. Other technical problems have frequently developed at the bronchial suture line because of the deficient blood supply of the transplanted bronchus, which must derive its blood supply from collaterals between the pulmonary and bronchial arteries. There is a high incidence of bronchial leakage and stenosis due to varying degrees of ischemic necrosis at the transplanted bronchus.

Lungs can be transplanted singly or along with the heart as a cardiopulmonary bilateral lung transplant. The latter procedure has been used on several patients and is preferred by some surgeons since the anastomoses are rather simple. Bronchial anastomoses are eliminated, and a simpler tracheal anastomosis is substituted. In addition, cardiopulmonary transplantation circumvents the possibility that overexpansion of the emphysematous contralateral lung will compress the freshly transplanted lung causing immediate malfunction. This complication has been reported in several human unilateral transplants but has not proved to be a problem in most cases.

Pulmonary transplantation has not received an adequate trial in man. Most of the patients died in the first few days

following transplantation. Many of the deaths were technical problems, such as leakage at the bronchial anastomoses. In the immunosuppressed patient, the transplanted lung might easily become infected, and pulmonary infections have frequently supervened. The problem here is that no single research group has embarked on an intensive experimental human program designed to define and solve the clinical and immunologic problems.

Kidney

The technical knowledge necessary to perform kidney transplants has been available since Carrel and Guthrie developed the techniques of vascular suture.

Between the years 1951 and 1953 Hume performed nine cadaver kidney transplants. Function was adequate to maintain these patients for a limited period; one patient survived for 6 months. Steroids were used in some of these patients, but apparently insufficient doses were used. In 1954 Murray et al. successfully transplanted kidneys between identical twins, and the technical feasibility of routine human renal transplantation was confirmed. The discoveries by Schwartz and Dameshek that 6-mercaptopurine was immunosuppressive in rabbits and the subsequent demonstrations by Calne and by Zukoski et al. that immunosuppression would prolong renal allografts in dogs led directly to the success of human renal allotransplantation. Renal transplantation is now the treatment of choice for most patients with renal failure.

RECIPIENT SELECTION AND INDICATIONS FOR TRANSPLANTATION

CRITERIA FOR SELECTION. The criteria for the selection of recipients of renal allotransplants have never been rigidly defined, but commonly accepted criteria include (1) age, (2) failure to respond to good conservative management, (3) absence of reversible features, (4) normal lower urinary outflow tract, (5) absence of major extrarenal complications (e.g., malignant tumor, systemic disease, cerebral or coronary artery disease), (6) absence of active infection, (7) absence of severe malnutrition, and (8) absence of pancytopenia. Some groups use socioeconomic and psychiatric screening parameters to choose prospective recipients.

At the University of Minnesota there is only one primary indication for renal allotransplantation and dialysis—namely, renal failure that cannot be corrected by conservative measures. We have found that most of the generally accepted contraindications to renal transplantation are unnecessarily exclusive. The only absolute contraindications are active infection or malignant disease that cannot be brought under control.

Renal transplantation has been carried out for almost every imaginable renal disease. Results of transplantation in most cases justify the indications, although certain precautions should be taken.

Congenital or hereditary diseases of the urinary tract are obvious indications without contraindication. Of particular note is the high degree of success with congenital obstruction and ureterovesical reflux and neurogenic bladders. It is possible to correct most such abnormalities or to substitute intestinal conduits for bladders that cannot be repaired.

Among the acquired diseases, most transplants are carried out for either chronic glomerulonephritis or chronic pyelonephritis. In fact, many patients do not present a classic history of either disease, and the kidney disease is so far advanced by the time biopsy is performed that the pathogenesis is indeterminate. Rather than assign a definitive diagnosis suggesting a cause, it is best to regard such patients as having end-stage renal disease of unknown cause. Among the more specific glomerulonephritides is Goodpasture's disease, in which antibodies to glomerular basement membrane can be detected by fluorescent techniques within the kidney. Such patients may or may not also have pulmonary hemorrhage and usually pursue a rather acute course to renal failure. It is generally agreed that serum titers of antiglomerular basement membranes should be performed and that the nephrectomy should precede transplantation in these patients. Transplantation should be delayed until the antiglomerular basement membrane antibody has reached a low level, and the patient should be maintained on dialysis for 6 months to 1 year following nephrectomy before transplantation.

The other glomerulonephritides are less well defined. One that is becoming increasingly well understood is related to low complement levels within the bloodstream and a proliferative membranoglomerulonephritis. Here, complement (β-C_1) can be detected in discrete fragments along the basement membrane without marked degrees of antibody deposition. Although the cause of this disease is not understood, it does not seem to be related to direct antikidney antibodies, so that delay in transplantation is not necessary. In the absence of well-defined disease, renal failure that follows an acute course complicated by a nonspecific glomerulonephritis should probably be treated by nephrectomy and a delay in transplantation, although prompt transplants have been performed with success in such cases.

Most children with a nephrotic syndrome recover spontaneously or with steroid or immunosuppressive therapy. Some patients, however, develop the nephrotic syndrome and progress toward terminal renal failure despite the use of steroids. Several of these patients have received transplants at the University of Minnesota. Both groups of patients have undergone either rapid renal failure or gradual reappearance of the previously existent nephrotic syndrome. In the absence of further information some caution should be utilized in performing transplantation in such patients.

Most patients with hypertensive nephrosclerosis present with gradual increase in hypertension and renal failure. A number of patients, however, have presented with sudden onset of malignant hypertension and renal failure. Emergency nephrectomy can occasionally be performed in such patients with resolution of the hypertension prior to transplantation.

Transplantation has been carried out in a number of patients with both benign and malignant tumors primarily arising within the kidney. Patients with benign tumors associated with tuberous sclerosis respond well to transplantation. It is best to maintain patients with malignant tumors on hemodialysis for several years prior to transplantation to avoid grafting patients with metastatic malignant disease. Although individual patients with diabetic end-stage renal disease have received renal transplants, no well-studied series has yet been reported. At the University of Minnesota, 45 patients with diabetes have received kidney transplants from related living donors. Good renal function is present in 28. No increased problems in management of the diabetes or infectious complications have been noted, and a gratifying cessation of the progression of gastroenteropathy and neuropathy, previously thought to be diabetic in origin, has occurred. It is possible that in such patients recurrent diabetic glomerulosclerosis will not develop for many more years, and further trials are certainly indicated.

Lupus erythematosus appears to involve the kidney by means of a complex nephritis. Anti-DNA antibodies combine with systemic DNA and are filtered out in the kidney, leading to renal damage. Extensive experience with transplantation for lupus erythematosus and renal disease has not been obtained, but it is generally felt to be a satisfactory procedure if other manifestations of lupus erythematosus have been brought under control by immunosuppressive drugs. In contrast, patients with polyarteritis may not be amenable to transplantation, although extensive trials have not been carried out.

A number of metabolic diseases (gout, oxalosis, cystinosis, hyperoxaluria, nephrocalcinosis, and amyloidosis) have very little in common except for the accumulation of abnormal deposits within the kidney leading to or associated with renal failure. Transplants in most of these diseases can be successful, although recurrence after oxalosis has been reported.

Patients with chronic obstructive pulmonary disease in addition to their renal disease require careful individual scrutiny. Such patients tolerate pulmonary infections poorly, and since pulmonary infections are the primary cause of death in patients with renal transplantation, careful selection of these patients is required. Heavy smokers should be allowed a long period to discontinue their smoking habit. Prolonged physical therapy for chronic pulmonary disease should also be carried out in order to evaluate the improvement that might be obtained prior to transplantation. This is of particular importance in chronic granulomatous diseases, such as histoplasmosis, coccidioidomycosis, and tuberculosis. Such diseases may remain latent and inactive prior to the institution of immunosuppression and then be exacerbated in the presence of the immunosuppressive drugs. Nevertheless, some patients with tuberculosis have received successful transplantations, and tuberculosis development following transplantation has not uniformly resulted in death or loss of graft.

The social and psychologic barriers to selection used by some groups seem capricious. It is extremely difficult to judge the psychologic and social stability of a patient who is dying of long-term renal disease. Similarly, one cannot exclude, out of hand, patients with coronary disease or cerebral vascular accidents. Patients with peptic ulceration frequently do quite well if surgical correction of the peptic ulcer disease is carried out prior to transplantation. Patients with severe liver disease, however, may be more susceptible to azathioprine toxicity. Liver disease therefore remains a relative contraindication.

In short, all transplantation centers are now rapidly expanding their indications for transplantation and finding that the number of contraindications has greatly diminished. Only 3 of the last 134 patients evaluated with terminal renal failure for transplantation at the University of Minnesota were refused either transplantation or dialysis. One patient was diabetic with paraplegia and had been bedridden for the previous 2 years; the second patient was a sixty-year-old man with severe emphysema, cirrhosis of the liver, and chronic glomerulonephritis, and the third patient, a fifty-six-year-old man, had active carcinoma of the bladder.

Patient selection is relatively easy, and the special committees used by some centers may not be necessary. Recipient selection at Minnesota is performed by the primary dialysis physician with consultation with the transplantation surgeons only if special problems exist.

WORK-UP OF POTENTIAL RECIPIENTS AND TIMING OF DIALYSIS. More important than the actual selection technique of the potential recipient is the choice of time for the institution of dialysis treatment. The conservative management of renal failure will not be discussed in detail here. In principle, homeostasis can be achieved by manipulation of the sodium, potassium, chloride, bicarbonate, and protein intake. An occasional dialysis may be necessary for exacerbations of renal failure secondary to infections in the urinary tract or elsewhere. The protein-limited (high-quality) diets described by Giodono and Giovanetti are essential. It is even possible to maintain patients in positive nitrogen balance over several months and even years on this diet. The main problem, however, has been patient motivation, and near-suicidal binges of eating are a constant problem over a long period.

Dialysis should be instituted prior to the development of uremic complications. Once hypertension, pericarditis, cardiac failure, severe bone disease, bleeding, malnutrition, severe anemia, and neuropathy appear, management is markedly complicated and rehabilitation compromised. Ideally, the conservative management of patients treated for progressive renal functional deterioration should be in conjunction with nephrologists associated with dialysis and transplant centers. In this way, the complication of severe uremia can be rapidly prevented by dialysis without the delays inherent in the referral process.

The main indication for the institution of dialysis has been a serum creatinine level greater than 15 mg/100 ml or a creatinine clearance less than 3 ml/minute despite meticulous conservative care. It is obvious that there are exceptions to this rule. Some patients, particularly patients with polycystic kidney disease, with serum creatinine levels greater than 15 mg/100 ml can be maintained well for months on dietary management. In other patients, especially diabetic patients, severe complications of uremia will develop long before the serum creatinine level reaches that level. The most pernicious of these complications is peripheral neuropathy. If there are signs of motor involvement, the patient should have dialysis and transplantation without delay, since very rapid progression of the disease can make it impossible ever to rehabilitate such a patient. Another indication for early dialysis-transplantation is uncontrollable hypertension, or hypertension that can be controlled only at the expense of severe orthostatic hypotension and other side effects. Severe anemia with anemic symptoms (dyspnea at the mildest exertion), severe bone disease (especially in children), and the failure to maintain his diet or carry on his social and family obligations all should lead to early dialysis and transplantation. There is little to be gained by a delay of 3 to 6 months, and lives may be lost in futile attempts at conservative management.

Since some of the complications of uremia may appear suddenly during conservative management, it is extremely important that the patient be fully evaluated prior to the institution of dialysis, if possible. In addition to the medical evaluation, this preparation should include interviews with the patient and his family by the business office of the hospital, the rehabilitation clinic, and social service in order to ameliorate the financial and social difficulties that may accompany dialysis and transplantation. Rehabilitation of the patient can be actively pursued even prior to the institution of dialysis.

PREPARATION FOR HEMODIALYSIS AND TRANSPLANTATION. The pretransplantation studies are listed in Table 10-3. Most of these studies are used by many transplant groups and for patients on dialysis. A few deserve special elaboration.

The urinary tract should be evaluated for patency of its outflow and absence of ureterovesical reflux. In general, a voiding cystogram suffices. That test makes it possible to determine that the urethra is unobstructed, that the bladder empties, that there are no abnormalities of the bladder wall, and that there is no ureteral reflux. Prostatic obstruction, urinary stricture, and bladder neck obstruction should be repaired prior to transplantation but only after the patient has been dialyzed for several weeks.

It is difficult or almost impossible to evaluate bladder emptying in the presence of ureterovesical reflux. Contraction of the bladder wall leads to reflux of the urine into the ureters, which then empty back into the bladder when the bladder wall is relaxed. It is necessary to remove both ureters at the ureterovesical junction prior to evaluation of the bladder for competence.

The upper gastrointestinal tract should be evaluated for the possibility of a preexisting peptic ulceration. These operations can usually be carried out conveniently at the time of pretransplant nephrectomy. Such precautions have almost completely eliminated upper gastrointestinal tract bleeding as a problem.

Electromyography is useful for documenting the progress or improvement of peripheral neuropathy. Because so many patients with uremia also have hearing deficits, periodic audiograms should be carried out.

Obviously dialysis frequently must be instituted prior to the completion of these studies. Most of the studies listed are primarily designed to prepare for transplantation. Dialysis is both a definitive therapy and the most impor-

Table 10-3. WORK-UP OF POTENTIAL RECIPIENTS
OF RENAL TRANSPLANTATION

1. General
   a. History and physical examination
   b. Chest x-ray
   c. ECG
   d. Electrophoresis
   e. (FBS)
2. Hematologic
   a. Hemoglobin
   b. Leukocyte count and differential count
   c. Platelet count
   d. Bleeding-clotting time
   e. Prothrombin time, partial thromboplastin time, thrombin
      time
3. "Allergic" potentially complicating
   a. Serum electrophoresis
   b. LE Test
   c. Antiglomerular basement antibodies
4. Renal
   a. Flat plate of abdomen (kidney size) (tomography)
   b. Creatinine clearance
   c. 23-hour protein excretion
   d. (Electrophoresis/urine, protein excretion selectivity)
   e. Electrolyte status in blood
   f. (Electrolyte status in urine)
   g. Urinalysis ×3
   h. Urine culture ×3
   i. Renal biopsy (nephrectomy specimen)
5. Signs of hyperparathyroidism
   a. Bone x-ray (hands, skull, clavical, lamina dura)
   b. Ca,PO$_4$, Mg, alkaline phosphatase
6. Hypertensive work-up
   a. Chest x-ray (heart size)
   b. ECG
   c. Ophthalmic examination
   d. Serial blood pressure
7. Urologic evaluation
   a. Voiding cystogram
   b. (Retrograde pyelography)
   c. (Cystometrography)
   d. (Bladder biopsy)
   e. (Bladder stimulation)
8. Upper gastrointestinal x-ray
9. (Colon x-ray in older patients)
10. Typing
    a. ABO
    b. Blood pedigree
    c. Tissue typing including serial cytotoxic antibody determinations
11. (Pulmonary function studies)
12. Infectious work-up
    a. Chest x-ray
    b. (PPD-fungal skin tests)
    c. Urine culture
    d. Blood culture
    e. Skin-nose-throat culture
    f. Feces culture
    g. (Sinus-teeth x-ray–ENT consultation)
13. Financial-social rehabilitation
    a. (Psychologic-psychiatric)

Note: The tests listed within parentheses are not administered routinely during the potential recipient work-up, but only when the circumstances so indicate.

tant part of the preparation for transplantation. It should not be delayed in order to complete other studies, the results of which no longer exclude the patient from treatment anyway.

Principles of Hemodialysis

Dialysis removes toxic products of small molecular size from the blood and reinstitutes acid-base balance and electrolyte homeostasis. Although such treatment will not relieve all the complications of uremia, it will prevent death in a large percentage of cases. Blood is passed through a tubing composed of a semipermeable membrane, so that dialyzable substances within the blood pass into the dialysis bath and dialyzable materials within the bath pass into the blood. Fluid can be removed (ultrafiltration) (1) by increasing the osmolarity of the dialysate bath (by adding glucose), (2) by constricting the outflow of blood from the dialyzer, or (3) by running dialysate at negative pressure to raise the filtration pressure.

Transplant dialysis is not an end in itself. It merely maintains the patient while he awaits transplantation, prepares him for the operations required, and retrieves him if the transplant is temporarily or permanently unsuccessful. Three requirements are necessary to perform dialysis: (1) access to a flow of blood, (2) a semipermeable membrane tubing, and (3) a dialysate bath of appropriate composition.

Access to Blood Flow. Indwelling Cannulae. The standard Quinton-Scribner Silastic Teflon cannula is the instrument most widely used for access to blood in dialysis. The technique currently used for insertion is shown in Fig. 10-41*A* and *B*. Either upper or lower extremities can be used for cannulation, but the upper extremity is preferable in order not to immobilize the patient while the wounds are healing. The ideal vessels are the radial artery and the cephalic or basilic vein on the nondominant arm.

The persistence of the cannulae within the vessels and the subsequent passage through the skin have predictable consequences—the vessels may clot, the cutaneous fistulae may become infected, and the shunt is in danger of bleeding. The clotting problem looms especially large after major surgical procedures.

Infectious complications at the shunt site are particularly dangerous before transplantation. *Staphylococcus aureus* is the most common infecting agent. Long-term treatment with synthetic penicillinase-resistant penicillin plus intensive local treatment with heat and elevation can cure these infections in most instances. Systemic gram-negative infections have been rare when using disposable dialyzers. Infections are best prevented by handling all shunts with sterile technique. Mask and glove precautions should be enforced whenever the shunt is opened or manipulated. The shunt should be removed as soon as possible after function of the transplanted kidney has been established.

Arteriovenous Fistulae. Because the problems of shunt care increase with time, external shunts are most satisfactory when transplantation is scheduled within a few weeks or months. In patients being dialyzed for prolonged periods while awaiting a kidney from a cadaver, the subcutaneous arteriovenous fistula described by Brescia et al. has been a major advance. Here an arteriovenous anasto-

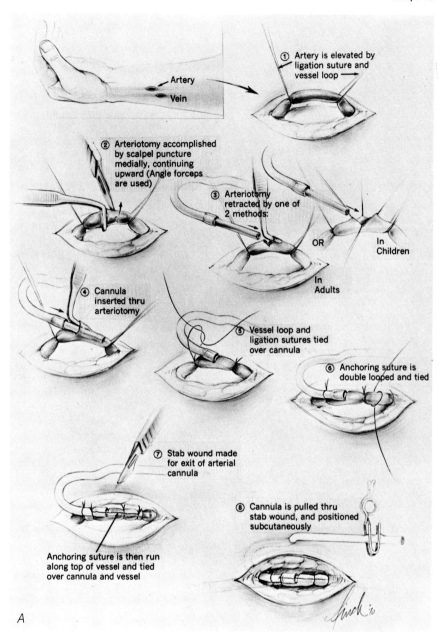

Fig. 10-41. Insertion of Scribner shunt (*A*) and connecting the two shunt limbs (*B*) (*.From C. M. Kjellstrand, R. L. Simmons, T. J. Buselmeier, and J. S. Najarian, Kidney: I. Recipient Selection, Medical Management, and Dialysis, in J. S. Najarian and R. L. Simmons (eds.), "Transplantation," p. 418, Lea & Febiger, Philadelphia, 1972.*)

mosis is performed, usually between the radial artery and the cephalic vein at the wrist (Fig. 10-42). The superficial veins become dilated, and blood can be obtained for passage through the dialyzer by the use of two large-bore needles inserted into the dilated venous system.

There are several advantages to this type of fistula: (1) no foreign bodies inviting infection pass through the skin except during dialysis; (2) the fistula has a lesser tendency to clot than does the Quinton-Scribner shunt; (3) the arteriovenous fistula can remain open in the posttransplant period, thereby facilitating dialysis if rejection occurs months or even years later; (4) the dilated veins are useful for the administration of any thrombogenic substance (e.g.,

antilymphoblast globulin) because of the rapid flow through the veins; and (5) it provides rapid access for the frequent blood samples required in the posttransplant period.

SELECTION AND EVALUATION OF LIVING DONORS

The principles of histocompatibility typing and matching have been described above. From the recipient's point of view it is generally preferable that the donor be a biologic relative. At the present time, histocompatibility typing cannot discern cadaver donors who will be more suitable than a relative. Even mismatched sibling and parent kidneys survive with better function and for more

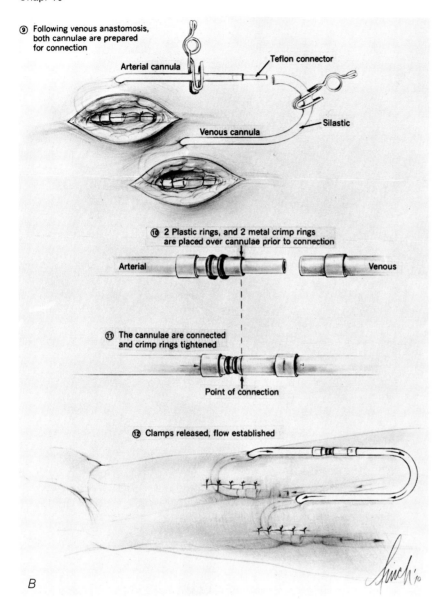

⑨ Following venous anastomosis, both cannulae are prepared for connection

Arterial cannula

Teflon connector

Venous cannula

Silastic

⑩ 2 Plastic rings, and 2 metal crimp rings are placed over cannulae prior to connection

Arterial   Venous

⑪ The cannulae are connected and crimp rings tightened

Point of connection

⑫ Clamps released, flow established

B

prolonged periods than do closely matched cadaver kidneys. Before the advent of histocompatibility typing, it was shown that kidneys from sibling donors functioned better than kidneys from parental donors. Because the genes governing the expression of histocompatibility antigens are situated at one (complex) locus, there will always be one major allelic difference between the parent and the offspring, whereas one-fourth of siblings will be identical, one-half will have one allelic difference, and one-fourth will have two allelic differences. The genetic relationship may be even more complex, since recent results from larger centers suggest that siblings', parents', and even aunts', uncles', and cousins' kidneys survive equally well—all better than matched cadaver transplants. A living related donor offers other advantages to the recipient: the delay between renal failure and rehabilitation is shorter,

posttransplant renal function is usually immediate, and there are fewer rejection episodes, so that smaller doses of immunosuppressive drugs are required.

The major blood group antigens (ABO) are strong transplantation antigens. Although a number of successful allotransplants have been carried out across isoantibody barriers, it is generally unwise to perform transplants into patients with known preformed isohemagglutinins against the donor blood type. The same rules apply to clinical transplantation that apply to transfusion; i.e., AB is the universal recipient and O the universal donor. When such blood type barriers are crossed, the most violent type of hyperacute rejection reaction may occur. There is no convincing evidence to suggest that minor blood group factors (Rh, Duffy, Kell) act as histocompatibility antigens.

The living related donor should be in perfect health to

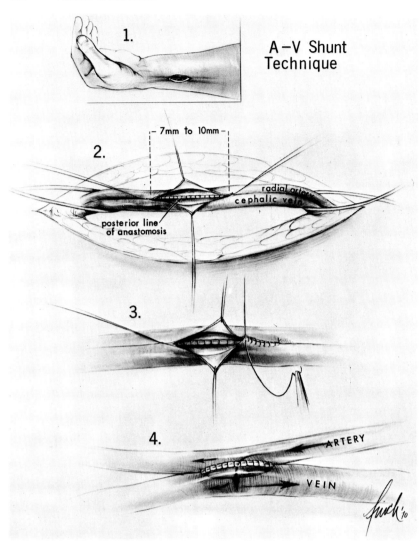

A–V Shunt Technique

1.

2.
— 7mm to 10mm —
radial artery
cephalic vein
posterior line
of anastomosis

3.

4.
ARTERY
VEIN

Fig. 10-42. Technique for constructing an arteriovenous anastomosis between radial artery and cephalic vein at the wrist. (*From C. M. Kjellstrand, R. L. Simmons, T. J. Buselmeier, and J. S. Najarian, Kidney: I. Recipient Selection, Medical Management, and Dialysis in J. S. Najarian and R. L. Simmons (eds.), "Transplantation," p. 418, Lea & Febiger, Philadelphia, 1972.*)

minimize any risks inherent in an operation of this magnitude. Only one death following renal donation from a healthy person has been reported. The utmost caution must be exerted not to harm or diminish the renal reserve of a healthy volunteer. Table 10-4 lists the examinations routinely carried out on volunteer related donors.

ETHICAL PROBLEMS. Selection of a related donor is made on the basis of histocompatibility testing when possible; often, however, there is only one volunteer. The ethical and social problems of donor selection have been extensively discussed elsewhere, but brief consideration is pertinent here.

In practice, the recipient is informed of the risks and benefits of receiving a kidney from a related donor. The recipient knows best which relatives he can approach and which he cannot. When a volunteer appears, he is blood-typed and tissue-typed. If he is acceptable on these grounds, the risk of donor nephrectomy is explained to him. The risk to life in an otherwise perfectly healthy patient has been estimated to be 0.05 percent. The long-

term risk has been estimated by actuarial statistics as equal to risk incurred by driving a car 16 miles every working day. Penn and Starzl have demonstrated that no long-term harm is done in the donation process. Although the risks are small, the pain, anxiety, and loss of work time are real.

It is difficult to conceive of a living related donor who is not subject to some family pressure to donate. That such pressures exist, however, is evidence that people have feelings of family and role obligations within the society. When a person freely volunteers to donate, both the benefits to the recipient and the risks to the donor are explained. No pressure is exerted to persuade or dissuade the potential donor. He is not subjected to extensive psychologic interviews or testing. The early studies of actual donors indicated a remarkably favorable psychologic response. Other studies indicate much ambivalence and conflict within the family. Further studies are needed to clarify the attitudes and feelings of people who donate or refuse to do so. On occasion, when the potential donor expresses anxiety concerning his donation, it is necessary to fabricate

Table 10-4. PROTOCOL FOR LIVING RELATED
DONOR WORK-UP

1. History and physical examination
2. Hematology: hematocrit, leukocyte count, differential count,
   platelet count
3. Coagulation: prothrombin time, partial thromboplastin time,
   thrombin time
4. Chemistry: serum Na^+, K^+, Cl^-, CO^{2-}, SGOT, bilirubin,
   uric acid, CA^{2+}, P, BUN, creatinine, fasting blood sugar,
   glucose tolerance test
5. Urine: urinalysis, 24-hour urine for creatinine clearance
6. Microbiology: clean catch urine culture $\times 2$
7. Immunology: blood type (major and minor), tissue typing,
   leukocyte cross match for recipient antidonor and leukocyte
   antibodies; VDRL; Australian antigen
8. X-ray: chest x-ray, PA and lateral; intravenous pyelogram
   (IVP), renal arteriograms
9. Isotope: bilateral renogram
10. Electrocardiogram

a medical excuse not to donate that can be used by the
otherwise medically and immunologically compatible
donor.

Sometimes it is necessary or advisable to use donors
under the age of twenty-one. This has frequently been
necessary for identical-twin transplants. The use of such
donors, however, should be restricted to those circumstances in which other donors are not available. A court
of law will also find it difficult to decide whether an adolescent should donate to his parents or siblings when family pressure may exist. Teen-aged donors have been used
when they insisted on donation and the court has agreed
to it.

Unrelated persons are not generally encouraged to donate, since the results are no better than that achieved with
cadaver donors. It is possible that a pool of living unrelated
donors may exist that could be typed and matched against
a similar recipient pool in order to obtain ideal donors
within unrelated populations. Such a system was tried at
the University of California but with results no better than
if cadaver donors were used. Prisoners, mental defectives,
and psychiatric patients are not generally used as donors
for the obvious reason that undue pressure might be exerted on these persons against their own best interests. The
purchase of organs, with its inevitable consequences, the
selling of living unrelated organs, or even the selling of
a cadaver organ must be discouraged.

SELECTION OF A CADAVER DONOR

The ideal cadaver kidney donor (1) is young, (2) has
remained normotensive until a short time before death,
(3) is free of transmissible infection and malignant disease,
and (4) has died in the hospital after observation for a
number of hours, during which time blood group and
tissue type has been determined and urinary function
assessed. Under these ideal conditions the donor kidneys
can be removed within minutes to minimize the warm
ischemia time. It is necessary, however, to compromise
with a number of these ideal principles: although the age
of the donor is not important and the kidney will even
recover from long periods of shock and anuria, not more
than 1 hour of warm ischemia time should elapse.

CRITERIA OF BRAIN DEATH. The procurement of cadaver organs for transplantation has raised some serious
moral, ethical, legal, and psychologic problems. The first
problem is to establish when death occurs. Since the decision is a clinical one, made by the physician in the interest
of the patient (potential donor), it should be based primarily on clinical criteria of irreversible brain damage—fixed
dilated pupils, absent reflexes, unresponsiveness to external
stimuli, and the inability to maintain vital functions such
as respiration, heartbeat, and blood pressure without artificial means. The decision should be made by physicians
who are not associated with the potential recipient in any
way, either as the referring physician or as a member of
the transplant team. The exact criteria vary among institutions and have been fully discussed by Schwab, Potts and
Bonazzi, the Harvard Committee, and Juul-Jensen.

Juul-Jensen established four criteria of brain death: (1)
The type of cerebral lesions must be established; the
donors must therefore be selected among neurosurgical
patients with severe trauma, vascular lesions, or tumors.
Neuroradiologic studies, arteriography revealing the absence of cerebral blood flow, and surgical exploration assist
in the diagnosis of irreversible brain damage. (2) The level
of consciousness must be that of deep coma, in which the
patient does not respond to any form of external stimulus.
Neurologic examination must reveal dilated and reaction-
less pupils, absence of corneal and pharyngeal reflexes, no
reaction to tracheal suction, absence of deep and plantar
reflexes, and hypotonia. The patient must be without
spontaneous respiration and must require controlled respiration. In this state, atropine will evidence no change in
cardiac rhythm.

The above two criteria have generally been sufficient for
most neurosurgeons to pronounce cerebral brain death
after a period of observation and knowledge of the cerebral disease. A recent autopsy study confirmed that the
brain damage in 24 consecutive cadaver donors was incompatible with recovery when these clinical criteria also
were satisfied. Even so, Juul-Jensen considers two more
criteria, (3) a negative caloric test and (4) an isoelectric
electroencephalogram (EEG), to be essential. Juul-Jensen
feels that the isoelectric EEG is essential but points out that
isoelectric EEGs have been described in anesthetized patients in hypothermia. He furthermore requires that the
tests be repeated with a 24-hour interval where the EEG
is recorded with normal amplification and double amplification with both a normal time constant and an increased
time constant.

These stringent EEG criteria are felt to be excessive by
most physicians; vital signs will frequently fail before an
isoelectric EEG will appear. A number of donors have been
unnecessarily lost because of delay in the event of a destroyed brain.

A falling blood pressure has been used as a criterion
of brain death, but it is frequently the result of dehydration
due to diabetes insipidis. This is aggravated by loss of
vasomotor tone, which produces hypotension. Almost all
patients with total brain death can be maintained for
prolonged periods with normal vital signs using plasma
and vasopressors; cardiac stimulants are rarely required.

Urinary output can likewise be maintained with hydration and diuretics. Even the head injury patient who has been anuric and in shock for many hours can be restored to hemodynamic stability by restoration of a normal blood volume.

All decisions regarding the death of the potential donor must be made by physicians who understand the criteria of brain death and who have had no contact with the potential recipients. Various administrative techniques have been used; the best require the determination of brain death to be made by a team of neurologists and neurosurgeons.

The principles of organ transplantation are described in a subsequent section. The advances in organ preservation have alleviated the urgency of cadaver transplantation. It is possible to harvest kidneys at the moment of death and preserve them in iced solutions for several hours until the transplant recipients are ready. Kidneys can now be routinely preserved by hypothermic perfusion for more than 24 hours (see subsequent section). The use of such machines has increased the availability of cadaver kidneys, because the kidneys can be transported for long distances. The development of preservation also allows for more careful typing, matching, shipping, and sharing of organs between various centers. If histocompatibility typing is ever of practical importance in cadaver transplantation, preservation techniques will be essential to move the harvested organs to the recipient.

ORGAN HARVEST

RELATED LIVING DONOR. The actual technique of the donor operation is not as crucial as those factors that maintain urinary output in the donated kidney and in the remaining donor kidney. An active diuresis in the donor at the moment of renal artery occlusion favors prompt function in the recipient. Conversely, a soft cyanotic kidney in spasm after a difficult dissection frequently is slow to put out urine even if the period of ischemia has been short. For these reasons, the urine output is monitored throughout the donor operation and should not fall below 1 ml/minute/kidney. The patient is hydrated during the night prior to operation, and both colloid (5 ml/kg/hour) and crystalloid solutions (5 ml/kg/hour) are administered during the operation, with constant attention to the central venous pressure and the urine output. Mannitol and furosemide are given shortly before the kidney is removed. In addition, systemic heparinization is carried out 5 minutes before the renal artery is occluded. The heparin is then counteracted with protamine.

The technique of donor operation is described in Fig. 10-43. It is carried out through a flank incision. The peritoneum is retracted, the ureter identified, and a length of ureter is dissected free. The ureter is then transected (preserving its blood supply from the renal pelvis) so that the urinary output of the donor kidney can be observed throughout the operation. The remainder of the ureter is dissected free up to the renal vein. A large lumbar vein, the ovarian or testicular vein, and the adrenal branch of the renal vein are doubly ligated on the left side. There are no major branches of the renal vein on the right side.

Dissection on the renal vein is carried down to the vena cava. The artery is not dissected free until the dissection of the renal vein is complete. The kidney is not removed until urinary output from the donor kidney itself is excellent. At that time the renal artery and vein are sequentially clamped and divided.

Minor complications of nephrectomy in healthy related donors are common, but serious complications are quite rare. There is almost immediate functional hypertrophy of the remaining kidney, so that about 70 percent of normal renal function is present in the average kidney donor. Prolonged follow-ups indicate that the health and life expectancy of the donor are not adversely affected by donation. Kohler's study of the survival of patients after unilateral nephrectomy for renal disease reached the same conclusion.

CADAVER DONOR. The technique of kidney harvest from a cadaver donor depends to a large degree on the status of the donor's circulation. If the cadaver is braindead but with intact circulation and urine output, nephrectomy can be performed as in living donors, but by the transperitoneal route. The circulatory function of the cadaver can also be maintained by closed heart massage or artificial circulatory devices during the harvest procedure.

If the donor dies suddenly, the kidneys must be removed more rapidly to minimize ischemia time. The donor is heparinized, and both kidneys are removed together by clamping the aorta and vena cava above the origin of the renal arteries and veins and pulling the kidneys up together, prior to transection of the aorta and vena cava below the origin of the renal vessels and the ureters in the pelvis. The operation need not be done hastily, for it requires only 10 minutes. Prompt cooling of the organs is required, and both kidneys can be perfused with iced crystalloid solution prior to storing them in the cold or perfusing them on preservation machines.

PREPARATION OF THE RECIPIENT FOR TRANSPLANTATION

NEPHRECTOMY. Removal of the patient's diseased kidneys is desirable to (1) control hypertension, (2) eliminate a potential or real source of infection, (3) remove ureters from patients with ureterovesical reflux, and (4) eliminate the patient's diseased kidneys as potential pathogenetic agents in the recurrence of the primary disease. The latter reason is of theoretic importance only, since the recurrence of the glomerulonephritis in the transplanted kidney is not known to be aggravated by the presence of the diseased kidneys. It is probably not necessary to remove the kidneys from most patients, but the decision should be carefully considered for all.

Many transplantation centers perform bilateral nephrectomy at the time of the transplantation. Others feel that it is better to stage the operations and perform the nephrectomy sometime prior to transplantation in order (1) to minimize the surgical stress at transplantation; (2) to minimize the surgical shock incurred, which might interfere with the function of the transplanted kidney; (3) to apply the minimal surgical stress when immunosuppressant drugs are utilized; (4) to completely eliminate urinary tract

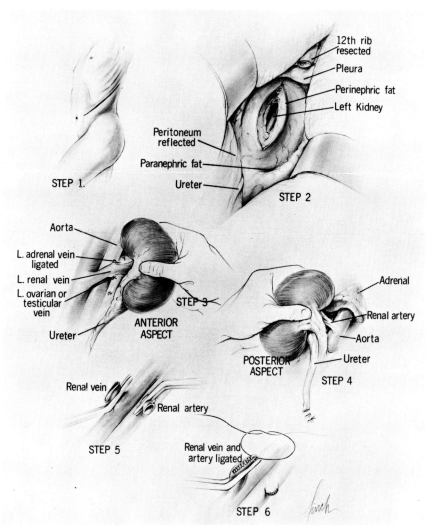

Fig. 10-43. Harvest of a kidney from a living related donor. (*From R. L. Simmons, C. M. Kjellstrand, and J. S. Najarian, Kidney: II. Technique, Complications, and Results, in J. S. Najarian and R. L. Simmons (eds.), "Transplantation," p. 445, Lea & Febiger, Philadelphia, 1972.*)

infection before immunosuppression is begun; and (5) to control hypertension prior to transplantation.

Splenectomy and/or thymectomy have also been performed in kidney recipients prior to transplantation. Thymectomy has fallen into disuse since its performance was associated with a high rate of morbidity without improvement of renal functional survival. Most groups still debate whether splenectomy contributes to the well-being of the recipient. There is no evidence that splenectomy increases the functional survival of the graft, although excision of a large portion of the bodies of lymphoid mass was the original indication for splenectomy. Splenectomy, however, seems to allow larger doses of immunosuppressants to be used without incurring leukopenia and thrombocytopenia.

When two-stage transplantation is carried out (i.e., nephrectomy preceding the transplantation by a week or

10 days), the postnephrectomy management is simple. Hyperkalemia is a recurrent postnephrectomy problem, but it can usually be prevented if a 20% glucose solution is administered prophylactically (with insulin if the patient has diabetes). Rectal ion-exchange resins may be required to control hyperkalemia. Dialysis can usually be postponed 2 or 3 days with these techniques. Delay in reinstituting dialysis is preferred to avoid any anticoagulation that might invite postoperative hemorrhage.

During preparation for transplantation, sepsis from any source must be scrupulously removed. Frequent sources of sepsis are (1) the hemodialysis cannulae, if present, (2) the bladder in patients with preexisting urinary tract infections, and (3) the skin of patients with uremic dermatitis. The bladder of the nephrectomized patient frequently becomes infected, and the bladder should be irrigated with neomycin several times weekly, prior to grafting.

Dialysis should be frequent and intense in the immediate pretransplantation period. Recipients of cadaver kidneys will have little preparation time prior to transplantation. Many patients will be maintained on systemic anticoagulants because of clotting problems in hemodialysis shunts; the anticoagulants must be discontinued, and vitamin K must be administered.

TECHNIQUE OF RENAL TRANSPLANTATION

The operative technique of renal transplantation used at the University of Minnesota is described in Figs. 10-44 and 10-45.

OPERATIVE MANAGEMENT. There must be no deficit in blood volume following vascular anastomoses. Hypovolemia interferes with the rapid resumption of renal function. Urine usually appears within a few minutes of completion of the vascular anastomoses in related living donor kidneys; mannitol and furosemide may be helpful in hastening the appearance of urine, a useful sign that there are no serious technical deficiencies.

Three methods are generally available for establishing urinary tract continuity. The preferred method involves ureteroneocystostomy. Pyeloureterostomy and ureteroureterostomy have also been recommended, but the incidence of urinary extravasation is far more common with that technique.

Renal biopsy at the time of transplantation can be useful where hyperacute rejection is suspected, but it is rarely

Fig. 10-44. Sites of anastomoses of renal vein to the side of the iliac vein. (*From R. L. Simmons, C. M. Kjellstrand, and J. S. Najarian, Kidney: II. Technique, Complications, and Results, in J. S. Najarian and R. L. Simmons (eds.), "Transplantation," p. 445, Lea & Febiger, Philadelphia, 1972.*)

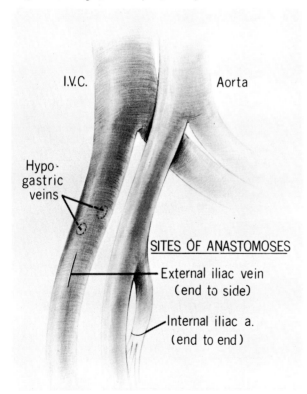

I.V.C.   Aorta

Hypo-
gastric
veins

SITES OF ANASTOMOSES

External iliac vein
(end to side)

Internal iliac a.
(end to end)

necessary in a primary transplant from a living related donor.

ANESTHESIA IN THE ANEPHRIC PATIENT. Certain precautions are necessary during any operation on an anephric patient: In particular, certain anesthetics are eliminated almost exclusively by the kidney and should not be used. These include the muscle relaxant gallamine triethiodide. Both curare and succinylcholine are metabolized by the liver, but both may also be accompanied by prolonged paralysis in the postoperative period. In the case of succinylcholine, a number of investigators have found that serum cholesterase is broken down during hemodialysis. In such patients, succinylcholine would be expected to have prolonged action. Conduction anesthesia is not adequate for the transplant operation. Most anesthesiologists use inhalation anesthesia (usually halothane) combined with muscle relaxants.

In the administration of anesthetics and fluids, it should always be assumed that the kidney will not function immediately after transplantation, even if dialysis is rarely required after transplantation. Similar thinking should be employed with regard to hyperkalemia in the uremic patient. Other concerns of the anesthesiologist are the loss of the hypertensive state after induction of anesthesia to normal levels and the low hematocrit in patients with chronic uremia. The hematocrit should be raised to 30 prior to transplantation; the normal decrease in blood pressure following induction of anesthesia is probably due to relaxation of the cardiovascular system in the face of uremic hypertension.

ROUTINE POSTTRANSPLANT CARE

The management of kidney allograft patients in the early posttransplant period does not differ radically from the management of other postoperative patients. Vital signs are monitored frequently in the early postoperative period, and the central venous pressure is utilized as a guide to blood volume. A Foley catheter is left in the bladder, and it is not irrigated unless clots are thought to be occluding the catheter. The urine output is measured at least very hour. The volume of urine should be replaced with intravenous fluids. A convenient replacement solution consists of one-half normal saline solution with 5% dextrose and water and 10 mEq of sodium bicarbonate per liter. Potassium need not be added to the intravenous fluids except in small children, whose urinary electrolytes should be replaced milliequivalent for milliequivalent. The urinary output in the early postoperative period may be enormous, due in part to tubular dysfunction but primarily to the overhydrated state of even the best-dialyzed patient. A creatinine clearance obtained on the evening of transplantation will confirm or contradict the presence or absence of obligatory diuresis associated with a high-output renal failure. High creatinine clearances are almost never associated with obligatory diureses. When high-output ischemic damage has been ruled out, fluid restriction can be practiced to keep from "chasing" the urinary output with intravenous fluids. The use of 1% dextrose and water with half-normal saline solution (as an intravenous infusion when urinary outputs are greater than 500 ml/hour) will diminish the osmotic diuresis due to glycosuria.

The Foley catheter can be removed almost any time after the first day. The tip of the catheter should be cultured at that time. Antibiotics may be necessary at this time to sterilize the urinary tract. Moderate hypertension is frequently seen in the early posttransplant period, and a low-sodium diet and low doses of antihypertensive medication (a-methyldopa, hydrochlorothiazide, or hydralazine) are useful to counteract this tendency. Antacids appear to be useful in preventing the appearance of gastrointestinal ulceration of patients on immunosuppressive drugs.

The patient is allowed out of bed and oral fluids are begun on the first postoperative day.

ROUTINE POSTTRANSPLANT LABORATORY DETERMINATIONS. A 2-hour creatinine clearance is determined in the second to fourth postoperative hours and once more in the sixth to eighth postoperative hours. These determinations are extremely useful in interpreting early oliguria. The hematocrit should be followed at 4-hour intervals, since rebleeding is a rare but severe complication frequently associated with oliguria and the onset of acute tubular necrosis (ATN) can occur.

A ^{131}I Hippuran renogram is usually performed soon after transplantation. Intravenous pyelography (IVP) is rarely necessary. Determinations of blood urea nitrogen (BUN), serum creatinine, and creatinine clearance suffice to estimate daily renal function. Serum electrolyte determinations can usually be discontinued after good renal function is established. Daily leukocyte and platelet counts are necessary to assay the state of the bone marrow during immunosuppression. Rarely, hyperglycemia and hypercalcemia are complications, and therefore blood sugar and calcium levels should be determined from time to time.

PROPHYLACTIC IMMUNOSUPPRESSION. The principles of immunosuppression have been described above. Standard immunosuppressive management at most clinical transplant centers consists of azathioprine with or without prednisone or ALG. A number of centers also use prophylactic irradiation of the graft. So many factors are involved in the success or failure of the transplant that the differences in immunosuppression methods used at different centers cannot easily be evaluated. The present regimen used at the University of Minnesota is typical. It is summarized in Table 10-5.

COMPLICATIONS OF RENAL TRANSPLANTATION

RENAL FAILURE. The most serious complication of renal transplantation is the failure of the graft to initiate or maintain function. Although the causes of failure can easily be defined, the differential diagnosis may, at the time, be impossible. The functional failure of the kidney is best examined in relation to the time after transplantation: The kidney may (1) never function, (2) have delayed onset of function, (3) fail to function after a brief or prolonged time, or (4) gradually lose its function over a period of months or years. In each phase, four general diagnoses should be considered: (1) ischemic damage to

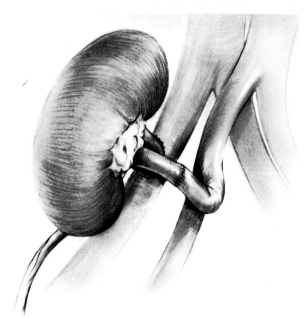

Fig. 10-45. Anastomosis of hypogastric artery to renal artery. (*From R. L. Simmons, C. M. Kjellstrand, and J. S. Najarian, Kidney: II. Technique, Complications, and Results, in J. S. Najarian and R. L. Simmons (eds.), "Transplantation," p. 445, Lea & Febiger, Philadelphia, 1972.*)

the kidney; (2) rejection of the kidney by reactions directed against histocompatibility antigens on the kidney; (3) technical complications; and (4) the development of renal disease, either a new disease or recurrence of the original.

The simplest and best assay for decreased renal function is the frequent determination of BUN and serum creatinine and the determination of creatinine clearance. Occasional renograms or intravenous pyelograms are also useful. The differential diagnosis of renal malfunction, however, may require retrograde pyelography, arteriography, and renal biopsy. On occasion, particularly with the patients with slow deterioration of renal function, the differential diagnosis may be impossible no matter what method of study is used.

Early Anuria and Oliguria

Early anuria or oliguria is a major diagnostic problem. The differential diagnoses must include (1) hypovolemia, (2) thrombosis of the renal artery or renal vein, (3) hyperacute rejection of the kidney, (4) ischemic renal damage (ACN), (5) compression of the kidney (by hematoma, seroma, or lymph), and (6) obstruction of the urinary flow.

Differential Diagnosis of Early Oliguria. The investigation of early posttransplant anuria should be rapidly performed in a strict sequence. The Foley catheter should first be irrigated and/or changed to remove any question of catheter obstruction. Unfortunately, whatever the cause of anuria, a clot can be obtained by bladder irrigation in the first posttransplant day. The clot may not be the primary cause of anuria, however, because blood will clot within the bladder if the urine is not copious enough to wash

Table 10-5. PROPHYLACTIC IMMUNOSUPPRESSION FOR RENAL TRANSPLANTATION AT THE UNIVERSITY OF MINNESOTA

A. Antilymphoblast globulin (ALG)
  1. 30 mg/kg intravenously daily for cadaver organ recipients for 2 weeks.
  2. 20 mg/kg intravenously daily for related organ recipients for 2 weeks.
B. Azathioprine (evening dose after checking leukocyte count)
  1. Preoperative dose is 5 mg/kg/day for 2 days.
  2. First and second postoperative days: 5 mg/kg.
  3. Third through sixth postoperative days: 4 mg/kg.
  4. Seventh postoperative day: 3 mg/kg; maintain at 2 to 3 mg/kg.
  5. Adjust at all times with respect to WBC, platelet count, and renal function.
  6. Caution: Reduce dosage to 1.5 mg/kg for severe renal functional impairment.
C. Prednisone
  1. Related kidney
    a. 0.25 mg/kg every 6 hr beginning 36 hr prior to transplant
    b. First and second postoperative days: 1 mg/kg/day.
    c. Third through sixth postoperative days: 0.75 mg/kg/day.
    d. Seventh through ninth postoperative days: 0.5 mg/kg/day.
    e. Reduce level slowly to achieve a maintenance dose of 0.15 to 0.25 mg/kg/day.
  2. Cadaver kidney
    a. 0.5 mg/kg every 6 hr on first 3 postoperative days (total dose 20 mg/kg).
    b. 1.5 mg/kg/day for the next 3 days.
    c. 1.0 mg/kg/day for 3 days.
    d. 0.75 mg/kg/day for 3 days.
    e. 0.5 mg/kg/day until discharge.
    f. Reduce dose slowly to achieve a maintenance dose of 0.3 to 0.4 mg/kg.
D. Methylprednisone
  1. 20 mg/kg/day intravenously on evening of transplantation and on first 2 postoperative days.

it out prior to coagulation. Therefore, even if a clot is present within the urinary catheter, the urine output should be monitored for the first 10 to 15 minutes after emptying the bladder to determine urine output adequacy.

If the obstructed catheter has not caused the oliguria, one must rule out hemorrhage and hypovolemia combined with compression or displacement of the kidney by the hematoma. Repeated hematocrit determinations in the posttransplant period will usually make such a diagnosis obvious. Concomitantly, there will be an increase in abdominal girth and inability to palpate the kidney in the pelvic fossa. Hypotension and tachycardia may also be present, and the central venous pressure will be low. A roentgenogram of the abdomen will reveal displacement of the intraperitoneal contents by a massive hematoma. The normal degree of ischemic damage to the transplanted kidney plus hypovolemia and compression of the kidney by a hematoma (and perhaps displacement and distortion of the renal vessels by the hematoma) all conspire to impair renal function. If anuria or severe oliguria is present, restoration of the blood volume will seldom suffice to restore renal function, even if furosemide or other diuretics are used. Many patients will require reexploration to control the bleeding point. After exploration, if the period of hypovolemia and renal compression has been

relatively brief and diuretics have been used during ischemia, prompt restoration of renal function usually occurs.

The diagnosis of bleeding is frequently apparent and obviates the need for the next step in the investigation sequence: an [131]I Hippuran renogram (Fig. 10-46*A* and *B*). The renogram will assess the blood flow to the kidney and the ability of the kidney to concentrate and excrete the Hippuran. The results are never diagnostic. If the vascular phase and concentration is near normal, however, the renal arterial and venous anastomoses are patent. Severe depressions of Hippuran uptake by the kidney should be promptly followed by a renal arteriogram. Arteriography should confirm patency of the renal arterial anastomosis and clarify the diagnosis of hyperacute rejection, in which case intravascular thrombosis of the kidney will be seen.

Technical Complications Causing Early Oliguria. Thrombosis of the renal arterial anastomosis is rare. Partial obstruction due to torsion or kinking of the vessels is more common and should be promptly repaired. When the renogram demonstrates poor concentration of the [131]I Hippuran, an arteriogram should be performed to detect correctable technical complications (Fig. 10-47*A* and *B*). Thrombosis of the renal vein occurs even more rarely than thrombosis of the renal artery. When it does occur, thrombosis of the artery ensues because the collateral venous circulation of the kidney has been interrupted by the transplant procedure. Partial thrombosis of the renal and iliac veins has occurred. Usually, this is accompanied by swelling of the ipsilateral lower extremity, fever, and evidence of pulmonary embolism.

Formerly, one of the most common, and most frequently fatal, complications following renal transplantation was urinary extravasation due to distal ureteral necrosis. Rejection was seldom at fault. The problem can generally be avoided by (1) shortening the ureter as much as possible; (2) avoiding tension at the ureteroneocystostomy site; (3) avoiding hematomas within the wound, which put tension on the ureter and also interfere with the developing collateral blood supply to the distal ureter; (4) avoiding transperitoneal "clotheslining" of the ureter by always placing the ureter in the retroperitoneal position where tension will be minimal and the collateral blood supply can develop. Urinary extravasation from ureteroureterostomies and from pyeloureterostomies occurs much more commonly than that from ureteroneocystostomies.

Urinary extravasation is a serious complication that leads to infection and frequently to death. It demands urgent reexploration with reimplantation of the ureter into the bladder, nephrostomy, or performance of a pyeloureterostomy to the host ureter. On occasion, the pelvis of the transplanted kidney may be involved, and nephrectomy may be required. Delay in definitive repair will frequently lead to infection, the development of mycotic aneurysms, loss of the kidney, and death.

Technical errors can become manifest long after the immediate posttransplant period. Arterial stenosis, venous thrombosis, and late ureteral leaks and strictures are frequently confused with rejection (Fig. 10-48). Prior to any antirejection treatment, technical problems should be ruled

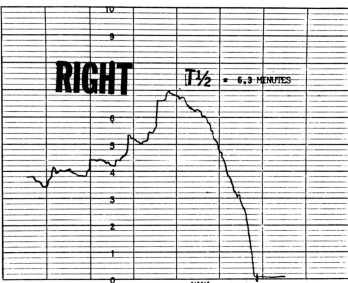

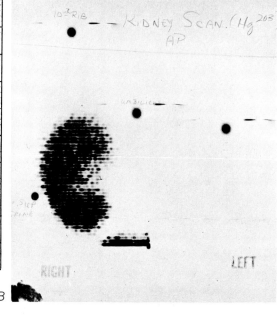

Fig. 10-46. Function of a homotransplanted kidney. *A.* A radiorenogram showing a half-life of 6.3 minutes and a completely normal-appearing curve. *B.* A scan of the same transplant showing excellent uptake in the kidney and the appearance of the radioactive material in the bladder. This transplant continued to have excellent function 5½ years later. (*From D. M. Hume, "Advances in Surgery," vol. II, Year Book Medical Publishers, Inc., Chicago, 1966.*)

out by arteriography, renography, or intravenous or retrograde pyelography.

Hyperacute Rejection. Hyperacute rejection of the kidney is almost surely mediated by humoral antibody, with the subsequent participation of the complement, coagulation, and kinin cascade systems. Platelets, PMNs, and vasospasm may also play a role. Hyperacute rejection occurs most frequently in patients who have demonstrable cytotoxic antibody directed against donor histocompatibility antigens. A lesser number of patients will reject renal allografts in the absence of demonstrable cytotoxic antibody, but a degree of subliminal sensitization that cannot be detected with current techniques may be present. Indeed, detectable cytotoxic antibody will appear and disappear at intervals in patients awaiting transplantation. The classic hyperacute rejection appears in patients who have received multiple transfusions or who have rejected a previous transplant. In these patients, the kidney will fail to regain its normal turgor and healthy pink color after anastomoses are established, despite patent anastomoses. Biopsy and histologic study at this time may reveal leukocytes in the glomerular capillaries, and intravascular renal thrombosis follows (Fig. 10-49). On rare occasions, the intravascular coagulation will be so severe that a consumptive coagulopathy with a bleeding diathesis is produced. Definite evidence of a hyperacute rejection should be treated by immediate nephrectomy. A less acute rejection may occur, however, and renal function may not fail until a day or two following transplantation.

Since the advent and improvement of in vitro cytotoxic cross-match tests, antibodies against donor leukocytes can be detected prior to operation. Although transplantation has been successful in recipients who have preformed antibodies against donor tissue, the likelihood of this success is decreased, and transplantation in the presence of a positive cross-match should not be performed. Patients awaiting cadaver renal transplantation may develop detectable cytotoxic antibodies against certain potential donors, but not against others. Terasaki et al. have shown that the incidence of success of transplants from any donor is reduced when such antibodies are found even if there are no detectable antibodies against the actual donor. Nevertheless, a large number of successful transplants have been carried out into patients with antibodies against antigens not possessed by the donor. Careful cross matching is therefore essential to any transplant program.

Acute Tubular Necrosis. The diagnosis of ischemic renal injury is one of exclusion. If all other causes of renal functional failure in the early posttransplant period have been ruled out, one must assume that the diagnosis is ATN and that the kidney should recover. "Acute tubular necrosis" is a misnomer, because biopsy of nonfunctioning viable kidneys frequently does not reveal necrosis of the tubules but merely hydropic changes within them. The term, in clinical parlance, refers to kidneys whose function is impaired secondarily to ischemic or other nonspecific or unknown causes. ATN, then, occurs most commonly in cadaver transplant recipients when the donor has undergone long periods of stress resulting in hypotension and oliguria. In addition, kidneys that sustain a period of warm ischemia preceding transplantation will fail to function immediately. The term "acute tubular necrosis" implies the expectation that function will return and that necrosis of the tubules is not too extensive. Kidneys with warm ischemic intervals greater than 1 to 2 hours should not be utilized for transplantation, because function will seldom return to normal. Cold ischemia is much better tolerated,

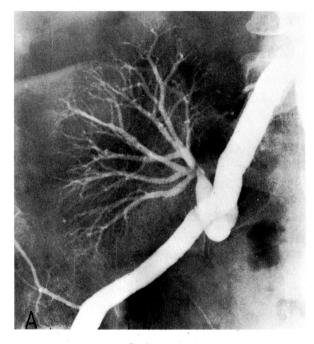
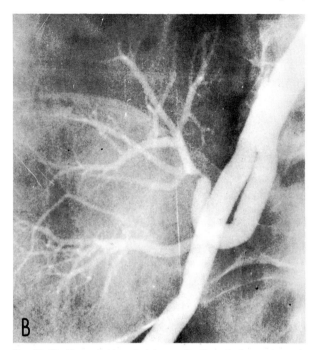

and preservation using hypothermic pulsatile perfusion is now routine.

Almost all transplanted kidneys have undergone some degree of damage secondary to trauma and ischemia. A second trauma (hypovolemia, hypoxemia, renal compression, bacteremia, allergic reactions to ALG) that normally might not result in ATN in normal kidneys may cause oliguria in transplanted kidneys. One must not diagnose rejection and institute massive steroid therapy in the early posttransplant period without ruling out the possibility that an additional insult to an already damaged kidney has occurred and that the diagnosis is not acute rejection but ATN.

The management of the patient with ATN is simple. Urinary flow will resume in almost all cases within 2 or 3 weeks, but anuria for as long as 6 weeks with total recovery has been observed. [131]I Hippuran renograms are useful in following improvement prior to resumption of urinary flow. A number of studies have shown that the long-term function of renal transplants is independent of the presence or absence of oliguria in the early posttransplant period. Dialysis is maintained intermittently during the period of oliguria.

Rejection

Technical errors may not become evident for several weeks postgrafting, and any trauma can aggravate the degree of ATN in a previously damaged kidney. Most renal failure appearing after the first posttransplant week, however, can be attributed to rejection.

As new immunosuppressants have been developed, the acute rejection episodes that formerly appeared in the first month following transplantation are seen less and less frequently. Nevertheless, the majority of patients will sustain at least one acute rejection episode during the first 3 to 4 months following transplantation. Clinical rejection

Fig. 10-47. Correctable arterial complications in the early posttransplant period. Oliguria was present in both patients. [131]I Hippuran revealed poor vascular phase. The arteriograms revealed (*A*) torsion distal to the renal arterial anastomosis, which was corrected by a reanastomosis, and (*B*) a suture that had caught the periadventitial tissues of the superior renal artery, kinking it. The defect was corrected by prompt lysis of the adventitial band. (*From R. L. Simmons, C. M. Kjellstrand, and J. S. Najarian, Kidney: II. Technique, Complications, and Results, in J. S. Najarian and R. L. Simmons (eds.), ''Transplantation,'' p. 445, Lea & Febiger, Philadelphia, 1972.*)

is rarely an all-or-nothing reaction, and the first episode seldom progresses to complete renal destruction. In fact, evidence from renal biopsy data would suggest that rejection is progressing at all times in almost all allograft recipients, regardless of their renal function. The functional changes induced by rejection appear to be in large part reversible; therefore, the recognition and treatment of the rejection episode prior to the development of severe renal damage is of extreme importance. Even with prompt treatment the creatinine clearance may be permanently impaired, however slightly, following each clinical rejection episode.

Differential Diagnosis of Renal Allograft Rejection. Classic renal rejection is characterized by oliguria, enlargement and tenderness of the graft, malaise, fever, leukocytosis, hypertension, weight gain, and peripheral edema. Laboratory studies have shown lymphocyturia, red cell casts, proteinuria, immunoglobulin fragments, fibrin fragments in the urine, complementuria, lysozymuria, decreased urine sodium excretion, renal tubular acidosis, and increased dehydrogenase in the urine. The level of the blood urea nitrogen increases, as does serum creatinine and lactic dehydrogenase, while the serum complement level is unstable. Creatinine clearance is obviously decreased; renograms will show slow uptake of the Hippuran and slow

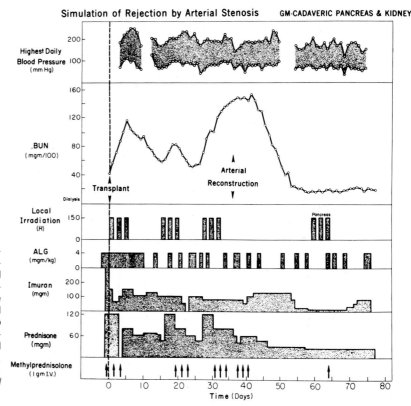

Fig. 10-48. Clinical course of a patient following cadaveric pancreas and kidney transplantation. The first episode of renal functional deterioration appeared to respond to anti-rejection therapy, but the second episode prompted renal arteriography, which revealed stenosis at the site of arterial anastomosis to the side of the iliac artery. Arterial reconstruction resulted in prompt restitution of normal renal function. (*From R. L. Simmons, M. B. Tallent, C. M. Kjellstrand, and J. S. Najarian, Renal Allograft Rejection Simulated by Arterial Stenosis, Surgery, 68:800, 1970.*)

urinary excretion. An intravenous pyelogram may be normal, or it may also show some increased blunting of the calices. The renal cortical blood flow is also decreased during rejection, and an arteriogram may show narrowing of the cortical vessels with irregularity of the distal vessels. The classic renal rejection responds to increased prednisone doses and local irradiation.

Unfortunately, almost all the above findings are also present in patients with several different maladies: obstruction or a leak of the ureter, hemorrhage with consequent ATN, infection, or partial obstruction of either the artery or the vein of the kidney. Biopsies of the kidney can be useful in attaining a true differential diagnosis, but frequently there are signs of rejection within the kidney that are simultaneous with urinary obstruction or infection. There seem to be no findings in typical acute allograft rejection that are specific, and the differential diagnosis depends on the experience and clinical acumen of the physician.

The most important parameter to follow is the serum creatinine level. Unlike the BUN, which is sensitive to a number of changes (steroid administration, fever, and high-protein diet), serum creatinine levels are relatively stable for each patient. The creatinine clearance is more sensitive, but it depends on a carefully timed collection of urine. The most reliable confirmatory test of renal functional deterioration (whatever the cause) is the radiorenogram. When compared with previous renograms, the early signs of rejection are a decreased excretory rate and a slight delay in the vascular phase. These changes are probably related to decreased cortical blood flow and may appear

prior to changes in serum creatinine. More sophisticated modes of evaluating the disturbances in renal blood flow that always occur in transplant rejection have been described, but they have not yet achieved widespread clinical acceptance.

The most reliable clinical signs of renal functional deterioration are a slight decrease in urinary output, slow

Fig. 10-49. Hyperacute rejection. A biopsy of the kidney transplant taken 90 minutes after transplantation. The glomerulus may be seen to be filled with polymorphonuclear leukocytes. These cells fill the small vessels of the cortex and aid in the rapid destruction of the endothelium.

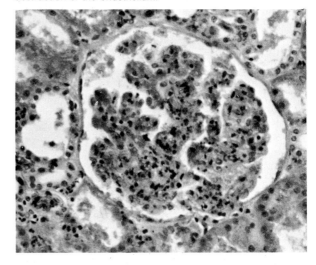

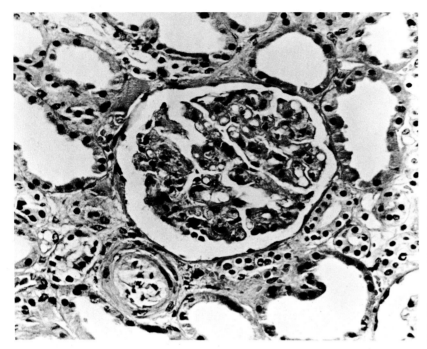

Fig. 10-50. Human allografted kidney 11 months posttransplant. The flattened, atrophic-appearing tubules are the most striking feature. The narrowed arteriole in the lower left quadrant of the picture suggests that the basis for the atrophy may be ischemia. The paucity of infiltrating host immune cells reflects both the patchy nature of the rejection reaction and the indolent pace imposed by relatively effective immunosuppression. (*From J. E. Foker, and J. S. Najarian, Allograft Rejection: III. The Pathobiology of Organ Rejection, in J. S. Najarian and R. L. Simmons (eds.), "Transplantation," p. 122, Lea & Febiger, Philadelphia, 1972.*)

weight gain, small increases in diastolic blood pressure, and edema of the lower extremity on the side of the graft. A peripheral leukocyte count and a serum creatinine level should be determined to confirm renal functional deterioration. A renogram and intravenous pyelogram should be promptly performed and compared with those obtained at the peak of renal function (usually prior to discharge from the hospital). In the face of poor renal function, tomograms during intravenous pyelography may outline a normal ureter. If ureteral obstruction cannot be ruled out, retrograde pyelography can be carried out, although it may be difficult to cannulate the ureteral orifice. Finally, arteri-

ography may reveal (1) characteristic changes of decreased concentration of dye flowing into the kidney, (2) decreased nephrogram effect, or (3) an irregularity of the cortical vasculature and intralobar vasculature characteristic of rejection.

Renal biopsy should be a definitive diagnostic tool. Both open biopsy and needle biopsy techniques have been described, and the histologic changes of rejection are characteristic (Figs. 10-18, 10-19, and 10-49 to 10-52). A normal kidney biopsy is diagnostic, but a biopsy that reveals renal damage may merely reflect acute rejection, a chronic ongoing process, exacerbation of the preexisting renal dis-

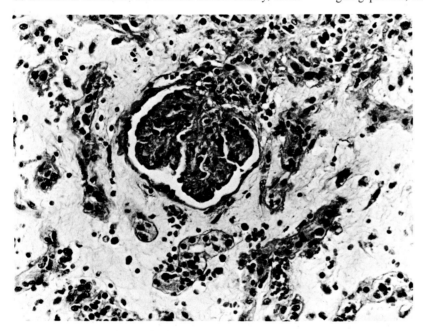

Fig. 10-51. Human renal allograft 27 months posttransplant. The interstitium dominates the morphologic features of this chronically rejected kidney. The area formerly occupied by tubule cells is largely replaced by ill-defined strands. The vacuolated appearance suggests the presence of edema. A modest round cell infiltrate, tubular atrophy, and occluded glomerular loops are also part of chronic rejection. (*From J. E. Foker, and J. S. Najarian, Allograft Rejection: III. The Pathobiology of Organ Rejection, in J. S. Najarian and R. L. Simmons (eds.), "Transplantation," p. 122, Lea & Febiger, Philadelphia, 1972.*)

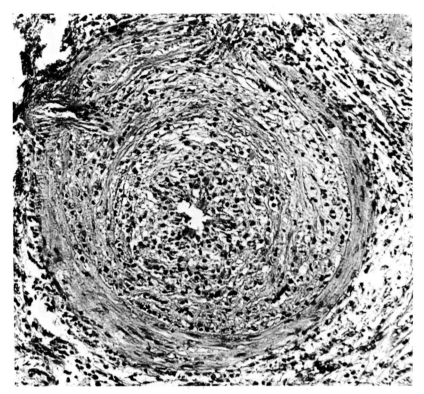

Fig. 10-52. Chronic rejection in a human renal allograft 11 months after transplantation. A small artery shows the result of endothelial cell damage and medial hypertrophy—a pinpoint lumen may be damaged endothelial cells. The bulk of the increase in vessel wall thickness, however, may be due to smooth muscle cell proliferation. The stimulus to cellular division among these cells may result from the immunologic activity on the elastic membranes of the vessel. *(From J. E. Foker and J. S. Najarian, Allograft Rejection: III. The Pathobiology of Organ Rejection, in J. S. Najarian and R. L. Simmons (eds.), "Transplantation" p. 122, Lea & Febiger, Philadelphia, 1972.)*

ease, or damage due to infection or radiation. Therefore, the interpretation of even classic rejection in such kidneys is difficult.

Infection and Rejection. Simmons et al. have recently shown that many apparent allograft rejection episodes are preceded or accompanied by rather mild bacterial or viral infections (Fig. 10-53). In each case, the infection, however mild, preceded the deterioration of the coincidence: (1) It is most likely that the infectious agent acts as a nonspecific adjuvant upsetting the immunologic balance that exists between donor organ and host. Endotoxins, tubercle bacilli, and other microbial agents and products have long been known to act as adjuvants to the immunologic responses. (2) It is also possible that antigens are produced by the infecting agent that cross-reacts with histocompatibility antigens, thus altering the specific unresponsive state. (3) A third possibility is that immune complex nephritis may result from the combination of the infecting agent and the antibodies elicited by the infection. Whatever the case, appearance of mild infection in a renal transplant recipient suggests that renal functional deterioration may follow. Conversely, the appearance of a rejection episode should prompt a search for underlying infection.

Treatment of Rejection. Most institutions have developed a standard rejection regimen for allografted kidneys (Table 10-6). This standard regimen can be repeated as many as three times within a 2-month period in patients for whom rejection appears to be unremitting. If it is repeated more often than that, infection may appear and be lethal. The decision to stop immunosuppression and resume the transplant is frequently subtle and difficult to make, particularly in patients who have deterioration of renal function over a period of months and years.

Williams et al. have classified prognoses into four groups, depending on the number of rejection episodes and the time that they occur. Group I includes those patients who had no rejection episodes and no proteinuria. Such patients had 100 percent long-term function. Group II includes those patients with one acute rejection episode; long-term function was 87 percent. Group III patients had two or more acute rejection episodes, and only 50 percent long-term function. Group IV patients had rejection episodes lasting over 30 days or rejection episodes within the first week or after the fourth month. The long-term function of related transplants in these patients was only 27 percent. Thus, the early onset of rejection episodes, their frequency in the early posttransplant period, or their appearance late following transplantation are relatively grave prognostic signs. In such patients it is relatively easy to make the decision to remove the grafted kidney in the face of recurrent rejection, because the chance of saving the kidney over the long term is poor and their lives may be saved by its removal at an early period.

Renal Failure Due to Recurrent Disease

Renal grafts between identical twins have been performed in man for 20 years. Even though such transplants do not encounter the severe immunologic barriers to success that allografts do, they have not been uniformly successful. Recipients of renal isografts whose original disease was glomerulonephritis frequently develop a lesion in the graft identifiable as glomerulonephritis. An original disease of

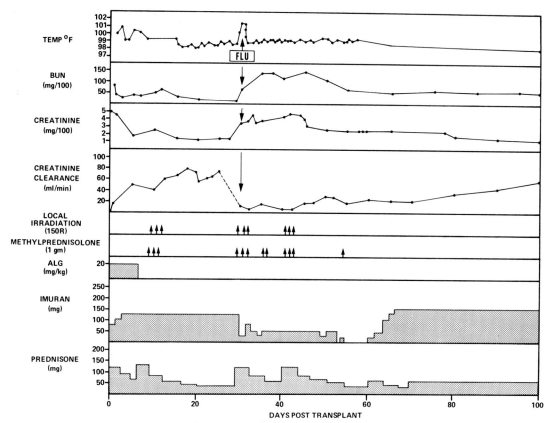

Fig. 10-53. The course of a patient whose "rejection episode" was preceded by an upper respiratory infection in both the patient and his wife. Despite prolonged and vigorous antirejection therapy, renal function returned to normal slowly. (*From R. L. Simmons, R. Weil III, M. B. Tallent, C. M. Kjellstrand, and J. S. Najarian, Do Mild Infections Stimulate Allograft Rejection? Transplant Proc, 2:419, 1970.*)

rapidly progressive glomerulonephritis is associated with the earlier and more frequent appearance of glomerular lesions on the isografts and subsequent progression to chronic renal failure. In contrast, a slowly progressive glomerulonephritis is correlated with lower instances of glomerular lesions in isografts and a greater opportunity for survival. Glomerulonephritis of the isograft rarely appears in recipients whose primary disease was not categorized as glomerulonephritis.

The recurrent disease in the isografts in some respects resembles the late-onset glomerular lesion of the allografted kidney; the nephrotic syndrome may occur in either situation. The glomerulonephritis of isografts is

Table 10-6. STANDARD ANTIREJECTION THERAPY AT THE UNIVERSITY OF MINNESOTA

1. Therapy
   a. Solumedrol: 20 mg/kg/day intravenously ×3.
   b. Prednisone: 2 mg/kg ×3 days; then 1.5 mg/kg ×3 days; then 1.0 mg/kg ×3 days; thereafter reduce prednisone slowly to a maintenance dose.
   c. Azathioprine: Regulate dose to prevent leukopenia; do not increase.
   d. Irradiate kidney transplant: 150 r every other day for 3 doses.
2. Adjuncts
   a. Reinstitute antacid therapy.
   b. Reinstitute oral nystatin (100,000 units twice daily) to prevent mucosal candidiasis.
   c. Reduce protein and fluid intake if renal function is significantly impaired.

associated with basement membrane and mesangial deposition of IgG, complement, and fibrinogen. The presence of preformed antiglomerular basement antibodies as well as immune complexes has been implicated in the pathogenesis of the recurrent disease. The high recurrence rate of glomerulonephritis in isografts and the apparent low rate in allografts is thought to be due to the relative universal use of immunosuppressive therapy in the latter group. Genetic predisposition to glomerulonephritis may also exist among the donor-recipient pairs in the isograft series.

Although experience is limited, prophylactic immunosuppression appears to have merit in the prevention and treatment of recurrent glomerulonephritis in isografts. There seems to be no relation to the time in which the recipient's diseased kidneys are removed and the time of transplantation. It is also not known whether the bilateral nephrectomy hastens the disappearance of antiglomerular antibodies or actually prolongs their circulatory life.

The general strategy is not to delay allotransplantation or isotransplantation after the nephrectomy of patients with proved glomerulonephritis unless the disease is of acute onset or there are high circulating titers of antiglomerular basement membrane (anti-GBM) antibody present. If the disease is of recent onset with rapid progression to failure, nephrectomy is performed and the titer of anti-GBM antibody followed until it falls to negligible quantities. At that time, transplantation should be carried out with immunosuppressive coverage in both isogenic and allogenic recipients. Patients with Goodpasture's disease respond well to this treatment.

Because of the nonspecific changes that can occur as consequences of chronic rejection treatment, there is still active debate about the incidence of recurrent nephritis in renal allotransplants. In patients with complex nephritis, either of unknown cause or secondary to lupus erythematosis, it is possible that precipitation of complexes on the transplanted kidney glomerular basement membrane will reactivate the disease. It is also possible that complexes of antibody will be filtered with streptococci, other bacteria, viruses, or ALG. Alternatively, direct binding of antibody with the GBM may take place, not only as a consequence of preexisting anti-GBM antibodies, but also secondary to GBM binding by ALG or by the development of Masugi nephritis. In general, however, most of the glomerular changes in allotransplants can be considered to be part of the rejection process.

COMPLICATIONS OF IMMUNOSUPPRESSIVE THERAPY. The complications of immunosuppressive therapy in recipients of organ allografts are difficult to distinguish from the complications of recurrent rejection. Patients who do not have rejection episodes generally do not suffer major complications of immunosuppressive therapy. Conversely, the patient who requires repeated large doses of prednisone to avoid further rejection episodes or who suffer diminished renal function in the presence of high doses of azathioprine will have potentially lethal complications. The major complications all relate to a relative inability to respond effectively to a large variety of pathogenic, and even to normally saprophytic, organisms. There may be, moreover, a decrease in the normal capacity to destroy mutant, potentially neoplastic cells.

Infection. Infection is the most common complication of immunosuppression and is the most common cause of death in transplant recipients. The Kidney Registry reports that sepsis was the primary cause of death in 47 percent of the renal allograft recipients who died, whereas rejection in the absence of sepsis accounted for less than 10 percent of the mortality. Most of the deaths early in the history of transplantation occurred in the first few months following transplantation, and the organisms responsible were highly pathogenic bacteria. As antibiotics have improved, there has been a relative increase in lethal infection due to organisms that are normally weakly pathogenic. As antibiotics eradicate the true pathogens, opportunistic organisms colonize the susceptible host. Some of these organisms include the protozoan *Pneumocystis carinii;* cytomegalovirus; the bacterium *Nocardia asteroides;* and the fungi *Candida albicans, Aspergillus fumigatus, Rhizopus oryzae* (mucormycosis), *Histoplasma capsulatum,* and *Cryptococcus neoformans* (Figs. 54 and 55).

Prevention of Infection. The incidence of severe, near-fatal infections can be reduced through a number of precautions: (1) The most important precaution is to eliminate all sources of infection prior to transplantation, especially those in the urinary tract and shunt site. Other sources of infection should be sought by routine preoperative cultures of nasopharynx, throat, sputum, urine, stool, and hemodialysis cannula sites. If any source is found, it should be eliminated by the appropriate use of surgical drainage or antibiotic therapy. (2) Technical problems clearly predispose to sepsis. Urinary extravasation frequently leads to wound infections. Abscesses deep to the transplant are difficult to drain, and mycotic aneurysms may develop at sites of anastomosis or in the iliac vessels. It is frequently necessary to remove the kidney to obtain control of the infection. (3) Recipients of cadaver renal transplants do less well than the recipients of living related donors, despite the use of histocompatibility typing in the selection of cadaver donors. Organs from unrelated donors elicit more frequent and more vigorous rejection reactions. They require such large doses of immunosuppressive drugs that the patient's resistance even to saprophytic organisms is eliminated. Consequently, if repeated rejection can be avoided, there is little danger that life will be lost because of infection. Rejection can be best avoided by using organs donated by living related donors whenever possible. (4) Almost all patients who die of infection develop leukopenia (especially neutropenia) at some time. Some bouts of leukopenia can be attributed to cytomegalovirus infections. Leukopenia can be prevented by careful reduction in azathioprine doses when the leukocyte count or platelet count falls and when renal function is lost for whatever reason. The use of other bone marrow depressants (chloramphenicol) should be scrupulously avoided in patients already on azathioprine therapy. (5) Gowns, masks, and gloves were formerly used to minimize infections in the initial postoperative care. Most transplant units have discontinued their use because they restrict access to the patient, impose psychologic stresses, and are probably ineffective against viral, fungal, or endogenous bacteria.

Malignant Tumors. Malignant tumors have been an unexpectedly frequent concomitant of clinical transplantation, although their frequency does not seem to be high enough to contraindicate the procedure. Tumors have come from two general sources: They have been inadvertently transplanted from cadaver donors in whom the cancer was unsuspected. These tumors can be cured merely by halting the immunosuppression and allowing rejection of both the organ and the tumor tissue.

The second and more common source of malignant tumors is primary tumors appearing in the immunosuppressed recipient. Prior to September 1972, 125 primary tumors had developed in 122 patients following renal transplantation. Seventy-six of the tumors were of epithelial origin (61 percent) and forty-nine (39 percent) were mesenchymal. The most common epithelial lesions were various skin cancers (27 cases, 36 percent), carcinomas of the cervix (11 cases, 14 percent), and carcinomas of the lip (11 cases, 14 percent). The remainder consisted of a wide variety of visceral carcinomas, many of high-grade malignancy.

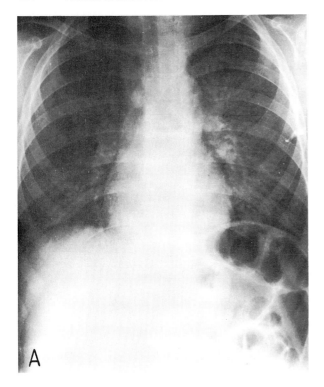

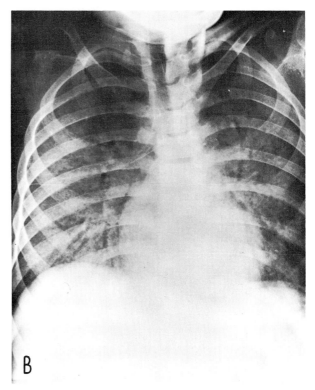

Fig. 10-54. An eight-year-old boy with *Pneumocystis carinii*. *A.* The air bronchogram is apparent even on this early roentgenogram, in which the alveolar infiltrate extends to the periphery of both lungs in characteristic fashion. Open-lung biopsy confirmed the diagnosis. *B.* Despite immediate institution of pentamidine therapy, the disease progressed to become even more characteristic, and the patient died 3 weeks later. (*From R. L. Simmons, C. M. Kjellstrand, and J. S. Najarian, Sepsis following Kidney Transplantation, in J. D. Hardy (ed.), "Critical Surgical Illness," p. 559, W. B. Saunders Company, Philadelphia, 1971.*)

Forty-two (86 percent) of the forty-nine mesenchymal tumors were solid lymphomas, of which the most prominent subgroup was reticulum cell sarcoma (30 cases, 61 percent). A most unusual feature of the lymphomas was their predilection for the central nervous system which occurred in 20 of 41 cases (49 percent).

The cancers occurred at an average age of thirty-six years. The mean time of appearance of the tumors after transplantation was 28 months (range 1 to 92 months). The possibility of transplantation of cancer from the donors was very small, as only 3 of the 137 donors had tumors. The rate of development of malignant disease in patients surviving renal transplantation may be as high as 6 percent, whereas the expected frequency in patients of these ages is 58 per 100,000 (0.058 percent). Superficial malignant lesions of the lip, skin, and cervix were frequently successfully treated by standard surgical techniques without exposing the allografts to risk by arbitrary reduction in immunosuppression. The deeper tumors could not be effectively treated by this approach and led to death in almost all cases. This increased incidence of malignant disease is presumably indicative of the loss of the immunologic surveillance mechanism that normally destroys mutant cells.

Cushing's Disease. Most transplant recipients on steroid therapy undergo a series of changes that are referred to as iatrogenic Cushing's syndrome. The rate of its development is a result of the dose of steroid and number of rejection episodes. The appearance of the face is altered by rounding, puffiness, and plethora: fat tends to be redistributed from the extremities to the trunk and face. There is also an increased growth of fine hair over the thighs and trunk, and sometimes the face. Acne may in-

crease or appear, and insomnia and increased appetite are noted; however, the underlying metabolic changes that accompany the obvious changes can be serious by the time the latter actually appear. The continuing breakdown of protein and diversion of amino acids to glucose increase the need for insulin and results in weight gain, fat deposition, muscle wasting, thinning of the skin with striae and bruising, hyperglycemia, growth suppression (in children), and sometimes the development of steroid diabetes, cataracts, and osteoporosis. In some patients a myopathy develops, the nature of which is unknown.

The cushingoid changes may on rare occasions represent such a psychologic problem that transplant nephrectomy will be necessary on that basis alone. Women are more severely affected physically, and the psychologic problems are greater. These problems can be enormous in children who grow less well and most particularly in small girls on chronic steroid therapy who seem to grow very little after age thirteen. The male psyche tolerates steroids better; the plethora and broad faces give most men a healthy look.

Steroid Diabetes. Steroid diabetes is an occasional complication of chronic steroid administration, even when the steroid doses are not high. This may represent exacerbation of the prediabetic state. The diabetes is frequently mild and may be controlled by oral hypoglycemic agents alone. The onset of diabetes, however, is frequently insidious, and the patient may have diabetic acidosis before the diabetic state is discovered and controlled.

Gastrointestinal Bleeding. Gastrointestinal bleeding due to reactivation of a preexisting ulcer or diffuse ulceration of the gastrointestinal tract is an almost uniformly fatal complication to renal allografts and frequently causes recipient death. The relative contribution of progressive uremia and repeated massive steroid administration in the pathogenesis of gastrointestinal hemorrhage is unknown, but when bleeding appears, it is severe and difficult to control by nonoperative means. Occasionally the intramesenteric arterial infusion of vasopressin and gastric cooling are effective.

During moderate doses of steroid therapy, episodes of gastrointestinal bleeding can be almost totally prevented by the use of antacids between meals. Magaldrate (Riopan) is a useful antacid since it is required in only small doses. In patients with recurrent rejection who require many episodes of high steroid dosage, antacid therapy must be intensified with each increase in steroid administration. Magnesium-containing antacids, however, are contraindicated in patients with poor renal function, since hypermagnesemia will result.

Other Intestinal Complications. Penn and Starzl reported a number of colonic complications, including diverticulitis, bleeding, and ulceration associated with immunosuppressive treatment. A syndrome of acute cecal ulceration with gastrointestinal bleeding has also been reported in transplant patients.

Cataracts. Cataracts are common in patients who have sustained several rejection episodes and high steroid doses. The cataracts, which develop slowly, appear to be independent of the absolute prednisone dosage.

Azathioprine Toxicity. The complications attributable to azathioprine primarily relate to depression of bone marrow function. Signs of hepatic dysfunction occasionally will require the reduction of azathioprine dosage (azathioprine has also been associated with temporary hair loss).

Thrombosis and Thromboembolic Phenomena. Thrombophlebitis may occur in the transplant recipient, particularly on the side of the graft where the venous anastomosis may become partially or completely thrombosed. This has occurred in patients who previously had steroid-resistant nephrotic syndrome and may be related to recurrence of the disease.

When attention is focused on the immunologic and infectious phenomena, thrombophlebitis and pulmonary embolism may be difficult to diagnose. Swelling of the leg on the side of the transplant site is a frequent sign of rejection associated with increases in weight, pulmonary infiltrates, and slight increases in serum creatinine. When the differential diagnosis is difficult, a femoral venogram is indicated. The diagnosis of pulmonary embolisms may also be difficult, and multiple pulmonary infiltrates should not be treated as fungal pneumonia based on sputum cultures alone.

Hypertension. Many of the patients who come to renal

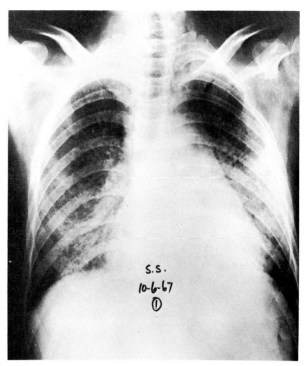

Fig. 10-55. A fourteen-year-old boy received a kidney from his mother 750 days prior to his chest roentgenogram. He had had a course characterized by multiple episodes of infection and rejection. Miliary nodules suddenly appeared in the lung, and the patient died. At autopsy miliary cryptococcosis was found in the lung, thyroid, liver, kidney, pancreas, spleen, lymph nodes, and bone marrow. (*From R. L. Simmons, C. M. Kjellstrand, and J. S. Najarian, Kidney: II. Technique, Complications, and Results, in J. S. Najarian and R. L. Simmons (eds.), "Transplantation," p. 445, Lea & Febiger, Philadelphia, 1972.*)

transplantation are already hypertensive. Hypertension can usually be controlled with dialysis and, if more refractory, with nephrectomy. Hypertension in most patients will develop soon after transplantation, but the posttransplant hypertension is mild and easily controlled with dietary salt restriction and drugs. The hypertension seems to be due not only to prednisone but also to failure to regulate the normal salt and water balance in the early posttransplant period. The transplanted kidney can secrete renin. The antihypertensive drugs can usually be stopped as maintenance levels of prednisone are reached. Hypertension returns with rejection, but significant hypertension may be due to renal arterial stenosis, and arteriography may be necessary for the differentiation.

Disorders of Calcium Metabolism. Patients frequently come to transplantation with renal osteodystrophy. Alterations in vitamin D metabolism and secondary hyperparathyroidism are prominent factors in the pathogenesis of skeletal disease. Long-standing acidosis may likewise be contributory. The resulting osteoporosis, osteomalacia, and osteitis fibrosa cystica in the child can lead to growth restriction, epiphysiolysis, skeletal deformities, and pathologic fracture. The bone disease in some cases can be

arrested with pharmacologic doses of vitamin D or aluminum hydroxide, or by total or subtotal parathyroidectomy.

Hemodialysis can correct the uremic state, but the bone
disease may actually progress if the stimulus to parathyroid
hormone secretion is not effectively eliminated. Great
attention should be directed toward keeping the dialysate
calcium concentration at a level (6 to 7 mg/100 ml) that
does not promote calcium loss from the blood. Again,
parathyroidectomy may be indicated if osteitis fibrosa
cystica is progressive and cannot be reversed by maintaining the calcium concentration in the serum at normal
or slightly elevated levels.

Parathyroidectomy performed in the patient with renal
failure or on hemodialysis may help to arrest progressive
bone disease. Frequently, however, the calcium levels will
remain high and will fall only after renal transplantation.
Conversely, if prompt transplantation from a related donor
is planned or if the cadaver list is short, transplantation
by itself will usually lead to the reversal of the hyperparathyroid state. The hypercalcemia of the immediate
posttransplant period can be managed with a high-
phosphate diet, low calcium intake, and furosemide diuretics. Even patients with flagrant osteitis fibrosa cystica
with metastatic calcification will respond to transplantation
alone without parathyroidectomy. Parathyroidectomy
seems primarily indicated for patients on chronic hemodialysis in whom transplantation is not planned.

Careful studies of calcium and phosphorus metabolism
after renal allotransplantation have been carried out by
Alfrey et al. They found that hypercalcemia, hypophosphatemia, and increased renal phosphate clearance were present in over 50 percent of their patients, suggesting the
diagnosis of hyperparathyroidism. Alfrey et al. however,
suggest that hypophosphatemia is an effect of steroid therapy and that the hypercalcemia is an effect of depletion
of body phosphate stores secondary not only to the effect
of steroids on phosphate stores but to the intense antacid
therapy with aluminum hydroxide. Posttransplant tertiary
hyperparathyroidism may then be an artifact that can be
reversed by the administration of phosphate-containing
antacids. In fact, posttransplant hypercalcemia is not associated with elevated parathyroid hormone levels, and
parathyroidectomy will rarely be indicated after successful
transplantation.

Musculoskeletal Complications. The most disturbing
complication of successful renal transplantation is avascular necrosis of the femoral heads and other bones. Its
occurrence is most closely correlated with the dosage of
steroid used. Transient rheumatoid symptoms precede
changes visible by radiography by several months. The
bone changes apparently occur secondarily to steroid os-
teopenia or osteonecrosis with resulting microfractures.
Alterations in lipid metabolism caused by fluctuating high
levels of steroids likewise appear to be important in explaining the pathogenesis. The treatment is for the most
part symptomatic. It is doubtful that bone lesions can
revascularize sufficiently to restore normal architecture in
the presence of maintenance steroids. Should symptoms
increase in the hip and bone destruction progress, replacement arthroplasty may be indicated.

Migratory arthralgia, myalgia, and tendonitis are common in our experience. It has been suggested that anti-
allotype antibodies may be a factor in joint and soft tissue
changes. Again, the treatment is symptomatic.

Occasionally the development of synovitis may occur
secondarily to the presence of fungal infections in the joint.
Associated skin lesions resembling erythema nodosum
should alert one to this possibility. Bacterial infection may
occur in joints as well as in the bursae; they must be
promptly recognized and surgically drained.

Serum sickness with arthralgias and arthritis can be seen
after ALG therapy and are usually controlled with antihistamines and steroids.

Pancreatitis. Pancreatitis may appear suddenly and unexpectedly in renal allograft recipients; it may occasionally
be fatal. Its cause is obscure, and it has been attributed
variously to corticosteroid therapy, cytomegalovirus, or
hepatitis virus. The clinical course is sometimes accompanied by increases in serum creatinine, which may or may
not be related to rejection. Most cases subside with conventional therapy and do not recur.

Erythremia and Anemia. The transplanted kidney is apparently fully capable of manufacturing and secreting
erythropoietin. During rejection, the serum level may be
increased. Erythremia also may appear, but apparently it
is not related to elevated erythropoietin levels.

Anemia usually is not present except in association with
uremia or immunodepression secondary to azathioprine
toxicity. A microangiopathic hemolytic anemia has also
been thought to be induced by the vascular changes within
the chronically rejecting organ.

RESULTS OF RENAL TRANSPLANTATION

TRANSPLANT REGISTRY RESULTS. The results presented here are those of the "Eleventh Report (1973) of
the ACS/NIH Human Renal Transplant Registry" (Figs.
10-56 to 10-58 and Table 10-7) All the data reported to
the registry are analyzed collectively. Although large numbers allow precise analysis, the reported results are neither
as good as those of the most experienced centers nor as
poor as those centers with the worst record. The report,
therefore, should be thought of as an average of performance achieved by groups reporting to the registry.

The data for calculations in this report were derived
from 12,389 transplants reported to the registry. These
include 7,476 transplants performed in the United States
and 4,913 reported from centers in Europe, Australia, and
Canada.

Cadaver donors are used more frequently, whereas parent and siblings are used as donors at approximately the
same rate as previously. Volunteer unrelated donors are
no longer being used.

It is clear from the data, pooled from first transplants
performed around the world, that the kidneys from living
related donors survive much better than do those from
cadaver donors. This has been a fairly consistent finding
throughout all the years of renal transplantation. It is also
clear that the improvements in results seen in the early
days following transplantation have now leveled off and
that the results of transplantation are not much better than

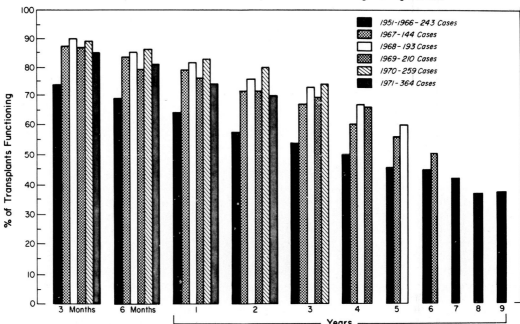

Fig. 10-56. (*From the "Eleventh Human Renal Transplant Registry Report," JAMA,* December 3, 1973.)

they were in 1968. The results of cadaver transplantation have improved slightly.

Table 10-8 (from an earlier registry report) also compares the results of transplantation from cadaver transplants performed since 1968 with those performed from

Fig. 10-57. (*From the "Eleventh Human Renal Transplant Registry Report," JAMA,* December 3, 1973.)

less closely related donors, including aunts, uncles, and cousins. The results from other related donors are certainly better than the results from unrelated donors but are less satisfactory than kidneys from siblings or parents. Some large centers have found, however, that aunts, uncles, cousins, and children are as satisfactory as siblings and parents.

Table 10-9 reports the results of renal transplantation according to the primary renal disease of the recipient. The

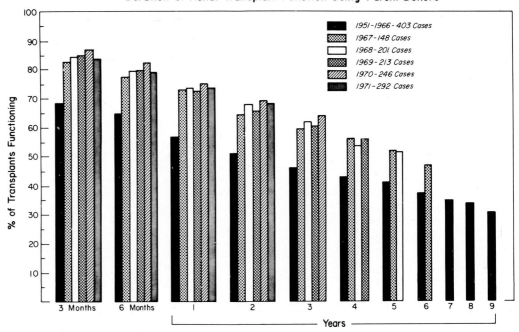

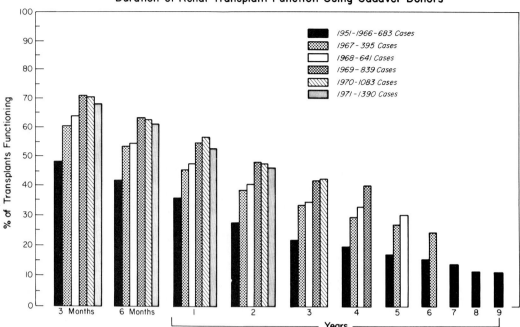

Fig. 10-58. (*From the "Eleventh Human Renal Transplant Registry Report," JAMA, December 3, 1973.*)

registry data suffers from an overwhelming preponderance of patients with a diagnosis of glomerulonephritis. This diagnosis is frequently based on the absence of evidence of infection in an end-stage kidney, the pathogenesis of which is indefinable. The diagnosis of glomerulonephritis does not, therefore, necessarily imply a specific disease.

The table reveals, however, that there are no great differences in survival or function among the different primary renal diseases. However, there are several exceptions to this rule; i.e., patients with familiar nephritis, who are

Table 10-7. CALCULATED PATIENT SURVIVAL AND TRANSPLANT FUNCTION, FIRST TRANSPLANT ONLY, BY DONOR SOURCE AND YEAR OF TRANSPLANT

Donor Source	Year of transplant	Sample size	1 year, %		2 years, %		3 years, %		4 years, %		5 years, %	
			Alive	Function	Alive	Function	Alive	Function	Alive	Function	Alive	Function
Sibling	1951–1966	243	68.5	64.1	62.2	57.3	58.5	53.1	56.1	49.3	54.1	46.2
	1967	144	84.6	78.4	77.7	71.3	72.9	66.2	66.3	59.5	63.0	55.6
	1968	193	89.0	81.3	83.8	75.5	81.4	72.3	77.6	66.2	71.4	59.4
	1969	210	82.5	76.2	78.2	71.3	76.9	68.4	73.7	65.6		
	1970	259	87.1	82.5	85.0	79.1	82.5	73.3				
	1971	364	85.8	73.8	81.7	69.6						
	1972	202	87.4	74.0								
Parent	1951–1966	403	61.2	56.4	56.6	50.2	52.9	45.4	51.0	42.7	50.4	40.7
	1967	148	74.9	72.2	69.1	63.9	64.6	58.4	63.0	55.5	60.8	51.7
	1968	201	79.2	72.5	75.2	67.3	71.0	61.0	66.5	52.8	66.5	51.4
	1969	213	80.8	71.7	75.3	65.0	70.6	59.3	67.4	55.3		
	1970	246	84.9	74.2	80.5	68.6	79.2	63.2				
	1971	292	86.6	72.9	82.4	67.7						
	1972	155	91.7	76.4								
Cadaver	1951–1966	683	42.0	35.6	34.0	27.8	28.7	22.3	25.9	19.5	23.2	16.3
	1967	395	56.0	45.3	49.1	38.7	44.7	33.9	40.3	29.1	39.3	26.6
	1968	641	58.3	47.5	51.3	40.3	46.1	34.9	44.1	32.2	42.6	29.4
	1969	839	66.2	54.9	59.9	47.7	55.2	42.0	53.6	39.7		
	1970	1,083	70.2	56.1	64.1	47.2	60.6	42.3				
	1971	1,390	69.6	52.8	64.7	46.6						
	1972	669	71.8	45.4								

Table 10-8. CALCULATED PATIENT SURVIVAL AND TRANSPLANT FUNCTION
BY DONOR SOURCE AND DATE OF TRANSPLANT

Donor type	Year of transplant	Sample size	1 year, %		2 years, %	
			Living	Function	Living	Function
Cadaver	1953–1966	640	42.6	36.0	35.2	28.6
	1967	344	56.8	45.3	49.5	38.3
	1968	534	57.2	45.0	49.5	36.9
	1969	644	66.7	54.0	60.6	46.6
	1970	408	70.2	52.5		
Aunts, uncles, cousins, grandparents	1953–1966	20	63.1	60.0	63.1	60.0
	1967	15	63.4	53.3	63.4	53.3
	1968	10	88.8	88.8	88.8	88.8
	1969	11	79.1	54.5	79.1	54.5
	1970	1				

SOURCE: Data taken from the "Ninth Report of the ACS/NIH Human Renal Transplant Registry."

usually children or adolescents, appear to have better survival. Far poorer survival rates are seen in patients with malignant hypertension and cancer of the kidney.

Table 10-10 reports results of all renal transplantations since 1955 grouped by recipient ages. The 2-year functional survival appears to depend largely on the age of the recipient. Although transplantation in children less than five years old does not appear to be highly successful, in the age range from six to forty years there is only a slight decline with increasing age. After age forty there is a sharp drop in survival in recipients of sibling transplantation, and after the age of fifty there is a sharp drop in the survival of recipients of cadaver transplants. The question may be raised whether older recipients should receive the kidneys of older donors. Registry data, however, can show no difference in functional renal survival in kidneys transplanted from cadavers of age eleven to twenty or cadavers of age forty to sixty.

TRANSPLANTATION IN CHILDREN. Renal failure in children is a common cause of death. Traditionally, young children have not been considered ideal candidates for renal transplantation, although excellent results have been reported by a number of investigators. The small caliber of vessels and active social behavior of children make their management on hemodialysis extremely difficult. Long-term immunosuppressive therapy is also thought to interfere with normal growth with resultant social problems. Long-term hemodialysis is seldom satisfactory, and a parent is almost always willing to donate a kidney. The Human Renal Transplant Registry statistics (Table 10-10) reveal that patients above the age of five do extremely well posttransplant, confirming the impression of several large pediatric transplant groups. Several infants have had transplants, and at least one has survived for more than 1 year. The growth of children following transplantation has been the subject of several studies. Most children with allografts grow slightly slower than normal. The adolescent growth spurt is absent in children with transplants and adolescent growth is particularly depressed in girls.

This early cessation of growth causes the typical appearance of girls with transplants who are short and more

Table 10-9. EFFECT OF PRIMARY RENAL DISEASE ON RESULTS OF
RENAL TRANSPLANTATION: CADAVER DONOR ONLY

Disease	Sample size	1 year, %		2 years, %	
		Living	Function	Living	Function
Glomerulonephritis	1,447	56.7	45.0	48.6	36.8
Pyelonephritis	404	57.6	45.4	52.2	39.0
Polycystic kidneys	166	63.2	52.6	54.2	44.1
Malignant hypertension	82	42.7	36.6	40.1	34.3
Familial nephritis	32	71.0	60.4	59.6	50.7
Congenital nonobstructive	30	54.4	46.6	54.4	46.6
Cancer of kidney	9	50.4	44.4	37.8	33.3
Lupus nephritis	5	57.1	40.0	57.1	40.0
Diabetic glomerulosclerosis	3	66.6	66.6	22.2	

SOURCE: Data from the "Ninth Report of the ACS/NIH Human Renal Transplant Registry."

Table 10-10. RESULTS OF RENAL TRANSPLANTATION BY
DONOR SOURCES AND RECIPIENT AGES

Donor type	Recipient age group	Sample size	1 year, %		2 years, %	
			Living	Function	Living	Function
Sibling	6–10	1	100.0	100.0	100.0	100.0
	11–20	68	87.4	84.6	83.3	76.7
	21–30	267	83.3	77.1	77.0	70.2
	31–40	285	82.1	75.5	78.6	70.9
	41–50	132	75.8	66.7	65.1	56.3
	51–60	16	65.0	65.0	53.1	53.1
Parent	0–5	6	30.0	30.0	30.0	30.0
	6–10	51	78.3	69.5	75.3	66.9
	11–20	415	73.6	67.1	67.8	58.9
	21–30	326	70.8	65.3	66.9	59.8
	31–40	105	59.9	54.8	58.5	53.6
	41–50	10	75.0	58.2	75.0	58.2
	51–60	1				
Cadaver	0–5	30	51.3	40.0	44.5	25.8
	6–10	40	52.7	42.5	45.2	36.3
	11–20	316	65.0	48.8	58.2	40.9
	21–30	659	60.6	47.7	53.8	40.5
	31–40	725	58.1	47.3	49.7	38.9
	41–50	576	51.8	43.1	45.0	36.3
	51–60	147	48.6	39.8	36.5	27.7
	61–99	7	18.1	18.1	18.1	18.1

SOURCE: Data from the "Ninth Report of the ACS/NIH Human Renal Transplant Registry."

cushingoid than the boys. Attempts to correlate the amount of first-year posttransplant growth with the kidney donor, renal function, or prednisone dosage have been unsuccessful. No such correlations can be made, even though it is generally felt that prednisone interferes with growth.

Sexual maturation in boys appears to be normal, although the period of observation has been short. Similarly, some girls have failed to menstruate at the usual age despite relatively normal renal function and only moderate doses of prednisone. Most girls have resumed menstruating if previously mature, or they undergo a normal menarche upon reaching age thirteen or fourteen.

MULTIPLE TRANSPLANTS. A number of studies have shown that second and third transplants are less successful than the first (Table 10-11). The rejection of one transplant will apparently sensitize the patient to a number of histocompatibility antigens that are shared by other potential donors within the population. The development of crossmatching techniques has increased the chances of finding a second donor to whom the recipient is not sensitized.

Table 10-12 summarizes the results of second transplants in patients who rejected the first transplant. Here it is clear that recipients of kidneys from related donors, after having lost the first such kidney, have a much better chance of maintaining function for 2 years in the second kidney than do patients who receive a cadaver kidney after rejecting one from a related donor. Similarly, patients who receive a transplant from a related donor after rejecting a cadaver transplant have a much better chance of success than those who receive a cadaver transplant after rejecting a first

cadaver transplant. There is no difference, however, between recipients of cadaver transplants, whether or not a cadaver transplant or one from a related donor was rejected the first time. Patients who lost the first kidney for technical reasons also seem to tolerate a second graft better than patients who rejected their first kidney graft.

REHABILITATION. The results of a survey performed at the University of Minnesota in December of 1970 are shown in Table 10-13. This survey included only patients surviving transplantation. Almost all the children had returned to their previous activities and were in school. By 1 year posttransplant, 90 percent of the adults were performing most of their customary activities. These figures support the generally held opinion that transplantation restores most patients with renal failure to good health.

Some problems do remain in the posttransplant patients, but uremic neuropathy, pericarditis, anemia, and malaise are relieved; however, cataracts, weakness, and musculoskeletal disorders are common. The sexual and reproductive functions of both males and females return to normal as soon as steroid doses are reduced to maintenance levels. Congenital defects in the offspring of patients on potentially teratogenic drugs have not proved to be a problem.

XENOGRAFTS

Xenografts between related species are rejected by the same immune mechanisms as are allografts. Xenografts

Table 10-11. RESULTS OF RENAL TRANSPLANTATION: COMPARISON
OF RESULTS OF MULTIPLE TRANSPLANTS

Transplant no.	Year of transplant	Sample size	1 year, %		2 years, %	
			Living	Function	Living	Function
1	1953–1966	1,488	52.8	47.1	46.8	40.7
	1967	656	68.0	58.6	61.8	51.5
	1968	906	68.7	58.1	63.0	51.5
	1969	1010	71.6	60.3	66.4	53.6
	1970	567	75.9	59.3		
2	1953–1966	113	37.4	32.3	28.7	24.0
	1967	55	63.9	43.6	55.6	34.5
	1968	96	53.6	40.7	47.2	33.7
	1969	100	59.2	43.7	49.8	34.7
	1970	52	64.3	50.3		
3	1953–1966	6	33.3	33.3	33.3	33.3
	1967	7	24.7	14.2	24.7	14.2
	1968	9	39.2	22.2	39.2	22.2
	1969	12	50.1	28.3	50.1	28.3
	1970	5	80.0	20.0		

SOURCE: Data from the "Ninth Report of the ACS/NIH Human Renal Transplant Registry."

between distant species are rejected by an additional mechanism—the reaction of the xenograft with preformed antibodies which then trigger the efficient complement and clotting cascades. In short, xenografts across distant species barriers are rejected like hyperacute rejections.

There is not much information about clinical xenografts, because, in general, they have not proved to be useful. Xenografts of calf skin have sometimes been used for burn dressings and appear to offer some advantage over other dressing material, although they are not as useful as allografts. Some xenograft calf heart valves have been placed in patients, although it seems likely that these will not be as successful as are allografts, and they might be expected to calcify and become incompetent over a period of years. One xenograft chimpanzee heart has been placed in a patient, but this functioned for only about an hour. Since allografted hearts are invariably rejected experimentally, it would be expected that cardiac xenotransplants would

suffer the same fate even more quickly. Renal xenografts using both chimpanzee and baboon donors have been done in a number of human beings, but this procedure has been abandoned. Surprisingly enough a few relatively long-term survivors were achieved with chimpanzee transplants which were considerably better tolerated than baboon transplants. Some testicular xenografts have been carried out in man in the past but have long since been abandoned. Bone and cartilage xenografts are still used from time to time but seem to offer no advantage over allografts.

The use of organs from nonhuman species for extracorporeal perfusion, both kidneys and livers, has been tried. Extracorporeal kidney xenograft perfusion has been done only occasionally and is probably not of great value. Extracorporeal allograft kidney perfusion may be of value in detecting cytotoxic antibodies in the recipient and to determine whether a particular transplant might be toler-

Table 10-12. RESULTS OF RENAL TRANSPLANTATION: RESULTS IN SECOND
GRAFTING FOLLOWING FAILURE OF A FIRST GRAFT

Donor relationship	Sample size	1 year, %		2 years, %	
		Living	Function	Living	Function
Transplant 1: related Transplant 2: related	23	90.3	81.4	84.1	70.5
Transplant 1: related Transplant 2: cadaver	87	51.3	37.3	43.1	28.7
Transplant 1: cadaver Transplant 2: related	30	70.0	62.9	65.6	58.9
Transplant 1: cadaver Transplant 2: cadaver	234	46.7	35.1	37.2	25.9

SOURCE: Data from the "Ninth Report of the ACS/NIH Human Renal Transplant Registry."

Table 10-13. REHABILITATION AFTER RENAL TRANSPLANTATION
AT THE UNIVERSITY OF MINNESOTA

Adults

Condition of patient	Time posttransplant, months			
	0–3	*3–6*	*6–12*	*12+*
Well and doing most things I did before illness	4 = 50%	4 = 50%	19 = 76%	39 = 78%
Well but not performing many customary activities . .	4 = 50%	2 = 25%	5 = 20%	6 = 12%
Up most of the day but quite restricted in activity . .	0	2 = 25%	1 = 4%	4 = 8%
Confined to a wheelchair or to bed	0	0	0	1 = 2%
	n = 8	*n* = 8	*n* = 25	*n* = 50

Children

Condition of patient				
Well and doing most things I did before illness	0	3 = 100%	4 = 80%	17 = 94%
Well but not performing many customary activities . .	0	0	1 = 20%	1 = 5%
Up most of the day but quite restricted in activity . .	0	0	0	0
Confined to a wheelchair or to bed	0	0	0	0
	n = 0	*n* = 3	*n* = 5	*n* = 18

ated if it were placed in the patient. This has been done on several occasions. The extracorporeal allografted kidney is capable of function, although it is difficult to keep the function going indefinitely because of the many technical problems encountered. Experiments are under way to determine whether human kidneys can be stored for periods of time in nonhuman primate hosts. Although this is an appealing possibility, it seems unlikely that it will succeed, since the nonhuman primate has been shown to be capable of rejecting the human kidney promptly. It may be possible, however, to obtain relatively long-term storage by giving the recipient a supralethal dose of total-body irradiation, which might permit him to keep the kidney for 2 or 3 days.

ORGAN PRESERVATION

The viable preservation of whole organs is one of the essential components of any transplantation program. Only cadaver donors can be used for some organs (heart and liver), and even when the organ is expendable (as in one of a pair of kidneys), the use of cadaver donors avoids the risks inherent in surgical removal of the organ from living persons. If tissue typing and matching ever achieves its true potential, it will be necessary to store the organ until these matching procedures can be carried out. Even more time-consuming procedures, such as tolerance induction, may soon be available to pretreat the recipient and make him unresponsive to specific histocompatibility antigens.

Sell listed those procedures which might be useful to carry out during organ preservation (Table 10-14).

Methods of Viable Organ Preservation

The main problem associated with organ preservation seems to be hypoxia. When the organ is removed from its physiologic state, it is deprived of its normal oxygenation. The two major approaches to organ preservation have been what might be called metabolic inhibition and metabolic maintenance.

Metabolic inhibition seeks to prevent the normal catabolic processes from causing severe or irreversible damage to the tissues during the period of preservation. It is currently best achieved by hypothermia, which protects the organ by slowing metabolic activity and decreasing oxygen need. Two techniques of cooling are currently available: (1) simple cooling of a kidney by immersing it in, or flushing it with, a cold solution, which allows many hours of preservation and is almost always used for shorter periods of time (1 hour) prior to transplantation of any organ, and (2) perfusion cooling, which allows longer periods of preservation.

Metabolic maintenance, the second approach to organ

Table 10-14. PROCEDURES DURING
ORGAN STORAGE

A. Evaluation of the organ
  1. Typing and matching
    a. ABO typing
    b. Lymphocyte typing
    c. Organ cell typing
    d. Mixed lymphocyte culture with the recipient
  2. Diagnosis of disease in the donor
    a. Malignant tumors
    b. Infections
    c. Degenerative conditions
  3. Determination of functional state
  4. Restoration of normal function
B. Preparation of the recipient
  1. Induction of tolerance
  2. Immunosuppression
  3. Surgical procedures
C. Logistical procedures
  1. Stockpile various sizes and types
  2. Transport to a distant recipient

preservation, attempts to sustain a level of metabolic activity as close to physiologic normalcy as is feasible. Usually it implies perfusion of the organ in vitro with a carefully controlled fluid medium, although tissue oxygenation may be attempted. In practice metabolic maintenance is always best combined with perfusion cooling. The best system, at present, utilizes a pulsatile pump and pooled homologous plasma passed through a membrane oxygenator (Figs. 10-59 and 10-60). Excellent transplantation results are obtained after perfusion as long as 72 hours. These moderately long preservation periods provide adequate time for accurate matching of donors and recipients.

Not all organs can be perfused equally well by the same approach. Certain precautions are necessary. It is necessary *to maintain optimal organ function* up to and beyond the moment of clinical death. For kidneys, adequate hydration and maintenance of systemic blood pressure are recommended. Manipulation of the organ also contributes to vasospasm, and so surgical dissection should be as rapid and efficient as possible. The *period of time* between the cessation of blood flow through the organ and the establishment of the organ in its new environment (warm ischemia time) is critical in preservation studies. *Temperature* is also important. Successful perfusion systems have incorporated hypothermia to reduce the need for oxygen and metabolic nutrients. *Oxygenation* is also critical. Oxygen dissolves in aqueous solution more readily at lower temperatures; a membrane oxygenator is incorporated into the system.

The *flow rate* necessary at 37°C can be substantially reduced when metabolic activity is lessened by hypothermia; flow rates of one-fifth to one-third of normal have been satisfactory. The *viscosity of the perfusion fluid* may have some influence on perfusion pressure and flow rate. The perfusion pressure is significant. If the flow rate is adequate to provide the nutrients and waste removal, then the absolute level of pressure is not critical, but excessive perfusion pressure invariably causes transudation of the perfusate, tissue edema, and, ultimately, obstruction to the flow. Another factor is *pulsation*. Perfusion results in less damage when the flow is pulsatile, particularly at normothermic temperatures. The necessity for pulsatile flow during hypothermic perfusion is less well documented. It is probably not necessary to maintain any *venous pressure gradient*. The *perfusate composition* has apparent significance. Whole plasma probably is the most physiologic perfusate and contains most of the nutrient ingredients, including fatty acids, which might be required for the metabolic activity of organs. Many other formulations have been tried, including dextran, albumin, other plasma expenders, tissue culture media, and balanced salt solutions. *Osmolarity* is important. Crystalloids are poor perfusates and lead to edema. The perfusate must be maintained at "normal" *pH* range of 7.35 to 7.45. CO_2 buffering may be necessary with the addition of 2.5 to 5 percent of this gas to the oxygenator. Extremes of alkalosis and acidosis can be prevented with the addition of HCl or $NaHCO_3$ as necessary. A number of *additives* to the perfusate have been tried. This includes membrane stabilizers, vasodilators, and anticoagulant. *Hyperbaric oxygenation*

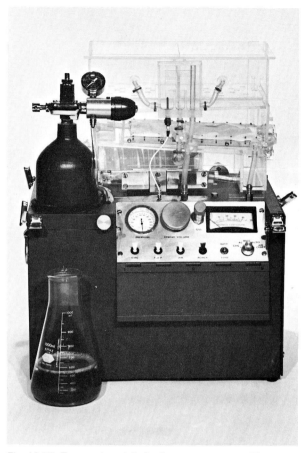

Fig. 10-59. Transport module for the organ cassette. The transport module measures 43 × 33 × 54 cm and weighs 30 kg. It operates on standard alternating current or independent battery power. The organ cassette is easily transferred to the hospital console after disengagement of pump, temperature, air, and heat-exchanger connections. (*From A. W. Moberg, E. A. Santiago, R. V. Mason, M. F. Mozes, R. A. Campos, and J. S. Najarian, Transportable Organ-Perfusion System for Kidney Preservation, Lancet, 2:1403, 1971.*)

has also been used to prolong the viability and storage time of organs in conjunction with hypothermia or a combination of hypothermia and perfusion. Hyperbaric oxygenations will probably play no significant role in organ preservation, or at least its effects may not prove to be additive to those of hypothermia and perfusion.

There is evidence that an adequate flow rate during perfusion is a good prognostic sign of the viability and transplantability of the organ. The most significant indication of inadequate flow rate is the swelling caused by fluid retention. This edema is usually the result of anoxia with subsequent lysosomal and cellular damage. However, poor perfusion itself can produce anoxia, so that a vicious cycle of edema-anoxia-edema can be started. Other possible causes of interstitial edema are perfusate osmolarity and excessive perfusion pressure. Even hypothermia alone may cause cellular swelling. Another important factor in the obstruction of flow is simple blockage of the microvasculature. The many causes of this blockage have been de-

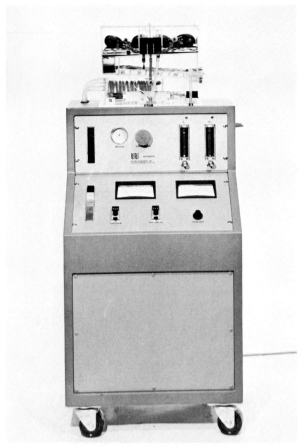

Fig. 10-60. Refrigeration console and organ cassette for the hypothermic pulsatile perfusion of kidneys during 24 to 72 hours of preservation. The organs rest within the organ cassette. The console provides the cassette with a pulsatile pump, a gas source for air, CO_2, O_2, and Freon refrigeration with constant temperature regulation. The simplified control panel is easy to operate; minimal supervision is required. Renal artery pressure and plasma flow is controlled by the stroke volume and pulse rate; pH is maintained by appropriate CO_2 and O_2 gas flows. (*From A. W. Moberg, E. A. Santiago, R. V. Mason, M. F. Mozes, R. A. Campos, and J. S. Najarian, Transportable Organ-Perfusion System for Kidney Preservation, Lancet, 2:1403, 1971.*)

scribed in detail and include bubbles in the perfusion system, fibrin, red cell agglutination, the adherence of platelets and leukocytes to endothelial cells, cell breakdown due to mechanically imperfect pumps, crystal formation, and even agglutination of bacteria. Some of this blockage can be prevented with adequate filtration, but even blood-derived perfusion media like whole plasma have been shown to contain aggregates that appear during hypothermic perfusion. This aggregated material has been identified as lipoprotein. Fortunately, these substances can be removed from plasma quite easily by freezing, which causes flocculation of the lipoprotein, and by subsequent filtration and/or ultracentrifugation to remove the aggregates.

One of the major problems in organ preservation research is the lack of methods to assay the functional state of organs in vitro and the consequent inability to measure the effectiveness of innovations in organ preservation techniques. Ultimately, of course, each preservation method must be tested by reimplantation of the organ. However, this is an all-or-none test requiring a large number of transplants in order to get statistically valid data. What is needed is an in vitro assay technique that can predict the transplantability of an organ and provide quantitative assessment of viability as the organ is subjected to the various preservation protocols. For practical purposes, such an assay should be utilized both before preservation (to determine whether postmortem changes have rendered the organ unfit for preservation) and immediately before transplantation (to determine whether the preservation efforts have been effective). As mentioned, the currently most popular technique involves the measurement of perfusate flow to the preserved kidney. However, studies of enzymes released from the graft appear promising.

Various pharmacologic agents have also been used as metabolic inhibitors. These include such drugs as magnesium sulfate, chlorpromazine, chloroquine, hydrocortisone, and diuretics such as mersalyl. Unfortunately, experiments utilizing such agents in addition to hypothermia show little additive effect. Most recently, however, allopurinal has been shown to protect against some of the anoxic damage to organs.

ORGAN FREEZING

Since hypothermic storage is the mainstay of most preservation systems, it would seem logical to extend hypothermia to subfreezing temperatures in order to produce total inhibition of metabolic activity. It has long been possible to successfully store individual tissue cells bathed in cryoprotective agents and frozen at controlled rates. Most recently Dietzman achieved kidney function in dogs after freezing the kidneys to $-20°C$. He found that several precautions were necessary. These included (1) a gentle surgical technique yielding kidneys that were producing large quantities of urine immediately prior to nephrectomy; (2) the use of plasma free of hemoglobin to wash the blood from the kidney; (3) the correct choice of cryoprotective agents such as dimethylsulfoxide or glycerin to protect the tissues from the damaging effect of freezing; (4) the addition of drugs capable of stabilizing membranes (methylprednisolone, isoproterenol) and inhibiting lysosomal enzymes (fluorophenylalanine); (5) the correct rate of freezing to control the rate of ice crystal formation and its ultimate size, and the control of thawing rate to maintain ice crystal size. Unfortunately, this research is still empiric, and general theoretic guidelines have not yet been clarified.

Storage of Nonviable Tissues by Freeze-drying

Tissue grafts have been used in human reconstructive surgery for several decades. A majority of these grafts are from connective tissue and do not require that the graft be viable to function adequately. A major constituent of most of these tissues is collagen, which seems to maintain its integrity (or at least its strength) even after long-term storage by freezing or freeze-drying. Many thousands of patients each year receive bone, fascia, dura, tendon, heart valve, or skin grafts in treatment of traumatic or surgical defects. The architecture of these grafts is used as a framework for reconstruction as the host slowly replaces the tissue.

These tissues are probably best preserved by freeze-drying, which consists of rapid freezing of the tissue and the application of vacuum for removal of the water from the frozen state to the vapor state without permitting it to become liquid. Such a process usually results in maintenance of morphologic structure and therefore maintains the strength and structural integrity of the tissue. The rapidity of the initial freeze is important, as slow freezing can result in the formation of large ice crystals which can disrupt the tissue. This is apparently not a severe problem in tissues which consist largely of collagen. However, other tissues, such as vascular grafts that contain elastic fibers, can show a disruption of these fibers due to crystal formation. In this instance, the most rapid freeze possible would be indicated to minimize crystal size. The graft is then dehydrated to a residual moisture of 5 percent. At this level it has been noted that tissues can subsequently be stored under vacuum at room temperature for years without further degradation or activation of metabolic processes. On reconstitution, it has been found preferable to inject water or saline solutions into a vacuum bottle containing tissue, so that the fluid can enter the tissue before it is exposed to air. Prior exposure to air apparently allows air molecules to enter the tissue and delays or prevents subsequent penetration of the water molecules necessary to rehydrate the tissue.

The usefulness of freeze-dried allografts is at least partly due to reduced antigenicity remaining in such grafts. The results of using freeze-dried allogeneic bone and autografting bone are not remarkably different. The dura has also been preserved by freeze-drying and functions extremely well when used to cover large cranial defects. Flexor tendon grafts of the hand have also been freeze-dried and used successfully, particularly when removed with their tendon sheaths intact. Many other freeze-dried tissues have been used with greater or lesser success. Cornea for non-penetrating lamellar transplants, fascia, cartilage, heart valve, and nerve have all been tried.

Similarly, freeze-dried grafts have served as temporary biologic dressings to cover large burn wounds. In these instances the nonviable, freeze-dried graft "takes" and is even revascularized. It remains in place for several weeks or months, before it is finally sloughed. These grafts can be applied repeatedly without sensitization or acceleration of sloughing. Skin grafts have proved to be the best biologic dressing to prevent infection and to promote maximum granulation tissue formation in open skin wounds.

References

General: books

Bloom, B. R., and Glade, P. R.: "In Vitro Methods in Cell-mediated Immunity," Academic Press, Inc., New York, 1971.

Fundenberg, H. H., Pink, J. R. L., Stites, D. P., and Wang, A. C.: "Basic Immunogenetics," Oxford University Press, New York, 1972.

Najarian, J. S., and Simmons, R. L. (eds.): "Transplantation," Lea & Febiger, Philadelphia, 1972.

Peer, L. A.: "Transplantation of Tissues," The Williams & Wilkins Company, Baltimore, 1959.

Rapaport, F. T., and Dausset, J., (eds.): "Human Transplantation," Grune & Stratton, Inc., New York, 1968.

Russell, P. S., and Monaco, A. P.: "The Biology of Tissue Transplantation," Little, Brown and Company, Boston, 1965.

Starzl, T. E.: "Experience in Renal Transplantation," W. B. Saunders Company, Philadelphia, 1964.

————: "Experiences in Hepatic Transplantation," W. B. Saunders Company, Philadelphia, 1969.

Woodruff, M. F. A.: "The Transplantation of Tissues and Organs," Charles C Thomas, Publisher, Springfield, Ill., 1960.

Yunis, E. J., Gatti, R. A., and Amos, D. B. (eds.): "Tissue Typing and Organ Transplantation," Academic Press, Inc., New York, 1973.

General: Articles

Albert, E. D., and Terasaki, P. I.: Histocompatibility Testing: Serology and Genetics of the HL-A System, in J. S. Najarian and R. L. Simmons (eds.), "Transplantation," p. 388, Lea & Febiger, Philadelphia, 1972.

Bach, F. H., and Bach, M. L.: Principles of Immunogenetics, in J. S. Najarian and R. L. Simmons (eds.), "Transplantation," p. 40, Lea & Febiger, Philadelphia, 1972.

Beer, A. E., and Billingham, R. E.: Immunobiology of Mammalian Reproduction, in F. J. Dixon and H. G. Kunkel (eds.), "Advances in Immunology," vol. 14, Academic Press, Inc., New York, 1971.

Castel, J.-G.: Medico-Legal Problems of Organ Transplantation, in J. S. Najarian and R. L. Simmons (eds.), "Transplantation," p. 325, Lea & Febiger, Philadelphia, 1972.

Celada, F.: The Cellular Basis of Immunologic Memory, in P. Kallos, B. H. Waksman, and A. DeWeck (eds.), "Progress in Allergy," vol. 15, S. Karger A. G., Basel, 1971.

Claman, H. N., and Mosier, D. E.: Cell-Cell Interactions in Antibody Production, in P. Kallos, B. H. Waksman, and A. DeWeck (eds.), "Progress in Allergy," vol. 16, S. Karger A. G., Basel, 1972.

Feldman, D.: Immunological Enhancement: A Study of Blocking Antibodies, in F. J. Dixon and H. G. Kunkel (eds.), "Advances in Immunology," vol. 15, Academic Press, Inc., New York, 1972.

Fisher, B.: The Present Status of Tumor Immunology, in C. E. Welch and J. D. Hardy (eds.), "Advances in Surgery," vol. 5, Year Book Medical Publishers, Inc., Chicago, 1971.

Foker, J. E., and Najarian, J. S.: Allograft Rejection: III. The Pathobiology of Organ Rejection, in J. S. Najarian and R. L. Simmons (eds.), "Transplantation," p. 122, Lea & Febiger, Philadelphia, 1972.

————, Simmons, R. L., and Najarian, J. S.: Allograft Rejection: I. The Induction of Immunity: The Afferent Arc, in J. S. Najarian and R. L. Simmons (eds.), "Transplantation," p. 63, Lea & Febiger, Philadelphia, 1972.

Good, R. A., and Finstad, J.: Structure and Development of the

Immune System, in J. S. Najarian and R. L. Simmons (eds.), "Transplantation," p. 26, Lea & Febiger, Philadelphia, 1972.

Hilgard, H. R., and Cole, L. J.: Related Topics in Immunology: I. Graft-versus-Host Rejections, in J. S. Najarian and R. L. Simmons (eds.), "Transplantation," p. 272, Lea & Febiger, Philadelphia, 1972.

Kaliss, N.: Circumventing Graft Rejection: II. Immunological Enhancement, in J. S. Najarian and R. L. Simmons (eds.), "Transplantation," p. 195, Lea & Febiger, Philadelphia, 1972.

Lundgren, G., Möller, E., and Möller, G.: Allograft Rejection: V. In Vitro Models of Graft Rejection, in J. S. Najarian and R. L. Simmons (eds.), "Transplantation," p. 164, Lea & Febiger, Philadelphia, 1972.

McKhann, C. F.: Related Topics in Immunology: III. Immunobiology of Cancer, in J. S. Najarian and R. L. Simmons (eds.), "Transplantation," p. 297, Lea & Febiger, Philadelphia, 1972.

Makinodan, T. and Price, G. B.: Circumventing Graft Rejection: V. Radiation, in J. S. Najarian and R. L. Simmons (eds.), "Transplantation," p. 251, Lea & Febiger, Philadelphia, 1972.

Monaco, A. P.: Circumventing Graft Rejection: IV. Antilymphocyte Serum, in J. S. Najarian, and R. L. Simmons (eds.), "Transplantation," p. 222, Lea & Febiger, Philadelphia, 1972.

Najarian, J. S., and Foker, J. E.: Allograft Rejection: II. The Expression of Immunity: The Efferent Arc, in J. S. Najarian and R. L. Simmons (eds.), "Transplantation," p. 94, Lea & Febiger, Philadelphia, 1972.

Nathenson, S. G.: Histocompatibility Antigens, in J. S. Najarian, and R. L. Simmons (eds.), "Transplantation," p. 51, Lea & Febiger, Philadelphia, 1972.

Natvig, J. B., and Kunkel, H. G.: Human Immunoglobulins: Classes, Subclasses, Genetic Variants, and Idiotypes, in F. J. Dixon and H. G. Kunkel (eds.), "Advances in Immunology," vol. 16, Academic Press, Inc., New York, 1973.

Santos, G. W.: Circumventing Graft Rejection: III. Chemical Immunosuppression, in J. S. Najarian and R. L. Simmons (eds.), "Transplantation," p. 206, Lea & Febiger, Philadelphia, 1972.

Saunders, J. B. deC. M.: A Conceptual History of Transplantation, in J. S. Najarian and R. L. Simmons (eds.), "Transplantation," p. 3, Lea & Febiger, Philadelphia, 1972.

Sell, K. W.: Tissue and Organ Preservation, in J. S. Najarian and R. L. Simmons (eds.), "Transplantation," p. 404, Lea & Febiger, Philadelphia, 1972.

Shons, A. R., Moberg, A. W., and Najarian, J. S.: Xenotransplantation, in J. S. Najarian and R. L. Simmons (eds.), "Transplantation," p. 729, Lea & Febiger, Philadelphia, 1972.

Simmons, R. L.: Related Topics in Immunity: II. Histocompatibility Antigens and Pregnancy, in J. S. Najarian and R. L. Simmons (eds.), "Transplantation," p. 285, Lea & Febiger, Philadelphia, 1972.

——— and Simmons, R. G.: Sociological and Psychological Aspects of Transplantation, in J. S. Najarian and R. L. Simmons (eds.), "Transplantation," p. 361, Lea & Febiger, Philadelphia, 1972.

Unanue, E. R., and Dixon, F. J.: Allograft Rejection: IV. Tissue Injury Produced by Antibody-Antigen Reactions, in J. S. Najarian and R. L. Simmons (eds.), "Transplantation," p. 145, Lea & Febiger, Philadelphia, 1972.

Voisin, G. A.: Immunological Facilitation: A Broadening of the Concept of the Enhancement Phenomenon, in P. Kallos, B. H. Waksman, and A. DeWeck (eds.), "Progress in Allergy," vol. 15, S. Karger A. G., Basel, 1971.

Weigle, W. O.: Circumventing Graft Rejection: I. Immunological Unresponsiveness, in J. S. Najarian and R. L. Simmons (eds.), "Transplantation," p. 174, Lea & Febiger, Philadelphia, 1972.

Transplantation Immunology

Amos, D. B., and Koprowski, H. (eds.): Cell-bound Council, in "Conference of the National Academy of Sciences–National Research Council" (Sponsored by Committee on Tissue Transplantation of the Division of Medical Sciences, National Academy of Sciences–National Research Council, p. 134. Wistar Institute, Philadelphia, 1963.

——— and Wakefield, J. D.: Growth of Mouse Ascites Tumor Cells in Diffusion Chambers: II. Lysis and Growth Inhibition by Diffusible Isoantibody, J Nat Cancer Inst, 22:1077, 1959.

Anderson, N. F., Delorme, E. J., and Woodruff, M. F. A.: Induction of Runt Disease in Rats by Injection of Thoracic Duct Lymphocytes at Birth, Transplant Bull, 7:93, 1960.

Argyis, B. F.: Thymus-Bone Marrow Interaction in Transplantation Immunity, Transplantation, 8:538, 1969.

Bach, F. H., and Kisken, W. A.: Predictive Value of Results of Mixed Leukocyte Cultures for Skin Allograft Survival in Man, Transplantation, 5:1046, 1967.

Billingham, R. E., and Brent, L.: Further Attempts to Transfer Transplantation Immunity by Means of Serum, Br J Exp Pathol, 37:566, 1956.

——— and ———: Simple Method for Inducing Tolerance of Skin Homografts in Mice, Transplant Bull, 4:67, 1957.

———, ———, and Medawar, P. B.: "Actively Acquired Tolerance" of Foreign Cells, Nature (Lond), 172:603, 1953.

——— and Silvers, W. K.: Studies on Homografts of Foetal and Infant Skin and Further Observations on the Anomalous Properties of Pouch Skin Grafts in Hamsters, Proc R Soc Lond [Biol], 161:168, 1964.

Bloom, B. R.: Biological Activities of Lymphocyte Products, in H. S. Lawrence and M. Landy (eds.), "Mediators of Cellular Immunity," p. 253, Academic Press, Inc., New York, 1969.

Boak, J. L., Christie, G. H., Ford, W. L., and Howard, J. G.: Pathways in the Development of Liver Macrophages: Alternative Precursors Contained in Populations of Lymphocytes and Bone-Marrow Cells, Proc R Soc [Biol], 169:307, 1968.

Boyse, E. A., Old, L. J., and Thomas, G.: A Report on Some Observations with a Simplified Cytotoxic Test, Transplant Bull, 29:435, 1962.

Brent, L., Brown, J., and Medawar, P. B.: Skin Transplantation Immunity in Relation to Hypersensitivity, Lancet, 2:561, 1958.

——— and Medawar, P. B.: Quantitative Studies on Tissue Transplantation Immunity: V. Role of Antiserum in Enhancement and Desensitization, Proc R Soc Lond [Biol], 155: 392, 1962.

Burnet, F. M.: "The Clonal Selection Theory of Acquired Immunity," Vanderbilt University Press, Nashville, Tenn., 1959.

——— and Fenner, F.: Genetics and Immunology, Heredity (Lond), 2:289, 1948.

Claman, H. N., Chapman, E. A., and Triplett, R. F.: Thymus–Marrow Cell Combinations: Synergism in Antibody Production, Proc Soc Biol Exp Med, 122:1167, 1966.

Clark, D. S., Foker, J. E., Good, R. A., and Varco, R. L.: Humoral

Factors in Canine Renal Allograft Rejection, *Lancet,* **1:**8, 1968.

Clark, J. M., and Weiss, L.: An Immunofluorescence Study of the In Vitro Interaction Between Lymphoid Cells and Target Cells, *J Immunol,* **103:**1006, 1969.

Cochrum, K. C., and Najarian, J. S.: Quantitation of Antigen Release from Renal Allografts, *Fed Proc,* **26:**572, 1967. (Abstract.)

Dutton, R. W., and Mishell, R. I.: Cellular Events in the Immune Response: The In Vitro Response of Normal Spleen Cells to Erythrocyte Antigens, in L. Frisch (ed.), "Cold Spring Harbor Symposia on Quantitative Biology (Vol. XXXII, Antibodies)," p. 407, Cold Spring Harbor Laboratory of Quantitative Biology, New York, 1967.

Egdahl, R. H., and Hume, D. M.: Immunologic Studies in Renal Homotransplantation, *Surg Gynecol Obstet,* **102:**450, 1956.

Feldman, J. D.: Ultrastructure of Immunologic Processes, *Adv Immunol,* **4:**175, 1964.

Fishman, M.: Antibody Formation in Tissue Culture, *Nature (Lond),* **183:**1200, 1959.

———: Induction of Antibodies In Vitro, *Annu Rev Microbiol,* **23:**199, 1969.

Foker, J. E., Clark, D. S., Pickering, R. J., Good, R. A., and Varco, R. L.: Mechanisms of Leukocyte Infiltration of Allografts: I. The Separation and Early Appearance of Two Components, *Surgery,* **66:**42, 1969.

George, M., and Vaughan, J. H.: In Vitro Cell Migration as a Model for Delayed Hypersensitivity, *Proc Soc Exp Biol Med,* **111:**415, 1962.

Globerson, A., and Auerbach, R.: Reactivation In Vitro of Immunocompetence in Irradiated Mouse Spleen, *J Exp Med,* **126:**223, 1967.

Goldstein, A. L., Asanuma, Y., Battisto, J. R., Hardy, M. A., Quint, J., and White, A.: Influence of Thymosin on Cell-mediated and Humoral Immune Responses in Normal Immunologically Deficient Mice, *J Immunol,* **104:**359, 1970.

Gorer, P. A.: Some Recent Work on Tumor Immunity, *Cancer Res,* **4:**149, 1956.

——— and Kaliss, N.: The Effect of Iso-antibodies In Vivo on Three Different Transplantable Neoplasms in Mice, *Cancer Res,* **19:**824, 1959.

Govaerts, A.: Cellular Antibodies in Kidney Homotransplantation, *J Immunol,* **85:**516, 1960.

Gowans, J. L.: The Fate of Parental Strain Small Lymphocytes in Fl Hybrid Rats, *Ann NY Acad Sci,* **99:**432, 1962.

———, McGregor, D. D., and Cowen, D. M.: The Role of Small Lymphocytes in the Rejection of Homograft Skin, in G. E. Wolstenholme and J. Knight, (eds.), "The Immunologically Competent Cell," p. 20, Little, Brown and Company, Boston, 1963.

——— and Uhr, J. W.: The Carriage of Immunological Memory by Small Lymphocytes in the Rat, *J Exp Med,* **124:**1017, 1966.

Greeves, M. F., Torrigiani, G., and Roitt, I. M.: Blocking of the Lymphocyte Receptors Site for Cell Mediated Hypersensitivity and Transplantation Reactions by Antilight Chain Sera, *Nature (Lond),* **222:**885, 1969.

Hall, B. D., and Doty, P.: The Configurational Properties of Ribonucleic Acid Isolated from Microsomal Particles of Calf Liver, in R. B. Roberts (ed.), "Microsomal Particles and Protein Synthesis," p. 27, Permagon Press, New York, 1958.

Hasek, M., Karakoz, I., Skamene, E., Chutna, J., Nouza, K., Bubenik, J., Nemec, M., and Sovova, V.: Protective Action of Homologous Serum Component on Graft Rejection, *Transplant Proc,* **1:**527, 1969.

Hildemann, W. H.: New Exceptions to the Immunogenetic Rules of Transplantation, in J. Dausset, J. Hamburger, and G. Mathé (eds.), "Advance in Transplantation," Munksgaard, Copenhagen, 1968.

Hume, D. M., and Egdahl, R. H.: Progressive Destruction of Renal Homografts Isolated from the Regional Lymphatics of the Host, *Surgery* **38:**194, 1955.

Interbitzen, T.: Histamine in Allergic Responses of the Skin, in J. G. Shaffer, G. A. LoGrippo, and M. W. Chase (eds.), "Mechanisms of Hypersensitivity," p. 493, Little, Brown and Company, Boston, 1958.

Jurezi, R. E., Thor, D. E., and Dray, S.: Transfer with RNA Extracts of the Cell Migration Inhibition Correlate of Delayed Hypersensitivity in the Guinea Pig, *J Immunol,* **101:**823, 1968.

———, ———, and ———: Transfer of the Delayed Hypersensitivity Skin Reaction in the Guinea Pig using RNA-Treated Lymphoid Cells, *J Immunol,* **105:**1313, 1970.

Kaliss, N.: Immunological Enhancement of Tumor Homografts in Mice: Review, *Cancer Res,* **18:**992, 1958.

Lawler, S. D., and Cohen, S.: Distribution of Allotypic Specificities on the Peptide Chains of Human Gamma Globulins, *Immunology,* **8:**206, 1966.

Lawrence, H. S.: Transfer Factor, in F. J. Dixon Jr. and H. G. Kunel (eds.), "Advances in Immunology," vol. II, p. 195, Academic Press, Inc., New York, 1969.

———: Transfer Factor, in H. S. Lawrence and M. Landy (eds.), "Mediators of Cellular Immunity," p. 145, Academic Press, Inc., New York, 1969.

McClusky, R. T., Benacerraf, B., and McClusky, J. W.: Studies on the Specificity of the Cellular Infiltrate in Delayed Hypersensitivity Reactions, *J Immunol,* **90:**466, 1963.

Mackaness, G. B., and Blanden, R. V.: Cellular Immunity, *Prog Allergy,* **11:**89, 1967.

Mannick, J. A., and Egdahl, R. H.: Transformation of Non-immune Lymph Node Cells to State of Transplantation Immunity by RNA, *Ann Surg,* **156:**356, 1962.

——— and ———: Endocrinologic Agents, in F. T. Rapaport and J. Dausset (eds.), "Human Transplantation," p. 472, Grune & Stratton, Inc., New York, 1968.

Medawar, P. B.: Second Study of Behavior and Fate of Skin Homografts in Rabbits: Report to War Wounds Committee of Medical Research Council, *J Anat,* **79:**157, 1945.

Merrill, J. P., Friedman, E. A., Wilson, R. E., and Marshall, D. C.: Production of "Delayed Type" Cutaneous Hypersensitivity to Human Donor Leukocytes as Result of Rejection of Skin Homografts, *J Clin Invest,* **40:**631, 1961.

Miller, J. F. A. P.: Immunological Function of Thymus, *Lancet,* **2:**748, 1961.

——— and Mitchell, G. F.: The Thymus and the Precursors of Antigen Reactive Cells, *Nature (Lond),* **216:**659, 1967.

Mitchison, N. A.: Passive Transfer of Transplantation Immunity, *Proc R Soc Lond [Biol],* **142:**72, 1954.

——— and Dube, O. L.: Studies on the Immunological Response to Foreign Tumor Transplants in the Mouse: II. The Relation between Hemagglutinating Antibody and Graft Resistance in the Normal Mouse and Mice Pretreated with Tissue Preparations, *J Exp Med,* **102:**179, 1955.

————: Discussion in Gowans, J. L.: Cell Populations Involved in Immune Responses, in M. Landy and W. Brown. (eds.), "Immunological Tolerance," p. 121, Academic Press, Inc., New York, 1969.

Monaco, A. P., Wood, M. L., and Russell, P. S.: Some Effects of Purified Heterologous Antihuman Lymphocyte Serum in Man, *Transplantation,* **5:**1106, 1967.

Murphy, J. B.: "Lymphocyte in Resistance to Tissue Grafting, Malignant Disease and Tuberculous Infection," Rockefeller Institute for Medical Research Monographs 21, p. 168, 1926.

Najarian, J. S., and Feldman, J. D.: Passive Transfer of Tuberculin Sensitivity by Tritiated Thymidine-labeled Lymphoid Cells, *J Exp Med,* **114:**779, 1962.

Nossal, G. J. V., Abbot, A., and Mitchell, J.: Antigens in Immunity: XIV. Electron Microscopic Radioautographic Studies of Antigen Capture in the Lymph Node Medulla, *J Exp Med,* **127:**263, 1968.

————, ————, ————, and Lummus, Z.: Antigens in Immunity: XV. Ultrastructural Features of Antigen Capture in Primary and Secondary Lymphoid Follicles, *J Exp Med,* **127:**277, 1968.

————, Shortman, K. D., Miller, J. F. A. P., Mitchell, G. F., and Haskin, J. S.: The Target Cell in the Induction of Immunity and Tolerance, in L. Frisch (ed.), "Cold Spring Harbor Symposia on Quantitative Biology (Vol. XXXII, Antibodies)," p. 369, Cold Spring Harbor Laboratory of Quantitative Biology, Cold Spring Harbor, New York, 1967.

O'Brien, T. F., and Coons, A. H.: Studies on Antibody Production: VII. The Effect of 5-Bromodeoxyuridine on the In Vitro Anamnestic Antibody Response, *J Exp Med,* **117:**1063, 1963.

Perey, D. Y., Cooper, M. D., and Good, R. A.: Normal Second Set Wattle Homograft Rejection in Agammaglobulinemic Chickens, *Transplantation,* **5:**615, 1967.

Prendergast, R. A.: Cellular Specificity in the Homograft Reaction, *J Exp Med,* **119:**377, 1964.

Raju, S., and Grogan, J. B.: Immunology of the Anterior Chamber of the Eye, *Transplant Proc,* **3:**605, 1971.

Rapaport, F. T., Dausset, J., Hamburger, J., Hume, D. M., Kaho, K., Williams, G. M., and Milgram, F.: Serologic Factors in Human Transplantation, *Ann Surg,* **166:**596, 1967.

Rich, A. R., and Lewis, M. R.: The Nature of Allergy in Tuberculosis as Revealed by Tissue Culture Studies, *Bull Johns Hopkins Hosp,* **50:**115, 1932.

Riesfield, R. A., Pellegrino, M. A., Ferrone, S., and Kahan, B. D.: Chemical and Molecular Nature of HL-A Antigens, *Transplant Proc,* **5:**447, 1973.

Scothorne, R. J., and McGregor, I. A.: Cellular Changes in Lymph Nodes and Spleen following Skin Homografting in the Rabbit, *J Anat,* **89:**283, 1955.

Sercarz, E., and Coons, A. H.: The Exhaustion of Specific Antibody Producing Capacity during a Secondary Response, in M. Hašek, A. Lengerová, and M. Vojtíšková (eds.), "Mechanisms of Immunological Tolerance," p. 73, Academic Press, Inc., New York, 1962.

Silverstein, A. M., and Kraner, K. L.: The Role of Circulating Antibody in the Rejection of Homografts, *Transplantation,* **3:**535, 1965.

Simmons, R. L., and Russell, P. S.: The Histocompatibility Anti-

gens of Fertilized Mouse Eggs and Trophoblast, *Ann NY Acad Sci,* **129:**35, 1966.

Snell, G. D.: Histocompatibility Genes of Mouse: II. Production and Analysis of Isogenic Resistant Lines, *J Natl Cancer Inst,* **21:**843, 1958.

Stuart, F. P., Saitoh, T., Fitch, F. W., and Spargo, B. H.: Immunological Enhancement of Renal Allografts in the Rat, *Surgery,* **64:**17, 1968.

Terasaki, P. I., and McClelland, J. D.: Microdroplet Assay of Human Serum Cytotoxins, *Nature (Lond),* **204:**998, 1964.

Ward, P. A., Chemotaxis of Mononuclear Cells, *J Exp Med,* **128:**1201, 1968.

Weaver, J. M., Algire, G. H., and Prehn, R. T.: Growth of Cells In Vivo in Diffusion Chambers: II. Role of Cells in Destruction of Homografts in Mice, *J Nat Cancer Inst,* **15:**1737, 1955.

Wilson, D. B.: The Reaction of Immunologically Activated Lymphoid Cells against Homologous Target Tissue Cells In Vitro, *J Cell Comp Physiol,* **62:**273, 1963.

Woodruff, M. F. A., and Anderson, N. A.: Effect of Lymphocyte Depletion by Thoracic Duct Fistula and Administration of Anti-lymphocyte Serum on Survival of Skin Homografts in Rats, *Nature (Lond),* **200:**702, 1963.

Liver Transplantation

Bergan, J. J., and ACS/NIH Organ Transplant Registry: "First Scientific Report," 1971.

Bieber, C. P., Stinson, E. B., Shumway, N. E., Payne, R., and Kosek, J. C.: Cardiac Transplantation in Man: VII. Cardiac Allograft Pathology, *Circulation,* **41:**753, 1970.

Brettschneider, L.: Liver: I. Experimental, in J. S. Najarian and R. L. Simmons (eds.), "Transplantation," p. 496, Lea & Febiger, Philadelphia, 1972.

Buckley, J. J.: Liver: II. Anesthesia, in J. S. Najarian and R. L. Simmons (eds.), "Transplantation," p. 517, Lea & Febiger, Philadelphia, 1972.

Calne, R. Y., White, H. J. O., Binns, R. M., Herbertson, B. M., Milard, P. R., Pena, D. R., Samuel, J. R., and Davis, D. R.: Immunosuppressive Effects of the Orthotopically Transplanted Porcine Liver, *Transplant Proc,* **1:**321, 1969.

————, ————, Yoffa, D. E., Maginn, R. R., Binns, R. M., Samuel, J. R., and Molina, V. P.: Observations of Orthotopic Liver Transplantation in the Pig, *Br Med J,* **2:**478, 1967.

Fortner, J. G., Beattie, E. J., Jr., Shiu, M. H., Kawano, N., and Howland, W. S.: Orthotopic and Heterotopic Liver Homografts in Man, *Ann Surg,* **172:**23, 1970.

Groth, C. G., Porter, K. A., Otte, J. B., Daloze, P. M., Marchioro, T. L., Brettschneider, L., and Starzl, T. E.: Studies of Blood Flow and Ultrastructural Changes in Rejecting and Nonrejecting Canine Orthotopic Liver Homografts, *Surgery,* **63:**658, 1968.

Halgrimson, C. G., Marchioro, T. L., Faris, T. D., Porter, K. A., Peters, G. N., and Starzl, T. E.: Auxiliary Liver Homotransplantation: Effect of Host Portacaval Shunt, *Arch Surg,* **93:**107, 1966.

Marchioro, T. L., Porter, K. A., Kickinson, T. C., Faris, T. D., and Starzl, T. E.: Physiologic Requirements for Auxiliary Liver Homotransplantation, *Surg Gynecol Obstet,* **121:**17, 1965.

Najarian, J. S.: Liver: III. Clinical Transplantation, in J. S. Najarian and R. L. Simmons (eds.), "Transplantation," p. 522, Lea & Febiger, Philadelphia, 1972.

Starzl, T. E.: "Experience in Hepatic Transplantation," W. B. Saunders Company, Philadelphia, 1969.

———: The Current Status of Liver Transplantation, *Hosp Prac,* **6:**47, 1971.

———, Brettschneider, L., Penn, I., Bell, P., Groth, C. G., Blanchard, H., Kashiwagi, N., and Putnam, C. W.: Orthotopic Liver Transplantation in Man, *Transplant Proc,* **1:**21, 1969.

——— and Marchioro, T. L.: Hepatic Transplantation, in F. T. Rapaport and J. Dausset (eds.), "Human Transplantation," p. 215, Grune & Stratton, Inc., New York, 1968.

Stuart, F. P., Torres, E., Hester, W. J., Dammin, G. J., and Moore, F. D.: Orthotopic Autotransplantation and Allotransplantation of the Liver: Functional and Structural Patterns in the Dog, *Ann Surg,* **165:**325, 1967.

Welch, C. S.: A Note on the Transplantation of the Whole Liver in Dogs, *Transplant Bull* **2:**54, 1955.

Cardiac Transplantation

Barnard, C. N.: A Human Cardiac Transplant, *S Afri Med J,* **41:**1271, 1967.

Campeau, L., Pospisil, L., Grondin, P., Dyrda, I., and Lepage, G.: Cardiac Catheterization Findings at Rest and after Exercise in Patients following Cardiac Transplantation, *Am J Cardiol,* **25:**523, 1970.

Carrel, A., and Guthrie, C. C.: The Transplantation of Veins and Organs, *Am Med,* **10:**1101, 1905.

Childs, J. W., and Lower, R. R.: Preservation of the Heart, *Prog Cardiovasc Dis,* **12:**149, 1969.

Cleveland, R. J., and Lower, R. R.: Transplantation of Canine Cadaver Hearts after Short-Term Preservation, *Transplantation,* **5:**904, 1967.

Cooley, D. A., Bloodwell, R. D., Hallman, G. L., and Nora, J. J.: Transplantation of the Heart: A Report of Four Cases. *JAMA,* **205:**479, 1968.

DeBakey, M. E., Diethrich, E. B., Glick, G., Noon, G. P., Butler, W. T., Rossen, R. D., Liddicoat, J. E., and Brooks, D. K.: Human Cardiac Transplantation: Clinical Experience, *J Thorac Cardiovasc Surg,* **58:**303, 1969.

Dong, E., Jr., Griepp, R. B., Stinson, E. B., and Shumway, N. E.: Review of Four Years Experience with Clinical Heart Transplantation at Stanford University Medical Center, *Transplant Proc,* **4:**787, 1972.

Ellis, R. J., Lillehei, C. W., and Zabriskie, J. B.: Detection of Circulating Heart-reactive antibody in Human Heart Transplants, *JAMA,* **211:**1505, 1970.

Griep, R. B., Stinson, E. B., Dong, E., Jr., Clark, D. A., and Shumway, N. E.: Hemodynamic Performance of the Transplanted Human Heart, *Surgery,* **70:**88, 1971.

Grinnan, G. L., Graham, W. H., Childs, J. W., and Lower, R. R.: Cardiopulmonary Homotransplantation, *J Thorac Cardiovasc Surg,* **60:**609, 1970.

Hardy, J. D., Chavez, C. M., Kurrus, F. D., Neely, W. A., Eraslan, S., Turner, M. D., Fabian, L. W., and Labeck, T. D.: Heart Transplantation in Man: Developmental Studies and Report of a Case, *JAMA,* **188:**1132, 1964.

Kahn, D. R., Reynolds, E. W., Jr., Walton, J. A., Kirsh, M. M., Vathayanon, S., and Sloan, H.: Human Heart Transplantation for Cardiomyopathy, *Surgery,* **67:**122, 1970.

Kontos, H. A., Thames, M. D., and Lower, R. R.: Responses to Electrical and Reflex Autonomic Stimulation in Dogs with Cardiac Transplantation Before and After Reinnervation, *J Thorac Cardiovasc Surg,* **59:**382, 1970.

Kosek, J. C., Bieber, C., and Lower, R. R.: Heart Graft Arteriosclerosis, *Transplant Proc,* **3:**512, 1971.

———, Hurley, E. J., and Lower, R. R.: Histopathology of Orthotopic Canine Cardiac Homografts, *Lab Invest,* **19:**97, 1968.

Lower, R. R.: Cardiac Transplantation without Complete Cardiac Denervation: The Role of the Afferent Receptors, *Am Heart J,* **72:**841, 1966.

———, Dong, E., Jr., and Shumway, N. E.: Long Term Survival of Cardiac Homografts, *Surgery,* **58:**100, 1965.

———, ———, and Glazener, F. S.: Electrocardiograms of Dogs with Heart Homografts, *Circulation,* **33:**455, 1966.

———, Stofer, R. C., Hurley, E. J., and Shumway, N. E.: Complete Homograft Replacement of the Heart and Both Lungs, *Surgery,* **50:**842, 1961.

———, and Shumway, N. E.: Homovital Transplantation of the Heart, *J Thorac Cardiovasc Surg,* **41:**196, 1961.

Mann, F. C., Priestley, J. T., Markowitz, J., and Yater, W. M.: Transplantation of the Intact Mammalian Heart, *Arch Surg,* **26:**219, 1933.

Milan, J. D., Shipkey, F. H., Lind, C. J., Jr., Nora, J. J., Leachman, R. D., Rochelle, D. G., Bloodwell, R. D., Hallman, G. L., and Cooley, D. A.: Morphologic Findings in Human Cardiac Allografts, *Circulation,* **41:**519, 1970

Schroeder, J. S., Popp, R. L., Stinson, E. B., Dong, E., Jr., Shumway, N. E., and Harrison, D. C.: Acute Rejection following Cardiac Transplantation: Phonocardiographic and Ultrasound Observations, *Circulation,* **40:**155, 1969.

Sewell, D. H., Kemp, V. E., and Lower, R. R.: The Epicardial ECG in Monitoring Cardiac Homograft Rejection, *Circulation,* **39** (*Suppl* 1):21, 1969.

Stinson, E. B., Griepp, R. B., Clark, D. A., Dong, E., Jr., and Shumway, N. E.: Cardiac Transplantation in Man: VIII. Survival and Function, *J. Thorac Cardiovasc Surg,* **60:**303, 1970.

Thomas, K. E., Linehan, J. D., and Lower, R. R.: Size Disparity in Dogs between Donor and Recipient in Cardiac Transplantation, *Surg Forum,* **21:**183, 1970.

Willman, V. L., Kaiser, G. C., Harades, Y., Cooper, T., and Hanlon, C. R.: Physiological Alterations following Transplantation of the Heart, *Adv Transplant Proc 1st Cong Transplant Soc,* 1968, p. 661.

Lung Transplantation

Arnar, O., Andersen, R. C., Hitchcock, C. R., and Haglin, J. J.: Reimplantation of the Baboon Lung after Extended Ischemia, *Transplantation,* **5:**929, 1967.

Blumenstock, D. A.: Transplantation of the Lung, *Transplantation,* **5:**917, 1967.

——— and Veith, F. J.: Lung (Clinical Transplantation.), in J. S. Najarian and R. L. Simmons (eds.), "Transplantation," p. 569, Lea & Febiger, Philadelphia, 1972.

Haglin, J. J., and Arnar, O.: Physiologic Studies of the Baboon Living on Only the Reimplanted Lung, *Surg Forum,* **15:**175, 1964.

Manax, W. G., Lyons, G. W., and Lillehei, R. C.: Transplantation of the Small Bowel and Stomach, in C. E. Welch (ed.), "Advances in Surgery," vol. II, p. 371, Year Book Medical Publishers, Inc., Chicago, 1966.

Mathe, G., Schwarzenberg, L., Amiel, J. L.: Bone Marrow, in J. S. Najarian and R. L. Simmons (eds.), "Transplantation," p. 588, Lea & Febiger, Philadelphia, 1972.

Metras, H.: Note préliminaire sur la greffe totale du poumon chez le chien, *C R Acad Sci [D]* (*Paris*), **231:**1176, 1950.

Norman, J. C., Covelli, V. H., and Sise, H. S.: Transplantation of the Spleen: Experimental Cure of Hemophilia, *Surgery,* **66:**1, 1968.

Rapaport, F. T., and Converse, J. M.: Skin Transplantation, in F. T. Rapaport and J. Dausset (eds.), "Human Transplantation," p. 304, Grune & Stratton, Inc., New York, 1968.

Ruiz, J. O., Uchida, H., and Lillehei, R. C.: Intestine (Clinical Transplantation), in J. S. Najarian and R. L. Simmons (eds.), "Transplantation," p. 646, Lea & Febiger, Philadelphia, 1972.

Waksman, B. H., Arbouys, S., and Arnason, B. G.: The Use of Specific "Lymphocyte" Antisera to Inhibit Hypersensitive Reactions of the "Delayed" Type. *J Exp Med* **114:**997, 1961.

White, R. J.: Experimental Transplantation of the Brain, in F. T. Rapaport and J. Dausset (eds.), "Human Transplantation," p. 692, Grune & Stratton, Inc., New York, 1968.

Kidney Transplantation

Advisory Committee to the Human Renal Transplant Registry: Ninth Report of the Human Renal Transplant Registry, *JAMA,* **220:**253, 1972.

Aldrete, J. A., Daniel, W., O'Higgins, J. W., Homatas, J., and Starzl, T. E.: Analysis of Anesthetic Related Morbidity in Human Recipients of Renal Homografts, *Anesth Analg* (*Cleve*), **50:**34, 1971.

Alfrey, A. C., Jenkins, D., Groth, C. G., Schorr, W. S., Gecelter, L., and Ogden, D. A.: Resolution of Hyperparathyroidism, Renal Osteodystrophy and Metastatic Calcification after Renal Homotransplantation, *N Engl J Med,* **279:**1349, 1968.

Asbury, A. K.: Recovery from Uremic Neuropathy, *New Engl J Med,* **281:**1211, 1971.

Beecher, H. K.: After the "Definition of Irreversible Coma," *N Engl J Med,* **281:**1070, 1969.

Belzer, F. O., Ashby, B. S., Gulyassy, P. F., and Powell, M.: Successful Seventeen-Hour Preservation and Transplantation of Human-Cadaver Kidney, *N Engl J Med,* **278:**608, 1968.

Bergentz, S. E., Olander, R., Kissmeyer-Nielsen, F., Olsen, T. S., and Hood, B., Hyperacute Rejection of a Kidney Allograft, *Scand J Urol Nephrol,* **4:**143, 1970.

Blaufox, M. D., Birbari, A. E., Hickler, T. B., and Merrill, J. P.: Peripheral Plasma Renin Activity in Renal-Homotransplant Recipients, *N Engl J Med,* **275:**1165, 1966.

———, Lewis, E. J., Jagger, P., Lauler, D., Hickler, R., and Merrill, J. P.: Physiologic Responses of the Transplanted Human Kidney: Sodium Regulation and Renin Secretion, *N Engl J Med,* **28:**62, 1969.

Bolton, C. F., Baltzan, M. A., and Baltzan, R. B.: Effects of Renal Transplantation on Uremic Neuropathy: A Clinical and Electrophysiologic Study, *N Engl J Med,* **284:**1170, 1971.

Bravo, J. F., Herman, J. J., and Smyth, C. J.: Musculoskeletal Disorders after Renal Homotransplantation: A Clinical and Laboratory Analysis of 60 Cases, *Ann Intern Med,* **66:**87, 1967.

Brescia, M. J., Cimino, J. E., Appel, K., and Hurwich, B. J.: Chronic Hemodialysis Using Venipuncture and Surgically Created Arteriovenous Fistula. *New Engl J Med* **275:**1089, 1966.

Bricker, N. S., Statopolsky, E., Reiss, E., and Avioli, L. V.: Calcium, Phosphorus, and Bone in Renal Disease and Transplantation, *Arch Intern Med,* **123:**543, 1969.

Calne, R. Y.: Cadaveric Kidneys for Transplantation, *Br Med J,* **2:**565, 1969.

Carbone, P. P., Sabesin, S. M., Sidrausky, H., and Frei, E., III: Secondary Aspergillosis, *Arch Intern Med,* **60:**556, 1964.

Clarke, S. E., Kennedy, J. A., Hewitt, J. C., McEvoy, J., McGeown, M. B., and Nelson, S. D.: Successful Removal of Thrombus from Renal Vein after Renal Transplantation, *Br Med J,* **1:**154, 1970.

Coolste, L. G., Bostrome, H., Magnusson, C., Skogsberg, G., and Werner, B.: Streptokinase Treatment of a Thrombosis at the Site of the Venous Connection of a Kidney Transplant, *Scand J Urol Nephrol,* **5:**80, 1971.

Dietzman, R. H., Rebelo, A. E., Graham, E. F., Crabo, B. G., and Lillehei, R. C.: Long-term Functional Success Following Freezing of Canine Kidneys, *Surgery,* **74:**181, 1973.

Dossetor, J. B., Zweig, S. M., Treves, S., and Ross, W. M.: The ^{131}I Ortho-iodohippurate Photoscan in Human Renal Allografts, *Canad Med Assoc J,* **102:**1373, 1970.

Faris, T. D., and Carey, T. A.: Arteriovenous Shunts for Hemodialysis, *Am J Surg,* **113:**679, 1967.

Fellner, C. H., and Schwartz, S. H.: Altruism in Disrepute: Medical versus Public Attitudes toward the Living Organ Donor, *N Engl J Med,* **284:**583, 1971.

Festenstein, H., Oliver, R. T. D., Hyams, A., Moorhead, J. R., Pirrie, A. J., Pegrum, G. C., and Balfour, I. C.: A Collaborative Scheme for Tissue Typing and Matching in Renal Transplantation, *Lancet,* **2:**389, 1969.

Figueroa, J. E., Cortez, L. M., DeCamp, P. T., and Ochsner, J. L.: Renal Vein Thrombosis after Transplantation, *Br Med J,* **1:**288, 1971.

Fletcher, E. W. L., Lecky, J. W., and Gonick, H. C.: Selective Phlebography of Transplanted Kidneys, *Clin Radiol,* **21:**144, 1970.

Glassock, R. J., Feldman, D., Reynolds, E. S., Dammin, G. J., and Merrill, J. P.: Human Renal Isografts: A Clinical and Pathologic Analysis, *Medicine* (*Baltimore*), **47:**411, 1968.

———, ———, ———, ———, and ———: Recurrent Glomerulonephritis in Human Renal Isograft Recipients: A Clinical and Pathologic Study, in J. Dausset, J. Hamburger, and G. Mathé (eds.), "Advance in Transplantation," p. 361, The Williams & Wilkins Company, Baltimore, 1968.

Greene, J. A., Jr., Vander, A. J., and Kowalczyk, R. S.: Plasma Renin Activity and Aldosterone Excretion after Renal Homotransplantation, *J Lab Clin Med,* **71:**586, 1968.

Halgrimson, C. G., Rapaport, F. T., Terasaki, P. I., Porter, K. A., Andres, G., Penn, I., Putnam, C. W., and Starzl, T. E.: Net Histocompatibility Ratios (NHR) for Clinical Transplantation, *Transplant Proc,* **3:**140, 1971.

Hall, M. C., Elmore, S. M., Bright, R. W., Pierce, J. C., and Hume, D. M.: Skeletal Complications in a Series of Human Renal Allografts, *JAMA,* **208:**1825, 1969.

Hamburger, J., and Crosnier, J.: Moral and Ethical Problems in Transplantation, in F. T. Rapaport and J. Dausset (eds.), "Human Transplantation," p. 37, Grune & Stratton, Inc., New York, 1968.

Hansen, H. E., and Sell, A: Isotope Renography Combined with Recording Isotope Cystogram in Patients with Renal Transplants, *Acta Med Scand,* **188:**205, 1970.

Harvard Medical School Committee: A Definition of Irreversible Coma: Report of the Ad Hoc Committee of the Harvard Medical School to Examine the Definition of Brain Death, *JAMA,* **205:**337, 1968.

Heale, W. F., Morris, P., Bennett, R. C., Mortensen, P. J., and Ting, A.: Leukocyte Antigens in Renal Transplantation: Eight Successful Renal Transplantations in the Presence of a Positive Cross-Match, *Med J Aust,* **2:**382, 1969.

Hinman, F., Jr., and Belzer, F. O.: Urinary Tract Infections and Renal Homotransplantation: I. Effect of Antibacterial Irrigations on Defenses of the Defunctionalized Bladder, *Trans Am Assoc Genitourin Surg,* **60:**46, 1968.

Hume, D. M.: Homotransplantation of Kidneys and of Fetal Liver and Spleen after Total Body Irradiation, *Ann Surg,* **152:**354, 1960.

———: Kidney Transplantation, in F. R. Rapaport and J. Dausset, (eds.), "Human Transplantation," pp. 110, 151, Grune & Stratton, Inc., New York, 1968.

———, Lee, H. M., Williams, G. M., White, H. J. O., Ferré, J., Wolf, J. S., Prout, G. R., Jr., Slapak, M., O'Brien, J., Kilpatrick, C. J., Kauffman, H. M., Jr., and Cleveland, R. J.: Comparative Results of Cadaver and Related Donor Renal Homografts in Man and Immunologic Implications of the Outcome of Second and Paired Transplants, *Ann Surg,* **164:**352, 1966.

Irby, R., and Hume, D. M.: Joint Changes Observed following Renal Transplants, *Clin Orthop,* **57:**101, 1968.

Jeannet, M., DeWeck, A., Frei, P. C., Grob, P., and Thiel, G.: A Cooperative Kidney Typing and Exchange Program, *Helv Med Acta,* **35:**239, 1969–1970.

Johnson, J. W., Hattner, R. S., Hampers, C. L., Bernstein, D. S., Merril, J. P., and Sherwood, L. M.: Secondary Hyperparathyroidism in Chronic Renal Failure: Effects of Renal Homotransplantation, *JAMA,* **215:**478, 1971.

Juul-Jensen, P.: "Criteria of Brain Death: Selection Donors for Transplantation," Munksgaard, Copenhagen, 1970.

Kincaid-Smith, P.: Histological Diagnosis of Rejection of Renal Homografts in Man, *Lancet,* **2:**849, 1967.

———: Modification of the Vascular Lesions of Rejection of Cadaveric Renal Allografts by Dipyridamole and Anticoagulants, *Lancet,* **2:**920, 1969.

Kjellstrand, C. M., Simmons, R. L., Buselmeier, T. J., and Najarian, J. S.: Kidney: I. Recipient Selection, Medical Management and Dialysis, in J. S. Najarian and R. L. Simmons, (eds.), "Transplantation," p. 418, Lea & Febiger, Philadelphia, 1972.

Kohler, B.: The Prognosis after Nephrectomy: A Clinical Study of Early and Late Results, *Acta Chir Scand* **91** [*Suppl* 94]:1, 1944.

Leadbetter, G. W., Monaco, A. P., and Russell, P. S.: A Technique for Reconstruction of the Urinary Tract in Renal Transplantation, *Surg Gynecol Obstet,* **123:**839, 1966.

Linn, B. S., Portal, P., and Snyder, G. B.: Complementuria in Renal Transplantation, *Life Sci,* **6:**1945, 1967.

Lucas, Z. J., Palmer, J. M., Payne, R., Kountz, S. L., and Cohn, R. B.: Renal Allotransplantation in Humans: I. Systemic Immunosuppressive Therapy, *Arch Surg,* **100:**113, 1970.

Merkatz, I. R., Schwartz, G. H., David, D. S., Stenzel, K. H., Riggio, R. R., and Whitsell, J. C.: Resumption of Female Reproductive Function following Renal Transplantation, *JAMA,* **216:**1749, 1971.

Moberg, A. W., Gewurz, H., Simmons, R. L., and Najarian, J. S.: Desensitization to Horse Globulin before Immunosuppressive Treatment, *Lancet,* **2:**214, 1970.

Mohandas, A., and Chau, S. N.: Brain Death: A Clinical and Pathological Study, *J Neurosurg,* **35:**211, 1971.

Moore, T. C.: Effective Use of Isoniazid and an Antihistamine in Clinical Renal Transplantation, *Surg Gynecol Obstet,* **133:**75, 1971.

Murphy, G. P., Mirand, E. A., and Grace, J. T.: Erythropoietin Activity in Anephric or Renal Allotransplanted Man, *Ann Surg.* **170:**581, 1969.

Murray, J. E., Merrill, J. P., and Harrison, J. H.: Renal Homotransplantation in Identical Twins, *Surg Forum,* **6:**432, 1955.

Najarian, J. S., Simmons, R. L., Kjellstrand, C. M., Vernier, R., and Michaels, A.: Renal Transplantation in Infants and Children, *Ann Surg,* **174:**583, 1971.

Olsson, C. A., Mannick, J. A., Schmitt, G. W., Idelson, B. A., Williams, L. F., Lemann, J., Harrington, J. T., and Nabseth, D. C.: Nephrostomy in Renal Transplantation, *Am J Surg,* **121:**467, 1971.

Pasternack, A.: Fine Needle Aspiration Biopsy of Human Renal Homografts, *Lancet,* **2:**82, 1968.

Penn, I., Halgrimson, C. G., Ogden, D., and Starzl, T.: Use of Living Donors in Kidney Transplantation in Man, *Arch Surg,* **101:**226, 1970.

———, and Starzl, T. E.: Immunosuppression and Cancer, *Transplant Proc,* **5:**943, 1973.

Pierce, J. C., and Hume, D. M.: The Effect of Splenectomy on the Survival of First and Second Renal Homotransplants in Man, *Surg Gynecol Obstet,* **127:**1300, 1968.

Quinton, W. E., Dillard, P. H., Cole, I. J., and Scribner, B. H.: Eight Months Experience with Silastic-Teflon Bypass Cannulas, *Trans Am Soc Artif Intern Organs,* **8:**236, 1962.

Rapaport, F. T., McCluskey, R. T., Hanaoka, T., and Shimada, T.: Induction of Renal Disease with Antisera to Group A Streptococcal Membranes, *Transplant Proc,* **1:**981, 1969.

———, Markowitz, A. S., and McCluskey, R. T.: The Bacterial Induction of Homograft Sensitivity: III. Effects of Group A Streptococcal Membrane Antisera, *J Exp Med,* **129:**623, 1969.

Schwab, R. S., Potts, F., and Bonazzi, A.: EEG as an Aid in Determining Death in the Presence of Cardiac Activity (Ethical, Legal and Medical Aspects), *Electroencephalogr Clin Neurophysiol,* **15:**147, 1963.

Schwartz, R. S., and Dameshek, W.: Drug Induced Immunological Tolerance, *Nature (Lond),* **183:**1682, 1959.

Shillito, J., Jr.: The Organ Donor's Doctor: A New Role for the Neurosurgeon, *N Engl J Med,* **281:**1071, 1969.

Skinner, D. B., Newman, M. H., and Squire, R. A.: Preservation and Transplantation of Dog Organs Maintained In Vivo for 24 Hours by Mechanical Ventricular Assistance, *J Surg Res,* **10:**287, 1970.

Simmons, R. L., Kjellstrand, C. M., Buselmeier, T. J., and Najarian, J. S.: Renal Transplantation in High Risk Patients, *Arch Surg,* **103:**290, 1971.

———, ———, and Najarian, J. S.: Kidney: II. Technique, Complications, and Results, in J. S. Najarian and R. L. Simmons (eds.), "Transplantation," p. 445, Lea & Febiger, Philadelphia, 1972.

———, Ozerkis, A. J., and Hoehn, R. J.: Antiserum to Lymphocytes: Interactions with Chemical Immunosuppressants, *Science,* **160**:1127, 1968.

Smellie, W. A. B., Vinik, M., Freed, T. A., and Hume, D. M.: Pertrochanteric Venography in the Study of Human Renal Transplant Recipients, *Surg Gynecol Obstet,* **127**:777, 1968.

Starzl, T. E.: "Experience in Renal Transplantation," W. B. Saunders Company, Philadelphia, 1964.

————, Groth, C. G., Terasaki, P. I., Putnam, C. W., Brettschneider, L., and Marchioro, T. L.: Heterologous Antilymphocyte Globulin Histoincompatibility Matching, and Human Renal Homotransplantation. *Surg Gynecol Obstet,* **126**:1023, 1968.

————, Halgrimson, C. G., Penn, L., Martineau, G., Schroter, G., Amemiya, H., Putnam, C. W., and Groth, C. G.: Cyclophosphamide and Human Organ Transplantation, *Lancet,* **2**:70, 1971.

————, Porter, K. A., Andres, G., Halgrimson, C. G., Hurwitz, R., Giles, G., Terasaki, P. I., Penn, I., Schroter, G. T., Lilly, J., Starkie, S. J., and Putnam, C. W.: Long-Term Survival after Renal Transplantation in Humans (with Special Reference to Histocompatibility Matching, Thymectomy, Homograft Glomerulonephritis, Heterogous ALG, and Recipient Malignancy), *Ann Surg,* **172**:437, 1979.

Stewart, J. H., Johnson, J. R., Sharp, A. M., Sheil, A. G. R., Wyatt, K. M., and Johnston, J. M.: Successful Renal Allotransplantation in Presence of Lymphocytotoxic Antibodies: Importance of Preoperative Cross-Matching, *Lancet,* **1**:176, 1969.

Sutherland, D., Frech, R. S., Weil, R., Najarian, J. S., and Simmons, R. L.: The Bleeding Cecal Ulcer: Pathogenesis, Angiographic Diagnosis, and Nonoperative Control, *Surgery,* **71**:290, 1972.

Swales, J. D., and Evans, D. B.: Erythraemia in Renal Transplantation, *Br Med J,* **2**:80, 1969.

Tallent, M. B., Simmons, R. L., and Najarian, J. S.: Birth Defects in a Child of a Male Kidney Transplant Recipient, *JAMA,* **211**:1854, 1970.

Terasaki, P. J., Kreisler, M., and Mickey, M. R.: Presensitization and Kidney Transplant Failures: I, *Postgrad Med,* **47**:89, 1971.

Tunner, W. S., Goldsmith, E. I., and Whitesell, J. C.: Human Homotransplantation of Normal and Neoplastic Tissue from the Same Organ, *J Urol,* **105**:18, 1971.

Weil, R. III, Simmons, R. L., Tallent, M. B., Lillehei, R. C., Kjellstrand, C. M., and Najarian, J. S.: Prevention of Urological Complications after Kidney Transplantation, *Ann Surg,* **174**:154, 1971.

West, T. H., Turcotte, J. G., and Vander, A. J.: Plasma Renin Activity, Sodium Balance, and Hypertension in a Group of Renal Transplant Recipients, *J Lab Clin Med,* **73**:564, 1970.

Williams, G. M., dePlanque, B., Lower, R., and Hume, D. M.: Antibodies and Human Transplant Rejection, *Ann Surg,* **170**:603, 1969.

————, White, H. J., and Hume, D. M.: Factors Influencing the Long-Term Functional Success Rate of Human Renal Allografts, *Transplantation, Suppl.* **51**:837, 1967.

Yashphe, D. J.: Immunological Factors in Nonspecific Stimulation of Host Resistance to Syngeneic Tumors, *Isr J Med Sci,* **7**:90, 1971.

Zukoski, C. F., Lee, H. M., and Hume, D. M.: The Prolongation of Functional Survival of Canine Renal Homografts by 6-Mercaptopurine, *Surg Forum,* **11**:470, 1960.

Transplantation of Organs Other than Kidney, Liver, Lung, and Heart

Barnicot, N. A.: The Local Action of the Parathyroid and Other Tissues on Bone in Intracerebral Grafts, *J Anat (Lond)* **82**:233, 1948.

Bortin, M. M.: A Compendium of Reported Human Bone Marrow Transplants, *Transplantation,* **9**:571, 1970.

Brooks, J. R., and Levy, J.: Endocrine Transplantation, in F. T. Rapaport and J. Dausset (eds.), "Human Transplantation," p. 271, Grune & Stratton, Inc., New York, 1968.

Congdon, C. C.: Bone Marrow Transplantation: Research in Marrow Grafting Has Generated Extensive New Information for the Hematologist, *Science,* **171**:1116, 1971.

D'Amico, R. A.: Ophthalmologic Aspects of Transplantation, in F. T. Rapaport and J. Dausset (eds.), "Human Transplantation," p. 332, Grune & Stratton, Inc., New York, 1968.

Flosdorf, E., and Hyatt, G. W.: The Preservation of Bone Grafts by Freeze Drying, *Surgery,* **31**:716, 1952.

Gittes, R. F.: Endocrine Tissues, in J. S. Najarian and R. L. Simmons (eds.), "Transplantation," p. 698, Lea & Febiger, Philadelphia, 1972.

Hardy, J. D., and Langford, H. G.: Surgical Management of Cushing's Syndrome: Including Studies of Adrenal Autotransplants, Body Composition and Pseudotumor Cerebri, *Ann Surg,* **159**:711, 1964.

Harris, G. W., and Jacobsohn, D.: Functional Grafts of the Anterior Pituitary Glands, *Proc R Soc Lond [Biol],* **139**:263, 1952.

Harris, J. E., and Rathbun, W. B.: Ocular Tissues, in J. S. Najarian and R. L. Simmons (eds.), "Transplantation," p. 613, Lea & Febiger, Philadelphia, 1972.

Kelly, W. D., Lillehei, R. C., Merkel, F. K., Idezuki, Y., and Goetz, F.: Renal and Pancreatic Allotransplantation in the Treatment of Diabetic Nephropathy in Man, in J. Dausset, J. Hamburger, and G. Mathé (eds.), "Advance in Transplantation," The Williams & Wilkins Company, Baltimore, 1968.

Lance, E. M.: Bone and Cartilage, in J. S. Najarian and R. L. Simmons (eds.), "Transplantation," p. 655, Lea & Febiger, Philadelphia, 1972.

Lillehei, R. C., and Ruiz, J. O.: Pancreas, in J. S. Najarian and R. L. Simmons (eds.), "Transplantation," p. 627, Lea & Febiger, Philadelphia, 1972.

Malt, R. A., and Harris, W. H.: Replantation of Limbs, in J. S. Najarian and R. L. Simmons (eds.), "Transplantation," p. 711, Lea & Febiger, Philadelphia, 1972.

————, and McKhann, C. F.: Replantation of Severed Arms, *JAMA,* **189**:716, 1964.

Peacock, E. E., and Madden, J. W.: Human Composite Flexor Tendon Allografts, *Ann Surg,* **166**:624, 1967.

Taylor, A. C.: Rates of Freezing, Drying and Rehydration of Nerves, *J Cell Comp Physiol,* **25**:161, 1945.

Woodruff, M. F. A.: "The Transplantation of Tissues and Organs," Charles C Thomas, Publisher, Springfield, Ill., 1960.

Chapter 11

Anesthesia

by **Nicholas M. Greene**

General Considerations

General Anesthesia

Inhalation Anesthesia
    Nitrous Oxide
    Cyclopropane
    Diethyl Ether
    Halothane (Fluothane)
    Methoxyflurane (Penthrane)
    Other Inhalation Anesthetics
Intravenous Anesthesia
    Barbiturates
    Narcotics
    Relaxants

Conduction Anesthesia

Spinal anesthesia
Epidural anesthesia
Nerve Block

Premedication

GENERAL CONSIDERATIONS

No presently available anesthetic agent or technique is ideal. Because no anesthetic agent is perfect, each anesthesia represents physiologic and pharmacologic trespass and inherently entails a certain risk. The magnitude of the risk depends upon the anesthetic agent, the method by which it is administered, and the circumstances under which it is employed. In an individual case the risk may be greater or smaller, but it cannot be completely eliminated.

The matter of anesthetic risk is not merely academic. All valid studies quantifying anesthetic risk in terms of mortality rates have demonstrated a remarkably consistent anesthetic death rate which averages approximately 1 in 1,600. This figure is based on *all* types of operative anesthesia, from the most "minor" to the most major, and applies in teaching university hospitals as well as in more general patient populations. To provide still more perspective, approximately 15 million anesthetics are now administered annually in the United States. If the published figures of anesthetic death rates are assumed to apply throughout the country, then the annual number of deaths associated with anesthesia in the United States is in the neighborhood of 9,000.

This major public health problem is not widely appreciated for two reasons: First, because deaths associated with anesthesia occur on the average of once in every 1,600 cases, the individual surgeon or anesthetist may not encounter a death associated with anesthesia for considerable periods of time. For example, the average surgeon performing 400 operations each year may not encounter such a death for four years. This, combined with the vagaries of human memory and clinical impression, may lead to the impression that deaths associated with anesthesia rarely if ever occur. The second major reason that the number of deaths associated with anesthesia is not widely recognized is related to the fact that all such deaths are, by definition, iatrogenic. Because serious medicolegal problems are immediately introduced each time a death associated with an anesthetic occurs, conscious or subconscious factors may make it exceptionally difficult to obtain reliable statistics or to analyze objectively the causes of death.

Because of the magnitude of the risk involved, the patient's safety must always be the first and most important consideration in any discussion of surgical anesthesia. True patient safety based upon sound physiologic and pharmacologic principles is not synonymous with the ability to "get away with" a calculated risk a certain number of times.

Bearing in mind the primacy of patient safety and the fact that no anesthetic agent or technique is without its disadvantages and dangers, it may be said that the selection of anesthetic agents and techniques in an individual clinical case depends upon five factors:

1. The condition of the patient. The presence or absence of concurrent conditions such as a full stomach, coronary artery disease, or asthma may contraindicate certain anesthetics.

2. The physiologic and pharmacologic effects of the various anesthetic agents. It is this aspect of anesthetic management which will be emphasized in the present chapter, noting that these effects are not necessarily the result of the anesthetic agent itself. A major portion of the physiologic trespass associated with anesthesia is due to factors such as mechanical effects of the apparatus used to administer the anesthetic, changes in blood-gas tensions, changes in fluid and electrolyte balance resulting from blood loss, creation of a surgical third space, and administration of intravenous fluids.

3. The site and type of surgical procedure to be performed. The anesthetic requirements for inguinal herniorrhaphy are different from those for pneumonectomy. Failure to recognize that the anesthetic should be tailored to the type of operation has led to inaccurate and dangerous generalizations as to anesthetic selection based solely upon

the patient's condition and the pharmacologic effects of the anesthetic agent.

4. The experience, training, and background of the person who is to administer the anesthetic. Not all persons who can administer an anesthetic are necessarily equally qualified to administer all types of anesthetics. It is frequently advisable for an anesthetist to administer the type of anesthetic with which he has had the most experience, hence that in which he has the most confidence, rather than to administer on rare occasions an anesthetic which theoretically may have certain advantages but with which he has had little experience.

5. The skill, training, and requirements of the surgeon. The anesthetic requirements for an appendectomy by an experienced surgeon who will accomplish the entire operation in 20 minutes are markedly different from those for a surgeon who is less experienced and who may require an hour and a half of anesthesia.

The most frequent factor, other than surgical experience, influencing the choice of anesthetic insofar as the surgeon is concerned is whether he will use electrocautery or not. The advantages of electrocautery, frequently cited but rarely quantified, are decreased operating time and decreased blood loss. These advantages, indisputable in certain instances, have not been verified in many types of surgery. The disadvantages of electrocautery relate primarily to the fact that nonexplosive anesthetics are usually more depressant to the patient's cardiovascular system and usually produce more physiologic derangement than do explosive inhalation anesthetics. This is especially true when deep levels of anesthesia are necessary, as during intraabdominal operations. In infants, the mechanical equipment and dangers of overdosage associated with nonexplosive anesthetics often may result in greater risk to the patient than the use of flammable but straightforward anesthetics such as open-drop ether.

Selection of anesthetic agent and technique based upon the preceding five factors will result in maximal patient safety. Convenience, surgical or anesthetic, should not play a significant role in selecting anesthetic agents, especially convenience measured in terms of minutes saved during induction of anesthesia. Similarly, what is most pleasant for the patient or what is acceptable to the patient should not be a primary consideration in selection of anesthetic agent or technique. Patient acceptability and surgical or anesthetic convenience may coincide with selection of the anesthetic which is also safest for the patient, but this should be regarded as fortuitous rather than the goal of selection of anesthetic agent and technique.

GENERAL ANESTHESIA

General anesthesia may be produced by anesthetics which are directly injected into the blood via the intravenous route or by anesthetics which are absorbed into the blood from the alveoli following inhalation. The advantages and disadvantages of inhalation general anesthesia as opposed to intravenous anesthesia and the physiologic and pharmacologic effects of the two techniques are such

that it is best to discuss the two methods separately. These methods, however, do have two things in common, the risk of overdosage and the risk of inadequate ventilation. The vast majority of cardiac arrests, if not all cardiac arrests due to general anesthesia, result from one or both of these two factors. Avoidance of overdosage may prove difficult under clinical conditions, especially in the hands of a novice, for two reasons: First, individual variations of patients' responses to general anesthetics are so great that reliable dose/response relationships do not exist. General anesthetics cannot be administered in a predetermined dosage based on milligrams of anesthetic per kilogram of patient's body weight without running the risk of serious overdosage in some patients and inadequate depth of anesthesia in others. Second, evaluation of depth of anesthesia is neither easy nor precise but instead highly subjective, clinical signs varying not only with each general anesthetic but also with each patient. The only method of quantifying depth of anesthesia is by electroencephalography, a technique suitable for research purposes but impractical for general clinical use. Signs such as pupillary size, eye motion, and character of respirations, as described by Guedel, apply only to ether and then only under select circumstances. The signs of depth of anesthesia with the more widely used present-day anesthetics are less well defined. Many anesthetics are such potent respiratory depressants, even in barely anesthetic concentrations, that respirations become an inadequate guide to depth of surgical anesthesia. Pragmatically, overdosage, whether absolute or relative, can be said to exist when arterial hypotension or (less frequently) cardiac arrhythmias are produced by a general anesthetic and is best avoided by repeated measurements of blood pressure. Electrocardiographic monitoring is of limited value as an index of depth of anesthesia or, for that matter, as a guide to the overall condition of the patient. It gives no indication of blood pressure or the adequacy of cardiac output, and it provides little information that cannot usually be more readily achieved by palpation of the pulse. Also, it may distract the anesthetist from more important duties such as maintenance of adequate ventilation.

There are three principal causes of inadequate ventilation during general anesthesia: obstruction of the airway, pharmacologic interference with normal respiratory mechanisms, and anesthetically induced abnormalities of gas exchange between alveoli and pulmonary capillary blood. Obstruction may occur at any level in the airway, from pharynx to bronchi, and may be caused by anything from the tongue falling back into the pharynx to laryngospasm, bronchospasm, or aspiration of blood, gastric contents, secretions, or foreign bodies. Airway obstruction must immediately be treated by correction of the cause, whether by manipulation of the soft tissues of the upper airway (elevation of the chin or entire mandible), by insertion of artificial pharyngeal or endotracheal airways, or by endotracheal suctioning. If left untreated, obstruction results in hypoxia and hypercapnia, i.e., asphyxia. *General anesthesia is contraindicated unless a patent airway can be assured at all times.*

Pharmacologic causes of inadequate ventilation include

interference with the normal neural or muscular mechanisms of respiration. These, together with anesthetically induced inadequacies of respiratory gas exchange secondary to abnormal alveolar ventilation perfusion ratios, are included in the subsequent discussion of the individual anesthetic agents. It must be emphasized that pharmacologic derangements of respiration are often subtle and difficult to recognize although they are potentially as dangerous as, or more dangerous than, the more obvious forms of inadequate ventilation due to obstruction. They are especially insidious because the classic signs and symptoms of hypoxia and carbon dioxide retention are notoriously unreliable during clinical anesthesia. Respiratory rate, clinical estimates of tidal volume, blood pressure, pulse rate, and color of the skin are all inaccurate indices of potentially dangerous levels of hypoxia or hypercapnia in a patient who is under general anesthesia. The only method by which abnormal blood levels of oxygen or carbon dioxide can be verified is by measurement of the tensions (i.e., partial pressures) of these gases in *arterial* blood using special electrodes. Such techniques are of major research value and of increasing clinical usefulness but not yet practical for the continuous measurement of blood-gas tensions during routine clinical anesthesia. Because of the difficulties inherent in estimating the adequacy of pulmonary ventilation and because of the dangers of inadequate ventilation compared with only minor and rather hypothetic disadvantages of hyperventilation, it is better to overventilate patients artificially during general anesthesia than to permit possible underventilation to occur. Hyperventilation is readily accomplished by intermittent manual compression of the anesthesia reservoir bag. Special mechanical ventilators are not required. Neither is an endotracheal tube invariably required. Although this may prove necessary or desirable, endotracheal intubation does not guarantee adequate alveolar ventilation or even airway patency.

Inhalation Anesthesia

The principle advantage of inhalation anesthetics is controllable reversibility. As what enters via the lungs exits via the lungs, the rate at which the inhalation anesthetic exits can be as readily controlled as the rate at which it enters. Therefore, the administrator of an inhalation anesthetic can control its duration of action. This control does not follow administration by intravenous or other parenteral routes, as all intravenous anesthetics require detoxication or excretion by processes over which the anesthetist has no control. The recent demonstration that inhalation anesthetics are metabolized by hepatic microsomal enzymes is clinically of no significance in terms of the ability of the anesthetist to alter anesthetic concentrations within the patient. The only inhalation anesthetic whose metabolism significantly alters its duration of central nervous system depression is trichloroethylene (Trilene), an anesthetic infrequently employed in modern practice.

Aside from controlled reversibility and the ability to alter excitability of neuronal tissue, inhalation anesthetics have no pharmacologic properties in common. Their effects are too diverse and individual to allow generalization.

NITROUS OXIDE

Although a perfect anesthetic agent does not exist at the present time, nitrous oxide probably comes closer than any other agent to being an ideal anesthetic. It is completely nontoxic. It has no clinically significant effect on respiration, on the cardiovascular system, on metabolism, on renal function, or on hepatic function. In addition, it is nonexplosive. But it has a major disadvantage: its pharmacologic weakness. Administration of 80% nitrous oxide with 20% oxygen will produce analgesia, and if premedication has consisted of adequate doses of analgesics or hypnotics, the patient may be maintained in light levels of anesthesia. However, if premedication is inadequate or if the patient is especially robust and muscular, it is impossible to progress beyond the stage of delirium with nitrous oxide–oxygen alone. Maintenance of the analgesic state with nitrous oxide–oxygen without progression into the stage of delirium is clinically so difficult to accomplish for more than moments in the absence of other, more potent central nervous system depressants that the use of this agent alone for the production of predictable states of analgesia is limited. Increasing the percentage of nitrous oxide inspired above 80% will result in slightly deeper anesthesia only at the cost of producing hypoxia.

Despite its weakness, nitrous oxide is useful and widely used in combination with other drugs, chiefly as a powerful yet rapidly reversible analgesic agent to supplement other anesthetics. That nitrous oxide is, in itself, a good analgesic agent is demonstrated by the fact that the analgesia obtained by inhaling 20% nitrous oxide is approximately equal to the analgesia obtained with 10 mg of morphine. The difference between the analgesia produced by morphine and that produced by nitrous oxide is that the latter is not associated with respiratory or cardiovascular depression and is rapidly reversible. As an analgesic, nitrous oxide is so extensively employed to supplement intravenous anesthetics (e.g., thiopental, or Pentothal) that "Pentothal anesthesia" almost invariably means thiopental–nitrous oxide–oxygen anesthesia, in which case nitrous oxide, not thiopental, is the primary anesthetic agent. Because of the effectiveness of nitrous oxide, the total amount of thiopental may be decreased by one-half or more, with the result that the severe depression which would be observed if thiopental alone were administered is not observed when nitrous oxide also is administered. Because of the effectiveness of nitrous oxide as a nondepressant analgesic, its use in low concentrations has been suggested for the production of postoperative analgesia. The utility of nitrous oxide for this purpose is limited by the leukopenia which its chronic administration produces, an action which has been used in the palliation of leukemia.

Two clinical situations exist in which nitrous oxide may have unexpected and potentially undesirable effects. Both situations are due to the fact that nitrous oxide is more soluble than nitrogen in blood. The first of these, diffusion anoxia, may occur when a patient who has been equilibrated on 80% nitrous oxide–20% oxygen spontaneously starts to breathe room air (80% nitrogen in 20% oxygen). The blood solubility differences between nitrous oxide and nitrogen being such that at equal partial pressures approximately thirty times more nitrous oxide than nitrogen is dissolved, when the patient starts to inhale room air there will be thirty times greater diffusion of nitrous oxide out of the bloodstream than of nitrogen into the bloodstream at the alveolar level. The net result is an increase in gas volume within the alveoli. Since intraalveolar pressure equals ambient pressure, the increased gas volume displaces oxygen molecules from the alveoli, with resulting transient hypoxemia. The phenomenon of diffusion anoxia may be prevented either by administration of nitrous oxide in concentrations of less than 60% or by increasing alveolar oxygen tension above approximately 200 mm Hg at the conclusion of the anesthesia.

The second situation in which the solubility of nitrous oxide in blood may cause clinical difficulties is in patients who are having pneumoencephalograms performed or in patients who have intestinal obstructions. During pneumoencephalography, air injected into the ventricles rapidly equilibrates with the blood surrounding it. If the patient is anesthetized with nitrous oxide during the pneumoencephalography, the anesthetic enters the ventricular air bubble at a faster rate than the nitrogen exits from it, with the result that the volume of the air bubble tends to increase. Since the air bubble during pneumoencephalography is within the cranium, an increase in volume cannot occur, and increased pressure results. If nitrous oxide anesthesia is employed, the contrast gas injected into the subarachnoid space should be nitrous oxide or carbon dioxide rather than room air. Comparable changes in gas pockets take place during administration of nitrous oxide to a patient whose gastrointestinal tract is filled with air, as in intestinal obstruction, as well as in a patient suffering from pneumothorax. In both these instances pressure within the air pocket will not increase but volume will, with possible detrimental results.

During the administration of nitrous oxide–oxygen, the degree of oxygenation of the arterial blood cannot be accurately estimated merely by observing the flows of oxygen and nitrous oxide being delivered by the anesthesia machine. The reasons for this are twofold: First, when nitrous oxide–oxygen is administered at a time when respirations are controlled by intermittent positive pressure, a progressive and significant decrease in arterial oxygen tension can take place even though oxygen tension in the inspired air remains constant. Reasons for this are discussed in the section dealing with muscle relaxants. Second, following equilibration with the anesthetic gases, the concentration of oxygen in the inspired air during nitrous oxide–oxygen anesthesia on a semiclosed system is influenced by the amount of oxygen being metabolically consumed. For example, if a patient consumes 250 ml of oxygen per minute and is anesthetized on a semiclosed circuit into which 1 liter each of oxygen and nitrous oxide are flowing per minute, after equilibration the patient will not be inhaling 50% oxygen, because over the period of 1 minute he will consume 250 ml of the 1,000 ml of oxygen being delivered in that minute. He will therefore be inhal-

ing approximately 42% oxygen. The importance of the metabolic requirements for oxygen as a determinant of the concentration of oxygen in the inspired mixture on semiclosed systems is a function of the total flow of anesthetic gases. The 250 ml of oxygen being metabolized per minute has little significant effect if the total flow rate into the anesthesia circuit is 8 liters per minute, but the same 250 ml will have a major effect if the total flow rate into the semiclosed system is only 1 liter per minute, e.g., 500 ml each of nitrous oxide and oxygen per minute. The concentration of oxygen in the inspired air when nitrous oxide is being administered is related not only to the percentage of oxygen being delivered to the anesthesia circuit but also to the total flow rates at which these gases are being delivered.

CYCLOPROPANE

Cyclopropane (C_3H_6) is an explosive anesthetic which produces surgical levels of anesthesia with 20 to 25 vol % of the agent in the inspired air, at which time there are approximately 16 to 20 mg cyclopropane per 100 ml of arterial blood. The noteworthy physiologic changes produced by cyclopropane may be divided into six categories: respiration, sympathetic tone, blood pressure, myocardial depression, myocardial irritability, and renal function.

Respiration is invariably depressed when cyclopropane is administered in concentrations adequate to provide surgical anesthesia. The depression is the result of an increased threshold of response of the respiratory center to carbon dioxide. Partly because the patient is inhaling a high concentration of oxygen, this respiratory depression is usually not great enough to result in anoxia or even hypoxia, but carbon dioxide may accumulate. Respiratory acidosis in the presence of normal oxygenation occurs not only during cyclopropane anesthesia but in any situation in which there is a moderate decrease in effective alveolar ventilation, as following the administration of narcotics or in patients with mild emphysema. In the absence of mechanical mixing, the rate of diffusion of gaseous molecules in a mixture of gases depends upon the physical properties of the gases and is inversely proportional to the square root of the molecular weights of the gases. Because the molecular weight of oxygen is less than that of carbon dioxide, oxygen diffuses approximately 20 percent faster in a mixture of gases in the absence of physical mixing, thus allowing maintenance of normal oxygen tensions at the alveolar-capillary interface but also allowing carbon dioxide to accumulate. The effect of cyclopropane on ventilation is so pronounced that surgical levels of anesthesia produced with this anesthetic are by definition accompanied by respiratory acidosis unless the patient is artificially hyperventilated. Unless respiratory acidosis is treated by artificial ventilation during the anesthesia, a state of severe hypotension may develop in the patient immediately after the operation. This so-called "cyclopropane shock" is characterized by a marked drop in systolic blood pressure and a bradycardia progressing in some cases to arrhythmia, including ventricular fibrillation.

Sympathetic tone is significantly increased by anesthetic concentrations of cyclopropane. This has been hypothesized to be due to depression of the inhibitory portion of the vasomotor center in the brainstem, resulting in a relative overactivity of the vasoexcitatory portion of the vasomotor center. The centrally induced increased sympathetic nervous system activity results in increased release of epinephrine from the adrenal medullae and of norepinephrine from postganglionic sympathetic sites. Consequently, cyclopropane anesthesia is associated with increased blood levels of catecholamines. These increased blood levels of epinephrine and norepinephrine may further accentuate the sympathetic response to cyclopropane reaching tissues hematogenously. For example, in an intact extremity the vasoconstriction resulting from the increased sympathetic activity during cyclopropane anesthesia is only partially reversed by sympathetic denervation. In the denervated state, the blood vessels of the extremity are still responding to the vasoconstrictors which are released from the rest of the body and hematogenously borne to the still functional effector organs in the denervated extremity.

Arterial blood pressure usually tends to rise during cyclopropane anesthesia because of the increased sympathetic activity, which results in contraction of smooth muscle on the arterial side of the circulation, and consequent increase in total peripheral vascular resistance. The elevation of arterial blood pressure is due primarily to the effect of the cyclopropane on the sympathetic nervous system and not to a respiratory acidosis. If respiratory acidosis is allowed to develop, the arterial blood pressure may be further elevated because of carbon dioxide retention, but arterial hypertension during cyclopropane administration is not a reliable indication of respiratory acidosis.

Cyclopropane, in common with most general anesthetic agents, exerts a negative inotropic effect on ventricular myocardial muscle. The decreased force of ventricular contraction may be readily demonstrated experimentally in a heart-lung preparation or in the presence of a total sympathetic block. With an intact sympathetic nervous system, the negative inotropism of cyclopropane is largely offset by the positive inotropic effect of the reflexly produced increase in sympathetic activity. The compensation is incomplete, however, and surgical levels of cyclopropane anesthesia in human beings are usually associated with a decrease in cardiac output. This in turn tends to counteract the effect of the increased peripheral vascular resistance on mean arterial blood pressure; i.e., the rise in blood pressure is not so great as would be expected if the peripheral vascular resistance increased to the same extent in the presence of a normal cardiac output.

The ability of cyclopropane to increase sympathetic nervous system activity and so maintain blood pressure has been considered one of the major advantages of this anesthetic agent, especially for the poor-risk patient. On the other hand, it has been suggested that the increased peripheral resistance associated with decreased cardiac output during cyclopropane may result in decreased tissue blood flow even though arterial blood pressure is maintained. The possibility that cyclopropane anesthesia may be associated with vasoconstriction sufficient to reduce tissue blood flow is supported by the observation that arterial lactate/pyruvate ratios and arterial excess-lactate

levels increase during cyclopropane anesthesia. However, proof of decreases in tissue oxygenation and demonstration of the site or sites in which this may occur have yet to be provided. This theoretical disadvantage of cyclopropane has not been shown to be of clinical significance, especially under the acute conditions prevailing in the operating room.

Cyclopropane increases the irritability of the ventricular myocardium, as well as decreasing the force of ventricular contraction. Increased ventricular irritability is clinically manifested by arrhythmias which can occur during cyclopropane administration. Premature ventricular contractions may progress to ventricular tachycardia or ventricular fibrillation. The effect of cyclopropane on the threshold of irritability of the ventricles is partly inherent in the agent itself, but it is also related to the increased sympathetic nervous system activity produced by the anesthetic agent. If cyclopropane anesthesia is associated with additional increases in sympathetic activity, the result can be dangerous ventricular arrhythmias. Therefore, any situation which increases further the blood levels of catecholamines during cyclopropane administration tends to make the anesthesia more dangerous. For these reasons, the administration of epinephrine, norepinephrine, or other vasopressors which have comparable effects on ventricular irritability is contraindicated during cyclopropane anesthesia. Hypoxia or respiratory acidosis also become more dangerous during cyclopropane anesthesia because they are associated with increased blood levels of catecholamines. In fact, the relation between adequate ventilation and ventricular arrhythmias during cyclopropane anesthesia is such that in clinical practice the most frequent causes of arrhythmias during such anesthesia are either hypoxia or carbon dioxide retention. For this reason, safe cyclopropane is synonymous with adequate ventilation. Because cyclopropane is such a potent respiratory depressant, safe surgical cyclopropane anesthesia becomes synonymous with controlled-respiration anesthesia. Cyclopropane anesthesia is contraindicated unless adequate alveolar ventilation and oxygenation can be assured. Parenthetically, since the effects of cyclopropane on myocardial irritability primarily involve the ventricles, cyclopropane is not necessarily contraindicated in the presence of arrhythmias of atrial origin. In fact, cyclopropane is widely employed as an anesthetic for mitral valvulotomies in patients who have atrial fibrillation, but it should be used cautiously if at all in patients who have ventricular arrhythmias or foci of ventricular ectopic beats.

Cyclopropane, like most other general anesthetics, decreases renal blood flow, glomerular filtration, and urinary output. With cyclopropane, this is due primarily to afferent arteriolar vasoconstriction, the filtration fraction remaining constant. The afferent arterial vasoconstriction is primarily a manifestation of the generalized increased sympathetic nervous system activity during this type of anesthesia. Evidence suggests that cyclopropane anesthesia is also associated with increased output of antidiuretic hormone, which further alters urinary output. The effects of cyclopropane on renal function may be further accentuated by surgical procedures themselves and by changes in fluid and electrolyte balance associated with the anesthetic state. The loss of fluid and electrolytes from the vascular space to the surgical third space, losses by gastrointestinal routes, and disturbance of blood osmolarity and electrolyte balance by the administration of fluids other than physiologic electrolyte solutions (especially 5% dextrose and water) all contribute further to the derangements of renal function which may be produced by the anesthetic agent.

DIETHYL ETHER

Ether (CH_3—CH_2—O—CH_2—CH_3) produces surgical levels of anesthesia with concentrations of approximately 2 vol % in the inspired air, corresponding levels in arterial blood being approximately 100 mg/100 ml. Recent innovations notwithstanding, ether remains a highly useful though often poorly appreciated anesthetic agent. Its primary advantage is its safety. This is based, first, on the fact that respiration is not depressed when surgical levels of anesthesia are present. Second, ether, if inadvertently administered in overdosage, produces respiratory arrest before cardiovascular collapse. Unlike the situation with many other general anesthetics, inadvertent ether overdosage may be corrected by artificial respiration. This is not possible with anesthetics in which cardiac arrest has occurred simultaneously with or preceding the respiratory arrest, in which case artificial ventilation must be associated with cardiac massage.

The disadvantages of ether are threefold: First, it is explosive. Second, it requires more skill for smooth clinical administration than do many inhalation anesthetics. Third, it has a series of disadvantages which may best be classified as "aesthetic." These include its unpleasant odor and its reputed tendency to produce nausea and vomiting. Actually, the incidence of nausea and vomiting following ether anesthesia is no greater than that following other anesthetic agents when comparable types of surgical procedures are performed and when comparable pre- and postoperative management is employed (especially in regard to narcotic administration). The pharmacologic advantages inherent in ether in terms of patient safety frequently outweigh its disadvantages, especially in the hands of the occasional or neophyte anesthetist. In pediatric cases ether anesthesia may obviate the complications associated with large and complicated mechanical apparatuses.

The pharmacology of ether may conveniently be considered according to its action in five areas: respiration, metabolism, cardiovascular function, adrenocortical function, and skeletal muscle function. Ether is the only general anesthetic agent which, when administered in concentrations adequate to produce surgical levels of anesthesia, is associated with spontaneous pulmonary ventilation adequate to maintain normal oxygenation and normal carbon dioxide elimination. Inadequate ventilation can occur during ether anesthesia if the anesthesia is unnecessarily deep, if airway obstruction is allowed to occur, or if a mechanically deficient anesthesia apparatus is used. The ability to maintain normal oxygenation is further accentuated by the fact that ether is potent enough to provide surgical anesthesia when inhaled in concentrations of less than 4%,

thereby allowing 96% oxygen to be administered. Therefore, during uncomplicated ether anesthesia, normal arterial and alveolar carbon dioxide tensions are to be expected. Carbon dioxide content of blood may change during ether anesthesia, not as a reflection of change in alveolar ventilation, but rather as a result of metabolic alterations.

The metabolic effects of ether anesthesia include a mild degree of metabolic acidosis, due primarily to an increase in blood levels of organic acids, notably lactate and pyruvate. This increase in fixed acids is mild (less than 5 mEq/L) and of doubtful clinical significance. The same increase in fixed acids may be observed in normal unanesthetized subjects in the course of their normal daily activities. The metabolic effects of ether anesthesia also include a hyperglycemia. The etiology of this is complex, including both increased rates of glucose production and decreased rates of glucose transport, utilization, and renal excretion. The effects of ether on acid-base balance and on blood glucose levels has led to the oft-repeated statement that ether is contraindicated in diabetic patients. Actually, ether is not necessarily contraindicated in the diabetic. The anesthetic management of the diabetic includes three objectives: preoperative control of the diabetes; conservative intraoperative management aimed at preventing either hypoglycemia or acidosis but not necessarily preventing glucosuria; and return of the patient to oral feedings and his usual insulin intake as soon as possible postoperatively.

Ether in concentrations adequate to provide surgical anesthesia produces either no change in cardiac output or an increase. The increase in cardiac output occurs despite the fact that ether is a direct myocardial depressant. This effect of ether is offset by the fact that ether, like cyclopropane, causes an increase in sympathetic nervous system activity. Also like cyclopropane, this increased sympathetic activity is centrally mediated, probably by a direct effect on the vasomotor center. In man, the increase in catecholamine levels associated with ether anesthesia is somewhat less pronounced than with cyclopropane anesthesia. This coincides with the fact that peripheral vascular resistance during ether anesthesia rarely increases and actually may decrease, because the direct depressant effect of ether on peripheral vascular smooth musculature offsets to some extent the vasoconstriction which otherwise would be expected to follow the increased sympathetic activity. The failure of peripheral vasoconstriction to occur or, in certain instances, the appearance of peripheral vasodilatation results in either no significant change in mean arterial blood pressure or a decrease during clinical anesthesia, despite the fact that cardiac output may be moderately increased.

Because ether is such a potent direct depressant on the cardiovascular system, its safety under clinical conditions is related to the integrity of the sympathetic nervous system. In the presence of a morphologically or pharmacologically impaired sympathetic nervous system, ether anesthesia is associated with prompt appearance of severe degrees of arterial hypotension, including cardiac arrest. Causes of impaired sympathetic nervous system activity include drugs such as reserpine which deplete tissue stores of catecholamines, antihypertensive drugs which either block ganglionic transmission within the sympathetic nervous system or alter the reactivity of the effector organs, and centrally acting drugs which depress the activity of hypothalamic autonomic centers.

In the absence of adequate adrenocortical function, ether anesthesia can be associated with acute and severe hypotension, as can other general anesthetic agents. The cause of the arterial hypotension during general anesthesia in patients with adrenocortical depression remains obscure but is probably related to the fact that catecholamines (and hence a functionally effective sympathetic nervous system) require adrenal corticosteroids as substrates. Because normal adrenocortical function is necessary for normal cardiovascular reactions during general anesthesia, it has been suggested that patients whose corticosteroid treatments have been discontinued prior to anesthesia and operation can develop arterial hypotension so readily that prophylactic corticosteroids should be administered. Although arterial hypotension during general anesthesia due to adrenocortical hypofunction secondary to previous prolonged steroid administration has been recorded, the incidence is extremely low. The prophylactic administration of steroids in large amounts to all patients who have had prior steroid therapy entails administration to many persons for whom it is not necessary and also results in further depression of borderline adrenocortical function. Since hydrocortisone for intravenous administration is readily available and can reverse states of adrenal hypofunction within minutes, it is no longer regarded as necessary or desirable to administer prophylactic steroids to these patients. Instead, hydrocortisone should be on hand for rapid administration when and if arterial hypotension which might be ascribed to this cause develops. Patients who have been given steroids chronically and who are still being maintained on this therapy at the time of surgical procedures and anesthesia should be kept on their maintenance doses, with conversion to parenteral administration if necessary. These patients often will not need increased amounts of steroids, but if they do, intravenous hydrocortisone may achieve a rapid therapeutic effect.

The depression of skeletal muscle function by ether is characterized by pronounced muscular relaxation accompanying surgical levels of ether anesthesia. No other general anesthetic agent is associated with equal surgical relaxation, a degree of which can be obtained without simultaneous hypotension or respiratory inadequacy. This effect was originally described as being primarily curare-like, with blocking at the myoneural junction. The present consensus is that the effect of ether on skeletal muscle tone probably involves several factors, including central synaptic depression, a complex competition at motor end-plate receptor sites, and perhaps a direct negative inotropic effect on muscle membranes.

HALOTHANE (FLUOTHANE)

Halothane (CF_3—CHBr—Cl) is an extremely potent inhalation anesthetic. Surgical anesthesia is maintained with concentrations in the inspired air of approximately 0.7 to 1.0 vol %, corresponding to arterial blood levels of 15 to 20 mg/100 ml. The advantages of halothane are that it is nonexplosive, that it is so potent that very high concentrations of oxygen (over 98%) may be administered with it, that it is rapid in onset, and that it is not unpleasant for the patient to inhale. The major disadvantages are that it is so potent that it can be administered only by experienced persons employing accurately calibrated vaporizers so that the concentration of halothane is always known and that it is frequently associated with arterial hypotension when administered in concentrations adequate to produce surgical anesthesia.

The potency of halothane is both an advantage and a disadvantage. The concentration required for maintenance of surgical anesthesia is approximately 0.7%, while the toxic concentration is approximately 1.5%. This narrow range of safe concentration necessitates not only special vaporizers but also placement of these vaporizers outside the anesthetic circuit to prevent accumulation within the anesthesia circuit. In clinical practice the advantage inherent in the high concentrations of oxygen which may be administered with halothane is offset by its wide use and, in some areas, routine combination with nitrous oxide-oxygen. The rationale behind combining an extremely potent anesthetic such as halothane with a weak anesthetic such as nitrous oxide is that the undesirable effects of halothane (e.g., arterial hypotension) may be avoided by the decrease in halothane concentration required to produce anesthesia following addition of nitrous oxide. Measurements of the effect of nitrous oxide on the concentration of halothane required to produce anesthesia indicate that 70 to 75% nitrous oxide in the inhaled air decreases the required concentration of halothane by 61%. Although the use of nitrous oxide to decrease halothane concentration does decrease the incidence of arterial hypotension, it does so at the cost of decreasing arterial oxygen tensions below those present when halothane is administered with 100% oxygen. Whether the benefit of nitrous oxide in decreasing halothane concentrations (and so diminishing the incidence of hypotension) is always offset by decreased oxygen tensions in arterial blood remains unclear. In terms of rate of oxygen delivery to the periphery, the decreases in cardiac output with halothane–100% oxygen mixtures might be less deleterious than when halothane is employed with 25 to 30% oxygen.

The hypotensive effect of halothane remains to be completely explained but probably involves several simultaneously operative factors. Central depression of the vasomotor center combined with a decrease in the force of myocardial contraction and impairment of ganglionic transmission produces both a decrease in cardiac output and a decrease in peripheral vascular resistance. Unlike cyclopropane and ether, the negative inotropism of halothane is not compensated by a reflex increase in sympathetic nervous system activity. Like cyclopropane, however, halothane increases the sensitivity of ventricular pacemakers. Thus, the use of epinephrine during halothane administration is generally contraindicated because of the danger of ventricular arrhythmias, including ventricular fibrillation. However, small amounts of epinephrine may be used, especially if adequate ventilation is provided and if the level of anesthesia is not too deep. If epinephrine is used, its risk should be appreciated, and it should be administered in small, accurately measured amounts.

Because halothane is a highly halogenated hydrocarbon, the possibility that it is a hepatotoxin has received considerable attention. Objective data remain difficult to obtain. Much of the literature on the subject, including numerous case reports, fail to establish cause-and-effect relationships and often further confuse the issue. Furthermore, most articles fail to deal with the fundamental question: What is the safety of halothane compared to other anesthetics? However, three points have become established concerning halothane and the liver: First, the massive National Halothane Study conclusively demonstrated that the frequency of postoperative hepatic dysfunction not related to shock, sepsis, hepatitis, etc., is no greater following halothane than it is following any other anesthetic, and may be even less. Second, otherwise inexplicable hepatic dysfunction following halothane is rare, occurring at most about once in 8,000 to 10,000 anesthesias, and not every case is fatal. Third, the rare appearance of otherwise unexplainable postoperative hepatic dysfunction following halothane probably represents a sensitization phenomenon, not hepatotoxicity.

Halothane does not predictably and replicably produce hepatic damage in man or experimental animals in the dose-related manner of carbon tetrachloride, for example. In human beings, halothane is associated with hepatic damage more frequently following repeated exposures than after a single exposure, although this can occur following an initial exposure. The hepatic reaction is often preceded by unexplained fever and accompanied by eosinophilia. It occurs more often in females than in males, more often in adults than in children. These characteristics suggest a sensitization reaction, substantiated beyond all doubt by the report from Klatskin and Kimberg of brief exposure under controlled conditions of a patient previously sensitized to halothane to subanesthetic concentrations of the anesthetic resulting in prompt and dramatic onset of liver damage. The in vivo demonstration of human sensitization has been further supported by the finding of Paronetto and Popper that halothane stimulates ^{3}H-thymidine uptake in lymphocytes of patients sensitized to halothane.

The occasional adverse response of the liver has been ascribed to the metabolism of as much as 20% of absorbed halothane in the liver, the resulting metabolites possibly producing hepatic damage either directly as hepatotoxins or indirectly by a sensitization reaction. To date, however, no pharmacologic, biochemical, or clinical data are available to prove this association. Most importantly, the safety of halothane as a clinical anesthetic cannot be judged solely by the incidence of associated hepatic damage. Substitution of another anesthetic for halothane may introduce risks greater than that of hepatitis. To replace halothane, with its low incidence of associated hepatitis, with an anesthetic associated with an incidence of ventricular fibrillation of 1 in 2,500 obviously accomplishes little in terms of overall patient safety; yet this is frequently advocated.

Therapeutic concentrations of halothane, like the majority of general anesthetics, decrease the sensitivity of the respiratory center to carbon dioxide. Recognition of this and the use of assisted or controlled respiration will circumvent this respiratory acidosis.

Finally, halothane is a potent depressant of uterine musculature. This has been used to provide anesthesia for relaxing contraction rings and for performing internal versions. On the other hand, the uterine-relaxing effect of halothane contraindicates its use for vaginal deliveries and cesarean sections by all but the most skilled physicians.

METHOXYFLURANE (PENTHRANE)

Methoxyflurane ($CHCl_2$—CF_2—O—CH_3), unlike halothane, is an ether but like halothane is highly halogenated and nonexplosive. Its anesthetic concentration in the inhaled air is approximately 0.7 vol %. The effect of methoxyflurane on the cardiovascular system is comparable to that of halothane, with perhaps a slightly decreased incidence and severity of arterial hypotension during surgical levels of anesthesia. Methoxyflurane and halothane differ in that there is no epinephrine hypersensitivity during methoxyflurane anesthesia.

Methoxyflurane is extremely soluble in lipids, as are all inhalation anesthetics. In methoxyflurane, however, the water-fat partition coefficient is so unusually high (approximately 1:800) that recovery of full consciousness, especially after long anesthesia, may be slow. The avoidance of abrupt and immediate return to full consciousness within moments after the end of the operation (as, for example, following cyclopropane) may be advantageous in certain circumstances. Such anesthetically induced analgesia makes the use of narcotics in the immediate postoperative period unnecessary.

One of the more striking properties of methoxyflurane is its low vapor pressure. Unlike ether, halothane, and the majority of other liquid anesthetics, it is not rapidly vaporized at room temperature, which constitutes both a major advantage and a minor disadvantage. The advantage is that inadvertent overdosage is unlikely, especially during the induction of anesthesia. Because of the low vapor pressure, however, induction of anesthesia with methoxyflurane alone can be relatively slow. This minor disadvantage can be offset by the judicious use of thiopental, cyclopropane, or other rapidly acting anesthetics to induce anesthesia prior to the administration of methoxyflurane.

High-output renal failure has been described after methoxyflurane anesthesia. The frequency of occurrence is related to duration of anesthesia and to patient obesity, which suggests that a dose-related response rather than a sensitization phenomenon is involved, although hepatic sensitization to methoxyflurane does occur. The renal toxicity of methoxyflurane probably results from the metabolism of the anesthetic itself, particularly the release of inorganic fluoride ions. Renal failure can be avoided by limiting the duration of administration and keeping the concentration as low as feasible.

OTHER INHALATION ANESTHETICS

In addition to older inhalation anesthetics of proved but limited clinical usefulness (divinyl ether, ethylene, trichloroethylene), today's anesthetist has available a number of compounds recently introduced. The result of systematic review of anesthetic activity in large series of hydrocarbons, the newer agents characteristically are halogenated ethers designed to have the advantages but not the disadvantages, including explosiveness, of diethyl ether while avoiding the histotoxicity and cardiovascular effects of halogenated agents such as chloroform. This felicitous pharmacologic goal has yet to be completely achieved. Fluroxene (Fluoromar) and ethylvinyl ether (Vinamar) are halogenated ethers which have been used long enough to assure that they possess no advantages over other inhalation anesthetics conspicuous enough to justify widespread popularity. Enflurane (Ethrane), another halogenated ether, has enjoyed a flurry of attention, but its association with abnormal electroencephalographic patterns has limited the enthusiasm of most clinicians. The recently introduced Forane is a halogenated ether with potential great enough to warrant thorough clinical evaluation. Only time will tell whether Forane is a true pharmacologic advance or just another "also-ran."

Intravenous Anesthesia

The primary advantage of intravenous anesthetics is convenience for the anesthetist and agreeableness for the patient. Convenience for the anesthetist consists of the rapid production of unconsciousness without the problems inherent in the somewhat longer and certainly more exacting induction of anesthesia by inhalation techniques. From the patient's point of view, the rapid onset of unconsciousness without exposure to odorous vapors and without the claustrophobic feeling of a mask applied to the face is a major advantage.

BARBITURATES

The intravenous agents most frequently used to produce surgical anesthesia are thiobarbiturates. Their popularity is based on the fact that they are "ultra-short-acting" barbiturates, i.e., rapid in onset and short in duration. Their pharmacologic actions, using thiopental (Pentothal) as a prototype, may be considered according to the cause of their "ultrashort action," with a brief comparison of their effects with those of inhalation anesthetics.

The rapid onset and apparently short duration of action of thiobarbiturates is a function primarily of increased lipoid solubility associated with the substitution of a sulfur atom for the oxygen atom in the barbituric acid ring. Thiopental (Pentothal) is structurally similar to pentobarbital (Nembutal), except that a sulfur atom has been substituted for the oxygen atom in the latter. The increased lipoid solubility, plus a pK which makes thiopental only slightly dissociated at a pH of 7.40, cause the rapid onset of action. The rate at which drugs cross the so-called blood-brain barrier is directly related to their lipoid solubility and inversely related to their degree of ionization.

These properties of thiopental combined with high cerebral blood flow result not only in an immediate onset of action (one circulation time) but also in an extremely short duration of action. Because the central nervous system has such a high flow compared to other areas of the body, more thiopental is delivered to it; this combined with high lipoid solubility produces a higher concentration in the central nervous system than elsewhere in the body immediately after administration of a single dose. With the passage of time other areas of the body with lesser blood flows gradually receive the barbiturate. In lean body mass, represented primarily by skeletal muscle, a concentration of thiopental develops after peak central nervous system concentrations have been achieved and in so doing produces a decrease in concentration of thiopental within the central nervous system. This hemodynamic redistribution of thiopental following a single intravenous injection is later followed by further redistribution to the areas of the body with the least blood flow, namely, adipose tissue. The buildup of thiopental in fatty depots throughout the body is relatively slow because of the low blood flow, but as time goes on the concentration in these areas becomes significant because of thiopental's high lipoid solubility in such tissues. As a result of this redistribution there is a relatively rapid reversal of the high central nervous system concentration following a single intravenous injection, and consciousness rapidly returns toward normal. This apparently ultrashort duration of action results not from a high rate of metabolism or excretion but from the dynamics of uptake and redistribution. The same sequence of events takes place, but to a less pronounced degree, following repeated intravenous injections of small amounts of the drug. The redistribution of thiopental within the body results in a regression of the state of central nervous system depression but does not result in its complete reversal until all the barbiturate has been metabolized or excreted.

The disadvantages of intravenous anesthetics are considerable. They are less rapidly and readily reversible than inhalation anesthetics. This is especially important when anesthesia is being induced by inexperienced personnel. The convenience of intravenous anesthetics to the anesthetist is also a disadvantage in that they can be administered by anyone skillful enough to perform a venopuncture.

The pharmacologic properties of thiopental are qualitatively comparable to those previously outlined for inhalation anesthetics, but with the additional disadvantage that when administered in equianesthetic doses thiopental is more depressant than true inhalation anesthetics. Thus thiopental is a cardiovascular and respiratory depressant. As a cardiovascular depressant, it acts directly on the myocardium to decrease the force of ventricular contraction. In addition it causes peripheral vasodilatation. Unlike cyclopropane or ether, but like halothane, thiopental is unassociated with any reflex increase in sympathetic tone to compensate for the cardiovascular depression. The hypotension which may accompany thiopental administration may be extreme, especially in patients in or bordering on oligemic shock. But the hypotension of thiopental does not have the saving grace of being associated with a state of true surgical anesthesia, as is usual with an agent such as halothane. The respiratory depression of thiopental resulting in an elevated threshold response of the respiratory center to carbon dioxide is unassociated with the production of a truly anesthetic state and so is of completely different clinical significance from that produced by, for example, cyclopropane.

Another major disadvantage of thiopental is that its depressant effects last longer than those observed with inhalation anesthetics. For example, the respiratory depression with cyclopropane is rapidly and completely reversed moments after its administration has been terminated, while the effects of intravenous anesthetics such as thiopental may linger on for hours. The complete metabolism or excretion of thiopental occurs at an extremely slow rate. Thus, although the greater part of the thiopental-induced anesthesia may be reversed within moments following a single injection, a long-lasting and subclinical degree of central nervous system depression may persist for many hours until the barbiturate has been metabolized in the liver and removed not only from the brain but also from the lean body mass and the fatty depots. The prolonged but subtle central nervous system depression following thiopental anesthesia is exemplified by the electroencephalographic changes, which may be detected for 18 hours following a brief period of thiopental anesthesia.

Thiobarbiturates today are mainly used to supplement other relatively weak anesthetics such as nitrous oxide or to induce general anesthesia prior to the administration of other more potent anesthetics such as ether or cyclopropane. When employed as a means of inducing general anesthesia, thiobarbiturates are best administered in "sleep" or hypnotic doses of 150 to 200 mg/70 kg of body weight and not in anesthetic doses (500 to 600 mg). Thiopental is contraindicated (as is any general anesthetic) in the presence of a full stomach or in other situations in which the patency of the patient's airway cannot be assured at all times.

NARCOTICS

Narcotics are not anesthetics. Nevertheless they are employed frequently and advantageously enough as adjuncts to anesthesia to warrant discussion in this chapter. Narcotics are primarily used in two situations: during general anesthesia produced by weak anesthetics such as nitrous oxide to provide more intense analgesia and during conduction anesthesia to provide relief of pain or discomfort. In such instances narcotics should be administered only intravenously. Intramuscular and subcutaneous injections are so slowly and erratically absorbed with such unpredictable onset and intensity of action that administration by such routes should be limited to premedication. When administered intravenously, narcotics must be given in repeated small doses rather than in a single therapeutic dose, to prevent development of transient dangerously high blood and brain levels.

The main disadvantage of narcotics as adjuvants to anesthesia is that some degree of respiratory depression and cardiovascular depression is inevitably produced whenever narcotics are employed in therapeutic amounts. As there is no significant difference in the degree of depression caused by the different narcotics *when administered in equianalgesic dosages,* the particular narcotic employed is not so important as its dosage. Meperidine (Demerol) has no advantage, for example, compared to morphine when the two are administered in equianalgesic dosages (100 mg of Demerol results in analgesia equivalent to that induced by 10 mg of morphine). Attempts to increase the usefulness of narcotics during anesthesia by administration of narcotic antagonists in the belief that respiratory depression will be alleviated without affecting analgesia have proved futile.

A frequent anesthetic use of narcotics involves induction of unconsciousness with a thiobarbiturate, following which analgesia is maintained during surgery with nitrous oxide and intermittent doses of narcotics, and skeletal muscles are relaxed with a relaxant such as curare. At the conclusion of surgery, the relaxant is pharmacologically reversed, as is the narcotic in certain instances. More accurately referred to as analgesia rather than anesthesia, this technique requires that the anesthetist successfully avoid the Charybdis of prolonged postoperative depression and the substantial Scylla of analgesia inadequate to prevent the patient from regaining awareness when total paralysis prevents him from signaling his distress. A variation of this technique uses Innovar in place of the narcotic. Innovar combines a hypnotic depressant, droperidol (Inapsine), with a highly potent analgesic, fentanyl (Sublimaze), in a ratio of 50:1. In common with all commercial preparations of two or more drugs with different actions, use of Innovar assumes that whenever sedation is required, a narcotic is required and vice versa and that both are always needed in the same arbitrarily determined proportions. This may be true much of the time but scarcely all the time. Techniques based on analgesia with paralysis are not for the novice. In experienced hands they may have advantages, but they always have the risks and limitations inherent in polypharmacy.

A completely different anesthetic use of narcotics involves their administration in amounts large enough to produce true anesthesia. Morphine is especially useful in this regard when given in doses of 2 to 3 mg/kg during cardiac surgery requiring cardiopulmonary bypass. Use of morphine in this manner is predicated on the assumption that respirations will be continuously controlled via an endotracheal tube in the immediate postoperative period, which is of considerable benefit to many cardiac patients.

Narcotics also are used during conduction anesthesia, whether spinal, epidural, or nerve block, either to supplement inadequate sensory blocking or to relieve patient discomfort if the conduction anesthesia wears off before the operation has been completed. The wisdom of using narcotics in either situation is often doubtful, because considerable depression is produced without real relief of pain. It is often wiser to give the patient a small amount of intravenous narcotic followed by a nondepressant, rapidly reversible analgesic such as nitrous oxide rather than try to provide true anesthesia with the narcotic alone. Intravenous narcotics in small amounts, however, are often of real value for patients undergoing lengthy procedures under conduction anesthesia, as the immobile patient with spinal anesthesia on an uncomfortable operating table for 4 hours becomes restless because of the physical discomfort of the unanesthetized portions of the body.

Intravenously administered tranquilizers, aside from any utility they may have in premedication, are limited adjuncts to general anesthesia. Occasionally they are given during conduction anesthesia to make the patient feel more comfortable. Whether their use is more effective than the separate or combined use of small, therapeutic amounts of intravenously administered barbiturates or narcotics is problematic.

Ketamine, although not a narcotic in the classic sense, produces profound analgesia combined with striking subjective dissociation from the environment. Administered intravenously or intramuscularly in the proper dosage, ketamine provides anesthesia adequate for superficial operations requiring no muscle relaxation without producing respiratory or cardiovascular depression. In fact, the arterial pressure frequently is elevated and the heart rate increased. Ketamine also has the important advantage of not relaxing muscles and soft tissue of the upper airway, as other narcotics and sedatives are prone to do. Therefore, airway obstruction is infrequent during ketamine anesthesia. However, it has the disadvantage of being occasionally associated with highly unpleasant hallucinations or subjective responses best described as nightmares. Since this adverse psychic response is particularly liable to occur in adults, ketamine is often restricted to children. As ketamine accentuates pharyngeal and laryngeal reflexes, it is usually contraindicated for operations on or about the mouth, lips, and nose because of the possibility of precipitating severe laryngospasm. It also rather sharply increases intracranial pressure and so is contraindicated in certain neurologic conditions.

RELAXANTS

Intravenously administered muscle relaxants allow profound muscular relaxation without deep levels of anesthesia. The avoidance of the adverse physiologic effects of deep general anesthesia by such means is not, however, without its disadvantages. These are related to the profound interference with normal respiration produced by all muscle relaxants when administered in amounts adequate to provide required degrees of muscular relaxation. The respiratory effects of muscle relaxants must be compensated for by artificial ventilation to maintain a normal arterial oxygenation and a normal carbon dioxide excretion as discussed above. This is not always readily achieved under clinical circumstances, and the clinical signs of respiratory acidosis or hypoxia are unreliable in the anesthetized patient.

An additional problem associated with the use of muscle relaxants is that their duration of action may exceed the duration of surgical procedures, with the result that a patient is apneic or hypoventilated after the operation and anesthesia have been completed. Although prolonged apnea following the use of muscle relaxants is not always due solely to their prolonged action, the apnea cannot always be reversed at will.

A third difficulty associated with the use of muscle relaxants is that the intermittent positive-pressure ventilation which their use necessitates may be associated with arterial hypoxemia even though alveolar ventilation adequate for removal of carbon dioxide is provided. Arterial hypoxemia may supervene despite amounts of oxygen in the inspired air adequate to maintain normal arterial oxygenation in the unanesthetized patient. The reason is that intermittent positive-pressure ventilation often is associated with derangements of normal alveolar ventilation/perfusion ratios, and certain alveoli are perfused with blood when they are not ventilated. The uneven alveolar ventilation, which to some extent inevitably follows the institution of positive-pressure respirations, results in an increased gradient in oxygen tension between alveoli and pulmonary venous (i.e., peripheral arterial) blood because of the continued perfusion of unventilated areas. For this reason it is necessary to provide at least 33% oxygen in the inspired air when artificial respiration is being carried on for long periods of time, as during nitrous oxide–oxygen anesthesia with muscle relaxants or halothane. The same events can occur in patients on controlled respiration for long periods of time, in the postoperative recovery room, and in intensive care units.

Muscle relaxants may be divided into two major categories depending on the method by which they produce muscle paralysis: those such as curare, which interfere with transmission of the nerve impulse at the myoneural junction by competing with acetylcholine for the motor end plate (nondepolarizing muscle relaxants), and those such as succinylcholine, which interfere with myoneural transmission by producing depolarization of the motor end plate, rendering it unresponsive. Agents such as curare are, by and large, longer acting than depolarizing agents. Curare, for example, shows significant regression from its peak action approximately 20 minutes after administration, the greater part of its action disappearing within approximately 40 minutes. Although curare is to a large extent ultimately excreted by renal mechanisms, its action is terminated after about 45 minutes primarily because of its redistribution throughout the body. Therefore, curare, like thiopental, may have a subtle subclinical effect persisting beyond its peak effect. Thus, curare has a cumulative effect, and a subsequent dose to produce muscular relaxation equal to that produced initially will be considerably lower than the first. Nondepolarizing agents such as curare can be antagonized by anticholinesterases such as neostigmine (Prostigmin). Available specific antagonists are advantageous when muscle relaxants of the curare type are employed, though reliance should not be placed upon antagonists to the exclusion of accurate dosage of minimum effective amounts.

Unlike curare, the depolarizing agent succinylcholine has a short duration of action, because it is metabolized by the enzyme pseudocholinesterase in approximately 8 minutes. However, after prolonged periods of administration the method by which succinylcholine produces neuromuscular block becomes more complex; it no longer resembles a depolarizing type of block so much as a non-depolarizing or curare type of block. This nondepolarizing phase of myoneural block occurs primarily after prolonged intravenous administration of dilute concentrations, is reversed by anticholinesterases, as is the block following curare. The original depolarizing block produced by a single injection of succinylcholine is not antagonized by anticholinesterases or by any other presently available agent.

Prolonged apnea following the use of muscle relaxants may be due to one or a combination of factors. It may be due to levels of pseudocholinesterases inadequate to metabolize succinylcholine, or it may be due to succinylcholine's action as a nondepolarizing blocker following prolonged periods of administration. The apnea is comparable to that observed following overdosage with curare or following inadequate elimination of curare, as in patients with renal failure. Differentiation of the type of neuromuscular block in cases of prolonged apnea is important, because although specific antagonists exist for the correction of one type, they prolong the apnea if administered in the other type. Differential diagnosis is most conveniently made by electrical stimulation of a peripheral motor nerve. Prolonged apnea due to a lack of pseudocholinesterase may be diagnosed by determination of plasma cholinesterase levels, but most laboratories are not prepared to perform such tests rapidly enough to be of clinical value. Clinically significant degrees of low pseudocholinesterase are primarily, if not entirely, genetically determined. The immediate relatives of a patient with this abnormality should have their pseudocholinesterase levels determined, so that abnormally low levels may be noted prior to any contemplated surgical procedure. Prolonged apnea may also occur after the use of relaxants for other reasons. Perhaps the most frequent single cause of prolonged apnea is hyperventilation so effective that there is no longer any chemical stimulus to initiate respiration, carbon dioxide tensions having been lowered and oxygen tensions increased. "Exhaustion" of the Hering-Breuer reflex, water intoxication, anesthetic overdosage, and altered levels of ionized calcium are but a few of the many additional causes of prolonged apnea.

Succinylcholine has been shown to be capable of triggering a potentially lethal and rapidly progressing condition referred to as *malignant hyperpyrexia*. Characterized by muscular rigidity instead of relaxation following injection, the body temperature is rapidly elevated as high as 107°F or higher within 30 minutes or less. Once established, this elevation is usually fatal because of associated neurologic damage, cardiovascular collapse, and profound metabolic derangements. Although rare, susceptibility to malignant hyperpyrexia is genetically determined and cannot reliably be discerned in advance, although it is often recorded in young muscular males. Management consists of prevention by monitoring rectal or esophageal temperature, prompt recognition of an atypical response to succinylcholine, and immediate aggressive pharmacologic and physical measures to lower temperature as rapidly as possible. It has been suggested that intravenous procaine amide effectively and rapidly reverses the hyperthermia.

CONDUCTION ANESTHESIA

Conduction anesthesia has the advantage of producing nonexplosive maximal sensory anesthesia and profound muscular relaxation without profound physiologic effects, *provided that the extent of anesthesia is limited*. The disadvantages of conduction anesthesia include the fact that if it is extensive, the resultant physiologic trespass may be greater than during well-administered general anesthesia. For example, the conduction anesthesia necessary for a gastrectomy is associated with physiologic changes more profound and potentially more dangerous than the changes accompanying a well-administered general anesthetic for the same operation, with or without muscle relaxants. On the other hand, the physiologic disturbance associated with conduction anesthesia for an operation such as hemorrhoidectomy is considerably less than that associated with general anesthesia for this procedure. The difference between the effects of extensive conduction anesthesia and conduction anesthesia limited in area is frequently unrecognized or forgotten but is one of the major considerations in evaluating the usefulness of this method. The inherent limitations of conduction anesthesia relate both to the anesthetist and to the surgeon. For conduction anesthesia to be smooth and successful, the anesthetist must have extensive experience and be highly skilled. Errors of omission or commission during conduction anesthesia not only are dangerous but are immediately (and painfully) apparent to all. The surgeon operating with conduction anesthesia must be gentle and silent to realize its full benefits.

Spinal Anesthesia

Spinal anesthesia consists of the injection of a local anesthetic into the subarachnoid space. The resulting anesthesia of somatic motor and sensory fibers is its raison d'être, but from a physiologic point of view the most important result of spinal anesthesia is the concurrent blocking of preganglionic sympathetic fibers. Almost all the profound physiologic changes which may be associated with spinal anesthesia are due to the effects of the sympathetic denervation. The sensory denervation produced by spinal anesthesia has little or no physiologic effect. The somatic motor denervation also has little physiologic effect, despite theories that somatic motor paralysis causes venous pooling, with a decrease in cardiac output. Succinylcholine is not associated with such changes, though the muscle relaxation is as profound as with spinal anesthesia. The physiologic effects of spinal anesthesia are also not due to any hypothetic ascent of the local anesthetic agent intracranially into the ventricular system to cause a direct depression of the vasomotor or respiratory centers.

Since the sympathetic nervous system block of spinal anesthesia is such an important determinant of the physiologic response to anesthesia, there are three aspects which deserve special emphasis. The first is that different types of nerve fibers are blocked by different concentrations of local anesthetic, smaller nerve fibers being blocked by lower concentrations of local anesthetic than larger fibers. The largest fibers in the human subarachnoid space being somatic motor fibers, these are the most resistant to local anesthetics. The next smaller fibers are somatic sensory fibers. The smallest fibers are the preganglionic fibers. These are blocked by concentrations of local anesthetic which have no effect on either sensory or motor nerve roots. Because the concentration of local anesthetic within the subarachnoid space decreases as the distance from the site of injection increases, a point is reached at which the concentration of local anesthetic in spinal fluid is no longer adequate to block somatic sensory fibers even though it is adequate to block sympathetic fibers. As a result, the sympathetic denervation of spinal anesthesia extends an average of two spinal segments beyond the level made anesthetic to pinprick. The physiologic response to spinal anesthesia may therefore be more profound than indicated by the extent of sensory denervation, especially if, as is sometimes the case, the zone of differential block extends beyond the usual two spinal segments to as much as six spinal segments. For the same reason, the level of somatic motor block during spinal anesthesia extends approximately two spinal segments below (i.e., caudal to) the level made anesthetic to pinprick. This is one reason why it is possible to have sensory anesthesia adequate for skin incision during appendectomy performed under spinal anesthesia without adequate muscular relaxation. The zone of differential anesthesia involving sympathetic, sensory, and motor nerves also explains why phrenic paralysis rarely occurs even during high spinal anesthesias, including those with cervical sensory levels.

The second factor concerning the sympathetic denervation associated with spinal anesthesia is related to the fact that the highest (i.e., most cephalad) preganglionic sympathetic fiber arises at the T_1 level. Because sympathetic block extends approximately two spinal segments higher than sensory block, complete sympathetic denervation will be present in patients who have spinal anesthesia with a sensory level at approximately T_3. In other words, spinal anesthesia with high sensory levels is associated with the physiologic changes inherent in total sympathetic denervation. As a corollary, since the vast majority of the physiologic effects of spinal anesthesia are due to the concurrent sympathetic block and since the sympathetic block is complete with sensory levels to T_3, the physiologic response to cervical levels of anesthesia is no greater than to high thoracic levels. A patient with a sensory block to the T_3 level has essentially the same physiologic response as a patient with a sensory level at C_5 or C_6.

The third important aspect of sympathetic block produced by spinal anesthesia relates to the fact that each preganglionic sympathetic fiber, after penetrating the dura and entering the paravertebral sympathetic chain, ascends and descends in the chain, synapsing with a number of postganglionic fibers which are distributed to the periphery in a nonsegmental fashion. A single preganglionic fiber may synapse with as many as 18 postganglionic fibers. Stimulation (or block) of a single preganglionic fiber accordingly produces a diffuse peripheral response extending over a large number of peripheral segmental dermatomes, a response which is not limited to the peripheral segmental dermatome corresponding to the spinal segmental level at which the sympathetic fiber was stimulated (or blocked). Therefore, the sympathetic response to spinal anesthesia may be surprisingly extensive peripherally.

Just as the sympathetic blocking of spinal anesthesia is the most important determinant of the physiologic response, the cardiovascular changes resulting from the sympathetic blocking represent the most important physiologic alteration during this type of anesthesia.

The sympathetic denervation produces peripheral arterial and arteriolar vasodilatation. In the presence of a fixed cardiac output, the resulting decrease in peripheral vascular resistance produces a decrease in mean arterial pressure. The decrease in resistance is, however, relatively modest, amounting to 12 to 15 percent even in the presence of a total sympathetic denervation. It also is limited because peripheral vascular resistance is not eliminated by the denervation. The major site of resistance is merely shifted more peripherally, and there is still resistance to flow through the postarteriolar capillary circulation. In the normal individual, approximately 60 percent of the total peripheral vascular resistance arises at the arteriolar level, approximately 40 percent arising at the postarteriolar level. Following sympathetic denervation, approximately 40 percent of the resistance is at the arteriolar level, and 60 percent at the postarteriolar level. Even maximal vasodilatation on the arterial side of the circulation does not eliminate resistance to flow at the tissue level. Since total peripheral vascular resistance decreases so modestly during even high levels of spinal anesthesia, arterial and arteriolar vasodilatation cannot be accepted as the cause of severe arterial hypotension during spinal anesthesia. A 10 to 15 percent decrease in systolic pressure during spinal anesthesia can be ascribed to a decrease in peripheral resistance, but the severe degrees of hypotension must be ascribed to another cause, a decreased cardiac output.

From a cardiovascular point of view the most important result of the sympathetic denervation of spinal anesthesia is the effect on venous circulation. Because veins are innervated by the sympathetic nervous system, spinal anesthesia also results in venodilatation in the denervated areas. There is, however, a major difference between the sympathetic denervation produced on the venous side of the circulation and that produced on the arterial side. Although vasodilatation is not maximal following denervation on the arterial side of the circulation, it can be and often is maximal on the venous side. The smooth muscle in the arterial side of the circulation and in the postarteriolar bed maintains a considerable degree of autonomous tone after removal of its sympathetic nervous supply, with the result that sympathectomy is rarely associated with maximal vasodilatation. There is little or no autonomous tone in veins, however, after their sympathetic denervation. Whether or not a vein is dilated following sympathetic denervation depends primarily upon the effects of gravity. If the sympathectomized vein is below the level of the right atrium, gravity causes the blood to pool in the dependent vein and venodilatation becomes maximal. On the other hand, if the sympathectomized vein is above the level of the right atrium, gravity causes the blood to drain out, and essentially no venodilatation occurs.

If a significant degree of peripheral venodilatation occurs during spinal anesthesia because the patient is in a position in which the greater part of the denervated peripheral circulation is below the level of the right side of the heart (e.g., in the head-up position), there will be a pronounced decrease in venous return to the right side of the heart and resultant decrease in cardiac output. This in turn will cause a severe arterial hypotension. Decreases in cardiac output, including those great enough to lead to cardiac arrest, during spinal anesthesia are almost always consequent to significant decreases in venous return to the right side of the heart.

The most frequent cause of impaired venous return to the heart during spinal anesthesia is the head-up position. The second most frequent cause is administration of spinal anesthetic to a patient with decreased blood volume. Since the safety of spinal anesthesia is related to maintenance of an adequate arterial blood pressure and cardiac output and since these are related to maintenance of normal venous return to the right side of the heart, the head-up position should be employed only very cautiously during high levels of anesthesia. Of course, this position should be employed to regulate the level of anesthesia when hyperbaric spinal solutions are being used, but if severe hypotension ensues or if an inadvertently high level of anesthesia is obtained, there should be no hesitation about putting the patient in the head-down position in order to assure adequate venous return and cardiac output. The head-down position may result in a higher level of anesthesia, but it will not result in cardiac arrest. Injudicious use of the head-up position during spinal anesthesia, under the misapprehension that limiting the spread of the anesthetic is the primary consideration, constitutes the major cause of cardiac arrest during spinal anesthesia.

Respiratory function during spinal anesthesia remains normal even during high levels of sensory block. The intercostal paralysis accompanying a high spinal anesthetic is compensated for by the diaphragm, especially in the presence of a relaxed abdominal musculature so that arterial carbon dioxide and oxygen tensions remain within normal limits. This occurs even during cervical sensory levels of anesthesia, because the phrenic nerves are highly resistant to the effects of local anesthetics. Respiratory arrest can occur during spinal anesthesia, but the most frequent cause is not phrenic paralysis but a centrally induced apnea consequent to decreases in cardiac output great enough to result in ischemic medullary paralysis. The association between respiratory arrest and cardiac output is exemplified by the vast majority of respiratory arrests during spinal anesthesia immediately preceding or following cardiac arrest. Furthermore, once resuscitation has restored cardiac output, the patient usually exhibits spontaneous respiration. Respiratory arrest due to phrenic paralysis during spinal anesthesia undoubtedly can occur, but it is infrequent and only exceptionally the cause of apnea. Misguided attempts to avoid respiratory arrest by use of the head-up position lead to more cardiac and respiratory arrests than does judicious use of the head-down position. Even if apnea due to phrenic paralysis were to occur during spinal anesthesia, artificial means of ventilation are

today such a standard part of every anesthetist's armamentarium that no harm will result. The same cannot be said for artificial means of maintaining cardiac output.

It is apparent from the above that the physiologic effects of high levels of spinal anesthesia are inevitably greater than with low levels of anesthesia. The difference in physiologic responses to high and low levels of spinal anesthesia is so great that from a practical and clinical point of view the two techniques should not be considered together. The advantage of low levels of spinal anesthesia is that profound sensory and muscular denervation can be achieved with relatively little other physiologic change. This is especially advantageous in patients with concurrent disease involving the cardiovascular or respiratory systems. The same cannot be said for high levels of anesthesia. The patient for whom a low spinal anesthesia is indicated during repair of an inguinal hernia because of concurrent disease, for example, is often the one for whom spinal anesthesia during cholecystectomy or gastrectomy is contraindicated because of concurrent disease. In modern practice there are few indications for the use of spinal anesthesia for surgical procedures above the level of the umbilicus, as the resulting total or near-total sympathetic denervation is too great a price to pay.

One potential drawback to spinal anesthesia is the association of the technique with postoperative headaches. So-called "spinal headaches" are especially frequent in the younger age groups and in females, the highest incidence being in obstetric patients. Although all the etiologic factors producing headaches following spinal anesthesia have not yet been completely defined, it has been demonstrated that the incidence of headache is related to the size of the needle used to perform the lumbar puncture. The use of 18-gauge needles is associated with postspinal headaches in as many as 20 percent of patients. On the other hand, the routine use of 24- or 25-gauge spinal needles is associated with postspinal headaches in less than 2 percent of patients. If a spinal headache does occur, it should be treated conservatively with hydration (by intravenous routes if necessary) plus mild analgesics. If the headache is severe or if imminent discharge from the hospital indicates more radical therapy, injection of saline solution into the lumbar epidural space will usually produce prompt and, for inexplicable reasons, permanent relief of the headache.

In modern practice the risk of possible neurologic complications from spinal anesthesia is more potential than actual. It is now apparent that the vast majority of neurologic complications associated with spinal anesthesia are the result of chemical contamination of the material being injected into the subarachnoid space. If the contaminating material is injected in a high concentration or if it is a strongly neurolytic substance such as alcohol or phenol, the resulting neurologic damage may be a chemical transverse myelitis which appears immediately and is irreversible. This is most frequently due to mistaken identification of ampules used to produce spinal anesthesia. On the other hand, if the contaminating material is injected in low concentrations or is only weakly neurolytic, the resultant neurologic deficit is more often a chronic adhesive arachnoiditis which may not become apparent for days or even weeks after the anesthesia but which, once it appears, progresses inexorably as the arachnoiditis spreads cephalad from the site of the injection. Since chemical contamination constitutes the most frequent single cause of neurologic complications associated with spinal anesthesia, the spinal set and drugs used should be not only bacteriologically sterile—a condition readily achieved by autoclaving—but also chemically sterile and free of all pyrogens and other contaminating substances, a condition achieved only by meticulously detailed preparation techniques. Not all neurologic deficits following spinal anesthesia are due to the anesthetic techniques. While the risk of neurologic or other complications with spinal anesthetics is negligible, it does exist. However, the risk of neurologic deficits following spinal anesthesia for operations on the lower extremities and perineum may well be less in the long run than that involved in the use of general anesthesia for such procedures.

Efficiency and safety in spinal anesthesia are best achieved by employing one or at most two local anesthetic agents and regulating their spread in the subarachnoid space solely by changing the position of the patient, keeping constant the specific gravity of the solution injected. A satisfactory local anesthetic of proved safety for spinal anesthesia is 1% tetracaine (Pontocaine). When mixed with equal volumes of 10% dextrose, a hyperbaric solution is achieved. The dosage of tetracaine will vary with the size of the patient and the extent and duration of anesthesia required but should not exceed 18 mg. The duration of tetracaine spinal anesthesia may safely be approximately doubled by the addition of 0.3 to 0.5 mg epinephrine.

Epidural Anesthesia

The physiologic response produced by the injection of local anesthetic agent into the epidural space is similar to that associated with spinal anesthesia in that sympathetic denervation is produced. But differences exist in the responses to the two techniques: First, the large amounts of local anesthetic agent used to produce epidural anesthesia may be absorbed and produce systemic effects on the cardiovascular system which add to the effects of the sympathetic block. The small amounts of local anesthetic employed in spinal anesthesia, on the other hand, produce no systemic effects. The physiologic response to epidural anesthesia also may be altered if epinephrine is injected with the anesthetic into the epidural space to prolong the duration of anesthesia. Epinephrine, even when administered in the pharmacologically ideal concentration of 1:200,000, can have peripheral systemic effects, whereas vasoconstrictors used intrathecally during spinal anesthesia are unassociated with such systemic responses.

The clinical advantage of epidural as opposed to spinal anesthesia is to a large extent a function of the degree of apprehension on the part of the patient, anesthetist, or surgeon regarding the dangers of neurologic complications following spinal anesthesia. The pharmacologic and actuarial basis of a psychologic advantage is dubious, epidural anesthesia is not without neurologic complications. Moreover, epidural injection of local anesthetic involves transfer of the local anesthetic across the dura into the subarachnoid space. Therefore, since epidural anesthesia is essentially spinal anesthesia, it is not clear why one is pharmacologically superior to the other with regard to the dangers of neurotoxic reactions. Properly performed epidural anesthesia does have the advantage of being associated with a lower incidence of spinal headache. But epidural anesthesia in clinical practice does not eliminate the danger of spinal headache, since the needle sometimes inadvertently may penetrate the dura instead of stopping in the epidural space during induction of this anesthesia. In large series of unselected cases, the incidence of spinal headache following routine use of 24-gauge needles for spinal anesthesia has been essentially the same as the incidence following epidural anesthesia complicated by occasional inadvertent perforation of the dura by the larger needles employed in epidural anesthesia.

There are two situations in which epidural anesthesia appears to have significant advantages over spinal anesthesia, the first being when rectal surgery is to be performed in the prone, jackknife position. In such a position it is clinically more convenient to produce caudal anesthesia with minimal patient manipulation and minimal physiologic effects from the anesthesia than to rely on spinal anesthesia, hypobaric or hyperbaric. Second, continuous epidural anesthesia with use of catheters has more to recommend it than does continuous spinal anesthesia when conduction anesthesia is to be continued for long periods of time.

Nerve Block

Nerve block, infiltration, and topical anesthesia are advantageous techniques but present technical complexities beyond the scope of the present chapter. The disadvantages of infiltration anesthesia arise from two sources: First, too much is expected of the anesthesia. A laparotomy cannot be performed under infiltration anesthesia alone. Second, the systemic toxicity of local anesthetics is often ignored when infiltration anesthesia is used. Toxic reactions to local anesthetics are the result of inadvertently high blood levels of local anesthetics. They are not the result of allergic reactions or hypersensitivity. The high blood levels may be the result of using total dosages exceeding the recognized safe limits, injection of the local anesthetic into highly vascular areas, or accidental intravenous injection.

Toxic reactions to local anesthetics may involve either the central nervous system, in which case they are characterized by twitching progressing to convulsions, or the cardiovascular system, in which case they are characterized by sudden hypotension. Treatment of the former previously consisted of the intravenous injection of small amounts of a barbiturate, but it has been conclusively demonstrated that intravenous diazepam (Valium) is superior to barbiturates in the management of central nervous system toxicity due to local anesthetics. Treatment of cardiovascular depression due to absorption of local anesthetics consists of placing the patient in the head-down position, followed by use of intravenous vasopressors. Oxygen should be administered in both cases. Safe dosage levels of local anesthetics depend upon the age, weight, and physical status of the patient and the speed and site of injection. A healthy 70-kg adult should not receive over 1.0 Gm of procaine or over 500 mg of lidocaine (Xylocaine) within 20 minutes. Tetracaime as a topical anesthetic for mucous membranes should not be administered in doses exceeding 40 mg.

Although nerve blocks and infiltration anesthesia have a definite role in surgery, the physiologic and pharmacologic effects of large amounts of local anesthetic injected into the operative area are often more adverse than the physiologic and pharmacologic effects of a well-administered general anesthetic. Present anesthesia techniques are such that *major* surgery is generally more safely and efficiently performed with techniques other than infiltration anesthesia. This is especially true in the poor-risk patient, in whom the systemic toxicity of a local anesthetic may be unusually difficult to handle. Major intra-abdominal surgery under infiltration anesthesia is especially contraindicated if the surgical diagnosis is not definite. The initiation of an exploratory laparotomy in a poor-risk patient under infiltration anesthesia all too frequently results in the necessity of inducing general anesthesia under the most adverse circumstances possible: a poor-risk patient in pain, often with a full stomach, with the abdomen open, and suffering from the adverse systemic effects of local anesthetics.

PREMEDICATION

The objectives of preanesthetic medication are, in order of decreasing importance, alleviation of anxiety, decreased reflex irritability, and decreased requirement for general anesthetic agents. Mental relaxation and detachment, not coma or unconsciousness, are the goals. The establishment of rapport between the anesthetist and the patient is more predictably able to produce the desired state of tranquility than is the use of drugs affecting the central nervous system. Nevertheless, drugs will continue to be used for psychic premedication. When pharmacologic agents are to be relied upon, those agents should be employed which produce the maximal desired effect with the greatest predictability and the fewest side effects. Evidence indicates that in the absence of pain, therapeutic amounts of barbiturates most frequently achieve the desired state of mental relaxation. Barbiturates, when employed for such purposes, also have the advantage of producing no respiratory depression. This is in contrast with the respiratory depression produced by narcotics in the absence of pain. Since maintenance of adequate ventilation during and after anesthesia is a frequent concern, it is often inadvisable to administer drugs preanesthetically which will further depress respiration. Barbiturates used in therapeutic amounts as premedicants also do not undermine the stability of the cardiovascular system to the same extent that narcotics do. Finally, normal persons without pain do not find the administration of a narcotic a pleasant experience; in fact, they show a high incidence of dysphoria rather than euphoria following narcotic administration. Barbiturates, on the other hand, do not have this effect.

The role of narcotics as premedicants is best limited to two major areas: First, narcotics should be administered preanesthetically to those patients who are in pain or who will experience pain prior to the induction of anesthesia. Second, narcotics are useful premedication for patients without pain but whose anesthesia is to be based upon a thiopental–nitrous oxide–narcotic–oxygen sequence, with or without muscle relaxants. In such cases, the preoperative narcotic is essentially part of the anesthetic management.

Tranquilizers have been used as premedicants with varying degrees of success. The disadvantage of routine preoperative tranquilizers is that many have diverse and frequent side effects in addition to their tranquilizing effects. This is particularly true of phenothiazine tranquilizers, which have adrenolytic, antihistaminic, parasympatholytic, and other actions. While nonphenothiazine tranquilizers such as diazepam (Valium) and hydroxyzine (Vistaril; Atarax) may not have such high incidences of undesirable side effects, their effectiveness in producing tranquility without physiologic trespass has not been demonstrated to be superior to barbiturates. The pharmacologic shotgun effect characteristic of many tranquilizers often represents a major disadvantage during subsequent general anesthesia. Tranquilizers have also been employed preoperatively to decrease the incidence of postoperative nausea and vomiting. The antiemetic effect of tranquilizers in such cases is unquestioned, but the incidence and severity of side actions such as arterial hypotension and prolongation of unconsciousness postoperatively detracts considerably from their usefulness. Since it has been demonstrated that any agent, including pentobarbital, which prolongs "sleep time" following general anesthesia will decrease the incidence of nausea and vomiting, the use of barbiturates as antiemetics is often more effective because of their lower incidence of side effects.

Finally, drugs may be administered preoperatively to decrease adverse reflex activity. Since the reflexes causing most concern are parasympathetic reflexes, in particular vagal cardiac and laryngeal reflexes, parasympatholytic agents are the most widely used. When employed in proper dosage, the incidence of bradycardia following certain types of anesthesia, notably halothane and cyclopropane, is lessened by the use of parasympatholytic agents. Whether the incidence of laryngospasm is significantly decreased by these agents is difficult to determine, since it is affected by so many factors, including the skill and training of the person administering the anesthetic. Parasympatholytic agents do have the advantage of decreasing the amount of salivation which occurs during certain types of inhalation anesthesia such as ether and divinyl ether (Vinethene).

Whether atropine or scopolamine is employed as the parasympatholytic agent is a matter of personal preference. The theoretic advantage of scopolamine in producing amnesia is offset in practice by the increased incidence of postoperative delirium in patients who have received the drug. When scopolamine is employed it should be administered in dosages equal to two-thirds the atropine dosage. Of all the drugs used for premedication, atropine and scopolamine are perhaps the most misused, in that they are either administered in doses incapable of producing the degree of parasympathetic block which is intended or they are administered when parasympathetic denervation is not required.

References

General

Beecher, H. K., and Todd, D. P.: A Study of Deaths Associated with Anesthesia, *Ann Surg,* **140:**2, 1954.

Dripps, R. D., Eckenhoff, J. E., and Vandam, L. D.: "Introduction to Anesthesia," W. B. Saunders Company, Philadelphia, 3d ed., 1969.

Greene, N. M., Bannister, W. K., Cohen, B., Keet, J. E., Mancinelli, M. J., Welch, E. T., and Welch, H. J.: Survey of Deaths Associated with Anesthesia in Connecticut, *Conn State Med J,* **23:**512, 1959.

Inhalation Anesthetics

Aprahamian, H. A., Vanderveen, J. L., Bunker, J. P., Murphy, A. J., and Crawford, J. D.: The Influence of General Anesthetics on Water and Solute Excretion in Man, *Ann Surg,* **150:**122, 1959.

Brewster, W. R., Jr., Isaacs, J. P., and Waino-Andersen, T.: Depressant Effect of Ether on Myocardium of the Dog and Its Modification by Reflex Release of Epinephrine and Norepinephrine, *Am J Physiol,* **175:**399, 1953.

Bunker, J. P., Forrest, W. H., Jr., Mosteller, F., and Vandam, L. D. (eds.): National Halothane Study, National Institutes of Health, National Institutes of General Medical Sciences, Bethesda, Md., 1969.

Cohen, E. N.: Metabolism of Volatile Anesthetics, *Anesthesiology,* **35:**193, 1971.

Deutsch, S., Linde, H. W., Dripps, R. D., and Price, H. L.: Circulatory and Respiratory Effects of Halothane in Normal Man, *Anesthesiology,* **23:**631, 1962.

Eastwood, D. W., Green, C. D., Lambdin, M. A., and Gardner, R.: Effect of Nitrous Oxide on the White-Cell Count in Leukemia, *N Engl J Med,* **268:**297, 1963.

Eger, E. I., II, and Saidman, L. J.: Hazards of Nitrous Oxide Anesthesia in Bowel Obstruction and Pneumothorax, *Anesthesiology,* **26:**61, 1965.

———, ———, and Brandstater, B.: Minimum Alveolar Anesthetic Concentration: A Standard of Anesthetic Potency, *Anesthesiology,* **26:**756, 1965.

Fink, B. R.: Diffusion Anoxia, *Anesthesiology,* **16:**511, 1955.

Greene, N. M.: "Inhalation Anesthetics and Carbohydrate Metabolism," The Williams & Wilkins Company, Baltimore, 1963.

Klatskin, G., and Kimberg, D. V.: Recurrent Hepatitis Attributable to Halothane Sensitization in an Anesthetist, *N Engl J Med,* **280:**515, 1969.

McArdle, L., and Black, G. W.: The Effects of Cyclopropane on the Peripheral Circulation in Man, *Br J Anaesth,* **35:**352, 1963.

Mazze, R. I., Trudell, J. R., and Cousins, M. J.: Methoxyflurane Metabolism and Renal Dysfunction, *Anesthesiology,* **35:**247, 1971.

Munson, E. S., Larson, C. P., Babab, A. A., Regan, M. J., Buechel, D. R., and Eger, E. I., II: Effects of Halothane, Fluroxene and Cyclopropane on Ventilation: A Comparative Study in Man, *Anesthesiology,* **27:**716, 1966.

Paronetto, F., and Popper, H.: Lymphocyte Stimulation Induced by Halothane in Patients with Post-halothane Hepatitis, *N Engl J Med,* **283:**277, 1970.

Price, H. L., and Price, M. L.: Has Halothane a Predominant Circulatory Action? *Anesthesiology,* **27:**764, 1966.

———, ———, and Morse, H. T.: Effects of Cyclopropane, Halothane and Procaine on the Vasomotor "Center" of the Dog, *Anesthesiology,* **26:**55, 1965.

Rehder, K., Forbes, J., Alter, H., Hessler, O., and Stier, A.: Halothane Biotransformation in Man, *Anesthesiology,* **28:**711, 1967.

Saidman, L. J., and Eger, E. I., II: Effect of Nitrous Oxide and of Narcotic Premedication on the Alveolar Concentration of Halothane Required for Anesthesia, *Anesthesiology,* **25:**302, 1964.

——— and ———: Change in Cerebro-spinal Fluid Pressure during Pneumoencephalography under Nitrous Oxide Anesthesia, *Anesthesiology,* **26:**67, 1965.

Stevens, W. C., Cromwell, T. H., Halsey, M. J., Eger, E. I., II, Shakespear, T. F., and Bahlman, S. H.: The Cardiovascular Effects of a New Inhalation Anesthetic, Forane, *Anesthesiology,* **35:**8, 1971.

Van Dyke, R. A., and Chenoweth, M. B.: Metabolism of Volatile Anesthetics, *Anesthesiology,* **26:**348, 1965.

Intravenous Anesthetics

Bendixen, H. H., Hedley-Whyte, J., and Laver, M. B.: Impaired Oxygenation in Surgical Patients during General Anesthesia with Controlled Ventilation: A Concept of Atelectasis, *N Engl J Med,* **269:**991, 1963.

Britt, B. A., and Kalow, W.: Malignant Hyperthermia: A Statistical Review, *Canad Anaesth Soc J,* **17:**293, 1970.

Churchill-Davidson, H. C.: A Portable Peripheral Nerve-Stimulator, *Anesthesiology,* **26:**224, 1965.

Corssen, G., Chodoff, P., Domino, E. F., and Kahn, D. R.: Neurolept Analgesia and Anesthesia for Open-Heart Surgery: Pharmacologic Rationale and Clinical Experience, *J Thorac Cardiovasc Surg,* **49:**901, 1965.

Lowenstein, E., Hollowell, P., Levine, F. H., Daggett, W. M., Austen, W. G., and Laver, M. B.: Cardiovascular Response to Large Doses of Intravenous Morphine in Man, *N Engl J Med,* **281:**1389, 1969.

Pender, J. W.: Dissociative Anesthesia, *JAMA,* **215:**1126, 1971.

Price, H. L.: A Dynamic Concept of the Distribution of Thiopental in the Human Body, *Anesthesiology,* **21:**40, 1960.

Conduction Anesthetics

Bonica, J. J., Akamatsu, T. J., Berges, P. U., Morikawa, K., and Kennedy, W. F., Jr.: Circulatory Effect of Peridural Block: Effects of Epinephrine, *Anesthesiology,* **34:**514, 1971.

Bromage, P. R.: Physiology and Pharmacology of Epidural Analgesia, *Anesthesiology,* **28:**592, 1967.

DeJong, R. H., and Heavener, J. E.: Local Anesthetic Seizure Prevention: Diazepam versus Pentobarbital, *Anesthesiology,* **36:**449, 1972.

Dripps, R. D., and Vandam, L. D.: Long-Term Follow-up of Patients Who Received 10,098 Spinal Anesthetics, *JAMA*, **156:**1486, 1954.

Greene, N. M.: "The·Physiology of Spinal Anesthesia," 2d ed., The Williams & Wilkins Company, Baltimore, 1969.

———: Neurological Sequelae of Spinal Anesthesia, *Anesthesiology*, **22:**682, 1961.

Ward, R. J., Bonica, J. J., Freund, F. G., Akamatsu, T., Danziger, F., and Englesson, S.: Epidural and Subarachnoid Anesthesia: Cardiovascular and Respiratory Effects, *JAMA*, **191:**275, 1965.

Premedication

Beecher, H. K.: "Measurement of Subjective Responses," Oxford University Press, New York, 1959.

Egbert, L. D., Battit, G. E., Turndorf, H., and Beecher, H. K.: The Value of Preoperative Visit by the Anesthetist, *JAMA*, **185:**553, 1963.

Chapter 12

Complications

by **Seymour I. Schwartz**

General Considerations

Wound Complications
Wound Dehiscence
Wound Infection
Wound Hemorrhage, Hematoma, and Seroma

Postoperative Parotitis

Postoperative Respiratory Complications
Respiratory Failure
Atelectasis
Pulmonary Edema

Cardiac Complications
Arrhythmias
Myocardial Infarction

Diabetes Mellitus

Fat Embolism

Psychiatric Complications
Special Surgical Situations
    Pediatric Surgery
    Surgery in the Aged
    Gynecologic Surgery
    Cancer Patients
    Cardiac Surgery
    Dialysis and Transplantation
    Intensive Care Delirium

Complications of Gastrointestinal Surgery
Vascular Complications
    Hemorrhage
    Gangrene
Mechanical Problems
    Stomal Obstruction
    Afferent (Blind) Loop Syndrome
    Intestinal Obstruction
    Inadvertent Gastroileostomy
Anastomotic Leak
External Fistulas and Stomal Complications
    Fistulas
    External Stomal Complications

GENERAL CONSIDERATIONS

Surgical care must encompass an appreciation and anticipation of postoperative complications which may result from the disease process per se, errors of omission, or errors of commission in technique. In regarding the patient postoperatively, any deviation from the anticipated norm for clinical evaluation and/or diagnostic findings should alert one to focus on complications of the disease and also to retrace the operative procedure. It is unusual, although certainly possible, that clinical and laboratory abnormalities may be caused by the chance occurrence of an unrelated disease during the postoperative period. Acute cholecystitis and appendicitis are two examples of diseases which may become manifest during the postoperative course of the patient. Routine care of a patient following surgical treatment includes repeated evaluation of the vital signs, i.e., temperature, pulse, blood pressure, and respiration. The extent of pain in the region of the incision and generalized discomfort are assessed, anticipating progressive improvement. The chest is auscultated for pleural rubs, bronchial breathing, and rales, while the abdomen is auscultated to determine the return of intestinal activity. The lower extremities are palpated in order to detect physical signs of deep venous thrombosis. The hematocrit and white blood cell count are measured at appropriate intervals to assess blood loss and continued infection, respectively. These determinations plus appropriate clinical chemistry determinations should be carried out when they are pertinent, not routinely.

TEMPORAL CONSIDERATIONS. Fever which presents shortly after surgical treatment in a patient who was previously afebrile is generally related to atelectasis or aspiration. Fever may also appear early in the postoperative course secondary to urinary tract infection, particularly if the patient has been catheterized. Fever of wound infection and leakage of an intestinal anastomosis or closure more frequently become evident on the fourth to seventh postoperative day. Hypotension in the early postoperative phase may be due to continued hemorrhage or the effects of depressive drugs which have been administered during the recovery period. Hypotension later in the postoperative course in a patient with sepsis should alert one to the possibility of endotoxin shock. The incidence of deep venous thrombosis and pulmonary embolism increases with duration of bed rest. Wound dehiscence usually does not become manifest until the fifth postoperative day.

WOUND COMPLICATIONS

Wound Dehiscence

Wound disruption, or dehiscence, generally refers to a separation of an abdominal wound, involving the anterior fascial sheath and deeper layers. The inaccuracy of computing the frequency of wound disruption is notorious; the incidence in the literature ranges from 0.5 to 3 percent, averaging 2.6 percent when all abdominal operations are considered collectively. The incidence is definitely related to age and is reported to be 1.3 percent for patients under forty-five years in contrast to 5.4 percent for those over forty-five years. There is a higher incidence in elderly, debilitated patients with poor nutrition and in the presence of significant ascites. Carcinoma is also associated with an increased incidence. In a collective review by Hartzell and Winfield, 22 percent of disruptions occurred when cancer was present, and 38 percent of dehiscences in Wolff's series were in cancer patients. Over 5 percent of laparotomies in patients in whom cancer was found are reported to have wound disruption in contrast to a 2 percent incidence when laparotomy demonstrates a benign condition. Other general factors which have been implicated include hypoproteinemia and atelectasis with its associated coughing, which, along with retching and hiccuping, increases the intraabdominal pressure and puts a strain on the incision. A lack of correlation between anemia and wound disruption has been reported. Obesity is definitely associated with an increased incidence.

Local factors involved in wound disruption include hemorrhage, infection, excessive suture material, and poor technique. Prompt wound healing is facilitated by a minimum of necrotic residue, bacterial contamination, and foreign material. Sutures should not be tied too tightly but should be positioned so that there is minimal peritoneal defect, since several theories suggest that wound disruptions start with a tiny wedge of omentum or bowel finding its way through such a defect, which is then enlarged.

Several series have suggested that the incidence of wound dehiscence is increased with vertical incisions. This has been related to the relative holding power of the fascia. The rectus abdominis sheath fascia runs horizontally, and therefore a transverse incision is in line with the fascial fibers, while a vertical paramedian incision transects the fascial fibers which act as a distracting force on the incision. It has been demonstrated that the pull on the fascial edges of a vertical incision is thirty times greater than that exerted on a transverse incision. A midline incision represents an exception, since there is marked decussation of the fibers with varying lines of forces. In reference to incisions for cholecystectomy, Pemberton and Manax noted no difference in incidences of dehiscence when vertical and transverse incisions were compared in a thoroughly randomized series. When an intestinal stoma or a drain is brought out through any incision, the incidence of wound dehiscence increases.

CLINICAL MANIFESTATIONS. Most disruptions are concealed in the deeper layers of the wound and do not manifest themselves until the fifth postoperative day, although the separation may, in fact, occur in the operating room or recovery room. The presenting sign is serosanguineous drainage from the wound, and if this occurs subsequent to the first 24 postoperative hours, it is virtually pathognomonic. Frequently, wound dehiscence becomes manifest when the skin sutures are removed and evisceration of intraperitoneal contents, either intestine or omentum, occurs. In some instances, wound disruptions remain concealed beneath an intact cutaneous closure and go unrecognized initially, only to become manifest later in the form of a postoperative ventral hernia.

TREATMENT. The management depends on the patient's condition. If the patient can tolerate the procedure, a secondary operative closure is indicated. The author prefers through-and-through horizontal mattress sutures placed superficial to the peritoneum or buried figure-of-eight monofilament stainless steel sutures to approximate the muscle and fascial layers. In some instances, it is preferable to treat the patient conservatively with an occlusive wound dressing and binder and to accept the complication of a postoperative hernia. If evisceration occurs, sterile moist towels should be applied to cover the extruded intestine or omentum, and the patient should be taken directly to the operating room. After general irrigation, the abdomen is closed with one of the two previously mentioned techniques.

The mortality associated with wound disruption depends on the patient's age and original pathologic condition; reported incidences range from 11 to 85 percent. The incidence of postoperative hernia in one large series was 31 percent.

Wound Infection

Postoperative wound infection results when bacteria within the wound multiply, exciting a local reaction and, frequently, a systemic response. Most wounds become infected in the operating room while they are open, but the presence of bacteria in the wound at the end of the surgical procedure does not usually result in a wound infection. The bacterium most frequently implicated is *Staphylococcus aureus.* Enteric organisms are the causative agents when bowel operation has been performed, and hemolytic streptococci account for about 3 percent of infections. Other common pathogens include enterococci, *Pseudomonas, Proteus,* and *Klebsiella.*

The reported incidence of wound infection has a wide range. In 1963, Howe and Mozden reported 350 major and 117 minor wound infections following 15,658 major operations. Barnes et al., in reporting "standardized operations," noted rates ranging from 1.7 to 9.4 percent for various procedures. The Public Health Laboratory Service of England and Wales reported an overall wound infection rate of 9.7 percent. In a combined study conducted by the Division of Medical Sciences, National Academy of Science-National Research Council, and reported in 1964, the overall incidence of infection in five participating hospitals varied from 3 to 11.1 percent. Clean atraumatic and uninfected operative wounds in which neither the bronchi, nor the gastrointestinal tract, nor the genitourinary tract was entered and which were elective, primarily closed, and undrained had an overall incidence of definite infection of 3.3 percent, while similar wounds which were either not elective, or not primarily closed, or drained mechanically through the incision or via a stab wound had a 7.4 percent incidence of wound infection. Operative wounds in which the bronchus, gastrointestinal tract, or oropharyngeal cavity were entered but without unusual contamination had an overall incidence of infection of 10.8 percent. Open, fresh traumatic wounds, operations with a major break in sterile technique, and incisions encountering acute nonpurulent inflammation were associated with an incidence of wound infections of 16.3 percent. Old traumatic wounds and those involving abscesses of perforated viscera had the highest rate of infection (28.6 percent).

A variety of factors other than the nature of the wound also influences the incidence of infection. Age is a definite factor; the rate of wound infection rises steadily from 4.7 percent in the fifteen- to twenty-four-year-old group to 10.7 percent in the sixty-five to seventy-four-year-old group. There is virtually no difference in sex and race. The presence of diabetes is associated with an increase in infection rate, but when this is adjusted for age, there is no statistical significance to this figure. Steroid therapy affects the wound infection rate adversely. An incidence of 16 percent for patients receiving steroids has been contrasted with 7 percent for those not on such drugs. Patients who are extremely obese also have a more than doubled rate of wound infection when compared with control groups. In the combined study, patients with severe malnutrition also displayed a markedly increased rate of wound infection, but this was distorted by other factors, which, if corrected, cast doubt on the widely held belief that malnourished patients are intrinsically more susceptible. Patients who harbor infections remote from the operative incision have an increased infection rate. The duration of operation exerts a profound influence on wound infection, the incidence rising steadily from 3.6 percent for procedures lasting less than 30 minutes to 18 percent for those lasting over 6 hours.

The urgency of operation only indirectly influences the wound infection rate. The type of closure also influences the rate indirectly. Although 7 percent of wounds primarily closed became infected, 15 percent of those not closed or incompletely closed became infected. The difference appears to result from the greater proportion of nonclean operations in the group without primary closure. When adjusted for wound classification, the infection rate of the two groups was essentially the same. Secondary wound closure, however, was associated with a 28 percent infection rate and skin graft closure with a 17 percent rate. The use of a drain was associated with an 11 percent infection rate, whereas undrained wounds had a rate of 5 percent, but it could not be concluded that the drains themselves were responsible for the infection. Patients hospitalized for fewer than 2 days preoperatively had an infection rate of 6 percent, whereas those hospitalized for periods greater than 3 weeks preoperatively had a rate of 14 percent, and this relationship could not be explained on the basis of other associated factors. The prophylactic use of antibiotics was paradoxically associated with a much higher wound infection rate in the combined series, and similar findings were reported by Schonholtz et al. for orthopedic cases. In contrast, Ketcham et al., in a double-blind study, reported a reduction of wound infection in patients with extensive cancer who were placed on prophylactic antibiotics. In addition, Polk and Lopez-Mayor noted that preoperative and early postoperative cephaloridine reduced the incidence of wound infection in patients in whom segments of stomach or intestine were opened.

The two factors of importance in the genesis of infection are breaks in surgical technique and the host parasite relationship. Two potential sources of contamination are the patient himself, particularly the gastrointestinal tract, and the environment of the operating room including the operating team. Carriers of *S. aureus* in the hospital population have become an increasing source. It has been demonstrated that patients who are nasal carriers of *S. aureus* have a higher incidence of wound infection than noncarriers.

CLINICAL MANIFESTATIONS. In a typical situation about 3 to 4 days following operation, there is some increase in pulse rate, and about the fourth postoperative day, a low-grade, intermittent fever is noted. Usually there is edema and redness of the wound, but the most important early sign is undue pain. In some types, marked thrombosis of surrounding blood vessels is an important feature. Wound dehiscence is usually not caused by infection per se unless the infection is neglected. The diagnosis is usually made on the fifth to seventh day, but this interval may be extended if the patient has been on antibiotics. At that time, the wound is commonly seen as a suppurative process, essentially an abscess. Systemic features of septicemia may be present.

TREATMENT. The most important prophylactic measure is excellent technique. In human volunteers, Elek and Conen have shown that the presence of suture material enhances the infective power of *S. aureus* 1,000 to 10,000 times. Therefore, fine sutures and accurate hemostasis should reduce the incidence. It is generally felt that prophylactic antibiotics do not contribute to a reduction in the incidence of wound infection.

Once diagnosed, the treatment consists of surgical drainage. The skin sutures should be removed and the wound irrigated with saline solution and lightly packed. As a general principle, antimicrobial drugs are not required unless the offending organism is *S. pyogenes* or hemolytic streptococci, which should be treated with penicillin for a period of at least 1 week. Also, patients with wound infections around the central area of the face should receive antimicrobial therapy to prevent intracranial extension. Finally, if the wound sepsis is associated with bacteremia or spreading cellulitis, antimicrobial therapy is also indicated.

See Chap. 5 for a discussion of specific infections, i.e., staphylococcal infections, streptococcal infections, anaero-

bic clostridial cellulitis, clostridial myonecrosis, streptococcal myositis, and tetanus.

Wound Hemorrhage, Hematoma, and Seroma (Accumulation of Serum)

Wound hemorrhage is generally related to an error in
technique in which hemostasis is not accomplished. There
is a higher incidence in patients with polycythemia vera,
myeloproliferative disorders, or coagulation defects and in
patients receiving anticoagulant therapy (see Chap. 3).
Postoperative hemorrhage usually becomes manifest with
a sensation of pressure or pain within the wound shortly
after the patient awakes from anesthesia. There may be
leakage of sanguineous or serosanguineous material at that
time. To control bleeding from the wound edges, pressure
may be applied initially, but if the bleeding continues,
additional sutures or reexploration of the wound may be
required.

The placement of drains in areas of anticipated wound
bleeding is usually not indicated. If the bleeding is trivial,
the drain is unnecessary, while if the bleeding is severe,
it will not evacuate the material. Drains are appropriately
used to evacuate serous fluid from underneath skin flaps,
such as that associated with radical mastectomy, in order
to prevent the vicious cycle in which an expanding serous
collection produces significant bleeding as it separates the
wound. If a large skin flap has been raised, it should be
anticipated that fluid will develop, and in order to facilitate
apposition between the subcutaneous tissue and deep fascia, the drainage should be effected. This obviates formation of a serous accumulation, a seroma.

Once a seroma develops, it should be aspirated initially;
if multiple aspirations are required, a polyethylene catheter may be inserted and attached to negative suction.
Prompt treatment is indicated, since the presence of contained serous fluid increases the incidence of subcutaneous
infection. The same situation pertains to a subcutaneous
hematoma, and drainage is required, since the blood
affords an excellent culture medium and also prevents
apposition between the two surfaces.

POSTOPERATIVE PAROTITIS

Postoperative parotitis is a serious complication and is
associated with a high mortality that is related to it and
to the primary disease with which it is associated. Recent
reviews indicate an incidence of 1:1,000 postoperative
cases, and there is a real recrudescence which is related
to the increasing age of the surgical population. The right
and left glands are involved equally, and in 10 to 15
percent of cases, the disease presents bilaterally. Seventy-
five percent of patients are seventy years or older, and the
overwhelming majority have associated diseases. Patients
having major abdominal surgical treatment, fractured hip,
debilitating diseases, and severe injury are among the most
commonly afflicted.

The factors which have been implicated in the etiology
include poor oral hygiene, dehydration, and the use of
anticholinergic drugs. In one large series, one-third of the
patients with acute suppurative parotitis had carcinoma,
and one-half had preexisting major infection elsewhere in
the body. In only one-third of the cases in this series the
acute suppurative process developed in the postoperative
period.

The pathogenesis is thought to be a transductal inoculation of the parotid, and the majority of infections are due
to staphylococci. The combination of poor oral hygiene
and lack of oral intake predisposes to bacterial invasion
of Stensen's duct. The inflammatory lesions of early parotitis are confined to an accumulation of cells within the
larger ducts. The parenchyma of the smaller ducts are
initially spared, but once penetration of the parenchyma
occurs, multiple abscesses form and later coalesce. If the
process continues, the purulent material penetrates the
capsule and invades the surrounding tissue along one of
three routes: downward into the deep fascial planes of the
neck, backward into the external auditory canal, or outward into the skin of the face.

CLINICAL MANIFESTATIONS. The interval between operation and the onset of parotitis varies from a few hours
to many weeks. The patient initially presents with pain
in the parotid region. The pain is usually unilateral but
may become bilateral in a short period of time. Initially,
inspection shows the gland to be slightly swollen, and
palpation demonstrates exquisite tenderness. The course
of postoperative parotitis is rapid and fulminating with
severe cellulitis developing on the affected side of the face
and neck. The temperature and leukocyte count may be
extremely high. Obstruction of the airway may necessitate
tracheostomy, and the abscess may rupture into adjacent
structures of the ear, mastoid, pharynx, or anterior and
posterior triangles of the neck. Parotitis is to be differentiated from benign postoperative swelling of the parotids,
which occurs more frequently in Negroes and may be
related to straining, belladonna, and neuromuscular depolarizing drugs.

TREATMENT. Prophylactic therapy consists of adequate
hydration and good oral hygiene which can be aided by
allowing the patient to take ice chips and stimulating
salivary flow. Prophylactic antibiotics are apparently of no
value.

Once the diagnosis is entertained, pus should be expressed from Stensen's duct and culture and sensitivity
tests performed. A broad-spectrum antibiotic which acts
against the staphylococci should be started while awaiting
results. In one series of 66 glands cultured, 64 contained
staphylococci. In some cases, these were combined with
streptococci, gram-negative bacilli, and pneumococci. If
there is considerable pain and the disease is less than 24
hours old, irradiation of the gland in small doses is indicated. Irradiation may provide symptomatic relief by reducing the secretions of the obstructed gland, but this type
of therapy does not affect the course of the disease as much
as antibiotics or surgical drainage.

Frequent observation of the patient is essential. If the
disease persists or progresses, drainage should be considered as early as the third day. If there is moderate improvement, drainage may be delayed for a day or two,

but in no circumstance should it be delayed beyond the fifth day. An incision is made anterior to the ear, extending down to the angle of the mandible, and flaps are reflected, exposing the gland. A hemostat is inserted through the capsule and opened in the direction of the course of the branches of the facial nerve. Multiple drainage sites are thus established, and the wound is packed lightly open. Deferring drainage until fluctuation is apparent is unwise. Stimulation of the salivary flow by massage of the gland or other means is contraindicated, once the inflammatory process is established.

PROGNOSIS. In a recent series, the mortality rate approximated 20 percent, but this was frequently related to the patient's basic disease. However, 36 percent of the patients who died demonstrated active parotitis. In 80 percent of patients treated with incision and drainage the parotitis was palliated or cured.

POSTOPERATIVE RESPIRATORY COMPLICATIONS

Respiratory Failure

The availability of techniques to measure the arterial P_{O_2} (Pa_{O_2}) has focused attention on respiratory failure in the postoperative period. Neely and associates, Moore et al., and Pontoppidan et al. have indicated that respiratory failure is a major cause in 25 percent of postoperative deaths and a major contributory factor in another 25 percent. Acute respiratory failure has been defined as a situation in which the Pa_{O_2} is below the predicted normal for the patient's age or the Pa_{CO_2} is above 50 mm Hg in the absence of metabolic acidosis. A broad spectrum of patients fall in this category; well over two-thirds have experienced surgery or trauma.

PATHOPHYSIOLOGY. Physiologic causes of acute respiratory insufficiency following surgery include (1) hypoventilation, (2) diffusion defects, (3) abnormalities in the ventilation/perfusion ratio, (4) shunting which is either anatomic or related to atelectasis, (5) reduction in cardiac output with concomitant persistent shunt, and (6) alteration in the hemoglobin level and/or dissociation curve.

A variety of measurements of ventilation and oxygenation have been applied, with multiple refinements. Those which are relatively routinely performed will be considered in this discussion. Ventilatory mechanics are evaluated by routine monitoring of the respiratory rate and determination of the vital capacity and inspiratory force. Ventilation, itself, is assessed by consideration of respiratory rate, tidal volume, and, more particularly, Pa_{CO_2}. A frequently employed refinement to assess CO_2 elimination is VD/VT, where VD is the physiologic dead space and VT is the tidal volume. This ratio is defined as that portion of the tidal volume which is ineffective in the removal of CO_2 from the blood. The technique involves collection of expired gas over several respiratory cycles for about 2 minutes and simultaneous measurements of Pa_{CO_2}. VD/VT is influenced by cardiac output, tidal volume, and the pattern of respiration.

The adequacy of intrapulmonary blood-gas exchange is determined by measuring the Pa_{CO_2} and the Pa_{O_2} in relation to the inspired P_{O_2}. The efficacy of oxygen exchange within the lung is expressed as the alveolar-arterial oxygen tension difference ($A-aDO_2$). Factors which influence the $A-aDO_2$ include the difference between the arterial and venous oxygen content; the mixed venous oxygen content, itself, which may reflect oxygen consumption; the cardiac output; the inspired oxygen concentration (Fi_{O_2}); the position of the oxygen hemoglobin dissociation curve; and the position of the Pa_{O_2} on the curve. Abnormalities in the ventilation/perfusion ratio ($\dot{Q}_S/\dot{Q}_T$) express right-to-left physiologic shunt. This ratio can be determined precisely by measuring the oxygen content of the pulmonary end-capillary arterial and mixed venous blood, but more frequently a nomogram can be used to define $\dot{Q}_S/\dot{Q}_T$ based on the measurement of Pa_{O_2} and pulmonary alveolar oxygen tension (PA_{O_2}), as shown in Fig. 12-1. As can be seen, small changes in the $\dot{Q}_S/\dot{Q}_T$ are more readily detected when the patient is breathing 100% oxygen for 20 or 30 minutes. Determinations are affected by alterations in the cardiac output and pH.

PATHOGENESIS. The major etiologic and contributory factors are conveniently considered under the categories listed in pathophysiology. Hypoventilation may be related to thoracic trauma; muscle weakness; and deleterious changes in the respiratory mechanics, which have been

Fig. 12-1. Analog-computed relationship between percent right-to-left shunt ($\dot{Q}_S/\dot{Q}_T \times 100$), arterial P_{O_2}, and inspired oxygen or alveolar oxygen tension (PA_{O_2}). The alveolar-arterial oxygen tension gradient can be obtained by drawing a horizontal line from the ordinate (arterial P_{O_2}) to the appropriate PA_{O_2} line. For example, when $\dot{Q}_S/\dot{Q}_T \times 100 = 20$, and $PA_{O_2} \times 680$ mm Hg, then the arterial P_{O_2} is approximately 175 mm Hg and the $A-aDO_2 = 680 - 175 = 505$ mm Hg. Note that below a right-to-left shunt value of 30, small changes in $Q_S/Q_T \times 100$ can produce drastic alterations in arterial P_{O_2} particularly when the subject is breathing high concentrations of oxygen. The curves were drawn assuming a hemoglobin concentration of 15 Gm/100 ml, an arterial pH of 7.40, an $A-V_{O_2}$ difference of 6 ml/100 ml, and a standard oxyhemoglobin dissociation curve. (From H. Pontoppidan et al., Adv Surg 4:163, 1970. Copyright 1970 by Year Book Medical Publishers, Inc., Chicago. Used by permission. Graphs kindly prepared by Dr. M. A. Duvelleroy.)

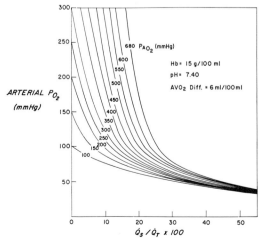

shown to exist for several days following thoracotomy and laparotomy. Diffusion defects may exist in patients who are chronic long-term smokers with consequent intra-alveolar septal thickening. The defects also may be related to the aspiration of gastric content, which is now appreciated to occur more commonly; an incidence of 10 percent has been reported for intubated patients undergoing elective surgery, and a higher percentage for patients undergoing emergency surgery. There is no evidence that tracheostomy protects against such aspiration. Oxygen, itself, has intrinsic toxicity, and when Fi_{O_2} is over 60%, destruction of respiratory epithelium may occur. Therefore, it is preferable to maintain patients with congestive heart failure and emphysema at Pa_{O_2} of 70 mm Hg with Fi_{O_2} of 60% rather than expose the airway to 100% oxygen for a long period of time. Fluid overload with pulmonary edema initially decreases compliance and ultimately impairs gas exchange (see below). Other intrapulmonary lesions which may contribute to interference with diffusion include microemboli, fat emboli, and pulmonary infection. Abnormalities of the ventilation/perfusion ratio ($\dot{Q}_S/\dot{Q}_T$) result when areas which are well perfused with blood are underventilated. Maintaining the patient in a supine position accentuates this maldistribution, and the pathophysiologic consequence of atelectasis is a significant abnormality in $\dot{Q}_S/\dot{Q}_T$. Other factors which alter the ventilation/perfusion ratio are obesity and upper abdominal surgery with consequent collapse of the basal aveoli. Both atelectasis and reduced cardiac output result in intrapulmonary shunting. A shift in the oxygen-hemoglobin dissociation curve to the left decreases oxygen delivery to the tissues. This may be caused by respiratory alkalosis and also by deficiency in 2,3-diphosphoglycerate, which results from transfusion of banked blood more than 3 days old.

The question has been raised whether "shock lung" per se exists and contributes to progressive pulmonary insufficiency. To date, the clinical experiences have been variously interpreted, but Collins' summary of combat casualties suggests that hemorrhagic shock, itself, represents an extremely infrequent cause of acute pulmonary insufficiency.

CLINICAL MANIFESTATIONS. Among the situations which should alert the observer to the development of the syndrome of postoperative pulmonary insufficiency are (1) congestive failure, (2) dyspnea, (3) cyanosis, (4) evidence of obstructive lung disease, and (5) pulmonary edema. Early in the evolution of the syndrome, the patient manifests hyperventilation associated with a reduction in Pa_{CO_2} below 35 mm Hg which precedes any significant reduction in Pa_{O_2}. Ultimately there is a reduction in Pa_{O_2} which becomes more significant when the patient does not respond to increases in Fi_{O_2}. Roentgenologic changes tend to occur late in the course of the condition and may represent the effects of therapy. These lesions are characteristically scattered, ill-defined, bilateral densities. A correlation exists between the extension of the densities and deterioration of pulmonary function.

TREATMENT. This should be mainly preventive and consists of ancillary measures and respiratory support. Antibiotics are indicated to treat established infections, and diuretics are useful in the management of pulmonary edema. Care is taken to avoid fluid overload of the patient, and the colloidal osmotic pressure of the plasma should be maintained at normal level. Normal hemoglobin level is also important. Respiratory support includes physical therapy; the importance of moving the patient in order to avoid ventilation-perfusion abnormalities is emphasized. Increase of the Fi_{O_2}, particularly to levels over 60%, requires constant monitoring in order to obviate severe oxygen toxicity of the lung.

The prophylactic use of artificial ventilation for respiratory support represents a major recent advance in the management of these patients. The indications for respiratory support have been categorized according to pathologic alterations (Table 12-1). Ventilatory support may be accomplished either through an endotracheal tube or a tracheostomy, since ventilation via a face mask or mouthpiece is rarely effective for more than short periods. Endotracheal intubation is considered the technique of choice when control of airway is urgently required.

The prolonged use of endotracheal intubation for ventilatory support is now gaining popularity as an alternative

Table 12-1. INDICATIONS FOR RESPIRATORY SUPPORT

		Acceptable range	Chest physical therapy, oxygen, close monitoring	Intubation, tracheostomy, ventilation
Mechanics	Respiratory rate	12–25	25–35	>35
	Vital capacity, ml/kg	70–30	30–15	<15
	Inspiratory force, cm H_2O	100–50	50–25	<25
Oxygenation . . .	$A - aDO_2$, mm Hg*	50–200	200–350	>350
	Pa_{O_2}, mm Hg	100–75 (Air)	200–70 (On mask O_2)	<70 (On mask O_2)
Ventilation	VD/VT	0.3–0.4	0.4–0.6	>0.6
	Pa_{CO_2}, mm Hg	35–45	45–60	>60†

* After 15 minutes of 100% O_2.
† Except in chronic hypercapnia.

to tracheostomy. Although endotracheal tubes are not tolerated as well as tracheostomy tubes and it is appreciated that prolonged intubation is associated with laryngeal swelling, 6 days in adults and up to 3 weeks in children are regarded as reasonable periods of prolonged endotracheal intubation. In general, intubation via a nasotracheal route is tolerated better than via the orotracheal route, but insertion may be more difficult. The major advantage of endotracheal intubation is that the mortality is low, the complications are minimal, and the hazards associated with tracheostomy are avoided.

Tracheostomy is now generally reserved for the patient who requires prolonged ventilatory support and, as is pointed out in Chap. 19, may be associated with the complications of stenosis which are generally related to cuff pressure. The introduction of low-pressure cuffs may reduce the incidence of this complication.

In general, ventilatory support is first accomplished using intermittent positive-pressure breathing (IPPB) in which expiration is unobstructed and intrapulmonary pressure returns to atmospheric level. The patient's blood gases are monitored while on ventilatory support, and if necessary the Fi_{O_2} is increased up to 60% to maintain the Pa_{O_2} at normal levels. If IPPB is ineffectual, positive end-expiratory pressure ventilation (PEEP) is instituted. PEEP results in increased functional residual capacity, reduced normal negative intrathoracic pressure with, at times, conversion to positive values, increased venous pressure, and decreased venous return to the heart. PEEP ventilation is particularly effective in causing a rise in Pa_{O_2} and a fall in physiologic shunt, and the greater amount of shunting across the lung, the greater the effect of this modality. PEEP ventilation is preferred for patients with profound hypoxemia, significant physiologic shunting, atelectasis, and high cardiac output. It is particularly appropriate for patients with massive chest wall injuries. PEEP is contraindicated for conditions characterized by normal oxygenation, hyperexpansion of the lung, and low cardiac output. In general, it is felt that the end-expiratory pressure should be maintained at 5 cm H_2O and should rarely be increased above 10 cm H_2O because of the danger of producing pneumothorax.

Prolonged artificial ventilation has been characterized by the formation of edema and deterioration of blood-gas interchange, which is generally manageable by water restriction and the administration of diuretic agents such as furosemide or ethacrynic acid. When there is objective evidence that lung function is adequate to permit transfer from artificial to spontaneous ventilation, a gradual weaning process is required. The patient on PEEP is initially converted to IPPB. Difficulty in weaning can be attributed to abnormalities in blood-gas exchange, pulmonary mechanics, reduction in cardiac output, and general muscle weakness. Weaning should be accomplished only with careful monitoring of blood gas and exchange; the pulmonary mechanics are indicated in Table 12-1.

Atelectasis

Atelectasis comprises 90 percent of all postoperative pulmonary complications, but a lack of definition and difficulty in diagnosis has resulted in a wide range of reported incidences varying between 1 and 80 percent depending on the type of operation and the reporting institution. The term "atelectasis" is derived from the Greek meaning "incomplete expansion" but is generally applied to the situation in which there are airless alveoli. Although collapse of alveoli may occur within definite anatomic units such as segments, lobes, or an entire lung, the most commonly encountered variety is platelike and subsegmental. Moersch reported atelectasis in 10 percent of operations on the thorax or upper abdomen and 4 percent of operations on the lower abdomen. Clendon and Pygott found 38 percent in patients undergoing abdominal surgical treatment and only 2.7 percent when operations were performed in areas other than the abdomen or thorax. Kurzweg indicated that atelectasis occurred in 3 percent of all operations, 10 to 20 percent of cases with abdominal surgery, and 20 to 30 percent of cases involving upper abdominal surgery. Becker et al., who took roentgenograms in a series of patients postoperatively, demonstrated that 51 percent of patients with upper abdominal surgical treatment had atelectasis. Three percent were lobar, fourteen percent segmental, and thirty-one percent platelike in distribution. When pulmonary function studies were used to determine the diagnosis, Beecher found evidence of collapse in 83 percent of laparotomies.

ETIOLOGY. The two major factors which have been implicated as causes of atelectasis are bronchial obstruction with distal gas absorption and hypoventilation or ineffectual respiration. The loss of chemical elements which stabilize the lung at low volumes by reducing alveolar surface tension, i.e., *surfactants,* recently has been implicated.

Obstruction of the tracheobronchial airway occurs secondary to changes in bronchial secretion, defect in the expulsion mechanism, and reduction in bronchial caliber. Subsequent to tracheobronchial obstruction by secretion, vomitus, blood, or tumor material, there is a period during which a change occurs in the composition of gases within the alveolus, following which the gas composition in the obstructed alveoli remains constant until absorption is complete. The rate of absorption is a function of the pressure difference between the gas in the alveoli and the gas in the blood, the absorption coefficient of the gas, and the rate and quantity of blood flow.

Obstruction of a large conductive airway certainly leads to atelectasis of the distal lung segment. However, there are many observations which cast doubt on bronchial obstruction as the sole or major causative factor in postoperative atelectasis. It is common to find atelectasis at autopsy with no obstructive plug. Conversely, it is uncommon for atelectasis to be accompanied by a definite plug, the removal of which leads to recovery. The excessive secretions associated with atelectasis might be a secondary effect rather than a cause. For atelectasis to occur on an obstructive basis, the obstruction must be complete; it seems unlikely that postoperative secretions could establish an obstruction in so short a time. Also, the fact that atelectasis can be prevented or relieved by hyperventilation suggests that the obstructive origin is improbable. Finally, Van Allen and Adams found that, in dogs breathing normally, bronchial occlusion did not result in atelectasis, and they felt that this was due to sufficient collateral respiration or circulation of gas to prevent collapse of the alveoli. Perhaps the strongest case against the etiologic necessity of airway obstruction is the demonstration by Griffo and Roos that the time course of atelectatic changes does not vary with the varying solubility of inspired gases.

Currently, many feel that atelectasis usually consists of small and diffuse lesions which are nonobstructive in origin and are due to inspiratory insufficiency. The concept of inspiratory failure was first demonstrated by Mead and Collier and subsequently expanded by several writers, particularly Bendixen and his associates. It has been shown that spontaneous or artificial ventilation at constant tidal volumes usually will result in decreased compliance, decreased lung volume, and increased shunting (venous admixture). These signs all suggest a decrease in the number of functioning alveoli and occur more rapidly than could be explained by the absorption of gases due to an obstructing lesion. The changes are almost completely reversible with pulmonary inflation beyond the tidal volume range or with intermittent deep breathing. Thus, atelectasis is thought to occur without airway obstruction as a result of a constant volume ventilation with volumes approximating normal tidal volume, and the process is reversible by hyperinflation. The validity of this etiologic concept is also debatable as evidenced by the findings of Brattstrom, who noted that before and after operation in patients with and without lung complications, the course of ventilation was essentially similar. There was no evidence of decreased effectivity of ventilation in the functioning alveoli nor of impaired pulmonary mixing.

The third major cause of alveolar collapse is related to the surface forces acting at the gas-liquid interface within the alveolar units. Normally, there is a film, surfactant, which has the property of reducing surface tension when the alveolar volume is decreased. Increased surface tension of this film encourages collapse or decrease in the size of the alveolus and makes it more difficult to inflate. Regional changes in the pulmonary circulation may alter the characteristics of surfactant. Clements postulates that deep breathing mobilizes surfactant from within the alveolar cell to augment or replace the aging surfactant on the alveolar surface, maintaining stability and preventing atelectasis.

Many factors predispose to the development of postoperative atelectasis. There is an increasing incidence in patients who smoke and those who suffer from bronchitis, asthma, emphysema, or other chronic lung diseases. Anesthesia and postoperative narcotics depress the cough reflex, while chest pain, immobilization, and splinting with bandages reduces the effective nature of the cough. The incidence of atelectasis is related to the duration and depth of anesthesia, and although higher incidences have been reported with general anesthesia than with regional anesthesia, when the same postoperative care was applied to the two groups, the difference disappeared. Nasogastric tubes have been implicated because of the increased secretions and predisposition toward aspiration. Bronchospasm is a predisposing factor, but severe bronchospasm is rarely encountered during clinical anesthesia. Congestion of the bronchial walls due to edema represents another source

of decrease in the bronchial lumen. As mentioned previously, there is a definite increase in atelectasis associated with upper abdominal as opposed to lower abdominal or extraabdominal surgical procedures. Transverse incisions are associated with a lower incidence of atelectasis when compared to vertical incisions in the same area.

CLINICAL MANIFESTATIONS. Atelectasis usually becomes manifest in the first 24 hours after an operation and rarely appears after 48 hours. There is usually a sudden onset of fever and tachycardia. Frequently, the pulmonary manifestations are so minor that they are not recognized. Early findings include rales located posteriorly in the bases, diminished breath sounds, and bronchial breathing. With massive involvement, there may be a shift of the trachea, mediastinum, and heart to the involved side, but this is not present with the more common subsegmental lesions. Pronounced dyspnea and/or cyanosis are relatively uncommon. Roentgenograms may demonstrate areas of consolidation, but in early cases bronchial breathing is detected more frequently than roentgenographic changes. Determination of blood gases indicating intrapulmonary shunting of blood provides the diagnosis. Characteristically with atelectasis and significant shunting, the arterial Pa_{O_2} is decreased while the arterial Pa_{CO_2} may be normal or decreased. The ventilation is normal or increased.

If atelectasis persists, the clinical manifestations are those generally associated with pneumonia. The temperature increases to a greater extent, and there is increasing tachycardia, dyspnea, and cyanosis. It is felt that the great majority of postoperative pneumonias begin as atelectasis, since atelectatic areas are poorly drained and represent good sites for infection. In some instances, however, pneumonia may result from the aspiration of infected material. Another consequence of atelectasis is the development of lung abscess, which also may be initiated by the aspiration of foreign material, such as teeth or blood during tonsillectomy and purulent material from putrid abscesses in the mouth. Aspiration of gastric contents also represents a possible cause of lung abscess.

TREATMENT. Prophylaxis begins preoperatively by having the patient cease smoking, if possible, for at least 2 weeks prior to operation and instructing the patient in deep abdominal breathing and productive coughing. Postoperative prophylaxis includes the minimal use of depressant drugs, the prevention of pain which may limit respiration, frequent changes of body position, deep breathing and coughing exercises, and early ambulation. Hyperinflation with its attendant alveolar distension and stimulation of coughing is the most important factor in the prevention and treatment of atelectasis. The usual IPPB units do not have the mechanism for instituting sighing or deep breathing, but manual inflation using an Ambu bag may accomplish this end. Becker et al. reported that the routine use of IPPB with bronchodilator and bronchodetergent drugs did not prevent the occurrence of atelectasis or accelerate its disappearance, once it was established.

Three groups of medications have been applied to the prophylaxis and therapy of atelectasis. These are (1) expectorants to provide more liquid and less viscous secretions, (2) detergents and mucolytic solutions to alter the surface tension of secretions and render their elimination more likely, and (3) bronchodilators used primarily by inhalation to provide increased size of the tracheobronchial tree and elimination of bronchospasm. The mucolytic agents, such as Mucomist or Alevaire, are indicated because inhaled air with a relative humidity lower than 70% inhibits ciliary activity and tends to desiccate secretions.

Once atelectasis becomes clinically manifest, coughing, clearing of secretions, and increase in depth of respiration may be stimulated by endotracheal suction with a soft rubber catheter or the instillation of 1 to 2 ml of saline solution directly into the trachea via an intracatheter polyethylene tube. If these measures are not successful, bronchoscopy may be required, and if multiple bronchoscopic aspirations are necessary, tracheostomy should be performed to facilitate subsequent aspiration.

Atelectasis, pneumonia, aspiration pneumonia, and lung abscesses are also discussed in Chap. 17.

Pulmonary Edema

Pulmonary edema may occur during or immediately after an operation. The increased use of massive blood transfusions, plasma expanders, and other fluids during operative procedures has resulted in an increased incidence of this complication. Circulatory overload represents the most common cause of pulmonary edema. Other factors which have been implicated include incomplete cardiac emptying, shift of blood from the peripheral to pulmonary vascular bed, negative pressure on the airway which increases the gradient between the transmural capillary pressure and the alveolar pressure favoring transudation, and injury to the alveolar membrane by noxious substances.

Although circulatory overload is most frequently due to infusion of fluid during operative procedure, it may also result from the absorption of solutions during irrigation of hollow viscera, such as the bladder, and is frequently associated with subclinical heart failure in those patients in whom pulmonary edema becomes manifest.

Incomplete cardiac emptying may be attributed to any anesthetic, narcotic, or hypnotic agent, since all are capable of decreasing myocardial contractility. Incomplete cardiac emptying may also be due to gross irregularities in rhythm. Pulmonary edema is rarely the result of this single factor, and there is usually elevated atrial and pulmonary blood pressure associated with incomplete cardiac emptying. Similarly, the etiologic mechanism of shift of blood to the pulmonary vascular bed is usually associated with other factors. Peripheral vascular beds may vasoconstrict, causing blood to shift centrally and result in pulmonary edema. A reflex mechanism of neurogenic origin which causes redistribution of blood from the periphery to the pulmonary bed has been reported to occur during manipulation of the brain.

Pulmonary edema caused by injury to the alveolar membrane is associated with the inhalation of noxious gases or vapors and the aspiration of gastric contents or chemicals, particularly kerosene, which are pulmonary irritants.

CLINICAL MANIFESTATIONS. The initial disturbance of pulmonary edema is thickening of the capillary and alveolar membranes. In the early stage, the principle effect is a reduction in diffusion, and unless increased oxygen tension is present, hypoxemia results. A reduction in lung compliance precedes evidence of carbon dioxide retention in the blood. Bronchospasm usually occurs and contributes further to reducing the compliance. As frank edema develops, a frothy pink-stained fluid appears in the alveoli, bronchi, and trachea, and at this time the problem is one of airway obstruction rather than diffusion. Clinically, bronchospasm and marked reduction in lung compliance in a patient being ventilated should provide premonitory evidence and anticipate the development of dyspnea and cough. A few scattered rales may appear early, but as the process intensifies, bubbling rales and rhonchi are heard all over the chest. The systemic blood pressure is usually raised initially but may be normal or reduced, and characteristically there is a marked tachycardia. Shock may appear with signs of peripheral circulatory failure, and death may occur from asphyxia.

TREATMENT. Therapy is directed at (1) providing oxygen, (2) allowing oxygen access to the alveoli by removing obstructive fluid, and (3) correcting the circulatory overload. Oxygen saturation can be restored by increasing the concentration of oxygen in inspired air. An increase in alveolar oxygen tension of 50 mm Hg, which can be achieved by a 7 percent increase in inspired oxygen, is sufficient to restore arterial oxygen tension to normal, even in the presence of the more severe diffusion defects. Hypoxemia, however, will persist even if pure oxygen is breathed unless the fluid is removed from the alveoli.

Measures to reduce the pulmonary capillary pressure include venous occlusion tourniquets, placing the patient in a head-up or sitting position to reduce the flow of venous blood to the heart, and phlebotomy. Since systemic vasoconstriction has been shown to be a precipitating cause, therapy may be indicated to reverse this mechanism. Spinal anesthesia has been applied successfully in the treatment of pulmonary edema, as has the ganglionic blocking agent Arfonad.

IPPB or PEEP (5 cm) must be used with caution, since it too may impair the efficiency of an already failing circulation. Drug therapy includes furosemide or ethacrynic acid for rapid diuresis and digitalis glycosides for situations where myocardial failure and lower output coexist (particularly in mitral stenosis) or where there is arrhythmia such as flutter or fibrillation. Morphine has been shown to be of value, though its mode of action remains unclear.

CARDIAC COMPLICATIONS

This section considers cardiac arrhythmias and myocardial ischemia and infarction related to surgery. A discussion of cardiac arrest and the postcardiotomy syndrome is presented in Chap. 19.

Arrhythmias

Although cardiac arrhythmias are frequently associated with operative repair of congenital and acquired lesions of the heart (see Chaps. 18 and 19), they represent a potential complication of any surgical procedure. As the age of the surgical population increases, one should encounter an increasing incidence of these disturbances.

INCIDENCE. The incidence varies and is somewhat determined by whether sinus tachycardia is included in the series. In a recent review, Reinikainen and Pontinen report that the incidence of cardiac arrhythmias occurring during extrathoracic operative procedures ranged between 30 and 100 percent. During thoracotomies carried out under general anesthesia, incidences as high as 77 percent have been recorded. Heart diseases increased the incidence; in one series, in 51 percent of cardiac patients as contrasted with 20 percent of other patients, arrhythmia developed during anesthesia. Kuner and associates, monitoring continuous electrocardiographic signals on magnetic tape for prolonged periods of time, found the incidence of cardiac arrhythmia during anesthesia to be 61.7 percent. The arrhythmias which they noted most frequently were wandering pacemaker, atrioventricular (AV) dissociation, and nodal rhythm and premature ventricular systoles. Relating intraoperative arrhythmias to type of anesthesia, Reinikainen and Pontinen recorded arrhythmias in 24 percent of patients in whom operations were carried out under local anesthesia. The majority of these were of vagal origin and caused by the occulocardiac reflex. There were also ventricular systoles due to emotional factors. Under epidural anesthesia, the incidence was 23.5 percent, and this was frequently related to blood pressure reduction. When general anesthesia was established with halothane, arrhythmias occurred during intubation in 29 percent and during maintenance of anesthesia in 13 percent of patients.

A study of over 3,000 noncardiac cases revealed 2.4 percent had abnormal postoperative electrocardiograms. The majority of patients were asymptomatic, and most of the abnormalities were conduction disturbances. Taylor reported postoperative arrhythmias in about 5 percent of cyclopropane administrations. Buckley and Jackson studied 100 patients immediately after surgical treatment and noted sinus tachycardia in 32 percent, sinus bradycardia in 2 percent, sinus arrhythmia in 3 percent, occasional ventricular contractions in 7 percent, and trigeminy in 1 percent. Arrhythmias occur much more frequently following thoracic surgical procedures, with paroxysmal fibrillation and atrial flutter or fibrillation representing the most common types. The time of onset is variable, 30 percent occurring on the first postoperative day and 60 percent with 72 hours of operation, though the onset has been noted as late as the eighteenth day. Wheat and Burford reported that 20 to 30 percent of patients recovering from thoracic operations exhibited cardiac arrhythmias. The site and extent of the procedure represented important factors. Arrhythmia occurred in 11 to 32 percent of cases following pneumonectomy and in only 5 percent following lobectomy or lesser resection procedures. When the thoracic lesions involved the vagus nerve, an increasing frequency was noted.

ETIOLOGY. Postoperative cardiac arrhythmias frequently have their genesis in the preoperative period. Atrial arrhythmias are usually due to vagal stimulation. Other provoking factors are hypotension, hypoxia, and hypercapnia, all of which may cause inhibition of the sinus node and activation of a local pacemaker situation within the region of the atria. The most important reason for ventricular arrhythmia is increased excitability of the ventricular muscle. This may be attributed to sympathomimetic drugs, such as epinephrine, increase in blood pressure, carotid sinus stimulation, and vagal inhibition. Certain antihypertensive drugs, such as reserpine and guanethidine, increase ventricular arrhythmia, and inadequate preoperative digitalization may also be responsible. It is generally held that some common anesthetic agents like halothane and cyclopropane produce sensitization of the myocardium, making it more responsive to the catecholamines, thus potentiating the development of arrhythmia. Muscle of the diseased heart is also more excitable, and hypercapnia provokes ectopic rhythm by decreasing pacemaker activity. Electrolyte disturbances, particularly alterations in potassium concentration, can cause ventricular arrhythmia. The vasovagal cardiac reflex has been implicated in arrhythmias which develop during intubation, surgical manipulation of the lung, and operations on the gallbladder and stomach. Positive-pressure breathing mechanisms may induce a high resistance in the pulmonary circulation, reduce venous return, and stimulate ventricular arrhythmia. Specific diseases which have been implicated as causes of arrhythmia during operative procedures are thyrotoxicosis and pheochromocytoma with its high catecholamine concentration in the plasma.

Important predisposing factors include the patient's age and the presence of preexisting heart disease, arteriosclerosis, or hypertension. The highest incidence of arrhythmias occurs in patients over sixty, and it has been shown that the diseased heart is definitely more excitable. Other determining factors include the type of anesthetic, the duration of surgical procedures, the need for intubation, and hyperventilation. The anesthetic agents most frequently implicated are halothane and cyclopropane, though arrhythmias occur with all types of anesthesia. Halothane is usually associated with bradycardia and AV dissociation, and when vasopressors are used in combination with halothane, there is an increased incidence of paroxysmal arrhythmia. Atropine also has been noted to cause AV dissociation during anesthesia and in patients undergoing breast and perineal surgery. There is a high incidence of sinus bradycardia during Pentothal induction. Serum electrolyte abnormalities during the postoperative course are contributory factors, particularly acidosis and hypokalemia. Hypercalcemia following parathyroid manipulation or with inappropriate intravenous calcium therapy may precipitate rapid ectopic atrial arrhythmia. Thoracic surgery is associated with an increased incidence of arrhythmias. During the postoperative period, myocardial infarction and pulmonary complications are frequently associated with ventricular arrhythmias.

TREATMENT. In view of the high incidence of arrhythmia in elderly patients undergoing thoracic surgical procedures, some have suggested prophylactic digitalization, and others have employed quinidine and procaine amide therapy preoperatively. Digitalization is particularly applicable in patients with frequent atrial premature systoles, while withholding of digitalis is indicated in the presence of sustained or intermittent paroxysmal nodal rhythms. Many have advised discontinuing all myocardial depressant agents, including quinidine and procainamide preoperatively, and withholding all cardiac drugs in the operating room, unless an arrhythmia compromises cardiac output. A bipolar electrode may be inserted preoperatively into the outflow tract of the right ventricle for emergency electronic pacing in patients with advanced second-degree heart block or third degree AV block.

Once an arrhythmia develops, if it is tolerated well by the patient, it may be simply observed, since a high percentage convert spontaneously. In general, therapy is directed at maintaining adequate cardiac output and coronary blood flow. Vasopressors may be administered to maintain the blood pressure while the definitive treatment is organized. If congestive failure threatens, digitalis is the treatment of choice. Digitalis is also the drug of choice in the presence of all supraventricular arrhythmias. For rapid digitalization, 1 mg of digoxin may be slowly given intravenously. Additional doses of 0.25 mg may be given orally, by intramuscular injection, or intravenously every 4 to 6 hours for three doses, if needed, before establishing maintenance therapy. However, paroxysmal and atrial tachycardia with block and nonparoxysmal nodal tachycardia may all be caused by inappropriate administration of digitalis. Although quinidine may convert atrial fibrillation to sinus rhythm, it does not represent the prime treatment in any real emergency. Cardioversion limits the applicability of quinidine to the prevention of arrhythmias. It is also unwise to administer calcium and depressant agents indiscriminately. If the arrhythmia is related to overdigitalization, potassium should be administered as 40 mEq of potassium chloride in 50 ml of solution, limiting the dose to 20 mEq/hour. Lidocaine, 1 mg/kg intravenously administered rapidly or as a continuous drip of 1 to 2 mg/mEq, is preferred for ventricular arrhythmias. It has the advantage over procainamide in that it causes less depression of myocardial contractility. Diphenylhydantoin (Dilantin) is effective as treatment for digitalis-induced supraventricular tachycardia and ventricular irritability. However, it may reduce myocardial contractility, increase AV block, and cause cardiac arrest. Propranolol, a beta-adrenergic blocker, is used for digitalis intoxication and for slowing ventricular rate in atrial flutter or fibrillation.

Sinus Tachycardia. By definition this disturbance in normal rhythm is not an arrhythmia. Sinus tachycardia is caused by increased sympathetic tone or decreased vagal tone frequently secondary to hypoxia, hypovolemia due to blood loss, and pain. Hypercapnia, dehydration, hyperthyroidism, and congestive heart failure are frequently associated with sinus tachycardia. A variety of drugs, including meperidine, atropine, and epinephrine, all increase the heart rate, as does digitalis intoxication. Treatment is directed at the cause.

Supraventricular Paroxysmal Tachycardia. This is usually characterized by the sudden onset of a regular heart rate ranging between 140 and 220 beats per minute. Rogers et al. reported an incidence of 0.2 percent during the postoperative period. The disturbance may be caused by digitalis or quinidine toxicity, myocardial infarction, congestive heart failure, thyrotoxicosis, and hypoxemia. The arrhythmia is more likely to occur in patients with a history of previous attacks.

The disturbance usually responds to carotid sinus stimulation, but immediate therapy is required only with extremely rapid ventricular rates. Depressive drugs may increase vagal tone via the carotid, and aortic sinus reflex stimulation associated with elevated blood pressure and phenylephrine hydrochloride is effective in about 80 percent of cases. Rapid digitalization may be needed, and intravenously administered diphenylhydantoin or propranolol or cardioversion may be used.

Atrial Flutter. While the atrial rate resulting from ectopic stimuli ranges between 200 and 400 per minute, the ventricular rate is dependent upon the degree of heart block which characteristically occurs. The ventricular rate decreases with carotid sinus pressure only to increase again when the pressure is released, in contrast to the permanent conversion of an atrial nodal paroxysmal tachycardia to sinus rhythm. Atrial flutter occurs more frequently in elderly patients with cardiovascular disease and in patients undergoing intrathoracic surgical treatment. Vagal nerve stimulation, hypotension, and hypoxemia have all been considered as etiologic factors. Continued atrial flutter frequently causes congestive heart failure, particularly when the ventricular rate is rapid.

Digitalis is the treatment of choice, and the flutter is usually converted to atrial fibrillation which will terminate when digitalis is withdrawn. Quinidine also has been used therapeutically. However, cardioversion is now the treatment of choice.

Paroxysmal Ventricular Tachycardia. This is a rare disorder which has serious implications, since it is associated with a damaged myocardium. The pulse rate is usually between 140 and 180. There is no effect with carotid sinus pressure, and there may be some irregularities of rhythm. Ventricular tachycardia may represent one of the first findings in a patient with myocardial infarction. This disorder of rhythm has also been precipitated by hypercapnia and may progress rapidly to ventricular fibrillation.

Cardioversion or lidocaine given intravenously are the treatments of choice. If the disorder is related to digitalis intoxication, diphenylhydantoin and correction of hypokalemia may be therapeutic.

Sinus Bradycardia. This refers to irregular rhythm with a rate less than 60 per minute. The low rate is normal in young athletic patients. The bradycardia may also be induced by drugs such as neostigmine, quinidine, procainamide, digitalis, methoxamine, and levarterenol. Arrhythmia usually does not require treatment unless there is evidence of reduced cardiac output, in which case atropine may be indicated.

AV Nodal Rhythm. This arrhythmia is usually a temporary disturbance caused by vagal inhibition of the sinus node and may be manifest only by a slow pulse, 40 to 50 per minute. A pronounced jugular venous thrust is characteristic and helps establish the diagnosis. The rhythm may be caused by carotid sinus pressure, endotracheal intubation, atropine, digitalis, and the vasopressor drugs. It usually corrects itself spontaneously, and no treatment is necessary.

AV Block. Incomplete block is an uncommon arrhythmia which is due to organic or surgically induced disturbance of the conduction pathway. Vagal stimulation, carotid sinus pressure, and vasovagal reflexes have also been implicated as have digitalis, quinidine, and morphine. The pulse is slow and regular, and the neck veins may demonstrate atrial pulsation. If the cause is reflex in origin, atropine is indicated, whereas if the condition is drug-induced, the drug should be withdrawn and potassium administered for digitalis intoxication.

Complete AV block results in a ventricular rhythm of between 30 and 60 beats per minute and occasionally follows trauma to the conduction system during heart operation or intraoperative and postoperative septal infarction. Surgically induced blocks are best treated by a pacemaker, while isopropylarterenol may be indicated in infarction to increase the contractility and rate.

Sinus Arrhythmia. This is more frequently noted in younger patients and children, and irregularity is characteristically associated with phases of respiration. It is occasionally seen in patients with digitalis toxicity. No treatment is required, though atropine will correct the abnormality, since it is related to vagal tone.

Sinoatrial Block. Either single beats drop out with regular sequence, or there are runs of two or three dropped beats. If the block is prolonged, nodal or ventricular escape occurs. The block is caused by increased vagal tone and depression of the sinus node impulse. It occurs during tracheobronchial suctioning, with carotid sinus pressure, and in hyperkalemia, and is associated with neostigmine administration. It may reverse itself spontaneously or with atropine administration.

Atrial Fibrillation. Atrial fibrillation with its characteristic irregular pulse most frequently appears postoperatively in arteriosclerotic patients subjected to thoracic surgical treatment. In early cases, the ventricular rate is usually rapid, but when digitalis has been given, a slow ventricular rate may be noted. In the absence of failure, no treatment is indicated, since spontaneous correction may occur. In the case of a paroxymal atrial fibrillation, which may precipitate congestive heart failure, digitalis therapy is indicated. Quinidine or electric cardioversion may be used when there is no associated failure.

Premature Contractions. These represent the most common irregularities of the pulse, and they may originate from any portion of the conduction system. The premature beat characteristically occurs earlier than expected and is followed by a pause due to failure of the ventricle to respond to the next normal impulse. The abnormality occurs in 2 to 8 percent of postoperative patients. The occurrence has been associated with changes in posture, drug therapy with ephedrine and epinephrine, digitalis toxicity, and myocardial infarction. Usually premature contractions have no clinical significance and require no therapy, though if they occur with disturbing frequency, quinidine or lidocaine is recommended unless there is congestive failure, in which case digitalis is the drug of choice, provided it does not represent a possible cause.

Myocardial Infarction

The magnitude of the problem of postoperative coronary occlusion is evidenced by the fact that Master and associates, in 1938, reported that 5.6 percent of attacks of coronary occlusion in patients hospitalized during a given period of time occurred after an operative procedure. The majority of patients who died suddenly during the operative and immediate postoperative period demonstrated coronary artery thrombosis or myocardial infarction at autopsy in another series. The reported incidence for postoperative myocardial infarction ranges between 0.1 and 1.2 percent of all surgical patients, and between 0.9 and 4.4 percent of all surgical patients over the age of fifty. The incidence rose to 6 percent in a group of men over fifty with histories of previous coronary occlusion, and this relationship was more pronounced when the previous occlusion occurred within 2 years of surgical treatment. Eleven unsuspected acute myocardial infarctions were detected by routine postoperative electrocardiograms taken on 1,000 patients in the recovery room.

Tarhan et al. recently assessed the significance of operative procedures under general anesthesia performed in patients who had previous myocardial infarction; 6.6 percent had another infarct in the first week after operation, and 54 percent of these died. Reinfarction occurred most frequently after operations on the thorax or upper abdomen. In over one-third of patients operated on within 3 months of infarction, reinfarction occurred. This rate decreased to 16 percent in patients at 3 to 6 months postinfarction and to 4 to 5 percent when infarction occurred more than 6 months prior to surgery.

CLINICAL MANIFESTATIONS. The majority of cases occur on the operative or the first 3 postoperative days, and although infarction has been associated with all anesthetics, the incidence is higher after general anesthesia for abdominal or pelvic surgical treatment. The most important precipitating factor is shock, either during the operation or in the early postoperative phase. The more prolonged the shock, the greater the risk of coronary thrombosis and myocardial ischemia. The electrocardiogram may show ST depression and T-wave flattening with the loss of as little as 500 ml of blood in patients with previous coronary occlusion.

The diagnosis may be difficult, because chest pain is often absent or obscured by narcotics. It is appropriate to consider routinely monitoring patients with previous infarction in an intensive care unit. In the study of Wroblewski and LaDue, chest pain occurred as a primary clinical manifestation in only 27 percent of patients, which is less than the 97 percent generally reported in patients in whom a coronary occlusion is not related to surgery. The sudden appearance of shock, dyspnea, cyanosis, tachycardia, arrhythmia, or congestive failure should alert one to the diagnosis. The triad of dyspnea, cyanosis, and arterial hypotension requires a differential diagnosis between cardiac and respiratory problems. The electrocardiogram may provide the diagnosis with a characteristic infarction pattern. However, this is not an unequivocal finding, since, in older patients, ST segment and T-wave changes may be associated with myocardial ischemia, and the same changes may be observed with postoperative shock. A study of arterial gases may provide a differential diagnosis in reference to respiratory problems. Left ventricular failure with edema is not generally accompanied by carbon dioxide retention, and, in contrast to airway obstruction and alveolar hypoventilation, there is usually a reduction in arterial carbon dioxide tension (P_{CO_2}) and respiratory alkalosis when cardiac failure accompanies myocardial infarction.

TREATMENT (See Chap. 4). Preoperative preparation of patients with signs of cardiac insufficiency should include digitalization for patients with enlarged hearts or histories of previous cardiac failure. Anemia, if present, requires treatment, and attention should be directed toward the regulation of fluid and electrolyte balance and hypovolemia. Operation is contraindicated for a period of at least 6 weeks and preferably 6 months following myocardial ischemia or infarction, except in an emergency. During the operation, a broad spectrum of factors which precipitate myocardial infarction should be avoided. These include anoxia, hypotension, hemorrhage, dehydration, electrolyte disturbance, and arrhythmias. The regulation of blood pressure during anesthesia is probably the most important measure in the prevention of myocardial ischemia and infarction. When the blood pressure falls significantly, in the absence of blood loss, the prompt correction of anoxia by adequate ventilation with oxygen and the administration of vasopressors is indicated. Digitalization may be required when shock is combined with heart failure. The administration of blood or fluid is indicated to maintain blood volume.

Treatment of myocardial infarction itself consists of relief of pain and anxiety using morphine and sedation. Relief of anoxia is accomplished with 33 to 50 percent oxygen delivered via a BLB mask or nasal catheter. Suctioning of the tracheobronchial tree may be required to clear obstructing secretions. Shock is treated by vasopressor agents. Promptness in instituting vasopressor therapy will increase the chances of its being effective. Rapid digitalization is applicable in treatment of shock when the myocardial insufficiency may be responsible for the severe hypotension. Digitalization is also indicated for the treatment of heart failure, which is a frequent manifestation of postoperative myocardial infarction. In addition to digitalization, parenteral diuretic therapy may be used in the treatment of cardiac failure. Some writers have advocated the use of anticoagulant therapy after the danger of excessive bleeding from an operative site ceases.

In 1952, Wroblewski and LaDue reported the mortality attributable to postoperative myocardial infarction to be 40 percent, which at the time was in keeping with the mortality rate for coronary occlusion unassociated with surgery. In contrast, Tarhan et al. and Mauney et al. reported that myocardial infarction after anesthesia and a major operation was more lethal than myocardial infarction alone.

DIABETES MELLITUS

Diabetes mellitus occurs in 2 to 3 percent of the general population with a higher rate among older people. In two series, the disease was discovered in the paraoperative period in 16 and 23 percent of patients. The most commonly associated operative procedures were complications of vascular disease, but in a high percentage of patients diabetes was discovered prior to an emergency procedure. Diabetic patients represent a special challenge during total surgical care, because the impairment of the homeostatic mechanism for glucose may result in ketoacidosis if untreated or hypoglycemia if overtreated and also because of the associated incidence of generalized vascular disease.

PATHOPHYSIOLOGY. Diabetes mellitus is characterized by hyperglycemia, usually accompanied by glycosuria. The basic defect is a lack of metabolically effective circulating insulin. The elevated blood sugar level is a result of deficient utilization on the part of peripheral tissues and an increased output of glucose by the liver. Excess glucose comes from dietary carbohydrates, liver glycogen, and glucose formed from protein and fat. In the course of metabolism, free fatty acids are released and metabolized in the liver to an end product of acetoacetate, which, by hydrogenation, is converted to β-hydroxybutyric acid or by decarboxylation to acetone. The three products are known collectively as *ketone bodies*. In diabetes, the breakdown of fatty acids is increased, and since the metabolism of the ketone bodies is limited, they accumulate in the bloodstream and are eliminated via the kidneys. Glycosuria itself produces an osmotic diuresis which is enhanced by the presence of ketone bodies and the associated loss of sodium and potassium. Evaluation of decompensated diabetes, therefore, includes not only measuring the blood glucose but also measuring acetone, electrolytes, and carbon dioxide–combining power of the serum.

The anesthetic agent may affect carbohydrate metabolism. Moderate elevation in blood glucose level occurs with cyclopropane and halothane; marked elevation occurs with ether, chloroform, and ethyl chloride; and only minor elevation is associated with nitrous oxide, and trichloroethylene anesthesia. The hyperglycemia is related to an increased breakdown of liver glycogen and a concomitant catabolism of muscle glycogen with the formation of lactic acid. Also, the anesthetic agents affecting glucose catabolism cause an exaggerated hyperglycemic epinephrine response and an increased resistance to exogenously administered insulin. It has been suggested that these phenomena are related to activation of the sympathoadrenal system.

The stress of surgical treatment aggravates hyperglycemia because of the increased secretion of epinephrine and glucocorticoids. Increased epinephrine secretion results in an increased breakdown of liver glycogen to glucose, which is released into the general circulation. The glucocorticoids also increase hepatic glucose output via mobilized protein and exert an anti-insulin effect by stimulating a circulating insulin antagonist. The effects of both epinephrine and glucocorticoids are offset to some extent by an increased secretion of endogenous insulin in the normal person but may require the administration of larger doses of insulin in diabetic patients.

MANAGEMENT. In the diabetic patient, essential laboratory studies include hemoglobin determination, white cell count, urinalysis for sugar and acetone, fasting and timed postprandial blood glucose determination, blood urea nitrogen, and, in older patients, serum cholesterol determination and electrocardiography. Diabetic patients should have a preference for an early place on the operative schedule to minimize the effects of fasting and ketosis. Preoperative medication should be kept to a minimum, since diabetic patients, particularly elderly ones, are sensitive to narcotics and sedatives and there is a danger of hypercapnia and hypoxia. The choice of anesthesia should be determined by the operative procedure and the preference of the anesthesiologist. It should not be influenced by the presence of diabetes. It is true, however, that spinal anesthesia has little tendency to evoke hyperglycemia apart from the stress of the operation; among the inhalation anesthetics, nitrous oxide, trichloroethylene, and halothane have the least effect on carbohydrate metabolism. The degree of control is assessed by serial determination of the blood sugar and urinalysis for glycosuria and acetonuria. In general, it is safer to permit mild glycosuria and minimal elevation of the blood sugar level in the paraoperative periods, particularly in the elderly and cardiac patients. In the patient with postoperative hypotension, blood glucose determination should be obtained to rule out hypoglycemia as an etiologic factor.

Mild diabetics frequently do not require insulin, and dietary control is sufficient. The cornerstone of all diabetic management is the dietary or parenteral intake. The preoperative diabetic intake should contain 140 to 200 Gm of carbohydrates, 60 to 100 Gm of protein, and adequate vitamins and minerals, and should furnish 1200 to 2100 kcal daily. If parenteral fluids are required, there is a theoretical advantage to the use of fructose or sorbitol, which can be utilized in amounts up to 50 Gm daily in the diabetic patient. The goal of the dietary or parenteral fluid regimen is to keep the patient free of acetonuria and without excessive hyperglycemia. The patients in whom diabetes is well controlled with oral agents should continue the use of these drugs until the day prior to operation, particularly if the medication is tolbutamide or phenformin. With longer-acting agents, such as chlorpropamide, the drug should be discontinued 72 hours preoperatively if the administration of insulin is contemplated. Galloway and Shuman stated that patients who take tolbutamide preoperatively usually require insulin during and immediately after major surgical treatment whereas patients receiving chlorpropamide usually do not require insulin during the immediate paraoperative period.

Insulin Therapy. A variety of programs for the administration of insulin have been proposed. One of the popular methods of treatment employs a regimen in which the daily carbohydrate requirement is divided into four equal doses and given parenterally as 5 to 10% dextrose in water every 6 hours. This initiation of the parenteral glucose infusion is accompanied by the subcutaneous injection of unmodified regular insulin in doses equal to approximately one-fourth the dose of insulin which the patient required prior to operation. Urine is checked regularly, and supplementary doses of crystalline insulin are given as indicated. Based on the extent of glycosuria, 4 to 10 units of additional insulin is provided for each unit of positivity. Larger doses may be indicated when acetonuria, severe stress,

infection, or marked hyperglycemia is present. The advantage of this method is that glucose and insulin are given at regular intervals permitting adjustment in the dose during the day. The major disadvantage is that inadvertent interruption of glucose infusion may result in hypoglycemia. With this regimen as with others, slight glycosuria is preferable provided there is no acetonuria.

For more labile diabetics and for patients in whom surgical treatment of great magnitude is anticipated, the use of short-term, unmodified insulin is preferable. In the case of the most labile patients, this regimen may be begun as early as 72 hours prior to operation and is sometimes continued well into the postoperative period. Although the caloric intake is generally less on the day of operation, the normal stress of anesthesia and the operative procedure usually more than compensate for the dietary deficiency. Some writers report having employed regular insulin directly in the intravenous glucose infusion, in doses ranging from 0.16 to 0.2 units/Gm of glucose, depending on the magnitude of the stress of surgical procedures and the fasting blood sugar level. Supplementary doses of 3 to 6 units of regular insulin are then given according to the glucose content of the urine. In general, however, the subcutaneous administration of insulin is preferred, since some of the insulin added to a solution may adhere to the walls of the bottle and tubing.

The second basic regimen is directed at patients who are under control with single-injection therapy employing long-acting insulin and in whom a complicated postoperative course is not anticipated. On the day of operation, the patient receives 50 Gm of glucose in 1,000 ml of solution, and at the time the intravenous solution is started, one-half the daily dose of insulin which previously was required is administered. Following operation and return to the recovery room or ward, the remainder of the usual daily dose of insulin is given subcutaneously. Thus, the amount of insulin given on the day of operation approximates that given the day before. On the day following operation, the usual dose of insulin is given in the morning prior to breakfast or at the time of starting an intravenous infusion. Modifications of this approach employ small doses of regular insulin subcutaneously during the postoperative period based on the extent of glycosuria. Supplementary doses of regular insulin are used if there is evidence of rapid deterioration of the metabolic status. In patients who have been treated with single daily injections and who are not under control prior to operation, conversion to a regimen of soluble insulin is indicated.

Management of Ketoacidosis. The preparation for surgical treatment of a patient with ketoacidosis is critical, and one should keep in mind that ketoacidosis itself may masquerade as a surgical emergency. The patient with frank diabetic coma is no candidate for surgical treatment regardless of the indication. Crystalline insulin should be used in all cases to establish control. Following the determination of the blood sugar level an appropriately large dose of crystalline insulin, occasionally higher than 200 units, is administered. A proportion of this may be given intravenously in an infusion of water and electrolytes. At this stage, the intravenous fluid should not contain glucose.

Serial determinations of the blood glucose at 2-hour intervals are carried out, and additional doses of crystalline insulin are given as indicated. There is an associated deficiency of dehydration and electrolyte abnormality which must be corrected, and the ordinary patient with advanced coma will require an average of 2 to 4 or more liters of fluid to overcome the dehydration. The serum potassium should be determined at 6- to 8-hour intervals and potassium added to the fluid in quantities of 40 mEq/L administered at a rate of no greater than 25 mEq/hour. Usually the need for potassium does not exceed 80 mEq. There is generally no need to add glucose to intravenous fluid unless the blood glucose level falls below normal. Lactate solutions are contraindicated in acidosis with shock, since the excretion of lactate may be impaired and lactic acidosis may be potentiated. Gastric atony is a frequent accompaniment of diabetic ketoacidosis, and suction is frequently required to minimize pulmonary aspiration. It is usually possible to correct ketoacidosis in sufficient time so that the patient's surgical status is not compromised.

Nonketotic Hyperglycemic Hyperosmolar Coma. Hyperosmolar dehydration and coma is a relatively uncommon syndrome which usually occurs in elderly diabetic or nondiabetic obese patients. The blood sugar level is frequently above 1,000 mg/100 ml, and ketone bodies are absent from the plasma and urine. Treatment consists of large amounts of hypotonic solutions plus insulin. Marked lowering of the blood sugar level may result with small doses of insulin, and it is recommended that a test dose of 10 units be given to determine responsiveness.

FAT EMBOLISM

Fat embolism is one of the important causes of increased morbidity and mortality in patients with fractures and extensive trauma. A distinction must be made between fat as a pathologically demonstrable phenomenon and fat embolism as a clinical entity. The presence of pulmonary fat embolism is a relatively common accompaniment of trauma, while the clinical entity is an infrequent occurrence. The pathologic entity of fat emboli in the pulmonary capillaries following trauma was described initially by Zenker in 1862. In World War I, Sutton estimated that 10 percent of the wounded suffered from fat embolism, and by 1931, 112 cases in which fat embolism was implicated as the cause of death had been reported. Mallory et al. reported that 65 percent of 60 patients who died of battle wounds in World War II, had pulmonary fat embolism, and a similar finding was noted in 39 percent of 79 patients dying from war wounds in the Korean conflict. In 1962, Sevitt described 100 cases of fat embolism, 82 percent of which were related to long bone fractures.

There are two peaks of age distribution: the second and third decades, when fractures of the tibia and fibula are most frequent, and the sixth and seventh decades, at which time fractured hips are common. The occurrence of the pathologic entity of fat embolization is correlated with the degree of injury and survival time. In a study of 300 accident victims, 80 percent of those dying immediately had embolization of varying degrees. In those living up to 6 hours after accident, fat embolism was found in 96 percent of autopsies, and 12 hours after a fatal accident from mechanical trauma, there was not a single case without fat embolism. Massive fat embolism occurred in 26 percent of the cases with one fracture and 44 percent of those with multiple fractures.

In addition to fat embolization associated with extensive trauma, the clinical syndrome has been reported in blast concussion, in burns, in severe infection, in closed-chest cardiac massage, with the use of extracorporeal circulation, and following renal transplantation and high-altitude flights.

PATHOGENESIS AND PATHOPHYSIOLOGY. There is disagreement as to whether the embolized fat originates from bone marrow and soft tissue or from circulating blood lipids. The most popular theory, which implicates mechanical causes, proposes that with trauma there is a liberation of liquid fat and intravasation of fat into the vascular channels. Bone, with its high fat content, vascularity, and rigidity, provides an ideal setting. It is theorized that the thin-walled intraosseous veins are prevented from collapsing by their adherence to the bony framework and permit the pressure generated by trauma to force fat into the general circulation. Supporting this theory is the fact that most of the cases of fat embolism occur after fracture of major long bones with high fat content and also the occasional finding that hematopoietic marrow fragments have been found within the lung as an accompaniment of fat embolization. Experimental work has demonstrated that if fat within marrow is stained with a dye and the bone subsequently broken, stained emboli may be detected in the lung within seconds.

The second theory is based on physicochemical changes in the circulating blood lipids. It is proposed that the normal emulsion of fat within the plasma is altered to allow coalescence of the chylomicrons into larger fat droplets with subsequent embolization. This is supported by the fact that emboli may be found in nontraumatic conditions and that the chemical makeup of the embolic fat more closely resembles circulating lipids than marrow or depot fat.

Circulating fat droplets larger than 7 μ in diameter are the offending elements. The lung usually acts as a very effective filter, as evidenced by the observation of Kuhne and Kremser that 95 percent of patients dying of injury had pulmonary involvement while only 23 percent demonstrated systemic fat embolism. Thus, in approximately three-fourths of the patients with fat embolism the lesion is confined to the lung. Pulmonary fat embolism produces disturbances within the lung itself and affects the resistance of blood flow through the pulmonary vascular bed. The cardiac effects are related primarily to the increased pulmonary vascular resistance and, to a lesser degree, to diffuse fat embolism within the myocardium itself. Since the increased resistance to pulmonary flow immediately follows diffuse pulmonary fat embolism, the heart is usually the first organ to be affected. If the heart is not able to compensate for the sudden increase in resistance to the flow, the patient may die a cardiac death; if the heart is able to compensate rapidly, the effects of its involvement may be overlooked. If the fat emboli pass through the pulmonary filter to reach the circulation, they may lodge in the cerebral vessels, accounting for central nervous system manifestations, and in the skin, producing the characteristic petechial changes. Although the kidneys are involved quite regularly when there is systemic fat embolism, they are usually not severely damaged.

CLINICAL MANIFESTATIONS. Although pathologic pulmonary fat embolization is a common occurrence, the clinical manifestations are rare. Symptoms characteristically occur within 12 to 48 hours but have been noted as late as 10 days following injury. The asymptomatic interval between injury and the onset of clinical manifestations has been referred to as the "latent period," but two-thirds of Killian's patients did not exhibit latency. Of 100 cases reported by Sevitt, 25 percent were symptomatic within 12 hours, 60 percent within 24 hours, and 85 percent within 48 hours.

The consequences of significant pulmonary fat embolization are related to its cardiac effects. These include tachycardia, hypotension, and fullness of the superficial veins secondary to increased venous pressure. Acute heart failure may occur. The direct pulmonary effects may be manifested by dyspnea, cyanosis, bubbly rales, and blood-tinged

Fig. 12-2. Pulmonary fat emboli. Note bilateral extensive ill-defined nodular densities situated primarily in peripheral lung fields. Patient was in an automobile accident and fractured his femur and two metatarsals. Twenty-four hours after admission fever developed, and 3 days later hemoptysis and mental confusion. Changes were seen roentgenographically on the fourth day after trauma. There were lipid bodies in the urine, and the serum lipase level was elevated. The patient was treated with antibiotics, heparin, and dextran, and the symptoms subsided 7 days after therapy.

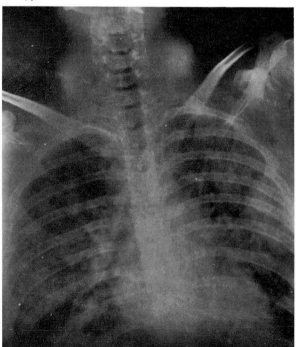

tracheobronchial secretions. Pulmonary embolization may present with similar findings but usually occurs later; a friction rub is more common, and evidence of venous thrombosis may be apparent.

The primary symptoms of fat embolism are frequently cerebral in origin and include confusion, disorientation, delirium, and acute psychoses, progressing to coma and stupor. Local weakness, spasticity, or decerebrate rigidity may be noted. Incontinence occurs relatively frequently, and most patients are febrile, with temperatures as high as 107°F. The cerebral manifestations must be differentiated from delirium tremens, cerebral contusion, and epidural hematoma. The lucid interval with cerebral contusion is usually absent, whereas it characteristically lasts 6 to 10 hours with epidural hematoma and 24 hours with fat embolism. Coma may be present immediately with cerebral contusion and evolves rapidly with fat embolism and slowly with an epidural hematoma. Decerebrate rigidity occurs early in fat embolism and is a terminal event with epidural hematoma. Tachypnea and tachycardia are characteristic of fat embolism, whereas the pulse and respiratory rate are slow with epidural hematoma.

The classic physical finding of fat embolism is the appearance of petechial hemorrhages in the capillary plexus of the dermis. They occur in a distinctive pattern over the shoulders, chest, axilla, and, rarely, the abdominal wall and extremities. They may also be noted in the subconjunctival region and on the palate. Petechiae occur as early as the second or third day and as late as the ninth day after injury and are present in 20 percent of patients found at autopsy to have fat embolism. A counterpart to the petechial hemorrhages is evident on funduscopic examination as emboli within the retinal vessels, and there may be streaks of hemorrhage throughout the retina and macular edema. Renal involvement usually does not produce severe damage, and both gross hematuria and impaired function are rare occurrences. Recently, an association with acute peptic ulceration has been noted.

DIAGNOSTIC STUDIES. A sudden and precipitous drop in the hemoglobin is frequently noted and has been related to hemorrhage within the pulmonary parenchyma. It may occur as early as the second or third day following injury, just prior to the onset of dyspnea, disorientation, and the appearance of petechial hemorrhages. Roentgenographic pulmonary changes are noted in about 36 percent of the cases, and when roentgenograms are taken at intervals following injury, they are helpful in establishing the diagnosis. The characteristic pattern is that of unevenly distributed areas of radiodensity, congestive hilar shadows, and increased bronchovascular markings with dilation of the right side of the heart (Fig. 12-2). Serial measurements of Pa_{O_2} offer a better index of the degree of pulmonary involvement. The electrocardiogram may reveal changes which reflect myocardial ischemia and right ventricular strain. These are usually noted 24 to 48 hours after injury. The important findings are the sudden appearance of a prominent S wave in lead I and prominent Q waves in lead III. Inversion of the T wave indicates severe overloading of the right ventricle. Depression of the RS-T segments suggests subendothelial ischemia. There may be a right bundle branch block. Arrhythmias are frequent. The electroencephalogram may indicate a diffuse slow wave pattern.

Detection of Fat. Lipuria occurs in the first few days following injury and is usually associated with a serious degree of fat embolism. Free fat in the urine has been demonstrated in over 57 percent of cases in one series. Examination of the urine is simple but must be precise. The collecting apparatus must be free of fat, and the bladder must be emptied completely, since the fat floats and the majority of globules remain in the bladder residue. The patient should be catheterized using a non-oily lubricant and the fluid collected in a volumetric flask. The meniscus may be skimmed, or, after centrifugation, the supranatant is smeared and stained with Sudan III. Deep-orange-colored droplets represent fat globules. Another method of demonstrating fat in the urine is the Scuderi "sizzle" test, which involves placing a wire loop containing the supranatant fluid over a flame and listening for a pop or sizzle produced by burning fat. The fat can be detected in concentrations as small as 1:1,000. Venous fat droplets have been demonstrated by a water-soluble fluorochrome dye, but the method is not generally available. The demonstration of fat in the sputum has little diagnostic value, since it is a common phenomenon following trauma. Biopsy of petechiae may establish the diagnosis, and frozen section is mandatory to determine the presence of fat. Needle biopsy of the kidney also has been applied to demonstrate fat globules.

Serum Lipase. A serum lipase level elevation occurs in about 50 percent of the cases, the rise usually beginning on the third day and reaching a maximum on the seventh or eighth day after injury. An elevation greater than 1 ml is significant, and this determination is considered by Peltier to be the best laboratory test between the third and seventh day. The serum lipase level can be suppressed by the administration of ethyl alcohol and augmented by heparinization. Once elevated, the level is thought to reflect the prognosis, and elevations greater than 2 ml are associated with a higher incidence of favorable outcome. In a patient with extensive trauma, an elevated serum lipase level in the first 48 hours is more suggestive of pancreatitis.

TREATMENT. Prophylaxis against potentiating fat embolization includes careful handling of the patient and early splinting of fractures. Vigorous applications of resuscitative measures are indicated to correct oligemic shock, since it has been demonstrated that fewer emboli may be lethal in the hypotensive than in the normotensive patient. Pulmonary manifestations are treated with oxygen therapy, rapid digitalization, and intensive endotracheal suction to minimize the accumulation of secretions. IPPB or PEEP are frequently indicated. Pa_{O_2} should be monitored and maintained between 80 and 100 mm Hg. Endotracheal intubation is preferred over tracheostomy, since the latter has been associated with a high mortality rate in these patients. Cerebral manifestations are treated with sedation and anticonvulsive therapy.

The efficacy of specific therapy remains inconclusive. Heparin in doses which do not have an anticoagulant effect will clear lipemic plasma and stimulate lipase activity. Twenty-five milligrams may be administered intravenously every 6 hours, or sublingual potassium heparin may be employed. Heparin is best used soon after injury when the clinical manifestations or laboratory findings first become apparent. In the presence of acute systemic toxicity or a rapidly rising lipase level, the drug should be discontinued. More recently, low-molecular-weight dextran (40,000) has been administered intravenously to counteract intravascular thrombosis when there is evidence of an increased erythrocyte sedimentation rate. One thousand milliliters is administered per 24 hours. Ethyl alcohol, which may decrease the rate of hydrolysis of neutral fat and slow the release of toxic free fatty acids, has been used. Presently, this applicability of alcohol is debatable. Ethyl alcohol also dilates pulmonary capillaries. It is best administered as 1,000 ml of 5% dextrose–5% ethanol intravenously every 12 hours for the first 3 days after injury. One hundred milligrams of corticosteroids every 6 hours in conjunction with assisted ventilation has been effective.

PROGNOSIS. Although a collective review of 57 cases demonstrated a fatality rate of 67 percent, this may not be representative, since the more severe cases are more likely to be diagnosed and many of the cases represented autopsy diagnoses. At the Birmingham Accident Hospital, a fatality rate of 12 percent has been reported for 25 cases diagnosed according to strict criteria (all had petechial rash). The presence of coma is a poor prognostic sign. The mortality rate for comatose patients ranges between 50 and 85 percent as compared with 0 to 13 percent for noncomatose patients. In the absence of cerebral effects, acute respiratory symptoms do not seem to carry a poor prognosis.

PSYCHIATRIC COMPLICATIONS

Severe psychiatric disturbances may occur any time during an illness, but their appearance in the postoperative period is particularly significant. The first account of postoperative psychiatric disturbance presented by a surgeon was that of Dupuytren who, in 1834, wrote that "the brain itself may be overcome by pain, terror, or even joy and reason leaves the patient at the instant when it is most necessary to his welfare that he should remain calm and undisturbed." In 1910, Da Costa indicated that the anticipated frequency for such complications is as high as 1 in 250 laparotomies, while Lewis, more recently, suggested an incidence of 1 in 1,500. Scott described 11 cases in 2,000 surgical procedures. In a 5-year survey of Belfast hospitals by Knox, the recorded incidence of severe psychiatric disturbance following surgical treatment was 1 in 1,600 operations. The validity of any of these figures, however, is open to question, since "postoperative psychosis" per se does not appear in the standard nomenclature and is frequently not coded on the patient's record, thus limiting the value of retrospective studies. Even more pertinent for surgical consideration is the study of Titchener et al., who evaluated 200 patients admitted to the surgical service of the Cincinnati General Hospital utilizing interview and the Minnesota Multiphasic Personality Inventory to substantiate a psychiatric diagnosis. Eighty-six percent of the sample had either distressing psychologic symptoms, disabling patterns of behavior, or both. It is true that the patients considered were in a municipal hospital and represented a lower socioeconomic group, but the figures of 21 percent having neuroses, 11 percent psychophysiologic reactions, 14 percent psychoses, 34 percent character behavior disorders, and 3 percent chronic brain syndrome are most impressive.

GENERAL CONSIDERATIONS. "Postoperative psychosis" cannot be considered as a distinct clinical entity. No single factor has been shown to be responsible, and the physical illness and operative procedure may merely bring to light a latent psychotic tendency. Both illness, particularly when prolonged, and surgical procedures represent threats to the integrity of the organism on somatic and psychologic grounds. In nearly every person informed of the need for a surgical procedure, some degree of anxiety arises. There may be fear of loss of life, of loss of body part, and of castration as with pelvic and hernia operations. The anxiety signal is assimilated and integrated by the patient in preparation for the surgical stress. Surgical intervention to cure, modify, or prevent illness is the beginning of a complicated and multifaceted process. The psychodynamic processes at work during the preoperative, postoperative, and convalescent periods may be classified as (1) psychophysiologic factors, (2) somatopsychic factors, and (3) psychosocial factors. Psychophysiologic factors represent processes originating from psychologic stress which act along neurogenic or humoral pathways to modify the healing process. A poorly functioning gastroenterostomy or marginal ulcer in a patient with emotional stress represents an example of this type. The somatopsychic factors have to do with the psychologic adaptation involved when the surgical procedure imposes a somatic defect, such as an ileostomy or colostomy. The psychosocial factors refer to the patient's concern with the effects of his physical illness or surgical procedure on his ultimate position in society. All these may interplay and contribute to anxiety, neurotic symptoms, severe depression, and frank psychosis.

CLINICAL MANIFESTATIONS. The time of occurrence of psychiatric derangement during illness is variable, and the duration of latent interval between surgical treatment and the psychologic disturbance may be days to weeks. Winkelstein and associates reported that, in the recovery room, patients who had been subjected to surgical procedures under general anesthesia exhibited a lack of concern about the operation and an absence of affective response, despite the fact that they were sufficiently oriented to be interviewed. After 24 hours the patients responded with these concerns and emotions which were so conspicuously absent in the immediate postoperative period. Both psychologic and pharmacologic factors are implicated in this response, since patients under spinal anesthesia exhibit immediate and overt emotional reaction.

The manifestations are extremely variable. Fear may be accompanied by depression or elation and overactivity. The clinical picture may be that of acute delirium with confusion and disorientation or merely a vague alteration in perception and mood. The manic type of reaction may incorporate psychomotor excitement, delirium, delusions, visual or auditory hallucinations, agitated depression, and feelings of persecution. The psychotic reactions which were observed in 44 of 200 patients in the Cincinnati series are indistinguishable from the range of psychoses observed under other circumstances. The acute brain syndrome, or delirium, was manifest in 20 patients.

Delirium may begin with an inappropriate remark or a dramatic agitated outburst and is frequently the first sign of continued mental deterioration leading to a chronic brain syndrome, particularly in an elderly patient. Therefore, delirium must be regarded as a potentially dangerous situation. It occurs most commonly in elderly patients who have lost closeness and support of family or friends and in patients who are immobilized for long periods of time.

Depressive reactions represented the second most important psychosis in surgical patients and occurred in 4.5 percent of patients in the Cincinnati series. The patient is characteristically uncooperative in an active way, or recovery may be impeded by listlessness, anorexia, and disinterest. The depressive reaction may be accompanied by physiologic changes; Moore et al. have demonstrated the effects of emotion on the pituitary-adrenal axis during the immediate and subsequent postoperative period. Suicide is a major risk in patients with depressive reaction.

Another category includes the paranoid psychotic disorder. Although it is not rare for schizophrenic reaction to have its onset in the surgical patient, no acute breaks of the schizophrenic type were noted among the 200 patients studied by Titchener et al. Generally, there is no contraindication to surgical treatment of patients with schizophrenia. Manic excitement is a particularly difficult problem in the management of surgical patients and requires the close cooperation of psychiatrist, surgeon, and anesthetist.

MANAGEMENT. The first step in the management of psychiatric disturbances occurring in the course of the surgical illness or following surgical procedures is that of anticipation. Although Knox has indicated that the incidence of postoperative psychosis was not related to the duration of preoperative hospital stay, the duration of illness, particularly when prolonged, does determine the patient's psychologic reaction to surgical experience. At the other end of the spectrum, sudden emergency operation often results in reactions marked by acute anxiety, nightmares, insomnia, irritability, and protective withdrawal from all stimuli. Age is an important factor, the highest incidence occurring in children under the age of two and in the elderly patients. In the latter group, this is particularly true of patients who have lost their proximity to and support of family and friends, and who have not developed a close relation with the hospital personnel. Knox has presented evidence of constitutional predisposition, and although 17 percent of his patients had had previous surgical treatment uncomplicated by psychiatric disturbances, 11 percent did have a previous psychiatric illness. Twenty-two percent of patients had a family history of mental illness of serious proportion. There is an increasing incidence of delirium in response to anesthesia and surgical treatment in patients who are alcoholic, while patients suffering from extensive trauma may have organic psychosis. Acidosis, acetonuria, hyperglycemia, and hepatic insufficiency may all cause postoperative mental aberrations, and cerebral hypoxia frequently results in behavioral changes. Medications, such as barbiturates, anticholinergics, and cortisone, also have been implicated.

There is an obvious need for integrating psychologic treatment with the management of surgical patients. As Titchener and Levine emphasize, it is not necessary, possible, or advisable for these needs to be turned over to psychiatrists, and it is frequently preferable that the measures be carried out by the surgeon in charge. Verbal communication between the surgeon and patient is the best means of overcoming emotional or mental difficulty. The anesthetist is regarded as an impersonal distant figure who carries out his task without emotional impact on the patient. The surgeon should become aware of the patient's feelings and attitudes and be appreciative of the effects of these factors on a patient's general well-being. Also, changes to increase the patient's positive adaptation to his illness should be constantly considered. The striking incidence of significant postoperative disturbance suggests the need for "mental check" to be incorporated into the usual postoperative surgical rounds. Efforts should be directed at removing toxic causes of the acute brain syndrome, removing undue stimuli without isolating the patient, and providing psychologic or pharmacologic tranquilization.

The physician's psychologic approach should include repeated reassurance of the patient. In some instances, specific counseling and directive treatment, which may require direct intervention in the patient's personal or family affairs and the assistance of the social service department, is indicated. The best prophylactic therapy, however, can be classified as supportive, in that the surgeon allows himself to be the object of dependency on the part of the patient. This relationship is fostered by interest on the part of the surgeon and trust on the part of the patient.

The provocative patient who emits anger or attempts to irritate others as a mechanism for covering fear or relieving guilt needs understanding of the emotional reason for the provocation and an attitude of firmness rather than anger from the physician. The attempt on the part of a patient to sign out against advice is a mechanism of expressing anger or fear and should be handled by the surgeon in such a way that the patient is allowed to change his mind without becoming embarrassed. In these and other situations, the patient may hide his real feeling behind an intellectual screen. For understanding himself, the patient must bring forth both the emotional and intellectual aspects of his personality.

Consultation with a psychiatrist is indicated in the case of any acute and severe emotional disturbance, and the referral should be candidly discussed between the surgeon and the patient. It is necessary for the patient to come to the conclusion that he requires expert help for his problems. Referral is also indicated for long-standing disturbances discovered during hospitalization and is frequently appropriate in patients with psychosomatic illness. Browning and Houseworth, in a study of patients with peptic ulcer, demonstrated that the removal of symptoms without altering the psychosomatic disorders led to the formation of a new spectrum of symptoms.

Special Surgical Situations

The very young and old patients are particularly vulnerable to the development of psychiatric complications following surgical treatment. Psychotic disturbances have been found in 2 to 3 percent of patients following cataract extraction. The combination of surgical procedure and the awareness of the implications of the illness is critical in the patient with cancer. Because of the high incidence of emotional disorders following surgical procedures, special consideration is indicated for mastectomy and gynecologic procedures, cardiac surgical treatment, dialysis and transplantation, and prolonged periods in an intensive care unit.

PEDIATRIC SURGERY

In children, severe anxiety states may be precipitated by the shock of operation. Levy reported that of a group of 124 children who had operations, 20 percent showed residual emotional disturbances. This occurred most frequently in the one- to two-year-old group; after the age of three there was a sharp decrease with age. The age distribution was attributed to a greater dependence on home and mother, and Levy went so far as to suggest postponement of elective surgical treatment until the child could comprehend something about the situation. Postoperative reactions consisted of negativism, disobedience, tantrums, defiance, destructive behavior, and dependency, as manifested by clinging to the mother or attendant. The responses have been related to a feeling of betrayal and the consequent desire for revenge and rebellion. When a child is suffering from fears engendered by an operation, a second operation usually intensifies the earlier fears.

Prophylactic therapy is important. The maturity of the child's emotional adaptation is more a factor in the response than the operation per se. Parental absence is frequently associated with emotional difficulty. Prugh and associates compared two groups, one treated without organized consideration for emotional needs and another in which these needs were considered and ample opportunity for play was provided. Moderate or severe anxiety reactions, immediately after leaving the hospital, were observed in 92 percent of the control group and in 68 percent of the experimental group, with a peak incidence in children under three. Three months after discharge, the incidence of persisting anxiety had fallen to 58 percent for the control group and 44 percent for the experimental group. The youngest children reacted more severely with apprehension, feeding disturbances, and depression. The pattern for the four- to six-year-old group was a tendency toward obsessive worries, phobias, and accentuated aches and pains. The six- to ten-year-olds manifested conversion symptoms, compulsive behavior, and restlessness.

SURGERY IN THE AGED

Elderly patients are more prone to become emotionally disturbed when confronted with new situations, especially if they have inadequate comprehension and a generalized feeling of insecurity. The operative procedure also presents an obvious physical threat to the integrity of the nervous system. Titchener and associates reported a 25 percent incidence of significant and, at times, irreversible change in cerebral function in the patients in their group over the age of sixty-five. Some degree of depression was observed in 90 percent of the older patients, and this was of a disabling nature in about 50 percent. Indifference of the family, friends, and society contributed to the evolution of a paranoid cycle.

Attempts should be directed at limiting the physical insult to the brain, and postoperative mental evaluation is indicated on a routine basis in order to detect the early changes of the organic brain syndrome and delirium. Efforts should be made to familiarize the patients with the hospital and personnel, and visitors should be encouraged to maintain a human contact and prevent withdrawal. Collaboration with a social worker is frequently indicated for long-term rehabilitation.

GYNECOLOGIC SURGERY

Removal of the breast and a variety of gynecologic procedures are highly represented in most series of postoperative psychosis. Hysterectomy is associated with emotional disturbance more frequently than other gynecologic operations, and the more the procedure antedates the menopause, the more the likelihood of associated psychologic disturbance. The loss of menstrual function is perceived by the woman as a blow to normal feminine esteem. Hollender reported that of 203 women admitted to psychiatric hospital, 9 had pelvic surgical treatment as a precipitating event, and this was in contrast to a total of 5 women admitted following operations of all other kinds. Lindemann noted that the relative frequency of restlessness, insomnia, agitation, and preoccupation with depressive thoughts was greater after pelvic operations than after cholecystectomy.

CANCER PATIENTS

The cancer patient is exposed to two major threats, disease and extensive surgical treatment. He is concerned with death or injury during operation and disruption of his pattern of living as a result of the effects of cancer or the surgical procedure. Patients with emotional problems involving self-destruction are particularly vulnerable to preoperative anxiety concerning death and mutilation. This may be manifest by anorexia, insomnia, tachycardia, fear, and panic. Acute depression with suicidal tendencies have been reported in anticipation of surgical procedures. Postoperatively, depression is related to an anticipated interference with valued activities. Sutherland and associates have demonstrated that colostomy imposed on almost all patients a new order of living, and the subjects were powerfully motivated to avoid social rejection. A rigid life arose from the fearful expectation of rejection because of the colostomy combined with the fear of death from cancer. There is a tendency toward seclusion, withdrawal, and nonparticipation. Spells of depression are frequent, and Sutherland and his associates are of the opinion that loss of an important bodily part or function is more depressing than the fear or expectation of death. The management of patients with carcinoma must be based on an appreciation that they frequently suffer a sense of isolation, guilt, and abandonment.

CARDIAC SURGERY

Serious psychiatric disturbances have been observed to occur with considerable frequency following mitral valvulotomy and open heart surgery. Fox and associates and Bliss et al. reported, respectively, a 19 and 16 percent incidence of serious emotional disturbance following mitral valve surgery. In contrast, Bolton and Bailey, in an evaluation of 1,500 consecutive patients, noted an incidence of psychosis of 3 percent with no relation to age, sex, severity of heart disease, duration of failure, or complications of surgical treatment. Kornfeld et al. reported a psychosis of an acute organic variety in 38 percent of 99 adult patients subjected to open heart surgery, while Egerton and Kay noted delirium in 25 of 60 adults following open heart surgery.

Manifestations generally occur after an initial lucid interval 3 to 5 days after operation and clear shortly after the patient is transferred from an intensive care unit to a standard hospital ward. Postoperative incapacitation and increased time on the heart-lung machine apparently are factors increasing the likelihood of delirium, while age and sex do not alter the incidence. Zaks has suggested that cardiac operation may produce organic brain damage, thus sensitizing patients and increasing the incidence of postoperative psychologic symptomatology. A prediction equation was successful in differentiating reactors from nonreactors. Using the ego strength variable of the Minnesota Multiphasic Personality Inventory, there is a significant inverse correlation between the reaction and the incidence of acute psychotic episodes following cardiac operation. The incidence of psychoses is greater in males, older patients, and those expressing minimal preoperative anxiety. A preoperative psychiatric interview reduces the incidence of postoperative psychosis by 50 percent.

Following operations on the heart, the patients with emotional disturbances manifest perceptual distortion, visual and auditory hallucinations, disorientation, and paranoia. Twenty-eight percent of adult patients subjected to open heart surgery, as reported by Egerton and Kay, had delirious states ranging in duration from several nights to several weeks, averaging 5 days. The delirious patients had no psychologic sequelae, and no relation could be established between the incidence of delirium and the duration of cardiac bypass, but open heart procedures were more likely to produce delirium than other intrathoracic operations. The writers felt that the precipitating factors for delirium included dehydration, hyponatremia, and the performance of a tracheostomy, while the predisposing factors included a familial history of psychosis, previous brain damage, overwhelming personal problems, and the presence of a rheumatic valvular lesion. Other psychiatric disturbances noted in patients following open heart surgery were disabling anxiety state, conversion hysteria, tension headaches, and, in a surprising 5 percent of the operative cases, exacerbation of peptic ulcer. The almost total absence of delirium and other emotional disorders in children is of particular interest and may be related to the fact that the concept of death as a permanent biologic process usually does not develop until the age of nine.

DIALYSIS AND TRANSPLANTATION

A variety of emotional disturbances has been observed in patients undergoing hemodialysis. The suicide rate is 300 times greater than for a comparable healthy population. Uremia, debilitating disease, and the repeated technical procedures which are performed all constitute etiologic factors. Wright et al. followed 11 patients on chronic dialysis and noted a number of stresses affecting them, such as unpredictability of well-being, tensions arising in the marital situation from guilt and anger, effects of separation on the families, and financial anxiety. Following each episode of dialysis, the main patient response was one of relief. Cramond and associates noted that their patients at first denied their illness and later realized that they had lost their health and independence and their futures were uncertain. This has been referred to as a "mourning reaction." From time to time the patients wished to be dead. They felt that life dependent on chronic dialysis was not worth living. Some patients passed from the mourning reaction to a state of active depression.

All patients undergoing dialysis become extremely dependent on the staff and emotionally attached to them. The patients often react emotionally to a sense of loss when any replacement of staff occurs. During the course of the dialysis program, regression occurs relatively frequently, and the patient becomes withdrawn and pretends to sleep. Insomnia and frightening dreams also occur, and the frequency with which emotional disturbances have been noted suggests that psychiatric assistance plays an important role in a dialysis program.

Two distinct groups of patients, the donors and recipients, must be considered in a renal homotransplantation program. Psychologic screening of the potential donors is indicated, and selection should be from individuals who are stable and who have mature judgment. Individuals with psychopathologic motives such as sacrifice or exhibitionism should be excluded, particularly when they are unrelated donors. It is to be emphasized that those who refuse to cooperate risk being rejected by the family and are frequently made to feel guilty. Therefore, when potential donors are rejected on psychiatric grounds, the rejection should be ascribed to a minor physical variation. In four of five cases, Cramond noted an ambivalent relationship between the donor and recipient. The donor experienced emotional and physical investment in the patient and, at times, sought to overprotect the patient. He felt that his sacrificial gift was in jeopardy if the patient behaved in a manner with which he did not approve.

The recipient has been shown to be aware of his obligation to the donor and resents the dependency relationship. At times feelings of shame and guilt must be considered. Kemph, in a follow-up of recipients of renal homotransplants, has noted periods of severe depression and concern with bodily damage and sexual damage. After the opera-

tion the donors also experience depression. Many expressed the feeling that they were not attentively supported by the hospital personnel.

Some recipients regard the operation as symbolic of rebirth and may undergo a religious conviction. In some recipients, a graft from a donor of an opposite sex is considered a threat to sexual identity. All recipients demonstrate anxiety in reference to injury of the grafted kidney. Although severe depressions and emotional reactions are uncommon, psychologic adjustment takes longer than a year to accomplish. When given a choice, patients who have rejected their kidney transplants have almost uniformly chosen a second transplant over return to dialysis.

INTENSIVE CARE DELIRIUM

Delirium manifested by a wide variety of behavior patterns, ranging from apathy to restlessness and combativeness, is a common occurrence in intensive care units. Both environmental and metabolic factors have been implicated. The former can be corrected by transferring the patient to a regular hospital ward or room as soon as possible. Katz et al. indicated a physiologic abnormality, such as hypoxemia or electrolyte or acid-base abnormality, as the cause in the great majority of patients.

COMPLICATIONS OF GASTROINTESTINAL SURGERY

The author has had the opportunity of reviewing all other chapters in the textbook and has included in this discussion those complications of gastrointestinal surgery which either demand special emphasis or are not covered in other sections. In general, the complications associated with surgery of a given organ system appear in the appropriate chapter.

For convenience, the gastrointestinal complications considered in this section are divided into (1) vascular complications, including hemorrhage and gangrene, (2) mechanical problems of gastroenterostomy and enteroenterostomy, including stomal obstruction, the afferent, or blind, loop syndrome, extrinsic obstruction and internal hernia, and inadvertent gastroileostomy, (3) leakage of an anastomosis, including the duodenal stump blowout, (4) external fistulas and stomal problems, and (5) damage to adjacent organs, including postoperative pancreatitis and jaundice.

Vascular Complications

HEMORRHAGE

Gastrointestinal hemorrhage which occurs subsequent to a gastrointestinal anastomosis may become manifest postoperatively by hematemesis, melena, hematochezia, or, most frequently, the passage of bright blood via a nasogastric tube positioned in the stomach. Bleeding from the suture line is most commonly associated with gastric surgery, occurring in approximately 1 percent of patients following gastric resection, with a higher incidence in those patients in whom operation is performed for a duodenal ulcer. Bleeding from the suture line is apt to occur either immediately after the operation or on the first postoperative day, but a second minor peak in incidence has been noted between the seventh and tenth postoperative days. Bleeding arising from the suture line on the first postoperative day is usually minimal or moderate and requires no specific therapy, but if it is continuous, the stomach should be aspirated and irrigated with ice-cold saline solution. Hemorrhage which does not stop following conservative measures constitutes an indication for laparotomy, at which time the suture line should be inspected. It may be preferable to enter the stomach above the line of anastomosis and ligate vessels from within. Bleeding later in the course of convalescence is usually due to sloughing from the suture line and generally responds to iced saline lavage. Significant hemorrhage from the suture line of small intestinal and large intestinal anastomoses is extremely rare. Upper gastrointestinal bleeding following a surgical procedure in a patient who is debilitated or in whom sepsis develops frequently indicates a stress ulcer (see Chap. 26).

GANGRENE

Gangrene is a rare complication of resection of a segment of gastrointestinal tract, since the intestine is supplied with a rich network of arteries. Necrosis of the gastric remnant has been reported following a high subtotal gastrectomy, particularly if the procedure incorporates ligation of the left gastric artery and concomitant splenectomy. Devascularization of the areas to be anastomosed should not occur following small intestinal surgical procedures if attention is directed toward the vascular supply. A precautionary measure is to slant the lines of incision so that more intestine is resected on the antimesenteric aspect. Small intestinal gangrene is more frequently due to mechanical strangulation, obstruction secondary to postoperative adhesions, volvulus, internal hernias, or vascular thrombosis. Gangrene of the segment of intestine may be apparent in the case of a colostomy in which an inadequate vascular supply has been provided.

In each instance, the recognition of gangrene requires resection of the gangrenous segment of intestine or stomach and reestablishment of intestinal continuity or a colostomy in bowel which is viable.

Mechanical Problems

STOMAL OBSTRUCTION

Although obstruction of the stoma may follow any intestinal anastomosis as a result of technical factors, postgastrectomy stomal obstruction represents the most common type and is frequently related to local edema. Factors which have been implicated in the etiology of edema include electrolyte depletion, hypochloremia, incomplete hemostasis, hypoproteinemia, leakage from the anastomosis, inadequate proximal decompression, and incorporation of too much tissue within the sutures. Other causes include rotation of the jejunum on its long axis, obstruction by the transverse mesocolon, particularly in an obese patient,

obstruction by a fatty omentum, effect of vagotomy, and, rarely, jejunogastric intussusception, which has been reported as a complication in slightly over 100 cases of Billroth II procedures.

Postgastrectomy stomal obstruction is a most troublesome complication, and the reported incidence has ranged between 1 and 3 percent. Magnuson and associates indicated an almost identical incidence of 3 percent subsequent to gastrectomy for gastric ulcer as compared with gastrectomy for duodenal ulcer. Hibner and Richards, in a review of 648 partial gastrectomies, noted an incidence of 4.6 percent for patients requiring further operative therapy, 4.1 percent for Billroth II operations, and 3.5 percent for Billroth I types. In most instances in their series, the efferent loop was obstructed by the transverse mesocolon.

Symptoms usually occur on the third to fourth postoperative day, at which time there is abdominal fullness and increased return from the nasogastric suction. If the patient has been on oral intake, nausea followed by vomiting of large quantities of bile-colored gastric fluid occurs. Instillation of barium or Gastrografin via the nasogastric tube may reveal stomal obstruction or a patent stoma with distal loop obstruction. The symptoms usually persist for only short intervals and cause little disability, but occasionally they are prolonged and then have severe metabolic effects.

Prophylaxis is directed at avoiding the factors which have been implicated. Therapy of established stomal obstruction consists of adequate decompression and replacement of fluids and nutrients, while waiting for the obstruction to become relieved spontaneously. The course may be prolonged, extending over a period of several weeks. If there is not relief after extended conservative management or if the patient's condition is deteriorating, operative intervention is indicated. Rarely, a simple release of adhesions may be therapeutic, but more often the anastomotic site requires revision, a procedure which is frequently difficult in view of the extensive reaction around the stoma. It is generally preferable to transect the proximal and distal loops of intestine at their entrance to and exit from the indurated mass. These are then anastomosed to one another, and the short segment of intestine and a cuff of stomach are removed with the gastroenterostomy. Continuity is reestablished with a long antecolic gastrojejunostomy.

AFFERENT (BLIND) LOOP SYNDROME

The blind loop syndrome is a consequence of small intestinal surgical procedures and is presented in Chap. 27. The present discussion is concerned with the afferent loop syndrome which represents a complication of subtotal gastrectomy with Billroth II gastroenterostomy. The afferent loop consists of duodenum and a segment of jejunum of variable length. Acute or chronic obstruction can occur at any point proximal to the gastrojejunostomy. The incidence is difficult to estimate and is dependent upon the criteria for diagnosis. Quinn and Gifford reported five cases in 500 gastrectomies, while Blomstedt and Dahlgren reported an incidence of 18 percent with mild to moderate symptoms (type I and type II). The symptom complex of partial obstruction of the afferent loop was reported by Magnuson et al. to occur following gastrectomy in 4.2 percent of patients with gastric ulcer in contrast to 0.9 percent of patients with duodenal ulcer.

PATHOGENESIS. Normally after partial gastrectomy, biliary and pancreatic secretions enter the afferent loop, pass through the gastrojejunostomy to mix with gastric juice, and then pass through into the efferent loop. During a 24-hour period, approximately 1 to 1.5 liters of secretion enters the afferent loop. The afferent loop syndrome is caused by partial and, rarely, total obstruction of flow from the afferent loop. The pressure within the duodenum and segment of jejunum rises, and the loop becomes dilated by bile and pancreatic juice. After the ingestion of food, particularly a fatty meal, the duodenal contents increase rapidly, thus explaining the postcibal nature of the syndrome. With incomplete obstruction, pressure within the intestine eventually becomes sufficient to overcome resistance, and the contents are emptied into the stomach, causing variable amounts to be vomited. With total obstruction, the loop no longer has any communication with the stomach, and vomitus is free of bile.

CLINICAL MANIFESTATIONS. The symptoms of partial obstruction of the afferent loop occur most commonly in the early postoperative period. Two-thirds of the cases occur during the first week, but in some instances the syndrome becomes apparent months to years following gastrectomy. The symptoms vary in intensity and are characterized by postcibal vomiting. Mild symptoms consist of eructation of a mouthful of green biliary fluid within an hour and a half after a meal. Vomiting is generally preceded by the sensation of fullness and, at times, pain in the epigastrium. In some instances, the symptoms of chronic obstruction persist for several months, and the amount of biliary vomiting and antecedent epigastric pain are appreciable. With persistence of partial obstruction, the stools become bulky and gray, and contain much fat. Roentgenographic examination may show passage of contrast material into the efferent loop, while the afferent loop, as a rule, fails to fill. Chronic partial obstruction is associated with anemia, and the vitamin B_{12} absorption test may provide the diagnosis. Urinary excretion of B_{12} is reduced or absent and is unaffected by the administration of intrinsic factor, in contrast to pernicious anemia. However, following a course of 3 to 5 days of tetracycline, B_{12} urinary excretion returns to normal.

In the rare situation of the acute complete obstruction of the afferent loop, the patient becomes acutely ill with severe epigastric pain, and bile is characteristically absent from the vomitus. A mass may be felt in the upper abdomen. The patient's condition may deteriorate rapidly, and shock may occur as a result of compromise of the circulation of the duodenal wall and/or perforation with generalized peritonitis. Roentgenograms are of little diagnostic assistance. There may be delayed emptying of contrast material from the gastric remnant, and no barium enters the afferent loop. The amylase level may be markedly elevated.

TREATMENT. Incomplete obstruction generally subsides on a conservative regimen. Capper and Welbourn collected 44 cases requiring surgical intervention and reported that 36 of them had a good outcome. Surgical decompression of the afferent loop may be accomplished by anastomosis between the afferent and efferent loops, by employing a Roux en Y anastomosis or converting a gastrojejunostomy to a gastroduodenostomy. In the case of acute total obstruction, early operation with decompression of the afferent loop is mandatory.

INTESTINAL OBSTRUCTION

Intestinal obstruction in the immediate postoperative period is most frequently due to ileus or fibrinous adhesions; however, a variety of mechanical causes should be considered. Internal herniation represents a complication of subtotal gastrectomy, generally following a Billroth II antecolic anastomosis. Internal herniation of the small intestine may also take place through improperly closed mesenteric rents or when the mesentery of the ileum or colon is not tacked to the peritoneum in the course of an ileostomy or colostomy. Closed-loop obstruction generally results and may rapidly progress to compromise the vascular supply with ultimate perforation. Operative reduction and repair of an internal hernia are required. Adhesions and/or volvulus may occur in the postoperative hospitalization and require surgical intervention for relief of obstruction. The incidence is particularly high following resection for congenital atresia in infancy, especially when the proximal dilated bowel is not resected. Postoperative intussusception, generally involving the small intestine, is also to be considered in the pediatric age group.

INADVERTENT GASTROILEOSTOMY

The error of anastomosing the stomach to the ileum rather than the jejunum is fortunately uncommon. In 1949, Moretz indicated that 27 cases were recorded in the literature. The situation results in a malabsorption syndrome which begins as soon as the patient is allowed to eat solid food. Diarrhea, weight loss, and inanition in the absence of abdominal pain are characteristic. The stool contains a high percentage of undigested food and a large quantity of unabsorbed fat. Fecal vomiting and hemorrhage occasionally occur, and an ulcer may develop at the site of the ileum, in which case abdominal pain may be present. The diagnosis can be established roentgenographically by demonstrating a rapid transit and short distal intestine. The error should be avoided by using the ligament of Treitz as a landmark in establishing a gastroenterostomy; in the absence of a ligament of Treitz an anomaly of rotation should be suspected, and the loop of intestine for anastomosis should be selected by tracing the duodenum distad or the small bowel proximally from the cecum. The preoperative management of patients with gastroileostomy requires a vigorous preparation, and a preliminary feeding jejunostomy is of value in these cases. A block resection of the gastroileostomy is advocated for patients who have had subtotal gastric resection, while, in the absence of gastric resection, the ileostomy may be taken down directly. A gastrojejunostomy and reconstitution of intestinal continuity are then performed.

Anastomotic Leak

Suture line leakage represents a potential complication of any intestinal anastomosis. The three prime etiologic factors are (1) poor surgical technique, (2) distal obstruction, and (3) inadequate proximal decompression. Leak from an enteroenterostomy becomes manifest as localized or generalized peritonitis. Small leaks with localized response may be treated by proximal decompression and administration of appropriate antibiotics, while large leaks and diffuse peritonitis frequently require surgical intervention. Fistulization may develop as a tract becomes established between the point of leakage and the skin. A leak from the line of anastomosis is a relatively rare complication following gastroenterostomy. Such leakage occurs more frequently when there has been impairment of the blood supply of the residual gastric pouch and a concomitant splenectomy has been performed. A common point at which leaks develop has been referred to as the "angle du mort," where the residual gastric pouch of a Hofmeister closure meets the line of anastomosis of the small intestine.

Duodenal stump leakage (blowout) is a more frequent and critical complication of gastric resection. A review of gastrectomies performed at the Mayo Clinic in 1956 revealed that 4.5 percent of patients subjected to the procedure for gastric ulcer had some evidence of leak, while 5.6 percent of patients in whom the same procedure was carried out for duodenal ulcer revealed similar evidence. In that study, drains had been inserted into the stump region, and in many patients increased drainage represented the evidence of a leak. Edmunds et al. indicate that a review of gastrectomies performed at the Massachusetts General Hospital from 1946 to 1959 showed that an incidence of dehiscence of the stump was 1.1 percent and the mortality due to this cause was 0.6 percent.

Duodenal stump leakage occurs most commonly after operation for a duodenal ulcer and frequently when gastrectomy is performed as an emergency procedure to stop hemorrhage. In a great majority of cases, the leak arises as a result of a technical error and failure of the suture line. A scarred and edematous duodenum predisposes to the complication, as does obstruction of the afferent loop and local pancreatitis. Complications of duodenal leakage include peritonitis, subhepatic abscess, pancreatitis, sepsis, and establishment of an external fistula with fluid and electrolyte abnormalities.

Specific measures can be taken to avoid this complication. Before embarking on a gastric resection, the surgeon should be as sure as possible that the duodenal stump can be safely closed. In the face of marked inflammatory disease in the duodenal region, vagotomy and gastroenterostomy definitely represent safer procedures. When resection has been undertaken and duodenal closure is difficult, catheter duodenostomy may be used as an adjunct. Rodkey and Welch reported that in 51 cases with difficult duodenal stump closures in whom planned duodenostomy was carried out, there was only one death, and only five patients had drainage from the fistula that lasted more than 48 hours after the catheter was removed. As a compromise between primary closure and planned duodenostomy, some surgeons have advised drainage of the right upper quadrant with a Penrose drain placed in the region of the duodenal stump in the hope that if perforation occurs, the contents will discharge along the tract. However, this does not provide the safety factor of planned duodenostomy, since the drain tract may wall off from the stump before the perforation becomes established.

Duodenal blowout is a major catastrophe which is most likely to occur between the second and seventh postoperative day and becomes manifest by sudden pain, elevation in temperature, pulse rate, and general deterioration of the patient's condition. Adequate drainage must be instituted at once and is best accomplished by an incision below the right costal margin and insertion of a large sump catheter which is passed down to the duodenal stump area, with constant suction applied. Attention must be directed toward fluid and electrolyte therapy, and a high caloric and nitrogen intake should be maintained. Fistula closure can be anticipated within 2 to 3 weeks. Another area in which leaks are a major concern is low colon anastomoses; incidences of 5 to 51 percent have been reported. The mortality rate in patients with major colon leaks is extremely high, and this has led to a resurgence of enthusiasm for protective transverse colostomy if the anastomosis appears compromised.

External Fistulas and Stomal Complications

FISTULAS

External fistulas may arise from stomach, small intestine, or colon. In a review of the experiences at the Massachusetts General Hospital from 1946 to 1959, it was reported that in 157 patients with external fistulas, 55 fistulas originated from stomach, duodenum, or gastrojejunal anastomosis; 46 from jejunum or ileum, with drainage of over 100 ml of intestinal content daily; and 56 from the lower ileum and colon. Surgical complications were the direct cause of 67 percent of these fistulas.

Gastric and Duodenal Fistulas

The incidence of gastrojejunal or duodenal stump fistulas following subtotal gastrectomy has been reported to be 1 to 2 percent, approximately one-quarter of which originated from the gastrojejunostomy. Suture line failure accounted for 82 percent of all gastroduodenal fistulas. The causes of fistulas arising from the gastrojejunostomy may be related to the suture line containing tumor, ischemia of the gastric stump due to high ligation of the gastric artery and vasa brevia, stomal obstruction, and pancreatitis or tension on the suture line. The causes of duodenal stump fistula have been referred to in the previous section on stump leakage. The complications of an established gastric or duodenal fistula include electrolyte abnormalities and malnutrition, sepsis, intraperitoneal abscesses and wound infection, jaundice, and pancreatitis.

Treatment. Intensive fluid, electrolyte, and nutritional therapy is frequently required, and quantitative control of imbalance is critical. The amount of drainage should be measured and analyzed, and these determinations plus the base-line requirements should provide a formula for replacement therapy (see Chap. 2). Sump suction is the most efficient method of managing the drainage, and protection of the skin from autodigestion is usually required. The majority of fistulas which close spontaneously do so in less than 2 months. Surgical intervention may be indicated to drain abscesses or to establish a feeding jejunostomy. An established gastric fistula may require resection and correction of distal obstruction if the latter is present. Fistulas arising at the gastrojejunostomy stoma may require re-resection and establishment of a new gastroenterostomy. Fistulas arising from the duodenal stump are not generally amenable to direct closure. The literature reveals that definitive procedures rarely have been employed for fistulas in this segment of the gastrointestinal tract, and the mortality rate of 55 gastric and duodenal fistulas treated at the Massachusetts General Hospital was 65 percent. These fistulas are readily managed with parenteral hyperalimentation. In the report of MacFadyen, et al. all duodenal fistulas closed spontaneously.

High Small Bowel Fistulas (See Chap. 27)

Seventy-two percent of the 46 fistulas in this group reported by Edmunds et al. represented surgical complications secondary to dehiscence of anastomoses or inadvertent injury during dissection or closure of an abdominal incision. Although jejunal and proximal ileal fistulas are frequently characterized by profuse drainage, the fluid loss is generally less than that associated with duodenal fistulas, and therefore fluid and electrolyte abnormalities occur less frequently. Malnutrition develops in about three-quarters of these patients, and sepsis is a major complication. Twenty-two percent of the patients reported by Edmunds et al. died of generalized peritonitis, and a large number of intraperitoneal abscesses developed. Skin digestion is a frequent occurrence, and many of these patients eventually develop a ventral hernia due to wound complications.

Treatment. Supportive management of small bowel fistulas is similar to that outlined for gastroduodenal fistulas. This includes maintenance of fluid and electrolyte balance and nutrition. Hyperalimentation may be applicable. In the case of a proximal jejunal fistula, a distal feeding jejunostomy is frequently indicated to permit adequate fluid and nutritional intake. Oral feeding of low-residue diets is feasible with ileal fistulas. Control of fluid loss and diarrhea may be accomplished with the use of Lomotil, Kaopectate, and opiates plus nonabsorbable antibiotics when indicated. Drainage is best controlled by sump suction, and protection of the skin in the region of the fistula is indicated.

Of 46 patients reported by Edmunds et al., definitive procedures were carried out in 50 percent. The operative procedures include direct attack on a fistula with resection both of the fistula and the segment of intestine from which it arises or an indirect attack through a clean abdominal incision with a bypass operation or complete exclusion of the fistula by means of end-to-end anastomosis of the proximal and distal intestine. The excluded loop is then decompressed completely through a large fistula by exteriorizing the ends of the intestine to prevent later blowout. In general, and particularly in the face of peritonitis, early direct attack on the fistula is safer and more satisfactory than exclusion procedures, and most fistulas can be operated on within 3 weeks of onset. In the series reported by Edmunds et al., only 1 patient of 17 treated by resection died, while the mortality rate of patients treated conservatively was 80 percent. Using hyperalimentation, MacFadyen et al. reported that over 70 percent of small bowel fistulas closed spontaneously. An average of 40 days of hyperalimentation was required.

Distal Ileal and Colonic Fistulas (See Chaps. 27 and 28).

These are generally caused by anastomotic leaks or inadvertent trauma to the segment of intestine. Anastomosis in the region of tumor or inflammation and distal partial obstruction are predisposing factors. Fluid and electrolyte abnormalities are uncommon, while the incidence of infection is extremely high. This includes peritonitis, intraperitoneal abscesses, and wound infections. Significant skin digestion and irritation are rare.

Treatment. The patients can generally be managed on a low-residue diet, using enteric or parenteral antibiotics when indicated, and rarely require sump suction. Spontaneous healing of fistulas in these regions is the rule rather than the exception, but defunctionalizing colostomies for descending colon fistulas or ileal transverse colostomies for ascending colon and distal ileal fistulas may be indicated. Medical management is generally indicated for about 6 weeks to permit any active inflammation to subside. If the inflammation persists after this time, a defunctionalizing procedure is indicated. Definitive surgical treatment is indicated for fistulas which fail to progress satisfactorily after 6 weeks. If the fistula is accompanied by generalized peritonitis, early emergency resection is indicated and frequently should be accompanied by a proximal defunctionalizing procedure. Definitive operations include a turn-in procedure or resection which may be coupled with a temporary protective colostomy or bypass. Seventy-nine percent of the patients in the experience at the Massachusetts General Hospital were cured. Seventy-five percent of patients with no operation experienced spontaneous cure. Lichtman and McDonald reported that 74 percent of chronic fecal fistulas treated by turn-in or resection were cured.

EXTERNAL STOMAL COMPLICATIONS (See Chap. 28).

Ileostomy

Ileostomy performed for ulcerative colitis is associated with a high incidence of complications related to technical factors, presence of disease, and the nature of the intestinal contents which are discharged. The location of ileostomy is critical to permit application of an effective collecting device, while the method of fixation of the ileal mesentery is important to prevent internal herniation. Formation of the ileostomy itself is important in reducing the incidence of complications. The technique of operative maturation by everting the mucosa reduces the incidence of serositis and peritonitis. Frozen section of the transected ileum is indicated, since ulcerative colitis may extend into the segment of ileum and result in improper function. The liquid nature of the ileostomy discharge requires that measures be taken to avoid excoriation of the skin, which is usually due to delayed application of the bag and a poor fit. When excoriation appears, it is generally wise to discontinue the use of cement and apply a soothing powder. The patient may be placed in a prone position on a frame so that the ileal contents are allowed to drain into a container and contact with the skin is avoided. The complication of prolapse, which requires revision, should be seen infrequently if the mesentery has been fixed. Fistulas which develop at or below the skin level are an indication for early revision of the ileostomy.

Cecostomy and Colostomy

Cecostomies generally demand more attention than colostomies, and frequent irrigation is indicated. Subsequent to removal of the cecostomy catheter, spontaneous closure is to be anticipated, but in unusual circumstances, surgical closure is required. Complications following colostomy include ischemia, gangrene, bleeding, wound abscesses, stenosis, or retraction of the stoma. In the case of a terminal colostomy, fixation during the operative procedure should prevent retraction. If either retraction or gangrene becomes evident, immediate operation is indicated to revise the colostomy using viable bowel of sufficient length.

References

General Considerations

Artz, C. P., and Hardy, J. D.: "Complications in Surgery and Their Management," W. B. Saunders Company, Philadelphia, 1967.

Wound Complications

Ad Hoc Committee of the Committee on Trauma, Division of Medical Sciences, National Academy of Sciences–National Research Council: Postoperative Wound Infections: The Influence of Ultraviolet Irradiation of the Operating Room and of Various Other Factors, *Ann Surg [Suppl]*, vol. 160, 1964.
Alexander, H. C., and Prudden, J.: The Causes of Abdominal Wound Disruption, *Surg Gynecol Obstet*, **122:**1223, 1966.
Barnes, J., Pace, W. G., Trump, D. S., and Ellison, E. H.: Prophylactic Postoperative Antibiotics: A Controlled Study of 1,007 Cases, *Arch Surg*, **79:**190, 1959.
Dineen, P.: A Critical Study of 100 Consecutive Wound Infections, *Surg Gynecol Obstet*, **113:**91, 1961.
————: Major Infections in the Postoperative Period, *Surg Clin North Am*, **44:**553, 1964.
Elek, S. D., and Conen, P. E.: The Virulence of *Staphylococcus pyogenes* for Man: A Study of the Problems of Wound Infections, *Br J Exp Pathol*, **38:**573, 1957.
Glenn, F., and Moore, S. W.: The Disruption of Abdominal Wounds, *Surg Gynecol Obstet*, **72:**1041, 1941.

Halasz, N. A.: Dehiscence of Laparotomy Wounds, *Am J Surg*, **116:**210, 1968.
Hartzell, J. B., and Winfield, J. M.: Disruption of Abdominal Wounds: Collective Review, *Int Abstr Surg*, **68:**585, 1939.
Howe, C. W., and Mozden, P. J.: Postoperative Infections: Current Concepts, *Surg Clin North Am*, **43:**859, 1963.
Ketcham, A. S., Lieberman, J. E., and West, J. T.: Antibiotic Prophylaxis in Cancer Surgery and Its Value in Staphylococcal Carrier Patients, *Surg Gynecol Obstet*, **117:**1, 1963.
Pemberton, L. B., and Manax, W. G.: Complications after Vertical and Transverse Incisions for Cholecystectomy, *Surg Gynecol Obstet*, **132:**892, 1971.
Polk, H. C., Jr., and Lopez-Mayor, J. F.: Postoperative Wound Infection: A Prospective Study of Determinant Factors and Prevention, *Surgery*, **66:**97, 1969.
Rees, V. L., and Coller, F. A.: Anatomic and Clinical Study of Transverse Abdominal Incision, *Arch Surg*, **47:**136, 1943.
Schonholtz, G. J., Borgia, C. A., and Blair, J. D.: Wound Sepsis in Orthopedic Surgery, *J Bone Joint Surg [Am]*, **44A:**1548, 1962.
Singleton, A. O., and Blocker, T. G., Jr.: The Problem of Disruption of Abdominal Wounds and Postoperative Hernia, *JAMA*, **112:**122, 1939.
Thomsen, V. F., Larsen, S. O., and Jepsen, O. B.: Post-operative Wound Sepsis in General Surgery: IV. Sources and Routes of Infection, *Acta Chir Scand*, **136:**251, 1970.
Thompson, W. D., Ravdin, I. S., and Frank, I. L.: Effect of Hypoproteinemia on Wound Disruption, *Arch Surg*, **36:**500, 1938.
Wolff, W. I.: Disruption of Abdominal Wounds, *Ann Surg*, **131:**534, 1950.

Postoperative Parotitis

Branson, B., Kugel, A. I., Stafford, C. E., and Morel, E. E.: The Re-emergence of Postoperative Parotitis, *Western J Surg Obstet Gynecol*, **67:**38, 1959.
Carlson, R. G., and Glas, W. W.: Acute Suppurative Parotitis, *Arch Surg*, **86:**659, 1963.
Hemenway, W. G., and English, G. M.: Surgical Treatment of Acute Bacterial Parotitis, *Postgrad Med*, **50:**114, 1971.
Krippaehne, W. W., Hunt, T. K., and Dunphy, J. E.: Acute Suppurative Parotitis: A Study of 161 Cases, *Ann Surg*, **156:**251, 1962.
Lary, B. G.: Postoperative Suppurative Parotitis, *Arch Surg*, **89:**653, 1964.
Petersdorf, R. G., Forsyth, B. B., and Bernake, D.: Staphylococcal Parotitis, *N Engl J Med*, **259:**1250, 1958.
Reilly, D. J.: Benign Transient Swelling of the Parotid Glands following General Anesthesia: "Anesthesia Mumps," *Anesth Anal (Cleve)*, **49:**560, 1970.

Postoperative Respiratory Complications

Adriani, J., Zepernick, R., Harmon, W., and Hiern, B.: Iatrogenic Pulmonary Edema in Surgical Patients, *Surgery*, **61:**183, 1967.
Ashbaugh, D. G., and Petty, T. L.: Positive End-expiratory Pressure: Physiology, Indications, and Contraindications, *J Thorac Cardiovasc Surg*, **65:**165, 1973.
Becker, A., Barak, S., Braun, E., and Meyers, M. P.: The Treatment of Postoperative Pulmonary Atelectasis with Inter-

mittent Positive Pressure Breathing, *Surg Gynecol Obstet,* **111:**517, 1960.

Beecher, H. K.: Measured Effect of Laparotomy on Respiration, *J Clin Invest,* **12:**639, 1933.

Bendixen, H. H., and Bunker, J. P.: "Ventilation and Postoperative Period," paper presented at The Second World Congress of Anaesthesiologists, Toronto, Sept. 6, 1960.

——, Hedley-Shyte, J., and Laver, M. B.: Impaired Oxygenation in Surgical Patients during General Anesthesia with Controlled Ventilation: A Concept of Atelectasis, *N Engl J Med,* **269:**991, 1963.

——, ——, and ——: Increased Physiologic Shunting during Anesthesia and Surgery, *Anesthesiology,* **24:**122, 1963.

Brattstrom, S.: Postoperative Pulmonary Ventilation with Reference to Postoperative Pulmonary Complications, *Acta Chir Scand Suppl* **195,** 1954.

Clements, J. A.: Surface Phenomena in Relation to Pulmonary Function (Sixth Bowditch Lecture), *Physiologist,* **5:**11, 1962.

Clendon, D. R. T., and Pygott, F.: Analysis of Pulmonary Complications Occurring after 579 Consecutive Operations, *Br J Anaesth,* **19:**62, 1944.

Collins, J. A.: The Causes of Progressive Pulmonary Insufficiency in Surgical Patients, *J Surg Res,* **9:**685, 1969.

Coryllos, P. N., and Birnbaum, G. L.: Studies in Pulmonary Gas Absorption in Bronchial Obstruction, *Am J Med Sci,* **183:**317, 1932.

Griffo, Z. J., and Roos, A.: Effect of O_2 Breathing on Pulmonary Compliance, *J Appl Physiol,* **17:**233, 1962.

Hamilton, W. K.: Postoperative Respiratory Complications, chap. 10 in "Clinical Anesthesia," 1/1965.

Joffe, N.: Roentgenologic Findings in Post-shock and Postoperative Pulmonary Insufficiency, *Radiology,* **94:**369, 1970.

Kurzweg, F. T.: Pulmonary Complications following Upper Abdominal Surgery, *Am Surg,* **19:**967, 1953.

Laver, M. B., and Bendixen, H. H.: Atelectasis in the Surgical Patient: Recent Conceptual Advances, *Prog Surg,* **5:**1, 1966.

Masson, A. H. B.: Pulmonary Edema during or after Surgery, pt. I, *Anesth Anal Current Res,* **43:**440, 1964.

——: Pulmonary Edema during or after Surgery, pt. II, *Anesth Anal Curr Res,* **43:**446, 1964.

Mead, J., and Collier, C.: Relation of Volume History of Lungs to Respiratory Mechanics in Anesthetized Dogs, *J Appl Physiol,* **14:**669, 1959.

Moersch, H. J.: Bronchoscopy in Treatment of Postoperative Atelectasis, *Surg Gynecol Obstet,* **77:**435, 1943.

Moore, F. D.: Postoperative Pulmonary Insufficiency: Anoxia, the Shunted Lung and Mechanical Assistance, in D. E. Harken (ed.), "Cardiac Surgery 2," *Cardiovasc Clin,* vol. 3, no. 3, F. A. Davis Company, Philadelphia, 1971.

——, Lyons, J. H., Pierce, E. C., Jr., Morgan, A. P., Jr., Drinker, P. A., MacArthur, J. D., and Dammin, G. J.: "Post-traumatic Pulmonary Insufficiency," W. B. Saunders Company, Philadelphia, 1969.

Neely, W. A., Robinson, T. W., McMullan, M. H., Bobo, W. O., Meadows, D. L., and Hardy, J. D.: Post-operative Respiratory Insufficiency, *Ann Surg,* **171:**679, 1970.

Overfield, W., and Powers, S. R., Jr.: Arterial Oxygen Tension: Significance in the Surgical Patient, *Surgery,* **71:**1, 1972.

Peters, R. M., Hilberman, M., Hogan, J. S., and Crawford, D. A.:

Objective Indications for Respiratory Therapy in Post-trauma and Postoperative Patients, *Am J Surg,* **124:**262, 1972.

Pontoppidan, H., Geffin, B., and Lowenstein, E.: Acute Respiratory Failure in the Adult: Trends in Treatment of Acute Respiratory Failure, *N Engl J Med,* **287:**690, 1972.

——, ——, and ——: Acute Respiratory Failure in the Adult: Assessment of Respiratory Function, *N Engl J Med,* **287:**743, 1972.

——, ——, and ——: Acute Respiratory Failure in the Adult: Effect of Mechanical Ventilation and Airway Pressures on Circulation and Blood Gas Exchange, *N Engl J Med,* **287:**799, 1972.

——, Laver, M. B., and Geffin, B.: Acute Respiratory Failure in the Surgical Patient, *Adv Surg,* **4:**163, 1970.

Van Allen, C. M., and Adams, W. E.: The Mechanism of Obstructive Pulmonary Atelectasis, *Surg Gynecol Obstet,* **50:**385, 1930.

—— and Lindskog, D. E.: Obstructive Pulmonary Atelectasis, *Arch Surg,* **21:**1195, 1930.

Webb, W. R.: New Mucolytic Agents for Sputum Liquefaction, *Postgrad Med,* **36:**449, 1964.

Cardiac Complications

Buckley J. J., and Jackson, J. A.: Postoperative Cardiac Arrhythmias, *Anesthesiology,* **22:**723, 1961.

Currens, J. H., White, P. D., and Churchill, E. D.: Cardiac Arrhythmias following Thoracic Surgery, *N Engl J Med,* **229:**360, 1943.

Dack, S.: Postoperative Myocardial Infarction, *Am J Cardiol,* **12:**423, 1963.

Dreifus, L. S., Rabbino, M. D., Watanabe, Y., and Tabesh, E.: Arrhythmias in the Postoperative Period, *Am J Cardiol,* **12:**431, 1963.

Krosnick, A., and Wassermann, F.: Cardiac Arrhythmias in Older Age Group following Thoracic Surgery, *Am J Med Sci,* **230:**541, 1955.

Kuner, J., Enescu, V., Utsu, F., Boszormenyi, E., Bernstein, H., and Corday, E.: Cardiac Arrhythmias during Anesthesia, *Dis Chest,* **52:**580, 1967.

Massie, E., and Valle, A. R.: Cardiac Arrhythmias Complicating Total Pneumonectomy, *Ann Intern Med,* **26:**231, 1947.

Master, A. M., Dack, S., and Jaffe, H. L.: Postoperative Coronary Artery Occlusion, *JAMA,* **110:**1415, 1938.

Mauney, F. M., Jr., Ebert, P. A., and Sabiston, D. C., Jr.: Postoperative Myocardial Infarction: A Study of Predisposing Factors, Diagnosis and Mortality in a High Risk Group of Surgical Patients, *Ann Surg,* **172:**497, 1970.

Merideth, J.: Cardiac Arrhythmias in the Postoperative Patient, *Surg Clin North Am,* **49:**1083, 1969.

Reinikainen, M., and Pontinen, P.: On Cardiac Arrhythmias during Anaesthesia and Surgery, *Acta Med Scand Suppl* 457, 1966.

Rogers, W. R., Wroblewski, F., and LaDue, J. S.: Supraventricular Tachycardia Complicating Surgical Procedures: Study of Contributing Causes, Course, and Treatment of This Complication in Fifty Patients, *Circulation,* **7:**192, 1953.

Sharnoff, J. G.: Postmortem Findings in 25 Cases of Sudden Heart Arrest in the Perioperative Period, *Lancet,* **2:**876, 1966.

Stein, I., and Caginalp, N.: The Postoperative Electrocardiogram, *Angiology,* **17:**323, 1966.

Tarhan, S., Moffitt, E. A., Taylor, W. F., and Giuliani, E. R.: Myocardial Infarction after General Anesthesia, *JAMA,* **220:**1451, 1972.

Taylor, I. B.: Cyclopropane Anesthesia: With Report of Results in 41,690 Administrations, *Anesthesiology,* **2:**641, 1941.

Wheat, M. W., Jr., and Burford, T. H.: Digitalis in Surgery: Extension of Classical Indications, *J Thorac Cardiovasc Surg,* **41:**162, 1961.

Wroblewski, F., and LaDue, J. S.: Myocardial Infarction as a Postoperative Complication of Major Surgery, *JAMA,* **150:**1212, 1952.

Diabetes Mellitus

Black, K.: Diabetes and the Surgical Patient, *Br J Clin Pract,* **20:**555, 1966.

Canary, J. J., Stoffer, R., Delawter, D. D., and Moss, J. M.: The Response of Tolbutamide-treated Patients to the Stress of Surgery, *Med Ann DC,* **28:**614, 1959.

Forsham, P. H.: Management of Diabetes during Stress and Surgery, in R. H. Williams (ed.), "Diabetes," chap. 36, Hoeber Medical Division, Harper & Row, Publishers, Incorporated, New York, 1960.

Galloway, J. A., and Shuman, C. R.: Diabetes and Surgery: A Study of 667 Cases, *Am J Med,* **34:**177, 1963.

Gastineau, C. F., and Molnar, G. D.: The Care of the Diabetic Patient During Emergency Surgery, *Surg Clin N Am,* **49:**1171, 1969.

Greenstein, A. J., and Dreiling, D. A.: Nonketotic Hyperosmolar Coma in the Postoperative Patient, *Am J Surg,* **121:**698, 1971.

Marble, A., and Steinke, J.: Physiology and Pharmacology in Diabetes Mellitus: Guiding the Diabetic Patient through the Surgical Period, *Anesthesiology,* **24:**442, 1963.

Packovich, M. J., Molnar, G. D., and Leonard, P. F.: Management of Diabetic patients during Surgery, *Surg Clin North Am,* **45:**975, 1965.

Weisenfeld, S., Podolsky, S., Goldsmith, L., and Ziff, L.: Adsorption of Insulin to Infusion Bottles and Tubing, *Diabetes,* **17:**766, 1968.

Fat Embolism

Ashbaugh, D. G., and Petty, T. L.: The Use of Corticosteroids in the Treatment of Respiratory Failure Associated with Massive Fat Embolism, *Surg Gynecol Obstet,* **123:**495, 1966.

Benoit, P. R., Hampson, L. G., and Burgess, J. H.: Value of Arterial Hypoxemia in the Diagnosis of Pulmonary Fat Embolis, *Ann Surg,* **175:**128, 1972.

Bergenz, S. E.: Studies on the Genesis of Posttraumatic Fat Embolism, *Acta Chir Scand Suppl* 282, 1961.

Cobb, C. A., and Hillman, J. W.: Fat Embolism, *Instruc Lect Am Acad Orthop Surg,* **18:**122, 1961.

———, LeQuire, V. S., Gray, M. E., and Hillman, J. W.: Therapy of Traumatic Fat Embolism with Intravenous Fluids and Heparin, *Surg Forum,* **9:**751, 1959.

Collins, J. A., Hudson, T. L., Hamacher, W. R., Rokous, J., Williams, G., and Hardaway, R. M., III: Systemic Fat Embolism in Four Combat Casualties, *Ann Surg,* **167:**493, 1968.

Evarts, C. M.: The Fat Embolism Syndrome: A Review, *Surg Clin North Am,* **50:**493, 1970.

Greendyke, R. M.: Fat Embolism in Fatal Automobile Accidents, *J Forensic Sci,* **9:**201, 1964.

Henzel, J. H., Smith, J. L., Pories, W. J., and Burget, D. E.: Fat Embolism: Diagnostic Challenge of a Potentially Lethal Clinical Entity, *Am J Surg,* **113:**525, 1967.

Jackson, C. T., and Greendyke, R. M.: Pulmonary and Cerebral Fat Embolism after Closed Chest Cardiac Massage, *Surg Gynecol Obstet,* **120:**25, 1965.

Killian, H.: Die traumatische Fettembolie, *Dtsch Z Chir,* **231:**97, 1931.

Kuhne, H., and Kremser, K. H.: Die klinische Bedeuting der traumatischen Fettembolie, *Beitr Klin Chir,* **195:**385, 1957.

Mallory, T. B., Sullivan, E. R., Burnett, C. H., Simeone, F., Shapiro, S. L., and Beecher, H. K.: The General Pathology of Traumatic Shock, *Surgery,* **27:**629, 1950.

Musselman, M. M., Glas, W. W., and Grekin, T. D.: Fat Embolism, *Arch Surg,* **65:**551, 1952.

Palmovic, V., and McCarroll, J. R.: Fat Embolism in Trauma, *Arch Pathol,* **80:**630, 1965.

Pazell, J. A., and Peltier, L. F.: Experience with Sixty-three Patients with Fat Embolism, *Surg Gynecol Obstet,* **135:**77, 1972.

Peltier, L. F.: The Diagnosis of Fat Embolism, *Surg Gynecol Obstet,* **121:**371, 1965.

Scuderi, C. S.: Fat Embolism: Clinical and Experimental Study, *Surg Gynecol Obstet,* **72:**732, 1941.

Sevitt, S.: "Fat Embolism," Butterworth Scientific Publications, London, 1962.

Sutton, G. E.: Pulmonary Fat Embolism, *Ann Surg,* **76:**581, 1922.

Psychiatric Complications

Altschule, M. D.: Postoperative Psychosis, *Surg Clin N Am,* **49:**677, 1969.

Bakwin, H.: Psychic Trauma of Operations, *J Pediatr,* **36:**262, 1950.

Bliss, E. L., Rumel, W. R., and Branch, C. H.: Psychiatric Complications of Mitral Surgery: Report of a Death after Electroshock Therapy, *Arch Neurol,* **74:**249, 1955.

Bolton, H. E., and Bailey, C. P.: Surgical Aspects in Psychosomatic Aspects of Cardiovascular Surgery, in A. J. Cantor and A. N. Foxe (eds.), "Psychosomatic Aspects of Surgery," chap. 3, Grune & Stratton, Inc., New York, 1955.

Browning, J., and Houseworth, J.: Development of New Symptoms following Medical and Surgical Treatment for Duodenal Ulcer, *Psychosom Med,* **15:**328, 1953.

Cramond, W. A.: Renal Homotransplantation: Some Observations on Recipients and Donors, *Br J Psychiat,* **113:**1223, 1967.

———, Court, J. H., Higgins, B. A., Knight, P. R., and Lawrence, J. R.: Psychological Screening of Potential Donors in a Renal Homotransplantation Programme, *Br J Psychiat,* **113:**1213, 1967.

———, Knight, P. R., and Lawrence, J. R.: The psychiatric Contribution to a Renal Unit Undertaking Chronic Haemodialysis and Renal Homotransplantation, *Br J Psychiat,* **113:**1201, 1967.

Da Costa, J. C.: The Diagnosis of Postoperative Insanity, *Surg Gynecol Obstet,* **11:**577, 1910.

Deutsch, H.: Psychoanalytic Observations in Surgery, *Psychosom Med,* **4:**105, 1942.

Donovan, J. C.: Some Psychosomatic Aspects of Obstetrics and Gynecology, *Am J Obstet Gynecol,* **75:**72, 1958.

Egerton, N., and Kay, J. H.: Psychological Disturbances Associated with Open Heart Surgery, *Br J Psychiat,* **110:**433, 1964.

Fox, H. M., Rizzo, N. D., and Gifford, S.: Psychological Observations of Patients Undergoing Mitral Surgery: Study of Stress, *Psychosom Med,* **16:**186, 1954.

Hackett, T. P., and Weisman, A. D.: Psychiatric Management of Operative Syndromes. I. The Therapeutic Consultation and the Effect of Noninterpretive Intervention, *Psychosom Med,* **22:**267, 1960.

———, and ———: Psychiatric Management of Operative Syndromes. II. Psychodynamic Factors in Formulation and Management, *Psychosom Med,* **22:**356, 1960.

Halper, I. S.: Psychiatric Observations in a Chronic Hemodialysis Program, *Med Clin North Am,* **55:**177, 1971.

Hollender, M. H.: A Study of Patients Admitted to a Psychiatric Hospital after Pelvic Operations, *Am J Obstet Gynecol,* **79:**498, 1960.

Katz, N. M., Agle, D. P., DePalma, R. G., and DeCosse, J. J.: Delirium in Surgical Patients under Intensive Care: Utility of Mental Status Examination, *Arch Surg,* **104:**310, 1972.

Kemph, J. P.: Renal Failure, Artificial Kidney and Kidney Transplant, *Am J Psychiat,* **122:**1270, 1966.

Knox, S. J.: Severe Psychiatric Disturbances in the Postoperative Period: A Five-Year Survey of Belfast Hospitals, *J Ment Sci,* **107:**1078, 1961.

Kornfeld, D. S., Zimberg, S., and Malm, J. R.: Psychiatric Complications of Open-Heart Surgery, *N Engl J Med,* **273:**287, 1965.

Layne, O. L., Jr., and Yudofsky, S. C.: Postoperative Psychosis in Cardiotomy Patients: The Role of Organic and Psychiatric Factors, *N Engl J Med,* **284:**518, 1971.

Levy, D.: Psychic Trauma of Operations in Children and a Note on Combat Neurosis, *Am J Dis Child,* **69:**7, 1945.

Lewis, A.: "The Relation between Operative Risk and the Patient's General Condition," Report 16, Congrès International de Chirurgie, Copenhague, 1955.

Lindemann, E.: Observations on Psychiatric Sequelae to Surgical Operations in Women, *Am J Psychiat,* **98:**132, 1941.

Meyer, B. C.: Some Psychiatric Aspects of Surgical Practice, *Psychosom Med,* **20:**203, 1958.

———, Brown, F., and Levine, A.: Observations on the House-Tree-Person Drawing Test Before and After Surgery, *Psychosom Med,* **17:**428, 1955.

Moore, F., Steinberg, R., Bull, M., Wilson, G., and Myrden, J.: Studies in Surgical Endocrinology: I, *Ann Surg,* **141:**145, 1955.

Prugh, D., Staub, E., Sands, H., Kirschbaum, R., and Lenihan, R.: A Study of the Emotional Reactions of Children and Families to Hospitalization and Illness, *Am J Orthopsychiatry,* **22:**70, 1953.

Sand, P., Livingston, G., and Wright, R. G.: Psychological Assessment of Candidates for a Haemodialysis Program, *Ann Intern Med,* **64:**602, 1966.

Scott, J.: Postoperative Psychosis in the Aged, *Am J Surg,* **10:**38, 1960.

Shea, E. J., Bogdan, D. F., Freeman, R. B., and Schreiner, G. E.: Haemodialysis for Chronic Renal Failure: IV. Psychological Considerations, *Ann Intern Med,* **62:**558, 1965.

Sutherland, A.: Psychological Impact of Postoperative Cancer, *Bull NY Acad Med,* **33:**428, 1957.

———, and Ohrbach, C.: Psychological Impact of Cancer and Cancer Surgery: II. Depressive Reactions Associated with Surgery for Cancer, *Cancer,* **6:**958, 1953.

———, ———, Dyk, R., and Bard, M.: The Psychological Impact of Cancer and Cancer Surgery: I. Adaptation to the Dry Colostomy: Preliminary Report and Summary of Findings, *Cancer,* **5:**857, 1952.

Titchener, J. L., and Levine, M.: "Surgery as a Human Experience: The Psychodynamics of Surgical Practice," Oxford University Press, Fair Lawn, N.J., 1960.

———, Zwerling, I., Gottschalk, L., Levine, M., Culbertson, W., Cohen, S., and Silver, H.: Psychosis in Surgical Patients, *Surg Gynecol Obstet,* **102:**59, 1956.

Weisman, A. D., and Hackett, T. P.: Psychosis after Eye Surgery: Establishment of a Specific Doctor-Patient Relation in the Prevention and Treatment of "Black-patch Delirium," *N Engl J Med,* **258:**1284, 1958.

Weiss, S. M.: Psychological Adjustment following Open-Heart Surgery, *J Nerv Ment Dis,* **143:**363, 1966.

Winkelstein, C., Blacher, R. S., and Meyer, B. C.: Psychiatric Observations on Surgical Patients in Recovery Room: Pilot Study, *NY J Med,* **65:**865, 1965.

Wright, R. G., Sand, P., and Livingston, G.: Psychological Stress during Haemodialysis for Chronic Renal Failure, *Ann Intern Med,* **64:**611, 1966.

Zaks, M. S.: Disturbances in Physiologic Functions and Neuropsychiatric Complications in Heart Surgery, in A. A. Luisada (ed.), "Cardiology: An Encyclopedia of the Cardiovascular System," vol. 3, McGraw-Hill Book Company, New York, 1959.

Complications of Gastrointestinal Surgery

Beal, J. M., and Moody, F. G.: Postoperative Complications of Duodenal Surgery, *Surg Clin North Am,* **44:**379, 1964.

Blomstedt, B., and Dahlgren, S.: The Afferent Loop Syndrome, *Acta Chir Scand,* **120:**347, 1961.

Burnett, W. E., Rosemond, G. P., Caswell, H. T., Beauchamp, E. W., Jr., Tyson, R. R., and Wright, W. C.: Studies on So-called Postgastrectomy Pancreatitis, *Ann Surg,* **149:**737, 1959.

Capper, W. M., and Welbourn, R. B.: Early Postcibal Symptoms following Gastrectomy, *Br J Surg,* **43:**24, 1955.

Colcock, B. P.: Leakage from the Duodenal Stump following Gastric Resection, *Lahey Clin Bull,* **13:**190, 1964.

Edmunds, L. H., Jr., Williams, G. M., and Welch, C. E.: External Fistulas Arising from the Gastro-intestinal Tract, *Ann Surg,* **152:**445, 1960.

Habif, D. V.: Immediate Complications of Surgery of the Small Intestine, *Surg Clin North Am,* **44:**387, 1964.

Hibner, R., and Richards, V.: Stomal or Small Bowel Obstruction following Partial Gastrectomy, *Am J Surg,* **96:**309, 1958.

Hoffman, W. A., and Spiro, H. M.: Afferent Loop Problems, *Gastroenterology,* **40:**201, 1961.

Johnson, C. L., and McIlrath, D. C.: Management of Patients with Enterocutaneous Fistulas, *Surg Clin North Am,* **49:**967, 1969.

Lichtman, A. L., and McDonald, J. R.: Fecal Fistula, *Surg Gynecol Obstet,* **78:**449, 1944.

MacFadyen, B. V., Dudrick, S. J., and Ruberg, R. L.: The Management of Gastrointestinal Fistulae with Parenteral Hyperalimentation, *Surgery,* 1973. (To be published.)

McGovern, J. B., and Gross, R. E.: Intussusception as a Postoperative Complication, *Surgery,* **63:**507, 1968.

Magnuson, F. K., Judd, E. S., and Dearing, W. H.: Comparison of Postgastrectomy Complications in Gastric and Duodenal Ulcer Patients, *Am Surg,* **32:**375, 1966.

Marshall, S. F., and Gerber, M. L.: Persistent Fecal Fistula, *Surg Clin North Am,* **30:**901, 1950.

Moore, H. G., Jr.: Complications of Gastric Surgery, in H. N. Harkins and L. M. Nyhus (eds.), "Surgery of the Stomach and Duodenum," chap. 11, Little, Brown and Company, Boston, 1962.

Moretz, W. H.: Inadvertent Gastro-ileostomy, *Ann Surg,* **130:**124, 1949.

Morgenstern, L., Yamakawa, T., Ben-Shoshan, M., and Lippman, H.: Anastomotic Leakage after Low Colonic Anastomosis. Clinical and Experimental Aspects, *Am J Surg,* **123:**104, 1972.

Pettersson, S., and Wallensten, S.: Leakage at Suture Lines after Partial Gastrectomy for Peptic Ulcer, *Acta Chir Scand,* **135:**229, 1969.

Quinn, W. F., and Gifford, J. H.: Syndrome of Proximal Jejunal Loop Obstruction following Anterior Gastric Resection, *Calif Med,* **72:**18, 1950.

Rodkey, G. V., and Welch, C. E.: Duodenal Decompression in Gastrectomy, *N Engl J Med,* **262:**498, 1960.

Rousselot, L. M., and Slattery, J. R.: Immediate Complications of Surgery of the Large Intestine, *Surg Clin North Am,* **44:**397, 1964.

Spencer, F. C.: Ischemic Necrosis of Remaining Stomach following Subtotal Gastrectomy, *Arch Surg,* **73:**844, 1956.

State, D.: Immediate Complications of Gastric Surgery, *Surg Clin North Am,* **44:**371, 1964.

Turner, F. P.: Postoperative Complications following Gastric Resection, *Am J Surg,* **101:**711, 1961.

Chapter 13

Physiologic Monitoring of the Surgical Patient

by Louis R. M. Del Guercio

Introduction

Physiologic Concepts and Monitoring

Instrumentation and Clinical Techniques
Physiologic Sensing
Respiratory Monitoring
Cardiovascular Monitoring
Cardiac Output Determinations
Monitoring of Tissue Metabolism

INTRODUCTION

Among the 14 definitions of the word "monitor" which appear in one dictionary, three appear applicable to medicine: "Something that serves to remind or give warning"; "A device or arrangement for observing or recording the operation of a machine or system, esp. an automatic control system"; and "To observe, record or detect an operation or condition with instruments that have no effect on the operation or condition."

This last definition offers the key to a basic problem of all patient monitoring, i.e., that the measuring system tends to change the measurements. The application of electrodes, cannulas, mouthpieces, and other paraphernalia definitely has psychologic and physiologic effects on the patient. From this it follows that the ideal monitoring system should be noninvasive and unobtrusive.

Another point to be stressed is that the most sophisticated and advanced electronic system can never substitute for close surveillance by an experienced and qualified health professional. Monitors in surgery are worthwhile only if they provide physiologic information about the patient which cannot be detected by the five senses of a physician or nurse. In addition, the transducers, signal processors, or readout devices should not so encumber the patient as to interfere with essential nursing care.

There is a tendency to think of monitoring in terms of complicated electronic devices and computers; in fact, the serial recordings of temperature, pulse, respiratory rate, and blood pressure are forms of clinical monitoring in common use for decades. These simple techniques served the surgeon fairly well until the advent of cardiopulmonary bypass and open heart surgery. At that point, it was recog-nized that clinician care of the patient, in the period following what could be considered at best a controlled physiologic insult, required a better assessment of the cardiovascular and respiratory status of the patient. Decisions regarding therapy had to be made rapidly on the basis of reasonably accurate measurements of physiologic variables.

This led in the early 1960s to the clinical use of central venous pressure and cardiac output determinations. The invention of the densitometer for the continuous recording of indicator dilution and of electrodes for the rapid determination of the partial pressures of oxygen and carbon dioxide in whole blood provided the technical impetus for the modern era of clinical monitoring.

Subsequently, many specialized diagnostic and treatment centers established within the hospital have included physiologic monitoring as an adjunct to patient care. Coronary care units, respiratory care centers, burn centers, neurosurgical intensive care units, pediatric and neonatal intensive care units, renal dialysis centers, and surgical intensive care units all utilize some forms of patient monitoring. Only in the coronary care unit, however, can it be statistically documented that lives are saved by monitoring. In this case, the electrocardiograph is an almost ideal monitor because it is safe, noninvasive, and specific for the physiologic aberration, cardiac arrhythmias, which kills most myocardial infarction victims.

The problem of monitoring for the surgical patient is much more complex, because there is as yet no known physiologic variable which can be used to warn against impending disaster. And although there are many systems in daily operation which on the basis of cardiac output, arterial pressure, central venous pressure, and blood-gas tensions provide assessment of cardiorespiratory function and oxygen transport, these techniques are primarily used when it is already obvious that the patient is in serious trouble. Such systems at the present time are generally invasive and are used intermittently to assess the response of a desperately ill patient to specific modes of therapy. There are many models of these "shock carts" currently available commercially.

The second type of surgical monitoring involves the continuous recording of one or two fundamental physiologic variables in order to show trends and changes which may warn of impending disaster. At the present time there is no system of this type in operation which has been proved to be practical for most surgical patients. Continuous rather than intermittent monitoring would be desirable for surgical patients if it could be performed inexpensively and noninvasively, because more information can be obtained from a variable which is measured in relation to time. Patterns and trends can be detected and compared with mathematical models obtained from studies of patients known to be in jeopardy. For example, it is believed by most experts that there is no such thing as cardiac arrest without antecedent events. Clinical studies have shown that long before cardiac standstill or ventricular fibrillation occurs, serious derangements of blood-gas tensions or hemodynamic variables can be demonstrated. Continuous monitoring of certain variables might reveal catastrophic trends.

But since cardiac arrest is a rare event, the need for surgical monitoring in the general population might be questioned, were it not for the National Halothane Study. That prospective statistical analysis of over 850,000 operations performed in 35 highly regarded hospitals revealed an overall 6-week mortality rate of 1.97 percent! This included ophthalmologic, plastic, and other low-death-rate operations. The overall need for surgical monitoring is mandated by that totally unacceptable mortality rate, which is higher than that for 1 year of combat service in World War II, Korea, or Vietnam!

PHYSIOLOGIC CONCEPTS AND MONITORING

One of the problems with patient monitoring today is that we tend to measure the variables which we *can* rather than the variables which we *should*. Thus far in the twentieth century, instruments have directed medicine rather than vice versa; we use the instruments which happen to be available. For example, the entire discipline of diagnostic cardiology developed around measurement of intracardiac pressure gradients and electric potentials rather than volume and flow relationships, because the strain gauge pressure transducer and electrocardiograph were the first instruments available. Monitoring to warn against surgical disaster or to record the proper operation of such a complex "automatic control system" as the human body must be based upon physiologic principles. Instruments and monitoring systems must be developed and designed to detect specific physiologic events known to be associated with surgical morbidity or mortality.

The overall physiology of oxygen transport, or the delivery of oxygen from the atmosphere to the mitochondria of the body cell mass, can be used as a model to assess the abilities of particular monitoring systems to detect critical events and trends. This process involves many organ systems and complicated feedback loops for regulation and compensation. It is imperative for the survival of the individual that the oxygen transport system continue in operation without interruption.

Even in the basal state, 4 ml of oxygen is required each

minute for each kilogram of body weight. Human beings can store only a 4- or 5-minute supply in the lungs and blood cells. With cessation of oxygen transport anywhere along the line serious defects of oxygen tension gradient develop within 2 minutes. Even the highly trained pearl divers of Northern Australia dive for less than 2 minutes, and they still manifest markedly elevated blood lactate levels and frequent cardiac arrythmias. The best of the diving mammals, the whale, cannot store proportionately more than twice the amount of oxygen stored by nondiving mammals such as man.

The upper airways serve to humidify and warm or cool the air entering the tracheobronchial tree during spontaneous respiration. The difference in temperature between inspired and expired air provides a basis for monitoring the rate of respiration in patients. Simple thermistor probes have been developed which are fixed in front of the external nares to record the passage of warmed expired air. It is not possible by this means to evaluate the adequacy of ventilation, but a simple noninvasive means of monitoring the respiratory rate and signaling respiratory arrest could be of value. Respiratory rate is regulated by changes in arterial oxygen content through the carotid and aortic body reflexes, and by changes in pH and carbon dioxide tension through brainstem chemoreceptors. Hyperpnea can be a relatively nonspecific warning sign suggesting hypoxia, increased metabolic demands, emotional excitement, or simply painful stimuli.

Table 13-1 traces the oxygen flow and partial pressure gradients from this point on. The critical importance of each stage is related to the oxygen stored beyond that point. For example, respiratory failure is tolerated far longer than circulatory arrest, because the circulatory system stores more than twice as much oxygen as the lungs. Cyanide kills quickly because it blocks the ability of the mitochondria to utilize oxygen. This is a point beyond which there is no oxygen reserve. Total body oxygen stores are about 1,500 ml. A monitoring system should detect a block of this most critical step, delivery of oxygen to the mitochondrion within the cell. At this point, oxygen stores are nil and the tension gradient is low.

The partial pressure of oxygen in the atmosphere is 159 mm Hg (20.84 percent of 760 mm Hg). As inspired air is rapidly humidified in the upper airways by the mucosa of the nasal turbinates, pharynx, and tracheobronchial tree, the partial pressure drops to 149 mm Hg due to the dilutional effect of the water vapor pressure at body temperature (47 mm Hg). As the alveoli are approached, the oxygen tension rapidly falls, because approximately 4 ml/Kg of body mass of that gas is removed from the alveoli each minute. The 45 mm Hg fall in oxygen tension is replaced by a similar rise in carbon dioxide tension in the alveoli. It is the rapid removal of oxygen from the alveoli by the unsaturated blood entering the pulmonary capillary bed which establishes this gradient. This is why it is possible to maintain adequate oxygenation for several minutes by flushing oxygen into a bronchoscope without any ventilation. Of course, the blood carbon dioxide level rises markedly. The energy cost of ventilation may represent a serious

Table 13-1. OXYGEN TRANSPORT AND MONITORING

Oxygen stores, ml	Oxygen tension gradient, mm Hg	Medium	Measurements
370	159 149 105	Atmosphere Airway Alveoli Interstitial fluid	Tidal volume, dead-space-to-tidal-volume ratio, lung compliance, work of breathing, functional residual capacity, end tidal CO_2, percent shunt, alveolar-arterial O_2 gradient, pulmonary transit time, blood gases
880	100 95 90	Pulmonary capillary Plasma Red cell membrane Hemoglobin Left side of heart Arteries Arteriole	Cardiac output, stroke volume, ejection fraction, ventricular function curves, systolic time intervals, central venous pressure, pulmonary wedge pressure, left ventricular end-diastolic pressure.
	90–40	Capillary	Oxygen consumption, effective oxygen transport, mixed venous oxygen levels, blood lactate concentration, tissue oxygen tension, muscle surface pH, far infrared emission spectroscopy.
56	40 38 20 10	Endothelium Extracellular fluid Pericapillary tissue cylinder Cell membrane	
240	6	Myoglobin	
0	5	Mitochondrion	

— Oxygen flow →

— Electron flow →

Oxygen + electrons +

       hydrogen ions ⟶ water

Cytochromes ⟶ 2 ATP
Ubiquinone
Flavoprotein ⟶ 1 ATP
Diphosphopyridine nucleotide (DPN)
Acetyl coenzyme A
Pyruvate
Glucose

problem to some postoperative patients. Many physiologic variables associated with ventilation and lung mechanics can be measured at the bedside if necessary; among these are tidal volume, minute ventilation, dead-space-to-tidal-volume ratios, compliance, and functional residual capacity. All these give an assessment of the efficiency of the lung, chest, and diaphragm in exchanging air in the alveoli.

The next stage in oxygen transport is truly remarkable. In 5 seconds, the entire output of the right side of the heart is spread out over an area the size of a tennis court and sucked back up into the left atrium. The blood pressure differential across this system is only 6 mm Hg, and all of the blood, during the brief time which the red cells spend in the pulmonary capillaries, normally reaches equilibrium with the oxygen in the alveoli. Only 90 ml of blood is in the capillaries at one time. Moreover, this remarkably efficient manifold system can dynamically expand within seconds to handle three times the normal blood flow without any sacrifice in oxygenation. Roughton has estimated that at normal flow rates each red cell takes 0.8 second to squeeze through two or three alveolar capillaries in succession. At high flow rates, during exercise or in hyper-

dynamic shock, the time spent in the capillary bed is reduced. When it is reduced below 0.35 second, there is insufficient time for the four heme positions of the hemoglobin molecule to take up oxygen, and unsaturation results. This situation can also occur when the cross-sectional area of pulmonary bed is reduced, as in pulmonary embolism, since a more rapid flow is forced past the remaining capillaries. Arterial hypoxemia is well known in pulmonary embolism.

It can be seen from Table 13-1 that oxygen flow from the alveoli to the hemoglobin within the red cell encounters a number of resistances: alveolar membrane, interstitial fluid, capillary membrane, plasma, red cell membrane, and the paracrystalline structure within the red cell. But since all these together are normally only a few microns thick, diffusion is rapid. Many things can go wrong with this efficient system, however, and opportunities for monitoring at this level have been recognized. The red cells normally leave the pulmonary capillaries with an oxygen tension of 100 mm Hg. When they arrive in the left side of the heart, the partial pressure has dropped to about 95 mm Hg because of the mixing effect of unsaturated blood from the bronchial and coronary circulation which empties into the left side of the heart. This shunted blood normally is 3 percent of the output of the right side of the heart.

The difference in the partial pressure of oxygen from the alveoli to the arterial blood is an important monitoring variable. It is called the *alveolar-arterial oxygen gradient.* It is most useful in assessing the efficiency of gas exchange in the lung and is an early indicator of incipient respiratory failure due to a variety of causes in surgical patients.

When the arterial oxygen tension falls below 60 mm Hg in a surgical patient without previous lung disease or intra-cardiac defects, the diagnosis of acute respiratory failure is made. An arterial oxygen tension below 30 mm Hg is generally incompatible with survival for more than a few hours. Several factors, singly or in combination, can produce this severe hypoxemia. Abnormal distribution of blood to sections of the lung containing closed or non-ventilated airways or alveoli will result in so-called physiologic shunting of unsaturated blood into the arterial circulation. Injury to the pulmonary capillary endothelium or pulmonary vascular congestion frequently leads to increased interstitial lung water, which not only increases the diffusion distance for oxygen but causes collapse of alveoli. Pulmonary surfactant, which normally prevents alveolar collapse by reducing surface tension at low lung volumes, may be depleted by hypoxemia and lack of metabolic substrates in acute disease. Thus the collapse of more alveoli creates a vicious cycle of increasing hypoxemia. The reduced lung volume and loss of compliance, or distensibility, are characteristic of a group of nonspecific respiratory distress syndromes associated with shock, trauma, and other clinical problems. They all result in serious venous admixture, so that as much as 50 percent of the output of the right side of the heart may bypass ventilated alveoli. In this circumstance, the alveolar-arterial oxygen gradient may be more than 600 mm Hg, resulting in an arterial oxygen tension of only 60 mm Hg. It is important to detect such a problem early, before irreversible damage is done. The use of a respirator with continuous positive-pressure breathing reduces the cost of respiratory work and decreases shunting by ventilating more alveoli.

Thus far, in dissecting the oxygen transport system as a guide to physiologic monitoring, only oxygen loading has been considered. Other problems can occur downstream related to bloodflow, hemoglobin deficiency, hemoglobin affinity, or cellular defects. These more or less reflect the classic forms of hypoxia described by Barcroft and later appended by Van Slyke: anoxic, stagnant, anemic, and histotoxic hypoxia.

In considering the physiology of body blood flow, two important points must be made: the cardiac output alone is not an indicator of myocardial contractility, and arterial blood pressure alone is not an indicator of blood flow. Myocardial contractility refers to the state of health of the heart muscle and the rate at which the muscle fibers can shorten circumferentially around the bolus of blood within the ventricles. As will be seen later, myocardial contractility is intimately involved with myocardial oxygen transport.

Cardiac output, the actual amount of blood ejected by the heart, is related to two other factors besides contractility: preload and afterload. The preload is the degree of muscle fiber stretch imposed by filling of the ventricles during diastole. According to Starling's law of the heart, this varies directly with cardiac output. The afterload is the impedance to cardiac ejection during systole imposed by vascular resistance, blood pressure, and blood viscosity. The stroke output of the heart varies inversely with the afterload. Any monitoring system designed to assess the state of the myocardium must include these factors. The Sarnoff ventricular function curve is a plot of stroke work (the product of stroke volume and mean aortic blood pressure) against ventricular end-diastolic pressure or end-diastolic volume. It provides a good evaluation of myocardial contractility because it includes consideration of afterload and preload.

One manifestation of the human body as an automatic control system is the fact that a major determinant of cardiac output is increased metabolic activity which produces peripheral vasodilation and a reduced cardiac afterload. Increased metabolic activity also increases the venous return and thus slightly increases cardiac preload. The peripheral arterioles under control of the autonomic nervous system largely control the systemic vascular resistance. The systemic blood pressure varies with the product of the total vascular resistance and the cardiac output. This is why it is impossible to evaluate blood flow on the basis of the blood pressure alone. One seldom used clue to the level of total peripheral resistance is the pulse pressure or the difference between systolic and diastolic blood pressure. As total peripheral resistance increases, the pulse pressure narrows because of increased outflow impedance from the arterial tree.

The varying distribution of the cardiac output to the different organs and body tissues is the body's most important defense in oxygen transport deficiency. During resuscitation from cardiac arrest, the cardiac index is slightly over 1 liter/minute with open-chest cardiac massage. Closed-chest massage produces half of that. The normal cardiac index is 3 liters/minute/m² of body surface area. Yet these low flows are frequent enough to keep the brain alive, because flow to all other tissues except the myocardium is drastically curtailed.

The brain is particularly sensitive to hypoxia. It has no oxygen reserves and constantly requires 15 percent of the resting cardiac output and 20 percent of the total basal oxygen consumption just to maintain its structural and physiologic integrity. The reasons for this will be discussed later. However, irreversible brain damage occurs in man when cerebral oxygen consumption is 50 percent reduced, while the kidneys can tolerate one-third the normal flow for over an hour without damage although they normally receive 25 percent of the cardiac output. In general, organs with low oxygen extraction ratios tolerate decreased blood flow fairly well. The kidneys normally extract only 10 percent of the oxygen available in their arterial blood supply, the heart extracts 70 percent, and the body as a whole extracts 25 percent. An arm or a leg can survive total tourniquet occlusion of its blood supply for over an hour without permanent damage, and the cornea of the eye survives several hours after death of the individual.

During acute hypoxia or circulatory crises, blood is preferentially sent to the heart and brain. Since flow is curtailed to tissues with a low priority such as the skin, skeletal muscles, and corneas as soon as hypoxia or low flow threatens, monitoring flow or oxygen tension in these tissues would provide an early warning.

Organs other than the heart, which normally extracts most of the oxygen from coronary artery blood, can compensate for low blood flow by extracting more oxygen from their venous oxygen reserves. Thus, the arteriovenous oxygen difference of the body or of an individual organ is a measure of the extent to which blood flow matches the metabolic demand for oxygen. In the normal resting state, the entire body consumes only 25 percent of the oxygen transported to it by the cardiac output. This is confirmed from all the organs after it has been mixed in the right side of the heart. Normal mixed venous blood is found to be 75 percent saturated with a partial pressure of 40 mm Hg. Levels lower than this indicate increased oxygen demands which cannot be met by increased cardiac output, decreased available arterial oxygen, or decreased cardiac output. Since most surgeons would like to be warned of any of these three circumstances, monitoring of mixed venous oxygen levels is becoming popular. Mixed venous oxygen tension during anesthesia responds to a fall in cardiac output before any change is noted in blood pressure, pulse rate, or central venous pressure. It would be useful to assess the oxygen supply to individual organs as well, particularly the brain. Cerebrospinal fluid from the cisterna magna of the brain responds promptly to hypoxemia or ischemia with a drop in oxygen tension, but this can hardly be considered a noninvasive approach.

Having considered the lungs, the heart, and major blood vessels, we now approach the business end of the oxygen transport system, where the partial pressure of oxygen rapidly drops from 90 to 40 mm Hg. The capillary bed of an organ is a rapidly changing dynamic system with precapillary sphincters under the control of tissue hypoxic feedback mechanisms as well as sympathetic and hemodynamic reflexes. When increased work, fever, inflammation, catecholamine stimulation, or increased thyroxine levels intensify the metabolic demands of an organ, precapillary sphincters relax and the capillary bed enlarges. A working skeletal muscle has ten to twenty times the number of functioning capillaries as a resting muscle. The myocardium has the most active set of sphincters and the most profuse capillary network of any organ. In the basal state, less than half the capillaries are open, but with increased demands the myocardial oxygen consumption can increase sixfold. Not only does more blood flow through the enlarged capillary bed, but the distance between open capillaries is reduced from 20 to 14 μ, so that oxygen has a shorter diffusion distance to the cells. This increased vascularity further reduces peripheral resistance and cardiac afterload in addition to that achieved by arteriolar dilatation. Up until this point, very little oxygen is lost from the arterial blood, but in the capillaries many factors combine to encourage oxygen unloading in the cylinder of tissue surrounding each capillary. The natural affinity of hemoglobin for oxygen is decreased by heat, hydrogen ions, carbon dioxide (Bohr effect), and red cell diphosphoglycerate (DPG). These agents act at a stereochemical level to help form a hemoglobin molecule which is more stable in its unsaturated state. The heat of working tissues, hypoxic acidosis, and carbon dioxide from cellular metabolism all tend to shift the oxyhemoglobin dissociation curve to the right where more oxygen is released at a higher tissue oxygen tension. The relative position of the oxyhemoglobin dissociation curve is identified by the P_{50} value, the partial pressure of oxygen at which the hemoglobin is half saturated at 37°C and pH 7.4. There is a biologic feedback mechanism which increases the red cell diphosphoglycerate in chronic hypoxic states, but like renal erythropoietin regulation, the mechanism is too slow to be of significance in clinical monitoring.

Red cell diphosphoglycerate may be of considerable clinical significance in patients requiring massive blood transfusions. Bank blood stored in standard acid citrate dextrose (ACD) solutions is rapidly depleted of diphosphoglycerate, reducing the P_{50} value from 26 to 11 mm Hg. Adequate oxygen release in the capillary bed can occur only at lower oxygen tensions, thus reducing the oxygen diffusion gradient in the tissue cylinder surrounding the capillary. The cells at the venous end of the capillary, where the oxygen tension is normally lower, are the first to suffer. For this reason, the periphery of the pericapillary cylinder at the venous end is called the *todlische Ecke,* or "deadly corner." This effect is best seen in centrilobular necrosis of the liver, wherein hypoxic cell death first occurs near the central venule.

Another frequently overlooked problem of hemoglobin affinity is carbon monoxide poisoning. Patients who have been burned in closed spaces may have serious defects of oxygen transport caused by carbon monoxide displacing oxygen from hemoglobin and poisoning mitochondrial cytochrome.

Since oxygen tension falls off with the square of the distance from the capillary, by the time oxygen diffuses through the pores of the cell membrane, the partial pressure of oxygen is about 6 mm Hg. Table 13-1 shows a value of 10 mm Hg outside the membrane. This does not mean that there is resistance to diffusion across the cell membrane but that, within the tissues, consumption of oxygen must occur in the cells in order to establish a gradient. Within the cell, myoglobin facilitates the passage of oxygen by serving as a sort of bucket brigade. As might be expected from what has been described in previous paragraphs, the cardiac muscle is richest in myoglobin. Myoglobin has a very high affinity for oxygen and releases it only at very low tensions, as needed. The actual utilization of oxygen occurs in complex intracellular organelles called *mitochondria.*

In the mitochondrion, an array of catalysts and cofactors comprising the Krebs cycle oxidize pyruvate produced by the anaerobic glycolysis of glucose. Anaerobic glycolysis of glucose yields only 50 kcal/mole, whereas the complete oxidation of glucose to carbon dioxide and water in the mitochondrion yields 686 kcal/mole of glucose. The higher animals cannot survive on the lower-energy-producing fermentative process alone. Some 1.2 billion years ago, organisms learned to protect themselves from the toxic oxygen molecules slowly building up in the primeval atmosphere by enzymatically catalyzing the reduction of oxygen to water while at the same time oxidizing the end products of cellular fermentation such as lactic acid. Trillions of generations later, the cells harnessed the extra energy thus released to the reconstitution of the high-energy phosphate bond of adenosine triphosphate (ATP). Vestiges of the earlier process are still found, even in human cells, in the form of other organelles called *peroxisomes.* Peroxisomes are believed to protect cells from excess oxygen by the enzymatic oxidation of amino acids and lactic acid. However, this oxidation is not coupled to energy storage.

Within the mitochondrion, the oxidation of pyruvate is carried out anaerobically by removal of electrons rather than the addition of oxygen. The electrons are passed along the respiratory chain, alternately oxidizing and reducing diphosphopyridine nucleotide (DPN), flavoproteins, ubiquinone, and cytochromes. At the final step cytochrome C passes two electrons to an oxygen atom, which combines with two hydrogen ions to form one molecule of water. An obligatory coupling of this process to the conversion of adenosine diphosphate (ADP) to ATP fulfills two functions. First, much of the high energy of the complete oxidation of glucose is stored for all forms of cellular work. Second, the rate of this oxidative phosphorylation is governed by the energy needs of the cell. The cell is protected from excess oxygen by the fact that only when ADP is present will oxygen be utilized to allow the establishment of an oxygen gradient across the cell membrane. As long as the intracellular oxygen tension is above 5 mm Hg, the rate-limiting factor of cellular respiration is the availability of ADP, not oxygen.

Certain agents, the best known of which is dinitrophenol, uncouple oxidation from phosphorylation permitting runaway oxidation without energy storage. This is a rapidly lethal process. Less well known is the uncoupling ability of certain bacterial endotoxins. Abnormally high oxygen consumption has been demonstrated just before death in patients with septic shock. Cyanide and carbon monoxide have the reverse effect on the cell; they block the transfer of electron from cytochrome C to oxygen.

Britton Chance has defined three cellular respiratory states. First, in the resting state, oxidative phosphorylation is limited by low levels of ADP and phosphates. Second, in the working state, most of the ATP has been converted to ADP, establishing a relatively high oxygen gradient from the capillary to the mitochondrion. Third, ADP and phosphate are in excess; if oxygen is not available for diffusion from the capillary, critical pyridine nucleotide reduction (CPNR) rapidly occurs. Critical levels of reduced DPN occur when oxygen tension in the mitochondrion falls to

0.1 mm Hg. This corresponds to a capillary oxygen tension of 4 mm Hg. The cell is forced to obtain energy from anaerobic glycolysis alone, thus building up an oxygen debt and conversion of pyruvate to lactic acid. Acidosis and elevated lactate levels can be detected in the peripheral circulation, but only if capillary perfusion is present to wash the cellular products into the venous circulation. This is why, in shock states, peripheral arterial pH may not accurately reflect intracellular pH. The autolytic wash-out products of critically hypoxic and injured cells have been monitored for decades on the false assumption that venous blood always equilibrates with ischemic tissue. A better approach would be to detect molecular signals at the cellular level. Progress in this direction will be reviewed later.

Voluntary muscle can build up an oxygen debt of 40 ml/kg of cell mass, compared to a resting oxygen requirement of 4 ml/kg/minute. The 10 billion neuron units of the human brain can tolerate no oxygen debt. When the cerebral arterial oxygen tension falls to 20 mm Hg, that within the neurons is only 0.2 mm Hg. At this level of hypoxia, half of the electron carrier, DPN, is in the reduced state. When 90 percent of DPN is in the reduced state, even the respiratory center ceases to function, and irreversible damage occurs. As long as some circulatory flow exists, even with severe hypoxemia, there is a chance to maintain the critical 0.1 mm Hg tension within the neuron. With complete circulatory arrest, however, the oxygen is quickly used up, and the neuron dies. The brain requires constant energy supplies just to maintain the unsteady state of polarization for the transmission of the network of impulses which is an integral part of the cerebral life process. This peculiar and critical requirement of the brain is related to modern information theory, which explains the energy requirements of complex information systems. Long before the critical state of cerebral hypoxia is reached, other symptoms and signs occur, such as restlessness, unconsciousness, Cheyne-Stokes respiration, and EEG abnormalities.

As other cells reach critical hypoxic states, they no longer have the energy to maintain important internal cell structures. One of these is the phospholipid lysosomal membrane which protects the cell from the necessary but potentially destructive enzymes contained within the lysosomes. When released into the cell, the powerful proteases, esterases, and phosphatases destroy the cell.

Britton Chance has lead the way in developing methods to study cellular hypoxia. His fluorometric instrument makes it possible to measure intracellular oxygen tensions between 0.03 and 2 mm Hg. This is accomplished by measuring the fluorescence emission of the reduced state of DPN when it is stimulated by ultraviolet light. Other techniques of detecting molecular signals at a distance for monitoring purposes are possible, among them stimulated emission of oxygen in the microwave range, far infrared emission spectroscopy (chemiluminescence), and surface reflectance spectroscopy. Though exciting, all these are a long way from validation and routine clinical use in man.

INSTRUMENTATION AND CLINICAL TECHNIQUES

Physiologic Sensing

Rushmer has classified the methods used to obtain information from the human body for monitoring purposes. The most obvious is the analysis of samples of tissue, blood, respiratory gases, urine, cerebrospinal fluid, or other body fluids. Here the assumption is that the sample in question is a representative aliquot of the state of the entire organ system.

In surgical monitoring, the most useful aspects of this approach include continuous or intermittent analysis of arterial or mixed venous pH, blood gases (P_{O_2}, P_{CO_2}), and lactate. As pointed out earlier, the blood lactate level can be considered an indicator of the adequacy of oxygen transport to the Krebs cycle in the mitochondria. Elevated blood lactate levels indicate anaerobic metabolism as long as there is enough tissue perfusion to "wash out" the acid metabolites. Blood lactate, increased from above 1.5 mEq/L to levels above 10 mEq/L, is a grave prognostic sign unless the trend is promptly reversed.

The disadvantage of the tissue and fluid sampling approach to monitoring is that it is invasive and therefore carries some risk of infection or blood loss. An invasive technique is always more expensive than a noninvasive one, because it requires more highly trained personnel for insertion, sterilization of parts, and surveillance to prevent accidents. A corollary to this rule is that the more invasive a device, the less likely is its use before it is too late.

Rushmer's two other monitoring categories are (1) techniques which utilize intrinsic energy sources within the body of the patient and (2) methods which direct extrinsic energy probes at or into the body, with analysis of the emerging energy. Many physiologic processes are characterized by the generation of dynamic potentials, tensions, pressures, and electromagnetic emissions which constitute the intrinsic energy sources available for surgical monitoring. Examples of this approach include electrocardiography, electroencephalography, thermography, infrared emission spectroscopy, and muscle surface pH metering.

The energy used for interrogating beams in extrinsic energy probe monitoring can be ultrasound, mechanical stimuli, or photons originating at any point along the electromagnetic spectrum from gamma rays to microwaves. Examples include ultrasonic echography, videodensitometry, nuclear magnetic resonance flow probes, and impedance plethysmography.

Shannon and Weaver's classic work on information theory can be used to show that, in general, the higher the frequency of the interrogating beam or intrinsic energy source, the more information capacity (bits per second) it has. For example, a gamma ray probe could be expected to detect more physiologic information than an ultrasonic probe. Other variables such as signal-to-noise ratio, of course, are important in determining the ultimate monitoring value of a particular system. A monitoring system employing extrinsic energy probes usually yields information with good spatial discrimination with regard to functional lesions, whereas devices which detect intrinsic energy usually provide an information-rich signal which often requires data processing for exploitation of its full information content.

The greatest need in the field of monitoring is for new sensors and transducers to detect critical states along the train of oxygen transport. Even very complicated occult signals from new sensing techniques can be made useful by modern spectral search systems. Computer programs are already available to examine and characterize more complex information in large amounts in order to analyze the fundamental properties of living systems.

Four guides to the development of new physiologic sensors are the following:

1. Detection of functional integrity of cells and cellular perfusion rather than the washout of autolytic products into the bloodstream.
2. A noninvasive mode; the device must not reduce the frequency of contact between the health professional and patient.
3. An information-rich signal originating from the desired organ system.
4. Extrinsic energy probes for spatial discrimination and intrinsic energy sources for a broader view of biologic activity.

A transducer is a device which converts energy from one form to another. A sensor is a device which detects an energy signal related to a particular state. In physiologic monitoring, a sensor is often a transducer, but not always. Electrocardiographic and electroencephalographic electrodes are sensors which do not convert energy from one form to another. The suitability of a sensing device for a particular clinical application is related to such factors as sensitivity, response time, linearity, and accuracy. The *sensitivity* is measured by the smallest change which is detectable by the device. The *response time* of an instrument is the period required to record a given change of input. *Linearity* refers to the constancy of the ratio of output signal to the measured variable. *Accuracy* is evaluated in terms of the ability to calibrate the instrument so that the output conforms precisely to the quantity of the measured variable. Accuracy is related to the error induced by unwanted variables such as temperature, pressure, and vibration.

Respiratory Monitoring

Respiratory monitoring can be very simple or extremely complex, depending on the trend or event to be warned against. The detection of a low-probability event such as respiratory arrest is easy compared to the on-line assessment of lung mechanics. Nevertheless, there is need for the former type of monitoring. One innovative and well-designed device provides an apnea alarm, using intrinsic energy sources. The Codman Apnea Alarm consists of a 10-compartment air mattress with sensors to detect the displacement of air associated with respiration. If the infant patient stops breathing, the alarm is set off. The advantages are low cost and lack of attachments to the subject. Unfortunately, no similar device is available for the adult patient.

Next in complexity is the measurement of blood gases. The widespread use of pressure-cycled or volume-controlled respirators in the postoperative period would not be safe without blood-gas monitoring. In order to take over the work of breathing, when the patient's own respiratory reflexes and servo-control mechanisms are overridden or suppressed by respiratory depressants, it is essential to know if ventilation and gas exchange suit the patient's requirements. Were it not for the invention of the Clark polarographic oxygen electrode and the Severinghaus potentiometric carbon dioxide electrode in the 1950s, the task of monitoring blood gases by the classic manometric technique of Van Slyke and Neill would have imposed enormous difficulties. The Clark electrode depends on the diffusion of oxygen from the blood sample through a gas-permeable plastic membrane surrounding a platinum polarographic electrode. The electrode current is proportional to the number of oxygen molecules, but careful calibration with water of known oxygen concentration is necessary because of variations in membrane permeability and electrolyte characteristics. The Severinghaus potentiometric electrode is a glass pH electrode with bicarbonate buffer within the gas-permeable plastic membrane. Diffusion of carbon dioxide from the blood sample to the electrode produces a change in pH, which is recorded.

There are several commercial apparatus available which include thermostatically controlled water baths, calibration equipment, and digital readout. It is impossible to care properly for many surgical patients today without access to a blood-gas and pH analyzer of this sort. Unlike blood chemistries or electrolytes, these determinations require, for reliability, a rapid turnaround time and rigid quality control. For this reason, the blood-gas laboratory is often located in proximity to the intensive care unit, recovery room, and operating room.

Continuous methods of blood-gas monitoring have been developed for on-line applications, but problems of calibration, quality control and expense reduce their utility over that of intermittent determinations. Mass spectrometry, which will be discussed later, shows promise as an accurate, rapid method for intermittent or continuous blood-gas monitoring.

Samples of arterial blood for these determinations can be obtained using an ordinary 20-gauge needle, by percutaneous puncture of the radial, brachial, or femoral arteries. The 5- or 10-ml glass or plastic syringe is first heparinized and then capped and placed in ice after the sample is drawn. Iced samples can be kept for 1 hour with a 1 percent drop in oxygen tension. Indwelling arterial and mixed venous lines can also be used as sampling sites, but the volume of blood contained in the catheter must first be discarded.

In assessing the process of gas exchange outlined in the upper part of Table 13-1, the decrement in oxygen tension from the alveolar level to the arterial blood is of considerable importance as a measure of the efficiency of oxygen exchange in the lungs. In normal man breathing room air, the alveolar-arterial oxygen tension gradient, abbreviated as $P(A-aDO_2)$, varies between 10 and 15 mm Hg. Half of this venoarterial admixture is caused by true shunting of desaturated blood into the left atrium, and the other half by ventilation-perfusion imbalance. When the patient with normal cardiorespiratory function breathes pure oxygen for 15 to 20 minutes, the alveolar-arterial gradient is approximately 40 mm Hg. Barometric pressure, less arterial carbon dioxide tension, less water vapor pressure, less the normal gradient yields a value of around 630 mm Hg for arterial oxygen tension while breathing pure oxygen. In this condition the gradient represents both anatomic shunting and perfusion of totally nonventilated alveoli. The effects of alveolar capillary diffusion barriers and ventilation-perfusion imbalance are eliminated by the high oxygen tension in all alveoli.

As mentioned earlier, an increased alveolar-arterial gradient on 100 percent oxygen is a very useful early warning sign for many postoperative pulmonary problems, among them atelectasis, pneumonia, interstitial pulmonary edema, septic shock lung, and posttraumatic pulmonary insufficiency. Although not very specific, it is very useful since an increase is easily determined at the bedside and occurs long before most radiologic changes are evident.

It is estimated that in normal resting man approximately 2 percent of total oxygen consumption is used to provide energy for breathing. In postoperative patients this may increase to 50 percent as a result of increased airway resistance and decreased compliance of the lung, chest wall, and diaphragm. Since much of this work can be taken over with proper use of a volume-cycled respirator, the clinical evaluation of respiratory resistance, compliance, and work has been the subject of much bioengineering research.

Patients with chronic obstructive lung disease, in whom the excess work of breathing is related primarily to expiratory rather than inspiratory effort, benefit little from respirator therapy alone. This situation generally should be detected in the preoperative state by standard pulmonary function testing, and the patient prepared for surgery by physiotherapy, bronchodilators, and antibiotics if infection is present.

Compliance is the change in pressure associated with each cubic centimeter increase in lung volume. When airway pressure is used, rather than the intrapleural pressure minus the intratracheal pressure, the compliance measurement includes that of the chest wall and diaphragm as well as the lungs. This is of little importance if the patient is entirely relaxed. However, in a postoperative patient, the difference between intraesophageal balloon or intrapleural pressure and aiway pressure must be used for meaningful results.

Volume is measured by integrating flow measured across a pneumotachograph at the airway. A *pneumotachograph* is a transducer which converts a pressure difference across a screen to an electric signal related to flow. Resistance is a function of the pressure necessary to overcome resistance at a given point in the respiratory cycle. Work per breath is the integral of the power expended during the respiratory cycle, where power is the transpulmonary pressure times flow.

The manual calculations for these variables of lung mechanics are much too tedious to be of clinical value, so a number of investigators have automated the procedures. Peters and coworkers have designed a mobile cart and digital computer programs for this purpose (Fig. 13-1). Analog voltages are transmitted from an infrared carbon dioxide analyzer, a polarographic oxygen monitor, a Fleisch pneumotachograph, and a differential pressure transducer. The temperatures of inspired and mixed expired air are used for correction of gas volumes. The apparatus can be used with patients on respirators or breathing spontaneously.

The commercial version of this cardiopulmonary measurement cart also provides a channel for indicator-dilution determination of cardiac output. Measured variables include air flow, transpulmonary pressure, inspired oxygen concentration, and mean expired oxygen and carbon dioxide concentrations. From these a small, dedicated computer derives variables associated with respiratory mechanics and gas exchange. These include tidal volume, rate, compliance, resistance, work, oxygen consumption, carbon dioxide output, respiratory quotient, alveolar-arterial oxygen gradient, shunt fraction and dead-space ratio. The results can be viewed on a cathode ray tube or as teletype copy. The prototype device has been in clinical operation for several years. An analysis of patients studied thus far indicated that multiple variables of lung mechanics were better predictors of the need for a respirator than single tests. The commercial version permits telephone transmission of digitized data to a dedicated small computer or a larger time-shared system.

Osborn and associates have used a similar approach but with the transducers built in at the bedside and reliance on continuous monitoring with sophisticated trend analysis. The pneumotachygraph is specially modified with a warm air flush between sampling periods to minimize water condensation and base-line drift. The device can be left on line for as long as 48 hours. Continuous gas samples from a side tube at the expiratory end of the pneumotachygraph are analyzed with a special ceramic oxygen cell and an infrared carbon dioxide analyzer. A digital computer is used to calculate the derived variables and determine trends. Their studies of postoperative patients have revealed wide swings in the pH and blood gases related to the loss of respiratory control or changing ventilation requirements. Sudden fluctuations in carbon dioxide tensions often lead to cardiac arrhythmias or hypotension. The most useful variable in this regard is end-expiratory carbon dioxide tension. The gradient is usually less than 5 mm Hg from arterial blood to end-expiratory gas in patients, with relatively normal dead space. Such a system reduces the number of arterial blood-gas determinations necessary for the management of seriously ill patients. It has also been shown to reduce morbidity and mortality of postoperative patients requiring respirator support.

Kinney's group uses a different method for continuous spirometric determinations. A specially constructed clear plastic chamber covers the head with a snug fit at the neck. This permits the measurement of gas exchange and lung mechanics in spontaneously breathing patients with a minimum of cooperation. Several other centers employ custom-tailored computer-based respiratory monitoring

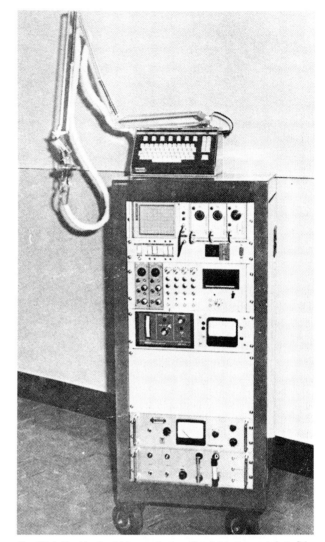

Fig. 13-1. Cart for bedside monitoring of variables associated with respiratory mechanics designed by Peters and associates. (*From R. M. Peters et al., Am J Surg, 124:262, 1972.*)

systems, usually developed in cooperation with a major research-oriented corporation or an engineering school. It is unlikely at the present time that the costs of such respiratory monitoring systems could be borne by even a large hospital on the basis of third-party payments. Nevertheless, the value of such systems for postoperative care of the high-risk patient has been proved.

Cardiovascular Monitoring

Most monitoring systems require access to arterial blood for sampling and direct pressure determinations. Monitoring, in many ways like politics, is the art of the possible. What is it possible to measure in the patient with consistent success and minimum risk? Maintaining an open arterial line without risk or discomfort requires skill and dedication to detail. The radial artery at the wrist is the site most frequently used because of safety and convenience. The

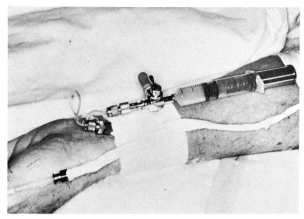

Fig. 13-2. Radial artery cannula with patency maintained by Sage electrolytic infusion pump. Note the sterile rubber nipple on the sidearm of the stopcock. A central venous catheter protected with adhesive tape is shown alongside the arm.

presence of a functioning ulnar arterial arcade must be checked by pressure occlusion of both arteries at the wrist with subsequent release of the ulnar to produce a palmar flush. It is dangerous to perform even a radial arterial puncture unless such evidence of ulnar collateral flow is present. For percutaneous catheterization or a cutdown and cannulation of the radial artery, the wrist should be attached to an arm board and moderately extended. Strict glove, mask, and sterile drape technique should be used, as with all intravascular cannulations. The standards established by Dudrick and associates for indwelling central venous catheters should be followed for arterial catheters as well. Sterility should be maintained by removing the protective dressing every 3 days, rubbing off skin oil with acetone, and applying iodine tincture to the surrounding skin and antibiotic ointment to the catheter exit site. The occlusive dressing should be small and fixed carefully to the skin, using compound tincture of benzoin for better adherence. Unused stopcock sidearms should be capped with sterile rubber or plastic nipples to prevent contamination. Cannula sepsis is an iatrogenic disaster which can largely be avoided by good technique.

The type of cannula chosen is important. The long Becton-Dickenson Teflon cannula is easily inserted and can be plugged with a plastic stylet when not in use. Other polyvinyl or polyethylene cannulas are available commercially. Patency is best maintained with a constant slow infusion of 2 units of heparin diluted in 5 ml of saline solution delivered in 24 hours. This can be accomplished with either a Sage electrolytic (Fig. 13-2) or a U.S. Catheter clockwork infusion pump. Both of these can be attached to the patient's arm to allow mobility.

Intermittent manual flushing to discharge clots is dangerous, since it has been demonstrated that as little as 3 ml may flush emboli back up into the cerebral circulation from a radial artery cannula. Other sites for indwelling arterial lines are the brachial or femoral artery, but these present the risk of distal ischemia and thrombophlebitis.

Catheterization of the central venous system or right side of the heart for manometry, injection of indicator, or mixed venous sampling is used as an integral part of many surgical monitoring systems. There are several routes of access to the central venous system (Fig. 13-3). In order of increasing risk these are the median basilic vein in the antecubital fossa, the external jugular vein, the internal jugular vein, and the subclavian vein. The femoral vein is seldom used because of contamination and thrombophlebitis. The median basilic vein directs the catheter directly into the subclavian vein and superior vena cava if the arm is extended laterally during the procedure, whereas the cephalic vein is difficult to negotiate at the shoulder. The external jugular vein is best approached with the neck extended, turned to the opposite side and lower than heart level (to fill the vein and prevent air embolism). The vein can also be steadied and distended by proximal pressure at the neck. As with the antecubital approach, venisection is best done before the vein is ruined with multiple puncture attempts. If there is difficulty passing the jugular-subclavian junction, the catheter may pass if the shoulder is depressed. The internal jugular vein can be cannulated percutaneously above the clavicle. The puncture is made immediately lateral to the pulsation of the common carotid artery through the lateral head of the sternocleidomastoid muscle. The distance to the proper position in the superior vena cava requires a catheter 8 in. long.

Puncture and catheter introduction into the subclavian vein involves a slightly greater risk of pneumothorax, but its ease of access makes it popular in emergency situations. As with the other sites, local anesthesia should be used as well as complete sterile precautions. Skin puncture is done just inferior to the clavicle at the junction of the middle and inner thirds, with the needle aimed at a point behind the manubrium. The catheter should not be threaded through or over the needle until venous blood is easily aspirated. When threaded through the needle, the catheter should never be withdrawn separately because of the danger of shearing if off with the sharp edge of the needle. Some commercial sets have protective sleeves which can be extended beyond the needle point to prevent cutting the catheter. A chest roentgenogram should always be obtained following central venous catheterization to check for pneumothorax and ascertain the position of the catheter tip. If a nonradiopaque catheter is used, it can be filled with contrast medium during the exposure. There are a number of commercial intravenous catheter sets available which are ingeniously designed to facilitate advancement of the catheter without contamination or kinking (Fig. 13-4). The Abbott set employs a reel device which is easily manipulated with one hand. The Sorenson catheter is housed in a longitudinally slit semirigid conduit with a sliding sleeve on the outside attached to the catheter inside through the slit. As the sleeve is advanced over the conduit, the catheter is pushed through the needle into the vein. These sets can also be used for arterial cannulations.

The proper interpretation of central venous pressure for monitoring surgical patients requires an understanding of *all* the factors which may cause elevated readings. Artifacts such as inaccurate zero level, blockage, or kinking should be excluded by observation of 1 to 2 cm pressure fluctuations with the respiratory cycle and careful sighting of the zero level at the midaxillary line. The zero level should correspond to the point of projection of the posterior leaflet of the tricuspid valve on the right chest wall. Noncardiac factors which increase central venous pressure are hypervolemia, vasoconstrictor drugs (metaraminol and mephentermine constrict the veins as well as arterioles), positive-pressure ventilation, pneumothorax, hydrothorax, flail chest, and mediastinal compression. If none of these factors exists, normal readings vary between 0 and 9 cm of water. A value above 15 cm of water is suggestive of inability of the right ventricle to handle venous return. By itself, it is not a measure of ventricular function or myocardial contractility, because afterload and ventricular work are unknown quantities. A high central venous pressure does serve as a warning that volume infusion should be continued with extreme caution. However, there are situations such as pericardial tamponade or pulmonary embolism where a high central venous pressure is essential to maintain an adequate cardiac output until definitive therapy is used to relieve the obstruction. The most logical use of central venous pressure as a guide to fluid replacement in seriously ill patients is the observation of the response to challenge with 100-ml increments of volume infusion. Infusion is stopped when a sharp rise in central venous pressure occurs.

The distinction between right and left ventricular failure is not possible without some indication of left atrial or left ventricular end-diastolic pressure. For this reason, various techniques have been developed for bedside monitoring of pressures in the left side of the heart. Cohn et al. have used a precurved polyethylene catheter which is threaded over a wire guide from the femoral artery into the left ventricle. Fluoroscopic control is not used, but the electrocardiograph is observed for premature ventricular beats which signal entry into the ventricle and subside when the catheter is withdrawn a few centimeters. In shock associated with myocardial infarction, the left ventricular end-diastolic pressure is elevated in the 12 to 44 mm Hg range even though the central venous pressure may be normal. Such monitoring has permitted more precise fluid replacement and inotropic drug adjustment in patients with left ventricular failure.

The great majority of clinical physiologists prefer to approach the problem of bedside left ventricular dynamics from the right side of the heart. In 1959, Zohman and Williams described flow-guided pulmonary artery catheterization. The location of the catheter tip, as it floated along with the bloodstream through the right side of the heart, is determined by characteristic intracardiac electrocardiographic patterns conducted back through the soft catheter in a column of 7.5% sodium bicarbonate acting as a salt bridge (Fig. 13-5). The pattern in the right atrium consists of a high, short inverted P wave, which becomes upright as the tricuspid valve is approached. The right ventricle pattern consists of a 7- to 9-mv downward QRS deflection. A standard low-voltage pattern is found in the pulmonary artery. If the catheter tip touches the endocardium, as it floats through, a contact pattern is produced. The catheter should then be withdrawn a short distance and allowed to advance again. In the atrium, the contact pattern is characterized by an elevation of the PQ segment. The ST segment is elevated in the ventricular contact pattern. These intracardiac potentials may not be indicative of actual injury, since they do not appear on simultaneously recorded precordial or peripheral leads. The safety

Fig. 13-3. Four routes of access to the central venous system. The direct line from the median antecubital vein to the superior vena cava makes this a safe approach, particularly with the arm extended. The cephalic vein empties into the subclavian vein at an acute angle, making central venous catheterization difficult. The external jugular vein is the next safest route. The arm should be at the side and the shoulder depressed to straighten the angle at which the external jugular enters the subclavian vein. The internal jugular vein can be cannulated by inserting the needle through the clavicular head of the sternocleidomastoid muscle, just lateral to the pulsation of the carotid artery. The subclavian cannulation over the first rib is shown. The danger of pneumothorax or hemothorax is greatest with this approach.

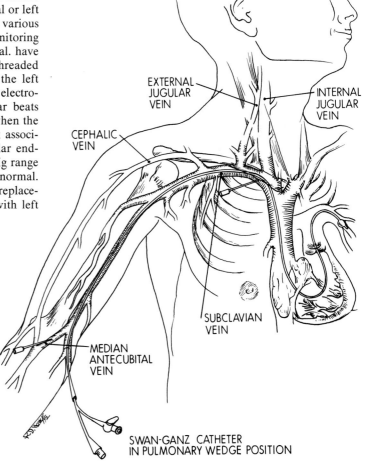

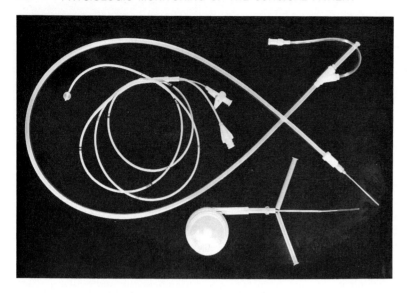

Fig. 13-4. Three popular types of monitoring catheters. The coiled Swan-Ganz balloon-tip catheter is designed to float into the pulmonary artery wedge position. The Sorenson catheter shown crossed in the photograph is contained in a conduit with a longitudinal slit to facilitate insertion into an artery or vein under sterile conditions. For similar purposes, the Abbott catheter is provided with a reellike device. The two halves of the sleeve which prevents shearing of the catheter are also shown.

of flow-guided catheterization of the right side of the heart depends upon avoiding arrhythmias by careful observation of the intracardiac patterns. The hazard of ventricular fibrillation due to stray 60-cycle current should be minimized by careful appraisal of the electrocardiograph and the grounding capacity of its power supply. In 1966 Del Guercio et al. reported on a number of patients with suspected pulmonary embolism shock studied by a modification of this technique (Fig. 13-6). Flow of the catheter was improved by a wind-sock effect created by heat curling the last 2 cm of catheter. The stylet kept it straight while it advanced through the veins.

More recently, a further advance of this approach was the commercial development of the balloon-tipped Swan-Ganz catheter (Fig. 13-4). With the balloon inflated, the catheter sails through the right side of the heart into a wedge position in the pulmonary artery in less than 1 minute. In the absence of pulmonary vascular disease, pulmonary capillary wedge pressure is a reliable guide to left atrial and, in turn, left ventricular end-diastolic pressure. Without the wedge position, the pulmonary artery end-diastolic pressure is an acceptable indicator of mean left atrial pressure. Central venous pressure alone has been found to be an unreliable index of left ventricular function, since filling pressure in the left side of the heart may rise sharply and pulmonary edema occur without significant increases in right atrial pressures.

Right-sided catheterization with flow-guided catheters also can be monitored by intracardiac pressure changes or mobile radiologic image intensifiers. The catheter through the right side of the heart also can be used for obtaining mixed venous blood samples, injecting indicator, and infusion of medications. Extreme caution should be exercised when drugs are infused directly into the central circulation, because high myocardial concentrations are quickly achieved. These catheters also make it possible to obtain bedside pulmonary angiograms in cases of pulmonary embolism shock.

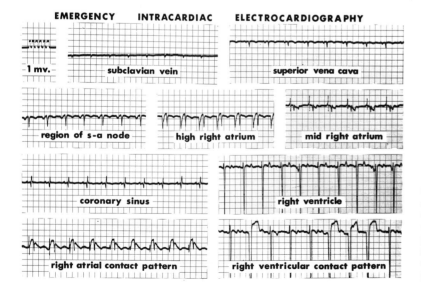

Fig. 13-5. Characteristic intracardial electrocardiographic patterns seen during flow-guided catheterization of the right side of the heart. The intracardiac potentials are conducted to the precordial lead through 7.5% sodium bicarbonate in the catheter. The catheter should be withdrawn slightly before advancing when contact patterns are seen.

As pointed out earlier regarding physiologic concepts of monitoring, the mixed venous oxygen level reflects the extent to which the body must call upon the blood oxygen stores in states of cardiovascular stress. The value of right atrial oxygen saturation monitoring during surgery has been demonstrated. Changes in cardiac output secondary to hemorrhage and other problems are reflected by early changes in right atrial oxygen saturations, usually before changes in arterial blood pressure, venous pressure, or heart rate. Changes in arterial oxygen content secondary to pulmonary shunting or decreased oxygen-carrying capacity also promptly affect mixed venous oxygen saturation. It was originally thought that pulmonary arterial samples would be necessary for this type of monitoring, but experience has shown that, in the stressed patient, right atrial or right ventricular samples correlate well with those from the pulmonary artery. Saturations below 50% from these sites are a bad prognostic sign and indicate either severe arterial hypoxemia or very significantly decreased cardiac output.

Border et al. originated a unique "no cost" bedside volumetric Vn Slyke device for determining the volumes percent of unsaturation of mixed venous blood (Fig. 13-7). It is assembled from a heparinized 10-ml syringe, a stopcock, and the barrel of a 1-ml tuberculin syringe. Exactly 10 ml of mixed venous blood is drawn into the larger syringe followed by approximately 1 ml of pure oxygen. The smaller syringe, filled with saline solution, serves as a monometer to record the volume of the oxygen bubble used to saturate the blood. If the meniscus falls to the 0.5-ml mark, it indicates that the mixed venous blood required 5 vol % of oxygen for saturation. This is about normal. If the arterial blood is 100% saturated, this value would be equivalent to the arteriovenous oxygen difference. This device makes it possible for everyone to practice clinical physiology at the bedside, with little expense.

Cardiac Output Determinations

In spite of various questions regarding accuracy in high- or low-flow states, the description of indicator-dilution curves from central circulation remains the basic method for monitoring cardiac output. The technique, which goes back to 1897, involves the injection of an indicator into the right side of the heart and continuous determination of its concentration as it mixes with the cardiac output somewhere downstream. Any indicator can be used, as long as it does not affect hemodynamics or disappear from the blood before the concentration is measured. It can best be understood as a variation of the Fick principle, where the known amount of indicator is equivalent to a fixed amount of oxygen consumption, and the mean concentration of indicator after mixing is equivalent to the arteriovenous oxygen difference. It follows, then, that the faster the volume of blood flow, the lower the arteriovenous oxygen difference and mean concentration of indicator. All methods for the calculation of cardiac ouput from both continuous and single bolus injection of indicator use this principle in analyzing the time-concentration curves to

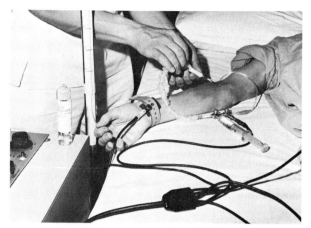

Fig. 13-6. Technique of flow-guided intracardiac ECG-monitored catheterization of the right side of the heart. The catheter is filled with 7.5% sodium bicarbonate, which forms a salt bridge. For purposes of illustration sterile drapes and gloves have been omitted.

obtain the mean concentration of indicator. The number of milligrams of indicator injected divided by the mean concentration of indicator gives the volume of flow during the time of the indicator-dilution curve. Since the cardiac output is usually expressed as flow per minute, the volume of flow during description of the curve is multiplied by 60 and divided by the number of seconds of duration of the curve.

Numerical integration of the curve obtained by the bolus injection of indicator, divided by the duration of the curve in seconds, provides the mean concentration of indicator for use in the cardiac output calculation. Before this can be done, however, the hump on the tail of the curve caused by recirculation of indicator through the systemic circulation must be excluded from the original curve. There are a number of ways of doing this, including semilogarithmic replots, nomograms, analog computers, and digital computer programs. Two nomograms have been designed by Cohn and Del Guercio which can be used as rapidly at

Fig. 13-7. Border's volumetric Van Slyke device for bedside determination of mixed venous unsaturation. Each 0.1-ml fall in the meniscus indicates 1 vol % unsaturation of blood. Normal is 4 to 5 vol %. When the arterial blood is fully saturated, this device indicates the arteriovenous oxygen difference. (*From J. R. Border et al., J Trauma, 6:176, 1966.*)

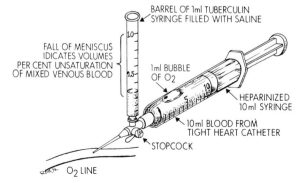

BARREL OF 1ml TUBERCULIN SYRINGE FILLED WITH SALINE

FALL OF MENISCUS IDICATES VOLUMES PER CENT UNSATURATION OF MIXED VENOUS BLOOD

1ml BUBBLE OF O2

HEPARINIZED 10ml SYRINGE

10ml BLOOD FROM TIGHT HEART CATHETER

STOPCOCK

O2 LINE

the bedside as computers. The most useful one is based upon the fact that clinical indicator-dilution curves closely follow a known mathematical function, the gamma function (Fig. 13-8). Two known points on the clinical curve are used to define the entire curve mathematically, and by matching points on the nomogram with a ruler, the cardiac output is calculated automatically. The correlation coefficient for this method compared with the standard semilogarithmic replot is excellent—.99.

Special-purpose analog computers are available from a number of manufacturers, usually as part of an entire densitometer system for sampling blood at a known rate and recording the concentration of indicator. The most commonly used indicator in clinical practice today is indo-

cyanine green dye. Usually 5 mg is injected into the central venous catheter as blood is withdrawn through a densitometer cuvette from an arterial line. The densitometer is a photoelectric device designed to record changes in concentration in terms of decreases in light transmission at the wavelength of maximum absorption by the green dye. Several commercial firms manufacture cardiac output densitometers for clinical use.

It is convenient to mount the densitometer with its control box and motor-driven withdrawal syringe on a mobile cart, along with blood pressure transducers, an electrocardiograph, and a multichannel recording device. As noted earlier, this mobile apparatus has been called a shock cart; it can be used to bring fairly complete cardiovascular assessment to the bedside, operating room, or emergency room, rather than transport a critically ill patient to a clinical laboratory. Intracardiac and arterial blood pressure tracings, indicator-dilution curves, and electrocardiograph tracings combined with arterial and mixed venous blood-gas data permit calculation of a number of derived cardiorespiratory variables of physiologic significance. Practical considerations in the design of a shock cart require a sturdy chassis with large wheels for mobility through elevator doors. There should be a waterproof work surface on top, since dilutions for calibration purposes are best done immediately. The instrument panel should be recessed out of harm's way, and the power cord

Fig. 13-8. Nomogram based on the indicator-dilution curve as a gamma function used for the rapid calculation of cardiac output at the bedside. First the number of seconds from appearance to the time of half maximum amplitude ($Tp/2$) is aligned on the proper scales with the time to the peak concentration (Tp). This line is extended to the far left scale and then back to the first scale parallel with the grid. This point then is aligned through Tp again to mark a point on vertical line 1. That point is then aligned with the peak deflection scale (Hp). The point at which it crossed vertical line 2 then is lined up with the calibration scale F and extended to read the cardiac output on scale Q. In practice, the cardiac output can be calculated in about 1 minute with this nomogram. (*From J. D. Cohn et al., J Lab Clin Med, 69:675, 1967.*)

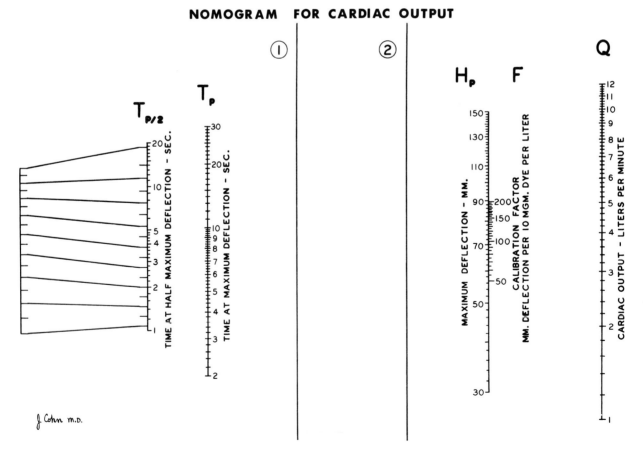

NOMOGRAM FOR CARDIAC OUTPUT

should be long and mounted on a reel of some sort. The multichannel recorder should be of the direct write-out type that does not require developing. It is also more convenient to have positioning arms for the support and alignment of the pressure strain gauges and the densitometer cuvette. Some of these units can be provided with built-in computers for calculation of the cardiac output and other derived cardiovascular variables. Others provide space for a programmable calculator to serve the same purpose.

Several small calculators with program cards specifically made up for shock-cart calculating are available. The primary data obtained from the recorder is entered on the keyboard, and the derived values are immediately printed out. One program is designed for calculation of cardiac output, cardiac index, stroke index, stroke volume, stroke work, and peripheral resistance. A second program permits computation of the total oxygen content of arterial and mixed venous blood, the arteriovenous oxygen difference, the total oxygen consumption, and an index of effective oxygen transport. This program also calculates the percentage of venoarterial admixture if the blood-gas samples are obtained after the patient has breathed 100% oxygen for 15 minutes.

It is most difficult to manage a patient in shock without some means of serial cardiac output measurement, and many systems have been developed to provide cardiac output measurements on demand. As in respiratory monitoring, some clinical physiologists have preferred to set up sophisticated shock centers with all the monitoring equipment built in at the bedside. For the average hospital, without outside research funds, the costs for sophisticated cardiovascular monitoring are borne by third-party payments, and as many patients as possible should have such service available to them if they need it. This is more easily accomplished with the shock cart than with the shock center.

When a seriously ill patient is undergoing hemodynamic assessment and blood-gas sampling, it is essential that a record be kept of the total volume of blood samples. Blood drawn during the description of the dye curves, the samples needed for calibration of the densitometer, and those for the arterial and mixed venous determinations may add up to a significant volume loss. For this reason, other systems have been constructed for cardiac output determination without blood loss. A fully automatic shock cart, designed by Cohn, has a programmed sequence of dye injection, blood sampling, air bubble monitoring, calibration, and reinfusion of the blood. Sterility is assured by a disposable tubing and cuvette package. This system can be used with infants and children, where blood loss would ordinarily be prohibitive.

Another approach to this problem uses fiberoptic oximetry to record the concentration of green dye right in the pulmonary artery after injection into the right atrium. A Swan-Ganz catheter was adapted with light-carrying glass fibers so that both oximetry for oxygen saturation measurement and densitometry for cardiac ouput determination could be carried out at the catheter tip. No arterial sampling is required when this technique is used.

It has long been known that fluid of a different temperature from that of the blood can be used as an indicator with delicate intravascular temperature probes replacing the densitometer. This method, called thermal dilution, is now employed by a clinical monitoring instrument used in a number of centers. Advantages over standard dye-dilution techniques are that blood is not withdrawn for sampling or calibration, that measurements can be repeated frequently, and that the lack of recirculation simplifies the calculation of cardiac output. Disadvantages include the requirement that a catheter be left in the right side of the heart and the spurious readings that occur when the thermistor touches the wall of the pulmonary artery.

There are other monitoring systems which involve the use of catheter-tip sensors. One measures pressure and electromagnetic flow velocity. When threaded retrograde into the left ventricle, this sensor permits the on-line recording of the left ventricular pressures, left ventricular pressure acceleration (dp/dt), intracardiac heart sounds, ascending aortic blood velocity, and ascending aortic blood acceleration. If the cross-sectional area of the aorta is known, total flow can be calculated. All these serve as very useful indices of left ventricular function, particularly following myocardial infarction. The problem of calibration of the electromagnetic flowmeter probe without a zero flow calibration point is a serious one, as it is for all clinical studies involving electromagnetic flowmeters.

A disposable, very thin polarographic oxygen-sensing electrode can be used for mixed venous oxygen tension monitoring. The miniature sensor is fabricated by dipcoating or painting the various insulators, diffusion membranes, and buffers directly onto the central wire electrode. Other similar devices are available complete with compact solid-state battery-powered recorders for use at the bedside.

The insertion of a long catheter from the radial artery up to the region of the aortic arch permits a detailed analysis of the aortic pulse contour. Warner has perfected this technique for clinical monitoring. Stroke volume is computed from the pulse contour on a beat-by-beat basis. This, combined with pressure variables, provides an almost instantaneous cardiovascular assessment. Unfortunately, McDonald et al. have pointed out, the method depends upon a stable vascular impedance, which is seldom the case in critically ill patients. For this reason, the technique is not in general use.

All the methods of estimating cardiac output described thus far are invasive to varying degrees and therefore present some risk and considerable expense because they require skilled personnel for their application. A number of promising noninvasive adaptations of the indicator-dilution principle are in clinical use. Included in this category are gamma densitometry (quantitative angiography), videodensitometry, isotope-dilution analysis, fluorescence excitation analysis, and magnetic fluid tracer dilution.

Information regarding flow rates, vascular volumes, distribution of pulmonary transit times, intracardiac and pulmonary shunting, and right or left ventricular ejection efficiency is theoretically contained in the shapes of indicator-dilution curves. With the conventional indocyanine green dye technique, sampling rates are too slow, and the injection and sampling sites are too far apart, for complete interpretation of the physiologic events that create the shape of the curve. Catheter lag between the sampling point and the densitometer cuvette also produces distortion of the curves and loss of potential information. Gamma densitometry, in which the indicator is a small bolus of radiopaque contrast medium and the blood vessels or cardiac chambers serve as the densitometer cuvettes, avoids these problems. Gamma rays or x-rays, projected through the cardiac silhouette, produce high-dynamic-response indicator time-concentration curves through the detection of changes in gamma photon density related, according to Beer's law, to the concentration of radiopaque indicator in the blood. In clinical practice, solid-state radiation detectors are placed behind the patient as in a portable x-ray unit. Five milliliters of Hypaque is then injected into the central venous catheter, and six simultaneous contrast dilution curves are recorded from the heart and great vessels. Analysis of these curves permits calculation of pulmonary circulation time, pulmonary blood volume, right and left ventricular ejection fraction, and other useful variables. More sophisticated interpretation requires electronic data processing for transfer function analysis.

Videodensitometry is similar in principle to gamma densitometry, except that an actual angiocardiogram is performed and recorded on magnetic tape. When played back on a television screen, the concentration of contrast medium is analyzed at any point in the heart and lungs by means of a movable electronic window. The advantages are that, at leisure, an infinite number of curves can be obtained from any point in the cardiac silhouette as the tape is played over and over. Disadvantages include great expense, lack of portability, and low signal-to-noise ratio requiring signal processing to obtain recognizable curves.

Isotope dilution analysis has made a great leap forward with the development of the Anger scintillation camera and other rapid-response isotope scanning devices. The ability to image and quantitate the distribution of a radioactive tracer second by second through the heart and lungs adds a new dimension of considerable value to surgical cardiovascular monitoring. High-photon-yield isotopes are injected intravenously and the gamma camera images recorded on magnetic tape. Later, specific areas can be analyzed to produce indicator-dilution curves which can be related to changes in size and position of the cardiac chambers. Jones et al. have produced good indicator-dilution curves for the right and left sides of the heart using an autofluoroscope. Spatial resolution and dynamic response, however, can never be as good as that obtained with the linear interrogating beams of radiation used in gamma densitometry. Furthermore, equipment for both isotope dilution and videodensitometry is expensive and bulky at present, and cannot be used for bedside studies.

Kaufman and associates have developed a highly innovative system for the bedside determination of cardiac output. Following the intravenous injection of a small amount of iodine containing radiographic contrast material, the iodine is caused to emit fluorescence in the gamma ray range by stimulation with an external gamma ray source. The stimulated emission of iodine is detected by a collimated silicon diode producing a characteristic indicator-dilution curve. The system is easily calibrated, and the radiation dose is low.

Another new method for the external noninvasive detection of indicator dilution has been described by Newbower. The indicator is a magnetic fluid tracer composed of fine ferromagnetic particles. The detection transducer is a simple set of air-core coils which easily measures the striking difference in magnetic susceptibility between the tracer and the background without the need for magnetic shielding. This novel approach has great potential because it does not involve ionizing radiation of any sort.

It is also possible to tag flowing blood in vivo by reversing the magnetic alignments of hydrogen nuclei in the water of the plasma by applying a powerful external magnetic field. These effects are detected further downstream by means of nuclear magnetic resonance. Nuclear magnetic resonance monitoring devices presently are under development. The technique is totally noninvasive.

It is obvious that noninvasive techniques for describing indicator-dilution curves will play a prominent role in surgical monitoring for years to come. Surgeons will be provided information regarding cardiac and circulatory function in their patients which will permit management of critical states on a firm physiologic basis.

The determination of systolic time intervals provides an external assessment of left ventricular function based entirely on intrinsic electrical and mechanical events. The methodology is gaining in popularity because it is physiologically sound and has been largely validated by extensive comparative clinical studies including catheterization of the left side of the heart.

Simultaneous recordings of the electrocardiogram, phonocardiogram, and external carotid pulse tracing are analyzed for the following time variables: total left ventricular systolic time (QRS complex to second heart sound), left ventricular ejection time (duration of carotid pulse upstroke), and preejection period (the difference between total left ventricular systolic and left ventricular ejection times). Although the calculations are straightforward, placement of the carotid pulse sensor and phonocardiogram microphone on the neck and chest is critical. With technical care in the performance of the recordings, remarkably good correlation with direct measures of the dynamics of the left side of the heart can be shown. Weissler et al. have found that the ratio of the preejection period to left ventricular ejection time (PEP/LVET) is relatively constant around 0.35 in patients with normal hearts. With failure of the left side of the heart, the PEP becomes longer and the LVET shorter, increasing the ratio. Serial studies reveal good correlation between the PEP/LVET ratio and left ventricular ejection fraction, end-diastolic volume, and end-diastolic pressure. This noninvasive approach, which requires inexpensive equipment, is useful for the continuous bedside monitoring of left ventricular function.

Alterations of left ventricular conduction, however, as

in left bundle branch block, prolong the PEP selectively with no apparent change in LVET. Changes in peripheral impedance or vascular runoff, as occur in septic shock, may alter the relation between the PEP/LVET ratio and cardiac performance. Few comparative studies have been done in clinical shock syndromes other than myocardial infarction shock, but at present systolic time internal recording looks as promising as aortic pulse contour analysis did 10 years ago.

The application of ultrasound to clinical monitoring is undergoing a period of rapid growth. Both industrial and academic sectors are developing methods for cardiovascular assessment based on interrogating beams of high-frequency sound waves (less than 1 mm wavelength). Ultrasonic energy can penetrate all tissues except bone and air-filled structures and provide good spatial resolution for diagnostic studies. Thus far, at the levels of energy needed for clinical work, there has been no suggestion of injury to living tissue, not even the fetus. The lack of hazard and the reasonable cost of the equipment required has led to more clinical studies than with any other technique aside from electrocardiography.

There are two basic methods of operation of ultrasound for diagnostic purposes—the pulse-echo mode (sonar) and the backscatter frequency shift mode (Doppler effect). In the former, the distance between the emitter and any sound-reflecting interface deep within the body is measured in terms of the transit time of bursts of ultrasound to and from the tissue. An A-scan device is held stationary against the body and a recording of the depth of structures in the path of the beam made on the basis of the known speed of sound in tissue. The B scan is produced if the ultrasonic emitter is traversed across the body while echo-ranging, in order to produce a picture of the tissue cross section.

Not only is ultrasound less harmful than ionizing radiation, but it is capable of revealing internal surfaces which are invisible to roentgen rays. These include the internal structures of the heart and blood vessels. In addition, devices using the Doppler principle can detect rapid motions within the body. This makes them useful for studies of peripheral blood flow and cardiac valve function.

In echocardiography for ultrasonic determination of cardiac chamber size and stroke volume, a transducer is applied to the chest over the cardiac area. Sound in the 1- to 5-megacycle frequency is delivered through the chest in on-off bursts about 1,500 times per second. Echoes are detected during the off periods and recorded in terms of time lag (distance). The distances between the intraventricular septum and the posterior endocardial wall of the left ventricle are recorded at end diastole and end systole. The calculations of end-diastolic and end-systolic volumes are made on the assumption that the shape of the chamber is a prolate ellipse. The results from a number of investigators are remarkable. The left ventricular volumes measured by echocardiography and by biplane angiocardiography were very similar over a wide range of values (correlation coefficient .97). The problem with this technique for surgical monitoring is that the operator must be highly skilled and experienced in aiming the transducer and recognizing on the scan the exact structures he wishes to measure. The device cannot be simply strapped on and left alone for 24 hours to record left ventricular function. Some method will have to be devised for the ultrasonic beam to "lock on" to the left ventricular wall reflections. This will not be an easy task.

The Doppler flowmeter has achieved considerable sophistication as a clinical tool in the past few years. Readout varies from a simple audible signal related to pulse velocity to signals combining vessel cross section and velocity to provide actual flow measurements. These techniques cannot yet be applied to aortic flow determination, but the entire field of ultrasonics offers many possibilities for the evolution of the perfect cardiovascular monitor.

The concept of measuring pulse volume on the basis of the electric properties of blood goes back 40 years, but practical instruments for measuring electric impedance related to movement of electrolyte of the electromagnetic field have only recently been developed. In the instrument developed by Kubicek et al., two electrodes are placed around the neck and two around the abdomen just below the chest. The volume of blood between the electrodes decreases as the stroke volume flows up the carotids and down the aorta. This produces a decrease in electric impedance in the thorax. Since this cyclic change in impedance, compared to total chest impedance, is equivalent to less than one part in a thousand, considerable electronic sophistication is required for its detection. Alternating current is sent through the outer electrodes, and the change in voltage between the inner electrodes measured during cardiac systole indicates the impedance change due to left ventricular ejection. The problem, of course, is that venous inflow occurs more or less continuously, so that a net stroke volume during maximum ejection is measured. Great hopes were held for thoracic impedance plethysmography as a relatively inexpensive noninvasive means of monitoring cardiac output and ventricular function. Unfortunately, electrode motion artifacts and lack of correlation with other methods for the estimation of cardiac output in nonsteady states have dampened enthusiasm for this class of instruments.

There is no more consistently accurate method of measuring cardiac output than a properly calibrated electromagnetic flowmeter placed firmly around the ascending aorta. In fact, this approach is accepted as the standard against which other cardiac output monitoring equipment is evaluated for accuracy. Until recently, electromagnetic flowmeters were used only during surgery for assessing vascular operations of various sorts. Now an extractable flowmeter probe is available for use in postoperative patients. It consists of a flexible electromagnetic transducer which can be wrapped around the ascending aorta and temporarily fixed in position with a removable retaining suture. When monitoring is no longer required, the retaining suture is released and the probe pulled out like a chest drainage tube. Calibration is not as easy as it is with probes of fixed dimensions or when zero flow readings can be obtained with the probe in position, but clinical studies

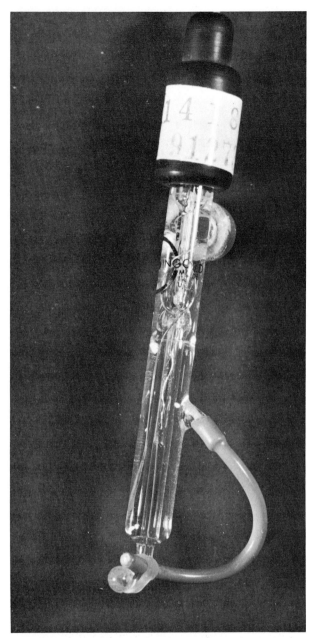

Fig. 13-9. Potentiometric electrode used to monitor muscle surface pH as an indicator of anaerobic metabolism related to inadequate perfusion. (*From N. P. Couch et al., Ann Surg, 173:173, 1971.*)

suggest that this is a practical method for cardiovascular monitoring following thoracotomy with access to the ascending aorta.

Monitoring of Tissue Metabolism

It was pointed out early in the chapter that a systems approach to monitoring would direct most effort toward a study of tissue metabolism. Under certain conditions,

such as hypoxemia or septic shock, a high cardiac output is no guarantee of adequate delivery of oxygen to the cells. Couch and colleagues have succeeded in developing a practical and simple solution to the problem of an early warning system for tissue hypoxia (Fig. 13-9). With an electrometer and right-angle pH electrode, skeletal muscle surface pH is continuously monitored. A 2-cm incision through skin, subcutaneous tissue, and fascia is required for placement of the electrode in gentle contact with the surface of the biceps muscle in adults and the quadriceps in children. Clinical monitoring by this technique has been continued for as long as 8 days.

The rationale for this approach is that with tissue deprivation of oxygen, oxidative phosphorylation ceases, and pyruvate is converted to lactic acid rather than carbon dioxide and water. Diffusion of the hydrogen ions and lactate across the cell membranes into the extracellular fluid is passive and rapid. Extracellular fluid acidosis related to anaerobic glycolysis precedes arterial pH depression because of a number of factors: in low flow states there is a delay of acid metabolite washout into the peripheral circulation; arterial pH will change only after the hemoglobin-, bicarbonate-, and phosphate-buffering capacity of the blood is exceeded; and metabolism of lactate by the heart and liver tend to reduce the peripheral lactate levels until late in shock. Skeletal muscle itself offers several advantages for surveillance of overall oxygen transport. Since it can tolerate hypoxia, its blood supply tends to get shut off early in critical states, and it tends to shift readily into anaerobic glycolysis and lactate production because of its high glycogen content. The surface of the muscle rather than the interior is monitored to avoid artifacts due to hematoma formation. Studies in man have shown that muscle surface pH is a sensitive indicator of muscle metabolism and as such is valuable as a practical monitoring instrument to alert against hypoxia of more vital tissues. The normal resting biceps pH is 7.38, slightly below arterial pH. When the normal oxygen gradient to the muscle cells is restored after the circulatory crisis is over, pH promptly returns to the normal resting level.

Couch's group has also done redox potential measurements of muscle as an indicator of balance between oxygen delivery and tissue needs. Redox potential of tissue reflects the overall balance of electron transfer which shifts toward the negative or reduced state with prolonged hypoxia. However, although the trends were found to be similar to the surface pH changes, absolute redox potential values were not as reliable indicators as pH changes. Muscle surface pH monitoring provides a good early warning of disaster during and after surgery. The small incision certainly can be justified in high-risk patients or those undergoing formidable operations.

Woldring et al. developed a mass spectrometer which accurately records partial pressures of oxygen, carbon dioxide, or other gases, sampled through plastic or rubber membranes mounted on a catheter tip. Using a mass spectrometer, Owens et al. measured intracerebral gas tensions continuously across a heparinized silastic membrane on a perforated cannula. Of course, the measurements represent the gas tensions in the extracellular fluid surrounding local tissue injury rather than intact cells. Other problems are related to changes in membrane permeability due to fibrin deposits and protein denaturation.

The quest for the perfect monitor of vital function is really just beginning, as investigators such as Chance learn about energy "spin-off" during bioenergetic exchange in the cells. More bioengineers are looking at the lower part of Table 13-1 to find noninvasive methods of scanning cellular bioenergetics. Huckabee has defined hypoxia as "the condition which exists when the supply of oxygen to the exterior of living cells is reduced to a rate insufficient for their current metabolic needs, with the result that various cellular oxidation-reduction systems must shift toward a more reduced state." Detection of this state by a safe external sensor is the ultimate goal.

A number of attempts in this direction are in progress. One involves the stimulation of intracellular oxygen molecules with modulated soft x-rays. The stimulated emission of oxygen is in the microwave area of the 0.5-cm band and can be detected externally with a suitable waveguide and amplifier system. This approach would offer some degree of spatial discrimination of tissue hypoxia in specific organs. Another experimental method is a cross between Chance's fluorescence emission technique and thermography. Energy transfers within living cells emit specific wavelengths of electromagnetic radiation according to quantum bioenergetic laws. Energy dissipation associated with inefficient anaerobic metabolism or uncoupling of oxidative phosphorylation should be detectable by suitable instrumentation. Such a system has been developed to detect and identify narrow band and line spectra associated with abnormal tissue states. These signals in a physiologic situation are superimposed on the broad band (black body) radiation of the skin or organ surface along with the far infrared spectral pattern of cellular water and carbon dioxide. The desired signals are somewhat analogous to the Fraunhofer lines of the solar spectrum due to absorption in the sun's mantle. The approach differs from conventional infrared thermography in that the strategy is to analyze the spectral pattern rather than to determine the energy level within a specified wavelength. A Fourier interferometer, which is about the size of a bread box, is used to scan the patient at the bedside. The recorded interferogram is then transmitted by a time-shared system over telephone lines to a computer for Fourier transform and signature analysis. Emission power spectral density tracings have been obtained from human limbs as well as other tissues and superficial carcinomas. Cross-correlation techniques have been used to establish significant differences. Alterations in infrared emission spectra reflect changes in tissue metabolism from analysis of the frequencies of radiation corresponding to molecular vibrations and rotations. Although highly experimental, this is a good example of monitoring at the business end of the oxygen transport chain.

References

Physiologic Concepts and Monitoring

Barcroft, J.: "The Respiratory Functions of the Blood," Cambridge University Press, London, 1925.

Brown, J. H. U. and Dickson, J. F., III: Instrumentation and the Delivery of Health Services, *Science,* **166:**334, 1969.

Bunker, J. P., Forrest, W. H., Jr., Mosteller, F., and Vandam, L. D. (eds.): "The National Halothane Study," National Institute of General Medical Sciences, Bethesda, 1969.

Chance, B.: Regulation of Intracellular Oxygen, *Proc Int Union Physiol Sci,* **6:**13, 1968.

Clark, L. C., Jr. and Lyons, C.: Electrode Systems for Continuous Monitoring in Cardiovascular Surgery, *Ann NY Acad Sci,* **102:**19, 1962.

Cohn, J. D. and Del Guercio, L. R. M.: Cardiorespiratory Analysis of Cardiac Arrest and Resuscitation, *Surg Gynecol Obstet,* **123:**1066, 1966.

Dammann, J. F.: Assessment of Continuous Monitoring in the Critically Ill Patient, *Dis Chest,* **55:**240, 1969.

Del Guercio, L. R. M., Feins, N. R., Cohn, J. D., Coomaraswamy, R. P., Wollman, S. B., and State, D.: A Comparison of Blood Flow during External and Internal Cardiac Massage in Man, *Circulation,* **32**(*Suppl* 1):171, 1965.

Dickens, F., and Neil, E.: "Oxygen in the Animal Organism," The Macmillan Company, New York, 1964.

Hershey, S. G., Del Guercio, L. R. M., and McConn, R.: "Septic Shock in Man," Little, Brown and Company, Boston, 1971.

Huckabee, W. E.: Relationships of Pyruvate and Lactate during Anaerobic Metabolism: II. Exercise and Formation of O_2 Debt. *J Clin Invest,* **37:**255, 1958.

Irving, L.: Respiration in Diving Mammals, *Physiol Rev,* **19:**112, 1939.

Maloney, J. V., Jr.: The Trouble with Patient Monitoring, *Ann Surg,* **168:**605, 1968.

Pontoppidau, H., Geffin, B., and Lowenstein, E.: Acute Respiratory Failure in the Adult. *N Engl J Med,* **287:**690, 1972.

Roughton, F. J. W.: The Average Time Spent by the Blood in the Human Lung Capillary and Its Relation to the Rates of CO Uptake and Elimination in Man, *Am J Physiol,* **143:**621, 1945.

Sarnoff, S. J., and Mitchell, J. H.: The Control of the Function of the Heart, in "Handbook of Physiology," vol. 1, The Williams & Wilkins Company, Baltimore, 1962.

Van Slyke, D. D.: The Carbon Dioxide Carriers of the Blood, *Physiol Rev,* **1:**141, 1921.

Physiologic Sensing

Collins, J. A., and Ballinger, W. F., II: "The Surgical Intensive Care Unit," *Surgery,* **66:**614, 1969.

Giles, A. F.: "Electronic Sensing Devices," William Clowes and Sons, London, 1966.

Johnson, H. A., Information Theory in Biology after 18 Years. *Science,* **168:**1545, 1970.

Rushmer, R. F. (ed.): "Medical Engineering: Projections for Health Care Delivery," Academic Press, Inc., New York, 1972.

Shannon, C. E., and Weaver, W.: "The Mathematical Theory of Communication," The University of Illinois Press, Urbana, 1959.

Respiratory Monitoring

Kinney, J. M., Morgan, A. P., Dominguous, F. G., and Gilder, K. J.: A Method for Continuous Measurement of Gas Exchange and Expired Radioactivity in Acutely Ill Patients, *Metabolism*, **13**:205, 1964.

Lewis, F. J., Shimizu, T., Scofield, A. L., and Rosi, P. S.: Analysis of Respiration by an On-Line Digital Computer System: Clinical Data following Thoraco Abdominal Surgery, *Ann Surg*, **164**:547, 1966.

———, Deller, S., Yokochi, H., Rosi, P. S., Quinn, M. L., Kite, M., and Rabin, S.: Automatic Monitoring in the Postoperative Recovery Room, *Surg Gynecol Obstet*, **130**:333, 1970.

Osborn, J. J., Badia, W., and Gerbode, F.: Respiratory or Cardiac Work and Other Analogue Computer Techniques, *J Thorac Surg*, **45**:500, 1963.

———, Beaumont, J. O., Raison, J. C. A., Russell, J., and Gerbode, F.: Measurement and Monitoring of Acutely Ill Patients by Digital Computer, *Surgery*, **64**:1057, 1968.

Peters, R. M.: Work of Breathing following Trauma, *J Trauma*, **8**:915, 1968.

——— and Hilberman, M.: Respiratory Insufficiency Diagnosis and Control of Therapy, *Surgery*, **70**:280, 1971.

——— and Stacy, R. W.: Automatized Clinical Measurement of Respiratory Parameters, *Surgery*, **56**:44, 1964.

Rosi, P. S., Yokochi, H., Deller, S., Quinn, M., Greenberg, A. G., Rabin, S., Blatt, S., Lewis, F. J., and Jacobs, J. E.: Noninvasive Automatic Patient Monitoring, *Surg Forum*, **20**:234, 1969.

Cardiovascular Monitoring

Bondurant, S. (ed.): Research on Acute Myocardial Infarction, *Circulation*, vol. 40, Suppl 4, 1969.

Border, J. R., Gallo, E., and Shenk, W. G.: Alterations in Cardiovascular and Pulmonary Physiology in the Severely Stressed Patient: A Rational Plan for the Management of Hypotension. *J Trauma*, **6**:176, 1966.

Cohn, J. N., Khatri, I. M., and Hamosh, P.: Diagnostic and Therapeutic Value of Bedside Monitoring of Left Ventricular Pressure, *Am J Cardiol*, **23**:107, 1969.

Dalton, B., and Laver, M. B.: Vasospasm with an Indwelling Radial Artery Cannula, *Anesthesiology*, **34**:194, 1971.

Del Guercio, L. R. M., Cohn, J. D., Feins, N. R., Coomaraswamy, R. P., and Mantel, L.: Pulmonary Embolism Shock: The Physiologic Basis of a Bedside Screening Test, *JAMA*, **196**:751, 1966.

Dudrick, S. J., Wilmore, D. W., Vars, H. M., and Rhoads, J. E.: Can Intravenous Feeding as the Sole Means of Nutrition Support Growth in the Child and Restore Weight Loss in an Adult? An Affirmative Answer, *Ann Surg*, **169**:974, 1969.

Friedman, E., Grable, E., and Fine, J.: Central Venous Pressure and Direct Serial Measurements as Guides in Blood-Volume Replacement, *Lancet*, **2**:609, 1966.

Ganz, W., and Swan, H. J. C.: Measurement of Blood Flow by Thermodilution, *Am J Cardiol*, **29**:241, 1972.

Garcia, E., Michenfelder, J. D., and Theye, R. A.: Right Atrial Oxygen Saturation Levels during Anesthesia and Surgery, *J Can Anaesth Soc*, **15**:593, 1968.

Kazamias, T. M., Gander, M. P., Ross, J., Jr., and Braunwald, E.: Detection of Left-Ventricular-Wall Motion Disorders in Coronary Artery Disease by Radarkymography, *N Engl J Med*, **285**:63, 1971.

Krauss, X. H., Verdouw, P. D., Hugenholtz, P. G., Hagemijer, F., and Polanyi, M. L.: Continuous Monitoring of O_2 Saturation in the Intensive Care Unit, *Circulation*, **45**(*Suppl* 2):178, 1972.

Lee, J., Wright, F., Barber, R., and Stanley, L.: Central Venous Oxygen Saturation in Shock: A Study in Man, *Anesthesiology*, **36**:472, 1972.

Lowenstein, E., Little, J. W., III, and Lo, H. H.: Prevention of Cerebral Embolization from Flushing Radial-Artery Cannulas. *N Engl J Med*, **285**:1415, 1971.

Owens, G., Belmusto, L., and Woldring, S.: Experimental Intracerebral PO_2 and PCO_2 Monitoring by Mass Spectrography, *J Neurosurg*, **30**:110, 1969.

Sheppard, L. C., Kouchoukos, N. T., Kurtis, M., and Kirklin, J. W.: Automated Treatment of Critically Ill Patients, *Ann Surg*, **168**:596, 1968.

Shubin, H., and Weil, M. H.: Efficient Monitoring with a Digital Computer of Cardiovascular Function in Seriously Ill Patients, *Ann Intern Med*, **65**:453, 1966.

Weinberg, D. I., Artley, J. L., Whalen, R., and McIntosh, H. D.: Electric Shock Hazards in Cardiac Catheterization, *Circ Res*, **9**:1004, 1962.

Woldring, S., Owens, G., and Woolford, D.: Blood Gases: Continuous In Vivo Recording of Partial Pressure by Mass Spectroscopy, *Science*, **153**:887, 1967.

Zohman, L. R., and Williams, M. H., Jr.: Percutaneous Right Heart Catheterization Using Polyethylene Tubing, *Am J Cardiol*, **4**:373, 1959.

Cardiac Output Determinations

Ashburn, W., L., Moser, K. M., and Guisan, M.: Digital and Analog Processing of Anger Camera Data and a Dedicated Computer Controlled System, *J Nucl Med*, **11**:680, 1970.

Bender, M. A., and Blau, M.: The Autofluoroscope, *Nucleonics*, **21**:52, 1963.

Cohn, J. D.: A Pump System for Performing Indicator-Dilution Curves without Blood Loss, *J Appl Physiol*, **26**:841, 1969.

——— and Del Guercio, L. R. M.: Nomogram for the Rapid Calculation of Cardiac Output at the Bedside, *Ann Surg*, **164**:109, 1966.

——— and ———: Clinical Applications of Indicator Dilution Curves as Gamma Functions, *J Lab Clin Med*, **69**:675, 1967.

Del Guercio, L. R. M.: Contrast Dilution Analysis, *Trans NY Acad Sci*, **33**:387, 1971.

Feigenbaum, H., Zaky, A., and Nasser, W. K.: Use of Ultrasound to Measure Left Ventricular Stroke Volume, *Circulation*, **35**:1092, 1967.

Franklin, D. L., Schlegel, W., and Rushmer, R. F.: Blood Flow Measured by Doppler Frequency Shift of Back-scattered Ultrasound, *Science*, **134**:564, 1961.

Ganz, W., and Swan, H. J. C.: Measurement of Blood Flow by Thermal Dilution, *Am J Cardiol*, **29**:241, 1972.

Hillenbrand, W. I.: Desk-top Computers and Electronic Calculators for Engineers, *Electronic Products*, June 1966, pp. 50–53.

Jones, R. H., Klaphaak, R. B., and Sabiston, D. C., Jr.: Anatomic Resolution in Dynamic Radionuclide Studies by Computer Identification or Radioactivity Fluctuation with Time, Proc 2d Symp Sharing Computer Programs Technology Nucl Med (*AEC Conf-720430*), 1972, p. 151.

Kaufman, L.: Clinical Applications of Silicon Lithium Radiation Detectors, *Proc IEEE Nucl Sci Symp*, December 1972.

Kubicek, W. G., Patterson, R. P., and Witsoe, D. A.: Impedance Cardiography as a Non-invasive Method of Monitoring Cardiac Function and Other Parameters of the Cardiovascular System, *Ann NY Acad Sci,* **170:**724, 1970.

McDonald, D. A., Kouchoukos, N. T., Shepard, L. C., and Kirklin, J. W.: Estimation of Stroke Volume and Cardiac Output from the Central Arterial Pulse Contour in Postoperative Patients, *Circulation,* **38**(*Suppl* 6):118, 1968.

Newbower, R. S.: Blood Flow Measurements with Magnetic Tracers, *Proc Conf Engineering Med Biol,* **14:**147, 1972.

Papp, R. L., and Harrison, D. C.: Ultrasonic Cardiac Echography for Determining Stroke Volume and Valvular Regurgitation, *Circulation,* **41:**493, 1970.

Pombo, J. F., Troy, B. L., and Russell, R. O., Jr.: Left Ventricular Volumes and Ejection Fraction by Echocardiography, *Circulation,* **43:**480, 1971.

Siegel, J. H., Fabian, M., Lankau, C., Levine, M., Cole, A., and Nahmad, M.: Clinical and Experimental Use of Thoracid Impedance Plethysmography in Quantifying Myocardial Contractility, *Surgery,* **67:**907, 1970.

———, Greenspan, M., Cohn, J. D., and Del Guercio, L. R. M.: A Bedside Computer and Physiologic Nomograms: Guides to the Management of the Patient in Shock, *Arch Surg,* **97:**480, 1968.

Sinclair, S., Duff, J. H., and MacLean, L. D.: Use of a Computer for Calculating Cardiac Output, *Surgery,* **57:**414, 1965.

Warner, H.: The Role of Computers in Medical Research, *JAMA,* **196:**944, 1966.

Weissler, A. M., Harris, W. S., and Schoenfeld, C. D.: Bedside Techniques for the Evaluation of Ventricular Function in Man, *Am J Cardiol,* **23:**577, 1969.

Williams, B. T., Barefoot, C., and Schenk, W. G., Jr.: A Removable Electromagnetic Flow Probe: Preliminary Report, *Rev Surg,* **3:**227, 1969.

Wood, E. H., Sturm, R. E., and Sanders, J. J.: Data Processing in Cardiovascular Physiology with Particular Reference to Roentgen Videodensitometry, *Mayo Clin Proc,* **39:**849, 1964.

Monitoring of Tissue Metabolism

Cohn, J. D., Del Guercio, L. R. M., Ito, K., Pan, C. H. T., and Moross, G.: Infrared Emission Spectroscopy from Human Limbs, *Proc 25th Conf Engineering Med Biol,* 1972, p. 55.

———, ———,———, ———, and ———: Infrared Spectral Analysis of Metabolic Function, *Fed Proc,* **31:**350, 1972.

Couch, N. P., Dmochowski, J. R., Van De Water, J. M., Harken, D. E., and Moore, F. D.: Muscle Surface pH as an Index of Peripheral Perfusion in Man, *Ann Surg,* **173:**173, 1971.

Del Guercio, L. R. M., Cohn, J. D., Ito, K., Moross, G. G., and Pan, C. H. T.: Non-invasive Assessment of Cellular Function and Organ Perfusion, *Proc 1972 Technicon Int Cong.* (In press.)

Owens, G., Belmusto, L., and Woldring, S.: Experimental Intracerebral PO_2 and PCO_2 Monitoring by Mass Spectroscopy, *J Neurosurg,* **30:**110, 1969.

Woldring, S., Owens, G., and Woolford, D. C.: Blood Gases: Continuous In Vivo Recording of Partial Pressures by Mass Spectroscopy, *Science,* **153:**885, 1966.

Chapter 14

Skin and Subcutaneous Tissue

by **Seymour I. Schwartz**

Physiology

Physical Properties
Functions of Skin

Pressure Sores

Hidradenitis Suppurativa

Cysts

Epidermal Inclusion Cyst
Ganglia
Sebaceous Cyst
Dermoid Cyst
Pilonidal Cyst and Sinus

Benign Tumors

Warts
Keratosis
Keloid
Vascular Tumors
    Capillary (Port Wine) Hemangioma
    Immature Hemangioma (Strawberry Mark)
    Cavernous Hemangioma
    Sclerosing Hemangioma
    Glomus Tumor
    Lymphangioma
Fat Tumors
    Lipoma
    Weber-Christian Disease
Neuromas

Malignant Tumors

Basal Cell Carcinoma
Squamous Cell Carcinoma
Sweat Gland Carcinoma
Other Malignant Tumors
    Fibrosarcoma
    Hemangiopericytoma
    Kaposi's Sarcoma
    Other Sarcomas

Melanoma and Other Pigmented Lesions

General Considerations
Benign Pigmented Lesions
Melanoma

PHYSIOLOGY

The skin, which is the largest organ in the body, represents more than a structure covering vital organs and separating them from the environment. It is a complex organ that possesses unique physical properties and physiologic functions.

Physical Properties

Both *tension* and *elasticity* are physical properties which are related to elastic fibers within the skin. Tension is the characteristic which accounts for the fact that the skin resists stretching by weak forces; the maximal deforming force which is resisted by the skin, expressed in dynes per centimeter, is a measurement of tension. Tension varies in different areas and is most marked where the skin contains dense elastic fibers, particularly in regions where the skin is thin. The direction of the tension also varies anatomically and forms the basis of the line system described by Langer in 1861. The tension of skin is greater in young than in elderly patients. Elasticity refers to the skin's ability to resume its original shape after an external force has been applied to cause deformation. This also varies with age, being less in the elderly and also in patients with edema.

Quantification of the physical properties of the skin has been made by determining the *tensile strength,* or the resistance of skin to tearing under tension. The average tensile strength of the adult skin, without fat, is approximately 1.8 kg/m². This is significantly reduced in infants up to three months of age, and the lowest values are found in the Ehlers-Danlos syndrome, which is characterized by a reduction of elastic fibers. In patients with Cushing's syndrome or those taking high doses of cortisone for prolonged periods of time, the tensile strength of skin is significantly less than normal, and there is also a low modulus of elasticity.

The electrical behavior of skin has been the subject of much investigation. The skin generates polarization currents which provide great resistance to external electric forces. The intensity of imposed current passing through the skin is therefore very low. The skin also offers a resistance to alternating currents by its property of impedence.

Functions of Skin

Important physiologic functions of skin include (1) percutaneous absorption, (2) an important role in the circulatory system, (3) serving as an organ of senses, (4) secretion of sweat, (5) providing an avenue for the insensible loss of water, and (6) contributing to thermal regulation.

PERCUTANEOUS ABSORPTION. This refers to the penetration of substances through the skin, permitting them to enter the bloodstream. It has been shown that radioactive water, applied either as a vapor or as a solution, appears both in the circulation and the urine. If the skin is warmed after exposure, the concentration in the urine increases rapidly. Electrolytes applied to the skin in aqueous solution either do not penetrate or may enter in small amounts via the appendages. The skin is impermeable to sodium and calcium when these are applied to the skin in the form of a chloride solution. However, there is some evidence that the iodide ion may enter the skin either because it increases the negative electric charge of skin or because it penetrates via appendages. When radioactive electrolytes are rubbed onto the skin, they are absorbed, and the absorption is increased if the skin is abraded or has been shaved.

Lipid-soluble substances are fairly rapidly and completely absorbed through the skin, and absorption appears to be faster if the substances are also soluble in water to some degree. In the latter instance, the penetration is so rapid that the rate of absorption is comparable to gastrointestinal absorption and even absorption of the material injected subcutaneously. The percutaneous absorption of phenol has been recognized for many years, and fatal poisoning may be associated with the application of carbolic acid to large areas of skin. Salicylic acid also penetrates with great ease from alcoholic and aqueous solutions as well as from ointments. Estrogenic hormones, testosterone, progesterone, and desoxycorticosterone all penetrate the intact skin rapidly. Hydrocortisone may be therapeutically effective by percutaneous application, while cortisone acetate applied locally is poorly absorbed. Water-soluble hormones, such as insulin, are not absorbed. Similarly, lipid-soluble vitamins are absorbed with ease, while water-soluble vitamins do not penetrate the skin. Heavy metals may be absorbed to some extent, and their absorption is dependent upon the formation of compounds in combination with the fatty acid of the sebum. This is particularly true of mercury.

Substances in the gaseous form, with the exception of carbon monoxide, penetrate the skin easily. Oxygen, nitrogen, and carbon dioxide are examples of gases which perfuse readily. Carbon tetrachloride is also readily absorbed through the skin, as demonstrated by experiments with ^{14}C-labeled compound. Recently, the absorption of pharmaceutic agents through the skin has been employed by using dimethyl sulfoxide as a vehicle. The applicability of this technique has not been totally defined.

CIRCULATION AND VASCULAR REACTIONS. The cutaneous vascular system is extremely complex and contributes significantly to the general circulation and vascular reactions. Direct visualization of flow in minute vessels can be carried out by observing the capillary circulation of the base of the nail. The color of the skin is dependent upon the quantity of blood in the subpapillary plexus of vessels, particularly in the Caucasian, while the skin temperature depends chiefly on the rate of flow through the whole skin. The range of pressure in human skin capillaries is between 12 and 45 mm Hg, and the average capillary pressure is equivalent to the colloid osmotic pressure of plasma proteins. Arteriovenous anastomoses of digital skin play an important role in temperature regulation and are implicated in the formation of the glomus tumor.

Local vascular responses may result from direct action on the vessel wall or its contractile elements. Local vasoconstriction follows gentle stroking. However, if the mechanical stimulus is of greater intensity than that which causes constriction, a red local reaction may develop secondary to dilatation of small vessels. Circumscribed superficial edema of the skin in areas responsive to stimuli is referred to as a "wheal" and is due to leakage of plasma from dilated blood vessels into the extracellular space. There are two distinct steps in the formation of the wheal: (1) local dilatation and (2) increased capillary permeability. Stimulation of the sympathetic fibers supplying the skin causes vasoconstriction of the cutaneous vessels, while interruption of these fibers results in dilatation of the small arteries and arterioles. The cutaneous circulatory system also responds to chemical agents. Acetylcholine causes vasodilatation, while norepinephrine and epinephrine are important vasoconstricting drugs. Pituitrin is also an active vasoconstrictor. Nicotinic acid and nitrites cause flushing and warmth, increased temperature, and increased blood flow. Ergot alkaloids act as vasodilators by their sympatholytic action, but the drugs also directly constrict the muscles of the peripheral arterioles, and the net effect is a decrease in blood flow.

SENSORY FUNCTION. The skin's sensory functions pertain to the modalities of pain (including itching), touch, and temperature. Skin consists of a mosaic of multiple sensitive spots, the relative density of which varies with the region of body. Cold sensitivity is probably mediated by Krause's end bulbs, whereas Ruffini's endings are probably receptors for warmth. Meissner's corpuscles and Merkel's discs are implicated in the tactile sensation, and the Pacinian corpuscles are involved in the sensation of pressure. Pain is mediated by free nonmyelinated endings, which are in a plexiform arrangement. Following injury to the skin, there is a widespread area of hyperalgesia which radiates from the point of injury. After traumatic injury of a peripheral nerve, causalgia, in which there is increased pain accompanied by cutaneous vasodilatation, may occur. Sympathectomy at the appropriate level in this case brings about almost complete relief.

SWEAT SECRETION. The skin contains two types of sweat glands, eccrine glands, which are small sweat glands, and apocrine, or large, sweat glands. The eccrine glands are distributed all over the body and are the true secretory glands which produce clear, aqueous sweat responsible for heat regulation. The apocrine glands in the human being are almost rudimentary structures. If the environmental temperature rises above 31 or 32°C (90°F), there is a sudden outbreak of visible sweating over the entire body. At lower environmental temperatures, the sweat glands secrete microscopically visible droplets in a periodic fashion. The insensible sweat secretion constitutes one part of the total insensible water loss.

The distribution of sweat glands is such that the highest number per square inch are located in the palms and soles and are also more dense on the dorsum of the hand, forehead, and trunk. There are fewer glands in the lower extremity than in the upper extremity. In most instances, sweating is almost exclusively the result of nervous impulses, but the glands are able to respond directly to application of heat if it is sufficiently intense. The nonnervous sweat response is strictly limited to the local area of stimulation. The nervous response is almost entirely mediated over sympathetic nerves and results from the pharmacologic action of parasympathetic substances. The nerve fibers to the sweat glands liberate acetylcholine at their endings upon stimulation. Atropine and other anticholinergics block the receptor sites so that they are unable to respond and thus interfere with secretion. Hyperhidrosis (increased sweating) may result from an abnormal increase in nerve impulses as in central nervous system lesions or emotional states. Increased tonicity of the sweat fibers may intensify the sweat response to normal nervous and nonnervous stimuli.

Primary hyperhidrosis usually presents as excessive sweating noted early in life. Mild cases can be managed with anticholinergic drugs and antiperspirant creams. Sympathectomy at T_2 to T_4 or T_5 abolishes eccrine sweating in the involved areas of the upper extremity. A modified Hurley-Shelley operation is used for axillary hyperhidrosis. The hair-bearing axillary skin is excised, and the ganglia at T_2 and T_3 are removed for accompanying hand sweating.

Eccrine sweat is a clear aqueous solution containing 99 percent water and 1 percent solids, half of which are inorganic salts and half organic compounds. Under normal circumstances, it is hypotonic, but at high rates of sweating it may approach isotonic concentration. Although the composition of sweat depends on material within the bloodstream, it is not a simple ultrafiltrate of plasma but represents an active secretion. The concentration of sodium and chloride is lower than that in plasma, while the concentration of potassium is somewhat higher. The concentration of chloride depends on many factors and is usually in the range of 15 to 60 mEq/L. The sodium concentration is almost always entirely equivalent to that of chloride and varies in a parallel fashion. Chloride and sodium concentrations rise with prolongation of sweating and with the rate of sweating and temperature of the skin. The chloride content of palmar sweat is greater than that from other parts of the body. The salt concentration of sweat also depends on the intake, and an adequate supply of drinking water depresses the concentration. The loss of potassium through the skin ranges between 2.7 and 3.1 mEq/L.

Nitrogen compounds are also lost transdermally, and the concentration of urea in sweat is twice as high as that in the blood. Creatinine is present in sweat in only a minute amount, and amino acids have also been noted. Ammonia is a primary constituent of sweat, and it can be concentrated by the sweat glands with nearly the same efficiency as the renal excreting unit. Large amounts of lactic acid and lactate have been demonstrated in sweat, particularly during heavy muscular exercise and in association with thermogenic sweat. The concentrations are ten to twenty times higher than that in the blood, and it is felt that the lactic acid originates from breakdown of glycogen within the sweat glands.

Sweat provides the skin with an "acid mantle." The average pH of freshly secreted sweat is 5.7 to 6.4. As the sweating progresses, the acidity decreases, but considerable amounts of acid are still lost with profuse thermal sweating. There is increasing acidity with evaporation of water from the sweat.

In contrast to the eccrine glands, which develop from the upper dermis, the apocrine glands are formed from follicular epithelium, as are sebaceous glands. Like sebaceous glands and hair follicles, the apocrine glands have major development during puberty. They are greater in number in females and respond to autonomic nervous stimulation rather than thermal stimulation. They function by producing a somewhat viscous milklike droplet.

INSENSIBLE WATER LOSS. Sweat secretion provides but one of two separate mechanisms contributing to insensible loss of water through continuous evaporation which occurs at all environmental temperatures. The other mechanism is that of loss through the epidermis which, unlike sweat secretion, is not affected by atropinization. Water loss through the epidermis is contrasted with sweat in that it does not contain salts or other solutes. The total insensible water loss through skin and lungs is constant under basal conditions and amounts to about 200 Gm/m^2/24 hours, 60 percent of which is cutaneous loss. Total cutaneous water loss in the adult man at rest without visible sweating is about 500 to 700 ml daily. The insensible loss from both the skin and the lungs shows a linear relationship to the basal metabolic rate. Water intake has no effect on cutaneous loss in the adult but does increase it in children. In hypothyroidism, the water loss is conspicuously low, whereas in thyrotoxicosis, total insensible perspiration is greatly increased.

THERMOREGULATION. The skin plays an important role in the regulation of body temperature. Heat is lost through the skin under the processes of radiation, convection, conduction, and evaporation. Sweating is a useful process only when the sweat can evaporate. It is therefore very efficient as a regulatory mechanism in a dry, hot environment, but with increased humidity the efficiency decreases markedly. Humidity begins to be of importance between 30 and 31°C (86 to 88°F) air temperature, at which point the difference between 50 and 100 percent relative humidity decides whether the person will be comfortable or hyperthermic. If heat production is raised or atmospheric temperature is raised, there is a shift of blood flow from the interior to the skin. The converse is also true, and this process is carried out reflexly.

Cold stimuli of a moderate degree result in the production of pallor. After the stimulus has ceased, there is reactive arterial vasodilatation. Cold stimuli of long duration are associated with livid discoloration as a result of paresis in the venous limbs of the capillaries. With extreme stimuli, there may be a reddish discoloration due to dilatation of the arterioles. The condition, however, is not associated with increased blood flow, and skin temperature does not rise. The reduction in temperature is also accompanied by interference with the utilization of oxyhemoglobin. Emersion foot, or "trench foot," occurs when the skin is exposed for long periods of time to cold water. There is vasoconstriction and capillary damage, and if the skin's temperature is returned to normal rapidly, reactive hyperemia and blistering result. Thrombosis may complicate the situation. It is therefore felt that exposure to the cold should be treated by gradual increase in temperature. The role of sympathectomy early in the course of frostbite has been debated, but there is some real evidence to indicate that it is applicable if carried out within 24 hours.

Heat exhaustion refers to a syndrome characterized by excessive loss of salt and water when people are exposed to high temperatures. A sweat retention syndrome has been recognized among troops in hot, humid climates, in which situation the personnel lose their ability to sweat and become moderately hyperthermic. Exhaustion, headache, palpitation, and dizziness are the characteristic manifestations.

PRESSURE SORES

Pressure on an area of skin for 2 or more hours, particularly in patients with impaired nutritional status, may result in sufficient ischemia to cause a decubitus ulcer. The ulceration usually occurs over bony prominences. Supportive therapy includes a nutritive diet, correction of anemia, and relief of pressure over the area. Routinely turning the patient and using special mattresses are effective. Surgical therapy requires sharp debridement to excise the ulcer and underlying fascia and necrotic material. The bony prominence frequently requires excision, with care to achieve hemostasis. The bone should be covered with muscle, and a large rotation flap of skin and fat provides the best skin coverage.

HIDRADENITIS SUPPURATIVA

This is a chronic acneform infection of the cutaneous apocrine glands, subcutaneous tissue, and fascia. It is generally confined to areas in which these glands are found, namely the axilla, areola of the nipple, groin, perineum, and circumanal and periumbilical regions. The disease was first described by Velpeau in 1839, and clinical manifestations vary with the duration of the lesion. At first, there is a slight subcutaneous induration, and as the tumor enlarges, the process advances to the skin, which becomes inflamed and adherent. Suppuration eventually develops, and cellulitis surrounds the abscess. At this stage, pain is often severe. Incision and drainage at this point results in a few drops of thick, viscous, purulent material. The process may subside after 2 or 3 days, only to recur. In the chronic stage, the patient presents with multiple painful cutaneous nodules which coalesce and are surrounded by fibrous reaction. The pathologic picture is similar to that seen in any acute pyogenic infection of the skin, but in-

volvement of the apocrine glands establishes the diagnosis. Culture of the pus yields a variety of saprophytic and pathogenic bacteria with a preponderance of staphylococci and streptococci.

Treatment consists of excision of the involved area or x-ray therapy for early cases. Cures can be achieved early in the course of the disease by improved hygiene and incision and drainage. In chronic cases, however, radical excision of all the pathologic tissue with split-thickness skin grafts for coverage affords the best opportunity for cure.

CYSTS

Epidermal Inclusion Cyst

When the epithelium of the skin is trapped subcutaneously, as a result of trauma or for other reasons, it may continue to grow and desquamate. This creates a cyst lined by epidermal cells and filled with keratin and desquamated cells. The lesions occur most frequently on the hand and are characterized by continued enlargement. Cure is effected by removal of the entire cyst and all its epithedial elements.

Ganglia

Ganglia are areas of mucoid degeneration of retinacular structures. They are tense, subcutaneous cystic masses occurring most commonly over the wrist and over tendon sheaths of the hands and feet. They grow very slowly and are usually associated with only minimal discomfort. The lesions consist of a wall of collagenous tissue which may or may not have synovial cells and contain thin clear collagenous material. They have been related to trauma, either accidental or occupational.

Treatment is by surgical excision which is usually performed after a tourniquet is applied to permit precise dissection. The ganglia which are closely adherent to a tendon sheath are relatively easy to remove, but those which communicate with the synovium of a joint require excision of the neck and base plate to protect against recurrence. Trauma to established ganglia usually results in rupture, but this is generally followed by recurrence.

Sebaceous Cyst

The ducts of ceruminous skin glands may be plugged or blocked for a variety of reasons. Sebaceous glands are most numerous on the face and in the midline of the trunk, and they are generally associated with hair follicles. They produce sebum, an oily material, which serves as a natural dressing for the hair and skin. If the exit of sebum is blocked, the material accumulates and a cyst is formed. The lesions, which are lined with glandular epithelium and surrounded by an area of compression fibrosis, gradually increase in size. They are usually painless and nontender but may become secondarily infected.

If infection is present, incision and drainage should be

performed followed by planned excision of the cyst as a second stage after the infection has totally disappeared. In the case of noninfected cysts, surgical excision of the entire cyst is indicated to prevent recurrence.

Dermoid Cyst

This is usually a congenital lesion which does not manifest itself until later in life. The dermoid cyst can be differentiated clinically from the sebaceous cyst in that it is cystic on palpation and does not exhibit a dimple or scar in the overlying skin. Dermoid cysts generally occur in the midline of the body, on the scalp over the occiput, on the nose, and in the abdominal, and sacral regions. They are considered to be occlusion cysts, taking their origin from an embryonic process. Although it has been suggested that malignant degeneration may occur, Conway indicates that no authentic case has been reported. Surgical excision is the treatment of choice.

Pilonidal Cyst and Sinus

These are common malformations which occur over the sacrococcygeal region. Their origin is associated with the neurenteric canal, and it is thought that their development is related to blockage of a congenital coccygeal sinus which is a vestige of this canal. This is substantiated by evidence that some of the pilonidal cysts and sinuses result from penetration of local skin by growing hairs. The ingrowth of such hairs sets the stage for cyst formation and repeated infection. The lesions may often be present from birth but are usually not manifest until the late adolescent or early adult years. The disease has been referred to as "jeep-driver's disease," and it is thought that the bumpy driving merely aggravates a congenital condition. Histologically, both the cysts and sinuses are lined with the stratified squamous epithelium.

The clinical manifestations vary from a barely perceptible dimple at the superior end of the buttock crease to an obvious sinus tract or cyst at this site. The sinus may chronically drain or become infected. The cyst also gradually increases in size and is susceptible to secondary infection. There have been rare reports of escape of cerebrospinal fluid from the pilonidal sinuses and equally rare instances of meningitis resulting.

TREATMENT. If the cyst is acutely infected, tender, and erythematous, incision and drainage are indicated. Secondary removal of the cyst or sinus is then planned after the infection has subsided. Elective surgical removal must be complete, and methylene blue may be injected as a guide to determine the extent of arborization of the sinus tract. Following excision of the sinus, closure may be accomplished either primarily or by granulation. If there is any infection, it is preferable to leave the wound open and allow it to heal by secondary intention. Primary closure incorporates fascial flaps, and a great variety of techniques are directed at moving the scar from the midline. In some instances, a very thin split-thickness graft (0.005 to 0.008 in.) may be used to achieve early closure and still permit the desirable contracture of the wound which accompanies the open technique.

BENIGN TUMORS

Warts

The common wart, or verruca vulgaris, is caused by a filterable virus and is both contagious and autoinoculable. Lesions may occur on any part of the body but are most common on the hand and the soles of the feet. They appear as circumscribed intraepidermal tumors which may be elevated or flat. Verruca plantaris (plantar wart) is the most troublesome variety and is located on the soles of the feet in the region of the metatarsal heads or over the os calcis. These warts may become quite tender and painful.

Verruca vulgaris may be treated by a variety of simple methods including caustic agents and x-ray therapy. In general, however, electrodesiccation under local anesthesia is the best primary treatment. Surgical treatment has been somewhat disappointing in view of the infectious nature of the lesion and the incidence of recurrence. The symptoms of plantar warts may be relieved by using pads to remove direct weight bearing from the wart area. Chemotherapy and surgical paring have also been used, and injection of local anesthesia into the base of the wart has achieved some success. It is difficult to evaluate therapy of these lesions, since the clinical course is extremely variable and spontaneous disappearance, formation of daughter warts, and recurrence challenge conclusions.

Keratosis

This represents hypertrophy of the epidermis and is considered a precancerous lesion. Clinical classification includes senile keratosis, arsenical keratosis, and seborrheic keratosis.

Senile keratosis develops most commonly in individuals with fair complexion and characteristically presents as multiple lesions in the sixth, seventh, and eighth decades. Lesions suspected of being malignant should be treated by surgical excision, since other methods of therapy which may be applied, including trichloracetic acid, electrodessication, and x-ray, all deny microscopic evaluation.

Seborrheic keratosis (Fig. 14-1) develops in middle-aged or older people as multiple lesions occurring chiefly on the trunk. They appear as thickened areas and may be yellow, gray, brown, or black. They are often great in number and may be confluent. The darker lesions have been mistaken for melanotic tumors. Histologically, they may be differentiated from senile keratoses, and they generally remain benign, though occasionally they may develop into basal cell carcinoma or, more rarely, squamous cell carcinoma. Treatment is usually conservative, employing electrocoagulation and curettage, but any rapid increase in size in indication for surgical excision.

Keloid

The term is derived from the Greek work meaning "crab's claw" and refers to a dense accumulation of fibrous tissue which extends above the surface of the skin and also

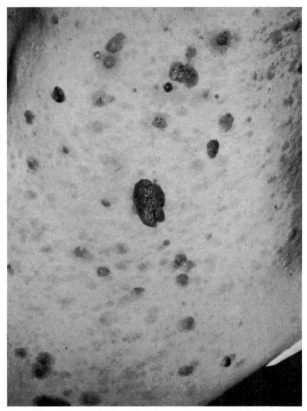

Fig. 14-1. Seborrheic keratosis: pigmented, greasy lesions which, when solitary, may be mistaken for melanotic tumors.

circumferentially in areas which were originally traumatized or incised and sutured. The color may vary from red to pink to white, and the lesion is notorious for its recurrence following surgical excision. There is an increased incidence in Negroes and dark-haired Caucasians and a predilection for the lesions to occur on the face, neck, and skin over the sternum.

Treatment consists of excision with closure. In order to reduce the amount of foreign body reaction, sutures should not be left buried. Radiation therapy has been applied with some success, but the use of corticotropins is the most efficacious method of preventing recurrence.

Vascular Tumors

CAPILLARY (PORT WINE) HEMANGIOMA

The lesion is made up of closely packed, dilated abnormal capillaries in the subpapillary, dermal, or subdermal region of the skin. Clinically, there is no elevation or contour change but rather a reddish or purplish patch of staining. Growth parallels that of the involved area. If the lesion is small, it may be treated by excision and closure with excellent results. Larger lesions, however, are most difficult to treat, since the entire dermis is involved and excision results in a contour defect and scar. The discoloration may be modified by tattooing, but repeated proce-

dures are neccessary, since the pigment is absorbed. Tattooing followed by the application of cosmetic preparations achieves the best approximation of normal skin color.

IMMATURE HEMANGIOMA (STRAWBERRY MARK) (Fig. 14-2)

This appears in infancy and undergoes a remarkable change with the growth of the child. The lesion generally enlarges, sometimes quite dramatically, during the first several months to 1 year, subsequent to which spontaneous regression usually occurs. Clinically, immature hemangiomas are raised and irregular, with some bright-red areas. They are compressible and may show superficial areas of opacity suggesting the beginning of regression. Regression takes the form of increasing opacity and whitening of the surface with progressive thickening and flattening. The hemangioma may become ulcerated if it is in an area subjected to trauma, but hemorrhage from these lesions is not common and is generally readily controlled by pressure. Such episodes of ulceration, minor hemorrhage, or superficial infection may actually hasten spontaneous resolution. Treatment in large part consists of reassuring the parents, and indications for surgical treatment, radiation, sclerosing agents, and local freezing and diminishing.

CAVERNOUS HEMANGIOMA

The lesions are full-sized in proportion to the child at birth and do not undergo changes with rapid growth or spontaneous regression. They consist of mature vessels and may include multiple arteriovenous communications. Cavernous hemangiomas frequently involve deep tissues, such as muscles and even the central nervous system. They may also be combined with lymphangiomatous elements. Rapidly growing tumors in childhood stop expanding or regress on a prednisone regimen. Treatment of established lesions is by wide surgical excision depending on the area of location.

SCLEROSING HEMANGIOMA

This is actually a subepidermal nodular fibrosis which occurs chiefly on the extremities and is related to trauma. It presents as a small nonpainful nodule, and the overlying epidermis may be pigmented in such a manner that the lesion is often mistaken for malignant melanoma. The treatment is surgical excision.

GLOMUS TUMOR

The glomus tumor is a benign, rare, and exquisitely painful small neoplasm of the skin and subcutaneous tissue occurring usually on the extremities and particularly in the nail beds of the hands and feet. The tumor is derived from the glomic end organ apparatus consisting of arteriovenous anastomoses which function normally to regulate the blood flow in the extremity. The organ contributes to the regulation of local and general body temperature through the dissipation or conservation of heat.

The tumors vary in structure but resemble the normal glomus unit and have often been referred to as *angio-*

myoneuroma. The layers of circular muscle of the vessels may be separated from the endothelium by collagenous membrane, or the endothelium may be bordered directly by the so-called "glomus epithelioid" cells. In some tumors, the blood vessels are so enlarged that they resemble true angiomas. The glomus cells are supplied by nonmyelinated nerve fibers, which account for the painful nature of the lesion. Although the tumor per se is benign, a malignant counterpart exists and is referred to as a *hemangiopericytoma*.

The lesion is usually single, but multicentric origin has been reported. The color varies from deep red to purple or blue, and there is variation in color with changes in temperature. The patients usually present in the fifth decade, but the tumor has been reported at all ages. The pain associated with the lesion is the most prominent symptom and may occur either spontaneously, with pressure, or in association with trauma. The pain, which is described as stabbing, lancinating, and radiating from the tumor, may be intermittent in character or may occur only when the lesion is touched. The glomus tumor is radioresistant, and wide excision is indicated for immediate and permanent relief.

LYMPHANGIOMA

Lymphangiomas, like hemangiomas, are congenital in origin. The most common type is deep and cavernous, consisting of lymph-filled spaces with thin-walled septums and some areas of fibrosis. A superficial variant presents as circumscribed lesions which appear as small blisters and slightly elevated skin patches. When deep lesions are present in the neck, mediastinum, and axilla, they are referred to as *cystic hygroma* (see Chap. 39). The treatment is surgical excision which, although frequently incomplete, is rarely associated with recurrence.

Fat Tumors

LIPOMA

This is an extremely common subcutaneous lesion which is composed of fat and is, at times, difficult to distinguish from the normal subcutaneous adipose tissue. Usually, however, there is a thin, fibrous capsule, and the lesion can be enucleated from surrounding normal fat. Benign lipomas occur more frequently over the back, between the shoulders, and on the back of the neck, and liposarcomatous transformation is extremely uncommon. Treatment is surgical excision.

WEBER-CHRISTIAN DISEASE

This is an uncommon inflammatory lesion of the subcutaneous fat characterized by painful reddened areas involving the panniculus. The diagnosis is made by biopsy and is based on the presence of inflammatory cells in the adipose tissue. Recently, it has been demonstrated that many of the lesions which were so classified represented facticial dermatitis or skin manifestations of fat necrosis associated with pancreatitis.

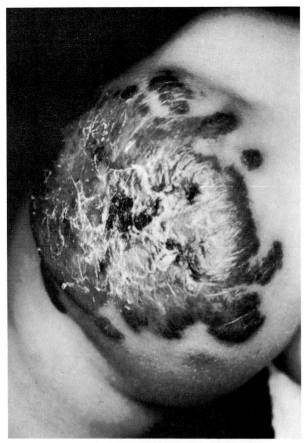

Fig. 14-2. Immature hemangioma (strawberry mark). Note opacification in the center. Lesion is undergoing spontaneous resolution.

Neuromas

These benign tumors involving the nerve tissue may be classified as neurilemmomas when the lesion arises from the sheath cell of Schwann or neurofibroma in which there are subcutaneous masses of neurofibromatous tissue. Neurilemmomas frequently arise from relatively small nerves and do not produce much pain. Treatment is surgical excision. Neurofibromas may be multiple and may be associated with von Recklinghausen's disease, including café au lait spots and scoliosis. Patients with neurofibromatosis are prone to develop meningiomas, gliomas, and pheochromocytomas, and eventual sarcomatous degeneration occurs in approximately 10 percent.

MALIGNANT TUMORS

Carcinoma of the skin occurs predominantly in exposed areas, most frequently in the weather-beaten skin of the aging sailor or farmer. It is generally a low-grade malignant tumor which may metastasize late, in which case the metastasis is usually to regional lymph nodes, so that curability is high compared with that of other tumors.

Basal Cell Carcinoma

This is a localized malignancy which grows slowly, at times taking 1 or more years to double in area. Basal cell carcinoma is more common than the squamous cell tumor, accounting for at least three-fourths of all cases in most clinical series. Lesions may be found over most areas of the body and are waxy, grayish yellow, or pink, often with telangiectasia below the surface. There is a predilection for the head and neck. In some instances, the tumors are darkly pigmented and difficult to distinguish from melanoma (Fig. 14-3). The lesions are firm but not indurated, and there is little sign of inflammation. As growth progresses, the skin is stretched, and the center of the lesion tends to necrose, resulting eventually in a flat ulcer. Basal carcinoma may extend deeper subcutaneously than is initially apparent, and extensive ulceration into the deep tissue without marked induration or infiltration has been referred to as *rodent ulcer*. If the tumor is not treated, it may erode into the deep structures including the skull, orbit, or brain. Less commonly, basal cell carcinoma may appear fungoid and grow large externally.

Squamous Cell Carcinoma

Squamous cell carcinoma tends to be more clearly defined than basal cell carcinoma. It grows more rapidly and may achieve in weeks the same size that the basal cell carcinoma reaches in months or years. Differential diagnosis between basal cell and squamous cell carcinoma can usually be made on the basis of site, appearance, history, type of skin, and presence of scars. However, only biopsy provides an accurate diagnosis.

The primary lesion of the squamous cell carcinoma is frequently surrounded by satellite nodules, and central ulceration may occur. The degree of induration around the lesion is significant. The center gradually deepens into a crater with an irregular base which is covered by crust. Small pearls may be expressed from the ulcer, and rolled margins surrounding the ulcer contribute to the lesion's resembling a small volcanic crater. Growth may be superficial, or the lesion may burrow into deeper tissue with

Fig. 14-3. Pigmented basal cell carcinoma. Note characteristics of melanotic tumor.

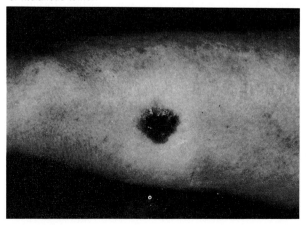

minimal effect on the cutaneous surface. Squamous cell carcinoma is more malignant than the basal cell variety and will metastasize to regional glands more rapidly.

Squamous cell carcinoma is particularly common in the lip at the vermillion border and in the folds of the paranasal area or in the axilla. Lesions occur more frequently in blond individuals with thin dry skin which is subjected to frequent irritation by rubbing or shaving. Squamous cell carcinoma is also particularly likely to originate in papillomas, senile warts, or cutaneous horns and develops at the site of postradiation dermatitis. The incidence is also higher in people exposed to arsenicals, nitrates, and hydrocarbons.

Sweat Gland Carcinoma

This rare tumor usually occurs in the sixth and seventh decades of life, but it has been reported in adolescents. Characteristically, a soft tissue mass has been present for many years. Therapy consists of wide local excision with consideration of lymphadenectomy, since regional lymph nodes are involved in about half the cases. Following treatment, the reported 5-year survival is 38 percent for all patients and 24 percent for those with lymph node involvement.

TREATMENT OF CARCINOMA. Both electrodesiccation and electrocoagulation have been used but are to be condemned, since they destroy more tissue than is needed, result in retardation of healing, and do not provide a diagnosis. Radiation therapy may afford good results in the treatment of basal cell carcinoma, whereas squamous cell carcinomas are generally more resistant.

Although there is wide disagreement, surgical excision generally shows rates of cure which are higher than those for radiation. The results of radiation are certainly not as good for basal cell carcinomas over 2 cm in diameter as those achieved with surgical excision. Radiation therapy is contraindicated for any lesion which has recurred following unsuccessful radiation or for lesions which have developed in tissue which has been scarred following burns, keratoses, or xeroderma pigmentosum.

Mohs has used an escharotic preparation which is applied to the surface of the skin; 24 hours later the area fixed by the preparation is removed and examined microscopically. From this evidence, decision is made as to the requirements for additional application. The procedure is repeated until marginal biopsy shows only healthy tissue. The advantage of this method is the possibility of eradicating small extensions of the central lesion with certainty, and the granulation tissue below the lesion heals rapidly. Mohs has achieved 93 percent cures for carcinoma of the skin in all locations on the surface of the body and 87.5 percent cures for carcinoma of the lip. Few surgeons have utilized this technique.

Surgical treatment for carcinoma of the skin should include complete excision of all malignant tissue and a sufficient margin of normal tissue. For smaller tumors, a margin of 0.5 cm laterally and in depth is usually sufficient, whereas for larger lesions, the margins must be significantly greater. Many of the larger lesions require planned reconstructive surgical procedures, frequently employing skin grafts. Prophylactic dissection of regional nodes is not practical and should be performed only if there is evidence of clinical involvement.

PROGNOSIS. This is difficult to evaluate, but recurrence rates are very low. Overall 5-year survival rates of 96 percent for basal cell carcinoma and 80 percent for squamous cell carcinoma have been reported. Sharp and Binkley reported on 983 cutaneous carcinomas of all types and found that a 14 percent recurrence rate followed surgical treatment, while 10 percent recurred following roentgen therapy and 17 percent following radium therapy. In contrast, Conway reported only one recurrence in 168 cases of basal cell carcinoma treated surgically as compared with a 7.2 percent recurrence rate following roentgen therapy.

Other Malignant Tumors

Since the skin has a mesodermal origin, it is logical that sarcomas should develop, and the skin represents the site of origin of 6 percent of all cases of sarcoma. Primary sarcomas vary in degree of malignancy and in histologic characteristics. Excision is associated with an overall incidence of recurrence of 61 percent.

FIBROSARCOMA

This occurs most commonly in women in the buttocks, thigh, and inguinal regions and particularly frequently in scars. The tumors are usually of relatively low-grade malignancy and are radioresistant. Wide surgical excision is the treatment of choice, but it is followed by a high incidence of recurrence. In one series, 56 percent survived 5 years without recurrence.

HEMANGIOPERICYTOMA

This is a malignant tumor of angioplastic origin and is considered a malignant variant of the glomus tumor. The lesions are extremely malignant, and the prognosis is poor, with only 27 percent surviving 5 years without evidence of disease. Surgical excision has proved unsatisfactory for larger tumors, and x-ray therapy is considered the treatment of choice.

KAPOSI'S SARCOMA

The etiology and pathogenesis of this lesion have not been resolved. It occurs more commonly in men. In Western countries there is a predilection for Jews, Italians, and Prussians. The tumor is prevalent in equatorial Africa and constitutes 9 percent of malignant tumors in Uganda. The tumor usually starts in the hands or feet as multiple plaques which are reddish to purple and may be flat, ulcerated, or polypoid. The lymph nodes may be involved and obstruction of the lymph nodes may result in lymphedema.

X-ray may retard the growth of the lesion, but wide surgical excision and, at times, amputation offer more promise. Patients with florid lesions respond well to actinomycin D (dactinomycin). The prognosis is poor, although some cases have survived for prolonged periods of time. In the terminal stages, the tumor extends to the mucous membranes and portions of the gastrointestinal tract.

OTHER SARCOMAS

A wide variety of other tumors having origin in different cells have been described. Dermatofibrosarcoma protuberans represents one tumor with relatively low-grade malignancy which generally occurs on the trunk. The tumors are radioresistant but respond to surgical excision, and 70 percent have been reported to be free of the disease for at least 5 years. Widespread dissemination is rare, but local recurrence may occur repeatedly.

Lymphangiosarcoma is almost always associated with chronic lymphedema. A recent review included 186 cases; 162 cases occurred postmastectomy an average of 10 years after surgery, with a range of 1 to 26 years. All patients had had radical mastectomy, and the overwhelming majority had received postoperative irradiation. Only 9 percent of the patients survived 5 or more years, and only 2 of 24 patients with nonpostmastectomy lymphangiosarcoma were alive at 5-year follow-up. Amputation gave significantly better results than radiation therapy.

MELANOMA AND OTHER PIGMENTED LESIONS

General Consideration

Since melanoma is a relatively uncommon disease, occurring in 0.0018 percent of the general population, while the average Caucasian adult has 15 to 20 nevi, it is obvious that removal of all moles is not advisable. On the other hand, about 25 percent of patients who have malignant melanoma recall having had a "mole" at the site of origin of the malignant lesion. Therefore, in dealing with pigmented lesions, the surgeon must be aware of characteristics which should arouse suspicion of malignancy or premalignancy.

Several pertinent facts regarding the predilection for malignant melanoma aid in the evaluation of pigmented lesions of the skin. Melanoma is rare before puberty. Females and males are affected with equal frequency. The lesions tend to occur in people with fair skin. The type of mole is important in assessing the likelihood of development of melanoma. The junctional nevus, either alone or as part of a compound nevus, has been implicated more frequently than the pure intradermal nevus. The blue nevus is rarely the source of melanoma, and the development of malignancy in the small congenital hairy nevus is even more unusual. The incidence of malignant melanoma in giant pigmented nevi has been reported as 10 to 17.5 percent. Nevi of the palms, soles, nail beds, genitalia, and mucous membranes retain functional elements that are more prone to be the source of melanoma than moles at other sites. The ratio of the number of moles at this site to melanoma substantiates this notion. There is probably a genetic predilection for the development of melanoma as evidenced by the studies of Harnly, who has created a strain of flies in which melanotic tumors develop spontaneously. Kassel et al. have also induced melanotic cancer in *Drosophila,* using as extract of human tumors.

Many theories concerning pigmented lesions that enjoyed acceptance in the past have recently proved to be unfounded. MacDonald has shown that there is probably no difference in incidence among races. It is also untrue that melanoma occurs more frequently in areas of highest total sunlight. Although endocrine dysfunction is related to pigmentation in Addison's disease, Cushing's syndrome, thyrotoxicosis, and diabetes, there is no relationship to the development of malignant melanoma. Castration, adrenalectomy, hypophysectomy, and hormone therapy have all failed to alter the course of metatastic melanoma. White and George et al. have recently refuted the notion that pregnancy adversely affects survival in women with melanoma. Repeated trauma and its role in malignant transformation of moles remains theoretic and unproved.

Benign Pigmented Lesions

These include the intradermal nevus, or common mole, the junctional nevus, compound nevus, juvenile melanoma, and freckles. The *intradermal nevus* is characterized by nests of melanoblasts which are confined to the dermis. The lesions are smooth or papillary and rarely occur on the soles or palms. The presence of hair is strong presumptive evidence of the diagnosis. In the case of the *junctional nevus,* the proliferation of melanoblasts originates in the basal layer of the epidermis and extends down into the dermis. The lesions are smooth, flat, or slightly raised. They occur on the genitalia, soles, palms, nail beds, and mucous membranes. The *compound nevus* is formed from junctional and intradermal elements. It is smooth, elevated, occasionally papillary, and hairless. *Juvenile melanomas* are nevi which occur prior to puberty, and although the microscopic picture is similar to that of melanoma, the lesions are clinically benign. They may be purplish red, brown, or black; they are generally smooth and hairless with irregular edges. The majority occur on the face and enlarge slowly. *Freckles* occur most commonly in blond and red-headed people on exposed portions of their bodies and represent pigment in the basal layer and upper dermis. They are not of clinical significance.

Fig. 14-4. Typical malignant melanoma. Note central darkly pigmented elevation and surrounding halo of superficial satellite extensions. Sudden change in appearance and growth brought the patient to his physician.

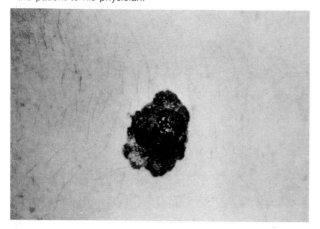

DIFFERENTIAL DIAGNOSIS. Although the classic mole has a characteristic appearance, the differential between benign pigmented skin lesions and melanoma may be quite difficult. Other lesions which cause particular confusion are (1) seborrheic and senile keratoses (Fig. 14-1) and (2) pigmented basal cell tumors (Fig. 14-3). Small intradermal hematomas may have an appearance similar to melanomas, and subungual hematomas have been mistaken for melanomas. High-speed dental drills may force silver fillings into the buccal mucosa, and the appearance mimics that of melanoma.

TREATMENT. If the pigmented lesion is considered to be a junctional nevus, excision is advisable. Various characteristics of any pigmented lesions are indications for excision. These include change in color or pigment distribution; development of erythema; change in size or consistency; change in the surface characteristic, i.e., scaling, oozing, bleeding, crustings or erosion; subjective symptoms such as pain, numbness, burning, itching, diffusion of pigment into normal skin; satellite nodules; and regional lymphadenopathy.

The *Hutchinson freckle* (lentigo maligna) is worthy of special note. This is a circumscribed precancerous melanosis of the face, generally occurring in elderly people. There are two stages of disease: In the macular stage, the lesion is smooth and light brown with irregular borders and uneven color. About one-third of the lesions then evolve into a tumor stage characterized by induration and all the histologic features of melanoma, but the behavior is not like melanoma. The prognosis is excellent when the lesion is excised from the face, but it is guarded when the lesion is found in other body areas, in which case it should be treated as a melanoma.

Excision of any suspicious lesion should be complete and should include a margin of normal skin.

Melanoma

The term, by definition, refers to a malignant lesion originating in the melanoblast of the skin, and therefore "malignant melanoma" represents a redundancy. The tumor may develop in any area of the skin or in the pigmented region of the eye. There is an almost equal distribution between the head and neck, lower extremity, and trunk, each accounting for approximately 25 percent of the cases. About 11 percent occur in the upper extremity, and the remainder involve the genitalia or represent cases in which the primary lesion is never determined. The typical skin lesion (Fig. 14-4) is darkly pigmented, smooth, firm, and nonhairy. Subungual melanomas are more frequent than pigmented nevi in the nail beds and may present difficulty in reference to differentiation from subungual hematoma and chronic paronychial infection (Fig. 14-5). All melanomas originate from the melanoblast at the dermal-epidermal junction, but the cell does not contain melanin at all times; therefore some lesions may not be darkly pigmented. The cells are characterized by a dopa-positive reaction.

TREATMENT. Incisional biopsy is performed only when the lesion is extremely large. Biopsy provides the definitive diagnosis and should indicate the depth of involvement.

When invasion does not extend beyond the papillary dermis, wide excision including the underlying fascia is generally sufficient. Inadequate excision has been associated with the development of satellite nodules (Fig. 14-6). When the tumor extends below the papillary dermis, a more aggressive approach is indicated.

The major argument in therapy centers around removal of the regional lymph nodes. Some advocate removing these nodes only when they are involved clinically, since there is significant morbidity associated with the procedure and statistical data do not demonstrate benefit. Others champion routine removal regardless of the clinical status in view of the accepted inaccuracy of clinical evaluation.

As a compromise, Knutson et al. recommend elective cervicofacial or axillary node dissection, in the absence of clinical involvement, for invasive lesions of the head and neck or upper extremity, since the consequent morbidity is minimal. Invasive melanomas of the trunk are treated with wide excision, and nodes are removed only if they are involved clinically, since lymphatic drainage is unpredictable. "Prophylactic" lymph node dissections generally are not advised for lower extremity lesions, since necrosis of skin flaps, delayed healing, infection, thrombophlebitis, edema, and satellitosis all contribute to a significant morbidity. The exception is a lesion which permits removal of the inguinal lymph nodes in continuity. Clinically palpable nodes should be excised (Fig. 14-7).

The appreciation of intermediate metastases between the primary tumor and regional nodes has led some writers to suggest aggressive amputation or, more recently, integumentectomy with removal of skin, subcutaneous tissue, and deep fascia from the foot to the inguinal ligament. In general, amputation is reserved for palliation of bulky, ulcerating, or painful lesions.

Groin Dissection (Fig. 14-8). The skin incision may be oblique and parallel to the inguinal ligament, or vertical, or S-shaped with an oblique limb running parallel to the inguinal ligament and the vertical limbs running parallel to the lateral margin of the rectus femoris muscles craniad and to the medial portion of the femoral triangle caudad. The oblique incision is associated with the lowest incidence of complications and delayed wound healing, since it cuts across the fewest anastomotic vessels in Camper's fascia. If the primary lesion is close to the line of incision or if the proposed skin incision is overlying a large lymph node which might be attached to the subcutaneous tissue, a wide ellipse can be removed beginning medial to the anterior superior iliac spine and continuing over the femoral triangle. The flaps are elevated by sharp dissection, and the superficial and deep inguinal dissection is begun. On the abdominal wall, the subcutaneous and fatty tissue is dissected cleanly from the aponeurosis of the external oblique down to the inguinal ligament. With genital primary melanomas, the presymphysial lymphatics and areolar tissue of the spermatic cord or round ligament must be included in the dissection. The lower flaps are retracted, the lateral margin is exposed first, and the superficial fascia and fascia lata are dissected off the bare sartorius muscle to the lateral margin of the femoral triangle. The femoral sheath is entered, and the femoral artery and vein are dissected clean of fatty tissue. The greater saphenous vein

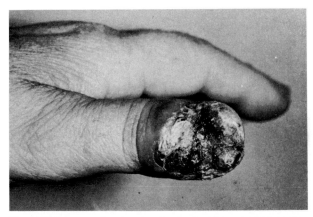

Fig. 14-5. Subungual melanoma. Lesion had been treated as an infection for nearly 1 year. Note pigmentation and replacement of nail. X-rays showed destruction of the distal phalanx. Axillary metastases were evident by this time.

is transected at two levels, first at the medial inferior portion of the transected tissue and second where the vein enters the femoral vein. Since the deep inguinal nodes lie in the areolar tissue about the femoral vessels, carrying the dissection down to the adventitial surface of the femoral artery and vein will include them in the dissected material. Mediad, the tissue is incised over the pectineus muscle, and eventually the specimen remains attached only by tissue passing into the femoral space medial to the femoral vein.

The illiac dissection represents a continuum of the inguinal dissection. The external oblique aponeurosis is incised, and a flap is established caudad down to the inguinal

Fig. 14-6. Recurrent satellite nodules. These followed inadequate excision of a malignant melanoma which was thought to be a simple nevus. Note the characteristic deep-black color and emergence of lesions from the subcutaneous tissues to and through the skin.

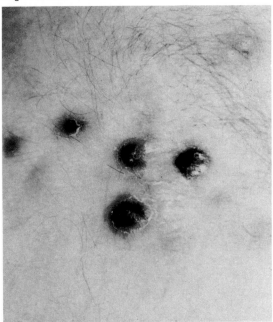

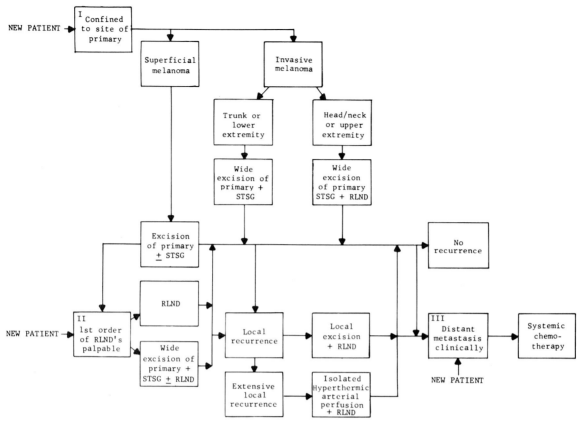

Fig. 14-7. Schematic diagram illustrating a treatment approach to melanoma patients. STSG, split-thickness skin graft; RLND, regional lymph node. (*From C. O. Knutson et al., Melanoma, Curr Probl Surg, The Year Book Medical Publishers, Inc., Chicago, December 1971.*)

ligament. The fibers of the transversus abdominis and internal oblique muscles are separated from the inguinal ligament. The ligamentous attachment of the transversalis fascia to the inguinal ligament is divided, and the epigastric artery and vein are ligated and transected at the level of the inguinal ligament. Following the division of muscle and fascial fibers along the inguinal ligament to the anterior superior iliac spine, the peritoneum is exposed and reflected from the lateral pelvic wall by blunt dissection. This permits visualization of the ureter and the iliac vessels. The endopelvic fascia is incised medial to the genitofemoral nerve from the inguinal ligament to above the bifurcation of the common iliac artery; the external iliac artery is rotated mediad, and the space between the artery and the muscle is dissected clear. The dissection then continues by reflecting the vascular sheath away from the external iliac artery and vein. The origin of the inferior epigastric arteries and veins will be exposed, and these are then transected. All the areolar tissue is swept down in a medial fashion. The medial chain of iliac lymph nodes is removed by dissection of the obturator fossa, retracting the external iliac vein laterally. In this dissection the bare muscle fibers of the internal obturator muscle are exposed, and the obturator veins must be transected. After the iliac dissection has been mobilized and freed from the margin of the inguinal-pectineal triangle, the inguinal ligament is elevated, and the iliac alveolar tissue and lymph nodes are delivered into the femoral triangle for completion of the en bloc dissection.

The lower abdominal wall is carefully reconstructed to avoid hernia formation, and the sartorius muscle transected and reflected mediad to cover the femoral artery and vein. Prior to closure of the subcutaneous tissue and skin, drainage is achieved with suction catheters.

Adjunctive Therapy. Systemic chemotherapy is used when there is recurrent or metastatic disease which precludes excision. Objective regression has been noted in about one-quarter of the patients receiving vinblastine or cyclophosphamide. Drug combinations appear promising; other effective agents include vincristine, hydroxyurea, and l-phenylalanine mustard (melphalan), BCNU (1,3-bis [2-chloroethyl]-1-nitrosourea), and DTIC (dimethyl-triazeno-imidazole-carboxamine).

Isolated regional artery perfusion with l-phenylalanine mustard or a combination of drugs has had striking results as treatment for multiple local metastases or inoperable satellitosis of an extremity. Some writers have applied perfusion as an adjunct to patients without clinical subcutaneous or cutaneous metastases. Recurrence rates lower than those associated with conventional surgical treatment have been reported. However, the complications of arterial perfusion therapy are of such magnitude as to argue against this approach, with suggestion that perfusion be withheld until recurrences are noted.

Recent attention has been directed to the host immune response. A correlation between a patient's prognosis and

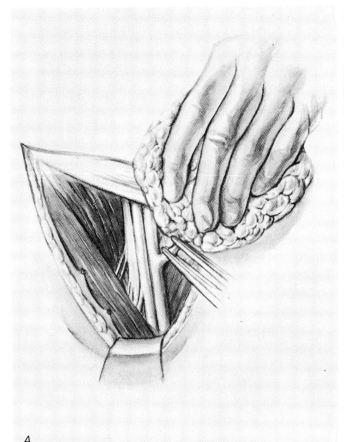

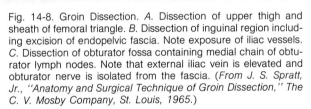

A

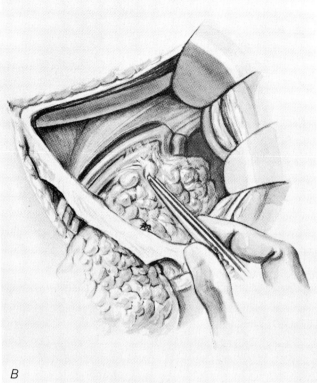

B

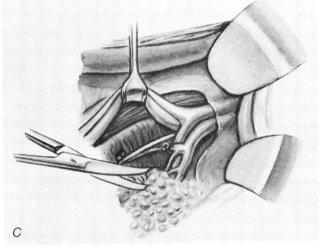

C

Fig. 14-8. Groin Dissection. *A.* Dissection of upper thigh and sheath of femoral triangle. *B.* Dissection of inguinal region including excision of endopelvic fascia. Note exposure of iliac vessels. *C.* Dissection of obturator fossa containing medial chain of obturator lymph nodes. Note that external iliac vein is elevated and obturator nerve is isolated from the fascia. *(From J. S. Spratt, Jr., "Anatomy and Surgical Technique of Groin Dissection," The C. V. Mosby Company, St. Louis, 1965.)*

his immune response to melanoma has been established. This response accounts for spontaneous regressions, which have been noted, and immunity to the tumor has been enhanced by active immunization with BCG (bacillus Calmette-Guérin) or autologous tumor cells.

PROGNOSIS. In a recent review of the Memorial Hospital (New York) experience with 1,483 cases available for follow-up, patients with grade 1 melanoma (primary melanoma only) had an overall 5-year survival of 80 percent. Patients with grade 2 (palpable regional lymph nodes) had a survival rate of 39 percent. There was a significant progressive mortality after 5 years. The data from the Ellis Fischel State Cancer Hospital are expressed as age-adjusted survivals. In a series of 230 patients, about 37 percent survived 5 years, while 30 percent lived for 10 years. The 5-year survival for women was better than that for men; this was related to the fact that the lesions in women were located in areas associated with better prognosis. Melanomas of the lower extremity had a 52 percent 5-year survival, while the 5-year survivals for the upper extremity and the trunk were 37 and 17 percent, respec-

tively. The 5-year age-adjusted survival when regional nodes were histologically positive was 27 percent, as compared to 46 percent for histologically negative nodes.

References

Physiology

Allen, A. C.: "The Skin: A Clinicopathological Treatise," 2d ed., Grune & Stratton, Inc., New York, 1967.

Ellis, H., and Morgan, M. N.: Surgical Treatment of Severe Hyperidrosis, *Proc Roy Soc Med,* **64:**768, 1971.

Harris, J. D., and Japson, R. P.: Essential Hyperhidrosis, *Med J Aust,* **2:**135, 1971.

Rothman, S.: "Physiology and Biochemistry of the Skin," The University of Chicago Press, Chicago, 1954.

Pressure Sores

Herceg, S. J., and Harding, R. L.: Surgical Treatment of Pressure Sores, *Pa Med,* **74:**45, 1971.

Hidradenitis Suppurative

Conway, H., Stark, R. B., Climo, S., Weeter, J. C., and Garcia, F. A.: The Surgical Treatment of Chronic Hidradenitis Suppurativa, *Surg Gynecol Obstet,* **95:**455, 1952.

Knaysi, G. A., Jr., Cosman, B., and Crikelair, G. F.: Hidradenitis Suppurativa, *JAMA,* **203:**19, 1968.

Cysts and Benign Tumors

Brasfield, R. D., and Das Gupta, T. K.: Von Recklinghausen's Disease: A Clinicopathological Study, *Ann Surg,* **175:**86, 1972.

Brown, S. H., Jr., Neerhout, R. C., and Fonkalsrud, E. W.: Prednisone Therapy in Management of Large Hemangiomas in Infants and Children, *Surgery,* **71:**168, 1972.

Conway, H.: "Tumors of the Skin," Charles C Thomas, Publisher, Springfield, Ill., 1956.

Dwight, R. W., and Maloy, J. K.: Pilonidal Sinus: Experience with 449 Cases, *N Engl J Med,* **249:**926, 1953.

Hvid-Hansen, O.: Treatment of Ganglions, *Acta Chir Scand,* **136:**471, 1970.

Mandel, S. R., and Thomas, C. C., Jr.: Management of Pilonidal Sinus by Excision and Primary Closure, *Surg Gynecol Obstet,* **134:**448, 1972.

Riveros, M., and Pack, G. T.: The Glomus Tumor: Report of Twenty Cases, *Ann Surg,* **133:**394, 1951.

Strahan, J., and Bailie, H. W. C.: Glomus Tumor: A Review of 15 Clinical Cases, *Br J Surg,* **59:**91, 1972.

Malignant Tumors

Ackerman, L. V.: "Surgical Pathology," The C. V. Mosby Company, St. Louis, 1964.

Conway, H.: "Tumors of the Skin," Charles C Thomas, Publisher, Springfield, Ill., 1956.

De Cholnoky, T.: Cancer of the Face: A Clinical and Statistical Study of 1062 Cases, *Ann Surg,* **122:**88, 1945.

El-Domeiri, A. A., Brasfield, R. D., Huvos, A. G., and Strong, E. W.: Sweat Gland Carcinoma, *Ann Surg,* **173:**270, 1971.

Epstein, E.: Sarcoma Involving the Skin, *Arch Dermatol,* **60:**1130, 1949.

Mohs, F. E.: "Chemosurgery in Cancer, Gangrene and Infections," Charles C Thomas Publisher, Springfield, Ill., 1956.

Pack, G. T.: End Results in the Treatment of Sarcomata of the Soft Somatic Tissues, *J Bone Joint Surg,* [Am], **36A:**241, 1954.

Paterson, R.: "The Treatment of Malignant Disease by Radium and X-rays, Being a Practice of Radiotherapy," Edward Arnold (Publishers) Ltd., London, 1948.

Sharp, G. S., and Binkley, F. C.: The Treatment of Carcinoma of the Skin, *Am J Roentgenol Radium Ther Nucl Med,* **67:**606, 1952.

Vogel, C. L., Templeton, C. J., Templeton, A. C., Taylor, J. F., and Kyalwazi, S. K.: Treatment of Kaposi's Sarcoma with Actinomycin-D and Cyclophosphamide: Results of a Randomized Clinical Trial, *Int J Cancer,* **8:**136, 1971.

Woodward, A. H., Ivins, J. C., and Soule, E. H.: Lymphangiosarcoma Arising in Chronic Lymphedematous Extremities, *Cancer,* **30:**562, 1972.

Melanoma and Other Pigmented Lesions

Allen, A. C., and Spitz, S.: Malignant Melanoma: A Clinicopathological Analysis of Criteria for Diagnosis and Prognosis, *Cancer,* **6:**1, 1953.

Daland, E.: Malignant Melanoma: Personal Experience with 170 Cases, *N Engl J Med,* **260:**453, 1959.

George, P. A., Fortner, J. G., and Pack, G. T.: Melanoma with Pregnancy: A Report of 115 Cases, *Cancer,* **13:**854, 1960.

Goldsmith, H. S., Shah, J. P., Kim, D. H.: Prognostic Significance of Lymph Node Dissection in Treatment of Malignant Melanoma, *Cancer,* **26:**606, 1970.

Greeley, P. W., Middleton, A. G., and Curtin, J. W.: Incidence of Malignancy in Giant Pigmented Nevi, *Plastic Reconstr Surg,* **36:**26, 1965.

Harnly, M. H.: Induced Hereditary Change in *Drosophila* by Injected Extracts of Neoplastic Flies, Mice or Humans, *Ann NY Acad Sci,* **100:**817, 1963.

Hueston, J. T.: Integumentectomy for Malignant Melanoma of the Limbs, *Aust NZ J Surg,* **40:**114, 1970.

Kassel, R., Burton, L., and Friedman, F.: Utilization of an Induced *Drosophila* Melanoma in the Study of Mammalian Neoplasia, *Ann NY Acad Sci,* **100:**791, 1963.

Knutson, C. O., Hori, J. M., and Spratt, J. S., Jr.: Melanoma, *Curr Probl Surg,* December, 1971.

Krementz, E. T., Creech, O., Ryan, R., and Reemtsma, K.: An Appraisal of Cancer Chemotherapy by Regional Perfusion, *Ann Surg,* **156:**417, 1962.

McBride, C. M.: Advanced Melanoma of the Extremities, *Arch Surg,* **101:**122, 1970.

MacDonald, E. J.: Epidemiology of Melanoma, *Ann NY Acad Sci* **100:**4, 1963.

Morton, D. L., Frederick, R. W., Joseph, W. L., Wood, W. C., Trahan, E., and Ketcham, A. S.: Immunological Factors in Human Sarcomas and Melanomas: A Rational Basis of Immunotherapy, *Ann Surg,* **172:**740, 1970.

Pack, G. T., and Davis, J.: Nevus Giganticus Pigmentosus with Malignant Transformation, *Surgery,* **49:**347, 1961.

Polk, H. C., Cohn, J. D., and Clarkson, J. G.: An Appraisal of Elective Regional Lymphadenectomy for Melanoma, in G. D. Zuidema and D. B. Skinner (eds.), "Current Topics in Surgical Research," vol. 1, Academic Press, Inc., New York, 1969.

Raven, R. W.: The Clinicopathological Aspects of Malignant Melanoma, *Ann NY Acad Sci,* **100:**142, 1963.

Spratt, J. S., Jr., Shieber, W., and Dillard, B. M.: "Anatomy and Surgical Technique of Groin Dissection," The C. V. Mosby Company, St. Louis, 1965.

Summer, W. C., and Foraker, A. G.: Spontaneous Regression of Human Melanoma: Clinical and Experimental Studies, *Cancer,* **13:**79, 1960.

White, L. P.: The Role of Natural Resistance in the Prognosis of Human Melanoma, *Ann NY Acad Sci,* **100:**115, 1963.

Chapter 15

Breast

by **Benjamin F. Rush, Jr.**

Embryology

Anatomy and Development

Examination

Diseases of the Breast

Neoplasms
    Incidence
    Etiology
    Natural History
    Diagnosis and Staging
    Differential Diagnosis (Benign Lesions)
    Breast Biopsy
    Histopathology
    Primary Treatment
    Prognosis
    Treatment of Recurrent Cancer
Infection
    Acute Infection
    Chronic Infection

The breast is man's insignia of membership in the class Mammalia. It is somewhat humbling to reflect that this badge of status had its origin as a modified sweat gland. In the male the breast is, with few exceptions, a dormant structure. In the female, from puberty to death, the breast is subjected to a constant dynamic role of physical changes related to the menstrual cycle, pregnancy, lactation, and the menopause. Associated with this active role are numerous malformations and dysfunctions which make diseases of the breast common clinical problems.

EMBRYOLOGY

The human breast makes its first appearance in the sixth week of embryonic development as an ectodermal thickening extending from the axilla to the groin, a distinct linear elevation called the *mammary ridge,* or *milk line.* Lens-shaped thickenings appear along the milk line, presaging the sites of developing breasts. In man the caudal two-thirds of the line disappears rapidly, and the pectoral thickening progresses with the ultimate formation of a breast primordium. Man shares this pectoral location of the breasts with other primates and with the elephant and sea cow, in contrast to the multiple breasts of the dog and pig and the inguinal location in the cow, goat, and whale.

In the fifth month of embryonic development the human primordial breast develops 15 to 20 solid cords which fan out beneath the skin in the underlying connective tissue. These primary milk ducts branch, and the ends develop club-shaped dilatations. During the seventh or eighth month the ducts hollow to develop lumina. During this same period the point in the skin corresponding to the nipple develops a small depression. At birth the breast is represented by a slight pit pierced by 15 to 20 openings into the primary milk ducts. The areola is a slight thickening in the skin which contains a few glands (of Montgomery). Shortly after birth the nipples become everted, and the areola is distinguished by a slight increase in pigmentation.

A few days after birth, bilateral or unilateral enlargement of the breast occurs in 70 percent of infants. In half the infants the swelling is accompanied by the secretion of a cloudy fluid similar to colostrum, the "witch's milk" of folklore. Histologically, these changes are associated with hypertrophy of the duct system, the appearance of acini, and an increased vascularity of the stroma. These alterations are considered an indirect effect of the high level of maternal estrogens in the infant's circulating blood. Following birth the falling estrogen level stimulates the hypophysis to produce prolactin, resulting in the mammary changes. These changes occur equally in male and female infants and regress spontaneously by the second or third week of life. Attempts to strip the breasts of their milk, as advocated by some superstitions, provoke the breasts to remain in the secretory state. Hyperplasia of the infant breast persisting over many months with persistent secretions has resulted from such manipulations.

CLINICAL CORRELATIONS. A number of developmental errors of the breast are of clinical importance. Most often observed is the persistence of one or more of the additional nipples in the milk line. These are commonly mistaken for moles. A rare anomaly is the occurrence of extramammary breast tissue, usually seen in the axilla or over the upper abdomen (Fig. 15-1), often not appearing until the tissue is stimulated by pregnancy and lactation. Excision of these supernumerary structures is the treatment of choice. Absence of one or both nipples or of one or both breasts also occurs, though rarely. While these conditions are serious cosmetic and functional defects, a more important functional deficiency is the often associated absence of the underlying pectoralis muscles and chest wall.

Occasionally the nipple fails to evert following birth and remains retracted or inverted throughout life. This is a

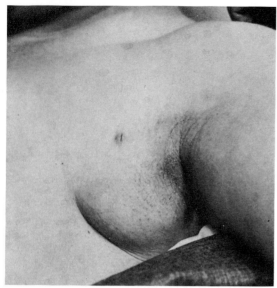

Fig. 15-1. Supernumerary breast.

serious functional problem when the patient attempts to nurse a child.

In some infants the collecting ducts fail to open onto the apex of the nipple, opening onto the areola instead. In a few instances collecting ducts are observed to empty onto the skin of the breast, failing entirely to traverse the nipple. These nippleless collecting ducts recapitulate the normal anatomy of the nippleless breast of the duckbill platypus.

ANATOMY AND DEVELOPMENT

Except for the neonatal period of hypertrophy and a period of slight hypertrophy occurring at puberty, the male breast undergoes little change throughout life. The female breast shows little change through infancy and childhood, but in the prepubertal period and throughout the remainder of life the breasts undergo numerous gross and microscopic changes (Fig. 15-2).

ADOLESCENCE. During the prepubertal period (from eleven to fifteen years) growth of the breast begins with the development of the prepubertal "bud." The areola becomes elevated and forms with the nipple a small conical protuberance. Histologically, the rudimentary primary ducts begin a rapid process of elongation and terminal branching, pushing down through the subcutaneous tissue toward the pectoral fascia and carrying with them sheaths of periductal connective tissue. A firm plaque of fibrous breast tissue forms as the lobes of the breasts develop, crowding out the subcutaneous fat. Roentgenograms of the breast at this period show a featureless, fibrous mass without trabeculae. Lobules do not form, however, until ovulation begins. Following ovulation at age fourteen to fifteen the breasts mature into their normal nulliparous form.

THE YOUNG ADULT. Anatomic Limits. The breast is suspended from the anterior chest wall, extending from the second to the sixth rib. The medial boundary is at the lateral border of the sternum, and the lateral border stretches to the anterior axillary line (Fig. 15-3).

Areola and Nipple. The areola in the young female is convex and lens-shaped, surmounted at its center by the nipple. The areola gains a slight amount of pigmentation during adolescence, and although its surface is hairless, a few hairs may appear at the skin of the periphery. Both the subareolar area and the nipple contain much smooth muscle. The fibers of the areola are arranged in concentric rings as well as radially and are inserted into the base of the dermis. They function to contract the areola and to compress the base of the nipple. The bulk of the nipple is made up of smooth muscle fibers arranged both circularly and longitudinally. The nipple is made erect, smaller, and firmer by contraction of these fibers, and this involuntary action serves to aid in emptying the intrapapillary ducts. This response is evoked by suckling or by tactile stimuli. Sir Astley Cooper, a pioneer in describing the anatomy and diseases of the breast, first pointed out that the nipple lies to the lateral side of the center line of the breast and that its axis points upward and outward. The teleologic assumption is that this arrangement is for the convenience of the suckling child.

Glandular Tissue. The functional portion of the breast is a modified cutaneous gland, an appendage of the skin. It is enclosed between the superficial and deep layers of the superficial fascia. The glandular portion of the breast spreads out widely as a layer over the chest wall beneath the integument. It is roughly circular in outline except at the upper outer quadrant, where the axillary tail of Spence extends toward the axilla (Fig. 15-3). The tip of the axillary tail intrudes through an opening in the deep fascia of the axilla, Langer's foramen, to lie well up within the axilla. Neoplasms or deformities in this tail are sometimes mistaken for enlarged axillary nodes.

Portions of the fibrous tissue of the breast parenchyma extend from the surface of the glandular breast anteriorly to intermingle with the superficial layer of the superficial fascia. Similar processes arise from the deep surface of the gland to cross the retromammary space and fuse with the pectoral fascia. The anterior ligaments were described by Cooper, who noted, "The breast is slung upon the fore part of the chest, for [the ligaments] form a movable but very firm connection with the skin so that the breast has sufficient motion."

Blood Supply and Venous Drainage. Three major arteries generously supply the breast with blood. The perforating branches of the internal mammary artery pass through the first, second, third, and fourth intercostal spaces just lateral to the sternum to penetrate and pass through the origin of the pectoralis major muscle and enter the medial edge of the breast, supplying more than 50 percent of the blood to this organ. The lateral thoracic artery arises from the axillary artery and courses down along the lateral border of the pectoralis minor muscle. Its external mammary branches provide the second largest source of blood to the breast. The third artery of importance is the pectoral branch of the acromiothoracic artery, also a branch of the axillary artery. The pectoral artery is given off by the acromiothoracic at the medial edge of the pectoralis minor muscle. In its course between the pectoralis major and minor muscles, the pectoralis artery gives off branches to the posterior surface of the breast. The superior branch of the axillary artery, the lateral perforating branches of the intercostal arteries, and branches of the subscapular artery also contribute minor amounts to the blood supply.

The mammary glands have a rich, anastomosing network of superficial subcutaneous veins. These veins become markedly dilated during pregnancy and may sometimes become quite prominent over an area of underlying neoplasm. The majority of the superficial veins drain to the internal mammary vein. In some individuals these veins drain into the superficial veins of the lower neck.

The deep veins of the mammary gland drain along routes roughly corresponding to the arterial blood supply. Thus one major route is through the anterior intercostal perforating veins to the internal mammary veins. Another is by way of multiple branches to the axillary vein. A third route is by way of posterior branches anastomosing with the intercostal veins. This last route has special significance, since the intercostal veins communicate with the vertebral veins. This anastomosis with the vertebral veins is offered by Batson as the explanation for the often capricious metastasis of mammary cancer to the vertebral bodies or even the sacrum or pelvis without the presence of metastatic deposits in the lung. He holds that the wide variation in pressure within the thoracic cavity induced by straining or coughing may change the flow patterns within the valveless anastomosing veins so that blood from the breast draining through the lateral perforators to the intercostal vessels is forced down along the vertebral plexus.

The Lymphatics. A generous lymphatic plexus drains the skin and glandular tissues of the breast (Fig. 15-4). The lymphatic vessels empty into two main depots represented by the axillary and the internal mammary lymph nodes. There are an average of 53 lymph nodes in the axillary fossa, arranged along the course of the arteries and veins. Lymph from the lower outer quadrant of the breast drains to the lateral and inferior axillary nodes, while lymph from the areola, the upper outer quadrant of the breast, and the axillary tail drains to the medial superior axillary nodes. Within the axilla, lymph passes from the lateral inferior to the medial superior nodes at the apex of the axilla. Lymph then courses through lymphatic channels under the clavicle to the supraclavicular lymph nodes and by major lymphatic trunks to the junction of the subclavian and jugular veins. On the right, lymph enters the blood directly through these lymphatic trunks as they join the veins. On the left these trunks may first join with the thoracic duct, which shortly communicates with the venous system.

The internal mammary lymph nodes are much fewer in number than the axillary nodes, averaging but three or four nodes on each side lying along the internal mammary vessels, usually in the first, second, and third interspaces. Despite the scarcity and tiny size of these lymph nodes, most of the lymph from the upper and lower inner quadrants of the breast drains by this channel. Lymph from the nipple and areola may drain to both the internal mammary and the axillary nodes. The internal mammary lym-

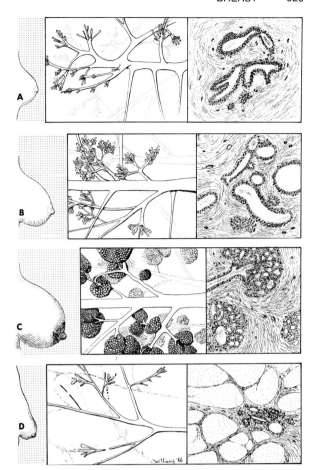

Fig. 15-2. Gross and microscopic appearance of breast at different stages of development. Central pictures show three-dimensional projection of microscopic structure. *A.* Adolescence. *B.* Pregnancy. *C.* Lactation. *D.* Postmenopausal period.

phatic trunks eventually empty into the great veins of the neck, usually by way of the thoracic duct or of the right lymphatic duct.

Histology of the Resting Mammary Gland. Each lobe of the mammary gland is an independent compound alveolar gland. The mammary gland is a conglomeration of a variable number of such independent glands, each with its own excretory duct which has its separate opening on the surface of the nipple. The excretory ducts measure from 0.4 to 0.7 mm in diameter at the nipple surface and run perpendicularly through the nipple to turn and radiate out toward the periphery of the breast. Beneath the areola they dilate into a short fusiform area called the *milk sinus.* Beyond the milk sinus the excretory ducts begin to subdivide into smaller and smaller branches forming the lobules of the lobe. Within the lobules the ducts subdivide further, forming terminal, elongated tubes, the alveolar ducts, which are covered by round evaginations, the alveolae. Lobules are peripheral and scanty in the nulliparous breast (Fig. 15-2*A*).

There is mild controversy as to whether alveolae are present in the resting mammary gland. Some claim that the resting gland is entirely a tubular structure and be-

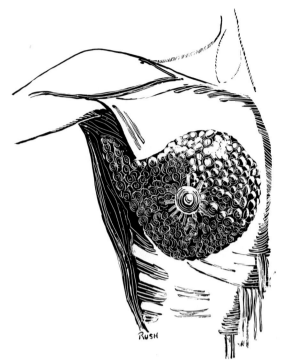

Fig. 15-3. Normal distribution of mammary tissue of adult female breast. Note long tail of Spence extending into axilla.

Fig. 15-4. Lymphatic drainage of breast. Nipple drains both laterally and mediado. Medial side of breast drains to small internal mammary lymph nodes.

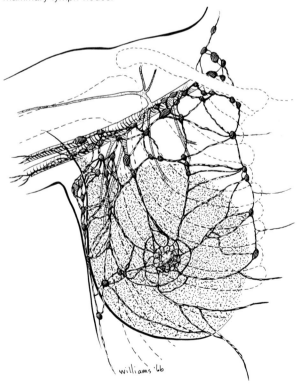

comes tuboalveolar only during pregnancy. The majority opinion is that a few alveolae are scattered through the lobules in the resting state.

The walls of the alveolae and the alveolar ducts consist of a prominent basement membrane surrounding a layer of myoepithelial cells, which in turn lie beneath a layer of low columnar glandular cells. The myoepithelial layer is thin and difficult to identify in the acini and the alveolar ducts but becomes more prominent in the more major lobular ducts. These cells take a spiral course about the larger ducts and probably play a role in propelling milk from the acini to the nipple during lactation.

The collecting ducts are lined with a double layer of cuboidal to columnar epithelium until the milk sinus is reached. Here the lining changes to squamous epithelium. This continues through the milk sinus to the surface of the nipple.

Each lobule is surrounded by a coating of dense, firm, interlobular connective tissue, which is an intimate part of the breast parenchyma. The lobules are separated by a looser coating of less dense fibrous tissue, the interlobular connective tissue. This layer represents the supporting stroma of the breast. These layers are easily recognized histologically, but grossly the various lobules are intimately and firmly bound together and cannot be dissected apart.

Cyclic Changes of the Breast. Beginning about the eighth day of the menstrual cycle the female breast gradually increases in size, the volume often increasing by 50 percent by the immediate premenstrual period. At this point the breast is tense and may be somewhat tender. Part of the increase in size is due to interlobular edema and increasing congestion of the vasculature. Ingleby and Gershon-Cohen state that there is also a proliferation of the parenchyma, with the appearance of new lobules. These lobules then regress and fibrose during menstruation. Congestion and edema subside, and the breast again reaches its smallest size on about the eighth day after the onset of menstruation.

PREGNANCY AND LACTATION. Implantation of the ovum initiates a profound change in the gross and histologic structures of the breast. Grossly there is a pronounced enlargement of the breast, progressing throughout pregnancy. The normal size may be increased as much as two or three times. The nipple and areola become more prominent and more deeply pigmented. The openings of Montgomery's glands on the areola become prominent and are called *Montgomery's tubercles.* Pigmentation may spread beyond the areola onto the skin, forming a "secondary areola." The veins are engorged, and striae are frequently visible in the skin.

Histologically, the epithelium of the lobular ducts and alveolar ducts proliferates, and new ducts covered with multiple alveolar outpouchings are generated. The total number of lobules increases greatly. By the end of the sixth month the glandular cells of the acini produce small amounts of a secretion, colostrum, which increases toward the end of pregnancy (Fig. 15-2C).

Two or three days after delivery, globules appear in the supranuclear cytoplasm of the acinar cells. These push toward the cell lumen, increasing in size. The cell becomes tall and more columnar. Finally the globule is extruded into the lumen, and the cell shrinks to a cuboidal form, to begin the process again. The acini become distended with milk, which is propelled to the nipple during nursing. This process continues as long as suckling continues. When lactation ends, the extralobular tissue involutes, leaving small areas of fibrosis, and the breast gradually returns to the resting state. It never returns to the nulliparous form, however, but has the contour of maturity. The areola recedes into the breast tissue, with only the nipple projecting. Some of the darker pigmentation of the nipple and areola and residual skin striae persist.

MENOPAUSAL CHANGES. Following menopause the mammary gland gradually involutes (Fig. 15-2D). This change is slow and progressive, with gradual disappearance of lobules. Senile involution does not lead to complete extinction of mammary tissue; some lobules always remain, but they are scattered and small. In many areas only the larger lobular and collecting ducts may be found. The parenchyma and stromal fibrous tissue gradually blend together into a homogeneous mass, and the original lobular structure is almost completely lost. As the glandular tissues recede, there is a gradual invasion of fat, which aids in maintaining the breast outline, although in very thin women the breasts may become quite flabby as glandular tissue is lost.

CLINICAL CORRELATION. Both breasts of the adolescent girl usually develop at the same pace. Occasionally development is out of phase, and one breast will develop much more rapidly than the other, leading to distressing asymmetry (Fig. 15-5). The difference in size is usually repaired with time but occasionally persists. Patients complaining of asymmetric breasts during the adolescent period are advised to wait until maturation is complete. If asymmetry persists, a plastic surgical procedure may be required to adjust the difference.

A slight swelling of the breasts is often seen in adolescent boys. This is called *gynecomastia* and is a physiologic response to the change in the hormonal milieu in the pubertal male (Fig. 15-6). This slight hypertrophy normally subsides spontaneously but occasionally persists, either unilaterally or bilaterally. Persisting gynecomastia in young manhood requires an evaluation to exclude the possibility of abnormal endocrine secretion. If no abnormalities are found, the small button of hypertrophied breast tissue may be removed surgically to repair an embarrassing cosmetic defect in a young man.

Occasionally the growth of the female breast at puberty fails to cease and the breasts become huge—so-called virginal hypertrophy (Fig. 15-7). Breasts weighing 40 to 50 lb and descending to the level of the genitalia are described. Spontaneous regression does not occur, and the only solution is plastic surgical repair. This rare defect is seen in pregnant females as well and requires the same treatment.

EXAMINATION

INSPECTION. Physical examination of the breasts should begin with the patient erect, usually sitting on the edge

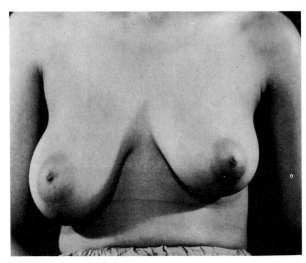

Fig. 15-5. Asymmetric breasts.

of the examining table. The breasts are observed for symmetry, dimpling of the skin, edema, deformity of outline, retraction of the nipple, or inflammation. Underlying masses will produce deformity or skin retraction, which is much more easily detected when the patient is erect and the breasts dependent. Haagensen suggests that the patient be allowed to lean forward to increase the breast dependency and further accentuate areas of deformity or dimpling.

PALPATION. Examination of the axillary and supraclavicular area is always part of a complete breast examination and is best done when the patient is erect. The axilla is examined with the humerus slightly abducted and the pectoralis muscle relaxes (Fig. 15-8B). The contents of the axilla are pressed gently against the rib cage, and the axilla is progressively palpated from apex to base. The apex of the axilla does not lie under the humeral head but anteriorly under the clavicle, where the axillary vein and artery pass under the clavicle to become the subclavian vessels.

Fig. 15-6. Gynecomastia.

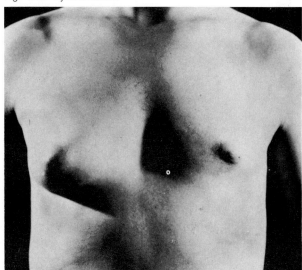

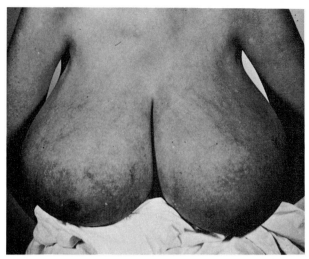

Fig. 15-7. Virginal hypertrophy. This growth occurred during 1 year in fifteen-year-old white girl and required plastic surgery for repair. (*Courtesy of Paul Weeks, M.D.*)

Palpation of lymph nodes at this level is of great importance in predicting the prognosis in a patient with cancer.

The supraclavicular area is palpated with the tips of the fingers, making sure that the fingers are pressed down well behind the clavicle to roll the supraclavicular structures against the scalene muscles. In a thin neck the transverse fibers of the posterior belly of the omohyoid are sometimes mistaken for an enlarged lymph node. This can be differentiated by observing that a medial and lateral margin to the supposed node cannot be felt, although an upper and lower border are easily detected. Following palpation of the axilla and supraclavicular area, the breasts are also palpated, although masses in the breasts are best felt when the patient is supine.

After inspection and palpation with the patient erect, the entire mammary gland is palpated carefully with the tips of the fingers with the patient in the supine position, with the arm first over the head and then at the side (Fig. 15-8). This should be done systematically and in the same way in each examination so that the examiner follows a definite pattern. One may begin at the upper inner quadrant, gradually inspecting the breast tissue from above downward until the medial portion of the breast has been examined. The areolar area is then palpated. If the patient has complained of secretions or blood from the nipple, the areola should be stroked toward the nipple to see if this symptom can be reproduced. The lateral portion of the breast is palpated starting at the upper outer quadrant and completing the examination at the lower outer quadrant. The tail of the breast should also be examined as it extends into the axilla.

By self-examination a woman can usually detect a smaller mass in her own breasts than can a physician if she knows the proper methods to use. Since cancer of the breast is one of the major neoplasms in females, instruction in self-examination is a valuable addition to the physician's examination of the breast. A patient is instructed to emulate the physician's pattern of inspection and examination.

She carries this out upon herself in both the erect and supine positions. Women thirty-five years of age and older should conduct such an examination at home once monthly.

MAMMOGRAPHY. Mammography represents a relatively recent addition to the methods of diagnosis of breast diseases. It requires special techniques and film, and a roentgenologist skilled in interpretation.

This technique is not a substitute for biopsy, which still provides definitive confirmation, but is a helpful adjunct in diagnosis. Mammography is especially useful in (1) follow-up examinations of the contralateral breast following radical mastectomy, (2) examination of an indeterminate mass which cannot be considered a dominant nodule, especially when there are multiple cysts or several vague masses and the indication for biopsy is uncertain, and (3) the large, fatty breast, when the patient has complaints but no nodules are palpated. Tumors cannot be easily felt in such breasts, but the mammogram is most accurate in the fatty breast.

A skilled radiologist can detect cancer of the breast with a false-positive rate of 11 percent and a false-negative rate of 6 percent. A fine stippling on the roentgenogram in the area of the lesion is almost pathognomonic of cancer. There is also a characteristic infiltration of the surrounding tissues; a typical skin thickening may be seen, and the density of the lesion itself is often helpful in interpretation (Fig. 15-9).

Radiography of the breast can detect some cancers which cannot be found in any other way. It has been estimated that the lead time for treatment of lesions discovered at this small size is 1 or 2 years compared to cancers discovered by conventional palpation of the breast. Axillary nodal involvement is very rare in these early lesions, and preliminary results of follow-up indicate that 5-year survival rates for such tumors may exceed 90 percent. This data has led to considerable activity in developing pilot mass screening programs for cancer of the breast which include mammography, careful physical examination, and thermography.

Xeroradiography of the breast is basically a radiographic technique which is carried out in exactly the same way as mammography, except that the image is recorded on a xerographic plate instead of the conventional x-ray transparency. Much less exposure to radiation is required, and the image obtained is much clearer and easier to interpret. Little training is required to interpret a xeroradiographic image compared to a conventional mammograph. Widespread use of the technique has been hampered by the extra expense of the equipment, but it seems likely that xeroradiography will see increasing use, especially in mass screening programs.

THERMOGRAPHY. The skin over malignant tumors of the breast is usually warmer than the surrounding areas. Using special heat scanners it is possible to delineate these "hot spots" on film. This method may help to differentiate malignant and benign tumors. Infection may be associated with a false positive, and, conversely, not all cancers are "hot," so false negatives may occur. The method is still too new to have a definite place in the diagnostic armamentarium but may find a role in mass screening programs.

DISEASES OF THE BREAST

Neoplasms

From the standpoint of morbidity and mortality, cancer is by far the most important clinical problem that concerns the breast today. Most benign neoplasms of the breast would have little clinical importance if it were not for the difficulty in differentiating them from cancer. To emphasize this relationship, benign neoplasms are discussed in the section on differential diagnosis of cancer.

INCIDENCE

Cancer of the breast is the commonest form of cancer in females. Almost 6 percent of all women will develop cancer of the breast in their lifetime. The lifetime incidence of cancer of all types in females is 27 percent; thus one out of every four women with cancer will have cancer of the breast. In the United States, 50,000 to 70,000 new cases of breast cancer occur annually, and about 20,000 women die of the disease each year. According to the excellent cancer registry systems in Connecticut and upper New York State, the age-adjusted incidence of new cases has been increasing steadily since the middle 1940s.

Worldwide figures show that the Dutch have the highest national mortality of cancer of the breast, with 24.19 patients per 100,000 population. The United States ranks ninth, with 21.38 cases per 100,000 population. The Japanese rank lowest among all nations with reliable statistics, with an incidence of 3.76 per 100,000 population. The factors leading to this wide range of incidence are unknown, although studies seeking an answer are in progress.

ETIOLOGY

Sex is certainly an important contributing factor in this disease, since it is very rare in males. Maleness is not a complete protection, however; there is 1 carcinoma of the breast in men for every 100 carcinomas of the breast in women.

The age of the patient is also important (Fig. 15-10). Breast cancer is almost unknown in the prepubertal female and is very rare under the age of twenty. From the age of twenty onward there is a gradually increasing incidence, which reaches a plateau between the ages of forty-five and fifty-five at about 125 new cases each year for every 100,000 females of that age range. After fifty-five the incidence begins to rise again quite sharply, so that the annual risk of developing breast cancer for women eighty to eighty-five is twice as high as for women sixty to sixty-five (312 versus 153 new cases per 100,000 women per year). Some suggest that the plateau of incidence during the menopausal age period reflects the effects of a changing hormonal pattern in women at this time.

Genetic factors play a role in the development of this cancer, though the genetic effect does not seem to be strong and more than one allelic gene must be involved. When

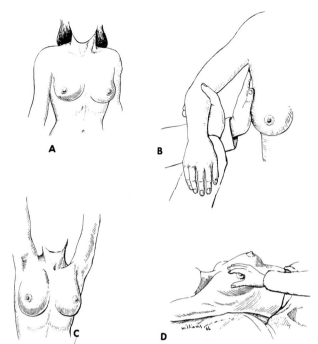

Fig. 15-8. Examination of breast. *A*. Observation with arms at side. *B*. Palpation of axilla. *C*. With arms raised. *D*. Palpation with patient supine.

the mother has had a breast cancer, the chance of cancer of the breast developing in the daughter is two to three times greater than would be expected in the general population, but no specific pattern of inheritance is evident. Some hypothesize that there is a genotype which has a predisposition to the formation of cancer but which must interact with some nongenetic agent before cancer develops.

Patients in whom breast cancer develops and who have positive family histories for the disease are generally younger and have a higher frequency of bilaterality than breast cancer patients with negative family histories. Blood type O, benign breast disease, and ovarian cysts and tumors also tend to be more common in patients with early diagnoses of breast cancer. Blood type A, diabetes, hypertension, and uterine disorders are more common in those who are older at the time of diagnosis.

Interlinked with factors of age, sex, national origin, and inheritance in the development of breast cancer is the important role played by hormonal environment. Some breast cancers are highly susceptible to changes in the patient's hormonal pattern and will regress for a time when hormones of various types are given. Mammary cancer can be induced in the mouse and rat by repeated injections of estrogens and in the rat by a combination of estrogen and progesterone. There is a vast literature concerning both experimental and clinical induction and extinction of tumors with hormonal agents. The exact role of hormones in human cancer still remains elusive. It is not known whether hormonal maladjustment is responsible for human breast cancer or what predisposing causes may be required to produce a susceptibility to hormonal change.

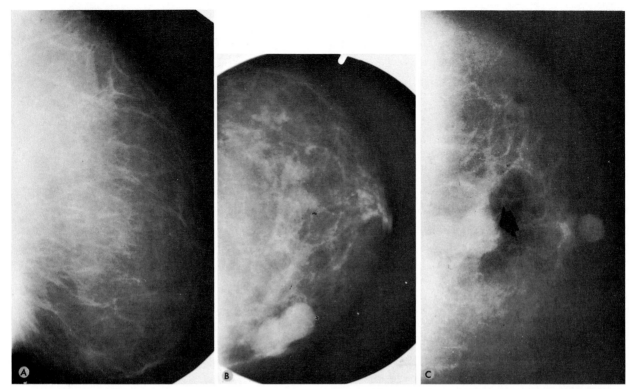

Breast cancer may well be multifactorial. Other interesting correlations with breast cancer include the incidence of coronary artery disease, which has a positive correlation with breast cancer death rates in 24 parts of the world. Hems has concluded that "early" breast cancer (age group forty to forty-four) appears to be genetically influenced, while "late" breast cancer (age group sixty-five to sixty-nine) is more closely associated with environmental fac-

Fig. 15-9. Mammography of breast. *A.* Normal postmenopausal patient with atrophy of lobular tissue and ducts and predominance of fatty supporting tissue. *B.* Multiloculated cyst in menopausal patient. *C.* Scirrhous carcinoma in menopausal patient, demonstrating sunburst pattern; characteristic calcifications not present in this case.

Fig. 15-10. Newly diagnosed breast cancer among women, 1958–1960: percentage distribution and incidence rates by age. Note plateau in incidence between ages forty-five and fifty-five.

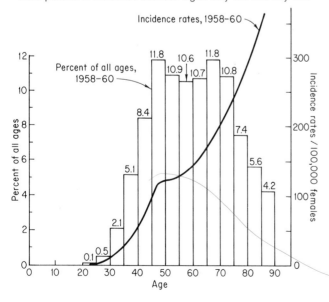

tors, such as diet. Among younger women, higher risk is associated with late first pregnancy, while among women over fifty years of age the risk appears to increase with weight and the relation of weight to height. Zippin and Petrakis have reported an association between wet cerumen, or earwax, and breast cancer rates in diverse population groups, and breast cancer mortality is closely associated with wet cerumen. Such an association is plausible since the mammary and ceruminous glands are histologically of the apocrine type and have many similarities in their secretions. Cerumen exists in two phenotypic forms, wet and dry, which are controlled by a pair of genes in which the allele for the wet type is dominant over that of the dry type. The dry is homozygous recessive and is highly prevalent in the mongoloid population of Asia and in American Indians. The wet type predominates in Western Europeans, Caucasian Americans, and Negro Americans. These findings support the hypothesis that genetic variations in the apocrine system may influence susceptibility to breast cancer.

It has long been known that breast cancer in mice is related to a viral factor transmitted in the milk. Considerable excitement has attended the recent discovery of particles in human milk with the same morphologic characteristics as those found to be associated with breast cancer in mice. These particles have been found in the milk from the breasts of 60 percent of American women with family histories of breast cancer compared to 5 percent of women without positive family histories. The milk of thirty-nine percent of Parsi women in India also were found to contain these particles. The group of Parsi women is of particular interest because of their endogamous history over the centuries, resulting in an inbred population. Breast cancer accounts for approximately half of the cancers among Parsi women in contrast with Connecticut women, for example, in whom breast cancer represents one-fourth of all cancers.

NATURAL HISTORY

A typical carcinoma of the breast is a scirrhous adenocarcinoma beginning in the ducts and invading the parenchyma (80 percent). Beginning in the upper outer quadrant (40 to 50 percent), it grows slowly, doubling its volume every 2 to 9 months in 70 percent of patients. Starting from a single cell, it takes 30 doubling times for a tumor to attain a size of 1 cm—the smallest tumor of the breast normally found on physical diagnosis. Thus even the fastest-growing tumor of the more common type may require 5 years before it becomes clinically palpable. The use of doubling times to calculate the preclinical course of tumors of the breast is subject to many errors, the most obvious being that growth rates are not always constant, varying with areas of necrosis within the tumor and hormonal changes in the patient. Laboratory and clinical observations indicate, however, that growth rates are more consistent than is usually appreciated. The concept of the origin of these tumors in a single cell with increase in size by doubling is a useful model and suggests the long occult period which probably is present in many tumors before they are diagnosed and treated.

As the tumor increases in size and invades the surrounding glandular tissue, the accompanying fibrosis tends to shorten Cooper's ligaments, producing the characteristic dimpling in the skin (Fig. 15-11). Cords of tumor cells grow out along lymphatics, ultimately invading the skin itself. This invasion is preceded by localized edema of the skin as many lymphatic avenues are blocked and drainage of fluid from the skin is impeded. Eventually tumor cells replace the skin, which breaks down to form an ulcer. The tumor increases in size, and new areas of skin invasion may occur, indicated by small satellite nodules adjacent to the ulcer crater. As involvement and destruction of the skin progresses, blood vessels are invaded, and tumor cells seed into the circulation, passing into axillary or intercostal veins to be scattered through the pulmonary circuit into the lungs or by way of the vertebral veins up and down the vertebral column. When this seeding is early and small in amount, the majority if not all of these cells may fail to implant and are destroyed by an unknown mechanism, perhaps immunity. Eventually, perhaps as the number of cells seeded into the circulation begins to rise, they implant and grow in favorable locations. These implants may occur in the vertebral bodies, pelvis, lungs, liver, or brain.

As the breast tumor extends toward the skin, tumor cells simultaneously pass along the lymphatic vessels from the upper outer quadrant to the axillary nodes, where they

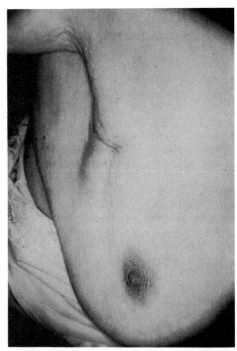

Fig. 15-11. Dimpling of skin over primary carcinoma of breast in upper outer quadrant. Slowly growing lesion in seventy-year-old patient; dimpling had been present for 2 years.

implant and grow. As the axillary nodes enlarge, they are at first shotty and fairly soft, then firm and hard as they are increasingly replaced by tumor. Eventually the nodes adhere to one another in a large conglomerate mass, and as the tumor breaks out of the lymphatic capsule the mass of nodes become fixed to the medial wall of the axilla. As the axillary nodes become choked with tumor, cells are passed along the chain to the supraclavicular nodes, which also enlarge. Other cancer cells pass by way of the right lymphatic trunk or the thoracic duct into the bloodstream, heart, and lungs. Systemic spread is the rule, and 95 percent of patients who die of uncontrolled breast cancer have distant metastases. Lung (65 percent), liver (56 percent), and bones (56 percent) are the commonest sites for these deposits.

Patients today are rarely allowed to proceed through all stages of carcinoma without some therapeutic intervention. Data are available, however, from the latter half of the 1800s and the first few years of this century indicating the normal course of events in untreated tumors. The excellent report in 1962 by Bloom and associates summarizes much of the data. They cite the experience of the Middlesex Hospital in London, where in 1791 a cancer charity was founded to which patients were admitted to "remain an unlimited time, until either relieved by art or released by death." From the well-preserved records of this charity it was possible to collect a series of 250 advanced cases of untreated breast cancer seen between 1805 and 1933 (Fig. 15-12). All the patients reported died in the hospital, and in every case an autopsy was performed. In the last 86 cases, histologic sections were available. The mean survival in this series and for over 1,000 untreated cases collected

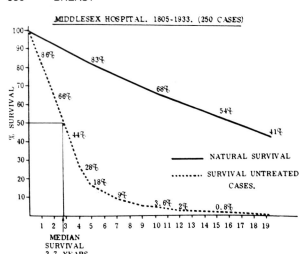

MIDDLESEX HOSPITAL. 1805-1933. (250 CASES)

Fig. 15-12. Survival of patients with untreated cancer of breast compared with natural survival. (*From H. J. G. Bloom, W. W. Richardson, and E. J. Harries, Br Med J, 5299:213, 1962, by permission.*)

from the literature was 38.7 months, with a range from 30.2 to 39.8 months. It must be noted that in all reports of untreated patients survival is calculated from the onset of the first symptom. Fifty percent of the patients died in 2.7 years (median survival); 18 percent survived 5 years, 3.6 percent 10 years, and 10.8 percent 15 years. The longest survivor in the group died in the nineteenth year after onset of symptoms. Histologic grading indicated that for 23 patients with grade 1 tumors the mean survival was 47 months. Autopsies indicated that 95 percent of the women died of their carcinoma, only 5 percent of intercurrent disease. Nearly three-fourths of the patients had ulceration of the breast at death, and in 21 percent this was very extensive, sometimes destroying the entire breast and excavating the chest wall. Bloom concluded that treatment of patients with breast cancer appeared to increase the length and improve the quality of survival.

DIAGNOSIS AND STAGING

The normal breast is a nodular structure by virtue of its lobular architecture, and this lobularity may be accentuated during the later portion of the menstrual cycle, pregnancy, or lactation. To the inexperienced examiner the normal nodularity may feel faintly suspicious throughout, although no obvious lesion can be felt. Palpation of the typical carcinoma of the breast normally leaves little doubt in the examiner's mind: the lesion is hard, almost cartilaginous; the edges are distinct, serrated, and irregular. This is true for the 75 to 80 percent of breast tumors associated with productive fibrosis. It is the remaining 20 to 25 percent of tumors, those associated with little fibrosis and those with a medullary or a colloid element or other less typical lesions, which form the spectrum of neoplasms most difficult to distinguish from benign lesions.

Physicians would prefer to have only the clues provided by the local mass to make the physical diagnosis of carci-

noma, for it is only when the mass is localized to the breast that one can assume an "early" lesion and expect the best possible chance of long survival. Too often the later signs of breast cancer are present to confirm the diagnosis. As indicated previously, these are skin dimpling or nipple retraction, satellite skin lesions, edema or ulceration, and ipsilateral enlarged axillary or supraclavicular nodes. Signs of even wider spread may be present such as a history of back or leg pain, an enlarged and nodular liver, or perhaps a complaint of dyspnea associated with physical findings or fluid in the chest.

The physical examination of a patient with breast cancer should include an attempt on the part of the examiner to classify and record the stage of the patient's disease specifically. Only consistent classification can make possible clear conclusions concerning prognosis and type of treatment. The problem of comparing the results of treatment from institution to institution and among different operators has been impaired for years by a lack of adequate classification or by varying standards of classification. At present a strong effort is being made to promote the adoption of a standard system devised by the American Joint Committee on Cancer Staging and End Results Reporting, based on a system proposed by the International Union against Cancer in 1958. This system of classification is called the T.N.M. Classification, the T standing for "tumor," the N for "nodes," and the M for "metastasis." The general outline used in breast cancer is as follows:

T—Primary tumor

T1   Tumor of 2 cm or less in its greatest dimension; skin not involved, or involved locally in Paget's disease

T2   Tumor over 2 cm in size or with skin attachment (dimpling of skin) or nipple retraction (in subareolar tumors); no pectoral-muscle or chest-wall attachment

T3   Tumor of any size with any of the following: skin infiltration, ulceration, peau d'orange, skin edema, pectoral-muscle or chest-wall attachment

N—Regional lymph nodes

N0   No clinically palpable axillary lymph node(s) (metastasis not suspected)

N1   Clinically palpable axillary lymph nodes that are not fixed (metastasis suspected)

N2   Clinically palpable homolateral axillary or infraclavicular lymph node or nodes that are fixed to one another or to other structures (metastasis suspected)

M—Distant metastasis

M0   No distant metastasis

M1   Clinical and radiographic evidence of metastasis other than to homolateral axillary or infraclavicular lymph nodes

Summary of clinical staging

Stage I   T1, N0, M0; T2, N0, M0

Stage II   T1, N1, M0; T2, N1, M0 (includes all N1, M0 except for T3)

Stage III   T3, N0, M0; T3, N1, M0; T3, N2, M0; T1, N2, M0; T2, N2, M0 and includes any combination of T1, T2, or T3 with N2 and M0

Stage IV   Any clinical stage of disease with distant metastasis (M1)

DIFFERENTIAL DIAGNOSIS (BENIGN LESIONS)

CHRONIC CYSTIC MASTITIS. Chronic cystic mastitis was first described in the medical literature in the last two decades of the nineteenth century, by Reclus (1883), Brissaud (1884), Schimmelbusch (1890), and König (1893). For a time the disease was known as either Reclus' or Schimmelbusch's disease, but use of these eponyms dwindled following the introduction of the term *chronic cystic mastitis* by König. He chose this term to describe a group of pathologic lesions found in the breast because he thought they were due to a "vicious cycle of secretion and irritation." While the disease is indeed chronic, it may not be cystic and is certainly not inflammatory, so this old name is at least two-thirds in error. Nonetheless, attempts to introduce more accurate or at least other nomenclatures have failed. Fibrocystic disease, fibroadenosis, mastopathy, nodular hyperplasia, cyclomastopathy, adenofibromatosis, mazoplasia, cystiphorous epithelial hyperplasia, adenocystic disease, and mammary dysplasia have all been offered, but chronic cystic mastitis is still the most widely used designation.

The term chronic cystic mastitis describes a family of lesions found in the breast. Pathologists disagree as to which lesions are legitimate family relations, so the morphology of the disease, like the terminology, appears rather fuzzy to the casual observer. Foote and Stewart have named 10 lesions often described as members of this group: cysts, papillomatosis, blunt duct adenosis, sclerosing adenosis, apocrine metaplasia, stasis and distension of ducts, periductal mastitis, fat necrosis, hyperplasia of duct epithelium, and fibroadenoma. These writers accept, however, only the first five of this group as being related lesions and forming part of chronic cystic mastitis; the others are held to represent different disease entities. They refer to the first five as the cystic and proliferative group, assuming that the proliferative lesions are responsible for the subsequent formation of cysts. A majority of pathologists accept this list, though some have argued for the inclusion of fibroadenoma. In addition, epithelial hyperplasia is usually accepted as part of the complex, with papillomas representing an advanced manifestation of hyperplasia.

The lesions of chronic cystic mastitis begin to appear in the breasts of a few women in their late twenties. The incidence is greater in the thirties and forties. Originally it was thought that the incidence of these lesions decreased after the menopause, but careful autopsy studies indicate that the lesions are common in the older age groups and may continue to increase in frequency with age. Frantz et al. found a 71 percent incidence of cystic and proliferative lesions in women over seventy years of age. Sandison noted epithelial hyperplasia of the ducts in 7 percent of women in their twenties and in 33 percent of women in their eighties. Rush and Kramer in 1963 reviewed step sections from the breasts of 20 women over seventy years of age. Approximately 100 sections were reviewed per patient, and with this close scrutiny two or more lesions of cystic mastitis were found in all patients. Moderately severe epithelial hyperplasia was found in 14 of the 20

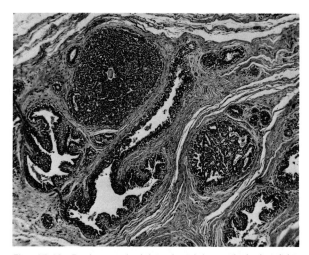

Fig. 15-13. Benign marked intraductal hyperplasia in eighty-eight-year-old female. (Hematoxylin and eosin; ×32). (*From B. F. Rush, Jr., and W. M. Kramer, Surg Gynec Obstet, 117:425, 1963.*)

(Fig. 15-13). A case may be made for considering the lesions of cystic mastitis somewhat as one considers arteriosclerosis: a pathologic process which varies in degree and in time of onset but which is found to some degree in all adult females as they age.

Most of the lesions making up the complex of chronic cystic mastitis are proliferative, and almost from the first recognition of this disease there has been a suspicion that these lesions may represent a premalignant condition. Follow-up studies of patients shown by biopsy to have chronic cystic mastitis uniformly indicate that cancer subsequently occurs three to five times more often in these patients than in the general population.

If one assumes that all women eventually develop some degree of chronic cystic mastitis, how can one conclude that the finding of chronic cystic mastitis on biopsy is associated with an increase in the incidence of cancer of the female breast compared to patients in the general population? A reasonable hypothesis is that patients in whom this complex develops early enough or severely enough to warrant biopsy do indeed represent a special group with a greater hazard of eventual cancer.

The lesions of chronic cystic mastitis which are most likely to present a problem in differential diagnosis and to require biopsy are cysts, fibroadenoma, ductal papilloma, and sclerosing adenosis.

CYSTS. The cystic component of chronic cystic mastitis is most prominent in patients in their thirties and forties. The cysts may vary in size from microcysts of 1 to 2 mm to large masses several centimeters in diameter (Fig. 15-14). They are felt in the breast substance as firm, round, fairly distinct masses, often with a rubbery feeling indicative of their cystic nature. Lesions in the anterior and dependent portions of the breast may be transilluminated. They are sometimes tender and, like many of the other lesions of this complex, may increase in size toward the end of the menstrual period.

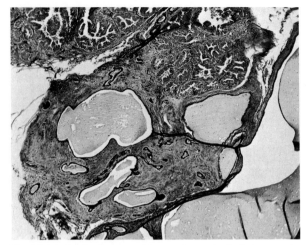

Fig. 15-14. Cystic disease with apocrine metaplasia in seventy-three-year-old female. (Hematoxylin and eosin; ×32.) (*From B. F. Rush, Jr., and W. M. Kramer Surg Gynec Obstet, 117:425, 1963.*)

If a lesion in a patient's breast is clearly suggestive of a cyst, aspiration is a good method for confirming the diagnosis. This technique should not be used unless the rules for its employment are clearly understood. The fluid obtained should be the characteristic clear, brown-green fluid of a cyst. When the cyst is aspirated dry, no underlying mass should be palpable. If a residual mass remains after aspiration or if the fluid is bloody, biopsy must be done. The patient should be followed at intervals for a month or two after aspiration; if the cyst reappears, biopsy is also indicated. Approximately half the cysts treated by aspiration will disappear, and fluid will not reaccumulate.

FIBROADENOMAS. These lesions are most common in the twenties and early thirties. They present as lobular but not serrated masses with a firm, rubbery consistency. Their edges are sharply defined. Most commonly solitary, they may occasionally be multiple. They are differentiated from cancer by the smooth rather than irregular lobulations and by the age group in which they occur. Although a skilled examiner can probably detect a fibroadenoma with an accuracy of 80 to 85 percent, biopsy is mandatory.

DUCTAL PAPILLOMA. The hallmark of the ductal papilloma is abnormal secretion from the nipple, which is often blood-stained. In 30 percent a small nodule, 3 or 4 mm in diameter, will be palpated in the major ducts underlying the areola. In the absence of a palpable nodule the papilloma's general position can often be detected by stroking the areola toward the nipple with the tips of the fingers, carefully working around the areola in a clockwise direction until an area is discovered which on pressure results in secretion from the nipple. A bloody nipple discharge may also be indicative of an intraductal carcinoma or even a deeper-lying infiltrating ductal carcinoma. The incidence of malignancy in the presence of this physical finding is 20 to 30 percent. Diagnosis is confirmed and treatment accomplished by excision of that portion of the collecting duct system shown on physical examination to be responsible for the secretion. Urban and Baker propose that the entire collecting duct system should be excised en bloc, since these lesions are often multiple and a partial excision of the duct system will often result in the retention of other lesions which will lead to further bloody secretions later.

SCLEROSING ADENOSIS. These lesions can sometimes result in an area of fibrosis within the mammary tissue which is firm and irregular and impossible to differentiate clinically from an ordinary scirrhous carcinoma. Biopsy is required to make the differential diagnosis.

OTHER BENIGN LESIONS. Fat necrosis, thrombophlebitis of the breast, and granular cell myoblastoma are three benign lesions of the breast which can be confused on physical examination with malignant growths. All three are uncommon. Fat necrosis is the most common of the group and is probably due to trauma, although only half the patients who have this lesion recall a trauma of the breast. The breasts are in an exposed position, however, and may be hurt at the time of a larger accident when the injury to the breast is overshadowed by more serious injuries. The lesions are always superficial and often near the areola. In 40 to 50 percent of patients with this lesion, accompanying ecchymoses are lingering stigmata of previous trauma. In one-third of the patients there is a history of pain or tenderness. Retraction of the skin over the lesion is seen in 50 to 60 percent. Retraction is due to the fibrosis and scarring in the fatty lobules which involve Cooper's ligaments. As the scarring progresses and matures, skin retraction, which may first be seen within two weeks of the original injury, becomes more prominent. The mass of subcutaneous scar tissue that forms is distinct, irregular, and often very firm. It is easy to understand how such a mass associated with skin retraction may be mistaken for carcinoma, and in every instance a biopsy specimen of the lesion must be examined histologically. In decades past, many unnecessary radical mastectomies were done in patients with fat necrosis. Today, the practice of routinely examining frozen sections of biopsy material prevents this tragedy.

Granular cell myoblastomas occur most commonly in the tongue but may also occur in the breast. The clinical importance of this rare tumor is that it can produce all the clinical signs of early cancer of the breast. The lesion is hard and relatively fixed to the breast tissue surrounding it. It sometimes causes dimpling of the overlying skin. Moreover, on gross examination of the specimen at operation the lesion looks and cuts like a scirrhous carcinoma of the breast. Only frozen sections can confirm that one is dealing with a benign rather than a malignant lesion.

Thrombophlebitis of a superficial vein of the breast, called *Mondor's disease,* may rarely be mistaken for a tumor because of the dimpling of the skin it produces. The tubular shape of the thrombosed vein and the accompanying tenderness usually indicate the diagnosis, but biopsy is often required for confirmation.

BREAST BIOPSY

Breast biopsy is a procedure with little risk. It can be done under local anesthesia; general anesthesia is the agent of choice, however, since a radical mastectomy is usually done immediately if the lesion proves malignant.

A curvilinear incision in the direction of the skin lines is made over the supicious mass. If the lesion is small, total excision is preferred, but if a large lesion is encountered, a small excisional biopsy of the main mass is done.

Needle biopsy of breast masses is done in some institutions and is very satisfactory if the pathologist is familiar with this type of material. Negative needle biopsies have no significance, however, since an adequate sample may not be obtained.

HISTOPATHOLOGY

Malignant neoplasms of the breast, with few exceptions, are adenocarcinomas. The histologic features of these lesions vary considerably, and a number of classifications are available. The following was proposed by Foote and Stewart:

HISTOLOGIC CLASSIFICATION OF CANCER OF THE BREAST

A. Paget's disease of the nipple
B. Carcinomas of mammary ducts
  1. Noninfiltrating
  2. Infiltrating
    a. Papillary carcinoma
    b. Comedocarcinoma
    c. Carcinoma with productive fibrosis
    d. Medullary carcinoma with lymphoid infiltrate
    e. Colloid carcinoma
C. Carcinomas of mammary lobules
  1. Noninfiltrating
  2. Infiltrating
D. Relatively rare carcinomas
E. Sarcoma of the breast

PAGET'S DISEASE OF THE NIPPLE. This constitutes 1 percent of all breast carcinomas but has attracted an inordinate amount of attention and speculation, since for many years there was confusion as to whether this lesion arose primarily in the skin or in the mammary ducts. It is now generally accepted that this is a primary carcinoma of the mammary ducts of the nipple which has subsequently invaded the skin. The lesion presents as a scaling, eczematoid, and quite innocent-appearing lesion of the nipple (Fig. 15-15). In most instances it has a slow natural history, and the skin lesion may be the only evidence of neoplasm for many years. Ultimately an underlying mass will develop if the lesion is untreated. Any eczematoid lesion of the nipple in a postmenopausal female which persists for more than a few weeks should be biopsied to exclude the possibility of Paget's disease. Adequate histologic studies of surgical specimens almost always reveal underlying carcinomas of the mammary ducts. Invasion of the skin by these cells produces the interesting Paget's cell, a large cell with clear cytoplasm and commonly with binucleation. This is associated with evidence of chronic inflammation and a surface crust. Robbins and Berg's study of 89 cases indicated that one-third of the patients showed noninfiltrating carcinoma, and in this group the survival rate was 100 percent at 5 years. The remaining patients had infiltrating carcinoma. The overall survival rate for the group was 64 percent, indicating a better

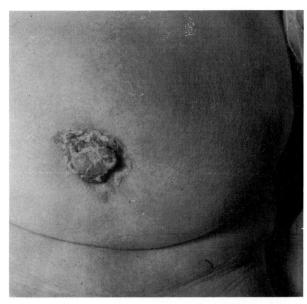

Fig. 15-15. Typical scaling eczematoid lesion of Paget's disease; frequently misdiagnosed and treated by salves and ointments, with long delay in proper diagnosis.

prognosis for this lesion than for the average carcinoma of the breast.

NONINFILTRATING CARCINOMAS OF THE MAMMARY DUCTS. These constitute 1 percent of carcinomas of the breast. It is unfortunate that more cancers are not seen at the noninfiltrating stage, since these lesions are carcinomas in situ and operation should result in 100 percent 5-year survival. That this is not the case, 5-year survival being about 90 percent, reflects the fact that the breast is a large organ and that lesions which appear to be noninfiltrating may in fact be infiltrating at some area which the pathologist has not examined. Foote and Stewart report that they have traced progression of intraductal carcinoma from benign papillary hyperplasia through atypism to noninfiltrating intraductal carcinoma and ultimately to infiltrating carcinoma throughout a breast specimen. They state that while this may be one route for the development of cancer of the breast, cancer may arise from normal intraductal cells directly. The differentiation of a noninfiltrating intraductal carcinoma from a benign hyperplasia may be difficult; areas of atypism can blend gradually from one state into the other. Histologically, the duct epithelium is usually seen to be thrown up into papillae which show a loss of cohesiveness and disorientation of cells, with pleomorphism and occasionally mitotic figures but without evidence of invasion of the basement membrane. A more dramatic form is the noninfiltrating comedocarcinoma, in which hyperplasia is more extreme, choking the entire duct for long distances with masses of cells. These lesions commonly develop central necrosis of the cells. A gross section of such a lesion will extrude small cores of tissue from the ducts very much as the core is extruded from a comedo when it is squeezed, thus giving rise to the term comedocarcinoma.

INFILTRATING PAPILLARY CARCINOMA. Presumably a later stage or a more aggressive form of the noninfiltrating papillary lesion, these carcinomas still tend to evolve slowly and have a better 5-year survival rate than the average carcinoma of the breast. They produce a mass rather soft to palpation compared with the typical hard, fibrous lesion usually associated with breast cancer. They may reach large size before metastasizing to the axilla. Dimpling and skin edema are less commonly seen, another index of the late infiltration of the lymphatics and of the failure to stimulate a fibrous response. Noninfiltrating papillary carcinomas are often seen in association with the infiltrating form.

Infiltrating comedocarcinomas comprise approximately 5 percent of all breast cancers. They are often found in association with other forms of adenocarcinoma that result in productive fibrosis, and the presence of comedocarcinoma together with other elements of carcinoma of the breast does not significantly alter the prognosis from the average.

INFILTRATING DUCT CARCINOMA WITH PRODUCTIVE FIBROSIS. This is the commonest form of breast cancer, constituting 78 percent of the specimens seen. There is a tremendous variation in the amount of fibrosis. The lesion has been termed *scirrhous carcinoma, fibrocarcinoma,* and *sclerosing carcinoma.* The desmoplastic response to the invading cancer cells accounts for the remarkable hardness of the average breast cancer. Grossly the lesions have uneven serrated edges. They cut with great resistance and often with a rather gritty feeling as the knife edge passes through them. Histologically the lesions may vary from scattered, well-differentiated adenomatous clusters and a massive amount of fibrostroma to dense cellular aggregates with only minor amounts of fibroplasia (Fig. 15-16). Electron microscopic examination of these tumors indicates that they originate in the myoepithelial cells of the mammary duct.

MEDULLARY CARCINOMAS. Five percent of carcinomas of the breast assume this pattern, and the diagnosis indi-

Fig. 15-16. Intraductal carcinoma with stromal invasion in eighty-three-year-old female. Field shows almost entire extent of this very early lesion. (Hematoxylin and eosin; ×32.)

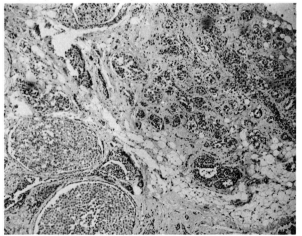

cates a favorable prognosis for the patient. Even in the presence of metastatic disease the prognosis remains favorable; the 5-year overall survival rate for the lesion is 85 to 90 percent. These lesions are soft, bulky, and often large. Necrotic areas of varying size are usually present. Occasionally one finds a lesion which is almost totally infarcted. On physical examination these tumors are freely movable, and smaller tumors are likely to be diagnosed clinically as cysts or fibroadenomas. Histologically the tumors are made up of large rounded or polygonal cells with an abundant cytoplasm arranged in broad or narrow plexiform masses anastomosing with one another. Electron microscopic and histochemical evidence suggests that these cells originate in the ductal epithelium. There is an abundant lymphoid infiltrate. Plasma cells are often seen and are sometimes very prominent. Axillary metastases occur less frequently than in the ordinary carcinoma of the breast but are not uncommon, occurring in about 40 percent. Metastasis frequently involves only a single node.

COLLOID CARCINOMA. This is an infrequent mammary cancer constituting about 1 percent of all breast cancers. The lesions contain a much greater amount of mucin than the usual adenocarcinoma and may be frankly gelatinous on cut section. Clinically these lesions are soft and ill defined and, like the medullary lesions, may be quite bulky before detection. Histologically the predominant picture is of large mucinous lakes in which epithelial aggregates float. Patients with these lesions have a better-than-average survival rate.

CARCINOMA OF THE MAMMARY LOBULES. This lesion arises in the mammary lobules from the cells of the acini and the terminal ducts. Most of the acini of a lobule are involved. Lobules may be of normal size or enlarged, with an unsystematic hyperplasia of the lining cells until the lumen is plugged. At the in situ stage of development these are the only changes, and simple mastectomy at this point should produce cure. The lesion subsequently becomes infiltrative and ultimately may give rise to regular scirrhous carcinoma.

Multicentricity and bilaterality are important features of lobular carcinoma. Eighty-eight percent of breast specimens removed for in situ lobular carcinoma show other in situ lesions scattered throughout the specimen. Examination of the contralateral breast has demonstrated in situ lesions in from 35 to 59 percent of specimens.

SARCOMA OF THE BREAST. Sarcomas of the breast are very rare. The commonest sarcoma seen is cystosarcoma phylloides, but only one in ten of these is truly malignant, the great majority being a benign variant of fibroadenoma. Great confusion is created because both the benign and malignant form are called "cystosarcoma." When Müller first described and named the lesion in 1838 he was aware of its predominantly benign nature. At that time "sarcoma" meant simply a fleshy tumor and did not carry the meaning of malignancy that it does today. Modern synonyms for the benign lesion are *giant intracanalicular or pericanalicular fibroadenoma* and *intracanalicular myxoma.* The malignant variant has been called *adenocarcinoma.*

Cystosarcoma phylloides occurs at an older average age

(forty), is larger, and has a more cellular stroma than fibroadenoma. When first seen clinically these tumors average 5 to 10 cm, have a firm and rubbery consistency, and may have a bosselated surface. In cut section the tumors have a discrete capsule. Small lesions present leaflike intracanalicular protrusions, and larger lesions have cystic spaces into which project densely packed polypoid masses.

The malignant variant metastasizes most commonly to the lungs, bones, and subcutaneous tissues. Axillary metastasis is so uncommon that simple mastectomy is an adequate procedure for both the benign and the malignant forms.

PRIMARY TREATMENT

The first historical reference to cancer of the breast appears in the Edwin Smith Surgical Papyrus (3000 to 2500 B.C.). The patient described is a man, but the description suggests most of the clinical features of breast cancer. The author concludes that "there is no treatment." References to cancer of the breast are scattered and brief over the following 2,500 years. Even in that large body of writings concerning Greek and Roman medicine, the Corpus Hippocraticum, direct reference to the treatment of breast cancer is absent, although it is clear that the condition was recognized.

Celsus, a Roman of the first century, spoke of operation and advised limiting it to early lesions: "None of these can be removed but the cacoethes [early lesion], the rest are irritated by every method of cure. The more violent the operations are, the more angry they grow." Galen, in the second century, inscribed one of the classic clinical observations:

> We have often seen in the breast a tumor exactly resembling the animal the crab. Just as the crab has legs on both sides of his body, so in this disease the veins extending out from the unnatural growth take the shape of a crab's legs. We have often cured this disease in its early stages, but after it has reached a large size no one has cured it without operation. In all operations we attempt to excise a pathological tumor in a circle in the region where it borders on the healthy tissue.

Although Galen spoke of operations for tumors, his system of medicine ascribed the disease to an excess of black bile, and logically excision of a local outbreak could not cure the systemic imbalance. The Galenic theories dominated medicine until the Renaissance. Most established physicians looked down on attempts at operative treatment as misdirected and futile. Only when it was again established that a cancer could arise in a part as a local disorder quite separate from a systemic imbalance could excision of the tumor be recognized as rational therapy. Morgagni's definitive study of gross pathology, appropriately entitled *The Seats and Causes of Disease,* supplied this new rationale. Today radical mastectomy is the standard treatment for operable cancer of the breast in the United States. This operation involves the removal of the entire breast with a generous portion of overlying skin, all the underlying pectoralis major and minor muscles, and the entire lymphatic and fibrofatty contents of the axilla (Fig. 15-17).

This procedure evolved slowly from simple amputation of the breast. LeDran in the eighteenth century repudiated Galen's humoral theory and stated that cancer of the breast was a local disease which spread by way of the lymphatics to the regional nodes. He removed enlarged axillary nodes in his operations on patients with breast cancer. In the nineteenth century, Moore of Middlesex Hospital, England, emphasized wide removal of the breast and felt that when there was neoplasm in the axilla, the axillary contents should be removed in one block together with the breast. In a presentation before the British Medical Association in 1877, Banks supported Moore's concepts and advocated that axillary nodes should always be removed in one block with the breast tissue whether there were palpable nodes present or not, since occult involvement of the axillary nodes was so often present.

As Lewison notes, it remained for Halsted, the new professor of surgery at a young school called The Johns Hopkins Medical School, to "culminate the operation and germinate the present modern method." Halsted proposed a standard procedure, removing all the structures in one block. His first operation was performed about 1882, and he reported 13 cases in 1890. The procedure was almost exactly as it is today except that the pectoralis minor muscle was not removed. In 1894 he reported more than 50 cases over the preceding 12 years. In the same year Herbert Willy Meyer of New York reported six patients operated upon by a technique he had evolved independently. This procedure, almost a duplicate of the Halsted mastectomy, added the removal of the pectoralis minor muscle. Halsted subsequently accepted this addition, and the modern radical mastectomy is often attributed to both these men. This procedure and the wide-block excision that it incorporated was soon adopted widely and for the following 50 years was the only operation used by the well-trained surgeon for treatment of breast cancer.

SELECTION OF PATIENTS. Operative treatment of breast cancer cannot be effective if disease has spread beyond the area removed by the operation. Distant spread to supraclavicular lymph nodes, lung, liver, or other sites is thus an absolute contraindication to the radical operation. Certain characteristics of the local lesion also indicate a high likelihood that operation would be futile. These generally accepted "criteria of inoperability" include fixation of the local breast lesion to the chest wall, fixation of the involved lymph nodes in the axilla, and inflammatory carcinoma of the breast. Haagensen compiled the following detailed list of criteria:

1. Extensive edema of the skin over the breast (Fig. 15-18)
2. Satellite nodules in the skin over the breast
3. Carcinoma of the inflammatory type (Fig. 15-19)
4. Parasternal tumor nodules
5. Proved supraclavicular metastases
6. Edema of the arm
7. Distant metastases
8. Any two or more of the following grave signs of locally advanced carcinoma:
   a. Ulceration of the skin

b. Edema of the skin of limited extent (less than one-third of breast skin involved)
c. Solid fixation of tumor to the chest wall
d. Axillary lymph nodes measuring 2.5 cm or more in transverse diameter
e. Fixation of the axillary nodes to the skin or deep structures of the axilla

Fig. 15-17. Technique of radical mastectomy. *A.* Willy Meyer elliptical incision. A_1 and A_2. Variations of mastectomy incision. *B.* Skin flaps developed and cephalic vein identified in order to delineate deltopectoral groove; tendinous insertion of pectoralis major muscle into humerus identified for transection. *C.* After transection of pectoralis major muscle, pectoralis minor insertion into coracoid process is defined. *D.* Pectoralis minor muscle transected and axilla being cleared of fatty tissue. *E.* Axillary vein cleared and all tributaries coursing caudad transected; long thoracic and thoracodorsal nerves identified and preserved; pectoralis major and minor muscle dissected with axillary fat and lymph nodes in medial direction. *F.* Dissection complete, showing chest wall including ribs and intercostal muscles cleared of pectoralis fascia, with sternum as medial limit of dissection. *G.* Incision closed and suction applied to obliterate dead space; with this technique, pressure dressing not needed.

If these criteria are strictly applied, 75 percent of breast cancers seen will be operable. Figures from Connecticut indicate that from 1940 to 1959 ninety-five percent of all new patients there under sixty-five were treated by operation. This suggests that these clinical criteria are not observed in many institutions.

Haagensen has proposed an even stricter method of evaluation, called the *triple biopsy.* The object is "to exclude all patients who have no chance of cure." Patients who would otherwise be eligible for radical mastectomy are selected for triple biopsy if they have palpable axillary lymph nodes, primary lesions larger than 3 cm, or tumors in the center or the inner quadrants of the breast. Biopsy of the breast lesion, highest axillary nodes, and internal mammary nodes is done. If occult cancer is found in any of these areas, the patient is treated by radiation. This procedure reduces the number of patients eligible for operation to 50 percent of those seen.

MacDonald introduced the term *biological determinism* into the consideration of cancer, meaning that the biologic nature of the tumor primarily determines the response to

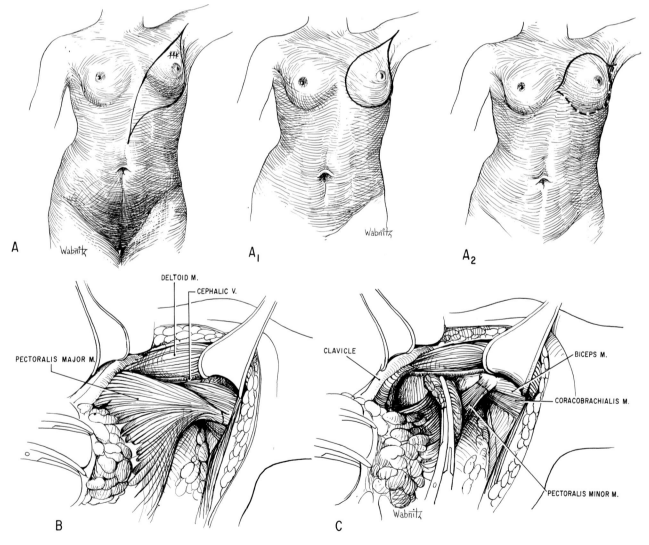

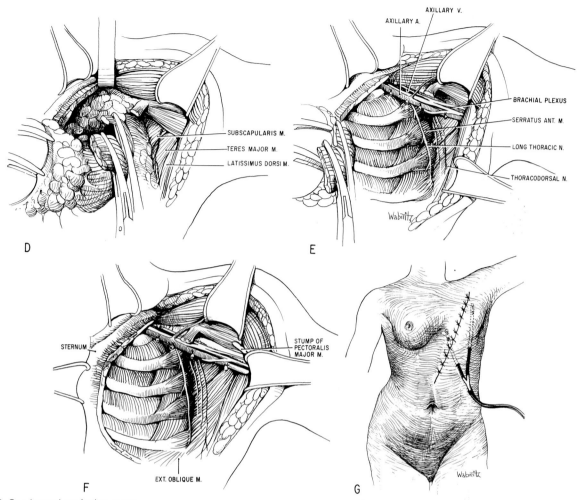

D

SUBSCAPULARIS M.
TERES MAJOR M.
LATISSIMUS DORSI M.

E

AXILLARY V.
AXILLARY A.

BRACHIAL PLEXUS
SERRATUS ANT. M.
LONG THORACIC N.
THORACODORSAL N.

F

STERNUM

STUMP OF
PECTORALIS
MAJOR M.

EXT. OBLIQUE M.

G

Fig. 15-17. See legend on facing page.

therapy. Concerning the breast he suggests that one-third of the lesions do not develop the propensity to metastasize, and while excision removes a disagreeable local growth, the procedure is not lifesaving since such a tumor would never be life-threatening. One-third of the lesions, he estimates, are incurable almost from inception, since they become generalized early, before they are clinically detectable, and no matter how early or how widely the tumor is excised, the procedure will not change the course of the disease. Finally, he assumes that in the remaining one-third of patients the systemic spread of the tumor is preceded by a long latent period in which the tumor reaches clinically detectable size before beginning to spread. In such patients early detection and excision of the tumor would be important, and treatment would have value in altering the course of the cancer. If this thesis is correct, a test to distinguish the different tumors, confining radical treatment to those of the last group only, would have great value. Such a test, as well as proof of this theory, remains to be provided.

The concept of biologic determinism would also explain much of the confusion that surrounds attempts to evaluate techniques of treatment by statistical methods. Butcher

compares this effort to attempting to evaluate a remedy for snakebite in a series of patients who fell into a pit of vipers, some poisonous, some benign, and some moderately toxic, with no way of knowing which patients were bitten by which snakes.

THE PROBLEM OF BILATERAL MASTECTOMY. Foote and Stewart have observed that "the most frequent precancerous lesion of the breast is a cancer of the opposite breast." Berg and Robbins noted that the incidence of occurrence of cancer in the contralateral breast following radical mastectomy was approximately 1 percent per year, so that the cumulative risk of cancer in the remaining breast among patients surviving radical mastectomy for 20 years was as high as 20 percent. As long ago as 1951, Pack published a plea for routine simple mastectomy of the remaining breast at the time of radical mastectomy for cancer. Presumably because of the psychologic blow to a woman who is asked to lose both her breasts, this approach has rarely been advocated by surgeons, and the usual routine after radical mastectomy has been to follow the contralateral breast with special care in the ensuing years. The recent recognition of the high risk of contralateral cancer in patients with in situ lobular carcinoma has

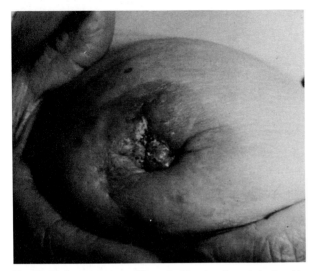

Fig. 15-18. Large cancer of breast with retraction of nipple, skin edema, and several satellite skin nodules.

caused a change in attitude toward this particular form of the disease. Currently recommended treatment for patients with either in situ or invasive lobular cancer of the breast is simple mastectomy of the contralateral breast. Should this recommendation be refused, the patient is requested at least to permit a biopsy of the remaining breast in an area which represents a mirror image of the area of cancer in the involved breast. If this biopsy reveals in situ lobular cancer, a simple mastectomy is carried out. If invasive lobular cancer is found, a radical mastectomy is done. If the biopsy is negative, a very careful follow-up is recommended with mammography and careful breast examination at least twice yearly.

Fig. 15-19. Inflammatory carcinoma of breast. Bright pink to red suffuses area of skin involvement, reflecting inflammatory response to extensive scattering of tumor cells in subcutaneous tissues. Large skin lesion above nipple is congenital pigmented nevus unrelated to the cancer.

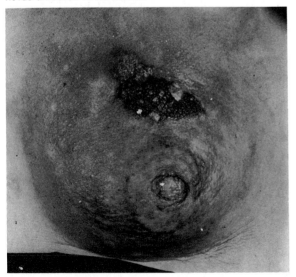

COMBINED RADIATION AND RADICAL MASTECTOMY. Once a patient is selected for radical mastectomy, a further consideration is the use of postoperative radiotherapy. Postoperative radiation in patients with proved axillary node metastasis is frequently employed, but the weight of evidence favors the view that survival is unaffected. Radiation is usually given over the axillary, the supraclavicular, and the internal mammary lymph nodes. Such therapy clearly reduces the incidence of postoperative local recurrence by as much as 15 percent, but whether survival is increased is uncertain, and reports from various series are conflicting.

Preoperative radiotherapy with orthovoltage radiation has not improved survival figures in the past. Current studies of preoperative high-voltage radiation therapy are in progress but are in too early a stage for interpretation.

OTHER METHODS OF TREATMENT. While radical mastectomy remains the dominant form of treatment for early cancer of the breast in the United States, in Great Britain, simple mastectomy plus radiation therapy has supplanted the radical procedure. McWhirter introduced this combined form of therapy in 1941. Estimating an operability rate of 55 percent and a 5-year survival of 45 percent, only 25 percent of patients (0.55 × 0.45) would benefit from operative management, a failure rate of 75 percent. He reasoned that the axillary dissection of a radical mastectomy benefited only 14 percent of patients. (These figures reflected the situation in 1941 but would be very low today.) A limited simple mastectomy plus radiation therapy could be brought to all patients and could be hoped to increase the total number of patients aided. He argued further that radiotherapy can destroy cancer in the axillary nodes, that radiation is better tolerated after simple mastectomy than after radical mastectomy, and that edema of the arm is virtually unknown after simple mastectomy and radiation. Five-year survivals by this technique have been very acceptable to the British and have been competitive with results of radical mastectomy.

Two methods of therapy of early breast cancer now under evaluation and not generally accepted are radiation alone and simple mastectomy alone. Baclesse of France is the only clinician with substantial long-term results of radiation therapy in breast cancer. He uses a rather unconventional prolonged period of therapy.

Several investigators feel that simple mastectomy alone is as effective an operation as radical mastectomy. Smith and Meyer, in 1959, concluded that survival was the same in patients treated by either radical or simple mastectomy. Crile, in a more recent study, came to the same conclusion and in addition implied that the removal of uninvolved axillary nodes had a deleterious effect on the spread of breast cancer. He advocated secondary removal of axillary metastasis after nodes become involved. Axillary dissections became necessary in one-third of his patients from a month to a year after the initial simple mastectomy, but he contended that this did not alter the 5-year end results.

The trend in clinical investigation is away from radical mastectomy toward evaluation of lesser procedures such as simple mastectomy, "modified" radical mastectomy with preservation of pectoral muscles, and radiation therapy.

However, a group of clinicians represented by Urban, Sugarbaker, and Dahl-Iversen advocate a more extensive operation which includes resection of the internal mammary lymph nodes in addition to conventional radical mastectomy. A segment of the anterior chest wall is removed en bloc with the radical mastectomy, including the underlying internal mammary nodes from the first to the fourth intercostal spaces. The rationale for this is the finding that 50 percent of internal mammary lymph nodes are involved by metastatic cancer when the axillary nodes are similarly involved. Thus it appears that radical mastectomy is futile in half the patients with axillary node involvement.

Operative mortality is very low for all the various types of mastectomy. Kennedy and Miller reported no deaths following 212 simple mastectomies. Handley and Thackray reported no deaths following 143 modified radical mastectomies. Butcher reported 0.7 percent mortality in 425 radical mastectomies. Haagensen and Cooley had no deaths in 556 radical mastectomies. In all the series cited above, any death of a patient up to 3 months after operation was considered an operative death. Even among patients with extended mastectomy, mortality is low: Sugarbaker reported 1 postoperative death in 250 patients with this procedure.

PROGNOSIS

The arguments for and against different forms of therapy in breast cancer are mainly statistical and are chiefly based on survival figures. Before an observer can appreciate this debate, a clear understanding of the data is required. The accurate comparison of results in different series demands that there be a common denominator. There is great variation in the base line of many published series, and astute investigation is often necessary to determine whether two sets of figures are truly comparable.

An older method of standard reporting required that all patients seen at an institution be reported in the final results, whether they were treated or not. This was called the "absolute," or "crude," survival figure. It had the advantage of indicating the effect of patient selection on the surgical, or "definitive," survival figures. Its disadvantage was that the total experience at different institutions varied greatly. Private hospitals and clinics have a much greater number of early and operable cases compared with cancer hospitals and charity institutions.

Recently, favorable attention has been given to methods of clinical evaluation of the stage of the tumor. By this method the results in patients at an equal stage of disease can be compared among institutions. An advantage of this approach is that since the evaluation is based on pretreatment clinical findings, it is possible to compare the results in patients treated by radiation, radical mastectomy, simple mastectomy, or extended radical mastectomy even though microscopic evaluation of lymph node involvement is available with some forms of treatment and not with others. Disadvantages are that judgment of the extent of involvement is subjective and classification depends greatly on the skill and consistency of the examiner. No standard method of staging is yet accepted very widely. In addition to the method of the American Joint Committee on Cancer Staging and End Results Reporting previously mentioned, there are the Columbia classification, the Manchester classification, and the Steinthal classification (Table 15-1).

New diagnostic methods, especially mammography, have provided a new group of lesions not previously considered by any of the staging methods. Termed by some "minimal breast cancer," these are in situ and microinvasive lesions so small that they are not detectable by conventional palpation of the breast. Current data indicate that 5-year survivals in this group may exceed 90 percent.

Table 15-1. CLINICAL CLASSIFICATIONS OF CANCER OF THE BREAST

Manchester	*Steinthal*	*Columbia*
Stage I: Growth confined to breast, skin involvement over and in direct continuity with tumor and small in relation to breast	*Stage I:* Cancer limited to breast	*Stage A:* No skin edema, ulceration, or solid fixation of tumor to chest wall; axillary nodes not involved
Stage II: As Stage I but with palpable mobile axillary lymph nodes	*Stage II:* Limited to breast and axillary nodes	*Stage B:* As Stage A but axillary nodes present, not larger than 2.5 cm and without fixation to skin or deeper structures
Stage III: Growth extending beyond body of breast: a. Skin invaded or fixed over large area b. Tumor fixed to underlying muscle; nodes may be present but are mobile	*Stage III:* Adjacent structures involved, e.g., pectoral muscle skin (if ulcerated), opposite breast, cervical lymph nodes, viscera, skeletal tissue	*Stage C:* Any *one* of five grave signs present: 1. Edema of skin of limited extent (less than one-third) 2. Skin ulceration 3. Solid fixation to chest wall 4. Massive involvement of axillary nodes 5. Fixation of axillary nodes
Stage IV: Growth spread beyond breast: a. Fixation of axillary nodes b. Tumor fixed to chest wall (not just muscle) c. Supraclavicular nodes involved d. Satellite metastasis to skin beyond area of tumor e. Secondary deposits in opposite breast f. Distant metastasis		*Stage D:* All other more advanced cancer of breast

The best way to evaluate methods of treatment would be cooperative programs among many institutions in which all factors were governed by the same rules and in which random selection of patients for the different methods of therapy was used. No such studies have been done for cancer of the breast, and other methods for comparing series must serve for the present.

NO TREATMENT. In 1951 Park and Lees in a statistical analysis of 5-year survival figures for breast carcinoma tried to show that the course of the disease was not affected by operation. They regarded the improvement in 5-year survival seen following operation as an artifact introduced by operating upon patients earlier in the natural course of the disease. There are now available a number of studies of large groups of patients with untreated breast cancer. Survival computed from the onset of symptoms averages 19 percent at 5 years, 2.5 percent at 10 years. If one computes survival from onset of diagnosis, a figure more comparable to the situation in surgical series, the 5- and 10-year survivals average 8.6 percent and 1.2 percent, respectively. Bloom et al. found that untreated patients with histologically low-grade (grade 1 of 3) neoplasms had survivals of 22 percent, 9 percent, and 0 at 5, 10, and 15 years, respectively. They compared these to survivals of 82, 56, and 37 percent at the same time intervals for lesions of comparable histologic grade in their own treated series (Fig. 15-12).

RADICAL MASTECTOMY. If survival data following radical mastectomy between 1915 and 1958 are examined, one may wonder why the procedure has received so much criticism. The absolute survival gradually increased from 30 to over 50 percent (Fig. 15-20). In California the incidence of patients with localized disease in different age groups has increased from 14–27 percent to 27–39 percent in county hospitals and from 39–44 percent to 43–48 percent in private hospitals (Fig. 15-21). The end-result group of the National Cancer Institute and a number of state tumor registries have reported small but steady increases in 5-year survivals in patients with both regional and localized disease since about 1950. These increases seem recently to have reached a plateau.

Survival for 5 years following radical mastectomy does not provide the same assurance against recurrence that it

does for some other cancers. The risk of death continues higher than for the general population for at least 25 years after the operation, although this risk gradually diminishes with time (Fig. 15-22). According to Berg and Robbins, change in risk over the postoperative period follows a log-normal curve. From this model it can be predicted that after operation the risk of recurrence and death will continue to decrease but will always be present, being about 1 percent in the decade from 30 to 40 years after operation and 0.5 percent from 40 to 50 years after operation. The 20-year survival rate after operation for patients without axillary lymph node involvement is 65 percent, and that for all patients with radical mastectomy is 41 percent [Berg and Robbins]. If patients are considered who have node involvement at the apex of the axilla, the middle, and the lower portion, the 20-year survival is 11, 30, and 39 percent, respectively. These figures illustrate how important the absence or the extent of lymph node involvement is in determining patient survival. The increasing number of patients with primary lesions of the breast without lymph node involvement is the most important factor in the improving survival rates today compared with 25 years ago.

In the past, not all observers believed that survival rates were improving. Shimkin argued that the incidence rates for breast cancer and the death rates from breast cancer in Connecticut and upper New York State were unchanged for two decades (1940–1960), indicating that no increase in cure rates has occurred (Fig. 15-23). On the other hand, Breslow cites figures of the California state tumor registry indicating that the mortality from cancer of the breast began to decline in that state in 1940 and has continued to drop significantly since that time. Gold and Roth write that "the results of radical mastectomy have changed little since the procedure was introduced by Halsted." They cite 5-year survival rates for his series of 75 percent when nodes were not involved and 25 percent when nodes were involved. In contast, current figures in large groups of pa-

Fig. 15-20. Absolute survival figures in different series following treatment by radical mastectomy. Note improvement in survival from original observations to 1955. (*From H. Vermund, Trends in Radiotherapy in Breast Cancer, Proc 5th Natl Cancer Conf Philadelphia, 1965, by permission.*)

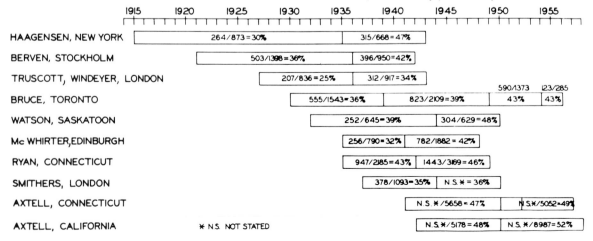

tients collected from entire states and areas indicate 5-year survivals of 80 to 85 percent when the axillary nodes are histologically negative and 50 to 55 percent when nodes are positive. In 1972 much of this confusion was cleared. Epidemiologic reports from Connecticut and Saskatchewan, Canada, have established a significant increase in the incidence of breast cancer over the past three decades, while the mortality rate in these areas has been decreasing (Fig. 15-24).

RADICAL MASTECTOMY INTEGRATED WITH PREOPERATIVE IRRADIATION. Preoperative irradiation in high doses to the primary and the node-bearing areas is currently being evaluated. The data of Fletcher and associates in 1964 indicate that this integrated therapy improves the 5-year survival rate, especially in patients with more advanced lesions, but there are not enough data available to confirm these findings.

SIMPLE MASTECTOMY AND RADIATION THERAPY. Absolute survival figures from McWhirter's original series agree fairly closely with those from series treated by radical mastectomy (Fig. 15-20). Comparison by clinical classification of patients treated by the McWhirter technique with patients treated by other methods also indicates fairly similar end results (Table 15-2). One of the rare randomized clinical studies was done by Kaae and Johansen, who compared simple mastectomy plus radiation therapy with extended radical mastectomy. The results in Stage A (Columbia classification) patients were 70 percent and 74 percent, respectively, and in Stage B patients 50 percent and 47 percent, respectively. From this it appears that treatment of node-bearing areas by radiation or by operation is equally effective. The chief criticisms of the Kaae and Johansen study have been (1) the unusually high proportion of Stage A cases (293 Stage A and 60 Stage B), in whom treatment of node-bearing areas would be least useful, and (2) the fact that the internal mammary node dissection done in the study was accomplished by picking out the nodes from the intercostal spaces instead of by en bloc dissection as in the United States.

RADIATION THERAPY ALONE. Baclesse, in the single extensive series of cases treated by radiation alone, reported 54 percent 5-year survival in the Columbia Stage A group and 67 percent 5-year survival in Columbia Stage B group. These figures again compare reasonably with similar groups treated by operative methods or by combined methods. Why Stage B patients did so well is unexplained. Since these results represent only one clinician and one institution, further study by others is needed.

Unique data concerning the use of radiation alone in the treatment of breast cancer were provided by Guttmann, who treated patients who had metastasis in the internal mammary, highest axillary, or supraclavicular nodes as demonstrated by Haagensen's triple-biopsy technique. A 2-million-volt x-ray was used, and the 5-year survival among 67 patients was 50 percent. Survival among 39 patients with involvement of both internal mammary and axillary nodes was 47 percent.

Some confusion has been generated in the recent years by surgeons who have advocated partial excision of the breast with only a small rim of surrounding normal breast.

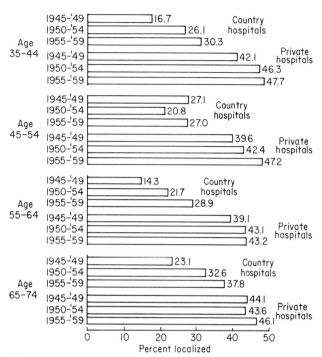

Fig. 15-21. Incidence of localized disease at time of diagnosis in California. Note greater increase in private than in county hospitals. (*From L. Breslow, Epidemiologic Considerations in Breast Cancer, Proc 5th Natl Cancer Conf Philadelphia, 1965, by permission.*)

This has been called by some "lumpectomy." It must be understood that this is not a primary or complete treatment. All such patients must receive radiation therapy to the breast and usually to the surrounding lymph nodes. It is known that at least 50 percent of all carcinomas of the breast have multicentric foci within the involved breast. While this is most prominent in lobular cancer, it occurs in all the other types as well. Simple excision of a portion of the breast is not a complete treatment and must be

Fig. 15-22. Mortality 20 years after treatment by radical mastectomy; 95 percent of expected mortality has been realized, and over 40 percent of treated patients are still surviving. (*From J. W. Berg and G. F. Robbins, Surg Gynecol Obstet, 122:1311, 1966, by permission.*)

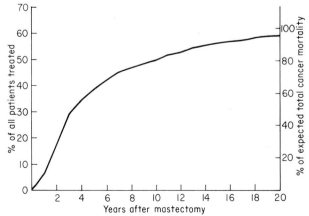

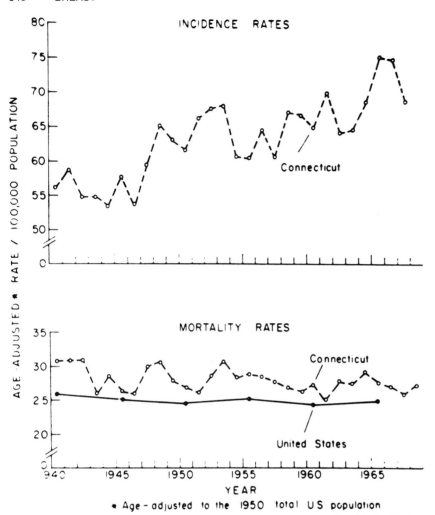

Fig. 15-23. Contrary to past reports data from large population groups now indicate an increasing incidence and a decreasing mortality rate for breast cancer. (*From S. J. Cutler, B. Christine, and T. H. C. Barcley, Cancer, 28:1376, 1971.*)

followed by further therapy. "Lumpectomy" should best be thought of as a simple excisional biopsy which must be followed by radiation if more extensive operation is not elected. In this case radiation is the therapeutic part of the regimen, whereas surgery has been restricted to its diagnostic function.

SIMPLE MASTECTOMY ALONE. In Rockford, Illinois, during World War II, many of the experienced surgeons in the community were called into service. The incidence of patients treated for carcinoma of the breast by simple mastectomy rose from 16 to 42 percent, as few of the remaining surgeons were able to perform the larger procedure. Following the war the incidence of simple mastectomy fell to 15 percent as more experienced surgeons returned. Smith and Meyer analyzed the results of this natural experiment, expecting to find that the long-term results would be worse for the war years. To their surprise they did not find this so. In fact, 5-year results were 53 percent survival for the patients with radical mastectomy and 54 percent with simple mastectomy. Shimkin et al. have reanalyzed these data and confirmed the results. The chief criticism of this study is the impossibility of eliminating selection as a major factor: were patients with

axillary node involvement or more advanced disease more likely to be sent either to the more experienced surgeons remaining in town for radical mastectomy or to Chicago for treatment?

Crile studied this problem by treating with simple mastectomy all patients on his service who were without clinical axillary node involvement. Other surgeons at the same clinic continued to do radical mastectomy. In this series, survival of Stage I (Manchester classification) patients at 5 years was 70 percent of 56 patients with simple mastectomy and 62.5 percent of 40 patients with radical mastectomy. This study unfortunately is too small to have significance, as Crile noted. More unfortunate is that 29 percent of the simple mastectomy group and 45 percent of the radical mastectomy group received radiation therapy postoperatively. In the author's opinion the experiment is compromised by the addition of this extra modality. Crile's treatment differs from all others in that the node-bearing areas are not treated. He argues that treatment of these areas diminishes the host's resistance to the tumor. But by the treatment of these areas with x-rays in almost one-third of his patients the point of his thesis is lost.

EXTENDED RADICAL MASTECTOMY. The best report of the results of this technique was published by Sugarbaker, who compared sequential series from his personal practice of 88 patients treated by conventional radical mastectomy and 158 treated by extended mastectomy. As would be expected, 5-year results in patients without node involvement were similar, 84 and 86 percent, respectively. In patients with involved nodes, survival at 5 years was 70 percent with the extended procedure and 33 percent with the conventional procedure. The major criticism of this report is that patients were treated in sequential blocks rather than concurrently as a randomized series. The same criticism can be directed to most other series, many of which lack any control group. In view of inconclusive results to date, this procedure has not been generally accepted.

SUMMARY. Most surgeons today perform radical mastectomy for cancer of the breast not because they know it is the best procedure but because they are unsure which procedure *is* best. Their adherence to the status quo is justified. The available data are vast, but there is not a single statistically valid study comparing various techniques with the exception of Kaae and Johansen's. Randomized concurrent studies are sorely needed and can be clinically justified. The National Institutes of Health has recently funded such a program under the supervision of Fisher. Until the results of this program are available, most United States surgeons will continue to rely on conventional radical mastectomy for the treatment of breast cancer. The conclusion can be drawn that treatment does favorably modify the course of cancer of the breast. Radiation or operation or both can accomplish this, but which modality or combination of modalities is best remains to be demonstrated.

TREATMENT OF RECURRENT CANCER

Prior to the 1940s recurrent cancer of the breast was treated either with radiation or operation or not at all. Radiation remains an extremely useful agent for painful osseous metastases and small subcutaneous lesions. Operation also may be useful for small local lesions. The basic

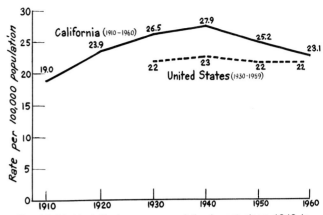

Fig. 15-24. Mortality from cancer of the breast since 1940 in California. Incidence rate remained stable while death rate decreased slowly. (*From L. Breslow, Epidemiologic Considerations in Breast Cancer, Proc 5th Natl Cancer Conf Philadelphia, 1965, by permission.*)

problem in the patient with recurrent cancer is most often wide dissemination, and the new systemic agents of hormone therapy and chemotherapy are the treatments of choice.

As these new agents became available over the past 25 years, the tendency of some was to treat recurrent lesions with everything simultaneously in the hope that something might work. There is no excuse for this shotgun approach today. Success or failure with each individual agent provides a valuable index to the next step in management. The first consideration in management is the patient's menopausal status.

THE PREMENOPAUSAL PATIENT. The first step in therapy is castration (Fig. 15-25). Remission of cancer with objective decrease in the size of lesions will occur in 30 to 50 percent of patients. Patients with such remissions will enjoy a significant increase in survival time. Kennedy has shown that the benefits of castration occur whether it is done at the time of the original radical mastectomy or at the time of recurrence. From the patient's standpoint there is great advantage in waiting for recurrence before castration is done. Unnecessary oophorectomy is thus avoided, since not all patients will require it. Important, too, is the opportunity to determine the hormonal sensitivity of the

Table 15-2. METHODS OF TREATMENT COMPARED BY COLUMBIA CLASSIFICATION STAGES

Author	No. of patients		Method	5-yr survival, %	
	A	B		A	B
Kennedy and Miller	115	34	Simple mastectomy	62	41
Handley and Thackray	77	58	Limited radical mastectomy	75	57
Butcher	216	135	Classic radical mastectomy	76	48
Haagensen I	228	122	Classic radical mastectomy	82.5	59
Haagensen II	116	16	Classic radical mastectomy	87.9	62.5
Dahl-Iversen and Tobiassen	277	61	Extended radical mastectomy	77	48
Williams and Curwen	68	57	Limited radical mastectomy and radiation	72	60
Kaae and Johansen	159	28	Simple mastectomy and radiation	70	50
Baclesse	50	86	Radiation only	54	67

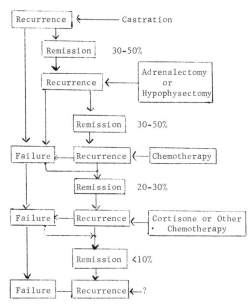

Fig. 15-25. Sequence of therapy in premenopausal female with inoperable or recurrent cancer of the breast.

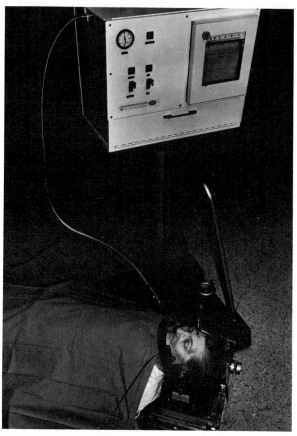

Fig. 15-26. Cryohypophysectomy. Patient is under local anesthesia. Insertion of cold probe into pituitary is by stereotaxic device. Ablation of gland is done with very low morbidity and mortality.

tumor. The response of a breast cancer to castration is still the only reliable index of "hormonal response." A patient who responds to this procedure and has a subsequent recurrence of tumor growth has a 30 to 50 percent chance of responding subsequently to adrenalectomy or hypophysectomy. Some human breast tumors take up and bind estradiol in tissue cultures. These tumors appear to respond well to hormonal ablation. This test has not been developed to the point of clinical usefulness, although it may have this potential.

If the patient refuses castration, testosterone (100 mg intramuscularly three times a week) may produce remission in 20 percent. The distressing masculinizing side effects—hirsutism, acne, lowering of the voice, and often increased libido—make this drug a poor second choice.

At one time there was much controversy as to which procedure, adrenalectomy or hypophysectomy, was the better. A national cooperative study indicates that neither is superior: they give identical response rates (30 to 50 percent), and the mortality (9 percent) and morbidity are approximately the same. The recent introduction of cryohypophysectomy, which can be done under local anesthesia, raises hope that this simpler procedure with lower mortality may be a better means for palliation. The cold probe is inserted through the nares and via the sphenoid sinus into the hypophysis (Fig. 15-26). The degree of cold and the duration of application determine the amount of tissue destruction. However, the procedure is still too new for complete evaluation.

Patients who have had recurrence following a good response to hypophysectomy or oophorectomy and adrenalectomy or who have failed to respond to oophorectomy are considered candidates for chemotherapy. The agent of choice has been 5-fluorouracil, which produces objective remissions in 20 to 30 percent of patients for an average period of 3 months. Other agents with modest remission

rates of 10 to 20 percent are cyclophosphamide and vincristine. Combinations of several agents given over more prolonged periods are now finding favor. Cyclophosphamide, prednisone, methotrexate, vincristine, and 5-fluorouracil used in combination have produced tumor response in 68 percent of patients in one series. Mean duration of response in one group of patients was 21 months.

THE POSTMENOPAUSAL PATIENT. The drug of choice in the postmenopausal patient with recurrent breast cancer

Fig. 15-27. Sequence of therapy in postmenopausal female with inoperable or recurrent cancer of the breast.

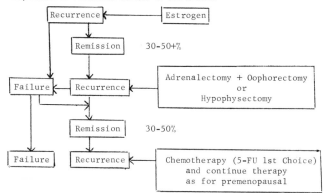

and systemic spread is estrogen (Fig. 15-27), usually administered as oral stilbestrol (15 mg/day). There is an obvious paradox in this, since the original hormonal management in these patients was designed to ablate estrogen-producing organs and to reduce the level of circulating estrogens, which were assumed to stimulate hormonally sensitive cancer. Whatever the theory, the current evidence shows estrogen to be very effective in suppressing the growth of breast tumor in the postmenopausal female. Its effectiveness increases with time following menopause, so that at 10 years postmenopause 50 percent or more of patients will have satisfactory remissions of their tumors. Some feel that the response to estrogens is a good index of the usefulness of surgical endocrine ablation. Kennedy reported that patients who respond to estrogen have a 70 percent chance of responding to hypophysectomy.

The chief side effect of estrogen is nausea. This is fleeting in most, but 10 percent of patients cannot tolerate the drug for this reason. All patients on estrogens who have an intact uterus must be warned that if the drug is stopped suddenly, a menstrual flow will follow. This can be most distressing to the eighty-year-old female, 35 years past her last period, if she is not prepared for the event.

Patients who fail to respond to estrogens or who have recurrences after a remission produced by estrogen and/or endocrine ablation are treated by chemotherapy or cortisone as described for premenopausal patients.

The orderly use of systemic agents may prolong life in some patients from a few months to several years. The physician must remember that this is palliative, not curative, therapy and there is usually no urgency in starting treatment. A few small skin nodules may be treated locally or observed for a time and treatment initiated only if growth appears rapid or symptoms supervene. There is no evidence that earlier introduction of these palliative measures produces better results than later treatment. If the cancer is sensitive, very large lesions often regress; if not, even the smallest lesions may be unaffected. The only urgency is in starting therapy in cases that have reached a near-terminal stage without hormonal or chemotherapeutic treatment.

Infection

ACUTE INFECTION

Bacterial infections almost always occur in the lactating breast in the first month or two following delivery. The portal of entry is an abrasion or fissure in the nipple. The best treatment is prevention, with the nursing mother carefully cleaning and drying her nipples after nursing. Because cleanliness is so important, infection more commonly occurs in patients from a lower socioeconomic stratum. It is also seasonal, being more common in the hot summer months.

The milk-containing ducts and acini of the lactating breast are a perfect culture medium, and infection, having gained access, often progresses rapidly through inflammation to suppuration. This is accompanied by extreme pain in the breast, and a good diagnostic sign of abscess is the patient's rapid withdrawal when the physician attempts to palpate the involved breast. The breast is red and the area of abscess indurated and firm. The tendency is to underestimate the size of the abscess on physical examination.

An abscess may be aborted by the use of systemic antibiotics and local radiation therapy. Treatment of abscess is by surgical drainage. Antibiotics will suppress the process for a time, but it will flare up again when they are discontinued. A curviliear transverse incision is made in the dependent portion of the breast and the gloved finger or a clamp used to break up the many septa which separate the cavity into loculations. A rubber drain is left in the wound. Culture of the pus usually demonstrates *Staphylococcus aureus*. Pain is relieved promptly by drainage, and the surrounding inflammation subsides rapidly.

CHRONIC INFECTION

Chronic infection of the breast is now rare. Tuberculosis is the major cause, and as the incidence of this disease has decreased, so have breast lesions caused by it. The genesis of breast tuberculosis is either pleural or, more commonly, the breaking down of a mediastinal node to involve one of the costal cartilages. Infection simmers in the cartilage for long periods, giving rise to lesions in the breast, which eventually form one or several fistulas to the skin. Antituberculosis drugs are now the primary treatment for this disease, but care of the breast lesion usually requires excision of the affected costal cartilage.

References

General

Geschickter, C. F.: "Diseases of the Breast," J. B. Lippincott Company, Philadelphia, 1943.

Haagensen, C. D.: "Diseases of the Breast," 2d ed., W. B. Saunders Company, Philadelphia, 1971.

Anatomy and Development

Batson, O. V.: The Function of the Vertebral Veins and Their Role in the Spread of Metastasis, *Ann Surg,* **112:**138, 1940.

Cooper, Sir A. P.: "The Anatomy and Diseases of the Breast," Lea and Blanchard, Philadelphia, 1845.

Ingleby, H., and Gershon-Cohen, J.: "Cooperative Anatomy: Pathology and Roentgenology of the Breast," University of Pennsylvania Press, Philadelphia, 1960.

Taylor, G. T.: Anatomy of the Breast with Particular Reference to Lymphatic Drainage, in W. H. Parson, "Cancer of the Breast," Charles C Thomas, Publisher, Springfield, Ill., 1959.

Examination of the Breast

Berger, S. M., and Gershon-Cohen, J.: Mammography of Breast Sarcoma, *Am J Roentgenol Radium Ther Nucl Med,* **87:**76, 1962.

Clark, R. L., Copeland, M. M., Egan, R. L., Gallagher, H. S., Geller, H., Lindsay, J. P., Robbins, L. C., and White, E. C.: Reproducibility of the Technic of Mammography (Egan) for Cancer of the Breast, *Am J Surg,* **109:**127, 1965.

Gershon-Cohen, J., and Berger, S. M.: Detection of Breast Cancer by Periodic X-ray Examinations: A Five-year Survey, *JAMA,* **176:**1114, 1961.

———, ———, and Klickstein, H. S.: Roentgenography of Breast Cancer Moderating Concept of "Biologic Predeterminism," *Cancer,* **16:**961, 1963.

——— and Ingleby, H.: Roentgenography of Unsuspected Carcinoma of Breast, *JAMA,* **166:**869, 1958.

Ingleby, H., Moore, L., and Gershon-Cohen, J.: A Roentgenographic Study of the Growth Rate of Six "Early" Cancers of the Breast, *Cancer,* **11:**726, 1958.

Snyder, R. E.: Mammography and Lobular Carcinoma In Situ, *Surg Gynecol Obstet,* **122:**255, 1966.

Treves, N., and Holleb, A. I.: Cancer of the Male Breast: A Report of 146 Cases, *Cancer,* **8:**1239, 1955.

Neoplasms

Auchincloss, H.: Significance of Location and Number of Auxillary Metastases in Carcinoma of the Breast: A Justification for a Conservative Operation, *Ann Surg,* **158:**37, 1963.

Baclesse, F.: Five-year Results in 431 Breast Cancers Treated Solely by Roentgen Rays, *Ann Surg,* **161:**103, 1965.

Berg, J. W., and Robbins, G. F.: Factors Influencing Short and Long-Term Survival of Breast Cancer Patients, *Surg Gynecol Obstet,* **122:**1311, 1966.

Bloom, H. J. G., Richardson, W. W., and Harries, E. J.: Natural History of Untreated Breast Cancer (1805–1933): Comparison of Untreated and Treated Cases according to Histological Grade of Malignancy, *Br Med J,* **5299:**213, 1962.

Branfield, J. R., Fingerhut, A. G., and Warner, N. E.: Lobular Carcinoma of the Breast—1969: A Therapeutic Proposal, *Arch Surg,* **99:**129, 1969.

Breslow, L.: Epidemiologic Considerations in Breast Cancer, *Proc 5th Natl Cancer Conf Philadelphia,* 1965.

Butcher, H. R., Jr.: Effectiveness of Radical Mastectomy for Mammary Cancer: An Analysis of Mortalities by the Method of Probits, *Ann Surg,* **154:**383, 1961.

———: Radical Mastectomy for Mammary Carcinoma, *Ann Surg,* **157:**165, 1963.

Crile, G., Jr.: Results of Simplified Treatment of Breast Cancer, *Surg Gynecol Obstet,* **118:**517, 1964.

——— and Hoerr, S. O.: Results of Treatment of Carcinoma of the Breast by Local Excision, *Surg Gynecol Obstet,* **132:**780, 1971.

Crowley, L. G., and MacDonald, I.: Delalutin and Estrogens for the Treatment of Advanced Mammary Carcinoma in the Postmenopausal Woman, *Cancer,* **18:**436, 1965.

Dahl-Iversen, E., and Tobiassen, T.: Radical Mastectomy with Parasternal and Supraclavicular Dissection for Mammary Carcinoma, *Ann Surg,* **157:**170, 1963.

Dao, T. L., and Nemoto, T.: An Evaluation of Adrenalectomy and Androgen in Disseminated Mammary Carcinoma, *Surg Gynecol Obstet,* **121:**1257, 1965.

Den Besten, L., and Ziffren, S. E.: Simple and Radical Mastectomy: A Comparison of Survival, *Arch Surg,* **90:**755, 1965.

Fairgrieve, J.: Selective Criteria for Surgical Removal of the Endocrine Glands in Advanced Breast Cancer, *Surg Gynecol Obstet,* **120:**371, 1965.

Fisher, B., Slack, N. H., Cavanaugh, P. J., Gardner, B., and

Ravdin, R. G.: Postoperative Radiotherapy in the Treatment of Breast Cancer: Results of the NSABP Clinical Trial, *Ann Surg,* **172:**711, 1970.

Fletcher, G. H., Montague, E., and White, E. C.: Evaluation of Preoperative Irradiation for Carcinoma for the Breast, *Proc 5th Natl Cancer Conf Philadelphia 1964,* 1965.

Foote, F. W., and Stewart, F. W.: Comparative Studies of Cancerous versus Noncancerous Breasts: I. Basic Morphology Characteristics, *Ann Surg,* **121:**6, 1945.

——— and ———: Comparative Studies of Cancerous versus Noncancerous Breasts: II. Role of So-called Chronic Cystic Mastitis in Mammary Carcinogenesis: Influence of Certain Hormones on Human Breast Structure, *Ann Surg,* **121:**197, 1945.

Freckman, H. A., Fry, H. L., Mendez, F. L., and Maurer, E. R.: Chlorambucil-Prednisolone Therapy for Disseminated Breast Carcinoma, *JAMA,* **189:**23, 1964.

Galante, M.: Minimal Breast Cancer: A Surgeon's Dilemma, *Cancer,* **28:**1516, 1971.

Gold, D., and Roth, E. J.: Current Operative Treatment of Carcinoma of the Breast and Its Rationale, *Am J Surg,* **110:**724, 1965.

Goldenberg, I. S.: Hormones and Breast Cancer: Historical Perspectives, *Surgery,* **53:**285, 1963.

———: Testosterone Propionate Therapy in Breast Cancer, *JAMA,* **188:**117, 1964.

———, Bailar, J. C., III, Hayes, M. A., and Lowry, R.: Female Breast Cancer: A Re-evaluation, *Ann Surg,* **154:**397, 1961.

———, ———, and Lowry, R.: Survival of Women with Hormonally Treated Breast Cancer, *Surg Gynecol Obstet,* **119:**785, 1964.

Green, R. B., Sethi, R. S., and Lindner, H. H.: Treatment of Advanced Carcinoma of the Breast, *Am J Surg,* **108:**107, 1964.

Guttman, R.: Radiotherapy in the Treatment of Primary Operable Carcinoma of the Breast with Proved Lymph Node Metastases: Approach and Results, *Am J Roentgenol Radium Ther Nucl Med,* **89:**58, 1963.

Haagensen, C. D., and Cooley, E.: Radical Mastectomy for Mammary Carcinoma, *Ann Surg,* **157:**166, 1963.

———, ———, Kennedy, C. S., Miller, E., Handley, R. S., Thackray, A. C., Butcher, H. R., Jr., Dahl-Iversen, E., Tobiassen, T., Williams, I. G., Curwen, M. P., Kaae, S., and Johansen, H.: Treatment of Early Mammary Carcinoma: A Cooperative International Study, *Ann Surg,* **157:**157, 1963.

Handley, R. S., and Thackray, A. C.: The Internal Mammary Lymph Chain in Carcinoma of the Breast: Study of 50 Cases, *Lancet,* **257:**276, 1949.

——— and ———: Conservative Radical Mastectomy (Patey's Operation), *Ann Surg,* **157:**162, 1963.

Hems, G.: Epidemiological Characteristics of Breast Cancer in Middle and Late Age, *Br J Cancer,* **24:**226, 1970.

Holleb, A. I., Montgomery, R., and Farrow, J. H.: The Hazard of Incomplete Simple Mastectomy, *Surg Gynecol Obstet,* **121:**819, 1965.

James, F., James, V. H. T., Carter, A. E., and Irvine, W. T.: A Comparison of In Vivo and In Vitro Uptake of Estradiol by Human Breast Tumors and the Relationship of Steroid Excretion, *Cancer Res,* **31:**1268, 1971.

Kaae, S., and Johansen, H.: Breast Cancer: A Comparison of

Simple Mastectomy with Postoperative Roentgen Irradiation by the McWhirter Method with Those of Extended Radical Mastectomy, *Acta Radiol Supp,* **155:**185, 1959.

————— and —————: Simple Mastectomy plus Postoperative Irradiation by the Method of McWhirter for Mammary Carcinoma, *Ann Surg,* **157:**175, 1963.

Karpas, C. M., Leis, H. P., Oppenheim, A., and Mersheimer, W. L.: Relationship of Fibrocystic Disease to Carcinoma of the Breast, *Ann Surg,* **162:**1, 1965.

Kaufman, R. J.: Medical Management of Breast Cancer, *Clin Bull Mem Hosp,* **2:**21, 1972.

Kay, S., and Poulos, N. G.: Evaluation of the Criteria of Operability of Carcinoma of the Breast, *Surg Gynecol Obstet,* **113:**562, 1961.

Kennedy, B. J.: The Role of Castration in Breast Cancer, *Arch Surg,* **88:**743, 1964.

—————: Diethylstilbestrol versus Testosterone Propionate Therapy in Advanced Breast Cancer, *Surg Gynecol Obstet,* **120:**1246, 1965.

—————: Hormone Therapy for Advanced Breast Cancer, *Cancer,* **18:**1551, 1965.

————— and Brown, J. H.: Combined Estrogenic and Androgenic Hormone Therapy in Advanced Breast Cancer, *Cancer,* **18:** 431, 1965.

————— and French, L.: Hypophysectomy in Advanced Breast Cancer, *Am J Surg,* **110:**411, 1965.

—————, Meilke, P. W., Jr., and Fortuny, I. E.: Therapeutic Castration versus Prophylactic Castration in Breast Cancer, *Surg Gynecol Obstet,* **118:**524, 1964.

Kennedy, C. S., and Miller, E.: Simple Mastectomy for Mammary Carcinoma, *Ann Surg,* **157:**161, 1963.

Kleinfeld, G., Haagensen, C. D., and Cooley, E.: Age and Menstrual Status as Prognostic Factors in Carcinoma of the Breast, *Ann Surg,* **157:**600, 1963.

Kraft, R. O., and Block, G. E.: Mammary Carcinoma in the Aged Patient, *Ann Surg,* **156:**981, 1962.

Kusama, S., Spratt, J. S., Jr., Donegan, W. L., Watson, F. R., and Cunningham, C.: The Gross Rates of Growth of Human Mammary Carcinoma, *Cancer,* **30:**594, 1972.

Landau, R. L., Ehrlich, E. N., and Huggins, C.: Estradiol Benzoate and Progesterone in Advanced Human-Breast Cancer, *JAMA,* **182:**632, 1962.

Leis, H. P.: The Hormonal Therapy of Advanced Carcinoma of the Breast, *J Int Coll Surg,* **36:**225, 1961.

Lewison, E. F.: "Breast Cancer and Its Diagnosis and Treatment," The Williams & Wilkins Company, Baltimore, 1955.

—————: The Problem of Prognosis in Cancer of the Breast, *Surgery,* **37:**479, 1955.

—————: The Results of Treatment of Breast Cancer at the Johns Hopkins Hospital 1941–1945 with a Discussion, *Surg Gynecol Obstet,* **107:**313, 1958.

—————: An Appraisal of Long-Term Results in Surgical Treatment of Breast Cancer, *JAMA,* **186:**975, 1963.

————— and Lyons, J. G., Jr.: Relationship between Benign Breast Disease and Cancer, *Arch Surg,* **66:**94, 1953.

————— and Neto, A. S.: Bilateral Breast Cancer at the Johns Hopkins Hospital: A Discussion of the Dilemma of Contralateral Breast Cancer, *Cancer,* **28:**1297, 1971.

Linden, G., Cline, J. W., Wood, D. A., Guiss, L. W., and Breslow, L.: Validity of Pathological Diagnosis of Breast Cancer, *JAMA,* **173:**143, 1960.

MacDonald, I.: Endocrine Ablation in Disseminated Mammary Carcinoma, *Surg Gynecol Obstet,* **115:**215, 1962.

—————: The Natural History of Mammary Carcinoma, *Am J Surg,* **111:**435, 1966.

McWhirter, R.: Treatment of Cancer of the Breast by Simple Mastectomy and Roentgenotherapy, *Arch Surg,* **59:**830, 1949.

Madden, J. L.: Modified Radical Mastectomy, *Surg Gynecol Obstet,* **121:**1221, 1965.

Missakian, M. M., Witten, D. M., and Harrison, E. G., Jr.: Mammography after Mastectomy: Usefulness in Search for Recurrent Carcinoma of the Breast, *JAMA,* **191:**1045, 1965.

Moore, D. H., Sarkar, N. H., Kramarksy, B., Lasfargues, E. Y., and Charney, J.: Some Aspects of the Search for a Human Mammary Tumor Virus, *Cancer,* **28:**1415, 1971.

Moore, F. D., Woodrow, S. I., Aliapoulios, M. A., and Wilson, R. E.: Carcinoma of the Breast: A Decade of New Results with Old Concepts, *N Engl J Med,* **277:**293, 1967.

Moore, S. W., and Lewis, R. J.: Carcinoma of the Breast in Women 30 Years of Age and Under, *Surg Synecol Obstet,* **119:**1253, 1964.

Murad, T. M.: A Proposed Histochemical and Electron Microscopic Classification of Human Breast Cancer According to Cell of Origin, *Cancer,* **27:**288, 1971.

Nelsen, T. S., and Dragstedt, L. R.: Adrenalectomy and Oophorectomy for Breast Cancer, *JAMA,* **175:**379, 1961.

Norris, H. J., and Taylor, H. B.: Carcinoma of the Breast in Women Less than Thirty Years Old, *Cancer,* **26:**953, 1970.

Oberman, H. A.: Sarcomas of the Breast, *Cancer,* **18:**1233, 1965.

Owen, H. W., Dockerty, M. B., and Gray, H. K.: Occult Carcinoma of the Breast, *Surg Gynecol Obstet,* **98:**302, 1954.

Pack, G. T.: Argument for Bilateral Mastectomy, *Surgery,* **29:**929, 1951. (Editorial.)

Papaioannou, A. N., and Urban, J. A.: Scalene Node Biopsy in Locally Advanced Primary Breast Cancer of Questionable Operability, *Cancer,* **17:**1006, 1964.

Papdrianos, E., Cooley, E., and Haagensen, C. D.: Mammary Carcinoma in Old Age, *Ann Surg,* **161:**189, 1965.

Park, W. W., and Lees, J. C.: Absolute Curability of Cancer of the Breast, *Surg Gynecol Obstet,* **93:**129, 1951.

Parson, W. H.: "Cancer of the Breast," Charles C Thomas, Publisher, Springfield, Ill., 1959.

Prohaska, J. V., Houttuin, E., and Kocandrle, V.: Mammary Carcinoma Metastes: Response to Bilateral Adrenalectomy and Oophorectomy, *Arch Surg,* **92:**530, 1966.

Richards, G. J., Jr., and Lewison, E. F.: Inflammatory Carcinoma of the Breast, *Surg Gynecol Obstet,* **113:**729, 1961.

Robbins, G. F., and Berg, J. W.: Bilateral Primary Breast Cancers, *Cancer,* **17:**1501, 1964.

—————, Brothers, J. H., III, Eberhart, W., F., and Quan, S.: Is Aspiration Biopsy of Breast Cancer Dangerous to the Patient? *Cancer,* **7:**774, 1954.

Rosen, P., Snyder, R. E., Foote, F. W., and Wallace, T.: Detection of Occult Carcinoma in the Apparently Benign Breast Biopsy through Specimen Radiography, *Cancer,* **26:**944, 1970.

Rubin, P.: "Carcinoma of the Breast," American Cancer Society, New York, 1967.

Rush, B. F., Jr., and Kramer, W. M.: Proliferative Histological

Changes and Occult Carcinoma in the Breast of the Aging Female, *Surg Synecol Obstet,* **117:**425, 1963.

Sandison, A. T.: An Autopsy Study of the Adult Human Breast: With Special Reference to Proliferative Epithelial Changes of Importance in the Pathology of the Breast, *Natl Cancer Inst Monogr* 8, June 1962.

Sanger, G.: An Aspect of Internal Mammary Metastases from Carcinoma of the Breast, *Ann Surg,* **157:**180, 1963.

Schmidt, M. L., Nemoto, T., Dao, T., and Bross, I. D. J.: Prognostic Factors Affecting Adrenalectomy in Patients with Metastatic Cancer of the Breast, *Cancer,* **27:**1106, 1971.

Sherlock, P., and Hartmann, W. H.: Adrenal Steroids and the Pattern of Metastases of Breast Cancer, *JAMA,* **181:**103, 1962.

Shimkin, M. B.: Cancer of the Breast: Some Old Facts and New Prospectives, *JAMA,* **183:**358, 1963.

————, Koppel, M., Connelly, R. R., and Cutler, S. J.: Simple and Radical Mastectomy for Breast Cancer: A Re-analysis of Smith and Meyer's Report from Rockford, Illinois, *J Natl Cancer Inst,* **27:**1197, 1961.

Shingleton, W. W., Sedransk, N., and Johnson, R. O.: Systemic Chemotherapy for Mammary Carcinoma, *Ann Surg,* **173:**913, 1971.

Silva, A. R. M., Smart, C. R., and Rochlin, D. B.: Chemotherapy of Breast Cancer, *Surg Gynecol Obstet,* **121:**494, 1965.

Smith, S. S., and Meyer, A. C.: Cancer of the Breast in Rockford, Illinois, *Am J Surg,* **98:**653, 1959.

Strax, P.: New Techniques in Mass Screening for Breast Cancer, *Cancer,* **28:**1563, 1971.

Subcommittee on Breast and Genital Cancer of the AMA: Androgens and Estrogens in the Treatment of Disseminated Mammary Carcinoma: Retrospective Study of Nine Hundred Forty-four Patients, *JAMA,* **172:**1271, 1960.

Sugarbaker, E. D.: Extended Radical Mastectomy: Its Superiority in the Treatment of Breast Cancer, *JAMA,* **187:**95, 1964.

Surgical Adjuvant Chemotherapy Breast Group: Breast Adjuvant Chemotherapy: Effectiveness of Thio-tepa (Triethylenethiophosphoramide) as Adjuvant to Radical Mastectomy for Breast Cancer, *Ann Surg,* **154:**629, 1961.

Tellem, M., Prive, L., and Meranze, D. R.: Four-quadrant Study of Breast Removed for Carcinoma, *Cancer,* **15:**10, 1962.

Treves, N., and Holleb, A. I.: Cancer of the Male Breast: A Report of 146 Cases, *Cancer,* **8:**1239, 1955.

Trimble, I. R., and Trimble, F. H.: Changes in the Treatment of Cancer of the Breast, *Surg Gynecol Obstet,* **114:**103, 1962.

Urban, J. A.: Bilaterality of Cancer of the Breast: Biopsy of the Opposite Breast, *Cancer,* **20:**1867, 1971.

———— and Baker, H. W.: Radical Mastectomy in Continuity with En Bloc Resection of the Internal Mammary Lymph-Node Chain: A New Procedure for Primary Operable Cancer of the Breast, *Cancer,* **5:**992, 1952.

Vermund, H.: Trends in Radiotherapy in Breast Cancer, *Proc 5th Natl Cancer Conf Philadelphia 1964,* 1965.

Whitney, D. G., Smith, R. F., and Szilagyi, D. E.: Meaning of Five-Year Cure in Cancer of the Breast, *Arch Surg,* **88:**637, 1964.

Williams, I. G., and Curwen, M. P.: Total Mastectomy with Axillary Dissection and Irradiation for Mammary Carcinoma, *Ann Surg,* **157:**174, 1963.

Wolfe, J. N., Cooley, R. P., and Harkins, L. E.: Xeroradiography of the Breast: A Comparative Study with Conventional Film Mammography, *Cancer,* **28:**1569, 1971.

Zippin, C., and Petrakis, N. L.: Identification of High Risk Groups in Breast Cancer, *Cancer,* **28:**1381, 1971.

Benign Lesions

Davis, H. H., Simons, M., and Davis, J. B.: Cystic Disease of the Breast: Relationship to Carcinoma, *Cancer,* **17:**957, 1964.

Frantz, V. K., Pickren, J. W., Melcher, G. W., and Auchincloss, H., Jr.: Incidence of Chronic Cystic Disease in So-called "Normal Breasts": A Study Based on 225 Postmortem Examinations, *Cancer,* **4:**762, 1951.

Grow, J. L., and Lewison, E. F.: Superficial Thrombophlebitis of the Breast, *Surg Gynecol Obstet,* **116:**180, 1963.

Urban, J. A.: Excision of Major Ducts of the Breast, *Cancer,* **16:**516, 1963.

Chapter 16

Tumors of the Head and Neck

by Benjamin F. Rush, Jr.

Historical Background

Diagnosis
Physical Examination
Diagnostic Studies

Lip
Benign Tumors
Hyperkeratosis
Carcinoma of the Lip

Oral Cavity
Benign Lesions
    Inflammatory Hyperplasia
    Cysts
    Peripheral Giant Cell Reparative Granuloma
    Peripheral Fibroma
    Granuloma Pyogenicum
    Salivary Tumors
    Hemangioma
    Granular Cell Myoblastoma
Hyperkeratosis
Malignant Tumors
    Tongue
    Floor of the Mouth
    Gingivae
    Hard Palate
    Buccal Mucosa

Oropharynx
    Tonsil
    Posterior Third of the Tongue
    Soft Palate
    Epiglottis

Larynx
Benign Tumors
    Polyps
    Vocal Nodules
    Retention Cysts
    Hyperkeratosis
    Papillomas
Malignant Lesions

Hypopharynx

Nasopharynx
Benign Lesions
    Hypertrophied Adenoids
    Juvenile Nasopharyngeal Hemangiofibroma

Malignant Lesions
    Epidermoid Carcinoma
    Lymphosarcoma

Nasal Cavity and Paranasal Sinuses

Benign Tumors
Malignant Tumors

Mandible
Odontogenic Tumors
    Follicular Cyst
    Radicular Cyst
    Ameloblastoma
Osteogenic Tumors

Salivary Glands

Tumors of the Neck
Inflammation
Malignant Tumors
Other Lesions
    Tumors of the Neck in Children

Chemotherapy

Operations of the Head and Neck
Radical Neck Dissection
    Combined Operation
    Bilateral Radical Neck Dissection
Parotidectomy
V Excision of the Lip
Maxillectomy
Total Laryngectomy
Partial Laryngectomy

Postoperative Care following Head and Neck Operations

HISTORICAL BACKGROUND

The head and neck are such public regions of the anatomy that one would expect ancient medical manuscripts to give considerable attention to tumors affecting these parts. Strangely, the ancient writers rarely mention such lesions. The Smith Papyrus (2300 B.C.) mentions wounds of the head frequently, but not a single tumor of the area is discussed. The Ebers Papyrus (1500 B.C.) contains references to "eating ulcer" of the gums and "illness of the tongue," but the descriptions are too brief to be adequately interpreted. Celsus (A.D. 178) is often credited with devising an operation for cancer of the lower lip. Martin notes that Celsus recognized and described cancer of the skin of the face, but his operation on the lower lip was for repair of a "mutilation," probably a war wound.

A perusal of *The Surgery of Theodoric* (A.D. 1267) in the translation of Campbell and Colton gives an interesting perspective of the personal experiences of a master surgeon of the era who had a profound knowledge of the writings of preceding centuries. Theodoric describes numerous lesions about the head and neck, mostly of minor significance, i.e., wens, "white pustules or spots which appear by the nose and over the cheeks," "lumps or swellings occurring on the head called horns," "nodes or wens which are formed on the eyelids," lipoma, pustules on the face, freckles, brown patches, wrinkles, and black and blue spots on the face. There is a lengthy section on "the scrofula." He had a much clearer concept of cancer than most of his contemporaries, but in his entire writing he does not mention the treatment of a single lesion of the lip or intraoral area.

This frequent failure to single out cancerous lesions in this area reflects the inability of our medical ancestors to differentiate grossly between chronic infections and cancer. Certainly some miraculous cures were achieved by ointments and spells applied to hard, round ulcers which, in fact, were chronic infections. An early, operable lesion was certain to be treated at length with salves and potions, and when it was evident beyond doubt that the treatment had failed, it was too late to do anything else.

Galen had established firmly the concept that cancer was a systemic disease, an oversupply of black bile. It made more sense by this concept to treat the systemic cause of the affliction by "proper balancing of the constitution" with bleeding or purging or hot and cold baths than it did to attack directly a symptom of the internal problem which happened to occur on the face or in the mouth. The beginnings of rational operations for cancer awaited the discovery of cancer's primary origin in the various organs and the ability to differentiate cancer grossly and microscopically from other confusingly similar diseases.

In addition to the problems of diagnosis, extensive cancer operations were impossible without anesthesia. Even minor operations about the head and neck were few when the patient had to be conscious to witness them. The gruesome habit of excising the tongue for torture and punishment is as old as man, but the first such excision for cancer is attributed to Marchette in 1664. Avicenna (980–1037) described excision of tumors of the lip, the wound being left open to heal by secondary intention, but the classic V excision for cancer of the lip was not described until the first part of the nineteenth century. Tracheotomy to relieve laryngeal obstruction was described by Galen and through the ages was occasionally used to prolong somewhat the lives of those with carcinoma of the larynx, but laryngectomy was not accomplished until the late nineteenth century.

With the advent of anesthesia and microscopic pathology in the mid-1800s, operative attack upon cancer in all areas moved swiftly forward. This was especially true of tumors of the head and neck, since they involved easily seen structures and were so readily diagnosed and the suffering of the untreated patients was so apparent. Surgeons of the German school introduced an array of new techniques for operations upon the tongue, gingiva, mandible, maxilla, and larynx. Partial laryngectomy was introduced by Gurdon Buck in 1853, and total laryngectomy for cancer was first accomplished by Billroth in 1873.

In general, the results of these new procedures were more horrifying than gratifying. Operations in a septic field and without antibiotics produced a postoperative complication rate close to 100 percent with cellulitis, sepsis, abscess, pneumonia, and death the common results. Mortality rates exceeded 50 percent. Moreover, the results of many of the early and unsophisticated operations were not much better than if the cancer had not been treated. Billroth's famous first laryngectomy left the patient with an open pharyngostome and esophagostome, so that he constantly drooled saliva over his neck and had to feed himself with a rubber tube during the entire 8 months that he survived operation.

Operative excision was usually confined to the primary lesion, and in many of the patients fortunate enough to survive the initial operation metastatic disease subsequently developed in cervical nodes. Kocher and Butlin recognized this problem early and recommended excision of the lymphatic contents of the anterior triangle of the neck together with the removal of the primary lesion in the mouth.

At the turn of the century Crile devised radical neck dissection, removing all lymphatic tissue in both the anterior and posterior triangles of the neck together with the jugular vein and the sternocleidomastoid muscle. The basic elements of his classic procedure remain valid to the present.

Patients were willing to risk the high morbidity and mortality of operations in this region because the relentless progress of untreated disease offered a slow death by asphyxia, malnutrition, and eventual hemorrhage. Even the slimmest chance of avoiding this terrible triad seemed worthwhile.

As Crile was developing his operation for treating the cervical lymph nodes, radiation therapy for cancer was introduced. This, it was quickly apparent, offered a preferable alternative to operation, especially for primary lesions of the skin and oral cavity. Until the end of the 1930s most radical operations for cancers of the head and neck were abandoned, and the primary therapy was radiation. Techniques of radiation therapy became more refined and more successful. External radiation replaced radium as the treatment of choice, and fractionated therapy replaced the use of single applications of radium or a single dose of external therapy. With each refinement the percentage of patients who were cured increased. It was soon found that metastatic deposits in the neck did not respond as well to radiation as to operation, and radical neck dissection remained in use. Occasionally, patients who failed to respond to radiation or who had recurrent cancers were submitted to one or another of the old radical procedures. But when these operations were performed in a heavily irradiated fibrotic field, wound breakdown and complications often resembled the results of surgical treatment of the prior century.

In the 1940s, the introduction of endotracheal anesthesia, liberal use of blood transfusions, and antibiotics markedly changed the ability of surgeons to operate in and about the oral cavity. Postoperative morbidity and mortality dropped to a reasonable level. Radiation therapy, so long dominant in the treatment of oral lesions, seemed at a plateau with much dissatisfaction concerning the morbidity of overtreatment. These factors led to a reevaluation of operation. Grant Ward of The Johns Hopkins Hospital and Hayes Martin of the Memorial Center for Cancer led in devising combined operations whereby the primary lesions and the cervical contents were removed in a single block.

Application of this principle improved substantially the prognosis of patients with head and neck carcinomas, especially large lesions involving the oral cavity, hypopharynx, and larynx. In some institutions the pendulum swung from almost exclusive use of radiotherapy to almost exclusive use of operation. Increasing application of these combined operations during the 1950s made possible an evaluation of their mortality, morbidity, and effectiveness. By the end of the decade the place for surgical control of head and neck lesions was much more clearly defined and accepted.

Because of the late development of operative therapy after the long period of dormancy during the radiation era, this field of surgery is still something of a frontier with rapid developments of new techniques and the evolution of new ideas and approaches.

In the meantime, radiation therapy also acquired new techniques. Supervoltage radiation, most commonly with cobalt 60, delivered higher doses of therapy with a decreased morbidity, especially sparing the patient's skin and leaving a field more suitable for operation when this was required. Radiotherapists and surgeons who previously tended to disparage the results of each other's methods and to advance their own techniques as the primary treatment for tumors suddenly found that there was considerable common ground for the two methods and that there were patients who frequently could benefit from both operation and radiation as a planned course of integrated treatment.

Detection of most lesions of the head and neck is relatively easy, since the majority are readily available to the eye and the examining finger. Even so, it is tragic to find how often malignant lesions of this area are overlooked, not only lesions more difficult to diagnose, as in the maxillary sinuses and hypopharynx, but lesions readily visualized, such as tumors of the floor of the mouth, tongue, and tonsil.

Physical Examination

SKIN. The skin (see Chap. 14) of the face and neck should be closely scrutinized, keeping in mind that basal and squamous carcinomas of the skin are the most com-

mon of all cancers and that the most common site for such lesions is the area of the head and neck. Seborrheic keratosis, senile keratosis, and patches of atrophic skin often appear side by side with skin neoplasms. Differential diagnosis may be difficult, and biopsy is often required. Pigmented lesions must be examined closely to determine the presence of bleeding ulceration or satellitosis indicating melanoma. All lumps should be palpated to observe their firmness, whether they have a cystic or solid quality and whether they are fixed to the underlying tissues.

ORAL CAVITY. The oral cavity is often neglected in the course of a complete physical examination. It is said that the internist looks at the top of the tongue depressor, the otolaryngologist looks at the tonsils, and the general surgeon may not look at all. There is no excuse for this neglect, since the oral cavity is a rich source of pathologic processes, not only of local lesions, but often of lesions reflecting pathologic conditions elsewhere in the body.

Proper examination requires the use of a tongue depressor, finger cot or glove, and good lighting. If the examiner is skilled with the use of a head mirror, this will provide ideal illumination. However, there are numerous electric headlights which work equally well and which can be used at different points in the office or at the bedside without requiring an elaborate setup.

With the patient's mouth open, the light is directed into the oral cavity. If the patient has dentures of any sort, they should be removed. The examiner begins by looking at the anterior floor of the mouth and the openings of Wharton's ducts. Then the floor of the mouth is observed, progressing posteriorly along the gingivolingual gutter to the tonsillar pillars on either side. The undersurface of the anterior and lateral tongue can also be observed. This is a good place to detect early jaundice.

The lower gingiva and teeth are examined next. The condition of the teeth and the presence or absence of sepsis are considered. The gingivobuccal gutters are often the hiding place of small malignant lesions and should be inspected thoroughly.

The buccal mucosa can be examined next. Patches of hyperkeratosis are often seen here. The examiner looks for the nipple indicating the opening of Stensen's duct. Pressure on the parotid should express saliva from the orifice. The position and mobility of the tongue are observed. A deviated tongue may indicate injury to the hypoglossal nerve or a previous stroke. Numerous longitudinal fissures reflect previous syphilis, a condition now rarely seen. Malignant lesions are normally found on the edges or at the tip of the tongue.

Occasionally, a patch of dirty fibers will occupy the surface of the tongue. This condition, called "hairy tongue," often occurs in a dry mouth with impaired salivary secretion. Vitamin deficiencies are reflected by an atrophy of the taste buds with a flat, smooth, erythematous mucosa.

The tonsils and soft palate are considered next. The presence or absence of the tonsils or tonsillar tags should be noted. If the patient gags, the posterior tonsillar pillars rotate toward the midline, better exposing the tonsillar fossa itself. The anterior tonsillar pillar is a common site

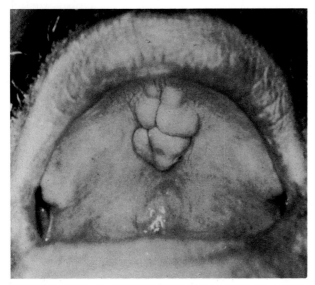

Fig. 16-1. Torus, a congenital lesion formed along the median raphe where the palatine processes of the maxilla join. These protuberances are normally smooth; the lobulation seen here is unusual.

for patches of hyperkeratosis, or sometimes for very early carcinomas. Inappropriate hypertrophy of one tonsil may reflect a lymphoma. Paralysis of one side of the soft palate is often seen in patients who have had a cerebrovascular accident. Large tumors in the nasopharynx may push the soft palate forward and down.

The examiner can complete his observations with inspection of the hard palate. A smooth or occasionally lobular elevation running down the midline of the palate is usually a torus, a harmless, congenital deformity (Fig. 16-1). Tori of the mandible also occur, projecting into the mouth bilaterally at the level of the canine tooth. They have no particular importance except to the frightened patient who may notice them for the first time in adulthood and mistake them for new growths. Occasionally, patients with atrophied lower alveoli following total loss of the lower teeth will have a spur which projects backward from the midline into the floor of the mouth. This represents a prominence of the symphysis made detectable by the absorption of the surrounding bone.

Palpation is equal in importance to inspection. Many early lesions of the oral cavity cannot be detected except by the sense of touch. This is especially true of lesions buried within the substance of the tongue or in the salivary glands. The gloved finger is passed over the tongue, the floor of the mouth, and the gingivobuccal gutters. Any mass encountered can be made more prominent by bimanual or bidigital palpation, pressing the mass inward from the cheek or submental area toward the oral cavity. If the patient can tolerate it, palpation of the lateral pharyngeal wall may reveal masses in the deep lobe of the parotid. If the index of suspicion is high concerning lesions in the nasopharynx or base of tongue, these areas should be palpated as well.

NECK. Inspection and palpation of the cervical area are done methodically, keeping in mind a distinct list of struc-

tures to be felt. These should include the larynx, thyroid, trachea, sternocleidomastoid muscle, lymph node–bearing areas, and salivary glands. The submental area is examined for the presence of enlarged lymph nodes and the size and consistency of the submaxillary glands. In the older patient they may hang low in the anterior cervical triangle as the enveloping fascia becomes lax with age. In this location they often are mistaken initially for enlarged lymph nodes. The presence of any enlarged or firm lymph nodes incorporated within the substance of the submaxillary gland should be noted. Bimanual palpation through the floor of the mouth helps greatly.

The angle of the jaw is a common site for enlarged lymph nodes or not infrequently of a tumor in the tail of the parotid gland. The anterior border of the sternocleidomastoid may overlap a cystic mass representing a branchial cleft cyst. Cystic or fluctuant masses in the posterior cervical triangle may represent a lipoma or a cystic lymphangioma.

The most important consideration in the adult is the presence of enlarged lymph nodes. A number of structures in the neck deceive the novice and at first appear to be enlarged lymph nodes when in fact they are normal structures. The carotid bulb is commonly so mistaken, especially in older patients in whom arteriosclerosis has diminished or obliterated the pulse at the bulb. The tip of the hyoid bone adjacent to the carotid bulb sometimes fools the unwary, unless they are clever enough to palpate for this structure bilaterally. The posterior belly of the omohyoid muscle as it crosses the posterior triangle in the thin patient can mimic a fusiform node until the examiner realizes that the ends of the apparent node cannot be felt. Also in thin patients the tips of the transverse process of the second cervical vertebra are felt posterior to the ascending ramus of the mandible and may seem like a lymph node until it is realized that the structures are bony in consistency and bilateral.

Masses in the thyroid are best felt if the examiner stands behind the patient and palpates the lobes of the gland between thumb and forefinger. A midline mass just above the isthmus of the thyroid may represent an enlarged lymph node, a pyramidal lobe of thyroid, or a thyroglossal duct cyst.

PARANASAL SINUSES. The paranasal sinuses are relatively inaccessible to physical examination. Neoplastic lesions often hide within these recesses and are not manifest until quite late. Bulging, particularly asymmetric bulging of one maxillary sinus, can best be appreciated by observing the cheeks from above either by having the patient lean toward the examiner or by standing above the patient and looking down (Fig. 16-2). Palpation of the maxillary, ethmoid, or temporal areas may elicit tenderness or a sense of fullness. Transillumination of the sinuses by a bright light placed within the oral cavity of a patient in a dark room may reveal opacification of one or more of the sinuses. This is a relatively crude method of examination compared to x-ray examination.

INDIRECT LARYNGOSCOPY. There is a common misconception that indirect laryngoscopy is an examination to be performed only by specialists. Hoarseness and throat pain are such common symptoms and cancer of the pharynx and larynx so frequent that indirect laryngoscopy should be part of the armamentarium of any physician and part of the routine general physical examination.

The patient is seated in a chair slightly higher than the chair or stool of the examiner. The examiner sits opposite him with his right thigh and knee parallel and immediately adjacent to the right thigh and knee of the patient. The patient should extend his neck, thrusting his chin straight forward, as though he had just finished sneezing. The patient's tongue is wrapped in a gauze sponge, and the examiner, if he is right-handed, grasps the tip of the tongue between the thumb and second finger of the left hand, using the first finger to elevate the patient's upper lip. The tongue is drawn forward, and the patient is instructed to breathe rapidly in short, quick breaths, to "pant like a dog." As long as the patient continues to breathe in this fashion, gagging is inhibited. The examiner inserts a medium to large laryngeal mirror, previously flamed to keep it from fogging, into the oropharynx and shines his headlight on the mirror, reflecting a spot of light down into the hypopharynx (Fig. 16-3).

If one is a novice with the head mirror, an electric head lamp should be used. With the mirror in the oropharynx and directed downward, the posterior third of the tongue, the lateral pharyngeal wall, the posterior pharyngeal wall, the epiglottis, the valleculae, and the pyriform sinuses can all be examined thoroughly. The epiglottis will usually hide most of the glottic opening, and only the posterior portions of the arytenoids may be seen at first. The patient is told to breathe deeply several times. This often throws the uvula forward until more of the glottic opening and a little of the subglottic space is seen. The patient is asked to attempt to enunciate an "ee" sound. This throws the epiglottis even farther forward and usually brings the entire glottis, including the anterior commissure, into view.

The false cords, aryepiglottic folds, and posterior epiglottis can now be examined. The movement of the cords is considered, to determine whether both are moving adequately and whether they meet in the midline. Paralysis of one cord may indicate a malignant lesion in the mediastinum or cervical area or may be related to previous operation or cerebrovascular accident. If nodules in the pharynx or posterior tongue are noted, they should subsequently be palpated. As the examiner acquires skill in this procedure, most of these examinations can be accomplished without local anesthesia. Topical anesthesia with lidocaine 1% (preferably) or Pontocaine 1% should be used by the beginner.

In one or two patients out of every twenty, examination is incomplete or impossible because of a hypersensitive gag reflex or an acquired or congenital malformation of the epiglottis which makes visualization of the glottis impossible. In such instances, direct laryngoscopy must be used. While direct laryngoscopy is the more sophisticated and complex procedure, indirect laryngoscopy actually gives a better overall picture of the larynx and pharynx. The chief reason for resorting to direct laryngoscopy other than the above is the necessity of biopsy of lesions deep in the larynx. Direct laryngoscopy is sometimes performed using

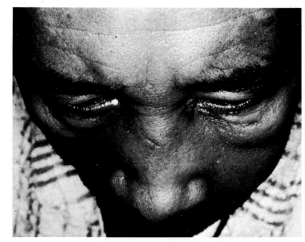

Fig. 16-2. Early swelling of the maxilla, seen best from above, as shown here. The patient had a space-occupying lesion within the sinus which was not as well appreciated in the frontal view.

a *suspension laryngoscope,* which, once the cords are visualized, can be fixed in place so that the operator does not have to use his hands to hold the laryngoscope. This technique can be combined with the use of an optical device which greatly magnifies the cords so that small irregulari-

Fig. 16-3. Laryngeal mirror examination of the larynx. Cross section of the oral cavity illustrates the relation of the mirror to the larynx. Insert: View seen by the examiner. Note the epiglottis hiding the anterior portion of the cords.

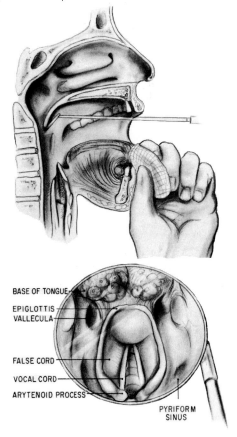

BASE OF TONGUE
EPIGLOTTIS
VALLECULA

FALSE CORD

VOCAL CORD

ARYTENOID PROCESS

PYRIFORM SINUS

ties and tiny lesions may be examined. Occasionally in patients with unexplained hoarseness this approach will reveal very early any localized benign and malignant changes.

NASOPHARYNGOSCOPY. The mirror used for indirect laryngoscopy may be turned over and directed upward. The examiner, standing at the patient's shoulder and depressing the tongue with a tongue blade, may shine his headlight on the mirror and gain a fairly spacious view of the nasopharynx. In most instances the space between the soft palate and posterior pharyngeal wall is too small for the nasopharynx to be adequately visualized in this fashion. If physical findings or the history so indicate, complete examination of the nasopharynx is done by inserting a soft rubber #10 French catheter through either nasal passage, drawing its tip out through the mouth and retracting the soft palate forward, revealing the entire nasopharynx for indirect examination by the mirror (Fig. 16-4). The torus tubarius, the openings of the eustachian tubes, the posterior surface of the soft palate, the posterior aspect of the nasal septum arching back toward the sphenoid sinus, and the posterior tips of the turbinates are seen. The normal lymphatic tissue of the adenoids may lend a granular appearance to some of the posterior and superior mucosal surfaces.

The direct nasopharyngoscope is an instrument which can be used in the office. It is a small instrument like a miniature cystoscope and has a Foroblique or right-angled lens. The diameter of the tube is 5 to 8 mm, and the visual field is quite small and easily obscured by mucus or blood.

Fig. 16-4. Mirror view of the nasopharynx. Soft palate is drawn forward, and the mirror in the oropharynx is directed upward. Insert: View seen in the mirror.

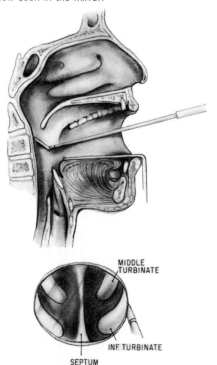

MIDDLE TURBINATE

INF. TURBINATE

SEPTUM

Use of this instrument is a valuable adjunct to indirect inspection of the nasopharynx and is particularly helpful in searching for small neoplasms.

Diagnostic Studies

ROENTGENOGRAPHY. Most of the bones of the face and neck are adjacent to air-filled cavities or are air-containing, creating an excellent situation for diagnostic roentgenograms. Lesions of the paranasal sinuses, nasal cavity, orbit, mandible, and larynx are readily revealed.

Arteriography. Injection of contrast medium into the vessels is a useful maneuver for evaluating tumors within the cranium or evaluating the arterial tree but has only rare indications for the evaluation of tumors in this region. The rare carotid body tumor can be nicely outlined by the use of radiopaque medium injected into the appropriate common carotid artery, and its appearance when examined in this fashion is pathognomonic. At times, arteriography is useful to outline the extent of a hemangioma of the face or oral cavity (Fig. 16-5).

Laminography. This technique is of great usefulness in examinations of the head and neck, especially for minute examination of the bony walls of the paranasal sinuses. Usually, the clouding of a paranasal sinus by tumor and by infection cannot be differentiated by x-ray unless obvious evidence of bone erosion is seen. Early detection of such erosions is best seen in laminographs. Tumors of the larynx are easily seen from above by indirect laryngoscopy, but their inferior extent is hidden from view unless the lesion is very small. Laminograms and lateral soft tissue views of the larynx play a useful role in revealing the extent of subglottic extension and often the degree of involvement of the pyriform sinuses, which may not otherwise be detectable (Fig. 16-6). Details of retropharyngeal and esophageal tumor spread can be seen on the lateral soft tissue view. Laryngograms are performed by the application of barium to the back of the tongue, cords, epiglottis, and all of the intrinsic larynx. A very clear examination of laryngeal structures can be obtained which offers excellent correlation with other diagnostic methods available.

BIOPSY. The vast majority of head and neck lesions can be easily biopsied in the office or clinic. The tools required are simple, and the procedure is short and uncomplicated. Lesions of the lip, skin, gingiva, floor of the mouth, tongue, and buccal mucosa can quickly be biopsied with a 4-mm dermatologist's skin punch. The area to be biopsied is cleansed with an antiseptic agent infiltrated with a small amount of local anesthesia, and the skin punch is pressed into the lesion to a depth of 4 to 6 mm, cutting a small disk of the tumor, and is withdrawn. The core of tissue which is still connected at its base is grasped with forceps, pulled up until the base is flush with the surface tissues, and cut off with a small pair of scissors. A silver nitrate stick thrust into the depth of the remaining cavity and mild pressure for a minute or two control bleeding in almost all instances. Lesions of the soft palate, tonsillar pillar, or posterior tongue which cannot be reached with a skin punch can often be biopsied easily and quickly with a cervical biopsy forcep; the techniques of anesthesia and hemostasis are essentially the same as described above.

If skill is obtained with indirect laryngoscopy, lesions of the lateral pharyngeal wall, pyriform sinus, epiglottis, and aryepiglottic folds can often be quickly biopsied in the office. While similar biopsies of the true and false cords sometimes can be achieved with skillful manipulation of the indirect mirror, such procedures are best carried out under direct laryngoscopy. Manipulation of biopsy forceps immediately above the cords is much more difficult for the patient to tolerate and may stimulate laryngeal spasm and bleeding at a site where aspiration of blood into the trachea is likely.

Biopsy of the primary lesion is always preferable, but sometimes although cervical nodes are enlarged, no primary tumor can be found. If so, needle biopsy of cervical nodes is indicated and is a rewarding procedure when the node contains metastatic squamous carcinoma. This neoplasm is easily diagnosed even with the smallest fragments of tissue. Nodes involved by lymphoma, on the other hand, are virtually impossible to diagnose by needle biopsy. Positive results of needle biopsy are useful and timesaving; the negative result of a needle biopsy has no significance and must be followed by open biopsy.

There has been much controversy concerning the tendency to spread tumor cells with the use of needle biopsies, and certainly it seems likely that tumor cells are spread into the needle tract by this manipulation. However, this is of greater theoretical than practical importance. Long experience with this technique at a number of major centers has not produced any gross difference in survival rates on long-term follow-up either in the head and neck or elsewhere. Open biopsy of a lymph node seems just as likely to scatter tumor cells, and even more widely.

VITAL DYES. Many cancers of the oral mucosa in their early stages are soft and superficial. They may have an erythematous appearance rather than a white color as usually thought and can easily escape detection even in a careful examination. If suspicion is aroused by a vaguely erythematous patch, the application of toluidine blue will aid in making the diagnosis. This technique will distinguish areas of dysplasia and carcinoma in situ as well as frank carcinoma of the mucosa. The method has its chief use in mapping out the full extent of dysplastic areas or areas of intraepithelial carcinoma.

CYTOLOGY. As used in the oral cavity exfoliative cytology is a superficial biopsy, since it does not reflect collection of fluid from the entire oral cavity but involves scraping a specific lesion with a spatula and spreading this scraping on a slide. Such cytologic examinations, therefore, require a specific area of suspicion compared to sampling of an entire anatomic area such as in the cervix or bronchial tree. If a specific lesion is present, it is best evaluated by an actual biopsy. The chief virtue of oral cytology is that the physician who cannot bring himself to use office biopsy techniques or who feels they are beyond his competence can still have the opportunity to obtain a histologic specimen from the lesion in question. Unlike biopsy, cytology has no significance when it is negative. Thus, cytol-

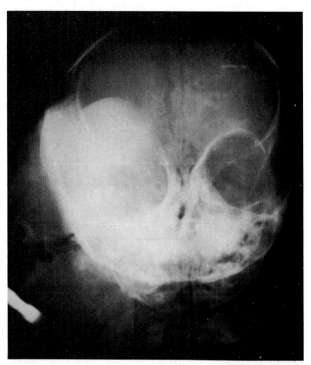

Fig. 16-5. Arteriographic demonstration of hemangioma of the oral cavity. On physical examination, only the cheek appeared involved. In the x-ray view, involvement of the lateral pharyngeal wall and oral cavity is noted. (*From B. F. Rush, Jr., Ann Surg, 164:921, 1966.*)

ogy will establish the presence of a lesion but cannot be relied on to rule that a questionable lesion is not malignant.

LIP

Squamous cell carcinomas of the lip are one of the common malignant tumors of the oral cavity, constituting 15 percent of all such lesions and 2.2 percent of all cancers. Basal cell carcinoma is much less frequent; only about 3 are seen for every 100 squamous cell carcinomas of the lip. Benign lesions which are occasionally seen in the lips include mucous cysts, tumors of the minor salivary glands, hemangiomas, lymphangiomas, venous lakes, fibromas, fissures, and hyperkeratosis.

ETIOLOGY. Like tumors of the skin, there is an important relationship between tumors of the lip and exposure to sunlight. About one-third of patients have a history of working outdoors, and the incidence of malignant squamous cancers of the lip increases progressively the farther south the latitude of the patient population being considered. Thus, in the United States the highest incidence is in Florida and Texas. Actinic rays are stronger at higher altitudes and in dryer air, and in areas having these features the incidence of lip (and skin) cancer is increased. Fishermen, sailors, and farmers are among the occupational groups with an increased incidence.

Complexion also plays a role. Susceptible types are fair-skinned, light, blond or ginger-haired, and blue-eyed,

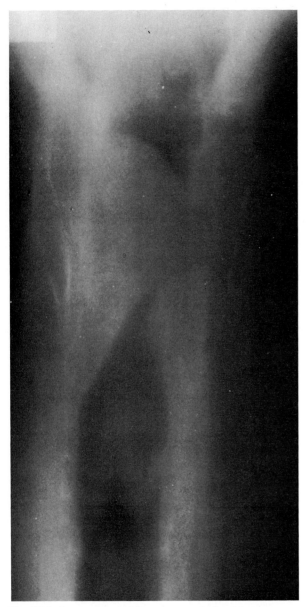

Fig. 16-6. Laminogram of the pharynx. Indirect laryngoscopy would show only the supraglottic portion of the tumor. The laminographic view indicates the large transglottic and subglottic component of the lesion. (*From B. F. Rush and R. H. Greenlaw (eds)., "Integrated Radiation and Operation in Cancer Therapy: A Symposium," Charles C Thomas, Publisher, Springfield, Ill., 1968.*)

with the kind of complexion that freckles and burns rather than tans on exposure to the sun. Resistant people have the opposite characteristics: they are brunet and dark-skinned; Negroes are rarely affected.

While there is a relation between lip cancer and tobacco, the exact cause for this is less apparent than in patients with lesions of the intraoral area, larynx, or lungs. The average cigarette smoker receives almost no carcinogen from his tobacco directly to the lips, since the smoke is drawn into the oral cavity and tracheobraonchial tree with-

out passing over the mucosa of the lips themselves. Some feel that the inmates of nursing homes and institutions are more prone to have carcinoma of the lip from cigarette smoking. Smokers in this population usually treasure their cigarettes, smoking them down to the smallest possible butt. Macerated, moist tobacco and heat are directly applied to the lips.

Reports in the literature implicating pipe smoking as a cause of lip cancer have been appearing since 1795, and the Advisory Committee to the Surgeon General on Smoking and Health has accepted the causal relationship as established. Pipestems of wood and clay which soak up tobacco tars directly and apply a "tar poultice" to the lips have been viewed with special suspicion. In any case, such stems are little used now, and indeed the incidence of cancer of the lip in the United States has been gradually decreasing over the past 30 years. One may speculate whether this reflects the decrease in pipe smoking, outdoor work, use of wood and clay pipestems, or a combination of these and other factors.

Cancer of the lip in women is very rare, occurring in only 1 woman for every 20 to 30 men.

Benign Tumors

The mucosa of the inner surface of the upper and lower lips is subject to the same benign lesions as those throughout the mucosa of the oral cavity. These are discussed in greater detail in the following section, Oral Cavity, and include such lesions as mucous cysts, hemangiomas, tumors of the minor salivary glands, hyperkeratosis, and inflammatory hyperplasia. Specific benign lesions that involve the exposed borders of the lips include venous lakes, pigmented spots, hemangiomas, and very rarely neuromas. Venous lakes are a telangiectasis, usually of the lower lip, occurring in older individuals as a small bluish spot. They appear to have no pathologic significance. The other three lesions all have interesting systemic correlations. Multiple pigmented spots of the lips may be associated with Peutz-Jeghers syndrome and denote the presence of multiple small intestinal polyps, which sometimes lead to bleeding and intussusception but are rarely malignant. Scattered small hemangiomas of the lip may be associated with similar lesions elsewhere in the oral cavity and gastrointestinal tract, those of Rendu-Osler-Weber disease. Neuromas of the lips, particularly at the commissures, suggest a neuroendocrine dysplasia, a fascinating syndrome associated with pheochromocytomas, medullary carcinoma of the thyroid, hyperparathyroidism, and hypertrophy of the gastrointestinal myenteric plexus.

Hyperkeratosis

This is a premalignant condition of the lips, usually associated with long exposure to sunlight. It typically occurs in a fair-skinned individual in his sixties or seventies who has a long history of outdoor employment. The normal distinct line marking the mucocutaneous border becomes indistinct and gradually retreats, indicating a metaplasia of the outer portion of the mucosa to a keratosquamous epithelium. The mucosa of the lip becomes paler, thinner, and more fragile. There may be perpendicular cracks and fissures. On this base, a white film indicative of early hyperkeratosis appears. This may grow gradually thicker and more exophytic as the condition progresses (Fig. 16-7) or may remain stationary for many years. Gradually, a small area of scabbing and ulceration occurs. This breakdown within the hyperkeratotic tissue represents a failure of the less resistant areas of hyperkeratosis to tolerate normal wear and tear. When such areas of ulceration appear, they continue to break down and heal and often give rise to carcinoma in situ and eventually invasive carcinoma. Persistent hyperkeratosis is a distinct premalignant lesion, and 35 to 40 percent of all carcinomas of the lip are preceded by this condition. Cancers arising on such a base can be prevented by excising the entire exposed mucosa of the lip, elevating the protected mucosa of the inner lip, and advancing it over the bed of the excised mucosa to form a new lining for the lip. This procedure is called a *lip stripping and resurfacing*.

Carcinoma of the Lip

Most cancers of the lip are squamous carcinomas. When basal cell carcinomas appear, they usually involve the skin of the lip beyond the vermillion border and probably should be considered with the cancers of the skin of the face. Ninety-three percent of the squamous cancers occur on the lower lip. These are usually low-grade, well-differentiated lesions, 80 percent being grade 1 or grade 2. The lesions most frequently start on the outer edge of the mucosa at the vermillion border and seem to favor the middle two-thirds of the lip somewhat more frequently than the commissures (Fig. 16-8).

The natural history of these lesions is of slow but relentless growth. Some grow to great size, destroying the entire lip without ever metastasizing, but the incidence of metastasis gradually increases with the increasing size of the tumors (Fig. 16-9). About 5 to 10 percent of all patients with lip cancer have cervical lymph node metastasis, and in half of these patients only one lymph node is involved. The normal spread of cancer from the lower lip is by way of lymphatics to the submental node on the side of the lesion. Metastases do not involve the opposite submental node unless the primary lesion crosses the midline. Lesions of the upper lip drain to lymph nodes in the anterior portion of the submaxillary gland.

An ulcer of the lip which fails to heal is soon detected by the patient or his friends, and in most urban populations such lesions quickly come to the attention of physicians. In rural populations it is surprising how long patients will carry these ulcerations before seeking medical aid.

Treatment for carcinoma of the lip has remained a topic of controversy between radiotherapists and surgeons for many decades. Recent controlled series comparing treatment by both modalities in randomly selected patients indicate that there is no statistical difference between the two methods in terms of cure rate. The choice for therapy must be made on other grounds. Small lesions of the lip

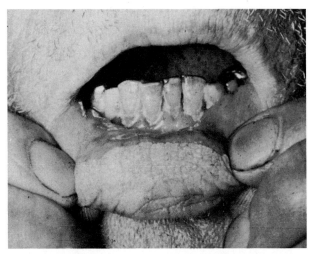

Fig. 16-7. Hyperkeratosis of lower lip. This degree of hyperkeratosis merits serious concern. The entire lower lip is involved and should be treated by excision (lip stripping) and advancement of the mucosa of the inner lip to cover the defect.

can usually be excised under local anesthesia with little or no hospitalization time. Good radiation therapy producing maximal regression with minimal residual scarring requires 2 to 4 weeks of outpatient therapy. Medium-sized lesions require the use of flaps from the upper lip or elsewhere for closure, and for these lesions radiotherapy often requires the same or less time and less morbidity. For very large lesions which have destroyed most of the lip and are associated with metastasis to the neck, subsequent repair of the lip will be required under any circumstance as well as probable radical neck dissection for removal of cervical nodes; for these major lesions an integration of radiation and surgical therapy may be used to improve cure rates, which are relatively low for either radiation or operation alone. A final consideration is that most carcinomas of the lip are related to solar radiation.

Fig. 16-8. Squamous carcinoma of lip. Any patient with a chronic ulcer of this sort should seek medical advice. The chance of cure at this early stage approached 100 percent.

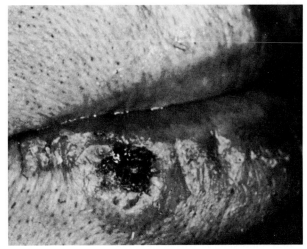

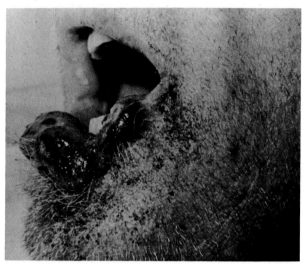

Fig. 16-9. Neglected carcinoma of the lip. A metastatic node is present along the line of the mandible. The chance of cure for this type of lesion is 50 percent or less.

Since radiotherapy increases the sensitivity of tissues to such exposure, it is best to avoid radiotherapy in patients who expect to return to outdoor occupations.

Prognosis for lip cancers of 1 cm or less is excellent, ranging from an 87 to 95 percent 5-year survival rate without recurrence. Neglected lesions, especially with associated cervical metastasis, do much more poorly, with a 5-year survival of 50 percent.

ORAL CAVITY

The oral cavity includes the buccal mucosa, upper and lower gingivae, anterior two-thirds of the tongue (that portion anterior to the circumvallate papillae), floor of the mouth, and hard palate.

INCIDENCE. Eight percent of all malignant tumors occur in this area, 95 percent of such tumors being squamous carcinomas. The risk of carcinomas developing here in a male is approximately 1 percent in a lifetime. The risk in females is far less: oral cancer develops in about 1 woman for every 10 males. Benign tumors of the oral cavity are common in both sexes.

ETIOLOGY. Some benign lesions have a specific cause, which will be discussed with the descriptions of the lesions below. Contributing causes to squamous carcinoma are smoking, a heavy intake of alcohol, poor oral hygiene, and syphilis. While cancer often occurs without the presence of any of these factors, they are associated with a majority of the lesions seen.

The *Report on Smoking and Health* by the Advisory Committee to the Surgeon General notes a suggestive relationship between smoking and oral carcinoma. This is especially true in pipe and cigar smokers, where oral cancer has the highest mortality ratio, 3.3,* of all causes of death compared with the nonsmoking population. There

*That is, 3.3 times as many pipe and cigar smokers died of oral cancer as did nonsmokers in the same age group. The mortality ratio for cancer of the lung in pipe smokers was 1:1, no different from that of the nonsmokers.

are a number of exotic cancers of the oral cavity which serve to indicate the relationship of tobacco to cancer. In Andhra Pradesh, a state in India, the habit of smoking a cigar (i.e., *chutta*) with the burning end inside the mouth is widespread. Carcinoma of the palate, called *chutta cancer,* is common. Presumably, repeated thermal trauma and/or tobacco smoke provide the carcinogenic agents.

In Uttar Pradesh and Bihar, a mixture of tobacco and slaked lime is habitually sucked by men of the districts. The quid is kept in the lower gingivolabial fornix for many hours during the day; a high incidence of carcinoma is found at this site. This has come to be called *khaini cancer,* from the name of the tobacco-lime mixture.

Betel-nut chewing is a common habit among the Indians, Javanese, and Malayans. The chew is made of a mixture of ground betel nut, slaked lime, and spices, such as ginger or pepper. These are wrapped in a betel leaf and chewed. The Indians add tobacco to their betel preparations and have a high incidence of oral cancer, whereas the incidence is low among the Javanese and Malayans, who consume their betel nut without benefit of the tobacco additive. Among betel nut–tobacco chewers, oral cancer comprises 36 percent of all cancers.

Alcoholism has a highly suggestive role in oral cancer. As many as 42 percent of all patients so afflicted have a history of alcoholism. As a corollary, cirrhosis of the liver is a common finding in patients with oral cancer, 20 percent having cirrhosis as compared to 9 percent in a control population. It has been proposed that alcohol acts as an adjuvant to the use of tobacco in producing oral cancer. This is a difficult point to prove, since finding a control population of patients who drink heavily but do not smoke is virtually impossible.

The roles of poor oral hygiene and oral sepsis, mentioned for decades as etiologic agents for oral cancers, are also difficult to evaluate. These conditions are seen most commonly in patients at the lower end of the social scale and in the ward population rather than in private practice. Oral hygiene is poor in this group, but it cannot be said whether poor hygiene or social level or other correlated factors are responsible.

Syphilis has a direct relation to cancer of one specific site in the oral cavity, the tongue. When syphilitic glossitis, a lesion of late syphilis, heals, it often leaves the tongue fibrotic and scarred with longitudinal fissures and thick hyperkeratotic plaques. It is on this base that lingual cancer develops (Fig. 16-10). In the days of Bloodgood (1921) 21 percent of American men with lingual cancer had syphilis. Willis still calls this condition "the most clearly established causative factor in European males."

Benign Lesions

Common benign tumors of the oral cavity are inflammatory hyperplasias and cysts. Less commonly seen are giant cell granulomas, salivary tumors, granular cell myoblastomas, dermoids, and hemangiomas.

INFLAMMATORY HYPERPLASIA

The oral mucosa is subject to a number of irritating conditions producing tumorlike projections which are not true neoplasms. Patients develop the nervous habit of sucking a portion of mucosa from the cheek, tongue, or lip between the teeth or through an interdental or edentulous space. The traumatized mucosa becomes edematous and prominent, and the irritation may be compounded by the patient who bites as well as sucks on the offending mucosal fold. Initially, the overlying mucosa is swollen, and eventually this undergoes metaplasia to squamous epithelium. The tissue underlying the elevated mucosa changes from edematous connective tissue to a denser and more fibrotic collection of collagen. At this stage the lesion may be termed a *fibroepithelial polyp* (Fig. 16-11). Similar lesions are often seen in the gingivobuccal gutter and on the palate in patients with ill-fitting dentures. Those lesions which occur along the vestibular mucosa next to the gingiva in this relation are sometimes called *epulis fissurata.* Another appropriate term, more descriptive of the later stages of these lesions when the fibrosis and scarring has advanced, is *irritation fibroma.* In the early inflammatory phase of these lesions, the overlying mucosa is friable and bleeds easily.

The chief responsibility of the examiner who has recognized the lesion is to reassure the patient that it is not malignant. Although these lesions are usually not ulcerated and are easily recognized, diagnosis should be confirmed by biopsy. Treatment is by correction of the causative factor, either by the design of new dentures or by discouraging the patient from manipulating and traumatizing the area involved. Excision may be necessary, but if the basic problem is not abolished, recurrence is prompt.

CYSTS

Mucous cysts are a common oral lesion occurring on the posterior surface of the lip, floor of the mouth, tongue, and buccal mucosa. These cysts arise from the salivary gland–bearing areas of the oral mucosa and were thought to be due to obstruction of the excretory duct of minor salivary glands. It has been found, however, that these cysts have no epithelial lining and that they result from a rupture of the excretory duct. Saliva spills from the defect in the duct and begins to collect in the tissues. At first it forms a diffuse lesion, but soon a circumscribed cyst with a wall of granulation tissue develops. These mucoceles measure from 1 or 2 mm to 1 or 2 cm in diameter and appear as elevated, translucent, bluish lesions of the mucosa (Fig. 16-12). They frequently rupture, discharging sticky mucoid material, and then recur as the laceration in the overlying mucosa heals. Treatment consists of wide surgical unroofing of the lesion.

A somewhat larger and more dramatic mucocele may result from obstruction and rupture of the major excretory ducts in the floor of the mouth, ducts of the lingual or submaxillary glands. Except for size, these lesions resemble in every way the lesions which result from obstruction of the minor salivary glands but have received the special name of *ranula.*

Dermoids may develop in the floor of the mouth and the base of the tongue along the midline. If neglected, these lesions grow slowly as they accumulate the sloughed-off cells, secretion, and hair of the epidermal lining. They present both as a swelling in the submental

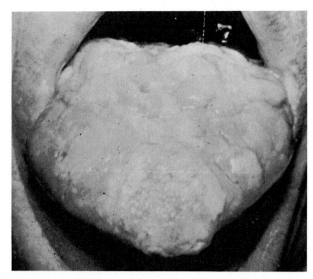

Fig. 16-10. Syphilis of the tongue. The dense, white patches are sometimes mistaken for "geographic tongue." Cancers of the dorsal surface often follow this condition.

triangle and an elevation of the floor of the mouth (Fig. 16-13). They will eventually elevate the floor of the mouth and tongue until it touches the palate and interferes with speech. Treatment consists of operative excision of the cyst, which may be done either intraorally or extraorally. The lesion has a definite, thick capsule and can be shelled out with ease from its relatively avascular midline location.

PERIPHERAL GIANT CELL REPARATIVE GRANULOMA

These benign tumors occur on the gingivae, affecting the maxillary or mandibular gingiva with equal frequency. Grossly, they appear as a slow-growing, reddish, smooth sessile tumor which bleeds easily. They often occur at an

Fig. 16-11. Irritation fibroma. The lesion seen here was caused by persistent sucking and irritation of mucosa through the edentulous space, which can be seen adjacent to this polyp. (*Courtesy of Sheldon Rovin, D.D.S.*)

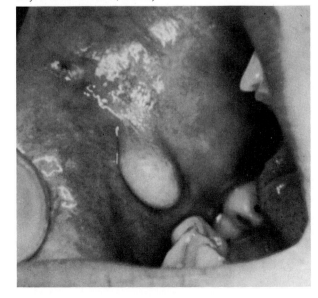

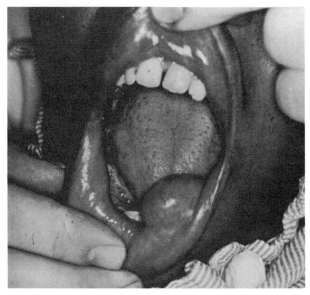

Fig. 16-12. Mucous cyst of the lip, the most common location for this lesion. This mucocele has resulted from rupture of a minor salivary gland duct with spillage of mucus into the surrounding tissue.

area of an interdental papilla (Fig. 16-14) but may also arise in edentulous patients. Histologically, the lesion is covered by stratified squamous epithelium. Endothelial and fibroplastic proliferations, multinucleated giant cells, and extracellular and intracellular hemosiderin are diagnostic microscopic criteria. Multinucleated giant cells are distributed unevenly throughout an area of rich fibroblastic proliferation. Some lesions show spicules of bone tissue. In general, the lesion closely resembles the giant cell tumor of bone seen in hyperparathyroidism. The descriptive term "peripheral" indicates that the lesion is of soft tissue, while the so-called "central" giant cell reparative granuloma is an intraosseous form found in the mandible or maxilla.

When these lesions arise in the mandible or maxilla,

Fig. 16-13. Dermoid of the mouth. This huge dermoid has elevated the floor of the mouth until the tongue is forced against the hard palate and in this illustration is out of sight behind the cyst.

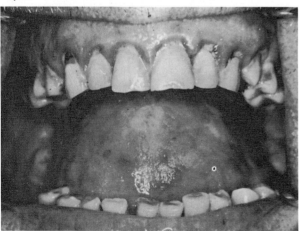

they may be confused with the giant cell tumors of long bones. The distinction between the two lesions must be made, since the oral lesions have no propensity for malignant transformation, as have the lesions seen elsewhere. Treatment of the soft tissue lesions is by complete excision. Inadequate removal may result in recurrence.

PERIPHERAL FIBROMA

These are also lesions of the gingiva and are in many respects similar grossly to the giant cell granuloma. They are usually firmer and under the microscope are made up of dense connective tissue. They may also contain bone spicules and may be calcified. One can speculate as to the relation of these lesions to the giant cell granuloma. They may represent a later stage of this lesion or may be a late stage of inflammatory hyperplasia. Excision is usually curative.

GRANULOMA PYOGENICUM

This is an elevated pedunculated or sessile lesion which may occur on the lips, tongue, buccal mucosa, or gingiva. It bleeds readily on being traumatized. Histologically it is made up of edematous, fibrous connective tissue with a prominent endothelial component arranged in lobules of varying sizes separated by bands of collagen. Numerous blood vessels are scattered throughout the tumor. No cause is known for the lesions of the lips, buccal mucosa, and tongue, but lesions of the gingiva are often associated with pregnancy. Thirty to forty percent of pregnant women show some degree of gingival enlargement. Of these, about 1 percent will have an isolated "tumor." These lesions in the pregnant female have been called "granuloma gravidarum." They appear about the third month of pregnancy and increase in size throughout the growth of the child in utero. They usually diminish in size and disappear following delivery, although with a subsequent pregnancy they may appear again in the same location. Lesions unassociated with pregnancy may be treated by excision. It is usually advisable to wait until the end of pregnancy to treat granuloma gravidarum.

SALIVARY TUMORS

Pleomorphic adenomas (mixed tumors) occasionally arise from any of the 400 to 700 minor salivary glands. Occurring most commonly on the lips, tongue, and palate, they can be found anywhere in the oral cavity where minor salivary glands are found. They are usually slow-growing, round masses of a rather rubbery consistency (Fig. 16-15). They have the potential of becoming malignant and if simply enucleated without adequate excision have a marked propensity for local recurrence. Treatment, therefore, is by wide local excision.

HEMANGIOMA

Capillary hemangiomas, not unlike the strawberry hemangioma of the skin, are sometimes seen in the mucous membranes of the oral cavity in infants. Like the lesions of the skin these lesions regress spontaneously, and unless they are so large that they interfere with function, they should be left to regress at their own pace. In most instances they will undergo involution by the end of the fifth year. Unlike the skin lesions they do not disappear completely and may still be seen as a small, dark lesion underneath the mucosa (Fig. 16-16). It is likely that the transparent nature of the mucosa reveals the sclerosed remnant in a manner that is not seen if the lesion is under the more opaque skin. The sclerosed hemangioma will remain visible throughout life but has no significance and does not require treatment. Rarely, large regional vascular malformations will involve the entire side of the mouth, including the tongue, gingiva, and buccal mucosa. Such lesions do not regress spontaneously. Their treatment is difficult, often requiring multiple plastic procedures to excise the hemangiomatous tissue and to return the contours of the mouth and oral cavity to normal.

GRANULAR CELL MYOBLASTOMA

This is a rare and interesting lesion which occurs most commonly within the muscle of the tongue, presenting as a small, firm spheroid mass detected best by manual palpation. These lesions have no malignant potential but may gradually increase in size with functional impairment. Treatment is by simple excision.

Hyperkeratosis

The gross finding of white patches on the oral mucosa elicits the diagnosis of leukoplakia from the clinician. "Leukoplakia" roughly translated means "white patches," so the physician need not feel too proud of his accomplishment; he has only managed to translate English into Latin. To some "leukoplakia" means a specific premalignant lesion. This meaning is not inherent in the original use of this term. Most pathologists adhere to a more rigid description of such lesions and describe the underlying microscopic changes: hyperplasia, keratosis, and dyskeratosis. White patches in the oral cavity may be associated with any of or all these basic changes (Fig. 16-17). Inflammation in this area often stimulates marked hyperplasia of cells, sometimes to the point where they resemble epidermoid tumors and are spoken of as *pseudoepitheliomatous hyperplasia.* Keratosis is a common response of the buccal mucosa and may appear in the presence of lichen planus, chronic dyscoid lupus, and Darier's disease, as well as be a possible forerunner of malignant change.

Dyskeratosis, the loss of normal stratification or orientation of cells together with irregularity in the size and shape of cells and abnormal staining characteristics, is a much more treacherous lesion and much more likely to precede malignant disease.

Hyperkeratosis is announced by the gradual development of whitened patches of the mucosa which appear first as a thin, white, translucent or opalescent film in the normal mucous membrane. No malignant or premalignant changes will be found at this point but only evidences of hyperplasia or keratosis. Later these lesions can become thickened and rougher; the white patches are now quite opaque. Palpation will reveal a definite change in the consistency of the mucosa. Microscopic examination may still show advanced hyperkeratosis and hyperplasia, but

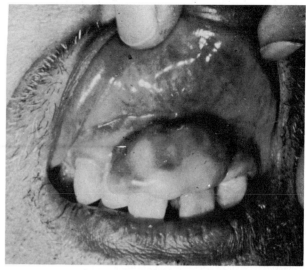

Fig. 16-14. Peripheral giant cell tumor. These often arise in interdental spaces as seen in photograph.

now areas of mild to marked dyskeratosis may be present as well. Eventually, areas of distinct carcinoma in situ will appear, and this can be followed in rapid order by microinvasion or the frank invasion of a well-developed cancer.

Obviously, the early appearance of hyperplasia and hyperkeratosis may or may not foreshadow malignant disease. Since there is no way of telling which is the case, patients with such lesions should be warned to avoid smoking or heavy intake of alcohol and should embark on a campaign of improvement of oral hygiene. Cancer will ultimately develop in 5 percent of such patients, and it is significant that about 50 percent of all oral cancers develop in patients with associated areas of hyperkeratosis and dyskeratosis. The thin, early lesions require only a warning, and a biopsy is not necessary, but thickened lesions may already contain carcinoma in situ and should

Fig. 16-15. Mixed tumor of palate. This is a benign lesion. Adequate removal to ensure prevention of recurrences includes resection of the underlying hard palate and gingiva.

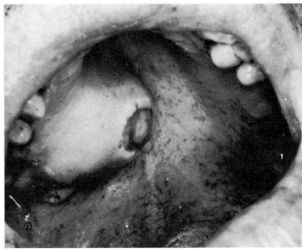

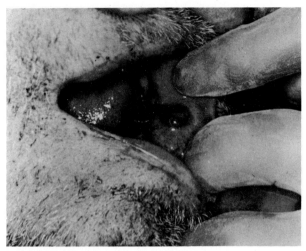

Fig. 16-16. Fibrosing hemangioma. Lesions in the mucosal area remain visible under the buccal mucosa, whereas similar lesions may not be discernible under the skin.

be biopsied in every instance and perhaps checked, as well, with vital dyes.

If a patch of dyskeratosis appears on biopsy to be particularly threatening and is limited in extent, local excision may be useful. More often, the extent of the lesion is so widespread that complete excision of the involved mucosa is impossible. Radiation therapy is contraindicated in these premalignant lesions. While the majority are associated with hyperkeratosis, which gives the whitish aspect to the surface, occasionally dyskeratosis and carcinoma in situ are the major elements. Such lesions may have a velvety erythematous appearance only slightly redder than the surrounding mucosa. These areas are difficult to detect, and toluidine blue may be very useful in mapping their true area.

Fig. 16-17. Hyperkeratosis of mucosa. The white mucosa in the gingivobuccal gutter of the patient is due to an ill-fitting denture causing hyperkeratosis, a normal response of the oral mucosa to irritation. (*Courtesy of Sheldon Rovin, D.D.S.*)

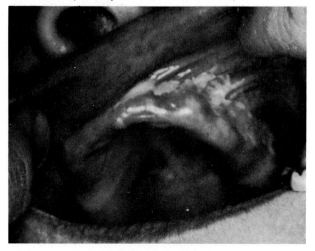

Malignant Tumors

PATHOLOGY. Low-grade epidermoid carcinomas make up the overwhelming majority of all carcinomas of the oral cavity, varying from highly differentiated tumors, difficult to tell histologically from inflammatory hyperplasia, to less well-organized but still obvious epidermoid tumors usually with associated squamous pearls. Highly undifferentiated and anaplastic lesions are rare. The few adenocarcinomas found are derived from minor salivary glands. The occasional adenoid cystic carcinomas and mucoepidermoid carcinomas seen also arise from salivary tissues.

In the Southern United States a very low-grade cancer, verrucous carcinoma, is occasionally seen. This is an exophytic, shaggy white lesion usually found in the gingivobuccal gutter of patients who are tobacco chewers or "snuff dippers." Unless treated by radiation, the lesion never metastasizes, although it frequently invades surrounding tissues, including the mandible.

In general, lesions of the oral cavity are better differentiated and less malignant than lesions occurring in the oropharynx.

TONGUE

Carcinoma of the tongue commonly begins at the tip or along the free borders. It often starts in an area of hyperkeratosis and gradually develops as an ulcerated lesion with a moderately exophytic undermined border. The area of ulceration is related to the rest of the tumor as the tip of an iceberg is to its main mass, and palpation of the tongue may indicate that invasion has occurred deeply throughout underlying muscle (Fig. 16-18). Carcinomas beginning in an area of syphilitic glossitis are exceptions to the normal pattern and occur on the dorsal glossal surface.

Cancer of the tip of the tongue (Fig. 16-19) metastasizes to submental nodes, often bilaterally, while lesions along the borders of the tongue metastasize to ipsilateral submandibular nodes and occasionally to nodes at the angle of the mandible.

These lesions are quick to metastasize, and 40 percent of patients have nodes in the neck when first seen. In another 40 percent nodes develop at some point during therapy or during follow-up. For this reason therapy is designed to attack not only the primary lesion but also the nodes of the ipsilateral neck, as well. Combined operation including wide resection of the oral lesion together with radical neck dissection has been our treatment of choice in the past. More recently we have been inclined to treat all larger lesions of the oral cavity with radiation therapy, following this with radical neck dissection and in continuity excision of any residual cancer. The horizontal ramus of the mandible must be resected together with the tumor if the oral cancer has come in contact with the periosteum of the mandible at any point. Such contact seeds the periosteal lymphatics with tumor cells and makes resection of bone mandatory. The determinate 5-year survival for cancer of the tongue is 32 to 40 percent. If no palpable lymph nodes are present, the 5-year survival rate is 53 percent.

FLOOR OF THE MOUTH

The floor of the mouth is that portion of the oral cavity between the tongue and the inner surface of the mandible. This crescentic area of the mucosa lies over the sublingual and submaxillary salivary glands and contains their excretory ducts. It is divided into two halves by the frenulum, a fold of mucosa lying in the midline and extending to the tongue.

Squamous carcinomas developing in this area tend to develop a "run-around" extending anteriorly and posteriorly around the rim of the mandible, and if they are neglected long enough, the entire floor of the mouth becomes involved. This pattern of growth results in common bilateral involvement at the anterior floor of the mouth (Fig. 16-20) with frequent bilateral cervical metastases. These lesions tend to be less well differentiated than lesions of the tongue or gingiva and rapidly invade the surrounding structures, especially the periosteum of the adjacent mandible and the tissues of the submaxillary space. Metastases occur first to the submaxillary lymph nodes and are frequent. Taylor and Nathanson observed that 60 percent of these patients had palpable cervical metastases on admission, and in 90 percent cervical lymph node involvement had developed within a year of diagnosis.

The primary symptoms of these neoplasms are often neglected for some time, since they are quite minimal. Eventually the patient complains of pain, swelling of the tongue, and difficulty in eating and speaking. Early lesions are usually discovered by the patient himself while inspecting his mouth or have been noticed by an alert dentist or physician. Rarely, very early lesions may be seen involving only the superficial mucosa.

Large lesions of the floor of the mouth require wide excision in continuity with resection of a portion of the mandible and radical neck dissection. The neck dissection is done whether lymph nodes are palpable or not, in view of the high incidence of positive cervical nodes. Operative therapy may be integrated with preoperative radiation in the larger lesions. The much less common superficial and in situ lesions can be treated by local excision only. The 5-year survival rates for cancers in this site are comparable with those for cancer of the tongue. James reports an average determinate survival of 37 percent, and the Tumor Registry of the Memorial Center for Cancer reports a 5-year survival rate of 39 percent.

GINGIVAE

Cancer of the gums is better differentiated and slower in its pattern of growth than lesions of the tongue and floor of the mouth. Patients first note a mass (Fig. 16-21) or slight tenderness of the gum, sometimes with loosening of teeth in the area of the tumor. This often leads them to consult their dentist, who, if he is not alert to the problem, may extract the teeth under the mistaken impression that the patient has an underlying abcess or cyst. As the lesion progresses, it ulcerates, bleeds, and interferes with mastication. As a neoplasm invades the underlying bone, it can involve the mandibular nerve with the appearance

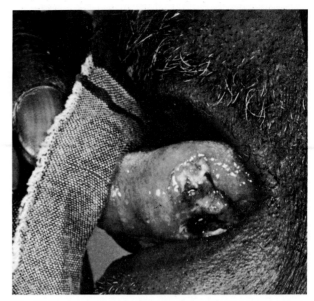

Fig. 16-18. Squamous carcinoma of the lateral border of the middle third of the tongue. The lesion is deeply invasive and much larger than the area of ulceration would indicate. The curled raised border is characteristic.

of numbness in the mental and submental areas. Extraction of a tooth often accelerates the invasion of the mandible.

Treatment of cancer of the lower gingiva requires resection of the involved mandible and overlying gum together with a radical neck dissection. Metastases from cancers at this site are usually to the submaxillary lymph nodes and are present in about half the patients at their first visit. Epidermoid cancers of the upper gingiva are less common and better differentiated than cancers of the lower gingiva. Metastases to cervical nodes are much less

Fig. 16-19. Squamous carcinoma of the tip of the tongue. An exophytic, fairly superficial lesion which histologically shows a well-differentiated structure. The prognosis for such a lesion is excellent.

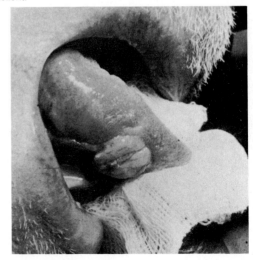

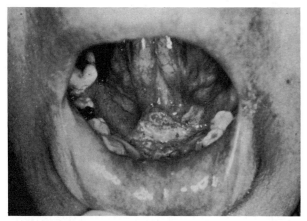

Fig. 16-20. Squamous carcinoma of the floor of the mouth. This lesion is in a typical location in the midline with spread in both directions around the curve of the mandible. It has invaded deeply into underlying structures.

common. Therefore, treatment is restricted to local excision. Radical neck dissection is deferred until there is evidence of palpable cervical node involvement.

The definitive 5-year survival rate following treatment for carcinoma of the gingiva averages 45 percent.

HARD PALATE

The hard palate is the U-shaped area enclosed by the upper gingiva and bounded posteriorly by the attachments of the soft palate. It consists of the palatine processes of the maxillary bones in its anterior two-thirds and of the horizontal portions of the palatine bones in its posterior third.

The most common malignant lesions of the hard palate are tumors of the minor salivary glands. Adenoid cystic carcinomas (Fig. 16-22) and adenocarcinomas occur in almost equal number; malignant mixed tumors are somewhat less frequent. Epidermoid carcinomas primary in the hard palate are rare, although carcinomas primary in the

Fig. 16-21. Carcinoma of the gingiva. The adjacent teeth are loose and easily removed. The underlying mandible is already invaded.

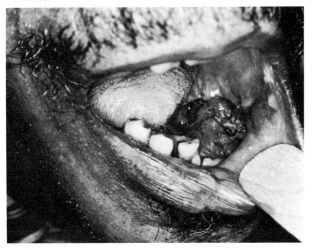

maxillary sinus will occasionally invade the hard palate and perforate into the oral cavity.

The primary symptom is a mass usually noted first by the patient himself. There is no tenderness or other associated symptom until fairly late in the course of the tumor. As in most salivary malignant tumors, growth is very slow and metastases occur quite late, so that involved cervical lymph nodes are not found initially. Salivary neoplasms respond poorly to radiation therapy, and primary treatment is excision. The chief fault in treatment is underestimation of the extent and potential of these lesions. They are usually fixed to the underlying periosteum, and adequate excision must include resection of the hard palate together with the tumor mass. An attempt to enucleate the tumor from the underlying bone almost ensures a local recurrence. Excision with a wide margin including the bony palate leaves a substantial palatal defect requiring repair either by surgical reconstruction or the use of an upper plate constructed by a prosthodontist with an obturator which will plug the defect.

Despite the phlegmatic nature of these tumors, complete excision and complete eradication of the lesions are often elusive. The lesions tend to be of a higher grade than malignant lesions of the major salivary glands. Five-year survival rates between 30 and 40 percent are reported, but the incidence of new disease between the fifth and fifteenth year is frequent.

BUCCAL MUCOSA

The lateral walls of the oral cavity are formed by the cheeks, which consist of the buccinator muscle covered on its inner surface by a layer of mucosa extending from the upper to the lower gingivobuccal gutters and from the lateral commissure of the lips anteriorly to the ascending ramus of the mandible posteriorly. Lymphatics from this area pass through the buccinator muscle and follow the facial vein to end in the submaxillary and upper cervical lymph nodes.

The natural evolution of epidermoid carcinoma of the buccal mucosa varies according to the grade of the tumor. About half of the lesions are rather undifferentiated and associated with ulceration, rapid invasion of the cheek, and sometimes even perforation of the skin and formation of an orocutaneous salivary fistula (Fig. 16-23). The majority of such lesions are accompanied by enlarged submaxillary lymph nodes when first seen.

A less aggressive form of buccal cancer is also encountered, especially in patients who are tobacco chewers and "snuff dippers." This is the so-called "verrucous carcinoma," which tends to occur in the gingivobuccal gutter and progresses very slowly, sometimes over a period of years. The tumor is locally invasive, but metastases have never been reported except in patients who have received previous irradiation. Verrucous lesions are easily recognized by their exophytic form and shaggy white appearance (Fig. 16-24). They may cover a wide area, sometimes the entire buccal surface, and have a propensity for bony invasion, often involving a large portion of the mandible or occasionally the maxilla.

Treatment of buccal carcinoma is dictated by the type

of lesion encountered. External radiation therapy alone does not eradicate the less well-differentiated lesions, although it has been combined with interstitial therapy with some success. The highly differentiated verrucous carcinomas are fairly radiosensitive but have a marked tendency to recur following an early gratifying regression. In addition, the distressing propensity of these lesions for developing a higher grade of malignancy with metastases after being exposed to radiation is a unique characteristic which has discouraged many from using radiation in treatment. Therefore, the initial therapy for verrucous lesions is wide excision. Since cervical metastases are not ordinarily found, an accompanying radical neck dissection is not done.

For the high-grade lesions, block dissection of the cheek with radical neck resection is the operative treatment of choice. Additional benefit may be derived from combining this with preoperative radiotherapy; this type of combined treatment is still undergoing evaluation. James reported 5-year survival rates in 181 patients with carcinoma of the buccal mucosa of all types as 54.4 percent. The prognosis for the well-differentiated lesions, such as the verrucous carcinoma, should be much better than this.

OROPHARYNX

The oropharynx is the region of the mouth posterior to the anterior tonsillar pillars and the circumvallate papillae of the tongue (Fig. 16-25). It contains the soft palate, tonsil and tonsillar fossa, posterior third of the tongue, anterior surface of the epiglottis, and surrounding pharyngeal walls. The most common site for malignant tumors in this area is the tonsil.

TONSIL

The most common benign lesion of the tonsil is, as every layman knows, inflammatory swelling. This can lead to confusion in diagnosing nonulcerated tumors of these organs. Common malignant lesions are high-grade epidermoid carcinomas (78 percent) and lymphosarcomas (16 percent). A large group of miscellaneous tumors are found, including hemangiomas, neurofibromas, and salivary gland tumors. High-grade epidermoid carcinomas in this area are often described as lymphoepitheliomas and transitional cell carcinomas. It is our feeling that these are simply microscopic variants of highly undifferentiated epidermoid carcinomas.

The frequent first symptom of carcinoma of the tonsil is a slight feeling of tenderness in the area, a typical sore throat. This is easily ignored by the patient for long periods until its persistence finally forces a consultation with the physician. Even then the evidence of a growing tumor may be overlooked and the patient treated for some time with mouthwashes and antibiotics. The lesion will appear grossly as a swelling of the tonsil with a central ulcer. Palpation reveals firmness and induration spreading well beyond the area of ulceration. Trismus and pain in the ear are common complaints. The metastatic spread from this area is to the tonsillar node at the angle of the man-

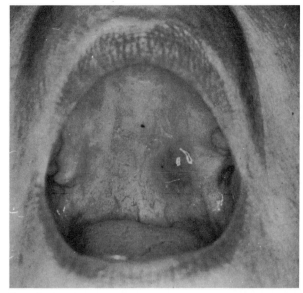

Fig. 16-22. Adenoid cystic carcinoma of the hard palate. Although this lesion is much smaller than the mixed tumor in Fig. 16-15, it is malignant. Treatment is by wide excision, including the underlying bone.

dible, so often enlarged in children who have tonsillitis. The tonsil is a common site for very tiny "occult" carcinomas, which lead to large cervical masses and must be inspected minutely when one is searching for a primary site for cervical metastases (Fig. 16-26). Lymphosarcomas of the tonsil usually present with a more bulky primary lesion and are not as inclined to ulceration. The primary lesions may be bilateral with involvement of both tonsils.

Treatment of tonsillar carcinoma either by radiation or operation has never been very satisfactory. Lymphosarcomas are quite radiosensitive and should be treated primarily by radiation. Carcinoma, on the other hand, yields poorly to either form of therapy. Still under evaluation,

Fig. 16-23. Carcinoma of buccal mucosa. A well-differentiated and slowly growing lesion which was neglected and mismanaged for many years. (*From B. F. Rush, Jr., Curr Probl Surg, May, 1967.*)

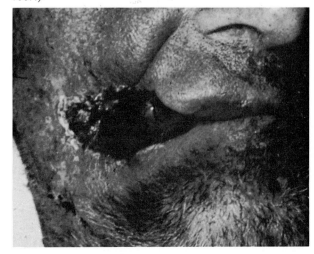

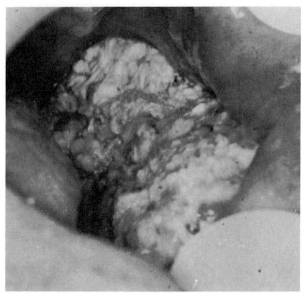

Fig. 16-24. Verrucous carcinoma. The shaggy white plaque along the gingivobuccal gutter is typical. The patient is seventy-five years old and has chewed tobacco for over 50 years.

integrated therapy with preoperative radiation to the tonsil followed by resection in continuity with a radical neck dissection may prove to produce the best results. The definitive 5-year survival following treatment of cancer of the tonsil is 25 percent.

POSTERIOR THIRD OF THE TONGUE

Tumors in the posterior third of the tongue differ markedly in their natural history from those in the anterior two-thirds. Whereas the anterior lesions tend to be well differentiated, remain confined to the primary site, or involve only high cervical nodes for long periods, lesions in the posterior third are of much higher grade, often being

Fig. 16-25. Oropharynx. The shaded area delineates the oropharynx. The nasopharynx is located above, and the hypopharynx and larynx are located below.

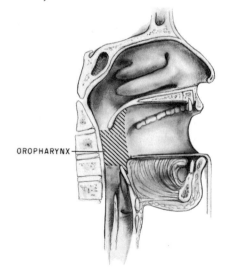

OROPHARYNX

classified as *lymphoepitheliomas,* or *transitional cell tumors.* They spread rapidly to the cervical nodes and often beyond to distant sites. A frequent initial symptom of carcinoma of the posterior third of the tongue is a large cervical lymph node accompanied by the complaint of pain on swallowing. Unfortunately, this is a fairly silent area, and lesions may attain considerable size before causing pain or dysfunction. Wide ulceration causes a malodorous breath and dysphasia. Weight loss is prominent. Treatment has been highly unsatisfactory in the past. Radiation therapy infrequently controls the primary lesion. Operation often results in total loss of the tongue, an overwhelming psychologic and functional deficit. Since these lesions are often across the midline, bilateral neck dissection must be combined with resection of the tongue. Initial experience with combined radiation and operation indicates that occasionally the lesions can be reduced in size sufficiently by preoperative radiation to permit a more conservative resection of the posterior tongue, leaving a functional anterior tongue behind.

SOFT PALATE

Malignant tumors of the soft palate are almost always epidermoid carcinomas. These tend to be well differentiated, slow-growing, and late to metastasize. They are generally superficial lesions spreading over the anterior surface of the soft palate and down the tonsillar pillars. Often it is difficult to determine whether the lesions arose in the tonsil or in the soft palate. Spread may be extensive, covering much of the soft palate, the tonsillar fossa, and the tongue. Pain and dysphagia are the usual first symptoms. Diagnosis by inspection and palpation is a simple matter, and biopsy is easily accomplished.

Response to radiation therapy is only fair. Resection is more likely to produce a cure but often leads to a difficult functional defect, since the patient is unable to close the nasopharynx and will tend to regurgitate food through the nose on swallowing. This is a situation where the clever prosthodontist can help greatly by installing an adequate extension on an upper plate which extends backward into the pharynx to seal the palatal defect. An even more convenient method of closing the palatal defect is to raise a flap from the posterior pharynx and swing it forward to close the defect at the time of the original operation. Prognosis is difficult to determine, since these tumors are usually classed in the literature with tumors of the tonsil or of the hard palate.

EPIGLOTTIS

Malignant tumors of the anterior surface of the epiglottis are usually exophytic and well differentiated and have a slow, natural evolution. Dysphagia and aspiration are early symptoms. Treatment by radiation therapy is quite successful. Hemilaryngectomy of the upper larynx above the cords has also produced good results. Patients who have had resection of the epiglottis must relearn swallowing, and this requires a reasonable level of intelligence. Senile patients or those with poor learning ability should be treated either by radiation or total laryngectomy.

LARYNX

When describing the site of tumors of the larynx, the terminology can be confusing and frustrating. According to current usage, the larynx is made up of those structures lying both above and below the true vocal cords. Thus, the mucosa of the larynx extends along the posterior surface of the epiglottis including its tip, along the aryepiglottic folds, and over the arytenoid cartilages posteriorly. It covers the inner surface of the aryepiglottic folds, the false vocal cords, and the ventricles. All of the larynx thus far described constitutes the supraglottic larynx, i.e., that which is above the true vocal cords. The glottic portion of the larynx is that portion made up of the true cords themselves. The mucosa lining the area underneath the true cords down to the lower border of the cricoid cartilage covers the infraglottic portion of the larynx.

In the past the area just described was called the "endolarynx," or the "intrinsic larynx," although the latter term gradually came to mean the true cords alone. Tumors taking their origin on the outside of the larynx for many years were designated as arising from the "extrinsic larynx." However, this term came to be used for supraglottic lesions as well, so this usage has now been abandoned. Lesions involving any portion of the exterior of the larynx are now spoken of as "hypopharyngeal" or, by some, "laryngopharyngeal."

INCIDENCE AND ETIOLOGY. Cancer of the larynx accounts for 1.62 percent of all cancers in men and only 0.14 percent of all cancers in woman; thus the ratio of incidence favors the male sex by over 11:1. The report of the Advisory Committee to the Surgeon General on Smoking and Health reviewed 10 retrospective studies and 7 prospective studies on the relationship of smoking to carcinoma of the larynx. There was a statistically positive relationship in every study. In the prospective studies the mortality ratios for smokers averaged 5.4 times greater for cigarette smokers than for nonsmokers and 2.8 times greater for cigar and pipe smokers than for nonsmokers. Laryngeal cancer mortality has increased somewhat over the past three decades, but the increase has been much less than that for lung cancer. It appears that the induction of carcinoma of the larynx cannot occur solely as a result of tobacco tars but that a further agent, or cocarcinogen, is needed. One such agent may be alcohol, since a high percentage (30 to 40 percent) of patients with carcinoma of the larynx are alcoholics and come from population groups where the risk of alcoholism is great, such as bartenders and entertainers. Cirrhosis of the liver is a common complaint among patients with carcinoma of the larynx; this may be a secondary relationship due to the frequency of alcoholism in this group.

CLASSIFICATION. As it has for other cancers, the American Joint Committee on Cancer Staging and End Results Reporting has developed a "TNM system" for carcinomas of the larynx. Because of differences in prognosis at different sites the committee has divided the larynx into its three major areas: the supraglottic (posterior surface of the epiglottis, aryepiglottic folds, arytenoids, false cords, ventricles); the glottic (right and left vocal cords and anterior

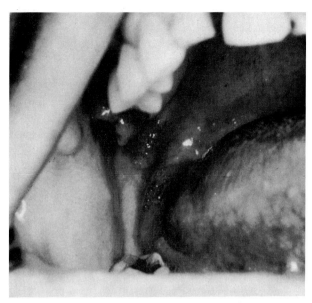

Fig. 16-26. Carcinoma of the anterior tonsillar pillar. These tiny lesions are invasive areas of carcinoma. Despite their size, the patient already had metastatic disease in the ipsilateral neck.

glottic commissure), and the subglottic (subglottic region exclusive of the undersurface of the true cords and down to the lower margin of the cricoid cartilage). About 56 percent of squamous epidermoid cancers of the larynx occur in the glottic region, 42 percent occur in the supraglottic region, and the remaining 2 percent are subglottic. The combination of topographic spread (T), nodal involvement (N), and distant metastasis (M) in a description of three separate anatomic sites results in a complex system, yet it is the most precise method whereby lesions can be classified and comparisons between institutions adequately made as to the results of treatment.

PATHOLOGY. Polyps, papillomas, granulomas, cysts, and areas of hyperkeratosis make up the common benign lesions of the cords. Rarely hemangiomas and chondromas of the laryngeal cartilages are seen. Ninety-nine percent of the malignant lesions of the larynx are epidermoid carcinomas, and most of these are of the ordinary cornifying (squamous cell) type. These lesions arise from the squamous epithelium of the cords themselves or from areas of metaplasia in the mucosa of the endolarynx. On the cord, carcinoma may be preceded by hyperkeratosis and stages of transition from hyperkeratosis to dyskeratosis, carcinoma in situ, and microinvasive carcinoma. Glottic cancers are usually very well differentiated, slow-growing, and late to metastasize. Supraglottic and infraglottic cancers are less well differentiated and more likely to have spread to lymph nodes when first seen.

DIAGNOSIS. Space-occupying lesions of the larynx produce initial symptoms through interference with phonation and respiration. Hoarseness, the usual first symptom, may be slight and intermittent but gradually becomes constant. What begins as a slight huskiness gradually progresses, until sounds are produced with difficulty. Respiratory obstruction is a later sign, although small lesions on the true cords will produce a greater degree of obstruction than somewhat larger lesions in supraglottic or infraglottic area. Obstruction progresses in severity until the patient may respire with visible effort, using his accessory muscles to force air through the cords, sometimes with audible stridor. At this point the patient's life is in jeopardy. At any moment the slightest additional swelling or edema can cut off breathing completely. The use of sedatives in patients at this phase of obstruction is fraught with danger. Under sedation the patient's tired muscles may fail, with a rapid shallowing of respiration, progressive anoxia, and cardiac arrest. The finding of a tumor on the cord associated with stridor, retraction, or the use of accessory muscles to breathe indicates immediate tracheostomy. It is far better to elect a tracheostomy done in the operating room than to be forced into an emergency tracheostomy on the ward or in the emergency room under much less favorable circumstances.

Late signs of malignant lesions of the larynx are a malodorous breath, pain on swallowing, weight loss, and hemoptysis.

Any patient who has persistent hoarseness for more than three or four weeks should have a careful inspection of his vocal cords by indirect laryngoscopy. If this reveals no pathologic conditions but hoarseness persists, then direct laryngoscopy should be used to examine the cords even more closely.

Benign Tumors

POLYPS

According to Holinger, 43 percent of all benign lesions of the larynx are simple polyps. These arise on the phonating edge of the cord at the junction between the anterior one-third and the posterior two-thirds (Fig. 16-27). Their

cause is obscure. Treatment is by removal with a cupped forceps at direct laryngoscopy.

VOCAL NODULES

The second most common benign tumor of the larynx, these are usually bilateral and, like polyps, occur at the junction of the anterior one-third with the posterior two-thirds of the cords. They are often called "singer's nodules" but certainly are not confined to singers and can occur in any occupational group. Treatment is by removal with the biopsy forceps.

RETENTION CYSTS

About half of these occur on the vocal cords, the remainder being found in the aryepiglottic folds, arytenoids, or epiglottis. They appear to occur as a result of the obstruction of small mucous glands. These lesions can reach considerable size and offer marked embarrassment to respiration.

HYPERKERATOSIS

Hyperkeratosis can affect the vocal cords as it does any of the mucosal areas of the lips, oral cavity, or pharynx. These lesions are evidence of a premalignant change and should be stripped off the cord with the use of the biopsy forceps. Patients who have developed hyperkeratosis should be followed at twice yearly intervals to guard against recurrence or the appearance of a frank carcinoma.

PAPILLOMAS

These multiple lesions are found most often on the true cords but may appear on any portion of the larynx or pharynx and even on the soft palate. While they are most commonly reported in children prior to adolescence, some

Fig. 16-27. Pedunculated polyp of the right vocal cord arising at the junction of the anterior and middle thirds. (*From P. H. Holinger et al., Ann Otol Rhinol Laryngol, 56:583, 1947.*)

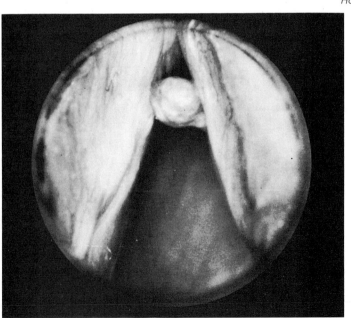
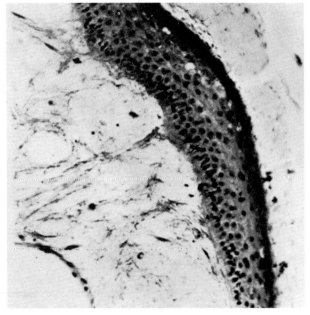

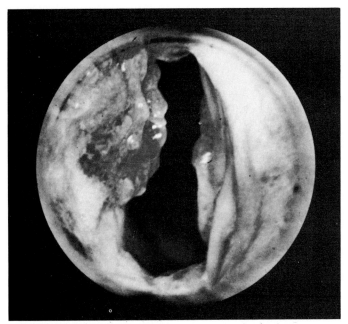

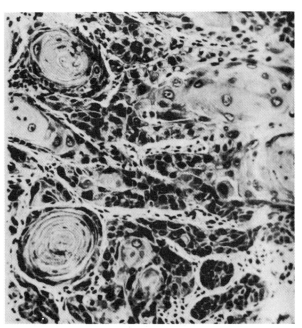

Fig. 16-28. Carcinoma involving the left side of the larynx and anterior commissure. (*From P. H. Holinger et al., Ann Otol Rhinol Laryngol, 56:583, 1947.*)

adults are also affected. Like warts, these tumors appear to be caused by viruses. Frequently the growths cover the mucosa of the cords in great profusion, causing severe respiratory embarrassment and requiring tracheostomy. They can persist for many years; during this period the patient often must continue to wear a tracheostomy tube while papillomas are cleared from his airway by frequent excisions through the laryngoscope. Repeated excision is the only effective treatment to date. The large number of other forms of therapy attempted indicates the generally unsatisfactory state of therapy. Eventually, after a period of months or years of repeated excisions, the lesions gradually disappear.

Malignant Lesions

Carcinoma of the true cords (Fig. 16-28) is a lesion which should be easily detected. It gives warning of its presence at an early stage through hoarseness and grows slowly enough so that early therapy should be rewarded by a 90 percent or better 5-year survival rate. In many urban areas over half of the lesions of the true cords are stage 1 lesions confined entirely to the cord. In contrast, some rural areas report that in only 5 percent of patients reaching the physician the lesions are still in stage 1. As the tumor grows, it extends off the cord, either up into the supraglottic area or less commonly inferiorly into the infraglottic region. Invasion occurs slowly but relentlessly, eventually with perforation of the thyroid cartilage and direct invasion of the soft tissues of the thyroid gland and of the neck.

If cancer remains confined to the true cords, a high percentage of 5-year survivals can be obtained following

treatment by radiotherapy alone. Holinger noted that in a series of 102 patients with cordal lesions treated with cobalt irradiation, only 9 patients had residual or recurrent cancer which required subsequent laryngectomy. None of the patients in this series died of carcinoma. Loss of the larynx is such a major functional and psychologic disability that if excellent results can be obtained by irradiation, this should be the treatment of choice.

Cancers which have invaded areas beyond the cord have a much different outlook. Involvement of cervical nodes becomes an important problem, and the ability to eradicate the disease by radiation alone is greatly decreased. For stage 2, 3, and 4 cancers, laryngectomy is mandatory. In addition, a radical neck dissection on the side of the lesion is usually performed, even though palpable nodes are not present. Using this approach, Norris has reported a 70 to 75 percent 5-year survival rate for stage 2 and 3 lesions of glottic and supraglottic origin. The very large stage 4 lesions do very poorly, with a 5-year survival rate of only 21 percent. Goldman et al. have combined radiation therapy and operation in treatment of advanced cancers of the larynx, and although the experience is still small, they feel that integration of the two modalities improves the long-term survival rate.

The major problem for the patient after laryngectomy is to regain a useful voice. About half of all such patients will learn to use effective esophageal speech, meaning they can communicate understandably with strangers and casual acquaintances. An additional 25 percent can make themselves understood to members of their family but find that their esophageal speech is too distorted to be useful in the general community. The remaining 25 percent of patients will be unable to conquer the technical problems of learning this method of conversation.

Esophageal speech is by far the most useful technique for speaking after laryngectomy, since it requires no additional paraphernalia and can be refined to the point where it very closely resembles the tone and expression of ordinary speech. It is produced by swallowing air and regurgitating it, creating a vibration in the pharynx—probably at the level of the cricothyroid muscle. The oral cavity modulates this tone just as it would a tone from the larynx.

For the 50 percent of patients who are partly or completely unable to learn esophageal speech, electric vibrating devices can be used to provide a tone in the oral cavity which is modulated by the patient's oral structures, giving a fairly reasonable method of communication.

HYPOPHARYNX

The hypopharynx is that area of the throat which surrounds the larynx. It is made up of the piriform sinuses on either side, the exterior portions of the aryepiglottic fold, and the lateral and posterior pharyngeal walls. It includes the mucosa overlying the posterior portions of the cricoid cartilage.

INCIDENCE. Cancer of the hypopharynx is three to four times as common as cancer of the larynx and constitutes 4.05 percent of all cancers in males. It is three times more common in men than in women. These tumors appear to be related to smoking. The correlation is stronger with pipe and cigar smoking than with cigarette smoking. Another etiologic factor is the Plummer-Vinson syndrome, found most commonly in Scandinavian women. This deficiency syndrome, now gradually disappearing, is clearly related to carcinoma of the hypopharynx and posterior tongue. At the Radiumhemmet in Stockholm carcinomas of the hypopharynx are seen more frequently in women than in men, and most of these cases are associated with a Plummer-Vinson syndrome.

PATHOLOGY. The great majority of these tumors are epidermoid carcinomas and compared with the oral cavity and endolarynx tend to be of a higher grade with a preponderance of grade 3 and 4 lesions. Better-differentiated forms are seen, however, most commonly on the exterior portions of the aryepiglottic folds and in the postcricoid area. Spread of the tumor occurs promptly and usually by way of the lymphatic channels which drain the hypopharynx, exiting between the lateral portion of the hyoid bone and the upper edge of the thyroid cartilage to travel with the superior thyroid artery to the midjugular chain of lymph nodes. Unlike most head and neck cancers, distant metastases are common with involvement of mediastinal nodes, lung, liver, and other distant viscera.

DIAGNOSIS. Since these lesions arise outside the endolarynx away from major paths of respiration and speech, hoarseness or dyspnea are uncommon findings until late in the growth of the tumor. Interference with swallowing, on the other hand, is the most common early symptom and is associated with choking and aspiration. Aspiration pneumonia may be the illness which first brings the patient to the physician. The lesions seem to have a long silent period and can grow to considerable size in the depths of the piriform sinus or on the pharyngeal walls before the first definite symptoms appear. Not uncommonly, the

first sign is the appearance of a midjugular cervical node. The better-differentiated lesions invade and ulcerate widely, so that a malodorous breath is a common associated finding. Diagnosis is confirmed by indirect laryngoscopy and biopsy through a laryngoscope.

TREATMENT. Until recent years this was a highly lethal tumor with few cures either by operation or by irradiation. The introduction of wide radical excision with removal of the larynx and hypopharynx and en bloc radical neck dissection increased the cure rate perceptibly. This may be another area where judicious combination of irradiation and operation can improve the cure rate even more. Five-year survival rates with the older form of therapy were no more than 10 to 15 percent. With more aggressive operative approaches, cure rates in the vicinity of 30 percent have been reported.

NASOPHARYNX

The nasopharynx is at the top of the pharynx, just underneath the base of the skull. The body of the sphenoid bone forms a roof for this cavity, while its floor is formed by the soft palate. There is no anterior wall as such except for the posterior openings of the nasal passage together with the posterior aspects of the nasal septum and the turbinates. The roof of the cavity slopes into the posterior wall made up of the basiocciput and the atlas and the overlying covering of muscle and mucosa. Each lateral wall contains the opening of a eustachian tube guarded by a small prominence, the torus tubarius. The only structure lying within the nasopharynx is the lymphoid tissue of the adenoids scattered on the posterior and superior walls.

INCIDENCE. These tumors are uncommon but not rare, constituting about $\frac{1}{2}$ percent of all cancers. They are somewhat more common in males than in females (2.4:1). There is an interesting relation to race. This is a frequent tumor in the Near East, among the Filipinos, Malays, and Dayaks, and especially among the Chinese. This cancer accounts for 30.4 percent of all cancers in males in Formosa. The incidence among the Chinese born in the Far East is more than thirty times greater than in this country, while the incidence among American-born Chinese is about six times as common as the incidence among the other racial groups here. This shift in pattern would suggest that both genetic and environmental causative factors are operating.

Benign Lesions

These include hypertrophied lymphatic tissue, juvenile nasopharyngeal hemangiofibroma, Rathke's pouch cyst, dermoids, and mixed tumors. Of these, hypertrophied adenoids occur commonly, and hemangiofibroma and Rathke's pouch cyst have a special predilection for this site.

Any enlarging, space-occupying lesion of the nasopharynx calls attention to itself by respiratory obstruction and nasal stuffiness. Obstruction to the eustachian tubes provokes earaches and often chronic ear infection. As the lesion encroaches on the soft palate, deglutition is disturbed with pain on swallowing or regurgitation of food and fluids into the nasopharynx and out of the nose.

HYPERTROPHIED ADENOIDS

The adenoids represent a portion of the large circle of lymphatic tissue surrounding the oral respiratory passageway at the level of the posterior tongue and tonsils. Chronic upper respiratory tract infections in infants and children often cause marked and persistent hypertrophy of some of this rim of tissue. In past decades resection of the adenoids and tonsils was one of the most common of operations in children. With the advent of the antibiotics the need for these procedures has diminished markedly. Nonetheless, in an occasional child a persistent hypertrophy of the adenoids will develop which disturbs his breathing pattern, causing mouth breathing, or more importantly will obstruct the eustachian tubes, leading to chronic ear infections with a threat to the child's hearing. These symptoms are adequate indication for operative excision.

JUVENILE NASOPHARYNGEAL HEMANGIOFIBROMA

Made up of a hard stroma of fibrous tissue, richly interlaced with capillaries and cavernous sinuses, this rare and interesting tumor appears to originate on the roof of the nasopharynx perhaps from the periosteum of the sphenoid bone (Fig. 16-29). It increases in size slowly but relentlessly and eventually begins to erode the anterior structures, obstruct the nasal passages and enter the maxillary sinus on one or both sides. The first symptom may be nasal obstruction but is usually epistaxis, which can be very profuse and even life-threatening.

This lesion is found exclusively in males, usually in the preadolescent or adolescent age groups. In some instances as the boy matures, the lesion appears to regress spontaneously. Just as often it persists, and hemangiofibromas of the nasopharynx have been described in males in their twenties and thirties, either persisting from childhood or appearing for the first time.

The progressive destruction of surrounding bone by pressure and the continuing threat of major hemorrhage require prompt treatment, preferably before the lesions grow too large. Radiation therapy is ineffective, and operative excision appears the only mode of treatment. There is a tendency toward local recurrence following excision, and these patients must be followed carefully for some years after operation.

Malignant Lesions

These are epidermoid carcinoma, lymphosarcoma, adenoid cystic carcinoma, cervical chordoma, sarcoma, and myeloma. The only lesions occurring with any frequency are epidermoid carcinoma and lymphosarcoma.

EPIDERMOID CARCINOMA

These develop from areas of metaplasia in the respiratory epithelium of the nasopharynx and are moderately to highly undifferentiated. There is a liberal amount of

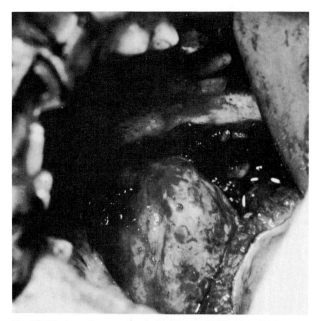

Fig. 16-29. Juvenile nasopharyngeal hemangiofibroma. A fibrous, highly vascular lesion on the posterior wall of the nasopharynx. This was first noted because of epistaxis. Exposure was obtained by an incision between the hard and soft palate with retraction of the soft palate downward.

lymphoid tissue in the nasopharynx, and frequently malignant epithelial cells are seen mixed with a prominent lymphoid stroma. This mixture of epidermoid and lymphoid cells gave rise to the term "lymphoepithelioma" introduced by Regaud and Schmincke. Many pathologists feel there is no place for this special term, since these tumors are probably highly anaplastic epidermoid carcinomas and the lymphoid element may not constitute an actual malignant part of the growth. Some feel that a large percentage of lymphoid intermixing indicates a more radiosensitive and more radiocurable tumor.

In addition to the obstructive symptoms described for benign tumors, the invasive qualities of malignant lesions produce a number of characteristic signs and symptoms. These lesions invade the roof of the nasopharynx entering the cavernous sinus with paralysis of the IIId, IVth, Vth, and VIth cranial nerves. The VIth nerve is usually paralyzed first; this is frequently accompanied by pain in the distribution of the supraorbital and infraorbital branches of the Vth nerve. The tumor reaches these nerves by spreading along the eustachian tube into the space between the pharynx and the maxilla, then extending upward through the suture line between the petrous portion of the temporal bone and the lateral wing of the sphenoid. Thus, the symptom complex is called the *petrosphenoidal syndrome*. Metastatic nodes in the retropharyngeal space tend to spread into the area along the base of the skull medial to the parotid gland, where they compress the IXth, Xth, XIth, and XIIth cranial nerves. This causes difficulties with deglutition from hemiparesis of the superior constrictor muscle, a perversion of the sense of taste in the posterior third of the tongue, and hypesthesia of the mucous mem-

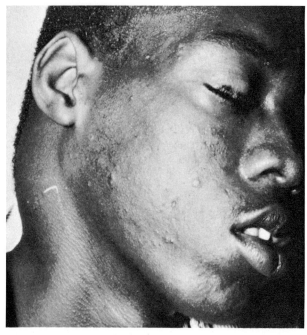

Fig. 16-30. Metastatic lymph nodes in the neck from lympho-sarcoma of the nasopharynx. Note the characteristic location behind and inferior to the ear.

branes of the soft palate, pharynx, and larynx. Paralysis of the trapezius muscle, the sternocleidomastoid, the soft palate, and one side of the tongue may also occur. These signs may be associated with Horner's syndrome from compression of the cervical sympathetic chain. Invasion of the orbit and displacement of the globe will cause double vision and proptosis.

Unfortunately, the nasopharynx is a silent area, and tumors here can reach considerable size before any symptoms are evident. The early signs of nasal obstruction or brief episodes of epistaxis are easily ignored. In two-thirds of the patients, by the time diagnosis is made, invasion of the sphenoid bone and base of the skull or nerve paralysis is present. Not infrequently, the primary growth will remain small, even microscopic, and is announced by its cervical metastases. These occur in a characteristic location, high in the neck behind the lower portion of the ear with additional involved nodes scattered along the path of the spinal accessory nerve as it courses down the trapezius muscle (Fig. 16-30). Cervical metastases are found in 50 percent of patients when first seen and are the presenting symptom in one-third.

There is no acceptable way of obtaining an adequate margin of resection when operating upon lesions of the nasopharynx, and the only operative procedure used is biopsy. Treatment of the primary lesion and usually of the metastases is by radiation therapy. Considering the advanced state of most of these lesions when first seen, the 5-year survival rate as a result of therapy is remarkably good, with an overall absolute survival of 28 percent. For the occasional patient who does not have evidence of cervical node metastasis at the beginning of treatment the 5-year survival rate is 55 percent.

LYMPHOSARCOMA

Lymphosarcomas of the nasopharynx tend to occur at the extremes of age in childhood and in the seventh and eighth decades. The majority of these lesions announce their presence by the occurrence of cervical node metastases, which are usually bulky with a rubbery consistency; the nodes mat together but are less inclined to be invasive and fixed than nodes involved by carcinoma. While lymphosarcoma may mimic all the symptoms produced by epidermoid carcinomas, they invade bone infrequently, and paralysis of nerves is much less common. If there is no evidence of spread beyond the area of the head and neck, the radiotherapist usually administers a high level of therapy in the vicinity of 6,000 rads of cobalt to both the nasopharynx and the cervical lymphatic tissues bilaterally. Five-year survival in these highly radiosensitive tumors is slightly better than for epidermoid carcinoma, averaging 35 to 40 percent.

NASAL CAVITY AND PARANASAL SINUSES

The position of the eight nasal sinuses surrounding the nasal cavity is often poorly appreciated. The maxillary sinuses lateral to the nasal cavities and beneath the orbits are the largest and most important of the sinus structures. The ethmoid air cells occupying the space between the orbit and the upper nasal cavity are much smaller and are less commonly involved by tumors. The frontal sinuses bilaterally above the orbits are the second largest set of sinuses. The paired sphenoid sinuses divided by a thin septum just below the pituitary and over the roof of the nasopharynx are the most remote of the sinuses. The frontal and sphenoid sinuses are rare primary sites for tumors.

INCIDENCE. Tumors of the nasal cavity and paranasal sinuses represent about 1 percent of all cancer seen. Malignant lesions are found here three times as commonly in men as in women. With the exception of the esthesioneuroblastoma no specific cause is known for lesions arising here.

Benign Tumors

Polyps of the nasal cavity and maxillary sinus are the most common growths seen. These are usually associated with chronic inflammation or, occasionally, allergy. Sometimes the underlying infection may be due to a tumor, so that the discovery of polyps should not be considered an adequate diagnosis until the possibility of an underlying tumor has been ruled out. While polyps can be eradicated by simple excision, they will usually re-form unless the basic pathologic condition leading to their growth has been determined and corrected. This may be allergy, septal deviation, or other factors which obstruct adequate drainage and promote infection.

Malignant Tumors

Of 293 patients with neoplasms of the nasal cavity and paranasal sinus examined at the Mayo Clinic approximately 50 percent had epidermoid carcinomas, 10 percent had lymphomas, and 20 percent had tumors which probably arose from minor salivary tissue. The remaining 20 percent had various soft tissue sarcomas such as fibrosarcoma, chondrosarcoma, neurofibrosarcoma, and osteogenic sarcoma. Among 648 patients seen in Sweden with epidermoid carcinomas arising from the paranasal sinuses, the average age ranged from fifty to seventy years, and the vast majority of the lesions arose in the maxillary sinus (Fig. 16-31). None of these tumors occurred in the sphenoid sinus and only one in the frontal sinus.

Tumors, whether benign or malignant, are announced by pain, nasal obstruction, and persistent nasal secretion. Fifty percent of the patients present with one or more of these three symptoms. Unfortunately, these are also the presenting symptoms of sinusitis; patients may be treated with antibiotics and other measures for long periods before the more serious nature of the disease is realized. Repeated epistaxis is more likely to suggest the presence of tumor but occurs in only 10 percent as a presenting symptom. Swelling or ulceration of the hard palate or gingiva, swelling of the cheek, or ocular symptoms are evidences of a much more advanced stage of tumor growth yet constitute the presenting symptom in 25 to 30 percent of patients (Fig. 16-32). Bone destruction seen on roentgenographic examination is almost certain evidence of a tumor and unfortunately is also a late sign. Absence of bone destruction does not rule out a malignant tumor. All tissue removed when polyps of the nose or maxillary sinus are treated or when the maxillary sinus is drained should be submitted for histologic examination. Not infrequently this is the first evidence of the presence of an underlying carcinoma and may be the only opportunity for diagnosis of such lesions at an early state.

TREATMENT. Electrosurgical therapy, radiation therapy, and operative excision have all been used to treat these tumors. Lymphomas are ordinarily treated by radiation alone. Epidermoid carcinomas of this site are refractory to either irradiation or operation. Integration of irradiation preoperatively with operative excision has been used for many years and has gained wide acceptance. This approach yields a 5-year survival rate of 30 to 35 percent for lesions of the maxillary sinuses. Cervical lymph nodes are involved late, and radical neck dissections are not done unless palpable nodes are present.

MANDIBLE

Tumors of the mandible arise from two main sources, from the tooth-forming (odontogenic) tissue and from bone.

Odontogenic Tumors

These neoplasms arise from ectodermal odontogenic tissue, mesodermal odontogenic tissue, or a mixture of both. They are invariably benign. The lesions most commonly seen are ectodermal odontogenic cysts: the follicular and radicular cysts. A rare and intriguing tumor is the ameloblastoma. Other odontogenic tumors are too rare to merit consideration here.

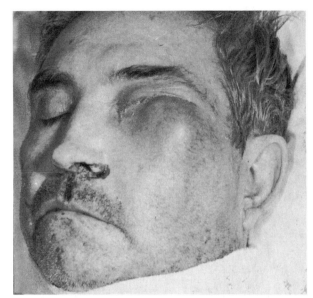

Fig. 16-31. Squamous carcinoma of the maxilla. The lesion had its origin in the upper portion of the maxillary sinus and invaded the floor of the orbit.

Fig. 16-32. Squamous carcinoma of the ethmoid sinuses. This lesion began in the left ethmoid and invaded the nasal cavity and right ethmoid sinus.

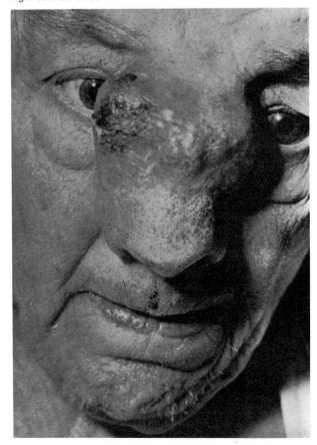

FOLLICULAR CYSTS

Some cysts are derived from the dental lamina and outer enamel epithelium of developing teeth. Remnants of this tissue sequestered during development may undergo proliferation and cystic change. Microscopically, they have fibrous walls usually lined by squamous epithelium. Occasionally remnants of odontogenic epithelium are present from which ameloblastomas may develop. Often the cyst envelops an unerupted tooth. A pathognomonic x-ray finding is the appearance of a smooth symmetric cyst in the mandible containing an unerupted tooth in its cavity. Clinically the tumor is found as a mass causing enlargement of the ramus of the mandible or the rim of the gingiva. Treatment is by intraoral excision, removing the top of the cyst and excising its entire lining membrane.

RADICULAR CYST

Infection of the dental pulp is the most common cause of this frequent cyst. A dental granuloma forms when epithelial remnants of the sheath about the tooth root are entrapped. Nests of epithelial tissue proliferate to line a central lumen usually at the apex of the infected tooth (Fig. 16-33). Cysts may vary in size from 1 to several centimeters. Microscopically, there is a dense, fibrous connective tissue lining covered internally by squamous epithelium. Frequently, a generalized inflammatory reaction in the cyst wall is seen. Treatment is by extraction of the tooth involved and excision of the cyst with its lining.

AMELOBLASTOMA

Although very uncommon, this is the most frequent solid tumor of the mandible. It usually appears in the body of the mandible at its junction with the ramus. Growth is slow, and the lesion is relatively asymptomatic, although it may expand the bone about it and eventually attain enormous size, encroaching on soft tissues of the face and neck (Fig. 16-34). Microscopically, the tumor presents interlacing strands and nests of odontogenic epithelium

Fig. 16-33. Roentgenogram of a radicular cyst. Note the root of the tooth from which the cyst took origin. (*Courtesy of Sheldon Rovin, D.D.S.*)

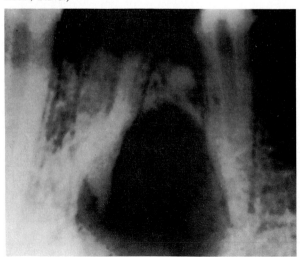

enmeshed in a connective tissue stroma with numerous areas of cystic degeneration. Treatment is by segmental resection of the portion of the mandible affected by the tumor including a centimeter or two of normal bone on either side. Unless the wide excision is accomplished, recurrence is common. The adjacent soft tissues need not be resected, and a good bed is usually left for reconstruction of the mandible.

Osteogenic Tumors

The mandible is affected by the same group of benign and malignant tumors which affect other bones in the body. Benign lesions include exostosis (torus mandibularis), fibrous dysplasia, Paget's disease, and giant cell tumor. Primary malignant lesions are multiple myeloma, Ewing's sarcoma, osteogenic sarcoma, chondrosarcoma (Fig. 16-35), and periosteal fibrosarcoma.

Giant cell tumors of the mandible are often referred to as *central* reparative giant cell tumors and are equivalent to the peripheral giant cell tumors of the gingiva. Although this lesion grows slowly and expands the surrounding bone, it never appears to have the malignant potential of giant cell tumors seen elsewhere in the skeleton and may have a different histogenesis. Microscopically, no distinction can be made between mandibular giant cell tumors and giant cell lesions of other bones. Treatment is usually by unroofing the tumor and curetting its tissue from the bony cavity.

SALIVARY GLANDS

Salivary tissue is found in the parotid gland, the submaxillary gland, the lingual gland, and the numerous salivary glands. The parotid gland is a unilobular structure which is bent in a U shape about the posterior portion of the mandible in such a way that the larger external portion of the gland is often called the *superficial lobe* and the smaller internal portion lying on the internal surface of the ascending ramus is called the *deep lobe*. The VIIth nerve exiting from the skull by way of the stylohyoid foramen crosses the space between the mastoid and the ascending ramus of the mandible and plunges into the parotid gland at the point where it turns the corner around the posterior edge of the ascending ramus. The VIIth nerve usually bifurcates within the substance of the parotid. Each bifurcation further subdivides, and the branches eventually lie between the parotid gland and the underlying masseter muscle. The relationship of the VIIth nerve to the parotid gland is of clinical importance, since tumors of the parotid lie most commonly in the external portion of the gland; on excising such tumors great care must be taken not to cut the branches or the main trunk of this nerve.

The submaxillary gland is an ovoid structure lying in the submaxillary fossa beneath the horizontal ramus of the mandible. It is bounded by the anterior and posterior portions of the digastric muscle, thus occupying most of the digastric triangle in the neck. The important relationships of this gland are to the ramus mandibularis, the lowest branch of the VIIth nerve which courses over the upper portion of the gland. Injury to this nerve blocks innervation of the inferior quarter of the orbicularis oris on the side of the nerve and deprives the patient of the ability to pucker his lips normally. The lingual nerve, deep to the upper inferior surface of the submaxillary gland, provides the gland with some small branches. In addition, the lingual nerve parallels the course of Wharton's duct, which conducts saliva from the submaxillary gland to the mouth. When the gland is removed, injury to the lingual nerve can occur either when Wharton's duct is clamped or when the gland is pulled down into the neck dragging the lingual nerve along by its nerve attachments.

The lingual gland is the smallest of the three major salivary glands. It lies beneath the mucosa of the anterior floor of the mouth.

The minor salivary glands are small deposits of salivary tissue which are scattered throughout the mucosa of the oral cavity, maxilla, and nasopharynx. The term "ectopic salivary tissue" is sometimes used but carries an incorrect connotation, since this salivary tissue is a normal finding in all individuals and is not the result of an error in development.

INCIDENCE. About $\frac{1}{3}$ percent of all malignant tumors occurs in the salivary tissues. These tumors are equally common in men and women. About 60 percent of these lesions occur in the parotid glands, which is not surprising, since this is the largest single collection of salivary tissues. The second largest concentration of tumors is found in the submaxillary gland and the third largest in the minor salivary glands. Tumors of the lingual glands are rare. No specific cause is known for any of the benign or malignant tumors of the salivary glands other than the occasional congenital or obstructive cyst. Women with malignant tumors of the salivary glands are known to have a higher incidence of cancer of the breast.

Benign Lesions. A variety of lesions may arise in salivary tissue.

Mixed Tumors. The most common lesion of the salivary glands is the mixed tumor (pleomorphic adenoma). Fifty percent of all tumors of the salivary glands and over eighty percent of all benign tumors are mixed tumors. These probably originate from adult glandular epithelium and, as their name implies, have an extremely diverse structural pattern. In 90 percent of the tumors one finds areas where the tumor grows in a network of strands made up of spindle and stellate cells not always connecting and sometimes lying entirely detached. In about a third of all cases this loose myxoid pattern predominates but is by no means the sole structural component. Half the tumors have pseudocartilaginous structures. Twenty percent show tissue closely resembling hyaline cartilage. Well-formed tubular structures are common and present a wide variety of patterns. The lining epithelium may be single-layered, conspicuously double-layered, stratified, or pseudostratified. Some areas of metaplasia into squamous epithelium may be seen, and well-differentiated squamous epithelium can be found in about a fourth of the cases.

Papillary Cystadenoma Lymphomatosum (Warthin's Tumor). These curious lesions occur only in parotid salivary

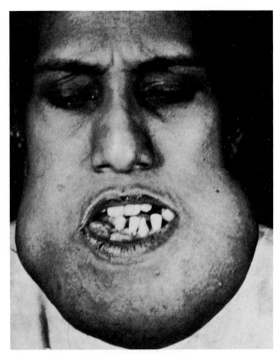

Fig. 16-34. Ameloblastoma. These lesions can grow to fantastic size, as shown here. Aside from the mass and functional disability, they are painless and never become malignant. (*Courtesy of Sheldon Rovin, D.D.S.*)

tissue and almost exclusively (95 percent) in males. About 10 percent of them are bilateral. Characteristically they are made up of a papillary epithelial component intermingled with well-developed lymphoid tissue commonly containing germinal centers. Their histogenesis is uncertain, but many feel they represent parotid duct tissue sequestered in lymph nodes within the parotid gland. They represent the second most common benign tumor of salivary tissue but

Fig. 16-35. Chondrosarcoma of the mandible. This is a slowly developing lesion and was present in this patient for 9 years before medical aid was sought. The pressure of the upper gingiva has caused the groove which is seen in the dorsal surface of the tumor. Even at this late date, the tumor had not metastasized, and the patient was still alive and well 5 years after resection. (*From B. F. Rush, Jr., and K. Trinkle, South Med J, 60:714, 1967.*)

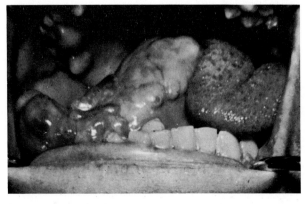

are a poor second to mixed tumors, which are at least eight times more common.

Mikulicz's Disease. This disease is characterized by a dense infiltration of lymphocytes occasionally arranged in follicles throughout the salivary tissue. This is accompanied by atrophy and disappearance of acinar tissue. Scattered throughout the lymphoid tissue are foci of epithelial and myloepithelial cells in close relationship to distal structures. The more popular modern term for this lesion is *benign lymphoepithelial lesion,* and many feel it represents a phase of the larger disease complex *Sjögren's syndrome.* The diffuse lymphocytic infiltrate, much as one sees in lymphomatous thyroiditis, suggests the possibility of an autoimmune disease. While several of or all the major salivary glands may be involved, a single parotid gland is the most frequent site (80 percent). The highest incidence of the disease is in patients between thirty-one and forty years of age.

Asymptomatic Enlargement of Salivary Tissue. This affectation is usually observed in both parotid glands but may involve all the major salivary glands. The characteristic microscopic findings are an increase in size of the glandular acini due to swelling of the individual acinar cells. There is an increase of the secretory granules, a fatty infiltration, and a moderate fibrosis. These changes seem associated with nutritional deficiencies and have been found in patients suffering from cirrhosis of the liver, kwashiorkor, and diabetes mellitus. It also has been found in whole populations suffering from malnutrition in India, in Greece during the occupation of World War II, and in the inmates of German concentration camps. Katsilambros believes that this is a fundamental response to a deficiency of vitamin A and has duplicated his findings in vitamin A–deficient rats.

Other Lesions. Cysts of the parotid glands are seen quite rarely and in some instances may represent cysts of the first branchial cleft. Hemangiomas in children have a predilection for the area of the parotid gland and sometimes persist into adulthood. Neurofibromas and lipomas of the parotid gland have been described.

Malignant Lesions. About 75 percent of all malignant salivary tumors arise from the parotid gland, and 25 percent of all parotid tumors are malignant. Ten percent of malignant salivary lesions arise in the submaxillary gland and an additional twelve percent in the minor salivary glands. The incidence of malignant lesions in the submaxillary and minor salivary glands compared to benign lesions is somewhat higher than in the parotid gland, averaging one-third to one-half of all lesions seen. Roughly one-third of the malignant lesions of salivary tissue arise from the acinar epithelium and are adenocarcinomas. Another third arise from the ductal epithelium as various forms of epidermoid carcinomas. The remaining third appear either as highly anaplastic and unclassified lesions or as malignant mixed tumors.

Epidermoid Carcinoma. The most frequent of these are the mucoepidermoid carcinomas originally identified as a special group by Stewart et al. in 1945. These interesting tumors are made up, as the name indicates, of epidermoid cells and mucus-containing cells. The name falls short of being completely descriptive, since there is a third cell called an "intermediate" cell, smaller than either of the other two, which closely resembles certain cells of the salivary gland duct. They are commonly seen in stratifications lining dilated ductlike structures. Stewart et al. suggest that this intermediate cell is capable of differentiation into mucinous cells or into epidermoid and even squamous cells.

Mucoepidermoid carcinomas are usually divided on the basis of the microscopic appearance into low-grade and high-grade tumors. Low-grade tumors contain a large portion of mucus-secreting cells, often with the presence of microcysts and large amounts of mucoid material which may leak diffusely through the tissues, generating variable degrees of inflammatory reaction. In the highly malignant tumors epidermoid and intermediate cells dominate the picture. Pseudoglandular formation is fairly frequent, and the growth pattern is commonly sheetlike or in coarse plugs.

Squamous cell carcinomas like mucoepidermoid carcinomas must certainly originate in the ductal epithelium, and the ability of salivary duct epithelium to undergo squamous metaplasia is well known. Stewart et al. suggest that most squamous cell carcinomas represent diffuse squamous cell overgrowth of tumors that were fundamentally mucoepidermoid. Microscopically, these lesions share the usual features of squamous cell carcinomas seen in the skin, oral cavity, and elsewhere. In this location, however, they are usually more malignant, and local and regional metastases are common.

Adenocarcinoma. *Adenoid Cystic Carcinoma (Cylindroma).* The chief histologic feature of these lesions is the arrangement of rather small, darkly staining cells with relatively low cytoplasm in anastomosing cords between which are acellular areas which may contain mucous, hyaline, or mucohyaline material. The cystic components of an adenoid cystic carcinoma usually stain positively with mucicarmine, indicating the presence of mucin. While the lesions are of sluggish evolution, metastases to cervical lymph nodes develop in 30 percent of the cases.

Acinar Cell Adenocarcinoma. These histologically distinct tumors are of low-grade clinical malignancy and fairly rare. They appear to arise from the acinar cells of salivary tissue and to be limited to the parotid gland. In the usual microscopic arrangement rounded or polygonal cells with a dark eccentric nucleus and a finely granular basophilic cytoplasm are packed closely together, sometimes in crude, acinar groups. While low-grade, these lesions are capable of metastasis both regionally and to distant locations.

Miscellaneous Adenocarcinomas. Adenocarcinomas may have a trabecular pattern and may be anaplastic or resemble adenocarcinomas of the gastrointestinal tract. These are usually highly malignant with a high degree of local invasiveness and regional and distant metastases.

Malignant Mixed Tumors. It is usually assumed that malignant mixed tumors arise from a neoplastic transformation of a previously benign mixed tumor. Patients who demonstrate these lesions are generally older than those with benign mixed tumors and have had a mass in the parotid for a longer period. Moreover, the malignant lesions are usually larger than the benign. In general, the microscopic picture is of a definite mixed tumor which contains within it malignant elements which may be adenocarcinomas, squamous cell carcinomas, or a malignant spindle cell alteration. The malignant component of a mixed tumor may so greatly overgrow the area of origin that it is extremely difficult to identify the previous benign mixed tumor.

NATURAL HISTORY. With the exception of the mixed tumor the common benign lesions of salivary tissue have no malignant potential. While the mixed tumor may have a very long history without malignant transformation and may grow for 20 to 30 years at a slow pace (Fig. 16-36), a rapidly growing and even anaplastic component can suddenly develop which markedly changes its course. On rare occasions mixed tumors have been found which have metastasized to local nodes without apparent histologic change and in their new location have pursued a slow course of growth. The most common pattern, however, is the development of a squamous cell carcinoma, adenocarcinoma, or other tumor which rapidly overgrows the original mixed tumor. Some very slowly evolving "chronic" carcinomas are known to develop from salivary tissue. Notable among these are the adenoid cystic carcinomas, which may develop their metastases 10, 15, and even 20 years after treatment of the primary tumor.

Many such tumors have been reported in which metastatic nodules in the lungs have been observed growing very slowly, at times appearing almost stationary for 10 and 15 years. The mucoepidermoid carcinoma, while not as slow-growing as the adenoid cystic carcinoma, is rather slowly progressive; however, this trait is offset by its great degree of local invasiveness, especially by perineural invasion. The chances for local recurrence are great even after wide local excision. Squamous cell carcinomas and adenocarcinomas of the salivary glands are almost always highly malignant, quick to invade and metastasize, and fatal in a high percentage of the patients affected.

DIFFERENTIAL DIAGNOSIS. Most tumors of the salivary glands appear as painless, slowly growing nodules (Fig. 16-37). Lesions of the parotid are bound by the heavy cervical fascia which splits on either side of the gland and invests it with a strong capsule. This dense covering obscures the actual size of the underlying tumor, and the surgeon may be surprised by the size and extent of a lesion at operation. Paralysis of the VIIth nerve is indicative of a malignant tumor and usually of a highly malignant lesion such as squamous carcinoma or adenocarcinoma. Mucoepidermoid carcinomas of the low-grade type or adenoid cystic carcinomas frequently spare the nerve until quite late in their course. Fixation of the gland to underlying structures and palpable nodes in the neck are also more commonly seen with the tumors of higher grade. Since there is nothing that can distinguish the benign mass in the salivary gland from an early malignant tumor, excision of the mass and histologic examination are indicated in every case.

TREATMENT. Benign mixed tumors, the most common solid tumors of salivary gland origin, are so easily disseminated that incisional biopsy is never indicated. In earlier

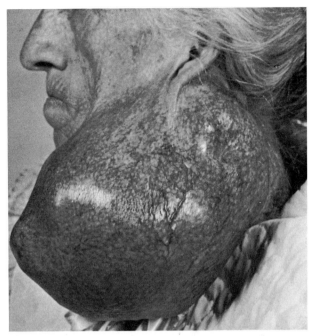

Fig. 16-36. Giant mixed tumor of the parotid. This lesion had been present for 29 years. It was still benign and was excised without evidence of recurrence in a 5-year follow-up. (*From B. F. Rush, Jr., and K. Trinkle, South Med J, 60:714, 1967.*)

decades the technique of choice for removal was enucleation. Follow-up of patients so treated indicated that local recurrence was late and slow to develop and occurred in as many as 50 percent. Attempt at excision of these lesions with a cuff of surrounding normal tissue was accompanied by a high rate of injury to one or more branches of the VIIth nerve.

Through these painful experiences the present method of therapy was developed. After isolation of the VIIth nerve, the superficial portion of the parotid gland is dissected from the underlying tissues and removed with the tumor contained within it, assuring against injury of

Fig. 16-37. Multilobulated mixed tumor of the parotid. The lesion presents in the upper pole of the superficial portion of the gland.

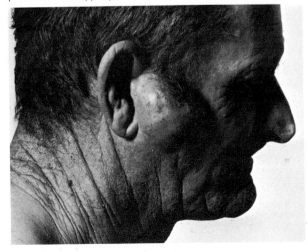

branches of the facial nerve and against dissemination and local recurrence of the tumor.

Frozen section of the lesion should be done at operation. If a low-grade malignant lesion such as an acinar cell adenocarcinoma, a low-grade mucoepidermoid carcinoma, or an adenoid cystic carcinoma is identified, the remainder of the gland and probably the VIIth nerve should be removed. If a high-grade lesion such as an anaplastic adenocarcinoma or squamous carcinoma is identified, a radical neck dissection should accompany the procedure. Aside from the problem of dealing with the VIIth nerve, the same general rules apply for lesions in the submaxillary gland.

Most of the tumors of salivary glands have a reputation for being poorly radiosensitive; however, the more malignant the lesion, the less likely this is to be true. Many high-grade mucoepidermoid carcinomas, squamous carcinomas, and even an occasional adenocarcinoma will demonstrate considerable sensitivity to x-ray therapy.

PROGNOSIS. Benign mixed tumors will recur in 40 to 50 percent of patients if improperly excised. If excision is by superficial lobectomy, the recurrence rate should be 5 percent or less. Five-year survival rates tend to be misleading, particularly in the chronic, slow-growing tumors. Adenoid cystic carcinoma has an 86 percent 5-year survival rate but a 57 percent 10-year survival. Malignant mixed tumor may have a 5-year survival of 87 to 90 percent and a 10-year survival of 60 to 70 percent.

TUMORS OF THE NECK

Palpable or visible cervical swellings are a common complaint. Two to three percent of all admissions to hospital surgical services are for this condition. About half of these lesions occur in the thyroid gland; the remainder are due to a wide range of malignant, congenital, or inflammatory swellings.

Inflammation

Inflammatory swelling in the adult neck is now a rare hospital problem. Skandalakis and coworkers, in reviewing 1,616 nonthyroid masses of the neck, found that only 3.2 percent were inflammatory, whereas 84 percent were neoplastic and 12 percent congenital or miscellaneous. The inflammatory lesions requiring hospitalization of adults are largely acute, often resulting from drainage from infection elsewhere. A common source is an infected tooth draining to the nodes in the submandibular area and causing an abscess. Only two patients in Skandalakis' entire series had tuberculous adenitis (scrofula). This was once the most common cause of neck masses, but with the tuberculin testing of cows and the pasteurization of milk, bovine tuberculosis has virtually disappeared in this country.

Malignant Tumors

The vast majority of cervical masses in adults are due to neoplasms. About 80 percent of these are metastatic from some other site, while the remainder occur from primary lesions in the neck. Primary cervical neoplasms occur either in the major salivary glands (40 percent) or are lymphomas primary in the cervical lymph nodes (60 percent). At one time it was proposed the squamous carcinomas arose primarily in the neck from the lining of branchial cleft cysts. This diagnosis was often made only to discover at a later date that the lesion was actually a metastasis from the oral cavity, nasopharynx, or laryngeal area. While there is some evidence that branchiogenic cysts become malignant, the reported, provable cases number only a handful.

A knowledge of the statistics quickly indicates that a clinician's first suspicion concerning any nonthyroid, cervical mass in adults is of a malignant tumor. He may also suspect that it is metastatic and from a site at some point above the clavicle, since 85 percent of all metastatic cervical lesions come from a supraclavicular site.

When a firm to hard cervical node which suggests malignancy is found, the first responsibility of clinicians is a thorough exploration of possible sites of origin. Cervical tumors appearing below and behind the ear and along the cervical chain are more likely to come from the nasopharynx or lateral pharyngeal walls. Swollen lymph nodes at the angle of the mandible or in the area of the submaxillary gland are most commonly from lesions in the tonsillar area, buccal mucosa, floor of the mouth, and gingiva. Swelling of the lymph nodes in the submental area should provoke a thorough examination of the tip of the tongue, lower lip, and anterior gingivobuccal gutter. Lymph nodes involved by neoplasm which appear in the middle third of the neck should cast suspicion first on the hypopharynx, piriform sinus, larynx, or thyroid.

Only when enlarged lymph nodes appear in the supraclavicular area does metastasis from below the clavicle become a major possibility. These may stem from carcinoma of the upper lobes of the lung or mediastinum or, in women, from carcinoma of the breast. The left supraclavicular nodes are frequently involved by malignant tumors metastatic from the abdomen (Virchow's node). Advanced adenocarcinoma of the stomach, pancreas, biliary tree, and even large bowel metastasize to this site.

If a thorough search of all sites reveals no possible source of a primary lesion, biopsy of the cervical node is usually carried out. If this confirms the clinical impression of malignancy, further attempts to find the primary lesion are indicated. This can include surgical exploration of the maxillary sinuses. If all avenues have been searched thoroughly and no primary lesion has been found, the problem of local treatment still remains. The best course is to treat the lesion to achieve cure. If operation is chosen, it should be a radical neck dissection; if radiation therapy is used, it should be a full course of therapy. Since lymph nodes involved by metastatic disease respond poorly to radiation, the treatment of choice is normally operation. In the presence of advanced lesions a combination of radiation and operation may be used.

If a group of these patients treated without a known primary lesion is followed for 5 years, 80 percent of the patients will ultimately manifest the primary lesion. In some instances this may subsequently be resected for cure. A few patients may die over this period without ever demonstrating the source for the metastatic lesion, and even at postmortem examination it may not be found. Even more interesting, about 20 percent of the patients survive 5 or more years with apparent "cure" of their metastatic lesion even though the presumed primary lesion has not been found or treated. In those patients who received radiation therapy, either together with operation or alone, it may be that the port included the primary lesion as well. In those patients who are treated by operation alone, the fate of the primary lesion remains a mystery. A few of these patients may represent true branchiogenic carcinoma, or possibly the primary lesion regresses spontaneously.

Other Lesions

A host of other tumors, found infrequently in the area of the neck, present problems in differential diagnosis. Dermoids occur in the midline, most commonly in the submental area and sometimes along the line of the clavicle. Sebaceous cysts are common, especially in men, and probably are related to the trauma of shaving.

Carotid body tumors (chemodectomas) are rare tumors of the paraganglionic tissue found at the carotid bifurcation. Another lesion with a slow evolution, it gradually increases in size over many years, enveloping the bifurcation and slowly compressing the adjacent nerves including the hypoglossal, vagus, and sympathetic chain. For many periods, the only symptom is the mass in the neck. Eventually nerve paralysis, dysphagia, and pain appear. Malignant transformation is rare, but early removal is indicated to avoid the late symptoms. Small lesions can be removed easily (Fig. 16-38), but advanced large tumors require resection of the carotid artery with the risk of subsequent hemiparesis.

TUMORS OF THE NECK IN CHILDREN

The order of frequency of masses in the neck in children differs markedly from that found in adults. Inflammatory lesions are by far the most common, often coming from related infections of the tonsils. The most common malignant lesion is the lymphoma, and the second most common is carcinoma of the thyroid. Congenital lesions, of course, are much more common in children than in adults.

CHEMOTHERAPY

In the past decade it has been discovered that certain types of neoplasms commonly found in the head and neck area can be cured by chemotherapy. Burkitt's lymphoma, a rare neoplasm in the United States but common in some parts of Africa, was the first such cancer. It became apparent that a predictable and consistent percentage of patients with this disease could be cured by the use of *systemic* chemotherapy alone. Recently we have also learned that squamous cancer of facial skin and of the lips, while in the in situ or microinvasive and superficial stages, can be

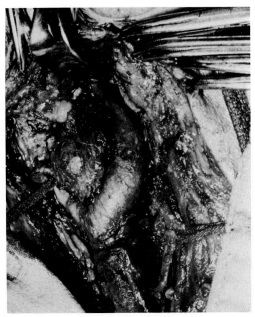

Fig. 16-38. Carotid body tumor of moderate size. The lesion lies between the internal and external branches of the carotid arteries; the adventitial layer binding it to the carotid bulb has been removed. (*From B. F. Rush, Jr., Ann Surg, 157:633, 1963.*)

cured by the topical application of 5-fluorouracil used as a cream or paste. These lesions are multiple and often tedious to eradicate by operation or radiation. A third head and neck lesion in which chemotherapy has become important is embryonal rhabdomyosarcoma, an uncommon lesion found in infants and children. Cure of this lesion occasionally has been obtained by combining radiation, chemotherapy, and operation.

Arterial infusion for the treatment of cancer in the head and neck area has received much attention. This involves the introduction of chemotherapy, usually methotrexate or 5-fluorouracil, into the external carotid artery via a catheter. The agents are administered either continuously or intermittently over 1 to several weeks. At present, this technique is known to produce a substantial to complete regression of the lesions in a large percentage of patients—as high as 50 percent in some series. Unfortunately, the response is usually transient, and the cancers return to continued growth within 2 to 3 months after treatment is discontinued. Long-term regression is uncommonly seen, and the period of regression obtained is rarely worth the morbidity and complications of the treatment itself. Nonetheless, these observations continue to tantalize clinical investigators seeking a clue which will lead to longer or even permanent remissions.

Combined forms of treatment for head and neck cancers, which include chemotherapy and immunotherapy as well as radiation and operation, have enjoyed marked clinical and investigative interest in the past 2 or 3 years. The more our knowledge of the natural history of tumor growth develops, the more rational and logical it appears to combine available treatment methods. In the next decade clinical research will be devoted to determining the best dose schedules and the best combinations of drugs and techniques.

OPERATIONS OF THE HEAD AND NECK

The most commonly performed major operation for cancer of the head and neck is radical neck dissection. This procedure was originally designed by Crile to eradicate the cervical lymphatic network, thereby eliminating sites of metastasis from cancer of the oral cavity, pharynx, paranasal sinuses, or other areas of the head and neck. In the early days of head and neck surgery radical neck dissections were usually performed after the primary lesion had been controlled through the use of radiation therapy. Today, we are more inclined to combine radical neck dissection with a simultaneous resection of the primary lesion. This is sometimes preceded by a course of radiation therapy to the primary area as part of a planned program of tumor treatment. Combined operations have been called by a number of terms including *composite resections* and *commando operations*. Other common operations in this area are superficial resection of the parotid gland, V excision of carcinoma of the lip, and resection of the maxillary antrum.

Radical Neck Dissection

Incisions for radical neck dissection are numerous and include a T-shaped incision originally used by Crile, a Y

Fig. 16-39. Common operative incisions for radical neck dissections. (*From B. F. Rush, Jr., Curr Probl Surg, May, 1966.*)

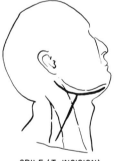

CRILE (T-INCISION)

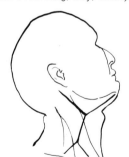

MARTIN (DOUBLE-Y INCISION)

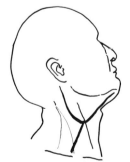

WARD (Y-INCISION)

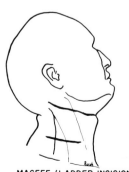

MACFEE (LADDER INCISION)

incision described by Ward, and a double Y incision described by Martin (Fig. 16-39). We prefer a hockey-stick-shaped incision with the ascending limb along the posterior border of the sternocleidomastoid muscle and the horizontal portion crossing the neck about 2 or 3 cm above the clavicle (Fig. 16-40). This last approach has the advantage of being outside areas of radiation when the neck has had previous exposure to radiation therapy and of being a simple linear incision avoiding small triangular-shaped flaps, which have a tendency to slough. The skin flap is reflected mediad, including the underlying platysma muscle, and dissection of neck structures begins in the posterior triangle, dissecting the fibroareolar tissue of this space away from the trapezius muscle and the underlying brachial plexus and scalene fibers. This portion of the dissection is carried mediad until the phrenic nerve lying on the anterior scalene muscle is identified.

The lower end of the sternocleidomastoid muscle is transected and the jugular vein identified and ligated. The accompanying vagus nerve next to the jugular vein in the carotid sheath is identified and spared. Dissection is then carried up the neck, gradually dissecting the lymph node chain free from underlying fascia and beneath the carotid artery. Just above the level of the carotid bulb the hypoglossal nerve is identified. In the upper portion of the neck the sternocleidomastoid muscle is again transected at the level of the mastoid together with the tip of the parotid gland. The submaxillary gland is dissected free from the digastric fossa and included with the specimen. The lingual nerve and artery in the depths of the submaxillary fossa are visualized and left intact. Care is taken to identify the ramus mandibularis, the tiny fiber of the VIIth nerve which innervates the lower lip, and to reflect this above the submaxillary gland so that its continuity is maintained. The spinal accessory nerve is usually sacrificed, being cut in the lower neck where it enters the trapezius muscle and in the upper neck where it enters the sternocleidomastoid muscle. The operation is completed with the transection of the jugular vein at the point where it leaves the base of the skull (Fig. 16-41). If a radical neck dissection alone is performed, the operation is ended at this point by closing the skin flaps. Multiperforated catheters are left underneath the flaps and are connected to suction. This helps to draw the flap firmly to the structures of the neck and eliminates the problem of fluid collecting under the flap.

COMBINED OPERATION

If a radical neck dissection is to be combined with the removal of structures within the oral cavity or tonsillar area, the contents of the neck dissection are left attached to the horizontal ramus of the mandible. The mandible is frequently divided. If the lesion is in the floor of the mouth or tongue, the horizontal ramus of the mandible may be resected. If the lesion is in the tonsillar fossa, the ascending ramus of the mandible is removed. If the lesion in the oral cavity is quite large, total removal of the hemimandible on the side of the lesion may be necessary. Resection of the mandible is done to remove bone involved by tumor and sometimes to obtain a closure of the oral cavity which would not be feasible without removing a portion of the bony framework. Mandibular resection can be done with the acceptable cosmetic and functional result, especially when the anterior portion of the mandible is preserved (Fig. 16-42). The more anteriorly the mandible is resected, the more likely there is to be facial deformity. If the primary site of the tumor is in the larynx or thyroid, then these structures may also be removed with the radical neck dissection. The mortality for radical neck dissection alone is less than 1 percent. If neck dissection is combined with en bloc excision of a primary lesion, then mortality rates range from 2 to 5 percent.

BILATERAL RADICAL NECK DISSECTION

Lesions that are in the midline of the oral cavity often spread bilaterally, and it is necessary to remove lymph nodes on both sides of the neck. Simultaneous bilateral neck dissections are feasible with an acceptable mortality; however, the postoperative course is likely to be prolonged, since there is a period of marked facial edema following this extensive resection which can persist for several weeks. Some operators will spare the jugular vein on one side when a bilateral neck dissection is done in order to decrease the amount of postoperative edema. Others stage the dissection, allowing a delay of several weeks before operating on the second side.

Parotidectomy

Most lesions in the superficial lobe of the parotid gland are removed by superficial parotidectomy. This operation is designed to give maximal safety in operating about the branches of the VIIth nerve (Fig. 16-43). The VIIth nerve pierces the parotid gland at its posterior margin and lies underneath the gland on the muscles of the face. A Y-shaped incision is made with the lower limb lying behind the angle of the mandible and the arms of the Y on either side of the lobe of the ear. Dissection is carried down to identify the main trunk of the VIIth nerve, which lies in the space between the mandible and the mastoid bone approximately one fingerbreadth below the external auditory meatus. Once the main trunk is identified, dissection is carried along the external surface of the nerve and its branches, gradually separating away the overlying portion of the parotid gland. Stensen's duct is identified at the most medial portion of the midpoint of the parotid gland and is ligated. This technique sometimes causes temporary weakness in the fibers of the VIIth nerve but prevents transecting any of the major trunks of the nerve. Recovery of function in all branches is ensured by the knowledge that they are intact and usually occurs within a week or two following completion of the operation.

V Excision of the Lip

Most cancers of the lower lip are removed with the use of V excision (see Chap. 51). Between one-fourth and one-third of the lower lip can be easily resected by simple excision without resulting in residual deformity or interference with function. While we refer to this excision as a V, a much better cosmetic result is obtained if the outline

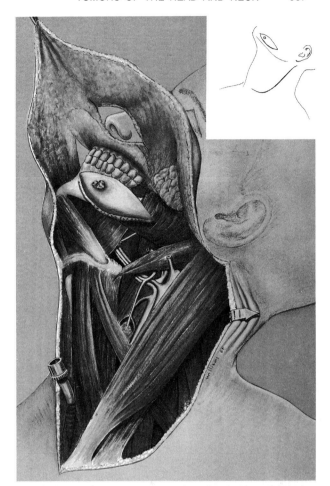

Fig. 16-40. Radical neck dissection through a hockey-stick incision (shown in insert) combined with an exposure of the mandible. The tumor has grown through the mandible and presented on the cheek so that a portion of the skin of the cheek has been left on the specimen. Structures of the neck are shown exposed and intact prior to the start of radical neck dissection. (*From B. F. Rush, Jr., Surg Gynecol Obstet, 121:353, 1965.*)

of the incision resembles that of a shield. A true V excision results in some flattening of the lower lip with a loss of normal eversion. If a shield-shaped incision is used, the lip will evert normally.

If the tumor involves more area than can be excised with a V excision, a flap is migrated from the upper lip. This involves outlining a V-shaped flap in the upper lip which is left attached at its lower medial corner and is then rotated into the defect in the lower lip. Using this type of closure excision of up to two-thirds of the lower lip can be accomplished without difficulty.

Maxillectomy

Cancer of the hard palate or the lower maxilla requires subtotal excision of the maxillary sinus. Cancer in the upper maxilla involving the orbital plate requires total excision of the maxillary sinus together with an exenteration of the orbital contents. While these excisions are

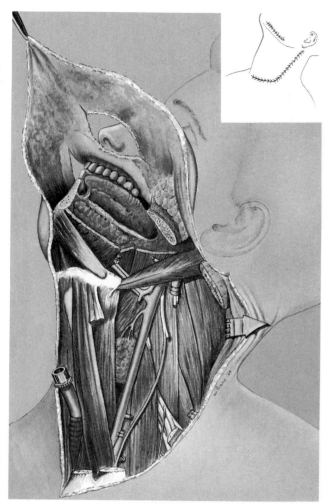

Fig. 16-41. Radical neck dissection completed, combined with excision of the horizontal ramus of the mandible. The jugular vein and sternocleidomastoid muscle have been removed. The phrenic nerve and the common carotid artery are seen coursing across the operative field. The closure of the neck incision is seen in the insert. (*From B. F. Rush, Jr., Surg Gynecol Obstet, 121:353, 1965.*)

basically mutilating, they can be accomplished with little visible external deformity. The Weber-Fergusson incision is used. This begins at the midpoint of the upper lip, extends to the columella of the nose, and is carried around the edge of the nose and up to the corner of the eye. A horizontal portion continues laterally from the inner canthus to a point just beyond the outer canthus and about 2 or 3 mm below the palpebral fissure. The skin and muscles of the cheek are undermined laterally, so that the entire cheek is turned outward, opening a door to the maxillary sinus. The bony attachments of the maxillary sinus are divided, including the midline of the hard palate, the zygoma, the pterygoid plates; if the orbital plate is to be removed, the bony walls of the medial and lateral orbit are also transected. When this is accomplished, the entire maxillary sinus can be lifted like a small box from its normal position. The inner surface of the Weber-Fergusson

flap is covered with a split-thickness skin graft, and the incision is closed. Because it falls in the normal skin lines and about the normal structures of the face, this incision is often difficult to detect after it has healed as long as the structures have been replaced precisely and in good apposition. This operation leaves a large defect in the hard palate on the side of the procedure. This is occasionally closed by subsequent operations, but more commonly a dental prosthesis with a large obturator which fits into the defect is constructed by the prosthodontist. This restores normal speech and relatively normal mastication for the patient.

Total Laryngectomy

Total laryngectomy is traditionally accomplished through a midline longitudinal incision. We have found definite advantages in accomplishing this procedure through a transverse incision in the lower neck very much like the typical thyroidectomy incision. The incision is made 4 cm above the clavicles and approximately 4 cm beyond the edge of the sternocleidomastoid muscles on either side; it is carried down through the platysma muscle, and the upper flap is then developed. The upper limit of dissection is approximately 1 cm above the hyoid, and at this point the entire group of strap muscles and the midportion of the hyoid are exposed. In cancer operations for glottic tumors of any size, all the anterior strap muscles are removed. Occasionally at the election of the operator in the presence of somewhat smaller lesions, the strap muscles on the side contralateral to the lesion may be preserved, or, rarely, the larynx is skeletonized with the preservation of strap muscles on both sides. In the ordinary instance, however, the sternothyroid and sternohyoid muscles are transected at the level of the cricoid, the digastric and mylohyoid muscles are separated from the hyoid above, and the body of the hyoid bone is cut at the junction of the attachments to the lateral wings on either side. The larynx is rocked laterally exposing the pharyngeal constrictors, which are cut at the lateral edge of the thyroid cartilages bilaterally. One can now enter the pharynx laterally, usually on the side opposite the tumor, so that proper visualization of the area can be obtained, and an adequate margin of excision of pharyngeal mucosa will be developed around the tumor. Once the pharynx is entered, it is possible for the surgeon to operate both outside and inside the pharynx. The remaining muscles of the tongue are severed from the hyoid, and the larynx is pulled forward. The vascular pedicles containing the laryngeal arteries and the superior laryngeal nerves are ligated bilaterally. An incision is made in the pharyngeal mucosa just posterior to the arytenoids, entirely circumscribing the point at which the larynx projects into the pharynx. As all pharyngeal mucosa is now separated from the larynx, the larynx is pulled forward, and a plane of dissection is developed between the larynx and the anterior esophageal wall. This dissection is carried inferiorly until the only remaining structure holding the larynx in place is the trachea. This is then divided obliquely around the site of the tracheostomy (if one has been done previous to the operation), or if an endotracheal tube has been used in anesthesia, this is now removed, and a tube is placed in the severed trachea so that anesthesia can be continued. After the larynx has been removed, the defect in the pharynx is closed transversely with an inverting Connell stitch. This is reinforced by interrupted sutures of 4-0 silk which are used to imbricate the constrictor muscles up and around the pharyngeal closure. This closure may further be reinforced by stitches which catch the platysma muscle and draw it down snugly along with the overlying skin. A generous circular portion of skin is removed in the lower midline; this measures about 3 to 4 cm in diameter with three-quarters of the circle lying above the transverse skin incision and one-quarter of the circle lying below. The beveled end of the trachea is then drawn up to the skin

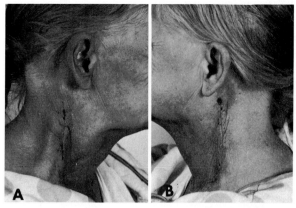

Fig. 16-42. Mandibular resection, 8 days after bilateral neck dissection and partial mandibulectomy on the left, with resection of a portion of the floor of the mouth and the anterior half of the tongue for carcinoma of the tongue. The portion of the jaw was replaced with a Steinmann pin. At 3 years postoperatively there still was no recurrence. Note that it is difficult to determine on which side the mandible was resected. (*From B. F. Rush, Jr., Curr Probl Surg, May, 1966.*)

Fig. 16-43. Superficial parotidectomy. *A.* Incision. *B.* Skin flaps established and fascia incised; greater auricular nerve transected and external jugular vein identified. *C.* External jugular vein transected; superficial lobe is being reflected anteriorly, and facial nerve with its mandibular and cervical branches are shown. *D.* Dissection continued anteriorly, demonstrating temporal, zygomatic, and buccal branches. *E.* Superficial lobe removed; if excision of the deep lobe is indicated, the facial nerve can be retracted craniad and the remaining parotid removed. *F.* Relationship of facial nerve and parotid gland. The nerve branches lie between the deep and superficial lobes of the parotid. (*Courtesy of Robert Chase, M.D.*)

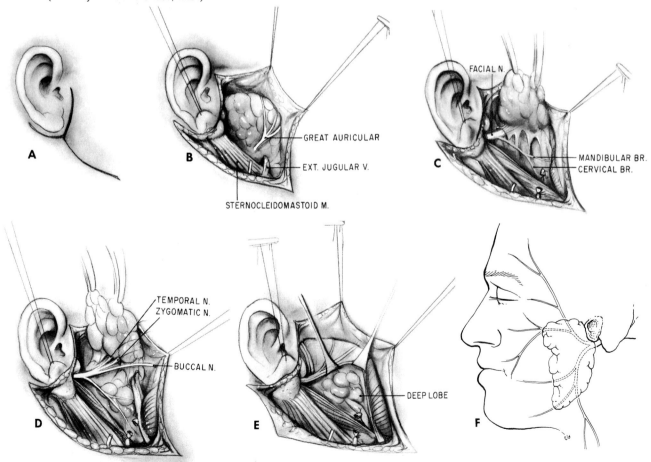

by interrupted sutures of nylon. Every attempt is made to obtain a delicate mucosa to skin closure, since the smaller the size of the scar at the junction between mucosa and skin, the less likely there is to be subsequent stenosis of the tracheal opening. The generous amount of skin excised tends to evert the trachea in a slightly "trumpet-like" manner, and this too ensures against subsequent stenosis. This type of trachea skin closure can be maintained without the use of an indwelling tracheostomy tube except for the first 24 hours or so postoperatively. The remainder of the wound is closed with interrupted sutures to the platysma muscle and skin. Two suction catheters are left in place on either side of the neck and are usually removed in 24 to 36 hours. The patient is maintained on postoperative feedings through a nasal tube made up of a #18 whistle-tip red rubber catheter inserted at the time of operation through the nose and into the esophagus before the pharyngeal defect is closed. This tube is sutured to the nasal columella. The patient is maintained on nasal tube feedings for about 10 days. A liquid diet is usually begun on the fifth or sixth day, and the patient may take solid food on the ninth or tenth day. The nasal tube is removed as soon as it is apparent that the patient can well maintain his own nutrition.

Partial Laryngectomy

In the past all lesions extending beyond the true cords have been treated by total laryngectomy. The functional importance of the voice and the great benefit of preserving it for the patient has led to an evaluation of cancer operations which do not remove the entire larynx. Ogura and Biller have led this effort and have proposed a number of new operations which involve removal of most or all of the larynx above the cords (supraglottic laryngectomy) or excision of most of one side of the larynx (hemilaryngectomy) for lesions which are confined enough in their growth to be suitable for this technique. This approach requires careful selection of patients who are young and flexible enough to overcome some of the swallowing and aspiration difficulties that often arise postoperatively. Since the resected margin around the tumor may be very limited, careful diagnostic techniques must be used to identify the outer margins. This technique is almost always combined with preoperative radiation therapy to ensure a lesser threat from residual cells at the periphery of the tumor which may be left by the surgeon. Using these techniques in patients with tumors advanced enough to cause fixation of the cord, Ogura and Biller have reported a 77 percent 3-year survival.

POSTOPERATIVE CARE FOLLOWING HEAD AND NECK OPERATIONS

Tracheostomy is performed at the time of operation in any patient in whom a portion of the mandible is removed or when there is extensive removal of oral structures. Postoperative edema plus the tendency for the larynx to shift position following sacrifice of many of its suspensory muscles predispose to aspiration and obstruction. Catastrophic anoxia may supervene rapidly, with little apparent warning. The tracheostomy tube must be aspirated frequently. This requires the presence of well-trained nursing personnel. If a patient appears to be accumulating unusual amounts of tracheal secretions, it is probable that saliva is being aspirated through an incompetent larynx. This can be controlled by diligent suctioning. In extreme instances, a cuffed tracheostomy may be required temporarily.

The patient with a tracheostomy has lost the usual humidifying effects of the nasal and pharyngeal passageways. The best way to provide humidity for the patient's trachea is to tie an umbilical tape about the neck above the tracheostomy and to hang a moistened 4 by 4 sponge over this tape very much in the manner that a towel is hung over a rail. The sponge must frequently be moistened, and after the first day or two the patient can be taught to moisten his own sponge and arrange it for himself.

There is no need to leave the tracheostomy in place for prolonged periods. As soon as the patient is found to be maintaining a dry, unobstructed airway and the skin flaps are sealed, the tracheostomy tube is covered with a piece of adhesive tape. This is done about 5 days postoperatively. If the patient tolerates the covering of the tracheostomy tube for 24 hours, it can be removed. This tube should always be removed in the morning, so that the patient can be observed during the daylight hours following removal.

Patients who have undergone combined resections have had extensive superficial operation, but the body cavities have been undisturbed, and the normal function of the gastrointestinal tract resumes almost immediately. A nasoesophageal tube consisting of a #16 French urethral catheter is left in place at the end of the operative procedure. The tip of the standard urethral catheter reaches to the lower third of the esophagus but does not traverse the esophagocardiac junction. Such tubes can be left in place for long periods without the risk of acid regurgitation and peptic esophagitis. The patient receives fluids intravenously on the day of operation, but on the first postoperative day nasal feedings of half-strength milk are given. On the second postoperative day a nasal formula consisting of a blenderized regular diet diluted with milk is begun. This is continued until the fifth or sixth postoperative day or until the patient shows evidence that he can tolerate an adequate diet by mouth.

Except for the different flora encountered, there is little difference in the principles of operating on the mouth and other areas in the gastrointestinal tract. This is a contaminated area, and numerous tissue planes are open to this contamination. All patients should be placed on appropriate antibiotics postoperatively. Ketcham et al. demonstrated in a controlled study the advantages of prophylactic antibiotics in these patients.

The mental stress in a patient undergoing an oral operation of any magnitude is considerable. He awakens unable to speak because of his tracheostomy. He is unable to control his saliva and finds that he is constantly aspirating small amounts of mucus. His neck and shoulder are completely numb and boardlike because of the section of all cervical sensory nerves on the side of the lesion, and while he has little or no sharp pain, he has a pounding and persistent headache due to the ligation of the jugular vein and concomitant rise of spinal fluid pressure. In a day or two he looks into the mirror and may not recognize the swollen, edematous, and possibly deformed face which stares back at him. It would be abnormal if he were not depressed under these circumstances. Support for the patient depends on good preoperative preparation. The patient must understand clearly what to expect in the postoperative period. Patients do not panic if they understand their problems and realize that most of their deficiencies are reversible as edema subsides and the tracheostomy tube is removed.

References

General

Advisory Committee to the Surgeon General on Smoking and Health, "Report on Smoking and Health," *Public Health Serv Publ,* 1103, 1964.

Arons, M. S., and Smith, R. R.: Distant Metastases and Local Recurrence in Head and Neck Cancer, *Ann Surg,* **154:**235, 1961.

Baker, H.: Oral Cancer: A Six Part Series, *CA,* pt. I: January–February, 1972; pt. II: March–April, 1972; pt. III: May–June, 1972; pt. IV: July–August, 1972; pt. V: September–October, 1972; pt. VI: January–February, 1973.

Conley, J. (ed.),: "Cancer of the Head and Neck," Butterworth Inc., Washington, 1967.

Gowen, G. F., and deSuto-Nagy, G.: The Incidence and Sites of Distant Metastases in Head and Neck Carcinoma, *Surg Gynecol Obstet,* **116:**603, 1963.

James, A. G.: "Cancer Prognosis Manual," American Cancer Society, Inc., New York, 1967.

Kark, W.: "A Synopsis of Cancer: Genesis and Biology," The Williams & Wilkins Company, Baltimore, 1966.

MacComb, W. S.: Treatment of Head and Neck Cancer, Janeway Lecture, 1960, *Am J Roentgenol Radium Ther Nucl Med,* **84:**589, 1960.

Moore, C.: Smoking and Cancer of the Mouth, Pharynx and Larynx, *JAMA,* **191:**107, 1965.

Rubin, P.: Current Concepts in Cancer: Cancer of the Head and Neck, *JAMA,* **221:**68, 1972. (First of a continuing series of articles.)

Rush, B. F., Jr., Chambers, R. G., and Ravitch, M. M.: Cancer of the Head and Neck in Children, *Surgery,* **53:**270, 1963.

———, Horie, N., and Klein, N. W.: Intra-arterial Infusion of the Head and Neck: Anatomical and Distributional Problems, *Am J Surg,* **110:**510, 1965.

——— and Trinkle, K.: The Management of Low-Grade, Neglected Neoplasms, *South Med J,* **60:**714, 1967.

Schottenfield, D.: Cancer of the Buccal Cavity and Pharynx: A Review of End Results of Primary Treatment in 2877 Cases 1949-1964, *Clin Bull Memorial Hosp,* **2:**51, 1972.

Taylor, G. W., and Nathanson, I. T.: "Lymph Node Metastases: Incidence and Surgical Treatment in Neoplastic Disease," Oxford University Press, London, 1942.

Willis, R. A.: "Pathology of Tumors," Butterworth & Co. (Publishers), Ltd., London, 1960.

Historical Background

Absolon, K. B., Rogers, W., and Aust, J. B.: Some Historical Developments of the Surgical Therapy of Tongue Cancer from the Seventeenth to the Nineteenth Century, *Am J Surg,* **104:**686, 1962.

Campbell, E., and Colton, J.: "The Surgery of Theodoric," Appleton-Century Crofts, Inc., New York, 1955.

Fletcher, G. H., and Jesse, R. H., Jr.: The Contribution of Supervoltage Roentgenotherapy to the Integration of Radiation and Surgery in Head and Neck Squamous Cell Carcinomas, *Cancer,* **15:**566, 1962.

Lip

Ashley, F. L., McConnell, D. V., Machida, R., Sterling, H. E., Galloway, D., and Grazer, F.: Carcinoma of the Lip: A Comparison of Five Year Results after Irradiation and Surgical Therapy, *Am J Surg,* **110:**549, 1965.

Blackerby, J. N., and Hamilton, J. E.: Carcinoma of the Lip, *Surgery,* **51:**591, 1962.

Ward, G. E.: Carcinoma of the Lips, *Md Med J,* **5:**23, 1956.

Oral Cavity

Fayos, J. V. and Lampe, I.: Treatment of Squamous Cell Carcinoma of the Oral Cavity, *Am J Surg,* **124:**493, 1972.

Helfrich, G. B., Nickels, M. E., El-Doomeiri, A., and DasGupta, T.: Management of Cancer of the Floor of the Mouth, *Am J Surg,* **124:**559, 1972.

Kraus, F. T., and Perez-Mesa, C.: Verrucous Carcinoma: Clinical and Pathologic Study of 105 Cases Involving Oral Cavity, Larynx, and Genitalia, *Cancer,* **19:**26, 1966.

Lash, H., Erich, J. B., and Dockerty, M. B.: Pathologic Study of 217 Cases of Epithelioma of the Tongue, *Am J Surg,* **102:**620, 1961.

Marchetta, F. C., Sako, K., and Murph, J. B.: The Periosteum of the Mandible and Intraoral Carcinoma, *Am J Surg,* **122:** 711, 1971.

Martin, H. E.: The History of Lingual Cancer, *Am J Surg,* **48:**703, 1940.

Niebel, H. H., and Chomet, B.: In Vivo Staining Test for Delineation of Oral Intraepithelial Neoplastic Change: Preliminary Report, *J Am Dent Assoc,* **68:**801, 1964.

O'Brien, P. H., and Catlin, D.: Cancer of the Cheek (Mucosa), *Cancer,* **18:**1392, 1965.

Rush, B. F., Jr.: Combined Procedures in the Treatment of Oral Carcinoma, *Curr Prob Surg,* May, 1966.

——— and Humphrey, L.: Primary Repair of Full Thickness Excision of the Cheek, *Am J Surg,* **114:**592, 1967.

Sandler, H. C.: Oral Cytology, *CA,* **16:**97, 1966.

Shedd, D. P., Hukill, P. B., Bahn, S., and Ferraro, R. H.: Further Appraisal of In Vivo Staining Properties of Oral Cancer, *Arch Surg,* **95:**16, 1967.

———, Von Essen, C. F., Bevin, A. G., and Greenberg, R. A.: Ten Year Survey of Oral Cancer in a General Hospital, *Am J Surg,* **114:**844, 1967.

Southwick, H. W., Slaughter, D. P., and Trevino, E. T.: Elective Neck Dissection for Intraoral Cancer, *Arch Surg,* **80:**905, 1960.

Stecker, R. H., Devine, K. D., and Harrison, E. G., Jr.: Verrucose "Snuff Dipper's" Carcinoma of the Oral Cavity: A Case of Self-induced Carcinogenesis, *JAMA,* **189:**144, 1964.

Thoma, K. H.: "Oral Surgery," The C. V. Mosby Company, St. Louis, 1963.

Yonemoto, R. H., Ching, P. T., Bryon, R. L., and Riihimaki, D. U.: The Composite Operation in Cancer of the Head and Neck (Commando Procedure), *Arch Surg,* **104**:809, 1972.

Oropharynx

Baker, R. R., and Weiner, S.: The Clinical Management of Tonsillar Carcinoma, *Surg Gynecol Obstet,* **121**:1035, 1965.

Barkley, H. T., Fletcher, G. H., Jesse, R. H., and Lindberg, R. D.: Management of Cervical Lymph Node Metastasis in Squamous Cell Carcinoma of the Tonsillar Fossa, Base of Tongue, Supraglottic Larynx and Hypopharynx, *Am J Surg,* **124**:464, 1972.

Keller, A. Z.: Cirrhosis of the Liver, Alcoholism and Heavy Smoking Associated with Cancer of the Mouth and Pharynx, *Cancer,* **20**:1015, 1967.

McIlrath, D. C., ReMine, W. H., Devine, K. D., and Dockerty, M. B.: Tumors of the Parapharyngeal Region, *Surg Gynecol Obstet,* **116**:88, 1963.

Perez, C. A., Ackerman, L. V., and Mill, W. B.: Malignant Tumors of the Tonsil: Analysis of Failures and Factors affecting Prognosis, *Am J Roentgenol, Radium Ther Nucl Med,* **114**:43, 1972.

Rush, B. F., Jr., Reynolds, G., and Greenlaw, R.: Integrated Irradiation and Operation in Treatment of Cancer of the Larynx and Hypopharynx: A Preliminary Report, *Am J Roentgenol Radium Ther Nucl Med,* **102**:129, 1968.

Larynx

Baker, R. R., and Cherry, J.: Carcinoma of the Larynx: Results of Therapy in 209 Cases, *Arch Surg,* **90**:449, 1965.

Carveth, S. W., Devine, K. D., and ReMine, W. H.: Laryngectomy with Radical Neck Dissection in Extensive Cancer of the Larynx, *Am J Surg,* **104**:705, 1962.

Clinical Staging System for Cancer of the Larynx, American Joint Committee on Cancer Staging and End Results Reporting, June, 1962.

Donegan, W. L.: An Early History of Total Laryngectomy, *Surgery,* **57**:902, 1965.

Flynn, M. B., Jesse, R. H., and Lindberg, R. D.: Surgery and Irradiation in the Treatment of Squamous Cell Cancer of the Supraglottic Larynx, *Am J Surg,* **124**:477, 1972.

Goldman, J. L., Cheren, R. V., Silverstone, S. M., and Zak, F. G.: Combined Irradiation and Surgery for Cancer of the Larynx and Laryngopharynx, in J. Conley (ed.), "Cancer of the Head and Neck," Butterworth Inc., Washington, 1967.

Holinger, P. H.: Cancer of the Larynx: Classification and Partial Laryngectomy, in J. Conley (ed.), "Cancer of the Head and Neck," Butterworth Inc., Washington, 1967.

Krause, L. G.: Clinical Review of Carcinoma of the Larynx: Experience of a Large Cancer Hospital, *Am J Surg,* **111**:206, 1966.

Norris, C. M.: Treatment of Cancer of the Larynx and the Hypopharynx, *Proc Natl Cancer Conf,* **5**:265, 1964.

Ogura, J. W., and Biller, H. F.: Preoperative Irradiation for Laryngeal and Laryngopharyngeal Cancer, *Laryngoscope,* **80**:802, 1970.

Ono, J., and Shigejo, S.: Endoscopic Microsurgery of the Larynx, *Ann Otol Rhinol Laryngol,* **80**:479, 1971.

Powell, R. W., Redd, B. L., and Wilkins, S. A., Jr.: An Evaluation of Treatment of Cancer of the Larynx, *Am J Surg,* **110**:635, 1965.

Shahrokh, D. K., Devine, K. D., and Harrison, E. G., Jr.: Statistical Evaluation of 115 Cases of Carcinoma of the Epiglottis (1943 to 1952), *Am J Surg,* **102**:781, 1961.

Smith, R. R., Caulk, R. M., Russell, W. O., and Jackson, C. L.: End Results in 600 Laryngeal Cancers Using the American Joint Committee's Proposed Method of Stage Classification and End Results Reporting, *Surg Gynecol Obstet,* **113**, 435, 1961.

Spalt, L., Greenlaw, R., and Rush, B. F., Jr.: Integrated Therapy for Carcinoma of the Larynx, in B. F. Rush, Jr. and R. H. Greenlaw (eds.), "Integrated Radiation and Operation in Cancer Therapy: A Symposium," Charles C Thomas, Publisher, Springfield, Ill., 1968.

Nasopharynx

Jesse, R. H.: Preoperative versus Postoperative Radiation in the Treatment of Squamous Carcinoma of the Paranasal Sinuses, *Am J Surg,* **110**:552, 1965.

Moench, H. C. and Phillips, T. L.: Carcinoma of the Nasopharynx: Review of 146 Patients with Emphasis on Radiation Dose and Time Factors, *Am J Surg,* **124**:515, 1971.

Thomas, J. E., and Waltz, A. G.: Neurological Manifestations of Nasopharyngeal Malignant Tumors, *JAMA,* **192**:103, 1965.

Nasal Cavity and Paranasal Sinuses

Kurohara, S. S., Ellis, F., Fitzgerald, J. P., Webster, J. H., Shedd, D. P., and Badib, A. O.: Role of Radiation Therapy and of Surgery in the Management of Localized Epidermoid Carcinoma of the Maxillary Sinus, *Am J Roentgenol Radium Ther Nucl Med,* **114**:35, 1972.

Rush, B. F., Jr., Knightly, J. J., and Jewell, W.: Transoral and Transverse Incision for Excision of the Maxillary Sinus, *J Surg Oncol,* **3**:53, 1971.

Tabah, E. J.: Cancer of the Paranasal Sinuses: A Study of the Results of Various Methods of Treatment in Fifty-four Patients, *Am J Surg,* **104**:741, 1962.

Mandible

Bernier, J. L.: "Tumors of the Odontogenic Apparatus and Jaws," Armed Forces Institute of Pathology, Washington, 1960.

Salivary Glands

Beahrs, O. H., Woolner, L. B., Caveth, S. W., and Devine, K. D.: Surgical Management of Parotid Lesions, *Arch Surg,* **80**:890, 1960.

Bhaskar, S. N., and Bernier, J. L.: Mikulicz's Disease, *Oral Surg,* **13**:1387, 1960.

Connell, H. C. and Evans, J. C.: Mucoepidermoid Carcinoma of the Salivary Glands, *Am J Surg,* **124**:519, 1972.

Foote, F. W., and Frazell, E. L.: "Tumors of the Major Salivary Glands," Armed Forces Institute of Pathology, Washington, 1954.

Grage, T. B., and Lober, P. H.: Benign Lymphoepithelial Lesion of the Salivary Glands, *Am J Surg,* **108**:495, 1964.

———, ———, and Shahon, D. B.: Benign Tumors of the Major Salivary Glands, *Surgery,* **50**:625, 1961.

Katsilambros, L.: Asymptomatic Enlargement of the Parotid Glands, *JAMA,* **178**:513, 1961.

Reynolds, C. T., McAuley, R. L., and Rogers, W. P., Jr.: Experience with Tumors of Minor Salivary Glands, *Am J Surg,* **111:**168, 1966.

Rosenfeld, L., Sessions, D. G., McSwain, B., and Graves, H., Jr.: Malignant Tumors of Salivary Gland Origin: 37-year Review of 184 Cases, *Ann Surg,* **163:**726, 1966.

Stewart, F. W., Foote, F. W., and Becker, W. F.: Mucoepidermoid Tumors of Salivary Glands, *Ann Surg,* **122:**820, 1945.

Stuteville, O. H., and Corley, R. D.: Surgical Management of Tumors of Intraoral Minor Salivary Glands: Report of Eighty Cases, *Cancer,* **20:**1578, 1967.

Winsten, J., and Ward, G. E.: The Parotid Gland: An Anatomic Study, *Surgery,* **40:**585, 1956.

Tumors of the Neck

Albers, G. D.: Branchial Anomalies, *JAMA,* **183:**399, 1963.

Hoffman, E.: Branchial Cysts within the Parotid Gland, *Ann Surg,* **152:**290, 1960.

Jesse, R. H., and Neff, L. E.: Metastatic Carcinoma in Cervical Nodes with an Unknown Primary Lesion, *Am J Surg,* **112:**547, 1966.

MacComb, W. S.: Diagnosis and Treatment of Metastatic Cervical Cancerous Nodes from an Unknown Primary Site, *Am J Surg,* **124:**441, 1972.

Marchetta, F. C., Murphy, W. T., and Kovaric, J. J.: Carcinoma of the Neck, *Am J Surg,* **106:**974, 1963.

Mooney, C. S., Jewell, W., Greenlaw, R., and Rush, B. F., Jr.: Simultaneous Bilateral Radical Neck Dissection following High Level Radiation Therapy, *J Surg Oncol,* **1:**335, 1969.

Rush, B. F., Jr.: Current Concepts in the Treatment of Carotid Body Tumors, *Surgery,* **52:**679, 1962.

————: Familial Bilateral Carotid Body Tumors, *Ann Surg,* **157:**633, 1963.

Skandalakis, J. E., Gray, S. W., Takakis, N. C., Godwin, J. T., and Poer, D. H.: Tumors of the Neck, *Surgery,* **48:**375, 1960.

Chemotherapy

Couture, J., and Deschenes, L.: Intra-arterial Infusion: An Adjuvant to the Treatment of Oral Carcinoma, *Cancer,* **29:**1632, 1972.

Donaldson, R. C.: Methotrexate plus Bacillus Calmette-Guerin and Isoniazid in the Treatment of Cancer of the Head and Neck, *Am J Surg,* **124:**527, 1972.

Freckman, H. A.: Results in 169 Patients with Cancer of the Head and Neck Treated by Intra-arterial Infusion Therapy, *Am J Surg,* **124:**501, 1972.

Ohnuma, T., Selawry, O. S., Holland, J. F., DeVita, V. T., Shedd, D. P., Hansen, H. H., and Muggia, F. M.: Clinical Study with Bleomycin: Tolerance to Twice Weekly Dosage, *Cancer,* **30:**914, 1972.

Williams, A. C.: Topical 5 FU: A New Approach to Skin Cancer, *Ann Surg,* **173:**864, 1971.

Operations of the Head and Neck

Frazell, E. L., and Moore, O. S.: Bilateral Radical Neck Dissection Performed in Stages: Experience with 467 Patients, *Am J Surg,* **102:**809, 1961.

Ketcham, A. S., Liebermann, J. E., and West, J. T.: Antibiotic Prophylaxis in Cancer Surgery and Its Value in Staphylococcal Carrier Patients, *Surg Gynecol Obstet,* **117:**1, 1963.

Lore, J. M.: "An Atlas of Head and Neck Surgery," W. B. Saunders Company, Philadelphia, 1962.

Madan, S. C., Rosenthal, S. P. and Bochetto, J. F.: Pneumomediastinum and Pneumothorax following Lower Neck Surgery, *Arch Surg,* **98:**153, 1969.

Martin, H., Del Valle, B., Ehrlich, H., and Cahan, W. G.: Neck Dissection, *Cancer,* **4:**441, 1951.

Moore, O. S., and Frazell, E. L.: Simultaneous Bilateral Neck Dissection: Experience with 151 Patients, *Am J Surg,* **107:**565, 1964.

Norris, C. M.: Composite Resections of Laryngeal and Supralaryngeal Cancer, in J. Conley (ed.), "Cancer of the Head and Neck," Butterworth Inc., Washington, 1967.

Royster, H. P., Noone, R. B., Graham, W. P., and Theogaraj, S. D.: Cervical Pharyngostomy for Feeding after Maxillofacial Surgery, *Am J Surg,* **116:**610, 1968.

Rush, B. F., Jr.: A Standard Technique for In-Continuity Incisions of the Head and Neck, *Surg Gynecol Obstet,* **121:**353, 1965.

Ward, G. E., Edgerton, M. T., Chambers, R. G., and McKee, D. M.: Cancer of the Oral Cavity and Pharynx and Results of Treatment by Means of the Composite Operation (in Continuity with Radical Neck Dissection), *Ann Surg,* **150:**202, 1959.

Wise, R. A., and Baker, H. W.: "Surgery of the Head and Neck," The Year Book Medical Publishers, Inc., Chicago, 1962.

Chapter 17

Chest Wall, Pleura, Lung, and Mediastinum

by **Herbert C. Maier and Seymour I. Schwartz**

Surgery of the Thorax
Anatomy
Pathophysiology
    Pulmonary Function
Clinical Manifestations of Pulmonary Disease
    Bronchoscopy
Anesthesia in Thoracic Surgery

Chest Wall
Congenital Defects
Pectus Excavatum
Pectus Carinatum
Hernias
Trauma
    Rib Fractures
Infection and Inflammation
    Infection of Costal Cartilages
    Osteomyelitis of the Sternum
    Abscesses
    Tietze's Syndrome
Tumors
    Chondroma
    Osteochondroma
    Fibrous Dysplasia
    Eosinophilic Granuloma
    Chondrosarcoma
    Osteogenic Sarcoma
    Ewing's Sarcoma
    Multiple Myeloma
    Solitary Bone Metastases
Radiation Necrosis

Pleura
Anatomy
Physiology
Transmediastinal Pleural Herniation
Spontaneous Pneumothorax
Pleural Effusion
Hemothorax
Empyema
    Acute Empyema
    Chronic Empyema
Tuberculosis
Chylothorax
Calcification

Tumors
    Primary Tumors
    Secondary Neoplasms

Diseases of the Lungs
Congenital Malformations
    Pulmonary Agenesis
    Hypoplasia of a Lung
    Vascular Anomalies of the Lungs
    Lobar Emphysema in Infancy
Cystic Disease of the Lung
    Congenital Cystic Disease
    Air Cysts
Trauma to Lung and Airways
    Foreign Bodies in the Airway
    Trauma to the Lung
    Traumatic Rupture of Bronchi or Trachea
Inflammation and Infection
    Bronchiectasis
    Lung Abscess
    Staphylococcal Pneumonia
    Lipoid Pneumonia
    Aspiration Pneumonia (Mendelson's Syndrome)
    Other Pneumonias
    Mucoviscidosis of Childhood and Mucoid Impaction
        of Bronchi in Adults
    Erosion of Lymph Node into Bronchus
    Tracheoesophageal and Bronchoesophageal Fistula
    Tuberculosis
    Mycotic Infections
    Hydatid Cysts of the Lung
    Boeck's Sarcoid
Solitary Pulmonary Nodule
Tumors of the Lung
    Benign Endobronchial Tumors
    Circumscribed Benign Tumors of the Interstitial Pulmonary Tissue
    Bronchial Carcinoid
    Adenoid Cystic Carcinoma (Cylindroma)
    Sarcomas of the Lung
    Carcinoma of the Lung
Diagnostic Operative Procedures
    Scalene Fat Pad Biopsy
    Mediastinoscopy and Biopsy
    Diagnostic Biopsy of the Lung

Pulmonary Resection
    Precautions during Operation
    Technique of Pulmonary Resection
    Postoperative Care
Trachea
    Tracheal Abnormalities of Infancy and Childhood
    Tracheal Lesions in Adults

Mediastinum

General Considerations
Mediastinitis
    Acute Mediastinitis
    Chronic Mediastinitis
Superior Vena Cava Obstruction
Mediastinal Lymphadenopathy
Lesions of the Thoracic Duct
Tumors of the Mediastinum
    General Considerations
    Superior Mediastinal Lesions
    Anterior Mediastinal Lesions
    Posterior Mediastinal Lesions
    Mediastinal Tumors without Specific Location
    Mediastinal Tumors in Infancy
    Tumors of the Costovertebral Region

SURGERY OF THE THORAX

Surgical therapy for diseases of the thoracic viscera had a very limited scope until the early part of the twentieth century. At a time when many major surgical procedures were already being undertaken for abdominal diseases, only occasional major operations were attempted for intrathoracic lesions. However, during the past half century tremendous strides have been made in the surgical therapy of all the intrathoracic organs. These advances became feasible in large measure because of the application of knowledge about the physiologic disturbances which opening the thorax entails. Developments in anesthesiology have permitted a satisfactory maintenance of the patient's respiratory and circulatory function while the surgeon performs the indicated procedures for the cure or palliation of a vast array of intrathoracic diseases. In order that surgery of the thorax may contribute its proper role in therapy, it is mandatory that the many ways in which the respiratory and circulatory function may be disturbed by intrathoracic disease are fully recognized. Then, when surgical intervention is undertaken, additional physiologic disturbances should be kept to a minimum, both during operation and in the postoperative period.

Anatomy

The anatomic structure of the thorax is designed to facilitate the ventilation of the lungs under a variety of circumstances and at the same time favor optimal conditions for the function of the cardiocirculatory system. The fact that there is normally a subatmospheric pressure in most portions of the thorax points to the importance of the thoracic wall and diaphragm in their respective roles in maintaining the pressure differential between the abdominal and thoracic portions of the trunk. The bony thoracic cage consists of the vertebral column, ribs, and sternum, which provide a firm, yet pliant, framework. This framework, together with the associated soft tissues, permits the coordinated motion necessary for pulmonary ventilation. The stability of the thoracic cage together with the elastic quality of the normal lung combine to create a negative intrathoracic pressure which is augmented by the normal respiratory excursions of the diaphragm. Not only is the rhythmic respiratory motion of the thoracic wall and diaphragm crucial to the ventilatory motion which provides gas exchange in the lungs, but also this fluctuating subatmospheric intrathoracic pressure facilitates the flow of blood in the veins within the chest and thus plays an important role in cardiocirculatory dynamics. Similarly, respiratory motion aids lymph flow.

The pleural serous cavities facilitate pulmonary mobility, which is so vital to adequate function of the lungs, and also play an important role in protecting the lung from serous fluid inundation in certain pathologic pulmonary states. Although a serous cavity is not an integral anatomic part of the lymphatic system, it may play a vital role in lymph homeostasis in the sick patient.

Since a stable chest wall is necessary for good ventilatory function and since opening into the pleural space may result in collapse of the lung due to loss of a negative intrathoracic pressure, it is apparent that when trauma impairs these anatomic necessities, serious physiologic disturbances may ensue.

The cartilaginous support of the trachea and bronchi maintains the patency of the air passages in the face of intrathoracic pressure fluctuations while, at the same time, the flexibility of the walls of the trachea and bronchi permits the mobility necessary for normal ventilatory motion.

The coordination which tends to occur between ventilatory motion and pulmonary blood flow results in remarkably little hypoxemia in the presence of many chronic localized pulmonary lesions. Moreover, the dual vascular system, i.e., pulmonary and bronchial arteries, which is present in the lungs results in some unusual physiologic and pathologic aspects which will be evident in the consideration of clinical conditions of the lungs and heart.

In man, in contrast to the dog, air or fluid in one pleural cavity does not traverse the mediastinal partition which separates the two pleural spaces, although anteriorly (retrosternally) and posteriorly (prevertebrally) the mediastinal reflections of the pleura of each side are in close proximity. Hence surgical access to the mediastinal structures without entry into either pleural cavity can be achieved only by approaches close to the midline. Similarly in the inferior portion of the thorax the pleural reflections extend downward into the costodiaphragmatic recesses, so that incisions or penetrations of the upper abdomen may result in entry into a pleural cavity (Fig. 17-1).

The mediastinum is that portion of the thoracic contents between the two pleural cavities. Although the heart and great vessels occupy most of the mediastinal space, a variety of other anatomic and pathologic structures, both congenital and acquired, may be found in this area. Hence a wide variety of tumors may occur in the mediastinum.

Some cervical and retroperitoneal fascial planes are continuous with those of the mediastinum, and thus air and fluid may dissect from one area into the other. Here again the negative pressure associated with inspiration can facilitate movement into the thorax.

Pulmonary and pleural disease may result in increases or decreases in the volume of either pleural space with resultant displacement of the mediastinal partition. When displacement of some magnitude occurs, especially if the change is rather sudden, impairment of the function of the mediastinal structures may ensue. The most compressible structures, i.e., veins and lymphatics, are most readily affected. Therefore cardiocirculatory disturbances are particularly frequent. The cartilaginous framework of the larger air passages lessens the vulnerability of the airway to compression, but in an infant a similar degree of pressure may be disastrous because of the greater compressibility of the trachea and bronchi in early life.

Clinical recognition of the segmental anatomy of the lungs with the pulmonary arterial branches accompanying the bronchi as they divide into smaller and smaller branches has permitted the development of segmental resection with resultant conservation of pulmonary tissue. Also in recent years there has been a fuller appreciation of the intimate functional interrelationship between the heart and the pulmonary vascular bed as well as the unique features of the dual circulation of the lungs. The vascular systems of the lungs obtained at surgical operations and at postmortem examination have been investigated by special techniques which fill the vascular systems with a colored plastic; after the plastic has hardened, the lung tissue is digested away, and the pattern of the vasculature is evident. Also angiograms, supplemented by pulmonary catheterization, have been of great value in clarifying anatomic and pathologic features of the pulmonary vasculature.

Pathophysiology

The respiratory function of the thorax is vital to the entire organism and is intimately coordinated with the circulation. The ventilatory component of respiration is concerned with the effective movement of air down the tracheobronchial tree to the alveoli, where the gaseous exchange with the blood in the alveolar capillaries occurs. Good respiratory function also requires an easy exit of the gases from the lungs during the expiratory phase of respiration. Thus normal ventilation of the lungs involves relatively effortless motion of the chest wall and diaphragm without undue resistance to gas flow through the air passages. It follows, therefore, that any pathologic condition which interferes with motion of the components of the thoracic cage or movement of the diaphragm will tend to reduce the ventilatory reserve. Also any narrowing of the trachea or bronchi will augment the resistance to the flow of gases and increase the effort necessary for respiration.

STABILITY OF CHEST WALL. Stability of the thoracic cage is one of the essential components of an adequate

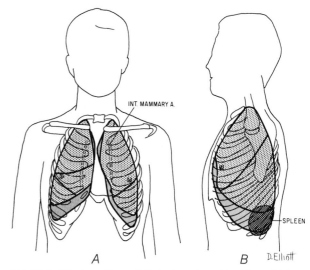

Fig. 17-1. Margins of lung (stippled area) and location of interlobar fissures. Shaded areas indicate outline of pleural spaces. Note depth of normal costophrenic sinus.

ventilatory mechanism. The ribs and sternum provide rigid struts which are moved in a coordinated manner by the intrinsic and accessory muscles of respiration. If any area of the chest wall is deprived of its bony stability, abnormal motion of that region of the thoracic cage will occur; this flail portion of the thoracic cage will sink in during inspiration because of the pressure differential between the outside and the inside of the thorax. Such paradoxic motion of the chest wall reduces the effective ventilation of the lungs and lessens the ventilatory reserve. When a large area of the rib cage is deprived of its stability, a crucial degree of ventilatory impairment may ensue. Hence either surgical or mechanical measures to improve chest wall stability are indicated, or temporary mechanical assistance of respiration is required.

DIAPHRAGM. The diaphragm also plays an important role in normal ventilation of the lungs. Impaired diaphragmatic mobility, as seen with fixation by a pleural inflammation, reduces the ventilatory reserve. Paralysis of a hemidiaphragm usually produces a paradoxic motion with respiration which results from the effect of the positive intraabdominal pressure exerted against the relaxed diaphragmatic musculature.

Normally there is a well-coordinated respiratory movement between the chest wall and diaphragm; augmented motion of one may compensate for reduced movement of the other. Therefore simultaneous impairment of mobility of chest wall and diaphragm as seen with extensive trauma or severe respiratory depression is particularly dangerous.

MOVEMENT OF AIR. The inspiratory phase of normal respiration is associated with the passage of sufficient air down the tracheobronchial tree to result in the mixing of inspired gas with the residual air which is present in the lungs. Normally the oxygen tension in the alveoli averages around 95 to 100 mg Hg. During expiration part of the carbon dioxide present in the alveoli is expelled from the lungs; normally the carbon dioxide tension in the alveoli is in the range of 35 to 45 mm Hg. Any increased resistance to the passage of the gases in and out of any segment or lobe of a lung due to bronchial obstruction usually results in a compensatory increase in ventilation of other portions of the lung. The full effect of bronchial obstruction on the degree of inflation of a pulmonary lobe will be determined by the degree of narrowing of the bronchial lumen in the inspiratory and expiratory phase of ventilation. If the bronchial narrowing is marked only during the expiratory phase (when the bronchial diameter is smaller than during inspiration), the involved lobe may become hyperinflated because of the trapping of gases. This is known as *obstructive emphysema* and may be either an acute or chronic process.

When the bronchial obstruction becomes essentially complete, either because of the obstructing lesion alone or because of an obstruction plus retained bronchial secretions, the portion of lung distal to the obstructed bronchus gradually becomes airless and is usually described as being *atelectatic.* The rapidity with which a lobe becomes atelectatic following complete bronchial occlusion depends on the nature of the trapped gases; oxygen is absorbed into the blood much more rapidly than nitrogen, and hence an unusually high oxygen content in the alveoli favors the more rapid development of atelectasis should bronchial obstruction occur. When a small segmental bronchus is occluded, airlessness of the distal segment of lung may not necessarily occur in the absence of inflammation or congestion because of the collateral ventilation which may occur from adjacent pulmonary segments through the pores of Kohn.

CIRCULATION. Decreased ventilation of a part or the whole of one lung soon leads to a reduced blood flow through the corresponding pulmonary artery and thus reduces or largely eliminates the arterial oxygen unsaturation which would otherwise readily occur. Because the time factor is important in the development of such vascular shunting, sudden occlusion of the main bronchus to one lung results in considerable unsaturation of the arterial blood, whereas chronic obstruction to a main bronchus may cause only a slight decrease in the arterial oxygen tension. The remarkable correlation between ventilation and circulation which is a constant occurrence in various physiologic and pathologic states of the lung provides a high degree of protection of the entire body against hypoxia. Chemical, neurovascular, and mechanical stimuli can all play a role in this important adaptive mechanism.

The dual blood supply of the lungs presents unique features. Normally the pulmonary arterial pressure is only a fraction of the bronchial arterial pressure. Although under normal conditions the pulmonary and bronchial arterial systems in the lungs are quite separate down to the arteriolar level, in pathologic states marked intercommunications between the two vascular systems may develop, especially in pathologic conditions of long standing. The marked circulatory alteration which can occur in long-standing pulmonary fibrosis and atelectasis is illustrated by the fact that occasionally in such chronic cases the blood flow in the pulmonary artery of the diseased lung is so reduced and the blood flow in the bronchial system so augmented as to result in a retrograde flow of blood in the main pulmonary artery of the involved lung. Since normally the pressure in the pulmonary artery is about a sixth of the systemic arterial pressure, sudden massive hemoptysis is more likely to result from erosion of a bronchial rather than a pulmonary artery. Likewise massive hemothorax in cases of penetrating thoracic trauma is more likely to result from injury to vessels in the chest wall than from pulmonary bleeding, in the absence of injury to the heart or great vessels.

Ventilation/Perfusion ($\dot{V}_A/\dot{Q}$)

In the normal upright lung a pattern of ventilation/perfusion inequality has been defined. The weight of the column of blood in the upright lung increases the perfusing pressure and blood flow at the base. The weight of the lung itself, by increasing pleural pressure, increases ventilation in the base but to a lesser extent than the increase in blood flow. Therefore, the ventilation/perfusion ratio decreases down the lung (Fig. 17-2).

This concept is important in managing a variety of postoperative and traumatized patients, but it is particularly meaningful following thoracic surgery. When the patient is in the lateral position, the dependent lung is in zone 3; i.e., venous pressure exceeds alveolar pressure. In the supine position the posterior portions of both lungs are in zone 3, while the head-down (Trendelenburg) position places most of both lungs in zone 3. By decreasing perfusion hypotension causes an increase in physiologic dead space, impairing carbon dioxide removal. Left ventricular failure with pulmonary edema leads to collapse of alveoli, which continue to be perfused with resultant increased hypoxemia. (See Chap. 12)

LYMPH FLOW. The lymphatic system of the lungs plays a vital role in maintaining homeostasis in the lungs. Lymphatic channels accompany the bronchi and pulmonary arteries. Lymphatic vessels are also found in the intersegmental septa accompanying the pulmonary veins and in the visceral, parietal, and diaphragmatic pleura. The various lymphatic networks drain into regional lymph nodes along the larger bronchi at the pulmonary hilus and into the mediastinum. The major portion of the lymph flow from the lungs usually drains cephalad via the right lymphatic duct, whereas the thoracic duct is the main channel for the passage of lymph and chyle from the infradiaphragmatic portions of the body. The lymphatics are the main channels by which fluid transudated from the vascular compartment is returned to the vascular system. Hence the lymphatics play a crucial role in keeping the aveoli free of excess fluid and avoiding edema of the lungs.

Since the lymphatic system has no intrinsic pumping mechanism, movement of lymph along lymphatic channels is largely promoted by the contraction and movement of adjacent structures. Although the thoracic duct has a muscular wall which is capable of contraction, most lymphatic vessels, including the right thoracic duct, which is the chief drainage route for lymph from the lungs, have a rather sparse musculature. The fluctuation in intrathoracic pres-

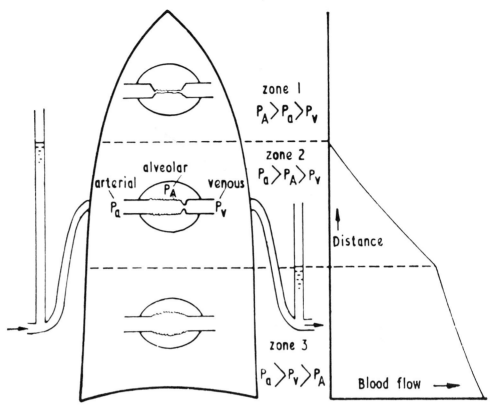

zone 1

$P_A > P_a > P_v$

zone 2

$P_a > P_A > P_v$

alveolar

arterial   venous

P_a P_A P_v

Distance

zone 3

$P_a > P_v > P_A$

Blood flow

Fig. 17-2. Scheme which accounts for the distribution of blood flow in the isolated lung. In zone 1, alveolar pressure exceeds arterial pressure, and no flow occurs, presumably because collapsible vessels are directly exposed to alveolar pressure. In zone 2, arterial pressure exceeds alveolar pressure, but alveolar exceeds venous pressure. Here the vessels behave like Starling resistors, and flow is determined by the arterioalveolar pressure difference, which steadily increases down the zone. In zone 3, venous pressure now exceeds alveolar pressure, and flow is determined by the arteriovenous pressure difference, which is constant down the lung. However, the pressure across the walls of the vessels increases down the zone, so that their caliber increases and so does flow. (*From J. B. West, "Ventilation/Blood Flow and Gas Exchange," 2d ed., Blackwell Scientific Publications, Ltd., Oxford, 1970.*)

sure associated with respiration appears to be an important factor in lymph transport from the lungs. Valves in the lymph vessels determine the direction of flow. Gravity may play a significant role in lymph distribution if a patient is kept in one position a long time without postural change. Similarly stasis tends to occur in the small pulmonary veins, and venous hypertension results in an increase in lymph formation. Hence the lung with impaired motion is prone to congestive complications.

Most lymph is returned to the vascular compartment by the lymphovenous communications near the base of the neck, the thoracic duct emptying into veins on the left side, and the right thoracic duct draining most of the thoracic lymph back into the venous compartment on the right side. Under abnormal conditions other lymphovenous channels which may be present but largely nonfunctioning may be-

come apparent. The negative phase of respiration which aids the filling of the large veins also facilitates the flow of lymph back into these veins. If the venous pressure is elevated, lymph flow is impaired.

PULMONARY FUNCTION

Although it is vital for the surgeon to have a good appreciation of the status of the respiratory function of the patient with thoracic disease, in most cases no detailed laboratory investigations of lung function are necessary for the care of the patient with localized pulmonary disease.

CLINICAL CORRELATION. Since one's response to daily activity can be a valuable gauge of respiratory function, a good clinical history is an essential screening method for determining whether a specific patient requires detailed study of lung function before the safety of the contemplated surgical procedure can be assessed. Is the patient aware of any shortness of breath? If so, is this a recent or long-standing symptom? Is the dyspnea rather constant, or does it appear to be related to allergic episodes? Is the shortness of breath related to chest wall pain which affects ventilatory motion? Are there any features of the clinical history that point to cardiocirculatory factors as the cause of the dyspnea?

The object of the various questions is to determine whether any shortness of breath, if present, appears to be caused by the pulmonary lesion to be treated surgically or whether the impaired lung function is in large measure due to a diffuse pulmonary condition such as emphysema or pulmonary circulatory factors. Also, if shortness of breath is present but caused by a pathologic condition which can be corrected by surgical intervention and the operative procedure should be expected to improve the respiratory function, the situation is very different from that in which a patient with dyspnea due to widespread pulmonary emphysema is being considered for a pneumonectomy with resultant further loss of lung tissue.

Pulmonary Function Tests

The development of various tests of cardiorespiratory function have added greatly to the understanding of the pathophysiology of lung disease and the effects of surgical procedures on the lungs and thoracic wall. However, the best use of such tests can be made only by the clinician who appreciates their limitations as well as their value. Such tests must not be regarded as a substitute for the detailed information on respiratory function which a good history and physical examination can supply, even though, at times, they may uncover some facet of lung dysfunction that was not suspected clinically.

VENTILATION. Vital capacity (VC) determinations alone are of limited value, as the vital capacity may be quite normal in a patient with obstructive emphysema who can move the gases in and out, though only slowly. By definition, vital capacity is the amount of gas which is expelled following a maximal expiration after a maximal inspiration. The timed vital capacity (TCV) provides more information, since it measures the speed with which ventilation can be effectively performed. Normally, 80 percent of the vital capacity is complete in the first second and almost 95 percent in the second second. An emphysematous patient with a normal vital capacity may complete only 40 percent in the first second and 60 percent in the second. The maximum breathing capacity (MBC) evaluates the activity of the muscles of respiration, the status of the airway, and the pulmonary parenchyma. It provides the best correlation with the degree of dyspnea, but it is a tiring test and requires patient cooperation. Spirometric tracings of the ventilatory effort may demonstrate a prolonged expiratory rate indicating obstructed air flow; whether this is due to bronchospasm can be shown by repeating the tracing after the patient has been given bronchspasmolytic medication. Determinations of the volume of residual air (RA) give information about the ability of the lungs to deflate, and lungs which do not deflate readily represent impaired ventilatory organs.

GAS EXCHANGE. Since ventilation is only one component of respiration, determinations of the gas exchange between the alveoli and blood in the pulmonary capillaries must be undertaken for any complete evaluation of respiratory function. Analysis of gases collected at the end of expiration gives information about the percentage of oxygen in the alveoli; this can be determined while the subject breathes room air and again when he breathes 100 percent oxygen. Also, the determination of the oxygen tension and cabon dioxide tension in arterial blood gives important information about the interchange of these gases between the alveoli and the blood. *Alveolar capillary block* is the pathologic state in which there is impairment in the passage of gases between alveoli and blood. Since carbon dioxide has an absorption coefficient about twenty-one times that of oxygen, the alveolar carbon dioxide tension is nearly equal to that of arterial blood, and there is no appreciable alveolar arterial gradient. In contrast, oxygen with a much lower absorption coefficient has an alveolar oxygen pressure which is 8 to 9 mm Hg higher than the partial pressure of arterial blood.

NEUROGENIC FACTORS. The nerve supply of the lung may play an important role in the contraction of the bronchial walls. A combination of neuromuscular and chemical factors enters into the dynamics of the tracheobronchial tree, and these factors may be influenced in various ways by pharmacologic agents. Similarly, contraction of the walls of the pulmonary blood vessels may be affected by neuromuscular mechanisms and hence alters the pulmonary blood flow either regionally or in general. Thus, neurogenic factors must be given recognition in assessing pulmonary function.

BRONCHOSPIROMETRY. By the use of double-lumen rubber catheters, the role played by each lung in ventilation and gas exchange may be established. Normally, 50 to 60 percent of the total ventilation as well as oxygen uptake and vital capacity is provided by the right lung. The procedure is particularly useful in patients with advanced bilateral cavitary tuberculosis and bilateral emphysema to determine the relative safety of pulmonary resection.

Clinical Manifestations of Pulmonary Disease

COUGH. Cough is an important sign of bronchial irritation and may be the first symptom of significant pulmonary disease. A history of cough is often ignored because of its common occurrence in smokers and in a host of pulmonary and other conditions of widely varying importance. A cough may be dry or productive. A productive cough may result from an abnormal amount of secretion of the bronchial glands as a result of bronchial irritation in the absence of any enlargement of the bronchi. A large amount of suptum of long duration suggests the possibility of bronchiectasis or pulmonary cavitation as the source of the expectoration. Also fistulous communications between the lungs and other organs such as the esophagus must be considered in special situations.

Since the cough reflex is not as readily elicited by stimulation of the smaller distal bronchi, absence of cough does not by any means eliminate the possibility of even a large lesion in the more peripheral parts of the lung.

WHEEZE. A wheeze should be regarded as a sign of disease of the respiratory tract. Since a diffuse wheeze is such a common occurrence among the many patients with allergic conditions of the lungs, a localized wheeze, which may have a different significance, is often ignored. Any localized wheeze not explained on the basis of tenacious secretion from bronchitis deserves investigation, as this sign points to localized bronchial narrowing. The likely cause of such a wheeze will vary widely but is influenced considerably by the age of the patient. In infancy and childhood, congenital lesions compressing the trachea or bronchi and aspirated foreign bodies must be especially considered. In later life, inflammatory strictures of the bronchus and tumors are important etiologic factors. In the older patient, bronchial carcinoma is a foremost consideration. Since a well-localized wheeze is usually caused by an abnormality in a bronchus of fair size, bronchoscopic examination is almost always indicated to clarify the diagnosis.

DYSPNEA. Dyspnea is a symptom which deserves great consideration in both the diagnosis and management of the patient with thoracic disease. A patient's complaint of dyspnea requires a careful evaluation of the cardiorespiratory function, because it usually indicates a potentially serious degree of disturbance which might be significantly aggravated by a major thoracic operation. Since the function of an entire lung can be gradually lost without the development of dyspnea, the presence of shortness of breath suggests the likelihood of a widespread impairment of respiratory function due to a pulmonary or cardiocirculatory pathologic condition, or a combination of both. Dyspnea may be due to decreased functional pulmonary volume, decreased alveolar ventilation, decreased diffusion of oxygen and carbon dioxide, or circulatory insufficiency. A detailed history of the time of onset, progression, and severity of the dyspnea aids in determining whether the shortness of breath is chiefly due to a chronic pulmonary emphysema or a diffuse congestion of the lungs from cardiocirculatory disease on one hand or can be explained entirely by a more localized respiratory lesion amenable to surgical correction.

CYANOSIS. Cyanosis often has a grave significance if it is caused by diffuse pulmonary disease, whereas certain patients with congenital pulmonary vascular anomalies or congenital heart disease may be cyanotic and yet not be in any obvious respiratory distress. Cyanosis caused by a right-to-left shunt may be of considerable magnitude and yet far less dangerous than a similar degree of arterial oxygen unsaturation produced by pulmonary disease which interferes with the transport of oxygen to the pulmonary capillaries. The degree of respiratory effort which the patient manifests gives some indication of the degree of tissue hypoxia provided that anoxia or hypercapnia have not damaged the respiratory drive. Cyanosis requires 5 Gm or more of reduced hemoglobin. In addition to the circulatory disorders, it may be related to polycythemia or pulmonary disease. Acute pneumonia is occasionally accompanied by cyanosis, as are chronic emphysema and fibrosis, in which instance clubbing of the fingers is occasionally noted.

PAIN. Since the lung contains no nerve fibers which carry pain impulses, extensive pulmonary disease which does not involve the pleura may be present in the absence of any pain. Inflammatory disease of the lung which is associated with pain indicates a pleural component to the pathologic process; the pleurisy may be either dry or associated with an effusion of varying amount. When a dry pleurisy progresses to a pleural effusion, the pain may lessen or disappear although the pleural inflammation is worsening. Hence, the evolution of the pain must be properly evaluated. A pleuritic pain due to infection is often aggravated

by deep respirations and varies considerably from time to time. Pain caused by infiltration of the chest wall by a malignant tumor such as carcinoma of the lung is often a rather constant pain and may antedate roentgenographic evidence of bone destruction by a considerable period. Osteomyelitis of a rib or suppurative chondritis may also be the cause of severe chest wall pain.

SPUTUM. From any patient who gives a history of raising sputum, this expectoration should be collected in a container for inspection by the clinician in addition to being sent to the laboratory for appropriate examinations. It should be noted whether the sputum is mucoid, blood-streaked, or purulent. A purulent sputum with foul odor points to a suppurative process. Hemoptysis may be associated with forceful coughing, bacterial pneumonia (particularly pneumococcal and *Klebsiellia*), and pulmonary infarction. Hemoptysis occurs in about 50 percent of patients with bronchiectasis. Small hemorrhages occur in the exudative stage of tuberculosis, and larger-vessel erosion may cause massive bleeding. Adenomas usually cause hemoptysis which may be profuse, while hemoptysis to some degree is present in about 30 percent of patients with bronchogenic carcinoma. Mitral stenosis is one of the most frequent cardiac causes.

BRONCHOSCOPY

The bronchoscope is an important instrument in both the diagnosis and therapy of thoracic disease. The bronchoscopic examination must be done by one familiar with the clinical, roentgenographic, and pathologic aspects of thoracic diseases if the maximal value is to be attained from this diagnostic measure. Similar knowledge should be possessed by those performing a therapeutic bronchoscopy in order to obtain the greatest benefit with the least disturbance to the patient. There are few procedures in which the skilled operator can be a greater boon to the patient if the procedure is required in a critically ill patient.

Although many prefer to employ general anesthesia for diagnostic bronchoscopy, the authors of this chapter are convinced that in adults topical anesthesia is usually the preferable method provided the operator is skilled in its use and does the bronchoscopy with gentleness. The patient who is scheduled for an operation within a day or so is less likely to have postoperative bronchial secretion problems if the tracheobronchial tree has not been irritated by unnecessary intrabronchial instrumental manipulation; therefore the extent of the bronchoscopic examination should be tailored to the individual case. When a bronchoscopy is performed for the removal of excessive bronchial secretions which could not be adequately removed by tracheal suction with a catheter, it is essential that the cough reflex not be obtunded by intratracheal topical anesthesia; otherwise an early reaccumulation of bronchial sections is likely.

A diagnostic bronchoscopy can give both direct and indirect evidence concerning the pulmonary and mediastinal pathologic condition. The larynx is also inspected in the course of the procedure. At bronchoscopy the character of the tracheal and bronchial mucosa is noted, and the sites of any inflammation, ulceration, or bleeding are recorded. Stenotic areas and tumors may be biopsied in order to establish a pathologic diagnosis. In cases of pulmonary carcinoma distortion of bronchi by extrinsic masses may be found together with a loss of bronchial mobility which point to probable mediastinal metastases. Secretions are removed for culture and cytologic study. Sputum is also studied the day following bronchoscopy, since higher yields of positive Papanicolaou smears have been reported.

Although a bronchoscopic examination may aid in determining the site of bleeding, it must be appreciated that blood seen coming from a lobar orifice does not necessarily indicate that the bleeding focus is in that lobe; the blood may have gravitated and even pooled in a portion of the bronchial tree other than the original site of bleeding.

When bronchoscopy is performed correctly and gently, there are few major complications. However, hemorrhage, perforation, bronchial spasm, and edema have all been reported. Bronchoscopy may represent definitive therapy for a foreign body within the major bronchi and the clearing of secretions which have resulted in atelectasis.

Anesthesia in Thoracic Surgery

In few fields of surgery is the skilled anesthesiologist a more important member of the team than in thoracic and cardiovascular surgery. When operating upon a patient with impaired pulmonary or cardiac function, it is essential that physiologic and pathologic derangements associated with the unconscious state be largely avoided by adequate ventilation and minimizing the cardiocirculatory disturbances which anesthetic agents may evoke. Whereas an adequate airway is vital to all patients, the margin of safety is reduced when a pathologic process has already narrowed the trachea or a main bronchus, or when a significant reduction in pulmonary function results from emphysema and some other pulmonary condition. The detrimental effects of a poor airway are often insidious; too often the presence of inadequate ventilatory exchange is not recognized until secondary metabolic and circulatory disturbances have occurred. Changes in blood pressure, alterations seen on the electrocardiogram, and changes in lung compliance will indicate to the alert physician that all is not well; it then behooves both anesthesiologist and surgeon to seek the causes of such changes and take immediate remedial action. Hypoxia or acidosis, or often both, precede the occurrence of cardiac arrest.

The circulatory support which infusion of fluids and plasma or blood can give a patient during a major operation is well established. But greater attention should be given to the volume of fluid which is most desirable for each individual patient. At present the volume of intravenous fluid given the patient undergoing pulmonary resection is frequently greater than desirable. Postoperative pulmonary complications are increased when unphysiologic amounts of intravenous fluids are administered.

Since the maintenance of a good airway is mandatory for an optimal physiologic state, it should be obvious that special precautions are necessary when operations are undertaken in a patient with tracheal obstruction. In an adult with tracheal stenosis it may be safest to insert the intratracheal tube past the obstruction under topical anesthesia, because the patient's respiratory obstruction may become rapidly worse under general anesthesia if an adequate airway is not quickly established. The endotracheal tube provides an adequate airway and prevents drowning by allowing rapid removal of purulent sections or blood. Endobronchial anesthesia may be performed by introducing a long, cuffed endotracheal catheter into one of the major bronchi. It is used when suppuration is present in one lung to isolate that lung from the other. It is particularly applicable for total pneumonectomy of a completely diseased lung or when significant hemoptysis is anticipated from the side to be resected.

CHEST WALL

Congenital Defects

Congenital defects of the thoracic wall may consist of abnormalities of the soft tissues or bony structures or a combination of both. Some extensive maldevelopments are associated with visceral defects which are incompatible with life.

RIB ANOMALIES. Rib anomalies vary from those that are of no clinical significance to extensive areas of deficient ribs, often associated with hemivertebrae, which lead to severe spinal curvature and impaired respiratory function (Fig. 17-3). Sometimes the rib deficiencies are associated with absence of soft tissue parts such as the pectoral muscles.

Congenital anomalies of the first rib or the presence of a cervical rib may result in compression of roots of the brachial plexus or of the subclavian artery with resultant pain or circulatory symptoms in the arm. Such symptoms as may develop usually become manifest in adult life. Unilateral or bilateral abnormalities may be found. Division of the scalene muscle often relieves the symptoms, but more frequently resection of the cervical rib is indicated (see Chap. 21).

STERNUM ANOMALIES. The sternum is normally formed by the fusion of two sternal bars. Varying degrees of incomplete sternal fusion result in a cleft sternum. Such a bifid sternum may be partial or complete. If not associated with true ectopia cordis such a cleft sternum can be corrected by a surgical procedure which brings the two halves of the sternum together. The operation is preferably performed in the neonatal period, especially if a complete sternal separation is present.

Ectopia cordis of varying degree may be associated with midline defects in the chest wall. Complete ectopia cordis is always associated with serious cardiac disease, and successful correction of complete ectopia cordis is a surgical rarity.

Pectus Excavatum

Pectus excavatum, also known as *funnel chest,* is a developmental deformity of the chest wall with varying degrees of depression of the sternum and curving inward of the medial portions of the adjacent costal cartilages. The deformity may be evident at birth and gradually become more marked as the child becomes older (Fig. 17-4). Children with this deformity usually have a small anteroposterior diameter of the entire chest cage and may have a tendency to kyphoscoliosis. A familial tendency toward the condition is often noted. The lower end of the sternum shows the most marked depression, and the level at which the sternal depression becomes evident varies widely. Also the associated extent and degree of costal cartilage depression may vary, and at times the deformity is asymmetric. In infants an inspiratory retraction of the lower sternum may be evident, and the role of the diaphragm in the maldevelopment is disputed. That portion of the diaphragm to which the inferior aspect of the pericardium is normally attached is in the retrosternal area, which is abnormally short in children with pectus excavatum; therefore the heart is displaced toward the left side. Even after satisfactory surgical elevation of the depressed sternum and costal cartilages, the cardiac displacement usually remains.

Many individuals with even marked degrees of pectus excavatum are free of definite symptoms, although some may tire easily or have some reduction in breathing capacity. A systolic murmur is often present. Normal hemodynamic responses are noted at rest and with supine exercise, but the cardiac output may be low during intense upright exercise. Psychologic problems are the outstanding reason for considering surgical intervention. Boys in particular are shy about being seen with the chest depression.

TREATMENT. Although surgical procedures to correct this deformity have been undertaken for several decades, the best method of treatment is still in dispute, because a high rate of recurrence of the depression has been noted many years after the operative procedure. The fundamental factors favoring recurrence have not been well clarified.

Operation is rarely recommended for patients under one

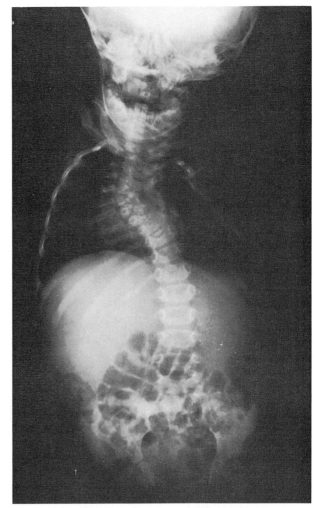

Fig. 17-3. Congenital absence of ribs and hemivertebrae. This resulted in chest deformity and impaired pulmonary function. Patient was treated by spine fusion.

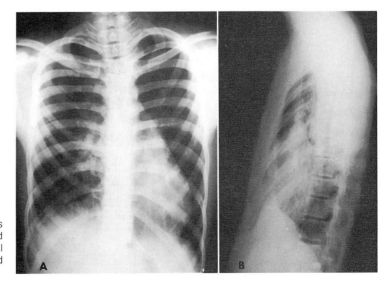

Fig. 17-4. Roentgenogram of young man with pectus excavatum. *A.* Note displacement of heart to left and abnormal slant of anterior portion of rib. *B.* Lateral x-ray demonstrates depressed stemum and narrowed chest cage.

year of age. The surgical procedures consist essentially of division and subperichondrial resection of the depressed cartilages together with transsection of the sternum at the level at which the depression begins. A wedge osteotomy of the sternum is performed at that level, so that the lower depressed portion of the sternum can be rotated upward. Struts to aid in holding the sternum in the elevated position are advocated by many surgeons. Excellent or acceptable results are achieved in over 80 percent of cases, and the operative morbidity is very low.

Pectus Carinatum

Pectus carinatum, or pigeon breast, is a rare deformity with a keellike protrusion of the sternum due to disproportionate rib growth or abnormal diaphragmatic pull. In some cases it is associated with congenital neuromuscular lesions or Marfan's syndrome. Surgical correction is occasionally warranted. Operative approaches generally consist of resection of the involved costal cartilages and the placement of sutures in the perichondrium to shorten them. Some have advised subperiosteal resection of the entire sternum from the second sternal segment downward, followed by suture of the pectoralis major muscles across the midline.

Hernias

A defect of the chest wall which permits herniation usually results in protrusion of a portion of lung, or pneumatocele, through the defect on straining or coughing. Congenital absence of ribs, extensive trauma to the chest wall, and surgical excision of a plaque of the chest wall may result in a lung hernia. Herniation due to disruption of a thoracotomy incision is rare if sutures of adequate strength are employed in closing the thoracotomy wound. Symptomatic hernias of the chest wall of small size may be repaired by mobilization of rib struts or segments of periosteum to buttress the defect. The paradoxic motion of large defects of the bony chest wall may be lessened by suturing a nonreactive plastic mesh or fascia lata into

Fig. 17-5. Paradoxic motion of chest wall, indicating mechanism by which a flail segment of chest wall disturbs thoracic ventilatory function. *A.* Inspiration. *B.* Expiration.

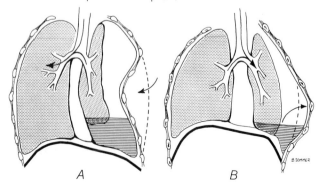

the defect. Full-thickness defects of the chest wall are best managed by the use of pedicle flaps.

Trauma

The management of thoracic injury is assuming a place of ever-increasing proportion as man seeks to go farther faster and also continues his engagement in warfare of many types and with a multitude of weapons. Moreover, the availability of many emergency measures now enable the seriously injured to survive the first few hours after sustaining major trauma; thus the physician and surgeon are afforded the opportunity to rehabilitate a large percentage of the injured. Since resuscitation is of major importance in the care of the severely injured, the management of the thoracic trauma together with the control of hemorrhage and treatment of shock merits top priority. The establishment of an adequate airway is the first consideration.

Since injuries to the chest commonly cause pulmonary and pleural complications and may cause trauma to structures in the mediastinum, the effects of injury of the chest wall are considered together with the injuries of the thoracic viscera later in this chapter. In many instances, the extent of damage to the thoracic cage may be a poor index of the severity of the injuries sustained by the intrathoracic organs. This is particularly true in the child with a compressible chest cage who may even be run over by a vehicle without sustaining any fractured ribs and yet have serious internal injuries. In penetrating injuries of the chest, the general examination and observation of the patient give the best clue to the potential severity of the lesions present.

RIB FRACTURES

Rib fractures are often associated with pulmonary complications even when little direct injury to the lung has occurred at the moment of trauma. Pneumonia is a particular threat in the elderly patient with rib fractures. If several ribs are fractured both anteriorly and posteriorly so as to result in a flail chest, the respiratory impairment may be severe at any age (Fig. 17-5). Treatment is directed at reducing the unphysiologic mechanics of ventilation: (1) by tracheostomy to decrease the dead space and resistance to air flow and (2) by the application of assisted ventilation, at times coupled with measures to lessen the abnormal mobility of the injured portion of the chest wall. In severe cases, the application of traction by locking towel clips around the rib has aided in the stabilization of the chest wall. It is felt that positive-pressure respiration provides adequate stabilization in most instances. In sternal fractures, as seen with steering wheel injuries, elevation and traction of the depressed sternum may be indicated. Such injuries are often associated with serious cardiac damage which may be detected by early electrocardiographic changes.

Intercostal nerve blocks are frequently helpful in reducing the pain associated with rib fractures and thus improving expansion of the lung. Pneumothorax, with or without hemothorax, is a common complication of rib fractures;

A   *B*

its treatment is discussed in the section on diseases of the pleura. At times a fragment of rib may be driven into the lung; early or late hemoptysis may result.

Compounded wounds of the chest wall, which may be sucking wounds, require debridement and closure with appropriate closed drainage of the pleural cavity. In penetrating wounds of the lower portion of the chest the possibility of associated injury to upper abdominal viscera requires serious consideration and often merits a thoracoabdominal exploration. Hemothorax associated with penetrating wounds of the thorax may reach major proportions if the intercostal or internal mammary vessels are lacerated (Fig. 17-6).

Infection and Inflammation

INFECTION OF COSTAL CARTILAGES

The special problems associated with infection of the costal cartilages are due to certain characteristics of hyaline cartilage as well as the anatomic arrangement of those cartilages forming the anterior thoracic wall. Hyaline cartilage does not contain any blood vessels or nerves and derives its nutrition from the lymph. Because of its avascularity, this tissue is very vulnerable to infection. When denuded of its perichondrium and left exposed in an infected wound, cartilage acts much like a foreign body. When only a portion of a cartilage is resected, the cut surface of the remaining segment is not covered by perichondrium. Similarly, removal of only one of two or more fused cartilages will leave an area denuded of perichondrium at the site of fusion. Whenever a piece of cartilage, any part of which is denuded of perichondrium, projects into an infected wound, a persistent sinus may occur. Only if infection is minimal or the exposed part of the cartilage is covered with viable tissue before the necrosis begins can sinus formation be avoided. In clean wounds, however, partial resection of cartilages is feasible.

Chondritis due to pyogenic organisms may occur as a result of wounds, as a direct extension from an adjacent infection, following operation for drainage of suppurative foci, and as a result of systemic infection. Staphylococci and streptococci are the most frequent pyogenic organisms found in costal chondritis. Tuberculous involvement of the cartilages is usually secondary to tuberculosis of adjacent structures, especially the pleura and the mediastinal lymph nodes. Various fungi, particularly *Actinomyces* and *Blastomyces,* may be the cause of chondritis. Extensive wound infection following radical mastectomy may result in costal chondritis and even osteomyelitis of the sternum. Pain is usually a prominent feature of chondritis.

Properly placed incisions will lessen the frequency of chondritis following operations for the drainage of intrathoracic or upper abdominal suppuration. When an empyma or pulmonary abscess requires drainage, it is advisable to resect a portion of rib rather than a cartilage, if such a procedure will provide an adequate approach. When the suppurative area lies beneath the cartilage, thus requiring its resection, several points should be borne in mind: If one of the upper five cartilages is to be resected,

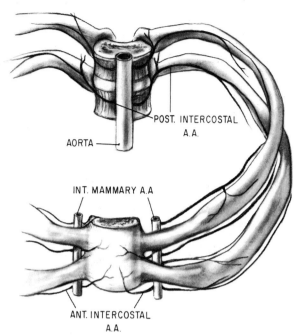

Fig. 17-6. Relationship between ribs and intercostal blood vessels. Posteriorly, the intercostal vessels are at the lower rib margin, whereas anteriorly the arteries are more within the intercostal spaces. These anatomic facts influence the vulnerability to injury.

the entire cartilage should be removed. Cartilage is often needlessly exposed because the surgeon does not determine the site of the costochondral junction before the rib segment is cut anteriorly. If a costal cartilage is partly resected in an infected wound and complete removal of the remainder of that cartilage is considered undesirable, the denuded part of the cartilage should be covered by perichondrium. If other tissue such as muscle is available, it also may be employed to cover the cartilage.

Infections of the costal arch of one side may extend to the opposite side, either through involvement of the xyphoid process or as a result of secondary osteomyelitis of the sternum. The xyphoid process is cartilaginous in early life but becomes partly ossified in adults. The risk of involvement of the xyphoid is greater when the structure is chiefly cartilaginous.

Following subperichondrial resection of a cartilage, osseous tissue may develop and result in the formation of a rigid structure. If the perichondrium is sacrificed in the removal of a cartilage, a permanently flaccid area in the chest wall will result. Unless care is taken to preserve the perichondrium, extensive removal of the cartilaginous structures of the chest wall will result in an undesirable instability of the thoracic cage.

OSTEOMYELITIS OF THE STERNUM

Osteomyelitis of the sternum as a result of septicemia is an uncommon occurrence; considerably more common is involvement of the sternum by direct extension of infection from adjacent areas or secondary to costal chondritis. Operative procedures which involve the sternum may result in an infected wound of the chest wall.

The clinical picture of osteomyelitis of the sternum resembles that of involvement of other bony structures. When the infection is due to pyogenic organisms, there are usually systemic signs of infection, combined with local tenderness, swelling, and perhaps fluctuation. Roentgenographic examination is usually of little aid in the early diagnosis of sternal osteomyelitis but is occasionally helpful in the more chronic stage of the disease. Lateral and oblique views are most satisfactory for visualization of the sternum. The absence of changes on the roentgenogram does not exclude an extensive osteomyelitic process. If the involvement of the sternum is due to the tubercle bacillus, there may be little pain or tenderness, and a cold abscess may be the presenting sign. A tuberculous abscess overlying the sternum does not necessarily indicate involvement of the underlying bone. The tuberculous process may have arisen in the mediastinum and broken through the interspace lateral to the sternum and then extended superficially to the midline. There may be difficulty in distinguishing between chronic osteomyelitis and a tumor of the sternum. When the sternum has been destroyed by a pyogenic or neoplastic process, the pulsation of the underlying great vessels may be transmitted to the skin and closely simulate an aneurysm.

TREATMENT. The treatment of sternal osteomyelitis consists of chemotherapy and resection of the involved portion of the sternum. Care must be taken to avoid injury to the pleura and the underlying mediastinal structures. The possibility of an anterior mediastinal abscess in association with substernal osteomyelitis must be borne in mind.

ABSCESSES

Abscesses of the chest wall may be secondary to an intrathoracic infection which penetrates into the thoracic parietes. Tuberculosis and fungus infections may be the etiologic factors (Fig. 17-7). Abscess of the thoracic wall also may be associated with osteomyelitis of the ribs or sternum, or a costal chondritis. Infection of the chest wall may result from penetrating trauma or following surgical procedures. At times abscesses of the thoracic wall are a complication of septicemia.

A *subpectoral abscess* may result from a suppurative adenitis in the lymph nodes underlying the axillary portion of the pectoralis muscles following infection in the arm or upper thoracic wall. Chills and fever with palpable fullness in the pectoral region are usually present. Surgical drainage of the abscess combined with appropriate chemotherapy is the indicated therapy.

A *subscapular abscess* is usually secondary to infection in the adjacent underlying portion of the thoracic cage.

TIETZE'S SYNDROME

Tietze's syndrome is a painful, nonsuppurative swelling, of unknown cause, of one or more costal cartilages. The second costal cartilage is frequently affected. The signs and symptoms may simulate those of a variety of conditions including cartilaginous tumors and chondritis. If symptoms persist or if a chondrosarcoma cannot be excluded, excision of the cartilage is warranted. The symptoms of

Tietze's syndrome are usually self-limited, but recurrence may be noted.

Tumors

Tumors arising primarily from structures of the chest wall may have their origins from either the soft tissues or bony structures of the thoracic cage. Soft tissue tumors include lesions of the skin and subcutaneous tissue or neurogenic tumors of the intercostal nerves. The latter are found along the lower margin of the rib (Fig. 17-8) and may distort the rib contour. Multiple neurofibromas are seen with neurofibromatosis. Neurofibrosarcoma also may occur, especially with neurofibromatosis. This discussion is limited to consideration of tumors arising in the cartilages and bones of the chest wall (see Chap. 46). Eight percent of all primary bone tumors occur in the bones of the chest, and ninety-five percent of thoracic bone tumors originate in ribs. The ratio of malignant to benign osseous tumors is somewhat greater in the chest wall than in the remainder of the body. Involvement of the ribs and sternum by a wide variety of metastatic growths is far more common than primary neoplasms of these bones, and rib lesions related to generalized metabolic diseases may be confused with neoplams.

Tumors of the chest wall generally become manifest by a swelling which may or may not be painful. At times tumors of the bony thoracic skeleton are detected on routine roentgenographic examinations or examinations performed because of pain (Fig. 17-9).

Chest wall tumors must be differentiated from other lesions which may present as masses in the thoracic wall. An indolent abscess such as may be seen with a tuberculous process arising in the pleura or intrathoracic lymph nodes may present as a nontender swelling without skin erythema. Similarly, fungus infections, such as with *Actinomyces,* may result in a chest wall mass. A careful history may aid in differentiating a chest wall hematoma from a neoplasm. A lesion suggesting metastatic disease, myeloma, lymphomatous processes, Paget's disease, or metabolic disorders may be identified by a complete bone survey. Needle biopsy of the mass or incisional biopsy is frequently indicated, since subsequent therapy will be dictated by pathologic findings. Aspiration biopsy is particularly helpful with multiple lesions.

TREATMENT. Most primary localized tumors of the chest wall require wide surgical excision. This may entail en bloc resection of the tumor-bearing area with a good margin of normal tissue, requiring subsequent reconstruction. The chest wall resection should include at least 5 cm of rib on either side of the tumor and, if malignancy is suspected, large segments of normal rib above and below the tumor. If there is fixation to the overlying chest wall, muscles, or skin, these should also be removed. Resection may include the pleura, intercostal muscles, and neuromuscular and vascular bundles. With deep invasion, the pleura should be entered at a distance from the tumor in order to determine whether there is involvement of the underlying parietal pleura or lung.

Reconstruction following resection of a major segment

of the chest wall aims at obtaining coverage and keeping enough rigidity to avoid paradoxic respiration. Usually the en bloc excision of three ribs and intercostal muscles with preservation of the pectoralis muscle and skin will not result in significant paradoxic motion. Pedicle grafts, particularly employing the latissimus dorsi, achieve good bulk coverage of large defects of the chest wall. Large segments of the sternum may be removed without affecting chest wall stability. If there is a question of stability, autogenous tibial bone grafts and bone shifts may provide support, or the ribs themselves may be used. Many prosthetic materials have been used to reconstruct the chest wall; these are frequently associated with a significant incidence of infection.

Radiosensitive tumors, such as Ewing's sarcoma, lymphosarcoma, and Hodgkin's disease, are best treated with radiation therapy. This has achieved symptomatic relief and regression of tumor size but rarely is curative.

CHONDROMA

Chondromas represent 25 to 30 percent of benign tumors of the chest wall. The majority of lesions occur anteriorly at the costochondral junction and become manifest during the second and third decades of life. Clinically, there may be difficulty in distinguishing between benign chondroma and the malignant chondrosarcoma (Fig. 17-10). The roentgenogram reveals a medullary lesion causing thinning of the cortex. If there is extension and involvement of the surrounding soft tissue, a malignant lesion is suggested. In view of the difficulty of distinguishing between chondroma and chondrosarcoma and because biopsy from one area may be misleading, treatment should consist of wide excision with a 4- to 5-cm margin of normal rib on either side and en bloc resection of the adjacent chest wall if necessary. Curettage is contraindicated in view of the high incidence of recurrence associated with this approach.

OSTEOCHONDROMA

Although this lesion occurs more commonly throughout the body than chondroma, it is much less prevalent in the bony thorax. Osteochondromas occur three times more commonly in males, are usually asymptomatic, and are characterized on roentgenogram by a lesion arising from the cortex with a distinct boundary between the tumor and the soft tissue.

Symptomatic osteochondroma always should be excised, and asymptomatic lesions in the adult should be removed. Prognosis is excellent.

FIBROUS DYSPLASIA

These bone cysts of the rib represent the most common chest tumors. Local swelling and tenderness are often noted, and attention may be drawn to the lesion following trauma. Fibrous dysplasia is a lesion of the young adult and generally involves the posterior portion of the rib. Roentgenogram reveals expansion and filling of the cortex with a central trabeculated appearance. Excision of the involved rib is indicated when the lesion cannot be distin-

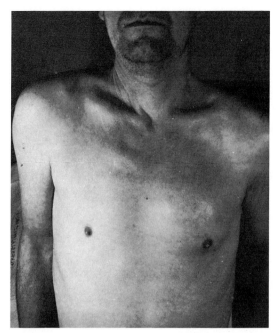

Fig. 17-7. Actinomycotic abscess extending into left side of anterior chest wall. Note swelling of anterior chest wall. Lesion was treated by surgical drainage and chemotherapy.

guished from a malignant growth and also since the tumor may grow to be very large.

EOSINOPHILIC GRANULOMA

This benign destructive process may occur in the ribs especially of children and young adults. Pain is often present, and there may be a history of antecedent trauma. Swelling and local tenderness may be noted; systemic

Fig. 17-8. Sarcoma of rib. Patient died of pulmonary metastases.

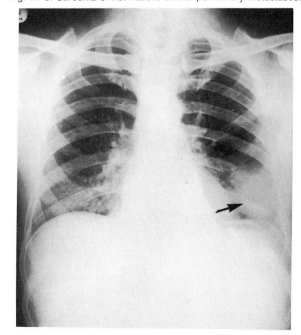

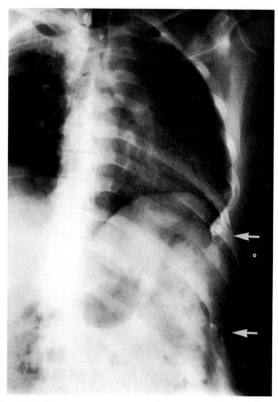

Fig. 17-9. Chondrosarcoma of sixth and ninth ribs. Preoperatively, lesions were thought to be benign. Patient was well several years after resection of both malignant lesions.

manifestations such as fever, malaise, leukocytosis, and eosinophilia may occur. A punched-out, rounded osteolytic area in the rib is noted on roentgenogram. Once the diagnosis is established by biopsy, the expected clinical course is generally benign. The tumor responds well to curettage or small doses of radiation.

CHONDROSARCOMA

Chondrosarcoma is the most common malignant tumor of the bony chest wall, approximately 50 percent in most series. The lesion is rarely seen in patients under the age of twenty, and the peak incidence occurs in the third and fourth decades. The tumor usually arises anteriorly at the costochondral junction, as is the case for the benign chondroma. Roentgenograms are usually distinctive in that chondrosarcoma destroys cortical bone and has mottled calcification. As microscopic diagnosis may be difficult, several areas of lesion should be biopsied. Treatment consists of radical excision (Fig. 17-11), since the lesion is radioresistant. In a series reporting results of radical resections, salvage rates of 25 to 30 percent 5-year survival have been reported.

OSTEOGENIC SARCOMA

Approximately 10 percent of all osteogenic sarcomas occur in the chest wall. The tumor may involve the ribs or sternum. Tumors of the sternum are almost always malignant, and the majority of these are either chondrosarcomas or osteogenic sarcomas. Osteogenic sarcomas occur most frequently in the second or third decades of life, with the patients complaining of rapidly enlarging, frequently painful masses. X-ray reveals an osteolytic lesion with extension to the soft tissues. It most frequently is a mixture of bony destruction and bone production, giving a "sunburst" appearance. Treatment is by radical excision, but the prognosis is extremely poor; osteogenic sarcomas occurring in the ribs have a lower 5-year survival than similar lesions occurring elsewhere in the body.

EWING'S SARCOMA

This is a highly malignant lesion which occurs chiefly in children and young adults and accounts for about 9 percent of all malignant tumors of the chest wall. About 14 percent of Ewing's sarcomas occur in the ribs, 6 percent arise in the scapula, and 3 percent arise in the clavicle. In contrast to other bony tumors of the chest wall, Ewing's sarcoma is frequently associated with systemic manifestations such as fever and malaise. The mass itself is characteristically warm and painful, suggesting infection. The characteristic radiologic appearance is that of onion-skin

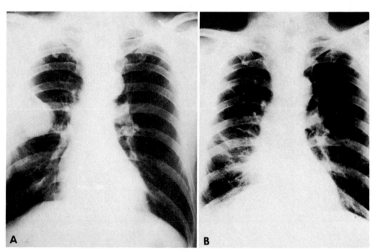

Fig. 17-10. Chondrosarcoma of rib. A. Preoperative. B. After wide surgical excision.

calcification caused by the tumor's elevating the periosteum. Since the tumor is highly radiosensitive and wide excision is not associated with a significant cure rate, radiation therapy is advised. Five-year survivals are rare.

MULTIPLE MYELOMA

The ribs are involved in about 44 percent and the clavicles in about 14 percent of cases of multiple myeloma. The sternum is involved in about 6 percent of cases. Unlike other bony tumors of the chest wall, this is a disease which predominates in the fifth or sixth decades of life. Roentgenograms reveal multiple osteolytic areas without evidence of new bone formation. Rarely an apparently solitary plasmacytoma may be the first manifestation of this systemic plasma cell dysplasia. Cure is rarely achieved by surgical excision; symptomatic relief is frequently obtained with antimetabolites.

SOLITARY BONE METASTASES

The ribs, vertebrae, and sternum are among the most frequent sites of bony metastases from a variety of carcinomas. Occasionally a single rib or the sternum may be involved by a metastatic lesion which may attain considerable size and stimulate a primary rib or sternal tumor both clinically and radiologically. A metastasis from a hypernephroma, in particular, may present such a picture (Fig. 17-12).

Radiation Necrosis

Radiation damage to the chest wall may result from intensive radiotherapy for malignant thoracic lesions, especially breast carcinoma. Fortunately such complications of radiation therapy are apparently becoming less frequent since greater knowledge of the late results of some types of radiation has been gained. If ulceration of the chest wall has occurred, there is usually considerable chronic penumonitis and fibrosis in the underlying lung (Fig. 17-13). The involved ribs may be very osteoporotic and undergo spon-

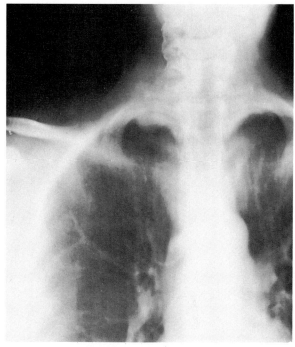

Fig. 17-11. Neurofibroma. Tomogram demonstrates small intercostal lesion at right apex.

taneous fracture. The costochondral junctions may dislocate. The chest wall may lose its stability. Radiation carcinoma may develop (Fig. 17-14A).

When ulceration has occurred, surgical excision of the involved portion of the chest wall is indicated (Fig. 17-14B). The entire thickness of the chest wall in the area of involvement must usually be excised. The defect is generally closed with a large pedicle flap in an airtight fashion. In women, pedicles formed from the opposite breast may be most advantageous, because some radiation reaction in the axillary line of the involved side may interfere with mobilization of a pedicle flap from the homolateral side.

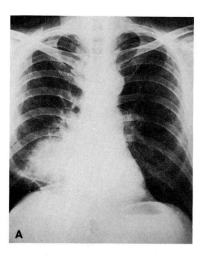

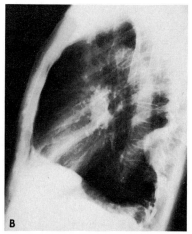

Fig. 17-12. Solitary metastasis to rib. A. Postero-anterior view demonstrating large metastasis from previously unrecognized hypernephroma of the kidney. B. Lateral view.

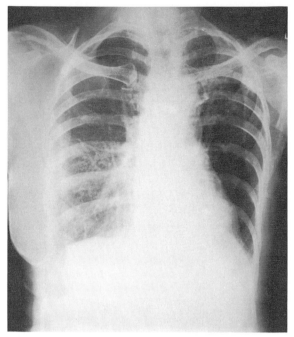

Fig. 17-13. Radiation pneumonitis and fibrosis of left lung with osteoporosis of ribs following therapy for carcinoma of the breast.

PLEURA

Anatomy

Embryologically the paired pleural cavities become separated from the central pericardial cavity by the development of the pleuropericardial membrane. For a time the pleural cavities are continuous with the peritoneal cavity, but normal development of the pleuroperitoneal membrane eventually separates these serous cavities. A failure of either of these membranes to develop properly leaves a defect which results in an abnormally persistent communication between pleural cavity and pericardial sac or between the peritoneal and pleural cavities.

The pleura covers the surface of the lung, lines most of the chest wall, and covers those portions of the diaphragm and mediastinum which are contiguous to the pleural space. Since the various portions of the pleura are continuous with each other, the pleural cavity is a closed space. The normally expanded lung projects so completely into all regions of this pleural cavity that ordinarily it is only a potential space. In abnormal states, however, the pleural cavity may contain fluid, gases, or masses of tissue which will compress the underlying lung to a varying degree.

The pleura consists of a very thin layer of connective tissue covered by a mesothelial layer. Elastic fibers and smooth muscle are also present. The pleura contains a generous vascular and lymphatic network and is also supplied with nerve fibers. The visceral pleura is an integral part of the outer surface of the lung, whereas the parietal pleura normally can be separated from the chest wall with relative ease.

The blood supply of the visceral pleura is derived from the *bronchial* vascular system of the lung. This fact can be of considerable clinical importance in certain pathologic states in which there is a decrease in the blood flow in the *pulmonary* vascular system of the lungs. Since there is a tendency for the bronchial circulation to increase when the pulmonary circulation is diminished, in some pathologic conditions there is a great tendency for the bronchial blood supply in visceroparietal adhesions to be exaggerated. This occurs in some types of congenital heart disease and certain pulmonary inflammatory conditions.

Physiology

Because of the inherent elastic recoil of the lungs, the intrapleural pressure within the normal intact thorax is subatmospheric. The intrapleural pressure fluctuates with the respiratory cycle, being more negative during inspiration than during expiration. Many factors, both physiologic and pathologic, may alter the intrapleural pressure. The depth and character of the respiratory movement, the status of the lungs, and the condition of the chest wall and diaphragm can all influence the intrapleural pressure readings. Measurements of the intrapleural pressure can

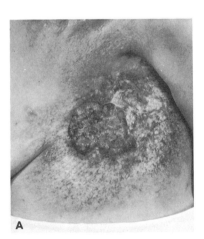

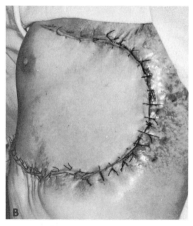

Fig. 17-14. Radiation necrosis and postradiation carcinoma of chest wall. *A.* Lesion, which followed therapy for breast carcinoma, prior to surgical excision. *B.* Appearance at end of operation with closure of defect by flap fashioned from opposite breast.

give valuable information concerning intrathoracic dynamics. It is customary to measure intrapleural pressure with a water manometer, since the pressures are low. In a normal person the pressure at the end of a quiet inspiration (namely, at the height of inspiration) might vary in the range of −4 to −8 cm of water, whereas at the end of a quiet (not strained) expiration the pressure might vary in the range of −2 to −4. In recording intrapleural pressure the extremes of manometric fluctuation between inspiration and expiration are noted; for example, a reading might be −6, −2, or the *mean* pressure (the average of the inspiratory and expiratory end pressures) may be stated as −4.

When a lung loses its elastic recoil, as in pulmonary emphysema, the intrapleural pressure is less negative than normally. Atelectasis with a reduction in lung volume, however, causes the intrapleural pressure to be more negative. When a pneumothorax occurs in a person with an essentially normal lung, there may be only slight changes in the pleural pressure as the lung partially collapses; the intrapleural readings still may be negative in spite of an extensive degree of lung collapse. In a chronic pneumothorax such as may be caused by a ruptured emphysematous bleb, a restrictive membrane may form over the visceral pleura while the lung is in a collapsed state. If the air leakage from the lung then ceases, the membrane over the pleura may interfere with pulmonary reexpansion, and a highly negative intrapleural pressure may be found in such a situation.

PLEURAL ABSORPTION AND TRANSUDATION. In the presence of a normal pleura, absorbable substances may be readily removed from the pleural space. The principles of absorption which apply to other serous cavities are applicable. The nature of the substance and the molecular and particle size influence the rate of uptake by the vascular and lymphatic channels. Experimental observations indicate that pleural absorption, especially of particulate matter, occurs chiefly via the parietal pleura. Pleural absorption is more rapid when respiratory motion is increased, as this results in an augmented vascular and lymphatic flow in the pleura.

Although normally no appreciable amount of fluid is found in the pleural cavity, it should be appreciated that this state of affairs merely represents an equilibrium between absorption and transudation. When a pleural transudate occurs, absorption of some substances from the pleura is still going on.

Changes in the character of the pleura may radically alter the rate of interchange of substances between the pleural cavity and the body as a whole. In general the vascularity of the membrane in contact with the pleural space together with the rate of lymphatic flow will influence the rate of absorption from the pleural space. A thick, avascular rigid pleural covering will greatly reduce the rate of absorption from the pleural cavity, whereas a hyperemic thin pleura in a dyspneic patient may be associated with maximal absorption from the pleural space. These facts should be borne in mind in a consideration of toxic absorption from an infected pleural cavity, and also in estimating the absorption of antibiotics or other agents in-

stilled into the pleural space. From these statements it should be obvious that studies of pleural absorption of antibiotics carried out in normal animals may have serious limitations in application to the patient with a chronically diseased pleural surface.

PLEURAL GASES. When air or other gas is introduced into or enters the pleural space, there is a gradual absorption of the gas into the blood. The rate of disappearance of the gas from the pleural cavity is influenced by the concentration of that gas in the blood and other factors. Oxygen is absorbed more rapidly than nitrogen. Therefore, when air is introduced into a closed pleural cavity, a subsequent analysis of the residual pleural gas will show a lower oxygen percentage and higher nitrogen concentration than are present in air. The carbon dioxide concentration is considerably increased because of a tendency for equilibrium to be established between the gas in the blood and the pleural cavity. Analysis of a sample of intrapleural air can be utilized in the diagnosis of obscure small bronchial air leaks in cases of chronic pneumothorax.

Transmediastinal Pleural Herniation

When there is a long-standing difference in the intrapleural pressure in the two pleural cavities, there is a gradual stretching of the mediastinal pleura in one or more of the so-called "weak places" in the mediastinal partition (Fig. 17-15). This bulging of mediastinal pleura tends to occur in those areas where the mediastinal structures do

Fig. 17-15. Pleural herniation through mediastinum. Shrunken left lung was caused by long-standing tuberculosis. Arrows point to upper retroesophageal mediastinal hernia and lower posterior mediastinal hernia.

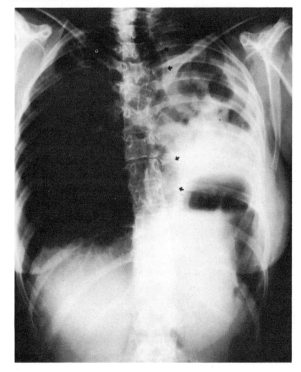

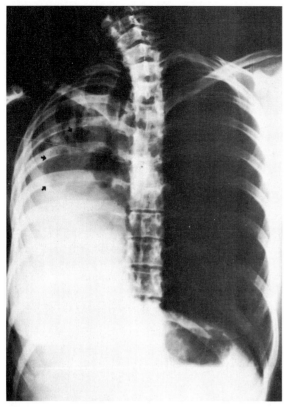

Fig. 17-16. Mediastinal herniation. Arrows indicate margin of left lung, which is herniated through anterior retrosternal area and to right hemothorax as a result of marked shrinkage of right lung from bronchostenosis.

not present a particular barrier to such protrusion. These areas are located retrosternally and also anterior to the vertebral column, where the pleural reflections of each pleural cavity are in close anatomic association. These bulgings of the mediastinal pleura of one side into the opposite hemithorax are called *herniations,* although some have criticized this terminology. Mediastinal herniation is always associated with some degree of lateral displacement of the mediastinal structures (Fig. 17-16). After pneumonectomy the occurrence of mediastinal herniation may be particularly obvious.

Spontaneous Pneumothorax

The term *spontaneous pneumothorax* is applied to cases in which a pneumothorax occurs as a result of rupture of the visceral pleura. The common causes of spontaneous pneumothorax are ruptured emphysematous blebs or bullae or rupture of subpleural tuberculous foci through the visceral pleura. Trauma may be involved as a possible exciting agent in some cases, but in many instances the pneumothorax occurs at a time when the person is not straining in any way. In some cases a spontaneous pneumothorax may occur in the presence of a pulmonary or mediastinal tumor. Rarely a spontaneous pneumothorax may occur with the menstrual period. Because of the recurrent nature of such pneumothoraces, a thoracotomy

may be indicated. Endometrial tissue may be found involving the right leaf of the diaphragm, and subpleural endometrial implants may be noted.

Until recent years the presence of a spontaneous pneumothorax was thought to indicate that the patient probably had pulmonary tuberculosis or was likely to develop tuberculosis in the future. It is now well established that in the apparently healthy patients (without roentgenographic evidence of tuberculosis) spontaneous pneumothorax is usually due to nontuberculous defects in the pleura and subpleural tissues. When a pneumothorax occurs spontaneously as a result of pulmonary tuberculosis, roentgen ray films usually show obvious tuberculosis of the lungs.

Sudden chest pain and shortness of breath of varying magnitude are the common symptoms. In some instances the symptoms may be so mild that the patient is unaware that any abnormal state exists, and the pneumothorax is detected by chance roentgenographic examination. At other times dyspnea may be severe because of the development of tension pneumothorax. Since emphysematous bullae are often bilateral, occasionally a patient sustains a pneumothorax on both sides concurrently.

The degree of pneumothorax produced by rupture of a bleb or bulla may vary widely; in some cases only a very small pneumothorax results, whereas at the other extreme an extensive tension pneumothorax may be found. The size and character of the visceral pleural defect and the nature and location of preexisting visceroparietal pleural adhesions may be factors in determining the size and chronicity of the pneumothorax. In some cases a pleural adhesion may be an initiating factor by causing pull on a weak place in the subpleural pulmonary tissues during coughing, sneezing, or straining. Such an adhesion in certain cases may be responsible for the visceral defect's being held open (Fig. 17-17), as indicated by the past experience with the cutting of such an adhesion by closed pneumonolysis with resultant closure of the tiny bronchial fistula.

Hemopneumothorax may also occur by a similar mechanism. In some such cases the hemorrhage from a blood vessel in the ruptured visceroparietal adhesion may be so extensive as to cause hemorrhagic shock. It should be realized that if a patient is seen shortly after the onset of symptoms of spontaneous pneumothorax and roentgenograms indicate the presence of fluid in the pleural cavity, this "fluid" is probably blood. A thoracentesis should be done at once to confirm this, and tube drainage should be established. Emergency thoracotomy to control the bleeding, remove the blood clots, suture the visceral pleural defect, and reexpand the lung is indicated in conjunction with transfusion in cases of massive hemopneumothorax.

TREATMENT. The treatment of spontaneous pneumothorax without pleural hemorrhage depends on the size and duration of the pneumothorax together with a consideration of its cause. A small asymptomatic pneumothorax requires no intervention. If more than a 25 percent pneumothorax is present, a rubber catheter for closed intercostal drainage, with or without suction, may be employed for several days. In most instances merely a water-seal type of drainage is satisfactory, although suction should be employed if the air leakage is considerable or the patient is threatened with respiratory insufficiency.

A thoracotomy is indicated in a few selected cases of spontaneous pneumothorax. When roentgenograms demonstrate one or more bullae or cystlike lesions in the lung, thoracotomy with resection of the cystic areas and pleurodesis is recommended. When the pneumothorax recurs after catheter drainage, thoracotomy is also indicated unless other factors such as preexisting respiratory insufficiency or other disease states render operation hazardous. If thoracotomy reveals numerous tiny visceral pleural blebs as the cause of the recurrent pneumothorax, a pleurectomy or pleurodesis which will result in diffuse adherence of the lung to the chest wall is the indicated procedure. It is highly desirable to get the lung adherent to the denuded chest wall as early as possible by adequate drainage of the pleural space in the early postoperative period.

When a spontaneous pneumothorax occurs as a result of rupture of a subpleural caseous tuberculous focus into the pleural space, the indicated treatment depends on the extent of the pulmonary tuberculous lesion, the time after occurrence of the pneumothrox that the patient is first seen, whether a pleural infection is already established, and the general condition of the patient. Antituberculous chemotherapy should be started at once; if the pneumothorax occurred while the patient was receiving antituberculous drug, consideration must be given to changing to more effective agents for that patient. If the tuberculous disease is unilobar and the patient is in good general condition and seen early, immediate lobectomy with chemotherapy may forestall the development of a tuberculous empyema. In most cases with widespread tuberculous disease closed intercostal drainage and chemotherapy is the preliminary treatment of choice.

Pleural Effusion

Pleurisy, or pleuritis, denotes an inflammation of the pleura. A "dry," fibrinous pleurisy will not be discussed here, since it is primarily a nonsurgical problem. When an effusion develops with the pleuritis, a variety of potential surgical implications, both diagnostic and therapeutic, may arise.

It has been customary to divide pleural fluids arbitrarily into two large groups: the transudates and exudates. Pleural exudates may be clear or cloudy, blood-tinged or frankly bloody. Examination of the exudate for the cellular content of the sediment may aid in diagnosis. Aspirated pleural fluid should always be cultured, because bacteria may be discovered on smear or culture in some fluids which appear clear, especially if the patient has received antibiotic therapy. Smears, cultures, and guinea pig inoculations for tubercle bacilli should be done. Careful examination of the sediment for tumor cells is indicated, especially when serosanguineous fluid is obtained. In many cases of nonbacterial involvement of the pleura, however, examination of the pleural fluid may fail to establish a diagnosis. Therefore pleural biopsy has been frequently employed as an aid to diagnosis. Closed pleural biopsy using an Abrams needle may be performed even in the

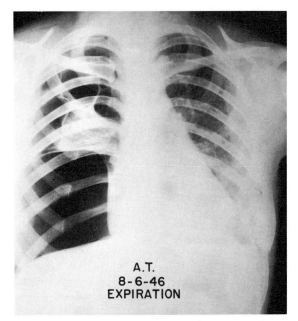

Fig. 17-17. Spontaneous pneumothroax with long-standing collapse of lung. Lung was completely reexpanded by surgical decortication.

absence of pleural fluid. In 60 to 80 percent of patients with tuberculosis and 40 to 60 percent of patients with neoplasia, a definitive diagnosis can be obtained from closed pleural biopsy.

In some cases a satisfactory pleural biopsy may be obtained with an ordinary large-bore needle. The use of special biopsy needles which core or punch out a bit of thickened pleura, however, will give better tissue for pathologic examination. In most cases in which a pleural biopsy is considered some pleural effusion is present and should be thoroughly examined.

TECHNIQUE OF THORACENTESIS. Attention to certain details may make a thoracentesis less disturbing to the patient and more informative to the physician. The size and length of the aspirating needles should be selected for the specific patient, bearing in mind the probable thickness of the chest wall and the anticipated character of the pleural fluid. A three-way stopcock may be employed with advantage between the needle and syringe, especially when the removal of considerable quantities of pleural fluid is anticipated, so as to avoid the undesired entrance of air into the pleural cavity.

The site of thoracentesis should be determined on the basis of a careful study of the roentgenograms of the chest and the physical findings with particular attention to the site of maximal dullness on percussion. Adequate posteroanterior and true lateral x-rays of the chest are required. Somewhat overexposed films or Bucky films may better differentiate intrapulmonary and pleural densities.

Errors in selecting the site of thoracentesis are frequently made because of a failure to correlate properly the roentgenographic findings with the patient's anatomic landmarks. There is a tendency to insert the needle lower than indicated. When a localized pleural effusion is paravertebral in location, aspiration is often carried out too far laterally.

As soon as the flow of fluid through the needle is satisfactory, a clamp should be placed on the needle at the skin level in order to avoid inadvertent shifting of the needle during the thoracentesis. Coughing during the aspiration is undesirable because of possible trauma to the lung by the needle point. An attack of coughing may require termination of the thoracentesis.

Pleural Effusion Secondary to Subdiaphragmatic Infection

Pleural effusion is a common finding in cases of subphrenic abscess. The development of pleural fluid in a patient who has had an intraabdominal inflammatory process or operative procedure which might lead to a suppurative complication should be investigated for possible subdiaphragmatic infection. If pulmonary infection or infarction has also been present, the pleural fluid might be secondary to either the lung or subdiaphragmatic lesion. Since such patients are often febrile, the question may well arise whether the pleural fluid is sterile or infected. In performing a thoracentesis in order to determine the nature of the fluid it is important to bear in mind that the diaphragm is often considerably elevated in such cases. Therefore the needle must be inserted fairly high in order to avoid confusion between fluid obtained from the plural space and that from a subphrenic collection. If a clear fluid is first aspirated and then the needle is advanced more deeply and a purulent fluid is obtained, it may well be that the first fluid came from the pleural cavity whereas the purulent fluid came from the subphrenic abscess. This is the means whereby improper needling may convert a sterile secondary effusion into an empyema.

Most pleural effusions secondary to subphrenic infections will subside following control of the infradiaphragmatic suppuration by antibiotics and surgical drainage. If the pleural effusion persists, it is likely that either the subphrenic infection has not been adequately treated or the previously sterile pleural effusion has now become an empyema.

Meigs' Syndrome

When an obscure pleural effusion occurs in a patient with an ovarian tumor, the question arises whether the two are related, whether the ovarian tumor is malignant and the pleural effusion due to intrapleural metastases, or whether one is dealing with Meigs' syndrome. In this syndrome the patient has a benign tumor of the ovary which may be associated with ascites and pleural effusion. The fluid is very rarely bloody. The pleural effusion disappears when the ovarian tumor is removed.

Pleural Effusion Secondary to Mediastinal Infection

In cases of acute mediastinitis secondary pleural effusions are common, and the effusion not infrequently is bilateral. With severe mediastinal infections a large accumulation of fluid may occur within 1 or 2 days, and thoracentesis may be urgently indicated in order to lessen respiratory embarrassment.

Hemothorax

The presence of blood in the pleural space is referred to as *hemothorax*. There is no sharp line of distinction between a bloody pleural effusion and a hemothorax. The common causes of hemothorax include trauma, pulmonary infarction, neoplasms, and surgical procedures. Occasionally blood in the pleural space may result from the spontaneous rupture of a pleural adhesion. Aneurysms of the aorta or other intrathoracic vessels may lead to a massive hemothorax. Endometriosis of the pleura is a very rare cause.

The fate of blood in the pleural cavity has been the subject of some controversy, and the outcome of a hemothorax may be influenced by associated factors. It has long been evident that the presence of much traumatized tissue or infection as seen with some shotgun and war wounds increases the likelihood of complications arising from the hemothorax; a fibrothorax may develop which seriously compromises the function of the lung. By contrast, the stab wound of civilian strife often results in a hemothorax which usually does not progress to a fibrothorax and often may disappear with surprisingly little residual pleural reaction.

Experimental studies have demonstrated that a blood clot placed in the pleural cavity of a dog is quickly fragmented and usually absorbed in a week provided the parietal pleura, which is the chief route of absorption, has not been damaged. Some of the red blood cells are resorbed intact into the lymphatics, whereas some of the red cells are lysed before absorption occurs.

Traumatic hemothorax may result from blunt trauma or from penetrating injuries. The bleeding may come from lacerated vessels of the chest wall or diaphragm, from the lung, or from the large vascular structures in the mediastinum. If physical examination and roentgenographic studies indicate the presence of fluid in the pleural cavity within a few hours after trauma, such "fluid" should be considered as largely blood.

TREATMENT. The treatment of a hemothorax will depend on the amount of blood in the pleural space and the rate of bleeding. With severe bleeding, emergency thoractomy is indicated in order to control the hemorrhage by appropriate surgical means. With moderate accumulations of blood in the pleural cavity and where intervention for control of a bleeding site is not necessary, a closed thoracotomy with intercostal tube drainage is indicated in order to evacuate the blood from the pleural cavity and obtain early and complete reexpansion of the lung. Lesser degrees of hemothorax may be treated by needle aspiration without air replacement.

Although some fever is not uncommon with a hemothorax in the absence of infection, a continued febrile course suggests the presence of secondary infection.

A hemothorax in which the blood is not resorbed may result in a marked fibrotic reaction over the pleural surface with severe impairment of pulmonary function by encasement of the lung. Decortication of the lung is indicated in such cases, but the results of such a decortication are more satisfactory if the procedure is not unduly delayed.

Empyema

ACUTE EMPYEMA

Empyema usually develops as a result of extension of infection from some contiguous structure. Prior to the introduction of effective chemotherapeutic agents against pyogenic infections, the vast majority of pleural empyemas was secondary to some type of pneumonia or pulmonary suppuration. In occasional instances empyema developed as a complication of septicemia. Other causes of empyema were infections extending upward from the abdomen, mediastinitis, perforations of the esophagus, penetrating trauma, and, intrathoracic surgical procedures. However, the introduction of chemotherapy and antibiotics has produced a vast change in the entire clinical picture of pleural infections. Because many cases of pneumonia are now controlled or have their course modified by antimicrobial agents, the development of a postpneumonic empyema is much less common today than it was prior to the late 1930s. Also, the bacteria encountered in cases of sepsis are now commonly of a somewhat different variety from that usually seen before the days of antibiotics.

Pneumococcal empyema associated with lobar pneumonia, which used to be one of the common types of empyema, is now rarely seen. Streptococcal empyema has also become relatively rare. Putrid empyema, usually caused by anaerobic organisms including streptococci, is less frequent. Today the most common type of empyema encountered in most places where antibiotics have been widely used is caused by *Staphylococcus aureus*. Other organisms cultured from infected pleural fluid in recent years include *Escherichia coli, Bacillus pyocyaneus,* and *B. lactis aerogenes.* The Friedländer bacillus continues to be an occasional cause of empyema, especially in the debilitated patient with chronic pulmonary disease.

The clinical manifestations of an empyema may be considerably altered in patients who have received antibiotic therapy. At present the recognition of pleural empyema is often delayed, because the use of antibiotics for the primary infection in the lung or elsewhere has partly controlled the virulence and spread of the infection. As a result the extension of the infection to the pleura may not be manifest by any sudden change in the clinical picture. An onset with acute pleuritic pain and the rapid development of a large pleural fluid collection in a toxic patient is now seen less often. The signs of the empyema may merge with those of the primary infection. In some cases an empyema is suspected because of an unexplained persistence of fever at a time when a pneumonic process has largely subsided.

A patient may have clear pleural fluid and the bacteriologic culture may fail to grow organisms, and yet a pleural infection, masked by antibiotic therapy, can still be present. Such patients are usually somewhat febrile, but, in some cases, the pleural infection may not become clinically manifest until some time after antibiotic therapy has been discontinued. Although microscopic examination of the sediment of the pleural fluid from such cases will show pus cells, these may not be present in sufficient numbers to confirm the diagnosis of empyema until a later date, after antibiotic therapy has been discontinued for some time. Empyema may occur as a complication of amebiasis. In some cases, a characteristic anchovy sauce type of pus may be obtained. The fluid should be examined for *Entamoeba histolytica.*

DIFFERENTIAL DIAGNOSIS OF ENCAPSULATED EMPYEMA AND INFECTED SOLITARY PULMONARY CYSTS. Large infected solitary cysts of the lung are often erroneously diagnosed as encapsulated empyema before operation, and at times the true condition is not even recognized during or after operation. A striking characteristic of an epithelialized pulmonary cyst is its failure to diminish appreciably in size over long periods of time despite adequate drainage (Fig. 17-18). The preoperative differentiation of a large infected pulmonary cyst and empyema is not always possible. Most epithelialized pulmonary cysts occur in children or young adults. Patients with a pulmonary cyst are likely to have had previous respiratory symptoms, and this history may date back to early life. The respiratory infections have usually been considered, in retrospect, as secondary to a preexisting congenital pulmonary abnormality. This interpretation, however, is not always correct, because in some cases the cyst is the result, rather than the cause, of the previous infection.

The roentgenographic examination is frequently of great aid in differentiating empyema and infected pulmonary cyst, but the two lesions cannot always be distinguished by this means. The contour of the fluid pocket is often of differential diagnostic value in that the outline of a cyst is spherical or oval in both posteroanterior and lateral projections, whereas the outline of an encapsulated empyema may be triangular or fusiform and conforms more to the contour of the thoracic cage or neighboring structures in the region it occupies. Little evidence of pleural thickening may be seen on the roentgenogram of a person with a pulmonary cyst even though the infection is of many months' standing. The combined thickness of the cyst wall

Fig. 17-18. Congenital cyst of lung simulating empyema. Note rounded contour of cavity persisting after tube drainage. Cyst had an epithelial lining and required excision.

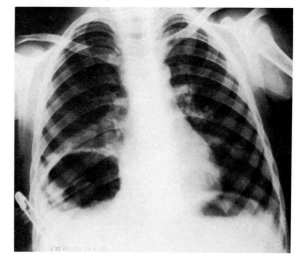

and pleura may be less than the thickness of the parietal pleura alone in cases of chronic empyema. If the infected cyst cavity is filled with air, the roentgenogram may show strands of pulmonary tissue traversing the cavity, and the correct diagnosis should then be suspected. The presence of other pulmonary cysts, either fluid-containing or air-containing, may give a clue to the correct diagnosis. It must be remembered, however, that an infected pulmonary cyst and empyema may coexist.

COMPLICATIONS OF EMPYEMA. Bronchopleural Fistula. An empyema, especially if neglected, may rupture into the lung with the establishment of a bronchopleural fistula. If the empyema is secondary to a suppurative process in the lung, however, a bronchopleural fistula, if present, would most likely be caused by rupture of the suppurative intrapulmonary lesion into the pleura rather than an extension of the process in the reverse direction. The development of a bronchopleural fistula may be heralded by the expectoration of a considerable quantity of purulent sputum, but if the fistula is small, such clinical findings may be lacking. Hemoptysis may occur at the time when the fistula becomes manifest.

Empyema Necessitans. An empyema which has been neglected may gradually burrow through the chest wall and present as an abscess of the chest wall. This complication is most commonly seen with tuberculous empyema. Extensive involvement of the chest wall may also occur with actinomycotic empyema and other rare fungus infections. Osteomyelitis of the ribs or costal chondritis may be an associated process. The process may dissect along the intercostal muscles and present anteriorly in the parasternal region where the external intercostal muscle is deficient; hence the empyema pocket may be located at some distance from the presenting external abscess.

Pericarditis. Pericarditis may result from the extension of infection from the adjacent pleura. Actual rupture of an empyema into the pericardium is very rare unless a surgical procedure or trauma has involved the pericardium.

Mediastinal Abscess. A mediastinal abscess may rarely be a complication of an empyema. Conversely, empyema is a common complication of mediastinitis.

Esophagopleural Fistula. Rarely an empyema will rupture into the esophagus. Tuberculosis or foreign body should be particularly suspected in such cases.

Osteomyelitis of Rib or Sternum and Costal Chondritis. Involvement of these structures of the chest wall in empyema cases is usually the result of chronicity of a pyogenic empyema, the presence of tuberculosis or fungus infection, or previous surgical intervention. If an empyema is located anteriorly and surgical drainage is required, it is desirable, if possible, to avoid the area of the costal cartilages because of the likelihood that a chondritis may ensue.

TREATMENT OF EMPYEMA. Thoracentesis. If an empyema is not associated with a bronchopleural fistula and the purulent material can be removed satisfactorily through a needle, a trial of therapy by thoracentesis is indicated in selected cases. As much of the purulent fluid as possible should be removed. Repeated taps may be necessary. The patient should be receiving systemically an antibiotic or chemotherapeutic agent known to be effective against the bacteria present in the pleural cavity. If the antibiotic used is suitable for intrapleural use, it also may be injected into the empyema cavity at the end of the thoracentesis. If adequate removal of the purulent material is not possible because the pus is thick or if the patient is infected with a pyogenic organism which is resistant to the antibacterial agents available, a thoracostomy for complete drainage should be performed. Also, if the patient continues to reaccumulate fluid, if bacteria continue to be cultured from the fluid, or if the patient fails to show clinical evidence of satisfactory improvement or remains febrile, thoracostomy should be undertaken unless one is dealing with a pure tuberculous empyema.

Closed Drainage of Empyema. Drainage of an empyema by insertion of a catheter through an intercostal space is indicated when adequate evacuation of the empyema fluid cannot be obtained by thoracentesis and yet an open thoracotomy is considered inadvisable because of fear of collapse of the lung (Fig. 17-19). A closed drainage is not usually recommended for a small or encapsulated empyema because of the difficulty in obtaining continuous complete drainage of the pleural exudate from such a

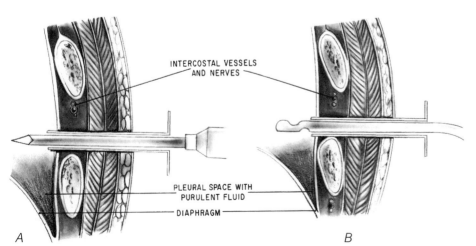

INTERCOSTAL VESSELS AND NERVES

PLEURAL SPACE WITH PURULENT FLUID

DIAPHRAGM

A   *B*

Fig. 17-19. Closed drainage of empyema. Catheter is inserted by means of a trochar and cannula. Tube is connected to a closed drainage system.

pocket by the closed method. Too often when a closed drainage is employed, the placement of the catheter or tube is not sufficiently dependent in the cavity to ensure complete evacuation of the empyema (Fig. 17-20), and chronicity may result. If the drainage tube is small, fibrin may repeatedly plug the tube. However, closed drainage (Fig. 17-21) has an important place in the management of larger empyemas at a time when an open thoractomy might result in collapse of the lung because of the lack of pleural adhesions limiting the empyema cavity. It is particularly indicated in the acutely ill toxic patient in whom the empyema is not satisfactorily managed by thoracentesis alone. The maximal results from closed drainage will be obtained if constant care is taken to ensure continued patency of the drainage tube. If roentgenograms show the presence of a fluid level within the empyema cavity, the drainage should not be deemed optimal. In such situations the advisability of an open thoracostomy to obtain complete dependent drainage should be considered.

Open Thoracostomy for Drainage of Empyema. The aim of open thoracostomy for drainage of an empyema is to obtain continued evacuation of the purulent exudate and at the same time facilitate the reexpansion of the lung so that the empyema cavity will become obliterated. It is therefore important that the proper site for thoracostomy be selected. Adequate roentgenographic studies are mandatory. Posteroanterior and true lateral chest films are the minimal requirement. Overexposed films or Bucky films may aid in distinguishing pulmonary from pleural densities. Careful physical examination with particular attention to the area of maximal dullness may be very helpful in selecting the general site for operation. Needle aspiration

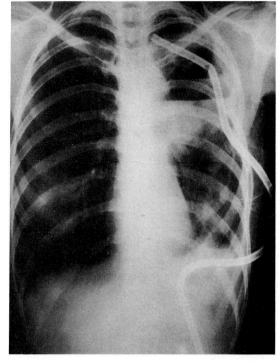

Fig. 17-20. Inadequate drainage of empyema following upper lobe lobectomy. Note that fluid levels are present. Drainage tube is positioned too far in and does not provide adequate drainage. Open thoracotomy and thoracoplasty resulted in eventual healing.

of the empyema determines the exact area in which the rib is to be resected.

Gentleness in the manipulation of instruments and correct injection of the local anesthetic agent permits a thoracostomy with rib resection for drainage of an empyema

Fig. 17-21. Pleural drainage systems. *A.* Water-sealed type of closed drainage. This is established for removal of fluids from pleural cavity. The tube from the pleural cavity goes to the tube under water. The other short tube in the stopper is opened and prevents any pressure accumulation within the bottle. *B.* Negative pressure pleural drainage system with application of suction at −10 cm H$_2$O.

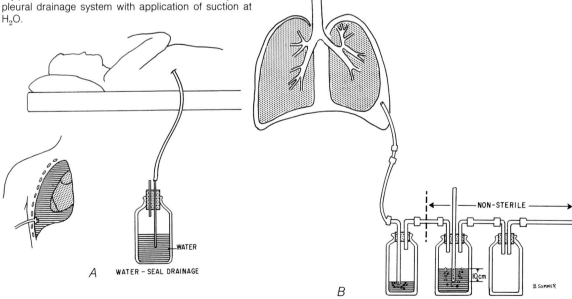

to be done under local anesthesia with minimal discomfort to the patient. If the patient is seriously ill with residual pneumonia or there is a bronchopleural fistula present, it is much safer to perform the thoracostomy under local anesthesia so that the protective cough reflex is not impaired. In some such cases the thoracostomy should be performed with the patient in the upright position because of the danger of flooding the lung via a large bronchopleural fistula when the patient is recumbent with the diseased side uppermost.

The site for rib resection is determined by exploratory needling to ascertain the dependent portion of the empyema cavity. A short segment of rib is then resected (Fig. 17-22). If the empyema underlies the rib bed as anticipated, induration and thickened pleura will be noted. If induration is absent, an error in site selection probably has been made. It is best to confirm the site of the empyema by again needling through the most indurated area of the exposed rib bed. Incision is then made into the empyema cavity. As soon as an opening has been made into the empyema space, a suction tip should be introduced into the cavity. This is particularly important if the patient has a large bronchopleural fistula, because when air from outside suddenly enters such an empyema, the pus may be concomitantly aspirated into the lung via the fistula. It is desirable that the tubing connected to the suction tip

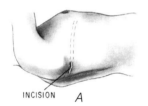

INCISION   *A*

contain a transparent plastic segment to permit observation of the nature of the material aspirated from the empyema cavity and whether any hemorrhage has been initiated. After all fluid has been aspirated from the empyema cavity, the opening should be enlarged slightly and the cavity inspected. It should be ascertained that the drainage site is in the proper dependent position. In some instances, another, more dependent rib may have to be resected or even another drainage site established. A biopsy of the empyema wall should be taken.

Treatment of Empyema Associated with Bronchopleural Fistula. The possible presence of a bronchopleural fistula should always be considered when a patient with pleural fluid collection raises more sputum than might be expected from the associated pulmonary or bronchial disease. A bronchopleural fistula should be particularly suspected if the patient tends to raise large amounts of sputum when lying on one side or the other, provided no large lung abscess is considered to be present.

In some cases, the roentgenographic demonstration of an air-fluid level in the empyema cavity may indicate the presence of the bronchial fistula provided no previously performed thoracentesis has permitted the entrance of air via the needle. The absence of air in the empyema cavity, however, does not rule out the presence of bronchopleural fistula.

When an empyema is complicated by the presence of a bronchopleural fistula, early adequate treatment is of paramount importance in order to avoid continuing damage to the lung as a result of leakage of the empyema fluid into the air passages. Since antibiotics have lessened the virulence and acute manifestations of empyema in general, the detrimental effects of failing to thoroughly evacuate an empyema cavity with associated bronchopleural fistula have been less obvious; this has led to a tendency toward

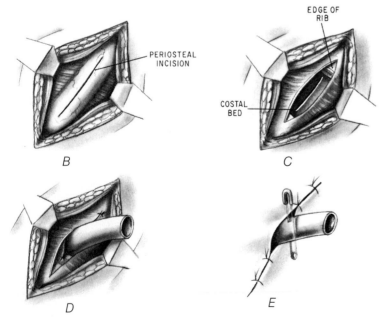

Fig. 17-22. Thoracostomy for open drainage of empyema. *A.* Incision positioned over posterior and inferior portion of empyema cavity. *B.* Exposed segment of rib and periosteal incision. *C.* Segment of rib has been excised subperiosteally. *D.* Drainage tube inserted into empyema cavity. *E.* Safety pin on tube to prevent loss of tube into pleural cavity.

a less vigorous approach to the problem. It is not uncommon now to see patients who are permitted to continue to cough up some empyema fluid for days or even weeks because only inadequate catheter drainage of the empyema has been established. A properly placed open thoracostomy (often with a rib resection) is a much safer way of accomplishing complete and continued evacuation of an empyema complicated by a bronchopleural fistula.

CHRONIC EMPYEMA

Chronic empyema may develop because an acute empyema was not recognized and properly treated. The use of antibiotics during a pulmonary infection or other suppurative process which may be the primary cause of an empyema may lead to an attenuation of the associated pleural infection without complete subsidence of the infection. The patient may become afebrile for a varying period of time. In some cases months or even years may elapse before clinical evidence of recurrent infection becomes manifest. The likelihood of a chronic empyema developing is enhanced if complete obliteration of the pleural cavity was not attained when the acute empyema was treated. This may occur following aspiration or closed or open drainage. Premature removal of a drainage tube is one cause of chronic empyema. Tuberculosis of the pleura also leads to chronicity. Disease of the lung or bronchi which interferes with pulmonary reexpansion favors the persistence of the empyema cavity. A bronchopleural fistula is an important cause of chronic empyema, especially following pulmonary surgical procedures.

The treatment of chronic empyema depends on the size of the empyema cavity, the rigidity of the walls of the pocket, and the ability of the lung to reexpand. In some cases only adequate open drainage is required. Decortication of the lung is one of the most useful procedures; it may greatly shorten the period of morbidity and lead to a much better final result from the standpoint of pulmonary function. If there is significant disease in the underlying lung, resection of a portion of the lung in conjunction with decortication may be required. In some instances this may have to be combined with a partial thoracoplasty to lessen the size of the space into which the decorticated lung must expand in order to obliterate the pleural cavity.

DECORTICATION OF THE LUNG. Decortication of the lung consists of the removal of a restrictive membrane or layer of tissue from the surface of the lung in order to improve pulmonary ventilatory motion. Decortication is usually performed surgically but in some instances may be effected by the employment of lytic agents intrapleurally when the covering over the lung is only a fibrinous exudate which has not yet developed into fibrous tissue.

Decortication of the lung may be indicated when it is deemed that the pulmonary function would be significantly improved by the removal of a restrictive layer over the lung (Fig. 17-23). Before deciding that a decortication is indicated, consideration must be given to whether the thickening of the patient's pleura would largely disappear spontaneously if an adequate period of time were permitted to elapse. An acute empyema may have a parietal pleura over 1 cm in thickness which can, in a period of months, regress to a thin, nonrestrictive layer. An edematous pleural covering may feel hard and thus be erroneously assumed to consist of dense fibrous tissue which would remain permanently unless removed surgically. Surgeons who have had limited experience in the treatment of acute empyema tend to think that many cases require decortication, whereas this procedure is usually not required in acute empyema if early adequate therapy has been instituted.

Tuberculosis

The most common form of involvement of the pleura in a patient with pulmonary tuberculosis is a fibrinous pleurisy which overlies the pulmonary lesion. Such a pleuritic reaction often results in the development of localized pleural adhesions which lessen the possibility of rupture of a subpleural tuberculous focus into the pleura space. Hence this type of a pleuritic reaction is beneficial in the same way that adhesions may protect the pleural cavity from other types of necrotizing pulmonary lesions.

A serofibrinous pleurisy may develop in cases of pulmonary tuberculosis. In some patients the parenchymal tuber-

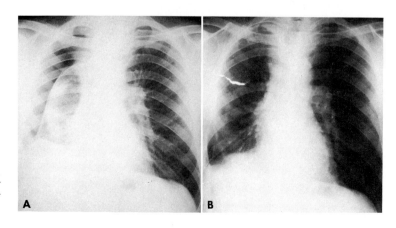

Fig. 17-23. Decortication for unexpanded lung. *A.* Unexpandable lung following pneumothorax for pulmonary tuberculosis. *B.* Reexpanded lung after pulmonary decortication.

culous lesion may be very small or obscured by the overlying pleural involvement. Malaise and fever may be the presenting symptoms. A cough which may or may not be productive may be present. If the effusion is large, dyspnea may be noted.

In many patients with a serofibrinous pleurisy the cause of the effusion is in doubt. Although in the past it was considered probable that most such effusions had a tuberculous origin, it is becoming more and more apparent that a wide variety of viral agents cause pleural effusions. Hence, there has been an increasing tendency in recent years to obtain a biopsy of the pleura by some technique so as to establish more accurately the exact nature of the pathologic process.

It is very important to recognize the possibility that one may be dealing with a tuberculous empyema, because the treatment differs from that of a pyogenic empyema. If an adequately evacuated empyema cavity continues to drain a considerable amount of pus, if the wall of the empyema is lined by unhealthy granulations, and if the patient's clinical progress is not satisfactory, the possibility of tuberculosis of the pleura should be considered. A biopsy of the pleura is then indicated.

An open drainage of a pure tuberculous empyema is contraindicated unless necessitated by a bronchopleural fistula. If thoracostomy and tube drainage is established in a tuberculous empyema, secondary infection of the tuberculous pleural cavity by a pyogenic organism may lead to a febrile downhill course. Prior to the days of antituberculous agents, a high mortality was associated with open drainage of a tuberculous empyema; now, active treatment with antituberculous drugs is generally effective. Pleural decortication may cure the tuberculous empyema if adequate pulmonary reexpansion can be obtained.

Fig. 17-24. Chylothorax. Note accumulation of fluid in pleural cavity, bilateral pulmonary fibrosis, and dilated pulmonary lymphatics.

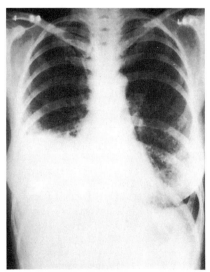

Chylothorax

Chyle may leak into the pleural cavity as a result of a variety of etiologic factors. The two most common causes of chylothorax are trauma and neoplasm. Other rare causes of chylous fluid in a pleural space are congenital anomalies of the lymphatics in the mediastinum or lung, thrombosis or other obstruction of the large veins of the upper portion of the body, and rare pulmonary lesions permitting the retrograde flow of chyle into the lung and hence into the pleural cavity (Fig. 17-24).

The trauma responsible for chylothorax may vary but in most instances results in a severence or rupture of the thoracic duct or one of its major branches. Penetrating injuries and inadvertent surgical severence of the thoracic duct may be the cause of chylothorax. Hyperextension of the spine is sometimes the apparent cause of ductal rupture. In a few cases a very minor stretching of the thoracic duct may be held responsible for its injury, but in some of these patients a further follow-up may disclose that an unrecognized neoplasm was actually present.

A variety of neoplasms may result in chylothorax. Lymphosarcoma is particularly likely to obstruct the thoracic duct, but metastatic carcinoma and occasionally rare tumors of the thoracic duct itself are responsible.

The management of chylothorax is influenced by the causative factor and the persistence of the chylous reaccumulation in the pleural cavity. In some cases the chylothorax will disappear after a few thoracenteses with the patient on a low-fat diet. Closed intercostal drainage of the pleural space which tends to favor sealing off the seepage from lymphatic channels by promoting full lung reexpansion may be effective. Care must be taken to avoid nutritional depletion of the patient by a large chyle loss. Radiation therapy has controlled chylothorax secondary to neoplasms. When these methods are unsatisfactory, thoracotomy with ligation of the thoracic duct low in the mediastinum is indicated.

Calcification

Calcification of the pleura usually results from a chronic pleuritis. It may be caused by an unabsorbed hemothorax of traumatic or other origin. It may follow a serous pleurisy or empyema of tuberculous cause. Occasionally a chronic nontuberculous empyema may lead to some pleural calcification. In some patients who had prolonged pneumothorax therapy for pulmonary tuberculosis which was associated with pleural effusion, calcification of the pleura later developed (Fig. 17-25).

In most instances there is considerable fibrous tissue over the pleural surface which contains calcium plaques, but in occasional cases localized calcium plaques may have relatively little adjacent pleural thickening. The calcium deposits may be deeply imbedded in a greatly thickened pleura, or some of the plaques may project irregularly from the shaggy wall of a chronic empyema cavity or lie free in the dependent part of the pleural space. Calcification tends to be more marked in the parietal than in the visceral surfaces. Sometimes an extensive sheet of calcium may be present.

The calcification of the pleura is usually not in itself the cause of symptoms, although the associated fibrous tissue often impairs pulmonary function by interfering with lung motion. Rarely a sharp calcium plaque erodes the visceral pleura and results in hemoptysis or hemothorax. The chief clinical importance of calcification of the pleura lies in its potential association with a chronic empyema of tuberculous or nontuberculous cause, often with a bronchopleural fistula. Healing cannot be expected after open drainage of an empyema with calcium plaques in the walls of the cavity unless it is feasible later to perform a decortication of the lung or a radical thoracoplasty and pleurectomy, which removes the calcium, which otherwise would continue to act as a foreign body.

Tumors

PRIMARY TUMORS

Although primary tumors of the pleura are uncommon, such neoplasms are now being encountered more frequently because of the increased use of chest radiography and surgical exploration of the thorax. The clinical, roentgenographic, and pathologic characteristics of these tumors vary.

Primary pleural tumors may be conveniently divided into localized and diffuse types. The localized type of tumor is usually benign and is either a fibroma or mesothelioma. Severe hypoglycemia, which may even progress to result in coma, may be caused by a large pleural mesothelioma or mesodermal tumor. The hypoglycemia is cured by surgical excision of the tumor.

Attachment to the visceral pleura is most common. Often the greater part of the mass is free in the pleural cavity with both visceral and parietal attachments. Primary pleural tumors occur in all decades of life. Malignant pleural mesothelioma is not uncommon in patients under twenty years of age in comparison to the extreme rarity of malignant pulmonary tumors in that age group. Asbestosis has been linked with some malignant mesotheliomas.

The following may aid in the recognition of the *localized benign pleural mesothelioma:* (1) the location of the tumor corresponds to the site of an interlobar fissure or periphery of lung; (2) symptoms are usually absent until the tumor attains large size, in contrast to the course in many bronchogenic neoplasms; (3) pulmonary osteoarthropathy of long duration is not uncommon, especially if the tumor is large and vascular. Surgical excision of the tumor is indicated, and the prognosis is very good, but there may be local recurrence.

The *diffuse malignant mesothelioma* often simulates pleural effusion. Fever may be present. Cough and sputum are not unusual. Hemoptysis occasionally is present. The roentgenographic findings are usually those of pleural effusion, sometimes encapsulated. Thoracentesis yields bloody fluid in varying quantity. The diagnosis may be established by microscopic examination of this fluid. Too

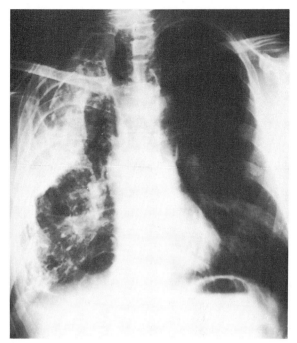

Fig. 17-25. Calcification of pleura following chronic tuberculous pleuritis.

often the material obtained is not sent to the laboratory because it is assumed to be frank blood. The prognosis of malignant mesothelioma is poor with either surgical or radiation therapy, and chemotherapy has been of limited value.

SECONDARY NEOPLASMS

Many neoplasms may be complicated by metastatic deposits on the pleura (Fig. 17-26). Although in most instances there are associated metastases in the lungs, in some cases the intrathoracic metastatic lesions may be apparently limited to the pleural cavity. In some patients the presenting evidence of illness may be shortness of breath caused by the associated pleural effusion, since the primary neoplasm has not yet caused any symptoms. When a serosanguineous fluid is found, the suspicion of neoplastic involvement should be very great, although a variety of other lesions, notably pulmonary infarction, can be responsible for blood-tinged pleural fluid. Cytologic examination of the sediment of the aspirated fluid is mandatory. Various diagnostic procedures to determine the primary site of the neoplasm are indicated, as such knowledge may determine the type and feasibility of therapy.

Pleural effusions caused by carcinomatous involvement of the pleura may tend to reaccumulate rapidly after thoracentesis. Closed intercostal tube drainage maintained for several days may permit reexpansion of the lung and result in obliteration of the pleural space, thus eliminating the problems and disadvantages of repeated aspirations. At times a thoracotomy and pleurectomy may be of benefit. Intrapleural instillation of cytotoxic agents is indicated in selected cases in addition to systemic treatment.

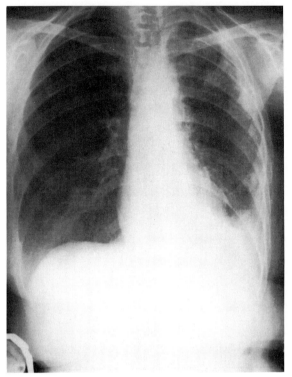

Fig. 17-26. Carcinoma of left pleura secondary to carcinoma of the breast. Treatment was by hormone therapy.

DISEASES OF THE LUNGS

Congenital Malformations

PULMONARY AGENESIS

Unilateral pulmonary agenesis (Fig. 17-27) may be compatible with long survival without symptoms provided other serious congenital anomalies are not present. The survival rate is much poorer in cases of agenesis of the right lung, but this is chiefly because associated cardiac abnormalities are more common. The changes in lung function as well as the physical and roentgenographic findings are similar to those seen after pneumonectomy performed in childhood, and the condition must be differentiated from atelectasis and hypoplasia of the lung.

Bronchoscopy, bronchography, and angiography are helpful diagnostic measures to demonstrate whether a rudimentary lung is present or whether complete agenesis of one lung exists.

HYPOPLASIA OF A LUNG

Varying degrees of hypoplasia of one lung may occur. Such lungs may have only one lobe with abnormalities of the bronchial distribution. Vascular anomalies are frequently found in such hypoplastic lungs; an abnormally large systemic vasculature may be associated with a hypoplastic pulmonary artery in such cases. If symptoms are present, dyspnea of varying degree may be noted. Hemoptysis may occur. At times the symptoms of vascular congestion in these abnormal lungs may simulate or predispose to secondary pulmonary infection. Roentgenograms may show a lung of diminished volume and abnormal vasculature. Angiocardiograms are a great aid in diagnosis, and may demonstrate that anomalous vessels traverse the diaphragm. The hypoplastic lung may have an arterial supply from anomalous branches of the aorta, or the lung may have anomalous pulmonary veins which drain into the inferior vena cava. Surgical intervention is indicated in certain carefully selected cases, usually because of hemoptysis or superimposed chronic infection, or because of associated congenital cardiac disease.

Pulmonary hypoplasia is a major cause of death of newborn infants with congenital diaphragmatic hernia. In those patients who survive, a degree of impaired function may be permanent.

VASCULAR ANOMALIES OF THE LUNGS

A variety of respiratory symptoms may be caused by vascular anomalies of the lungs, but in some cases there are no obvious symptoms. Angiograms are usually indicated in addition to the standard roentgenographic examinations. Barium studies of the esophagus may reveal various characteristic types of esophageal indentation by anomalous arteries.

ABSENCE OF MAIN PORTION OF PULMONARY ARTERY TO ONE LUNG. This may result in one lung receiving its entire circulation from enlarged bronchial arteries (Fig. 17-28). Such a lung may be prone to infection, and hemoptysis may occur because of the congestion resulting from the enlarged systemic blood supply. The involved lung has a reduced volume. Surgical reestablishment of the pulmonary circulation to such a lung may be feasible in early life.

SEQUESTRATION OF THE LUNG. This is a term that has been applied to a congenital maldevelopment of pulmonary tissue associated with anomalous systemic arteries (Fig. 17-29). In many instances the abnormal pulmonary tissue does not have a connection with the bronchial tree of the adjacent lung, and cyst formation is common. Secondary infection is a common complication of this congenital lesion and is the most common cause of symptoms. The cysts are most often located just above the diaphragm and most commonly on the left side. Both extralobar and intralobar sequestration of the lung may occur (Fig. 17-30). Surgical excision with due attention to the anomalous blood vessels is the therapy of choice.

ANOMALOUS ORIGIN OF A PULMONARY ARTERY. The pulmonary artery to one lung may arise from the aorta instead of the main pulmonary trunk and thus lead to an abnormally high pressure in the pulmonary artery to that lung which may result in pulmonary congestion and edema, with cardiac failure. Surgical transplantation of the anomalous vessel to the pulmonary artery, with or without a prosthetic bridge, is indicated.

An aberrant left pulmonary artery may arise from the pulmonary artery to the right side of the trachea and pass posteriorly between the trachea and esophagus, resulting in obstruction to the lower trachea or right main stem bronchus. Surgical correction may be achieved by dividing the aberrant pulmonary artery and reanastomosing it in front of the trachea.

CONGENITAL CYSTIC ADENOMATOID MALFORMATION. This usually presents in infancy as a large pulmonary mass containing cystic cavities which often displaces the mediastinum toward the opposite side. Tall mucoid epithelium lines the cystic spaces. Often the infant is born prematurely, and dyspnea occurs early. Early surgical excision of the involved lobe of lung is indicated. The prognosis is better in older children.

HYPERLUCENT LUNG. The term *hyperlucent lung* has been applied to a condition in which the roentgenogram shows hyperlucency of the lung due chiefly to a decrease in pulmonary vasculature. The reduced pulmonary blood flow may be associated with some degree of pulmonary hypoplasia but more often is the result of acquired chronic pulmonary infection.

PULMONARY ARTERIOVENOUS FISTULA. A pulmonary arteriovenous fistula consists of a cavernous hemangioma with direct communication between a pulmonary artery and pulmonary vein. This leads to the shunting of a variable amount of blood from the pulmonary arterial system to the pulmonary veins without traversing the capillary bed. The condition is usually congenital, and the lesions may be single or multiple. Many persons with such anomalous pulmonary vessels have other evidence of multiple hemangiomas; the lips and nasal mucous membrane are common sites of involvement. A familial history of multiple hemangiomas is not uncommon.

When a considerable amount of the venous blood from the pulmonary artery is shunted directly into the pulmonary veins, varying degrees of oxygen unsaturation of the systemic arterial blood develop. Since in some large pulmonary arteriovenous aneurysms even more than half of the pulmonary blood flow may be shunted through the anomalous channels, varying degrees of cyanosis may be noted in severe cases. With small fistulas, cyanosis may not be present. In contrast to an arteriovenous fistula in the systemic circulation, cardiac enlargement and hypertrophy are usually absent even in large arteriovenous aneurysms in the pulmonary circuit. The pulmonary artery pressure is usually normal in spite of the increase in pulmonary blood flow. Cor pulmonale is very rare and is seen only with numerous arteriovenous fistulas.

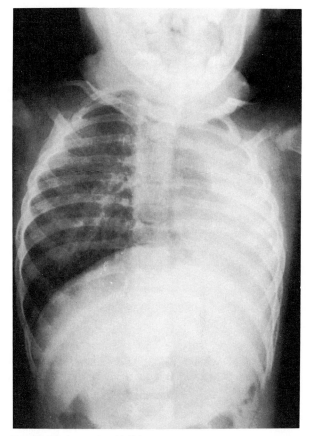

Fig. 17-27. Agenesis of left lung.

Clinical manifestations usually depend upon the size and number of the pulmonary arteriovenous shunts. Many small lesions are asymptomatic. Some are incidental roentgenographic findings and may appear as small circumscribed densities in the lung field simulating the appearance of a tumor. Hemoptysis may occur. When a large arteriovenous shunt is present, cyanosis and the symptoms associated with secondary polycythemia may appear. Cyanotic patients usually have a considerable increase in the hemoglobin, red cell count, and hematocrit. The plasma

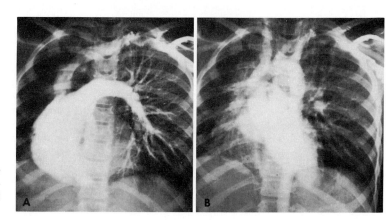

Fig. 17-28. Absence of main portion of pulmonary artery to one lung. *A.* Angiogram fails to demonstrate any right pulmonary artery. *B.* Enlarged bronchial circulation to right lung is visualized.

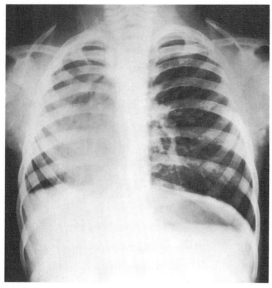

Fig. 17-29. Hypoplastic right lung with hypoplastic right pulmonary artery and anomalous systemic arteries from abdominal aorta. Girl was dyspneic at age twelve but became asymptomatic after anomalous arteries were ligated.

volume is usually not increased. In some roentgenograms, an enlarged pulmonary arterial shadow leading to the otherwise circumscribed area of density in the lung field indicates the probable diagnosis. Angiocardiograms are diagnostic and often indicate that multiple lesions are present. Secondary brain abscess and bacterial endocarditis are occasional complications. Polycythemia vera and con-

Fig. 17-30. Intralobar sequestration. Surgical specimen has been injected with radiopaque medium via large anomalous systemic artery. This demonstrates a very vascular wall over the bronchogenic cavity.

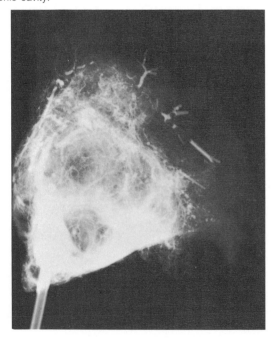

genital heart disease are the conditions most likely to be confused with pulmonary arteriovenous fistula.

The treatment of a solitary pulmonary arteriovenous fistula is surgical. Most lesions can be successfully removed by segmental resection or lobectomy. After removal of the lesion, all clinical manifestations usually regress to normal, but occasionally other fistulas become manifest later. When multiple small hemangiomas are present, surgical intervention is usually not advisable.

PULMONARY LYMPHANGIECTASIS. Dilatation of the lymphatic channels in the lungs and pleurae may be congenital or acquired. In the congenital cases the abnormality of lymphatic development is often rather widespread, and the changes present in the lung may be only a part of a generalized process. Sometimes the congenital lymphatic maldevelopment is associated with other congenital defects. Cystic formation in the lungs may accompany the lymphangiectasis. In the acquired pulmonary lymphangiectasis other pulmonary changes such as pulmonary fibrosis are usually a prominent feature and may obscure the dilatation of the lymphatics. A cystic type of emphysema and marked hypertrophy of the smooth muscle in the lungs are other features frequently noted together with an inflammatory component which may be primary or secondary.

Although in almost all reported cases of pulmonary lymphangiectasis which have been recognized so far in infancy the patients have died, there is mounting evidence that patients with lesser degrees of lymphangiectasis may be relatively asymptomatic in infancy, the pulmonary disease becoming manifest only at an older age. When symptoms are present in the neonatal period, dyspnea is usually the presenting symptom; the respiratory difficulty may be pronounced and present from birth. The roentgenographic pulmonary findings may be difficult to interpret. Pleural effusion may be present a few hours after birth. Chylothorax may be secondary to pulmonary and pleural lymphangiectasis. Surgery is indicated if pulmonary lymphangiectasis is of limited distribution or if pleural effusion does not respond to thoracentesis.

LOBAR EMPHYSEMA OF INFANCY

One cause of dyspnea in infancy is the development of emphysema in a portion of a lung unassociated with obstruction of a bronchus by an anomalous vessel, inhaled foreign body, or infection. The pathologic process often has a lobar distribution but on occasion may involve less than a lobe or the greater portion of the entire lung. A variety of etiologic factors have been thought to explain different cases; congenital deficiency of the cartilage in the lobar bronchus and a diffuse structural deficiency in the involved portion of lung have been described.

CLINICAL MANIFESTATIONS. Respiratory difficulty is usually first noticed when the infant is several weeks of age and may rapidly reach a serious stage. The radiographic appearance of the lung is quite diagnostic; the lung on one side shows marked hyperinflation in all phases of respiration and mediastinal displacement to the opposite side. Unless the findings of auscultation are interpreted in relation to the roentgenographic findings, lobar obstructive emphysema of one side may be incorrectly diagnosed as atelectasis of the opposite side; that is, obstructive emphysema is confused with compensatory emphysema (Fig. 17-31). Breath sounds tend to be absent over the lung with obstructive emphysema, while the contralateral lung, which is compressed by the shifted mediastinum, reveals prominent breath sounds. With compensatory emphysema breath sounds are usually present.

TREATMENT. The treatment of lobar obstructive emphysema is surgical excision of the involved lobe or segment. The operation may be an emergency procedure, because the respiratory difficulty may progress to a critical stage in a short space of time. The operation permits the remaining lung tissue, which preoperatively was compressed by the hyperinflated lobe, to expand and resume function. Usually the prognosis is good; occasionally the condition recurs in another lobe.

Cystic Disease of the Lung

The term *cystic disease of the lung* has been applied to a wide variety of pulmonary lesions characterized by the presence of air- or fluid-containing spaces within the lung. Most lesions designated as cysts of the lung are not congenital but are acquired secondary to infection, partial bronchial obstruction, and obstructive emphysema.

The use of the term "pulmonary cyst" without due regard for the pathologic characteristics of such cavities is unsatisfactory. The mechanics of the cavity formation and the structural characteristics of the cavity wall determine the distinctive clinical features of the various types of cystlike pulmonary conditions. Rational treatment can be applied only when the factors which differentiate the various types of lesions are evaluated.

The formation of a cavity in the lung depends on (1) a developmental abnormality, (2) destruction of pulmonary tissue by an inflammatory process, or (3) hyperinflation of a small defect in the pulmonary parenchyma, or a combination of these processes. Persistence of intrapulmonary cavities may be due to one or more of the following factors: (1) positive intracavitary pressure, (2) progressive destructive process within the lung, (3) loss of expansibility of surrounding pulmonary tissue, (4) elastic properties of the pericavitary tissue, or (5) epithelialization of the cavity wall.

The various factors just enumerated determine whether a given pulmonary cavity is likely to disappear spontaneously, whether the cavity can obliterate itself after drainage or whether excision of pulmonary tissue is necessary. A cavity which owes its size chiefly to hyperinflation by a check-valve mechanism of the communicating bronchus may have a very different clinical course from that of a cavity produced by destruction of pulmonary tissue.

The following types of lesions have been included under the term "pulmonary cysts"; the diagnosis and treatment of each type will be discussed in the section dealing with the particular pathologic entity.

1. Congenital pulmonary cysts.
2. Pneumatoceles: nonepithelialized positive-pressure cavities produced by the hyperinflation of a defect in the pulmonary parenchyma resulting from pulmonary disruption or infection.

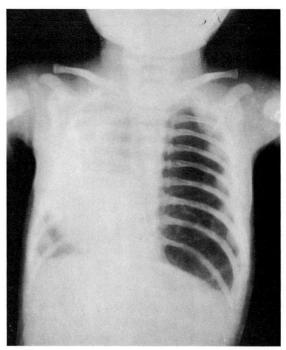

Fig. 17-31. Obstructive emphysema of lingular portion of left lung. Note marked mediastinal displacement to right. Treatment by emergency resection of involved segment during infancy was successful.

3. Emphysematous bullae: nonepithelialized pulmonary cavities produced chiefly by the disruption of interalveolar septa.
4. Pulmonary blebs: localized collections of air within the pleural interstitial tissue.
5. Cystic bronchiectasis: a cystlike dilatation of the bronchi which may be congenital but is usually acquired secondary to infection.
6. Acquired intrapulmonary cavities originally caused by the destruction of pulmonary tissue by infection due to pyogens or fungi. The cavity may or may not be epithelialized.
7. Parasitic cysts.

CONGENITAL CYSTIC DISEASE OF THE LUNG

This is relatively rare (Fig. 17-32) and is due to embryologic maldevelopment of the lungs. Congenital cysts may be single or multiple, fluid- or air-containing. Such cysts are sometimes associated with anomalies of lobar development of the lung together with anomalies of the pulmonary or bronchial vessels. The cyst may have an epithelial lining. If such cysts become distended, dyspnea and cyanosis may be present. Frequently the first symptoms, which may occur in childhood or later, are those of secondary infection, to which such lesions are prone. The larger lesions may simulate a pneumothorax (Fig. 17-33) or encapsulated empyema. Surgical excision of true congenital cysts is usually indicated.

AIR CYSTS

Pneumatoceles, emphysematous bullae, and *pulmonary blebs* are types of air cysts. Pneumatoceles are often a temporary roentgenographic finding following pulmonary infections which are prone to cause areas of localized

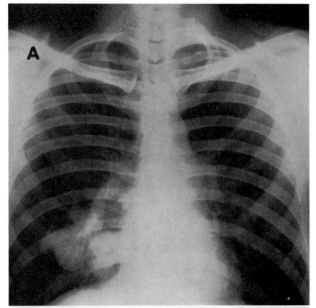

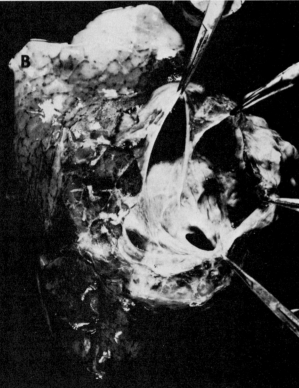

Fig. 17-32. Multilocular bronchogenic cysts of right lower lobe. *A.* Roentgenographic appearance. *B.* Open cysts and operative lobectomy specimen.

obstructive emphysema. Such air spaces are most common with certain types of pneumonia in infancy and childhood, although a similar air cyst is occasionally seen with pneumonia in adults. Emphysematous bullae and pulmonary blebs are usually found in adult patients with varying degrees of diffuse emphysema.

CLINICAL MANIFESTATIONS. Air cysts may be asymptomatic, but not infrequently because of a check-valve mechanism of the communicating bronchus the cyst becomes hyperinflated and may assume a huge size. These balloon cysts may encroach on the remaining pulmonary tissue to a sufficient degree to cause respiratory insufficiency. The physical signs vary and are rarely diagnostic.

ROENTGENOGRAPHIC FINDINGS. These are the most important diagnostic studies. The fluid cysts appear on the roentgenogram as round or oval areas of increased density. If the cyst communicates with a bronchus, a fluid level may be present. The air-filled cavities appear as round or oval areas of increased radiolucency. The location and contour of the area of radiolucency may serve to differentiate an intrapulmonary cavity from a localized pneumothorax. In expansile cysts there may be evidence of compression of the surrounding pulmonary parenchyma. The large positive-pressure cysts may occupy almost an entire hemithorax and may even displace the mediastinum markedly toward the opposite side. This latter type of cyst is frequently incorrectly diagnosed as a tension pneumothorax. The two conditions can usually be differentiated radiographically. In the case of a huge cyst there is no prominence at the pulmonary hilus representing collapsed lung, and the costophrenic sinus contains compressed pulmonary tissue.

DIFFERENTIAL DIAGNOSIS. In pulmonary emphysema there is fragmentation of the elastic tissue with rupture of the interalveolar septa. In most cases of pulmonary emphysema the number of alveolar septa which rupture in a given area is sufficient to produce only a small cavity. The disruption of the interalveolar septa may be fairly uniform throughout the lung, although there is a tendency for the process to be pronounced in certain areas, especially along the border of the lung and in the pulmonary apices. In cases of diffuse emphysema, the roentgenogram shows increased radiolucency throughout the pulmonary field. If, on the other hand, extensive disruption of the interalveolar septa occurs in a localized portion of the lung, a large cavity, called a *bulla,* is produced. One or more such bullae may be present. The cavity is lined by the walls of the surrounding alveoli, and there is no true epithelial lining. The bullous cavity has a rather poor communication with the bronchial tree by means of one or more small bronchi. The bulla shows on the roentgenogram as an area of even greater radiolucency than the surrounding emphysematous lung. If the bulla is large, there may be an absence of pulmonary markings in that region. In some instances the outline of the bulla may be clearly defined on the roentgenogram, but frequently the borders are indistinct.

In infants and children especially, pneumatoceles may attain huge size. One or more pneumatoceles may occupy almost an entire hemithorax and markedly compress the surrounding pulmonary tissue. Some pneumatoceles may disappear in a few weeks, while others persist and often fluctuate in size over a period of months or years, although the patient is asymptomatic.

TREATMENT. The pneumatocele may disappear spontaneously after it has been present even for months. A pneumatocele usually requires no surgical treatment, in contrast to congenital pulmonary cysts and huge abscess cavities from which it must be differentiated. Pulmonary bullae and pleural blebs may at times compress the adjacent lung tissue, thus causing impairment of the pulmonary function beyond that caused by the associated pulmonary emphysema alone (Fig. 17-34). The surgical resection of such bullae and blebs can be expected to be beneficial only if their removal improves the function of the remaining portion of lung. If operation is undertaken when the adjacent lung tissue cannot expand, there is a considerable risk of postoperative complications and mortality. Therefore these patients require thorough investigation of pulmonary function with a study of the blood gases, prior to any decision as to the wisdom of surgical intervention. In properly selected cases considerable improvement in lung function may follow operation. All efforts to lessen prolonged air leakage from the transected emphysematous pulmonary tissue should be made by the most atraumatic suturing of the abnormal lung tissue.

Trauma to Lung and Airways

FOREIGN BODIES IN THE AIRWAY

ETIOLOGY. Inhaled foreign bodies are an important cause of respiratory difficulty in infancy and childhood, and are an occasional etiologic factor in adults, especially after general anesthesia or other episodes of unconsciousness. The mentally ill patient may harbor a variety of foreign objects. Foreign bodies which are not radiopaque are a particular threat, because the chest roentgenogram taken for evaluation of respiratory symptoms or signs may not indicate their presence. A large foreign body lodged in the upper esophagus may cause respiratory symptoms by tracheal compression, especially in infants. Foreign bodies may be of a great variety, especially in infants and in mentally ill adults. In addition to those objects which human beings might ordinarily handle, such plant substances as timothy seeds which some persons may habitually place in their mouths may be etiologic agents of a severe chronic pneumonitis, as is an aspirated peanut.

CLINICAL MANIFESTATIONS. In infancy respiratory distress is often a presenting feature. Cough with signs and symptoms of bronchial obstruction may be noted in any age group. The degree of secondary pneumonitis depends on the nature of the foreign body, the extent of bronchial obstruction, and the duration of its presence. Hemoptysis may occur. The lack of any definite history in the case of an infant does not rule out a foreign body as the cause of airway obstruction. Adequate roentgenograms are essential. The findings at first will vary from obstructive emphysema to atelectasis with, later, pneumonitis. A bronchoscopic examination is indicated in all suspected cases.

TREATMENT. Endoscopic removal is usually feasible unless a small object has migrated into a peripheral bronchus. Early removal of foreign bodies, before secondary suppuration has occurred, is indicated. A foreign body in the trachea requires emergency treatment. Some small foreign bodies in the peripheral parts of the lungs may

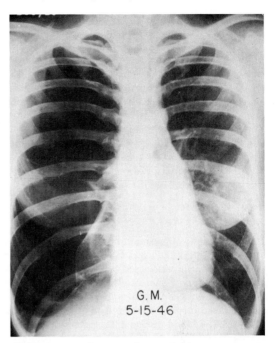

Fig. 17-33. Large pulmonary air cyst. Lesion occupies almost entire right hemothorax and was erroneously regarded as a pneumothorax.

be removed by thoracotomy and possible bronchotomy, but not every nonirritating small fragment which is not causing symptoms requires surgical removal. An aspirated peanut or timothy seed which cannot be removed by bron-

Fig. 17-34. Giant bulla of right lung. There is associated diffuse pulmonary fibrosis and emphysema. Much improvement is respiratory function followed excision of the cyst.

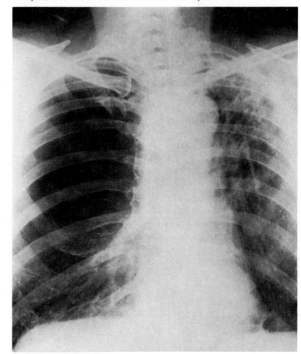

choscopy should be removed by early thoracotomy and bronchotomy in view of the inflammatory reaction provoked by these objects.

Retained foreign bodies in the bronchi are a cause of pulmonary abscess and bronchiectasis. Depending on the degree of pulmonary damage at the time when the foreign body is removed endoscopically, the secondary suppurative process in the lung may largely resolve or require a limited pulmonary resection. At times granulation tissue surrounding an irritating foreign body may obscure the foreign body from endoscopic identification, and the foreign body as the etiologic factor of the pulmonary suppuration may be recognized only at the time of a pulmonary resection.

TRAUMA TO THE LUNG

With both blunt and penetrating injuries of the chest trauma to the lung may occur. Contusion and hematoma of the lung may be associated with varying degrees of edema and secondary pneumonitis. In severe penetrating injuries of the lung emergency thoractomy may be required for the control of bleeding and repair of extensive lacerations. At times pulmonary resection may be necessary. Pulmonary infection frequently results from the retention of secretions and blood in the bronchi, and therefore antibiotic therapy is often indicated in conjunction with measures to improve the bronchial drainage. Severe trauma to the lung may damage the blood supply and occasionally result in pulmonary gangrene. The "wet lung" is a serious complication of severe injury to the chest wall and intrathoracic viscera. Assisted respiration may be of vital importance in pulmonary trauma, and adequate oxygen therapy is also important. It is extremely difficult to differentiate destroyed lung from tissue which will recover

Fig. 17-35. Segmental bronchi. *A.* Anteroposterior view. *B.* Oblique view. *C.* Right lateral view. *D.* Diagram of saccular bronchiectasis of right lower lobe, left lower lobe, and lingula of left upper lobe.

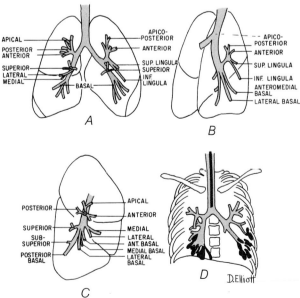

if early thoracotomy is performed. Therefore, one should be very conservative in considering pulmonary resection for blunt trauma.

TRAUMATIC RUPTURE OF BRONCHI OR TRACHEA

Severe blunt trauma or, occasionally, penetrating injury to the thorax may result in rupture of a bronchus or the trachea. Such rupture may occur with surprisingly little evidence of chest wall injury, especially in the child with a compressible thorax. A pneumothorax with evidence of a large continuing air leak via a thoracotomy tube should lead to consideration of tracheal or bronchial rupture. Deep cervical emphysema is a reliable clue. Bronchoscopic examination is usually indicated. In cases with severe respiratory distress a tracheostomy may have already been done as a resuscitative measure. However, tracheostomy alone is not recommended except for patients with fracture of tracheal cartilage, larynx, or cricoid cartilages. A thoracotomy is indicated for immediate primary suture repair of tracheal or bronchial rupture.

At times complete rupture of a bronchus is not recognized at the time of injury and is manifest later by atelectasis of the lung. Repair of such a bronchial disruption is indicated and may be feasible even many months after the injury if secondary pulmonary suppuration has not developed. Such a lung can be reexpanded with the resultant return of considerable pulmonary function.

Inflammation and Infection

BRONCHIECTASIS

Bronchiectasis is an abnormal state of bronchial dilatation which tends to involve certain segmental bronchi (Fig. 17-35). The condition is most commonly the result of chronic infection in the lungs and bronchi, but occasionally bronchiectasis is due to congenital malformation of the bronchial tree. The significant dilatation occurs in the distal portions of the bronchi, which normally should be tapering into smaller and smaller branches. The bronchial lesions are associated with widely varying degrees of pulmonary inflammatory and fibrotic changes depending on the nature, severity, and duration of the pathologic process. Bronchiectasis may occur distal to bronchial obstruction of varied causes or develop as a result of chronic infection in the lungs without any proximal bronchial stenosis.

It is important to differentiate bronchiectasis from *bronchiectasia;* the former implies an essentially irreversible pathologic process, whereas bronchiectasia refers to a bronchial dilatation which may or may not be reversible. Bronchial dilatation distal to a bronchial obstruction may be reversible; the chances of avoiding irreversible bronchial dilatation depend on the duration of the bronchial obstruction and the degree and nature of infection distal to the obstruction. Because infection distal to a bronchostenosis is of prime importance in producing bronchiectasis, significant bronchiectasis may not develop if effective antibiotic therapy is given while the bronchial obstruction is present. Prior to the advent of effective chemotherapy, in most patients with bronchostenosis of any prolonged duration significant bronchiectasis usually developed. Since antibiotics have become available, bronchial obstruction of many months' duration does not always result in irreversible bronchiectasis.

ETIOLOGY. Bronchiectasis secondary to a bronchial obstruction may be seen with benign and malignant bronchial tumors, foreign bodies in the bronchi, ulcerative bronchial stenosis, broncholiths, trauma, and compression of the bronchus by extrabronchial lesions. In all these situations the therapy is directed at the primary lesion causing the bronchial stenosis to which the bronchiectasia or bronchiectasis is secondary. Therefore the discussion of the therapy of such secondary bronchiectasis is dealt with in those sections discussing the primary lesion. In some instances the secondary bronchiectasis may still be present after the bronchostenosis itself has been satisfactorily treated; in such cases the bronchiectasis would be managed as indicated in this section.

Bronchiectasis may also result from severe infection of the pulmonary parenchyma with resultant chronic inflammation and fibrosis. The etiology of the infection is of importance, as it may influence the therapy. The bronchiectasis which is secondary to pulmonary tuberculosis requires separate consideration in therapy and is discussed in the section on the surgery of pulmonary tuberculosis. Most cases of bronchiectasis which are not secondary to a localized bronchostenosis are the result of pneumonia. The incidence of such bronchiectasis is much lower now in many parts of the world since antibiotic treatment has become available for pneumonia.

CLINICAL MANIFESTATIONS. Chronic cough with purulent sputum of varying amounts is usually present. At times, the sputum may have a bad taste or foul odor. If there is little purulent expectoration, the term "dry bronchiectasis" has been applied. Hemoptysis of widely varying amounts may also be noted. In some patients, hemoptysis may be of considerable magnitude and represent the chief symptom. In females with dry bronchiectasis, the hemoptysis frequently occurs at the time of the menstrual period.

The presence or absence of dyspnea depends on the extent of bronchiectasis, its duration, and the degree of associated pulmonary fibrosis and emphysema. The patient's general health often appears normal, and weight loss is usually absent except in advanced cases with severe infection and reduction in pulmonary function with associated chronic hypoxemia. The patient with bronchiectasis is prone to recurrent attacks of pneumonia, although the incidence of such episodes has been considerably reduced by antibiotic therapy.

The location of chronically dilated infected bronchi will influence considerably the magnitude of symptoms and the need for surgical therapy. It is the dilated bronchi located in a dependent position which are most likely to cause trouble because of the tendency of infected bronchial secretions to stagnate in such dependent bronchi. Dilated bronchi in an upper lobe tend to drain spontaneously and hence are usually less symptomatic than similarly dilated bronchi in the basilar segments of the lower lobes. The magnitude of the bronchial dilatation is also often related to the severity of symptoms; the big dilatations of a saccular bronchiectasis are likely to be associated with more sputum and a poorer prognosis than when only a tubular bronchial dilatation is present.

DIAGNOSTIC FINDINGS. A patient with chronic cough and expectoration due to bronchiectasis may show no obvious abnormal roentgenographic findings on the routine film if examined at a time without much pneumonitis. A bronchogram is necessary for the diagnosis of bronchiectasis (Fig. 17-36). This examination will reveal both the character and distribution of the bronchiectasis if proper visualization of the entire bronchial tree is obtained with contrast medium. Both lungs should be studied. Repeated sputum examinations for tubercle bacilli are important in order to differentiate pyogenic bronchiectasis from the primarily tuberculous bronchiectasis.

DIFFERENTIAL DIAGNOSIS. When a segment or lobe of lung is involved by an inflammatory process, the regional peribronchial lymph nodes are likely to become enlarged. If a cluster of such enlarged nodes surrounds a bronchus, narrowing of the bronchial lumen by a combination of lymph node compression and bronchial mucosal edema may cause obstruction and atelectasis of the segment or lobe of lung. Because this anatomicopathologic situation

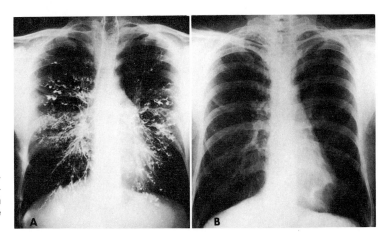

Fig. 17-36. Bronchiectasis. *A.* Bronchogram demonstrating diffuse bilateral congenital cystic bronchiectasis. *B.* Roentgenogram without contrast medium shows only some emphysema and faint outline of the cystic bronchiectasis.

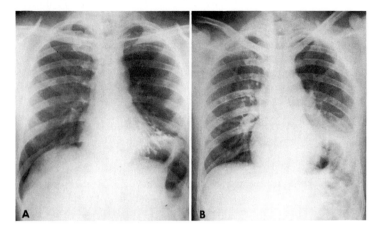

Fig. 17-37. Shrunken left lower lobe with bronchiectasis. *A.* Note compensatory hyperaeration of left upper lobe. *B.* Appearance shortly after left lower lobectomy. Note elevated diaphragm on that side.

is particularly likely to exist in the right middle lobe, the term "middle lobe syndrome" has been applied to this condition. It should be appreciated, however, that an essentially similar process occurs in other portions of the lungs although somewhat less frequently. If this type of bronchial obstruction with infection persists, bronchiectasis may develop, but if the obstruction is lessened by subsidence of the peribronchial lymph node swelling, reaeration of the lobe may occur before bronchiectasis is established. Although most cases of "middle lobe syndrome" are not due to bronchogenic tumor, similar clinical and roentgenographic findings may be seen with a carcinoma involving the area of the orifice of the right middle lobe bronchus. A bronchoscopic examination is an important measure to aid in the differentiation of the two conditions.

It is important to distinguish a bronchiectasis due to a pyogenic infection from that associated with pulmonary tuberculosis. The latter is most commonly seen in cases of chronic tuberculosis involving one or both upper lobes, but at times the tuberculous process is in a lower lobe. When tuberculous bronchiectasis is present, a considerable period of therapy with antituberculous agents should precede any surgical excision. Many patients with dilated

bronchi in an upper lobe with healed tuberculosis are quite asymptomatic and require no surgical intervention.

TREATMENT. When bronchiectasis is causing symptoms and the disease process is sufficiently localized, resection of the bronchiectatic portion is warranted (Fig. 17-37). A lobectomy or a segmental resection, or a combination of both, may be indicated after an adequate period of antibiotic therapy. At times a staged resection of portions of each lung or a pneumonectomy (Fig. 17-38) is feasible. The presence of associated pulmonary emphysema with the resultant decrease in pulmonary function may limit the feasibility of pulmonary resection, especially if the symptoms can be ameliorated by antibiotic therapy. Postural drainage of the bronchial tree can afford considerable palliation and also be of value in preoperative preparation. Studies of the bronchial flora may indicate the best antibiotic regimen.

LUNG ABSCESS

A pulmonary abscess is a suppurative focus within the lung associated with necrosis. Although inflammatory processes such as pneumonitis and bronchiectasis may show microscopic evidence of abscess formation, only

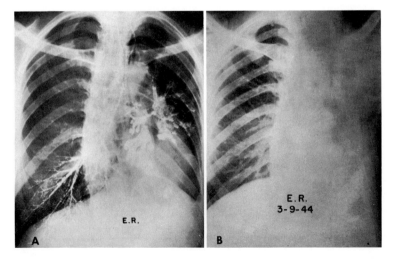

Fig. 17-38. Bronchiectasis of left lung. *A.* Preoperative bronchogram. Bronchospirometry revealed that left lung accounted for only 4 percent of total oxygen uptake. *B.* Roentgenogram following pneumonectomy and thoracoplasty.

those lesions in which the abscess is a predominant gross pathologic finding are classified clinically as pulmonary abscesses. When necrosis of tissue is the outstanding feature of the lesion, the term *gangrene of the lung* has been used. Most cases of gangrene of the lung can be considered to be pulmonary abscesses in which vascular thrombosis is a prominent feature.

ETIOLOGY AND PATHOGENESIS. Whenever the defensive mechanisms provided by the upper air passages are interfered with, the threat of pulmonary infection and abscess arises. Staphylococci, streptococci, Friedländer bacillus, *E. coli, Hemophilus influenzae, Pseudomonas aeruginosa, Actinomyces,* and various anaerobes are among the pathogenic bacteria commonly found. The pus from a pulmonary abscess often yields several types of bacteria, and more than one may play an etiologic role. This point should be borne in mind in the choice of antimicrobial therapy. Following chemotherapy the bacterial flora may change, because the reduction or elimination of the predominant organisms favors the emergence of secondary invaders. Thus fungi have become of greater etiologic importance since antimicrobial therapy. Coagulase-positive staphylococci have assumed a prominent role as the etiologic agent of pulmonary abscesses among hospitalized patients, especially among those with tracheostomy, or after a prolonged period of chemoprophylaxis with antimicrobial drugs. A pyogenic pulmonary abscess can develop as a complication of tuberculous bronchostenosis (Fig. 17-39).

The bacteria responsible for a pulmonary abscess may reach the lung through aspiration down the tracheobronchial tree, via the blood, or by penetrating trauma or extension of an adjacent suppurative focus. Infected material aspirated from the upper air passages, especially in persons with poor dental hygiene, may lodge in a small branch bronchus and produce an acute inflammatory process. Partial obstruction of a bronchus favors retention of secretion and suppuration in the corresponding bronchopulmonary segment. Tumors of the bronchus, foreign bodies, and various stenotic bronchial lesions frequently are responsible for abscess formation. Infected pulmonary emboli or secondary infection of any infarct may produce a lung abscess. Suppuration may also result from secondary infection of a pulmonary hematoma or from penetrating trauma. Pulmonary abscess may result from the extension of a suppurative focus from beneath the diaphragm into the adherent basal portion of the lung. Amebic abscess or perforating lesion of the esophagus may cause an abscess of the lung by direct extension. Obstructive lesions of the esophagus may cause abscesses in the lung by aspiration. Multiple pulmonary abscesses may occur as a complication of septicemia.

The location of pulmonary abscesses varies depending on the etiologic factors. Abscesses produced by aspiration are most common in those portions of the lung that are dependent in the recumbent position. The apical portions of the lower lobes and the posterior segments of the upper lobes are the most frequent sites of such abscesses. Pulmonary abscesses secondary to infarction are more common in the basal portions of the lower lobe. Abscess secondary

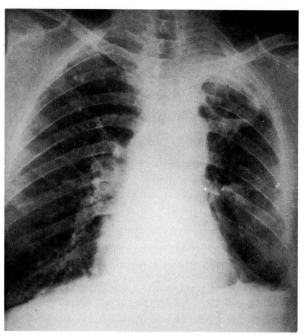

Fig. 17-39. Pyogenic pulmonary abscess as a complication of tuberculous bronchostenosis. Note old tuberculous lesions. Patient was treated by lobectomy.

to bronchial obstruction by tumor may occur in any portion of the lungs.

The nature of the predominant bacteria and the degree of local vascular thrombosis determine the extent of the abscess formation. The pathologic findings vary from lesions with a large area of pneumonia surrounding one or more pulmonary abscesses of varying size to necrosis of a large segment of lung tissue resulting from a pyogenic process with much vascular thrombosis. Foul pus usually indicates the presence of anaerobic infection. The degree of bronchial communication will determine the ease with which purulent material may drain from a pulmonary abscess and air may enter the cavity. With good bronchial drainage and antibiotic therapy in the acute phase, the abscess may progressively diminish in size and heal with only a residual fibrous scar. Edema and granulation tissue in the bronchus often interfere with bronchial drainage. If a pulmonary abscess becomes chronic, an increasing amount of fibrosis develops in the adjacent lung tissue, and bronchiectasis of varying extent is usually found.

A cavity resulting entirely from destruction of lung tissue must be differentiated from a small suppurative defect that is enlarged owing to localized obstructive emphysema. In staphylococcal pneumonia of infancy and childhood, the occurrence of such cavities is particularly common. Very few of these lesions fail to disappear under appropriate antimicrobial therapy.

CLINICAL MANIFESTATIONS. Pulmonary abscesses are more frequent in persons with oral sepsis and in those subject to spells of unconsciousness. Epileptics and persons with severe alcoholism are particularly prone to pulmonary suppuration. Aspiration into the lungs may also occur during general anesthesia, but this is becoming less frequent owing to improvements in anesthesiology. The symptoms at the onset of the illness are usually considered to be due to an acute bronchitis or pneumonia with cough, malaise, and fever. Chest pain is frequently present because of the development of pleuritis over the area of pulmonary involvement. Chills and night sweats may occur.

The patient with an acute lung abscess usually appears acutely ill. Dyspnea is usually not prominent except with massive involvement. In the absence of pleural complications, the physical signs may be meager. Slight dullness and rales may be noted. Early in the course of the disease, a localized pleural friction rub may be present. Localization of the site of the abscess, if pleural pain and chest wall tenderness are absent, is often difficult by physical examination alone. Auscultatory signs of cavitation are often absent. Clubbing of fingers is common in the subacute and chronic abscess. Leukocytosis is common, and anemia often develops with persisting infection.

The possibility of an abscess of the lung should be considered when a patient who is acutely ill begins to expectorate pus. It is of greatest importance to differentiate a primary pulmonary abscess from suppuration distal to a bronchial neoplasm. If the history does not suggest the possibility of aspiration of infectious material into the lungs or an embolic origin and the area of involvement corresponds to a bronchial segment, the possibility of a primary neoplasm is very real. Purulent expectoration of long duration is often due to bronchiectasis, but a chronic lung abscess must also be considered.

The nature of the sputum may warn the clinician that the process is not a simple pneumonia. Purulent expectoration is often present after the first few days, but when an abscess has developed distal to a bronchial obstruction, purulent sputum may be late in appearing or not be manifest because of interference with bronchial drainage. Foul sputum is typical; its occurrence will depend on the nature of the organisms, and it is less common if antimicrobial therapy has been employed in the early stages of the pneumonitis. Hemoptysis of varying amount may occur with a pulmonary abscess, and occasionally there are massive hemorrhages when much gangrene is present. The untreated pulmonary abscess often leads to progressive loss of weight and strength, with anemia. A pulmonary abscess distal to a bronchogenic carcinoma often causes little malaise, because the infection is less virulent.

DIAGNOSTIC FINDINGS. Roentgenographic studies are an important aid in the diagnosis of pulmonary abscess, but the findings may not be diagnostic. When the films demonstrate an intrapulmonary cavity, particularly with an air fluid level, and the patient is expectorating foul sputum, the diagnosis of abscess is quite certain. If the sputum is not foul, bacteriologic examination may differentiate between a pyogenic abscess and tuberculosis. An intrapulmonary cavity may be erroneously considered to be a lung abscess when it is actually an excavated carcinoma. The wall of a neoplastic cavity is usually of irregular thickness, and a patient with such a condition often does

not have purulent sputum. If poor bronchial drainage from a lung abscess exists, the roentgenogram may fail to demonstrate the presence of a pulmonary cavity because of the failure of air to enter the abscess. In such cases, the abscess appears as an area of homogeneous density on the film, and roentgenographic differentiation from a pneumonic area is difficult. In chronic cases, bronchograms may differentiate bronchiectasis from a chronic pulmonary abscess. Posteroanterior and lateral roentgenograms of the chest should be taken weekly during the acute phase of the illness. Bucky films and tomograms may aid in the visualization of cavitation. If the suppurative process does not respond to antimicrobial therapy as anticipated, the possibility of bronchial obstruction must be reconsidered.

Bronchoscopic examination is indicated for both diagnostic and therapeutic purposes. By bronchoscopy a foreign body, neoplasm, or bronchial stenosis may be visualized if the lesion is not too peripheral in location. Bronchoscopy also may facilitate bronchial drainage, and the cultures of the secretion obtained at bronchoscopy will give more reliable bacteriologic data than the examination of sputum that is contaminated with mouth organisms.

COURSE. The course of a pulmonary abscess developing after aspiration is considerably influenced by the adequacy of bronchial drainage. If the purulent material drains into the larger bronchi and can be expectorated, spontaneous healing may occur. Such drainage of purulent material into the bronchial tree does at times result in bronchogenic spread of infection into other portions of the lung, although spillover abscesses are relatively uncommon with antimicrobial therapy. A pulmonary abscess may rupture into the pleural space and produce a pyopneumothorax, or the infection may extend to the pleura without gross rupture and result in empyema. Occasionally, a lung abscess ruptures into the esophagus or some other adjacent organ. Brain abscess, either single or multiple, may be a hematogenous complication of pulmonary abscess.

TREATMENT. The initial treatment of pulmonary abscess hinges on whether the lesion is secondary to a bronchial obstruction. Therefore, early bronchoscopic examination is indicated. Antimicrobial therapy with broad-spectrum agents should be started at once in all cases. When the abscess is secondary to a neoplasm, pulmonary resection is indicated after a brief period of preoperative preparation with antimicrobial drugs. Suppuration distal to a bronchial stenosis is treated by surgical excision of the involved portion of the lung. Multiple hematogenous lung abscesses require prolonged intensive antimicrobial therapy and adequate treatment of the primary focus.

Antimicrobial therapy is the chief measure employed for an acute primary pulmonary abscess. Bacteriologic examination of the sputum or bronchial secretions obtained at the time of bronchoscopy may aid in the selection of the best agent for the individual patient, but it is important to realize that in most cases more than one bacterium plays an etiologic role. Most pulmonary abscesses respond well to penicillin therapy. If there is reason to suspect that a penicillinase-producing strain of staphylococci is playing an etiologic role, one of the penicillinase-resisting penicillins, such as methicillin, should be substituted. With massive lung gangrene, it is advisable to use a multiple drug regimen consisting of penicillin and streptomycin or chloramphenicol. The drug susceptibilities of the organisms should be determined. Because of the possibility of development of drug resistance and changing bacterial flora, it may be advisable to culture the secretions again in a few weeks and repeat the drug-susceptibility tests. Such examinations may indicate that a different drug should then be employed, but the drug regimen should not be altered solely on the basis of drug susceptibility tests if the lesion appears to be responding to a particular chemotherapy. Prolonged treatment for several weeks or even a few months is usually indicated in order to avoid relapse. Clinical improvement is usually noted within a few days of the institution of drug therapy, and surgical drainage of an acute pulmonary abscess is rarely necessary. Postural drainage may be helpful.

The degree of response of a pulmonary abscess to antimicrobial therapy and the amount of pulmonary damage will determine whether surgical treatment is indicated. If the pulmonary cavity disappears and no significant pneumonitis or bronchiectasis remains, only medical measures are necessary. If cavitation persists or clinical improvement is not maintained, surgical excision of the diseased part, usually by lobectomy or segmental resection, is indicated. The risk is low and the results are good if the suppuration is localized.

STAPHYLOCOCCAL PNEUMONIA

Pneumonia due to *S. aureus* deserves special mention because of its frequency, morbidity and mortality, and related surgical problems. Staphylococcal pneumonia in infancy and childhood has assumed a more prominent place among pulmonary infections since antibiotics have reduced the morbidity of certain other types of bacterial infection and thus have resulted in the emergence of resistant organisms, of which *S. aureus* is a prominent example. Staphylococcal pneumonia is also a serious complication of tracheostomies, especially if the most exacting aseptic technique is not observed in the management of tracheal aspiration. In infancy, lung abscesses may simulate areas of obstructive emphysema, and since they usually resolve spontaneously, surgical intervention is rarely required. These abscess-related pneumatoceles must be distinguished from congenital lung cysts with an epithelial lining, as the latter lesion usually requires excision. The primary treatment of staphylococcal pneumonia is by effective antibiotics, but complications, such as empyema and pneumothorax, may require drainage.

LIPOID PNEUMONIA

Lipoid pneumonia may be of either exogenous or endogenous origin. The *exogenous* type is seen most frequently as a result of the prolonged use of oily nose drops or the use of mineral oil for constipation. The elderly patient with impaired gag reflex is particularly prone to the insidious aspiration of oil into the lower respiratory tract. Malnour-

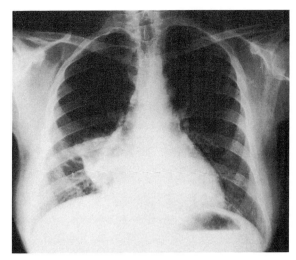

Fig. 17-40. Lipoid pneumonia caused by oily nose drops. Original clinical diagnosis was carcinoma.

ished infants are also vulnerable to lipoid pneumonia. Chronic cough and expectoration may be noted. Dyspnea may result from the secondary pulmonary fibrosis in patients with diffuse lesions. Roentgenograms may show patchy infiltrations, either unilaterally or bilaterally, but in some adults a localized granuloma that simulates a carcinoma may be present (Fig. 17-40). Since the clinical and roentgenographic features often simulate other pulmonary lesions, a good history is essential to alert the physician to the possibility of lipoid pneumonia. Examination of the sputum or the bronchial secretions obtained at bronchoscopy while the patient is on a fat-free diet may suggest the diagnosis. Sudan stains of the sputum are indicated. Surgical intervention is warranted only when neoplasm is suspected or secondary infection of a localized lesion causes significant symptoms.

Endogenous lipoid pneumonia develops following injury to pulmonary tissue, probably as a result of chronic interstitial inflammation of the lung. Cholesterol and other lipoid deposits are prominent features. Clinically and roentgenographically the lesion may be difficult to distinguish from other types of chronic pneumonitis or from bronchogenic carcinoma. Surgical excision is usually required for clarification of the diagnosis.

ASPIRATION PNEUMONIA (MENDELSON'S SYNDROME)

Aspiration of gastric contents accounts for 11 percent of anesthetic deaths. It also occurs in unanesthetized, unconscious patients undergoing emergency endotracheal intubation, tube feeding, or cardiac resuscitation, and in patients with esophageal disease. The most important factor in determining the degree of pneumonitis is the pH of the aspirated gastric content. With a pH of gastric juices less than 1.2, patchy areas of atelectasis and frank necrosis occur immediately. Severe pneumonitis with hemorrhagic consolidation ensues within 24 hours. In the experimental animal it has been shown that even if the bronchial aspirate is neutralized within a few minutes, the damage cannot be avoided.

The clinical manifestations are dependent upon the volume and nature of the aspirate. Small amounts of gastric content may be aspirated without a change in the clinical picture. The manifestations attending aspiration of large amounts of gastric juice are characteristic. There may be an immediate fall in systemic arterial pressure, and the right atrial and pulmonary arterial pressure may also fall progressively. There also may be an immediate fall in oxygen tension. Two hours after the aspiration there is onset of cyanosis, dyspnea, tachypnea, tachycardia, and hypotension. The sputum is frothy and blood-tinged. Auscultation of the lung reveals the signs of bronchospasm with rales and rhonchi throughout both lung fields. Roentgenograms show soft mottling throughout both lung fields.

Treatment of aspiration pneumonitis consists of immediately clearing the tracheobronchial tree by bronchoscopic aspiration. The previously accepted concept of copious pulmonary lavage with saline or sodium bicarbonate has been shown to be ineffectual and actually harmful. It is preferable to use small amounts (2 to 5 ml) of saline solution with prompt removal to clear the aspirate and bronchial secretions. This should be performed at frequent intervals until ventilation is improved. Oxygen is indicated, and positive pressure ventilation with 100% oxygen via an endotracheal tube generally is required. Arterial gases should be monitored. The protective effect of steroids is debated, but at present it is reasonable to treat the patient with 8 mg of dexamethasone, followed by 2 to 4 mg every 6 hours for 48 hours, and gradually tapering the drug off over the next 72 hours.

OTHER PNEUMONIAS

With the more frequent use of immunosuppressive agents in the treatment of certain neoplasms and for organ transplantation, previously unrecognized types of pneumonia, caused by previously unrecognized pathogens, are increasingly being encountered. Some of these infections, such as *Pneumocystis carinii* pneumonia, do not respond to the commonly employed antibacterial agents but may respond well to a specific drug such as pentamidine. Hence it has become necessary to establish diagnosis in such cases by percutaneous needle biopsy or, if this is not diagnostic, by open lung biopsy.

MUCOVISCIDOSIS OF CHILDHOOD AND MUCOID IMPACTION OF BRONCHI IN ADULTS

Mucoviscidosis causes a relatively common serious pulmonary condition in childhood. The abnormal secretion of bronchial glands which is a part of this systemic disease results in bronchitis, bronchiectasis, pulmonary fibrosis, and emphysema, and occasionally a lung abscess. The diagnosis is established by demonstrating the abnormal sodium loss from the skin by the classic sweat test. Intensive medical treatment, including antibiotics and pancreatic extract, has greatly improved the life expectancy of these children, and in some carefully selected cases a lobectomy of a particularly diseased portion of the lung may be helpful. It is now recognized that in some adults with

chronic bronchial disease a similar latent pathologic process of lesser severity may be present.

Whenever an adult has a tenacious secretion which blocks a bronchus, the condition must be differentiated from the many other pathologic causes of bronchial obstruction. When the bronchial mucosal glands secrete an abnormal amount of mucus which tends to solidify and chronically plug a bronchial lumen, the roentgenographic findings may simulate those found with a bronchial neoplasm. Mucoid impaction may be suspected when such findings occur in asthmatic patients or when several scattered areas of obstruction to small bronchi are demonstrated roentgenographically. Mucolytic agents inhaled or instilled into the bronchi may clear up such mucoid impactions. Long-standing mucoid impaction of bronchi may lead to broncholithiasis.

EROSION OF LYMPH NODE INTO BRONCHUS

A peribronchial lymph node may erode into a bronchus either because of an active granulomatous process within the lymph node or because an irregularly calcified portion of a lymph node behaves like a migrating foreign body. Varying degrees of bronchostenosis may ensue with the development of a distal pneumonitis which may progress to abscess formation. The clinical and roentgenographic findings often simulate those of bronchogenic carcinoma, but the occurrence of a massive hemoptysis or sudden hemoptysis of some magnitude due to erosion into a bronchial artery should suggest the correct diagnosis, because a similar type of severe hemoptysis is not common with most bronchogenic carcinomas at an early stage. Bronchoscopic and tomographic examinations may aid in differential diagnosis, but in some cases the correct diagnosis is established only after thoracotomy.

Such lymphadenopathy is usually caused by tuberculosis or the calcifications of histoplasmosis. The right middle lobe is a relatively frequent site for bronchostenosis secondary to peribronchial lymphadenopathy. Lobectomy is often the treatment of choice in adults, usually combined with antituberculous therapy, at least until laboratory tests have ruled out a tuberculous process in the involved nodes. It is important to differentiate this condition from bronchogenic carcinoma, so that extensive pulmonary resection is avoided. In some cases only the offending node needs to be removed by thoracotomy if operation is undertaken before suppurative bronchiectasis has developed distal to the site of bronchial erosion. In children with primary tuberculosis, lymph node compression of a bronchus is not infrequent; here medical treatment with adequate antituberculous chemotherapy is usually effective.

BRONCHOLITH. When a calcified mass from a node is extruded into the bronchial lumen, it may be called a *broncholith* (lung stone). Asymptomatic patients may be treated conservatively. Bronchoscopic removal of such a broncholith is feasible in two-thirds of cases; the remainder of symptomatic patients should be treated by bronchotomy. Rarely inspissated bronchial secretion may calcify with resultant formation of multiple broncholiths, which may be coughed up at times.

TRACHEOESOPHAGEAL AND
BRONCHOESOPHAGEAL FISTULA

Most infants with a congenital tracheoesophageal fistula have an associated esophageal atresia (see Chap. 39). When a congenital tracheoesophageal fistula is present in the absence of esophageal obstruction (H fistula), recurrent pulmonary infection due to aspiration into the lungs is the presenting feature. Cough related to feedings may be noted. The recognition of the cause of the pulmonary infections is often delayed because the diagnosis is not considered or because adequate roentgenographic and endoscopic examinations are not carried out. Early surgical closure of the fistula is indicated.

Occasionally a congenital bronchoesophageal fistula may be of small size or the fistulous opening covered by a mucosal flap so that little aspiration into the lungs occurs and the pulmonary infection may not become manifest until adult life. In such cases surgical closure of the fistula, often with resection of the pulmonary tissue with irreversible suppuration, is indicated.

Most cases of acquired tracheoesophageal fistula are secondary to carcinoma, especially of the upper thoracic esophagus. Fistulas may also follow trauma caused by foreign bodies, penetrating wounds, or severe blunt trauma. When caused by a small foreign body, endoscopic removal of the foreign body may result in closure of the fistula. Other nonneoplastic fistulas usually require closure by thoracotomy.

Acquired bronchoesophageal fistulas may result from carcinoma of either the esophagus or the lung. However, a granulomatous lesion in the mediastinal lymph nodes is an important cause of such a fistula which can be cured by adequate surgical intervention combined with medical therapy. Caseation of subcarinal lymph nodes due to tuberculosis, histoplasmosis, and other fungal diseases are prominent etiologic factors. As recurrent pulmonary symptoms, including hemoptysis, may dominate the clinical picture, the fistulous tract to the esophagus may go unrecognized (Fig. 17-41). A granulomatous process seen in the bronchus on bronchoscopy is a frequent finding. The fistulous tract may be too small to be readily demonstrated by roentgenographic studies with contrast media.

TUBERCULOSIS

A proper appreciation of the role that surgical treatment may play in the management of pulmonary and pleural tuberculosis can be attained only if certain basic concepts in the pathology of a tuberculous lesion are borne in mind. Also much is added to an understanding of the present-day place of surgery if a brief history of the surgical treatment of tuberculosis is appreciated. The advent of effective chemotherapy has revolutionized the therapy of tuberculosis and reduced the number of cases requiring surgical intervention in addition to the medical therapy. However, an intelligent management of the patient with tubercle bacilli resistant to the best antituberculous chemotherapeutic agents requires knowledge of how the disease is likely to behave when chemotherapy cannot be relied upon.

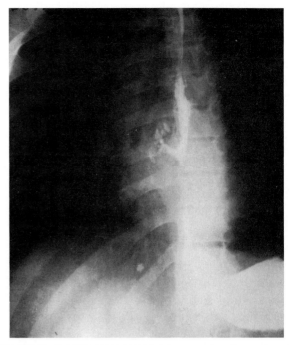

Fig. 17-41. Bronchoesophageal fistula secondary to erosion of calcified node into right bronchus and esophagus. Barium in esophagus outlines fistulous tract leading to calcified nodes. Histoplasmosis was the probable cause. Cure was effected by excision of fistula and lobectomy.

HISTORICAL BACKGROUND. Historically the early surgical experience with the drainage of a tuberculous abscess was unfavorable. Unless the tuberculous infection was relatively inactive and the patient's resistance to the disease especially good, the tuberculous abscess which was drained by surgical incision usually did not heal, sinus formation was common, and secondary infection was prone to develop. Such was especially likely to occur if a tuberculous empyema was subjected to open thoracotomy. Hence it was long recognized that it was important to distinguish between a pyogenic and a tuberculous empyema, as the treatment of the two types of pleural infection differed. Although today chemotherapeutic agents may protect the patient with a thoracotomy performed in the presence of an acute tuberculous empyema, it is important to realize that surgical intervention is not the primary therapy for uncomplicated acute tuberculous empyema.

When surgical treatment was first being employed for pulmonary pyogenic abscesses, it was soon learned that if active pulmonary tuberculosis was present, a spread of the disease and usually a fatal outcome ensued. Therefore prior to the advent of effective antituberculosis therapy those patients with pulmonary tuberculosis who required more than bed rest and general medical measures for control of the pulmonary disease were treated by collapsing of the involved lung in order to favor closure of the tuberculous cavity in the lung and thus lessen the chances of bronchogenic spread of the active tuberculous process. If collapse of the diseased lung could not be obtained by a therapeutic pneumothorax, surgical procedures to obtain collapse of the most diseased portion of the lung were undertaken provided the disease was sufficiently localized and limited to permit such intervention.

A variety of surgical procedures aiming at collapse of the diseased portion of the lung were performed. A closed pneumonolysis was employed if a pneumothorax could be established, but visceroparietal adhesions over the diseased portion of the lung prevented adequate collapse of the very area most needing collapse. In closed pneumonolysis a thorascope and a cautery were inserted through cannulae and the offending adhesions divided with the cautery under direct vision *provided* that the adhesions were of sufficient length to permit their division without any injury to the adjacent diseased lung. When a closed pneumonolysis was not feasible and the pneumothorax not adequate for control of the pulmonary lesions, other measures were employed. In some, temporary phrenic nerve interruption or pneumoperitoneum were applied in order to reduce the volume of the lung by elevation of the diaphragm. A large tuberculous cavity unsatisfactory for collapse procedures because of a positive intracavity pressure was sometimes drained surgically through the chest wall by a cavernostomy; this might be combined with a thoracoplasty in order to maintain cavity closure.

The chief surgical procedure employed in the period between 1930 and 1950 for the control of cavitary pulmonary tuberculosis was the collapse of the cavitary area by extrapleural thoracoplasty. In this operation long lengths of ribs were removed over the area of disease with the result that this portion of the chest wall, now deprived of its rigid component, would retract inward due to the underlying negative pressure of the thoracic contents. The ribs were resected subperiosteally, so that some regeneration of the ribs in the collapsed position would occur and thus a permanently flail chest wall would be avoided. The operation was usually done in stages in order to lessen the risk of bronchogenic spread of the tuberculosis and minimize the paradoxic motion of the decostalized portion of the chest wall in the postoperative period.

An extrapleural thoracoplasty results in a permanent sinking inward of the decostalized portion of the chest wall. When the posterolateral portions of the upper ribs are resected, the thoracic deformity which results is less than one would anticipate from the appearance of a postoperative chest x-ray; this is because the shoulder girdle with the clavicle maintains the contour of the shoulder. Some sinking in of the chest wall below the clavicle may be noted. When a more extensive removal of ribs is carried out, greater deformity of the thoracic cage becomes noticeable. All efforts were made by postural exercises to lessen the tendency to lateral curvature of the spine, which may affect the function of the entire chest cage. Since in these procedures no tuberculous tissue was excised, it is obvious that a certain degree of resistance to the tuberculosis had to be present in the patient if arrest of the disease was to occur. These surgical procedures were ancillary to general medical treatment; this is even more pertinent today, when medical therapy has so much more to offer.

PRESENT TREATMENT. It has always been necessary to properly time the surgical intervention if maximal results were to be attained. Operations performed too early before activity of the tuberculous infection has lessened may result in spread of the disease, whereas required operations unduly delayed favor chronicity and delayed rehabilitation. Surgical intervention for pulmonary tuberculosis is indicated when the tuberculous process is not arrested by antituberculous chemotherapy and yet the pulmonary involvement is sufficiently limited to permit adequate postoperative pulmonary function (Fig. 17-42). As additional antituberculous drugs become available and as a greater percentage of cases are arrested by medical therapy, fewer cases require excision of residual active foci. A full knowledge of the value and limitations of the various antituberculous drugs, such as streptomycin, isoniazid, and para-aminosalicylic acid, should be acquired by any surgeon who performs operations for pulmonary tuberculosis, because the indications for surgical intervention and the proper timing of indicated operations and the selection of the best surgical procedure for a specific patient can be made only by one cognizant of the relative roles of medications and surgical treatment in the management of this disease.

When a pulmonary lesion of uncertain cause is resected and found on pathologic examination to be of probable

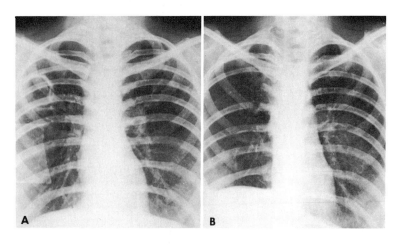

Fig. 17-42. Lobectomy for pulmonary tuberculosis. *A.* Tuberculous cavity in right upper lobe. *B.* Roentgenogram following right upper lobectomy.

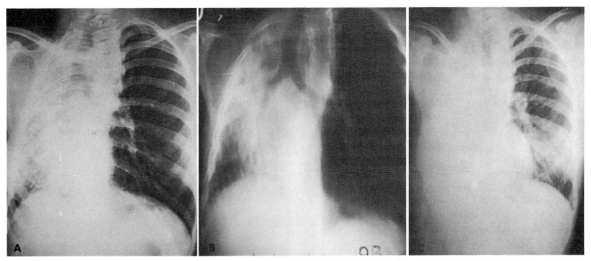

Fig. 17-43. Pneumonectomy for pulmonary tuberculosis. Destroyed right lung was associated with mediastinal displacement. *A.* Posteroanterior roentgenogram. *B.* Tomogram. *C.* Roentgenogram following pneumonectomy.

tuberculous cause, adequate postoperative antituberculous chemotherapy should be instituted promptly in order to lessen the risk of any spread of the tuberculous process. The duration of such chemotherapy would be influenced by the degree of activity of the tuberculous process as indicated by the pathologic and bacteriologic examinations of the excised tissue.

Since the search for better antituberculous agents continues, it may be anticipated that more agents will be added in the future. The problem of the development of bacterial resistance to a drug is especially prominent when dealing with a chronic disease requiring long-term therapy. It has long been evident that if two antituberculous agents are given concurrently from the beginning, bacterial resistance of the tubercle bacilli is delayed.

If a patient is scheduled for a pulmonary resection after a considerable period of antituberculous therapy and especially if the sputum is still positive for tubercle bacilli, it is highly desirable that an additional antituberculous drug which that patient has not previously received should be given in conjunction with the surgical treatment (Fig. 17-43). By such a program the possibility of tuberculous complications following surgical treatment is reduced, since the patient is far more certain of receiving effective chemotherapy at a time when tubercle bacilli might be implanted into the pleural cavity or spread via the bronchial route. As some of these drugs are hepatotoxic or nephrotoxic on long-term usage, it may be desirable to limit their use to a period of a month or so postoperatively and then continue with the two antituberculous drugs that are considered best for long-term treatment.

In most cases of proved active pulmonary tuberculosis with sputum positive for tubercle bacilli, the patient is treated for several months with two or three antituberculous drugs in combination in order to ascertain whether the pulmonary disease can be arrested by medical treatment. In the patient with a solid circumscribed caseous lesion which may simulate a tumor, early surgical excision may be indicated, because it is unknown whether the mass in the lung is a carcinoma or tuberculoma. This patient should be protected from a spread of any tuberculosis by receiving antituberculous chemotherapy in conjunction with the operation, and this chemotherapy should be continued for months after operation if the excised lesion has been demonstrated to be an active tuberculous focus. It must also be appreciated that a new discrete mass appearing in the lung of an older adult under adequate chemotherapeutic treatment for tuberculosis may well be a carcinoma and not merely another tuberculous lesion; hence such a mass may also require early surgical resection.

A persistence of the positive sputum after several months of adequate antituberculous chemotherapy may warrant surgical resection if the active disease is localized to a portion of one lung. If the disease is bilateral and more widespread, a longer trial with various antituberculous agents is usually advisable before deciding that surgical intervention is advantageous. With bilateral disease of considerable extent, a reduction in pulmonary function may be anticipated from the pulmonary fibrosis and other changes which the tuberculosis may cause even in the healing process. Therefore in such cases the ultimate surgical therapy may be restricted to the excision of the most diseased area with cavitation, with the expectation that the prolonged use of chemotherapy will aid the arrest of the noncavitary tuberculous foci.

Whereas in the era prior to antituberculous chemotherapy a persistence of cavitation usually meant that tubercle bacilli were being discharged from the lung, now many a patient with a residual cavity after a chemotherapeutic course of treatment may no longer have positive sputum. In some such treated patients active tuberculous granulations disappear from the lining of the cavity. Hence one now speaks of the "open healed cavity." Actually it is often not really known how complete the recession of the tuberculous process is unless the lesion has been resected and examined. It is known, however, that patients with a residual cavity but persistently negative sputum may do quite well clinically if carefully followed with a long-term pro-

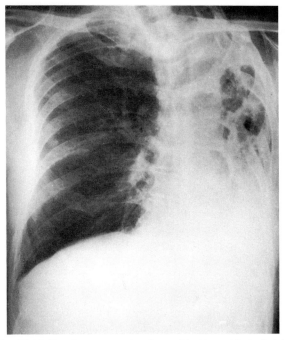

Fig. 17-44. Roentgenogram showing residual bronchiectasis following tuberculosis. Patient had severe bronchiectasis in left lung, which was partially collapsed by a thoracoplasty performed for tuberculosis. Patient was much improved following pneumonectomy. There is emphysema of the right lung.

gram of chemotherapy, provided that other detrimental factors such as diabetes are not also present. Thus, it is understandable that there is at present no uniform opinion as to how many of the patients with a residual cavity but

Fig. 17-45. Cut section of lung removed because of bronchiectasis secondary to tuberculous stenosis of main bronchus.

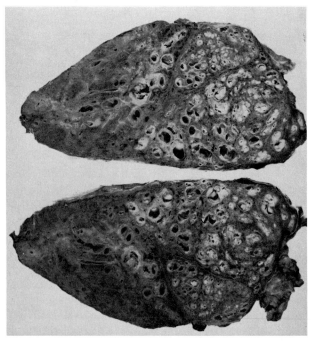

negative sputum should have the cavitary area of the lung resected in order to ensure a safer future.

Some patients whose sputum becomes negative after thoracoplasty or antituberculous chemotherapy have significant cough and expectoration due to the residual bronchiectasis. Some of these patients are greatly benefited by pulmonary resection, which in some cases requires a pneumonectomy (Figs. 17-44 and 17-45).

MYCOTIC INFECTIONS

Mycotic infections of the lung have assumed a greater importance in recent years because of (1) emergence of fungal disease in patients receiving antibiotic therapy for bacterial infection, (2) the use of steroids, (3) the employment of antimetabolites for neoplasms and immunosuppressive therapy for transplantation, and (4) greater dissemination of certain types of mycotic infections previously largely limited to certain geographic areas. In some instances it may be difficult to differentiate between saprophytic and pathogenic fungi, because their presence in sputum and bronchial secretion does not necessarily indicate a pathogenic role. In some fungal infections the organisms must be demonstrated in the tissue in order to prove their pathogenicity. Some granulomatous lesions previously assumed to be tuberculous have been shown more recently to be caused by fungi; histoplasmosis is the outstanding example. Therefore, thorough bacteriologic examination of granulomas which warrant surgical excision is indicated in order to attempt to establish the true etiologic agent.

HISTOPLASMOSIS. Although this infection caused by the fungus *Histoplasma capsulatum* has been recognized as an important medical problem only since 1945, it is now known to occur in large areas in various parts of the world. In the United States the Mississippi and Ohio River Valleys and some river valleys in Eastern states are areas with a high incidence of infection. The clinical manifestations of histoplasmosis are similar to those of tuberculosis in many respects. Disseminated and localized forms of the disease are encountered. As the organism, found in soil with much bird manure, is inhaled into the lungs, an inflammatory response similar to that in tuberculosis is seen. The infection extends to the regional lymph nodes, where calcification is common. Multiple pulmonary calcifications are most frequently due to histoplasmosis.

The acute disseminated form is uncommon, especially considering the high percentage of persons in some areas who show a positive histoplasmin skin test. Pathologically histoplasmosis is a parasitism of the reticuloendothelial system with a tissue response of granulomatous inflammation accompanied by giant cells and tubercle formation. Healing in most cases results in a Ghon type of complex.

Only a small number of cases of histoplasmosis require any surgical therapy. Enlarged calcified hilar lymph nodes may compress or erode a bronchus and cause bronchiectasis. Chronic cavitary disease in the lung may require resection under coverage with amphotericin B. Chronic mediastinal fibrosis is a rare development with poor prognosis.

COCCIDIOIDOMYCOSIS. Coccidioidomycosis is a fungal

infection caused by the inhalation of *Coccidioides immitis* from the air in certain endemic areas, chiefly in the Southwestern part of the United States. Although coccidioidin skin tests have demonstrated that a considerable portion of the population in endemic areas have acquired an asymptomatic primary infection from this fungus, in most persons an immunity to the fungus develops, and clinically demonstrable lesions develop in only a small percentage. The evolution of coccidioidomycosis closely resembles that of pulmonary tuberculosis. Although a serious diffuse type of the disease occurs occasionally, the usual pathologic lesions are evident in the lungs and lymph nodes. A diffuse pulmonary infiltration of a pneumonic type is most likely in those who become ill. Persistent pulmonary cavitation and granulomatous lesions which simulate pulmonary neoplasms may be encountered. Although most antibiotics are ineffective against coccidioidomycosis, amphotericin B is of value, but its usefulness is somewhat limited by its nephrotoxic effect.

Asymptomatic pulmonary cavities in patients with proved coccidioidomycosis usually require no surgical intervention. The surgical indications for persistent localized pulmonary lesions parallel those which are applied at present to pulmonary tuberculosis. Resection is indicated for giant cavities, those with persistent secondary infection, and when rupture occurs with pleural complications such as empyema or nonexpansile lung. Solid granulomatous lesions are fortunately relatively uncommon, because differentiation of such a lesion from a pulmonary carcinoma may be possible only after surgical resection. An older-adult heavy cigarette smoker with known coccidioidomycosis and a discrete pulmonary density on radiography should have surgical excision of the lesion without delay, because carcinoma is a strong possibility.

ACTINOMYCOSIS. Actinomycosis may infect the lungs and the thoracic cage (Fig. 17-46). Such infection is caused by an organism which stands midway between the true bacteria and the more complex molds. In many the pathogenic organism is the *Actinomyces israelii*. Although cervicofacial and abdominal infections are more common, thoracic infection may occur as the primary lesion or by extension from the neck or abdomen. Thoracic actinomycosis was usually fatal prior to the advent of sulfonamides and antibiotics.

The pulmonary disease appears as a pneumonic suppurative process which may at first appear similar to suppurative pneumonia or lung abscess caused by other agents. Hemoptysis may occur. Actinomycosis of the lung has a tendency to extend through the pulmonary tissue to the pleura with resultant pleuritis and empyema. Such a pleural infection due to actinomycosis has a great tendency to burrow into the chest wall, over a wide area (Fig. 17-7), and cause osteomyelitis of the ribs and a suppurative chondritis. Whenever involvement of the chest wall is a prominent feature in the presence of empyema, actinomycosis should be seriously considered as a pathogenic factor; such involvement is usually more acute than the thoracic cage involvement of tuberculosis. Multiple draining sinuses may occur through the skin. Surgical drainage of the pleural and chest wall abscesses together with vigor-

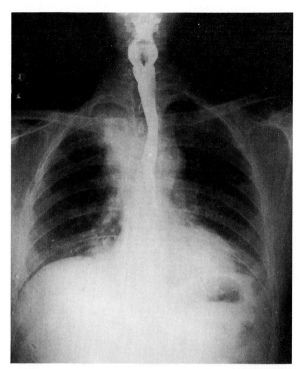

Fig. 17-46. Pulmonary actinomycosis simulating carcinoma of the lung. Patient was well 15 years after thoracotomy and chemotherapy.

ous and prolonged chemotherapy with penicillin or other antibiotics, perhaps combined with sulfonamides, is now an effective therapeutic program. Early medical therapy will usually prevent the development of such surgical conditions. Chronic pulmonary actinomycotic abscesses, often with other pathogenic organisms, may require surgical resection combined with chemotherapy (Fig. 17-47).

NOCARDIOSIS. This infection is caused by the organism *Nocardia asteroides*. Symptomatically and roentgenologi-

Fig. 17-47. Bilateral actinomycosis treated by left pneumonectomy and chemotherapy. There was no recurrence of infection after 20 years.

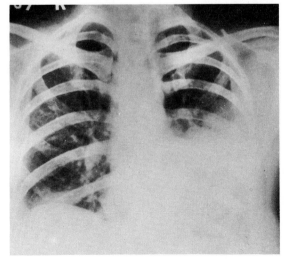

cally the disease may be confused with tuberculosis or actinomycosis. Cough productive of foul sputum, dyspnea, or hemoptysis may occur. *N. asteroides,* like *Mycobacterium tuberculosis,* is acid-fast. Chest wall sinuses as seen with actinomycosis are uncommon, although subcutaneous abscesses may occur. Sulfadiazine and antibiotics are the therapeutic agents advocated. Surgical drainage of abscesses or resection of undiagnosed lesions may be indicated.

ASPERGILLOSIS. Pulmonary symptoms caused by the fungus *Aspergillus fumigatus* were rare before the antibiotic era. This organism is normally a saprophyte which is widely distributed in nature. As a pathogen it causes some avian disease, and until recently the rare human cases were often acquired from such sources. Although a hemorrhagic pneumonitis may occasionally occur, aspergillosis usually appears as a chronic pulmonary infection often associated with bronchiectasis, lung abscess, or pulmonary fibrosis and especially as an invader of a chronic pulmonary cavity. Whenever a residual pulmonary cavity persists, such as in a patient with tuberculosis after conversion of the sputum by antituberculous therapy, fungi may form a mycelium mass within the pulmonary cavity. Such a mycelium "ball" within the cavity may give the characteristic roentgenographic finding of a rounded density within the cavity with a rim of air surrounding the "ball" within the cavity. Hemoptyses, sometimes severe, may occur. Limited pulmonary resection is the treatment of choice.

BLASTOMYCOSIS. Both the North American and South American varieties of blastomycosis may cause pulmonary lesions of a granulomatous type. The pulmonary findings may resemble those seen with tuberculosis, but at times a solitary circumscribed granulomatous lesion may simu-

Fig. 17-48. Hydatid cyst of lung. Note large cyst in right lung and small cyst at left apex.

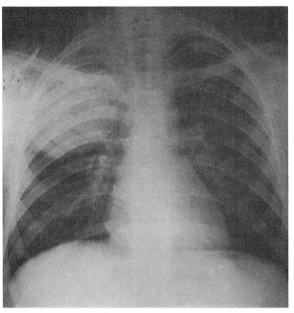

late a neoplasm. Other blastomycotic lesions, especially skin lesions, may be present, and investigation of these may aid in establishing a definite diagnosis. Appropriate chemotherapy is the primary method of treatment, but surgical excision may occasionally be indicated.

CRYPTOCOCCOSIS (TORULOSIS). This subacute and chronic fungus infection may occur as an opportunistic infection in patients with such debilitating diseases as lymphoma and collagen diseases and in patients receiving prolonged treatment with antimetabolites, antibiotics, and steroids. Chronic granulomatous lesions in the lungs may warrant resection, because the lesion simulates a neoplasm or because dissemination with meningitis is feared. Resection is curative in 90 percent of cases. A spinal tap is mandatory. Amphotericin B is the most effective of the antifungal drugs against the infection and should be employed in cases of disseminated disease. The toxicity of this drug, however, limits its use. A less toxic oral medication, 5-fluorocystosine, may be effective.

HYDATID CYSTS OF THE LUNG

Echinococcus disease is common in some countries bordering on the Mediterranean Sea, in parts of South America, and in Australia and New Zealand. People from these areas of the world may travel elsewhere and then have the disease become manifest. The parasite gains entry into the portal bloodstream and usually lodges in the liver but may pass directly into the lung. Pulmonary hydatid cysts (Fig. 17-48) are treated by thoracotomy and single-stage enucleation of the cyst, with great care taken to avoid pleural contamination and the anaphylactic reaction which may ensue if cyst contents should spill. Infected hydatid cysts in the lung are best treated by pulmonary resection. Hydatid cysts may rupture into the bronchus, pleura, or pericardium (Fig. 17-49). Massive pleural involvement may result from transdiaphragmatic rupture of hepatic hydatids; this requires thoracoabdominal drainage together with adequate treatment of the hydatid cysts in the liver (see Chap. 30).

BOECK'S SARCOID

Sarcoidosis frequently involves the hilar lymph nodes, and there is often an associated diffuse involvement of the lungs. This granulomatous process may be apparently localized to one anatomic area or have widespread manifestations. Many patients with prominent bilateral hilar lymphadenopathy are largely asymptomatic, but some may have cough and some constitutional symptoms. As involvement of the cervical lymph nodes is a common finding, cervical node biopsy is indicated when intrathoracic Boeck's sarcoid is suspected. At times a mediastinotomy or even a thoracotomy with hilar lymph node biopsy and lung biopsy may be required to establish a definite diagnosis. The condition is to be distinguished from tuberculosis and lymphoma. A Nickerson-Kveim skin test may be helpful. Definitive treatment, if necessary, is nonsurgical and may employ steroid therapy for symptoms. Spontaneous

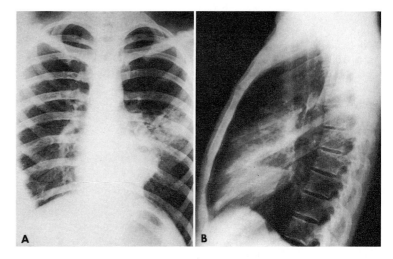

Fig. 17-49. Paracardiac hydatid cyst which ruptured into lingular portion of lung. *A.* Posteroanterior view. *B.* Lateral view demonstrating fluid level and ruptured cyst. Lesion was treated by removal of the cyst and resection of lingular portion of the lung.

regression has been reported with recovery in 35 percent and improvement in 32 percent. The mortality rate averages 14 percent.

Solitary Pulmonary Nodule

Often a small mass in the lung is discovered on roentgenographic examination in a person with no pulmonary symptoms. The density may be caused by a very wide variety of pathologic lesions with a widely varying prognostic significance. Such roentgenographic shadows may be caused by (1) tumors which range from very benign to highly malignant, (2) granulomas due to tuberculosis, histoplasmosis, and many other mycotic infections, (3) congenital lesions of the bronchopulmonary and vascular structures of the lung, and (4) an additional wide variety of acute and chronic pathologic lesions which may have a roughly rounded shape. The term "coin lesion" has been applied to small, discrete rounded densities seen in roentgenograms of the lungs. This term is obviously a poor one to indicate the presence of a spherical mass, and furthermore some apply this term to densities which are not even well rounded or sharply circumscribed. The term "solitary pulmonary nodule" is satisfactory provided the extreme variation that may be present in its pathologic nature is fully appreciated.

The age of the patient, where he has lived, the history and physical examination, skin tests, and laboratory tests may point toward a statistically likely diagnosis. The review of previously taken chest roentgenograms may be of great help. Often only pathologic and bacteriologic examination of the surgically excised nodule provides a final answer, but this does not mean that every such density seen on a roentgenogram is an indication for surgical excision. Judgment is necessary to decide which type of management is safest for a specific individual. The age of the patient will greatly influence the likelihood of a solitary pulmonary nodule's being a neoplasm. In the older adult excision of such nodules is usually indicated, because a high percentage are carcinomas.

Tumors of the Lung

BENIGN ENDOBRONCHIAL TUMORS

Benign tumors which arise from the bronchial wall and project into the lumen of the bronchus without significant extension into the adjacent extrabronchial structures are rare. A benign tumor derived from one or more of the component structures of the bronchus may be a polyp, fibroma, lipoma, chondroma, leiomyoma, osteoma, or lymphoma. Bronchial carcinoid tumors (adenomas) should be considered as a separate group because of their tendency toward extrabronchial invasion, although occasionally a bronchial carcinoid may be almost entirely an endobronchial lesion.

CLINICAL MANIFESTATIONS. If a tumor is small and does not obstruct the bronchus to any marked degree, symptoms may be absent. A dry cough may be one of the earliest complaints. When the tumor arises in one of the larger branches of the bronchial tree, wheezing may be noted when the bronchial lumen is partly obstructed. Many patients with these signs and symptoms are erroneously diagnosed as having asthma.

DIAGNOSTIC STUDIES. A roentgenogram of the chest may be negative in the presence of wheezing. Fluoroscopy, however, may indicate partial bronchial obstruction by demonstrating interference with the emptying of air from a portion of the lung. The involved lobe remains more radiolucent on full expiration than the normal portions of the lung, which can deflate to a normal degree. If the main bronchus to an entire lung is partially obstructed, fluoroscopy may demonstrate displacement of the mediastinum toward the contralateral side on expiration, and failure of the diaphragm on the side of the bronchial obstruction to ascend normally with expiration. This phenomenon is due to the trapping of air in the involved lung. The same findings can be demonstrated by roentgenograms of the chest taken in deep inspiration and full expiration. If the tumor obstructs only a small bronchus, these findings may be absent. In some cases the tumor may cast a shadow on the routine roentgenogram of the chest, but tomographic x-rays are of greatest help. Bronchograms may also aid in diagnosis. Bronchoscopy is the chief diagnostic method for endobronchial tumors of the larger bronchi and should be performed in cases of localized wheezing even when the radiographic findings are negative. As the bronchial obstructions become more complete, atelectasis, often with secondary pneumonitis, supervenes.

COMPLICATIONS. Frequently a diagnosis of endobronchial tumor is not made until after secondary suppuration has occurred. The clinical picture of a pneumonia is then the presenting feature. Such a pneumonitis usually responds to antibiotics, but the clinical benefit may be more marked than the roentgenographic evidence of clearing of the pulmonary infiltration. The omission of repeated roentgenograms during the course of a pneumonitis is often responsible for the failure to recognize that the pneumonitis is chronic because it is secondary to a bronchial lesion. Early diagnostic bronchoscopy is indicated in any case in which there is a suspicion that the pulmonary infection might be secondary to bronchial obstruction.

TREATMENT. The proper treatment for benign endobronchial tumors varies according to the size of the involved bronchus and the associated pulmonary changes. If a diagnosis is made before significant infection has developed distal to the site of bronchial obstruction, local endoscopic removal of the tumor may result in cure. Because it may be difficult to determine bronchoscopically how far the base of the growth extends into the bronchial wall, it is usually not possible to be certain whether the lesion has been completely removed. For this reason patients should be closely followed and repeated bronchoscopies performed. Often transthoracic bronchotomy and local surgical excision of the involved segment of bronchus with plastic repair is the best therapy when the tumor arises in a large bronchus. If the endobronchial tumor is located in one of the smaller branch bronchi not visible bronchoscopically and no tissue for biopsy can be obtained, a definite diagnosis usually cannot be made preoperatively. In such cases conservative resection of the involved portion of the lung is indicated. Even in those cases in which the tumor can be removed bronchoscopically, pulmonary suppuration secondary to the bronchial obstruction may have caused sufficient bronchiectasis to require removal of the involved portion of the lung.

CIRCUMSCRIBED BENIGN TUMORS OF THE INTERSTITIAL PULMONARY TISSUE

The vast majority of pulmonary tumors arise from the bronchial wall. Circumscribed benign tumors unassociated with a bronchus are rare. Included in this group are hamartoma, leiomyoma, lymphocytoma, neurofibroma, and plasmocytoma. The exact diagnosis is often not established until the tumor has been removed surgically. Since tumors in the pulmonary parenchyma usually do not obstruct any large bronchus, the symptoms of bronchial obstruction and secondary suppuration are often absent. If the tumor is small, there may be no symptoms, and the lesion may be a chance finding on a routine chest roentgenogram or at autopsy. There may be a cough which is

often nonproductive. Hemoptysis and chest pain are infrequent. Definite preoperative differentiating of benign tumors of the pulmonary interstitial tissue from bronchogenic carcinoma is usually not possible, as a carcinoma of the lung may be just as sharply circumscribed on the roentgenogram as a benign tumor. Lobectomy, either partial or total, will usually suffice; pneumonectomy is rarely necessary.

HAMARTOMA. This is one of the more common of the circumscribed benign tumors of the pulmonary parenchyma. The term *hamartoma* is derived from a Greek word which means "to err." The tumor is due to a malformation in which there is an abnormal mixing of various normal components of the organ. Since these intrapulmonary hamartomas consist largely of cartilage, they have usually been called "chondromas," but the presence of other structures within the tumor makes the term "chondroma" unsatisfactory. The characteristic hamartoma of the lung is a solid tumor which consists of benign mesodermal and epithelial elements. Amid the cartilage one finds cystlike spaces lined by columnar epithelium. Smooth muscle, mucous glands, and fat are also usually present. The connective tissue may be myxomatous in type. Bone is occasionally present. In contrast to true chondromas, which arise from the bronchial cartilages, the hamartoma is usually located near the periphery of the lung, where no large bronchi are present. In some instances the tumor may be directly beneath the visceral pleura or may even project above the pulmonary surface. The adjacent lung tissue is usually normal. The roentgenographic appearance simulates that of other pulmonary lesions, but the characteristic "popcorn" calcification should suggest the diagnosis. At operation it is important for the surgeon to recognize the true nature of the lesion, as enucleation or local excision is adequate therapy. Malignant degeneration is apparently a very rare occurrence in hamartomas of the lung.

BRONCHIAL CARCINOID

Bronchial carcinoid is the term most widely used to designate a tumor of slow growth found chiefly in the larger bronchi. These carcinoids frequently have been designated as benign tumors, but the dangerous potentialities of the growth make such a term misleading. Because of the marked difference in their clinical course and prognosis carcinoids must be differentiated from typical epidermoids and adenocarcinomas of the lung. Among so-called "bronchial adenomas" three types of tumors may be recognized: (1) the bronchial carcinoid, which is the most common and has a good prognosis if properly treated; (2) the bronchial cylindroma (adenoid cystic carcinoma), a malignant tumor which has an uncertain prognosis but which may grow slowly over a period of years; (3) the mucoepidermoid bronchial adenoma, which is uncommon and usually does not recur after adequate removal.

Bronchial carcinoid tumors are usually found in the main stem bronchus or projecting from a lobar orifice (Fig. 17-50). Occasionally the tumor arises from a smaller branch bronchus, and only rarely is it located near the periphery of the lung. Carcinoid tumors of the tracheal wall are uncommon, but occasionally those arising in a bronchus may extend secondarily into the trachea or project across the carina. The gross appearance usually enables one to differentiate these lesions from typical carcinomas of the bronchus, but some tumors which grossly simulate adenomas may prove on microscopic examination to be rapidly growing carcinomas. Since the clinical manifestations of carcinoid tumors and other "adenomas" are chiefly those of obstruction caused by their endobranchial portion, these tumors have been classified frequently as endobronchial lesions, but in most instances a portion of the tumor extends outside the bronchial wall. The endobronchial portion of the tumor usually has a rounded, smooth surface. Obvious ulceration is usually absent, even in cases with a history of repeated hemoptyses.

CLINICAL MANIFESTATIONS. Carcinoid tumors of the bronchus occur somewhat more frequently in females than in males. This is in marked contrast to squamous carcinoma of the bronchus. The majority of carcinoids are recognized in the age period between twenty and forty years. Since carcinoid tumors are usually very vascular, the frequent occurrence of hemoptysis is easily understood. Bleeding varies considerably in frequency and amount; occasionally it is severe. Cough is frequently present, and wheezing may be noted. Not infrequently symptoms are minimal until suppuration develops. The classic carcinoid syndrome (see Chap. 27) may be caused by these tumors. A sudden onset of chest pain, fever, and cough may lead to a diagnosis of pneumonia. If the acute infection does not subside quickly in the usual manner and particularly if serial x-rays show a persistent density in the pulmonary field, the possibility of bronchial obstruction as a forerunner of the infection must be considered (Figs. 17-51 and 17-52). Bronchoscopy should then be done. Many cases of bronchial carcinoid are treated as recurrent pneumonia without recognition of the presence of the tumor. Empyema which fails to heal may be secondary to pulmonary suppuration distal to a bronchial obstruction. The possibility of carcinoid tumor's being a cause of bronchial obstruction in any age group should be remembered. In

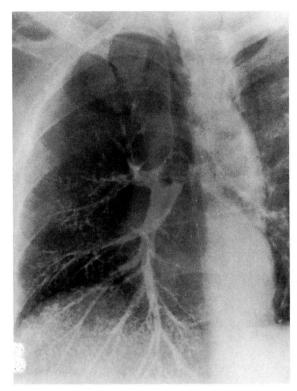

Fig. 17-50. Bronchogram in patient with bronchial carcinoid. Note filling defect in right main bronchus. Patient was treated by transthoracic bronchotomy and excision of lesion without sacrifice of pulmonary tissue.

children the bronchial obstruction may be erroneously attributed to tuberculous lymph nodes eroding the bronchial tree.

DIAGNOSTIC STUDIES. A negative roentgenogram of the chest does not rule out the presence of carcinoid tumor. A tumor in a large bronchus may cast no shadow distinguishable from the other hilar densities. Tomograms may demonstrate the endobronchial portion of the carcinoid tumor as well as aid in determining the size of the extrabronchial part. Bronchoscopy often defines the lesion.

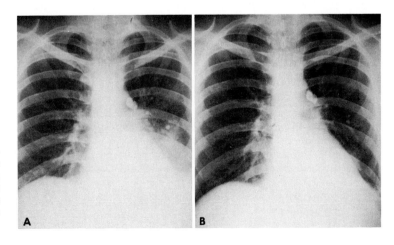

Fig. 17-51. Bronchial carcinoid of left lower lobe bronchus. A. Roentgenogram at time of secondary pneumonitis. B. Roentgenogram following clearing of pneumonitis. Diagnosis might have been missed if bronchoscopy had not been performed in spite of clearing pneumonitis. Calcified node in this case was asymptomatic.

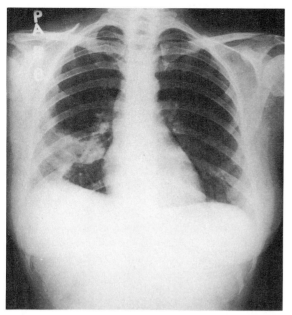

Fig. 17-52. Bronchial carcinoid with distal pneumonitis. The more central portion of the density is the tumor mass.

Bronchoscopy is one of the most important investigative procedures in the diagnosis of a carcinoid tumor. Since about 90 percent of these tumors occur in the larger bronchi, in contrast to bronchogenic carcinoma, which may occur in any portion of the lung, endoscopic examination is far more conclusive in the diagnosis of carcinoid than of bronchogenic carcinoma. The few cases of carcinoid tumor which are not within the range of bronchoscopic vision will be seen as rounded areas of density on the roentgenogram. The gross appearance on bronchoscopy is usually quite characteristic. The tumor appears as a rounded, reddish or purplish mass with a smooth, non-ulcerated surface. If the site of attachment of the bronchial wall is visible, it may be noted to be either pedunculated or sessile. A pedunculated tumor may move up and down with respiration. Purulent material may be aspirated by bronchoscope from a point distal to the obstruction, but caution is indicated in the manipulation of the growth because of its vascularity. Biopsy of a vascular carcinoid occasionally results in severe bleeding. Urinary 5-HIAA and serum catecholamines should be determined.

TREATMENT. The treatment of bronchial carcinoid tumors varies with the extent of the pulmonary pathologic process present in the particular case. Bronchoscopic treatment is advised only in those cases in which other diseases contraindicate transthoracic surgical therapy. Since it is impossible by bronchoscopic visualization to evaluate degree of infiltration of the tumor into the bronchial wall, the success of bronchoscopic removal can be determined only by repeated examinations and biopsies of suspicious areas. In cases where the location of the tumor is such that a total pneumonectomy might seem necessary, transthoracic bronchotomy and plastic repair of the bronchus

may conserve much pulmonary tissue if secondary bronchiectasis has not yet occurred. Lobectomy is usually the treatment of choice if secondary infection has caused lobar bronchiectasis.

ADENOID CYSTIC CARCINOMA (CYLINDROMA)

Cylindromas may resemble bronchial carcinoid tumors grossly but have a different microscopic appearance. In some reports in the literature, both tumors have been called bronchial adenomas. In an occasional case, microscopic examination may reveal some parts which have the appearance of a bronchial carcinoid tumor, whereas other portions of the same tumor may have the characteristics of a cylindroma. Designation as adenoid cystic carcinoma correctly indicates that this growth is truly malignant and should be treated as a cancer. Cylindromas arise in, or extend into, the trachea more frequently than adenomas and are definitely more invasive. Cylindromas are considerably less common than bronchial carcinoid tumors except in the trachea.

The lesions are made up of cells which are small and regular but often hyperchromatic. The cells often show a tubular formation. The main differentiation from adenomas is the presence of a kind of mucus which sometimes stains with mucicarmine. There may also be a rather marked myxomatous connective tissue. Cylindromas of the trachea resemble tumors of the salivary glands.

TREATMENT. Treatment of cylindromas is radical surgical excision similar to that employed for cancers. Because of their greater tendency to extend into the mediastinum and trachea, the results will be less satisfactory than with bronchial carcinoid tumors unless the diagnosis is established before the lesion is advanced. Radiation therapy is not recommended for carcinoids but can be of real value in the therapy of an inoperable cylindroma. Although its histologic appearance would suggest that a cylindroma is radioresistant, some of these tumors respond quite satisfactorily to a radiation therapy. It is important to realize that a cylindroma may show evidence of recurrence after many years. Thus very long periods of follow-up are required for an analysis of therapeutic results.

SARCOMAS OF THE LUNG

These are rare primary pulmonary neoplasms. Primary lymphosarcoma of the lung is not distinguishable from bronchogenic carcinoma radiologically but has a much better prognosis than the latter following surgical excision (Fig. 17-53). Secondary involvement of the lung by lymphosarcoma and Hodgkin's disease is much more frequent than primary pulmonary lymphosarcoma.

Sarcoma of the lung may present as an endobronchial lesion. A fibrosarcoma sometimes is difficult to distinguish from a granulomatous process. Sarcoma of the pulmonary parenchyma also occurs. Here, too, definite differentiation from "inflammatory tumor" of the lung may be uncertain even after complete pathologic study. These latter lesions may occur in children as well as adults. Fever is occa-

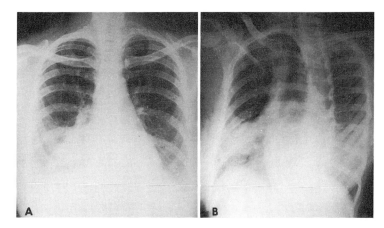

Fig. 17-53. Sarcoma of right middle lobe. *A.* Postero-anterior roentgenogram. *B.* Oblique roentgenogram. Patient was well 15 years after lobectomy.

sionally present. Further data are needed before the true nature of these masses is established. Surgical excision, usually by lobectomy, is the treatment of choice.

CARCINOMA OF THE LUNG

Bronchogenic carcinoma is by far the most important primary pulmonary neoplasm, although metastatic cancer in the lungs is also common. Well over 90 percent of all primary pulmonary tumors are malignant. That those who smoke many cigarettes are statistically more likely to develop a bronchogenic carcinoma seems unquestionable on the basis of much data from many sources and geographic areas of the world. Various other factors, including inherited traits, may play a role in determining whether a cancer develops in a particular individual as a result of the chronic irritation produced by heavy smoking. Exposure to radioactive substances and certain chemicals such as chromate compounds account for the high incidence of cancer of the lung in special occupations. The effects of industrial vapors and the irritants in the atmosphere of urban areas remain to be evaluated. An analysis of etiologic factors must take into consideration the possibility that different types of primary pulmonary neoplasms may well have varied and multiple causes.

Bronchogenic carcinoma has shown a startling increase in incidence during the past few decades. It has become the most common cause of death from cancer among males in some parts of the world and is much more frequent among males, with a ratio of about 6:1. Most persons with bronchogenic carcinoma are over forty-five years of age, but some cases, especially of adenocarcinoma and undifferentiated carcinoma, occur in a younger age group (Fig. 17-54).

PATHOLOGY. Bronchogenic carcinoma may be of various histologic types. Squamous or epidermoid, undifferentiated, large cell, small cell, or oat cell cancers, and adenocarcinoma are common types. An alveolar cell or bronchiolar tumor may occur occasionally.

Bronchogenic carcinoma arising in a bronchus of large or intermediate size often produces sufficient bronchial narrowing to cause a secondary pneumonitis, bronchiectasis, or abscess in the corresponding portion of the

bronchial tree. The neoplasm also extends into the pulmonary tissue or may involve other adjacent structures. The pleural cavity, mediastinum, chest wall, base of the neck, and diaphragm may be invaded by direct extension depending upon the primary location of the tumor (Fig. 17-55). Metastases in the mediastinal lymph nodes are frequent, and infiltration of the wall of the esophagus, pericardium, and heart may occur. Metastases in the opposite lung occur much more frequently with adenocarcinoma and undifferentiated carcinoma than with the squamous cancer. Extrathoracic metastases to the cervical lymph nodes, liver, and brain are of particular clinical

Fig. 17-54. Adenocarcinoma in right upper lobe of thirty-two-year-old woman. Clubbing of fingers and joint pain indicated that the solitary nodule was probably a neoplasm and not a tuberculous lesion.

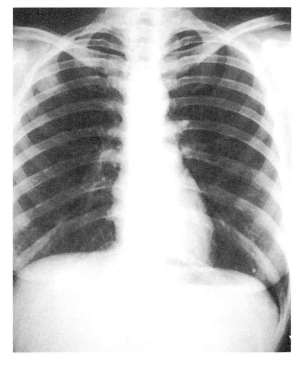

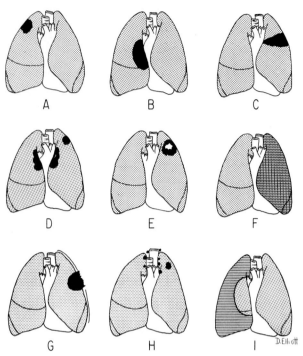

Fig. 17-55. Diagrammatic representation of varied roentgenographic (and resultant clinical) features of bronchogenic carcinoma as influenced by location. *A.* Peripheral carcinoma. *B.* Paramediastinal carcinoma. *C.* Carcinoma causing segmental atelectasis. *D.* Peripheral primary carcinoma with large hilar metastases. *E.* Excavated carcinoma simulating abscess. *F.* Main bronchial carcinoma causing atelectasis over entire lung. *G.* Peripheral carcinoma involving chest wall. *H.* Multifocal neoplastic tumor. *I.* Pleural effusion masking pulmonary lesion.

importance. Adrenal metastases are common with bronchogenic carcinoma, but Addisonian syndrome develops in very few patients. Anaplastic growths may show widespread metastases.

CLINICAL MANIFESTATIONS. The symptomatology of bronchogenic carcinoma is influenced considerably by the location of the growth in reference to the bronchial tree (Fig. 17-56). Relatively small tumors in a main bronchus may cause a cough which may be nonproductive at first.

In contrast, a carcinoma which involves only a bronchus of small size in the peripheral portion of a lung may be asymptomatic (Fig. 17-57) until it attains considerable size. Therefore, the complete absence of symptoms is entirely consistent with a diagnosis of carcinoma of the lung. Cough is the most common symptom of carcinoma of the lung, but since most persons with primary pulmonary carcinoma are heavy smokers who have a chronic cough antedating the disease, the significance of this symptom may not be appreciated. Mucoid or mucopurulent sputum, sometimes with blood streaking, may appear. Hemoptysis may be the initial symptom. Localized wheezing may indicate partial bronchial obstruction. Fever may be present as a result of secondary pneumonitis, but septic manifestations and chills are rare. Dyspnea is usually a late symptom. Chest pain, unless inconstant and of minor degree, often indicates extension of the carcinoma into the chest wall, base of the neck, or mediastinum. Weakness and appreciable weight loss are also signs of advanced disease unless produced by secondary pulmonary suppuration. Hoarseness of recent onset usually indicates involvement of the recurrent laryngeal nerve and is most common with carcinoma of the left upper lobe. Pain in the shoulder, often radiating down the arm, is common with bronchogenic carcinoma of the pulmonary apex and may be the first symptom. This may be accompanied by Horner's syndrome. A pleural effusion, sometimes serosanguineous, may be the first manifestation of a pulmonary cancer.

In some patients with bronchogenic carcinoma a large part of the neoplastic mass may extend outside the lung and invade adjacent structures. When the upper portion of the mediastinum is thus involved, the presenting symptoms may be swelling of the neck and face with venous engorgement caused by neoplastic compression or invasion of the superior vena cava. Dyspnea from tracheal compression and dysphagia from esophageal involvement may be present. Occasionally the earliest recognized symptoms may be from a brain metastasis. A small percentage of persons with bronchogenic carcinoma have joint symptoms simulating those of rheumatoid arthritis. The associated clubbing of the fingers which this group of patients with pulmonary osteoarthropathy manifest should lead to a careful radiographic search for an intrathoracic neoplasm. As such persons may have a small peripheral bronchogenic

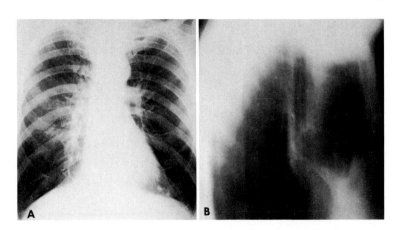

Fig. 17-56. Carcinoma of right middle lobe simulating inflammatory lesion. *A.* Note that posteroanterior film merely shows some increase in right hilar shadows. *B.* Lateral tomogram shows collapsed middle lobe.

carcinoma, pulmonary symptoms may be slight or absent for a considerable time. The periarticular swelling and tenderness disappear dramatically following excision of the pulmonary tumor.

Some patients with pulmonary and pleural tumors may manifest a variety of metabolic and hormonal derangements which are not necessarily due to metastases. Hypercalcemia mimicking hyperparathyroidism is occasionally seen, especially with large tumors. Neuromuscular disorders related to the lung cancer may be erroneously diagnosed as a sign of metastatic involvement. Hyponatremia and disturbances of the antidiuretic hormone may be noted. Cushing's disease is sometimes seen, especially with the oat cell carcinoma. Excessive serotonin excretion by oat cell tumors is encountered. Hypoglycemia is seen with some large pleural tumors.

There are often no physical signs of pulmonary cancer in the earlier stages. Localized wheezing may indicate the presence of a lesion causing partial bronchial obstruction. Such wheezing may disappear as the obstruction becomes more complete. Dullness may result from the pulmonary consolidation distal to the bronchostenosis or from a large peripheral tumor. Rales of an associated pneumonitis and various alterations in breath sounds are sometimes noted. Signs of pleural effusion usually indicate neoplastic involvement of the pleura secondary to the pulmonary neoplasm.

The life expectancy in untreated primary pulmonary cancer varies considerably. Although many patients die within a year of the onset of notable symptoms, others may survive for a somewhat longer period. In rare instances the growth may be radiographically demonstrable for a few years before symptoms develop.

DIAGNOSTIC FINDINGS. Roentgenographic examination of the chest is the most important diagnostic step in the detection of tumors in the lung (see Fig. 17-55). Since pulmonary cancer is often in an advanced stage before significant symptoms are recognized, routine roentgenographic studies at half-yearly intervals are necessary if one hopes to discover such neoplasms early. Although the film may thus alert the physician to the presence of a pulmonary lesion, the roentgenographic appearance alone may

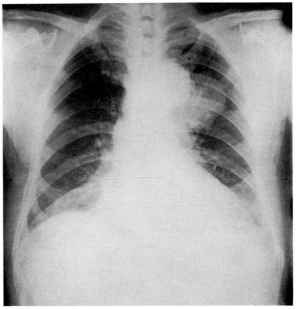

Fig. 17-57. Bronchogenic carcinoma in lower portion of left lower lobe. Note fibrosis at right apex due to healed tuberculosis.

not permit a positive diagnosis in the earlier phases of the disease in many instances. Moreover, in some cases of bronchogenic carcinoma the lesion may escape detection because of its small size or its location close to the hilus of the lung or obscuration by the cardiac shadow or dome of the diaphragm. Special radiographic techniques such as tomography are sometimes helpful (Fig. 17-58). The data obtained by roentgenography should be interpreted in conjunction with the information gained from the history, physical examination, and special laboratory studies. Bronchoscopic examination is indicated in all except the very peripheral lesions and permits the visualization and biopsy of tumors in the larger bronchi. The cytologic study of the bronchial secretions obtained by bronchial brushings, at bronchoscopy, and from sputum may demonstrate tumor cells even though the neoplasm is not visible

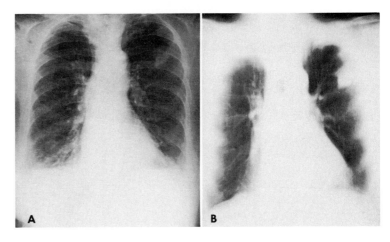

Fig. 17-58. Tomography. *A.* Small bronchogenic carcinoma superimposed on anterior end of left third rib. *B.* Tomogram defining lesion.

through the bronchoscope. Negative bronchoscopic findings do not rule out a neoplasm; in fact, the carcinoma in its earlier stages is not visible endoscopically in the vast majority of cases.

DIFFERENTIAL DIAGNOSIS. Among the nonneoplastic pulmonary lesions which can simulate cancer of the lung are solitary tuberculous lesions, chronic lung abscess, bronchial erosion by lymph nodes, lipoid and interstitial pneumonia, and pulmonary infarction. The scattered infiltration usually seen in the tuberculous lesions permits radiographic differentiation from a tumor in most instances. If only a solitary rounded tuberculous focus is seen on the roentgenogram, the appearance may be similar to that of a benign tumor or peripheral carcinoma. Since noncavitary tuberculous lesions do not necessarily produce a sputum with tubercle bacilli, only pathologic examination of the surgically excised nodule will establish the diagnosis (Fig. 17-59). Chronic lung abscess may be confused clinically and radiographically with either a centrally excavated carcinoma or abscess distal to a bronchogenic cancer. Erosion of the wall of a bronchus by a diseased or calcified lymph node may cause severe hemoptyses and the signs of an endobronchial lesion. Bronchoscopy, bronchography, and tomography aid in differentiation, but doubt may remain prior to surgical exploration. Lipoid pneumonia may be suspected from a history of use of oily nose drops or mineral oil inhalation due to impaired gag reflex. Unless the possibility of lipoid pneumonia is considered preoperatively, the surgeon may needlessly sacrifice lung tissue because of inability to distinguish chronic

Fig. 17-59. Carcinoma in patient with tuberculosis. Mass in right upper lobe enlarged while patient was receiving chemotherapy for proved tuberculosis, chiefly in the left lung. Right upper lobectomy confirmed the suspected diagnosis of bronchogenic carcinoma. Patient was well 12 years later.

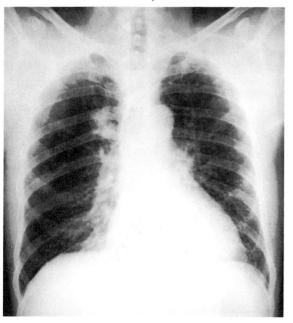

lipoid pneumonia from carcinoma on gross examination. Pulmonary infarction must be carefully differentiated from neoplasm, since surgical exploration is not indicated and is more hazardous in thromboembolic conditions.

Since the lungs are one of the most frequent sites of metastases from various primary neoplasms in other organs, the differentiation of primary pulmonary cancer from metastases is most important. Metastases are less likely to cause bronchial symptoms or hemoptysis. If the neoplasm is solitary and involves a bronchus, a primary bronchogenic carcinoma is most probable. When multiple nodules are present in the lungs, the pulmonary lesions are usually metastatic. Alveolar carcinoma of the lung, however, may be multicentric. A solitary nodule in the lung field might be either a primary or metastatic lesion. If physical and radiologic investigation of other portions of the body fail to demonstrate a primary neoplasm elsewhere, the pulmonary mass should be treated as a primary lung tumor (Fig. 17-60). Since multiple primary tumors are not rare, a solitary mass discovered in the lung of a person who previously had a primary cancer elsewhere should not lead to the assumption that the lung lesion is necessarily a metastasis (Fig. 17-61).

Alveolar carcinoma may present clinical and radiologic features which differ from bronchogenic carcinoma and simulate a diffuse inflammatory lesion or metastatic carcinoma. Severe dyspnea without obstruction of any major bronchus may be noted. Some cases of alveolar carcinoma have a profuse bronchorrhea with large amounts of watery sputum. Cytologic studies of the sputum are valuable.

TREATMENT. The indicated therapy for bronchogenic carcinoma will be influenced by the location and extent of the primary lesion, the presence and location of metastases, and the patient's general condition and respiratory reserve. A careful history is the best guide to possible metastatic disease outside the thorax; pain, weight loss, weakness, dyspnea, dysphagia, or recent hoarseness are all symptoms which suggest an unfavorable outlook. Roentgenographic findings of mediastinal involvement and bronchoscopic evidence of distortion or loss of mobility of the tracheobronchial tree may also suggest possible inoperability. Because of the frequency of mediastinal and cervical metastases diagnostic surgical exploration of these areas are often recommended. A most careful examination of the lower part of the neck for possible lymphadenopathy is indicated, because the biopsy of such lymph nodes may prove extrathoracic extension of the carcinoma and indicate the futility of pulmonary resection. Mediastinoscopy, either via a cervical approach or through a small parasternal incision, has many advocates as a means of establishing the extent of neoplastic invasion. Evidence of a paralyzed vocal cord, which indicates recurrent nerve involvement and pleural effusion, with positive cytology, generally precludes curative resection.

When pulmonary resection is decided upon, lobectomy or pneumonectomy with removal of adjacent lymph nodes is usually performed. In the earliest years of resectional surgery for cancer of the lung it was customary to perform a pneumonectomy. Experience has shown, however, that if the tumor can be completely removed by a lobectomy, the removal of additional lobes of the lung is unlikely to add significantly to the cancer cure rate, whereas the morbidity and mortality, both early and late, is significantly greater when the entire lung is removed. This is particularly true when the right lung is involved. Therefore in some cases of right upper lobe carcinoma, when the tumor encroaches on the main bronchus, segmental resection of the right main bronchus together with the upper lobe is advocated, the middle and lower lobe being saved by a bronchial reconstruction procedure. For large central lesions with submucosal extension to the carina or lateral tracheal wall, tracheal sleeve pneumonectomy with tracheobronchial anastomosis may be performed.

Radiation therapy is not indicated if the primary lesion has been removed with an adequate margin and the regional lymph nodes are negative. Radiation therapy may be employed for symptomatic relief of pain accompanying thoracic wall involvement or to reduce the size of the nonresectable tumor which obstructs the bronchus and results in atelectasis and pneumonitis. Dramatic effects have been reported with the use of radiation therapy and diuretics in patients with manifestations of superior vena cava obstruction. To date, chemotherapeutic agents have not proved helpful in the treatment of bronchogenic carcinoma.

An analysis of the disposition of 1,000 cases of carcinoma of the lung revealed that 22.5 percent were inoperable, 33.5 percent were explored but the lesion was not resectable, and 9 percent died in the hospital. Approximately one-quarter of the patients whose tumors were excised survived without evidence of recurrence for 5 years or longer. When the tumor is confined to the lung and there are no lymph node metastases, a 40 percent 5-year survival has been reported. Recently, encouraging results have been reported for patients with mediastinal metastases treated by resection and irradiation. There is an interesting suggestion that patients in whom empyema develops following resection have a better prognosis for long-term survival. Ninety percent of patients whose lesions are not resectable die within a year.

Treatment of Pulmonary Metastases. In selected patients with a solitary pulmonary metastasis the solitary metastatic lesion should be resected; a conservative type of resection

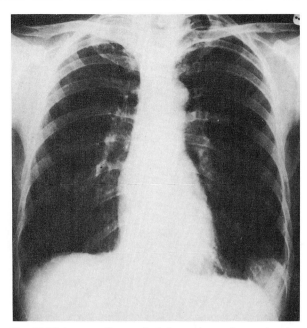

Fig. 17-60. Large solitary metastatic carcinoma from colon. Lesion simulated a primary pulmonary neoplasm and was treated by lobectomy.

is recommended. Prior to resection of the metastatic lesion, it should be ascertained that there is no evidence of residual or recurrent neoplasm at the primary site. If the patients are properly selected, the long-term results of the resection of a single pulmonary metastatic lesion may approach that obtained with resection of bronchogenic carcinoma (Fig. 17-62).

Diagnostic Operative Procedures

SCALENE FAT PAD BIOPSY

The procedure involves the excision of a deep cervical and paratracheal fat pad in the supraclavicular fossa of patients in whom cervical lymph nodes are not palpable. The operation is not routinely employed for peripherally

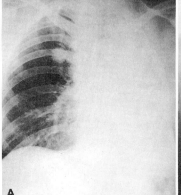
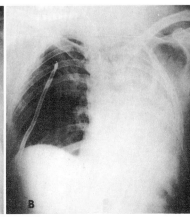

Fig. 17-61. Second primary carcinoma. A. A second primary carcinoma in right lung appearing several years after left pneumonectomy for bronchogenic carcinoma. B. Roentgenogram following segmental resection from right lung.

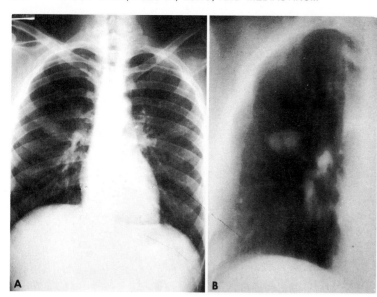

Fig. 17-62. Resection for metastatic carcinoma to the lung. *A.* Patient with paraosteal sarcoma of humerus and metastasis in right lung which appeared 2 years after arm was amputated. *B.* Tomogram shows tumor mass which was obscured by rib. Lesion was resected and patient was well 5 years later.

located lesions of the lung and is generally applicable if there is questionable resectability and with hilar or mediastinal node enlargement. The yield of positive tissue diagnosis in patients with carcinoma of the lung is reported to be less than 25 percent, but the presence of positive nodes in this location is indication that a curative pulmonary section cannot be accomplished. Scalene fat pad biopsy provides a diagnosis in approximately 80 percent of patients with Boeck's sarcoid and is an excellent diagnostic procedure if this condition is considered.

The operation is occasionally performed bilaterally to increase the diagnostic yield. However, in general, a right scalene fat pad biopsy is performed for lesions of the right lung, the left lower lobe, and the lingula, while a left scalene fat pad biopsy is performed for lesions of the left upper lobe. The operation is usually carried out under local anesthesia through a low-lying neck incision which courses parallel to the clavicle. The sternocleidomastoid muscle is retracted forward, or its posterior fibers are divided. The deep cervical fascia is incised, and the fat pad overlying the scalenus anterior muscle is mobilized. Dissection is carried out to the junction of the internal jugular vein and subclavian vein, taking care to avoid the phrenic nerve. The procedure, in effect, removes paratracheal and high superior mediastinal nodes for biopsy.

MEDIASTINOSCOPY AND BIOPSY

This is a procedure which permits biopsy of the lymph nodes in the upper mediastinum and is employed to aid in establishing the diagnosis of a variety of intrathoracic diseases. As is the case with scalene node biopsy, highest yields are obtained with sarcoidosis and other granulomatous processes. Mediastinoscopy is also employed to assess the operability of bronchogenic carcinoma without resorting to thoracotomy. In many instances it has sup-

planted scalene fat pad biopsy because of increased yield in patients with bronchogenic carcinoma.

Although some prefer to perform the procedure by resecting the second costal cartilage, the more usual approach is through a cervical incision with dissection downward along the paratracheal fascia. Insertion of a flat laryngoscope into the wound provides illumination and visualization of the area.

DIAGNOSTIC BIOPSY OF THE LUNG

The principle of most surgical treatment of the lungs is the excision of the diseased portion of pulmonary tissue. In another group of pulmonary diseases, the only goal of the surgical intervention is to obtain a sufficient piece of lung with pathologic tissue to establish the exact nature of a diffuse pulmonary pathologic process. In these instances, the surgical procedure is undertaken entirely as a diagnostic measure. Subsequent therapy may then be medical, hormonal, or a radiotherapeutic modality.

A biopsy of the lung may be required to differentiate multiple small pulmonary metastases from focal areas of pulmonary fibrosis of varied causes. Among the latter are the occupational causes of pulmonary fibrosis such as berylliosis, silicosis, asbestosis, farmer's lung, and other, less common industrial hazards. Chemical analysis of the biopsied portion of lung tissue may be necessary to determine the offending agent. In some cases, the cause of the pulmonary fibrosis may remain obscure.

Since many of the patients in whom a lung biopsy is undertaken for diagnostic reasons are short of breath because of the effects of the diffuse pulmonary lesion and often have associated pulmonary emphysema, it is highly desirable that the procedure be associated with minimal risk of even minor complications which would result in a further reduction in respiratory function. Needle biopsy under fluoroscopic control frequently will provide the diagnosis. If thoractomy is required, the chest wall incision should be of a type associated with minimal chest wall pain and little impairment of ventilatory motion; the technique should assure immediate reexpansion of the lung and entail little pleural reaction. These goals are usually best attained by an anterior intercostal incision of only sufficient size to permit an edge of a pulmonary lobe to be drawn with relatively atraumatic clamps up into the wound. The multitoothed clamps originally designed for vascular surgical procedures are eminently satisfactory for this purpose. Techniques which minimize the risk of significant leakage of air from the lung in the postoperative period should be utilized.

Pulmonary Resection

The risk of morbidity and mortality following a lobectomy or pneumonectomy may be dependent in no small measure on the patient's preoperative cardiorespiratory status. The question to be answered is what degree of permanent reduction in respiratory capacity is to be anticipated. When a patient has bilateral pulmonary disease, a detailed evaluation is necessary to assess whether the lung requiring removal may be contributing a significant portion of the total respiratory function. In some patients, although a pneumonectomy is contraindicated, a less extensive operation, such as lobectomy combined with a bronchoplastic procedure, may be feasible. Such a situation is frequently encountered in the elderly patient with carcinoma of the lung who has a significant degree of diffuse pulmonary emphysema.

The risk of any pulmonary resection may be greatly increased by partial tracheal obstruction or compression of the bronchi near the carina. Careful auscultation of the lungs and adequate bronchoscopic examination should alert the surgeon to such a situation. The presence of much sputum usually means that further preoperative preparation with appropriate antibiotics is indicated prior to operation. Except in emergency situations, it is best not to undertake a resection when the patient is expectorating blood in more than very minimal amounts. Clotted blood in the airway can readily become a life-threatening hazard. Minimizing the physiologic burden of the operation itself is particularly critical in patients with marginal reserve.

PRECAUTIONS DURING OPERATION

Few lung resections are emergency procedures. It follows that the operation should not be undertaken on the planned day if something occurs that renders the patient a poorer risk than he or she might be a few days or a week later. Unexplained fever or a change in general condition just prior to the time of a scheduled operation may be such a factor. An unfavorable reaction to preoperative medication may increase the operative risk. But the single most important and most frequent reason for postponing the operation is the occurrence of a period of hypoxia during anesthesia. This may be caused by difficulty in introducing the intratracheal tube and may be associated with some trauma to the upper air passages.

One of the greatest and most widespread fallacies in thinking is the notion that if the color of the patient returns to normal and the pulse and electrocardiographic findings revert to normal after a period of severe hypoxia, the patient has completely recovered from the detrimental episode. It should be appreciated that many complications which become manifest hours or days later if a major surgical procedure is superimposed on such a hypoxic episode can be traced back to such an error in judgment.

Although the assignment of duties among the members of the surgical team may vary, it is important that while the patient is still in the supine position, both sides of the chest be auscultated so as to be certain that the intratracheal tube is in proper position and not placed so far down as to interfere with unrestricted ventilation of each lung. The operation should not be started until it is ascertained by the anesthetist that the patient's ventilatory and circulatory status is optimum.

Throughout the operation any abnormal manifestation should be reported by anesthetist and surgeon to each other. It is easier for the surgeon to tell that the blood is not adequately oxygenated when he makes a skin or muscle incision than it is for the anesthetist to determine the color of the blood by the skin appearance. At other times during the operation, however, the anesthetist may note cyanosis when the surgeon is unaware of it. When the chest is open, the alert surgeon may be aware of secretions in the air passages before they are obvious to the anesthetist. Such secretions should be aspirated as soon as detected.

Close cooperation between surgeon and anesthetist is also required in the management of any cardiac arrhythmias or impairment of cardiac contraction. Whenever such circulatory abnormalities occur, interruption of all surgical manipulation may facilitate and hasten the return to a normal circulatory status. Minimizing traction on the hilus of the lung, avoiding unnecessary manipulations, and allowing a few minutes rest period before resuming surgical maneuvers after the electrocardiogram or blood pressure has shown cardiocirculatory abnormalities will lessen operative risks. The experienced surgeon will almost always recognize warning signs of trouble in pulmonary surgical procedures before serious cardiocirculatory failure occurs.

Undue traction on the main bronchus must be avoided. Such traction may impair the ventilation of the opposite lung by tracheal or bronchial angulation or by displacement or partial occlusion of the end of the endotracheal tube. The anesthetist should report immediately to the surgeon any change noted in the ease of pulmonary ventilation. The threat of hypoxia during operation is constant. Bronchial secretions, blood in the airway, and mechanical obstruction may quickly lead to severe degrees of hypoxia. Whenever bleeding into the tracheobronchial tree occurs, it is mandatory that the blood be aspirated quickly before clots, which are difficult to remove, have formed.

Much evidence has become available in recent years to indicate the ever-present possibility of respiratory acidosis in the patient undergoing lung resection. Respiratory acidosis is primarily due to inadequate alveolar ventilation.

It is true, however, that in some clinics such a degree of ventilation is now employed that the patient may actually have respiratory alkalosis. This too is undesirable. Present knowledge and equipment should permit us to keep the patient in a normal hydrogen ion range.

Since removal of an entire lung results in a drastic reduction in the available pulmonary vascular bed, it is of paramount importance that no circulatory overload be created by the injudicious intravenous administration of fluids. Since giving the patient some blood by transfusion during the operative procedure is usually indicated and since some additional fluid is usually administered by the anesthetist as a vehicle for various anesthetic agents, the patient is likely to receive more than 1,000 ml of fluid intravenously during operation. If more than 1,000 ml of blood is given during the pneumonectomy, the total volume of fluid infused may reach undesirable quantities. In the patient undergoing pulmonary resection and especially if major portions of the pulmonary vascular bed are removed, it would seem much safer to err on the side of having the patient slightly dehydrated rather than overhydrated. With modern anesthetic techniques, the incidence of postoperative nausea and vomiting has been significantly reduced, and many patients may be permitted to take fluid by mouth shortly after recovery from anesthesia.

In the performance of a pneumonectomy it is highly desirable to obtain a good, relatively airtight closure of the thoracic wall at the conclusion of the operation. If the deeper layers of the thoracotomy incision are not closely approximated and air can readily be forced out of the pleural space into the tissues of the chest wall, several undesirable sequelae may occur: The extrusion of air from the pleural space will result in mediastinal displacement toward the side of the pneumonectomy, and the dissection of air along fascial planes of the chest wall and into the neck can occasionally become sufficiently severe to cause compression of the great veins.

TECHNIQUE OF PULMONARY RESECTION

POSITION AND INCISION. Although thoracic incisions should be modified to meet special situations dictated by variations in the pathologic features, experience has demonstrated that certain operative approaches have a wide utility. Most operations undertaken for lung resection, with the exception of the less extensive procedure required for a lung biopsy, are best performed through a posterolateral incision with the patient in the lateral decubitus position. Although this position of the patient increases the demands on the skill of the anesthesiologist in overcoming some physiologic disadvantages which this position imposes, these drawbacks are usually offset by the greater safety of this approach.

This lateral decubitus position may be undesirable, however, whenever large amounts of bronchial secretion liberated from the uppermost diseased lung might tend to flow downward into the dependent lung. This is a special danger in the rare instances where lung resection must be undertaken in the face of active pulmonary hemorrhage.

Blood in the airway which may clot before it is aspirated by the anesthesiologist is a potentially great threat, as it may suddenly plug the main bronchus of the opposite lung and cause a sudden fatality or at least an episode of severe hypoxia which is highly detrimental. Therefore, modified positions of the patient which lessen the threat of the gravitation of material into the opposite lung are indicated in these special circumstances. The prone or supine position of the patient on the operating table, with modifications in the site of surgical incision, may be best under these special circumstances. An alternate method is the use of a special type of endobronchial tube such as the Carlens tube which, if properly placed, may prevent blood or secretions from crossing over into the other lung; these special methods require experienced personnel for their satisfactory use.

The posterolateral thoracotomy incision is so placed that it permits sufficient upward displacement of the scapula in operative procedures involving the upper lobe where resection of the fifth or sixth rib or a fifth intercostal incision may be elected (Fig. 17-63). When a lower lobe lobectomy is planned, a seventh rib approach may be satisfactory unless, as in the case of carcinoma, a more extensive resection such as pneumonectomy is found to be necessary because of the extent of the neoplastic process. Resection of either the fifth or sixth rib in cases of a planned pneumonectomy is usually best. Incisions made through the bed of a resected rib are preferred in cases of pneumonectomy, because such openings into the pleural cavity can be closed in a more airtight fashion than intercostal incisions (Fig. 17-64A). This is a distinct advantage in lessening the tendency of air from the empty pleural space to be forced into the tissues of the chest wall on coughing in the postoperative period.

RESECTION. Following entry into the pleural cavity such division of pleural adhesions as may be necessary for the insertion of a rib spreader is first accomplished. Then, after adequate spreading of ribs, the pathologic findings are assessed. The portion of lung to be resected is freed of visceroparietal adhesions so as to gain better exposure of the pulmonary hilus. When secretions or blood from the diseased portion of the lung threaten maintenance of a good airway, early occlusion of the bronchus is desirable in order to lessen the risk of aspiration into other parts of the lungs. Usually the hilar dissection consists of division of the mediastinal pleura, dissecting out those pulmonary arterial branches which require ligation (Fig. 17-64B) and division and then dissecting out the corresponding pulmonary veins. Most of the bronchial arterial supply is not interrupted until the bronchus is transected, since these vessels are largely in intimate relationship to the bronchus.

When cancer is being resected, some surgeons consider it important to occlude the pulmonary veins early, in the belief that this lessens the risk of liberation of cancer cells into the bloodstream during the operation. If the veins are occluded early when a large inflow of blood into the lung is still possible, the lung may distend with blood and be less compressible. In those pathologic conditions in which a greatly augmented bronchial arterial supply has developed, it is desirable to interrupt some of this inflow before or quickly after the pulmonary veins are ligated, since this bronchial arterial flow is returned via the pulmonary veins.

Safe ligation of the hilar blood vessels is achieved by rigid observation of the following principles: (1) an adequate length of the vessel must be isolated (Fig. 17-64C); this often means dissecting out the branches distad (Fig. 17-64D); (2) an adequate length of vessel stump must be present distal to the ligature site; dividing the vessel close to the ligature is never safe, especially if the vessel is large (Fig. 17-64E); (3) inappropriately large-sized ligatures should be avoided, as they cannot be tied with the same snugness that can be attained with the proper-sized thread; the size of thread employed is adjusted to the size of the structure being managed.

The history of pulmonary resection indicates the importance of obtaining healing of the transected bronchus, since the development of a postoperative bronchopleural fistula has been a most important cause of postoperative morbidity and mortality. Although various surgeons may employ somewhat different techniques, the observance of the following principles are the fundamental considerations: (1) the bronchus should be free of disease at the site of transection; (2) a good blood supply to the edge of the transected bronchus is important; undue stripping of the peribronchial tissues is undesirable; (3) the blood supply should not be jeopardized by too many sutures or sutures tied too tightly, or sutures of a type which strangulates tissue (Fig. 17-64F); and (4) a flap of tissue overlying the bronchial stump may be beneficial (Fig. 17-64G).

DRAINAGE. All lobectomies, segmental resections, wedge resections, and lung biopsies should have a closed drainage of the pleural space established at the end of the operation. This permits drainage of air and fluid from the pleural cavity and favors early reexpansion of the remaining lung tissue. Suction is preferred by many surgeons, although this is not routine. Drainage of the empty pleural space following pneumonectomy is not advised.

Segmental Resection

When the nature and extent of the pulmonary pathologic process is such that adequate treatment of the disease is possible with removal of only one or two segments of a lobe of lung, a segmental resection may be elected. This may be done in order to minimize the sacrifice of functioning pulmonary tissue. It must be appreciated, however, that problems with full reexpansion of the residual portion of lung and pleural complications postoperatively can markedly impair the respiratory function of the remaining portion of the lung. Therefore in many instances of essentially unilateral disease it may be better to do a lobectomy rather than a segmental type of resection which would leave behind only one more segment of lung.

The anatomic basis of a segmental resection of a portion of a pulmonary lobe is the segmental distribution of the bronchi with their accompanying branches of the pulmonary artery. The branches of the pulmonary veins are located in the intersegmental plane. Bronchi do not traverse the intersegmental plane, and therefore blunt sepa-

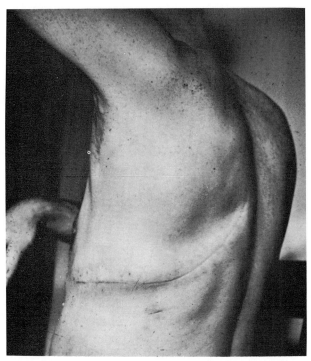

Fig. 17-63. Healed posterolateral thoracotomy incision. Site of drainage tube is a short scar in axillary line below main incision.

ration of the lung tissue in this plane should not result in major air leakage. The small branches of the pulmonary vein can be dealt with individually as a segment of the lung is teased bluntly away from the adjacent segment.

The amount of immediate and delayed air leakage which follows a segmental resection of lung tissue will depend on how well the surgeon had adhered to the anatomic intersegmental plane and minimized trauma to the adjacent remaining segment, and also on how free the lung is of fibrosis and emphysema. Blunt dissection of a normal intersegmental plane may result in surprisingly little air leakage, whereas fibrosis and emphysema of the lung may render such a type of resection prone to a high incidence of postoperative morbidity due to continued air leakage into the pleural space.

Wedge Resection

When a small mass lies close to the pleural surface of the lung, it may be feasible to remove the mass intact with a small margin of adjacent pulmonary tissue by a wedge resection of that portion of the lung. The technique of wedge resection is also a good method of obtaining a piece of lung tissue for the diagnosis of a diffuse pulmonary lesion. Subpleural granulomas in particular are an indication for wedge resection. In some cases a very small peripheral tumor of unknown histologic nature may be removed by a wedge resection and then immediately examined by frozen-section technique to ascertain the pathologic diagnosis, which will then indicate whether additional pulmonary tissue should be resected.

The multitoothed vascular clamps originally designed

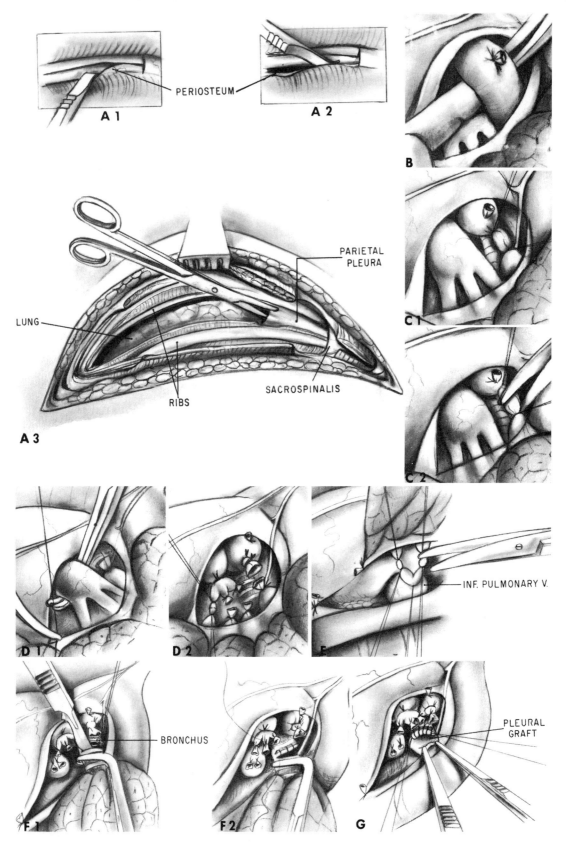

PERIOSTEUM

A 1

A 2

B

PARIETAL
PLEURA

LUNG

SACROSPINALIS

RIBS

A 3

C 1

C 2

D 1

D 2

INF. PULMONARY V.

E

BRONCHUS

F 1

F 2

PLEURAL
GRAFT

G

for resection of a coarctation of the aorta are especially good for the performance of a wedge resection. A pie-shaped piece of lung is isolated by the application of two such clamps at right angles to each other. It is desirable that the ends of the two clamps should be close together. If this is not feasible, it usually indicates that the pulmonary lesion is too large or too deep within the lung for a satisfactory wedge resection; a segmental resection or lobectomy is then a better and safer procedure.

In the performance of a wedge resection it is essential that the surgeon have control of the pulmonary tissue at the apex of the wedge, because the main pulmonary arterial branch and bronchus to the area to be resected will tend to be in this region. If the cut vessel and bronchus retract centrally out of control, blood in dangerous amounts may flow into the severed bronchus and flood the bronchial tree without evidence of much bleeding in the operative field. Control of the apex of the wedge to be resected may be secured by placing and tying a mattress suture through-and-through the lung at that central point. The wedge of lung to be removed is secured by cutting the lung a sufficient distance peripheral to the multitoothed clamps, so that a row of mattress sutures on an atraumatic needle can be inserted and tied before the clamps are removed. When the pulmonary tissue is emphysematous, great care in minimizing trauma to the lung tissue is especially important, because otherwise continued air leakage from the lung may be a disturbing postoperative problem which increases morbidity.

Bronchial Surgery

Transthoracic Bronchotomy. This procedure may be employed for removing impacted foreign bodies and for treating a lesion in one of the larger bronchi which cannot be satisfactorily managed by endoscopic means. Plastic repair of a benign stricture which has not responded to peroral dilatation is occasionally feasible; retrograde dilatation and disruption of such a stricture via a bronchotomy opening distal to the stricture site is occasionally indicated. Care must be taken not to produce undesirable narrowing of the bronchus in the process of suturing the opening into the bronchus; a pleural flap over the suture line is highly desirable.

◀ Fig. 17-64. Resection of lung. A. Opening into pleural cavity. 1, Periosteum incised over the rib; 2, subperiosteal resection being performed; 3, pleura opened through bed of resected rib. B. Freeing of pulmonary artery from adjacent structures. C. Ligation and division of pulmonary artery. 1, Artery doubly ligated with an adequate distance between the two ligatures; 2, artery transected between two ligatures; D. Peripheral dissection of pulmonary artery to increase safety factor. 1, Branches of pulmonary artery and main pulmonary artery identified; 2, branches individually double-ligated and transected. E. Division of pulmonary vein. Double ligatures are on inferior pulmonary vein which is to be transected. F. Transection of bronchus. This is performed after ligation of pulmonary arteries and veins. Diagram indicates bronchial transection during a left pneumonectomy. 1, Clamp is applied to bronchus distad, and as the bronchus is transected, the proximal end is closed with interrupted sutures in order to avoid a widely open bronchus with its associated ventilatory disturbance; 2, progression of bronchial transection. G. Pleural flap placed over sutured bronchial stump.

Bronchoplastic Reconstruction. This is employed in cases in which a segment of a bronchus requires resection. Either an end-to-end anastomosis may be performed, or a bronchial defect may be repaired by utilizing a flap fashioned from adjacent tissue.

POSTOPERATIVE CARE

The fundamental principles of the postoperative care of all surgical patients apply to the thoracic patient, but because of the reduction in respiratory function which most of these patients have, related to either disease or the physiologic alterations imposed by the surgical procedure, details in management can play a vital role in reducing postoperative morbidity and mortality.

Combating respiratory depression is of great importance in the patient whose pulmonary function is reduced by disease, because otherwise detrimental hypoxia will occur. During operation the action of the depressant drugs used as anesthetic agents is combated by manual or mechanical assisted ventilation. After operation such augmentation of ventilation is usually discontinued except in patients in a precarious state. Thus, at a time when the effect of the anesthetic agents has not yet been completely eliminated, respiratory depression is common. Even though the respiratory rate may be satisfactory, the amplitude of ventilation is often inadequate at this time.

MEDIASTINAL POSITIONING AND ADJUSTMENT OF INTRATHORACIC PRESSURE. Among the factors requiring particular attention in patients subjected to pneumonectomy, the proper position of the mediastinum in the immediate postoperative period deserves special consideration. When the mediastinum is left displaced toward the contralateral side for even a brief time at the conclusion of a pneumonectomy, a number of physiologically adverse conditions are permitted to exist. A displaced mediastinum indicates an abnormal intrathoracic pressure, which places an additional burden on the cardiovascular system of a patient who has been required to make important physiologic adjustments to compensate for ligation of one main pulmonary artery. Although the sudden shunting of the entire right ventricular output through a single lung in the good-risk patient is not accompanied by demonstrable radical pressure alterations in the cardiovascular system, the magnitude of this remarkable readjustment in circulatory dynamics should not be forgotten.

There has been a regrettable failure to appreciate the importance of accurate adjustment of intrathoracic pressure after pneumonectomy. Manometric recordings of the intrapleural pressure should be taken as soon as the patient is placed in the supine position at the conclusion of the operation; when necessary, the proper amount of air to achieve a normal mean intrapleural pressure of about -4 to -6 cm of water should be withdrawn or introduced. The aim of adjusting the intrapleural pressure is to leave the mediastinum in its normal position, so that the remaining lung will not be compressed or overinflated in the early postoperative period. When satisfactory intrapleural pressure readings cannot be obtained because of the abnormal character of the expiratory phase of respiration in some patients coming out of anesthesia, a roentgenogram of

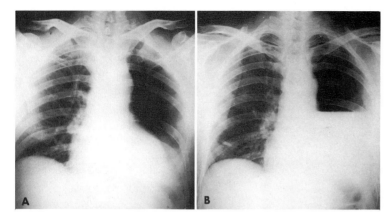

Fig. 17-65. Postpneumonectomy roentgenogram. *A.* One day after pneumonectomy. Left hemithorax contains much air and little fluid. Mediastinum is in normal position. *B.* A few days later there is absorption of air as fluid in the left side of the chest gradually fills the hemithorax.

the chest should immediately be taken to determine the mediastinal position.

Clinical guides which may be employed to determine the position of the mediastinum in the days following operation include (1) palpation of the trachea in the cervical region, (2) palpation and auscultation to determine the position of the apex of the heart, and (3) a roentgenogram of the chest. The last is by far the most reliable. Whereas deviations of the trachea may be quite apparent in some cases of massive atelectasis of an entire lung, one may be unimpressed by tracheal shift in some cases of pneumo-

Fig. 17-66. Roentgenogram following left pneumonectomy and thoracoplasty.

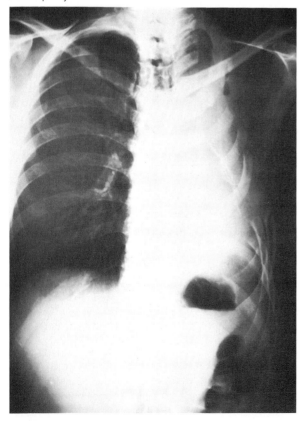

nectomy with considerable mediastinal shift. The heart may be displaced to a significant degree without the cervical trachea's showing obvious deviation. In some patients it may be possible to determine the site of the apical impulse of the heart with considerable reliability, whereas in others the location of the heart may not be readily ascertained. This is particularly true in barrel-chested, emphysematous patients, and these constitute the majority of those undergoing pneumonectomy for carcinoma.

The roentgenogram of the chest must be properly taken in order to give the most reliable information (Fig. 17-65). Unless a true anteroposterior view is obtained, an erroneous interpretation of the position of the mediastinum may be made. In instances of even slightly oblique projections, the mediastinum may appear more or less displaced than is truly the case. When the policy of avoiding even slight degrees of mediastinal displacement in the first few days after pneumonectomy is closely adhered to, the incidence of pulmonary edema in the remaining lung and cardiocirculatory complications will be considerably lower than reported in many publications. Whenever a cardiac arrhythmia develops in the postoperative period, a bedside roentgenogram of the chest should immediately be taken and studied in order to ascertain whether the mediastinum is in good position. If displacement to the contralateral side is present, this should be corrected by the removal of air or fluid, or both, from the pneumonectomy space until it has been demonstrated by another roentgenogram that the mediastinal displacement has been corrected. If the mediastinum is displaced toward the side from which the lung was removed, air should be introduced into the empty pleural space under manometric control and roentgenographic confirmation of proper correction obtained. If atrial fibrillation has developed, an electrocardiogram should be made and appropriate drug therapy instituted at once. Although cardiac arrhythmias are common in elderly patients undergoing pneumonectomy for carcinoma, the occurrence and duration of this complication can be lessened by avoiding mediastinal displacement (Fig. 17-66).

RESPIRATORY DISTRESS. Ordinarily the patient who has had a lung removed should not feel that he is short of breath while inactive in the first few days after operation. Appropriate positioning of the patient is directed at minimizing ventilation/perfusion abnormalities. The oxygen which is routinely given for the first 1 to 3 days may contribute to this lack of sense of dyspnea. Respiratory distress or a feeling of tightness in the chest should be regarded as an abnormal state. It is most commonly caused by retained tracheobronchial secretions or an unfavorable intrathoracic pressure. Restlessness is often the first sign of hypoxia and demands correction of its cause. It is most important to avoid heavy sedation of the patient who is restless as a result of anoxemia, since such management may seriously aggravate an already dangerous situation.

ANATOMIC AND PHYSIOLOGIC ADJUSTMENT AFTER LOBECTOMY AND PNEUMONECTOMY. After a lobectomy the remaining lobe or lobes, if relatively normal, will hyperinflate and obliterate the pleural space, which may be somewhat smaller as a result of compensatory elevation of the diaphragm (Fig. 17-67) and sometimes slight shift of the mediastinum. If the remaining lobe is abnormal and compensatory hyperinflation is limited, the pleural space may have to be reduced in size by an extrapleural thoracoplasty. Occasionally after a right pneumonectomy, if the left lung has obstructive emphysema, severe dyspnea and cor pulmonale may ensue unless a thoracoplasty is performed (Fig. 17-68). Usually after a left pneumonectomy for cancer no thoracoplasty to diminish the mediastinal displacement is necessary.

A right as well as a left pneumonectomy performed in childhood may cause no dyspnea when adult years are reached in spite of the marked anatomic distortions which may be present (Fig. 17-69). Also no circulatory disturbances may be noted in spite of the dextrocardia.

HYPOVENTILATION IN THE POSTOPERATIVE PERIOD. Many investigations have demonstrated the frequent occurrence of hypoventilation in surgical patients in the early postoperative period. The same dose of narcotic or sedative which is satisfactory on the first or second postoperative day may be responsible for significant depression of respiration with its secondary hypoxia, and often subsequent hypotension, if given in the early postoperative hours. Therefore, half the usual dose is often best for the first injection. Too often hypotension which is predominantly due to poor ventilation is treated by increasing the blood volume by infusions or transfusions which may increase pulmonary congestion.

In spite of voluminous documentation of the important role of adequate spontaneous respirations in assuring good cardiovascular function, respiratory depression by injudicious dosage in the early postoperative hours is a frequent occurrence. Many studies have shown that the oxygen tension in the blood of patients shortly after the termination of anesthesia is below normal. Oxygen therapy is frequently indicated in the early postoperative hours. Whereas oxygen therapy may correct the hypoxia, it does not eliminate the possibility of pulmonary complications which the hypoventilation may foreshadow. Hypoventilation is associated with blood stasis in the dependent portions of the lung and a diminished lymphatic drainage from the lungs; both these factors favor the development

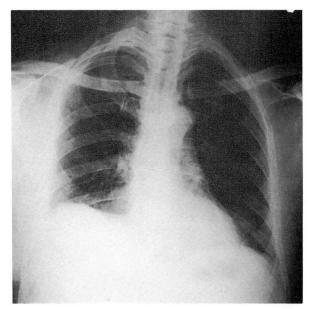

Fig. 17-67. Roentgenogram after recovery from right upper lobe lobectomy for carcinoma. Note elevation of diaphragm.

of patchy atelectasis and ventilation/perfusion abnormalities with intraparenchymal shunting of blood. That it is desirable for the surgical patient to reestablish normal breathing as quickly as possible after operation has long been evident. Restlessness is often a sign of hypoxia, for

Fig. 17-68. Obstructive emphysema following pneumonectomy. Roentgenogram of patient several years after right pneumonectomy for carcinoma. The undesirable degree of overdistension at the left lung was due to obstructive emphysema. Thoracoplasty was of some benefit.

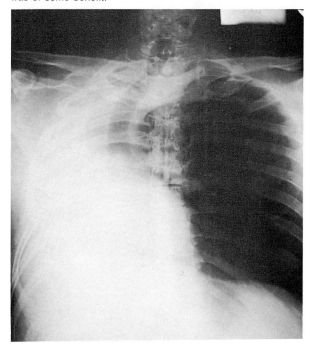

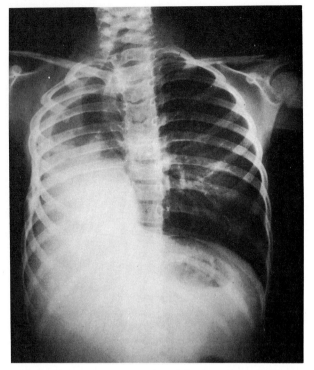

Fig. 17-69. Anatomic distortion following pneumonectomy. Roentgenogram was made several years after right pneumonectomy for multiple lung abscesses in childhood. Note tracheal displacement and herniation of left lung into right hemithorax. Patient was asymptomatic.

which proper oxygenation, not more sedation, is the logical therapy.

Whereas the great value of assisted respiration, manual or mechanical, is well established, it is not as physiologic as the patient's own normal respiratory effort. Hence, it should be our goal to leave the normal ventilatory drive essentially unimpaired. When that goal cannot be attained, the respiratory effort should be supported without delay by assisted respiration and oxygen therapy.

Trachea

TRACEAL ABNORMALITIES OF INFANCY AND CHILDHOOD

The importance and pathology of lesions of the trachea are greatly influenced by the age of the patient. Because of the small size of the infant's trachea, even small degrees of narrowing of the lumen may be of grave clinical significance. A wide variety of inflammatory swellings of the tracheal mucosa may lead to respiratory difficulty of varying degree, and hence there is a great tendency to ascribe respiratory difficulty in infancy to a tracheobronchitis. Aspirated foreign bodies may lodge in the trachea. A careful history obtained from the infant's nurse or parents may aid in differentiating acute tracheobronchitis from dyspnea caused by congenital malformations. Among the latter conditions are maldevelopments of the trachea and

especially tracheal and bronchial obstruction by anomalous vessels such as a double aortic arch. Roentgenograms which delineate the tracheal air column may be helpful but at times are difficult to interpret. Delineation of the esophagus with contrast medium may yield informative x-rays, because vascular anomalies which compress the trachea often produce a characteristic indenting of the esophagus (see Chap. 18).

Examination of the larynx aids in distinguishing laryngeal from tracheal causes of respiratory obstruction. In an infant with subcutaneous hemangiomas, a subglottic or tracheal hemangioma may be the cause of respiratory difficulty in the first few months of life. Maldevelopment of components of the foregut may lead to cysts, such as those of the bronchogenic type, which may compress either the trachea or esophagus, or both (see Tumors of the Mediastinum, below).

A tracheal cause for respiratory difficulty should be considered whenever the physical findings point to a bilateral obstruction and roentgenograms of the lungs do not demonstrate pulmonary findings which explain the physical findings. Bronchoscopy is an important diagnostic procedure in selected cases, but it must be appreciated that even slight trauma to an inflamed tracheal mucosa in an infant may cause a serious degree of respiratory obstruction. Tracheoesophageal fistula unassociated with esophageal atresia may cause recurrent respiratory infections due to aspiration.

TRACHEAL LESIONS IN ADULTS

Acute inflammatory processes are much less likely to cause serious narrowing of the trachea in adults than in children. Tuberculous involvement of the trachea may progress to stricture formation, but such a development is now rare with adequate antituberculous chemotherapy before the pulmonary disease is advanced. The trachea may be injured by blunt or penetrating trauma with resultant dyspnea which may be severe. Examination of the neck may reveal the crepitation of air in the paratracheal tissues, and roentgenography may disclose cervical and mediastinal emphysema. Surgical repair, usually combined with tracheostomy, is then indicated.

Tumors are an important cause of tracheal narrowing in adults. These may be mediastinal masses which compress the trachea or neoplasms primary in the tracheal wall (Fig. 17-70). Because wheezing is a common finding with lesions which narrow the trachea, asthma is often incorrectly diagnosed in such cases. The absence of any history of asthma in earlier life should lead to a consideration of nonallergic causes of wheezing. Bronchoscopy is the essential diagnostic procedure. All tumors of the trachea, whether histologically benign or malignant, threaten life. Adenoid cystic carcinoma (cylindroma), carcinoid adenomas, polyps (both inflammatory and neoplastic), and carcinoma may occur in the trachea. Except for inflammatory polyps which may be removed bronchoscopically, tumors of the trachea should be treated by tracheal resection unless the lesion is inoperable because of metastasis or extent of the neoplasm. In some cases, a small tumor may be resected and tracheal continuity may be reestablished

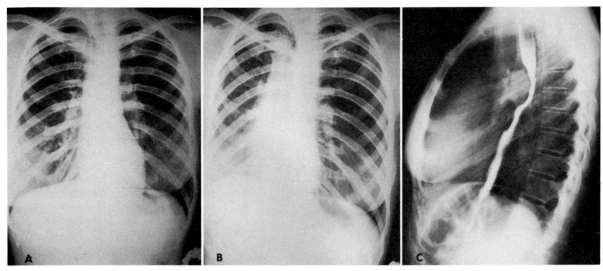

Fig. 17-70. Carcinoma of trachea with esophageal involvement. *A.* Roentgenogram on inspiration is not revealing. *B.* Expiratory film shows mediastinal shift to right because of tumor partially blocking left main bronchus. *C.* Esophagogram shows esophageal involvement.

by direct end-to-end anastomosis after thorough mobilization of the trachea. In other cases, prosthetic material may be employed to bridge the gap. It is mandatory that a rigid framework be provided, so that the trachea does not collapse on inspiration. Retained secretions, granulation tissue, and strictures may be postoperative problems. Roentgen ray therapy may afford long palliation in inoperable cases of adenoid cystic carcinoma.

Strictures of the trachea may follow a poorly executed tracheostomy or the prolonged presence of a tube in the trachea. In recent years the widespread use of cuffed endotracheal and tracheostomy tubes in the treatment of respiratory insufficiency and failure has resulted in the later development of tracheostenosis in a significant percentage of the critically ill. Clinical and experimental evidence has definitely demonstrated the mechanism by which such tracheal stenosis is produced. The inflated cuff on the tube causes an ischemia of the compressed tracheal mucosa; the greater the pressure in the balloon and the longer the time that the cuff is inflated, the greater the likelihood of damage to the tracheal wall. The pathologic process may vary from edema and superficial ulceration to the development of granulation tissue. The late effect of such ulceration of the tracheal wall not infrequently results in the development of tracheal stenosis which is caused by the replacement of the granulation tissue by fibrosis with marked narrowing of the tracheal airway. In rare instances the ischemia may be so pronounced that necrosis through the entire thickness of the tracheal wall ensues, and a tracheoesophageal fistula may result. The fibrous tracheal stenosis is often not responsive to conservative management and is best treated by resection of the stenotic area of the trachea and an end-to-end anastomosis. A considerable length of the trachea can be surgically resected and an end-to-end anastomosis performed if the lower portion of the trachea and main bronchi are freed.

The incidence of tracheal stenosis due to cuffed tubes can be significantly reduced by greater attention to the following factors: (1) the degree of pressure in the balloon, (2) whether the balloon is intermittently deflated, (3) the total length of time the balloon is inflated, and (4) the type of balloon used. Fortunately intratracheal tubes and tracheostomy tubes are now available with balloons which lessen the degree of ischemia of the tracheal mucosa when properly employed.

Dilatation or plastic reconstruction is indicated for such a tracheal obstruction. In dealing with all types of tracheal obstruction, it is important to realize that a trachea may be narrowed considerably without causing very obvious difficulty but that only a slight further decrease in the size of the airway, as may result from some edema, may be life-threatening or rapidly fatal.

TRACHEOSTOMY. The important role of tracheostomy in high obstructions to the airway has long been known. The value of tracheostomy as a route for removal of excessive recurrent bronchial secretions is well established. Bronchoscopic aspiration, transnasal tracheal suction, and transoral intubation of trachea with an intratracheal tube all have their place, but a tracheostomy may be superior in a given patient. At times, a tracheostomy permits better artificial ventilation of the lungs in the patient who has sustained extensive chest trauma or has severe respiratory or cardiocirculatory insufficiency. However, certain complications which may be associated with the employment of a tracheostomy must be borne in mind if the procedure is to be assigned its most beneficial place. In spite of apparently aseptic techniques used in the care of a tracheostomy, some patients develop serious pulmonary infections with bacteria often resistant to most antibiotics. A tracheostomy negates some of the defense barriers which the upper air passages normally provide.

Technique. Local anesthesia is generally employed, and a vertical incision extending from the cricoid cartilage to the suprasternal notch provides optimal exposure. Division and ligature of the thyroid isthmus may be required to expose the tracheal rings. The opening into the trachea is made in the midline at the level of the second ring and frequently extends across the third ring. A dilator keeps the tracheal edges apart while the tube is inserted. The wound is not sutured.

Postoperative Care. This includes frequent cleaning of the inner cannula to prevent encrustation. A clean tube may be inserted daily after the first 48 hours when a tract has been established. In anticipation of permanent removal of the tracheostomy tube, the lumen should be corked for 48 hours. After the tube is removed, a dressing is placed over the wound, which heals by granulation.

MEDIASTINUM

General Considerations

The mediastinum is the central compartment within the thorax between the two pleural cavities. Fascial planes within the mediastinum are continuous with anatomic planes in the cervical region above and with retroperitoneal areas caudad. Thus infections from one region may dissect into adjacent areas. Such dissection into the mediastinum may be facilitated by the negative intrathoracic pressure. The heart and great vessels occupy a large part of the mediastinum; hemorrhage from these vascular structures may cause large hematomas within this area. Disease of the great vessels may produce compression of other mediastinal structures such as the trachea and esophagus. Lesions of the esophagus may cause various types of inflammatory reactions in the mediastinum. Injury to the trachea may cause air to dissect along the mediastinal tissue planes.

Displacement of the mediastinum may result from pleural or pulmonary disease which alters the volume of a pleural cavity. Since lateral mediastinal displacement is usually caused by pleural and pulmonary conditions, this is discussed in connection with the pleural and pulmonary diseases which are the etiologic factors. Displacement of mediastinal structures may be localized to a limited portion of the mediastinum as seen with fibrotic contraction of the upper lobe of one lung. The entire mediastinum may be displaced with a large tension pneumothorax which displaces the mediastinal structures toward the opposite side; atelectasis of an entire lung results in the mediastinum's moving toward the side with the airless lung. Mediastinal displacement may result in cardiovascular disturbances such as tachycardia and arrhythmias, especially if there is a significant disturbance in respiratory function.

MEDIASTINAL EMPHYSEMA (PNEUMOMEDIASTINUM). The importance of the presence of air in the mediastinum is related to its cause. When caused by leakage of air from the trachea, bronchus, or esophagus, it is a sign of potentially grave import. Such mediastinal emphysema may indicate traumatic rupture of the trachea or a bronchus such as occurs with severe blunt trauma or penetrating injuries to the chest. Mediastinal emphysema due to rupture or injury of the esophagus may signal the development of a life-threatening mediastinitis. Mediastinal em-

physema secondary to intrapulmonary rupture with the dissection of air along the hilar structures into the mediastinum may be of widely varying severity and clinical importance; when severe it may be relieved by surgical incision into the tissue planes of the lower cervical region which are in continuity with the distended fascial planes within the mediastinum.

The presence of air in the neck as revealed by the characteristic crepitation of subcutaneous emphysema should lead to the suspicion of mediastinal emphysema, especially if there has been thoracic trauma or possible injury to the esophagus by esophagoscopy or a foreign body. Roentgenographic studies designed to detect air in the mediastinum are indicated in the attempt to make an early diagnosis of mediastinal emphysema in those conditions in which the presence of mediastinal air has serious implications. Extensive mediastinal emphysema is associated with respiratory difficulty of varying severity, which, when severe, may cause serious secondary circulatory insufficiency.

MEDIASTINAL HEMATOMA. Hematoma may occur in the mediastinum as a result of severe blunt trauma as well as penetrating injuries. In such cases, cardiac contusion and trauma to the great vessels must be suspected. Partial traumatic rupture of the aorta, which may lead to an aortic aneurysm, is being recognized with increasing frequency after severe vehicular injury. The treatment of a mediastinal hematoma is directed at the source of bleeding.

Mediastinitis

ACUTE MEDIASTINITIS

ETIOLOGY. Acute suppurative mediastinitis is most commonly seen as a result of injury to the esophagus in the cervical or thoracic region. Cervical infections may extend along the tissue planes into the mediastinum. Mediastinitis secondary to a cervical cellulitis has become much less frequent since the advent of antibiotics and better treatment of cervical inflammatory processes. Likewise, a mediastinitis secondary to osteomyelitis of the vertebrae or sternum is a rare occurrence. However, anterior mediastinitis as a complication of median sternotomy is being reported with increasing frequency. Occasionally, retroperitoneal infections extend upward into the mediastinum. Mediastinitis may be a complication of surgical procedures, especially on the esophagus. A suppurative process in mediastinal lymph nodes may cause a mediastinal abscess of an acute or more chronic nature. Mediastinitis is rarely seen as a complication of pleural empyema or pericarditis, whereas pleural effusion, often bilateral, is a very common complication of acute mediastinitis.

Acute mediastinitis may result from so-called "spontaneus" rupture of the esophagus (see Chap. 25). Such a rupture is usually due to vomiting which results in sudden forceful ejection of a considerable volume of gastric contents into the lower esophagus with resultant splitting of the esophageal wall. In some cases, the material which leaks from the esophagus dissects along the mediastinum, but usually there is an associated rupture of the mediastinal pleura, commonly on the left side, with inundation of the pleural cavity with air and gastric contents.

CLINICAL MANIFESTATIONS. A history of possible injury to the esophagus, such as may occur with a swallowed foreign body or by an esophagoscopy, should alert one to the possibility of mediastinal infection. Dilatations of esophageal strictures are a particular hazard. The sudden onset of chest pain often associated with fever and chills after esophageal instrumentation should result in immediate investigation for signs of mediastinitis. Roentgenograms of the chest may demonstrate air in the mediastinal tissue planes or a widening of the mediastinum. Subcutaneous emphysema in the neck is diagnostic but may be absent in lower thoracic esophageal perforations. A low thoracic mediastinitis will often cause upper abdominal pain and tenderness and thus be confused with an acute process in the upper part of the abdominal cavity. If chest pain is the main feature of the symptomatology, a coronary thrombosis may be suspected. Pericarditis may occur secondary to a mediastinitis. Also an acute mediastinitis may cause inflammatory changes in the paramediastinal portion of the lungs.

TREATMENT. Recent years have witnessed the appearance of articles either championing a nonoperative treatment of acute esophageal performations or else advocating early surgical intervention in all cases of suspected esophageal perforation, as was usually recommended in the past. In general, for lacerations of the thoracic esophagus, thoracotomy, closure of the laceration, and transpleural drainage are indicated. Some patients with instrumental perforation of the cervical esophagus will recover if only aggressive antibiotic and medical measures are employed. If surgical intervention is delayed in some cases, however, the chance of preventing a fatality can be lost. What must be considered is the nature and extent of the injury to the esophagus. Where there is contamination of the mediastinum by an esophageal perforation caused by a small sharp foreign body which is removed endoscopically, the perforation may quickly close off and is in a potentially different category from a condition in which continued leakage of esophageal contents into the mediastinum is likely. A completely reliable way of ascertaining in which category a particular case falls is not at hand, but several factors deserve consideration: Knowledge concerning the type and apparent extent to esophageal injury must be considered. Radiographic evidence of air in the mediastinum or other evidence of esophageal leakage should favor surgical drainage in addition to massive antibiotic therapy. Failure to demonstrate esophageal extravasation on radiographic examination with the patient swallowing an inert radiopaque fluid does not definitely prove that the perforation has sealed off.

Because of the rapid dissection of an inflammatory process along the mediastinum, a mediastinotomy often does not provide good dependent drainage of the mediastinal infection. When a cervical approach is used for an upper esophageal perforation, a supplementary posterior upper thoracic mediastinotomy may become necessary. In the performance of all posterior thoracic mediastinotomies

for infection, the part of rib or ribs to be resected should be a small segment close to the vertebral column, and every effort should be made to avoid entry into the pleural cavity by directing the dissection toward the midline. Only soft drains should be used because of the risk of pressure necrosis of vessels in the infected wound.

In all cases of postemetic rupture of the esophagus, emergency thoracotomy is mandatory. Suturing of the esophageal tear is indicated unless the patient is first seen a few days after rupture has occurred, in which case preliminary drainage procedure may be performed. Mediastinotomy is indicated when a peptic ulcer in the esophagus perforates into the mediastinum. Early drainage and closed antibiotic irrigation is the best method of treating mediastinitis following sternotomy.

CHRONIC MEDIASTINITIS

Since diffuse suppurative mediastinitis is usually rapidly fatal unless successfully handled in the acute phase, most cases of chronic mediastinitis are either localized inflammatory processes or nonpyogenic reactive lesions. A granulomatous process, often with involvement of mediastinal lymph nodes, is an important cause of chronic mediastinitis. The tubercle bacillus and fungus infections, particularly histoplasmosis, are important etiologic agents.

CLINICAL MANIFESTATIONS. The symptomatology will vary depending on the chronicity and location of the inflammatory process, and may be obscured by an associated pneumonitis, empyema, or pericarditis. There may be chest pain, some fever, chronic cough, and signs of chronic infection. The physical and other findings may be determined by the location of the chronic inflammatory process. In the upper mediastinum constriction of the superior vena cava (Fig. 17-71) may ensue with the development of characteristic signs and symptoms. At times other vascular structures, particularly thin-walled veins, may be compromised. Constriction of the pulmonary veins may lead to cardiocirculatory signs and symptoms. A prevertebral abscess, as seen with tuberculous involvement of the spine, may also result in a chronic mediastinitis.

TREATMENT. Treatment often consists of a combination of appropriate antibiotic therapy with the surgical drainage of any localized abscess or the excision of necrotic ganulomatous lymph node masses.

Fibrous Mediastinitis

Fibrous mediastinitis may result from a chronic inflammation of the mediastinum; most often such infections are due to chronic infection in mediastinal lymph nodes. In other cases the diffuse fibrotic change in the mediastinal connective tissue is of unknown cause. It may be associated with a similar process in the retroperitoneal area. The development of dense connective tissue can interfere with the function of the structures passing through the involved area by limiting their mobility. The usual mobility of the tracheobronchial tree in the mediastinum with respiration is impaired. The dense fibrous tissue may also limit the normal mobility of the esophagus as well as cause traction diverticula. The large veins in the mediastinum may be constricted and even become occluded because of second-

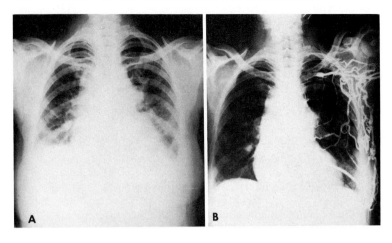

Fig. 17-71. Chronic mediastinitis with thrombosis of the vena cava. *A.* Posteroanterior roentgenogram. *B.* Angiogram outlining collateral circulation including large phrenic vessel.

ary thrombosis; the superior vena cava and the pulmonary veins may be affected. Constriction of the pulmonary veins may result in findings suggestive of cardiac lesions causing left atrial hypertension. Apparently the lymphatics are abnormal in fibrous mediastinitis, but whether this is entirely secondary or whether disease of the lymphatics plays an etiologic role awaits clarification.

Surgical experience in the management of fibrous mediastinitis is quite limited and not comparable to that which has accumulated in the treatment of retroperitoneal fibrosis, where much can be accomplished by release of the ureters from the constricting effect of the dense fibrous tissue.

Superior Vena Cava Obstruction

Pathologic processes which cause a marked obstruction of the superior vena cava produce a set of signs and symptoms which has been designated as the *superior vena cava syndrome.* The features of the syndrome may vary some-

Fig. 17-72. Superior vena cava obstruction. Note dilated veins over chest wall.

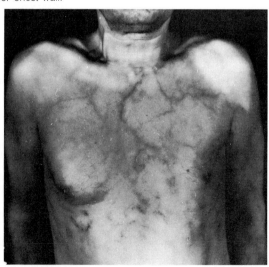

what depending on the cause of the obstruction of the vena cava and the rapidity with which the venous obstruction develops. Invasive malignant tumors, usually anaplastic lung cancers, are the most common cause of the superior vena cava syndrome. Primary thrombosis of the superior vena cava is occasionally responsible. A chronic fibrous mediastinitis or a granulomatous lesion may cause constriction of the vena cava.

CLINICAL MANIFESTATIONS. Depending on the rapidity of the development of the vena cava obstruction there will be varying degrees of edema of the neck, head, and arms with evidence of venous stasis. Tearing from the eyes is a frequent early symptom which is often misdiagnosed as due to allergy. When the vena cava is occluded gradually, the collateral venous system which develops to drain the venous blood from the upper part of the body may be the striking feature (Fig. 17-72), since many of these collateral channels are subcutaneous. The blood in the upper portion of the body is returned via the collateral vessels to the inferior vena cava (Fig. 17-71).

TREATMENT. Acute obstruction of the superior vena cava secondary to tumor should be treated aggressively by intravenous administration of diuretics and early therapy with radiation, which has been associated with dramatic temporary relief. Since malignant tumor represents the most common cause of the syndrome, it must be appreciated that cervical lymphadenopathy may be related to lymph stasis rather than metastatic involvement. Cervical exploration is often unsatisfactory as a result of the elevated venous and lymphatic pressure.

In rare cases of superior vena cava obstruction due to a benign process, venous shunt employing a prosthetic graft may be used to bypass the area of localized obstruction.

Traumatic Asphyxia

This is a condition produced by a violent and sustained compression of the thorax which results in a venous hypertension due to sudden mechanical obstruction of the superior vena cava. A marked bluish discoloration of the face and neck with striking conjunctival and occular congestion is characteristic. There may be associated vascular disturb-

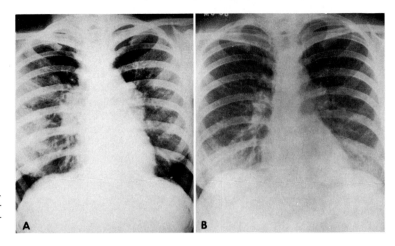

Fig. 17-73. Sarcoid of hilar lymph nodes and lungs. *A.* Prior to establishment of diagnosis by thoracotomy. *B.* Several years later after spontaneous regression of lesions.

ance in the central nervous system. Fractures of ribs and sternum are sometimes present. Oxygen and supportive therapy with the treatment of any concomitant injuries are indicated.

Mediastinal Lymphadenopathy

Enlargement of the mediastinal lymph nodes may be caused by a wide variety of etiologic agents. An acute nonsuppurative lymphadenitis may be associated with an inflammatory process in adjacent viscera; this rarely progresses to abscess formation. Various granulomatous processes may result in a chronic lymphadenopathy; tuberculosis, sarcoidosis (Fig. 17-73), and fungus infections are the most common etiologic agents. Caseation or necrosis of such lymph node masses may cause involvement of adjacent organs, as discussed under Chronic Mediastinitis. The diagnosis of the pathologic features of the lymphadenopathy may be aided by a cervical lymph node biopsy, but in some cases a mediastinotomy is necessary in order to establish the diagnosis and guide therapy. Involvement of mediastinal nodes by metastatic cancer is very common; the primary lesion may be in the lungs, breast, and many other sites.

Lesions of the Thoracic Duct

Congenital maldevelopment of the lymphatic system may result in anomalies of the thoracic duct. Pleural effusion and chylothorax in the neonatal period may result. Although injury to the thoracic duct may occur at birth, undoubtedly some cases of chylothorax attributed to birth injury in the past were caused by developmental deficiencies of the lymphatic system, often of a diffuse nature.

Because of the protected anatomic position of the thoracic duct in the depths of the thorax and adjacent to the vertebral column, injury to the thoracic duct by penetrating trauma is unlikely unless the trauma is so extensive as to make survival improbable. Rupture of the thoracic duct apparently may occur, however, from sudden hyperextension of the spine; chylothorax may then ensue. One should

be cautious in attributing a chylothorax to rupture of the thoracic duct by minimal trauma; later evidence may indicate that neoplastic obstruction of the thoracic duct was the true etiologic factor.

Since the advent of frequent extensive surgical procedures within the mediastinum, operative division of a lymphatic channel of appreciable size has become a more common occurrence. In such cases it is often unknown whether the main thoracic duct or minor lymph channel has been severed. If the site of the lymph leak can be identified and the leakage stopped by suture at the time of surgical injury, this should be done. Often, however, the source of the lymph seepage into the wound is not obvious, and in most such cases a persistent chylothorax will not develop if the pleural space is well drained and the lung quickly expanded postoperatively.

Tumors of the thoracic duct such as lymphangiomyoma are rare; chylothorax may be the presenting feature.

Tumors of the Mediastinum

GENERAL CONSIDERATIONS

Tumors of the mediastinum must be differentiated from paramediastinal pulmonary lesions, aneurysms, dilated blood vessels, a dilated esophagus filled with fluid, esophageal neoplasms, certain lesions of the sternum and vertebral column, diaphragmatic hernias, and also cardiac lesions. Since paramediastinal pulmonary lesions frequently involve the mediastinum and, conversely, mediastinal lesions may involve the lung secondarily, it is not always possible to determine the exact site of origin prior to the diagnosis by thoracotomy and histologic evaluation.

ANATOMY. The mediastinum is defined as the space between the lungs bounded by the posterior aspect of the sternum, the anterior surface of the spine, the two pleural pulmonary areas, and the diaphragm. It should be noted that no portion of the mediastinum lies posterior to the anterior aspect of the vertebral bodies. The mediastinum has been arbitrarily divided into an anterior and posterior division. This has a clinical application, since certain tumors have predilections for given areas. The anterior and posterior divisions are divided by a frontal plane passing in front of the trachea and its bifurcation. Since the tracheal air column can be seen in a lateral roentgenogram, this method of localization is readily applied clinically. As the depth of the upper portion of mediastinum is small, it is more practical to consider the area which lies cephalad to the superior border of the fifth thoracic vertebra as the superior mediastinum rather than divide this particular area into anterior and posterior portions.

CLINICAL MANIFESTATIONS. The signs and symptoms of mediastinal tumors depend on the location of the mass, its size, its invasiveness, whether it has become secondarily infected, and whether the tumor has produced metabolic effects. Many benign mediastinal tumors cause no symptoms for long periods of time.

The location of the tumor in relation to the tracheobronchial tree is critical. A slowly enlarging invasive tumor of the anterior mediastinum may attain large size without causing symptoms, while a small tumor in close proximity to the trachea or main bronchus may produce pronounced respiratory symptoms such as dyspnea and pulmonary infection. With the exception of the instance in which the mediastinal neoplasm attains huge size, respiratory symptoms are usually due to narrowing of the trachea or bronchus. The respiratory symptoms caused by mediastinal tumor may include dyspnea, wheezing, and cough. The cough may be dry or productive of mucus, pus, or even blood. Rupture of a cyst into a part of the tracheobronchial tree may occur, and the expectoration of hair or sebaceous material is diagnostic of a dermoid cyst or teratoma. Hemoptysis may occur with both benign and malignant tumors. Although mild pain may be noted with many mediastinal neoplasms, a constant boring pain is suggestive of an invasive lesion.

Compression of vascular structures of sufficient degree to produce symptoms is uncommon with benign tumors but is frequent with malignant neoplasms. Although benign tumors may markedly displace vessels as demonstrated by angiocardiography and operative findings, the flexibility of these arteries and great veins usually prevents much obstruction unless the walls of the vessels are invaded by tumor. Rarely, direct cardiac compression by benign neoplasms may be the cause of clinical manifestations. Secondary thrombosis of a large vessel compressed by a benign tumor is rare.

The signs and symptoms suggestive of an invasive malignant lesion are recurrent pain of considerable severity; manifestations of vascular obstruction, particularly of the superior vena cava; weakness; and weight loss. However, it may be impossible to differentiate clinically between a benign and malignant lesion.

Metabolic manifestations of certain mediastinal neoplasms may aid in diagnosis. Rarely, an intrathoracic goiter is associated with hyperthyroidism. The signs and laboratory findings of primary hyperparathyroidism indicate the presence of a parathyroid adenoma, which is more frequently found in the cervical region. Thymic tumors are occasionally associated with myasthenia gravis. Hypertension may, on rare occasions, be secondary to an intrathoracic pheochromocytoma. A mediastinal chorio-epithelioma in the male may produce a positive Aschheim-Zondek test. Malignant tumors such as anaplastic carcinomas, Hodgkin's disease, and lymphomas may be associated with a generalized hypermetabolic state.

TREATMENT. Since it is usually not possible to establish a precise diagnosis in reference to malignancy and since small asymptomatic benign tumors may enlarge or become infected and cause difficulty, surgical excision of most localized mediastinal tumors is recommended. In some diffuse malignant infiltrating tumors, radiotherapy and chemotherapy are the therapeutic modalities of choice, but such therapy should be decided upon only after a diagnosis has been established, except in a situation where serious respiratory or vascular obstruction is already present and all clinical indications point to a rapidly growing malignant lesion which is probably radiosensitive. In such cases it may be preferable to reduce the size of the tumor prior to establishment of a diagnosis. In these patients, a needle biopsy may be feasible and provide enough tissue for diagnosis. After a course of radiotherapy, the advisability of surgical intervention may be reconsidered.

In the patient with severe dyspnea from tracheobronchial obstruction, the advisability of surgical procedure is dependent on the nature of the lesion. If the lesion is apparently resectable, this constitutes an indication for emergency thoracotomy with special precaution taken to establish an adequate airway prior to the induction of general anesthesia. Cervical exploration for lymph node biopsy may frequently be indicated in a patient with mediastinal mass to establish the diagnosis, but if the neck is swollen as a result of vena cava obstruction, cervical exploration may be ill advised.

SUPERIOR MEDIASTINAL LESIONS

THYROID. The most common mediastinal tumor found in the superior segment in adults is an intrathoracic goiter. Most thyroid masses within the chest are downward extensions of a cervical component, and the intrathoracic or substernal extension may be appreciated on careful palpation when the patient swallows or by correlation with radiologic findings. Substernal extensions of a cervical thyroid may be unilateral or bilateral and often cause varying degrees of compression and displacement of the trachea which can be demonstrated on films of proper exposure.

Occasionally, an intrathoracic goiter may be present without an obvious mass in the cervical region (Fig. 17-74). Examination of the patient with a substernal thyroid often discloses prominent veins over the upper thorax on the side of the mass. If symptoms are present, they usually include some slight difficulty in breathing, although occasionally severe compression of the trachea may lead to stridor. An annoying dry cough may be present, and, in a few cases, difficulty in swallowing is noted when the mass presses upon and distorts the esophagus. In such cases, aspiration pneumonitis may occur. Pain is usually absent and hyperthyroidism is rare with intrathoracic goiters.

Fluoroscopic examination frequently demonstrates that the mass moves with deglutition. The lesions are usually thyroid adenomas arising from the lower posterior portion of the gland, and the right side is more commonly involved. Carcinoma of an entirely intrathoracic thyroid mass is rare.

Surgical removal is indicated to relieve tracheal compression. If the lesion is a downward extension of a cervical mass, it is best removed through the neck, but when no cervical component is palpable, a transthoracic excision is indicated.

BRONCHOGENIC CYSTS. Although this lesion may occur along the trachea or esophagus in the superior mediastinum, it is much more common in other portions and will be discussed to a greater extent below. The paratracheal bronchogenic cyst usually appears as a rounded mass generally on the right side of the trachea and may closely simulate an intrathoracic goiter (Fig. 17-75). However, the upper margin of the shadow does not usually extend into the cervical region as evidenced on a posteroanterior chest film. In infants severe or moderate respiratory distress is characteristic and indicates early excision. Elective removal is appropriate for other patients.

PARATHYROID ADENOMA. Parathyroid adenoma may occur in the superior mediastinum but in most instances is too small to be demonstrated on a chest roentgenogram. Thorough mediastinal exploration for parathyroid adenoma is indicated whenever meticulous surgical exploration of the cervical region has been negative in a patient with evidence of primary hyperparathyroidism. Parathyroid adenomas have occurred within the thymus. The sternum-splitting incision gives the best approach.

ANTERIOR MEDIASTINAL LESIONS

The most common lesions in this region, i.e., anterior to the root of the lung, are dermoid cysts and teratomas, thymic tumors (Fig. 17-76), lymphosarcoma (Fig. 17-77), Hodgkin's disease (Fig. 17-78), and pleuropericardial cysts (Fig. 17-79). Bronchogenic cysts can also occur in this location but are far more common in the posterior half of the mediastinum. In the region of the diaphragm, a pleuropericardial cyst may be located in the cardiophrenic angle but must be differentiated from the retrosternal diaphragmatic hernia of Morgagni, pericardial fat pads, and liver herniation.

DERMOID CYSTS AND TERATOMAS. Since these tumors antedate the birth of the patient, early films usually demonstrate the lesion. Dermoid cysts often appear as a sharply defined rounded mass on x-ray and show calcium within the wall. If the cyst has ruptured into the lung, there may be a history of expectorating hair or sebaceous material and accompanying hemoptysis. The more solid teratoma is less likely to rupture into the lung but may undergo malignant changes.

THYMIC TUMORS. These constitute the most common type of tumor found in the anterior mediastinum (Fig. 17-76). A variety of pathologic lesions including thymic cysts are encountered, and at times it is difficult to differentiate between benign and malignant tumors. Therefore, the practice has developed of calling the tumor "thymoma" without specifying whether it is clearly benign or malignant. At times the gross pathologic features, i.e., whether the tumor is encapsulated or infiltrating, are more

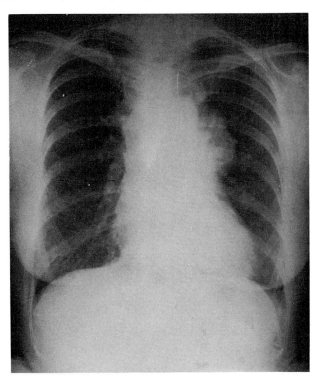

Fig. 17-74. Intrathoracic adenomatous goiter. Roentgenogram demonstrates anterior mediastinal tumor in patient with previous excision of nodular goiter from neck.

helpful in separating the benign from the malignant thymomas than is microscopic evaluation alone. Both Hodgkin's disease and lymphosarcoma may involve the thymus, and cellular origin of the neoplasm may be difficult to determine.

Fig. 17-75. Roentgenogram of infant with respiratory difficulty due to bronchogenic cyst compressing trachea and displacing esophagus.

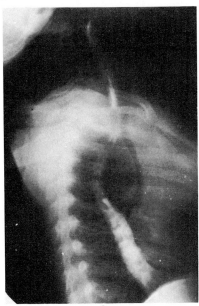

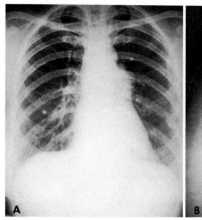
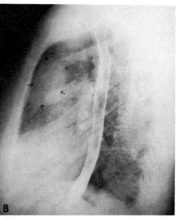

Fig. 17-76. Thymoma. *A.* Posteroanterior film showing mass in left hilar region. *B.* Lateral film demonstrating retrosternal position of mass.

A percentage of thymic tumors are associated with myasthenia gravis, which may or may not be improved by excision of the lesion. The results of thymectomy for myasthenia gravis are more favorable in younger women with disease of short duration and particularly those without an obvious thymic lesion. Recent articles have reported as many as 80 percent of patients to have improved following thymectomy. The improvement may be delayed as long as several years. Rather than the previously used median sternotomy, cervical thymectomy has been advised for these patients. Occasionally, thymic tumors are associated with a regenerative anemia, which is sometimes improved following thymectomy.

LYMPHOSARCOMA AND HODGKIN'S DISEASE. These diseases may present as mediastinal masses in the anterior mediastinum and at the root of the lung (Fig. 17-77). When the mass lies anterior to the pericardium, it is difficult to differentiate it from a thymic tumor. Most cases of lymphosarcoma show gross invasion of the adjacent tissue, and complete surgical removal is not possible. Radiation therapy is indicated for lymphosarcoma and Hodgkin's disease, but exploration of the mediastinum is frequently required to establish the diagnosis. Occasionally, the mass may be encapsulated and the tumor removed intact with good prognosis (Fig. 17-77).

PLEUROPERICARDIAL CYST. This represents a relatively common mediastinal lesion. The thin-walled cysts contain clear fluid and are usually found in close proximity to the pericardium (Fig. 17-79). The evidence strongly points to the origin as being a pinching off of the pericardial coelom, since, in most instances, they are the lesions associated with a diverticulum of the pericardial sac. Many patients have no symptoms or only slight discomfort, although an occasional patient may complain of attacks of tachycardia. The usual indication for surgical excision is failure to establish the exact nature preoperatively. If aspirated, the cyst usually refills with fluid within a few months.

POSTERIOR MEDIASTINAL LESIONS

Although it is customary to refer to tumors of the costovertebral area as posterior mediastinal lesions, it should be noted that anatomically, the mediastinum is defined as lying in front of the vertebral bodies and being bound on either side by the mediastinal pleura. Therefore, tumors lying lateral and posterior to the vertebral bodies are not truly located within the mediastinum. Since tumors of the mediastinum proper are of a different type, this differentiation has practical clinical significance.

BRONCHOGENIC CYSTS. This is one of the most common tumors found in the posterior part of the mediasti-

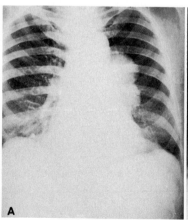
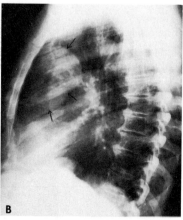

Fig. 17-77. Encapsulated lymphoma of anterior mediastinum. *A.* Posteroanterior roentgenogram showing mass in left hilus. *B.* Lateral roentgenogram defining mass.

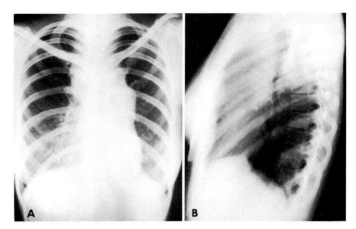

Fig. 17-78. Bilateral mediastinal Hodgkin's disease. *A.* Posteroanterior roentgenogram. *B.* Lateral roentgenogram. Anterior mediastinal mass is not sharply delineated.

num, if mediastinal lymph nodes are left out of consideration. The bronchogenic cyst represents a developmental aberration in the budding of the tracheobronchial tree. Not infrequently, the cyst retains some attachment to the tracheobronchial tree, but in some instances the cyst has been completely sequestrated. Bronchogenic cysts are usually lined by a ciliated columnar epithelium, and the wall of the cyst usually contains glands, smooth muscle, and cartilage. The wall may be only a few millimeters in thickness; the bulk of the mass is produced by a thick mucilaginous material within the cyst. The lesions tend to enlarge gradually over a period of years and may become secondarily infected. Because of their close proximity to the bronchi, pressure on the air passages may be produced. In infancy, a relatively small cyst, located near the tracheal bifurcation, may produce stridor and even cause fatal respiratory obstruction (Fig. 17-75).

HILAR LYMPHADENOPATHY. The various pathologic processes which involve the hilar lymph nodes may produce a mass in the posterior mediastinum. Included in this group are Hodgkin's disease, lymphosarcoma, reticulum cell sarcoma, tuberculomas, and rarer granulomas. If the roentgenogram shows bilateral processes with irregular nodularities in the region of the hilus of each lung, disease of the mediastinal nodes is to be strongly suspected. Sarcoidosis is another cause of lympoid enlargement, but it is also associated with pulmonary lesions which aid in the differential diagnosis. All patients with suspected hilar adenopathy should be examined particularly for cervical lymph nodes which might be biopsied to provide a diagnosis.

DUPLICATION CYST OF THE ESOPHAGUS. This usually enlarges fairly rapidly and causes symptoms in childhood. Part of the wall of the duplication cyst may be an integral portion of the esophagus, and surgical removal can be difficult. The lesions usually present on the right side of the esophagus, and the lining of the cyst may be gastric, enteric, or esophageal.

THORACIC DIVERTICULA. These originate from the intestine and may extend through the diaphragm and present as a mediastinal tumor, usually on the right side. Symptoms may be produced by these lesions, particularly in children, and are related to the accumulation of gas or material within the thoracic portion of the diverticulum. An acid secretion from the mucosal lining may produce pain, ulceration, and hemorrhage. Since the diverticulum drains its acid contents into the duodenum or jejunum, massive gastrointestinal bleeding may occur. The possibility of this lesion should be considered when the combination of posterior mediastinal tumors and severe gastrointestinal lesions are encountered in a child.

CHORDOMA. This rare tumor is derived from a remnant of the notochord and presents as a lesion attached to the vertebral bodies. Complete surgical removal is usually not feasible, and recurrence and metastases are common.

Fig. 17-79. Pleuropericardial cyst. Mass merges with left cardiac border.

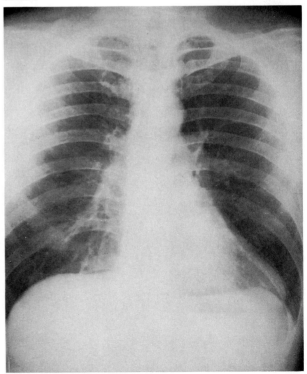

MEDIASTINAL TUMORS WITHOUT SPECIFIC LOCATION

A variety of mediastinal tumors which arise from tissues occurring in any portion have no characteristic location, and it is therefore extremely difficult to make a preoperative diagnosis. Included in this group are tumors of connective tissues, such as *fibromas* and *sarcomas. Lipomas* may also occur in various portions of the mediastinum, but these lesions provide a clue to diagnosis in that there is a tendency for a part of the mass to extend into the cervical region, into the chest wall, or through the diaphragm. A lipoma may also present as an hourglass tumor of the spine. The lesion can reach huge size before causing symptoms from compression. *Liposarcoma* of the mediastinum is very rare. Occasionally, a tumor of vascular origin may be encountered in the mediastinum, and many of these are malignant. A *hemangioma* of the mediastinum should be considered when a mass of calcified thrombus is suggested by roentgenographic examination. *Plasma cell tumors* are extremely rare. Masses of ectopic hematopoietic tissue may also simulate a mediastinal tumor. *Mestatic involvement* of the mediastinum by carcinoma or sarcoma is a common occurrence, and these lesions can occasionally attain great size.

MEDIASTINAL TUMORS IN INFANCY

Neurogenic tumors occur more commonly in children than in adults. Because some tumors in children may require urgent care, special consideration is warranted. In infancy and early childhood, mediastinal tumors which compress the trachea or main bronchi deserve particular attention, because a correct diagnosis may lead to early surgical therapy, which may be lifesaving. Such mediastinal tumors must be differentiated from other conditions causing respiratory difficulty such as laryngeal lesions, tracheobronchitis, aspirated foreign body, and vascular anomalies and circulatory conditions which compromise the airway.

CYSTS OF FOREGUT ORIGIN. These may cause respiratory difficulty in early life. Since the foregut develops into the tracheobronchial tree and esophagus, it is easy to understand that some cysts and tumors of congenital origin arising from the foregut may contain both respiratory and alimentary tract elements. The term *bronchogenic cyst* has been applied to cysts which have a wall composed of tissues common to a bronchus. Duplication cysts represent duplications of the alimentary tract, and those in the chest adjacent to the esophagus are usually lined with gastric mucosa which is often capable of secreting acid. In some cases a mixture of tissue elements from both the respiratory and alimentary tract are found in the same cyst. Foregut cysts are occasionally associated with developmental abnormalities of the notochord which result in congenital vertebral lesions. When located in the upper portion of the chest, such cysts may cause respiratory difficulty in infancy or childhood (Fig. 17-75). Masses lower in the mediastinum may become symptomatic at a later date. Surgical excision is the indicated treatment for foregut cysts.

NEUROBLASTOMA. Neuroblastoma is a relatively common type of mediastinal tumor in children. This malignant tumor often involves regions other than the mediastinum, but when the tumor is limited to the mediastinum and especially if the child is under one year of age, the prognosis is much better than usual. Surgical excision combined with radiotherapy, and perhaps chemotherapy, is the therapy of choice.

LYMPHATIC CYSTS AND LYMPHANGIOMAS. These may occur in various parts of the mediastinum. Cervical cystic hygromas of childhood may extend downward into the upper mediastinum (see Chap. 39). These cystic lesions may cause some compression of mediastinal structures and be the cause of respiratory difficulty. The lymphangiomas vary from a circumscribed to a diffuse type; complete surgical excision of the diffuse type may not be feasible or always necessary, whereas excision of a circumscribed lymphangioma is usually the procedure of choice. Mixed

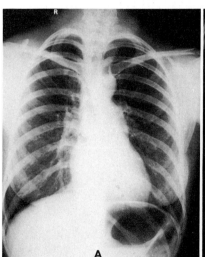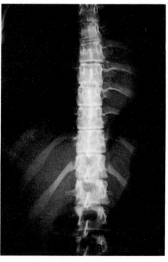

Fig. 17-80. Neurofibroma. *A.* Posteroanterior x-ray barely shows lateral margin of tumor projecting to the left at the upper cardiac border. *B.* Markedly overexposed film shows the paravertebral neurogenic tumor.

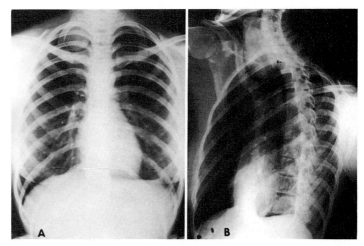

Fig. 17-81. Upper thoracic meningocele. *A.* Postero-anterior roentgenogram showing lesion in upper right chest. *B.* Oblique view with lesion defined.

lymphangiomatous and angiomatous lesions also may occur.

HEMANGIOMA. Hemangioma of the mediastinum is uncommon but may be the cause of respiratory difficulty in infancy. Hemangiomas within the airway, such as in the subglottic region or trachea of infants, may require urgent treatment by tracheostomy and small amounts of radiotherapy. Multiple hemangiomas, including cutaneous hemangiomas, are often also present. Circumscribed hemangiomas of the mediastinum are treated by surgical excision.

TUMORS OF THE COSTOVERTEBRAL REGION

Tumors of the costovertebral region of the thorax consist essentially of tumors arising from the nerve structures located in that area and tumors derived from components of the chest wall.

NEUROGENIC TUMORS. These are the most important neoplasms found in this location. Although similar neurogenic tumors are occasionally encountered in the true anatomic mediastinum, they are much more common in the costovertebral region. Among the neurogenic tumors are neurofibroma, neurilemmoma, neurosarcoma, ganglioneuroma, neuroblastoma, sympathicoblastoma, and paraganglioma, of which the pheochromocytoma is a special type. Characteristically, all these tumors lie against the posterior chest wall, as best seen on lateral roentgenograms. Tumors of the sympathetic nerve trunk are slightly more anterior. Symptoms may be absent, but pain may be radicular in distribution. Compression of the airway is rare except with large malignant neuroblastomas. The ganglioneuroma is the most common type of benign tumor requiring excision in later childhood, whereas, among adults, neurilemmoma and neurofibroma are more frequently encountered (Fig. 17-80).

PHEOCHROMOCYTOMAS. These may occur in the mediastinum along the course of the sympathetic trunk in the paravertebral region. They usually become manifest as a result of hypertension produced by the secretion of norepi-nephrine (see Chaps. 23 and 37). Often, they are also associated with retroperitoneal pheochromocytomas, especially if there is a familial history of these or if the lesion is manifest in childhood. The tumor is usually small but may be visualized on chest roentgenograms using oblique projection or laminography. Surgical excision is indicated and precautions are necessary during the operation to prevent excessive release of catecholamines.

INTRATHORACIC MENINGOCELE. This lesion presents with clinical roentgenographic pictures simulating neurogenic tumor (Fig. 17-81). Roentgenograms may demonstrate changes in the vertebral column, and the patient may have neurofibromatosis. If the diagnosis is suspected and aspiration if performed, spinal fluid will be obtained. The diagnosis can be confirmed by the injection of nonirritating radiopaque substance either into the sac or the spinal canal and demonstrating the migration of the substance from one area to another. If the sac is enlarging or causing symptoms, surgical removal is indicated, although recurrence following operation has been reported.

CHONDROMA AND CHONDROSARCOMA. These lesions are occasionally encountered in the costovertebral region. Surgical excision is difficult in this region, and the behavior of the tumor is comparable to similar lesions in other portions of the chest wall.

References

General

Aviado, D. M.: "The Lung Circulation," vols. 1 and 2, Pergamon Press, New York, 1965.

Bendixen, H. H., Egbert, L. D., Hedley-Whyte, J., Laver, M. B., and Pontoppidan, H.: "Respiratory Care," The C. V. Mosby Company, St. Louis, 1965.

Drinker, C. K.: "Pulmonary Edema and Inflammation," Harvard University Press, Cambridge, Mass., 1945.

Felson, B.: "Fundamentals of Chest Roentgenology," W. B. Saunders Company, Philadelphia, 1960.

Fischer, J. W., and Dolehide, R. A.: Total Cardiac Failure in

Persons with Thoracic Deformities, *Arch Intern Med,* **93:**687, 1954.

Gibbon, J. H., Jr., Sabiston, D. C., Jr., and Spencer, F. C.: "Surgery of the Chest," 2d ed., W. B. Saunders Company, Philadelphia, 1969.

Laver, M. B., Hallowell, P., and Goldblatt, A.: Pulmonary Dysfunction Secondary to Heart Disease: Aspects Relevant to Anesthesia and Surgery, *Anesthesiology,* **33:**161, 1970.

Levine, M. I., and Mascia, A. V.: "Pulmonary Diseases and Anomalies of Infancy and Childhood," Hoeber Medical Division, Harper & Row, Publishers, Incorporated, New York, 1966.

Rubin, E. H., and Rubin, M.: "Thoracic Diseases," W. B. Saunders Company, Philadelphia, 1961.

Spencer, H.: "Pathology of the Lung," The Macmillan Company, New York, 1962.

Von Hayek, H.: "The Human Lung," Hafner Publishing Company, Inc., New York, 1960.

West, J. B.: "Ventilation/Blood Flow and Gas Exchange," 2d ed., Blackwell Scientific Publications, Ltd., Oxford, 1970.

Chest Wall

Avery, E. E., Morch, E. T., and Benson, D. W.: Critically Crushed Chests, *J Thorac Cardiovasc Surg,* **32:**291, 1956.

Barrett, N. R.: Primary Tumors of Rib, *Br J Surg,* **43:**113, 1955.

Beall, A. C., Jr., Crawford, H. W., and DeBakey, M. E.: Considerations in the Management of Acute Traumatic Hemothorax, *J Thorac Cardiovasc Surg,* **52:**351, 1966.

Beiser, G. D., Epstein, S. E., Stampfer, M., Goldstein, R. E., Noland, S. P., and Levitsky, S.: Impairment of Cardiac Function in Patients with Pectus Excavatum, *N Engl J Med,* **287:**267, 1972.

Groff, D. B., III, and Adkins, P. C.: Chest Wall Tumors, *Ann Thorac Surg,* **3:**260, 1967.

Haller, J. A., Jr., Peters, G. N., Mazur, D., and White, J. J.: Pectus Excavatum: A 20 Year Surgical Experience, *J Thorac Cardiovasc Surg,* **60:**375, 1970.

Hochberg, L. A., and Rivkin, L. M.: Benign Neurogenic Tumors of the Chest Wall, *Ann Surg,* **138:**104, 1953.

Hood, R. M.: "Management of Thoracic Injuries," Charles C Thomas, Publisher, Springfield, Ill., 1968.

Howell, J. F., Crawford, E. S., and Jordan, G. L., Jr.: Flail Chest: Analysis of 100 Patients, *Am J Surg,* **106:**628, 1963.

Hughes, R. K.: Thoracic Trauma, *Ann Thorac Surg,* **1:**778, 1965.

Jones, R. J., Samson, P. C., and Dugan, D. J.: Current Management of Civilian Thoracic Trauma, *Am J Surg,* **114:**289, 1967.

Kaufman, P. A.: Subcutaneous Phlebitis of the Breast and Chest Wall, *Ann Surg,* **144:**841, 1956.

Kayser, H. L.: Tietze's Syndrome, *Am J Med,* **21:**982, 1956.

Latham, W. D.: Operative Treatment for Post-radiation defects of the Chest Wall, *Am Surg,* **32:**700, 1966.

Lester, C. W.: Surgical Treatment of Protrusion Deformities of the Sternum and Costal Cartilages (Pectus Carinatum, Pigeon Breast), *Ann Surg,* **153:**441, 1961.

Maier, H. C.: Infections of the Costal Cartilages and Sternum, *Surg Gynecol Obstet,* **84:**1038, 1947.

——— and Bortone, F.: Complete Failure of Sternal Fusion with Herniation of Pericardium: Report of a Case Corrected Surgically in Infancy. *J Thorac Cardiovasc Surg,* **18:**851, 1949.

Martin, L. W., and Helmsworth, J. A.: Management of Congenital Deformities of the Sternum, *JAMA,* **179:**82, 1962.

Moghissi, K.: Long-Term Results of Surgical Correction of Pectus Excavatum and Sternal Prominence, *Thorax,* **19:**350, 1964.

Munnell, E. R.: Herniation of the Lung, *Ann Thorac Surg,* **5:**204, 1968.

Pascuzzi, C. A., Dahlin, D. C., and Clagett, O. T.: Primary Tumors of the Ribs and Sternum, *Surg Gynecol Obstet,* **104:**390, 1957.

Pontius, J. G., Clagett, O. T., and McDonald, J. R.: Costal Chondritis and Perichondritis, *Surgery,* **45:**852, 1959.

Ravitch, M. M.: The Operative Treatment of Congenital Deformities of the Chest, *Am J Surg,* **101:**588, 1961.

Sabiston, D. C.: The Surgical Management of Congenital Bifid Sternum with Partial Ectopic Cordis, *J Thorac Cardiovasc Surg,* **35:**118, 1958.

Schmidt, F. E., and Trummer, M. J.: Primary Tumors of Ribs, *Ann Thorac Surg,* **13:**251, 1972.

Strug, L. H., Glass, B., Leon, W., and Salatich, M.: Severe Crushing Injuries of the Chest, *J Thor Cardiov Surg,* **39:**166, 1960.

Teitelbaum, S. L.: Twenty Years' Experience With Intrinsic Tumors of the Bony Thorax at a Large Institution, *J Thorac Cardiovasc Surg,* **63:**776, 1972.

Threlkel, J. B., and Adkins, R. B.: Primary Chest Wall Tumors, *Ann Thorac Surg,* **11:**450, 1971.

Vieta, J. O., and Maier, H. C.: Tumors of the Sternum: Collective Review, *Surg Gynecol Obstet,* **114:**513, 1962.

Watkins, E., Jr., and Gerard, F. P.: Malignant Tumors Involving the Chest Wall, *J Thorac Cardiovasc Surg,* **39:**117, 1960.

Pleura

Andrews, N. C.: Surgical Treatment of Chronic Empyema, *Dis Chest,* **47:**533, 1965.

Barker, W. L., Neuhaus, H., and Langston, H. T.: Ventilatory Improvement following Decortication in Pulmonary Tuberculosis, *Ann Thorac Surg,* **1:**532, 1965.

Berne, A. S., and Heitzman, E. R.: The Roentgenologic Signs of Pedunculated Pleural Tumors, *Am J Roentgenol Radium Ther Nucl Med,* **87:**892, 1962.

Bessone, L. N., Ferguson, T. B., and Burford, T. H.: Chylothorax, *Ann Thorac Surg,* **12:**527, 1971.

Bloomer, W. E., Giammona, S., Lindskog, G. E., and Cooke, R. E.: Staphylococcal Pneumonia and Empyema in Infancy, *J Thorac Surg,* **30:**265, 1955.

Burford, T. H., Parker, E. F., and Samson, P. C.: Early Pulmonary Decortication in Treatment of Post-traumatic Empyema, *Ann Surg,* **122:**163, 1945.

Christiansen, K. H., Morgan, S. W., Karich, A. F., and Takaro, T.: Pleural Space following Pneumonectomy, *Ann Thorac Surg,* **1:**298, 1965.

Clagett, O. T., McDonald, J. R., and Schmidt, H. W.: Localized Fibrous Mesothelioma of the Pleura, *J Thorac Cardiovasc Surg,* **24:**213, 1952.

Collins, H. A., Daniel, R. A., Jr., and Diveley, W. L.: Parietal Pleurectomy for Spontaneous Pneumothorax, *Am Surg* **29:**844, 1963.

Donahoe, R. F., Katz, S., and Mathews, M. J.: Pleural Biopsy as an Aid in the Etiologic Diagnosis of Pleural Effusion: Review of the Literature and Report of 132 Biopsies, *Ann Intern Med,* **48:**344, 1958.

Emerson, J. D., Boruchow, I. B., Daicoff, G. R., Bartley, T. D., and Wheat, M. W., Jr.: Empyema, *J Thorac Cardiovasc Surg,* **62:**967, 1971.

Godwin, M. C.: Diffuse Mesotheliomas, with Comment on Their

Relation to Localized Fibrous Mesotheliomas, *Cancer,* **10:**298, 1957.

Jensik, R., Cagle, J. E., Jr., Millroy, F., Perlia, C., Taylor, S., Kofman, S., and Beattie, E. J., Jr.: Pleurectomy in Treatment of Pleural Effusion Due to Metastatic Malignancy, *J Thorac Cardiovasc Surg,* **46:**322, 1963.

Kergin, F. G.: An Operation for Chronic Pleural Empyema, *J Thorac Cardiovasc Surg,* **26:**430, 1953.

Lambert, C. J., Shah, H. H., Urschel, H. C., Jr., and Paulson, D. L.: The Treatment of Malignant Pleural Effusions by Closed Trocar Tube Drainage, *Ann Thorac Surg,* **3:**1, 1967.

Langston, H. T., Barker, W. L., and Graham, A. A.: Pleural Tuberculosis, *J Thorac Cardiovasc Surg,* **54:**511, 1967.

LeRoux, B. T.: Empyema Thoracis, *Br J Surg,* 52:89, 1965.

Lillington, G. A., Mitchell, S. P., and Wood, G. A.: Catamenial Pneumothorax, *JAMA,* **219:**1328, 1972.

Maier, H. C., and Barr, D.: Intrathoracic Tumors Associated with Hypoglycemia, *J Thorac Cardiovasc Surg,* **44:**321, 1962.

Maloney, J. V., and Spencer, F. C.: The Nonoperative Treatment of Traumatic Chylothorax, *Surgery,* **40:**121, 1956.

Meyer, P. C.: Metastatic Carcinoma of the Pleura, *Thorax,* **21:**437, 1966.

Mills, M., and Baisch, B. F.: Spontaneous Pneumothorax: A Series of 400 Cases, *Ann Thorac Surg,* **1:**286, 1965.

Price-Thomas, C., and Drew, C. E.: Fibroma of the Visceral Pleura, *Thorax,* **8:**180, 1953.

Samson, P. C.: Empyema Thoracis: Essentials of Present-Day Management, *Ann Thorac Surg,* **11:**210, 1971.

Scerbo, J., Keltz, H., and Stone, D. J.: A Prospective Study of Closed Pleural Biopsies, *JAMA,* **218:**377, 1971.

Sensenig, D. M., Rossi, N. P., and Ehrenhaft, J. L.: Decortication for Chronic Nontuberculous Empyema, *Surg Gynecol Obstet,* **117:**443, 1963.

Stafford, E. G., and Clagett, O. T.: Postpneumonectomy Empyema, *J Thorac Cardiovasc Surg,* **63:**771, 1972.

Stiles, Q. R., Lindesmith, G., Tucker, B. L., Meyer, B. W., and Jones, J. C.: Pleural Empyema in Children, *Ann Thorac Surg,* **10:**37, 1970.

Symbas, P. N., Nugent, J. T., Abbott, O. A., Logan, W. D., Jr., and Hatcher, C. R., Jr.: Nontuberculous Pleural Empyema in Adults: Role of a Modified Eloesser Procedure in Its Management, *Ann Thorac Surg,* **12:**69, 1971.

Thomas, D. F., Glass, J. L., and Baisch, B. F.: Management of Streptococcal Empyema, *Ann Thorac Surg,* **2:**658, 1966.

Williams, K. R., and Burford, T. H.: The Management of Chylothorax related to Trauma, *J Trauma,* **3:**317, 1963.

Lung

Anderson, R. P., Leand, P. M., and Kieffer, R. F., Jr.: Changing Attitudes in the Surgical Management of Pulmonary Tuberculosis: Analysis of 425 Consecutive Patients, *Ann Thorac Surg,* **3:**43, 1967.

Armer, R. M., Shumacker, H. B., and Klatte, E.: Origin of the Right Pulmonary Artery from the Ascending Aorta: Report of a Surgically Corrected Case, *Circulation,* **24:**662, 1961.

Arrigoni, M. G., Woolner, L. B., Bernatz, P. E., Miller, W. E., and Fontana, R. S.: Benign Tumors of the Lung: Ten-Year Surgical Experience, *J Thorac Cardiovasc Surg,* **60:**589, 1970.

———, Bernatz, P. E., and Donoghue, F. E.: Broncholithiasis, *J Thorac Cardiovasc Surg,* **62:**231, 1971.

Baker, D. C., Jr., Papper, E. M., and Lang, R. R.: Foreign Bodies in the Tracheo-Bronchial Tree Causing Obstructive Emphysema: A Clinical Study, *Laryngoscope,* **73:**1099, 1963.

Baker, R. R.: The Clinical Management of Bronchogenic Carcinoma, *Johns Hopkins Med J,* **121:**401, 1967.

Baldwin, E. deF., Harden, K. A., Greene, D. G., Cournand, A., and Richards, D. W., Jr.: Pulmonary Insufficiency: A Study of 16 Cases of Large Pulmonary Air Cysts or Bullae, *Medicine (Baltimore),* **29:**169, 1950.

Batson, J. F., Gale, J. W., and Hickey, R. C.: Bronchial Adenomata: A Clinical Resumé, *Arch Surg,* **92:**623, 1966.

Battersby, J. S., and Kilman, J. W.: Traumatic Injuries of the Tracheobronchial Tree, *Arch Surg,* **86:**644, 1964.

Baum, G. L., Racz, I., Bubis, J. J., Molho, M., and Shapiro, B. L.: Cystic Disease of the Lung: Report of 88 Cases with an Ethnologic Relationship, *Am J Med,* **40:**578, 1966.

Beall, A. C., Bricker, D. L., Crawford, H. W., and DeBakey, M.: Surgical Management of Penetrating Thoracic Trauma, *Dis Chest,* **49:**568, 1966.

Belanger, R., LaFleche, L. R., and Picard, J.-L.: Congenital Cystic Adenomatoid Malformation of the Lung, *Thorax,* **19:**1, 1964.

Bergh, N. P., Rydberg, B., and Schersten, T.: Mediastinal Exploration by Technic of Carlens, *Dis Chest,* **46:**399, 1964.

Bernhard, W. F., Malcolm, J. A., and Wylie, R. H.: Lung Abscess: A Study of 148 Cases Due to Aspiration, *Dis Chest,* **43:**620, 1963.

Bignall, J. R., Martin, M., and Smithers, D. W.: Survival in 6086 Cases of Bronchial Carcinoma, *Lancet,* **1:**1067, 1967.

Blesovsky, A.: Pulmonary Sequestration: A Report of an Unusual Case and a Review of the Literature, *Thorax,* **22:**351, 1967.

Borrie, J.: "Lung Cancer: Surgery and Survival," Appleton-Century-Crofts, Inc., New York, 1965.

——— and Lichter, I.: Surgical Treatment of Bronchiectasis: Ten-Year Survey, *Br Med J,* **2:**908, 1965.

Boyden, E. A.: The Intrahilar and Related Segmental Anatomy of the Lung, *Surgery,* **18:**706, 1945.

———: Developmental Anomalies of the Lungs, *Am J Surg,* **89:**79, 1955.

———: Bronchogenic Cysts and the Theory of Intralobar Sequestration: New Embryologic Data, *J Thorac Surg,* **35:**604, 1958.

Brattstrom, S.: Postoperative Pulmonary Ventilation with Reference to Postoperative Pulmonary Complications, *Acta Chir Scand [Suppl],* vol. 195, 1954.

Brown, M. D., and Reidbord, H. A.: Congenital Pulmonary Lymphangiectasis, *Am J Dis Child,* **114:**654, 1967.

Byrd, R. B., Divertie, M. B., and Spittell, J. A., Jr.: Bronchogenic Carcinoma and Thromboembolic Disease, *JAMA,* **202:**1019, 1967.

Cameron, J. L., Mitchell, W. H., and Zuidema, G. D.: Aspiration Pneumonia, *Arch Surg,* **106:**49, 1973.

Canetti, G.: Present Aspects of Bacterial Resistance in Tuberculosis, *Am Rev Resp Dis,* **92:**687, 1965.

Carter, R.: Pulmonary Sequestration, *Ann Thorac Surg,* **7:**68, 1969.

———, Wareham, E. E., Bullock, W., K., and Brewer, L. A.: Intrathoracic Fibroxanthomatous Pseudotumors, *Ann Thorac Surg,* **5:**97, 1968.

Chatrath, R. R., El Shafie, M., and Jones, R. S.: Fate of Hypoplastic Lungs after Repair of Congenital Diaphragmatic Hernia, *Arch Dis Child,* **46:**633, 1971.

Christoforidis, A. J., and Browning, R. H.: Pulmonary Tuberculosis Associated with Carcinoma of the Lung, *Arch Intern Med,* **103:**231, 1959.

Churchill, E. D.: The Segmental and Lobular Physiology and Pathology of the Lung, *J Thorac Surg*, **18:**279, 1949.

———, Sweet, R. H., Scannell, J. G., and Wilkins, E. W., Jr.: Further Studies in the Surgical Management of Carcinoma of the Lung, *J Thorac Surg*, **36:**301, 1958.

Clagett, O. T., and Woolner, L. B.: Surgical Treatment of Solitary Metastatic Pulmonary Lesions, *Med Clin North Am*, **48:**939, 1964.

Cleary, A. P., Ellis, F. H., Jr., and Schmidt, H. W.: Problems Associated with Aspiration of Grass Heads (Inflorescences), *JAMA*, **171:**1478, 1959.

Cliffton, E. E., Gupta, T. D., and Pool, J. L.: Bilateral Pulmonary Resection for Primary or Metastatic Lung Cancer, *Cancer*, **17:**86, 1964.

Cockett, F. B., and Vass, C. C. N.: The Collateral Circulation to the Lungs, *Br J Surg*, **38:**97, 1950.

Collins, H. A., Guest, J. L., and Daniel, R. A.: Primary Lung Abscess, *J Thorac Cardiovasc Surg*, **47:**383, 1964.

Cooley, J. C., Ginsberg, R. L., Olsen, A. M., and Kirklin, J. W.: Foreign Body Bronchiectasis, *J Thorac Cardiovasc Surg*, **31:**615, 1956.

Cotton, R. E., and Jackson, J. W.: Localized Amyloid "Tumors" of the Lung Simulating Malignant Neoplasms, *Thorax*, **19:**97, 1964.

Delarue, N. C., and Strasberg, S. M.: The Rationale of Intensive Preoperative Investigation in Bronchogenic Carcinoma, *J Thorac Cardiovasc Surg*, **51:**391, 1966.

Deverall, P. B.: Tracheal Stricture following Tracheostomy, *Thorax*, **22:**572, 1967.

Dillon, M. L., and Postlethwait, R. W.: Carcinoma of the Lung, *Ann Thorac Surg*, **11:**193, 1971.

Ecker, R. R., Libertini, R. V., Rea, W. J., Sugg, W. L., and Webb, W. R.: Injuries of the Trachea and Bronchi, *Ann Thorac Surg*, **11:**289, 1971.

Faber, L. P., Pedreira, A. L. S., Pevsner, P. H., and Beattie, E. J., Jr.: The Immediate and Long-Term Physiologic Function of Bilateral Reimplanted Lungs, *J Thorac Cardiovasc Surg*, **50:**761, 1965.

Fain, W. R., Conn, J. H., Campbell, G. D., Chavez, C. M., Gee, H. L., and Hardy, J. D.: Excision of Giant Pulmonary Emphysematous Cysts: Report of 20 Cases without Deaths, *Surgery*, **62:**552, 1967.

Feinstein, A. R.: Symptomatic Patterns, Biologic Behavior and Prognosis in Lung Cancer: Practical Application of Boolean Algebra and Clinical Taxonomy, *Ann Intern Med*, **61:**27, 1964.

Fennessy, J. J.: Bronchial Brushing, *Ann Otol*, **79:**924, 1970.

Ferencz, C.: Congenital Abnormalities of Pulmonary Vessels and Their Relation to Malformations of the Lung, *Pediatrics*, **28:**993, 1961.

Foreman, S., Weill, H., Duke, R., George, R., and Ziskind, M.: Bullous Disease of the Lung: Physiologic Improvement after Surgery, *Ann Intern Med*, **69:**757, 1968.

Foster, E. D., Muneo, D. D., and Dobell, A. R. C.: Mediastinoscopy: A Review of Anatomical Relationships and Complications, *Ann Thorac Surg*, **13:**273, 1972.

Gaensler, E. A., Moister, M. V. B., and Hamm, J.: Open Lung Biopsy in Diffuse Pulmonary Disease, *N Engl J Med*, **270:**1319, 1964.

Garzon, A. A., Gourin, A., Seltzer, B., Chiu, C.-J., and Karlson, K. E.: Severe Blunt Chest Trauma: Studies of Pulmonary Mechanics and Blood Gases, *Ann Thorac Surg*, **2:**629, 1966.

Geelhoed, G. W., Levin, B. J., Adkins, P. C., and Joseph, W. L.: The Diagnosis and Management of Pneumocystis Carinii Pneumonia, *Ann Thorac Surg*, **14:**335, 1972.

Gotsman, M. S., and Whitby, J. L.: Respiratory Infection following Tracheostomy, *Thorax*, **19:**89, 1964.

Greenberg, E., Divertie, M. B., and Woolner, L. B.: Review of Unusual Systemic Manifestations Associated with Carcinoma, *Am J Med*, **36:**106, 1964.

Grillo, H. C.: The Management of Tracheal Stenosis following Assisted Respiration, *J Thorac Cardiovasc Surg*, **57:**52, 1969.

Greenberg, J. J., and Wilkins, E. W., Jr.: Resection of Bronchogenic Carcinoma Involving Thoracic Wall, *J Thorac Cardiovasc Surg*, **51:**417, 1966.

Guest, J. L., Yeh, T. J., Ellison, L. T., and Ellison, R. G.: Pulmonary Parenchymal Air Space Abnormalities, *Ann Thorac Surg*, **1:**102, 1965.

Guttmann, R.: Results of Radiotherapy in Cancer of the Lung Classified as Inoperable at Exploratory Thoracotomy, *Cancer*, **17:**37, 1964.

Hajdu, S. I., Huvos, A. G., Goodner, J. T., Foote, F. W., Jr., and Beattie, E. J., Jr.: Carcinoma of the Trachea: Clinicopathologic Study of 41 Cases, *Cancer*, **25:**1448, 1970.

Hardy, J. D., and Alican, F.: Lung Transplantation, *Adv Surg*, **2:**235, 1966.

Hatch, D.: Ventilation and Arterial Oxygenation during Thoracic Surgery, *Thorax*, **21:**310, 1966.

Haynes, A. L., Clagett, O. T., and McDonald, J. R.: Tumor-forming Amyloidosis of the Lung, *Surgery*, **24:**120, 1948.

Higgins, G. A., Jr., and Wolf, J.: Chemotherapy and Lung Cancer: Present Status, *J Thorac Cardiovasc Surg*, **51:**449, 1966.

Hinshaw, H. C., and Garland, L. H.: Pulmonary Diseases of Occupational Origin, in H. C. Hinshaw, and L. H. Garland (eds.), "Diseases of the Chest," W. B. Saunders Company, Philadelphia, 1963.

Houk, V. N., Kent, D. C., and Fosburg, R. G.: Unilateral Hyperlucent Lung: A Study in Pathophysiology and Etiology, *Am J Med Sci*, **253:**406, 1967.

Hughes, F. A., Jr., Pate, J. W., and Campbell, R. E.: Bronchogenic Carcinoma: Comparison of Natural Course and Treatment with Resection, X-Radiation, and Nitrogen Mustards, *J Thorac Cardiovasc Surg*, **39:**409, 1960.

Hughes, R. K.: Thoracic Trauma: A Collective Review, *Ann Thorac Surg*, **1:**778, 1965.

Hutchin, P., and Lingskog, G. E.: Acquired Esophagobronchial Fistula of Infectious Origin, *J Thorac Cardiovasc Surg*, **48:**1, 1964.

Jenski, R. J., Faber, L. P., Milloy, F. J., and Goldin, M. D.: Tracheal Sleeve Pneumonectomy for Advanced Carcinoma of the Lung, *Surg Gynecol Obstet*, **134:**231, 1972.

Jeresaty, R. M., Knight, H. F., and Hart, W. E.: Pulmonary Arteriovenous fistulas in Children: Report of Two Cases and Review of Literature, *Am J Dis Child*, **111:**256, 1966.

Jones, J. C., Almond, C. H., Snyder, H. M., and Meyer, B. W.: Congenital Pulmonary Cysts in Infants and Children, *Ann Thorac Surg*, **3:**297, 1967.

Kennedy, J. H., and Rothmann, B. F.: Surgical Treatment of Congenital Lobar Emphysema, *Surg Gynecol Obstet*, **121:**253, 1965.

Kent, E. M., and Blades, B.: The Surgical Anatomy of the Pulmonary Lobes, *J Thorac Cardiovasc Surg,* **12:**18, 1942.

Klassen, K. P., and Andrews, N. C.: Biopsy of Diffuse Pulmonary Lesions, *Ann Thorac Surg,* **4:**117, 1967.

Larson, R. E., Bernatz, P. E., and Geraci, J. E.: Results of Surgical and Nonoperative Treatment for Pulmonary North American Blastomycosis, *J Thorac Cardiovasc Surg,* **51:**714, 1966.

Laurenzi, G. A., Turino, G. M., and Fishman, A. P.: Bullous Disease of the Lung, *Am J Med,* **32:**361, 1962.

Law, S. W., Jenkins, D. E., Chofnas, I., Bahar, D., Witcomb, F., Barkley, H. T., and DeBakey, M. E.: Surgical Experience in Management of Atypical Mycobacterial Infections, *J Thorac Cardiovasc Surg,* **46:**689, 1963.

LeRoux, B. T.: Intrathoracic Foreign Bodies, *Thorax,* **19:**203, 1964.

Lewis, F. J., and Welch, J. A.: Respiratory Mechanics in Postoperative Patients, *Surg Gynecol Obstet,* **120:**305, 1965.

Liebow, A. A., Hales, M. R., and Lindskog, G. E.: Enlargement of the Bronchial Arteries and Their Anastomoses with the Pulmonary Arteries in Bronchiectasis, *Am J Pathol,* **25:**211, 1949.

Macartney, J. N.: Pulmonary Aspergillosis: A Review and a Description of Three New Cases, *Thorax,* **19:**287, 1964.

McNeill, T. M., and Chamberlain, J. M.: Diagnostic Anterior Mediastinotomy, *Ann Thorac Surg,* **2:**532, 1966.

Maier, H. C.: The Pulmonary and Pleural Lymphatics, *J Thorac Cardiovasc Surg,* **52:**155, 1966.

Maloney, J. V., Jr., Franks, R., Makoff, D., and Sherman, P. H.: Biopsy of the Scalene Lymph Nodes and the Right Thoracic Duct Lymph Node for the Diagnosis of Pulmonary Disease, *J Thorac Cardiovasc Surg,* **47:**438, 1964.

Mannix, E. P., and Haight, C.: Anomalous Pulmonary Arteries and Cystic Disease of the Lung, *Medicine* (*Baltimore*), **34:**193, 1955.

Martini, N., Hajdu, S. I., and Beattie, E. J.: Primary Sarcoma of the Lung, *J Thorac Cardiovasc Surg,* **61:**33, 1971.

Mathey, J., Binet, J. P., Galey, J. J., Evrard, C., Lemoine, G., and Denis, B.: Tracheal and Tracheobronchial Resections: Technique and Results in 20 Cases, *J Thorac Cardiovasc Surg,* **51:**1, 1966.

Mayer, E., and Maier, H. C.: "Pulmonary Carcinoma," New York University Press, New York, 1956.

Mendelson, C. L.: The Aspiration of Stomach Contents into the Lung during Obstetrical Anesthesia, *Ann J Obstet Gynecol,* **52:**191, 1946.

Miller, D. R.: Benign Tumors of Lung and Tracheobronchial Tree, *Ann Thorac Surg,* **8:**542, 1969.

Moncrief, M. W., Cameron, A. H., Astley, R., Roberts, K. D., Abrams, L. D., and Mann, J. R.: Congenital Cystic Adenomatoid Malformation of the Lung, *Thorax,* **24:**476, 1969.

Moskowitz, M., Kim, Y. I., and Freihoffer, A.: To Brush or Not to Brush: Is There Really a Question, *Chest,* **59:**648, 1971.

Moss, H. B.: The Hazards of Tracheostomy, *J Indiana Med Assoc,* **59:**446, 1966.

Moyer, J. H., Glantz, G., and Brest, A. N.: Pulmonary Arteriovenous Fistulas: Physiologic and Clinical Considerations, *Am J Med,* **32:**417, 1962.

Murphy, D. R., and Owen, H. F.: Respiratory Emergencies in the Newborn, *Am J Surg,* **101:**581, 1961.

Murphy, J. D., and Davis, J. M.: Pulmonary Resection for Tuberculosis: A Five to Ten Year Follow-up Study, *J Thorac Cardiovasc Surg,* **32:**772, 1956.

Neptune, W. B., Woods, F. M., and Overholt, R. H.: Reoperation for Bronchogenic Carcinoma, *J Thorac Cardiovasc Surg,* **52:**342, 1966.

————, Kim, S., and Bookwalter, J.: Current Surgical Management of Pulmonary Tuberculosis, *J Thorac Cardiovasc Surg,* **60:**384, 1970.

Neville, W. E., Hamouda, F., Andersen, J., and Dawn, F. M.: Replacement of the Intrathoracic Trachea and Both Stem Bronchi with a Molded Silastic Prosthesis, *J Thorac Cardiovasc Surg,* **63:**569, 1972.

Oakley, C., Glick, G., and McCredie, R. M.: Congenital Absence of a Pulmonary Artery, *Am J Med,* **34:**264, 1963.

Oyamada, A., Gasul, B. M., and Hollinger, P. H.: Agenesis of the Lung: Report of a Case with a Review of All Previously Reported Cases, *Am J Dis Child,* **85:**182, 1953.

Paulson, D. L., Shaw, R. R., Kee, J. L., Mallams, J. T., and Collier, R. E.: Combined Preoperative Irradiation and Resection for Bronchogenic Carcinoma, *J Thorac Cardiovasc Surg,* **44:**281, 1962.

Peters, R. M., Wilcox, B. R., and Schultz, E. H., Jr.: Pulmonary Resection in Children: Long-Term Effect on Function and Lung Growth, *Ann Surg,* **159:**652, 1964.

Pinkerton, J. A., Lawler, M. W., and Foster, J. H.: Pulmonary Nocardiosis, *Am Surg,* **37:**729, 1971.

Portin, B. A., Rasmussen, G. L., Stewart, J. D., and Andersen, M. N.: Physiologic and Anatomic Studies Thirty-five Months after Successful Replantation of the Lung, *J Thorac Cardiovasc Surg,* **39:**380, 1960.

Potter, R. T., Laforet, E. G., and Strieder, J. W.: Resectional Surgery for Pulmonary Tuberculosis: Analysis of Series of 420 Resections Performed between 1947 and 1957, *Am Rev Resp Dis,* **93:**30, 1966.

Potts, W. J., and Riker, W. L.: Differentiation of Congenital Cysts of the Lung and Those following Staphylococcal Pneumonia, *Arch Surg,* **61:**684, 1950.

Prather, J. R., Eastridge, C. E., Hughes, F. A., Jr., and McCaughan, J. J., Jr.: Actinomycosis of the Thorax: Diagnosis and Treatment, *Ann Thorac Surg,* **9:**307, 1970.

Ravitch, M. M., and Hardy, J. B.: Congenital Cystic Disease of the Lung in Infants and in Children, *Arch Surg,* **59:**1, 1959.

Raynor, A. C., Capp, M. B. P., and Sealy, W. C.: Lobar Emphysema of Infancy, *Ann Thorac Surg,* **4:**374, 1967.

Rees, G. M., and Paneth, M.: Lobectomy with Sleeve Resection in the Treatment of Bronchial Tumours, *Thorax,* **25:**160, 1970.

Reichle, F. A., and Rosemond, G. P.: Mucoepidermoid Tumors of the Bronchus, *J Thorac Cardiovasc Surg,* **51:**443, 1966.

Ribaudo, C. A., and Grace, W. J.: *Pulmonary Aspiration, Am J Med,* **50:**510, 1971.

Roberts, W. C., and Sjoerdsma, A.: The Cardiac Disease Associated with the Carcinoid Syndrome (Carcinoid Heart Disease), *Am J Med,* **36:**5, 1964.

Roehm, J. O. F., Jr., Jue, K. L., and Amplatz, K.: Radiographic Features of the Scimitar Syndrome, *Radiology,* **86:**856, 1966.

Rubin, E. H., and Rubin, M.: Lung Biopsy for Diffuse Pulmonary Lesions: Value and Limitations, *Dis Chest,* **46:**635, 1964.

Ryland, D., and Reid, L.: Pulmonary Aplasia: A Quantative Analysis of the Development of the Single Lung, *Thorax,* **26:**602, 1971.

Schuster, S. R., Schwachman, H., Harris, G. B. C., and Khaw, K.-T.: Pulmonary Surgery for Cystic Fibrosis, *J Thorac Cardiovasc Surg,* **48:**750, 1964.

Sealy, W. C.: Nonmetastatic Extrapulmonary Manifestations of Bronchogenic Carcinoma, *Surgery,* **68:**906, 1970.

Siderys, H., and Pittman, J. N.: Percutaneous Needle Biopsy of the Lung in Cases of Superior Sulcus Tumor, *J Thorac Cardiovasc Surg,* **53:**716, 1967.

Smith, R. A.: Bronchial Carcinoid Tumours, *Thorax,* **24:**43, 1969.

————: Long-Term Clinical Follow-up after Operation for Lung Carcinoma, *Thorax,* **25:**62, 1970.

Smith, W. G.: Needle Biopsy of the Lung, *Thorax,* **19:**68, 1964.

Steele, J. D.: The Solitary Pulmonary Nodule: Report of a Cooperative Study of Resected Asymptomatic Solitary Pulmonary Nodules in Males, *J Thorac Cardiovasc Surg,* **46:**21, 1963.

———— (ed.): "Treatment of Mycotic and Parasitic Diseases of the Chest," Charles C Thomas, Publisher, Springfield, Ill., 1964.

Stemmer, E. A., Calvin, J. W., Steedman, R. A., and Connolly, J. E.: Parasternal Mediastinal Exploration to Evaluate Resectability of Thoracic Neoplasms, *Ann Thorac Surg,* **12:**375, 1971.

Sternberg, W. H., Sidransky, H., and Ochsner, S.: Primary Malignant Lymphomas of the Lung, *Cancer,* **12:**806, 1959.

Struve-Christensen, E.: Bilateral Primary Bronchogenic Carcinoma, *Acta Chir Scand,* **131:**375, 1966.

Sutaria, M. K., Polk, J. W., Reddy, P., and Mohanty, S. K.: Surgical Aspects of Pulmonary Histoplasmosis, *Thorax,* **25:**31, 1970.

Takaro, T.: Mycotic Infections of Interest to Thoracic Surgeons, *Ann Thorac Cardiovasc Surg,* **3:**71, 1967.

Taylor, E. R.: Pulmonary Cryptococcosis, *Ann Thorac Surg,* **10:**309, 1970.

Thomford, N. R., Woolner, L. B., and Clagett, O. T.: The Surgical Treatment of Metastatic Tumors in the Lungs, *J Thorac Cardiovasc Surg,* **49:**357, 1965.

Thompson, D. T.: Conservative Resection in Surgery for Bronchogenic Carcinoma, *J Thorac Cardiovasc Surg,* **53:**159, 1967.

Thorn, N. A., and Transbøe, I.: Hyponatremia and Bronchogenic Carcinoma Associated with Renal Excretion of Large Amounts of Antidiuretic Material, *Am J Med,* **35:**257, 1963.

Tildon, T. T., and Hughes, R. K.: Complications from Preoperative Irradiation Therapy for Lung Cancer, *Ann Thorac Surg,* **3:**307, 1967.

Tillotson, J. R. and Lerner, A. M.: Characteristics of Pneumonias Caused by *Esherichia coli, N Engl J Med,* **277:**115, 1967.

———— and ————: Bacteroides Pneumonias: Characteristics of Cases with Empyema, *Ann Intern Med,* **68:**308, 1968.

Titus, J. L., Harrison, E. G., Clagett, O. T., Anderson, M. W., and Knaff, L. J.: Xanthomatous and Inflammatory Pseudotumors of the Lung, *Cancer,* **15:**522, 1962.

Turkington, R. W., Goldman, J. K., Ruffner, B. W., and Dobson, J. L.: Bronchogenic Carcinoma Simulating Hyperparathyroidism, *Cancer,* **19:**406, 1966.

Urschel, H. C., Paulson, D. L., and Shaw, R. R.: Mucoid Impaction of the Bronchi, *Ann Thorac Surg,* **2:**1, 1966.

Vieta, J. O., and Maier, H. C.: The Treatment of Adenoid Cystic Carcinoma (Cylindroma) of the Respiratory Tract by Surgery and Radiation Therapy, *Dis Chest,* **31:**493, 1957.

Villegas, A. H., and Sala, C. A.: Pulmonary Actinomycosis of Pseudotumoral Form, *J Thorac Cardiovasc Surg,* **49:**677, 1965.

Wahner, H. W., Hepper, N. G. G., Andersen, H. A., and Weed, L. A.: Pulmonary Aspergillosis, *Ann Intern Med,* **58:**472, 1963.

Waldhausen, J. A., and Abel, F. L.: Circulatory Effects of Pulmonary Arteriovenous Fistulas, *Surgery,* **59:**76, 1966.

Wangel, A. G., and Deller, D. J.: Malabsorption Syndrome Associated with Carcinoma of the Bronchus, *Gut,* **6:**73, 1965.

Webb, W. R., Elston, W. C., and Bowlin, J. S.: Evaluation of Extensive Unilateral Resections for Tuberculosis, *J Thorac Cardiovasc Surg,* **47:**809, 1964.

Weill, H., Ferrans, V. J., Gay, R. M., and Ziskind, M. M.: Early Lipoid Pneumonia: Roentgenologic Anatomic and Physiologic Characteristics, *Am J Med,* **36:**370, 1964.

Weinberg, M., Jr., Agustsson, M. H., D'Cruz, I. A., Bicoff, J. P., Behravesh, M., Raffensperger, J. G., and Fell, E. H.: Stenosis of the Branches of the Pulmonary Artery, *J Thorac Cardiovasc Surg,* **47:**40, 1964.

Weiss, L., and Ingram, M.: Adenomatoid Bronchial Tumors: A Consideration of the Carcinoid Tumors and the Salivary Tumors of the Bronchial Tree, *Cancer,* **14:**161, 1961.

Wilkins, E. W., Jr., and Head, J. M.: Pulmonary Neoplasms: Surgical Experience at Massachusetts General Hospital, *Postgrad Med,* **37:**584, 1965.

Wolcott, M. W., Harris, S. H., Briggs, J. N., Dobell, A. R. C., and Brown, R. K.: Hydatid Disease of the Lung, *J Thorac Cardiovasc Surg,* **62:**465, 1971.

Wolf, J., Spear, P., Yesner, R., and Patno, M. E.: Nitrogen Mustard and the Steroid Hormones in the Treatment of Inoperable Bronchogenic Carcinoma, *Am J Med,* **29:**1008, 1960.

Zavala, D. C., Bedell, G. N., and Rossi, N. P.: Trephine Lung Biopsy with a High-Speed Air Drill; Results of 50 Biopsies in 47 Patients, *J Thorac Cardiovasc Surg,* **64:**220, 1972.

————, Rossi, N. P., and Bedell, G. N.: Bronchial Brush Biopsy; a Valuable Diagnostic Technique in the Presurgical Evaluation of Indeterminate Lung Densities, *Ann Thorac Surg,* **13:**519, 1972.

Mediastinum

Barrett, N. R.: Idiopathic Mediastinal Fibrosis, *Br J Surg,* **46:**207, 1958.

Burke, W. A., Burford, T. H., and Dorfman, R. F.: Hodgkin's Disease of the Mediastinum, *Ann Thorac Surg,* **3:**287, 1967.

Downs, A. R., and Schoemperlen, C. B.: Intrathoracic Pheochromocytoma, *Can J Surg,* **9:**180, 1966.

Drake, C. T., Marshall, L. W., Meyers, S. N., and Shields, T. W.: Ectopic Hematopoietic Tissue Masquerading as a Mediastinal Tumor, *Ann Thorac Surg,* **1:**736, 1965.

Effler, D. B., and Groves, L. K.: Superior Vena Cava Obstruction, *J Thorac Cardiovasc Surg,* **43:**574, 1962.

Eraklis, A. J., Griscom, N. T., and McGovern, J. B.: Bronchogenic Cysts of the Mediastinum in Infancy, *N Engl J Med,* **281:**1150, 1969.

Failor, H. J., Edwards, J. E., and Hodgson, C. H.: Etiologic Factors in Obstruction of the Superior Vena Cava, *Proc Staff Meetings Mayo Clin,* **33:**671, 1958.

Gray, J. M., and Hanson, G. C.: Mediastinal Emphysema: Aetiology, Diagnosis, and Treatment, *Thorax,* **21:**325, 1966.

Grosfeld, J. L., Weinberger, M., Kilman, J. W., and Clatworthy, H. W.: Primary Mediastinal Neoplasms in Infants and Children, *Ann Thorac Surg,* **12:**179, 1971.

Hirst, E., and Robertson, T. I.: The Syndrome of Thymoma and

Erythroblastopenic Anemia, *Medicine (Baltimore)*, **46:**225, 1967.

Jimenez-Martinez, M., Arguero-Sanchez, A., Perez-Alvarez, J. J., and Mina-Castaneda, P.: Anterior Mediastinitis as a Complication of Median Sternotomy Incisions: Diagnostic and Surgical Considerations, *Surgery,* **67:**929, 1970.

Kark, A. E., and Kirschner, P. A.: Total Thymectomy by the Transcervical Approach, *Br J Surg,* **58:**321, 1971.

Katz, R. I., Joseph, W. L., and Mulder, D. G.: Surgery of the Thymus: Collective Review, *Ann Thorac Surg,* **6:**591, 1968.

Kunkel, W. M., Jr., Clagett, O. T., and McDonald, J. R.: Mediastinal Granulomas, *J Thorac Cardiovasc Surg,* **27:**565, 1954.

Leigh, T. F., and Weens, H. S.: "The Mediastinum," Charles C Thomas Publisher, Springfield, Ill. 1959.

LeRoux, B. T.: Primary Intrathoracic Neural Tumors, *Thorax,* **15:**339, 1960.

McNamara, J. J., Messersmith, J. K., Dunn, R. A., Molot, M. D., and Stremple, J. F.: Thoracic Injuries in Combat Casualties in Vietnam, *Ann Thorac Surg,* **10:**389, 1970.

Maier, H. C.: Bronchiogenic Cysts of the Mediastinum, *Ann Surg,* **127:**476, 1948.

———: Hemangiomas of the Subglottic Region, Trachea, and Mediastinum in Infancy and Childhood, *Ann Thorac Surg,* **3:**514, 1967.

Mulder, D. G., Braitman, H., and Herrmann, C., Jr.: Surgical Management in Myasthenia Gravis, *J Thorac Cardiovasc Surg,* **63:**105, 1972.

Nathan, M. T.: Cysts and Duplications of Neurenteric Origin, *Pediatrics,* **23:**476, 1959.

Nelson, W. P., Lundberg, G. D., and Dickerson, R. B.: Pulmonary Artery Obstruction and Cor Pulmonale Due to Chronic Fibrous Mediastinitis, *Am J Med,* **38:**279, 1965.

Oldham, H. N.: Mediastinal Tumors and Cysts, *Ann Thorac Surg,* **11:**246, 1971.

Papatestas, A. E., Alpert, L. I., Osserman, K. E., Osserman, R. S., and Kark, A. E.: Studies in Myasthenia Gravis: Effects of Thymectomy; Results of 185 Patients with Nonthymomatous and Thymomatous Myasthenia Gravis, 1941–1969, *Am J Med,* **50:**465, 1971.

Ross, J. K.: A Review of the Surgery of the Thoracic Duct, *Thorax,* **16:**12, 1961.

Sakulsky, S. B., Harrison, E. G., Dines, D. E., and Payne, W. S.: Mediastinal Granuloma, *J Thorac Cardiovasc Surg,* **54:**279, 1967.

Sandor, F.: Incidence and Significance of Traumatic Mediastinal Haematoma, *Thorax,* **22:**43, 1967.

Sellors, T. H., Thackray, A. C., and Thomson, A. D.: Tumours of the Thymus: A Review of 88 Operation Cases, *Thorax,* **22:**193, 1967.

Voorhees, M. L., and Gardner, L. I.: Studies of Catecholamine Excretion by Children with Neural Tumors, *J Clin Endocrinol Metab,* **22:**126, 1962.

Weimann, R. B., Hallman, G. L., Bahar, D., and Greenberg, S. D.: Intrathoracic Meningocele, *J Thorac Cardiovasc Surg,* **46:**40, 1963.

Wychulis, A. R., Payne, W. S., Clagett, O. T., and Woolner, L. B.: Surgical Treatment of Mediastinal Tumors: 40-Year Experience, *J Thorac Cardiovasc Surg,* **62:**379, 1971.

Chapter 18

Congenital Heart Disease

by **Frank C. Spencer**

Introduction

Classification
Pathophysiology
Clinical Examination
Principles of Operative and Postoperative Care
 of Infants

Obstructive Lesions

Pulmonic Stenosis
  Stenosis of the Pulmonary Artery
Congenital Aortic Stenosis
  Supravalvular Aortic Stenosis
  Hypertrophic Subaortic Stenosis
Coarctation of the Aorta
Vascular Rings

Left-to-right Shunts (Acyanotic Group)

Atrial Septal Defects
  Secundum Defects
  Anomalous Drainage of Pulmonary Veins
  Ostium Primum Defect
  Persistent Atrioventricular Canal
Ventricular Septal Defect
Patent Ductus Arteriosus

Right-to-left Shunts (Cyanotic Group)

Tetralogy of Fallot

Complex Malformations

Transposition of the Great Vessels
Tricuspid Atresia

Rare Malformations

Cor Triatriatum
Congenital Mitral Stenosis
Aortic-Pulmonary Window
Ruptured Aneurysm of Sinus of Valsalva
Truncus Arteriosus
Single Ventricle
Ebstein's Anomaly
Anomalies of the Coronary Arteries
  Anomalous Origin of Left Coronary Artery
    from Pulmonary Artery
  Coronary Arteriovenous Fistula
Corrected Transposition

INTRODUCTION

With the declining incidence of rheumatic fever, congenital heart disease has become the most common form of heart disease seen in children. In several studies the frequency has been found to be about 3 cases of congenital heart disease occurring in every 1,000 live births. The frequency is about ten times greater in members of the same family than in the normal population, and a convenient approximation of risk of occurrence in younger siblings of a child with congenital heart disease is about 2 percent. In most patients the etiologic factors are unknown.

Rubella occurring in the first trimester of pregnancy is one of the few infectious diseases known to cause congenital heart disease; this disease produces the well-recognized syndrome of mental deficiency, deafness, cataracts, and congenital heart disease, usually a patent ductus arteriosus. Mongolism is another type of congenital malformation associated with a high incidence of congenital heart disease. Usually congenital heart disease occurs as an isolated malformation resulting from defective embryonic development without known cause.

The surprisingly short period of time during which cardiac development occurs in uterine life should be emphasized, for virtually all the fetal heart structures are formed between the third and eighth week of pregnancy, a time interval of only 5 weeks. Atrial or ventricular septal defects result from incomplete formation of the respective septa, while transposition and other anomalies of the aorta result from abnormalities in the spiral division of the primitive bulbus cordis. Although there are six branchial aortic arches, all atrophy with the exception of the fourth left arch, remaining as the aorta, and the sixth left arch, remaining as the ductus arteriosus. Malformations with vascular rings arise from different remnants of these embryonic branchial arches.

Fetal circulation has several distinctive features, which may persist in association with congenital heart disease in adults. In embryonic life the lungs are collapsed, with a high vascular resistance, and pulmonary blood flow is small. Most of the blood returning through the inferior vena cava to the right atrium goes through the foramen ovale into the left atrium and thence to the left ventricle. Also, most of the blood expelled from the right ventricle into the pulmonary artery is shunted through the ductus arteriosus into the descending thoracic aorta. At birth, with expansion of the lungs, there is a fall in pulmonary vascular resistance, although the vascular resistance does not decrease to that normally found in older individuals for the first few years of life. There is a corresponding persistence in early years of life of the fetal histologic structure of the pulmonary arteries, characterized principally by prominent smooth muscle in the media of the arterial wall. Persistence of the fetal histologic structure of the pulmonary arterioles has been associated with pulmonary hypertension in small children.

With expansion of the lungs, the ductus arteriosus normally closes in the first few days after birth. It remains patent in only a small percentage of individuals, but this is one of the most common forms of congenital heart disease. The foramen ovale is a slitlike channel which is automatically sealed when left atrial pressure becomes higher than right atrial pressure and normally permits the flow of blood only from the right atrium to the left atrium and not in a reverse direction. Patency of the foramen ovale, constituting an innocuous defect, remains throughout adult life in at least 10 to 20 percent of patients. With elevation of right atrial pressure, the foramen ovale may be stretched open and create a right-to-left shunt from the right atrium to the left atrium, resulting in cyanosis from shunting of unoxygenated blood. This characteristically occurs in patients with pulmonic valvular stenosis when right ventricular failure develops, with subsequent elevation of right atrial pressure to exceed left atrial pressure.

Although a large number of congenital heart defects have been recognized and classified, in a large pediatric cardiac clinic seven malformations will be found to comprise the majority of abnormalities seen. Ventricular septal defect, with or without pulmonic stenosis, is by far the most common, representing 20 percent or more of all patients. The other six malformations, each occurring in 10 to 15 percent of patients, are atrial septal defect, pulmonic valvular stenosis, aortic valvular stenosis, patent ductus arteriosus, coarctation of the aorta, and transposition of the great vessels. The frequency of different defects varies somewhat with the age of the patient studied; transposition of the great vessels is a much more common disease in the newborn, as many do not survive beyond six months of age.

Classification

Congenital heart disease may be conveniently classified by the type of anatomic abnormality present, which in turn produces a distinct physiologic disturbance and similarly has prognostic significance regarding feasibility of surgical correction: (1) obstructive lesions predominantly restrict the flow of blood, with corresponding increased work loads on the obstructed ventricular chamber; (2) left-to-right shunts occur through uncomplicated septal defects; (3) right-to-left shunts result from combination of a septal defect with obstruction to ventricular emptying; (4) complex malformations, as the name indicates, are more extensive disturbances of the structure of the heart from gross errors in development which cannot presently be corrected by available surgical methods and in some instances probably require cardiac transplantation.

Pathophysiology

Four stages in the severity of congenital heart disease often can be recognized. Initially, there may be only abnormal physical findings. In milder forms of congenital heart disease, such as trivial pulmonic valvular stenosis, there may never be any sign of heart disease except the characteristic systolic murmur. In the second stage of evolution, physiologic disturbances can be measured by cardiac catheterization, such as pressure gradients across stenotic pulmonic or aortic valves, increased blood flow through shunts occurring through atrial or ventricular septal defects, or elevation in pulmonary artery pressure as pulmonary hypertension evolves. Sooner or later, these physiologic signs of impaired function result in corresponding anatomic changes, manifested principally by cardiac enlargement with associated hypertrophy of the right or left ventricle, as best measured by the electrocardiogram and roentgenogram. With the development of pulmonary hypertension, histologic changes occur in the media and intima of the pulmonary arterioles. Only in the fourth stage do the overt symptoms of cardiac failure appear. This late appearance of symptoms is an important consideration in evaluating children with congenital heart disease, for parents are normally apprehensive about consenting to complex diagnostic studies or operative procedures on a child who seems, to the inexperienced eye, to have little disability. Postponing therapy until a child is disabled to a point that is clinically obvious may result in irreversible changes in ventricular muscle, for severe hypertrophy of the right or left ventricle does not always regress completely following surgical correction of the basic cause, such as pulmonic or aortic stenosis.

The three main physiologic disturbances resulting from congenital heart disease are (1) obstruction to emptying of the ventricles, (2) left-to-right shunts with increase in pulmonary blood flow and corresponding decrease in systemic blood flow, and (3) right-to-left shunts producing oxygen unsaturation of the arterial blood. Each of these physiologic disturbances is considered in detail in subsequent sections. With all forms of congenital heart disease there is an increased susceptibility to bacterial endocarditis, because the anatomic malformation creates a localized turbulent flow of blood predisposing to local deposition of bacteria migrating in the circulation.

OBSTRUCTIVE LESIONS. The most common disorders are pulmonic valvular stenosis, aortic valvular stenosis, and coarctation of the aorta. These impede emptying of the involved ventricular chamber, resulting in what has been termed "systolic" overloading and corresponding concentric hypertrophy of the ventricle. As the ventricular response is predominantly concentric hypertrophy, cardiac enlargement cannot be detected by clinical means, and often the chest roentgenogram is only slightly abnormal. The electrocardiogram is a most useful guide, however, in indicating the degree of ventricular hypertrophy evolving. With progressive hypertrophy angina pectoris may occur, with susceptibility to arrhythmias and even sudden death. Cardiac failure is a late and often preterminal manifestation.

LEFT-TO-RIGHT SHUNTS. As pressures in the left atrium and left ventricle are normally greater than those in the right atrium and right ventricle, a defect in either the atrial or ventricular septum results in a shunt of oxygenated blood from the left side of the heart to the right side. This causes pulmonary congestion from an increase in pulmonary blood flow and often a corresponding decrease in systemic blood flow. Cyanosis, of course, does not occur. With the increase in pulmonary blood flow there is a tendency to develop pulmonary hypertension, varying both with the type of defect and with the individual patient. The most common defects producing left-to-right shunts are atrial septal defects, with or without anomalous pulmonary veins, ventricular septal defects, and patent ductus arteriosus.

Pulmonary Congestion. A shunt becomes physiologically significant when the pulmonary blood flow is one and one-half times to twice as great as the systemic blood flow. Large shunts may produce a pulmonary blood flow three to four times greater than systemic blood flow, with a calculated pulmonary blood flow of even 10 to 15 liters/minute/square meter of body surface. The resulting pulmonary congestion produces a susceptibility to bacterial infection; recurrent bouts of pneumonia may occur in the first few years of life. Beyond early childhood, however, high pulmonary blood flows may be associated with surprisingly little disability for a period of time. With the increase in pulmonary blood flow there is a corresponding enlargement of the involved ventricle (right ventricle with atrial septal defect, left ventricle with patent ductus arteriosus, both ventricles with ventricular septal defect), resulting in so-called "diastolic" overloading of the ventricle, with cardiac dilatation rather than hypertrophy. The dilatation can be more easily recognized on clinical examination and on the chest roentgenogram than its counterpart, concentric hypertrophy. The changes in the electrocardiogram are often less prominent than those seen with concentric hypertrophy. Cardiac failure tends to occur somewhat earlier in the course of the disease than with concentric hypertrophy, and the prognosis with medical therapy is somewhat better than that for predominantly obstructive lesions.

Pulmonary Hypertension. With the increase in pulmonary blood flow there is a tendency to develop pulmonary hypertension. Although the mode of development has been a subject of intense study in recent years, many factors remain unknown. An excellent analysis of the functional pathology of the pulmonary vascular bed was published by Edwards in 1957. Pulmonary hypertension may result from an increase in pulmonary blood flow, from histologic changes in the pulmonary vascular bed with corresponding anatomic restriction of distensibility of the pulmonary vessels, or from pulmonary venous obstruction. It should be emphasized that the most important consideration in evaluating the pulmonary circulation is the pulmonary vascular resistance, not the systolic pulmonary arterial pressure per se. Pulmonary hypertension resulting from an increase in pulmonary blood flow subsides as soon as the cardiac defect producing the increase in blood flow is corrected. Pulmonary hypertension due to decrease in distensibility of the pulmonary vascular bed from histologic changes is often irreversible, however, and surgical therapy may be of limited value or even contraindicated. Hence, in evaluating pulmonary hypertension, the significant physiologic measurement is the degree of change in the pulmonary vascular resistance, as calculated from the relation between flow and pressure, and not the absolute level of the pulmonary artery pressure per se.

Normally pulmonary arterioles are very distensible and can accommodate an increase in pulmonary blood flow up to three times normal values without any increase in pressure. Further distensibility is limited by the fibrous tissue in the adventitial sheath surrounding the arterioles. In infants and young children with pulmonary hypertension the prominent histologic change in the pulmonary arterioles is hypertrophy of the smooth muscle of the media of the arteriolar wall, which is similar to that normally found in embryonic life. Some feel that the histologic changes represent merely a failure of involution of the normal fetal pattern. In older children and adults, thickening of the intima occurs also, with associated fibrosis, and has a more serious prognosis, for such histologic changes are often irreversible and do not improve even after the underlying cause has been corrected.

More significant than increase in pulmonary blood flow, however, is the pressure under which blood is propelled into the pulmonary artery, for pulmonary hypertension is much more frequent with ventricular septal defects than with atrial septal defects producing comparable increase in pulmonary blood flow. In general, the incidence of hypertension with secundum atrial septal defects in children is about 5 percent, with atrioventricular canal defects about 10 percent, and with ventricular septal defects about 25 percent, as reported by Nadas.

In addition, there is an individual variation in susceptibility to development of pulmonary hypertension, for some children with a large ventricular septal defect and a large increase in pulmonary blood flow will not develop any change in pulmonary vascular resistance, while others with a smaller septal defect will develop significant pulmonary hypertension at an early age. Finally, there are unexplained variations in pulmonary hypertension for which no known cause can at present be discerned. In some children pulmonary hypertension is apparently present from birth and remains for several years without any change. In others pulmonary hypertension found at birth may be seen to have regressed spontaneously when the patient is studied at repeat cardiac catheterization some years later. In most patients, however, pulmonary hypertension gradually increases in severity, although during the first decade of life the increase is slow in the majority of patients.

The earliest age at which pulmonary vascular changes become irreversible is unknown. Dammann has stated that some patients with ventricular septal defect apparently have irreversible pulmonary hypertension by six years of age, whereas such changes in patients with atrial septal defect usually occur at a much later age. Patients with a patent ductus arteriosus or an aortic-pulmonary window may develop irreversible changes even earlier than at six years, causing an immediate fatality when an aortic septal defect is surgically divided.

Restriction in Systemic Blood Flow. With large left-to-right shunts there is a corresponding restriction in systemic blood flow and retardation in normal growth and development. This is more prominently seen in children with a patent ductus arteriosus or an atrial septal defect. The appearance of frail, underweight children with atrial septal defect has been termed the *gracile* habitus. Although mental retardation is slightly more common in children with congenital heart disease, beyond this association there is no evidence that congenital heart disease retards mental development, and unfortunately correction of the cardiac defect does not result in any improvement in mental function. There is, however, often a substantial increase in growth and weight once the cardiac defect has been corrected.

RIGHT-TO-LEFT SHUNTS. Right-to-left shunts of unoxygenated venous blood directly into the systemic circulation, producing arterial unsaturation and cyanosis, result from the combination of an intracardiac septal defect with obstruction to normal flow of blood into the pulmonary artery. The classic example is the tetralogy of Fallot, a combination of ventricular septal defect and pulmonic stenosis. Other cyanotic disorders include the more complex malformations, such as transposition of the great vessels, tricuspid atresia, truncus arteriosus, and total anomalous drainage of the pulmonary veins. Right-to-left shunts produce a large number of physiologic disturbances because of the anoxia resulting from chronic oxygen unsaturation of the arterial blood. These are considered in detail in the following paragraphs. It should be emphasized that all these disturbances result from deficient oxygen transport to tissues of the body. With right-to-left shunts there is no increase in cardiac output, and often the pulmonary blood flow is less than normal. Hence cardiac failure is rare with an uncomplicated right-to-left shunt, in contrast to its inevitable eventual occurrence with left-to-right shunts.

Cyanosis. This is the most prominent feature of a right-to-left shunt. The degree of cyanosis depends upon both the degree of anoxia and the blood hemoglobin concentration, for the visible intensity of cyanosis is determined by the number of grams of reduced hemoglobin in the circulation. It has been estimated that about 5 Gm of reduced hemoglobin is required to produce visible cyanosis. Normally in the capillaries about 2.25 Gm of reduced hemoglobin is present, so with an average hemoglobin concentration of 15 Gm/100 ml of blood, a decrease in arterial oxygen from the normal range of 92–95% to 75% is needed to produce visible cyanosis. In the presence of anemia, however, a more severe degree of anoxia is required to produce visible cyanosis, while with polycythemia and hemoglobin concentrations of 20 Gm/100 ml of blood or more, severe cyanosis may represent less serious anoxia.

Cyanosis has been conveniently grouped into "central" and "peripheral" types. Peripheral cyanosis results simply from a decrease in cardiac output with sluggish regional flow of blood through the capillary circulation, as a result of which more oxygen is extracted and a greater amount of reduced hemoglobin is present. This type of cyanosis occurs with conditions producing a low cardiac output, such as mitral stenosis, and varies with the condition of the patient. It is usually more prominent in certain regions of the body, such as the tips of the fingers, the lips, or the lobes of the ears. Central cyanosis results either from a defect in oxygenation of blood in the lungs or from an intracardiac shunt. Cyanosis resulting from pulmonary insufficiency can usually be recognized from its prompt improvement when the patient breathes 100% oxygen, increasing the efficiency of pulmonary ventilation. In the catheterization laboratory it can be recognized from the finding that oxygen saturation of blood in the left atrium is less than 95%. Cyanosis from pulmonary insufficiency occurs only with severe pulmonary congestion from cardiac failure or far advanced pulmonary vascular disease.

An intracardiac shunt, permitting direct entry of unoxygenated blood into the systemic circulation, is the cause of central cyanosis in most patients. The intensity of the cyanosis is related to the degree of pulmonary blood flow, for ultimately cyanosis depends upon the relative proportions of unoxygenated and oxygenated blood in the arterial circulation. Even though a large intracardiac shunt is present, an increase in pulmonary blood flow to produce a larger amount of oxygenated blood can substantially reduce cyanosis and improve oxygen transport. This was dramatically demonstrated by Blalock with the systemic-pulmonary artery anastomosis for tetralogy of Fallot.

Two distinctive changes which inevitably result with chronic cyanosis are clubbing of the digits and polycythemia. The triad of cyanosis, clubbing, and polycythemia is a familiar one in children with congenital heart disease. Clubbing of the digits, or hypertrophic osteoarthropathy, is an unusual change in the appearance and structure of the digits, consisting of a rounding of the tips of the fingers and toes, as well as a thickening of the ends, associated with deposition of fibrous tissue. In addition, there is a development of pronounced convexity of the fingernails. Histologically, the fingers have increased numbers of capillaries, with a large number of tiny arteriovenous aneurysms. Clubbing is usually not prominent until a cyanotic child is one to two years of age, but in some instances of severe anoxia it may evolve within several weeks. It usually gradually subsides following correction of the intracardiac defect.

Polycythemia is a fortunate physiologic response of the bone marrow to chronic anoxia, as an increase in red cell and hemoglobin concentration increases the ability of the blood to transport oxygen. Hematocrit readings of 60 to 70 percent are frequent with chronic cyanosis, and readings exceeding 80 percent are found in extreme cases. There is a parallel rise in viscosity of the blood, with restriction to the flow of blood as the hematocrit reading increases. Once the hematocrit reading exceeds 75 to 80 percent, the increased viscosity constitutes a significant hazard, for transitory dehydration in an infant with a hematocrit reading above 80 percent may precipitate cerebral venous thrombosis and permanent neurologic injury, apparently from formation of thrombi in the viscous blood.

Limitation of Exercise Tolerance. Limited tolerance of exercise, with dyspnea on exertion, is characteristic of cyanotic heart disease, for the circulation is unable to increase oxygen transport with exercise. The severity of a disability, or its progression, can be conveniently measured in terms of the patient's ability to walk a measured distance. Associated with exertional dyspnea is squatting, a phenomenon first emphasized by Taussig. The cyanotic child quickly learns that dyspnea on walking can be lessened by assuming a squatting position. Physiologic studies indicate that squatting produces an increase in peripheral vascular resistance, with a corresponding increase in pulmonary blood flow. Squatting is most commonly seen in tetralogy of Fallot, less frequently in other cyanotic conditions.

Neurologic Damage. Periodic episodes of unconsciousness, termed *cyanotic spells,* are grave signs of cerebral anoxia. They often appear in the third to fourth month of life in severely cyanotic children, and are rarely seen after the fifth to sixth year of life. They characteristically occur at different times, not always associated with exertion, and evolve as episodes of crying, deepening cyanosis, and coma, lasting a few minutes to a few hours. Such episodes are extremely grave, for although recovery may ensue promptly, the spells are recurrent, and any spell may either terminate fatally or result in permanent neurologic injury. Emergency surgical treatment to improve the oxygen saturation is indicated when possible.

Another cause of neurologic injury in cyanotic children is brain abscess, for which there is increased susceptibility especially in children with tetralogy of Fallot. The increased susceptibility is partly related to direct access of bacteria in the venous circulation to the arterial circulation through the right-to-left shunt. This is probably not the entire explanation, however, for a similar increased frequency does not occur in other cyanotic conditions. A localized infarct with subsequent bacterial infection may explain the evolution in some patients. Another rare cause of cerebral injury is paradoxic embolism through an intracardiac defect, in which a thrombus migrating in the venous circulation, which would normally produce a pulmonary embolus, traverses an intracardiac defect and lodges in the cerebral circulation as an embolus. From these various causes, permanent neurologic injury, most often seen as hemiplegia, is not uncommon in children with chronic severe cyanosis.

Other Changes. In older children with severe cyanosis there is a striking increase in bronchial circulation, apparently a compensatory response to increased blood flow to the lungs. The myriads of collateral vessels, often constituting a mass of varicosities in the mediastinum, are principally of surgical significance because of the risk of bleeding during operation. They may be associated with epistaxis in some children, but hemoptysis is rare because the pulmonary blood flow is usually less than normal, even though the bronchial circulation is greatly increased.

Finally, with chronic polycythemia in children older than ten to fifteen years of age, some ill-defined defects in blood coagulation occur, with abnormalities in several aspects of the blood-clotting mechanism. Clinically this may result in mild gastrointestinal bleeding, but the major significance is the increased susceptibility to hemorrhage following surgical procedures.

Clinical Examination

HISTORY. In obtaining the history of a patient with congenital heart disease, the presence of abnormal factors during pregnancy, especially during the first trimester, should be noted. Rubella in the first trimester has been emphasized because of the high incidence of cardiac and other defects. In some disorders, notably hypertrophic muscular aortic stenosis, there is a definite familial history of the disorder. Also, with the majority of patients with congenital heart disease there is about a 2 percent associated occurrence of congenital heart disease in other members of the same family. In most patients, however, no etiologic factors can be found.

The age at which a cardiac murmur was detected for the first time should be carefully noted, and the reliability of this observation should be estimated. Similarly the time of appearance of cyanosis is of significance, whether at birth or subsequently during infancy. Variations in the appearance of cyanosis, as well as its location, are also important. In some patients cyanosis may be recognized at birth, then disappear for months or years, and finally appear again.

Intolerance of exercise, manifested by dyspnea on exertion, is a common symptom and a convenient indication of the severity of the disorder in patients with right-to-left shunts. Squatting can be readily identified by the parents. Symptoms of lesser degrees of restriction in physical capacity, such as undue fatigability or inability to participate in exercise, should be noted, although the ability of many children with large left-to-right shunts to participate vigorously in athletics is impressive. Feeding habits and the pattern of weight are also important features to determine.

Previous neurologic episodes such as cyanotic spells, cerebral embolism, brain abscess, or other signs of cerebral injury should be noted.

Finally, episodes of infection occurring as pneumonia, bacterial endocarditis, or rheumatic fever should be ascertained.

PHYSICAL EXAMINATION. Abnormalities in growth and development should be particularly assessed, because these are among the most common signs of cardiac disease. Cyanosis, with clubbing or polycythemia, may be obvious or may require close scrutiny for detection. On examination of the heart, any deformity of the left costal cartilages, indicating long-standing cardiac enlargement, should be noted. Palpation for a thrill is particularly important, for its presence almost uniformly indicates significant underlying cardiac disease. Cardiac size should be estimated, although this is difficult in small children and infants and is best determined by the roentgenogram. Systolic murmurs are commonly found but often are of no diagnostic significance. Basal systolic murmurs occur with pulmonic stenosis, aortic stenosis, patent ductus in infants, and coarctation of the aorta. A murmur along the left sternal border is particularly prominent with ventricular septal defect. With systolic murmurs the type of murmur, location, and transmission are of particular importance. Diastolic murmurs are infrequent in infants, but when present they are significant. They may occur from aortic insufficiency with prolapse of an aortic cusp, with pulmonic insufficiency from long-standing pulmonary hypertension, or in association with a systolic murmur as the continuous murmur of a patent ductus arteriosus. The cardiac sounds, especially the second sound at the base, may be of importance in certain conditions. The pulmonic second sound is increased with pulmonary hypertension, decreased or absent with pulmonic stenosis or atresia. Variation in splitting of the second sound may be recognized by experienced observers and is of diagnostic importance, especially with atrial septal defect. Disturbances of rhythm are infrequent. The gallop rhythm with its ominous prognosis is seen in terminal forms of cardiac disease.

Examination of the lungs may detect rales from cardiac failure in large left-to-right shunts, but characteristically no abnormalities are found in the lungs with right-to-left shunts producing cyanosis. The hallmark of congestive failure in children is hepatic enlargement, occurring with surprising rapidity and regressing rapidly as failure improves. Hence estimation of the presence and extent of hepatic enlargement is of particular importance. Often hepatic enlargement precedes the detection of audible rales, in contrast to adult forms of cardiac disease. Similarly, edema is often less prominent clinically than hepatic enlargement.

Fig. 18-1. Chest roentgenogram of child with tetralogy of Fallot, showing typical cardiac silhouette (sabot-shaped heart). Features include heart of normal size with prominent apex from right ventricular hypertrophy. There is increased concavity at base of heart because pulmonic stenosis produces decrease in size or absence of shadow normally seen from pulmonary artery. Vascularity of lung fields may be normal or decreased. (*Courtesy of Dr. Raymond M. Abrams, Department of Radiology, New York University Medical Center.*)

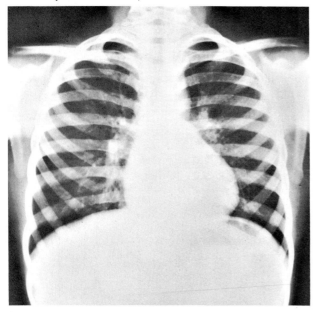

In the extremities, the presence and quality of the radial, femoral, and pedal pulses should be noted. Faint pulses are characteristic of aortic stenosis. With coarctation, radial pulses are prominent while femoral pulses are weak or absent. Easily palpable, bounding pulses are characteristic of defects producing an abnormal exit of blood from the aorta during diastole, such as patent ductus arteriosus, aortic insufficiency, or a ruptured aneurysm of the sinus of Valsalva. These are associated with an increase in pulse pressure, usually due to a decrease in diastolic pressure. Normally the systolic blood pressure in infants is in the range of 70 to 90 mm Hg, rising to about 100 mm Hg in the first five years of life and subsequently to the normal adult level of 120 mm Hg in the next few years. Diastolic pressures are usually in the range of 55 to 60 mm Hg.

Examination of the digits is pertinent with cyanosis, because clubbing is an inevitable accompaniment of long-standing cyanosis.

LABORATORY STUDIES. The diagnostic tripod for congenital heart disease is composed of the clinical examination, the chest roentgenogram, and the electrocardiogram; these three modalities are equally important in arriving at the correct diagnosis. In the roentgenogram, contour of the heart, cardiac size, and vascularity should be particularly noted. Infrequent abnormalities include pleural effusion and notching of the ribs in coarctation of the aorta. Cardiac size is best estimated from the cardiothoracic ratio; a ratio greater than 0.5 indicates cardiac enlargement. In infants a cardiac shadow with a transverse diameter greater than 5.5 cm indicates cardiac enlargement. In oblique views with fluoroscopy, cardiac enlargement involving the atria, right ventricle, left ventricle, or both ventricles may be estimated. Enlargement of the left atrium occurs with mitral insufficiency, ventricular septal defect, patent ductus arteriosus, or any form of left ventricular failure. Left ventricular enlargement is characteristic of aortic disease, mitral insufficiency, coarctation of the aorta, patent ductus arteriosus, ventricular septal defect, or tricuspid atresia. Right atrial enlargement is especially prominent in Ebstein's malformation and also occurs in tricuspid atresia, atrial septal defect, and pulmonic stenosis. Selective enlargement of the right ventricle is frequent with pulmonic stenosis, pulmonary hypertension from any cause, atrial septal defect, and ventricular septal defect.

Changes in cardiac contour may be characteristic in certain conditions. The sabot-shaped heart of tetralogy of Fallot results from hypertrophy of the right ventricle in association with a small pulmonary conus (Fig. 18-1). The egg-shaped heart of transposition of the great vessels (Fig. 18-2) is caused by enlargement of the right ventricle and right atrium, with a narrow shadow at the base from the anteroposterior relation between the aorta and the pulmonary arteries. With total anomalous drainage of the pulmonary venous return, a figure-of-eight abnormality (Fig. 18-3), composed of a large left superior vena cava in the upper mediastinum separate from the cardiac shadow, is characteristic.

The size of the pulmonary vessels and the pulmonary vascularity are also important. This is best determined by fluoroscopy, where the vigor of the pulsations can be observed. Defects with an increased pulmonary blood flow and pulmonary hypertension can be easily differentiated from conditions associated with a normal or a decreased pulmonary blood flow.

The electrocardiogram is the best guide to the presence of ventricular hypertrophy. Selective hypertrophy of the left ventricle, as in aortic valvular stenosis, or selective hypertrophy of the right ventricle, as in pulmonic valvular stenosis, can be recognized and also correlated with the degree of stenosis. Bundle branch block, typically seen as a right bundle branch block with an atrial septal defect, also occurs in certain conditions.

Cardiac catheterization combined with cineangiography provides the most precise method of evaluating congenital heart disease and has been responsible for many significant advances in both diagnosis and therapy. With cardiac catheterization, intracardiac pressures can be determined, abnormal shunts of blood can be recognized, and the ratio between pulmonary and systemic blood flow determined. Direct passage of the catheter into an abnormal chamber, such as a patent ductus arteriosus, may provide visual confirmation of the diagnosis. Mitral or aortic insufficiency are best evaluated by cineangiography. Dye-dilution curves, obtained by selective injection of dye into different chambers, are particularly useful for recognition of right-to-left shunts.

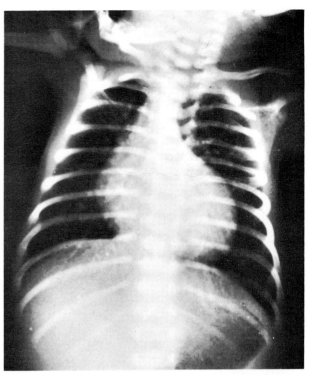

Fig. 18-2. Chest roentgenogram of child with transposition of great vessels, showing egg-shaped heart with large ventricular silhouette and small "waist," which results from abnormal location of aorta directly anterior to pulmonary artery. (*Courtesy of Dr. Raymond M. Abrams, Department of Radiology, New York University Medical Center.*)

Fig. 18-3. *A.* Chest roentgenogram of child with total anomalous drainage of pulmonary veins through left superior vena cava. Shadow in left upper mediastinum is due to dilated left superior vena cava. *B.* Angiogram demonstrates left superior vena cava emptying into greatly dilated left innominate vein. This x-ray appearance is pathognomonic of total anomalous drainage of pulmonary veins into left superior vena cava. (*Courtesy of Dr. Raymond M. Abrams, Department of Radiology, New York University Medical Center.*)

In the normal heart the right atrial systolic pressure does not exceed 5 mm Hg, while left atrial pressure is in the range of 5 to 10 mm Hg. In the normal right ventricle systolic pressure ranges from 15 to 30 mm Hg, while in the left ventricle pressures average 80 to 130 mm Hg

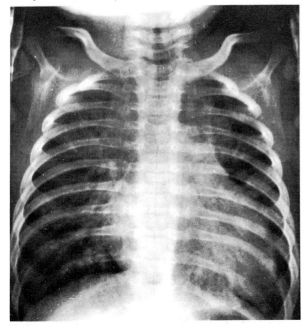

A

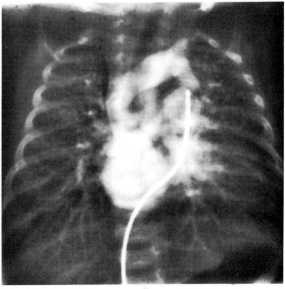

B

systolic and 5 to 10 mm Hg diastolic. Continuous pressure recordings as a catheter is withdrawn from one cardiac chamber to another can readily detect the presence of stenosis; pulmonic stenosis can be measured as a catheter is withdrawn from the pulmonary artery to the right ventricle, and aortic stenosis as a catheter is withdrawn from the left ventricle into the aorta. Combined right- and left-heart catheterization is usually done with the introduction of a catheter through a systemic vein into the right side of the heart, combined with introduction of another catheter from a peripheral artery into the aorta and across the aortic valve into the left ventricle to obtain information from both the right and left sides of the heart simultaneously.

All variations from the normal pulmonary and systemic flow of 3 liters/minute/square meter of body surface may occur with intracardiac shunts. A rise in oxygen saturation of 1 vol % between cardiac chambers is usually sufficient evidence to diagnose an intracardiac left-to-right shunt. A pulmonary blood flow one and one-half to two times greater than systemic blood flow is associated with mild physiologic disturbances and is on the borderline of indications for surgical correction, while defects producing greater pulmonary blood flows are uniformly recommended for operation. From the combination of pulmonary blood flow and pulmonary pressure, pulmonary vascular resistance can be calculated, which with pulmonary hypertension is the most significant physiologic measurement deciding prognosis.

Although the method is not frequently used clinically, the most precise physiologic evaluation of the degree of valvular stenosis is obtained by calculation of the functional cross-sectional area of the stenotic valve orifice, as elucidated by Gorlin and Gorlin in 1951. A normal mitral valve has a functional cross-sectional area of about 5 cm^2; mitral stenosis with an area of less than 1.5 cm^2 is functionally significant. In the aortic valve, normally with a cross-sectional area of 3 to 4 cm^2, a stenosis producing an opening of less than 0.8 cm^2 is functionally significant. Similarly, in the pulmonic valve, with a normal cross-sectional area of 2 to 4 cm^2, a stenosis producing an opening of less than 0.8 cm^2 is functionally significant.

Principles of Operative and Postoperative Care of Infants

Certain principles of management specifically pertain to infants undergoing cardiovascular surgery. For general principles of operative monitoring, extracorporeal circulation, cardiac massage, and defibrillation, Chap. 19 on acquired heart disease should be consulted.

OPERATIVE MANAGEMENT. Four important aspects of operative care which are frequently overlooked are temperature control, fluid administration, prevention of air emboli, and serial blood-gas monitoring. Temperature control is essential in infants, especially in air-conditioned operating rooms, because body temperature will quickly decrease to 32 to 34° C when the infant is anesthetized and shivering mechanisms abolished. Constant recording of the temperature with an electric esophageal or rectal probe is mandatory, and some method of warming the infant, either a mattress or hot-water bottles, should routinely be employed.

Fluids must be administered with unusual precision; a 3-kg infant in cardiac failure should have no more than 20 to 40 ml of fluid in excess of measured losses during an operative procedure.

The danger of air embolism is frequently overlooked in cyanotic infants with right-to-left shunts, in whom air emboli can bypass the heart and lungs to enter the cerebral or the coronary circulation. With intravenous therapy, much care is required to prevent small air emboli, which almost routinely occur with the usual intravenous therapy during an operation. Only a few small bubbles, if lodged in a coronary artery, can precipitate ventricular fibrillation.

Serial measurement of the pH and the oxygen and carbon dioxide tensions of central venous blood, usually at 20- to 30-minute intervals during an operation, is perhaps the most essential part of monitoring. Metabolic and respiratory acidosis are extremely frequent in seriously ill infants and may quickly become intensified with compression of the lung, ineffective cardiac contraction, or hypovolemia. A pH of central venous blood below 7.30 should be promptly corrected by appropriate ventilation, bicarbonate infusion, cessation of anesthesia, or other measures to increase cardiac output. In the author's experience, changes in pH always well antedate cardiac arrest or ventricular fibrillation. With serial monitoring of blood-gas tensions during operation, desperately ill anoxic children may tolerate procedures which ordinarily would terminate in cardiac arrest or fibrillation.

POSTOPERATIVE CARE. Four important principles are constant observation, monitoring of the electrocardiogram, routine measurement of blood-gas tensions, and respiratory therapy.

Constant observation of the seriously ill infant by experienced staff on a 24-hour basis is mandatory. This includes observation of adequacy of ventilation, blood-gas tensions, fluid therapy, and arrhythmias appearing on the electrocardiogram. For experienced staff to be "on call" is totally inadequate, for in infants ventricular fibrillation can appear virtually without warning and can be corrected only if therapy can be started within 1 to 3 minutes. With a policy of constant observation, fibrillation has been corrected with subsequent recovery in infants who otherwise would surely have succumbed to transitory ventricular arrhythmias following operation.

Serial measurement of blood-gas tensions by analysis of blood samples withdrawn through a central venous catheter introduced through the saphenous vein into the inferior vena cava is the best measurement of adequacy of ventilation and circulation. Venous carbon dioxide tensions above 45 mm Hg promptly develop with inefficient ventilation, and pH values below 7.30 quickly occur with either metabolic or respiratory acidosis. These changes far antedate any obvious clinical alteration in pulse or blood pressure and accordingly permit more effective therapy. Whether changes in pH and gas tensions are due to metabolic or respiratory causes can be determined by clinical evaluation and by gas analysis of peripheral arterial blood.

Proper ventilation is perhaps the most difficult postoperative problem in the infant following a thoracotomy. Secretions are difficult to remove, the tracheobronchial passages are so small that instrumental manipulation is difficult and can precipitate occlusive edema, and infants quickly develop cardiac arrest with transient anoxia or respiratory acidosis. Management of such problems has not been completely perfected, and inability to correct such respiratory problems remains one of the major causes of mortality in infants following operation.

The following methods of management have been found useful, but the mode of application varies widely with individual patients. Adequate humidity, with the infant kept in a dense mist right from the time of operation, is essential. An endotracheal tube may be left in place for an indeterminate length of time following operation to assist ventilation and removal of secretions. Some have left endotracheal tubes in position for days or weeks, but the author prefers a much shorter period, usually less than 24 hours. When an endotracheal tube is left in position, it may require changing every 6 to 12 hours if inspissated secretions occlude the tip of the tube.

Translaryngeal aspiration of the trachea, accomplished with a laryngoscope to permit direct introduction of a soft catheter between the vocal cords into the trachea, is a valuable technique. It must be done by experienced personnel; otherwise trauma and edema of the vocal cords will quickly develop. It is simpler than bronchoscopy, less traumatic, and can be repeated frequently. Tracheostomy should be avoided if possible because of the many complications inherent in tracheostomy in infants. Early removal of the tracheostomy tube may permit healing of the trachea without difficulty, but often the tube cannot be removed for several months. The proper respirator for infants is still evolving, though significant advances have been made; adult mechanical ventilators are too insensitive for the small tidal volumes required in the infant. The rapid respiratory rate of the infant, in combination with small tidal volumes, makes pressure-sensitive devices unreliable. The author's preference is for a piston-type respirator, delivering a fixed tidal volume, rather than a pressure-sensitive ventilator. Stewart et al. have recently reported favorable experiences with a type of continuous positive-pressure ventilator developed by Gregory in 1971. This has been especially useful for 1 to 2 days after operation.

OBSTRUCTIVE LESIONS

Pulmonic Stenosis

HISTORICAL DATA. In 1948 Brock and Sellors independently performed the first successful valvulotomies for pulmonic valvular stenosis, using a valvulotome through a transventricular approach. In 1954 Swan and Zeavin, applying the newly developed technique of hypothermia and venous-inflow occlusion, introduced a transarterial approach to perform valvulotomy under direct vision. Operation with extracorporeal circulation has since be-

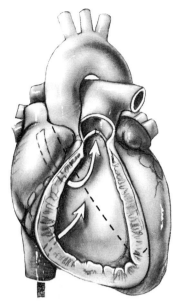

Fig. 18-4. Pulmonic valvular stenosis with fused valve cusps creating central stenotic opening. Annulus of pulmonic valve ring is normal. (*Adapted from W. H. Cole and R. M. Zollinger, "Textbook of Surgery," Appleton-Century-Crofts, Inc., New York, 1963, 8th ed., p. 935.*)

come the preferred technique, because a more precise surgical procedure can be performed and additional anomalies which are frequently encountered can be adequately treated.

INCIDENCE AND ETIOLOGY. Pulmonic stenosis is a common disease, representing about 10 percent of all patients with congenital heart disease. However, only 25 years ago pulmonic stenosis was considered a very rare disease. Taussig, in her monograph in 1947, wrote that she had not had an opportunity to study a proved case herself. The present widespread recognition of this disorder well indicates the advances in techniques of diagnosis, stimulated to a great extent by the evolution of effective methods of surgical therapy.

There are no known significant etiologic factors.

PATHOLOGIC ANATOMY. Pulmonic stenosis results, in 85 to 95 percent of patients, from stenosis of the pulmonary valve (Fig. 18-4). Two unusual forms of pulmonic stenosis are found in a small percentage of patients: infundibular stenosis (Fig. 18-5) and peripheral stenosis of the pulmonary artery.

Pulmonary valvular stenosis results from fusion of the three semilunar cusps of the pulmonic valve to form a dome with a central opening usually 1 to 3 mm in diameter. In infants with severe obstruction only a pinpoint orifice may be present, while in milder forms the orifice may be 7 to 10 mm in diameter (Fig. 18-6). It has been estimated that the pulmonary valve orifice must be reduced to about one-third of normal size before significant physiologic obstruction results. Normally the three valve cusps are well formed, although variation in size is frequent. In most patients the cusps are of normal thickness and mobility, and the fused commissures can be readily identified.

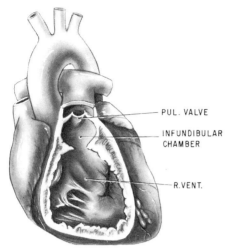

Fig. 18-5. Types of subvalvular or infundibular pulmonic stenosis. Infundibular stenosis may result in a discrete chamber between stenotic area and pulmonic valve. (*Adapted from W. H. Cole and R. M. Zollinger, "Textbook of Surgery," Appleton-Century-Crofts, Inc., New York, 1963, 8th ed., p. 936.*)

Variants include a bicuspid valve or, rarely, a fused dome-like structure with a central opening and only vestigial commissures. Usually the annulus of the pulmonic valve is of normal diameter. The pulmonary artery is also normal initially, but in later years poststenotic dilatation of varying degree evolves. As in other areas in the arterial circulation with focal stenotic lesions, the mechanism of development of poststenotic dilatation, as elucidated by Holman in 1954, is related to the increased lateral pressure resulting from deceleration of high-velocity flow through

Fig. 18-6. Pulmonic valvular stenosis exposed at operation following incision of pulmonary artery. Dome-shaped structure produced by fusion of valve cusps, with small central opening, is clearly shown. Suction tip has been placed in distal pulmonary artery.

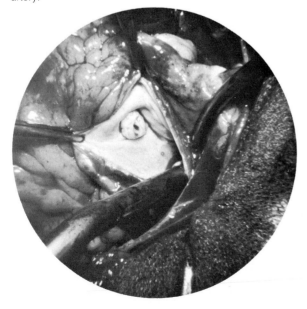

a small orifice. Other factors influence the evolution of poststenotic dilatation, however, for the degree of dilatation is not related to the severity of the stenosis. Occasionally an asymptomatic patient in the fourth or fifth decade is seen following the detection of a mediastinal mass on a chest roentgenogram, who on later study will be found to have mild pulmonic stenosis with extensive poststenotic dilatation.

Compensatory hypertrophy of the right ventricle to eject blood through the stenotic orifice occurs regularly. In severe, chronic stenosis the massive ventricular hypertrophy, exceeding 1 cm in thickness, may significantly reduce the lumen of the right ventricular cavity, constituting an additional element of obstruction to the flow of blood.

Infundibular stenosis, occurring in 5 to 10 percent of patients with pulmonic stenosis, consists of a discrete fibrous diaphragm with a 3- to 6-mm central opening in the outflow tract of the right ventricle located 2 to 5 cm proximal to the pulmonic valve. The most frequent location is at the site of the crista supraventricularis. With infundibular stenosis, an "infundibular chamber" exists in the right ventricle between the site of stenosis and the pulmonic valve (Fig. 18-7). Detection of this chamber on cardiac catheterization or angiography readily confirms the diagnosis.

A patent foramen ovale is present in at least 50 percent of patients with pulmonic stenosis. This often is a slitlike opening which is apparently stretched open from the increased right ventricular pressure and dilatation of the right atrium. Rarely, a larger typical atrial septal defect, 1 to 3 cm in diameter, is present. Other associated abnormalities such as patent ductus arteriosus are rarely seen.

Aberrant forms of pulmonic stenosis are occasionally encountered, representing more severe malformations in development of the right side of the heart. These include, in addition to valvular stenosis, hypoplasia of the pulmonic annulus, extensive hypertrophy of the right ventricular muscle, and varying degrees of hypoplasia of the tricuspid valve. Apparently such malformations exist as transitional ones in a spectrum of malformations, with isolated pulmonic valvular stenosis at one end of the spectrum and tricuspid atresia at the other.

PATHOPHYSIOLOGY. The physiologic disturbance is obstruction to flow of blood from the right ventricle with resulting hypertrophy of the right ventricle. Initially the severity of the obstruction is related to the diameter of the stenotic orifice. Right ventricular pressures of 75 to 100 mm Hg are found with moderate pulmonic stenosis, while severe obstruction results in right ventricular pressures of 100 to 200 mm Hg, and levels as high as 270 mm Hg have been recorded. With growth of the patient, two additional elements of obstruction occur. One of these is progressive hypertrophy of the right ventricle, until subsequently the contraction of the hypertrophied muscle of the right ventricular outflow tract also constitutes an obstruction to the flow of blood. The other factor is a relative one related to the growth of the child with corresponding increase in the flow of blood. Hence a 3- to 4-mm opening tolerated by an infant may produce serious symptoms in a child of twelve to fourteen years.

With the obstruction to the flow of blood, over one-half the patients have a patent foramen ovale with a right-to-left shunt producing unsaturation of the arterial blood. When the shunt through the foramen ovale is large, visible cyanosis develops, followed by polycythemia and clubbing. The usual clinical story is a progressive increase in cyanosis over a period of years, insidiously appearing in early childhood and gradually increasing in severity.

Overt cardiac failure seldom occurs in children except in infancy. In infants with a pinpoint opening in the pulmonary valve, severe failure may constitute an emergency indication for pulmonic valvulotomy to prevent immediate death. Cardiac failure gradually becomes more common in older children and young adults, as cardiac reserve is progressively limited.

CLINICAL MANIFESTATIONS. Symptoms. Dyspnea on exertion is the dominant symptom, increasing in severity as the cardiac reserve fails. Easy fatigability is common but less precise. Dizziness and/or syncope are occasionally seen; chest pain is infrequent. The history of the development of cyanosis may be characteristic. Cyanosis may have been noted in infancy, due to a right-to-left shunt through a foramen ovale, which subsequently disappeared as the foramen ovale closed. In later years, as right ventricular pressure increases and atrial dilatation occurs, the foramen ovale is gradually stretched open, resulting in the insidious appearance and progression of cyanosis as the right-to-left shunt progressively increases in magnitude. With chronic cyanosis, clubbing and polycythemia appear.

Sudden death in childhood has been reported in isolated cases but fortunately is rare. Symptoms of overt cardiac failure are rarely seen in children except in infancy but may be present in adults with severe stenosis.

Physical Examination. The characteristic finding is a harsh, loud systolic murmur heard best in the second left intercostal space and widely transmitted to the neck and adjacent areas. The murmur is of the ejection type, the peak intensity varying with the severity of the stenosis. Usually in infancy it can be clearly detected, although in advanced failure it may be faint. The pulmonic second sound is characteristically weak or absent. Diastolic murmurs are almost never heard. With increasing cardiac hypertrophy, the forceful contractions of the right ventricle can be palpated along the left sternal border. Cyanosis is present in varying degrees in patients with a patent foramen ovale and when chronic is associated with polycythemia and clubbing.

Signs of cardiac failure, with hepatomegaly and edema, are usually found only in adults with severe obstruction.

LABORATORY FINDINGS. The chest roentgenogram characteristically shows cardiac enlargement confined to the right ventricle, although this is not marked until cardiac reserve fails. In older patients the poststenotic dilatation of the pulmonary artery, often unusually prominent in the left pulmonary artery, is a characteristic feature of the disease, especially in association with normal or decreased vascularity of the peripheral lung fields. Changes in cardiac size are of particular importance, because, as emphasized by Taussig, cardiac enlargement regularly precedes the onset of symptoms, which in turn are followed by overt

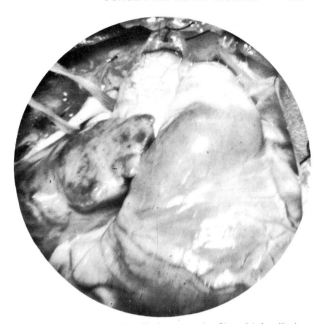

Fig. 18-7. Heart with infundibular stenosis. Site of infundibular stenosis is visible as area of constriction in outflow tract of right ventricle. Infundibular chamber, consisting of dilated right ventricular muscle, is located between infundibular stenosis proximally and pulmonary vein distad.

congestive failure. In infants, marked cardiac enlargement may occur within only a few months.

The electrocardiogram is of great value in assessing the severity of the obstruction, for signs of right ventricular hypertrophy are regularly present. With severe disease a right ventricular strain pattern with changes in the ST segment and T waves becomes apparent.

Cardiac catheterization and angiography are needed to define precisely the severity of the condition and the associated abnormalities. With moderate disease, a right ventricular systolic pressure of 100 mm Hg or more, associated with a systolic gradient across the stenotic pulmonary valve of 80 to 90 mm Hg, is frequent. With severe disease, systolic ventricular pressures may even exceed 200 mm Hg. The presence of a foramen ovale can be detected by noting oxygen unsaturation in the arterial blood and can be confirmed by dye-dilution curves obtained by selectively injecting dye into different cardiac chambers. Differentiation from a ventricular septal defect, constituting a tetralogy of Fallot, can often best be made by catheterization. It should be noted that a right ventricular pressure exceeding systemic pressure almost always indicates an intact ventricular septum, although unusual exceptions have been recorded. On angiography the degree of stenosis of the right ventricular outflow tract by the hypertrophied muscle should be noted and particular care taken to detect any signs of a focal infundibular stenosis with a distal infundibular chamber. Such a localized stenosis can also be recognized from a continuous pressure recording as a cardiac catheter is withdrawn from the pulmonary artery into the right atrium. Gilbert and associates have correlated the ratio between the diameter of the stenosed right ventricular outflow tract and the stenosed pulmonary valve, with subsequent regression of right ventricular hypertension after adequate valvulotomy. Less satisfactory results were obtained in patients in whom the right ventricular outflow tract was narrowed to less than one-half the diameter of the pulmonic valve ring.

Angiograms should be carefully analyzed for focal pulmonic arterial stenoses in the distal pulmonary arteries. Such stenoses have been recognized with increasing frequency with improvements in angiography.

DIAGNOSIS. The diagnosis can usually be made with certainty in the presence of a loud systolic murmur with a weak pulmonic second sound, combined with roentgenographic evidence of enlargement of the right ventricle and electrocardiographic signs of right ventricular hypertrophy. An atrial septal defect or pulmonary hypertension may be confused with pulmonic stenosis, but the quality of the pulmonic second sound is a helpful guide. Ebstein's anomaly of the tricuspid valve is a rare malformation which can simulate pulmonic stenosis; catheterization and angiography are required to establish the correct diagnosis.

Differentiating pulmonic stenosis from tetralogy of Fallot is a common problem when right-to-left shunting of blood through a foramen ovale has produced cyanosis. Cyanosis is usually a more prominent feature of the history with tetralogy of Fallot; cardiac enlargement and failure also are unusual with the latter. Cardiac angiography is required to confirm the diagnosis.

TREATMENT. Indications for Operation. With mild pulmonic stenosis associated with a heart of normal size and no signs of hypertrophy of the right ventricle on the electrocardiogram, no treatment has been found necessary. Johnson and associates recently described the benign course of trivial pulmonic stenosis in a significant group of patients followed over many years. Surgical therapy should be carried out when either symptoms or signs of cardiac enlargement are present. With signs of right ventricular hypertrophy, cardiac catheterization should be carried out to assess the need for operation. Operation is usually recommended if the systolic pressure gradient across the stenotic pulmonary valve is greater than 50 mm Hg. It should be emphasized that the severity of the obstruction often increases with growth of the child, so a physiologically insignificant stenosis in a young child may become more significant in later childhood.

Operative Technique. Except in some emergency operations in infants, the preferred technique is valvulotomy performed with extracorporeal circulation, using a median sternotomy incision. The closed technique with a valvulotome has been used less frequently and is almost never used at New York University, as bypass techniques have become standardized and reliable, even in infants. The great advantage for extracorporeal circulation, of course, is that a much better valvulotomy can be performed and any additional abnormalities corrected. If a closed technique is used, the valvulotome developed by Potts (Fig. 18-8) is preferred, the valvulotome being introduced through the right ventricle. After the valve is incised, a dilator is inserted to stretch the margins.

Using cardiopulmonary bypass, bypass is instituted, the heart is electrically fibrillated, and a left ventricular vent is inserted. Usually the aorta is occluded for 10 to 15 minutes to obtain a dry, quiet field. The pulmonary artery is incised for about 3 cm with a longitudinal arteriotomy which extends down into a pulmonary valve sinus. The edges of the stenotic valve then can be exposed with traction and the fused commissures incised along the center of the commissural raphe with a small knife (Fig. 18-9). The commissural incisions should be carried completely to the wall of the pulmonary artery. The subcommissural areas are carefully examined, and any obstructing bands are divided. Careful incision of the commissures seems the best safeguard against pulmonic insufficiency, although mild to moderate pulmonic insufficiency seems to be of little physiologic significance.

Graduated Hegar dilators are useful for calibrating the size of the valve ring. If the pulmonic annulus can be enlarged to accommodate a #16 or #18 Hegar dilator, corresponding to a cross-sectional area greater than 2 cm², the obstruction will have been significantly relieved. Frequently the pulmonary artery is somewhat hypoplastic. If so, our preference has been to widen it with a small patch of pericardium sewn into the arteriotomy so that the final diameter of the enlarged pulmonary artery is at least 2 cm.

In recent years we usually have preferred to open the right ventricle as well with a short transverse ventriculotomy in the outflow tract. Hypertrophied muscle can be excised, and any fibrous obstructions can be removed. Placing the ventriculotomy about 4 cm proximal to the pulmonic annulus permits visualization of the base of the pulmonary valve cusps and the commissures from within the ventricle. Any subcommissural areas of fusion then can be divided. This approach considerably facilitates operative correction of all significant obstructions, usually resulting in a systolic pressure gradient between the right ventricle and pulmonary artery of less than 30 mm Hg.

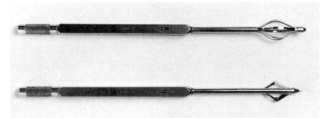

Fig. 18-8. Dilator and valvulotome developed by Potts for pulmonic valvulotomy. Calibrated swivel mechanism permits precise opening or closing of instruments.

No significant impairment of cardiac function has been recognized to result from the ventriculotomy.

A foramen ovale, if present, is sutured. This can be done directly through a small incision in the right atrium. If the ventricle has been opened, the tricuspid leaflets can be retracted and the septum exposed sufficiently to suture a small opening without making a separate atriotomy. After the various incisions have been sutured, permitting blood to drain briefly through the left ventricular vent ensures that no air emboli have been trapped in the left side of the heart. Following electrical defibrillation, bypass is slowed and stopped.

In the past considerable care was taken to avoid opening the right ventricle, because significant muscular hypertrophy disappears within 1 to 2 years after valvulotomy in most patients. This is not invariably true, however, and will not occur if a fibrous obstruction is present. Because of the benign consequences of a ventriculotomy, we generally have come to prefer ventriculotomy at the time of operation in the majority of patients with significant right ventricular hypertrophy.

A separate category is the patient with isolated infundibular stenosis from a fibrous obstruction or an anomalous muscle bundle. These can be recognized by catheterization and also by angiography. Correction at operation is not difficult; opening the right ventricle with a transverse incision and excising the area of obstruction suffices.

A difficult problem is encountered in the unusual patient in whom a hypoplastic valve ring contributes significantly to the stenosis. Fortunately this is rare. The condition can be relieved only by incising the valve ring for a short distance onto the ventricle and widening the orifice with a patch graft of pericardium. This is necessary only if the valve ring is smaller than 1.4 to 1.5 cm, depending upon the size of the child. Of course, pulmonic insufficiency is produced, but it is well tolerated.

Postoperative Course. With the exception of emergency operations in infants, the operative risk is very low, approaching 1 to 2 percent, and most patients have an uneventful convalescence. There have been no operative deaths at New York University during operations for uncomplicated pulmonic stenosis since 1963.

After recovery from operation, symptomatic improvement is usually prompt. A systolic murmur almost always remains audible, and a faint diastolic murmur of no known physiologic significance frequently can be heard. The electrocardiogram will show signs of gradual regression of right ventricular hypertrophy, although such changes may require 1 to 3 years to evolve completely. Often there is little change in the heart size as seen on the chest roentgenogram, unless cardiac dilatation from failure was present before operation. If significant right ventricular hypertension remains after valvulotomy, cardiac catheterization should be performed after 6 months to 1 year to evaluate the degree of residual hypertension. In the majority of patients the systolic pressure in the right ventricle will subsequently be found to be less than 50 mm Hg.

A study of a group of 108 patients reported by Tandon and associates included only 10 percent with significant

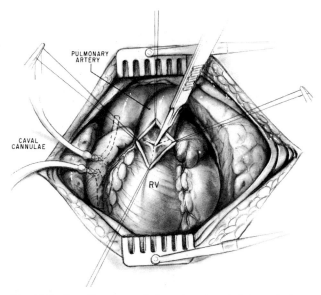

Fig. 18-9. Operative approach for pulmonic valvulotomy during cardiopulmonary bypass. Pulmonary artery is opened with longitudinal arteriotomy, after which fused valve commissures are incised with knife. Vertical sternotomy, rather than transverse one shown here, is usually employed.

residual abnormalities on the electrocardiogram or roentgenogram. Postoperative catheterization studies performed upon 22 patients demonstrated only 1 with significant hypertension in the right ventricle.

STENOSIS OF THE PULMONARY ARTERY

Focal stenosis of the pulmonary artery or its peripheral branches, either single or multiple, has been appreciated since the development of selective angiocardiography. Formerly thought to be a rare condition, it is now recognized with increasing frequency, often in association with other cardiac defects. A review by Franch and Gay in 1963 reported experience with 11 patients and found 90 previous cases in the medical literature.

The physiologic limitation from stenosis of a pulmonary artery depends upon the severity of the stenosis and the artery involved. Usually no limitation is present unless multiple stenoses involving both pulmonary arteries are present. The condition can be differentiated from the usual pulmonic valvular stenosis by the presence of a normal pulmonic second sound and by the finding in many patients of a continuous murmur over the hemithorax where the pulmonic stenoses are located. If the stenotic areas can be located with precise angiography, plastic reconstruction with patch grafts of pericardium can be carried out. Several such cases have been reported; one of the first such operations was reported by McGoon and Kincaid in 1964.

The author performed a similar operation in association with surgical correction of a tetralogy of Fallot in a thirteen-year-old boy who, on angiography before operation, was found to have complete obstruction of the origin of the left pulmonary artery. At surgical exploration a 2- to 3-mm area of stenosis, involving the proximal 1 cm of the origin of the left pulmonary artery, was corrected by longitudinal incision and insertion of a patch graft of pericardium.

Congenital Aortic Stenosis

HISTORICAL DATA. Adequate surgical treatment of congenital aortic stenosis was not possible until the development of extracorporeal circulation. In 1955 Swan and associates and Lewis independently performed valvulotomy under hypothermia, but this approach was quickly discarded in favor of the more precise approach possible with cardiopulmonary bypass. By 1958, Spencer et al. had reported successful operation upon 12 children without any mortality.

INCIDENCE AND ETIOLOGY. Congenital aortic stenosis is a common congenital cardiac anomaly, representing 8 to 10 percent of all patients with congenital heart disease. For unknown reasons it is three to four times more frequent in males than in females. By contrast, congenital aortic regurgitation is an extremely rare lesion. The four patients with isolated congenital aortic regurgitation reported by Frahm and associates in 1961 were the first reported in whom the diagnosis was firmly established during life.

There are no known causative factors associated with valvular or subvalvular aortic stenosis. Only in the unusual forms of supravalvular or diffuse muscular stenosis are there associated factors suggesting a genetic basis for the disease. Rheumatic fever is rarely a cause of isolated aortic stenosis; it usually causes associated disease of the mitral valve.

PATHOLOGIC ANATOMY. In valvular stenosis the valve cusps are often well formed but are fused along the commissures to produce an opening varying from 2 to 6 mm in diameter. The pattern of fusion of the commissures is similar in many patients. The commissure between the right and left coronary cusps is often the least developed, the valve functioning as a bicuspid valve. Commissural fusion between the right and noncoronary cusps is usually moderate, and fusion between the left and noncoronary cusps is usually the least extensive. The valve cusps are usually thicker than normal cusps but have adequate mobility. Calcification is common in adults but is almost never seen before seventeen to eighteen years of age. In most patients the aortic annulus is of normal diameter, but mild poststenotic dilatation of the ascending aorta is common (42 percent of 100 patients reported by Braunwald et al.). Fortunately, only in a minority of patients are the more bizarre, extreme forms of valvular stenosis seen, with a hypoplastic annulus, unusual valve cusps with absence of commissures, and associated hypoplasia of the left ventricle.

Subvalvular stenosis usually occurs as a narrow ring of fibrous tissue 1 to 2 cm proximal to the aortic valve cusps. The orifice varies from 4 to 8 mm. The aortic outflow tract is usually of normal diameter proximal and distal to the stenotic ring, although muscular hypertrophy may be prominent in older patients. In some patients the base of the aortic cusps is immediately adjacent to the stenotic ring

and must be protected from injury during surgical excision of the stenosis. Two other anatomic relations are of particular importance during surgical excision. Beneath the noncoronary cusp where the stenotic ring is attached to the ventricular septum, the conduction bundle is present and may easily be injured. Beneath the left coronary cusp the ring is attached to the base of the aortic leaflet of the mitral valve, which is also susceptible to injury.

Associated cardiac malformations are found in 15 to 20 percent of patients, being more frequent with valvular stenosis than with subvalvular stenosis. The most frequent associated conditions are patent ductus, coarctation, ventricular septal defect, and pulmonic stenosis.

PATHOPHYSIOLOGY. The physiologic limitations from aortic stenosis are directly related to the severity of obstruction. Mild stenosis can occur with typical findings which are of no physiologic significance. Conversely, severe obstruction can cause death from congestive heart failure in infants or sudden death in older children. The severity of the stenosis can be quantitated only by left heart catheterization; it is usually expressed in terms of the peak systolic gradient between the left ventricle and the ascending aorta. A gradient of less than 40 mm Hg is usually associated with such mild disability that operation is not recommended. In such patients cardiac output should be measured as well as the pressure gradient in order to calculate the functional cross-sectional area of the aortic valve. A functional cross-sectional area less than 0.5 cm^2/m^2 of body surface should usually be surgically corrected. Systolic pressure gradients of 50 to 75 mm Hg are usual with aortic stenosis of moderate severity, while gradients exceeding 100 mm Hg may be found with severe stenosis.

Depending upon the degree of stenosis, there is resulting hypertrophy of the left ventricle. Cardiac failure may occur in infants and is often fatal: 19 of 25 infants with cardiac failure reported by Peckham et al. died from their illness. The stenosis in infants is almost always valvular, not subvalvular, and is often associated with additional cardiac malformations.

Between the ages of two and ten there are usually few or no signs of impairment of function of the left ventricle. In older children symptoms representing limited cardiac reserve and a restriction in coronary or cerebral blood flow become increasingly common, although overt congestive heart failure is rare. Sudden death may occur in children, apparently from ventricular fibrillation. The frequency of sudden death varies with different reports. Braverman and Gibson reported 6 deaths in 73 patients, an 8.2 percent mortality rate. Nadas estimated the incidence of sudden death in his group of 250 patients as 7.5 percent. The lowest incidence of sudden death was reported by Peckham et al., who observed only 4 deaths in a group of 300 patients, approximately 1 percent. The occurrence of sudden death has not always correlated with clinical signs of severity of obstruction, so the risk of this tragedy cannot be predicted with certainty.

In young adults calcification of the fused valve cusps occurs with increasing frequency and probably approaches 100 percent in the third and fourth decades. Calcification adds the element of rigidity to the obstruction formerly originating only from the small size of the orifice. Consequently patients in the third or fourth decades may be seen with severe symptoms who have a history of a cardiac murmur during childhood without symptoms. It is likely that many such cases, misdiagnosed as rheumatic aortic stenosis in the past, in reality represent calcification of a mild congenital aortic stenosis.

CLINICAL MANIFESTATIONS. Symptoms. Many young children with significant aortic stenosis are asymptomatic. The most common symptoms are fatigue, dyspnea, angina pectoris, and syncope. These were found in 30 to 50 percent of a group of 100 patients studied by Braunwald et al. In most of these patients the systolic gradient was greater than 50 to 70 mm Hg.

Physical Examination. The four principal physical findings are a basal systolic murmur, palpable thrill, forceful left ventricular impulse, and narrow pulse pressure. The systolic murmur is a harsh, ejection-type murmur usually heard best in the second right interspace and is widely transmitted to the neck and arms. In infants and young children it may be loudest to the left of the sternum. A thrill can be felt in over 80 percent of patients. The left ventricular impulse is usually forceful and heaving. The pulse pressure was found to be decreased from the normal value of 30 mm Hg in 38 percent of 300 patients studied by Peckham and associates but was considered normal in 54 of 67 patients studied by Nadas.

An early diastolic murmur can be heard in about 20 percent of patients but is usually of no physiologic significance. For unknown reasons, it is considerably more frequent with subvalvular stenosis than with valvular stenosis.

LABORATORY FINDINGS. The electrocardiogram is the most sensitive guide to the severity of aortic stenosis but has distinct limitations. The usual abnormalities are signs of left ventricular hypertrophy, subsequently followed by depression of the ST segment and inversion of T waves. In about 75 percent of patients in whom the gradient exceeded 50 mm Hg, a left ventricular strain pattern was present. The limitations of electrocardiography have been emphasized by Braunwald and associates, for in some patients with severe obstruction the electrocardiogram may show few abnormalities.

The chest roentgenogram is frequently normal. In about one-half the patients slight enlargement of the left ventricle can be recognized, with a cardiothoracic ratio greater than 50 percent. Mild dilatation of the ascending aorta may be detected in 30 to 40 percent of patients. Calcification of the stenotic valve is rarely found except in adults.

Cardiac catheterization is usually performed to determine whether operation is indicated. The critical determination is measurement of the systolic gradient between the left ventricle and the ascending aorta. With gradients of less than 50 mm Hg, cardiac output should be determined to permit calculation of the functional cross-sectional area of the aortic valve. It may be possible to differentiate valvular from subvalvular stenosis by noting changes in pressure as a catheter is withdrawn from the apex of the left ventricle into the aorta, but this information is of little value to the surgeon, as the two areas are immediately adjacent to each other and can be easily identified at operation. Usually on catheterization the pulmonary artery pressure, left atrial pressure, and cardiac output are normal. The left ventricular pressure is elevated when severe stenosis with early cardiac failure is present.

DIAGNOSIS. The diagnosis can be made with confidence in the presence of the characteristic murmur, thrill, left ventricular impulse, and narrow pulse pressure. Confirmation can be obtained from the chest roentgenogram and electrocardiogram, reserving cardiac catheterization to assess the severity of the obstruction. In infants, when the murmur is loudest to the left of the sternum, catheterization may be required to differentiate from ventricular septal defect or pulmonic valvular stenosis.

TREATMENT. Infants in congestive heart failure should usually be operated upon with a pump-oxygenator once the diagnosis has been established. The mortality from nonoperative therapy is extremely high, 19 of 25 patients having died in a series reported by Peckham et al. Before operation, catheterization is required to differentiate the condition from coarctation of the aorta or the hypoplastic left heart syndrome. The surgical mortality is high and extensive data are not available, but surgical therapy offers the best chance of survival.

In most children operation is considered because of mild symptoms or the presence of changes in the electrocardiogram. A final decision can be made after left heart catheterization; operation is usually performed if the peak systolic gradients are greater than 40 to 50 mm Hg.

Operative Technique. Operation is performed with cardiopulmonary bypass, using a median sternotomy incision. The venae cavae are cannulated through the right atrium for venous return, and the ascending aorta is cannulated for arterial infusion. After bypass is established, the temperature is lowered to about 30°C, and a vent is inserted into the apex of the left ventricle to aspirate blood from the operative field. Subsequently the ascending aorta is clamped and opened with a curved incision, which is extended down into the noncoronary sinus but does not go to the base of the sinus. Extending the incision into the depth of the noncoronary sinus may increase exposure but theoretically may result in prolapse of the noncoronary cusp when the aortic circumference is narrowed by suture of the aortotomy.

Coronary perfusion should be available, but usually this is not required, as the operative procedure can be completed in 10 to 20 minutes.

Calibrated Hegar dilators are useful for measuring the diameter of the stenotic orifice both before and after commissurotomy. If an orifice admitting a #16 or #18 Hegar dilator can be obtained by commissurotomy, corresponding to a cross-sectional area nearly 2 cm², the obstruction will have been adequately relieved. Even a larger opening is preferable, of course, if this can be obtained without risking the production of aortic insufficiency. Measuring the stenotic orifice before commissurotomy provides a good guide to the length of commissural incision necessary to obtain the desired opening.

With valvular stenosis, the fused commissures are grad-

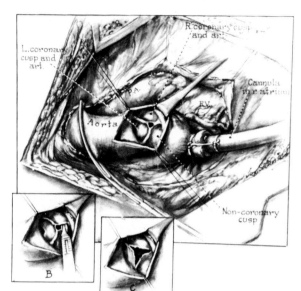

Fig. 18-10. *A.* Operative exposure of congenital aortic stenosis. Stenotic aortic valve has been exposed through longitudinal aortotomy. Fused commissures between three aortic cusps are clearly seen, with small central opening. *B* and *C.* Commissurotomy performed with knife, with center of fused commissures carefully incised and incision avoided in areas where commissures are not well developed. (*Reprinted by permission of The C. V. Mosby Company, St. Louis, from F. C. Spencer, C. A. Neill, and H. T. Bahnson, The Treatment of Congenital Aortic Stenosis with Valvulotomy during Cardiopulmonary Bypass, Surgery, 44:116, 1958.*)

ually incised with a small (#15) knife blade, the fused commissure being incised exactly along the center of the fibrous raphe in order to have a thick margin on each of the two cusps which are thus separated (Fig. 18-10). Attempted division of the fused commissures with scissors will often result in division of the area to one side of the area of fusion and increase the likelihood of insufficiency. As far as possible, the incision of the commissures should be limited to areas where the commissures are well formed. When necessary, the commissural incisions may be carried completely to the aortic wall or, if not necessary, can be stopped 1 to 3 mm away. With the classic bicuspid valve, the commissure between the right and left coronary cusps is not well developed, and only a 2- to 4-mm incision or no incision at all may be made in this area, leaving the valve as a bicuspid valve. It is better to relieve the stenosis incompletely than to produce severe aortic insufficiency. In most patients, however, a stenosis can be adequately relieved by selective incision of the fused commissures without producing significant insufficiency. In one group of 23 patients studied, limited incision of the commissures was performed in 15 and obtained a satisfactory reduction in pressure gradient. The technique of commissurotomy is emphasized in some detail, for most difficulties with aortic insufficiency following aortic valvulotomy have resulted from inept valvulotomies rather than from the pathologic anatomy.

With subvalvular stenosis the valve cusps can be carefully retracted and the fibrotic ring excised. The tissue between the base of the valve cusps and the fibrotic ring must be clearly visualized to avoid injury of the base of the aortic valve cusps. The ring may consist of thin fibrous tissue, easily removed, or it may be a thick fibrotic structure requiring excision with a knife and rongeur. The surgical anatomy is of crucial importance in this area, for only in a narrow zone constituting less than 20 percent of the circumference of the stenotic ring can excision be safely carried into the underlying ventricular wall. This corresponds to the area beneath the commissure between the right and left coronary cusps (Fig. 18-11). Radical excision of the fibrotic ring beneath the left coronary cusp will perforate the aortic leaflet of the mitral valve, producing severe or fatal mitral insufficiency. Radical excision beneath the noncoronary cusp and part of the right coronary cusp will injure the ventricular septum, creating either a complete heart block or ventricular septal defect. The most useful instrument for excising the stenotic ring is a right-angled rongeur with a swivel for rotating the instrument to an appropriate angle (Fig. 18-12). With good exposure, an unhurried approach, and appropriate instruments, a stenotic area can be regularly excised satisfactorily.

The aortotomy is sutured with two continuous sutures of 4-0 or 5-0 silk, placed as simple over-and-over sutures. A small opening is left for removal of air. Following closure of the aortotomy, induced electrical ventricular fibrillation is carefully maintained with electrodes on the heart. The heart is then allowed to fill with blood by stopping the suction on the left ventricular vent, after which it is gently massaged to expel air from the ventricle and the aorta through the small opening remaining in the aortotomy. While compressing the right coronary artery digitally, the aortic clamp is cautiously removed and any remaining air expelled through the aortic vent site, which can later be sutured.

Following removal of the aortic clamp and meticulous removal of air from the heart, the heart can be defibrillated. Subsequently the left ventricular vent is removed and bypass slowed and stopped.

Following bypass, with a systemic pressure over 100 mm Hg, the residual gradient across the aortic valve can be measured by needle puncture of the left ventricle and the aorta. The residual gradient should be less than 40 mm Hg, and it is often very small.

Postoperative care is little different from that for thoracotomy for other conditions. Arrhythmias or mild congestive failure may occur, but are infrequent.

The risks of operation are small and the results good. Nadas reported that only 2 of 54 patients with uncomplicated aortic stenosis died following operation. Some have expressed pessimism and dissatisfaction with operations for aortic stenosis, but the experience of the author has been most favorable. In a series exceeding 50 patients over the past several years, there have been no deaths among those with valvular stenosis, a satisfactory reduction in systolic gradient was achieved in almost all, and only a few have slight aortic insufficiency. Two deaths followed operation for subvalvular stenoses, one from operative injury of the ventricular septum and the other from cardiac

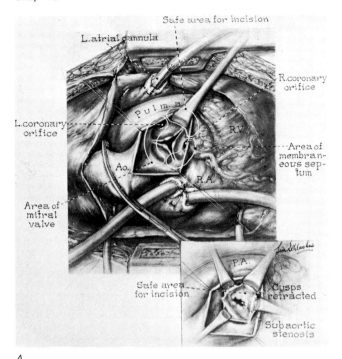

A

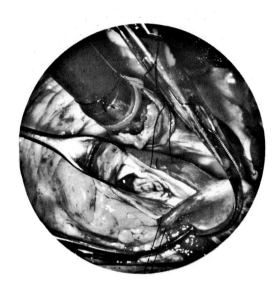

C

Fig. 18-11. *A.* Operative exposure of congenital subaortic stenosis. Valve cusps are normal. Insert shows membranelike subaortic stenosis exposed by retraction of valve cusps. (*From Am Surg, 26:210, 1960.*) *B.* Diagram of pertinent surgical anatomy with subaortic stenosis. Beneath noncoronary cusps and part of left coronary cusp is aortic leaflet of mitral valve. Beneath part of right coronary cusp is membranous septum. Only in area beneath commissure between right and left coronary cusps is limited zone where underlying ventricular muscle can be safely excised. Failure to observe these landmarks can result in injury to mitral valve or to membranous septum with conduction bundle. *C.* Subaortic stenosis exposed at operation. Aorta has been opened with longitudinal aortotomy and retractor inserted to retract normal aortic cusps. Diaphragmlike subaortic stenosis can be clearly seen with small pinpoint central opening. (*Reprinted by permission of C. V. Mosby Co. from F. C. Spencer, C. A. Neill, and H. T. Bahnson, The Treatment of Congenital Aortic Stenosis with Valvulotomy during Cardioplumonary Bypass, Surgery, 44: 117, 1958.*)

B

failure several days after operation in an older patient with advanced fibrosis of the left ventricle. Both deaths occurred several years ago.

Postoperative Course. Electrocardiographic changes may show improvement in some patients after recovery from operation, but in others little change may occur. The failure to show electrocardiographic improvement may indicate that operation should have been performed earlier than is customary. Changes in heart size on the chest roentgenogram are usually negligible. Usually a systolic murmur is audible, and a faint diastolic murmur without any signs of significant aortic insufficiency may be heard.

The long-term prognosis for these patients is yet unknown, although some patients have now survived for over 15 years after operation and recurrence of the stenosis has not been observed. That the thickened aortic cusps may progressively develop aortic insufficiency, requiring valvular replacement, is a distinct but unpredictable possibility. Another hypothetic question is whether the performance of valvulotomy will lessen the tendency for calcification of the abnormal cusps to develop in later years. The long-term prognosis for patients in whom the electrocardiogram shows persisting changes after operation, even though the gradient has been abolished, is also unknown.

SUPRAVALVULAR AORTIC STENOSIS

Supravalvular aortic stenosis is the rarest form of aortic stenosis, although it has been recognized with increasing frequency in recent years. The first successfully treated patient was reported by McGoon and Kirklin in 1956, and

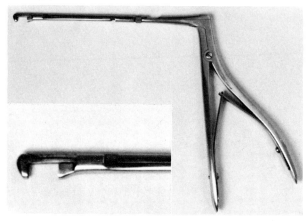

Fig. 18-12. Right-angled sharp rongeur used for excision of subaortic stenosis. Swivel mechanism permits rotation of instrument to obtain proper exposure.

10 years later Rastelli et al. reported surgical experience with 16 patients. At that time a total of 88 cases were found in the medical literature, 51 of which had been treated surgically. In most patients there are no known etiologic factors. Both sexes are equally involved. In about 20 percent of patients there is a peculiar facies consisting of a broad forehead, heavy cheeks, protuberant lips, and pointed chin. This facies is similar to that found with idiopathic hypercalcemia of infancy, and experimental induction of hypercalcemia in rats may produce a vascular lesion resembling supravalvular aortic stenosis. Most but not all patients with the characteristic facies are mentally deficient.

There is considerable variation in the type of aortic obstruction in different patients. In a review of 68 cases, Peterson et al. found three types: membranous, 9 cases; diffuse hypoplastic, 14 cases; hourglass, 45 cases (Fig. 18-13). The diffuse hypoplastic type has not been satisfactorily treated surgically. Most successful operations have been with the hourglass type, in which constriction of the aorta is found as a shelflike thickening and hypertrophy of the plica at the upper margin of the sinuses of Valsalva. The outer diameter of the aorta may be normal or reduced. The stenotic ridge has thickened intima and hypertrophy of the media, with an increase in fibrous and elastic tissue.

Associated abnormalities are frequent. In about one-third of the patients abnormalities of the aortic valve cusps are present, frequently consisting of adherence of part of one of the free margins of the cusps to the aortic wall, which, when extensive, can result in aortic regurgitation. The coronary arteries are abnormal in over one-half the patients. Often the right coronary artery is markedly dilated and tortuous, with hypertrophy of the media and intima which produce narrowing of the lumen. Focal stenotic lesions of the branches of the aortic arch and of the peripheral branches of the pulmonary arteries have also been found.

The usual symptoms are either angina or syncope, as with other forms of aortic stenosis. Death usually either has been sudden, suggesting an arrhythmia, or has resulted from congestive heart failure. Physical examination provides no clues to the diagnosis except when the typical facies, first described by Williams and associates in 1961, is present. A precise diagnosis can be established only by aortography.

A satisfactory operation can be accomplished in the localized type of stenosis by widening the stenotic area by the insertion of a patch of Dacron or pericardium. Complete excision of the stenotic ridge is not possible because of the attachment of the aortic valve cusps (Fig. 18-14). Although some have reported sudden death of patients after such an operation, a report by Rastelli et al. in 1966 stated that 15 of 16 patients survived operation, and in subsequent follow-up evaluation 13 of the 15 were considered to have had a good result (Fig. 18-15).

HYPERTROPHIC SUBAORTIC STENOSIS

In recent years an unusual form of aortic stenosis, which results from diffuse hypertrophy of the left ventricular muscle, has been recognized with increasing frequency. The condition was first noted by surgeons operating upon a patient for aortic stenosis who could find no focal point of obstruction when the arrested heart was explored. When the heart is contracting, however, a strong obliteration of the outflow tract of the left ventricle can be visualized and also palpated with an examining finger.

The disease is basically a myopathy involving the left ventricle, with secondary obstruction of the left ventricular outflow tract. The hypertrophy is not uniform throughout the left ventricle but is especially marked in the septum, in some patients producing obstruction of the right ven-

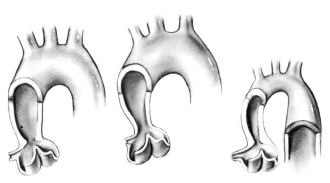

LOCALIZED   DIFFUSE

Fig. 18-13. Different types of supravalvular aortic stenosis, obstruction varying from localized constriction near aortic valve to diffuse hypoplasia of ascending aorta. (*Adapted from G. C. Rastelli et al., J Thorac Cardiovasc Surg, 51:878, 1966.*)

tricular outflow tract as well. There is a familial history, in 30 to 40 percent of patients, of puzzling forms of heart disease in other members of the family, often terminated by sudden death at an early age. In one group of 27 patients reported by Braunwald et al., a positive familial history was found in 10. Often there is no sign of heart disease in childhood, with symptoms and physical findings appearing in later years, apparently as the hypertrophy of the left ventricle progresses. Pathologically, the heart shows massive ventricular hypertrophy with virtual obliteration of the lumen. The histologic structure of the hypertrophied muscle fibers is not distinctive. Although little is known of the natural history of the disease, the usual course has not been a favorable one, with death occurring at an early age.

The symptoms differ little from those of patients with the usual form of aortic stenosis, including syncope, angina, and dyspnea. On physical examination a systolic murmur, of medium intensity near the apex but not prominent at the base of the heart in the aortic area, may first arouse suspicion that a valvular stenosis is present. The chest roentgenogram will usually show some enlargement of the left ventricle, while the electrocardiogram shows left ventricular hypertrophy with depression of the ST segment and inversion of the T waves.

Diagnosis is best established by cardiac catheterization and angiography. On catheterization a gradient can usually be demonstrated over an area in the proximal outflow tract of the left ventricle. The systolic gradient may vary from 50 to 150 mm Hg, the average value being 80 to 90 mm Hg. An increase in the pressure gradient can characteristically be produced by the infusion of isoproterenol, apparently resulting from a more forceful contraction of

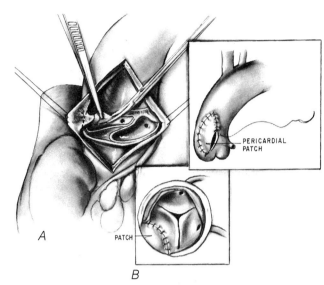

Fig. 18-14. Operation for localized supravalvular aortic stenosis. Stenotic area is widened by making longitudinal aortotomy and inserting pericardial patch. Partial excision of stenotic membrane is also shown. (*Adapted from G. C. Rastelli et al., J Thorac Cardiovasc Surg, 51:875, 1966.*)

the left ventricle. Cardiac angiography will show striking hypertrophy of the left ventricle, with a small lumen.

Operation is indicated in the presence of symptoms when there is a systolic gradient of more than 50 mm Hg. Although operation can relieve the left ventricular obstruction, it of course does not alter the basic disease of diffuse progressive ventricular hypertrophy.

At operation the outflow tract is widened by radical excision of a wedge of left ventricular muscle. This is best done beneath the commissure between the right and left coronary cusps. The excision must be deep, often more

Fig. 18-15. *A.* Operative photograph of the unusual lesion of supravalvular aortic stenosis. The waistlike narrowing of the ascending aorta just above the aortic valve can be clearly seen. *B.* Operative photograph of correction of supravalvular aortic stenosis by insertion of a Dacron patch to widen the area. The aortic valve gradient was reduced from 80 to near 30 mm Hg.

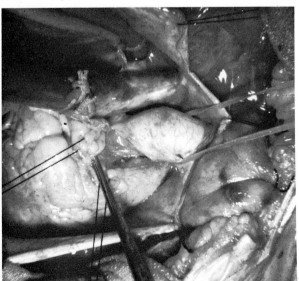

A

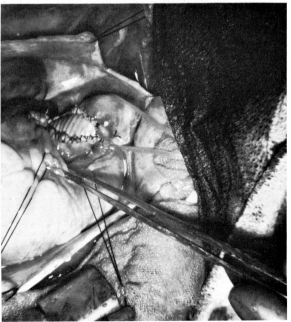

B

than 1 cm, and carried down almost to the apex of the ventricle; otherwise the obstruction is inadequately relieved. A variety of approaches have been used, varying from simple myotomy, to excision of muscle through an aortotomy, to excision through a combined aortotomy and left ventriculotomy. The author has preferred a radical excision of muscle performed through the aortotomy, making certain that the excision has been carried down to the apex of the left ventricle. To accomplish this through an aortotomy requires excellent exposure, a dry, still heart, and a significant amount of time. Others, including both Kirklin and Barratt-Boyes, have preferred a combined approach through the aorta and a short left ventriculotomy. Whatever approach is used, following proper excision of muscle, subsequent pressure gradients show virtual elimination of the gradient existing beforehand.

In a group of 16 patients reported by Frye et al., 13 of 14 survived resection of left ventricular muscle, and all were improved. Postoperative study of four patients showed a satisfactory reduction of the gradient in each. Barratt-Boyes has reported a much larger series of patients, including catheterization studies over a year later which indicated that surgical abolition of the gradient had been sustained. The long-term prognosis then becomes that of the underlying cardiac myopathy.

Coarctation of the Aorta

HISTORICAL DATA. In 1928 the characteristic features of coarctation of the aorta were outlined by Abbott in her classic analysis of 200 cases, including postmortem examinations. In 1944 and 1945 Blalock and Park, Gross, and Crafoord and Nylin all independently contributed to the first successful surgical treatment of coarctation by excision and direct anastomosis. Subsequently Gross provided a strong impetus to the study of vascular grafts by successfully using aortic homografts for patients with coarctation in whom direct anastomosis could not be performed.

INCIDENCE AND ETIOLOGY. Coarctation is one of the most common congenital abnormalities, occurring in 10 to 15 percent of patients with congenital heart disease. It is approximately twice as frequent in males as in females.

The exact cause of coarctation is unknown, but proximity of the coarctation to the ligamentum arteriosum has supported the most popular theory, that coarctation is an aberrant extension of the same fibrotic process that converts a patent ductus into a ligamentum arteriosum. Some observations indicate that a coarctation may increase in severity with time as a result of progressive thickening of the intima.

PATHOLOGIC ANATOMY. In most patients the coarctation is located as a diaphragmlike constriction in the first 2 to 4 cm of thoracic aorta distal to the left subclavian artery. Usually there is a 1- to 3-mm lumen, although complete occlusion may be present. On histologic examination the intima and media are both found to be markedly thickened. In older patients fibrosis and calcification may be found in the adjacent aortic wall. Usually the ligamentum arteriosum is attached to the medial surface of the aorta at the site of coarctation, although it may be

inserted slightly above or below. The ligamentum clearly anchors the coarctation in this area, for when surgically divided, the two ends retract sharply, indicating the degree of tension previously exerted.

The aorta distal to the coarctation is usually dilated, more so in older patients; rarely it develops into an aneurysm. The mode of development of poststenotic aneurysms throughout the arterial circulation has been a subject of many experimental studies. The phenomenon is related to the kinetics of the flow of blood, abruptly changing from a flow at high velocity through the area of coarctation to an area of low velocity immediately beyond. A striking feature of coarctation, becoming more prominent in older patients, is the large, dilated intercostal arteries which enter the distal aorta. As these vessels dilate, there is progressive thinning of the arterial wall, frequently resulting in the development of small aneurysms in adult patients.

The proximal aorta between the coarctation and the left subclavian artery is usually smaller than the distal aorta and may be hypoplastic, requiring excision along with the coarctation to relieve the obstruction completely.

Much discussion and classification has centered about the relation between patency of the ductus arteriosus and an associated coarctation. In the majority of patients with coarctation the ligamentum arteriosum enters at the site of coarctation or slightly proximal to it. In about 10 percent of patients a patent ductus arteriosus, rather than a ligamentum, is present, constituting a left-to-right shunt which places some additional strain on the heart. This is the so-called "adult," or "postductal," type of coarctation.

In a small percentage of patients, 70 to 80 percent of whom die in the first few months of life, a coarctation is present with a large patent ductus arteriosus continuing directly into the descending thoracic aorta distal to the coarctation. This has been termed a "preductal," or "infantile," type of coarctation. There are several factors contributing to the severity of this malformation. Frequently severe additional cardiac malformations are present, such as ventricular septal defect or transposition of the great vessels. If collateral circulation around the coarctation is well developed, the flow of blood from the distal aorta goes from the aorta through the patent ductus to the pulmonary arteries and creates pulmonary congestion. Conversely, if pulmonary vascular resistance is increased to systemic levels, the flow of blood is in the reverse direction, from the pulmonary artery to the distal aorta, creating cyanosis in the lower half of the body. This latter condition is seldom encountered in older patients, because few patients survive beyond infancy.

The striking clinical characteristics of coarctation of the aorta are related to the growth of collateral circulation around the site of obstruction. These tributaries predominantly arise from the subclavian arteries and anastomose with the intercostal and epigastric vessels to enter the distal aorta. The development of collateral circulation through the intercostal arteries results in the characteristic "notching" of the ribs seen on the chest roentgenogram in patients over eight to ten years of age, virtually pathognomonic of coarctation.

A variety of unusual forms of coarctation are occasionally seen. The coarctation may be associated with hypoplasia of the proximal aorta, extending up to the left subclavian or rarely as far proximally as the innominate artery. These are termed *interruptions of the aortic arch.* Atypical sites of coarctation also are seen in the distal aorta, involving the lower thoracic aorta or even the upper abdominal aorta down to the level of the origin of the renal arteries.

Associated congenital anomalies vary with the type of patients studied. In infants who die with coarctation of the aorta, a high percentage of associated anomalies is found, including aortic stenosis, ventricular septal defect, hypoplasia of the left side of the heart, and endocardial fibroelastosis. In older patients, the most common anomaly is a patent ductus arteriosus, found in 10 to 15 percent of patients. A bicuspid aortic valve is also frequently encountered. Ventricular septal defects or atrial septal defects are uncommon in older patients.

PATHOPHYSIOLOGY. In infants, left ventricular failure may result from the obstruction to emptying of the left ventricle created by the coarctation. In infants this is often fatal if untreated. Subsequently, enlarging collateral circulation partly relieves the obstruction; thus congestive failure is rare after the first year of life until late childhood or early adult life.

In infants with a preductal coarctation, severe symptoms are present, with pulmonary congestion, cardiac failure, and cyanosis. These disabilities cause death in the majority of infants unless effective surgical therapy can be performed. The disabilities result from the coarctation, the large patent ductus entering the distal aorta, and the other associated cardiac malformations so frequently present, such as ventricular septal defect, fibroelastosis, or even transposition of the great vessels.

The hypertension from the coarctation causes rapid degenerative changes in the proximal aorta at such a rate that children in their early teens may have severe fibrosis that complicates surgical repair. Although some patients may live until the fifth or sixth decade, the average life expectancy is between 30 or 40 years. Formerly, approximately 25 percent of untreated patients died from rupture of the aorta, 25 percent from cardiac failure, 25 percent from rupture of intracranial aneurysms, and 25 percent from superimposed bacterial endocarditis.

CLINICAL MANIFESTATIONS. Symptoms. Many children are asymptomatic for long periods of time despite severe hypertension and the progressive degenerative changes occurring in the aorta. When symptoms are present, headache, dizziness, and epistaxis are the most common. Dyspnea on exertion or occasionally chest pain may be mentioned. Claudication in the lower extremities is infrequent despite the restriction of peripheral blood flow.

Physical Findings. The combination of hypertension in the upper extremities and absence or decrease of pulses in the lower extremities in a child immediately suggest the diagnosis of coarctation. In less severe forms measurements of the blood pressure in the upper and lower extremities may be required to confirm the diagnosis. Normally the blood pressure in the lower extremities is slightly higher than in the upper. Prominent pulsations are usually

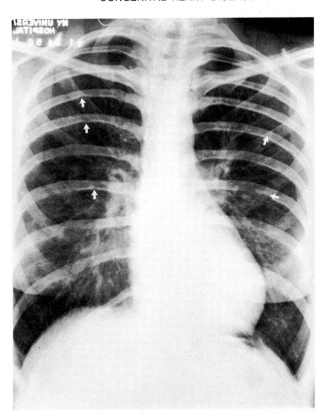

Fig. 18-16. Chest roentgenogram in patient with coarctation of aorta, demonstrating classic notching of ribs from enlarged intercostal arteries. This roentgen appearance is virtually pathognomonic of coarctation of aorta, as it is rarely produced by any other condition. (*Courtesy of Dr. Raymond M. Abrams, Department of Radiology, New York University Medical Center.*)

visible in the neck, and examination of the muscles of the shoulder girdle, especially the latissimus dorsi and suprascapular muscles, will often reveal visible and palpable pulsations. Auscultation over these sites may detect a bruit. A systolic murmur, the origin of which is often obscure, is usually widely audible over the left hemithorax. It may result from the coarctation, an associated abnormality of the aortic valve, or dilated, tortuous arteries.

LABORATORY STUDIES. The chest roentgenogram in older patients may automatically establish the diagnosis by demonstrating bilateral notching of the ribs (Fig. 18-16). Notching of the ribs from other causes is extremely rare. Left ventricular hypertrophy also may be evident. In older patients a "reverse-three" sign may be visible in the left upper mediastinal border: the dilated left subclavian artery superiorly and the dilated aorta distal to the coarctation inferiorly, with an indentation between the two. The electrocardiogram shows signs of left ventricular hypertrophy or strain.

Aortography is not necessary for routine diagnosis but is a helpful guide in planning surgical correction and always should be employed with atypical findings. In most patients the diagnosis can be made with confidence from the clinical findings in combination with the roentgenogram and the electrocardiogram. Cardiac catheterization should be performed if additional anomalies are suspected, usually aortic stenosis from a bicuspid aortic valve.

TREATMENT. The ideal age for operation is between five and seven years, preferably before the child begins to attend school. Although postponing operation until age ten to twelve has been recommended in the past to permit more growth of the aorta, there is little evidence that much value is gained. In addition there are some disadvantages. There is the emotional trauma to the child attending school with a known cardiovascular anomaly. Also several cases of hemiplegia developing in childhood have been reported, probably from rupture of an intercostal aneurysm. In general, there is little justification for postponing the operation beyond the age of five to seven years after the diagnosis has been established, even though the patient is asymptomatic.

In adults there is apparently no upper age limit beyond which resection carries a prohibitive risk: Brom has reported only one death in 39 patients operated on in the fourth and fifth decades. Degenerative changes in the aorta, as well as developing intercostal aneurysms, greatly complicate operation in older patients and often require the use of a prosthetic graft.

In infants there is an increasing tendency to employ operation promptly, often urgently, when congestive failure is severe. Occasionally this requires operation within the first few weeks of life. The author favors this aggressive surgical approach, for the risk of operation has become much less with improvements in surgical techniques, anes-

Fig. 18-17. Excision of coarction of aorta. *A.* Chest is opened with posterolateral incision in fourth intercostal space. *B.* Once chest has been opened and lung retracted, site of coarctation is often visible where aorta is angulated inward toward mediastinum just distal to left subclavian artery. This is site where ligamentum arteriosum is inserted. *C.* After incision of mediastinal pleura overlying coarctation, vessels are isolated proximal and distal to coarctation and ligamentum arteriosum is mobilized and divided. Recurrent laryngeal nerve, often not seen during operative procedure, is displaced mediad with vagus nerve. *D.* After division of ligamentum arteriosum, vascular occlusion clamps are applied to aorta proximal and distal to site of coarctation. Often it is necessary to apply proximal clamp to aorta between left carotid and left subclavian arteries, separately occluding left subclavian artery, in order to excise widely the narrowed segment of aorta. *E.* End-to-end anastomosis is constructed with continuous or interrupted sutures of silk. *F.* After completion of posterior row of anastomosis, interrupted sutures are often used in anterior row in young children to permit growth of anastomosis. *G.* Final view of completed anastomosis.

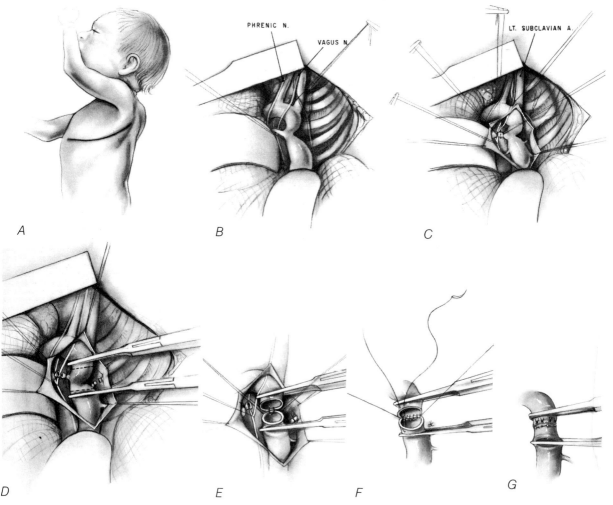

A   *B*   *C*

D   *E*   *F*   *G*

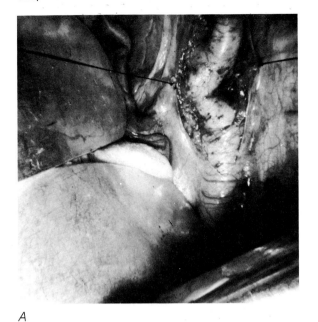

A

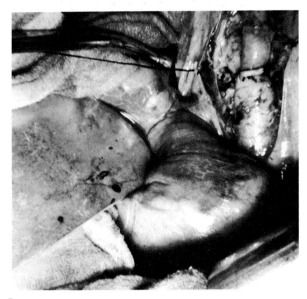

B

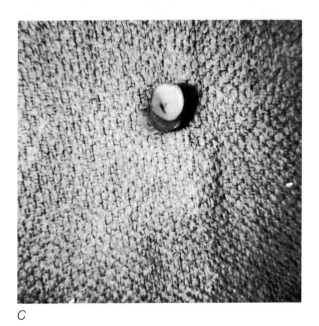

C

Fig. 18-18. *A.* Typical coarctation of aorta in child. Dilated sub-clavian artery is visible at top of field. At area of coarctation, aorta is angulated into mediastinum, where ligamentum arteriosum is inserted. *B.* Aortic anastomosis performed after excision of co-arctation. Anastomosis is made at point of origin of left subclavian artery. *C.* Resected coarctation of aorta, showing narrow lumen which was present.

thesia, and supportive care, while death from congestive failure is especially frequent in this group, almost all of whom have associated cardiac anomalies. With an associated ventricular septal defect and a large increase in pulmonary blood flow, banding of the pulmonary artery may be done at the same time that the coarctation is resected.

Operative Technique. A left posterolateral thoracotomy in the fourth intercostal space is used, usually dividing the fourth rib posteriorly in older patients (Fig. 18-17). After the lung is retracted inferiorly, the coarctation is usually obvious, with the indentation mediad at the site of insertion of the ligamentum arteriosum, and large, tortuous intercostal arteries entering the distal aorta (Fig. 18-18).

After incision of the mediastinal pleura, the vagus nerve is retracted mediad; the aorta proximal to the left subclavian artery, the left subclavian artery, the ligamentum arteriosum, and the distal aorta are serially mobilized and encircled with tapes. The recurrent nerve coursing around the ligamentum arteriosum is usually not seen if dissection is kept close to the aorta but should be identified and protected if more extensive dissection is performed. Injury of the thoracic duct may also occur if dissection is not kept next to the aorta. If the aorta is sharply angulated, division of the ligamentum will provide sufficient mobility. This may be done before the aorta is occluded; otherwise the ligamentum may be divided at the same time that the coarctation is excised. Dissection of the distal aorta is the greatest hazard in the operation because of friable intercostal arteries. In older patients, intercostal aneurysms occur. Such aneurysms were found in 45 of 487 patients operated upon by Gross and associates. Division of dilated intercostal arteries should be avoided wherever possible, both because of their friability and because of the uncertain relation between the anterior spinal artery nourishing the spinal cord and the intercostal arteries. Usually the aorta can be mobilized sufficiently beyond the intercostal arteries. The intercostals are then individually isolated and can be separately occluded during performance of the anastomosis.

Once the vessels have been adequately mobilized, occluding vascular clamps are applied to the left subclavian artery, the proximal aorta, and the distal aorta, following which the coarctation is excised. The principle decision at this time is how much of the proximal aorta between the coarctation and the origin of the left subclavian artery should be excised, for frequently this segment is appreciably smaller than the distal aorta. The author prefers in the majority of patients to excise all of this segment, performing the proximal anastomosis at the level of origin of the left subclavian artery to obtain a wide lumen. Brom has presented good evidence in support of this policy, trying to obtain an anastomosis at least 4 cm in diameter. In children the aorta has sufficient elasticity so that surprisingly long segments, as much as 5 cm, can be excised and a primary anastomosis performed (Fig. 18-19).

The anastomosis is usually performed with continuous or figure-of-eight sutures of 4-0 or 5-0 synthetic suture posteriorly, with interrupted or mattress sutures anteriorly. In smaller children, interrupted or mattress sutures are used throughout to provide the best opportunity for subsequent growth of the anastomosis.

Before the aorta is occluded, the question should be routinely asked, "How adequate is the collateral circulation?" This will vary with the age of the patient, the severity of the coarctation, and other factors. Flow through collateral circulation is decreased greatly by occlusion of the left subclavian artery and also if distal intercostal vessels are occluded. If the collateral circulation is inadequate, there will be significant hypotension in the distal aorta and an increased risk of paraplegia. Brewer et al. have recently described reported clinical experiences with paraplegia, occurring in varying degrees as frequently as in 1 patient in 200 following operation. Hughes and Reemtsma also have studied the problem and have recommended a temporary aortic shunt if distal aortic pressure is low after the aorta is occluded.

For similar reasons the author routinely has the time during which the aorta is occluded periodically measured and announced, with the objective of having the aorta occluded for little longer than 20 minutes, which is a safe period of occlusion for even a normal aorta. If a longer period of occlusion is anticipated, as during insertion of a vascular graft, pressures should probably be measured in the aorta distal to the occlusion clamps to be certain that collateral circulation is adequate. Fortunately, there have been no neurologic complications following repair of coarctation at New York University since 1963.

After the vascular clamps are removed and aortic flow reestablished, blood pressure is measured proximal and distal to the anastomosis to confirm that no significant gradient remains. In children the diameter of the anastomosis is also measured, preferably obtaining an opening

Fig. 18-19. *A.* Preductal coarctation exposed at emergency operation on thirteen-day-old infant. Large patent ductus equal in diameter to descending aorta is present. Proximal to patent ductus is coarctation of aorta with narrow proximal aortic segment and narrow subclavian artery. *B.* Appearance after excision of coarctation and suture of patent ductus arteriosus. Anastomosis was constructed proximally at point of origin of left subclavian artery from aorta.

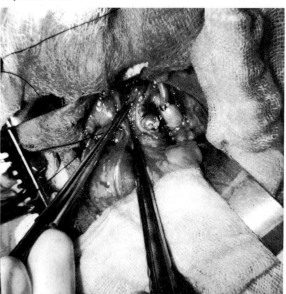

A   *B*

larger than 40 mm in circumference, as recommended by Brom. Subsequently the mediastinal pleura is approximated over the aorta before the thoracotomy incision is closed.

The frequency of insertion of a vascular graft, rather than an anastomosis, has varied with different groups. Such a graft is needed with a long narrow segment or with associated intercostal aneurysms. Schuster and Gross inserted grafts in 70 patients, 14 percent of their series, with excellent results over periods of observation as long as 12 years. Crafoord and Nylin employed grafts in only 1 percent of patients, while Brom reported the use of grafts in about 5 percent.

Postoperative Course. Antibiotics are given routinely during operation and for 4 to 5 days thereafter. Patients are ambulatory within 3 to 4 days and usually discharged in 10 to 12 days.

Blood pressure is measured frequently during the first few days after operation. In some a mild paradoxic hypertension, first described by Sealy et al., may occur. This should be treated with appropriate antihypertensive medication, usually reserpine. If untreated, a number of complications can occur, including intermittent abdominal pain, probably a mesenteric arteritis which has even resulted in intestinal necrosis in its extreme form. The pathologic process is apparently a result of sudden perfusion at a high pressure of visceral arteries which previously had been functioning under a low perfusion pressure. If hypertension is treated promptly, such complications are usually minimal. Brom reported the abdominal pain syndrome in 16 of 548 patients, none of whom required laparotomy.

With present techniques, the risk of operation is small and long-term results are excellent. In the series of 487 resections reported by Schuster and Gross, operative mortality was 4 percent. On long-term follow-up, 4 percent of the patients had systolic pressures above 150 mm Hg, 36 percent had values between 130 and 150 mm Hg, and 60 percent had pressures below 130 mm Hg. Crafoord and Nylin reported experiences with 249 patients, with a 4.5 percent mortality, and Brom reported experiences with 530 patients and a mortality of slightly greater than 3 percent. In a long-term evaluation of 350 patients, Brom found only 42 with some residual hypertension. At New York University, of patients operated upon beyond the first year of life, there has been no mortality and no significant complications since 1963.

Vascular Rings

HISTORICAL DATA. Although the clinical significance of vascular rings was recognized by Abbott in her classic survey of congenital heart disease in 1932, surgical therapy was first successfully used with the division of a double aortic arch by Gross in 1945. Gross has subsequently made many superb contributions to diagnosis and therapy of vascular rings, classifying and illustrating with clarity and precision the various anomalies which have been found.

INCIDENCE AND ETIOLOGY. Vascular rings are fairly common among patients with congenital heart disease. Nadas reported seeing over 50 such patients during a period of 10 years. Embryologically, the vascular rings result from variation in the formation of the aorta and pulmonary artery from the sixth embryonic aortic arches. In view of the fact that six aortic arches exist in the embryo, it is surprising that such abnormalities are not even more frequent. In embryonic life six pairs of aortic arches appear and disappear as the heart migrates caudad. The first two arches disappear before the fifth and sixth have developed, and the fifth never fully develops. Only the third, fourth, and sixth are significant in normal development. Ultimately the right common carotid artery arises from the third arch and the innominate from the right fourth. The left fourth contributes to the transverse aortic arch, while the ductus arteriosus originates from the sixth aortic arch.

PATHOLOGIC ANATOMY. Five types of vascular anomalies of clinical significance have been recognized: (1) double aortic arch; (2) right aortic arch with left ligamentum arteriosum; (3) retroesophageal subclavian artery; (4) anomalous origin of innominate artery; and (5) anomalous origin of left common carotid artery. The last two conditions, anomalous origin of the innominate or of the left common carotid artery, are rare malformations in which the origin of the artery from the aortic arch is such that the trachea is compressed. Briefly, surgical correction can be achieved by mobilizing the vessel and suturing it in a more normal position. The other three conditions are considered here in more detail.

A double aortic arch, with one limb anterior to the trachea and the other limb posterior to the esophagus (Figs. 18-20 and 18-21), is usually the most severe malformation, producing symptoms in early infancy. Usually one limb is smaller than the other. Often the thoracic aorta descends on the right rather than on the left.

A right aortic arch with a retroesophageal ligamentum arteriosum is an important anomaly, often producing symptoms in later childhood (Fig. 18-22). A retroesopha-

Fig. 18-20. Double aortic arch with small anterior and large posterior limb. *A.* Anterior view of double aortic arch with small anterior limb. *B.* Exposure after division of small anterior arch between left carotid and left subclavian artery, followed by displacement of carotid artery anteriorly toward sternum. (*Adapted from R. E. Gross, "The Surgery of Infancy and Childhood," W. B. Saunders Company, Philadelphia, 1953, p. 917.*)

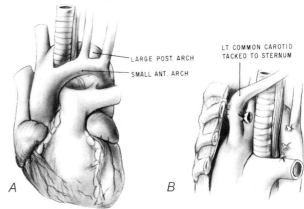

LARGE POST. ARCH
SMALL ANT. ARCH

LT. COMMON CAROTID TACKED TO STERNUM

A   *B*

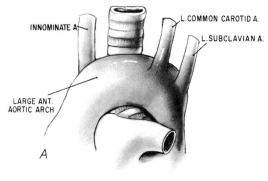

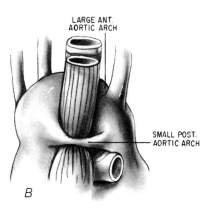

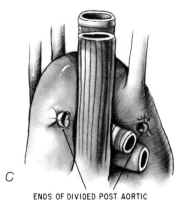

Fig. 18-21. *A.* Double aortic arch with large anterior arch. *B.* Small posterior arch, compressing esophagus. *C.* Appearance after division of small posterior arch. (*Adapted from R. E. Gross, "The Surgery of Infancy and Childhood," W. B. Saunders Company, Philadelphia, 1953, p. 918.*)

geal subclavian artery, usually consisting of a right sub-clavian artery originating beyond the left subclavian artery and coursing posterior to the esophagus to the right arm, is a common anomaly but usually does not cause symptoms (Fig. 18-23).

CLINICAL MANIFESTATIONS. Symptoms from vascular rings are usually due to respiratory obstruction from compression of the trachea. Less frequently, there is difficulty in swallowing from compression of the esophagus.

Symptoms. Infants with a double aortic arch often develop respiratory difficulty in the first few months of life and become seriously ill. Episodes of serious respiratory distress, with "crowing" respirations, are common. During these attacks the infant prefers to lie in hyperextension, and there is visible retraction of the intercostal and supra-clavicular spaces with inspiration. Feeding may precipitate such episodes, perhaps from flexing of the neck, and attempts at feeding may be interrupted by vomiting, and cyanosis, probably from aspiration. Because of the feeding difficulties, infants soon become underweight and mal-nourished.

Symptoms developing after infancy are more gradual in onset, with intermittent episodes of respiratory compression, at times precipitated by a respiratory infection. Mild difficulty in swallowing may be present, but this is seldom prominent. Recurrent pneumonic infections occur, perhaps from aspiration. The mildest clinical picture is seen with the retroesophageal subclavian artery, which may cause only mild or intermittent dysphagia for long periods of time. Some patients may be symptomatic in infancy and spontaneously recover with growth.

Physical Examination. The physical examination is within normal limits unless respiratory distress is present. During such episodes, the infant remains with the back arched and the neck extended. Attempts to flex the neck may precipitate severe dyspnea and cyanosis. Stridor is usually obvious. There are no abnormalities in the heart or peripheral circulation.

LABORATORY STUDIES. The chest roentgenogram is normal unless aspiration pneumonia is present, and the electrocardiogram is normal. Examination of the esophagus with a barium swallow usually establishes the diagnosis by demonstrating a typical area of compression from the retroesophageal vessel, usually at the level of the third or fourth thoracic vertebra. Such a finding is virtually all that is needed to establish the diagnosis of a vascular ring. To determine whether the ring is responsible for the symptoms may require further study. Tracheal compression may be defined with a tracheogram. In the anterior view, compression may be noted laterally, but the lateral tracheo-gram provides the best evidence for the vascular ring, demonstrating anterior compression of the trachea a short distance above the carina. The demonstration of anterior compression of the trachea combined with posterior compression of the esophagus firmly establishes the diagnosis of a vascular ring. Aortography can further delineate the abnormal vessels.

TREATMENT. Since a vascular ring has no physiologic significance, no treatment is needed in the absence of symptoms. If symptoms are mild, their origin may be uncertain, and an observation period is required to be sure that other difficulties are not responsible. If obvious respiratory compression is present, operation should be performed promptly, however, because death from aspiration can occur.

Operative Technique. The preferred operative approach is through a left lateral thoracotomy, usually the fourth intercostal space. An important feature of the operation is to dissect the aortic arch completely and identify the innominate artery, the left common carotid artery, and both subclavian arteries. Opening the pericardium will

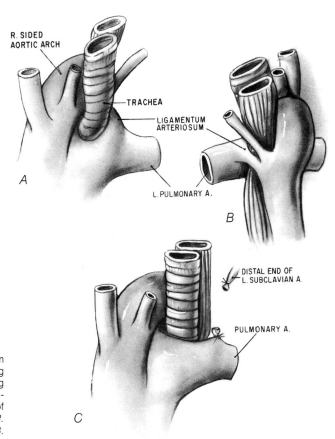

Fig. 18-22. *A.* Right aortic arch with left posterior ligamentum arteriosum. *B.* Posterior view of ligamentum arteriosum extending from right aortic arch to left pulmonary artery, compressing esophagus. Small left subclavian artery arising close to ligamentum arteriosum is also present. *C.* Appearance after division of ligamentum arteriosum and subclavian artery. (*Adapted from R. E. Gross, "The Surgery of Infancy and Childhood," W. B. Saunders Company, Philadelphia, 1953, p. 923.*)

facilitate identification of these vessels. The vagus nerve should be traced to the recurrent laryngeal nerve and, usually, the ligamentum arteriosum divided. Removal of part of the thymus gland will facilitate exposure. It should be emphasized that operative correction is more than simple division of an abnormal ring, because fibrosis surrounding the adventitia of the abnormal vessel may cause continued compression unless the vessels are widely mobilized and all possible compression relieved.

With a double aortic arch, the smaller of the two arches should be divided. Usually, with a left descending aorta,

the anterior arch is smaller and should be divided between the left common carotid and left subclavian artery, after which the mobilized anterior arch can be sutured to the posterior surface of the anterior chest wall to prevent compression of the trachea. If the posterior arch is smaller, it can be divided behind the esophagus. With a right descending thoracic aorta, almost always the posterior arch is the smaller of the two.

With a right aortic arch and a retroesophageal ligamentum arteriosum, division of the ligamentum arteriosum may be all that is necessary. In some patients the left

Fig. 18-23. *A.* Retroesophageal subclavian artery, anomalous vessel arising from aortic arch distal to left subclavian artery. *B.* Appearance after division of anomalous vessel with retraction of distal stump to right of trachea. (*Adapted from R. E. Gross, "The Surgery of Infancy and Childhood," W. B. Saunders Company, Philadelphia, 1953, p. 932.*)

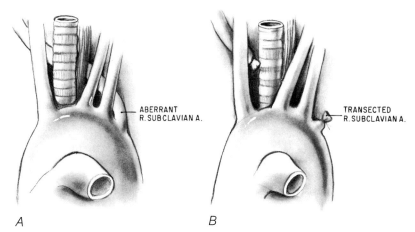

subclavian artery may be in a retroesophageal location and should also be divided. A nubbin of aorta, constituting an aortic diverticulum, has been found in a retroesophageal location in some patients and may require amputation to relieve compression.

With a retroesophageal subclavian artery as an isolated anomaly, simple division of the artery is all that is necessary. Division of this artery through a cervical incision, followed by reimplantation into the right carotid artery, has been reported.

Postoperative Course. Postoperative care consists primarily of careful attention to respiration, with the infant kept in a highly humidified atmosphere and tracheal secretions aspirated. Tracheostomy should be avoided if at all possible. If serious tracheal compression was present before operation, serious difficulties may develop after operation if extensive dissection around the trachea was necessary, creating postoperative edema. In such cases the patient may require unusually vigilant care for 24 to 72 hours because of edema of the trachea. After recovery from operation, symptoms promptly disappear without further disability. The risk of operation is primarily related to the age of the patient and the severity of compression of the trachea. Excellent results in a group of 70 patients have been reported by Gross, who had only 5 postoperative deaths, all of which occurred in a group of 26 infants with double aortic arches.

LEFT-TO-RIGHT SHUNTS (ACYANOTIC GROUP)

Atrial Septal Defects

A variety of malformations involve the atrial septum or the pulmonary veins and result in a left-to-right shunt of blood from the systemic to the pulmonary circulation. These include atrial septal defects of the secundum type, anomalous drainage of the pulmonary veins, ostium primum defects, and atrioventricular canal malformations. These defects are serially considered below. The physiologic disturbance is identical with secundum-type atrial defects and with anomalous pulmonary veins, consisting simply in a left-to-right shunt. With ostium primum defects and atrioventricular canals, mitral and tricuspid insufficiency are present in addition to the left-to-right shunt.

SECUNDUM DEFECTS

HISTORICAL DATA. Several ingenious attempts were made to close atrial septal defects by closed techniques from 1947 to 1953, but only following the successful closure of an atrial septal defect by Lewis in 1953 under direct vision with inflow occlusion and hypothermia did a method of surgical closure become firmly established. In the same year Gibbon employed the pump-oxygenator successfully for the first time in man to suture an atrial septal defect. In subsequent years a large number of patients were successfully operated upon by using hypothermia to permit interruption of the circulation for 5 to 10 minutes, but extracorporeal circulation is now the pre-

ferred technique because of the additional time available to close the septal defect and also to correct any additional malformations which may be encountered.

INCIDENCE AND ETIOLOGY. Atrial septal defects are among the most common cardiac malformations, representing 10 to 15 percent of all cases of congenital heart disease. They are approximately twice as frequent in females as in males. Embryologically, the secundum defects result from failure of the septum secundum to develop completely.

PATHOLOGIC ANATOMY. Atrial septal defects vary widely in size and location. A "high" defect near the entrance of the superior vena cava is commonly referred to as a sinus venosus type of defect and is usually associated with anomalous entry of the superior pulmonary veins into the vena cava. The majority of secundum defects are located in the midportion of the atrial septum. "Low" defects are near the point of entry of the inferior vena cava, and caution must be taken in closing such defects to avoid compromising the entry of the inferior vena cava into the right atrium. Defects vary from as small as 1 cm in diameter to virtual absence of the atrial septum, but most are 2 to 3 cm. A foramen ovale should not be considered an atrial septal defect, for it is a normal opening in 15 to 25 percent of adult hearts. Because of its slitlike construction, a normal foramen ovale allows shunting of blood only from right to left. In some patients the atrial septum is fenestrated with multiple defects.

Anomalous pulmonary veins entering the right atrium are frequent, occurring in 15 to 20 percent of patients with atrial septal defects. An unusual variant of atrial septal defect is seen when a secundum defect occurs in association with mitral stenosis, the so-called Lutembacher's syndrome. The mitral stenosis retards flow of blood from the left atrium to the left ventricle and results in an enormous shunt of blood through the septal defect, with massive dilatation of the pulmonary arteries.

PATHOPHYSIOLOGY. An atrial septal defect results in a left-to-right shunt of blood from the left atrium to the right atrium because of the pressure-volume characteristics of the left and right ventricles. The thick-walled left ventricle is less distensible than the right ventricle; with a closed atrial septum, left atrial pressure is normally 8 to 10 mm Hg, while right atrial pressure is 4 to 5 mm Hg. This difference in distensibility of the two ventricles results in a left-to-right shunt when an atrial septal defect is present. However, during infancy and the first few years of life the structure of the right ventricle more closely resembles the left ventricle, and usually only a small shunt is present. For this reason atrial septal defects are commonly not recognized during the first few years of life.

Depending upon the size of the atrial defect, as well as the difference in distensibility of the two ventricles, the size of the left-to-right shunt may vary from as little as 1 liter to as high as 20 liters/minute. Most septal defects have a pulmonary blood flow two to four times greater than the systemic blood flow. The great reduction in systemic blood flow may result in retardation of normal growth and development, with the so-called gracile habitus seen in some children with a large atrial septal defect. The increase in pulmonary blood flow increases susceptibility to pneumonia and also causes dyspnea on exertion. For unknown reasons patients are susceptible to rheumatic fever, but fortunately bacterial endocarditis is rare. Arrhythmias of different types are also frequently seen.

With the increased pulmonary blood flow, pulmonary vascular resistance in children is usually less than normal, but it gradually increases. Pulmonary hypertension is found in less than 5 percent of children with this condition but occurs in 20 to 25 percent of adult patients as fibrotic changes develop in the pulmonary vessels. Cardiac failure is similarly unusual in children but becomes more frequent in the second and third decades. It has been estimated that the average life span of an untreated patient with an atrial septal defect is about 40 years.

CLINICAL MANIFESTATIONS. Symptoms. Symptoms are uncommon in the first few years of life because the shunt may be small until the right ventricular hypertrophy of embryonic life has subsided. Frequently children with large shunts are physically active and completely free of symptoms. In a report of 275 surgically treated patients with hemodynamically significant atrial defects, Sellers et al. found 113 asymptomatic. The most frequent symptoms are fatigue, palpitations, and exertional dyspnea. Slow growth and development may also be noted by the parents. In adults overt signs of congestive heart failure gradually appear, often with the first pregnancy.

Physical Examination. A soft systolic murmur is usually audible in the second or third left intercostal space. In the first few years of life this murmur may be scarcely detectable or may be diagnosed as a functional murmur. The murmur arises at the pulmonary valve from the increased flow of blood through the valve. The second pulmonic sound is characteristically widely split, and "fixed" splitting (not varying with respiration) is characteristic of the disorder. Slight to moderate cardiac enlargement is present with large defects. With large defects the cardiac enlargement may produce a distinct prominence of the left costal cartilages. The physical habitus of such patients is often thin, with long, narrow bones and limited muscular development—the gracile habitus.

LABORATORY FINDINGS. The chest roentgenogram shows mild to moderate cardiac enlargement limited to the right ventricle. The pulmonary artery is prominent, with increased vascularity in the lung fields. The electrocardiogram typically shows a right axis deviation with a right bundle branch block. Mild but not severe right ventricular hypertrophy is usually evident.

On cardiac catheterization the diagnosis can be confirmed by finding a rise in oxygen saturation of 1.5 to 2.0 vol % between the superior vena cava and right atrium. During catheterization the presence of anomalous veins should be noted, although the diagnosis cannot always be established with certainty. The right ventricular systolic pressure in children is usually 30 to 40 mm Hg. With large shunts there may be a 20 to 40 mm Hg gradient across a normal pulmonary valve as a result of the large flow of blood. Selective angiography with injection of dye into the pulmonary artery may disclose opacification of the right atrium as dye flows from the left atrium through the

defect. Dye-dilution curves can similarly localize the area of shunting of blood.

DIAGNOSIS. Diagnosis in infancy is virtually impossible on clinical grounds, because the systolic murmur is not distinctive. In older children the diagnosis can be made with reasonable certainty from the combination of a soft systolic murmur with fixed splitting of the pulmonic second sound. These physical findings, combined with the chest roentgenogram and electrocardiogram, provide firm support for the diagnosis. Differentiation from anomalous pulmonary veins is virtually impossible without cardiac catheterization. A left axis deviation on the electrocardiogram immediately suggests that an ostium primum malformation is present.

TREATMENT. Indications. Since many children are asymptomatic, operation is frequently recommended on the basis of clinical findings and laboratory determination of the size of shunt present. Operation is usually performed if the pulmonary blood flow is one and one-half to two times greater than the systemic blood flow. The only contraindication to operation is the presence of severe pulmonary hypertension with an elevated pulmonary vascular resistance, fortunately almost unknown in children. In adults, if the pulmonary vascular resistance has increased to where pulmonary blood flow is only slightly greater than systemic flow, operation is hazardous, and patients who survive often show little benefit. However, if pulmonary blood flow is still significantly increased despite the presence of pulmonary hypertension, operation may be very beneficial, although the operative risk is considerably greater than with uncomplicated atrial septal defect and improvement does not occur to an equal degree in all patients.

Frequently patients are first seen for operation in the fifth or even the sixth decade. A number of such patients have been safely operated upon with significant symptomatic improvement. The main determinant of the risk of operation is not the age of the patient but the increase in pulmonary vascular resistance. As long as the pulmonary blood flow is more than twice the systemic blood flow, benefit can be anticipated from closure of the defect.

Operative Technique. All patients are operated upon with extracorporeal circulation. A sternotomy or a right thoracotomy in the fourth intercostal space may be employed. Once cardiopulmonary bypass has been instituted, the author prefers to induce ventricular fibrillation before opening the heart in order to prevent any risk of air embolism; otherwise in a small percentage of patients serious neurologic defects can result from trapping of air in the left atrium during closure of the defect. Usually the aorta is also occluded just before the atriotomy is made.

Once ventricular fibrillation has been instituted, the atrium is opened widely and the margins of the defect identified (Fig. 18-24). In 70 to 85 percent of patients closure can be done with a simple continuous over-and-over suture. In some patients the margins of the defect are friable, and closure is best done with a prosthetic patch. A variety of such patches have been successfully used; the author prefers knitted Dacron or pericardium. Normal entry of the pulmonary vein is confirmed before the defect

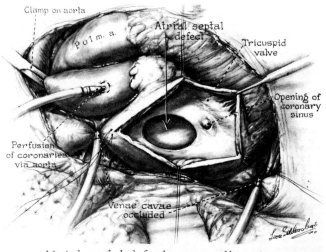

Atrial septal defect as seen thru
incision in r. atrium

Fig. 18-24. Atrial septal defect of secundum type exposed at operation. Operation illustrated was performed under hypothermia several years ago with perfusion of aorta with oxygenated blood. Such operations are now performed with cardiopulmonary bypass. Large oval opening in atrial septum superior to coronary sinus is type usually found with secundum-type defects.

is closed. Therapy for anomalous veins is described in the following section. The patch is usually inserted with a continuous suture approximating the margin of the patch to the margins of the defect. Care is taken, as the last sutures are tightened, to be certain that blood flows freely from the left atrium to avoid trapping any air in the left atrium. Subsequently, after bypass has been stopped, closure of the defect can be confirmed by aspirating blood from the superior cava and pulmonary artery and demonstrating similar oxygen concentration in the two samples. Left atrial pressure also is measured and serially monitored if elevated.

Postoperative Course. Postoperative convalescence is uncomplicated and recovery from any signs of cardiac disability is prompt in the usual patient with uncomplicated atrial septal defect.

The risk of operation with extracorporeal circulation is surprisingly small. Several groups have reported series of more than 100 patients operated upon with a mortality of 1 to 3 percent. Gerbode et al. reported one death in 77 patients, and Sellers et al. a 1.8 percent mortality in uncomplicated atrial defects in a group of 275 patients. In the author's experience with more than 100 secundum defects, no deaths have occurred in the past decade.

ANOMALOUS DRAINAGE OF PULMONARY VEINS

Partial and total anomalous drainage of the pulmonary veins are distinct clinical entities and are presented separately in the following sections. The physiologic handicap from partial drainage of the pulmonary veins resembles atrial septal defect, while total anomalous drainage is a much more serious physiologic derangement, often fatal in the first few months of life.

Partial anomalous drainage is frequent, occurring in 10 to 20 percent of patients with atrial septal defect. Total anomalous drainage, however, is much less common.

HISTORICAL DATA. Although anomalous pulmonary veins have been recognized at postmortem examinations

for decades, emphasis was focused on clinical features by the analysis by Brody of 106 cases in 1942. Before open cardiac surgery was possible, only a few cases of successful surgical correction were reported. One of the first of these was reported in 1951 by Muller, who successfully implanted an anomalous left pulmonary vein into the left atrium. Subsequently, with operations performed under hypothermia, partial anomalous drainage of pulmonary veins, usually into the right atrium or superior vena cava, could be corrected by changing the position of the atrial septum. Successful correction of total anomalous pulmonary venous drainage, however, was accomplished only with extracorporeal circulation. A modification of the technique reported by Cooley and Oschner in 1957 has subsequently proved to be the most useful.

PARTIAL ANOMALOUS DRAINAGE OF PULMONARY VEINS. Pathologic Anatomy. Anomalous drainage of the right pulmonary veins occurs approximately twice as frequently as that involving the left. Anomalous right pulmonary veins usually enter the superior vena cava inferior to the point of entry of the azygos vein, the right atrium, or the inferior vena cava. Anomalous left pulmonary veins commonly enter a persistent left superior vena cava or innominate vein or, more rarely, the coronary sinus. Partial anomalous drainage usually involves only the veins from one lung, but a few unusual examples of partial drainage of pulmonary veins from both lungs have been described. One of the most detailed reports of the pathologic anatomy of anomalous pulmonary veins was published by Blake et al. in an analysis of data from the Armed Forces Institute of Pathology. In a group of 113 patients with anomalous pulmonary venous return, a total of 27 different variations were found, emphasizing the wide variation in physiologic derangement which occur.

Anomalous right pulmonary veins entering the superior vena cava are almost always associated with a characteristic high atrial septal defect at the point of entry of the superior vena cava, which has been termed a sinus venosus defect because of its embryologic origin. Pulmonary veins entering the right atrium are also usually associated with an atrial septal defect of the secundum type. Only rarely are anomalous pulmonary veins found with an intact atrial septum. Pulmonary veins entering the inferior vena cava usually communicate through a single channel with the inferior vena cava near the diaphragm.

An unusual variant of anomalous right pulmonary veins entering the inferior vena cava, in association with other anomalies, has been described as a "scimitar" syndrome, a term emphasizing a characteristic radiologic appearance resulting from the shadow of the anomalous vein parallel to the right border of the heart. Although this roentgenographic appearance is suggestive, other abnormalities may have a similar appearance. The malformation is often associated with defective development of the right lung and anomalous origin of the pulmonary arteries from the aorta. The physiologic disturbance is not severe, because the amount of blood shunted through the hypoplastic lung is small.

Pathophysiology. With partial anomalous drainage of the pulmonary veins, the volume of blood shunted is usually less than 50 percent of normal pulmonary blood flow, because less than one-half the pulmonary veins are involved. Hence the abnormal physiology is a left-to-right shunt identical to that of an atrial septal defect.

Clinical Manifestations. The symptoms and signs are identical to those of an atrial septal defect, and clinical separation of the two entities is not possible. Cardiac catheterization is the only method for establishing a precise diagnosis. Direct entry of an anomalous vein by the cardiac catheter may be diagnostic, especially if the vein is entered from the superior vena cava. In the right atrium, one often cannot be certain whether or not the catheter has traversed an atrial septal defect before entering the pulmonary vein. Selective dye-dilution curves, with dye injected separately into the two pulmonary arteries, can establish the diagnosis because of the difference in circulation times from the lung with normal pulmonary veins and with anomalous pulmonary veins.

Treatment. A single anomalous pulmonary vein, usually from the right upper lobe entering the superior vena cava, is physiologically harmless and does not require treatment. More extensive malformations are usually operated upon in conjunction with closure of an atrial septal defect. Anomalous veins entering the right atrium can be corrected by changing the position of the atrial septum at the time the septal defect is closed so that the pulmonary veins enter the left atrium (Figs. 18-25, and 18-26). Pulmonary veins entering the superior vena cava in association with a sinus venosus defect can be corrected by the application of a prosthetic patch, preferably of pericardium, to shunt blood into the left atrium (Fig. 18-27). Anomalous veins entering the inferior vena cava are usually treated by division of the aberrant channel and direct implantation into the left atrium.

TOTAL ANOMALOUS DRAINAGE OF PULMONARY VEINS.
Pathologic Anatomy. Darling et al. have classified anatomically the types of total anomalous drainage of pulmonary veins according to location. Supracardiac drainage occurs

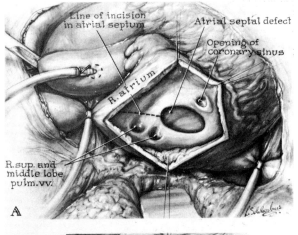

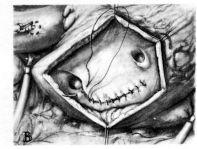

Fig. 18-25. Atrial septal defect with anomalous drainage of right pulmonary veins into right atrium. By enlargement of defect it was possible to shift atrial septum so that closure could be performed with diversion of pulmonary veins into left atrium. Prosthetic patch can be used if it is not possible to shift atrial septum. (*Reprinted by permission of C. V. Mosby Co. from H. T. Bahnson, F. C. Spencer, and C. A. Neill, Surgical Treatment of Thirty-five Cases of Drainage of Pulmonary Veins to the Right Side of the Heart, J Thorac Surg, 36:787, 1958.*)

in 55 percent of cases, paracardiac in 30 percent, and infracardiac in 12 percent. Multiple sites of entry are found in 3 percent.

With the supracardiac type of drainage, the most common point of entry of the anomalous veins is into a left vertical vein which in turn enters the left innominate vein. Rarely, the common anomalous venous trunk may drain directly into the posterior aspect of a right superior vena cava. With paracardiac drainage, the anomalous veins may enter the right atrium directly or, more rarely, may drain into the coronary sinus. With infracardiac drainage the pulmonary venous blood usually enters the inferior vena cava through a common channel traversing the diaphragm to connect with a hepatic vein or the portal vein.

Pathophysiology. Life is possible with total anomalous pulmonary venous drainage only as long as an atrial septal defect, often only a foramen ovale, is present. In addition, pulmonary venous hypertension often exists because of constriction of the point of entry of the anomalous pulmonary veins into the systemic venous system, which in turn results in pulmonary hypertension. With adequate communication between the anomalous pulmonary veins and the systemic venous circulation and a large atrial septal defect, patients may do surprisingly well for a period of

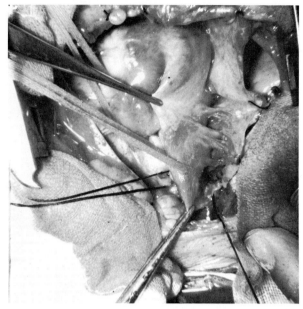

Fig. 18-26. Operative photograph of sinus venosus defect. The umbilical tape encircles the vena cava above the point of entry of the anomalous pulmonary veins. Three separate anomalous pulmonary veins are shown entering the superior vena cava. When the atrium was opened, a classic atrial septal defect was found at the point of entry of the superior vena cava into the left atrium. The anomaly was corrected with a large pericardial patch, diverting blood from the anomalous veins through the atrial defect into the left atrium.

time, the disability resembling that from a large atrial septal defect. This fortunate situation occurs in about 20 percent of patients. In the majority (80 percent) severe pulmonary hypertension is present; half these patients die in the first 3 months of life, and most within the first year. Cardiac failure develops with great rapidity, and cyanosis, varying with the degree of pulmonary blood flow, is frequent.

Clinical Manifestations. The dominant findings are a seriously ill infant with congestive failure, cyanosis, and rap-

idly progressive cardiac enlargement. In infants a murmur may not be audible. Hepatic enlargement is frequent.

The chest roentgenogram may be diagnostic when there is significant dilatation of the left vertebral and left innominate veins, creating a characteristic double contour on the x-ray termed a "snowman" appearance (Fig. 18-3).

Occasionally, with severe pulmonary venous obstruction, pulmonary congestion may be so severe in the infant as to suggest miliary tuberculosis. Diagnosis can be confirmed by cardiac catheterization. The hallmark of the physiologic disturbance in total anomalous pulmonary venous drainage is an almost identical oxygen content of the right atrium, pulmonary artery, and femoral artery because of complete mixing of oxygenated and unoxygenated blood in the right atrium before entering the left atrium through an atrial septal defect. Pulmonary hypertension is common. Also, the right atrial pressure is usually greater than the left atrial pressure.

Treatment. Infants with total anomalous pulmonary venous drainage are extremely ill and often must be operated upon under emergency circumstances. Enlarging the atrial septal defect in the catheterization laboratory by the balloon septostomy technique of Rashkind may provide valuable palliation until surgical correction can be done. El-Said et al. recently published data supporting this approach in the first few weeks of life.

When the venous drainage is into a left vertical vein, the surgical correction includes creation of a long (2.5- to 3-cm) side-to-side anastomosis between the anomalous pulmonary veins and the left atrium (Fig. 18-28), followed by closure of the atrial septal defect and ligation of the

Fig. 18-27. A. Sinus venosus type of atrial septal defect located near junction of superior vena cava with right atrium. Defect is partly obscured by crescentic lower margin. Anomalous pulmonary veins from right upper lobe enter superior vena cava near its juncture with right atrium. B. Prosthetic patch can be applied to encompass both atrial septal defect and ostia of anomalous pulmonary veins, avoiding undue constriction of point of entry of superior vena cava into right atrium. C. Final view of prosthetic patch which excludes anomalous veins and atrial septal defect from right atrium. (Adapted from C. D. Benson, et al., "Pediatric Surgery," vol. I, Year Book Medical Publishers, Inc., Chicago, 1962, p. 439.)

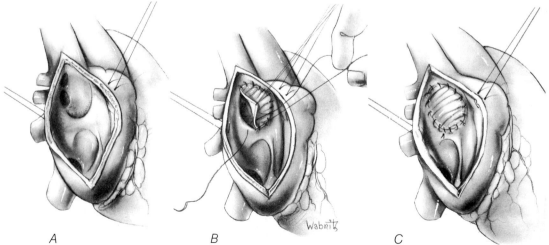

A   B   C

left vertical vein. If the anomalous veins enter the right atrium or the coronary sinus, surgical reconstruction can be more simply performed (Fig. 18-29).

Beyond the first year of life operative risk is small, approaching that of atrial septal defect, if there is not a great increase in pulmonary vascular resistance. Operations in infants, however, retain a high operative mortality, exceeding 50 percent. For this reason a few such patients have been operated upon with the technique of deep hypothermia and temporary circulatory arrest, with results substantially better than those previously reported with a pump-oxygenator. Further experience is needed to determine the most effective approach for these seriously ill patients.

OSTIUM PRIMUM DEFECT

The significant clinical differences between atrial septal defects of the ostium primum type and those of the secundum type became evident only when closure of such defects became possible with open heart surgery. Primum defects are relatively infrequent, occurring in 4 to 5 percent of patients with defects in the atrial septum. One of the first papers to emphasize clinical differentiation of the two conditions was published in 1956 by Blount and associates.

Ostium primum defects are often found in children with mongolism, occurring in 20 to 30 percent. Except for this unusual association, no other etiologically significant factors are known.

A primum defect results from incomplete formation of the mitral and tricuspid valves and the atrial and ventricular septa from the embryonic endocardial cushions. In embryonic life the endocardial cushions develop as dorsal and ventral partitions to separate the single atrium and ventricle of the embryo and join with the ventricular and atrial septa to form the normal four cardiac chambers. A synonym for ostium primum defects and the more severe associated malformation, atrioventricular canal, is *endocardial cushion defect,* partial (ostium primum) or complete (atrioventricular canal).

PATHOLOGIC ANATOMY. The two significant defects are a cleft in the anterior leaflet of the mitral valve and a low, crescent-shaped defect in the atrial septum (Fig. 18-30A). The sicklelike superior border of an ostium primum defect can be easily recognized on palpation at the time of surgical correction. The cleft in the anterior leaflet of the mitral valve may be partial, extending for a short distance from the ventricular septum, or complete, separating the mitral valve leaflet into anterior and posterior halves.

Chordae tendineae are usually attached to the margins of the cleft and in some fortunate patients may prevent significant mitral insufficiency. In other patients, usually those with more severe malformations, abnormal chordae tendineae are present.

An associated partial or complete cleft in the tricuspid valve is also frequently seen. Conduction abnormalities from fibrosis or distortion of the conduction bundle, characteristically located along the posterior rim of the septal defect, are common.

Primum defects are anatomically distinguished from the more severe atrioventricular canal malformation by the

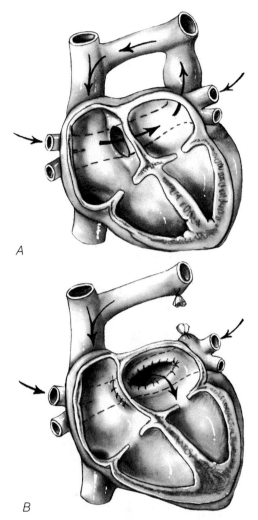

A

B

Fig. 18-28. *A.* Abnormal physiology with anomalous drainage of pulmonary veins into left superior vena cava. All pulmonary venous blood flows through left innominate vein into large right superior vena cava and can enter systemic circulation only through atrial septal defect, usually foramen ovale. *B.* At operation, wide opening is made between posteriorly located common pulmonary venous trunk and left atrium, after which opening in atrial septum is closed and left superior vena cava divided. *(Adapted from C. D. Benson et al., "Pediatric Surgery," vol. I, Year Book Medical Publishers, Inc., Chicago, 1962, p. 446.)*

presence of distinct, separate mitral and tricuspid valve rings and an intact ventricular septum. With an atrioventricular canal malformation there is an additional defect in the ventricular septum, as well as extensive abnormalities of the mitral and tricuspid valve leaflets.

PATHOPHYSIOLOGY. The physiologic abnormalities are a left-to-right shunt combined with mitral insufficiency. When mitral insufficiency is minimal, the malformation is identical with that of atrial septal defect of the secundum type. When mitral insufficiency is severe, left ventricular failure and pulmonary hypertension appear early in life and produce a much more severe impairment of cardiac function than is seen in secundum-type septal defects.

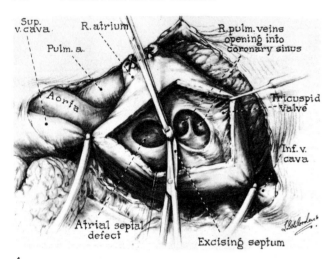

A

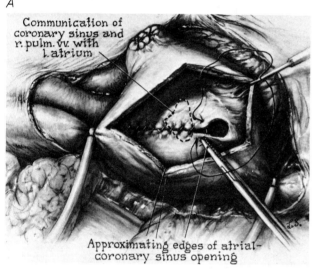

B

Fig. 18-29. *A.* Total anomalous drainage of pulmonary veins into coronary sinus. With this anomaly, atrial septal defect, usually foramen ovale, must be present to maintain life. It is possible to correct anomaly by excision of septum between foramen ovale and dilated coronary sinus. *B.* After excision of septum between foramen ovale and coronary sinus, resulting opening can be closed by suture of atrial septum, thus diverting all pulmonary venous blood, as well as blood draining from coronary sinus, into left atrium.

Increase in pulmonary vascular resistance with associated pulmonary hypertension may develop but is more frequent with atrioventricular canals.

CLINICAL MANIFESTATIONS. Symptoms. A variety of clinical profiles occur, varying with the degree of mitral insufficiency. When mitral insufficiency is minimal, the clinical picture is similar to that of atrial septal defect of the secundum type. Before the advent of precise diagnostic techniques, ostium primum defects were often first recognized at operation. With significant mitral insufficiency, cardiac failure with pulmonary congestion, dyspnea, recurrent bouts of pneumonia, and retardation of growth may be prominent in the first years of life.

Physical Examination. On physical examination moderate cardiac enlargement is often found, with a thrill near the apex. A harsh apical systolic murmur from mitral insufficiency is usually present and should arouse suspicion of an ostium primum defect. An additional systolic murmur may be heard along the left sternal border. The intensity of the pulmonic second sound is often increased. With

cardiac failure, signs of pulmonary congestion and hepatic enlargement are found. Growth is frequently retarded.

LABORATORY FINDINGS. The chest roentgenogram usually shows moderate cardiac enlargement, involving both the right and the left ventricle. Increased pulmonary vascularity is also common. The most useful diagnostic guide is provided by the electrocardiogram, which shows both right and left ventricular hypertrophy, with a left axis deviation. In the vectorcardiogram the inscription in the frontal plane is in a counterclockwise loop, a finding almost pathognomonic of ostium primum defect. Conduction defects with prolongation of the P-R interval are frequent. These electrocardiographic abnormalities are due primarily to the conduction defect and not to the associated left ventricular hypertrophy.

On cardiac catheterization a left-to-right shunt is found at the atrial level; frequently the catheter will enter the left atrium or left ventricle. The pulmonary blood flow is frequently two to three times greater than systemic flow. Mitral insufficiency, suggested by prominent V waves in

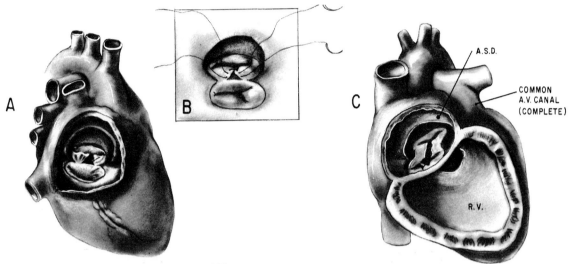

Fig. 18-30. *A.* Ostium primum type of atrioventricular canal. There is a cleft in anterior mitral leaflet, but ventricular septum is intact. *B.* Method of repair of cleft valve with interrupted sutures to produce competent mitral valve. Classic crescent-shaped atrial septal defect superior to valve ring is shown. *C.* Appearance of complete atrioventricular canal, showing complete division of mitral and tricuspid valves in association with atrial septal defect and ventricular septal defect. *(Adapted from D. C. McGoon et al., Am J Cardiol, 6:598, 1960.)*

the left atrial pressure tracing, is best confirmed by injection of contrast media into the left ventricle.

DIAGNOSIS. The diagnosis usually can be made with reasonable certainty from the clinical picture of a child with cardiac enlargement, a left-to-right shunt with an apical systolic murmur, and an electrocardiogram showing left axis deviation with a frontal-plane counterclockwise loop in the vectorcardiogram. Differential diagnosis should exclude ventricular septal defect and atrial septal defect of the secundum type.

TREATMENT. In most patients operative correction of the defect should be performed between the ages of four and six years. Rarely, an adult is seen in the third or fourth decade with a history of little disability from a primum defect, but such patients are those in whom mitral insufficiency has been minimal and the clinical course has been more similar to the benign secundum-type defect. In most patients the combination of a left-to-right shunt with mitral insufficiency results in progressive cardiac enlargement and failure in childhood.

Operative Technique. Operation is performed with extracorporeal circulation, using a median sternotomy incision. The three principal objectives are correction of the mitral insufficiency, closure of the septal defect, and avoidance of the production of heart block from injury to the conduction bundle along the posterior margin of the septal defect. It must be emphasized that incomplete correction of the mitral insufficiency can be disastrous. Closure of the septal defect with residual severe mitral insufficiency may produce severe or fatal pulmonary edema, because decompression of the left atrium into the right atrium has been abolished by closure of the defect.

At operation the right atrium is widely opened, and the

septal defect, cleft in the mitral valve, associated cleft in the tricuspid valve, and ventricular septum are carefully examined. Initially the cleft in the mitral valve is closed with interrupted sutures of silk placed from the ventricular septum out to the free margin of the mitral orifice (Fig. 18-30*B*), the points of insertion of the chordae tendineae being carefully noted. Usually a left ventricular vent is inserted through the apex of the left ventricle to avoid production of air embolism once the mitral valve has been rendered competent by closure of the cleft. Additional protection from air embolism is gained by using induced ventricular fibrillation during most of the operation. After repair of the cleft mitral valve, the septal defect is repaired with a prosthetic patch of pericardium inserted with interrupted silk sutures. Along the posterior rim near the conduction bundle the sutures are inserted superficially to the left of the rim of the defect along the annulus of the mitral valve, the electrocardiogram being checked after the sutures are inserted to avoid producing a conduction injury. A defect in the tricuspid valve is frequent but usually is not amenable to repair by direct suture. Air should be completely evacuated from the left atrium as closure of the septal defect is completed.

Postoperative Course. If adequate correction of the mitral insufficiency is accomplished and production of heart block avoided, postoperative recovery is usually uneventful and similar to that for closure of other septal defects. A conduction injury is a grave complication and should be treated at operation by the temporary insertion of a pacemaker. If a complete heart block should persist, a permanent pacemaker should be inserted before the patient is discharged from the hospital. Some patients have a residual systolic murmur, and some of these will be found on subsequent study to have significant mitral regurgitation. Reoperation for such regurgitation has been reported. The functional results in the majority of patients, however, are satisfactory. Long-term data, extending over a period of years, are not yet available to indicate the ultimate outcome of the malformed valves. The operative mortality, as with other cardiac defects, has steadily decreased with cumulative experience and is now near 5 percent. At New York University since 1963, there have been no deaths or complete heart blocks following operation.

A few years ago an unusual syndrome of severe hemolytic anemia was recognized in a small percentage of patients following repair of an ostium primum defect. This striking clinical picture resulted from residual mitral insufficiency accidentally oriented so that the regurgitant jet of blood struck the prosthetic patch closing the septal defect and intermittently dislodged fibrin from the surface of the patch with each systolic jet. Although rare, such a syndrome should be recognized, for reoperation and closure of the residual insufficiency is curative.

PERSISTENT ATRIOVENTRICULAR CANAL

This malformation is a more extensive error in development of the endocardial cushions, consisting of a large common defect involving both the atrial and ventricular septa, and extensive defects in the mitral and tricuspid valves (Fig. 18-30C). These are often connected across the incomplete septa to form large common valve leaflets in the anterior and posterior portions of the heart. The great variation in valve deformities in these patients was well described by Rastelli et al. in an analysis of 30 postmortem specimens. The physiologic defect is a left-to-right shunt at both the atrial and ventricular levels, resulting in cardiac failure in early life as well as pulmonary vascular obstruction and pulmonary hypertension. The severity of the malformation depends upon the extent of the mitral insufficiency and the size of the ventricular septal defect. In infants with severe deformities the course is a severe one, with death in the first few months of life, while patients with less severe lesions do reasonably well for the first few years of life.

An atrioventricular canal, rather than an ostium primum

Fig. 18-31. Common types of ventricular septal defect. Most common is type B, with defect lying just proximal to crista supraventricularis. Type A defects are located immediately proximal to pulmonic valve. Type C defects are located beneath septal leaflet of tricuspid valve. Type D defects are in muscular part of ventricular septum and are often multiple. (*Adapted from J. W. Kirklin et al., J Thorac Surg, 33:45, 1957.*)

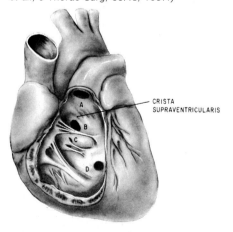

CRISTA
SUPRAVENTRICULARIS

defect, may be suspected from the malignant clinical course of severe cardiac failure and cardiac enlargement in the first one or two years of life. Diagnosis is established principally by cardiac catheterization and angiography, demonstrating both a ventricular septal defect and mitral insufficiency.

Formerly, results of operative correction were very poor, with mortality exceeding 75 percent in infants. For this reason prosthetic valves have been employed in a few infants, but with unimpressive results. In the past few years, modifications of the technique of surgical correction developed by Rastelli et al. and by McGoon et al. have reduced operative mortality substantially, to the range of 10 to 15 percent in patients over two years of age. Details of the technique will not be given here, but a large prosthetic patch is inserted to the underlying ventricular septum, after which the mitral valve is reconstructed and attached to the patch at an appropriate level. The tricuspid valve is usually not reconstructed. Significant long-term data are not yet available.

Ventricular Septal Defect

HISTORICAL DATA. A description by Roger in 1879 of two patients with ventricular septal defect led to the eponymic designation *Roger's disease* and emphasized the asymptomatic nature of the disease when the ventricular septal defect is small. Further contributions to clinical characterization of the syndrome were made by Abbott in 1932, by Taussig in 1947, and later by Selzer and by Wood. Surgical closure became possible with the development of the pump-oxygenator in 1955.

INCIDENCE AND ETIOLOGY. There are no known significant etiologic factors, although ventricular septal defect is a common form of congenital heart disease, constituting 20 to 30 percent of all cases in various cardiac clinics.

PATHOLOGIC ANATOMY. Five types of ventricular septal defect have been recognized, depending upon the location in the ventricular septum: membranous septum defect; defect anterior to the crista supraventricularis near the pulmonic valve; posterior ventricular septum defect; low muscular defect; and left ventricular–right atrial defect. Defects in the membranous septum are by far the most frequent (85 to 90 percent of patients), the other types being seen only infrequently.

Defects in the membranous septum (Fig. 18-31, type B) are located posterior to the crista supraventricularis. With small defects a rim exists superiorly, while large defects are extremely close to the base of the septal leaflet of the tricuspid valve on the right and the mitral valve on the left. The bundle of His, of critical importance to the surgeon, is located at the posterior and superior rim of the defect, where it bifurcates into the right and left conduction bundles. The septal defects are located beneath the right aortic cusp or beneath the junction of the right aortic and septal cusps. Often these cusps are easily visible through the defect and must be protected from injury during surgical repair. The degree of dextroposition of the aorta varies widely. With some defects the aortic valve is not visible at all. At the other extreme are those defects in which the aorta partly arises from the right ventricle. This type is common with tetralogy of Fallot.

Anterior ventricular septal defects (Fig. 18-31, type A) occur anterior to the crista supraventricularis near the pulmonic valve. Surgical closure is simple because the defect is a safe distance from the conduction bundle. Posterior ventricular septal defects (Fig. 18-31, type C), are posterior to the papillary muscle of the conus and beneath the tricuspid valve. Often the rim is partly or completely muscular. Exposure is awkward but can be accomplished with appropriate retraction. Muscular ventricular septal defects (Fig. 18-31, type D) are located inferiorly in the ventricular septum and are often multiple. In the most extreme form, the "Swiss cheese" type of septum, there are multiple tiny serpentine communications which make complete surgical closure difficult or perhaps impossible. Left ventricular–right atrial defects are the rarest of all, consisting of a communication between the left ventricle and the right atrium through the membranous septum superior to the annulus of the tricuspid valve. Such defects are small but are associated with a large shunt because of the great difference in pressure between the left ventricle and right atrium. Once these defects are recognized, closure by direct suture is simple.

The size of ventricular septal defects varies from as small as 0.3 cm to greater than 3 cm. A diameter of 0.8 to 1 cm is a convenient one for separating "small" and "large" septal defects, for those smaller than 1 cm are often associated with a pulmonary blood flow less than twice systemic blood flow and few cardiac abnormalities. "Small" defects are seen in about 25 percent of patients. Defects larger than 1 cm, corresponding to about one-half the diameter of the aortic valve orifice, are regularly associated with more severe physiologic disturbances.

Histologic changes in the pulmonary vasculature are an important part of the pathologic anatomy, for these are related to the evolution of pulmonary hypertension. Young children with pulmonary hypertension have prominent smooth muscle in the media of the pulmonary arterioles, resembling that found in the pulmonary vasculature during fetal life. In subsequent years, with continued pulmonary hypertension, proliferative changes appear in the intima, becoming more prominent in late childhood and early adult life. The intimal proliferative changes apparently represent a permanent increase in pulmonary vascular resistance, with irreversible pulmonary hypertension. Though the pathogenesis of pulmonary hypertension has been studied intensely, the sporadic appearance and erratic course among different patients with similar defects remains a mystery.

Associated anomalies with ventricular defects are common. These include patent ductus arteriosus, coarctation of the aorta, atrial septal defect, mild infundibular stenosis of the right ventricle, and aortic insufficiency from prolapse of an aortic valve cusp into the ventricular septal defect. Recognition of the additional anomalies is an obviously important part of preoperative diagnosis and planning prior to surgical correction.

PATHOPHYSIOLOGY. Since normally the systolic left ventricular pressure is about four times greater than the systolic right ventricular pressure, a ventricular septal defect results in a left-to-right shunt of blood from the left ventricle into the pulmonary circulation, producing a pulmonary blood flow greater than systemic blood flow. The size of the left-to-right shunt varies with both the size of the defect and the pulmonary vascular resistance. In a small number of patients, a discrete infundibular stenosis also restricts the size of the shunt. With a septal defect less than 1 cm in diameter, the pulmonary blood flow may be only about $1\frac{1}{2}$ times systemic blood flow, and few physiologic changes result. With septal defects greater than 1 cm in diameter and a pulmonary blood flow more than twice systemic flow, a strain on cardiac function becomes obvious. With huge septal defects, pulmonary blood flow may be four to five times greater than systemic flow, producing severe pulmonary congestion and heart failure.

The two major changes from a ventricular septal defect are cardiac failure and pulmonary hypertension. In infancy severe cardiac failure develops if a large defect is present. This may be fatal in some unless surgical therapy, either closure of the defect or banding of the pulmonary artery, is performed. After the first year of life, chronic pulmonary congestion may persist with large defects, resulting in recurrent pulmonary infections and limitation of growth and development. Death from congestive heart failure is unusual in children after the first year of life. In adults, however, congestive heart failure is frequent.

Pulmonary hypertension from progressive sclerosis of the pulmonary vascular bed is the other major pathologic change. As mentioned earlier, the principal histologic changes are in the pulmonary arterioles, with hypertrophy of the smooth muscle of the media and proliferation of the intima. These evolve slowly during childhood, becoming more prominent in the late teens and early adult life. Rarely, such changes may progress to an "irreversible" degree in the first few years of life. The cause of this great variability is unknown.

As pulmonary vascular resistance increases to approach systemic vascular resistance, definite changes in blood flow result, for right-to-left shunting through the defect appears in association with the predominant left-to-right shunt. This right-to-left shunt produces unsaturation of the peripheral arterial blood. When the pulmonary vascular resistance and the systemic vascular resistance are nearly equal, a *balanced shunt* results. Ultimately, when pulmonary vascular resistance has risen to exceed systemic vascular resistance, the right-to-left shunt is predominant, resulting in cyanosis, clubbing, and polycythemia. This advanced inoperable disease, formerly termed the Eisenmenger syndrome, is now recognized as simply the end stage of progressive pulmonary hypertension from a large left-to-right shunt. It usually results from a ventricular septal defect but can also occur from a neglected patent ductus arteriosus, atrial septal defect, or other malformations. With severe pulmonary hypertension, death usually occurs at about forty years of age from cardiac failure, respiratory infection, or hemoptysis. The natural course of disease in these patients has been well documented by Wood.

Three other variants of ventricular septal defect occur. Spontaneous closure occurs in a significant percentage of small defects, more frequently than previously thought. This may explain the rarity with which patients are seen in adult life with small defects. Closure apparently occurs from progressive fibrosis and contraction.

An increased susceptibility to bacterial endocarditis has been long recognized with ventricular defects and is the only known physiologic handicap from a small one. The susceptibility results from the jet of blood through the defect striking the right ventricular wall; bacterial fungations form here. The estimated frequency of the disease varies widely, from 15 to 30 percent, but the risk emphasizes the importance of prophylactic chemotherapy.

Patients with mild infundibular stenosis and a ventricular septal defect are in the midportion of the spectrum of malformations extending from ventricular septal defect at one end to tetralogy of Fallot at the other. The clinical picture varies with severity of the infundibular stenosis. As long as the infundibular stenosis is mild, pulmonary blood flow exceeds systemic blood flow, and the patient is acyanotic. However, if infundibular stenosis is more severe, with a systemic blood flow greater than pulmonary blood flow, cyanosis develops. Cases in this intermediate zone are often termed *acyanotic* tetralogies of Fallot.

The ultimate life expectancy of patients with a ventricular septal defect is unknown, but it appears that average life expectancy of patients with a pulmonary blood flow more than twice the systemic blood flow is near forty years of age. Death is from pulmonary hypertension, cardiac failure, or endocarditis.

CLINICAL MANIFESTATIONS. Symptoms. Patients with a small ventricular septal defect (0.3 to 0.8 cm in diameter) are often asymptomatic and enjoy unrestricted physical activity. Those with larger defects are usually symptomatic. Dyspnea on exertion with easy fatigability is most common, often accompanied by frequent pulmonary infections. Severe cardiac failure is usually seen only in infants or in adults, although chronic pulmonary congestion may occur throughout early childhood. Hemoptysis occurs only in older children or adults with severe pulmonary hypertension. In these unfortunate patients it is a frequent cause of death in the third and fourth decades.

Physical Findings. A loud, harsh, pansystolic murmur is typically present along the left sternal border in the third and fourth intercostal spaces. Frequently a thrill is palpable. The pulmonic second sound varies with pulmonary vascular resistance and may even be palpable when pulmonary vascular resistance is markedly elevated. Intensity of the systolic murmur also varies with the pulmonary vascular resistance, diminishing in many patients as the pulmonary vascular resistance increases. In some patients there is a paradoxic variation between signs and symptoms: pronounced physical findings with a loud murmur and thrill in an asymptomatic child, but a murmur of less intensity without a thrill with severe pulmonary hypertension.

Retardation of growth may be obvious, accompanied by

rales from chronic pulmonary congestion and hepatic enlargement. Some cardiac enlargement is regularly present. When severe, it may produce a visible deformity of the left costal cartilages. Basal diastolic murmurs are infrequent but can originate from two sources: A murmur of aortic insufficiency can develop from prolapse of an aortic cusp into the underlying ventricular septal defect. Alternately, a murmur resulting from pulmonic insufficiency may appear with far advanced pulmonary hypertension.

LABORATORY FINDINGS. The chest roentgenogram with a small ventricular septal defect is usually normal. With larger defects, enlargement of both ventricles becomes visible, especially as pulmonary vascular resistance increases. When the pulmonary blood flow is significantly increased, there is visible enlargement of the pulmonary artery and its tributaries, pulmonary congestion, and enlargement of the left atrium.

The electrocardiogram varies with both the pulmonary blood flow and the pulmonary vascular resistance. With a small defect it is normal. A large pulmonary blood flow produces left ventricular hypertrophy, while an increase in pulmonary vascular resistance induces right ventricular hypertrophy. Often hypertrophy of both ventricles is evident, and the axis of the electrocardiogram varies with the relative degree of ventricular hypertrophy. Predominant right ventricular hypertrophy and a right axis deviation appear with severe pulmonary hypertension.

Cardiac catheterization confirms the diagnosis and assesses the extent of the left-to-right shunt and the pulmonary vascular resistance. A rise in oxygen saturation of more than 1 vol % between the right atrium and the right ventricle establishes the diagnosis, and calculation of the ratio between the pulmonary blood flow and the systemic blood flow will indicate both the size of the shunt and the pulmonary vascular resistance. At times the catheter may actually traverse the septal defect. Selective angiography, usually by injection of dye directly into the left ventricle from a catheter advanced from the aorta across the aortic valve, can opacify the defect.

DIAGNOSIS. The diagnosis is suggested by the loud systolic murmur along the left sternal border, often with a thrill. Similar physical findings may be present with aortic stenosis in infancy, infundibular pulmonic stenosis, or an ostium primum defect. An atrial septal defect usually has a softer systolic murmur near the base of the heart. Confirmation of the diagnosis requires cardiac catheterization, although the changes in the chest roentgenogram and electrocardiogram are helpful.

TREATMENT. Indications for Operation. In infancy, operation is considered only with severe congestive failure and failure to gain weight. Fortunately, this occurs in only a small percentage of patients. Formerly, when operation was done, banding of the pulmonary artery was preferred. As this significantly increases the risk of later closure of the defect, direct closure in infants, especially after six months of age, is being done more often.

Beyond infancy, operation should be performed when the pulmonary blood flow is more than one and one-half to two times greater than normal. Postponement of operation results in cardiac hypertrophy, possibly produces pulmonary vascular changes, and risks bacterial endocarditis. The preferred age for such operations has been about five or six years, but with the very low operative risk in the absence of pulmonary hypertension there has been a progressive tendency to operate at an earlier age, especially if there are any symptoms or retardation of growth. If pulmonary hypertension is present, operation is preferred between one and two years of age to avoid permanent injury to the pulmonary vasculature.

Operation has not often been recommended in asymptomatic patients with a normal roentgenogram and pulmonary blood flow only about 1½ times systemic blood flow. These patients, however, have a permanent susceptibility to bacterial endocarditis, and with the increasing safety of operative closure of ventricular defects, such children will probably be operated upon more frequently in the future.

When pulmonary vascular resistance approaches systemic vascular resistance, with the development of a right-to-left shunt producing cyanosis and clubbing, the condition becomes inoperable: The surgical mortality rate is great, with little improvement in the elevated pulmonary vascular resistance in surviving patients. The absolute criteria of inoperability vary with different institutions, but generally the risk is great and benefit small once pulmonary vascular resistance is greater than one-half systemic resistance.

Technique of Operation. Operation is usually performed through a median sternotomy incision with extracorporeal circulation. The presence of a patent ductus arteriosus, a commonly associated defect in infants, must be carefully determined. This usually can be done by preoperative catheterization and angiography. If uncertainty remains, the ligamentum arteriosum should be dissected from an intrapericardial approach before the ventricle is incised. In selecting the ventriculotomy site, probably the most important consideration is to avoid division of *any* obvious coronary arteries. The course of the anterior descending coronary artery is carefully marked beforehand. This consideration is more significant than whether a transverse, longitudinal, or oblique ventriculotomy is made. The author has employed all types and prefers a transverse or oblique one but always avoiding division of any obvious coronary artery. If a longitudinal ventriculotomy is made, it should be located near the anterior descending coronary artery in order to devascularize as small an area of myocardium as possible.

Rarely, the arrangement of the coronary arteries is such that a satisfactory ventriculotomy cannot be made. Hence a transatrial approach through the tricuspid valve must be used. With severe pulmonary hypertension and increased pulmonary vascular resistance a transatrial approach is also preferred, in order to preserve function of the right ventricle following operation. This approach, however, is more awkward.

During bypass, a vent is inserted into the apex of the left ventricle to aspirate blood from the operative field. Intermittent cardiac ischemia is employed by clamping the aorta for 10 to 12 minutes, at a temperature of 30 to 32°C, to still the heart and identify the anatomic features surrounding the defect. Longer periods of ischemia are not

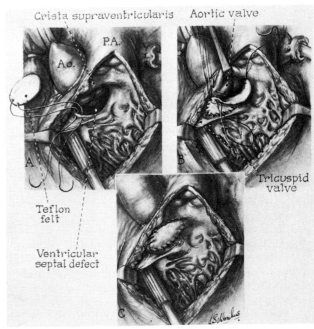

Fig. 18-32. *A.* Ventricular septal defect exposed through longitudinal ventriculotomy. Cusps of aortic valve are clearly visible through large defect. Closure is carried out with prosthetic patch of Teflon felt. First sutures are inserted in posterosuperior margin where conduction bundle is located. Often sutures are placed to right of margin of defect, through base of septal leaflet of tricuspid valve. Heart is beating while sutures are inserted, in order to observe conduction disturbances on electrocardiogram. *B.* Subsequent sutures around margins of defect may be interrupted or continuous sutures. In aortic valve area, care is taken to insert sutures directly into aortic annulus, avoiding injury to valve cusps. *C.* Final position of prosthetic patch.

employed, however, for monitoring of the electrocardiogram is a most important safeguard against production of complete heart block. This is the most serious complication associated with closure of a ventricular septal defect and can best be avoided by observing the electrocardiogram during insertion of sutures. Surgical repair is undoubtedly facilitated by induction of cardiac arrest, but one cannot be totally certain that a heart block is being avoided if the electrocardiogram is not monitored. On the author's service there have been no complete heart blocks in the past decade.

After identification of the septal defect, usually in the membranous septum posterior to the crista supraventricularis, closure is done with an oval patch of knitted Dacron inserted with 10 to 15 mattress sutures of 4-0 silk or synthetic sutures, which are placed circumferentially about the rim. About 3 mm of tissue are included in each suture (Fig. 18-32). Posteriorly, the sutures are inserted through the base of the septal leaflet of the tricuspid valve and to the right of the posterior margin of the defect, especially at the posterior superior angle where the conduction bundle is located. A useful surgical guide for avoiding the conduction bundle, described to the author by Barratt-Boyes, is to identify the fibrous trigone located at the bottom of the noncoronary aortic sinus, inspecting this area through the ventricular septal defect with a dry, still operative field. The conduction bundle passes through this fibrous trigone and is often visible as well as palpable, after which the portion to the left ventricle travels to the left. Projecting an imaginary line between the fibrous trigone and the papillary muscle of the conus and subsequently inserting sutures to the right of this line avoid injury to the conduction bundle. This can be confirmed by observing the electrocardiogram after the sutures are inserted but before the prosthetic patch is tied in position.

Superiorly, sutures are inserted into the aortic annulus for security, clearly visualizing the aortic cusps to avoid injury. Following insertion of the patch, adequacy of closure, as well as the presence of additional defects, is checked by temporarily occluding the aorta, aspirating air, and forcefully injecting saline solution retrograde through the left ventricular vent into the left ventricle. If this technique is carefully carried out, the ventricular septum is forcefully distended, and additional defects can be identified. This technique, thus far unpublished, has been a valuable adjunct and has identified additional defects in several patients.

Subsequently, after closure of the ventriculotomy and stopping cardiopulmonary bypass, oxygen content of blood samples from the right atrium and pulmonary artery are compared to confirm elimination of all left-to-right shunts.

Rarely, ventricular septal defects occur in other locations, as mentioned earlier. These areas should be routinely examined at operation. The retrograde saline solution injection test is especially useful, however, and has proved much more reliable than inspection or palpation.

The combination of ventricular septal defect with aortic insufficiency from prolapse of an aortic valve cusp is rare. The lesion is often a progressive one from continued herniation of an aortic valve cusp, usually the right coronary cusp, into the underlying ventricular septal defect. Surgical correction, though not always totally effective, usually can be done without insertion of a prosthetic aortic valve, even though some aortic insufficiency remains. A detailed report of the author's experience with this condition, in association with Bahnson and Weldon who employed a similar technique at their universities, was published in 1973 (Fig. 18-33).

Postoperative Course. A temporary pacemaker wire is routinely left in the ventricle before the thoracotomy incision is closed. If bradycardia appears, with a rate lower than 70 to 80 per minute, pacing is done for 1 to 2 days, as necessary. Transitory conduction disturbances often subside within 24 to 48 hours. A report some years ago by Lillehei et al. indicates the grim prognosis with complete heart block. If a complete heart block persists for as long as 3 weeks after operation, a permanent pacemaker should be inserted before the patient is discharged from the hospital, for the risk of sudden death is great even though the patient is asymptomatic.

Digitalis is usually given after operation, as some degree of right ventricular failure is common, especially if significant pulmonary hypertension was present. In most patients convalescence is uneventful.

The risk of operation increases if pulmonary vascular resistance is increased, but with earlier diagnosis and treatment such complicated problems are fortunately becoming rare. With normal pulmonary vascular resistance, postoperative mortalities as low as 1 to 2 percent have been reported. Similar results have been obtained at New York University. However, when the pulmonary vascular resistance is significantly elevated, the risk of operation rises, approaching 15 to 30 percent if pulmonary vascular resistance is as much as one-half systemic resistance.

Following recovery from operation, patients without an increase in pulmonary vascular resistance have a dramatic regression of all signs of cardiac disease. Heart size and the vascularity of the lung fields both return to normal. A right bundle branch block usually persists on the electrocardiogram as a consequence of insertion of sutures to the right of the margin of the septal defect. Life expectancy is probably that of a normal person. In patients with increased pulmonary vascular resistance, there may be regression in some. In general, the pulmonary vascular resistance decreases in about one-third of the patients, remains stationary in about one-third, and actually increases in the remainder, probably representing an inherent disease in the pulmonary vasculature separate from that due to the previous left-to-right shunt.

Patent Ductus Arteriosus

HISTORICAL DATA. Gibson, in Edinburgh, first reported in 1900 the classic clinical findings of a patent ductus arteriosus, but it was not until 1937 that Strieder first attempted ligation of the ductus in a patient with bacterial endocarditis. This patient died on the fourth postoperative day, but the following year Gross successfully ligated the patent ductus of a seven-year-old girl.

INCIDENCE AND ETIOLOGY. Patent ductus arteriosus is one of the most common forms of congenital heart disease, occurring once in about every 4,000 births and constituting about 15 percent of all cases of congenital heart disease. For unknown reasons it is two to three times more frequent in females than in males.

The patent ductus arteriosus, which develops as an embryologic remnant of the sixth left aortic arch, is an important normal fetal pathway connecting the pulmonary artery at its bifurcation to the aorta just beyond the origin of the left subclavian artery. Through this channel in embryonic life blood bypasses the collapsed lungs, flowing directly from the pulmonary artery into the aorta. With the expansion of the lungs at birth, the ductus normally closes within a few days, remaining in older patients as the fibrotic ligamentum arteriosum. The physiologic stimuli responsible for closure of the ductus have been studied in detail. Apparently changes in oxygen tension of the arterial blood exert a profound stimulus on the closure. The most important cause of closure, however, is probably related to the distinctive histologic structure of the wall of the ductus, which is different from that of either the pulmonary artery or the aorta. As the ductus closes, the wall of the ductus contracts, the internal elastic membrane fragments, and smooth muscle projects into the lumen as progressive fibrosis obliterates the patent channel.

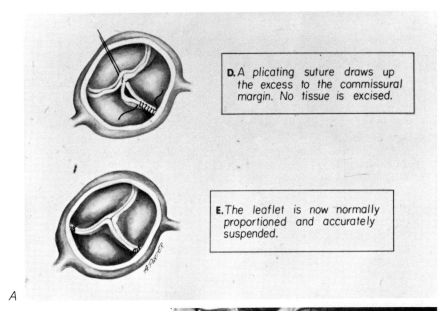

D. A plicating suture draws up the excess to the commissural margin. No tissue is excised.

E. The leaflet is now normally proportioned and accurately suspended.

A

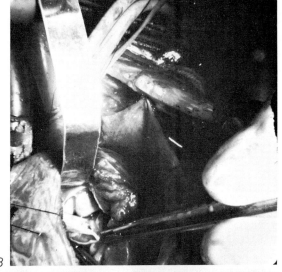

B

Fig. 18-33. *A.* Diagram of concept of one method of repair of the prolapsed valve cusp, developed by Weldon at Washington University in St. Louis. *B.* Operative view of the prolapsed aortic cusp through a right ventriculotomy, showing the cusp prolapsing into the ventricular septal defect. Partial occlusion of the ventricular septal defect by the prolapsing cusp is one reason that the left-to-right shunt is not large. *C.* Pre- and postoperative aortograms showing massive aortic insufficiency before operation and no insufficiency whatever several months later.

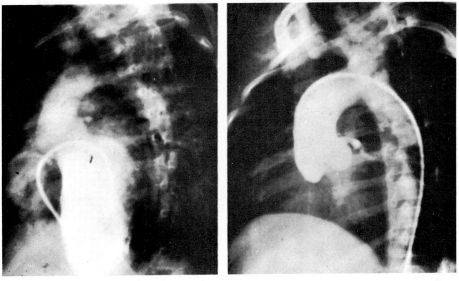

C

If rubella occurs during the first trimester of pregnancy, a well-recognized syndrome of congenital defects can occur, including mental retardation, cataracts, and a patent ductus. For the majority of patients, however, the cause of persistent patency is unknown.

PATHOLOGIC ANATOMY. The diameter of a ductus ranges from as small as 2 to 3 mm to greater than 1 cm. Usually it is 5 to 7 mm. The length is usually slightly greater than the width, although in some cases the ductus is unusually short, creating some technical hazard at the time of surgical correction (Fig. 18-34).

Associated anomalies occur in approximately 15 percent of cases; the most common are ventricular septal defect and coarctation of the aorta.

PATHOPHYSIOLOGY. Depending upon the diameter of the ductus, a varying amount of blood is shunted from the aorta to the pulmonary artery, constituting a left-to-right shunt. In a large ductus, the shunt may constitute 50 to 70 percent of the output from the left ventricle, with resulting decrease of blood flow to other tissues and retardation of development. With such large shunts, the pulmonary blood flow may reach levels as high as 10 to 15 liters/minute. The symptomatology is directly proportional to the size of the shunt.

A large patent ductus in infants may result in serious or even lethal heart failure. However, after the age of two years heart failure is rare until adult life, although symptoms of limited cardiac reserve may occur.

In infancy the high pulmonary vascular resistance of fetal life subsides gradually in the first 1 to 2 years after birth. During this time only a systolic murmur may be audible. In some infants the increased pulmonary blood flow from the ductus causes the pulmonary vascular resistance to remain elevated and even increase, with resulting pulmonary hypertension. Usually the pulmonary vascular resistance will decrease to normal levels following surgical division of the ductus, but in older patients only a partial regression toward normal levels may occur. With a long-neglected patent ductus pulmonary resistance may, rarely, increase to exceed systemic vascular resistance, resulting in a "reversed" ductus, with blood flowing from the pulmonary artery to the descending thoracic aorta to produce cyanosis in the lower half of the body. Fortunately this is now almost unknown, for diagnosis and treatment are carried out at an early age.

An unusual feature of a patent ductus is susceptibility to development of bacterial endocarditis from viridans streptococci. Although this is most common in the second or third decade, it may occur rarely in children. It has been estimated that in untreated cases such an infection would ultimately develop in 20 to 25 percent of patients. The localization of the infection apparently is related to turbulent blood flow where blood forcefully ejected from the aorta through the ductus strikes the wall of the pulmonary artery. The fungations of bacterial endocarditis usually begin in this location, with septicemia initially limited to the lungs until systemic spread occurs. Fortunately such infections can usually be promptly controlled with antibiotic therapy.

With the dual tendency to develop either heart failure or bacterial endocarditis, it has been estimated that the life expectancy of a seventeen-year-old patient with a patent ductus is approximately one-half that of a normal individual.

CLINICAL MANIFESTATIONS. Symptoms. In infants a large patent ductus may cause serious heart failure, but many older children are asymptomatic. When symptoms are present, the most common are palpitations, fatigue, and dyspnea. More definite symptoms of congestive heart failure are usually seen only in adult patients. In the female these often appear during the first pregnancy.

Physical Examination. The hallmark of a patent ductus is the continuous murmur. This murmur is one of the most distinctive signs in clinical medicine, and usually a patent ductus can be diagnosed with confidence simply on this basis. Because of the continuous quality of the murmur it is often described as a "machinery" murmur. It is a harsh, rasping sound, accentuated in systole and diminishing in diastole. It is best heard in the second left intercostal space but is normally widely transmitted over the chest and into the neck. In many patients the murmur is so loud that it is associated with a palpable thrill. Often in infants either no murmur or only a systolic murmur can be heard until the age of one or two years, after which a continuous murmur may be detected for the first time. The absence of the diastolic component of the murmur during infancy is due to persistent elevation of the pulmonary vascular resistance, which limits flow of blood through the ductus during diastole.

A wide pulse pressure is usually found with a large

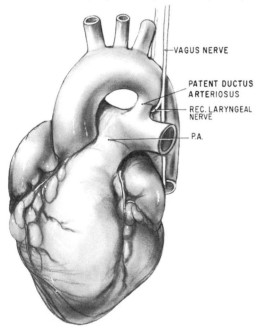

Fig. 18-34. Patent ductus arteriosus as regularly found just distal to left subclavian artery between aorta and pulmonary artery. It is encircled by recurrent laryngeal nerve, a useful surgical landmark in isolating patent ductus in mediastinal tissues. (*Adapted from R. E. Gross, "The Surgery of Infancy and Childhood," W. B. Saunders Company, Philadelphia, 1953, p. 807.*)

VAGUS NERVE

PATENT DUCTUS ARTERIOSUS

REC. LARYNGEAL NERVE

P.A.

ductus, resulting from a decrease in diastolic pressure. In the extremely large ductus the diastolic pressure may approach very low levels and be associated with peripheral vascular findings similar to those of severe aortic insufficiency.

Cyanosis is never present with an uncomplicated patent ductus. The presence of cyanosis indicates either an associated cardiac anomaly, such as tetralogy of Fallot, or a marked increase in pulmonary vascular resistance, either from progressive sclerosis of the pulmonary arteriolar bed or from congestive heart failure. The severity of the arterial hypoxia which can result from heart failure in infants often has not been recognized. Arterial oxygen saturations as low as 75% may occur with the severe pulmonary congestion of heart failure.

LABORATORY FINDINGS. With a small patent ductus the chest roentgenogram may be normal. With a larger ductus the pulmonary conus is prominent, the left ventricle is enlarged, and the pulmonary vascular markings are increased, all indicating a large left-to-right shunt. On fluoroscopy a "hilar dance" may be observed. The electrocardiogram is often normal with a small ductus but will show left ventricular hypertrophy with a larger one. Cardiac catheterization can readily localize the left-to-right shunt to the pulmonary artery and differentiate the condition from a ventricular septal defect or an atrial septal defect. Often with appropriate manipulation the cardiac catheter can be passed through the patent ductus, visually confirming the diagnosis. Aortography is the most definitive diagnostic measure, visually demonstrating the flow of dye from the aorta through the ductus into the pulmonary arteries (Fig. 18-35). It is of particular value with severe pulmonary hypertension, when only a systolic murmur may be audible.

DIAGNOSIS. In most patients the diagnosis can be made with confidence from the clinical findings combined with the chest roentgenogram and the electrocardiogram. Cardiac catheterization or aortography should be employed when atypical features are present. This usually occurs in infants with severe pulmonary hypertension or with associated cardiovascular anomalies.

There are several rare conditions which may produce a continuous murmur simulating a patent ductus arteriosus and requiring cardiac catheterization and angiography for differentiation from a patent ductus. These include an aortic-pulmonary window, a ventricular septal defect with a prolapsed cusp causing aortic insufficiency, a ruptured aneurysm of the sinus of Valsalva, and a coronary arteriovenous fistula. Most of these conditions create a physiologic left-to-right shunt and hence a continuous murmur simulating a patent ductus.

TREATMENT. In most patients over two to three years of age, a patent ductus should be surgically corrected as soon as convenient after the diagnosis has been made. The operative risk is low and the results are excellent. In infants, operation should be performed if serious heart failure is present.

The only contraindication to operation, rarely seen, is cyanosis. Cyanosis may be due to an associated cardiac anomaly such as tetralogy of Fallot, in which case the

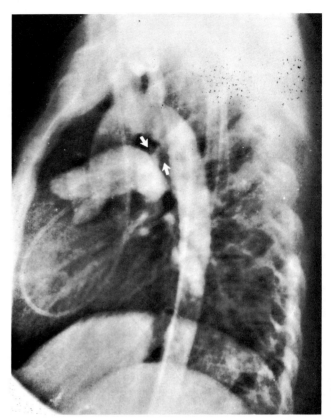

Fig. 18-35. Aortogram performed by injection of dye into aorta demonstrates patent ductus arteriosus, as indicated by arrows, with opacification of pulmonary artery. (*Courtesy of Dr. Raymond M. Abrams, Department of Radiology, New York University Medical Center.*)

patent ductus is an important ancillary source of blood flow to the lungs. Cyanosis can also develop with a reversed ductus when pulmonary vascular resistance has increased to exceed systemic vascular resistance, as a result of which blood flows from the pulmonary artery to the aorta and creates cyanosis in the lower half of the body. A reversed ductus cannot be safely closed, for the patent ductus partly decreases the pulmonary hypertension, shunting blood from the pulmonary artery to the aorta. Attempted surgical closure usually results in immediate death. Fortunately, with early operations for patent ductus, such advanced pulmonary vascular disease is almost unknown.

With bacterial endocarditis, intensive antibiotic therapy will effect cure in most patients; operation can then be more safely performed several weeks later. If the endocarditis cannot be controlled with antibiotic therapy, operation should be undertaken as a last resort, although operations upon a friable, infected ductus have a high mortality rate from hemorrhage or subsequent infection.

Operative Technique. Operation may be satisfactorily performed with either a left anterolateral thoracotomy in the third intercostal space or a posterolateral thoracotomy in the fourth intercostal space. A posterolateral thoracotomy provides a more extensive operative field and is pre-

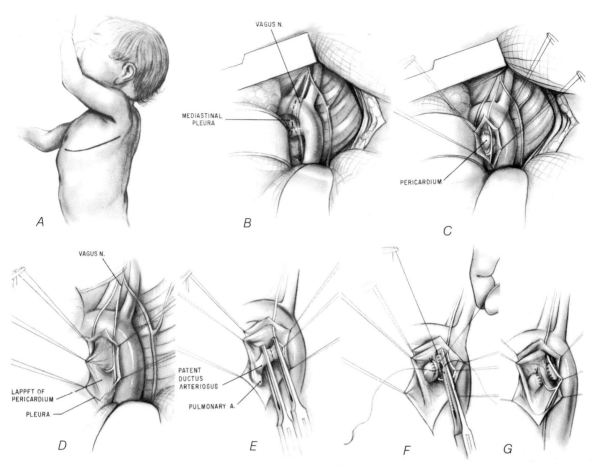

Fig. 18-36. Division of patent ductus arteriosus. *A.* Chest is opened with left posterolateral incision in fourth intercostal space. *B.* Once lung has been retracted, mediastinal pleura is incised longitudinally parallel to vagus nerve. *C.* Initial dissection is along vagus nerve to expose widely the recurrent laryngeal nerve originating from vagus and passing beneath ductus. Wide exposure of recurrent laryngeal nerve is essential part of operative procedure. *D.* After dissection of recurrent laryngeal nerve, lappet of pericardium overlying ductus is freed by sharp dissection proximally to expose pulmonary artery. *E.* Subsequently ductus is encircled, and vascular occlusion clamps are applied. *F.* Ductus is gradually divided and sutured, employing two rows of sutures. *G.* Final view of divided ends of ductus with recurrent laryngeal nerve well exposed.

ferred. The author's preferred operative technique is shown in detail in Fig. 18-36.

A difficult and dangerous technical problem may develop with patients in the third and fourth decade in whom pulmonary hypertension is present and sclerosis or even calcification of the ductus has appeared. In such patients laceration of the friable ductus at its junction with the pulmonary artery quickly results in fatal hemorrhage. Such problems are best approached with a temporary left atrial–femoral artery bypass. Once bypass has been instituted the aorta can be safely clamped above and below the ductus, which can then be occluded with a single clamp near its junction with the aorta. Subsequent division of the ductus at its point of origin from the aorta can be followed by suture of the two ends.

Ligation of a patent ductus with multiple ligatures, as developed by Blalock, is now rarely used but is a safe and effective technique. It should not be used for a short, wide ductus, especially with elevated pressure in the pulmonary artery. The original technique included four separate ligatures, initially placing two purse strings at the aortic and pulmonary artery ends of the ductus, and subsequently interposing two transfixion ligatures on the remaining portions of the ductus between the two purse-string sutures.

In 1971 the author treated a sixty-five-year-old patient with congestive failure and extensive calcification of both the aorta and a large patent ductus. Even simple appli-

cation of vascular clamps to the calcified vessels seemed unduly hazardous. Accordingly, the ductus was effectively obliterated with multiple mattress sutures placed through Teflon felt surrounding the ductus. The patient has subsequently remained well.

For the vast majority of patients, simple division and suture is preferred. A useful technical point is the application of a partial occlusion vascular clamp onto the aorta a few millimeters from the ductus, rather than placing the clamp on the ductus itself. This variation avoids the problem of a short ductus and greatly simplifies operative division and suture.

Postoperative Course. With an uncomplicated ductus, the operative risk is surprisingly small. As early as 1953 Gross reported experience with 611 patients, with a mortality rate of less than 0.5 percent in those with neither cardiac failure nor infection before operation. Similar figures were described by Jones in a total series of 909 patients. When patent ductus is associated with other abnormalities, a condition encountered in infants with cardiac failure, operative mortality is higher. At New York University there has been no mortality or serious complications following division of an uncomplicated patent ductus in several years.

Convalescence following operation is usually uneventful, most patients leaving the hospital within 7 to 10 days. A functional systolic murmur may remain audible in a few patients. This may be related to a localized irregularity in the wall of the pulmonary artery where the ductus was present. The electrocardiogram usually returns to normal within a few months. From data now available from over 25 years' experience, it appears that cardiac function becomes normal once the ductus has been surgically obliterated.

RIGHT-TO-LEFT SHUNTS (CYANOTIC GROUP)

Tetralogy of Fallot

HISTORICAL DATA. Tetralogy of Fallot was described as long ago as 1671 by Stensen, but it was not until 1888 that the combination of abnormalities regularly present was emphasized by Fallot. Effective therapy first became possible in 1944, when Blalock dramatically demonstrated that much benefit could be obtained by anastomosis of the subclavian artery and pulmonary artery to create an artificial ductus arteriosus. This operation was developed following the suggestion of Taussig, who had noted an increase in symptoms in infants when a patent ductus arteriosus spontaneously closed. Thereafter the operation was referred to as the *Blalock-Taussig procedure*. It constitutes one of the milestones in cardiac surgery. Subsequently over 1,500 such procedures were performed at the Johns Hopkins Hospital, and experience with these operations led to the development of many other aspects of cardiac surgery. Subsequent contributions were made by Potts et al., who developed an aortic-pulmonary side-to-side anastomosis, especially applicable to infants, and by Brock, who introduced partial excision of the infundibular obstruction. With the development of extracorporeal circulation, correction of the tetralogy first became possible in 1954–1955 and is now the preferred operation.

INCIDENCE AND ETIOLOGY. Tetralogy of Fallot is one of the most common cyanotic malformations, constituting over 50 percent of all cases of cyanotic heart disease. In cyanotic children who survive beyond the first 2 years of life, a tetralogy of Fallot is present in 70 to 75 percent. There are no known etiologic factors.

PATHOLOGIC ANATOMY. The four features of the tetralogy from which the name originates are obstruction of the outflow tract of the right ventricle, a ventricular septal defect, dextroposition of the aorta, and hypertrophy of the right ventricle. The right ventricular obstruction is severe enough to increase right ventricular systolic pressure to equal left ventricular systolic pressure. The ventricular septal defect is large (2 to 3 cm), approximately equaling the diameter of the orifice of the aortic valve. Right ventricular hypertrophy is the natural consequence of the severe obstruction to emptying of the right ventricle; dextroposition of the aorta is an anatomic variant of probably little physiologic significance.

The right ventricular obstruction may be an infundibular stenosis, a valvular stenosis, or a combined lesion (Fig. 18-37). Often it is a localized obstruction, although less frequently a diffuse stenosis of the entire right ventricular outflow tract is present. In one series of patients, Brock found a localized infundibular stenosis in slightly less than 50 percent of patients, a valvular stenosis in 35 percent, and a combined lesion in 22 percent. The pulmonary artery is often smaller than normal, while the diameter of the aorta is larger than normal. When a localized infundibular stenosis is present, an "infundibular chamber" exists between the right ventricle proximal to the stenosis and the pulmonary valve distad.

The ventricular septal defect is almost always located proximal to the crista supraventricularis and is usually 2 to 3 cm in diameter. The aortic cusps are readily seen through the defect, varying with the degree of dextroposition which is present.

With the decrease in pulmonary blood flow, there is striking enlargement of the bronchial arteries and other routes of collateral circulation to the lungs, creating extensive varicosities throughout the mediastinum and chest wall. In some older children with severe cyanosis, a progressive occlusive disease also develops in the peripheral pulmonary arteries. Absence of the left pulmonary artery has been found in a small number of patients, and in others one or more focal stenoses may be found in either one or both the pulmonary arteries. The frequency of these additional malformations is not yet known, because they have been recognized only with the advent of selective angiocardiography.

Anomalous coronary arteries are also frequent, especially in the outflow tract of the right ventricle, where they are of particular surgical significance. A right aortic arch, for unknown reasons, occurs in about 25 percent of patients. An atrial septal defect is also frequent, at times referred to as part of a pentalogy of Fallot, although the malformation differs little physiologically from the tetralogy. It is noteworthy that although a patent ductus arteriosus may be essential to life, it gradually closes in almost all patients during the first few months of life, often with a disastrous increase in the severity of anoxia.

PATHOPHYSIOLOGY. Physiologically, a tetralogy of Fallot is a combination of a large ventricular septal defect with an obstruction in the right ventricular outflow tract of sufficient severity to elevate right ventricular systolic pressure to equal left ventricular systolic pressure. Venous blood entering the right ventricle then is shunted directly into the aorta to produce cyanosis. In addition to cyanosis, the malformation decreases pulmonary blood flow and hence limits the ability of the lungs to absorb oxygen. The

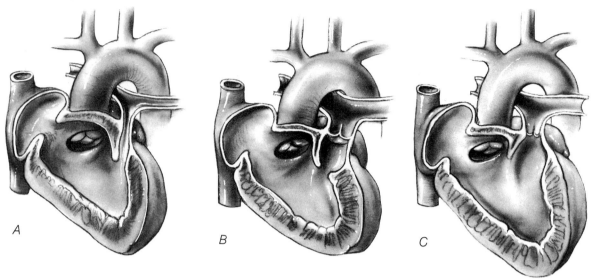

basis for the severe intolerance of exercise. The large
ventricular septal defect has a separate influence, in that
right ventricular pressure almost never exceeds left ventricular pressure, in contrast to isolated pulmonic valvular
stenosis. Hence cardiac enlargement and cardiac failure are
rare. Only a few unusual patients have been reported in
whom the malformation was such that right ventricular
pressure exceeded left ventricular pressure.

The severity of the anoxia varies with the degree of
reduction in pulmonary blood flow. Arterial oxygen saturations of 70 to 85% are seen in older children, but in
younger children, who may not survive through infancy
without operation, astonishingly low arterial oxygen saturations are encountered. Saturations of 30 to 35% may be
seen in patients who can walk only a short distance, and
levels of 20 to 25% are found in some infants who are
unable to walk. Saturations as low as 10% have been
recorded, usually associated with loss of consciousness
from cerebral anoxia. With exercise, there is often a precipitous fall in arterial oxygen saturation, decreasing from
a resting level of 70% to 20 to 25%, which clearly indicates
the physiologic basis for exertional dyspnea.

Chronic anoxia produces compensatory polycythemia
and, subsequently, clubbing of the extremities. Polycythemia is seldom apparent until after two years of age, but
later hematocrit readings varying from 60 to 75 percent
are common. Wide variations in hematocrit readings are
found, ranging from normal with mild tetralogies to readings as high as 85 to 90 percent in the most severe forms.

The degree of cyanosis increases significantly in the first
few years of life, for visible cyanosis is proportional to the
number of grams of unsaturated hemoglobin in the peripheral circulation and not to the actual oxygen concentration. Hence severe cyanosis is visible only after polycythemia has developed. The time of appearance has been
used by Nadas for a convenient grouping of the clinical
course of the disease. About one-third of patients are
cyanotic at birth, another one-third become cyanotic in the
first year of life, and one-third develop cyanosis only sub-

Fig. 18-37. Different types of right ventricular obstruction in tetralogy of Fallot. *A.* Combined obstruction from hypoplasia of pulmonic annulus in association with diffuse stenosis of outflow tract
of right ventricle. This type of diffuse stenosis is commonly found
and often requires insertion of prosthetic patch to widen annulus.
B. Localized stenosis of infundibulum of right ventricle, with
"infundibular chamber" distal to this which is proximal to normal
pulmonic valve. *C.* Pulmonic stenosis of valvular type in association with normal right ventricular outflow tract. (*Adapted from C.
D. Benson et al., "Pediatric Surgery," vol. I, Year Book Medical
Publishers, Inc., Chicago, 1962, p. 463.*)

sequently in childhood. Patients who are cyanotic at birth
have severe anoxia and often do not survive infancy unless
operation is performed. Patients who become cyanotic in
the first year of life have a milder course but are seriously
disabled, while those who develop cyanosis in later years
may have little incapacity and little polycythemia—a so-
called "pink" tetralogy. These patients, of course, have
only moderate reduction in pulmonary blood flow.

The main threat to life in the first years of life is a
cerebral vascular accident, either from cerebral thrombosis
or from a localized infarct from anoxia. In severe cases,
cyanotic "spells" are seen in which the infant becomes
deeply cyanotic and comatose. Spontaneous recovery usually occurs, but death or hemiplegia may ensue.

Brain abscess is another serious, often lethal, complication to which patients are peculiarly susceptible. The
right-to-left shunt, bypassing the lungs and providing direct access for bacteria into the venous blood to the arterial
circulation, is the most convenient explanation of the high
incidence of brain abscess, although localized cerebral
infarcts may also play a role in etiology.

Cardiac failure is extremely rare with the tetralogy, and
its presence always brings into question the accuracy of
the diagnosis. It is seen in a few adults in the second or
third decade but is virtually unknown in children. There
is also a susceptibility to bacterial endocarditis, as with
other cardiac malformations.

Life expectancy without treatment is relatively short.
Infants cyanotic at birth formerly seldom lived beyond the
first decade. Those becoming cyanotic in the first year of

life might survive to early adult life, while those becoming cyanotic in later years would occasionally survive into the third or fourth decade or, rarely, beyond. In older, chronically cyanotic patients, other physiologic signs of chronic anoxia appear, with disturbances in the blood-clotting mechanism and secondary hemorrhage in the gastrointestinal tract.

CLINICAL MANIFESTATIONS. Symptoms. Almost all patients are symptomatic. Dyspnea and cyanosis, markedly aggravated by exertion, are the outstanding features. Two additional characteristics are cyanotic spells and squatting. Cyanotic spells are episodes of sudden increase in intensity of cyanosis, followed by unconsciousness, usually with spontaneous recovery within a few minutes or hours. Such episodes, representing acute cerebral anoxia, may be fatal or may result in hemiplegia. They are frequent in infants but seldom occur in older children, probably because symptomatic infants seldom survive without treatment. Squatting is an impressive characteristic, for children learn quickly to relieve dyspnea by assuming a squatting position. The physiologic benefit from squatting, apparently a redistribution of blood flow, is not clear. Walking for short distances, interrupted by squatting, is a well-recognized hallmark of the tetralogy. Hemoptysis is a rare symptom, occurring usually in older children with marked varicosities of the bronchial circulation.

Physical Examination. On physical examination the obvious features are cyanosis of varying severity and clubbing of the digits. The heart usually has a normal size, rate, and rhythm. A systolic murmur of grade II to III intensity is commonly present along the left sternal border at the third or fourth intercostal spaces, and a thrill is present in about one-half the patients. With severe pulmonic stenosis or pulmonary atresia, the murmur may be faint or even absent because of absence of flow through the pulmonic orifice. The second pulmonic sound is weak or absent, while the aortic second sound is increased above normal intensity.

LABORATORY FINDINGS. The chest roentgenogram shows a heart of normal size with an unusual contour, termed the *coeur en sabot,* or sabot-shaped heart (Fig. 18-1). This indicates the characteristic enlargement due to selective hypertrophy of the right ventricle, combined with a concavity in the area where the pulmonary artery is normally located. The lung fields often show decreased vascularity.

The electrocardiogram is always abnormal, showing right ventricular hypertrophy of varying severity with right axis deviation.

Cardiac catheterization demonstrates several characteristic features. A slight left-to-right shunt may be detected at the ventricular level in mild cases, but often no left-to-right intracardiac shunt is present. A large right-to-left shunt is indicated by arterial unsaturation. This can also be confirmed by dye-dilution curves. The right ventricular systolic pressure is usually identical with the left ventricular systolic pressure, while pulmonary artery pressure is decreased below normal levels, resulting in a large systolic pressure gradient between the right ventricle and pulmonary artery. The pulmonary blood flow is decreased,

varying with the severity of the disorder. The degree of decrease in pulmonary blood flow will be found to parallel the severity of the arterial oxygen saturation. The hematocrit reading is usually between 60 and 75 percent, with a range from 45 to 90 percent.

Selective angiocardiography is of great importance in planning surgical correction, for the location of the right ventricular obstruction, either infundibular, valvular, or diffuse, can be outlined. The presence of associated abnormalities in the pulmonary arteries should be particularly noted. Simultaneous opacification of the aorta and pulmonary arteries when dye is injected into the right ventricle is typical of tetralogy of Fallot (Fig. 18-38).

DIAGNOSIS. The diagnosis can usually be made with certainty from clinical examination combined with roentgenogram and electrocardiogram. The important clinical features are cyanosis with severe exertional dyspnea and squatting. The important physical findings are a heart of normal size with a systolic murmur. Roentgenographic findings demonstrate a heart of normal size with decreased vascularity of the lung fields, while the electrocardiogram shows right ventricular hypertrophy.

Other cyanotic conditions to be distinguished from the tetralogy include tricuspid atresia, transposition of the great vessels, and pulmonic valvular stenosis with a patent foramen ovale. Tricuspid atresia can be best differentiated

Fig. 18-38. Cardiac angiogram in patient with tetralogy of Fallot, demonstrating large ventricular septal defect. Dye has been injected through catheter in right ventricle. Dye flows through large ventricular septal defect into left ventricle. Pulmonic stenosis which was present is not visible on this angiogram. (Courtesy of Dr. Raymond M. Abrams, Department of Radiology, New York University Medical Center.)

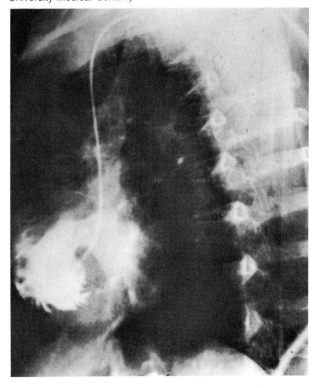

by the electrocardiogram, which characteristically shows a left axis deviation. Transposition may be recognized by the cardiac enlargement and vascular lung fields, although cardiac catheterization may be required. Pulmonic valvular stenosis with a patent foramen ovale is diagnosed by the presence of cardiac enlargement with signs of cardiac failure. The most important feature in differentiating the tetralogy from other cyanotic malformations is the fact that the heart with a tetralogy is of normal size.

TREATMENT. Indications for Operation. Infants with cyanotic spells from anoxia require emergency operation to prevent death or hemiplegia; some type of shunt procedure should be performed. The side-to-side anastomosis between the ascending aorta and the right pulmonary artery, developed by Waterston, is almost always possible unless the right pulmonary artery is absent. In small infants it is usually the procedure of choice, creating a stoma 3 to 4 mm in diameter. Simplicity of closure of the shunt at the time of subsequent surgical correction is also an attractive feature. (Fig. 18-39). However, a serious hazard is that the difference between an adequate shunt and an excessively large shunt, producing serious or even lethal cardiac failure, is small. An aortotomy near 4 mm in length is usually satisfactory, but all reports of such anastomoses in infants describe difficulties from excessively large shunts.

For this reason, the subclavian-pulmonary anastomosis is preferable when the subclavian artery is large enough.

The subclavian artery may occasionally be used in infants and almost always after the first three to four months of life (Fig. 18-40).

The Potts operation of aortic-pulmonary side-to-side anastomosis performed through a left thoracotomy provides a satisfactory shunt but is avoided because of the technical difficulties of dismantling such a shunt at the time of subsequent corrective surgery (Fig. 18-41).

Except when cyanosis and hypoxia are disabling, operative correction is best postponed until the age of four to five years. Some groups are now cautiously exploring the possibility of definitive surgical correction at whatever age operation becomes necessary, even in the first year of life, thus avoiding the necessity for two operative procedures. The complexities of open operative repair in the first two years of life, however, are significant, and so this approach remains somewhat experimental.

Technique of Corrective Operation. A median sternotomy incision is preferred. If a previous shunt operation has been performed, the anastomosis is isolated before extracorporeal circulation is begun and subsequently occluded during bypass before the heart is opened. Once the pericardium has been opened, the outflow tract of the right ventricle is carefully examined for anomalous coronary arteries, selecting an incision in the right ventricle to avoid dividing any such arteries. Only rarely is the anatomy of the coronary circulation such that a ventriculotomy cannot be safely performed. In such instances the approach may

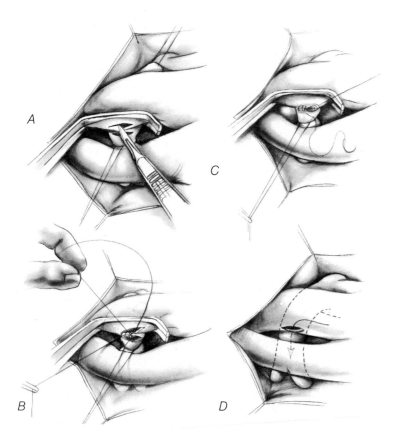

Fig. 18-39. Side-to-side anastomosis between ascending aorta and right pulmonary artery. *A.* Tangential clamp has been applied to ascending aorta, which is then incised for 4 to 5 mm. Corresponding incision is then made in right pulmonary artery, which has been occluded with proximal and distal ligatures. *B.* Posterior row of anastomosis is constructed with continuous suture of 5-0 silk. *C.* Anterior anastomosis may be done with interrupted or continuous sutures. *D.* Diagram of final anastomosis, depicting flow of blood from aorta into pulmonary artery. (*Adapted from D. A. Cooley and G. L. Hallman, "Surgical Treatment of Congenital Heart Disease," Lea & Febiger, Philadelphia, 1966, p. 128.*)

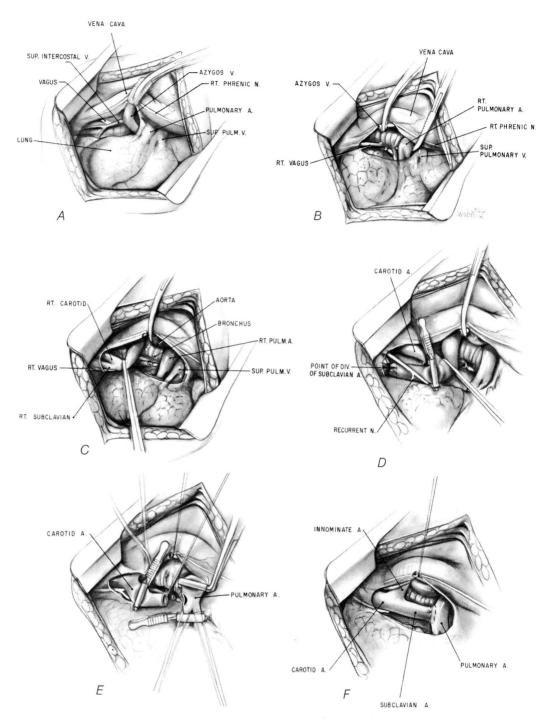

Fig. 18-40. Blalock procedure. *A.* Dissection is begun by isolation of azygos vein, followed by incision of mediastinal pleura in front of pulmonary artery. *B.* Pulmonary artery is isolated in hilum, dissecting artery distally to beyond point of origin of upper lobe branch. Medially, artery is freed well into mediastinum in order to permit displacement of artery superiorly during construction of anastomosis. Traction on stump of divided azygos vein retracts superior vena cava to expose pulmonary artery in mediastinum. *C.* Subclavian artery is mobilized at apex of thorax, mobilizing carotid artery and subclavian artery down into mediastinum. Wide mobilization of carotid artery greatly facilitates subsequent performance of anastomosis. Vagus and recurrent nerves are protected during this dissection. *D.* After mobilization of carotid and

subclavian arteries, tributaries of subclavian arteries are ligated, vertebral artery being ligated separately to avoid retrograde flow of blood from vertebral artery distad into arm, producing subclavian "steal" abnormality. *E.* After division of subclavian artery, longitudinal arteriotomy is made in pulmonary artery. Adventitia is carefully cleared from subclavian artery before performance of anastomosis. *F.* Appearance of completed anastomosis. Anterior row of anastomosis is usually made with interrupted sutures of 5-0 silk to permit growth of anastomosis. With wide mobilization of carotid artery superiorly and pulmonary artery inferiorly, satisfactory anastomosis can be accomplished with sublclavian artery as short as 1 to 1.5 cm in length. Vein graft is rarely necessary.

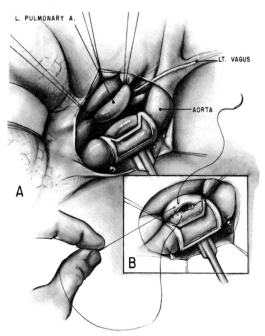

Fig. 18-41. Potts type of aortic-pulmonary anastomosis. *A.* Partial-occlusion clamp has been applied to aorta, and segment of pulmonary artery has been occluded by traction on ligatures. *B.* After approximation of two vessels, side-to-side anastomosis is constructed. Size of anastomosis is critical, an aortic incision 4 mm long being used in infants and one 6 mm in older children. This type of anastomosis is avoided whenever possible because of difficulties in dividing it during subsequent corrective surgery with cardiopulmonary bypass.

be through the right atrium, detaching part of the tricuspid valve, but this approach is far more complicated than that through the ventricle.

The five potential zones of obstruction to flow of blood to the lungs should be considered for surgical correction, the location, the severity, and number varying with each patient. These include fusion of the pulmonary valve leaflets; a hypoplastic pulmonic annulus; varying degrees of infundibular stenosis in the right ventricle, either fibrous or muscular; hypoplastic main pulmonary artery; or hypoplastic distal pulmonary arteries. Precise selective angiocardiograms are of great value before operation in identifying these zones of obstruction.

The preferred ventriculotomy is an oblique one placed about 4 cm from the pulmonic valve and curving downward about 1 cm from the anterior descending coronary artery. A left ventricular vent is used to aspirate blood from the operative field.

Hypertrophied right ventricular musculature is radically excised, especially the large muscle bundles of the crista supraventricularis. Excision is carried out to the base of the pulmonic valve cusps.

A separate incision is usually made in the pulmonary artery to permit incision of the fused valve commissures, as well as any subcommissural stenosis. The zones of incision of the fused commissures can be visualized through the ventriculotomy and extended if inadequate. Adequate

correction of the infundibular obstruction is simple in some patients but very difficult in others. However, employing a transverse ventriculotomy, combined with a radical excision of hypertrophied ventricular muscle almost always makes it possible to correct the obstruction without the insertion of a prosthetic patch in the wall of the right ventricle.

A critical zone of obstruction is a hypoplastic pulmonic valve ring. If an opening can be created that will accommodate a #16 Hegar dilator, representing a diameter of 16 mm or a cross-sectional area slightly less than 2 cm², obstruction is satisfactorily, though not completely, relieved. A smaller opening may be acceptable in small children. Otherwise the pulmonary arteriotomy is extended across the pulmonic annulus and onto the ventricle for 1 to 2 cm. Care is taken not to extend the incision far down onto the ventricle. With the approach described, incision of the pulmonic annulus, creating pulmonic insufficiency, is required in only 10 to 15 percent of patients (Fig. 18-42).

Following correction of the infundibular obstruction, the ventricular septal defect is closed. The technique is identical to that described previously for ventricular septal defect. Circumferential mattress or figure-of-eight sutures, usually 4-0 silk or synthetic sutures, are inserted, each suture encompassing 3 to 4 mm of tissue. Care is taken in the region of the posterosuperior margin of the ventricular septal defect to avoid the conduction bundle by inserting sutures into the right side of the ventricular septum, often through the base of the septal leaflet of the tricuspid valve. With good illumination and a dry, quiet field, the fibrous trigone at the base of the noncoronary aortic sinus can be palpated or even visualized. This is a valuable landmark, for the conduction bundle passes through this fibrous trigone and lies to the left of an imaginary line projected between the trigone and the papillary muscle of the conus. Hence, sutures placed to the right of this imaginary line safely avoid injury of the conduction bundle. Intermittent aortic occlusion for 5 to 10 minutes at a temperature of 30 to 32°C is employed while the sutures are inserted, after which the electrocardiogram is observed to be certain that conduction is adequate. With electrocardiogram monitoring, there has been no permanent heart block in any patient in the author's experience in the past decade. After the sutures are inserted, they are threaded through a knitted Dacron patch of appropriate size, which is then tied in position. Adequacy of closure is confirmed by retrograde injection of saline solution through the left ventricular vent while the aorta is temporarily clamped, first removing all air from the left ventricle. This has been found a useful guide to confirm adequacy of closure.

If the diameter of the pulmonary artery is less than 2 cm, it is widened to an appropriate degree by sewing a pericardial patch into the pulmonary arteriotomy and extending the patch down to the pulmonic valve ring but avoiding the production of pulmonic insufficiency. The ostia of the distal pulmonary arteries are closely examined, and any localized obstruction is also corrected.

After subsequent closure of the ventriculotomy, taking the usual precautions to remove all air from the cardiac chambers, extracorporeal circulation is stopped, and intracardiac pressures are measured to confirm that the right ventricular obstruction has been corrected. The right ventricular systolic pressure should be reduced to less than 60 to 70 percent of left ventricular systolic pressure. If right ventricular pressure is still elevated beyond this level, the ventriculotomy is usually reopened and more extensive correction of the obstruction performed. Otherwise fatal depression of cardiac output from right ventricular failure may occur in the early postoperative course. In most patients, following bypass, a satisfactory result is obtained with a systolic pressure near 100 mm Hg, a right ventricular systolic pressure between 35 and 50 mm Hg, and a pulmonary artery systolic pressure of 20 to 25 mm Hg.

Postoperative Course. Following operation, particular attention is required in the first 24 hours to intrathoracic bleeding, because older cyanotic patients have an increased hemorrhagic tendency from the long-standing polycythemia. Transfusion of fresh frozen plasma, often combined with platelet transfusions, is the best therapy. Close observation is necessary to avoid intrathoracic accumulation of blood with cardiac tamponade. Reoperation is often necessary if more than 1 liter of blood drains from the thoracotomy tubes in the first 24 hours after operation.

Adequacy of cardiac output is monitored by observing blood pressure, blood-gas concentrations in mixed venous blood, and urine output. Blood is transfused in sufficient amounts to keep central venous pressure near 12 to 15 mm Hg if necessary, possibly at higher levels. If cardiac output is inadequate despite these measures, small amounts of isoproterenol or epinephrine are infused (1 to 2 μg/minute). Acidosis is not a significant problem if cardiac output remains adequate. Assisted ventilation may be required for a few hours but seldom for longer.

Some degree of right ventricular failure is commonly encountered, both from the ventriculotomy incision and the radical resection of hypertrophied muscle. Hence, digitalis is routinely given, combined with bedrest and restriction of sodium intake.

The risk of operation varies with the age of the patient and the degree of cyanosis, reflecting the severity of the right ventricular obstruction. The risk is only 3 to 5 percent in older children but larger in smaller ones with severe cyanosis. The excellent monograph by Kirklin et al. contains much data regarding experiences with tetralogy of Fallot. Large clinical series showing low operative mortality have also been published by Kirklin et al., Malm et al., and Shumway et al.

Following recovery from operation, dramatic improvement is obvious. Cyanosis is, of course, absent, and exercise tolerance within a few months approaches that of a normal individual. If cardiac failure is significant following operation, convalescence may be slow for several weeks. Some cardiac enlargement may remain, but long-term studies show that most patients have excellent cardiac function. The tolerance for pulmonic insufficiency which results if the pulmonic annulus is incised and a prosthetic patch inserted is surprisingly good. Ultimate prognosis in such patients is uncertain, though some have now survived for over 15 years with continuing good results. Some groups have inserted homograft valves at the time of oper-

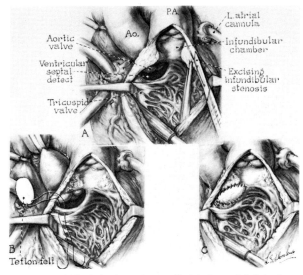

Fig. 18-42. *A.* Pathologic anatomy with tetralogy of Fallot, showing ventricular septal defect, through which aortic valve cusps are usually visible. Infundibular stenosis in this patient consisted of hypertrophied infundibular muscle. Pulmonic valve was normal. In many patients pulmonic valve is stenotic. *B.* After excision of infundibular stenosis, ventricular septal defect is closed with prosthetic patch of Teflon felt. Sutures along posterosuperior rim are inserted cautiously to avoid injury to conduction bundle. These are usually placed with heart contracting in order to monitor electrocardiogram. Often sutures are inserted to right of margin of defect to avoid conduction bundle. *C.* Final insertion of prosthetic patch. Interrupted rather than continuous sutures are frequently used.

ation to avoid pulmonic insufficiency, but there is not sufficient evidence to warrant this as a routine procedure.

COMPLEX MALFORMATIONS

Transposition of the Great Vessels

HISTORICAL DATA. The clinical syndrome of transposition of the great vessels was clearly described by Taussig in 1938. The first surgical procedure to achieve significant benefit, creation of an atrial septal defect, was reported by Blalock and Hanlon. Another palliative surgical procedure, no longer used, was developed by Baffes, who transposed the inferior vena cava and the right pulmonary veins. Senning, in 1957, first completely corrected transposition of the great vessels by repositioning the atrial septum, but mortality was prohibitively high. Subsequently Mustard, in 1964, developed a method of reconstructing the atrial cavity which has produced the best clinical results to date.

INCIDENCE AND ETIOLOGY. Transposition of the great vessels is one of the most frequent causes of cyanotic heart disease in the newborn, constituting 30 to 40 percent of all cases. It is the most common cause of cardiac failure in the newborn. As many patients die in infancy, it is much less common after the first two years of life.

Transposition of the aorta and pulmonary arteries results

from abnormal division of the bulbar trunk in embryologic development, occurring between the fifth and seventh uterine week. Etiologic factors are unknown. It is about four times more frequent in males than in females.

PATHOLOGIC ANATOMY. With transposition of the arteries, the aorta originates from the right ventricle and the pulmonary artery from the left ventricle (Fig. 18-43). As a result of these abnormal locations, venous blood returning through the venae cavae to the right atrium enters the right ventricle and is then propelled directly into the aorta. Oxygenated blood returning from the lungs through the pulmonary veins to the left atrium enters the left ventricle and is then expelled through the pulmonary artery again to the lungs. This dual, parallel circulatory arrangement is obviously incompatible with life without communication between the pulmonary and systemic circulations. Three possible communications exist, a patent ductus arteriosus, an atrial septal defect or foramen ovale, or a ventricular septal defect. One or more of these, of course, must exist for the infant to survive even a few hours after birth. Normally a patent ductus is present for a few weeks after birth in over one-half the patients. A foramen ovale is frequently found, and a ventricular septal defect occurs in 50 to 70 percent of patients, varying with the type of clinical material analyzed.

Associated anomalies are common. One of the most frequent of these, pulmonic stenosis, occurs so commonly as to constitute a well-defined variant of the syndrome, because the prognosis is unusually favorable in such patients. A wide variety of other anomalies may occur, including coarctation of the aorta, pulmonary atresia, and dextrocardia.

One of the most distinctive anomalies is a variant of transposition termed the *Taussig-Bing syndrome,* in which the aorta originates from the right ventricle, but the pulmonary artery originates opposite a large ventricular septal defect, "overriding" the ventricular septum and hence receiving blood from both the right and left ventricles. This malformation is a distinctive one, though uncommon, in that cardiac enlargement is not severe and prognosis is more favorable.

PATHOPHYSIOLOGY. The two basic physiologic handicaps with transposition are severe anoxia from inability to transport oxygen from the lungs to the tissues of the body and progressive cardiac failure. The severe and rapidly progressive cardiac failure results partly from a high cardiac output and partly from the fact that the coronary arteries are filled with unoxygenated blood with resulting myocardial anoxia. The relative severity of the anoxia and the cardiac failure varies with the nature of the intracardiac communications and valvular stenoses. Nadas has found in his group of patients that cardiac failure was present at birth in 80 percent. Because of the severe cardiac failure and anoxia, physical development is severely retarded.

Transposition is a lethal condition, and a high percentage of patients die within the first 1 to 3 months of life. Mustard et al. estimated that 90 percent of their patients died within 7 months. A survey by Hanlon and Blalock in 1948 found only six patients reported in the literature at that time who had lived beyond ten years of age.

Nadas has conveniently grouped patients into four clinical categories related to prognosis. Those with an intact ventricular septum do poorly because of inadequate mixing of the pulmonary and systemic circulations. Similarly, those with a large ventricular septal defect do badly because of excessive pulmonary blood flow. Pulmonary hypertension in this group of patients is also associated with a poor prognosis. The most favorable prognosis is associated with a ventricular septal defect combined with pulmonic stenosis. This combination which permits mixing of the pulmonary and systemic circulations through the ventricular septal defect, while the pulmonic stenosis prevents excessive pulmonary blood flow with pulmonary congestion and secondary pulmonary hypertension.

CLINICAL MANIFESTATIONS. Symptoms. A high percentage of infants are cyanotic at birth (80 percent in Nadas' series), and cardiac failure is similarly frequent. Cyanosis appears in most other patients in the first year

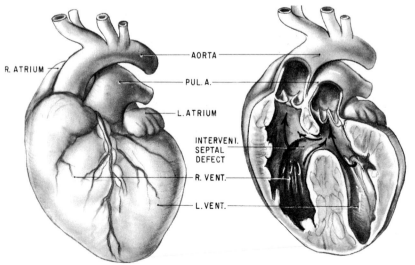

Fig. 18-43. Transposition of great vessels, with aorta arising from right ventricle and pulmonary artery from left ventricle. Ventricular septal defect permits communication between pulmonic and systemic circulations; otherwise condition would be incompatible with life after birth. (*Adapted from H. B. Taussig, "Congenital Malformations of the Heart," 3d ed., Harvard University Press, Cambridge, 1960, p. 149.*)

R. ATRIUM
AORTA
PUL. A.
L. ATRIUM
INTERVENI. SEPTAL DEFECT
R. VENT.
L. VENT.

of life. There is a corresponding severe retardation of growth and development, and anoxic spells of unconsciousness are frequent. Mental development, however, is not impaired. The most prominent symptoms are cyanosis and dyspnea. In children who survive beyond the first two years of life, clubbing and polycythemia appear.

Physical Findings. Cyanosis is frequently obvious on inspection and is often severe. In older children clubbing and polycythemia are similarly evident. Signs of congestive failure are almost always found, with cardiac enlargement, hepatomegaly, and pulmonary congestion. A systolic murmur is usually present but is variable and not diagnostic. It can result from any of the different intracardiac communications which may be present. Severe retardation of physical development is obvious in older infants.

Absence of a murmur, often indicating absence of an intracardiac communication, indicates a particularly unfavorable prognosis because of inadequate communication between the pulmonary and systemic circulations.

LABORATORY FINDINGS. The chest roentgenogram shows cardiac enlargement, often with a distinctive silhouette, and pulmonary congestion. The contour of the heart has been described as "egg-shaped" and results from the prominent right ventricle projecting into the left side of the chest and the dilated right atrium bulging into the right side. The base of the cardiac shadow, termed the "waist," may be unusually narrow because of the location of the aorta directly in front of the pulmonary artery, rather than the conventional side-to-side relationship seen in the normal cardiac shadow (Fig. 18-2).

The electrocardiogram consistently shows severe right ventricular hypertrophy. Left ventricular hypertrophy varies with the pulmonary blood flow or with the presence of pulmonary valvular stenosis.

Careful cardiac catheterization reveals several distinctive features: All four chambers can be entered in only 60 to 75 percent of patients because of the malformations. The systolic pressure in the right ventricle is the same as in the aorta, while that in the left ventricle varies with the size of the ventricular septal defect and the presence of pulmonic stenosis. The oxygen saturation in the pulmonary artery is increased, and a hallmark of the condition is the fact that oxygen saturation in the pulmonary artery is greater than that in the femoral artery. Varying degrees of arterial oxygen unsaturation are regularly found, ranging from as low as 12% to as high as 85%. Angiocardiography provides the best means for confirming the diagnosis, for it classically demonstrates the anterior origin of the aorta from the right ventricle, with the more faintly visualized pulmonary artery lying posterior to the aorta.

DIAGNOSIS. The diagnosis of transposition can be immediately considered in a seriously ill, cyanotic infant with cardiac enlargement and congestive heart failure. In older children the retardation of physical development is striking. It must be differentiated from tetralogy of Fallot, tricuspid atresia, and total anomaly of venous return. Tetralogy of Fallot is readily identified in many patients by the normal cardiac size and the absence of cardiac failure. Tricuspid atresia is easily recognized by the characteristic left axis deviation on the electrocardiogram. Total

anomalous drainage of the pulmonary veins may require cardiac catheterization to establish the diagnosis with certainty.

TREATMENT. Indications for Operation. For several reasons transposition may be classified into four broad groups, as follows: (1) Intact ventricular septum, patent foramen ovale; (2) ventricular septal defect; (3) ventricular septal defect and pulmonic stenosis; and (4) complex transposition, one of the previous three forms in association with other severe defects such as coarctation of the aorta.

The most urgent problems are seen with an intact ventricular septum, for the only communication between the pulmonary and systemic circulations is through the foramen ovale. In these patients, balloon septostomy provides dramatic, though not permanent, improvement. In the other groups, balloon septostomy is of considerably less value.

Because of the high fatality rate in the first month of life, some type of surgical procedure must be done to increase communication between the pulmonary and systemic circulations at the time the diagnosis is established in the catheterization laboratory. The simplest procedure is the balloon septostomy, enlarging the foramen ovale or atrial septal defect present by passing a deflated balloon catheter through the defect into the left atrium, inflating the balloon, and forcefully pulling the inflated balloon across the septum to enlarge the opening. This ingenious technique was developed by Rashkind and has greatly helped in the initial treatment of these seriously ill infants. In most instances, balloon septostomy probably should be routinely done at the time of cardiac catheterization to establish the diagnosis.

When balloon septostomy is ineffective, an atrial septal defect may be created by the Blalock-Hanlon technique. With the attractive simplicity of balloon septostomy, this procedure is now performed much less frequently than in the past. The operative procedure is illustrated in Fig. 18-44. A right thoracotomy is performed, after which the pericardium is opened and the superior and inferior pulmonary veins are isolated. The atrial septum is identified at the point of entry of the right pulmonary veins and a vascular clamp applied to isolate a segment of both the right and left atria at this point. Parallel incisions are then made in the right atrium and pulmonary vein through the septum, after which the two incisions are connected and a portion of the septum is incised, creating a defect 1 to 2 cm in diameter. Although this procedure has provided dramatic palliation in many patients for 6 to 12 months, results are often not sustained, but there is an increasing tendency to attempt total correction if balloon septostomy is inadequate.

In patients with a large ventricular septal defect resulting in flooding of the lung fields from excessive pulmonary blood flow, banding of the pulmonary artery may be performed. Conversely, if pulmonic stenosis is present with severe reduction in pulmonary blood flow, a palliative subclavian-pulmonary anastomosis may be done. It is noteworthy that there is little risk of pulmonary hypertension in patients following palliation.

Corrective Operations. All the previously described pro-

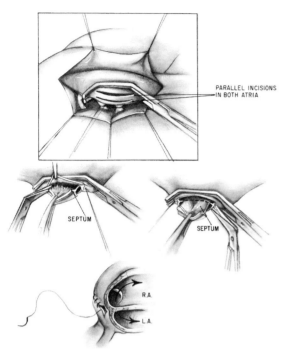

PARALLEL INCISIONS
IN BOTH ATRIA

SEPTUM

SEPTUM

R.A.

L.A.

Fig. 18-44. Creation of atrial septal defect (Blalock-Hanlon Technique). Right pulmonary veins are mobilized and occluded by traction on ligatures. Pulmonary artery and right main bronchus are also occluded to avoid congestion of lungs during occlusion of pulmonary veins. Tangential occlusion clamp is applied to right and left atria, enclosing atrial septum. Separate incisions are then made in right atrium and left atrium. Exposed atrial septum is then removed, temporarily releasing clamp in order to withdraw more septum from between its jaws and create larger defect. After excision of this septum, incision is sutured, creating large atrial septal defect. (*Adapted from D. A. Cooley et al., Arch Surg, 93:704, 1966.*)

cedures are palliative only. If the ventricular septum is intact, many patients do reasonably well with a large atrial septal defect up to two to three years of age, and then total correction may be undertaken. In patients with ventricular septal defects, however, operation must be employed at an earlier age unless banding of the pulmonary artery is performed. Otherwise irreversible changes in the pulmonary vascular bed may develop before two years of age.

Almost all currently used operative procedures construct channels in the atria to transmit blood to the left ventricle from which the pulmonary artery arises, and pulmonary venous blood to the right ventricle from which the aorta arises. Attempts to transpose the aorta and pulmonary artery to their normal positions have thus far been unsuccessful, partly because of the abnormal location of the pulmonary arteries. The theoretical concept of surgical transposition of the atria was advanced by Albert and first successfully done by Senning. However, consistent good results were not obtained until the significant work of Mustard, who repositioned the atrial septum with a pericardial graft. This procedure has now been performed in

a large number of patients, with an operative mortality as low as 5 to 10 percent.

A significant advance in cardiac surgery has been made in recent years by application of the techniques of deep hypothermia and circulatory arrest to perform corrective cardiac surgery in infants. Some of the earliest reports were by Merendino and associates, but some of the most extensive experience has been by the group headed by Barratt-Boyes. Although few long-term data are yet available, it has been convincingly demonstrated that total operative correction of transposition can be performed successfully in the first few months of life. The exact technique, as well as the limitations and hazards, of deep hypothermia and circulatory arrest are still under investigation, but clearly the correction of many severe cardiac anomalies, previously fatal in the first few months of life, is now becoming possible. Experiences with a small group of patients in whom total correction was done with a conventional pump-oxygenator technique have been reported. Which technique is preferable has yet to be determined.

Tricuspid Atresia

PATHOLOGIC ANATOMY. Tricuspid atresia is a rare form of congenital heart disease (Fig. 18-45) affecting 3 to 8 percent of children with cyanotic heart disease. However, series of 50 to 80 cases have been analyzed and reported from different cardiac centers. The basic abnormality is atresia of the tricuspid valve. Often only a dimple is found in the right atrial cavity where the tricuspid valve orifice is normally located. Several other cardiac malformations are associated with tricuspid atresia, and the severity of the disease varies with the associated malformations. The right ventricle is always underdeveloped, even absent, its place being taken by a solid mass of hypoplastic muscle. In other patients it exists as a small chamber, either a blind sac or one communicating with the left ventricle through a ventricular septal defect. The pulmonary artery and pulmonary valve are atretic with severe right ventricular hypoplasia, the pulmonary circulation being maintained through the ductus arteriosus. When a small right ventricular cavity is present, a normal pulmonary valve may be found. The ventricular septum is intact with right ventricular hypoplasia, but with a rudimentary ventricular chamber a septal defect is usually present. There is often an associated transposition of the great vessels. Edwards and Bargeron have described four anatomic variants of tricuspid atresia, differing in the presence of a ventricular septal defect, pulmonic stenosis, or transposition of the great vessels. An atrial septal defect must, of necessity, be present to maintain life. This may consist of a foramen ovale stretched open by a high right atrial pressure, a small atrial septal defect, or virtual absence of the atrial septum.

PATHOPHYSIOLOGY. The basic physiologic disturbance results from complete mixing of systemic venous blood and pulmonary venous blood in the left atrium, as blood returning to the right atrium is diverted by the hypoplastic tricuspid orifice through the atrial septal defect into the left atrium. The severity of the resulting cyanosis varies

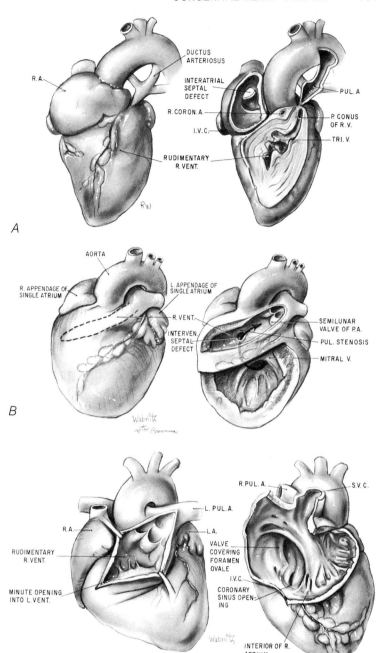

Fig. 18-45. *A.* Tricuspid atresia with rudimentary right ventricle, pulmonary atresia, and vestigial pulmonary artery which does not communicate with hypoplastic right ventricular cavity. *B.* Tricuspid atresia in which pulmonary artery is normally formed and arises from rudimentary right ventricular cavity. Small ventricular septal defect is present, permitting flow of blood from normal left ventricular cavity through rudimentary right ventricular cavity into pulmonary artery. *C.* Tricuspid atresia with rudimentary right ventricle in which normal pulmonary artery with normal pulmonic valves arises from rudimentary right ventricle. Right atrial cavity is dilated, with absence of tricuspid valve. (*Adapted from H. B. Taussig, "Congenital Malformations of the Heart," 2d ed., Harvard University Press, Cambridge, 1960, pp. 77–79.*)

with the pulmonary blood flow. Cyanosis and anoxia are severe with pulmonary atresia, while they may be minimal with an adequate pulmonary blood flow. The hypoplastic right ventricle which is uniformly present is the most valuable clue to the diagnosis. An additional significant physiologic disturbance is the elevated right atrial pressure resulting from flow of systemic venous blood through the atrial septal defect and into the left ventricle. The right atrial pressure may be elevated 5 to 10 mm Hg if only a foramen ovale is present, resulting in hepatic enlargement and other signs of right-sided heart failure.

CLINICAL MANIFESTATIONS. Symptoms. The disease is a severe one, and most infants die in the first few months of life as the patent ductus arteriosus closes, unless an operation is performed. The severity of the malformation varies with the degree of reduction in pulmonary blood flow, which in turn is related to the degree of hypoplasia of the right ventricle. The patients are usually cyanotic at birth and have exercise intolerance, retarded development, and frequent anoxic spells of unconsciousness. Hemiplegia may develop after a severe anoxic spell. Death occurs during an anoxic episode or results from congestive heart failure. In older children endocarditis may occur.

The prominent symptoms are cyanosis and dyspnea with intolerance to exercise, squatting, and limited growth and development.

Physical Examination. On physical examination there is slight to moderate cardiac enlargement. A moderate systolic murmur along the left sternal border is present in about one-half the patients but is of no diagnostic significance. It presumably arises either from flow through the atrial septal defect or possibly from flow through a stenotic pulmonic valve. Absence of a murmur often indicates an unusually poor prognosis. The second heart sound is unusually "pure" because the pulmonic second sound is weak or absent. A particularly significant diagnostic finding is hepatic enlargement and other signs of right-sided failure, especially in association with absence of any signs of pulmonary congestion or left-sided failure.

LABORATORY FINDINGS. The chest roentgenogram regularly shows cardiac enlargement, and on fluoroscopy it may be possible to detect that the enlargement is predominantly in the left ventricle. There is decreased vascularity in the lung fields. The electrocardiogram is the most important diagnostic tool, for left ventricular hypertrophy and left axis deviation are uniformly present, in contrast to the classic right ventricular hypertrophy of most forms of cyanotic heart disease. There are often unusually tall, peaked P waves, indicating right atrial hypertrophy in association with a small atrial septal defect or foramen ovale. On cardiac catheterization there is a right-to-left shunt at the atrial level, with some elevation of the right atrial pressure. The right atrial pressure is higher than the left atrial pressure if only a foramen ovale is present. Characteristically it is impossible to advance the catheter into the right ventricle because of the tricuspid atresia. Selective angiocardiography establishes the diagnosis by demonstrating flow of blood from the right atrium to the left atrium and into the left ventricle. Some caution is required, however, in interpreting angiographic studies, because in infants streaming of blood through a foramen ovale may give a false indication of absence of the tricuspid valve.

DIAGNOSIS. Diagnosis can usually be established from the combination of clinical cyanosis with left ventricular hypertrophy shown on the electrocardiogram. The usual differential diagnosis is from tetralogy of Fallot or from transposition of the great vessels, with the electrocardiogram and other clinical features providing the best diagnostic clues.

TREATMENT. As the malformation is often incompatible with life once the ductus arteriosus closes, emergency operations in infants undergoing cyanotic spells are often necessary. In children who survive infancy, the presence of cyanosis and severe retardation of growth are the usual indications for operation. In selecting an operative procedure, signs of hepatic enlargement and right-sided failure should be closely noted, because congestive failure often will be intensified if a shunt operation is performed to increase pulmonary blood flow.

Operative Procedures. Only palliative operative procedures have been successful, because of the severity of the malformation. Brock, in 1964, reported one unsuccessful attempt to partly correct the malformation by enlargement of the ventricular septal defect. Palliative operations to increase pulmonary blood flow may be of great help in patients with a decrease in pulmonary blood flow. Caution in selecting patients for such an operation is necessary, however, because of the right ventricular failure. Cardiac catheterization may be of value in evaluating this risk, for right atrial pressure elevated above left atrial pressure indicates a greater risk of cardiac failure, as only a foramen ovale is present, in contrast to patients with a large defect in the atrial septum.

In infants, the preferred operation is anastomosis between a systemic artery and a pulmonary artery to increase pulmonary blood flow. Most experience has been with the Potts type of operation, performing an emergency aorta-left pulmonary artery side-to-side anastomosis. The incision in the aorta should be only about 4 mm in length in order to avoid production of congestive heart failure (Fig. 18-41).

Recently experiences with an intrapericardial anastomosis between the side of the ascending aorta and the right pulmonary artery have indicated that this may become a preferred operative procedure because it can be performed more quickly and with less dissection of mediastinal tissues (Fig. 18-39). However, extensive data with the procedure are not yet available. With right atrial hypertension and only a foramen ovale, consideration should be given to operative enlargement of the atrial septal defect, although data evaluating the effectiveness of this procedure are not available because it is usually performed in conjunction with a shunt operation.

In infants over six months of age, the preferred operation is anastomosis of the superior vena cava to the right pulmonary artery, as popularized by Glenn (Fig. 18-46). This has the great advantage of not adding any strain to the functioning left ventricle and hence does not carry the risk of congestive heart failure. In infants younger than six months of age, the superior vena cava operation has had a high mortality from cerebral complications, because the pulmonary vascular resistance in infants may significantly obstruct cerebral blood flow. Edwards et al. have reported a technique of delayed ligation of the azygos vein in infants which has greatly reduced mortality in their experience.

Postoperative Course. The risk of operation in infants is significant because of the severity of the malformation; an operative mortality of 20 to 35 percent is common. In those who survive operation, long-term evaluation has shown an improvement in 60 to 70 percent. The results are not so good as those obtained with shunt operations for tetralogy of Fallot. Somewhat better results have been obtained with the superior vena cava—pulmonary artery operations in older children. Glenn et al. stated in 1965 that eight patients followed from 1 to 4 years after operation had all sustained improvement.

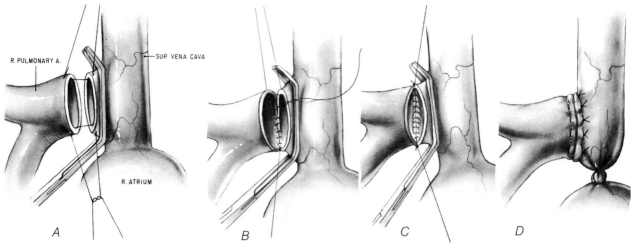

Fig. 18-46. Anastomosis between superior vena cava and right pulmonary artery. *A.* Tangential clamp has been applied to superior vena cava to include origin of azygos vein. Right pulmonary artery has been divided, and end-to-end anastomosis will be constructed. *B.* Posterior row of anastomosis is constructed with continuous 5-0 silk suture. *C.* Completed posterior row of anastomosis. *D.* Anterior row of anastomosis is constructed with interrupted sutures to permit growth of anastomosis. After removal of occluding clamps, superior vena cava is doubly ligated at point of juncture with right atrium. (*Adapted from W. W. L. Glenn, N Engl J Med, 259:117, 1958.*)

RARE MALFORMATIONS

Cor Triatriatum

Cor triatriatum is a rare malformation. In 1960 a review by Niwayama found only 36 cases, and in 1965 McGuire et al. stated that only about 10 cases had been recognized in adult patients.

PATHOLOGIC ANATOMY. The anomaly results from incomplete absorption of the embryonic common pulmonary vein into the left atrium, so that it remains as an additional cardiac chamber superior and posterior to the normal left atrium. The pulmonary veins enter this accessory chamber, which communicates with the left atrium through a tiny opening, often only 3 to 4 mm in diameter. The mitral valve and atrial appendage are normal. The foramen ovale almost always opens into the left atrium and not into the accessory chamber.

CLINICAL MANIFESTATIONS. The disease is a severe one, with rapid progression of pulmonary congestion, pulmonary hypertension, and heart failure. Over 50 percent of affected infants do not survive the first year of life. Symptoms are identical to those of mitral stenosis, although in the few older patients who have been studied, hemoptysis has been an unusually prominent feature. On physical examination a typical diastolic rumbling murmur of mitral stenosis is usually not present, although a systolic murmur is audible. The absence of a typical murmur, combined with the presence of a sinus rhythm, should raise the suspicion that something other than mitral stenosis is present. A forceful impulse may be palpable in the left parasternal area because of marked right ventricular hypertrophy.

LABORATORY FINDINGS. The roentgenogram shows pulmonary congestion with enlargement of the right ventricle, and the electrocardiogram shows right ventricular hypertrophy. The diagnosis can be established at catheterization by the finding of elevated pulmonary artery pressure as well as an increased wedge pressure (often 25 to 30 mm Hg), *combined with a normal pressure in the left atrium.* Selective angiocardiography will disclose the accessory chamber superior and posterior to the normal left atrium.

TREATMENT. Operation should be performed as soon as the diagnosis is established, because most patients succumb to cardiac failure at an early age. Although a successful operation was performed by Lewis and one by Vineberg in 1956, the collective review published in 1960 by Niwayama found a total of only five successful operations at that time. In 1964 Grondin et al. reported experiences with six cases, four of whom had been operated upon, with three survivors.

The operative procedure is theoretically a simple one, consisting of enlarging the small opening between the accessory atrium and the normal left atrium. It should ideally be performed with cardiopulmonary bypass, to permit extensive excision of the obstructing membrane. The few reported survivors have been asymptomatic.

Congenital Mitral Stenosis

Congenital mitral stenosis is a rare lesion with frequently results in congestive heart failure and death in the first year of life. Ferencz et al., in 1954, found 34 patients previously reported and described nine additional cases. Nadas has studied five cases, and Daoud and associates in 1963 described experiences with seven. In 1967 Tsuji et al. stated that 131 cases had been reported. Two additional patients who had been successfully operated upon were described, making a total of 41 patients operated upon with 21 known survivors.

PATHOLOGIC ANATOMY. A diffuse abnormality of the mitral valve is often present, with thick, rubbery leaflets, ill-defined commissures, and short, thickened chordae. The deformity of the valve is such that surgical attempts at commissurotomy have often resulted in the production of fatal mitral insufficiency, and probably some patients can be treated effectively only by the insertion of a prosthetic valve. The obstruction to flow of blood leads to marked enlargement of the left atrium, pulmonary congestion and pulmonary hypertension, right ventricular hypertrophy, and subsequently cardiac failure. Other anomalies are frequent, especially patent ductus arteriosus and coarctation of the aorta.

CLINICAL MANIFESTATIONS. Symptoms often appear in infancy, with dyspnea, pulmonary congestion, and repeated pneumonic infections. In milder forms of stenosis, symptoms may appear only in later childhood. On physical examination an apical diastolic rumbling murmur is almost always found and provides the best clue to the diagnosis. A thrill is also frequent. An associated systolic murmur, probably from concomitant mitral insufficiency, is common. Sinus rhythm is usually present.

LABORATORY FINDINGS. The main abnormality on the chest roentgenogram is enlargement of the left atrium, with some associated enlargement of the right ventricle. The electrocardiogram will demonstrate right ventricular hypertrophy and right axis deviation. On cardiac catheterization the diagnosis can be confirmed by the finding of an elevated pulmonary artery pressure and pulmonary capillary pressure. Selective angiography may outline the dilated left atrium.

TREATMENT. Operation in infancy or early childhood should be attempted only to forestall impending death from pulmonary congestion. It is likely that the best results can be obtained with the use of a pump-oxygenator, permitting selective incision of the deformed valve, but significant data are not available. In some patients prosthetic valvular replacement will almost surely be necessary. Almost all patients who have survived operation to date have been more than five years of age at operation.

Aortic-Pulmonary Window

Several terms have been applied to this rare anomaly, including *aortopulmonary fenestration, aorticopulmonary fistula,* and *aortic septal defect.* It is an unusual lesion and has been recognized only with the development of diagnostic and surgical techniques for patent ductus arteriosus. In a group of 100 patients with a diagnosis of patent ductus arteriosus, 1 will usually be found to have an aortic-pulmonary window. A comprehensive report by Skall-Jensen in 1958 found 62 cases in the medical literature. One case was successfully treated by ligation by Gross in 1948, and another was treated by division and suture by Scott and Sabiston in 1951 (Fig. 18-47), but correction with extracorporeal circulation is now the preferred procedure. Three such patients were reported by Cooley et al. in 1957. In 1962, Morrow and associates found 71 reported cases, 27 of whom had been operated upon.

PATHOLOGIC ANATOMY. Embryologically, the defect results from incomplete development of the spiral septum dividing the primitive truncus arteriosus into the aorta and the pulmonary artery. Persistent truncus arteriosus is a more severe malformation of similar cause but represents incomplete development of both the spiral septum in the truncus arteriosus and the bulbar septum in the bulbus cordis. In persistent truncus arteriosus there is both a ventricular septal defect and a failure of formation of the separate aortic and pulmonic valves, while in aortic-pulmonary window the aortic and pulmonic valves are normally formed, although a separate ventricular septal defect has been found in some patients.

The opening, or "window," between the aorta and the pulmonary artery may vary in diameter from 5 to 30 mm. It may be located proximally near the ostia of the coronary arteries and the pulmonic valve, or it may be as much as 2 cm distal to these structures.

Fig. 18-47. Aortic-pulmonary fistula, showing large communication between aorta and pulmonary artery near base of heart. (*Adapted from H. W. Scott and D. C. Sabiston, J Thorac Surg, 25:26, 1953.*)

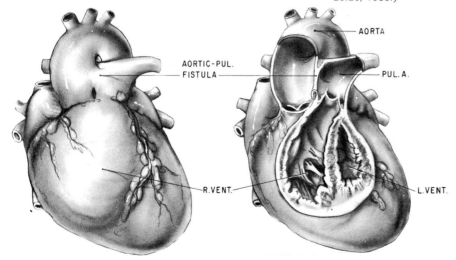

AORTA

AORTIC-PUL. FISTULA

PUL. A.

R.VENT.

L.VENT.

PATHOPHYSIOLOGY. The defect produces a large left-to-right shunt similar to that of a patent ductus arteriosus. The course is a more malignant one, however, because the shunt is usually larger than that seen in the usual patent ductus, resulting in the rapid development of pulmonary hypertension, increase in pulmonary vascular resistance, and cardiac failure.

CLINICAL MANIFESTATIONS. The clinical findings may be identical to those found in patent ductus arteriosus, with a continuous murmur, wide pulse pressure, left ventricular enlargement, and pulmonary congestion. Often only a systolic murmur is present, however, because of severe pulmonary hypertension. Usually the condition is diagnosed as patent ductus arteriosus until cardiac catheterization, angiography, or surgical exploration discloses the correct diagnosis.

LABORATORY FINDINGS. At catheterization the findings are identical to those with a patent ductus arteriosus unless the cardiac catheter can be manipulated through the defect into the aorta, in which case the catheter takes a characteristic course to enter either the ascending aorta or the innominate artery; in patent ductus arteriosus, the catheter enters the aorta distal to the left subclavian artery and usually goes into the descending thoracic aorta. This observation of the course of the catheter can visually establish the diagnosis.

Angiography can also confirm the diagnosis, demonstrating dye flowing from the aorta into the pulmonary artery near the aortic valve rather than in the usual location distal to the left subclavian artery.

DIAGNOSIS. Differential diagnosis must exclude persistent truncus arteriosus, ventricular septal defect with a prolapsed aortic cusp, and patent ductus arteriosus. The exact diagnosis can be made only upon cardiac catheterization and angiography.

TREATMENT. Usually operation should be performed as soon as the diagnosis has been established, because irreversible changes in pulmonary vascular resistance develop rapidly. There is a paucity of data about the natural history of the disease because of its rarity and recent recognition, but irreversible changes in the pulmonary arterioles have been seen as early as three or four years of age. The author has had one three-year-old patient who died within a few hours from elevated pulmonary vascular resistance following an uncomplicated division and suture of a large aortic-pulmonary window with extracorporeal circulation, and Gross has reported similar experiences with two patients.

Operation almost always should be performed with extracorporeal circulation because of the unpredictable variation in friability of the vascular structures. Once cardiopulmonary bypass has been established, the aorta can be occluded distal to the window, lowering the pressure in the pulmonary artery.

The window may then be divided and the aortic and pulmonary openings sutured. If possible, tangential vascular clamps may be applied to the aorta and pulmonary artery at the site of the window before it is divided, but simple division is usually preferable. The main precaution is evacuation of air from the aorta before circulation is reestablished. Shumway has reported an alternate technique of opening the pulmonary artery and suturing the opening without dividing it.

The risk of operation is proportional to the increase in pulmonary vascular resistance and is probably in the range of 15 to 20 percent. Gross has operated upon seven patients with two fatalities, both in patients who had an elevated pulmonary vascular resistance. Following recovery from operation, prognosis is apparently as favorable as that found with patent ductus arteriosus.

Ruptured Aneurysm of Sinus of Valsalva

This unusual entity produces a distinct syndrome which can be readily diagnosed and effectively treated. Before the advent of extracorporeal circulation it usually caused death from cardiac failure within 1 to 2 years after onset. An aneurysm of the sinus of Valsalva can result from syphilis or other infections; at present most are congenital in origin.

A detailed review by Sawyer et al. in 1957 found 47 patients with congenital aneurysms, but the natural increased interest in diagnosis and therapy which followed the first successful surgical closure in 1956 has led to more widespread recognition. Paton and associates stated in 1965 that since the first operation performed, there had been reports of 91 additional patients operated upon and at least 60 other cases had been described.

PATHOLOGIC ANATOMY. The normal sinus of Valsalva is composed of an aortic valve cusp medially and the aortic wall laterally, which joins the annulus fibrosus of the aortic valve ring inferiorly. In embryonic development the developing ventricular septum inferiorly meets the spiral septum superiorly which separates the aorta and the pulmonary arteries. Incomplete merger of these two structures results in a ventricular septal defect in the membranous septum. An aneurysm of the sinus of Valsalva results from a less severe malformation of the same type, for the media of the aortic wall does not extend down to the annulus of the aortic valve ring. As might be expected, however, an associated ventricular septal defect is often found.

The right coronary sinus is involved in about 70 percent of patients, and rupture occurs into the right ventricle. The noncoronary sinus is involved in about 20 percent of patients, with rupture occurring into the right atrium. Involvement of the left coronary sinus is rare, and rupture into the left atrium or left ventricle is very unusual.

CLINICAL MANIFESTATIONS. Until rupture occurs, an aneurysm of the sinus of Valsalva does not cause any disability, and diagnosis can be made only accidentally during aortography performed for other reasons. The average age at rupture is thirty-one years, although a few such instances have been reported in childhood. Rupture usually occurs without known cause and is soon followed by cardiac failure. Once cardiac failure develops, life expectancy without surgical correction is about 1 year.

At the time of rupture there may be transitory pain in the chest, subsequently followed by dyspnea and palpitation, although in some patients the first symptom is

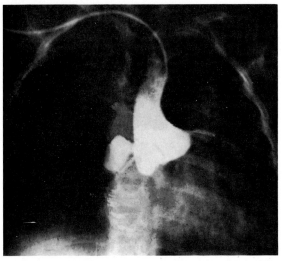

Fig. 18-48. Aortogram confirms diagnosis of ruptured aneurysm of sinus of Valsalva by demonstrating flow of dye from region of aortic sinuses to right atrium. (*Courtesy of Dr. Raymond M. Abrams, Department of Radiology, New York University Medical Center.*)

dyspnea. Subsequently other symptoms of congestive heart failure appear. On physical examination, the important abnormality is the characteristic parasternal murmur, often accompanied by a palpable thrill. The murmur may be continuous or may be a to-and-fro murmur with a somewhat louder component in diastole. It is often located somewhat lower than the usual murmur of a ductus arteriosus, being heard in the third, fourth, or fifth parasternal

Fig. 18-49. Diagram of unusual type of ruptured aneurysm of sinus of Valsalva. Aneurysm arose from left coronary cusp and developed fistulous tract before rupture into right atrium. Operative closure was performed by opening aorta and closing opening directly. (*From Ann Surg, 152:965, 1960.*)

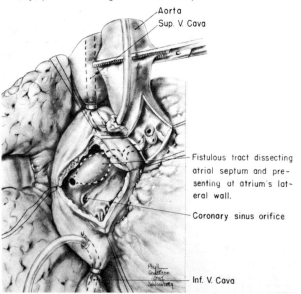

Aorta

Sup. V. Cava

Fistulous tract dissecting atrial septum and presenting at atrium's lateral wall.

Coronary sinus orifice

Inf. V. Cava

spaces to the right or left of the sternum, depending upon the point of rupture of the aneurysm. The murmur is unusually superficial in location and is widely transmitted. These unusual qualities may lead to the suspicion that it is not arising from the usual patent ductus arteriosus. Other physical findings, including a wide pulse pressure, cardiac enlargement, and pulmonary congestion, resemble those of a patent ductus arteriosus.

LABORATORY FINDINGS. Cardiac enlargement and pulmonary congestion are noted on the roentgenogram, and cardiac hypertrophy on the electrocardiogram. On cardiac catheterization, a left-to-right shunt can be identified at the atrial or ventricular level. Diagnosis is best established by selective aortography, demonstrating the leakage of dye from the aorta into the involved cardiac chamber (Fig. 18-48). The differential diagnosis must exclude patent ductus arteriosus and aortic-pulmonary window.

TREATMENT. Operative correction should be performed as soon as the diagnosis has been established. This is done with extracorporeal circulation through a median sternotomy incision. The basic objective at operation is to close the defect in the aortic wall at the mouth of the aneurysm by attaching the aortic media superiorly to the aortic ring below (Fig. 18-49). Although initially operations were usually performed by approaching the lesion through the right atrium or right ventricle, excising the fistulous sac and suturing the opening, a transaortic approach, as suggested by Shumacker et al., permits a more precise closure, assuring adequate repair of the aortic wall without any risk of injury to the aortic valve cusps. A concomitant ventricular septal defect may frequently be found and repaired at the same operation. The operative risk is small and the results have been excellent.

Truncus Arteriosus

Truncus arteriosus is a rare malformation resulting from failure of division of the fetal arterial channel into the aorta and pulmonary arteries and the left and right ventricles. Therapy of this condition is a good example of the rapid changes in cardiac surgery. When the first edition of this book was written in 1969, only palliative therapy was possible. Since that time McGoon and associates have developed a technique of surgical correction with an aortic homograft which has been successfully applied to a significant number of patients.

PATHOLOGIC ANATOMY. In this condition the entire circulation, including the coronary arteries, the pulmonary arteries, and the systemic arteries, arises from a common arterial trunk. There is always a ventricular septal defect, and a single ventricle occurs in 15 to 20 percent of patients. Only one semilunar valve is present, usually with four cusps, although the number may vary from two to six. The pulmonary arteries may arise from the aorta as a single pulmonary artery, from which the right and left pulmonary arteries originate, or the two pulmonary arteries may originate separately.

"Pseudotruncus" has been used by some to describe a condition in which a single large artery originates from the base of the heart, but the pulmonary arteries are absent and pulmonary blood flows through enlarged bronchial vessels. Others consider the condition as pulmonary atresia or a variant of severe tetralogy of Fallot. "Hemiotruncus" is a term which has been applied to a condition which is physiologically quite different from the truncus arteriosus condition. This is a very rare malformation in which one pulmonary artery originates from the aorta while the other arises normally from the right ventricle. Hence there is an abnormality only in the pulmonary circulation to one lung, and the physiologic derangement is much less than in truncus arteriosus.

PATHOPHYSIOLOGY. The disability with this condition is a severe one, with 50 to 60 percent of infants dying in the first year of life, usually from congestive heart failure. As blood entering the aorta is a mixture of blood from the systemic circulation and the pulmonary circulation, oxygen unsaturation is always present in the arterial blood, the degree varying with the volume of pulmonary blood flow. If large pulmonary arteries originate from the aorta, initially there is a large pulmonary blood flow with minimal cyanosis. Subsequently there is an inevitable rise in pulmonary vascular resistance, with diminution in pulmonary blood flow and increase in cyanosis. If pulmonary blood flow is greatly diminished, as in "pseudotruncus," cyanosis is severe.

CLINICAL MANIFESTATIONS. Disability is evident in infancy, with cyanosis and dyspnea on exertion and retardation of growth and development. On physical examination, loud systolic and diastolic murmurs are audible over the base of the heart, often as a to-and-fro murmur rather than a true continuous murmur. In older children, continuous murmurs may be best heard over one or both lungs, originating from collateral circulation to the lungs; as emphasized by Taussig, this is virtually diagnostic of the malformation. The second heart sound is "pure" and increased in intensity.

LABORATORY FINDINGS. The chest roentgenogram and electrocardiogram show both right and left ventricular enlargement. Cardiac catheterization will demonstrate a left-to-right shunt in the ventricle with a systolic pulmonary artery pressure equal to aortic systolic pressure. The abnormal vessels can be outlined with selective angiography, but precise studies are required to demonstrate with certainty the exact point of origin of the pulmonary arteries.

In acyanotic children the condition must be differentiated from patent ductus arteriosus or an aortic-pulmonary window. With severe cyanosis, pulmonary atresia, tricuspid atresia, and transposition of the great vessels must be considered.

TREATMENT. The operation developed by McGoon et al. consists of construction of a new pulmonary artery with a homograft of ascending aorta, containing an aortic valve. Employing extracorporeal circulation, the pulmonary arteries are detached from the aorta. The right ventricle is then opened in the outflow tract, excising a small segment to make an adequate opening. The ventricular septal defect is then closed so that the aorta originates only from the left ventricle. The homograft with the aortic valve is then attached to the opening in the right ventricle, and distally is connected to the right and left pulmonary arteries, creating a new pulmonary artery.

Operative mortality has been surprisingly low in patients in whom pulmonary vascular resistance is not significantly increased. To date the only late complication has been calcification of the homograft, thus far of no physiologic significance. A similar operative procedure has been performed in which the new pulmonary artery is constructed of Dacron and an aortic homograft valve inserted to function as a new pulmonic valve.

Single Ventricle

A single ventricle is a rare, severe malformation for which only palliative therapy is possible. Nadas found only 10 cases in a group of 577 patients.

PATHOLOGIC ANATOMY. The anomaly consists of a single functioning ventricular chamber into which both atrioventricular valves enter. Connected to the functioning ventricle is a rudimentary outlet chamber located in the position normally occupied by the outflow tract of the right ventricle. From this rudimentary chamber one or both of the great vessels may arise. Transposition of the aorta and pulmonary artery occurs in over one-half the patients. The clinical profile varies widely, depending upon whether or not the arteries are transposed and whether the artery arising from the rudimentary outlet chamber is of normal diameter or hypoplastic.

PATHOPHYSIOLOGY. The two physiologic characteristics are admixture of oxygenated and unoxygenated blood in the common ventricle before entering the aorta, and pulmonary hypertension resulting from origin of the pulmonary artery and the aorta from the same ventricle. The degree of cyanosis depends upon the pulmonary blood flow.

CLINICAL MANIFESTATIONS. Infants with an increased pulmonary blood flow, occurring when the aorta arises from the rudimentary outlet chamber and the pulmonary artery from the functioning ventricle, may be acyanotic but disabled from pulmonary congestion and cardiac failure. Conversely, with a decreased pulmonary blood flow from a hypoplastic pulmonary artery, cyanosis may be severe and the clinical picture dominated by signs of anoxia. Much variation between these two extremes is seen because of other anomalies frequently present. A single ventricle per se is most unusual, for concomitant cardiac malformations are frequent.

The disability is severe and associated with cardiac failure or cyanosis. In a group of 85 patients reviewed by Campbell and associates, over one-half died in the first year of life, although 18 lived to be twenty years of age. On physical examination variable systolic murmurs and cardiac enlargement are found, but variation in the murmurs precludes any diagnostic significance.

LABORATORY FINDINGS. The roentgenogram demonstrates cardiac enlargement, and the electrocardiogram shows left or right ventricular hypertrophy. Great variation is present, depending upon the relation of the aorta and pulmonary artery to the common ventricle and the rudimentary outlet chamber. The best diagnostic information is obtained on cardiac catheterization, with a rise in oxygen concentration of 4 to 5 vol % noted when a catheter is advanced from the atrium into the common ventricle. Similar pressures may be found in the aorta and pulmonary artery. Selective angiography may demonstrate the rudimentary outlet chamber.

TREATMENT. Effective treatment is not possible. Banding of the pulmonary artery has been attempted in a few patients with a marked increase in pulmonary blood flow. In cyanotic patients with a marked decrease in pulmonary blood flow a systemic–pulmonary artery anastomosis may be of benefit, but cardiac failure often results. Although a few patients may survive to adult life, the prognosis is guarded.

Ebstein's Anomaly

This peculiar and unusual anomaly was described by Wilhelm Ebstein in 1866 following postmortem examination of a nineteen-year-old cyanotic youth who had died with signs of tricuspid insufficiency. Although the anomaly is uncommon, with improvement in cardiac diagnostic techniques it has been recognized with increased frequency. Vacca and associates in 1958 found the total number of cases reported to be 108. The cause is unknown.

PATHOLOGIC ANATOMY. The anomaly consists of a downward displacement of part of the tricuspid valve, creating a third chamber in the right side of the heart. Usually the anterior leaflet of the tricuspid valve arises normally from the tricuspid annulus and may be abnormally large and prominent. It has been described as saillike. The septal and posterior leaflets, however, are not attached to the normal tricuspid annulus but arise from the wall of the right ventricle at a varying distance from the true annulus. These two cusps may be small and adherent to the wall of the ventricle, with little functional ability (Fig. 18-50). The segment of right ventricular wall between the true annulus of the tricuspid valve and the origin of the displaced leaflets is then functionally a part

of the right atrium and has been termed the *atrialized* ventricle. The wall of this part of the ventricle may be unusually thin. The foramen ovale is usually patent, and often an atrial septal defect is also present.

The malformation varies widely in severity, depending upon the relative size of the atrialized ventricle above the tricuspid valve and the functioning right ventricle below the abnormal valve. The anatomic spectrum of malformations which may be seen has been well illustrated by Taussig.

PATHOPHYSIOLOGY. The main physiologic disturbance is inadequate cardiac output from the right ventricle. This is probably due to both the tricuspid insufficiency and the paradoxic contraction of the atrialized segment of the right ventricle. Less significant causes are the small size of the functioning right ventricle and the frequent arrhythmias. With the low cardiac output and tricuspid insufficiency, the right atrium becomes massively dilated, and cyanosis of moderate degree is usually present because of a right-to-left shunt through the foramen ovale. The cyanosis tends to become more severe in later years of life, probably because of progressive right ventricular failure.

CLINICAL MANIFESTATIONS. The clinical course is often a severe one, although some adults survive for many years. Analysis of reported cases has found that about 40 percent of patients die in the first decade and 30 percent in the next. Death occurs from congestive failure in about one-

Fig. 18-50. *A.* Normal heart showing septal and posterior leaflets of tricuspid valve. *B.* Pathologic anatomy in Ebstein's malformation, with displacement of diminutive septal and posterior leaflets down into normal right ventricular cavity. Large anterior leaflet is not shown. *C.* Abnormal pathologic anatomy in Ebstein's malformation. There is large "saillike" anterior leaflet with hypoplastic septal and posterior leaflets, which are often displaced downward into ventricle, creating third cardiac chamber interposed between right atrium and functioning right ventricle. (*Adapted from K. L. Hardy et al., J Thorac Cardiovasc Surg, 48:931, 1964.*)

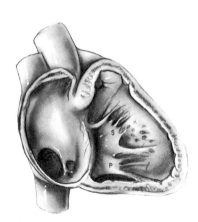

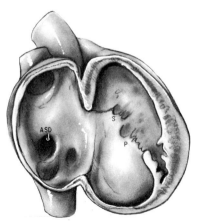

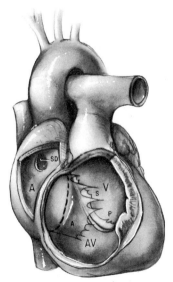

A   B   C

third of patients, and at least another third may die suddenly from an arrhythmia.

The predominant symptoms are fatigue, with gradual increase in exertional dyspnea and cyanosis over the years. Symptoms may be present in some patients during early childhood, while in others they appear only after the first decade. Signs of right-sided failure gradually become more evident. Physical examination discloses soft, blurred systolic and diastolic murmurs along the left sternal border, with muffled heart sounds and signs of feeble, ineffective cardiac contractions. The cardiac size is usually increased. The findings have been appropriately compared to those with a large pericardial effusion. Cyanosis and clubbing may be found but are usually not severe.

Nadas has stated that the auscultatory findings are pathognomonic of the condition. He emphasizes three findings: a slow cardiac rate with a triple or quadruple rhythm, a systolic murmur of tricuspid regurgitation, and frequently a low-pitched diastolic murmur.

LABORATORY FINDINGS. The roentgenogram may be remarkable for the great enlargement of the right side of the heart, including a huge right atrium and the atrialized part of the right ventricle. The pulmonary artery segment is often small, and the vascularity in the lung fields is less than normal. On fluoroscopy, feeble cardiac contractions are frequently seen. The electrocardiographic findings are also considered to be typical. Conduction disturbances with prolonged P-R interval and partial right bundle branch block are common. Right ventricular hypertrophy is absent after infancy, but the left chest leads show average potentials.

Cardiac catheterization may be unusually hazardous; deaths from arrhythmias have occurred in several laboratories. Alertness to the possibility, however, in combination with use of electric defibrillators, has greatly decreased the risk of catheterization. With catheterization, a right-to-left shunt at the atrial level, with resulting arterial unsaturation, is found in 25 to 50 percent of patients. Interestingly enough, the contour of the right atrial pressure wave may not be strikingly abnormal, perhaps because of the damping effect of the large cavity of the right atrium on the blood regurgitating through the incompetent tricuspid orifice. The abnormal course of the cardiac catheter in the atrialized part of the right ventricle can be of diagnostic significance, and with selective angiography, the huge right atrium can be outlined. Diagnosis can usually be made with certainty on the basis of the typical physical findings, combined with the abnormalities observed on the roentgenogram and electrocardiogram and those found at cardiac catheterization.

TREATMENT. Until recently only palliative therapy has been possible. In a few patients, pulmonary blood flow has been increased by a superior vena cava–right pulmonary artery anastomosis, but good results have not been consistently obtained. The usual difficulty is not cyanosis but inadequate output from the right ventricle. Recent surgical attempts to eliminate the paradoxic contraction of the atrialized part of the right ventricle and to restore competency to the tricuspid valve have produced good results in a few patients. A suggestion by Hunter and Lillehei to exclude the atrialized ventricle from the circulation by approximating the true tricuspid annulus with the area on the right ventricular wall from which the displaced septal and posterior leaflets originate has been carried out by Hardy and associates in one patient in 1963 and by Bahnson and associates in two patients. Replacement of the abnormal valve with a prosthetic valve has been performed by Barnard, and Timmis and associates have combined prosthetic replacement with elimination of the atrialized ventricle in one patient.

At New York University four patients have been operated upon by replacing the diseased tricuspid valve with a ball-valve prosthesis and partly or completely excluding the atrialized portion of the right ventricle, as suggested by Timmis. Two patients have an excellent result, one patient over fifty years of age died several months later from continued arrhythmias, and one other patient died postoperatively from a low cardiac output (Fig. 18-51). It seems from data currently available that prognosis for repair of Ebstein's anomaly is more favorable than that considered in the past, but there is still a paucity of reported surgical experiences. It is hoped that the susceptibility to sudden death from arrhythmias will be eliminated by operative procedures performed before severe cardiac hypertrophy has developed.

Anomalies of the Coronary Arteries

ANOMALOUS ORIGIN OF LEFT CORONARY ARTERY FROM PULMONARY ARTERY

The first case of this unusual malformation was described by Abrikosov in 1911, but little clinical interest evolved until Bland et al. in 1933 described the clinical features of the syndrome and emphasized its similarity to myocardial infarction in adults. Over 50 cases were reviewed by Keith in 1959. A significant advance was made by Sabiston et al. in 1959 when they conclusively demonstrated retrograde flow of blood from the anomalous left coronary artery into the pulmonary artery, a theoretical possibility previously mentioned by several investigators. Subsequently, in two older children, four and five years of age, the ideal operation was accomplished by Cooley and associates, who detached the coronary artery from the pulmonary artery and connected it to the aorta by means of an interposed graft (Fig. 18-52).

PATHOLOGIC ANATOMY AND PHYSIOLOGY. The disease is a severe one, and the majority of affected children die in the first year of life. The left ventricle is usually grossly dilated, with a thin fibrotic wall showing multiple areas of infarction. Other abnormalities are secondary to chronic congestive failure. Apparently the serious physiologic handicap from origin of the left coronary artery from the pulmonary artery is the low perfusion pressure and not the low oxygen content of blood in the coronary artery, because even more severe degrees of oxygen unsaturation in severely cyanotic children do not produce gross injury to the muscle of the left ventricle. The demonstration that the flow of blood may be retrograde through the coronary artery into the pulmonary artery indicates that the anomaly

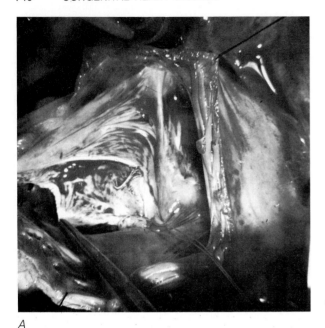

A

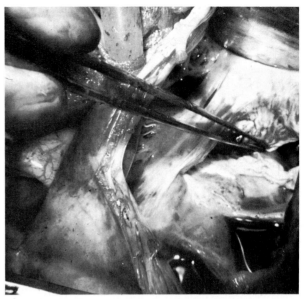

B

Fig. 18-51. *A*. Operative photograph of the tricuspid valve in a forty-five-year-old patient with Ebstein's disease. The large "sail" anterior leaflet is demonstrated. *B*. In contrast to the large anterior leaflet, the posterior and septal leaflets are displaced downward into the right ventricle and are rudimentary and nonfunctional, which is characteristic of the Ebstein malformation.

Fig. 18-52 (*Below*). *A*. Anomalous left coronary artery arising from pulmonary artery. *B*. Vein graft is used to anastomose coronary artery to aorta. This theoretically ideal operation has rarely been accomplished as yet. (*Adapted from D. A. Cooley et al., J Thorac Cardiovasc. Surg, 52:805, 1966.*)

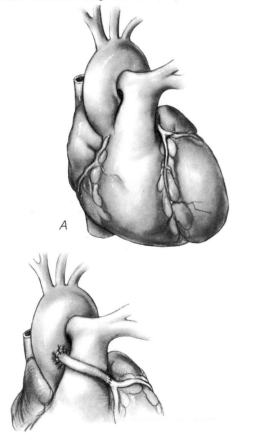

A

B

actually siphons oxygenated blood away from the ischemic myocardium. Retrograde flow is proved by finding a higher oxygen content in blood in the coronary artery than in the pulmonary artery, and also by demonstrating a *rise* in pressure in the coronary artery when its origin from the pulmonary artery is occluded. Survival of a few patients beyond infancy apparently results from an abundant collateral circulation with the right coronary artery, so that the left ventricle is supplied with blood first entering the right coronary artery and then flowing through collateral channels into tributaries of the left coronary artery. Anomalous origin of the *right* coronary artery from the pulmonary artery is apparently an innocuous condition and compatible with normal longevity.

CLINICAL MANIFESTATIONS. Dyspnea and other symptoms often appear in the first 3 months of life. Characteristically, acute episodes may occur with feeding, between which the infant is completely normal. During these episodes there may be colicky pain, tachypnea, cyanosis, pallor, and sweating, apparently a syndrome resembling angina pectoris. Subsequently, with chronic congestive failure, tachypnea becomes a chronic symptom. On examination, obvious cardiac enlargement is found, with muffled heart sounds. Frequently no murmurs are audible.

LABORATORY FINDINGS. The chest roentgenogram will confirm the extensive enlargement of the left ventricle, and cardiac angiography will demonstrate that the enlargement is predominantly dilatation of the left ventricle, often with an unusually thin wall. The electrocardiogram may be diagnostic, demonstrating inversion of the T waves and prominent Q waves in certain precordial leads. In older children, cardiac catheterization will detect a small left-to-right shunt at the level of the pulmonary artery. Aortography may graphically confirm the diagnosis. The diagnosis is suggested by opacification of a normal right coronary artery at the base of the aorta without opacification of the left coronary artery; subsequent films may show filling of the left coronary artery through tributaries of the right coronary artery, confirming the diagnosis.

TREATMENT. Patients who remain asymptomatic in the first year of life, presumably because of abundant collateral circulation through the right coronary artery, have a more gradual onset of symptoms and are the best candidates for definitive reconstruction of the coronary artery, as demonstrated by Cooley et al. Unfortunately, this group of patients constitutes the minority. Infants in whom symptoms develop in the first few months of life seldom survive; thus ligation of the anomalous coronary artery should probably be done unless direct arterial reconstruction appears feasible in these small children. Unfortunately, ligation virtually precludes the possibility of subsequent direct reconstruction. A study by Likar and associates of 27 patients who underwent ligation of the anomalous artery included 20 infants, 11 of whom died after operation. With the extensive experience with coronary bypass operations, direct reconstruction will surely be used more frequently in the future.

CORONARY ARTERIOVENOUS FISTULA

Information concerning this unusual anomaly was crystallized in 1960 by Gasul and associates in their collective review of 52 cases.

PATHOLOGIC ANATOMY AND PHYSIOLOGY. The abnormality consists of a direct communication between a coronary artery and a cardiac chamber through one or more abnormal openings. Usually the coronary fistula opens into the right atrium or right ventricle, constituting a left-to-right shunt. Rarely it enters the left atrium or left ventricle, causing signs of mild aortic insufficiency. With the increased blood flow through the arteriovenous fistula there is dilatation of the coronary arteries, which become progressively elongated and tortuous (Fig. 18-53). Astonishing degrees of dilatation, with vessels 1 to 2 cm in diameter, have been reported.

When the fistula opens into the right side of the heart, the resulting left-to-right shunt is small, but with subsequent dilatation of the parent artery the shunt may eventually become large enough to cause significant cardiac enlargement.

CLINICAL MANIFESTATIONS. Although the arteriovenous fistula may cause myocardial ischemia from blood preferentially flowing through the fistula rather than through the myocardial capillaries, this is uncommon. Several patients with minor hemodynamic disability have been reported living normal lives without symptoms. When the fistula is large, however, significant cardiac symptoms appear, both from the left-to-right shunt and from the myocardial ischemia.

The most common symptoms are fatigue and dyspnea. On physical examination the significant finding is a continuous murmur that seems unusually loud and superficial, especially in combination with absence of symptoms and

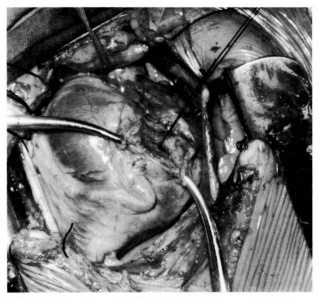

Fig. 18-53. Arteriovenous fistula of right coronary artery. Enlarged, tortuous right coronary artery is clearly visible over surface of right ventricle. Fistulous communication directly into right ventricle was found, as illustrated by ligatures, and ligated.

minimal signs of cardiac disability. The location of maximal intensity of the murmur varies with the site of the fistula; it usually is at a lower level than that of the typical patent ductus arteriosus.

LABORATORY FINDINGS. The chest roentgenogram may be normal or may show only slight cardiac enlargement. Similarly, the electrocardiogram may be normal or may show minimal signs of ventricular hypertrophy. Cardiac catheterization can detect the site of the left-to-right shunt and thereby identify the chamber into which the fistula empties. The most definitive study is coronary arteriography, outlining both the site of the fistula and the course of the abnormal vessels. The degree of dilatation and tortuosity in some patients is most impressive.

TREATMENT. If a patient is asymptomatic with no signs of cardiac disability, operation is not urgent. Some have been managed simply by continued observation. However, as the usual course is continued enlargement of the fistula, with progressive hemodynamic disability, elective repair is preferable in most instances (Fig. 18-54).

A 1971 review by Oldham et al. well summarized clinical experiences. In a review of over 200 reported cases, including their own personal experiences with 12 cases, 183 of the fistulas entered the right side of the heart, and only 17 entered one of the chambers of the left side. A significant point facilitating surgical treatment is the fact that almost all fistulas had a single, rather than multiple, point of entry into the heart. The shunt was seldom large, with the pulmonary blood flow usually increased to about twice normal. Congestive heart failure appeared in two age groups, either in infancy or after forty years of age. The latter group probably resulted from progressive enlargement of the fistula. However, in the overall series there

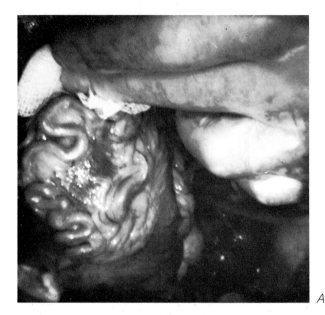

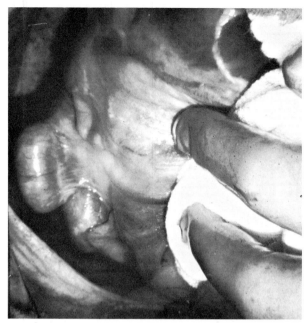

B

was a history of congestive heart failure in only 14 percent of the patients, and angina in 7 percent.

Precise coronary angiography has greatly facilitated treatment. The single point of entry of the fistula can be identified by angiography. Surgical dissection in this area can often locate the abnormal vessel and occlude it but preserve continuity of the involved coronary artery. Of 116 reported cases undergoing operation, only four deaths have occurred.

Corrected Transposition

This unusual anomaly has been studied in detail in recent years, principally because of the influence of its unusual anatomic features on the surgical treatment of associated cardiovascular malformations. The clinical features of the syndrome were well summarized by Anderson et al. in their report of 14 patients in 1957. An additional group of 33 cases was reported by Schiebler and associates in 1961.

PATHOLOGIC ANATOMY AND PHYSIOLOGY. In this malformation the aorta and pulmonary artery are transposed to lie in a relation exactly the opposite of that normally occurring. The aorta arises from the anterior left border of the heart and the pulmonary artery from the right and posterior area of the heart (Fig. 18-55). The ventricle from which the aorta arises has the anatomic characteristics of a normal trabeculated right ventricle, and that from which the pulmonary artery arises resembles a left ventricle. The atrioventricular valves are similarly reversed, with the tricuspid valve opening into the aortic ventricle and the mitral valve opening into the pulmonary ventricle. Venous drainage into the atria, however, is normal; so despite the abnormal anatomic relations, the circulation is normal. Venous blood returns to the right atrium, flows through the mitral valve into an anatomic "left" ventricle, and is expelled into the pulmonary artery. From the lungs blood returns through the pulmonary veins to the left atrium,

Fig. 18-54. *A.* Operative photograph of the tortuous coronary vessels with a coronary arteriovenous fistula in a woman in the fifth decade who was virtually asymptomatic. *B.* Operative photograph of the site of entry of the fistula into the right ventricle near the apex of the heart. This was eliminated by simple ligature.

flows across a tricuspid valve into an anatomic "right" ventricle, and is expelled into the aorta. The anatomic relations of the coronary arteries are also reversed, the right coronary artery arising anteriorly and the left coronary artery posteriorly and the noncoronary sinus being located at the anterior left border of the heart.

The significance of the malformation is primarily in the high incidence of associated abnormalities, for some additional malformation is almost always present. Nadas has stated that at least 50 percent of patients with this condition have mitral insufficiency, perhaps as a result of the tricuspid valve being poorly designed to withstand systemic ventricular pressures. A ventricular septal defect is common, and a wide variety of other malformations may be seen. Conduction defects are frequent. Approximately one-third of the patients have a first- to third-degree heart block, and another third have different types of arrhythmias, such as paroxysmal atrial tachycardia.

CLINICAL MANIFESTATIONS. The symptoms are principally determined by the associated malformations. In the unusual case of "pure" corrected transposition, there are no symptoms except for those resulting from the cardiac arrhythmias. Physical examination similarly discloses no abnormalities, except that the cardiac second sound to the left of the sternum is unusually loud because it originates from closure of the aortic valve.

LABORATORY FINDINGS. On the roentgenogram there is an unusual contour at the base of the heart from the unusual relation of the great vessels, but often this is not distinctive enough to be diagnostic. The electrocardiogram is almost always abnormal and is one of the best diagnostic

NORMAL

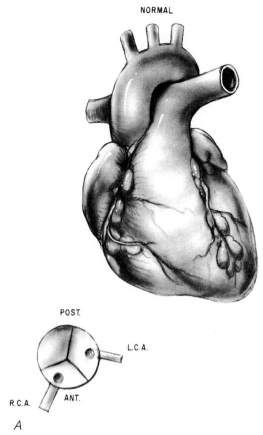

POST.

L.C.A.

R.C.A.   ANT.

A

CORRECTED TRANSPOSITION

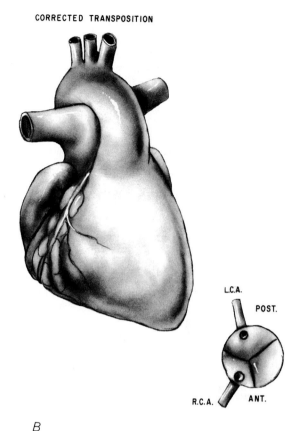

L.C.A.

POST.

R.C.A.   ANT.

B

Fig. 18-55. *A.* Normal cardiac anatomy with pulmonary artery arising from right ventricle and aorta from left ventricle. Comparison with *B* shows that in corrected transposition, relative positions of aorta and pulmonary artery are reversed. *B.* In corrected transposition of great vessels, aorta arises anteriorly from ventricle that has anatomic characteristics of right ventricle. Pulmonary artery arises posteriorly and to right of aorta—reverse of normal anatomic arrangement. Insert depicts origin of coronary arteries in corrected transposition. (*Adapted from A. S. Nadas, "Pediatric Cardiology," W. B. Saunders Company, Philadelphia, 1964, p. 714.*)

guides. Conduction disturbances, arrhythmias, and unusual patterns of ventricular hypertrophy in the precordial leads may all suggest the diagnosis. Diagnosis can be firmly established by angiography, which will demonstrate the aorta to the left of the pulmonary artery.

TREATMENT. The importance of the condition is predominantly related to the anatomic implications inherent in the surgical correction of associated lesions. With ventricular septal defect there is a high incidence of conduction defects, so the risk of complete heart block during closure of the septal defect is significant. Similarly, ventriculotomy must be so planned as to avoid division of any major coronary arteries. If a tetralogy of Fallot is present, correction of the infundibular stenosis may be difficult or impossible because of the unusual position of the coronary vessels. In the absence of other defects, older patients in the past have died from mitral insufficiency, but this can now be treated by prosthetic mitral valve replacement.

References

General

Abbott, M. E.: "Atlas of Congenital Cardiac Disease," The American Heart Association, New York, 1936.

Benson, C. D., Mustard, W. T., Ravitch, M. M., Snyder, W. H., and Welch, K. J. (eds.): "Pediatric Surgery," 2d ed., Year Book Medical Publishers, Inc., Chicago, 1971.

Breckenridge, I. M., Oelert, H., Graham, G. R., Stark, J., Waterston, D. J., and Bonham-Carter, R. E.: Open Heart Surgery in the First Year of Life, *J Thorac Cardiovasc Surg,* **65:**58, 1973.

Cooley, D. A., and Hallman, G. L.: "Surgical Treatment of Congenital Heart Disease," Lea & Febiger, Philadelphia, 1966.

Dammann, J. F., Jr.: Pulmonary Hypertension in C. D. Benson et al. (eds.), "Pediatric Surgery," 2d ed., vol. 1, Year Book Medical Publishers, Inc., Chicago, 1971.

Edwards, J. E.: Functional Pathology of the Pulmonary Vascular Tree in Congenital Cardiac Disease, *Circulation,* **15:**164, 1957.

Gorlin, R., and Gorlin, S. G.: Hydraulic Formula for Calculation of the Area of the Stenotic Mitral Valve, Other Cardiac Valves, and Central Circulatory Shunts: I, *Am Heart J,* **41:**1, 1951.

Gross, R. E.: "The Surgery of Infancy and Childhood," W. B. Saunders Company, Philadelphia, 1953.

Keith, J. D., Rowe, R. D., and Vlad, P.: "Heart Disease in Infancy and Childhood," 2d ed., The Macmillan Company, New York, 1967.

Nadas, A. S.: "Pediatric Cardiology," 2d ed., W. B. Saunders Company, Philadelphia, 1963.

Stewart, S., III, Edmunds, L. H., Jr., Kirklin, J. W., and Allarde, R. R.: Spontaneous Breathing with Continuous Positive Airway Pressure after Open Intracardiac Operations in Infants, *J Thorac Cardiovasc Surg,* **65:**37, 1973.

Taussig, H. B.: "Congenital Malformations of the Heart," 2d ed., Harvard University Press, Cambridge, Mass., 1960.

Pulmonic Stenosis

Brock, R. C.: Pulmonary Valvulotomy for the Relief of Congenital Stenosis: Report of Three Cases, *Br Med J,* **1:**112, 1948.

Engle, M. A., Holswade, G. R., Goldberg, H. P., Lukas, D. S., and Glenn, F.: Regression after Open Valvotomy of Infundibular Stenosis Accompanying Severe Valvular Pulmonic Stenosis, *Circulation,* **17:**862, 1958.

Gilbert, J. W., Morrow, A. G., and Talbert, J. L.: The Surgical Significance of Hypertrophic Infundibular Obstruction Accompanying Valvular Pulmonic Stenosis, *J Thorac Cardiovasc Surg,* **46:**457, 1963.

Holman, E.: On Circumscribed Dilation of an Artery Immediately Distal to a Partially Occluding Band: Poststenotic Dilatation, *Surgery,* **36:**3, 1954.

Johnson, L. W., Grossman, W., Dalen, J. E., and Dexter, L.: Pulmonic Stenosis in the Adult: Longterm Followup Results, *N Engl J Med,* **287:**1159, 1972.

Nadas, A. S.: Pulmonic Stenosis: Indications for Surgery in Children and Adults, *N Engl J Med,* **287:**1196, 1972.

Sellors, T. H.: Surgery of Pulmonic Stenosis, *Lancet,* **1:**988, 1948.

Spencer, F. C., and Bahnson, H. T.: Intracardiac Surgery Employing Hypothermia and Coronary Perfusion Performed on 100 Patients, *Surgery,* **46:**987, 1959.

Swan, H., and Zeavin, I.: Cessation of Circulation in General Hypothermia, *Ann Surg,* **139:**385, 1954.

Tandon, R., Nadas, A. S., and Gross, R. E.: Results of Open Heart Surgery in Patients with Pulmonic Stenosis and Intact Ventricular Septum: A Report of 108 Cases, *Circulation,* **31:**190, 1965.

Stenosis of the Pulmonary Artery

Franch, R. H., and Gay, B. B.: Congenital Stenosis of the Pulmonary Artery Branches, *Am J Med,* **35:**512, 1963.

McGoon, D. C., and Kincaid, O. W.: Stenosis of Branches of the Pulmonary Artery: Surgical Repair, *Med Clin North Am,* **48:**1083, 1964.

Wallsh, E., Reppert, E. H., Doyle, E. F., and Spencer, F. C.: "Absent" Left Pulmonary Artery with Tetralogy of Fallot, *J Thorac Cardiovasc Surg,* **55:**333, 1968.

Congenital Aortic Stenosis

Braunwald, E., Goldblatt, A., Aygen, M. M., Rockoff, S. D., and Morrow, A. G.: Congenital Aortic Stenosis: Clinical and Hemodynamic Findings in 100 patients, *Circulation,* **27:**426, 1963.

Braverman, I. B., and Gibson, S.: The Outlook for Children with Congenital Aortic Stenosis, *Am Heart J,* **53:**487, 1957.

Frahm, C. J., Braunwald, E., and Morrow, A. G.: Congenital Aortic Regurgitation: Findings in Four Patients, *Am J Med,* **31:**63, 1961.

Peckham, G. B., Keith, J. D., and Evans, J. R.: Congenital Aortic

Stenosis: Some Observations on the Natural History and Clinical Assessment, *J Can Med Assoc,* **90:**639, 1964.

Spencer, F. C., Neill, C. A., and Bahnson, H. T.: The Treatment of Congenital Aortic Stenosis with Valvulotomy during Cardiopulmonary Bypass, *Surgery,* **44:**109, 1958.

———, ———, Sank, L., and Bahnson, H. T.: Anatomical Variations in 46 Patients with Congenital Aortic Stenosis, *Am Surg,* **26:**204, 1960.

Supravalvular Aortic Stenosis

Morrow, A. G., Waldhausen, J. A., Peters, R. L., Bloodwell, R. D., and Braunwald, E.: Supravalvular Aortic Stenosis, *Circulation,* **20:**1003, 1959.

Peterson, T. A., Todd, D. C., and Edwards, J. E.: Supravalvular Aortic Stenosis, *J Thorac Cardiovasc Surg,* **50:**734, 1965.

Rastelli, G. C., McGoon, D. C., Ongley, P. A., Mankin, H. T., and Kirklin, J. W.: Surgical Treatment of Supravalvular Aortic Stenosis: Report of 16 Cases and Review of Literature, *J Thorac Cardiovasc Surg,* **51:**873, 1966.

Williams, J. C. P., Barratt-Boyes, B. G., and Lowe, J. B.: Supravalvular Aortic Stenosis, *Circulation,* **24:**1311, 1961.

Hypertrophic Subaortic Stenosis

Barratt-Boyes, B. G.: "Symposium on Congenital Cardiac Malformations and Their Treatment, Auckland, New Zealand, February 1972." (In press.)

Bigelow, W. G., Trimble, A. S., Auger, P., Marquis, Y., and Wigle, E. D.: The Ventriculomyotomy Operation for Muscular Subaortic Stenosis: A Reappraisal, *J Thorac Cardiovasc Surg,* **52:**514, 1966.

Braunwald, E., Brockenbrough, E. C., and Morrow, A. G.: Hypertrophic Subaortic Stenosis: A Broadened Concept, *Circulation,* **26:**161, 1962. (Editorial.)

Frye, R. L., Kincaid, O. W., Swan, H. J. C., and Kirklin, J. W.: Results of Surgical Treatment of Patients with Diffuse Subvalvular Aortic Stenosis, *Circulation,* **32:**52, 1965.

Kelly, D. T., Barratt-Boyes, B. G., and Lowe, J. B.: Results of Surgery and Hemodynamic Observations in Muscular Subaortic Stenosis, *J Thorac Cardiovasc Surg,* **51:**353, 1966.

Kirklin, J. W.: "Symposium on Congenital Cardiac Malformations and Their Treatment, Auckland, New Zealand, 1972." (In press.)

Coarctation of the Aorta

Abbott, M. E.: Coarctation of the Aorta of the Adult Type: II. A Statistical Study and Historical Retrospect of 200 Recorded Cases, with Autopsy, of Stenosis or Obliteration of the Descending Arch in Subjects above the Age of Two Years, *Am Heart J,* **3:**392, 1928.

Blalock, A., and Park, E. A.: The Surgical Treatment of Experimental Coarctation (Atresia) of the Aorta, *Ann Surg,* **119:**445, 1944.

Brewer, L. A., III, Fosburg, R. G., Mulder, A. G., and Verska, J. J.: Spinal Cord Complications following Surgery for Coarctation of the Aorta: A Study of 66 Cases, *J Thorac Cardiovasc Surg,* **64:**368, 1972.

Brom, A. G.: Narrowing of the Aortic Isthmus and Enlargement of the Mind, *J Thorac Cardiovasc Surg,* **50:**166, 1965.

Crafoord, C., and Nylin, G.: Congenital Coarctation of the Aorta and Its Surgical Treatment, *J Thorac Surg,* **14:**347, 1945.

DeBakey, M. E., Garrett, H. E., Howell, J. F., and Morris, G. C.: Coarctation of the Abdominal Aorta with Renal Arterial Stenosis: Surgical Considerations, *Ann Surg,* **165:**830, 1967.

Gross, R. E.: Coarctation of the Aorta: Surgical Treatment of One Hundred Cases, *Circulation,* **1:**41, 1950.

Hughes, R. K., and Reemtsma, K.: Correction of Coarctation of the Aorta: Manometric Determination of Safety during Test Occlusion, *J Thorac Cardiovasc Surg,* **62:**31, 1971.

Schuster, S. R., and Gross, R. E.: Surgery for Coarctation of the Aorta: A Review of 500 Cases, *J Thor Cardiovasc Surg,* **43:**54, 1962.

Sealy, W. C., Harris, J. S., Young, W. G., and Callaway, H. A.: Paradoxical Hypertension following Resection of Coarctation of the Aorta, *Surgery,* **42:**135, 1957.

Vascular Rings

Gross, R. E.: Arterial Malformations Which Cause Compression of the Trachea or Esophagus, *Circulation,* **11:**124, 1955.

Mahoney, E. B., and Manning, J. A.: Congenital Abnormalities of the Aortic Arch, *Surgery,* **55:**1, 1964.

Shumacker, H. B., Jr., and Burford, T. H.: Unusual Sequel to Operative Intervention for Vascular Ring, *J Thorac Cardiovasc Surg,* **65:**124, 1973.

Atrial Septal Defects: Secundum Defects

Gerbode, F., Harkins, G. A., Ross, J. K., and Osborn, J. J.: Experience with Atrial Septal Defects Repaired with the Aid of Cardiopulmonary Bypass, *Arch Surg,* **80:**846, 1960.

Gibbon, J. H., Jr.: Application of a Mechanical Heart and Lung Apparatus to Cardiac Surgery, *Minn Med,* **37:**171, 1954.

Sellers, R. D., Ferlic, R. M., Sterns, L. P., and Lillehei, C. W.: Secundum Type Atrial Septal Defects: Results with 275 Patients, *Surgery,* **59:**155, 1966.

Spencer, F. C., and Bahnson, H. T.: Intracardiac Surgery Employing Hypothermia and Coronary Perfusion Performed on 100 Patients, *Surgery,* **46:**987, 1959.

Anomalous Drainage of Pulmonary Veins

Bahnson, H. T., Spencer, F. C., and Neill, C. A.: Surgical Treatment of 35 Cases of Drainage of Pulmonary Veins to the Right Side of the Heart, *J Thorac Cardiovasc Surg,* **36:**777, 1958.

Blake, H. A., Hall, R. C., and Manion, W. C.: Anomalous Pulmonary Venous Return, *Circulation,* **32:**406, 1965.

Brody, H.: Drainage of the Pulmonary Veins into the Right Side of the Heart, *Arch Pathol,* **33:**221, 1942.

Cooley, D. A., Hallman, G. L., and Leachman, R. D.: Total Anomalous Pulmonary Venous Drainage, *J Thorac Cardiovasc Surg,* **51:**88, 1966.

———, and Ochsner, A., Jr.: Correction of Total Anomalous Pulmonary Venous Drainage: Technical Considerations, *Surgery,* **42:**1014, 1957.

Darling, R. C., Rothney, W. B., and Craig, J. M.: Total Pulmonary Venous Drainage into the Right Side of the Heart: Report of 17 Autopsied Cases Not Associated with Other Major Cardiovascular Anomalies, *Lab Invest,* **6:**44, 1957.

El-Said, G., Mullins, C. E., and McNamara, J. J.: Management of Total Anomalous Pulmonary Venous Return, *Circulation,* **45:**1240, 1972.

Gott, V. L., Lester, R. G., Lillehei, C. W., and Varco, R. L.: Total

Anomalous Pulmonary Venous Return: An Analysis of 30 Cases, *Circulation,* **13:**543, 1956.

Muller, W. H.: Surgical Treatment of Transposition of Pulmonary Veins, *Ann Surg,* **134:**683, 1951.

Ostium Primum Defect and Persistent Atrioventricular Canal

Blount, S. G., Jr., Balchum, O. J., and Gensini, G.: Persistent Ostium Primum Atrial Septal Defect, *Circulation,* **13:**499, 1956.

Braunwald, N. S., and Morrow, A. G.: Incomplete Persistent Atrioventricular Canal, *J Thorac Cardiovasc Surg,* **51:**71, 1966.

Castaneda, A. R., Nicoloff, D. M., Moller, J. H., and Lucas, R. V., Jr.: Surgical Correction of Complete Atrioventricular Canal Utilizing Ball-Valve Replacement of the Mitral Valve: Technical Considerations, *J Thorac Cardiovasc Surg,* **62:**926, 1971.

Cooley, D. A., and Hallman, G. L.: "Surgical Treatment of Congenital Heart Disease," Lea & Febiger, Philadelphia, 1966.

Gerbode, F., Sanchez, P. A., Arguero, R., Kerth, W. J., Hill, J. D., and deVries, P. A.: Endocardial Cushion Defects, *Ann Surg,* **167:**486, 1967.

Levy, M. J., Cuello, L., Tuna, N., and Lillehei, C. W.: Atrioventricularis Communis, *Am J Cardiol,* **14:**587, 1964.

McGoon, D. C., DeShane, J. W., and Kirklin, J. W.: The Surgical Treatment of Endocardial Cushion Defects, *Surgery,* **46:**185, 1959.

Neill, C. A.: Postoperative Hemolytic Anemia in Endocardial Cushion Defects, *Circulation,* **30:**801, 1964.

Rastelli, G. C., Kirklin, J. W., and Titus, J. L.: Anatomic Observations on Complete Form of Persistent Common Atrioventricular Canal with Special Reference to Atrioventricular Valves, *Mayo Clin Proc,* **41:**296, 1966.

———, Weidman, W. H., and Kirklin, J. W.: Surgical Repair of the Partial Form of Persistent Common Atrioventricular Canal, with Special Reference to the Problem of Mitral Valve Incompetence, *Circulation,* **31:**31, 1965.

Ventricular Septal Defect

Bloomfield, D. K.: The Natural History of Ventricular Septal Defect in Patients Surviving Infancy, *Circulation,* **29:**914, 1964.

Cartmill, T. B., DuShane, J. W., McGoon, D. C., and Kirklin, J. W.: Results of Repair of Ventricular Septal Defect, *J Thorac Cardiovasc Surg,* **52:**486, 1966.

Cooley, D. A., and Hallman, G. L.: "Surgical Treatment of Congenital Heart Disease," Lea & Febiger, Philadelphia, 1966.

Hallman, G. L., Cooley, D. A., and Bloodwell, R. D.: Two-stage Surgical Treatment of Ventricular Septal Defect: Results of Pulmonary Artery Banding in Infants and Subsequent Open-Heart Repair, *J Thorac Cardiovasc Surg,* **52:**476, 1966.

———, ———, Wolff, R. R., and McNamara, D. G.: Surgical Treatment of Ventricular Septal Defect Associated with Pulmonary Hypertension, *J Thorac Cardiovasc Surg,* **48:**588, 1964.

Lillehei, C. W., Anderson, R. C., Eliot, R. S., Wang, Y., and Ferlic, R. M.: Pre and Postoperative Cardiac Catheterization in 200 Patients Undergoing Closure of Ventricular Septal Defects, *Surgery,* **63:**69, 1968.

———, Sellers, R. D., Bonnabeau, R. C., Jr., and Eliot, R. S.:

Chronic Postsurgical Complete Heart Block: With Particular Reference to Prognosis, Management, and a New P-Wave Pacemaker, *J Thorac Cardiovasc Surg,* **46:**436, 1963.

McGoon, D. C.: Closure of Patent Ductus during Open-Heart Surgery, *J Thorac Cardiovasc Surg,* **48:**456, 1964.

Spencer, F. C., Doyle, E. F., Danilowicz, D. A., Bahnson, H. T., and Weldon, C. S.: Longterm Evaluation of Aortic Valvuloplasty for Aortic Insufficiency and Ventricular Septal Defect, *J Thorac Cardiovasc Surg,* **65:**15, 1973.

Walker, W. J., Garcia-Gonzalez, E., Hall, R. J., Czarnecki, S. W., Franklin, R. B., Das, S. K., and Cheitlin, M. D.: Interventricular Septal Defect: Analysis of 415 Catheterized Cases, *Circulation,* **31:**54, 1965.

Wood, P.: The Eisenmenger Syndrome, *Br Med J,* **2:**701, 1958.

Patent Ductus Arteriosus

Blalock, A.: Operative Closure of the Patent Ductus Arteriosus, *Surg Gynecol Obstet,* **82:**113, 1946.

Dammann, J. F., Jr.: Berthrong, M., and Bing, R. J.: Reverse Ductus, *Bull Johns Hopkins Hosp,* **92:**128, 1953.

Gross, R. E.: "The Surgery of Infancy and Childhood: Its Principles and Techniques," W. B. Saunders Company, Philadelphia, 1953.

——— and Hubbard, J. P.: Surgical Ligation of a Patent Ductus Arteriosus: Report of First Successful Case, *JAMA,* **112:**729, 1939.

Jones, J. C.: Twenty-five Years Experience with the Surgery of Patent Ductus Arteriosus, *J Thorac Cardiovasc Surg,* **50:**149, 1965.

Touroff, A. S. W., and Vesell, H.: Subacute Streptococcus Viridans Endarteritis Complicating Patent Ductus Arteriosus: Recovery following Surgical Treatment, *JAMA,* **115:**1270, 1940.

Tetralogy of Fallot

Bahnson, H. T., Spencer, F. C., and Neill, C. A.: Surgical Treatment and Follow-up of 147 Cases of Tetralogy of Fallot Treated by Correction, *J Thorac Cardiovasc Surg,* **44:**419, 1962.

Blalock, A.: Surgical Procedures Employed and Anatomical Variations Encountered in the Treatment of Congenital Pulmonic Stenosis, *Surg Gynecol Obstet,* **87:**385, 1948.

——— and Taussig, H. B.: The Surgical Treatment of Malformations of the Heart in Which There Is Pulmonary Stenosis or Pulmonary Atresia, *JAMA,* **128:**189, 1945.

Brock, R. C.: Pulmonary Valvulotomy for the Relief of Congenital Pulmonary Stenosis: Report of Three Cases, *Br Med J,* **1:**1121, 1948.

Cooley, D. A., and Hallman, G. L.: "Surgical Treatment of Congenital Heart Disease," Lea & Febiger, Philadelphia, 1966.

Ebert, P. A., and Sabiston, D. C.: Surgical Management of the Tetralogy of Fallot: Influence of a Previous Systemic-Pulmonary Anastomosis on the Results of Open Correction, *Ann Surg,* **165:**806, 1967.

Kirklin, J. W.: "Tetralogy of Fallot," W. B. Saunders Company, Philadelphia, 1971.

———, Wallace, R. B., McGoon, D. C., and DuShane, J. W.: Early and Late Results after Intracardiac Repair of Tetralogy of Fallot, *Ann Surg,* **162:**578, 1965.

Lillehei, C. W., Levy, M. J., Adams, P., and Anderson, R. C.: Corrective Surgery of Tetralogy of Fallot: Longterm Follow-up by Postoperative Recatheterization in 69 Cases and Certain Surgical Considerations, *J Thorac Cardiovasc Surg,* **48:**556, 1964.

Malm, J. R., Blumenthal, S., Bowman, F. O., Jr., Ellis, K., Jameson, A. G., Jesse, M. J., and Yeoh, C. B.: Factors That Modify Hemodynamic Results in Total Correction of Tetralogy of Fallot, *J Thorac Cardiovasc Surg,* **52:**502, 1966.

Potts, W. J., Smith, S., and Gibson, S.: Anastomosis of the Aorta to a Pulmonary Artery: Certain Types in Congenital Heart Disease, *JAMA,* **132:**627, 1946.

Shumway, N. E., Lower, R. R., Hurley, E. J., and Pillsbury, R. C.: Results of Total Surgical Correction of Fallot's Tetralogy, *Circulation,* **31:**I-57, 1965.

Wolf, M. D., Landtman, B., Neill, C. A., and Taussig, H. B.: Total Correction of Tetralogy of Fallot: Follow-up Study of 104 Cases, *Circulation,* **31:**385, 1965.

Transposition of the Great Vessels

Baffes, T. G., Riker, W. L., Boer, A. D., and Potts, W. J.: Surgical Correction of Transposition of the Aorta and the Pulmonary Artery, *J Thorac Cardiovasc Surg,* **34:**469, 1957.

Barratt-Boyes, B. G.: "Symposium on Congenital Cardiac Malformations and Their Treatment, Auckland, New Zealand, February 1972. (In press.)

Blalock, A., and Hanlon, C. R.: The Surgical Treatment of Complete Transposition of the Aorta and the Pulmonary Artery, *Surg Gynecol Obstet,* **90:**1, 1950.

Cooley, D. A., Hallman, G. L., Bloodwell, R. D., and Leachman, R. D.: Two Stage Surgical Treatment of Complete Transposition of the Great Vessels, *Arch Surg,* **93:**704, 1966.

Cornell, W. P., Maxwell, R. E., Haller, J. A., and Sabiston, D. C.: Results of the Blalock-Hanlon Operation in 90 Patients with Transposition of the Great Vessels, *J Thor Cardiovasc Surg,* **52:**525, 1966.

Edwards, W. S., Bargeron, L. M., and Lyons, C.: Reposition of Right Pulmonary Veins in Transposition of Great Vessels, *JAMA,* **188:**522, 1964.

Glenn, W. W. L., Ordway, N. K., Talner, N. S., and Call, E. P.: Circulatory Bypass of the Right Side of the Heart, *Circulation,* **31:**172, 1965.

Hanlon, C. R., and Blalock, A.: Complete Transposition of Aorta and Pulmonary Artery: Experimental Observations on Venous Shunts as Corrective Procedures, *Ann Surg,* **127:**385, 1948.

McGoon, D. C.: Intraventricular Repair of Transposition of the Great Arteries, *J Thorac Cardiovasc Surg,* **64:**430, 1972.

Merendino, K. H., Jesseph, J. E., Herron, P. W., Thomas, G. I., and Vetto, R. R.: Interatrial Venous Transposition, *Surgery,* **42:**898, 1957.

Moss, A. J., Maloney, J. V., Jr., and Adams, F. H.: Transposition of the Great Vessels, *Ann Surg,* **153:**183, 1961.

Mustard, W. T.: Progress in the Total Correction of Complete Transposition of the Great Vessels, *Vasc Dis,* **3:**177, 1966.

———, Keith, J. D., Trusler, G. A., Fowler, R., and Kidd, L.: The Surgical Management of Transposition of the Great Vessels, *J Thorac Cardiovasc Surg,* **48:**953, 1964.

Senning, A.: Surgical Correction of Transposition of the Great Vessels, *Surgery,* **45:**966, 1959.

———: Surgical Correction of Transposition of the Great Vessels, *Surgery,* **59:**334, 1966.

Tricuspid Atresia

Brock, R. C.: Tricuspid Atresia: A Step Toward Corrective Treatment, *J Thorac Cardiovasc Surg,* **47:**17, 1964.

Edwards, W. S., and Bargeron, L. M.: The Superiority of the Glenn Operation for Tricuspid Atresia in Infants and Children, *J Thorac Cardiovasc Surg,* **55:**60, 1968.

Glenn, W. W. L., Ordway, N. K., Talner, N. S., and Capp, E. P.: Circulatory Bypass of the Right Side of the Heart: Shunt between Superior Vena Cava and Distal Right Pulmonary Artery; Report of Clinical Application in 38 Cases, *Circulation,* **31:**172, 1965.

Cor Triatriatum

Grondin, C., Leonard, A. S., Anderson, R. C., Amplatz, K. A., Edwards, J. E., and Varco, R. L.: Cor Triatriatum: A Diagnostic Surgical Enigma, *J Thorac Cardiovasc Surg,* **48:**527, 1964.

McGuire, L. B., Nolan, T. B., Reede, R., and Dammann, J. F.: Cor Triatriatum as a Problem of Adult Heart Disease, *Circulation,* **31:**263, 1965.

Niwayama, G.: Cor Triatriatum, *Am Heart J,* **59:**291, 1960.

Congenital Mitral Stenosis

Daoud, G., Kaplan, S., Perrin, E. V., Dorst, J. P., and Edwards, F. K.: Congenital Mitral Stenosis, *Circulation,* **27:**185, 1963.

Ferencz, C., Johnson, A. L., and Wiglesworth, F. W.: Congenital Mitral Stenosis, *Circulation,* **9:**161, 1954.

Tsuji, H. K., Shapiro, M., Redington, J. V., and Kay, J. H.: Congenital Mitral Stenosis: Report of Two Cases and Review of the Literature, *J Thorac Cardiovasc Surg,* **53:**850, 1967.

Aortic-Pulmonary Window

Cooley, D. A., McNamara, D. G., and Latson, J. R.: Aorticopulmonary Septal Defect, *Surgery,* **42:**101, 1957.

Gross, R. E.: Surgical Closure of an Aortic Septal Defect, *Circulation,* **5:**858, 1952.

Morrow, A. G., Greenfield, L. J., and Braunwald, E.: Congenital Aortopulmonary Septal Defect: Clinical and Hemodynamic Findings, Surgical Technique, and Results of Operative Correction, *Circulation,* **25:**463, 1962.

Putnam, T. C., and Gross, R. E.: Surgical Management of Aortopulmonary Fenestration, *Surgery,* **59:**727, 1966.

Scott, H. W., and Sabiston, D. C.: Surgical Treatment for Congenital Aortico-pulmonary Fistula, *J Thorac Cardiovasc Surg,* **25:**26, 1953.

Skall-Jensen, J.: Congenital Aortico-pulmonary Fistula: A Review of the Literature and Report of Two Cases, *Acta Med Scand,* **160:**221, 1958.

Ruptured Aneurysm of Sinus of Valsalva

Gerbode, F., Osborn, J. J., Johnston, J. B., and Kerth, W. J.: Transaortic Approach for the Repair of Ruptured Aneurysms of the Sinus of Valsalva, *Ann Surg,* **161:**946, 1965.

Lillehei, C. W., Stanley, P., and Varco, R. L.: Surgical Treatment of Ruptured Aneurysms of the Sinus of Valsalva, *Ann Surg,* **146:**459, 1957.

Paton, B. C., MacMahon, R. A., Swan, H., and Blount, S. G.: Ruptured Sinus of Valsalva, *Arch Surg,* **90:**209, 1965.

Sawyer, J. L., Adams, J. E., and Scott, H. W.: Surgical Treatment for Aneurysms of Aortic Sinuses with Aorticoatrial Fistula, *Surgery,* **41:**126, 1957.

Shumacker, H. B., King, H., and Waldhausen, J. A.: Transaortic Approach for the Repair of Ruptured Aneurysms of the Sinus of Valsalva, *Ann Surg,* **161:**946, 1965.

Spencer, F. C.,Blake, H. A., and Bahnson, H. T.: Surgical Repair of Ruptured Aneurysm of Sinus of Valsalva in Two Patients, *Ann Surg,* **162:**963, 1960.

Truncus Arteriosus

Cooley, D. A., and Hallman, G. L.: "Surgical Treatment of Congenital Heart Disease," Lea & Febiger, Philadelphia, 1966.

McGoon, D. C., Wallace, R. B., and Danielson, G. K.: The Rastelli Operation: Its Indications and Results, *J Thorac Cardiovasc Surg,* **65:**65, 1973.

Single Ventricle

Campbell, M. G., Reynolds, G., and Trounce, J. R.: Six Cases of Single Ventricle with Pulmonary Stenosis, *Guys Hosp Rep,* **102:**99, 1953.

Ebstein's Anomaly

Bahnson, H. T., Bauersfeld, S. R., and Smith, J. W.: Pathological Anatomy and Surgical Correction of Ebstein's Anomaly, *Circulation,* **31**(*Suppl 1*):3, 1965.

Barnard, C. N., and Schrire, V.: Surgical Correction of Ebstein's Malformation with Prosthetic Tricuspid Valve, *Surgery,* **54:**302, 1963.

Hardy, K. L., May, I. A., Webster, C. A., and Kimball, K. G.: Ebstein's Anomaly: A Functional Concept and Successful Definitive Repair, *J Thorac Cardiovasc Surg,* **48:**927, 1964.

Hunter, S. W., and Lillehei, C. W.: Ebstein's Malformation of the Tricuspid Valve, *Dis Chest,* **33:**297, 1958.

Timmis, H. H., Hardy, J. D., and Watson, D. G.: The Surgical Management of Ebstein's Anomaly, *J Thorac Cardiovasc Surg,* **53:**385, 1967.

Vacca, J. B., Bussmann, D. W., and Mudd, J. G.: Ebstein's Anomaly: Complete Review of 108 Cases, *Am J Cardiol,* **2:**210, 1958.

Anomalous Origin of Left Coronary Artery from Pulmonary Artery

Bland, E. F., White, P. D., and Garland, J.: Congenital Anomalies of Coronary Arteries: Report of an Unusual Case Associated with Cardiac Hypertrophy, *Am Heart J,* **8:**787, 1933.

Cooley, D. A., Hallman, G. L., and Bloodwell, R. D.: Definitive Surgical Treatment of Anomalous Origin of Left Coronary Artery from Pulmonary Artery, *J Thorac Cardiovasc Surg,* **52:**798, 1966.

Keith, J. D.: Anomalous Origin of the Left Coronary Artery from the Pulmonary Artery, *Br Heart J,* **21:**149, 1959.

Likar, I., Criley, J. M., and Lewis, K. B.: Anomalous Left Coronary Artery Arising from the Pulmonary Artery in Adults: A Review of the Therapeutic Problems, *Circulation,* **33:**727, 1966.

Sabiston, D. C., Neill, C. A., and Taussig, H. B.: The Direction of Blood Flow in Anomalous Left Coronary Artery Arising from the Pulmonary Artery, *Circulation,* **22:**591, 1960.

Coronary Arteriovenous Fistula

Effler, D. B., Sheldon, W. C., Turner, J. J., and Groves, L. K.: Coronary Arteriovenous Fistulas: Diagnosis and Surgical Management; Report of Fifteen Cases, *Surgery,* **61:**41, 1967.

Gasul, B. M., Arcilla, R. A., Fell, E. H., Lynfield, J., Bicoff, J. P., and Luan, L. L.: Congenital Coronary Arteriovenous Fistula: Clinical, Phonocardiographic, Angiocardiographic, and Hemodynamic Studies in Five Patients, *Pediatrics,* **25:**531, 1960.

Hallman, G. L., Cooley, D. A., and Singer, D. B.: Congenital Anomalies of the Coronary Arteries: Anatomy, Pathology, and Surgical Treatment, *Surgery,* **59:**133, 1966.

Oldham, H. N., Jr., Ebert, P. A., Young, W. G., and Sabiston, D. C., Jr.: Surgical Management of Congenital Coronary Arteriovenous Fistula, *Ann Thorac Surg,* **12:**503, 1971.

Corrected Transposition

Anderson, R. C., Lillehei, C. W., and Lester, R. G.: Corrected Transposition of the Great Vessels of the Heart: A Review of 17 Cases, *Pediatrics,* **20:**626, 1957.

Schiebler, G. L., Edwards, J. E., Burchell, H. B., DuShane, J. W., Ongley, P. A., and Wood, E. H.: Congenital Corrected Transposition of the Great Vessels: A Study of 33 Cases, *Pediatrics,* **27:**851, 1961.

Chapter 19

Acquired Heart Disease

by **Frank C. Spencer**

Introduction: Clinical Manifestations

Pathophysiology

Physiology of Extracorporeal Circulation

Postoperative Care and Complications following Extracorporeal Circulation

Cardiac Arrest and Ventricular Fibrillation

Mitral Stenosis

Mitral Insufficiency

Aortic Stenosis

Aortic Insufficiency

Tricuspid Stenosis and Insufficiency

Multivalvular Heart Disease

Cardiac Trauma

Foreign Bodies

Cardiac Tumors

Myxoma
Metastatic Neoplasms
Sarcoma
Rhabdomyoma
Miscellaneous Tumors

Coronary Artery Disease

Ventricular Aneurysm

Pericarditis

Acute Pyogenic Pericarditis
Chronic Constrictive Pericarditis

Heart Block and Pacemakers

Cardiac Transplantation, Assisted Circulation, and Artificial Hearts

Cardiac Transplantation
Assisted Circulation and Artificial Hearts

INTRODUCTION: CLINICAL MANIFESTATIONS

With the development of prosthetic cardiac valves, the scope of surgical therapy for heart disease was greatly enlarged. An additional major advance was the development of bypass grafting for coronary artery disease, starting in the year 1967–1968 and now widely employed, although indications, techniques, and long-term results are still under intense investigation. Present frontiers include corrective operations for severe cardiac malformations in infancy, cardiac transplantation, and the development of an artificial heart. This steadily expanding scope of cardiac surgery requires that the surgeon become familiar with features of cardiac disease that have traditionally been the province of the cardiologist. Accordingly, basic clinical features of cardiac disease, which classically are found only in a textbook of cardiology, are briefly presented in this section. The objective is not to train a surgeon as an amateur cardiologist but to enable the surgeon to be familiar enough with the clinical manifestations of cardiac disease to recognize gross abnormalities and to appreciate further the great importance of having a cardiologist as an integral part of a cardiac surgical team. Unless a cardiologist works closely with a cardiac surgeon, many surgical mishaps can occur which otherwise might be prevented or promptly treated, such as arrhythmias or myocardial infarction.

The five major methods of evaluating a patient with heart disease can be conveniently grouped as history, physical examination, electrocardiogram, radiologic studies, and special diagnostic tests, especially cardiac catheterization and cineangiography. In this introductory section the major characteristics of cardiac disease, as elicited by the history, physical examination, and laboratory studies, will be briefly described. For additional details, a textbook of cardiology should be consulted.

HISTORY. It is particularly important to determine the degree of disability present and its rate of progression. These considerations are especially pertinent to a decision as to the advisability of surgical intervention, especially if the contemplated operative procedure would require insertion of a prosthetic mitral or aortic valve. The hazard of thromboembolism with prosthetic valves, though decreased to the range of 2 to 4 percent since about 1970, still limits their use to patients seriously disabled or to those developing marked cardiac enlargement.

Dyspnea, fatigue, edema, and *cyanosis* are all usually manifestations of decreased cardiac output and congestive heart failure. *Pain* is an especially prominent feature with coronary artery disease. *Palpitation* and *syncope* occur with many forms of heart disease, especially with disturbances of rhythm. *Hemoptysis* can result from either cardiac or pulmonary causes. Each of these disorders will be briefly discussed.

Dyspnea on exertion is an extremely common symptom with heart disease, resulting from pulmonary congestion from elevation of left atrial pressure with increased physical activity. The degree of exertion required to cause dyspnea, especially with any changes in recent months, should be carefully noted. Other clinical manifestations of pulmonary congestion include cough, orthopnea, paroxysmal nocturnal dyspnea, or frank pulmonary edema. In considering the possible causes of dyspnea, it should be remembered that probably the most common cause is an anxiety syndrome, not heart disease. This can usually be determined by careful examination. *Fatigue,* probably a reflection of decrease in cardiac output, is a more subtle sign of limited cardiac function than dyspnea and may be the only complaint when the patient has subtly restricted his physical activities to avoid dyspnea. Patients following a sedentary existence can tolerate serious cardiac disease for long periods of time without having any other symptoms from a significant underlying hemodynamic disturbance.

Cyanosis may appear with acute pulmonary congestion but is usually variable and not a reliable guide to the type or severity of cardiac disease. It is a more reliable and significant finding in patients with congenital heart disease. *Edema* is a late symptom of congestive heart failure, for it can be detected clinically only after 10 lb or more of extracellular fluid have accumulated. Few symptoms may result from the presence of edema except for generalized aching and discomfort from the increased weight of the legs.

Chest pain is a particularly significant symptom which must be closely analyzed. Angina pectoris is one of the most frequent causes and, in perhaps 75 percent of patients, can be readily diagnosed from the characteristic symptoms. It usually occurs as a substernal pain or constriction provoked by exercise, eating, emotion, or exposure to cold. The discomfort commonly lasts 1 to 4 minutes and may be immediately relieved by sublingual administration of nitroglycerin. In perhaps 20 to 25 percent of patients a bizarre discomfort develops with radiation of pain to numerous unusual locations, such as the ear, the right hand, or the epigastrium. In such patients establishing the correct diagnosis may challenge the most experienced cardiologist and require laboratory evaluation with exercise electrocardiography or coronary arteriography.

Other frequent causes of chest pain include myocardial infarction, dissecting aneurysm, pericarditis, or pulmonary infarction. As with dyspnea, anxiety is a frequent cause for a precordial discomfort described as pain or "tightness," and its frequency must be appreciated in considering the differential diagnosis. Other noncardiac conditions which may be easily confused with angina pectoris are diseases of the esophagus or, less frequently, biliary disease.

Palpitation is a generalized term for the patient's becoming aware of cardiac contractions. Rarely this occurs in a thin-chested individual without cardiac disease. Usually it results from increased force of left ventricular contraction as a result of underlying heart disease or from a cardiac arrhythmia, such as an extrasystole. Its significance is re-

lated to the underlying disease or disturbance which produces the discomfort. *Syncope* may result from several cardiac diseases, the most important of which are aortic stenosis, heart block, mitral stenosis, tetralogy of Fallot, or rarely pulmonary hypertension. It is a particularly ominous symptom in patients with aortic stenosis, for the life expectancy of such patients is brief unless surgical therapy is performed. In evaluating the significance of syncope, the possibility of epilepsy or cerebrovascular disease must be considered.

Hemoptysis, an alarming symptom, often results from pulmonary disease. The four most frequent disorders are tuberculosis, bronchogenic carcinoma, bronchiectasis, or pneumonia. The two cardiac conditions most commonly associated with hemoptysis are mitral stenosis and pulmonary infarction. Patients with fulminating pulmonary edema may expectorate a pink, frothy sputum as a result of rupture of pulmonary capillaries into the alveoli, but the frothy sputum of pulmonary edema can be easily distinguished from the blood clots expectorated with frank hemoptysis.

PHYSICAL EXAMINATION. The general body habitus of the patient should be carefully noted. A number of unusual genetic syndromes are associated with cardiac disease. Most of these are described in recent textbooks of cardiology. The Marfan syndrome is a familiar example of a disorder of connective tissue which may cause either a dissecting aneurysm or aortic insufficiency.

The prominence of the neck veins is a guide to venous pressure. With a normal venous pressure of 2 to 10 mm Hg, the internal jugular vein is visible for only 2 to 3 cm above the level of the clavicle. With obviously distended veins, venous pressure should be measured accordingly. In patients with tricuspid valvular disease, the experienced cardiologist can detect prominent *a* waves in the jugular pulse generated from forceful contractions of the right atrium. Peripheral edema can be best noted in the legs, but in patients confined to bed edema may be more prominent in the flanks or buttocks.

Much information can be obtained from a careful examination of the peripheral pulse and the blood pressure. A disturbance of cardiac rhythm, such as atrial fibrillation, can be recognized from the pulse and then investigated more thoroughly by auscultation of the heart and study of the electrocardiogram. Pulsus alternans, a rhythmic alternation between a forceful pulse and a weak one, is a significant sign of serious left ventricular failure. A small, weak pulse is found with cardiac disease associated with a low cardiac output, increased peripheral vascular resistance, and a narrow pulse pressure. This may occur with myocardial failure, aortic stenosis, mitral stenosis, or cardiac tamponade. A forceful, bounding pulse results when there is an increased cardiac output with a wide pulse pressure and decreased peripheral vascular resistance. This is classically seen with aortic insufficiency but is also a prominent feature in any disease associated with a decreased peripheral vascular resistance, such as patent ductus arteriosus, peripheral arteriovenous fistula, hyperthyroidism, or pregnancy.

Inspection and palpation of the precordium is another

important part of the cardiac examination. Some cardiologists have almost discarded percussion of the cardiac shadow because of the wide range of normal findings among persons of different habitus and have found more significant information by careful inspection and palpation. Cardiac pulsations should be observed for their location, timing, amplitude, and distribution. Normally, the apical impulse is near the midclavicular line and can be detected as a moderately forceful tapping sensation in early systole over an area 2 to 3 cm in diameter. With left ventricular hypertrophy, as with aortic stenosis or insufficiency, both the size and vigor of the left ventricular impulse are increased. With right ventricular hypertrophy, a prominent parasternal impulse, which some cardiologists consider a better index of right ventricular hypertrophy than the electrocardiogram, can be felt. In the presence of marked dilatation of the heart from congestive heart failure, palpation becomes less reliable because of the diffuse nature of the cardiac impulse.

Characteristic thrills develop with certain types of valvular disease. The more common of these are the thrill in the aortic area from aortic stenosis, a similar one in the pulmonic area with pulmonic stenosis, and less frequently a diastolic thrill at the apex with mitral stenosis.

Auscultation is a very important part of the cardiac examination, because some serious disorders, such as mitral stenosis or aortic insufficiency, can be firmly diagnosed best by detection of the characteristic murmur. In auscultation the cardiac sounds should be carefully analyzed and any murmurs identified. A convenient method for beginning the examination is to identify the first and second sounds by auscultation at the base of the heart. Normally the second sound, produced by closure of the aortic and pulmonic valves, is of a higher pitch and shorter duration than the first sound, produced by seating of the mitral and tricuspid valves. If uncertainty exists, simultaneous palpation of the carotid pulse will identify the two sounds. Splitting of the pulmonic second sound is a familiar characteristic of conditions which increase pulmonary blood flow, especially atrial septal defect.

In defining the characteristics of a murmur, the timing, duration, intensity, and location are of particular significance. Aortic and pulmonic stenosis each produce so-called "diamond-shaped" murmurs, representing an early rise and late decline in intensity. Mitral insufficiency, by contrast, produces a loud apical systolic murmur without the characteristic sharp decrease heard in aortic stenosis. The diastolic murmur of aortic insufficiency is usually best heard along the left sternal border, while the typical diastolic murmur of mitral stenosis may be sharply localized at the cardiac apex. Murmurs of tricuspid stenosis and insufficiency often are similar to the more frequently encountered murmurs of mitral stenosis or insufficiency, except that they also may be audible near the lower end of the sternum and can be accentuated during inspiration. Confirmation of the diagnosis usually requires cardiac catherization. A murmur of ventricular septal defect is usually a harsh holosystolic murmur near the lower border of the sternum, while the murmur of an atrial septal defect

originates near the pulmonic valve as a result of the increased pulmonary blood flow. The classic murmur of patent ductus arteriosus is a continuous murmur best heard in the left second or third intercostal space.

Functional murmurs are especially common in conditions with an increase in cardiac output, such as hyperthyroidism, anemia, or pregnancy. In general these are short systolic murmurs which may be audible at the apex or in the pulmonic area. Their differential diagnosis, which may necessitate cardiac catheterization, is beyond the scope of this presentation.

Two infrequent findings on auscultation are a pericardial friction rub or a gallop rhythm. A friction rub is particularly common after cardiac operations and may be unassociated with any other clinical signs, originating from resorption of fluid in the pericardium. In other patients it may indicate the so-called "pericardiotomy syndrome," which frequently occurs following cardiac surgical procedures. A gallop rhythm is of particular importance, because its presence usually indicates serious disease of the myocardium, such as myocardial infarction or impending cardiac failure.

ELECTROCARDIOGRAPHY. The electrocardiogram will be mentioned only briefly, for its proper interpretation requires the careful analysis of an experienced cardiologist. Disorders of cardiac rhythm are extremely common following cardiac surgical procedures, and a wide variety of rhythms can occur in a patient over a period of several hours. In analysis of the electrocardiogram, the cardiac rate, rhythm, and electrical axis should be noted. It is particularly useful for detection of hypertrophy of either the right or left ventricle. Conduction defects, such as right or left bundle branch block, can be diagnosed only by electrocardiography. With serious coronary artery disease, either as chronic coronary artery disease or with acute myocardial infarction, the electrocardiogram may provide the only positive laboratory findings.

RADIOLOGY. The chest roentgenogram provides many valuable guides in evaluation of cardiac disease. Determination of heart size is of basic importance, for cardiac enlargement immediately establishes the presence of cardiac disease. Alterations in cardiac contour occur with different diseases. Normally the right border of the heart is formed by the superior vena cava and the right atrium, and the left border by the aorta, pulmonary artery, and left ventricle. Selective enlargement of any of the four cardiac chambers is best recognized by oblique or lateral views. In the left anterior oblique position, enlargement of the left ventricle can be recognized as a posterior shadow against the spine, while an enlarged right ventricle can be seen bulging anteriorly into the retrosternal space. Enlargement of the left atrium is best recognized in the lateral view, by simultaneous opacification of the esophagus with barium, as it produces a characteristic concave indentation of the esophagus. Enlargement of the right atrium, bulging into the right hemithorax, can be easily seen in the usual posteroanterior view.

In analysis of the cardiac shadow, detection of calcification is of particular importance. Calcification of the aortic or mitral valves is very common with long-standing rheumatic disease. With constrictive pericarditis most patients will have visible areas of calcification.

Analysis of the pulmonary circulation provides many valuable guides to the status of the circulation. Pulmonary venous congestion develops when left atrial pressure is chronically elevated above the upper limit of normal of 10 mm Hg. With severe mitral stenosis, a typical picture of engorged pulmonary veins may be readily recognized. When severe left atrial hypertension is present, edema forms in the lungs in both the alveoli and the interstitial tissues. Edema accumulating in the interlobar planes forms transverse linear opacities on the chest roentgenogram which are perpendicular to the surface of the pleura, the so-called "Kerley lines." Their presence usually indicates a left atrial pressure exceeding 20 mm Hg.

The prominenence of the pulmonary arteries is also of particular significance. Marked enlargement of the pulmonary arteries may occur with either an increase in pulmonary blood flow or an increase in pulmonary vascular resistance with pulmonary hypertension. Normally, the central pulmonary arteries are three to five times larger than the peripheral arteries. With an increase in pulmonary blood flow, as with an atrial septal defect, both the central and peripheral pulmonary arteries are symmetrically enlarged. With an increase in pulmonary vascular resistance and pulmonary hypertension, the central pulmonary arteries may become strikingly enlarged, while the peripheral pulmonary arteries do not distend, producing a striking disproportion in the size of the two vessels. An estimation of the pulmonary blood flow by fluoroscopy is of particular importance in the presence of congenital heart disease. Wide variations are seen, ranging from the avascular lung fields with tetralogy of Fallot to the plethoric lung fields of ventricular or atrial septal defect.

CARDIAC CATHETERIZATION AND CINEANGIOGRAPHY. These two techniques have greatly advanced the precision of diagnosis of cardiac disease. Only by these studies can many cardiac disorders be properly diagnosed and quantitatively analyzed. It is our practice to perform cardiac catheterization and angiography upon virtually every patient undergoing cardiac surgical treatment to assess the hemodynamic disturbance, confirm the diagnosis, and detect any associated cardiac disease. This liberal policy has provided numerous dividends in the care of patients both during and following operation.

Cardiac catheterization, by obtaining oxygen concentration and pressure in different cardiac chambers, can establish the diagnosis of an intracardiac shunt, such as an atrial or ventricular septal defect, or the presence of a valvular stenosis, such as pulmonic stenosis, mitral stenosis, or aortic stenosis. The presence of cardiac failure, as indicated by an elevation of left atrial pressure, or pulmonary hypertension can also be measured. It is not of great value for analysis of aortic or mitral insufficiency, except to detect the development of cardiac failure.

Cineangiography, however, provides the best method for analysis of aortic or mitral insufficiency, visually demonstrating the amount of dye refluxing through the incompetent valve. In patients over forty years of age, simultaneous coronary arteriography by the Sones technique is routinely done to evaluate the presence of associated coronary atherosclerosis,

The combination of cardiac catheterization and cineangiography in a well-equipped cardiac catheterization laboratory is an essential component of any cardiac surgical unit.

PATHOPHYSIOLOGY

A detailed analysis of the pathophysiology of mitral and aortic disease is presented in those respective sections. Accordingly, only a brief discussion of certain broad principles of pathophysiology of acquired heart disease is presented here.

As stated earlier, the degree of incapacity of a patient with cardiac disease should be carefully evaluated in deciding that an operation should be performed. Many patients with aortic or mitral disease can function well for years and should be treated by nonoperative methods until the disease has progressed to an incapacitating stage. The reason for this conservatism, which may change in the future, is the significant frequency of thromboemboli with prosthetic cardiac valves. Hence, an operation which entails insertion of a prosthetic cardiac valve should be postponed as long as a patient can carry out his normal activities with appropriate medical therapy. One exception to this policy is the presence of progressive cardiac enlargement. As very large hearts of 750 to 1,000 Gm may not decrease after operation, surgery is being performed earlier in some patients with only moderate symptoms but with progressive cardiac enlargement.

Conversely, it is important to realize that with present surgical techniques an operation almost always can be performed, even though advanced, severe cardiac failure is present. The immediate risk of operation is increased, but possibilities for rehabilitating a patient are fairly good, even though he is bedridden with severe edema from far advanced congestive failure. The most important principle in operating upon such patients is to be certain that all existing valvular pathologic conditions are corrected, for multivalvular disease is common with intractable congestive failure. In some patients replacement of three cardiac valves, the mitral, aortic, and tricuspid, is necessary.

With mitral stenosis, different considerations apply, because many such patients can be effectively treated by commissurotomy. Accordingly, operation should be planned whenever the diagnosis is made if any symptoms are present. Surgical therapy should be especially considered once atrial fibrillation has occurred because of the risk of thromboembolism. Before either anticoagulant or surgical therapy was available, approximately 25 percent of patients with mitral stenosis ultimately died from cerebral embolism.

With aortic stenosis or insufficiency, once symptoms such as dyspnea, syncope, or chest pain have appeared, operation should be performed quickly, because sudden death is a real possibility. This is particularly true with aortic stenosis. Sudden death of patients with aortic stenosis either contemplating or scheduled for operation still occurs with distressing frequency.

Pulmonary hypertension is of considerably different significance with acquired heart disease than with congenital heart disease. With ventricular septal defect an elevated pulmonary vascular resistance may or may not decrease following closure of the defect. With pulmonary hypertension from mitral stenosis, however, even in its more severe forms with a pulmonary artery systolic pressure exceeding 100 mm Hg, improvement almost invariably occurs following adequate correction of the stenosis.

The heart size and presence of congestive failure are important indices of long-term rehabilitation following successful cardiac valvular surgical treatment. Unfortunately in most patients disabled by the disease significant cardiac enlargement has developed. A small percentage of patients with mitral disease following valvular replacement will have permanent cardiac disability, requiring careful limitation of physical activities and administration of diuretics. Whether this permanent disability reflects a rheumatic myocarditis or a permanent injury to the myocardium from long-standing valvular disease is unknown. Similarly, with aortic valvular disease and severe cardiac enlargement, sometimes to weights of 700 to 900 Gm, sudden death remains an ominous possibility following operation, especially in the first year. Death is probably due to a disturbance of rhythm from the severely hypertrophied left ventricle. As mentioned earlier, the probable solution for this group of patients is performance of operation at an earlier date, which will surely be done when cardiac valvular prostheses are completely free from the risk of thromboembolism.

PHYSIOLOGY OF EXTRACORPOREAL CIRCULATION

HISTORICAL DATA. The pioneering imagination and efforts of Gibbon were largely responsible for the development of extracorporeal circulation. In 1932, Gibbon initiated laboratory investigations which continued for over 20 years until the first successful open heart operation in man was performed by him in 1953. Subsequent developments were rapid, with the brief use of cross circulation by Lillehei and associates at the University of Minnesota in 1954, followed a short time later by the development of the bubble oxygenator by DeWall, who was working in the group with Lillehei. Kirklin and associates at the Mayo Clinic first began routine, successful use of the Gibbon oxygenator in 1955. The disc oxygenator, widely used today, was developed in Sweden by Björk and Crafoord and introduced to the United States by Kay and Cross.

PUMPS. The majority of heart-lung machines utilize a simple roller pump, originally developed by DeBakey. The resulting flow is almost nonpulsatile, with a pulse pressure of about 15 mm Hg. A variety of other pumps have been employed, with no clear demonstration of any advantages over the simple roller pump. A recurrent physiologic question has been the importance of a pulsatile flow in the normal circulation. Available experimental data indicate that over long periods of time a pulsatile flow may be of importance, but for periods of 1 to 4 hours a nonpulsatile flow seems adequate. The gradual increase in vasomotor tone which occurs during extracorporeal circulation may be a physiologic response to nonpulsatile perfusion.

OXYGENATORS. In the past 3 years a disposable bubble oxygenator has become the most widely used type (Fig. 19-1). Earlier a disc or screen oxygenator were more popular. Improvements in bubble oxygenators to a point where perfusion for as long as 4 to 6 hours may be done has made the disposable feature an important one. Several membrane oxygenators recently have been used clinically; thus far they are little better and are more cumbersome and more expensive than disposable bubble oxygenators.

PRIMING SOLUTIONS. Originally heart-lung machines were primed with heparinized blood collected within 24 hours before the time of operation, adding 20 mg heparin for each 500 ml blood used. Citrated blood (first demonstrated by Maloney and associates) is now used almost routinely, except in small infants. In recent years there has appeared to be some advantage to hemodilution with a variety of substances, such as dextrose-water, Ringer's lactate, dextran, and other solutions. A modified Ringer's lactate solution closely approximating the electrolyte composition of blood, is probably the most physiologic of this group. Our present technique is to prime the pump-oxygenator with about 1,500 ml whole blood and 1,500 ml modified Ringer's lactate to which serum albumin has been added. A popular technique with a bubble oxygenator, which can be filled with about 1,500 ml fluid, is to use only a dextrose or Ringer's lactate solution, avoiding the use of blood completely.

TECHNIQUE OF PERFUSION. Heparin, 3 mg/kg body weight, is given before the venous and arterial cannulae are inserted. Venous blood is aspirated by gravity or pump drainage through large cannulae inserted into the right atrium, except in some children and young adults, and advanced into the venae cavae. Oxygenated blood is returned to the arterial circulation, usually through a cannula directly inserted into the ascending aorta. Once widely popular, femoral artery cannulation has been almost abandoned to avoid the rare but lethal complication of retrograde dissection of the aorta. Perfusion is done at a flow rate of about 2,500 ml/m^2/minute, providing a flow rate between 4 and 5 liters/minute for adults of normal size. Oxygen flow rates through the oxygenator are adjusted to produce an arterial oxygen tension near 100 mm Hg. Temperature is controlled with a heat exchanger in the circuit and is often lowered to 30 to 32°C. This moderate hypothermia increases the tolerance of the heart to ischemia produced by temporary occlusion of the ascending aorta in order to permit better visualization of intracardiac structures. Intracardiac blood is aspirated with a suction apparatus and returned to the oxygenator.

During perfusion a number of modalities are monitored. Arterial pressure is monitored with a catheter previously inserted into a peripheral artery. Venous pressure in the superior vena cava is carefully observed to be certain that there is no obstruction to return of blood from the brain. The electrocardiogram and electroencephalogram are also

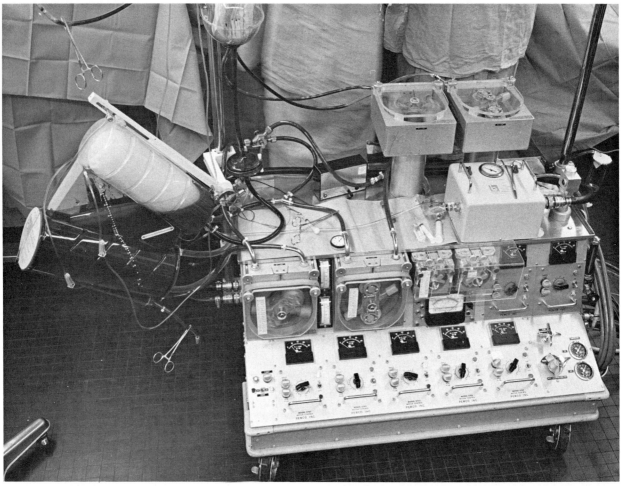

Fig. 19-1. Photograph of heart-lung machine, showing the Bentley bubble oxygenator with DeBakey roller pumps. The filters in the coronary suction return are also visible.

monitored. Mean arterial pressure usually decreases sharply with the onset of perfusion, apparently from vasodilatation, and then subsequently rises to levels varying between 50 and 80 mm Hg. The importance of the actual level of mean arterial pressure, as long as flow rate is adequate, is debated. In recent months we have preferred to maintain a mean perfusion pressure near that existing before bypass.

Oxygen and carbon dioxide tensions are periodically measured in the venous blood returned to the oxygenator and the oxygenated blood returned to the patient. Preferably the arterial oxygen tension should be near 100 mm Hg and the carbon dioxide tension 30 to 35 mm Hg. Venous blood returning to the heart-lung machine with the described flow rate will usually have an oxygen saturation greater than 50 percent. With flow rates and oxygen saturations in this range, metabolic acidosis of significant degree does not occur.

Heparin is gradually metabolized by the body; so, additional heparin is given each hour of perfusion in a dose of 1 mg/kg body weight. During perfusion the lungs are kept stationary in a partially inflated position with intermittent periods of inflation. Mannitol, 0.5 to 1 Gm/kg, is given at the beginning of the operation to produce an osmotic diuresis of urine during perfusion.

Termination of Perfusion. As perfusion is stopped, left atrial pressure is measured and blood transfused from the heart-lung machine until a left atrial pressure adequate to maintain cardiac output is obtained. The left atrial pressure needed will vary according to that existing before bypass. This technique has been found a better guide to adjustment of blood volume than either blood volume measurement or careful, balanced measurements of blood withdrawn versus blood transfused. Heparin is then neutralized with protamine. The amount of protamine given is calculated from the total amount of heparin given, estimating that heparin is metabolized at a rate near 15 percent of the original dose per hour. Protamine-heparin neutralization is calculated as 1 milligram protamine for each milligram heparin. A protamine titration is then done. Additional small amounts of protamine are frequently needed.

TRAUMA FROM PERFUSION. Definite trauma to the blood results from extracorporeal circulation, primarily from the exposure of blood to gas in the oxygenator and from the use of suction to aspirate intracardiac blood. At present tolerance for extracorporeal circulation is in the range of 6 to 8 hours; some patients undergo a very long perfusion with surprisingly few metabolic defects, but others show definite signs of physiologic injury after 6 hours of perfusion. Experimental studies of the capillary microcirculation during perfusion have found a progressive sludging of the blood elements, producing stasis and obstruction to capillary blood flow. The concentration of hemoglobin in the plasma is an index of hemolysis occurring during perfusion and may rise 40 to 50 mg/hour perfusion, the amount varying with the volume of urine secreted during perfusion. Some derangement of the clotting mechanisms invariably occurs and is reflected by an increased bleeding tendency afterward even though heparin activity has been neutralized. The coagulation defects, usually from multiple sources, subside within 6 to 12 hours. Fat embolism also has been demonstrated, although the significance is uncertain. Denaturation of plasma proteins occurs from the trauma at the gas-blood interphase and is probably responsible for some of the subtle physiologic changes with long perfusions.

In the past 2 to 3 years several studies have demonstrated microaggregates in the blood in the oxygenator, which can be partly removed with special filters in the pump circuit. Filters of different porosity are now widely used clinically, but their importance is yet uncertain.

The clinical counterparts of trauma with long perfusions have manifestations in different organs. A bleeding tendency develops, the degree varying with the duration of perfusion and the degree of trauma. This subsides within 12 to 18 hours. A mild degree of renal insufficiency is common after long perfusions, varying with flow rate during perfusion, blood trauma, and acidosis. Fortunately this is usually reversible. Varying degrees of respiratory insufficiency can develop with long perfusions. The cause is not completely clear and is probably related to multiple factors. Postoperatively, some patients require mechanical ventilation for a few hours but seldom for more than 8 to 12 hours. The central nervous system also becomes injured with long perfusions, as a result of which a variety of generalized neurolgic signs may appear. One of the most interesting of these is a psychosis, appearing unpredictably in a few patients, with all the symptoms of a severe toxic psychosis; fortunately this subsides within 2 weeks after operation.

RISK OF PERFUSION. At present the risk of extracorporeal circulation for 1 to 2 hours is extremely small, in the range of 1 percent. This low risk represents an astonishing achievement, especially when compared with the fact that as late as 1950 to 1952 the entire concept of extracorporeal circulation was purely hypothetic. Perhaps the most common complication is the development of serum hepatitis, related to the amount of blood used to prime the oxygenator and perform the operation. With longer periods of perfusion, the risk of perfusion per se gradually increases, though perfusion for as long as 6 hours is well tolerated in some patients. In a few patients with severe respiratory insufficiency, partial perfusion with extrathoracic cannulation and a membrane oxygenator has been performed for as long as 7 to 8 days.

POSTOPERATIVE CARE AND COMPLICATIONS FOLLOWING EXTRACORPOREAL CIRCULATION

Postoperative care following extracorporeal circulation involves problems which are not encountered following other surgical procedures. Part of the complications arise from the use of extracorporeal circulation, involving several units of blood and moderate trauma to the blood, the degree varying with the duration of extracorporeal circulation as well as with the type of oxygenator. In general, extracorporeal circulation for 2 to 4 hours is well tolerated, periods of 4 to 6 hours may have moderate but reversible complications, while periods for 6 to 9 hours approach the physiologic limits compatible with survival with present pump-oxygenators. The complications are also related to the type of disease which is treated by open cardiotomy and often occur in patients with chronic congestive failure with the attendant impaired function of many organ systems.

GENERAL PROCEDURES. Following these operations, as with most major surgical procedures, temperature, pulse, blood pressure, and respirations are frequently measured. Intraarterial pressure recording is often used for 24 to 48 hours, because residual vasoconstriction following extracorporeal circulation may make auscultatory methods for blood pressure measurement difficult and unreliable. Central venous pressure is routinely measured. In addition, during the past few years, small polyvinyl catheters frequently have been left in the left atrium and pulmonary artery for 24 to 48 hours to measure oxygen and carbon dioxide tensions in left atrial and mixed venous blood, as well as to measure pulmonary artery and left atrial pressures. The oxygen saturation of mixed venous blood, representing the ability of the respiratory and circulatory systems to supply oxygen requirements, is a particularly useful guide, especially in seriously ill patients. Left atrial pressure may be of more value than central venous pressure, especially with isolated left ventricular failure. Pulmonary artery diastolic pressure in most patients parallels left atrial pressure and may be substituted for direct measurement of left atrial pressure.

Chest roentgenograms are frequently made to evaluate hemothorax, pleural effusion, or atelectasis. The electrocardiogram is regularly monitored on an oscilloscope for varying periods of time because of the frequency of cardiac arrhythmias. Hematocrit, serum electrolyte concentrations (sodium, potassium, carbon dioxide, and chloride), and blood urea nitrogen (BUN) levels are serially measured.

Antibiotics are regularly given in large amounts during the operative procedure and for different lengths of time after operation. Although routines for antibiotic therapy vary widely among different institutions, we have preferred to administer oxacillin, 4 to 8 Gm daily, for approximately

4 to 7 days following insertion of valvular prostheses. Digitalis is given routinely to patients who previously have been in congestive failure. Anticoagulant therapy is regularly used with valvular prostheses and continued for varying periods of time. It is usually begun 5 to 7 days after operation.

SPECIFIC COMPLICATIONS. Bleeding Syndromes. Although heparin is routinely neutralized with protamine following extracorporeal circulation, it is important to realize that blood-clotting mechanisms are abnormal for 8 to 12 hours following bypass. Unusually diligent care is required following extracorporeal circulation to obtain hemostasis before incisions are sutured, necessitating much more attention than after usual operations. The exact basis for the deficient clotting mechanisms is not certain, since detailed studies of the different components of the blood responsible for normal clotting show some derangement of several components, without any specific correctible factor. Residual heparin activity, the so-called "heparin rebound phenomenon," probably occurs very rarely. When serious defects of blood coagulation persist after operation, transfusion with fresh frozen plasma, platelets, or fresh blood represents the most effective therapy. Fortunately, the clotting derangements are transitory and will disappear in the majority of patients within a few hours.

Because of the bleeding tendency, unusual care is required to measure blood loss serially and transfuse appropriate amounts of blood. Careful attention to the oscillation of fluid within the chest tubes in the pleural cavities is a most useful bedside guide, because a freely oscillating chest tube indicates that clotted blood is not accumulating within the thorax. Percussion of the chest is the most useful bedside technique for detecting a hemothorax.

With the extensive bleeding, the possibility of cardiac tamponade from blood clots accumulating in the pericardium should be considered. The usual findings with cardiac tamponade include hypotension, elevated venous pressure, and a wide mediastinal shadow on the chest roentgenogram. In doubtful cases reoperation may be required to confirm or exclude the diagnosis. In most patients the right or left pleural cavity is opened at operation to lessen the subsequent risk of cardiac tamponade.

The usual blood loss following operation is in the range of 400 to 800 ml, although this varies widely among individual patients. A blood loss exceeding 1 liter usually indicates active intrathoracic hemorrhage requiring reoperation. With improvements in pump-oxygenators and surgical technique, the frequency of reoperation for postoperative hemorrhage has greatly decreased.

Cardiac Failure. *Low-Cardiac-Output Syndrome.* In the early period of open heart surgery, a low-cardiac-output syndrome frequently developed. With increasing experience, however, the syndrome has progressively decreased in frequency and is now rarely encountered except in association with specific causes, most of which can be prevented. The normal cardiac output is near 3 liters/m²/minute. Following cardiac surgical procedures, there may be a decrease to 2 liters/m²/minute with moderate cardiac failure or to as low as 1 to 1.5 liters/m²/minute with severe depression of cardiac function. With low car-

diac output and deficient perfusion of different organs, a number of metabolic disturbances appear. There is hypotension, vasoconstriction, oliguria, and metabolic acidosis. After varying periods of time, ranging from a few hours to 1 to 2 days, death may result from either progressive hypotension or cardiac arrest.

Although a number of complex hypotheses were developed to explain the low-output syndrome, it is now realized that most of the causative factors are preventable. Even with advanced cardiac failure, the majority of patients will maintain an adequate cardiac ouput following operation if the entire underlying valvular pathologic condition is corrected and significant injury to the heart does not occur during operation. Failure to correct the valvular pathologic condition completely, especially before the advent of satisfactory prosthetic cardiac valves, was a frequent cause of cardiac failure. A second frequent cause was hypovolemia.

Although a number of methods to adjust blood volume have been used following extracorporeal circulation, including blood volume determinations and careful fluid balance measurements, the most reliable technique has been transfusion of fluid to elevate the central venous pressure or left atrial pressure to normal or moderately high levels. Preoperatively, many patients with aortic or mitral valvular disease may have a mean left atrial pressure of 15 to 20 mm Hg, and at times even higher levels (20 to 40 mm Hg). As this pressure represents the pressure distending the left ventricle in diastole and hence determining stroke volume and cardiac output, transfusion to similar levels may be required following operation to maintain a satisfactory cardiac output. In retrospect, failure to transfuse adequate fluid was a frequent unrecognized cause of the low-output syndrome.

Coronary air emboli, transection of coronary arteries during a ventriculotomy, or prolonged cardiac ischemia from temporary aortic occlusion are all insults which can depress cardiac function but can be avoided in carefully executed operative procedures. In the case of congenital heart disease, a greatly increased pulmonary vascular resistance, as with a ventricular septal defect and pulmonary hypertension, can severely impair cardiac function after operation and in some patients can result in death. Fortunately, with acquired valvular disease an irreversible increase in pulmonary vascular resistance almost never occurs.

An inadequate cardiac output can be suspected if hypotension, oliguria, or acidosis develops. Acidosis following operation is virtually unknown in the presence of an adequate cardiac ouput, for the acidosis results from production of lactate, pyruvate, and similar anions by anaerobic metabolism. A more precise method for evaluating the low-cardiac-output syndrome is either by direct measurement of cardiac output or by measurement of oxygen saturation of mixed venous blood obtained from the pulmonary artery through an indwelling catheter implanted at operation. The oxygen saturation of mixed venous blood, normally greater than 60 percent, is only an approximation of cardiac output, for it varies with the adequacy of ventilation, the blood volume, the hematocrit, and temperature. However, the oxygen saturation is an extremely useful guide, because it reflects how well the circulation is supplying the oxygen requirements of the body tissues. An oxygen saturation in the range of 50 to 60 percent indicates a moderate deficiency in oxygen transport, while a saturation in the range of 40 to 50 percent represents a serious deficiency and may be associated with a fatal outcome unless corrected.

Therapy of the low-cardiac-output syndrome includes transfusion of fluid to elevate the central venous pressure to an appropriate level, usually 10 to 12 mm Hg, or the left atrial pressure to 15 to 20 mm Hg. Acidosis which has developed can be corrected by infusion of sodium bicarbonate (50 to 200 mEq). If a low cardiac output remains despite transfusion of appropriate fluid, cardiac inotropic drugs, such as epinephrine or isoproterenol, may be cautiously administered, usually in the range of 1 to 3 μg/minute in adult patients. Premature use of inotropic drugs and vasopressors, such as norepinephrine or metaraminol, in the past perhaps accentuated the severity of the low-cardiac-output syndrome because hypovolemia was not recognized and was further masked by elevation of the blood pressure.

If respiratory insufficiency is present, as manifested by dyspnea or abnormalities in the oxygen and carbon dioxide tensions of arterial blood, artificial ventilation may be required. This is usually done initially by insertion of an endotracheal tube following appropriate sedation of the patient. If ventilation is required longer than 24 to 48 hours, a tracheostomy is usually performed. Digitalis, usually digoxin, should be administered to full therapeutic doses, although the immediate effect on cardiac output is often not significant.

Cardiac Arrhythmias. Minor arrhythmias, such as atrial fibrillation or a nodal rhythm, are very common after open heart surgical procedures. An important feature of postoperative care is constant, 24-hour-a-day, visual monitoring of the cardiac rhythm on an oscilloscope for 2 to 3 days following operation. Only by constant visual observation can serious arrhythmias be promptly detected, because such arrhythmias may develop in the presence of a normal cardiac output and without any other signs of circulatory failure.

Tachycardia, either as a sinus rhythm or rapid atrial fibrillation, may result from inadequate amounts of digitalis. Ventricular extrasystoles are the most common serious arrhythmia, because their appearance may herald the developing of more serious arrhythmias, such as bigeminy, ventricular tachycardia, or ventricular fibrillation. Digitalis toxicity is probably the most frequent cause of ventricular arrhythmias, resulting from varying sensitivity to digitalis after operation in relation to changes in plasma potassium concentration. Hypokalemia is particularly frequent, because patients in cardiac failure preoperatively may have significant depletion of body stores of potassium from chronic diuretic therapy.

Mild disturbance of cardiac rhythm from digitalis toxicity will subside following restriction of digitalis and administration of supplemental potassium. Intravenous lidocaine, 1 mg/minute, can be used in urgent circumstances

for temporary control of arrhythmias, although the drug is quickly metabolized. In selected arrhythmias the beta-blocking drug propranolol is of great value. Procainamide, in doses varying from 2 to 6 Gm/day, is also useful for more lasting control. In serious circumstances with ventricular tachycardia or other rhythms refractory to other forms of therapy, electric shock may be necessary.

Chronic Cardiac Failure. When the patient becomes ambulatory a few days after operation, fluid retention commonly becomes evident, especially if sodium intake is not carefully restricted. This can be easily detected by noting the appearance of edema in the flanks, hips, and legs. Weighing the patient daily is an important part of routine postoperative care. The edema usually responds promptly to diuretic therapy and restriction of sodium, but some patients with severe chronic cardiac failure before operation may require long periods of care before edema no longer develops.

Respiratory Insufficiency. Some disturbance of pulmonary function is very common following extracorporeal circulation. The frequency varies widely with different groups and also at different periods of time. The simplest numerical expression of the pulmonary dysfunction is indicated by the alveolar-arterial oxygen gradient, representing impaired diffusion of oxygen from the alveoli into the pulmonary venous blood. There are undoubtedly many causes of the pulmonary dysfunction, some of which are not well understood. Overtransfusion with resulting elevation of left atrial pressure and pulmonary congestion is one of the most frequent causes. Inadequate removal of pulmonary secretions, with resulting atelectasis and infection, is another. Microemboli or fat emboli are less well understood possible causative factors.

In some centers tracheostomy and assisted ventilation for 1 to 4 days are frequently employed with seriously ill patients, while in other centers tracheostomy is seldom done. In recent years our experience has been to decrease greatly the use of routine tracheostomy and mechanical ventilation, because of difficulties with humidification and infection if a tracheostomy is performed. Ventilation through an indwelling endotracheal tube for 24 to 48 hours has much decreased the need for tracheostomy. The most effective measures for avoiding pulmonary congestion following operation are the familiar ones of humidification of inspired gas, usually with an oxygen mask, and diligent removal of tracheobronchial secretions, including frequent turning of the patient with coughing and deep breathing. Nasotracheal aspiration with a catheter is frequently performed in the first 48 hours following operation. Bronchoscopy is rarely necessary.

Postoperative Fluids. Fluids are usually restricted to a moderate degree during the first 3 days following operation, about 800 ml/m² body surface being administered during the first 24 hours after operation and about 1,000 ml/m² body surface for subsequent 24-hour periods during the next 2 days. Fluid restriction is necessary because of the risk of pulmonary congestion from excessive fluid intake. A curious symptom following extracorporeal circulation is acute thirst, perhaps a reflection of peripheral vasoconstriction following the nonpulsatile circulation of cardiopulmonary bypass. Unless fluids are restricted, a patient may drink large amounts of fluid, with resultant serious edema. Oral intake is usually prohibited for at least 24 hours after operation because of the risk of gastric dilatation with vomiting and aspiration.

Renal Function. Hourly urine output is carefully measured for 1 to 2 days after operation, preferably keeping the average urine output greater than 30 ml/hour. A transitory elevation of BUN level to 25 to 35 mg/100 ml is commonly seen after complex operative procedures, although the frequency has much decreased with the use of hemodilution priming of the pump-oxygenator, as well as the routine administration of mannitol to promote an osmotic diuresis during perfusion. The renal injury may be produced by deficient perfusion, excessive hemolysis, or a transfusion incompatibility. Significant renal failure often presents a high-output renal failure, with daily secretion of 1 to 2 liters of dilute urine, associated with progressive elevation in BUN level. The degree of renal insufficiency in such circumstances can be most simply evaluated by performance of a simple urea clearance test, comparing the simultaneous urea concentration in the blood and the urine. Normally, urea should be concentrated at least fifteen to twenty times greater in the urine than in the blood; a urea concentration less than ten times greater in the urine than in the blood usually represents a severe degree of renal insufficiency.

If serious renal insufficiency evolves, peritoneal dialysis is employed at an early stage, often within 2 to 3 days after operation with BUN levels of 75 to 90 mg/100 ml. Postponement of peritoneal dialysis, with progressive increase of BUN concentration above 100 mg/100 ml, may be associated with serious or even fatal cardiac arrhythmias. As the risk of arrhythmias cannot be predicted for an individual patient, the routine use of early dialysis has been of significant benefit. With frequent dialysis, recovery from the renal injury almost always takes place.

Fever. There is almost always some fever following extracorporeal circulation, temperatures of 38 to 39°C being very common in the first 1 to 3 days after operation. In some patients, unexplained fevers of 39 to 40°C may develop, probably as a result of minute areas of atelectasis. Contamination of the heart-lung machine with pyrogens was a frequent cause of fever in the early experiences with open heart operations but with disposable oxygenators now occurs rarely. Significant fever, with its detrimental effects on metabolic requirements, can be most simply controlled by the use of a hypothermia mattress beneath the patient through which cold fluid can be circulated at appropriate intervals.

Fever persisting beyond a few days after operation is commonly found to be due to atelectasis or a pleural effusion. Another frequent cause of fever is the so-called "pericardiotomy syndrome," which may develop in any patient in whom the pericardium has been opened at operation, even if extracorporeal circulation has not been employed. This puzzling syndrome, the cause of which still remains unknown despite numerous investigations, may be associated with sustained fever, a pericardial friction rub, and pericardial and pleural effusions. The white blood cell count may be increased in some patients, while in others it is normal or decreased to 5,000 to 7,000 white blood cells per cubic millimeter. In a minority of patients abnormal lymphocytes appear, the recognition of which greatly facilitates the diagnosis. Most patients respond promptly to administration of 50 to 60 mg prednisone daily, which is frequently employed for both a diagnostic and therapeutic test. Prednisone is given for 3 to 4 days and then stopped to see if fever recurs. Recurrences are not uncommon and may require administration of smaller amounts of prednisone, 10 to 20 mg daily, for several days.

Urinary tract infection is another frequent cause of postoperative fever and can be easily recognized by microscopic examination of the urine and appropriate bacterial cultures. With fever continuing more than a few days after operation, the dread question of bacterial endocarditis must always be considered. The diagnosis can be established or excluded only by serial blood cultures, which should routinely be done with persistent unexplained fever. Fortunately in recent years bacterial endocarditis has become extremely rare. With routine use of large amounts of methicillin both during and following cardiac operations, staphylococcal endocarditis has almost disappeared. Rarely a fungal endocarditis, usually organisms of the *Candida* group, appears and is often lethal. Prolonged use of antibiotics probably increases the susceptibility to a fungal infection.

Central Nervous System. Probably the most common cause of injury to the central nervous system following extracorporeal circulation is air embolism associated with incomplete evacuation of air from the cardiac chambers. It is extraordinarily difficult to remove all intracardiac air, because air pockets may be loculated in pulmonary veins, the left atrium, or the left ventricle. Rarely air accumulating in the right side of the heart with a functioning right ventricle may be propelled through the pulmonary vascular bed into the left side of the heart. Prevention of air embolism is more difficult when previous operations have been performed, producing adhesions which fix the heart in the pericardial cavity and limit manipulation and massage of the heart at the end of perfusion to displace air pockets. Another cause of focal neurologic injury is calcium emboli, especially in patients with calcific aortic stenosis in whom extensive fragmentation of the calcific valve may occur as it is removed, often piecemeal, with rongeurs. Thrombi in the left atrium, usually in patients with chronic mitral stenosis, are another cause of emboli unless they are carefully removed. Fortunately, all these forms of cerebral injury are avoidable with a carefully planned and executed procedure.

With extracorporeal circulation for 5 to 6 hours or longer, especially when associated with significant trauma to the blood from extensive use of intracardiac suction, a diffuse depression of cerebral function may occur, almost always subsiding without residual neurologic injury in a few days. The exact cause of this difficulty is unknown but is probably sludging of blood elements in cerebral capillaries with focal areas of circulatory stasis. Fat emboli have been long considered as a possible cause, but their significance remains uncertain.

A curious postperfusion psychosis may develop in some patients, with all the emotional symptoms of a psychotic syndrome. Intensive therapy with appropriate sedation and physical restraints to avoid bodily harm is necessary. Fortunately such emotional disturbances almost always subside within 2 weeks after operation. They probably also result from diffuse disturbances in cerebral microcirculation.

With focal injuries to the central nervous system, convulsions are frequent and should be anticipated in therapy. With severe injuries, a tracheostomy is usually performed to facilitate removal of bronchial secretions and assist ventilation. In a seriously ill, comatose patient, a sustained convulsion with anoxia can precipitate a serious or fatal cardiac arrhythmia. This can be avoided if a tracheostomy with mechanical ventilation is performed prophylactically. Convulsions usually can be controlled satisfactorily with appropriate amounts of diphenylhydantoin (Dilantin) or phenobarbital. With neurologic injuries fever of 39 to 40°C is common but can be controlled simply by the use of a hypothermia mattress. A massive neurologic injury may be fatal, but less severe ones are seldom permanent. Although intensive care may be necessary for 3 to 4 weeks, virtually complete recovery usually results.

Gastrointestinal Disturbances. A mild paralytic ileus is frequent for the first 24 hours after operation, and for this reason patients are usually not allowed fluids by mouth for this period of time. Otherwise, gastric dilatation with the risk of vomiting and aspiration can occur. After this period of time, gastrointestinal disturbances are infrequent. Rarely, in seriously ill patients, a stress ulcer with serious gastrointestinal hemorrhage can develop. However, the routine use of a bland (antiulcer) diet, combined with antacid medications for the first few days after operation, has greatly decreased the frequency of this ulcer. Perforation of a stress ulcer is a rare and often fatal complication.

Anemia. Often following operation there is a daily decrease in hematocrit to levels of 28 to 32 percent. Blood transfusion in appropriate amounts is usually given for severe anemia, while oral therapy with iron is sufficient for most patients. Although anemia can result from many causes, it is usually not due to continuing loss of blood but to an accelerated rate of blood cell destruction, probably from trauma to the red blood cells during extracorporeal circulation.

Anticoagulant Therapy. Although policies vary at different cardiac centers, most patients with prosthetic valves are routinely started on anticoagulants in the first week following operation. Since 1971, with the use of cloth-covered valves, anticoagulant programs have varied widely among different centers, and the overall frequency of major thromboembolism is only 1 to 3 percent. At New York University sodium warfarin is used only for 3 to 4 weeks for aortic prostheses but indefinitely for mitral and tricuspid prostheses. Because of the small but definite risk of fatal cerebral hemorrage, dosage levels have been decreased to maintain a prothrombin level near 20 seconds, rather than the previous level of 25 to 30 seconds. Most patients require about 5 mg of warfarin daily.

CARDIAC ARREST AND VENTRICULAR FIBRILLATION

Cardiac arrest and ventricular fibrillation are considered together in this section because either of these catastrophes produce immediate cessation of the circulation. An injury causing generalized cardiac depression, such as anoxia, is more likely to lead to cardiac arrest, while agents increasing myocardial irritability, such as digitalis intoxication, are more likely to produce ventricular fibrillation. Diagnosis and treatment for the two conditions are, however, very similar.

HISTORICAL DATA. By first successful cardiac resuscitation was performed in 1901 by Igelsrud in Norway, but for many years this remained an isolated therapeutic triumph. The first successful case of electrical defibrillation was reported by Beck in 1947. In 1960 a dramatic advance in cardiac resuscitation occurred when Kouwenhoven, Jude, and Knickerbocker, working as a group at the Johns Hopkins Hospital, first introduced the concept of closed-chest massage. The same group also contributed greatly to the simultaneous development of methods of closed-chest defibrillation. The applicability of closed-chest cardiac massage and defibrillation has greatly enlarged the feasibility of cardiac resuscitation and has made it a responsibility of every physician to become familiar with these techniques.

PATHOGENSIS. Etiology. A great many agents may cause cardiac arrest. The more frequent of these will be briefly mentioned.

Coronary Thrombosis. Coronary thrombosis, with or without myocardial infarction, may induce either cardiac arrest or ventricular fibrillation and is a frequent cause of cardiac arrest refractory to all forms of therapy.

Anoxia. The depressant effect of anoxia on the myocardium is a frequent major underlying factor in producing cardiac arrest. This can occur from many causes, including depression of respiration, airway obstruction, and aspiration of gastric contents.

Drugs. Several drugs may produce either ventricular fibrillation or cardiac arrest when excessive amounts are used or when an abnormal sensitivity to the drug is present. Digitalis is one of the most prominent of this group, for the sensitivity of the myocardium to digitalis varies with the serum electrolyte concentrations, especially potassium.

Serum Electrolyte Abnormalities. Either deficiency or excess of potassium can cause cardiac arrest. The effects of the abnormal potassium concentration are significantly influenced by the existing concentration of calcium ions, and also by the presence of acidosis or alkalosis.

Anesthesia. Almost any anesthetic agent in excessive amounts will depress the myocardium and precipitate cardiac arrest. Statistical surveys have disclosed that cardiac arrest occurs in approximately 1 in every 1,500 operations.

Bradycardia. A profound bradycardia, with a heart rate below 60 beats per minute, may result in ventricular extrasystoles, subsequently followed by ventricular tachycardia or fibrillation. This is frequently seen in patients with a complete heart block unless the heart rate is increased by electrical or chemical stimulation.

Cardiac Catheterization. Ventricular fibrillation is an infrequent but well-recognized complication of cardiac catheterization or angiocardiography, usually developing during manipulation of the cardiac catheter into different cardiac chambers.

Reflex Mechanisms. On many occasions cardiac arrest has developed in association with some event which stimulated the vagus nerve. Such episodes include endotracheal suctioning, insertion of a gastric tube, or vomiting. It is doubtful that a vagal reflex per se can ever arrest a normal heart. In the laboratory, normal hearts can be arrested for only a few seconds even with continuous electrical stimulation of the vagus nerve. It is probable in clinical circumstances that only a myocardium seriously injured from other causes will be arrested or fibrillated during some event which stimulates the vagus nerve.

Pathophysiology. The cerebral anoxia resulting from cessation of circulation produces significant brain injury within 3 to 4 minutes, depending upon the temperature. Periods of anoxia for 6 to 8 minutes may produce extensive but reversible brain damage, whereas longer periods regularly cause irreversible brain injury. Myocardial anoxia is, of course, also present but is of little clinical significance as compared to the central nervous system injury.

DIAGNOSIS. Since brain injury will develop following 3 to 4 minutes of cardiac arrest, it is imperative that a diagnosis be made rapidly and therapy begun. The physician considering a diagnosis of cardiac arrest should either confirm or exclude it within 30 to 60 seconds and act accordingly. In most patients the diagnosis can be simply

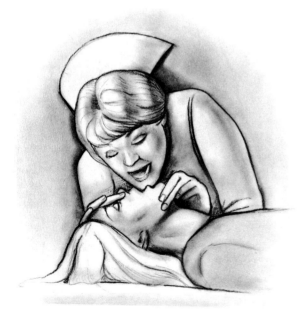

Fig. 19-2. Technique of mouth-to-mouth ventilation. The chin of the patient must be held forward with one hand to prevent obstruction of the nasopharynx by backward displacement of the tongue. The nostrils need to be occluded with the other hand. The head should be extended on the cervical spine to avoid obstruction in the nasopharynx.

made. There is an abrupt disappearance of peripheral pulses, most easily confirmed by palpation of the femoral or carotid arteries. Loss of consciousness quickly occurs, as well as absence of respiratory activity except for a few agonal gasps. Auscultation of the chest readily demonstrates that no cardiac sounds are audible. Complex diagnostic maneuvers which require larger amounts of time should be avoided. It should be emphasized that the *electrocardiogram is of little value for the diagnosis of cardiac arrest,* for electrical activity can continue on the electrocardiogram for some minutes after effective cardiac contractions have ceased. The main value of the electrocardiogram is to demonstrate the presence of ventricular fibrillation, because cardiac arrest can be differentiated from ventricular fibrillation only by the electrocardiogram or by direct inspection of the myocardium.

The most common differential diagnosis from cardiac arrest is the presence of extreme bradycardia with hypotension, as in someone who has fainted or developed anaphylactic shock from a hypersensitivity syndrome. Usually differentiation is not difficult, for although profound peripheral vascular collapse is present, there is some respiratory activity and not a total loss of consciousness.

TREATMENT. Ventilation. The most urgent first step in treatment of cardiac arrest is to provide adequate oxygenation (Fig. 19-2). It is futile to begin cardiac massage without ventilation of the lungs, although under the pressures of extreme circumstances, this obvious fact is often overlooked. Ventilation is most readily accomplished by mouth-to-mouth insufflation of the lungs. This can be begun immediately and continued until less laborious methods can be arranged. Most cardiac resuscitation kits include a laryngoscope and an endotracheal tube which can be inserted by any physician with moderate experience. Until an endotracheal tube can be inserted, however, mouth-to-mouth ventilation should be continued. Attempts to perform a hurried tracheostomy should not be made unless there is an obstruction at the larynx. Tracheostomy under emergency circumstances can be surprisingly difficult and quickly waste the precious few minutes available for preserving cerebral function.

Cardiac Massage. Closed-chest massage should be used in the majority of patients. Its efficacy depends upon intermittent compression of the heart between the sternum and the vertebral column, with lateral motion of the heart limited by the pericardium. For performing cardiac massage, the patient must be on a firm surface, such as the floor or a board under his shoulders. Certain points of technique are essential. The heel of the hand should be applied over the lower third of the sternum with the other hand above it to depress the sternum intermittently for 3 to 4 cm (Fig. 19-3). Sternal compression should be brisk, depressing the sternum sharply and then releasing it to permit cardiac filling. Compression of the sternum at a lower level near the xyphoid process may injure the liver, while compression more superiorly or laterally over the chest will result in multiple fractures of the ribs. Massage should be at a rate of about 60 per minute; more than one person is usually required, since the person performing massage will fatigue quickly. The amount of force applied

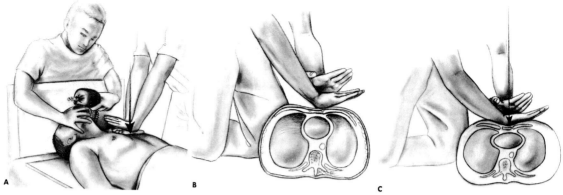

Fig. 19-3. *A.* Closed-chest massage. The heel of the hand should be used to compress intermittently the lower portion of the sternum toward the vertebral column. The effectiveness of the compression should be monitored by palpation of a peripheral pulse by another member of the team. Artificial ventilation must be performed at the same time. *B.* Cross section of chest showing the anatomic basis for closed-chest massage. The heart is seen suspended in the midthorax between the sternum anteriorly and the vertebral column posteriorly. The pericardium must be intact for closed-chest massage to be effective. *C.* Compression of the heart as the sternum is depressed downward toward the vertebral column.

should be gauged by palpation of a peripheral pulse, usually the femoral. Some caution is required to be certain that a regurgitant pulse in the femoral vein is not confused with a pulse in the femoral artery, because a strong retrograde pulse wave can be propagated down the vena cava during massage. Massage should be continued for as long as cardiac resuscitation remains feasible, especially if cerebral function is intact. A definite time limit cannot be given beyond which cardiac massage should be abandoned, although most successful cardiac resuscitations are accomplished within a few minutes. On one occasion we participated in a successful cardiac resuscitation which required 2 hours and 20 minutes of direct massage before a fibrillating heart could be successfully defibrillated. The patient was still well 10 years later.

Open cardiac massage, performed through a lateral thoracotomy in the left fourth or fifth intercostal space, is seldom needed. It should, however, be used if there is an open pericardium, cardiac tamponade, or massive intrathoracic hemorrhage.

Drugs and Fluids. Epinephrine, sodium bicarbonate, and calcium are the most useful agents. Epinephrine, 1 to 2 ml of 1:10,000 dilution, may be injected directly into the heart or into a peripheral vein. Calcium, 3 to 4 ml of a 10% solution, is a similarly powerful stimulant of myocardial contraction. Acidosis is especially common with cardiac arrest and may require vigorous therapy to restore a normal pH before effective cardiac contractions can be obtained. Sodium bicarbonate, in amounts as large as 200 to 300 mEq, may be required if severe acidosis is present. Rapid intravenous infusion of fluids, up to 1 liter or more, is usually of value, especially if hypovolemia was present before cardiac arrest occurred. An intravenous infusion of vasopressors, usually 1 to 4 μg/minute of norepinephrine or epinephrine, is frequently of value. Other drugs, such as atropine or digitalis, are usually of little benefit.

Defibrillation. In the presence of ventricular fibrillation, which can be confirmed only by the electrocardiogram or by direct inspection of the myocardium, electrical defibrillation is required. This can be accomplished in the closed chest by applying electrodes over the base and apex of the heart or by applying one large electrode posteriorly near the vertebral column and a smaller electrode anteriorly near the cardiac apex (Fig. 19-4). Defibrillation can

be done with either alternating or direct current, although studies in recent years have indicated that direct current defibrillation is preferable (approximately 400 joules). With an open chest, direct defibrillation can be easily accomplished by application of electrodes to the heart and administration of an appropriate electric impulse, usually 110 to 120 volts for 0.1 second. The usual cause of failure to defibrillate is either an anoxic or an acidotic myocar-

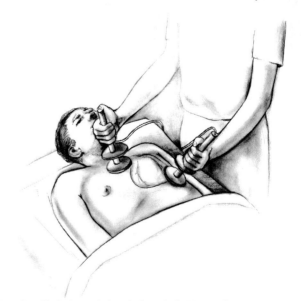

Fig. 19-4. Technique of closed-chest defibrillation. One electrode paddle is applied at the apex of the heart and the other at the base. The most common errors are inadequate electrical contact between the electrodes and the skin or inadequate amounts of current.

dium. Vigorous massage before application of the electric shock may be required to oxgenate the myocardium sufficiently. Acidosis can be corrected with bicarbonate. Injection of epinephrine may also stimulate myocardial tone and enhance subsequent defibrillation. Unless a coronary thrombosis has occurred, it should be possible to defibrillate almost all fibrillating hearts, although the ensuing cardiac arrest may be refractory to therapy. Inability to defibrillate is usually due to one or more correctible causes, such as inadequate electric stimulus, inadequate application of electrodes, anoxic myocardium, or acidosis.

Therapy following Cardiac Resuscitation. Following restoration of an adequate heartbeat, careful note should be made of the presence of injury to the central nervous system. This is usually indicated by continuing coma. Patients with significant brain injury are best treated by mild hypothermia, lowering the body temperature to 33 to 34°C and maintaining this temperature for 3 to 4 days. There are abundant experimental data indicating that this mild degree of hypothermia will significantly enhance recovery from cerebral injury. Hypothermia should be begun soon, because hyperthermia to 39 to 40°C often develops within 2 to 4 hours.

Continuous visual monitoring of the cardiac rhythm with an oscilloscope is essential, because arrhythmias are frequent and some can progress to ventricular fibrillation unless promptly treated. Intravenously administered lidocaine, 1 mg/minute, and procainamide are both very useful drugs for suppressing cardiac arrhythmias. Adequacy of cardiac output and ventilation can be monitored by periodic measurment of arterial and central venous blood-gas concentrations (P_{O_2}, P_{CO_2}, and pH).

Fluid therapy should be carefully regulated, depending upon the blood volume and the renal function. Excessive fluids may intensify cerebral edema. Adequacy of ventilation should be carefully assessed, because anoxia can readily precipitate another episode of cardiac arrest. In comatose patients, a tracheostomy is usually performed, and frequent assisted ventilation with a mechanical respirator is performed for 2 to 3 days.

PROGNOSIS. Unless a myocardial thrombosis or some other irreversible injury is present, the majority of patients in whom cardiac arrest has developed may be effectively treated if the correct diagnosis is made promptly.

When a reversible cardiac injury is present, as with overdose of an anesthetic agent, cardiac resuscitation is almost uniformly possible if begun quickly. Similarly, ventricular fibrillation from a variety of mechanisms can be promptly and effectively treated by external defibrillation if defibrillation is done before severe myocardial anoxia has developed. The usual cause of failure of defibrillation is the presence of an underlying myocardial thrombosis.

MITRAL STENOSIS

HISTORICAL DATA. A valiant effort to treat mitral stenosis by excising a portion of the valve with a valvulotome was made by Cutler and Levine in 1923, but the resulting

mitral insufficiency caused a prohibitive operative mortality. Souttar, in 1925, performed a digital commissurotomy in one patient. Thereafter surgical efforts virtually ceased for over 20 years until the year 1948–1949 when Harken et al. and Bailey independently demonstrated the value of digital commissurotomy. These early commissurotomies, often limited in extent, frequently produced striking clinical improvement, even though mitral stenosis frequently recurred within 5 years. A transventricular mitral dilator developed around 1957 produced a more extensive commissurotomy and was widely adopted. In recent years the increasing safety of cardiopulmonary bypass has made commissurotomy under direct vision the procedure of choice in most centers, though some groups still obtain excellent results with a closed commissurotomy. When a closed commissurotomy is undertaken, the heart-lung machine is usually kept on a standby basis in the operating room to permit use of cardiopulmonary bypass if closed commissurotomy becomes hazardous or unsuccessful. When the mitral valve has been virtually destroyed by fibrosis and calcification, effective commissurotomy is not possible, and replacement with a prosthetic valve is necessary.

ETIOLOGY. All evidence indicates that mitral stenosis is almost always due to rheumatic fever, even though a definite history of rheumatic fever can be obtained in only about 50 percent of patients. Congenital mitral stenosis is very rare, less than 200 cases having been reported. After the initial episode of rheumatic fever, symptoms of mitral stenosis may not appear for 10 or more years but may develop as soon as 3 years in some patients and as late as 25 years in others. Selzer and Cohn, in an excellent review of clinical characteristics of mitral stenosis, have suggested that scarring of the mitral valve from rheumatic fever may cause turbulent flow of blood which in turn causes progressive scarring and contraction over many years; this would explain the appearance of severe mitral stenosis 20 to 30 years after the last known bout of rheumatic fever.

PATHOLOGY. Although rheumatic fever produces a pancarditis, involving pericardium, myocardium, and endocardium, the most serious permanent injury results from the endocarditis. Permanent myocardial injury following recovery from acute myocarditis is ill defined and apparently seldom of clinical significance. Endocarditis produces ulceration of the endocardium along the edges of the valve leaflets where they normally appose in systole. Tiny, 1- to 2-mm nodules of fibrin and platelets accumulate and may progress to fusion of the leaflets at the commissures. A more serious injury evolves from extensive valvulitis with fibrosis and contraction of the body of the leaflets, compounded in subsequent years with calcification and decreasing leaflet mobility. Inflammation of the chordae tendineae similarly leads to fibrosis with contraction, thickening, and fusion. With severe disease the chordae contract to such an extent that the valve leaflets are pulled down to appose the tips of the underlying papillary muscles.

In many patients mitral stenosis gradually increases in severity over many years, at times more than 20. Previously these progressive changes were considered due to clinically silent episodes of rheumatic fever. A more plausible current hypothesis is that the changes are hemodynamic in origin, resulting from turbulent flow of blood originally produced by the initial inflammation and scarring.

The possibilities of surgical correction of mitral stenosis vary greatly with the nature of the valve injury. When simple fusion of the commissures is the only lesion, mitral commissurotomy is highly successful. With concomitant fibrosis and rigidity of the leaflets, commissurotomy is less effective. If the chordae tendineae have contracted and fused to make the leaflets immobile, commissurotomy is futile. With such advanced pathology replacement of the diseased valve with a prosthesis is necessary.

PATHOPHYSIOLOGY. A normal mitral valve has a cross-sectional area between 4 and 6 cm². Reduction of the cross-sectional area to 2 to 2.5 cm² constitutes the mildest form of mitral stenosis. Typical auscultatory findings are present, but the patient is often asymptomatic (Class I). Further reduction to the range of 1.5 to 2.0 cm² produces some symptoms (Class II disability); these are more severe with a cross-sectional area in the range of 1 to 1.5 cm². Patients with a cross-sectional area of less than 1 cm² are usually seriously disabled (Class IV). A valve area near 0.4 cm² is said to be the minimal size compatible with life.

Three significant physiologic events result from mitral stenosis—increase in left atrial pressure, decrease in cardiac output, and increase in pulmonary vascular resistance. Increase in left atrial pressure (normally less than 10 to 12 mm Hg) is the immediate consequence of mitral stenosis. The degree of elevation of left atrial pressure varies with three factors: (1) the cross-sectional area of the mitral orifice, (2) cardiac output, and (3) cardiac rate. These three factors represent physical laws determining pressure-flow relations through a stenotic orifice, namely, cross-sectional area of orifice, total volume of flow, and duration of time during which flow occurs. When left atrial pressure rises to exceed oncotic pressure of plasma (25 to 30 mm Hg), transudation of fluid across the pulmonary capillaries will occur. The result of this transudation depends upon the capacity of the pulmonary lymphatics to transport the additional fluid. When the fluid load exceeds the capacity of the lymphatic circulation, pulmonary edema results. Clinically, therefore, left atrial pressure and concomitant pulmonary symptoms vary with the degree of mitral stenosis, the cardiac output as influenced by exercise or emotion, and the length of diastole determined by cardiac rate.

As the oncotic pressure of plasma is 25 to 30 mm Hg, about that of a column of blood 12 to 14 in. high, pulmonary congestion in the upright position may be much greater in the lower lobes of the lung than in the upper, for the average thorax is about 20 in. high. A patient with only basilar rales in the upright position may develop extensive pulmonary congestion when supine, with cough, dyspnea, or frank pulmonary edema. Hence, the pathogenesis of paroxysmal noctural dyspnea.

The cardiac output is fixed at a low level by the rigid stenotic orifice. With exercise, cardiac output cannot be increased significantly, and dyspnea results. The general fatigue and limitation of physical activity with mitral stenosis is a clinical reflection of this physiologic inability to increase cardiac output.

The degree to which pulmonary vascular resistance increases with mitral stenosis varies greatly among different patients. The cause for the variation is unknown. Some, with severe mitral stenosis, have little change, while in others vascular resistance increases to levels fifteen to twenty times greater than normal. This increased resistance is primarily a result of vasoconstriction in the pulmonary arterioles, ultimately intensified by hypertrophy of the media and intima. In far advanced cases recurrent pulmonary emboli may create additional obstruction, but this is uncommon. Fortunately, in the vast majority of patients, the increased vascular resistance either decreases greatly or disappears following surgical correction of the mitral stenosis.

Two other serious disabilities which appear with chronic mitral stenosis are atrial fibrillation and systemic embolization. Atrial fibrillation is the usual ultimate consequence of the atrial hypertrophy produced by chronic left atrial hypertension. Fibrillation produces some decrease in cardiac output and also is often a prelude to more serious arrhythmias. The most serious consequence, however, is the development of thrombi, usually in the ineffectively contracting left atrial appendage. The frequency of thrombi varies both with the duration of mitral stenosis and the presence of atrial fibrillation. Ultimately thrombi develop in 15 to 20 percent of patients, after which episodes of arterial embolism appear with increasing frequency. Before either anticoagulant therapy or operation was possible, cerebral embolism caused death in 20 to 25 percent of patients dying from mitral stenosis.

CLINICAL MANIFESTATIONS. Symptoms. The most important symptom is *dyspnea*. This appears whenever mean left atrial pressure exceeds 30 mm Hg long enough to produce significant transudation of fluid into the pulmonary capillaries. Characteristically, it first appears with extreme exertion and subsequently, with more severe stenosis, occurs with lesser degrees of exertion. It may also appear with emotion or other circumstances which increase cardiac output.

Several other symptoms subsequently appear, all developing as a result of recurrent pulmonary congestion. A chronic *cough*, worse in the evenings in the recumbent position, is frequent, reflecting basilar congestion. *Orthopnea* and *paroxysmal nocturnal dyspnea* similarly reflect the influence of the upright position on the localization of pulmonary congestion. In the upright position, congestion may be limited to the lower lobes but becomes more diffuse in the supine position. Mobilization of peripheral edema from the lower extremities when the patient is supine intensifies the degree of pulmonary congestion. *Hemoptysis* is a frequent symptom, varying from expectoration of blood-tinged sputum to massive amounts of bright red blood, in unusual circumstances exceeding 1 liter. Fortunately such severe hemoptysis, although an alarming symptom, subsides spontaneously. Episodes of *pulmonary edema* occur when pulmonary congestion greatly exceeds the capacity of the pulmonary lymphatics. In contrast to hemoptysis, pulmonary edema may be fatal unless quickly and effectively treated.

When pulmonary vascular resistance rises to produce pulmonary hypertension, failure of the right side of the heart appears, manifested by venous distension, hepatic enlargement, and peripheral edema.

As mentioned earlier, atrial fibrillation develops eventually in most patients. Initially it may be transient, but ultimately in most patients chronic atrial fibrillation is the most common rhythm.

Arterial embolism is a constant threat, especially with atrial fibrillation, although emboli can occur with a sinus rhythm. Emboli evolve from stasis in the dilated left atrium, especially in the atrial appendage. Rarely, huge thrombi 5 to 10 cm in diameter may fill much of the left atrium and partly obstruct the ostia of the pulmonary veins.

Angina pectoris develops in about 10 percent of patients. The basic cause is unclear, for it is usually not due to associated coronary atherosclerosis. Possible mechanisms include a low cardiac output, impaired blood flow during diastole because of tachycardia, and recurrent small emboli to the coronary arteries.

Physical Examination. A patient with chronic, severe mitral stenosis may be thin and frail, with the muscular wasting characteristic of a chronic illness. Dilated neck veins are visible if congestive failure is present. Rubor and/or cyanosis are often seen over the fingers or lips. These signs reflect a chronic severe restriction in cardiac output, resulting in blood flowing slowly through peripheral capillary beds. Rales are frequently audible over the lung bases.

On examination of the heart, the cardiac size and the quality of the apical impulse are of particular importance. Often with pure mitral stenosis, the cardiac size is normal, and the apical impulse is normal or decreased in intensity. A forceful, heaving left ventricular impulse immediately suggests that associated disease, such as mitral insufficiency or aortic valvular disease with resulting ventricular hypertrophy, is present. With increased pulmonary vascular resistance, palpation of the left parasternal area may find a "lift," resulting from contraction of a hypertrophied right ventricle. The pulse rhythm may be regular but is usually atrial fibrillation.

The three significant auscultatory findings with mitral stenosis are the diastolic rumble, an opening snap, and an increased first sound. The apical diastolic rumble, at times sharply localized to an area at the apex only 2 to 3 cm

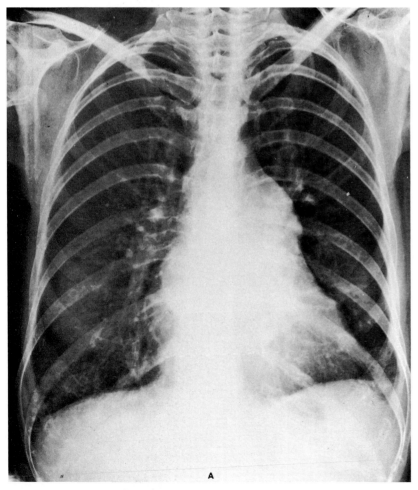

Fig. 19-5. *A.* Chest roentgenogram of a patient with mitral stenosis showing a heart of normal size. The prominent pulmonary artery along the left cardiac border is characteristic of this condition. The enlarged left atrium can be seen as a double density behind the shadow normally formed by the right atrium.

in diameter, is the hallmark of mitral stenosis. It may be of grade I or II intensity in some patients, while in others it is unusually loud with a palpable thrill. The intensity of the murmur, however, does not correlate with the severity of the stenosis. Rarely "silent" mitral stenosis is present without an audible murmur. This results from a calcified, fibrosed valve with little mobility. The increased first sound, the origin of which is not certain, is another distinctive feature and is often the first auscultatory abnormality detected. The opening snap, closely following the second sound, is the third distinctive feature. In many patients careful auscultation can immediately establish the diagnosis of mitral stenosis by finding the triad of an opening snap, followed by a diastolic rumble, and an accentuated first sound.

A short apical systolic murmur may be heard in patients with pure mitral stenosis without any associated mitral insufficiency. Loud pansystolic murmurs, however, which are transmitted to the axilla usually indicate associated mitral insufficiency. A systolic murmur from tricuspid insufficiency may be confused with one arising from mitral insufficiency. The systolic murmur of tricuspid insufficiency, although audible at the apex with hypertrophy of the right ventricle, is usually heard equally well near the sternum and may be accentuated with deep inspiration.

Laboratory Studies. The initial change in mitral stenosis is dilatation of the left atrium (Fig. 19-5). Hence, detection of slight degrees of enlargement of the left atrium is of particular importance in establishing the diagnosis. Once it has been determined that the left atrium is enlarged, however, there is little correlation between the actual size of the left atrium and the severity of the mitral stenosis. Left atrial enlargement is best detected with a lateral chest roentgenogram exposed during oral administration of barium to outline the esophagus. Characteristically, the middle third of the esophagus is displaced backward to form a slight concave curve. With additional degrees of enlargement, the dilated left atrium may be visible as a double shadow in the posteroanterior roentgenogram, forming a separate dense shadow behind the normal shadow of the right atrium. The left border of the cardiac shadow also shows characteristic changes with mitral stenosis, for the normal concavity between the shadow of the aortic knob and the left ventricle becomes obliterated as both the left atrium and the pulmonary artery enlarge to produce a "straight" left heart border. The overall cardiac size may be normal, but lateral views can demonstrate enlargement of the right ventricle when pulmonary vascular resistance has increased. Calcification of the mitral valve is visible with chronic disease in older patients.

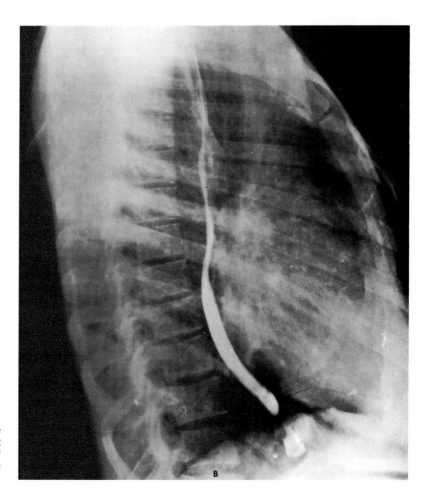

Fig. 19-5. *B*. Lateral roentgenogram of the same patient shows enlargement of the left atrium, producing a concave displacement of the esophagus, which has been filled with barium.

Careful roentgenographic scrutiny of the lung fields is of particular importance, for several abnormalities occur. Engorged pulmonary veins can be unusually prominent, often with a greater degree of dilatation in the veins to the upper lobes. With pulmonary hypertension the pulmonary arteries are also enlarged. With chronic, severe left atrial hypertension, dilated pulmonary lymphatics become visible as transverse lines across the lower lung fields, "Kerley lines," indicating significant left atrial hypertension.

The electrocardiogram is normal in some patients. The earliest change is an increased P wave from hypertrophy of the left atrium. Unfortunately, this is not consistent, and different studies have reported variation in the frequency of P-wave abnormalities from as low as 20 to 30 percent to as high as 70 to 80 percent. Only with increase in pulmonary vascular resistance does right ventricular hypertrophy produce distinct electrocardiographic changes, with the development of a right axis deviation. Hence, the electrocardiogram often is an inaccurate guide to the severity of the mitral stenosis. It is of particular value, however, in differential diagnosis, for signs of left ventricular hypertrophy immediately suggest some disease in addition to mitral stenosis, usually mitral insufficiency or aortic valvular disease.

Cardiac catheterization is an important method for evaluating the severity of mitral stenosis, as well as for detecting the presence of additional valvular disease, such as mitral insufficiency or aortic valvular disease. Left atrial pressure is usually estimated from the pulmonary capillary "wedge" pressure, although alternatively the left atrium can be entered directly with a catheter, usually by puncture of the atrial septum. The left atrial pressure in isolated mitral stenosis is increased from the normal range of 5 to 10 mm Hg to levels of 20 to 30 mm Hg with severe stenosis, producing a diastolic pressure gradient between the left atrium and left ventricle of 10 to 20 mm Hg. It is important to realize that the left atrial pressure varies not only with the severity of the stenosis, but also with the cardiac output and the cardiac rate. Hence, evaluation of an isolated determination must include assessment of these additional factors. The most precise measurement is mathematical calculation of the cross-sectional area of the mitral valve, determined by the pressure gradient and the cardiac output. Angiography may demonstrate rigidity and limited mobility of the valve leaflets but is not of great diagnostic value. It is of particular value, however, in determining the presence of mitral insufficiency by noting the reflux of dye after injection into the left ventricle. Coronary arteriography is gradually becoming an important part of the evaluation at cardiac catheterization, especially in patients over forty years of age in whom coronary atherosclerosis may be present.

DIAGNOSIS. A diagnosis of mitral stenosis can usually be made with certainty on physical examination, upon finding the triad of an opening snap, an apical diastolic rumble, and an increased first sound. These abnormalities often occur in association with a normal left ventricle, an enlarged left atrium, signs of pulmonary congestion, pulmonary hypertension, and right ventricular hypertrophy.

The differential diagnosis should include associated mitral insufficiency, tricuspid insufficiency, or aortic valvular disease.

TREATMENT. Indications for Operation. Operation is usually recommended for any patient with symptoms, because the risk is small (1 to 3 percent) and the slight but definite hazard of cerebral embolism is always present. If peripheral embolism has occurred, operation should be performed as soon as the patient has recovered from the embolic episode, for sooner or later emboli almost always recur. Until operation is performed, continuous anticoagulant therapy should be employed.

Fortunately, mitral stenosis almost always can be successfully operated upon, no matter how far advanced the disease or how severe the pulmonary hypertension. The immediate risk of operation is increased with far advanced disease, but surviving patients nearly always show remarkable improvement, with a significant decrease in, or complete disappearance of, pulmonary hypertension.

General Considerations. Since 1971 at New York University almost all mitral valve operations have been performed with cardiopulmonary bypass. The "closed" commissurotomy, performed blindly with the index finger introduced through the left atrial appendage, has been virtually abandoned. For some years mitral operations were performed with the heart-lung machine on a "standby" basis: a closed commissurotomy is attempted first, but if it is unsatisfactory, cardiopulmonary bypass is employed. For several reasons, an "open" operation with cardiopulmonary bypass is now preferred. The risk of bypass is very small, approaching 1 percent. The hazard of emboli from thrombi in the atrium or calcium in the mitral valve is much less than with blind, digital commissurotomy. Of even greater importance, perhaps, is that a more effective commissurotomy can be performed as the commissures can be clearly separated, underlying fused chordae separated, and a wide mitral orifice obtained without producing mitral insufficiency. Not all cardiac centers agree with this policy, however, and some continue to report excellent short-term results with the classic digital commissurotomy.

Technique of Open Mitral Commissurotomy. A median sternotomy incision is employed in almost all cases unless a previous sternotomy incision has been made, in which case a left thoracotomy is used. A sternotomy is preferred because of ready access to the heart, including palpation of the mitral and tricuspid valves, cannulation of the aorta and venae cavae, as well as access to the aortic valve if needed. Once cardiopulmonary bypass is established, body temperature is lowered to 30°C and the heart fibrillated. The left atrium is opened with a longitudinal incision in the interatrial groove, anterior to the point of entry of the right pulmonary veins. By extending the atriotomy beneath the superior vena cava above and the inferior vena cava below, adequate exposure of the mitral valve can be obtained. Usually the aorta is intermittently occluded for periods of 10 to 15 minutes to attain a dry, quiet heart. Before the aortic occlusion clamp is intermittently released, a small catheter vent is placed in the ascending aorta through a stab wound to remove accumulated air.

Any thrombi in the atrium or atrial appendage are carefully removed before the mitral valve is approached. The atrial appendage, a potential source of postoperative emboli, is routinely amputated, either by closure of the orifice from within the atrium or by amputating the appendage outside the heart (Fig. 19-6).

The fused commissures of the mitral valve are best exposed by inserting sutures into both the aortic and mural leaflets for traction. By applying *horizontal*, not vertical, traction on the two leaflets, the fused commissures can be clearly visualized. The commissure is then carefully separated with a knife, often with a right-angled clamp held open below the commissure to identify chordae arising from the underlying papillary muscle and inserting on the adjacent leaflets. Division of any chordae is scrupulously avoided. A technical problem frequently encountered is fusion and contraction of the chordae beneath the commissures, often with the fused commissures virtually attached to the papillary muscle. In such instances the papillary muscle is carefully split with a knife for as much as 1 cm, carefully preserving the chordae to each leaflet. This, of course, greatly increases the efficacy of the commissurotomy and is one of the attractive features of routine open operation.

Following commissurotomy the atriotomy is partly closed, leaving an opening large enough for subsequent introduction of the index finger to palpate the mitral valve. This opening is temporarily occluded with two mattress sutures tightened with snares. Following removal of air from the heart, it is defibrillated and bypass subsequently slowed, often stopped altogether. With the heart beating forcefully enough to generate a systemic systolic pressure of at least 100 mm Hg, the finger is reintroduced into the left atrium and the mitral valve palpated for insufficiency. Any insufficiency present can be corrected by appropriate sutures or annuloplasty. This technique, employed in a large number of patients, has virtually eliminated the production of significant insufficiency with commissurotomy. Previously insufficiency occurred in a significant percentage of operations, in as many as 15 to 20 percent of cases with instrumental commissurotomy according to published reports. Correction of the mitral stenosis is confirmed by measurement of left atrial and ventricular pressures by needle puncture to demonstrate elimination of the end-diastolic pressure gradient.

Following operation convalescence is usually benign, and the patient is discharged in 10 to 12 days. If atrial fibrillation is present, an attempt is made to convert it to a sinus rhythm. This is usually successful if chronic atrial fibrillation, with hypertrophy of left atrial musculature, has not been present.

Technique of Mitral Valve Replacement. An approach with a sternotomy incision similar to that for open commissurotomy is used. Mitral replacement, rather than commissurotomy, is almost always necessary if both insufficiency and stenosis are present. It is frequently needed for mitral stenosis with extensive calcification in the valve if the calcification is in the commissures, while calcification in the leaflets does not preclude effective commissurotomy. When replacement is done, the valve is excised by incising

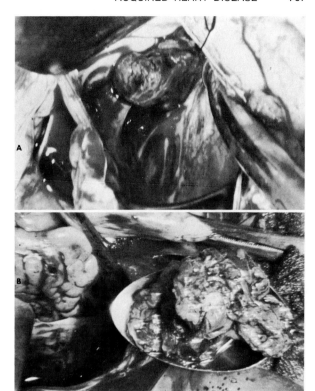

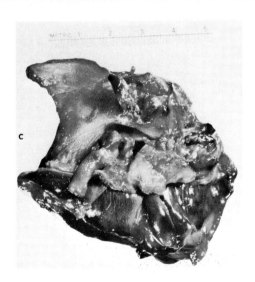

Fig. 19-6. Open mitral commissurotomy. *A.* The left atrium has been incised and the edges retracted. A small thrombus is present in the midportion of the field, demonstrating the pathologic condition which frequently causes cerebral embolism with mitral stenosis. *B.* Large clot found within the left atrium. With cardiopulmonary bypass functioning, the left atrium has been opened widely. The laminated clot is being removed with a large spoon. A clamp occluding the ascending aorta to avoid embolization of clot is visible at the top of the illustration. *C.* Large laminated clot removed at operation from a patient with mitral stenosis. The inability to detect the presence of such a clot before operation is the most cogent reason that all mitral commissurotomies should be performed with a pump-oxygenator as a "standby," to be employed if such a clot is found.

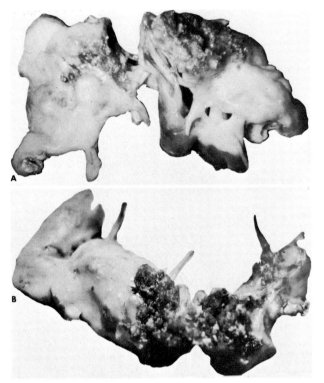

Fig. 19-7. *A.* Excised mitral valve with severe calcification. When such calcification is present, satisfactory function can rarely be restored to the valve. *B.* Calcified mitral valve removed from another patient in whom prosthetic replacement of the mitral valve was necessary.

it a few millimeters from the annulus with a circumferential incision, which often removes the entire valve intact (Fig. 19-7). Underlying papillary muscles are divided near their apexes. A ball-valve prosthesis is used almost routinely, though excellent results also have been reported with a disc prosthesis. The ball-valve prosthesis has the advantages of longer experience in its use and less likelihood of prosthetic failure, which has been more frequent with a disc prosthesis. The problem of a small left ventricle with mitral stenosis has been avoided by careful selection

of a valve of appropriate size. Rarely an obstructing collar of muscle in the wall of the left ventricle has been excised to avoid possible protrusion of muscle into the cage of the prosthesis. With these precautions a ball-valve prosthesis has functioned well. Some have proposed that ventricular function is better with a disc than with a ball-valve prosthesis, but data demonstrating a significant difference are meager (Figs. 19-8 and 19-9).

The prosthesis is inserted with a series of 12 to 18 mattress sutures of Dacron, with a pledget in each mattress suture to avoid the suture's cutting through a friable annulus (Fig. 19-10). Before pledgeted mattress sutures were routinely employed, significant postoperative insufficiency from suture leaks continued to occur, but the routine use of pledgets has virtually eliminated this complication. An alternative technique, widely and effectively used by others, is to insert 25 to 30 simple interrupted sutures. Care is taken to insert the sutures in the annulus, but no deeper, to avoid injury to the coronary sinus, the circumflex coronary artery, or the conduction bundle. Once the prosthesis has been tied in position, the motion of the ball in the cage is carefully checked to be certain that no muscle bundles in the ventricular cavity protrude into the cage and restrict motion of the ball. With this important precaution, so-called postoperative thrombosis of a prosthetic valve has not been seen.

As the atriotomy is closed, air is removed from the heart with the conventional Foley catheter left across the mitral valve, but in addition the apexes of both the left ventricle and the ascending aorta are vented to remove air, as the simple use of the Foley catheter is not completely effective in removing air emboli. A catheter vent in the ascending aorta, rather than the needle vent previously used, has been found far more effective for prevention of air embolism.

Fig. 19-8. *A.* Starr-Edwards mitral prosthesis. This prosthesis is completely covered with cloth and uses a steel ball. It is hoped that the complete covering of the prosthesis with cloth will decrease the incidence of thromboembolism. *B.* Mitral valve prosthesis with a Silastic ball used prior to 1967. In contrast to the prosthesis in *A*, the Teflon cloth does not cover the metallic ring and struts. *C.* Disc prosthesis. The disc prosthesis has a wider opening than a ball-valve prosthesis, and the cage does not protrude as far into the ventricle.

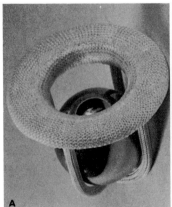
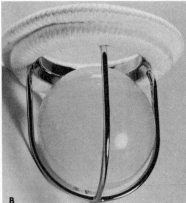
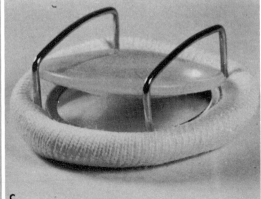

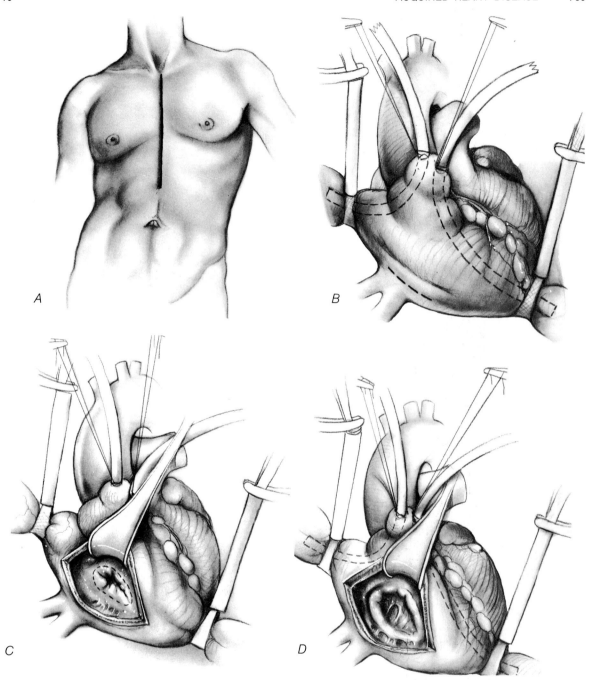

Fig. 19-9. Insertion of mitral valve prosthesis. A. A median ster-notomy is the preferred incision, providing ready access to all areas of the heart. B. Cannulae are introduced through the atrial wall into the venae cavae. Normally these are not snared with encircling tapes unless a patent foramen ovale is encountered which causes aspiration of air from the opened left atrium into the right atrium. C. The mitral valve is exposed with an incision in the left atrium anterior to the point of entry of the right pulmo-nary veins. Exposure is facilitated by intermittent occlusion of the aorta, which will arrest and stop the heart, and also decrease the amount of blood in the operative field. D. The mitral valve with the papillary muscles is completely excised, leaving a small rim of annulus. The cavity of the left ventricle is carefully in-spected and a prosthesis of appropriate size chosen, making certain that the cage of the prosthesis can be readily accommo-dated in the ventricular cavity. E. A Starr-Edwards ball-valve prosthesis, cloth-covered and with a steel ball, is preferred. It is inserted with 12 to 15 mattress sutures of #0 Dacron. Often the mattress sutures are buttressed with Teflon felt on the ven-tricular surface (not shown). F. Following insertion of the valve, a Foley catheter is placed across the valve to keep the valve incompetent and avoid air embolism. G. Final view of the valve in position before closure of the atriotomy. H. The atriotomy incision is closed around the Foley catheter, after which the heart is allowed to fill with blood and displace air. Subsequently the Foley catheter is removed, which permits the left ventricle to contract normally. (Figure continued on next page.)

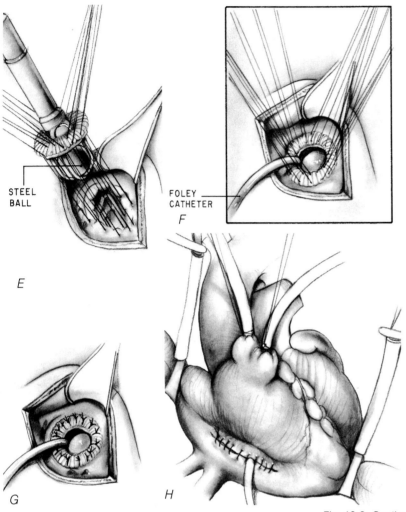

STEEL
BALL

FOLEY
CATHETER
F

E

G   H

Fig. 19-9. Continued.

Convalescence is usually benign except in patients with long-standing congestive failure where the cardiac output may be low for 1 to 2 days and require careful supportive care. Antibiotics are given for 5 to 7 days. Anticoagulation with sodium warfarin is begun about 4 days after operation and maintained with a prothrombin time near 20 seconds, a significantly lesser degree of anticoagulation than the former prothrombin levels near 30 seconds. This more conservative approach has less risk of anticoagulant hemorrhage but has not been associated with an increase in frequency of thromboembolism. Acetylsalicylic acid, 0.6 Gm twice daily, is also given for 1 to 2 years for possible inhibition of platelet aggregation. The frequency of thromboembolism has been small, in a range of 2 to 4 percent. With aortic prostheses, it has been possible to use anticoagulation for the first 4 weeks after operation, but stopping anticoagulants with mitral prosthetic valves has promptly resulted in a sharp increase in thromboembolism, and so currently anticoagulants are continued permanently.

Most patients improve promptly after operation, obtaining the full therapeutic benefit within 3 to 6 months. During this time careful attention to salt intake and body weight is necessary, for renal excretion of sodium remains impaired for several weeks.

Within 6 months after operation most patients have little physical restriction of activity. However, a few, with chronic congestive failure and cardiac enlargement beforehand, continue to have some permanent limitation, apparently from irreversible myocardial injury before operation.

Different types of tissue valves have been used for mitral replacement, but their durability remains uncertain. The valves used include aortic homograft valves, inserted in an inverted position, porcine heterograft valves, and fascia lata valves. Tissue valves are strikingly free from thromboembolism, but recurrence of mitral insufficiency within 1 to 2 years after operation has been too frequent to be acceptable. This has been particularly true with porcine heterograft valves and fascia lata valves, though both types are still under active experimental study.

PROGNOSIS. Following an adequate mitral commissurotomy that does not produce insufficiency, long-term prognosis is very good. As the valve is not normal, long-term function will probably be determined by the degree of fibrosis in the leaflets and the chordae. If these fibrotic changes are extensive enough to produce significant turbulent flow of blood, eventual stiffening and calcification of the leaflets are likely. However, if disease is predominantly in the commissures, excellent long-term function may be expected. Formerly a recurrence rate of mitral stenosis as high as 30 to 40 percent within 5 years after operation was reported, but this group included a significant percentage of patients in whom commissurotomy was initially ineffective, either because of technique or because calcification and fibrosis prevented effective reconstruction, for which prosthetic replacement is now done.

With commissurotomy as now performed, recurrence at 5 years is probably near 10 percent, far less than that estimated in the past. In a group of patients operated upon by the author at the University of Kentucky between 1961 and 1966, reported in a larger series by Bryant and Trinkle in 1971, the recurrence rate was well under 10 percent. Similarly, Higgs and associates in 1970 and Morrow and Braunwald in a careful study of 45 patients from a series of 226 undergoing mitral commissurotomy found that true restenosis occurred in only 5 patients. As stated earlier, the frequent "restenosis" reported previously was often simply an ineffective commissurotomy. Valve complications which do occur at a later date, either restenosis or insufficiency, are probably due to fibrosis of the valve leaflets from turbulent flow of blood, much as that seen in a congenitally bicuspid aortic valve, and are not a result of recurrent rheumatic fever.

Following prosthetic replacement of the mitral valve, the risk of endocarditis is small but permanent. Hence, prophylactic antibiotics should be routinely employed when episodes of transient bacteremia can be anticipated, as with dental extraction or cystoscopy. Thromboembolism remains a small but definite hazard. For this reason anticoagulants are used permanently, as described in the earlier paragraphs. A detailed report by Starr in 1971 of all experiences with mitral valve replacement, beginning with the first model prosthetic valve in 1961, confirms the durability of prosthetic mitral replacement (Figs. 19-11 and 19-12).

MITRAL INSUFFICIENCY

HISTORICAL DATA. A number of ingenious attempts to treat mitral insufficiency surgically by a closed approach were made before cardiopulmonary bypass became clinically feasible in 1955. Since that time an open approach with cardiopulmonary bypass has been uniformly used. Prosthetic replacement of the insufficient valve is usually necessary, especially if calcification of the valve has occurred. In some patients with mobile valve leaflets it may be possible to correct the insufficiency with an annuloplasty. Long-term results following annuloplasty in selected cases have been reported by Merendino and by Reed et al.

ETIOLOGY. Mitral insufficiency is usually rheumatic in

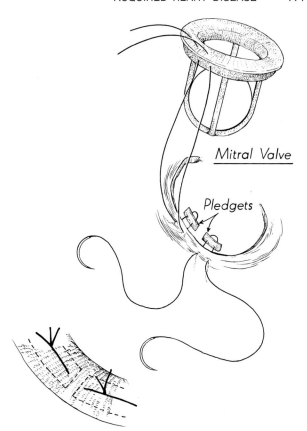

Fig. 19-10. Technique for suturing a mitral valve prosthesis with Dacron pledgets seated below the mitral annulus.

origin, although a definite history of rheumatic fever can be obtained only in somewhat over one-half of the patients. Unusual causes of mitral insufficiency include bacterial endocarditis, rupture of chordae tendineae usually from other causes, or papillary muscle dysfunction from extensive occlusive disease of the coronary arteries. Bacterial endocarditis can be suspected when protracted fever is associated with the development and persistence of the systolic murmur of mitral insufficiency, but the diagnosis can be proved only by identification of the bacterial organism in serial blood cultures. Rupture of chordae tendineae is an unusual but important cause of mitral insufficiency in older patients. Clinically it simulates rheumatic mitral insufficiency closely, but the acute onset in an older patient without previous signs of cardiac disease should suggest the diagnosis. Papillary muscle dysfunction is usually associated with obvious extensive disease of the coronary arteries, causing either cardiac dilatation and failure or myocardial infarction. Since about 1969 an increasing number of cases of "floppy valve" syndrome have been reported. This is a condition in which the leaflets and chordae thin and elongate, permitting herniation of the billowing leaflets into the atrium during systole. The condition apparently is a degenerative disease of connective tissue.

PATHOLOGIC ANATOMY. The basic changes with rheu-

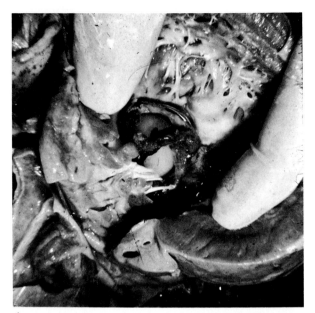

A

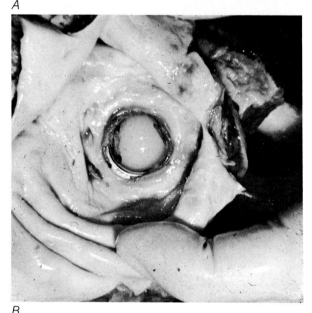

B

Fig. 19-11. *A*. Autopsy photograph of a Starr-Edwards valve prosthesis inserted before 1966, showing the tendency for original model of the prosthetic valve to develop extensive thromboembolism. Surprisingly enough the patient had had no clinical signs of emboli although myriads of scars were found in the kidneys at autopsy. Death occurred 7 years after operation, following a pulmonary infection. Thrombi extending from the ring of the prosthesis down the struts to the apex are clearly seen. *B*. Atrial view of valve, showing thrombi over approximately two-thirds of the metallic ring. Development of such thrombi was the principle reason for the development of cloth-covered prosthetic valves.

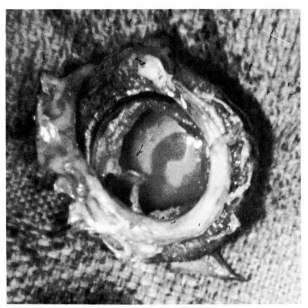

Fig. 19-12. Operative photograph of a Kay-Shiley disc prosthesis removed over 2 years after insertion because of recurrent emboli. Extensive thrombi, easily detached from the metallic surface of the prosthesis, are present. Development of these thrombi, intermittently dislodging into the circulation, is the principal reason for the development of cloth-covered prostheses.

matic fever have been described under Pathology in the preceding section, Mitral Stenosis. Several alterations in the normal mitral valve, either singly or in combination, may produce mitral insufficiency. These include fibrosis and retraction of the valve leaflets, extensive calcification limiting mobility of the valve leaflets, fibrosis and contraction of the chordae tendineae, rupture of the chordae tendineae, or dysfunction of the papillary muscles. Although seldom a primary cause, dilatation of the mitral annulus develops with mitral insufficiency and accordingly intensifies the insufficiency over a period of time as progressive dilatation of the annulus occurs. The reason that rheumatic endocarditis produces mitral stenosis in one patient and mitral insufficiency in another is unknown and may be fortuitous.

PATHOPHYSIOLOGY. The basic physiologic change is systolic elevation of left atrial pressure as blood regurgitates through the incompetent mitral valve during ventricular systole. The ventricular pressure spike is commonly to levels of 30 to 40 mm Hg, but levels as high as 80 to 90 mm Hg have been recorded. In diastole the left atrial pressure drops sharply to approach the left ventricular diastolic pressure, although a small gradient usually remains because of the large blood flow through the mitral valve during diastole. Mean left atrial pressure is usually 15 to 25 mm Hg. The mitral regurgitation produces enlargement of the left atrium, although for unknown reasons the degree of left atrial enlargement varies greatly among different patients and is not proportional to the degree of regurgitation. In some patients with significant regurgitation only slight left atrial enlargement is present, while in others giant left atria evolve, enlarging to contact the right chest wall. In contrast to mitral stenosis, pulmonary vascular changes appear rather late in the course of the disease, perhaps as a result of a large left atrium absorbing much of the kinetic energy of the regurgitating blood without sustained elevation of left atrial pressure. Fortunately, the dilated left ventricle with mitral insufficiency may function adequately for surprisingly long periods of time, maintaining the left ventricular diastolic pressure near the normal range of 8 to 12 mm Hg until eventually left ventricular failure appears.

As there is little stasis of blood in the left atrium, in contrast to mitral stenosis, left atrial thrombosis and arterial embolism are much less frequent in mitral insufficiency then in mitral stenosis.

CLINICAL MANIFESTATIONS. Symptoms. In some patients mild mitral insufficiency may be present without significant disability. This results from minimal rheumatic injury to the mitral leaflets, producing a systolic murmur but few other hemodynamic alterations. Such patients have an increased susceptibility to bacterial endocarditis, but in the absence of symptoms or cardiac enlargement additional therapy is not needed. With more significant mitral insufficiency, the most common symptoms are fatigue, dyspnea on exertion, and palpitation. Often these symptoms remain mild for long periods of time, despite impressive physical signs of mitral insufficiency and cardiac enlargement. Eventually left ventricular failure and increase in pulmonary vascular resistance both develop and intensify the cardiac disability. Respiratory symptoms then become prominent, with increasing dyspnea, cough, and paroxysmal nocturnal dyspnea, all of which are essentially similar to those occurring with mitral stenosis and are described in more detail in that section.

Physical Examination. The two characteristic features of mitral insufficiency are the apical systolic murmur and the increased force of the apical impulse. The systolic murmur is heard best at the apex, which is often displaced downward and to the left from enlargement of the left ventricle. It is well transmitted to the axilla. The quality is of a harsh, blowing type. With severe insufficiency, the murmur is pansystolic, appearing immediately after the first sound and continuing until the second sound. The intensity of the murmur does not correlate with the severity of the regurgitation, but the pansystolic characteristic does. Murmurs not extending completely through systole are seen with less serious degrees of regurgitation. The systolic murmur is a highly characteristic feature of mitral insufficiency and is absent only in most unusual circumstances. A diastolic murmur is usually present in addition, resulting from increased flow across the mitral valve as a result of blood regurgitated into the atrium during systole. The absence of an opening snap and the normal quality of the first heart sound both suggest that the diastolic murmur is due to increased flow of blood rather than anatomic mitral stenosis.

The apical impulse is typically forceful, prolonged, and diffuse, occupying an area 3 to 4 cm². The first heart sound is usually normal, although it has been reported as decreased or absent, usually from confusion with the early onset of the systolic murmur. Atrial fibrillation is frequent with chronic disease.

Laboratory Examinations. The chest roentgenogram will show enlargement of both the left ventricle and the left

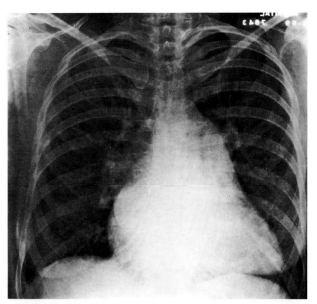

Fig. 19-13. Chest roentgenogram of a patient with mitral insufficiency. The distinctive features include an enlarged cardiac shadow with a prominent pulmonary artery. The shadow of the left atrium is visible in the right border of the cardiac shadow behind the shadow of the right atrium. The pulmonary vascular markings are prominent.

atrium (Fig. 19-13). As mentioned earlier, in some patients for unknown reasons a giant enlargement of the left atrium occurs, with an atrial chamber extending to the right chest wall and producing a grotesque deformity of the cardiac shadow. Calcification of the regurgitant valve is infrequent, although with combined lesions of stenosis and insufficiency, calcification is common. Visible changes in the pulmonary vasculature are often minimal except with advanced disease.

The electrocardiogram is unfortunately variable and may not contribute greatly to assessment of the severity of the disease. In about 50 percent of patients there is definite left ventricular hypertrophy. Significant insufficiency may be present, however, with a normal electrocardiogram, or in some patients a right axis may develop as a result of pulmonary vascular changes. Atrial fibrillation is frequent.

Mitral insufficiency is best quantified by cardiac catheterization with cineangiography. Only by injection of dye into the left ventricle, with evaluation of the degree of reflux into the atrium, can the degree of insufficiency be best estimated. This is far superior to complex studies with indicator dilution dye curves. The left atrial pressure tracing with mitral insufficiency is greatly altered, usually with a prominent V wave developing from regurgitation of blood during systole. During diastole the left atrial pressure decreases sharply to approach left ventricular diastolic pressure, but usually some gradient remains throughout diastole because of increased flow of blood across the mitral valve.

Diagnosis. The diagnosis of mitral insufficiency can be made with reasonable certainty from the characteristic

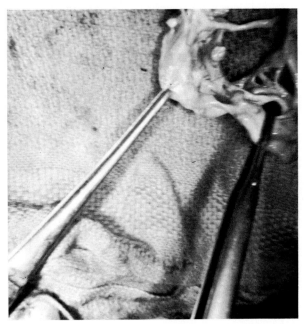

Fig. 19-14. Operative photograph of mitral valve showing rupture of a major chordae, creating severe mitral insufficiency. In some such patients, plication of the mitral leaflet will obviate mitral replacement.

systolic murmur radiating to the axilla in association with evidence of left ventricular hypertrophy obtained by palpation, the chest roentgenogram, or the electrocardiogram. The degree of severity of the insufficiency is best quantitated with cineangiography. When multivalvular disease is present, cardiac catheterization and angiography are needed to delineate the relative severity of the different valvular lesions.

TREATMENT. Indications for Operation. An acceptable operation for mitral insufficiency was not routinely available until the pioneering work of Starr and Edwards first developed a mitral valve prosthesis in 1961. With the mitral prostheses available between 1961 and 1966, the 5-year survival was only about 50 percent. Great improvements have been made in the prostheses, principally the concept of covering most of the valve surface with cloth. This cloth becomes covered with a translucent layer of compacted fibrin less than 1 mm thick that is very (though not totally) resistant to thromboembolism. Because of the limitations of the prosthesis, operation is recommended only for progressive disability resistant to customary medical therapy.

Medical therapy includes appropriate use of digitalis, diuretics, and restriction of sodium intake in the presence of heart failure. Arrhythmias, usually atrial fibrillation, require frequent therapy, both to control tachycardia and to attempt conversion of the arrhythmia to a sinus mechanism.

Technique of Operation. The technique for mitral valve replacement was described under Mitral Stenosis and will not be repeated in detail here. In general, operation is performed through a median sternotomy, occasionally a

right thoracotomy. The main precautions during mitral replacement are to anchor the prosthetic valve adequately in position to prevent subsequent partial dislodgment with recurrent mitral insufficiency and to avoid air embolism. Until recent years the prevalence of the two complications cited resulted in an operative mortality of 15 to 20 percent. Following operation anticoagulant therapy is begun on the fifth or sixth postoperative day and continued indefinitely.

In 10 to 15 percent of patients a mitral annuloplasty may be employed, rather than prosthetic replacement of the valve. Such patients are usually younger, with a dilated mitral annulus and mobile valve leaflets with little or no calcification. Several techniques of annuloplasty have been described, with the objective of producing a small, competent mitral orifice. In general, heavy sutures are used, often including more of the annulus of the mural leaflet rather than the aortic leaflet, because the aortic leaflet often has more mobility than the smaller mural leaflet. When annuloplasty can be satisfactorily performed, excellent long-term results may be obtained. Unfortunately, in many patients the insufficiency cannot be completely corrected at the first operation; also, it may recur at a later date.

Ruptured chordae tendineae causing mitral insufficiency create a special surgical problem, varying with the number and location of the chordae ruptured (Fig. 19-14). McGoon has described a technique of plication of the flail mitral leaflet which is applicable in some patients. Kay and Egerton have described other methods of repair, including suture of the flail leaflet directly to the underlying papillary muscle. In some patients excision of the valve with prosthetic replacement is necessary.

PROGNOSIS. Recovery from operation is usually followed by excellent rehabilitation. There is subsidence of pulmonary vascular changes and of signs of cardiac failure. For unknown reasons, however, cardiac function does not return to completely normal values, perhaps because of the rigid ring of the prosthesis in the mitral annulus or because of irreversible myocardial injury from long-standing mitral insufficiency. Most patients have few, if any, restrictions on physical activity. (For specific data following prosthetic valve replacement, see Prognosis, under Mitral Stenosis.)

Careful long-term management is required to supervise anticoagulant therapy, to detect any signs of malfunction of the prosthesis, and to protect from endocarditis during episodes of transient bacteremia by using prophylactic antibiotics.

AORTIC STENOSIS

HISTORICAL DATA. Effective treatment of aortic valve disease first became acceptable in 1961 with the development of satisfactory prosthetic valves by Starr and Edwards and by Harken and associates. Earlier attempts to correct aortic valvular disease by cusp replacement with prosthetic cusps of Teflon cloth or by extensive debridement of calcific material from calcified valve cusps initially gave satisfactory results in many patients, but a high failure rate within 1 to 2 years following operation led to abandonment of these techniques as soon as a satisfactory prosthetic valve became available.

As with all prosthetic valves, the major limitation is thromboembolism. With the improvements in prosthetic valves in the past few years, especially with the use of cloth covering, thromboembolism has decreased to a range of 1 to 3 percent. Endocarditis following transient bacteremia remains a small but definite risk.

Tissue valves are virtually free of thromboembolism but in many patients gradually fibrose over a period of years to produce progressive aortic insufficiency. The best results are with homograft valves, tried and discarded by many but used preferentially by several experienced groups—those of Kirklin, Shumway, Barratt-Boyes, and Ross. Heterografts have a much higher failure rate but are still under evaluation by some groups. Fascia lata valves gave excellent initial results and have been studied for several years by Senning. Again, however, late fibrosis and contraction in a variable number of patients have been disappointing.

ETIOLOGY. A definite history of rheumatic fever can be obtained in 30 to 50 percent of patients, and undiagnosed rheumatic fever is probably a frequent cause in the remainder. The presence of mitral valve disease in 30 to 50 percent of patients with aortic stenosis indicates the frequency of previous rheumatic fever. In a significant percentage of patients, calcification superimposed upon a mild congenital aortic stenosis is probably the causative mechanism, for in almost all untreated patients with congenital aortic stenosis calcification in the aortic leaflets develops after thirty years of age. The development of calcification adds the element of rigidity of the valve cusps to the obstruction already present from the congenital fusion. It is likely that calcification progressively increases over long periods of time, gradually producing a more severe obstruction. Hence, a calcified bicuspid valve is a not uncommon operative finding in a sixty-year-old patient with a history of a heart murmur since childhood but no symptoms until 2 or 3 years before operation.

In patients in the seventh and eighth decades, an aortic systolic murmur is extremly common, resulting from mild fibrosis and minimal calcification of the valve leaflets. Usually, however, this form of atherosclerosis in the elderly does not produce significant physiologic obstruction.

PATHOLOGY. The basic pathology of rheumatic fever has been detailed under Mitral Stenosis. The pathologic process with aortic valvulitis is similar, with ulceration of the endocardium developing over the valve leaflets where the margins normally appose in diastole. Tiny, beadlike vegetations form and produce fusion of the commissures as healing takes place. Fibrosis and stiffening of the leaflets may develop as well as fusion of the commissures, both features producing obstruction to the flow of blood. In subsequent years superimposed calcification of the diseased leaflets, probably from turbulent flow of blood, regularly occurs and creates further rigidity of the valve cusps.

Mitral valve disease, either stenosis or insufficiency, is found in a high percentage of patients with aortic disease, indicating the underlying rheumatic cause. In older pa-

tients coronary atherosclerosis may be present, although the incidence is no greater than that in the normal population. When extensive coronary atherosclerosis is present in association with aortic stenosis of only moderate severity, it may be difficult to determine which of the two lesions is responsible for the symptoms.

PATHOPHYSIOLOGY. The normal aortic valve has a cross-sectional area of 2.5 to 3.5 cm^2. Moderately severe aortic stenosis is present when the valve orifice has been narrowed to a cross-sectional area of 0.8 to 1 cm^2, which is associated with a systolic gradient of about 50 mm Hg at a moderate cardiac output. Severe aortic stenosis exists if the cross-sectional area has been reduced to 0.5 to 0.7 cm^2, which requires a systolic pressure gradient near 150 mm Hg to produce a moderate cardiac output. When stenosis of such severity is present, increases in ventricular systolic pressure are very ineffective in producing further increases in cardiac output. A left ventricular systolic pressure of 250 mm Hg is near the maximum that a left ventricle can sustain for any period of time.

With the increased cardiac work imposed by the stenosis, there is progressive concentric ventricular hypertrophy but little cardiac dilatation, as a result of which the heart size may be near normal on the conventional chest roentgenogram. The cardiac output is often normal, though the left ventricular diastolic pressure is frequently elevated above the normal of 10 mm Hg, especially during exercise, because of the extensive muscular hypertrophy. Left atrial pressure may be temporarily elevated, but sustained elevation of left atrial pressure with production of pulmonary edema is a late and often a preterminal manifestation. Similarly, pulmonary vascular disease is infrequent. In contrast to mitral stenosis, a patient with aortic stenosis may have relatively few symptoms for a long period of time, but when cardiac decompensation with pulmonary congestion appears, a fatal outcome often ensues within a few months.

The quality of the pulse is frequently altered with aortic stenosis because of the restriction to ventricular ejection. The typical changes include a pulse wave of low amplitude, a slow rate of rise, and a rounded peak.

Myocardial ischemia, manifested as angina pectoris, is frequent in aortic stenosis from a combination of factors. These include increase in left ventricular work, myocardial hypertrophy with resulting fewer capillaries per gram of myocardium, decreased aortic pressure in diastole, during which the majority of coronary blood flow usually occurs, and in some patients superimposed atherosclerosis. Because of the myocardial ischemia, aortic stenosis is a most treacherous lesion, for sudden death is *always* a possibility. The risk varies with the severity of the disease but is always present, even with mild aortic stenosis. It is much more frequent with aortic stenosis than with any other form of acquired valvular heart disease.

CLINICAL MANIFESTATIONS. Symptoms. Characteristically there is a prolonged latent period in the development of aortic stenosis. For perhaps 10 to 20 years classic physical findings may be present with slight dyspnea on exertion as the only symptom. The turning point in the illness is heralded by the appearance of one or more of three symptoms: angina pectoris, syncope, or left ventricular failure. Sudden death, which accounts for about 20 percent of fatalities from aortic stenosis, becomes much more of a threat once these symptoms are present, although sudden death is an ever-present hazard in any patient with aortic stenosis. Once angina or syncope appears, the average life expectancy for the untreated patient is 3 to 4 years. Left ventricular failure is an even more serious symptom, death usually occurring within 1 to 2 years, although great variations are seen among different patients, ranging from periods as short as 1 week to as long as 10 years.

Syncope develops in about one-third of the patients. In a minority of patients syncope may result from a conduction abnormality, arising from involvement of the atrioventricular node by calcium spicules deposited on the stenotic valve. Usually syncope develops with effort, and it is commonly associated with angina pectoris. Once left ventricular failure has developed, syncopal attacks may be precipitated by very little effort and are of the gravest significance.

Angina pectoris develops in about two-thirds of the patients, representing myocardial ischemia from an inadequate cardiac output. With protracted angina, small areas of muscle necrosis may evolve, ultimately represented as myocardial fibrosis; infrequently large areas of silent infarction occur.

Left ventricular failure is a grave development and demands immediate therapy. Many patients do not survive long enough to develop associated right ventricular failure. Atrial fibrillation, developing as a consequence of prolonged elevation of left atrial pressure, is similarly a grave event, as it indicates an advanced stage of left ventricular failure.

Physical Examination. The classic physical finding with aortic stenosis is the systolic diamond-shaped ejection murmur produced by blood forced through the stenotic orifice. The murmur is usually heard best in the aortic area to the right of the sternum but in some patients is loudest at the cardiac apex. The intensity of the murmur varies from grade II to grade IV but has no correlation with the severity of the stenosis. Loud murmurs are associated with a palpable thrill and are readily transmitted to the carotid arteries. The aortic second sound is soft but can be detected in 70 to 80 percent of patients. A grade I to II diastolic murmur of aortic insufficiency can often be heard along the left sternal border.

The apical impulse has distinctive features. It is usually in a normal position, for cardiac size is not increased. Palpation of the apical contraction detects a prolonged heave but not a forceful thrust such as is found with ventricular dilatation from aortic or mitral insufficiency. In many patients the blood pressure is normal. Only with advanced stenosis is the pulse pressure significantly lowered to less than 30 mm Hg.

Laboratory Studies. The chest roentgenogram often demonstrates a heart of normal size. Gross cardiac enlargement, resulting from ventricular dilatation and failure, is associated with an ominous prognosis. Mild degrees of left atrial enlargement are often found. Calcification of the

aortic valve should be almost routinely visible in patients over thirty-five years of age. If calcification is not found, the validity of the diagnosis should be seriously questioned.

With advanced disease the electrocardiogram will show signs of left ventricular hypertrophy, including increased voltage of the QRS complex, in association with ST-segment and T-wave abnormalities. With less advanced stenosis, however, the changes may be much less specific, and in some dangerously ill patients the electrocardiogram is virtually normal. In older patients the prevalence of ST-segment and T-wave abnormalities from coronary artery disease makes correlation of the electrocardiogram with the severity of the aortic stenosis difficult. A left bundle branch block is occasionally seen in some patients with advanced stenosis.

Cardiac catheterization to determine the pressure gradient between the left ventricle and the aorta is required to estimate the severity of the stenosis. With mild aortic stenosis, a systolic pressure gradient of only 30 to 40 mm Hg is found, while severe stenosis may have a pressure gradient exceeding 100 mm Hg. Actually, the severity is best correlated with the cross-sectional area of the valve, calculated from simultaneous measurement of pressure gradient and cardiac output. In most patients simple determination of the gradient is sufficient if the patient is in a resting, basal state. At the time of catheterization the presence of mitral disease can also be determined, as well as associated aortic insufficiency. When feasible, coronary arteriography should be done in association with aortography to detect associated coronary vascular disease.

Diagnosis. A diagnosis of aortic stenosis can usually be made with certainty from detection of the characteristic ejection-type systolic murmur in the aortic area, associated with findings of left ventricular hypertrophy. Supportive evidence can be obtained from the chest roentgenogram, demonstrating calcification of the aortic valve and often a heart of normal size. The electrocardiogram will usually show variable degrees of left ventricular hypertrophy.

The diagnosis can be confirmed by cardiac catheterization, which also provides the only precise method of measuring the severity of the stenosis. In some patients with aortic systolic murmurs, especially those in the seventh and eighth decades, catheterization will demonstrate that significant obstruction is not present.

TREATMENT. Indications for Operation. Once a clinical diagnosis of aortic stenosis has been made, usually cardiac catheterization should be performed to measure the severity of the obstruction. Subsequent management of the patient depends upon the symptoms, the severity of the obstruction, and the degree of cardiac hypertrophy. Operation is usually recommended with a gradient exceeding 50 mm Hg, though some such patients are virtually asymptomatic.

Once syncope, angina, or congestive heart failure has appeared, operation should be performed promptly because of the high incidence of sudden death.

Technique of Operation. Detailed preoperative care is not often necessary. If diuretic therapy has been employed, supplemental potassium is usually given before operation to avoid postoperative hypokalemia and arrhythmias. Patients are usually hospitalized 2 to 3 days in advance of the scheduled operation.

A median sternotomy incision is usually employed, with cannulation of the venae cavae for withdrawal of venous blood from the patient to the pump-oxygenator and cannulation of the ascending aorta for return of arterial blood from the pump-oxygenator to the patient (Fig. 19-15). Before bypass is instituted, left atrial pressure is measured to indicate the degree of left ventricular failure. The preoperative left atrial pressure is a convenient guide to postoperative infusion of fluids, because left atrial pressure reflects the diastolic filling pressure of the left ventricle. With severe cardiac failure a mean left atrial pressure of 20 to 30 mm Hg may be present, and following operation elevation of left atrial pressure to similar levels by infusion of fluids may be required for a short time to maintain an adequate cardiac output.

Once cardiopulmonary bypass has been instituted, a vent is placed in the apex of the left ventricle to aspirate blood. The ascending aorta is then occluded distad and incised with an oblique incision which extends proximally into the noncoronary sinus. Perfusion of the left and right coronary arteries is then instituted following cannulation with Silastic coronary cannulae of appropriate size. Perfusions at 100 to 150 ml/minute are used in each artery, depending upon the size of the left ventricle (Fig. 19-16).

The stenotic aortic valve is then completely removed (Fig. 19-17). Only in a small percentage of cases is simple fusion of the valve commissures found which can be treated by commissurotomy. In most patients there is extensive destruction of the valve cusps with superimposed calcification; complete removal has been found the only satisfactory therapy (Fig. 19-18). Removal of the calcified valve requires great care to avoid losing fragments of calcium into the left ventricle which could subsequently be embolized into the peripheral circulation. A gauze pack is routinely placed in the ventricle before removal of the valve is begun. Subsequent removal of the pack often reveals several fragments of calcium which have been dislodged during removal of the valve and would otherwise have been lost in the left ventricle.

Following removal of the diseased valve, a prosthetic ball valve (Starr-Edwards type) of appropriate size is selected (Fig. 19-19). It is important that the valve fit easily into the aortic lumen, choosing one that is neither too large nor too small. Once the appropriate valve has been chosen, 12 to 15 mattress sutures of 2-0 Dacron are placed in the valve annulus and inserted into the prosthetic valve. Each mattress suture is buttressed with a small pledget of Dacron cloth to avoid tearing of the sutures through the annulus (Fig. 19-20). During seating of the valve, care is taken to seat the valve well below the coronary ostia and to avoid any tilting of the valve in its final position. Following closure of the aortotomy, air is displaced from the left ventricle, the coronary cannulae are removed, effective cardiac contraction is restored, and bypass gradually is slowed and stopped (Fig. 19-21).

Coronary perfusion is maintained throughout operation at a flow rate of 250 to 300 ml/minute and a temperature of 30 to 32°C, interrupting perfusion for 5 to 10 minutes when necessary for adequate exposure. Cardiac contractions may continue throughout the procedure, or ventricular fibrillation may develop. There is some evidence that subendocardial perfusion is inadequate in hypertrophied hearts during ventricular fibrillation. Therefore, some groups attempt to keep the ventricle contracting throughout operation by electrically defibrillating the heart if fibrillation occurs.

Following bypass, blood is transfused to elevate left atrial pressure to a level adequate to maintain a satisfactory cardiac output. The actual mean left atrial pressure required varies with that existing before bypass but is usually between 10 and 20 mm Hg. The left atrial pressure has been found a more valuable guide for postoperative fluid infusion than measurement of blood volume or blood loss.

Postoperative Care. After initial adjustment of blood volume following operation, convalescence may be uneventful. Arrhythmias are among the more frequent complications. Because they are serious and even fatal, early detection by 24-hour monitoring of the cardiac rhythm with an oscilloscope in a cardiac intensive care unit is necessary. Arrhythmias are often related to changes in electrolyte concentration, such as decreased potassium concentration and varying sensitivities to digitalis. The most frequently employed therapeutic measures include supplemental potassium, intravenously administered lidocaine for short-term therapy, procainamide, or propranolol.

Anticoagulant therapy is begun with sodium warfarin 4 days after operation, keeping the prothrombin time in the conservative range of 20 to 25 seconds. Elevation of the prothrombin time to 25 to 30 seconds has resulted in serious hemorrhage in a few patients, especially in the early postoperative course. With cloth-covered prostheses, warfarin is given only for about 1 month after operation, as the greatest risk of thromboembolism is during this period of time. It is stopped thereafter, and acetylsalicylic acid, 0.6 Gm twice a day, is given for 1 to 2 years to inhibit platelet aggregation, for such aggregates rather than fibrin appear to be the most frequent cause of thromboembolism with cloth-covered prostheses. Some groups do not employ any anticoagulants whatever following operation.

Within 3 to 4 months after operation the majority of patients are asymptomatic, with a normal range of physical activities. Careful long-term medical supervision is essential, however, especially in patients with marked cardiac hypertrophy. Actually there is a greater risk of death during the first year after leaving the hospital than from the operation itself. With severely hypertrophied hearts, arrhythmias remain a constant problem for months or longer and may be fatal if not treated. A mild degree of salt restriction and diuretic therapy may also be required if cardiac enlargement was severe beforehand. The rate of increase of physical activity should be determined from the patient's symptoms, heart size, and signs of left ventricular hypertrophy on the electrocardiogram.

PROGNOSIS. The average operative morality for aortic valve replacement is in the range of 5 to 8 percent. It may

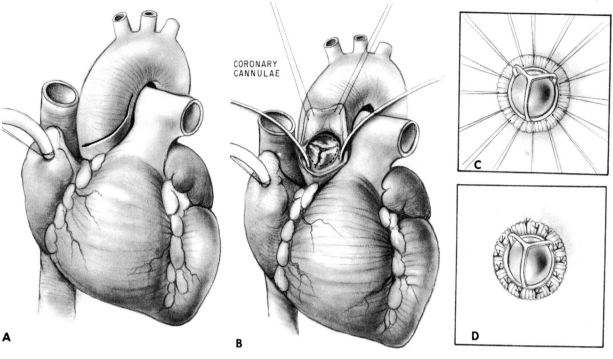

CORONARY
CANNULAE

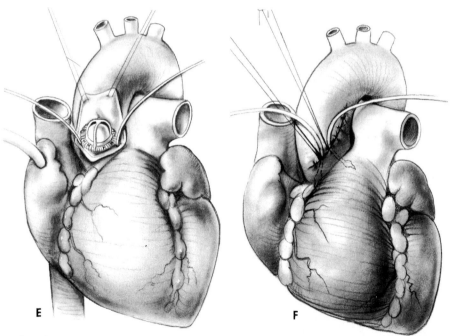

Fig. 19-15. Insertion of aortic valve prosthesis. A. Cardiopulmonary bypass is instituted following cannulation of the right atrium with a single large cannula. Usually the ascending aorta is cannulated for arterial return (not shown). The aorta is opened with an oblique incision, initially begun about a centimeter above the right coronary artery. B. The right and left coronary arteries are cannulated with Silastic coronary cannulae, held in position with purse-string sutures about the coronary ostia. Coronary perfusion is then begun at a rate of 200 to 250 ml/minute in each coronary artery. The aortic valve is then excised, with care to avoid the loss of any calcific fragments into the ventricle which might subsequently embolize. C. The Starr-Edwards ball valve which is normally used. D. Valve sutured in position. E. Final position of the valve. Care is taken, as the valve is tied in position, to seat the valve well below the coronary ostia, actually farther below than is shown here. F. The aortotomy is closed around the coronary cannulae, encircling each one with a mattress suture. Subsequently the contracting heart is allowed to fill with blood and expel air from the heart before the cannulae are removed.

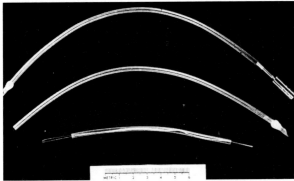

Fig. 19-16. Silastic coronary cannulae used to cannulate the coronary arteries at operation for coronary perfusion. Once the cannulae are inserted, slight tension is applied through the snare shown here to a purse-string suture of 4-0 silk which has been sutured about the coronary ostium. If a short left coronary artery is present, the tip of the cannula is amputated back to the ball to avoid inadvertent perfusion of only one tributary of the left coronary artery.

be much higher in patients with far advanced disease from cardiac failure or less than 5 percent in good-risk patients. Probably the major factor influencing operative mortality is the ability to perfuse the coronary arteries effectively during operation, though some groups report good results with aortic replacement performed without coronary perfusion as long as myocardial ischemia lasts less than 45 to 50 minutes. In 1965 McGoon et al. reported an impressive series of 100 consecutive aortic replacements without *any* operative mortality.

Most patients show a surprising degree of recovery following operation, and many subsequently have virtually

Fig. 19-17. A. Stenotic aortic valve exposed during cardiopulmonary bypass through a transverse aortotomy. The valve orifice has been almost obliterated by calcification and apposition of the cusps. B. Calcified aortic valve in another patient exposed through a transverse aortotomy. Fusion has produced a small eccentric rigid ostium which is both stenotic and insufficient.

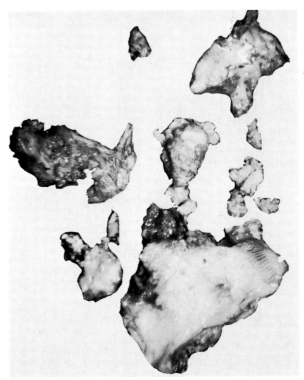

Fig. 19-18. Calcified fragments removed with rongeurs from a patient with severe aortic stenosis. The multiplicity of such fragments emphasizes the grave risk of embolization of calcified material during aortic valve replacement with reduction of severe or fatal neurologic injury. Careful packing of the ventricle with gauze before removal of the calcified valve is essential.

no limitation of physical activity. With severe cardiac enlargement, however, there remains a risk of sudden death, even beyond 1 year after operation. This is probably due to arrhythmias, for the cause is often not found at postmortem examination.

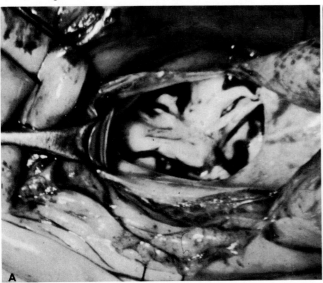

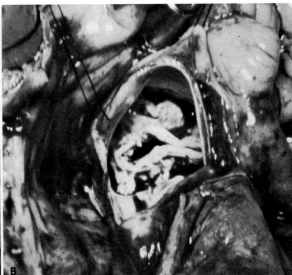

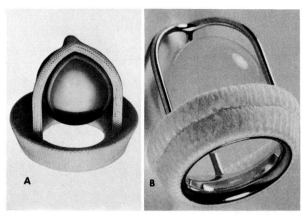

Fig. 19-19. *A.* The Starr-Edwards aortic ball-valve prosthesis developed in the latter part of 1967. The prosthesis is completely covered with Teflon cloth. A metal ball is used. *B.* The Starr-Edwards ball valve prosthesis used prior to 1967. The ball is composed of Silastic. The Teflon cloth, in contrast to the valve shown in *A*, only partially covers the metal surfaces of the prosthesis.

AORTIC INSUFFICIENCY

ETIOLOGY. The most common cause of aortic insufficiency is rheumatic fever. A definite history of this illness can be obtained from 60 to 70 percent of patients. In the past, syphilis was a frequent cause, but it is now rare. Bacterial endocarditis produces insufficiency from destruc-

tion and perforation of valve cusps. Though formerly operation was strenuously avoided until the bacterial infection had been controlled, operation is now being performed much earlier, at times within the first 7 to 14 days of the illness in patients with life-threatening insufficiency. This is only possible, of course, if effective antibiotic therapy is used.

A dissecting aneurysm produces insufficiency by dissection of the aortic wall with detachment and prolapse of the valve cusps. Usually the noncoronary cusp is involved most. Diseases producing dilatation of the aortic annulus create insufficiency by preventing effective coaptation of the valve cusps in diastole. This is typically seen in the Marfan syndrome and also in less well defined diseases in which there is an isolated unexplained dilatation of the aortic annulus and ascending aorta. A similar pathologic process develops in a small percentage of patients with rheumatoid arthritis. Not infrequently a patient is seen with a "floppy valve," a connective tissue degeneration of the valve cusps resulting in elongation and prolapse without any signs of infection or fibrosis. Congenital aortic insufficiency is fairly rare and is seen almost only in young children.

PATHOLOGY. Normal function of the aortic valve depends upon sufficient mobility and length of the cusps so that the centers of the three cusps appose in diastole. With fibrosis and retraction of the cusps, varying degrees of distortion produce an incompetent valve (Fig. 19-22). It is probable that the turbulent blood flow produced by the

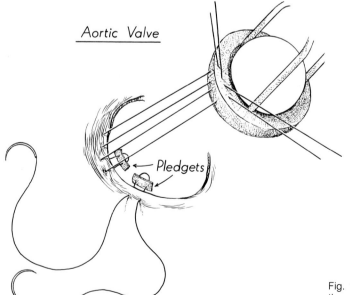

Fig. 19-20. Schematic representation of technique for suturing the aortic valve with Dacron pledgets seated below the aortic annulus.

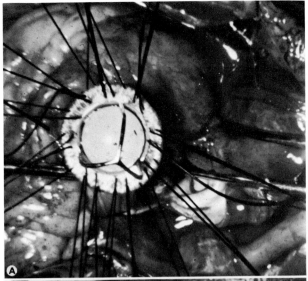

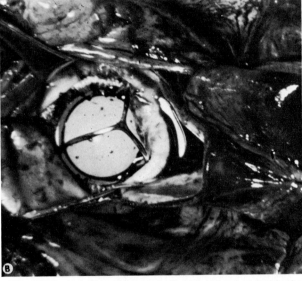

Fig. 19-21. *A.* A Starr-Edwards ball valve being inserted in the operation shown in Fig. 18-15*B* following excision of the calcified valve. The operation was performed in 1963. The patient has done well since that time. *B.* The aortic ball valve in position.

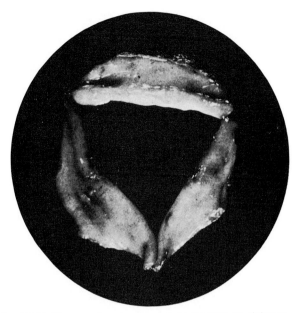

Fig. 19-22. Three aortic valve cusps removed from an eighteen-year-old boy with rheumatic aortic insufficiency. The contracted free margins of each cusp are clearly shown, illustrating the mechanism of production of aortic insufficiency from contracture and retraction of the free margins of the aortic valve cusps.

initial distortion of the cusps results in progressive fibrosis, stiffening, and eventual calcification, all of which result in a gradual increase in the degree of insufficiency. In the Marfan syndrome and other diseases associated with dilatation of the aortic annulus, the basic disturbance is stretching of the aortic valve ring, as a result of which the valve cusps, histologically normal, can no longer meet centrally (Fig. 19-23).

The cardiac response to blood regurgitating into the left ventricle in diastole is an increase in left ventricular stroke volume, accomplished by dilatation of the heart. Progressive dilatation of the left ventricle gradually evolves. This response is quite different from that occurring with aortic stenosis, where there is concentric muscular hypertrophy but little increase in ventricular diastolic volume.

PATHOPHYSIOLOGY. Surprisingly large volumes of blood can regurgitate through an incompetent orifice of less than 1 cm^2 because of the large differential in diastolic pressure between the aorta and the left ventricle. The actual amount of blood regurgitating with each cardiac cycle can be only approximated by existing techniques, such as dye-dilution measurements. The initial adjustment of the heart is an increase in diastolic fiber length and a corresponding increase in stroke volume. There is no elevation in left ventricular diastolic pressure until cardiac failure appears near the end of the course of the disease. In the absence of elevation of left ventricular diastolic pressure, there is accordingly no increase in left atrial pressure or pulmonary congestion. Hence, in contrast to patients with mitral disease, symptoms of pulmonary congestion appear only in the terminal stages once left ventricular failure has occurred.

The amount of blood regurgitating during diastole varies not only with the size of the incompetent orifice but also with the degree of peripheral vasodilatation and the heart rate. Tachycardia has a somewhat beneficial effect, for diastole is shortened and less time is available for blood to regurgitate into the ventricle. Peripheral vasodilation apparently is a compensatory mechanism by which peripheral resistance and the amount of blood regurgitating into the ventricle are decreased. It is often a prominent clinical finding.

With advanced aortic insufficiency and marked dilatation of the left ventricle, some mitral insufficiency may develop from dilation of the annulus of the mitral valve.

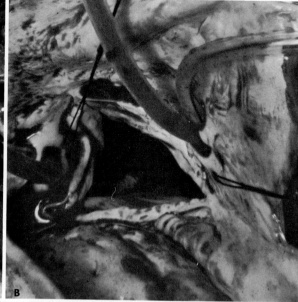

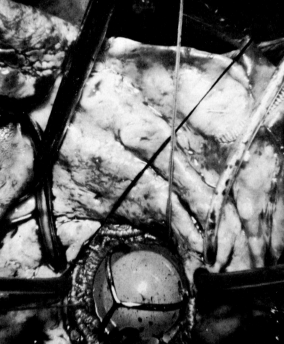

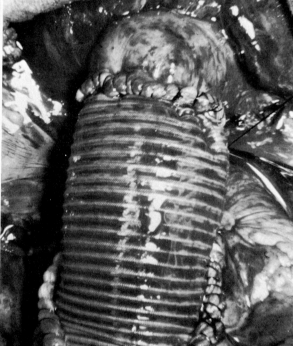

Fig. 19-23. *A.* Aneurysm in the ascending aorta in a patient with the Marfan syndrome. Marked dilatation of the proximal ascending aorta has developed, stretching the aortic annulus and producing aortic insufficiency. The distal ascending aorta, proximal to the innominate artery, is nearly normal in diameter and has been encircled with an umbilical tape. The left innominate vein is retracted at the top of the field. *B.* With the patient on cardiopulmonary bypass, the aorta has been clamped and the aneurysm opened. The aortic annulus is shown with the stretched leaflets producing total insufficiency. Silastic coronary cannulae have been inserted into each coronary ostium for coronary perfusion while reconstruction is performed. *C.* A Starr-Edwards ball valve in position which has been inserted following excision of the insufficient valve leaflets. The coronary perfusion cannulae are still in position. *D.* Following insertion of the aortic valve, the ascending aorta was reconstructed with a short prosthesis of Dacron cloth. The distal suture line is just proximal to the origin of the innominate artery.

When severe cardiac failure is present, with elevation of left ventricular end-diastolic pressure above 20 mm Hg, clinical findings of aortic insufficiency may actually decrease, for the total volume of blood regurgitating during diastole decreases as the left ventricular diastolic pressure rises.

CLINICAL MANIFESTATIONS. Symptoms. Although there is considerable variability among different patients, in general the symptom-free period after the appearance of aortic insufficiency averages about 10 years. With the onset of symptoms, death occurs in about 5 years, but the variability is great. Although in a large group, about 40 percent of patients will be dead within 10 years and over 50 percent within 20 years, another 25 percent may live for 20 years with very few symptoms. The terminal illness is usually a progressive downhill course from increasing cardiac failure, but sudden death occurs in about 5 percent.

The earliest symptom is palpitations because of the forceful contractions of the dilated left ventricle. Dyspnea on exertion is another early symptom, gradually increasing as the disease progresses. Angina pectoris is common in the later stages from myocardial ischemia, developing from the decreased coronary blood flow during diastole as well as the large size of the left ventricle. Peripheral vasomotor phenomena, including episodes of severe sweating and intolerance to heat, are common.

Physical Examination. The cardiac rhythm is usually normal. With significant aortic insufficiency palpation readily discloses a prominent cardiac impulse, located downward and to the left of the normal location because of dilatation of the left ventricle. The hallmark of aortic insufficiency is the high-pitched, decrescendo diastolic murmur along the left sternal border. The murmur starts immediately after the second sound and may be confused with it. The length of the murmur correlates approximately with the severity of the insufficiency; those lasting only through early diastole represent less severe degrees of regurgitation. Having the patient lean forward while listening along the left sternal border makes the murmur more audible. With faint high-pitched murmurs, having the patient stop breathing momentarily is helpful. If the murmur is loudest to the right of the sternum, dilatation of the aortic ring, as in the Marfan syndrome, is likely. As mentioned earlier, with advanced cardiac failure and increase in the left ventricular diastolic pressure, the intensity of the diastolic murmur may decrease to actually become inaudible in terminal stages. A systolic murmur of the ejection type, moderate in intensity, is frequently heard, arising from increased volume of blood expelled from the left ventricle, not from anatomic aortic stenosis.

Examination of the peripheral arterial circulation reveals many positive findings. The pulse pressure is increased, partly from an increase in systolic pressure, but principally from a decrease in diastolic pressure from the normal range near 80 mm Hg. The diastolic pressure may be as low as 40 mm Hg, but true diastolic pressure is never less than 30 to 35 mm Hg, as measured by direct arterial puncture. Auscultatory findings of a diastolic pressure of zero results from dilatation of peripheral arteries. The

exact level of diastolic pressure does not correlate closely with the severity of the aortic insufficiency. For example, a blood pressure of 130/65 mm Hg may be present with either moderate or severe insufficiency. This lack of correlation is due to the influence of peripheral resistance. With vasodilatation, diastolic pressure may be low without marked regurgitation, while with severe vasoconstriction diastolic pressure may be higher but with severe regurgitation.

With significant insufficiency, peripheral pulses are easily visible, forceful, and bounding. "Pistol shot" sounds are readily heard with the bell of the stethoscope over peripheral arteries. A wide variety of other auscultatory phenomena have been described, all of which indicate vasodilatation and a hyperactive peripheral circulation.

Laboratory Studies. The chest roentgenogram usually shows enlargement of the left ventricle, with the apex displaced downward and to the left. Serial chest roentgenograms over months or years is the best method for evaluating progression of the disease. Lateral views are required to appreciate fully the degree of enlargement of the left ventricle because of its posterior location. The electrocardiogram may be normal with early aortic insufficiency, but with more advanced disease and the appearance of symptoms there are signs of left ventricular hypertrophy with abnormalities in the ST-T segments. The cardiac rhythm is usually sinus. Atrial fibrillation is rare. Its presence suggests either terminal aortic insufficiency or concomitant mitral valve disease.

Cardiac catheterization may show no abnormalities in the early stages of the disease when left ventricular diastolic pressure is normal. With cardiac failure and elevation of the left ventricular diastolic pressure to 15 to 20 mm Hg, there is corresponding elevation of left atrial pressure. The best method for quantitating the degree of insufficiency is aortography, injecting dye into the ascending aorta and visually estimating the degree of reflux into the ventricle. Though subjective, this method is quite satisfactory for most clinical decisions.

DIAGNOSIS. A diagnosis can be readily made when the characteristic diastolic murmur is heard along the left sternal border. Quantitation of the degree of insufficiency, however, is more difficult. Mild insufficiency exists when only a murmur is audible without any changes in pulse pressure. Such patients may be treated optimistically, as their only serious risk is that of developing bacterial endocarditis. With more significant insufficiency, a diastolic murmur extending throughout diastole is audible in association with a decrease in diastolic blood pressure and prominent peripheral pulses. Cardiac enlargement as well as changes in the electrocardiogram of left ventricular hypertrophy are usually present.

A significant surgical problem exists regarding the degree of aortic insufficiency when concomitant mitral valve disease requires operation. In such patients a decision needs to be made whether or not to replace the diseased aortic valve as well as the diseased mitral valve. Aortography is the best method for estimating the degree of insufficiency but is not totally accurate. A final decision must be made at operation, approaching the heart through a median sternotomy incision and noting the amount of blood regurgitating through the aortic valve after the mitral valve has been removed.

TREATMENT. Surgical treatment is recommended ordinarily only when symptoms become significant. In some patients progressive enlargement of the left ventricle develops with surprisingly few symptoms, and probably these patients should be operated upon to avoid extreme degrees of left ventricular hypertrophy, with heart weights approaching 900 to 1,000 Gm. Once symptoms become significant, surgical therapy should be prompt because of the rapid downhill course of the disease in most symptomatic patients.

When operation is performed, we prefer prosthetic replacement with a cloth-covered ball valve of the Starr-Edwards variety (Fig. 19-24). With small aortic roots, the disc valve of the Bjork-Shiley type is useful. Tissue prostheses, such as homografts, are described in the preceding section, Aortic Stenosis. They have been widely and effectively used by several groups.

TRICUSPID STENOSIS AND INSUFFICIENCY

ETIOLOGY. Organic disease of the tricuspid valve is almost always due to rheumatic fever. It virtually never occurs as an isolated lesion, but only in association with extensive disease of the mitral valve. With mitral disease the frequency of associated tricuspid disease is near 10 to 15 percent, although an incidence as high as 30 percent has been reported.

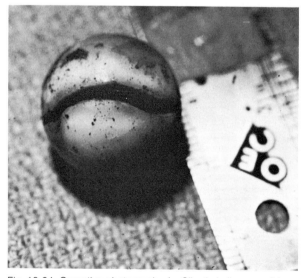

Fig. 19-24. Operative photograph of a Silastic ball removed from an aortic valve prosthesis, inserted before 1966. Development of a diastolic murmur fortunately led to reoperation before fatal embolization of the fragmented silastic ball occurred. With improvement in Silastic ball prostheses this complication has been virtually unknown since 1966.

Tricuspid insufficiency is the more common lesion encountered, while pure stenosis is infrequent. Often both stenosis and insufficiency are present.

Functional tricuspid insufficiency is actually more common than insufficiency from organic disease. It develops from dilatation of the tricuspid annulus and right ventricle as a result of pulmonary hypertension and right ventricular failure. The hypertension is usually a consequence of mitral valve disease with elevated left atrial pressure.

A more recent etiologic factor in isolated tricuspid disease is bacterial endocarditis among heroin addicts. This presents many very special problems because of the repeated infections which such patients tend to sustain.

PATHOLOGY. With tricuspid stenosis the pathologic changes are similar to those found with the more familiar mitral stenosis. There is fusion of the commissures to form a small central opening 1 to 1.5 cm in diameter. As right atrial pressure is normally only 4 to 5 mm Hg, significant tricuspid stenosis may be present with a valve orifice considerably larger than that seen with mitral stenosis.

Tricuspid insufficiency results from fibrosis and contraction of the valve leaflets, often in association with shortening and fusion of chordae tendineae. Calcification is rare. With dilation of the tricuspid annulus the valve leaflets appear stretched, but otherwise are pliable and seemingly normal even though serious regurgitation is present. An unexplained fact, however, is that such valves may not regain competence after correction of mitral valve disease and restoration of pulmonary artery systolic pressure to normal.

PATHOPHYSIOLOGY. With tricuspid stenosis the mean right atrial pressure is elevated to 10 to 20 mm Hg. The higher pressures are found with a tricuspid valve orifice smaller than 1.5 cm² and a mean diastolic gradient between the atrium and ventricle of 5 to 15 mm Hg. When mean right atrial pressure remains above 10 mm Hg, edema and ascites usually appear.

Moderate degrees of tricuspid insufficiency may be tolerated surprisingly well because the regurgitant blood is dissipated into the systemic veins with little adverse influence on circulation except for a decrease in cardiac output. This is in striking contrast to mitral insufficiency, where the regurgitating blood produces pulmonary congestion. The significance of tricuspid insufficiency alone is difficult to evaluate because it is almost always seen in association with the more serious mitral valve disease. However, rarely tricuspid insufficiency results from an isolated traumatic injury. Such patients may tolerate the disease well for many years, the only physiologic disturbance being elevation of venous pressure and a decrease in cardiac output.

CLINICAL MANIFESTATIONS. Symptoms. The symptoms of tricuspid valve disease are similar to those of failure of the right side of the heart resulting from the associated mitral valve disease. Prominent features include elevation of venous pressure with edema, ascites, and hepatomegaly. As similar findings occur from failure of the right side of the heart without disease of the tricuspid valve, the concomitant presence of tricuspid disease may be easily overlooked. The general effects of tricuspid disease are to increase the severity of failure of the right side of the heart. Otherwise the clinical course is similar to that seen with isolated mitral stenosis or insufficiency.

Physical Examination. The characteristic murmur of tricuspid stenosis is best heard as a diastolic murmur at the lower end of the sternum. It is a low-pitched murmur of medium intensity and can easily be overlooked as it is well localized at the lower end of the sternum. During inspiration the intensity of the murmur increases as the volume of blood returning to the heart is temporarily increased by an increase in intrathoracic negative pressure. Tricuspid insufficiency produces a prominent systolic murmur at the lower end of the sternum and also at the cardiac apex, where it may be confused with the systolic murmur of mitral insufficiency. The murmur is often seen in association with an enlarged pulsating liver and prominent engorged peripheral veins. A prominent jugular pulse, especially when the cardiac rhythm is sinus, may be the best clue to unsuspected tricuspid disease.

Laboratory Studies. The chest roentgenogram and electrocardiogram may show enlargement of the right side of the heart, but this does not differentiate tricuspid disease from cardiac enlargement caused by pulmonary hypertension secondary to mitral disease. Cardiac catheterization and cineangiography are the most precise ways of establishing the diagnosis. At catheterization the presence of tricuspid stenosis can be established by measuring the diastolic gradient between the atrium and the ventricle. As the gradient may be quite small (5 to 7 mm Hg), careful measurements are necessary.

With serious tricuspid insufficiency, the contour of the right atrial pressure tracing is altered by the regurgitating of blood during systole. If the right atrium is large, however, significant regurgitation may be present with little alteration in contour of the right atrial pressure tracing; so a normal pressure tracing does not exclude significant insufficiency. Cineangiography is the best method for detecting insufficiency, noting the degree of reflux of dye into the atrium when dye is injected into the ventricle.

DIAGNOSIS. The diagnosis can be made with reasonable certainty if the characteristic systolic or diastolic murmurs are audible at the lower end of the sternum, especially in association with an enlarged, pulsating liver. Confirmatory studies are best obtained by catheterization and angiography. A good surgical routine at the time of mitral valve operation is to palpate the tricuspid valve through the right atrium before bypass is started to confirm or exclude the presence of tricuspid disease.

TREATMENT. Tricuspid disease is surgically treated at the time of correction of more serious mitral disease. Rarely the aortic valve is also involved; so replacement of three cardiac valves is necessary. There is not a uniform opinion about the necessity for treating minor to moderate degrees of tricuspid insufficiency secondary to pulmonary hypertension from mitral disease. Some have felt that correction of mitral valve disease, followed by regression of the pulmonary hypertension, would decrease the degree of tricuspid insufficiency to clinically unimportant levels. Braunwald and associates reported results with operation

upon 23 patients with tricuspid disease, 4 of whom had an annuloplasty while 19 had no therapy other than correction of the mitral disease. Fairly good clinical results were obtained. With extensive tricuspid insufficiency, however, almost all surgeons have concluded that tricuspid replacement or annuloplasty, should be performed at operation because a significant impairment of cardiac output from untreated tricuspid insufficiency jeopardizes the patient's opportunity for recovery following mitral replacement.

Tricuspid stenosis may be treated by simple commissurotomy, usually opening the commissure between the anterior and septal leaflets and the commissure between the posterior and septal leaflets, but leaving the fused commissure between the anterior and posterior leaflets. Opening of this commissure usually produces insufficiency. Hence, following commissurotomy the valve functions as a bicuspid one.

With organic disease of the tricuspid valve producing tricuspid insufficiency, surgical correction has been ineffective except with prosthetic replacement. The choice varies among different cardiac centers between a disc and a ball-valve prosthesis, because there is some hazard with a ball-valve prosthesis of impingement of the cage of the prosthesis on the ventricular septum (Fig. 19-25). Some have reported late thrombosis of a tricuspid ball-valve prosthesis occurring several months after operation, presumably from decrease in size of the right ventricle with resulting impairment of motion of the ball within the cage of the prosthesis. However, if a ball-valve prosthesis of appropriate size is carefully selected and any obstructing bands of ventricular muscle are excised, good results have been obtained. At New York University we have routinely employed a ball-valve prosthesis since 1970.

During insertion of the prosthetic valve, along the septal leaflet where the conduction bundle is located between the coronary sinus and the ventricular septum, sutures are placed through the base of the septal leaflet rather than through the annulus to avoid injury of the conduction bundle and production of heart block (Fig. 19-26). As arrhythmias are frequent after operation, two pacemaker wires are routinely left in the ventricle.

When moderate tricuspid insufficiency is present with pulmonary hypertension and the leaflets of the tricuspid valve appear normal, an annuloplasty is frequently performed. However, the durability of the annuloplasty remains uncertain, and there is less enthusiasm for annuloplasty now than a few years ago. The difficulties with annuloplasty probably are related to the fragile nature of the annulus of the tricuspid valve, especially near the commissure between the anterior and septal leaflets. Late results with prosthetic replacement of the tricuspid valve are quite good, for clinically detectable pulmonary emboli are virtually unknown. Small emboli which may go to the lungs are probably resorbed without any clinical sequelae.

Starr et al. have reported a series of 40 patients with tricuspid replacement with a 10 percent operative mortality and a 7 percent late mortality. At New York University in 1972 a survey was made of a series of 267 patients

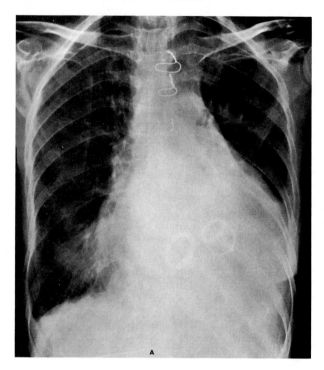

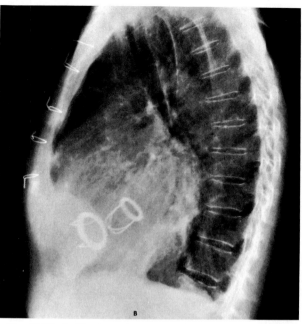

Fig. 19-25. *A.* Chest roentgenogram of a patient following prosthetic replacement of the mitral and tricuspid valves. The mitral valve has been replaced with a Starr-Edwards ball-valve prosthesis. A Kay-Shiley disc prosthesis was used for the tricuspid valve. *B.* Lateral-roentgenogram showing the mitral and tricuspid valves in position.

undergoing valve replacement with cloth-covered ball-valve prostheses. In over 1,500 patients operated upon between 1967 and 1971, results following tricuspid replacement were quite good.

An astonishing observation of some physiologic importance concerning tricuspid function is the finding reported by Arbulu and associates that total excision of the tricuspid valve *without replacement* could be tolerated for at least short periods of time. These observations were made in treating the difficult problem of tricuspid valve endocarditis in heroin addicts, where repeated septic injections had resulted in endocarditis of the tricuspid valve. Chemotherapy in such instances has often been futile, and prosthetic replacement has frequently resulted in reinfection.

These writers made the significant observation that the valve could simply be excised with fair cardiac function for at least several months. At the time of their report, the longest survival without a tricuspid valve was 10 months after operation. The long-term course remains

Fig. 19-26. Technique for suturing the tricuspid valve prosthesis with Dacron pledgets seated below the tricuspid annulus. The pledgets are used in all areas except the area of the partially resected septal leaflet, which is used as an autogenous pledget to avoid the conduction bundle and the production of heart block.

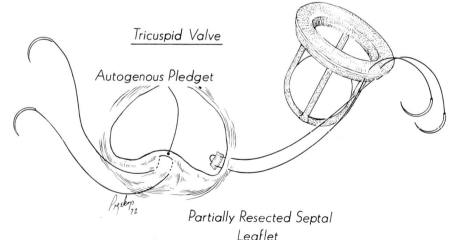

Tricuspid Valve

Autogenous Pledget

Partially Resected Septal Leaflet

uncertain. However, as a two-stage procedure for the treatment of endocarditis, the method seems to be the one of choice. By excision of all diseased valvular tissues, the endocarditis can be cured, and then prosthetic replacement can be done electively a few months later.

MULTIVALVULAR HEART DISEASE

With rheumatic heart disease, more than one cardiac valve is frequently involved. The physician must remain alert to this possibility, for prominent signs of disease of one valve can readily mask disease of additional valves. For this reason, cardiac catheterization and cineangiography are used to evaluate the function of all four cardiac valves to determine stenosis or insufficiency. In addition, at the time of operation other valves can be inspected or palpated. This is one of the great advantages of the sternotomy incision, which provides ready access to all cardiac chambers. The precise recognition of multivalvular disease is of considerable therapeutic importance, for widespread clinical experience has demonstrated that failure to correct all significant valvular disease at the time of operation significantly increases the surgical mortality.

A variety of clinical syndromes can be produced by different combinations of valvular disease. Often the clinical diagnosis can be only suspected and must be decided either by cardiac catheterization and angiography or operative exploration. The more common types of multivalvular disease will be briefly mentioned.

AORTIC DISEASE WITH FUNCTIONAL MITRAL INSUFFICIENCY. With dilatation of the left ventricle from cardiac failure due to aortic insufficiency, rarely from aortic stenosis, dilatation of the mitral annulus can produce a functional mitral insufficiency without intrinsic disease of the mitral valve. Such insufficiency may regress following repair of the aortic lesion, or it may be corrected by annuloplasty at operation, narrowing the annulus to normal dimensions by placing sutures at the stretched commissures. Replacement of the stretched but normal mitral valve is not often necessary. Usually the procedure can be decided by palpation of the mitral valve in the functioning, beating heart by introducing a finger into the left atrium through a stab wound in the intraatrial groove, just before cardiopulmonary bypass is started.

AORTIC STENOSIS AND MITRAL STENOSIS. When these two stenotic lesions coexist, the clinical signs of mitral stenosis often overshadow those of aortic stenosis, for the volume of blood entering the left ventricle is restricted by the stenotic mitral valve. Hence, functionally severe aortic stenosis may be present with minimal physical findings and a systolic pressure gradient between the left ventricle and aorta or only 20 to 40 mm Hg. Calculation of the cross-sectional area of the aortic valve by simultaneous measurement of cardiac output will quantitate the degree of aortic stenosis present. In uncertain instances, at the end of operative correction of the mitral stenosis, the aortic valve should be examined, either by pressure measurements or by inspection. Overlooking significant aortic ste-

nosis at the time of correction of mitral stenosis can easily result in death early in the postoperative period.

AORTIC INSUFFICIENCY AND MITRAL STENOSIS. With prominent aortic disease, an underlying mitral stenosis can easily be masked because the classic diastolic rumble of mitral stenosis is overshadowed by the prominent aortic murmurs. Cardiac catheterization will usually detect significant mitral stenosis beforehand. If uncertainty remains, however, the mitral valve may be readily palpated or inspected through a short incision in the left atrium at the time of surgical correction of aortic valve disease.

MITRAL STENOSIS WITH TRICUSPID DISEASE. When signs of mitral disease are prominent, tricuspid disease can be easily overlooked. As mentioned earlier, the most significant clinical signs of tricuspid disease are a systolic or diastolic murmur at the lower end of the sternum, especially one accentuated during inspiration. Often the jugular veins are prominent with systolic pulsations, in combination with an enlarged, pulsating liver. These clinical signs, however, are not precise. Catheterization and angiography may establish the diagnosis, but again the technique is not totally reliable. The pressure gradient with significant tricuspid stenosis may be small, and tricuspid insufficiency can be assessed by angiography only by introducing a catheter across the triscupid valve to inject dye into the right ventricle, a procedure which in itself may produce some tricuspid insufficiency. For these reasons, routine palpation of the tricuspid valve at the time of operation on the mitral valve is preferred. This is technically simple and quickly confirms or excludes the presence of tricuspid disease.

TRIVALVULAR DISEASE. In some unfortunate patients, significant disease of the mitral, aortic, and tricuspid valves is present. Such patients are usually in far advanced cardiac failure with generalized cardiomegaly. Hence, detection and surgical correction of all three valvular lesions is of critical importance if the patient is to survive operation. Attempting to shorten and simplify the operative procedure by not correcting all three diseased valves is usually unsatisfactory. Triple valve replacement, however, is an operative procedure of significant complexity and magnitude and retains a mortality in the range of 15 to 25 percent, primarily because patients requiring triple valve replacement are usually critically ill with far advanced chronic congestive failure and extensive cardiomegaly. In such patients cardiac function often improves only slowly over weeks or even months after operation (Fig. 19-27).

CARDIAC TRAUMA

HISTORICAL DATA. In 1896 Rehn first successfully sutured a stab wound of the heart, but for over 20 years this remained principally an isolated historic achievement until developments in anesthesia, blood transfusion, and other surgical advances made thoracotomy progressively safer, especially after 1940. In 1943 Blalock and Ravitch recognized that many patients survived a penetrating in-

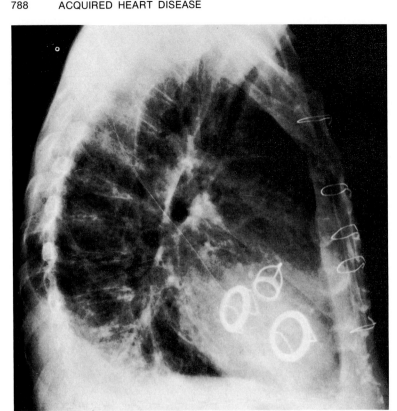

Fig. 19-27. Lateral roentgenogram in a patient with prosthetic replacement of the mitral, tricuspid, and aortic valves. The mitral and tricuspid valves were replaced with Kay-Shiley disc prostheses, while the aortic valve was replaced with a Starr-Edwards ball-valve prosthesis.

jury of the heart because pericardial tamponade developed and prevented exsanguination. Their introduction of pericardial aspiration as a form of definitive treatment greatly lowered mortality from penetrating cardiac injuries. Improvements in diagnosis, resuscitative therapy for shock, anesthesia, and operative technique have all contributed to lower mortality from cardiac injuries in recent years.

ETIOLOGY. Patients with penetrating cardiac injuries who are still alive when first seen by a physician usually have stab wounds from a small instrument such as an ice pick or small knife. Less common are similar injuries from low-velocity bullets, but injuries from high-velocity bullets or large knives are often immediately fatal after exsanguination. Nonpenetrating cardiac injuries result from blunt trauma to the chest wall, the most frequent of which is the "steering wheel" injury from contusion of the chest wall by impact against the steering wheel in an automobile accident.

PATHOLOGY. Because of its anterior position, the right ventricle is the cardiac chamber most frequently injured with penetrating wounds. In surviving patients most wounds are penetrating rather than perforating wounds, which are often immediately fatal from exsanguination. Nonpenetrating crushing injuries usually cause diffuse contusion of the myocardium. With nonpenetrating injuries of severe force, however, actual cardiac lacerations occur, and these are usually fatal. Rarely, a surviving patient is seen with a laceration of the tricuspid valve, the right atrium, or even the ventricular septum.

PATHOPHYSIOLOGY. The three principal physiologic disturbances following a cardiac injury are intrathoracic hemorrhage, pericardial tamponade, and cardiac failure. Hemorrhage of varying degree, of course, is present with every cardiac injury. The clinical signs are usually obvious with profound shock; death often occurs before definitive treatment can be started. Cardiac tamponade is frequently the dominant physiologic injury in surviving patients because patients surviving long enough for therapy often do so because tamponade has delayed or stopped the bleeding from the cardiac laceration. Tamponade quickly occurs because the normal pericardium can accommodate only 100 to 250 ml of blood. As the intrapericardial pressure rises with continuing tamponade, there is a progressive fall in cardiac output. Careful experimental studies by Isaacs found that elevation of intrapericardial pressure to 17 cm saline solution virtually stopped cardiac output unless venous pressure was elevated by infusion of fluid. This restriction of cardiac output results from prevention of diastolic filling of the ventricles, not from impaired venous flow into atria from the venae cavae.

Impaired cardiac function from the penetrating injury per se is unusual. It is seen only with the rare instance of injury of specific structures, such as a major coronary artery, a heart valve, or the cardiac conduction bundle.

CLINICAL MANIFESTATIONS. Symptoms. Patients with a cardiac injury may collapse immediately in profound shock or develop shock more gradually over a period of 1 to 2 hours. The clinical appearance of some patients with tamponade is initially deceptive, for they may appear only moderately ill and then collapse suddenly with an imperceptible blood pressure. This rapid change is due to the fact that once the pericardial cavity becomes distended, only 5 to 10 ml additional fluid is sufficient to raise the intrapericardial pressure to the critical zone of 17 to 18 cm saline solution, where cardiac output falls to very low levels.

The most frequent symptoms are the familiar ones of shock, including weakness, thirst, and restlessness. Chest pain is seldom severe. An unusual degree of restlessness, at times with the patient wildly rolling about, in contrast to the usual quiet, apathetic state of patients in hemorrhagic shock, perhaps results from cerebral anoxia produced by both arterial hypotension and venous hypertension.

Physical Examination. If tamponade is not present, the findings are those of hemorrhagic shock, hypotension with collapsed peripheral veins, and intense vasoconstriction. Tamponade is immediately suggested by finding hypotension combined with venous hypertension, indicated by visible, dilated neck and arm veins. The chest roentgenogram often shows little cardiac enlargement with tamponade, because the pericardium does not distend easily. A hemothorax is common, especially if there is concomitant injury of the lung or if the laceration is large enough for blood to drain from the pericardium into the pleural space. Particular care should be taken in examining the film for the presence of a small foreign body. The electrocardiogram is often normal, except for the rare patient with injury of a coronary artery or the conduction bundle. Fluoroscopy, once a popular technique for evaluating tamponade, has been virtually abandoned because of the time required and the lack of precision. Accurate measurement of central venous pressure, an important early measurement in the treatment of any patient with hemorrhagic shock, may quickly establish or exclude tamponade. A venous pressure above 10 cm saline solution suggests the diagnosis, while one above 15 cm is virtually diagnostic.

DIAGNOSIS. With the combination of arterial hypotension and venous hypertension, combined with other clinical findings, cardiac tamponade can be diagnosed with considerable accuracy. The differential diagnosis includes venous hypertension from overtransfusion, cardiac failure, or pulmonary embolism. If tamponade is a possibility, the pericardium should be aspirated promptly, at times within 5 to 10 minutes after the patient is first seen in the emergency department. Aspiration both confirms the diagnosis and partially relieves the tamponade.

In urgent instances where death is imminent and the presence of tamponade uncertain, a subxiphoid incision can be made in the linea alba and the pericardial cavity entered by making a small opening in the diaphragm immediately behind the xiphoid process. This can be quickly done and the pericardial cavity digitally explored. This is particularly helpful when large clots in the pericardium make needle aspiration ineffective.

The diagnosis of chronic or subacute cardiac tamponade is difficult. The question may arise several days after a penetrating thoracic injury which initially was not thought to have entered the pericardium. It more commonly arises after cardiac surgery, usually several days after operation when the question of intrathoracic bleeding no longer exists. As with acute tamponade, the clinical findings are a decreased cardiac output with hypotension and elevation of venous pressure. The usual condition to be differentiated from chronic tamponade is cardiac failure, more rarely pulmonary embolism. Several years of experience have indicated the great variation in clinical signs with chronic tamponade and the unreliability of such findings as a paradoxic pulse, changes in intensity of cardiac sounds, or size of the cardiac silhouette on the chest roentgenogram. The safest approach seems to be the realization that in the presence of decreased cardiac output and elevated venous pressure tamponade cannot be excluded with 100 percent certainty except by thoractomy. Simply being aware of these diagnostic limitations is particularly important in treating a patient for supposedly congestive failure who does not respond to the usual therapy of digitalis and diuretics. In uncertain instances the pericardial cavity must be explored, either by needle aspiration, subxiphoid digital aspiration, or formal thoracotomy.

TREATMENT. With shock from penetrating cardiac injuries, therapy includes intravenous infusion of fluids, administration of catecholamines to stimulate myocardial contractility, pericardial aspiration, and thoracotomy. Appropriate amounts of fluid, 1 to 3 liters of electrolyte or blood, should be infused rapidly to elevate venous pressure and thus enhance cardiac filling, despite the elevated intrapericardial pressure. Cardiac filling results from the difference between venous pressure and intrapericardial pressure; hence, elevation of venous pressure by intravenously infused fluids will partly correct the impaired myocardial filling from the elevated pericardial pressures. For patients in extremis with bradycardia and impending cardiac arrest, probably from impaired coronary blood flow, catecholamines such as epinephrine or isoproterenol may be useful for short periods of time.

When a moribund patient with possible tamponade is first seen, pericardial aspiration should be done immediately. One of the most dramatic experiences in surgery is to aspirate as little as 10 to 15 ml blood from the pericardium of a moribund patient with an imperceptible blood pressure and see a prompt rise in blood pressure to 70 to 80 mm Hg and a return of consciousness. Aspiration is best done through a subxiphoid approach, inserting a 16- or 18-gauge needle slowly upward in the angle between the xiphoid process and the left costal margin. Ideally, the electrocardiogram should be monitored for an arrhythmia during the procedure. As the needle is angled upward, a sense of resistance can be noted as the diaphragm and pericardium are traversed. Varying amounts of blood may be obtained, ranging from as little as 10 ml to as much as 300 to 400 ml. The blood obtained from the pericardium may not clot, while blood obtained from inadvertent puncture of the heart, usually the right ventricle, does.

As mentioned earlier, when tamponade is likely but

aspiration is ineffective, a prompt subxiphoid digital exploration should be done, making a short incision in the linea alba, separating the diaphragm behind the xiphoid process, and digitally entering the pericardium. The technique is well described by Berger et al.

Immediate thoracotomy should be considered and the operating room notified as soon as a patient is seen with a penetrating cardiac injury, because of the unpredictability of either continued hemorrhage or tamponade. Final decision about thoracotomy can be made after initial response to intravenously administered fluids.

Some patients with massive hemorrhage from cardiac wounds are near death on arrival in an emergency department and are often seen alive only because they were injured not far from the hospital. In such patients immediate thoracotomy in the emergency room, often with minimal aseptic technique, may be lifesaving. Once hemorrhage has been controlled by digital pressure or temporary suture, resuscitation can proceed in a more orderly fashion, usually followed by closure of the incision in the operating room. Since 1970, at Bellevue Hospital, several such patients have recovered uneventfully after immediate thoracotomy who clearly would not have survived otherwise.

Separate from the necessity of immediate thoracotomy for massive hemorrhage is the question of elective thoracotomy for penetrating cardiac injuries with tamponade. Data clearly indicate that 60 to 70 percent of the patients with tamponade can be safely treated by serial aspiration. In 1959 Isaacs reported that in a group of 60 patients with cardiac injuries treated at The Johns Hopkins Hospital, 40 had symptoms of tamponade for which aspiration was successful treatment in 75 percent; there was only one death in this group. However, there has been a gradual trend in recent years to perform thoracotomy upon virtually all patients with penetrating injuries and tamponade. The risk of thoracotomy is very small, probably no more than 1 to 2 percent, and the likelihood of delayed bleeding and recurrent tamponade small.

Sugg et al. in 1968 presented convincing data that routine thoracotomy gave overall better results in most institutions than selective thoracotomy for patients judged to have continuing hemorrhage or recurrent tamponade. In 1971 Beall et al. described a similar trend at Baylor University, where thoracotomy is now done almost routinely, rather than repeated pericardiocentesis.

Myocardial contusion from blunt thoracic trauma should be treated much as an acute myocardial infarction, with bed rest and serial observations with blood-enzyme measurements and the electrocardiogram. Complete recovery after a period of weeks can be expected in most patients. Rarely blunt injury may be associated with signs of intrapericardial bleeding from a laceration. Such instances are unusual, but because of the unpredictable nature of the laceration a pump-oxygenator should be available, and attachment of the pump-oxygenator to the femoral vessels in the thigh before the chest is opened should be considered. Without the pump-oxygenator, fatal hemorrhage may occur when the pericardium is opened if the laceration is too extensive to be promptly controlled by digital pressure. A recent report by Drapanas dramatically illustrates the utility of the pump-oxygenator in such injuries.

COMPLICATIONS. In the absence of injury of a discrete cardiac structure, recovery in most patients following suture of a cardiac laceration is uneventful. Formerly in those treated by serial aspiration alone, 15 to 20 percent developed a pericardiotomy syndrome with fever and effusion, lasting for several days to a few weeks but eventually resulting in complete recovery. Septic pericarditis from bacterial infection is very rare, and constrictive pericarditis has occurred as a late complication in only a few patients.

Foreign Bodies

Foreign bodies remaining in the heart after injury have naturally attracted much interest because of the unusual circumstances and the profound psychologic influences of having a missile embedded in the heart. Following World War II, Harken published a careful analysis of extensive experiences with foreign bodies, defining the complications and the indications for removal at that time. A reevaluation of the problem was published by Holdeger et al. in 1966. Data clearly indicate that symptomatic foreign bodies smaller than 1 cm are innocuous and can be safely left alone. Larger foreign bodies or those associated with a pericardial effusion or signs of pericarditis are best removed. Occasionally foreign bodies migrate in the circulation, moving from a large vein to the right ventricle or to a pulmonary artery.

In 1966 Bland and Beebe published a significant report of the 20-year course of 40 patients with foreign bodies remaining in the heart after World War II. All patients survived. A major complication occurred in only 1 patient, in whom a shell fragment in the left pulmonary artery moved to the right pulmonary artery and eroded the bronchus. The electrocardiogram became normal in all but 2 patients. Only 1 patient, who had a distinct injury of the aortic valve, had persistent cardiac enlargement. However, the emotional disability was impressive, apparently related to the strain of living with a condition of uncertain prognosis. Almost all patients were seriously concerned, and 5 were incapacitated with anxiety neuroses. Because of this significant emotional disability and the safety of current cardiac surgical procedures, most foreign bodies of significant size should be electively removed.

CARDIAC TUMORS

Metastatic neoplasms are the most common cardiac neoplasms, occurring in 4 to 12 percent of the autopsies performed on patients with neoplastic disease. The most frequent primary cardiac tumor is *myxoma*, comprising 50 to 60 percent of all primary cardiac neoplasms. *Sarcomas* are found in 20 to 25 percent of cases, and *rhabdomyomas* in 10 to 15 percent. Benign but extremely rare neoplasms include fibromas, angiomas, lipomas, teratomas, and cysts.

The clinical significance of cardiac tumors is similar to that of many other cardiac lesions in that accurate diagnosis and successful treatment first became possible with the development of extracorporeal circulation. Before 1950 cardiac tumors were usually first diagnosed at autopsy. Several excellent reviews have previously summarized the pathologic findings and clinical features. A classic analysis was published by Yater in 1931, and a detailed French monograph was published by Mahaim in 1945. In 1949 Whorton described the clinical findings in 100 sarcomas of the heart, and in 1951 Prichard reviewed 150 lesions, most of which were metastatic in origin.

In 1953 Steinberg et al. reported the diagnosis of an atrial myxoma in three patients by angiocardiography. An unsuccessful attempt was made to remove the myxoma in one of the patients studied by Steinberg et al., and in 1952 another unsuccessful attempt was made by Bahnson. Both these efforts preceded the development of open heart surgery. The first successful removal of an atrial myxoma was performed by Crafoord in 1954, using extracorporeal circulation. Other successful reports quickly followed, and in 1967 Thomas et al. stated that there had been 126 attempted excisions of atrial myxomas, either planned or inadvertent, 85 of which had been successful.

Myxoma

Sixty to seventy-five percent of cardiac myxomas develop in the left atrium, almost always from the atrial septum near the fossa ovalis. Most other myxomas develop in the right atrium. Less than 20 have been found in either the right or left ventricle. The curious predilection for a myxoma to develop from the rim of the fossa ovalis in the left atrium has been studied by several observers, but a satisfactory explanation has not been found.

Myxomas are apparently true neoplasms, although their similarity to an organized atrial thrombus led to considerable debate over whether they represented a true neoplasm or not. Their occurrence in the absence of other organic heart disease, histochemical studies demonstrating mucopolysaccharide and glycoprotein, and a distinct histologic appearance all indicate that myxomas are true neoplasms.

PATHOLOGY. The tumors are usually polypoid, projecting into the atrial cavity from a 1- to 2-cm stalk attached to the atrial septum. The maximal diameter varies from 0.5 to 10 cm. Careful histologic study of the point of origin of the myxoma from the atrial septum has demonstrated that only the superficial layer of the septum is involved, and invasion of the septum does not occur. Frequently myxomas grow slowly, some patients having symptoms for 10 to 20 years. There is no tendency to invade other areas of the heart, and metastases have not occurred. The consistency of a myxoma is of surgical significance, for extreme friability has been found in some tumors, resulting in fatal embolization when the tumor was digitally manipulated.

Histologically, a myxoma is covered with endothelium and composed of a myxomatous stroma with large stellate cells mixed with fusiform or multinucleated cells. Mitoses are infrequent. Lymphocytes and plasmacytes are regularly found. Hemosiderin, a result of hemorrhage into the tumor, is also common.

PATHOPHYSIOLOGY. A myxoma may cause no difficulty until it grows large enough to obstruct the flow of blood through either the mitral or tricuspid valve, or fragments to produce peripheral emboli. The rarity of embolization is surprising, for an astonishing degree of to-and-fro motion of a myxoma swinging on a small pedicle with each cardiac contraction may occur. This has been vividly demonstrated by angiographic and fluoroscopic studies.

Because of its rarity, myxoma is almost always confused with a more frequent cardiac condition. Left atrial myxomas simulate mitral stenosis or insufficiency or idiopathic pulmonary hypertension. Right atrial myxomas are confused with tricuspid valvular disease or constrictive pericarditis. Because of the polypoid nature of the myxoma, intermittent obstruction of the mitral or tricuspid valve may occur, with resulting variation in symptoms, but this has not been observed frequently enough to be of much diagnostic significance.

CLINICAL MANIFESTATIONS. The clinical course of the patient with a myxoma may be protracted, with a variety of erroneous clinical diagnoses. The rate of development and variation in symptoms depend upon the growth of the tumor with the associated obstruction to cardiac filling and obstruction at the valve orifice. There are no characteristic symptoms or signs from which a precise diagnosis can be made. The usual findings are those of mitral valvular disease, with progressive dyspnea, cough, and subsequent cardiac failure with hepatic enlargement and edema.

In a few patients unusual signs of a generalized systemic disease have developed, with recurrent fever, weight loss, malaise, and abnormalities in serum proteins gradually evolving over 1 to 3 years. Why these symptoms should occur with a myxoma is not known.

Peripheral emboli occur in a minority of patients and in some are the first sign of a myxoma. A few instances have been described in which the diagnosis was first made as a result of histologic examination of a surgically removed embolus, recognizing the characteristic myxomatous structure.

On physical examination patients with a left atrial myxoma may have either a diastolic murmur suggesting mitral stenosis or a systolic murmur simulating mitral insufficiency. With a right atrial myxoma, hepatic enlargement and edema characteristic of constrictive pericarditis are frequent.

The electrocardiogram is often normal unless pulmonary hypertension from long-standing mitral valve obstruction has produced right ventricular hypertrophy. The chest roentgenogram may show enlargement of the left atrium with pulmonary congestion. Rarely on fluoroscopy calcification is visible. Selective angiocardiography is the only method of making a precise diagnosis in most patients. With good opacification of the atria, a characteristic filling defect may be identified with considerable accuracy. Unless good opacification of the atrium is obtained, however, an erroneous diagnosis can be made because of incomplete filling of the atria. Often the diagnosis cannot be differentiated from an organized thrombus in the left atrium.

Differential diagnosis includes more frequent cardiac lesions, such as mitral stenosis or insufficiency, pulmonary

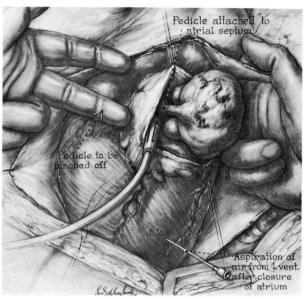

Fig. 19-28. Pedunculated atrial myxoma removed at operation in 1957. The patient has remained free of cardiac symptoms since that time. (*Reprinted from H. T. Bahnson, F. C. Spencer, and E. C. Andrus, Diagnosis and Treatment of Intracavitary Myxomas of the Heart, Ann Surg, 145:915, 1957, by permission of J. B. Lippincott Company, Philadelphia.*)

hypertension, constrictive pericarditis, rheumatic fever, or bacterial endocarditis.

TREATMENT. Operation should be performed upon all patients once the diagnosis has been established. Extracorporeal circulation is routinely employed because of the grave risk of dislodging emboli into the arterial circulation.

A sternotomy or a right lateral thoracotomy are preferred to approach the left atrium through an incision in the interatrial groove. Once extracorporeal circulation has been established, ventricular fibrillation may be induced to avoid the risk of embolism of tumor fragments. Palpation of the lesion is avoided. Once the atrium has been opened and the lesion exposed, it can be readily excised, with careful removal of the small segment of atrial septum where the stalk of the tumor is attached. How much atrial septum should be removed is debatable. Most surgeons have obtained good results by simple excision of the base of the stalk of the myxoma. Gerbode et al., however, have reported one patient in whom a recurrence developed requiring reoperation 3 years later; they prefer excision of a small segment of atrial septum, closing the resulting atrial septal defect with a patch of prosthetic material.

Following operation the prognosis is excellent for complete recovery. Complete regression of severe pulmonary hypertension has been reported in several patients. One of the earliest cases, a fifty-seven-year-old patient operated upon in 1956, was well and asymptomatic 8 years later (Fig. 19-28).

Metastatic Neoplasms

Cardiac metastases have been found in 4 to 12 percent of autopsies performed for neoplastic disease. Although they have occurred from primary neoplasms developing in almost every known site of the body, the most frequent have been carcinoma of the lung or breast, melanoma, and lymphoma. Cardiac metastases involving only the heart are very unusual. Similarly, a solitary cardiac metastasis is infrequent; usually there are multiple areas of involvement. Cardiac involvement is particularly common with leukemia or lymphoma, developing in 25 to 40 percent of patients. All areas of the heart are involved with equal frequency except the cardiac valves, perhaps as a result of the absence of lymphatics in the valves.

Most patients have no symptoms of heart disease, even though large areas of myocardium are involved by an infiltrating neoplasm. A pericardial effusion, which is hemorrhagic in about 15 percent of patients, is the most frequent abnormality. This was found in 45 of 217 patients studied by Gassman and associates, but only 3 of these had cardiac tamponade. Symptoms from cardiac failure are the most common disability, but these developed in only 17 of the 217 patients in Gassman's series. Recurrent arrhythmias are infrequent. The electrocardiogram is similarly nonspecific, usually showing T-wave changes, although a wide variety of conduction abnormalities have been reported.

The diagnosis can be suspected in a patient with malignant disease in whom a hemorrhagic pericardial effusion develops. Identification of malignant cells in fluid aspirated from the pericardium can establish the diagnosis. Thoracotomy should be avoided if possible, because no effective treatment is available and death usually occurs from generalized metastatic disease within a few months. The cardiac involvement per se is seldom a significant factor in the terminal illness.

Sarcoma

Sarcomas of the heart constitute about 25 percent of all primary cardiac neoplasms. In 1962 Dong et al. reported that 178 cases had been described. Spindle cell and round cell sarcomas are the most frequent, but the entire range of mesenchymal tumors has been reported, including leiomyosarcoma and fibrosarcoma. The right atrium and right ventricle are the most frequent sites of involvement, usually with a diffuse infiltrating tumor that does not involve the cardiac valves. Valvular obstruction or embolization, in contrast to atrial myxoma, is infrequent. Metastatic spread to the mediastinum is frequent, with death occurring 1 month to 3 years after onset of symptoms. Symptoms usually evolve from obstruction of the venae cavae, pericardial effusion, or arrhythmias from invasion of the conduction system.

Sarcomas developing in the pericardium, usually mesotheliomas, are rare lesions that grow rapidly and cause symptoms from obstruction of the venae cavae. Invasion of the myocardium develops in the late stages of the tumor.

The diagnosis of a primary cardiac malignant tumor can

be suspected in a patient in whom an unexplained hemorrhagic pericardial effusion develops, especially in association with a bizarre cardiac shadow on the roentgenogram. Thoracotomy is usually required to establish the diagnosis. Only rarely is effective therapy possible. Scannell and Grillo, in 1958, reported one fortunate experience in a child in whom exploration for pericardial effusion found a localized fibrosarcoma in the right atrial wall which was successfully excised. In 1966, we removed an angiosarcoma of the right side of the heart, invading the tricuspid valve, along with a large segment of right atrial wall. Reconstruction was with a pericardial patch graft, reattaching the tricuspid valve to the reconstructed annulus. Postoperative radiotherapy was given, following which the patient lived for 18 months before dying of widespread metastatic disease.

Rhabdomyoma

A cardiac rhabdomyoma is a rare lesion which is not a true tumor but is probably a focal arrest in maturation of cardiac muscle. Seventy such patients were reviewed by Prichard in 1951. The nodules have been termed *nodular glycogenic degeneration,* being interpreted as an example of localized glycogen storage disease. It is uncertain whether they are hamartomas or merely localized manifestations of glycogen storage disease.

The cardiac lesions may be solitary or multiple nodules, or may present as diffuse infiltration of the cardiac muscle. The nodules are not encapsulated but merge imperceptibly with the surrounding healthy myocardium. The lesions do not grow, and metastases do not occur.

On histologic examination, the nodules are composed of tubular muscle cells with large vacuoles in which the nuclei appear suspended by threads of cytoplasm, like spiders in a web, giving origin to the term "spider cell." About one-half of the patients have tuberous sclerosis of the brain. The clinical significance of the cardiac lesions is uncertain, for disability is usually due to the associated tuberous sclerosis. Sudden death has been reported in some patients who, at postmortem examination, were found to have a rhabdomyoma. Isolated instances of obstruction of the outflow tract of the right ventricle from a large rhabdomyoma requiring surgical excision have been reported.

Miscellaneous Tumors

Unusual benign lesions of the heart include fibromas, lipomas, angiomas, teratomas, and cysts. Fewer than 50 examples of each of these types of lesions have been reported. Fibromas have been found most frequently in the left ventricle, often as 2- to 5-cm nodules within the muscle. Sudden death, probably from a cardiac arrhythmia, has been reported with such tumors and may be the reason that only 18 percent of the reported tumors have been found in adults.

Lipomas are usually asymptomatic tumors found projecting from the epicardial or endocardial surface of the heart in older patients. Only about 30 such cases have been reported. Angiomas are commonly small, focal vascular malformations of no clinical significance, except four that have been found associated with a heart block. Pericardial teratomas and bronchogenic cysts are rare lesions that may cause symptoms from compression of the right atrium and obstruction of venous return. About 30 such patients have been reported in the surgical literature, most of them children. Some of the larger cysts, up to 10 cm in diameter, may produce grotesque deformities from extensive invagination of the right atrial wall.

CORONARY ARTERY DISEASE

HISTORICAL DATA. For well over 30 years different investigators have attempted to increase the blood supply of a heart ischemic from coronary atherosclerosis. Beck pioneered these efforts by attempting to develop vascular adhesions around the heart to introduce additional blood supply and to redistribute blood flowing through patent coronary vessels. Many unusual, imaginative, and sometimes bizarre procedures were tried. These included abrasion of the epicardium, painting the epicardium with phenol, insertion of talc or asbestos into the pericardial cavity, and wrapping omentum around the heart. Unfortunately, consistent benefit could not be demonstrated from any of these procedures, and virtually all have been abandoned. Perhaps the fundamental biologic reason for failure is the natural tendency for vascular adhesions to progressively fibrose and become more avascular with time.

In 1946, Vineberg developed a new concept for revascularizing the heart when he found that an internal mammary artery implanted in a tunnel in the myocardium of a dog would remain patent in a high percentage of cases. The operation of implantation of the internal mammary artery into the wall of the left ventricle in man was begun by Vineberg in 1950 and has been consistently employed by him since that time. Objective analysis of the results of arterial implantation was not possible until the development of coronary arteriography by Sones in the year 1958–1959. Demonstration by Sones that the implanted artery remained patent in the majority of patients and in some patients connected with regional coronary arteries provided a stimulus to further investigation of methods of arterial implantation. Subsequently between 1960 and 1967 different arterial implants were extensively tried in several centers, but with the subsequent introduction of the bypass operation the procedure has greatly decreased in popularity and has been virtually abandoned in most institutions. The limited, often negligible, physiologic improvement in most patients is related to the fact that even though the artery remains patent in over 90 percent of patients, it often carries only a small amount of blood, as little as 5 to 10 ml/minute, to the myocardium. An occasional patient develops significant collateral circulation following implantation, and isolated instances have been reported in which the implanted artery clearly was of substantial benefit, carrying as much as 50 ml of blood per minute and causing obvious severe myocardial ischemia when temporarily interrupted. The reason for the wide variation in the development of collateral circulation after implantation has never been satisfactorily determined.

From 1956 to 1959 initial attempts were made with coronary endarterectomy to remove directly localized areas of obstruction caused by atherosclerotic plaques. Longmire and Cannon, Bailey, and others attempted such procedures, but results were discouraging because of a high operative mortality and a high rate of subsequent occlusion. Subsequent performance of such procedures with cardiopulmonary bypass, often combined with a pericardial roof patch, was satisfactory in a small percentage of patients but disappointing in many.

The development of the bypass operation for coronary occlusive disease from 1967 to 1968 was a dramatic achievement, for this represented the first such operation in which it was possible to immediately increase the blood flow to the myocardium. Most of the basic clinical investigations of the technique of bypass grafting evolved from studies in three centers in the United States during this period. Favaloro, discouraged with the limited application of endarterectomy and pericardial patch grafting, began using longer and longer segments of saphenous vein to bypass occlusive disease in the right coronary artery, eventually demonstrating that grafts could be effectively interposed between the aorta proximally and the termination of the right coronary artery at the posterior descending coronary artery distad. Johnson first showed that similar grafts could be effectively used for the left coronary artery, a most significant achievement, for previously all direct operative procedures upon the left coronary artery had had a prohibitive operative mortality well over 50 percent. At New York University, Green et al., following extensive experimental studies, first began direct anastomoses between the left internal mammary artery and the anterior descending coronary artery, using an end-to-side anastomosis. This procedure was not widely used by others for 2 to 3 years, but has greatly increased in popularity in the past 2 years. The dramatic, virtually instantaneous relief of angina with bypass techniques led to performance of the procedure in thousands of patients in the past several years.

However, despite this widespread popularity, much remains unknown about the long-term results. For this reason there is considerable debate at present about indications and contraindications for bypass grafting, a question that will require several years' accumulation of data to answer.

ETIOLOGY AND PATHOGENESIS. Atherosclerosis is the cause of coronary occlusive disease in almost all patients. It is extremely common in the American male; autopsy studies of men killed in the Korean conflict who were between twenty and thirty years of age found some coronary atherosclerosis in 30 to 40 percent. The frequency gradually rises in men to approach 70 to 80 percent by seventy years of age. For a detailed analysis of the different theories concerning the cause of coronary disease, as well as its widely varying incidence according to race, sex, and other factors, recent monographs on epidemiology of atherosclerosis should be consulted.

The basic lesion is a segmental atherosclerotic plaque, often localized within the first 5 cm of the origin of the coronary arteries from the aorta. Involvement of the tributaries of the major coronary arteries, as well as the arterioles, is often minimal. This segmental localization makes bypass procedures possible. The atherosclerotic plaque is composed of focal deposits of lipid alternating with areas of fibrosis, perhaps a histologic reaction to the deposition of lipids. In older lesions spotty areas of calcification develop. Areas of intramural hemorrhage are visible in some lesions and often seem to precipitate thrombosis of the stenosed vessel.

The myocardial ischemia produced by coronary atherosclerosis results in a number of grave complications: sudden death, angina pectoris, myocardial infarction (with or without coronary thrombosis), and congestive heart failure. Any one or all of these events may occur unpredictably in a patient with coronary atherosclerosis.

Of these four, angina pectoris occurs most frequently. Patients experience a periodic discomfort, usually substernal, appearing typically with exertion, after eating, or with extreme emotion. Characteristically these symptoms subside within 3 to 5 minutes or may be dramatically relieved by sublingual nitroglycerin. In about 25 percent of patients, the symptoms are less typical and may have unusual areas of radiation to such remote areas as the teeth, the shoulder, the hand, or the epigastrium. Establishing a diagnosis of angina in such patients is difficult, perhaps impossible, without angiography, for results of the physical examination are usually normal. Differential diagnosis includes anxiety states, musculoskeletal disorders, and reflux esophagitis.

There is a constant risk of sudden death with angina pectoris; 5 to 10 percent of patients die each year. Often postmortem examination does not show any acute cause of death, such as myocardial infarction or coronary thrombosis. In such instances death is probably due to an acute disturbance of rhythm with terminal ventricular fibrillation.

Myocardial infarction, with or without thrombosis of a diseased coronary artery, is another frequent and often fatal complication. For a detailed discussion of myocardial infarction, a textbook of cardiology should be consulted. Surgical procedures for acute myocardial infarction have been tried in a few instances, but thus far the procedures remain experimental, with a high operative mortality.

In some patients congestive heart failure develops and may become the principle disability, eventually causing death. Congestive failure may or may not be preceded by angina or a myocardial infarction. Probably congestive failure is a result of myriads of tiny myocardial infarctions, eventually destroying over one-third of left ventricular muscle mass. What determines angina as the dominant symptom in one patient and congestive failure in another is unknown. Repeated tiny emboli from an ulcerated atherosclerotic plaque have been suggested as one possible mechanism. Once congestive failure has developed, revascularization of the heart with bypass operations has been disappointing, for objective signs of improved cardiac function have been small in a few and negligible in most. Probably this unfortunate group of patients may be best treated by cardiac transplantation when advances in immunology make organ transplantation more feasible.

DIAGNOSIS OF ANGINA PECTORIS. The history is the most important method for making the diagnosis, for usually there are no abnormal physical findings. With unusual symptoms, especially the absence of pain induced by exertion and relieved by nitroglycerin, laboratory studies are needed.

The electrocardiogram is normal at rest in about 70 percent of patients. Evaluation of changes in the electrocardiogram with graded exercise is a useful and widely used test, noting signs of ischemia in the cardiogram with increasing exercise, but the exact reliability of this technique remains somewhat controversial. By far the most exact method for determining the presence and severity of coronary artery disease is selective coronary arteriography (Fig. 19-29). Coronary arteriography provided the first method for accurately determining the extent and severity of coronary disease in individual patients. Not only the presence of disease but progression and response to therapy over months or years can be evaluated by serial arteriograms. Since the introduction of arteriography, little over a decade ago, thousands of such procedures have been performed, although at this time there are inadequate laboratory facilities to meet clinical demands.

OPERATIVE PROCEDURES FOR CORONARY ARTERY DISEASE. Coronary Bypass Operations. *Indications and Contraindications.* There is considerable uncertainty at present about indications for bypass grafting for angina. It is well established that operation can be performed in good-risk patients with a mortality of less than 5 percent, and it is followed by almost immediate and complete relief of angina in the majority of patients. However, the long-term influence of grafts is yet unknown. There is a disquieting thrombosis rate near 20 percent within the first year after operation, though apparently substantially less in the subsequent 1 to 2 years. Not enough time has yet elapsed to determine the protection provided by the grafts from myocardial infarction or death.

For this reason bypass grafting is widely used for patients with disabling angina unresponsive to conventional medical therapy, and also for angina of increasing intensity, so-called preinfarction angina, for this is often a forerunner of acute myocardial infarction. At New York University most operations have been performed for patients in these two categories.

More uncertain is the use of bypass grafts for patients with mild, nonincapacitating angina or on a prophylactic basis in patients with few or no symptoms but with previous myocardial infarction and extensive occlusive disease seen on subsequent coronary arteriography. In such patients the operation would provide protection from future myocardial infarctions, a very plausible hypothesis if the grafts remain patent for several years but one that has not yet been proved.

Severe congestive failure is a definite contraindication to operation, for the mortality is high and improvement small in surviving patients.

When a patient is considered for operation, coronary arteriography must be performed to determine the areas of obstruction, the size and patency of vessels beyond the area of obstruction, and the function of the left ventricle. Atherosclerotic obstruction is physiologically significant if the diameter of the vessel is narrowed more than 50 percent, corresponding to a reduction in cross-sectional area greater than 75 percent. The size and patency of vessels beyond the area of obstruction is also of importance, for patency rates after bypass grafting have been better with larger arteries in the range of 2 to 3 mm, as compared to 1 to 2 mm. However, ability to visualize vessels beyond an area of obstruction is a function of collateral circulation; so, the angiographic evaluation is not precise. In some patients dissection at operation will find an adequate vessel beyond an area of obstruction not visualized by angiography, because the flow of the injected dye was linked by sparse collateral circulation.

Multiple areas of obstruction are common. Nearly 50 percent of patients with severe angina have involvement of all three major coronary arteries, the anterior descending, the circumflex, and the right coronary.

Ventricular function, judged by contractility of the left ventricle during ventriculography, is a crucial part of preoperative evaluation, as it indicates the degree of previous muscle injury. In patients with normal ventricular function, operative risk is less than 5 percent and the likelihood of improvement great. At the other extreme, severe impairment of ventricular function with congestive failure, representing infarction of areas of myocardium and replacement by scar, indicates an operative risk as high as 20 to 30 percent and far less likelihood of improvement.

Attempts have been made to quantitate the degree of impairment of ventricular function by measurement of ejection fractions, angiographically estimating the percentage of blood in the ventricle which is ejected during systole. Though an imprecise measurement, reduction of ventricular function to where the ejection fraction is less than 0.20 indicates a virtually inoperable condition.

Left ventricular end-diastolic pressure in patients with normal ventricular function is normal, less than 10 to 12 mm Hg. Some increase occurs with moderate failure, but the level of elevation varies so much with the medical management of congestive failure preceding catheterization that the actual value found at catheterization is not of precise prognostic value. Elevation beyond 20 to 25 mm Hg, however, indicates a poor prognosis.

Operative Technique. Coronary bypass opeations are usually performed during extracorporeal circulation with the heart stilled either by inducing ventricular fibrillation or by ischemic arrest produced by temporary occlusion of the ascending aorta. Before bypass is started, a long segment of saphenous vein is removed from the thigh or leg, taking 15 to 20 cm of vein for each graft to be performed. It is reversed before insertion because of venous valves, attaching the distal end to the aorta. During bypass with the heart fibrillating, the left ventricle is decompressed with a vent to avoid overdistension. The patent coronary artery beyond the area of obstruction is then dissected, and an arteriotomy about 1 cm long made. Care is taken to avoid dissecting the coronary artery from its bed, for inclusion of the surrounding soft tissue in the subsequent anas-

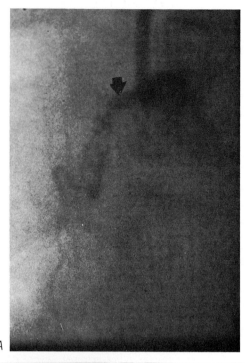

A

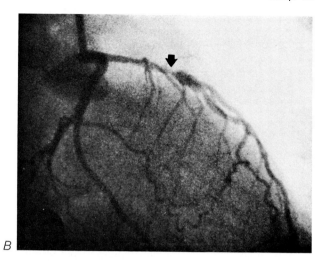

B

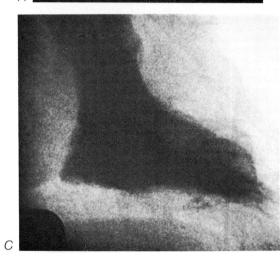

C

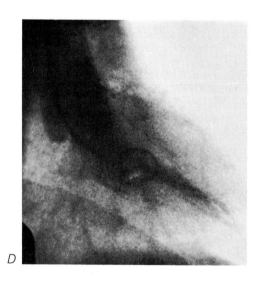

D

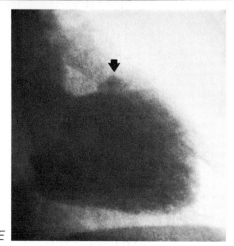

E

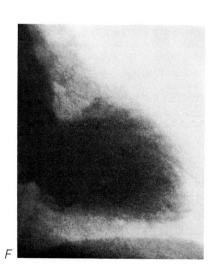

F

tomotic suture line greatly aids hemostasis. The vein–coronary artery anastomoses are performed end-to-side with interrupted and continuous sutures of 6-0 or 7-0 synthetic suture material. Three- to four-power optical magnification is routinely employed and greatly facilitates the performance of these small anastomoses. Following completion of the distal anastomosis, the vein graft is attached in gentle curves to the epicardium over the surface of the heart and then connected to the aorta proximally, usually with a 1-cm aortotomy. In some instances a small wedge of aortic wall is removed. Our usual preference is for a 1-cm longitudinal aortotomy (Fig. 19-30).

One theoretic objection to the use of vein grafts is the discrepancy in size between the vein and the artery, which results in turbulent flow. For example, if a 6-mm vein is anastomosed to a 2-mm artery, the rate of blood flow in the vein will be only one-ninth of that in the artery because of the difference in cross-sectional area. For this reason there has been an increased tendency to use veins from the leg, with a diameter near 4 mm, rather than larger veins from the thigh. However, significant data regarding influence of the size of veins on long-term patency rates are not available.

Because of the frequency of multiple areas of occlusion, double or triple bypass grafts are used in most patients, usually attaching each graft separately to the aorta. At New York University between 1971 and 1973 during the performance of over 500 bypass procedures, nearly 50 percent of patients have had a triple bypass. With the techniques described, a graft can be attached to a vessel on almost any surface of the heart, the most difficult being the posterior wall of the left ventricle near the termination of the circumflex coronary artery. With optical magnification, grafts can be attached to vessels as small as 1 mm internal diameter. This fact, combined with the ability to attach grafts to any area of the heart, makes it possible to perform bypass grafts in the majority of patients with angina, well over 90 percent of patients seen. The conditions are technically inoperable when there are multiple areas of occlusion throughout the length of the artery, fortunately an unusual pattern of involvement.

Once the bypass grafts have been constructed, rate of blood flow is measured with a flowmeter. Though accuracy in the operating room is sometimes questionable, these

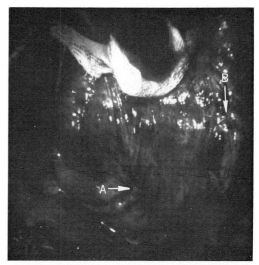

Fig. 19-30. Operative photograph showing bypass grafts inserted to both the posterior descending coronary artery on the *left* (point A) and a marginal branch of the circumflex on the *right* (point B). The heart has been retracted upward to demonstrate the posterior surface. This illustrates that bypass grafts can be attached to virtually any area of the heart.

measurements are of particular prognostic value, for there is good correlation between rate of flow and long-term patency. A mean flow rate of less than 20 ml/minute is associated with a high rate of subsequent occlusion, while high mean flow rates, greater than 70 to 80 ml/minute, have a much better prognosis. The flow rate, of course, varies with the size of the distal artery and the patency of the distal vascular bed. Patency rates have not been good with grafts attached to vessels as small as 1 mm in diameter, probably because of the small rate of flow.

Following operation careful observation in a cardiac intensive care unit is necessary to maintain adequate ventilation and cardiac output and to detect arrhythmias. Arrhythmias are quite frequent following operation but can be controlled by appropriate measures. These include infusion of lidocaine, procainamide, digitalis, propranolol, and electrical cardioversion. In most patients convalescence is comparatively uneventful, with the patient leaving the hospital in 10 to 14 days. A pericardiotomy syndrome, with fever, pleural effusion, and pleural or pericardial friction rubs, occurs in a small percentage of patients but responds well to administration of prednisone in small amounts for several days.

Angiographic studies performed within 1 to 2 weeks after operation have found a patency rate well above 90 percent. However, angiograms performed 6 to 12 months later have found occlusion of 20 to 25 percent of vein grafts. Though extensive data are not yet available, with periods of observation now between 3 and 4 years in small numbers of patients the rate of occlusion beyond the first year after operation apparently is small. Several factors may cause early or late thrombosis in a vein graft. These include technical factors at the time of operation in the construction of the anastomoses or ischemic injury to the

Fig. 19-29. *A.* Right coronary artery, left anterior oblique projection. There is total obstruction of the vessel immediately distal to its aortic origin (arrow). A network of collateral vessels on the anterior surface of the right atrium and the right ventricle is apparent. *B.* Left coronary artery, right anterior oblique projection. There is severe narrowing of the left anterior descending coronary artery (arrow) distal to the origin of the second septal branch. *C.* Left ventricle in right anterior oblique projection in diastole. There is a normal contour of the chamber. *D.* Same ventricle in systole showing excellent contraction of all areas of the ventricle. *E.* Left ventricle in diastole, right anterior oblique projection. There is increased rounding of the ventricle and bulging of the anterolateral wall. A localized bulge on the superior portion of the anterolateral wall is evident (arrow). *F.* The same ventricle in systole. The degree of left ventricular contraction is generally markedly impaired.

vein during removal from its bed, such as excessive removal of adventitia or other mechanical trauma. As mentioned earlier, the size of the coronary artery grafted and the rate of flow through the vein graft both correlate reasonably well with late patency. A progressive fibrosis has been seen in some vein grafts, usually segmental in location, which progresses to complete obliteration within a few months. This curious histologic response at times is observed in one vein graft but not in others in the same patient. It probably represents segmental ischemic or mechanical injury to the vein at the time of operation or else injury from turbulent flow of blood. Other factors influencing thrombosis of vein grafts include turbulent blood flow producing intimal proliferation at the anastomotic sites, pericardial adhesions, and theoretically progressive coronary atherosclerosis. The last factor has not been documented, however, because of the short period of observation.

With the natural concern about the significant rate of thrombosis of vein grafts, arterial grafts have been used with increasing frequency. The left internal mammary–anterior descending coronary anastomosis was first developed by Green and Tice and has been used consistently by Green since (Fig. 19-31). Since 1970 there has been increasing use of the internal mammary artery by several groups because of the long-term patency rates above 90 percent, a much more favorable finding than that with vein grafts. Unfortunately the internal mammary artery is small, and the rate of flow of blood is not as great as with vein grafts. However, the size of the internal mammary closely approximates that of the coronary artery in many patients. Another objection is the fact that use of the internal mammary is much more restrictive than that with free vein grafts. It is possible to attach the right internal mammary artery to the anterior descending, and the left internal mammary artery to the circumflex, but the right internal mammary will not reach to the termination of the right coronary on the posterior surface of the heart. For this reason, Edwards has rotated the splenic artery up from the celiac axis to connect to the right coronary artery posteriorly. A search for other arterial grafts continues, and at this time a few experiences with the radial artery have been verbally reported but not published. At present the feasibility of bypass grafting has been thoroughly established, but undoubtedly the best technique for grafting will require long periods of comparison of data with different methods.

The critical question with coronary bypass grafting is, of course, the long-term protection from myocardial infarction and death. This will require several years of careful study. Efforts are being made by the National Institutes of Health to coordinate observations among different cardiac centers over a period of years. It is encouraging that in the more than 800 patients undergoing bypass grafting at New York University there have been no known late deaths from coronary disease in patients in whom there were functioning double or triple grafts. Death has occurred following operation when the bypass grafts became occluded several months later, but in those with patent grafts the protection thus far from myocardial infarction has been significant.

Other Operative Procedures. It is significant that when the previous edition of this textbook was published, most of the discussion of surgical procedures concerned implantation of a systemic artery into the myocardium, the Vineberg procedure. In the intervening years, with the dramatic results obtained with the bypass operation, the popularity of arterial implants has waned sharply. Almost none have been performed at New York University since 1970, primarily because bypass grafts can be used in the majority of patients. The implanted artery remains patent in the majority of patients, a range of 80 to 90 percent, but the amount of blood flowing through the implanted artery seems to be small in most. Hence, the degree of improvement in myocardial ischemia is disappointingly small. A few unusual exceptions have been cited where at repeat operation months or years later when disease developed in other areas, direct flow measurements of an implanted artery found blood flow as high as 50 ml/minute.

Endarterectomy, either with carbon dioxide gas or with mechanical strippers, is employed particularly on the right coronary artery but in selected instances on the left. The procedure now is done almost always in conjunction with bypass grafting to improve flow rates through the graft. Operative procedures for acute myocardial infarction, performing bypass grafting within hours after the vessel has become occluded, are under evaluation. Experimentally, total ischemia to an area of myocardium produces irreversible necrosis within less than 1 hour; so the potential value of bypass grafting is to improve blood flow to critically ischemic areas which have not yet undergone necrosis. Excision of myocardial infarcts has been studied experimentally and in a few instances clinically, but mortality remains too high for clinical application at present.

Intestinal bypass procedures to decrease absorption of cholesterol and to stop or even reverse the coronary atherosclerotic process have been cautiously but hopefully evaluated primarily by Buchwald and Varco and by others.

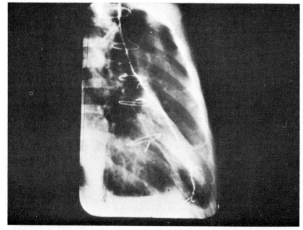

Fig. 19-31. Angiogram performed several months after left internal mammary–left anterior descending coronary bypass, showing a good flow from the internal mammary artery into the anterior descending coronary and its branches.

Results are somewhat encouraging, but significant data are not yet available. Such observations require several years.

VENTRICULAR ANEURYSM

HISTORICAL DATA. A few early attempts to excise ventricular aneurysms by a closed technique were made before the development of pump-oxygenators, but a precise, safe surgical technique with a pump-oxygenator was first employed by Cooley et al. in 1958. Initially the operation was rarely done; by 1962 a total of only 28 cases operated upon had been reported. By 1965 Effler et al. reported that 61 patients with such aneurysms had been operated upon at the Cleveland Clinic. With coronary bypass, excision of such aneurysms has become commonplace, usually combined with bypass grafting. By 1971 the Cleveland Clinic group alone had performed over 300 such procedures.

ETIOLOGY. Almost all aneurysms develop as a complication of myocardial infarction (Fig. 19-32). The reported frequency with which an aneurysm develops after an infarction varies from 10 to 15 percent.

PATHOLOGY AND PATHOPHYSIOLOGY. Most of the aneurysms which have been surgically treated have been located in the anterior portion of the left ventricle in the area supplied by the anterior descending coronary artery. Aneurysms of the posterior portion of the ventricle, an area supplied by the circumflex artery, have seldom been operated upon. It has been suggested that large aneurysms seldom arise in the posterior part of the left ventricle because of the attachments of the papillary muscles in this area, for a large infarction involving the attachments of the papillary muscles is usually fatal. Calcification may develop in the wall of a chronic aneurysm, but this is not common. Lower recently described several uncommon types of ventricular aneurysms.

An aneurysm with an expansile wall can impair function of the left ventricle, since energy developed during contraction of the left ventricle is dissipated into expanding the wall of the aneurysm. This may be recognized by fluoroscopy. The resulting decrease in cardiac function can increase the severity of congestive heart failure. Mural thrombi often develop in the aneurysm and may be a source of systemic embolization, although this is not frequent. Also, the aneurysm may enlarge and rupture, fortunately an uncommon complication. Rupture occurred in only 2 of 65 cases studied at autopsy by Abrams et al. Death in most patients with a left ventricular aneurysm is from further complications of the underlying coronary atherosclerosis, usually a subsequent myocardial infarction.

Prognosis of patients with an untreated left ventricular aneurysm was found by Schlichter et al. to be grim; 75 percent of the patients died within 3 years after the myocardial infarction. In contrast, a study of 65 patients by Abrams et al. found a much more favorable prognosis; the 5-year survival rate following myocardial infarction was 69 percent, and in only 14 percent of the patients was death considered to be a complication of the aneurysm. The patients studied by Abrams et al., however, had small

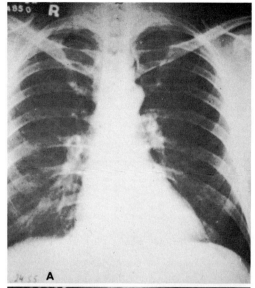

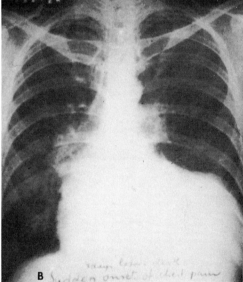

Fig. 19-32. Ventricular aneurysm. *A.* Chest roentgenogram showing a heart of normal size 2 days following an acute myocardial infarction. *B.* Chest roentgenogram showing cardiac enlargement from a large left ventricular aneurysm which progressively enlarged before a fatal episode of cardiac arrhythmia.

aneurysms in the posterior portion of the left ventricle, with an average diameter of 4 cm, which may explain the discrepancy in the two reports.

CLINICAL MANIFESTATIONS. No significant findings can be obtained from the patient's history or on physical examination to suggest the development of a ventricular aneurysm. The chest roentgenogram may show a suspicious bulge in the area of the left ventricle, but with small aneurysms the roentgenogram may appear normal. The electrocardiogram shows only the changes of coronary artery disease with a previous myocardial infarction. Small aneurysms are probably often not recognized, and in only

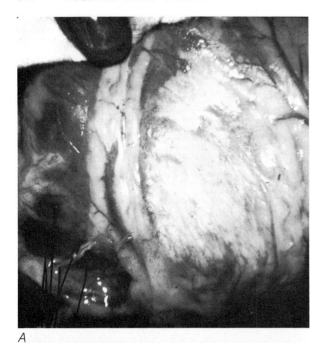

A

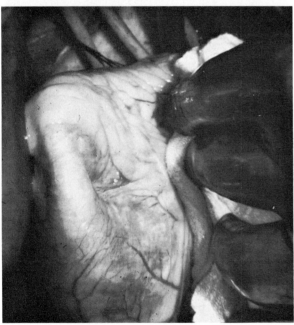

B

Fig. 19-33. *A*. Operative photograph of left ventricle, showing advanced destruction of the left ventricle from multiple myocardial infarcts. The heart has been turned upward so that the posterior surface of the left ventricle is exposed. *B*. During cardiopulmonary bypass, when suction was applied to the left ventricle, the ventricle collapsed readily, demonstrating that most of the ventricular muscle had been replaced by scar. The patient did not survive operation, and in retrospect it appears that the condition was probably inoperable because of extensive destruction of left ventricular muscle.

4 of the 65 cases studied by Abrams et al. was the diagnosis made before autopsy. The size of the aneurysm ranged up to 8 cm, with an average diameter of 4 cm, and all were located in the posterior portion of the ventricle.

Diagnosis can be made principally by cineangiography, outlining the size, location, and expansile nature of the aneurysm. Simultaneous coronary arteriography is of significant value, indicating the extent of the coronary artery disease and the consequent risk of operation. Preferably the cardiac output should be measured at the time of cardiac catheterization, in order to evaluate subsequent improvement of the patient following operation. In equivocal cases evaluation by cineangiography and catheterization should form the basis for a decision to excise the aneurysm. It seems probable that small left ventricular aneurysms are of negligible physiologic significance, while larger ones significantly impair cardiac function. Operation should be postponed for a minimum of 3 months after the preceding myocardial infarction because of the friability of the ventricular muscle.

TREATMENT. Technique of Operation. A sternotomy incision is preferred. Dissection of adherent pericardium over the aneurysm, usually obliterating the major portion of the pericardial cavity overlying the left ventricle, is postponed until cardiopulmonary bypass is started. Once bypass is established, the heart is fibrillated and a cannula inserted in the right interatrial groove into the left atrium and advanced across the mitral valve into the left ventricle. Suction through this cannula will decompress the aneurysm and facilitate dissection (Fig. 19-33). At this time the aneurysm is incised in its central portion and widely opened, carefully removing any laminated clot. If pericardial adhesions are extensive, the wall of the aneurysm is simply divided a short distance from the pericardial adhesions, leaving this part of the aneurysmal wall in situ and thus avoiding troublesome bleeding. Similarly, the wall of the aneurysm is divided about 2 cm from its junction with left ventricular muscle. When the opening of the aneurysm is sutured, most of the suture line includes the scar at the point of junction, and there is little compromise of the adjacent left ventricular muscle and no reduction in size of the left ventricular cavity (Fig. 19-34).

At New York University the frequency with which the wall of the aneurysm includes the area of the anterior descending coronary artery has been significant, for the scar may extend over into the ventricular septum. Preservation of the anterior descending coronary artery, often occluded proximally, may not be significant in some patients because the ventricular muscle supplied by the anterior descending coronary artery has been previously infarcted, but in other patients significant tributaries arise from this artery, especially to the ventricular septum. For this reason, before the aneurysm is excised, the anterior descending coronary artery is opened proximally and a probe inserted distad. With the inlying probe as a guide, sutures are placed between the anterior descending coronary artery and the aneurysm to define the margin of excision near the artery and thus avoid incorporating this vessel in the suture line. If bypass grafting is to be done, the bypass graft is attached to the artery while the aneurysm is opened. Subsequently the wall of the aneurysm is closed with two or three rows of continuous sutures, placing these through Teflon felt to reinforce the closure. Air is removed subsequently from the heart and the ventricle defibrillated.

This technique avoids several hazards associated with excision of an aneurysm. Extensive bleeding is avoided by not dissecting adhesions. There is no danger of reduction in size of the ventricular cavity or loss of functioning ventricular muscle from incorporation in the suture line to close the aneurysm, and the anterior descending coronary artery is revascularized. With these guidelines and precautions, operative excision has a very low mortality, and convalescence is usually uneventful. If the other coronary vessels, the right and the circumflex, are involved, bypass grafts are also inserted to these vessels.

PROGNOSIS. Substantial improvement has been reported following excision of large ventricular aneurysms. Actually this is the only cardiac operation in which preoperative congestive failure has been greatly improved by the surgical procedure. Disruption of the suture line with recurrence of the aneurysm has not been reported. In 1964 Cooley et al. reported experiences with 37 patients, with eight hospital deaths and five subsequent deaths. Thirteen patients at that time were living more than 3 years after operation, and substantial improvement had occurred in most of these. Catheterization studies before and after operation in seven patients showed an increase in cardiac output and regression of pulmonary hypertension, confirming the physiologic benefit following excision of large aneurysms. Most patients undergoing excision of a left ventricular aneurysm now often have concomitant bypass grafting; so the benefit from excision of the aneurysm per se cannot be easily determined.

PERICARDITIS

Acute Pyogenic Pericarditis

A purulent infection of the pericardium has been reported for many centuries, and some of the earliest operations in thoracic surgery involved resection of costal cartilages to drain a purulent pericarditis. In recent years, with the widespread availability of antibiotics, purulent pericarditis has become a rare disease, and few institutions have experiences with more than a few cases. In 1961 Boyle and associates reviewed 414 cases reported in the

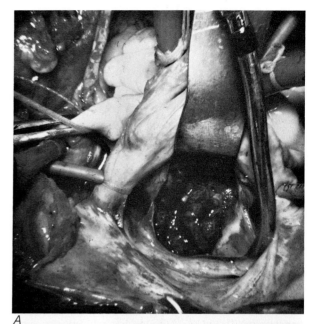

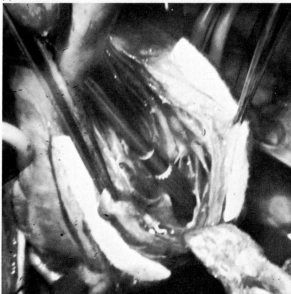

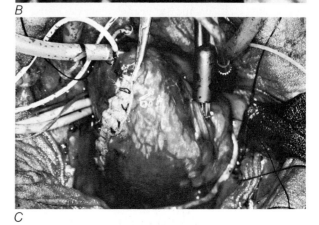

Fig. 19-34. *A.* Photograph of left ventricular aneurysm involving ▶ the posterior part of the left ventricle, an unusual location. *B.* The aneurysm has been excised, and the interior of the left ventricle is being inspected. The suction tip is within the ostium of the mitral valve, showing the proximity of the aneurysm to the mitral valve. The unusual occurrence of these aneurysms may be related to the fact that myocardial infarction in this area is often fatal because of concomitant mitral insufficiency. *C.* Completed repair of the aneurysm with a long suture line buttressed with Teflon felt. A coronary bypass graft is visible at the top of the field which was inserted into a branch of the circumflex coronary artery.

literature and added 11 of their own. At that time their group of 11 patients constituted one of the largest single series ever reported.

Formerly pneumococcal pericarditis was one of the most common types and developed in association with a pneumonic infection in the lungs. Such infections are now infrequent. Staphylococcal infection, by contrast, usually occurs as a complication of generalized septicemia from a septic focus in another area of the body. Less frequent forms of pericarditis include a streptococcal pericarditis, now rarely seen, and infection with such unusual organisms as *Hemophilus influenzae* or *Salmonella.*

An unrecognized, untreated purulent pericarditis usually terminates fatally. The clinical picture is that of an acute septic course, which soon includes signs of a pericardial effusion and may progress to cardiac tamponade. Simply considering the possibility of the disease is probably the main factor in making a correct diagnosis. Once the diagnosis has been considered, needle aspiration of the pericardial cavity can confirm or exclude it.

Treatment is with parenteral administration of appropriate antibiotics, combined with serial pericardial aspiration and instillation of antibiotics directly into the pericardial cavity. In patients not responding to therapy, surgical drainage may be required, but this has not always been necessary.

Chronic Constrictive Pericarditis

HISTORICAL DATA. The first successful pericardiectomy was performed by Rehn in 1913, although the theoretical basis for the operation had been suggested some years before. Subsequently, the first pericardiectomy in the United States was performed by Churchill in 1929. Initial operations were limited in scope, partly because of differences in philosophy as to what part and how much of the constricted pericardium should be removed. In the 1960s routine performance of a radical pericardiectomy became widely accepted with considerable improvement in results.

ETIOLOGY. In most patients the cause is unknown. Possibly the disease represents the end stages of an undiagnosed viral pericarditis. Tuberculosis was formerly thought to be the most frequent cause, but in recent years it has been responsible for less than 20 percent of cases in most series. Rarely, a traumatic hemopericardium can evolve to a constrictive pericarditis.

PATHOLOGY AND PATHOPHYSIOLOGY. The pericardial cavity is obliterated by dense scar tissue which encases and constricts the heart. In chronic cases areas of calcification develop in the fibrous tissue, resulting in an additional element of constriction.

The physiologic handicap from pericardial constriction is limitation of diastolic filling of the ventricles. Several sequelae result: Stroke volume is decreased with a resulting decrease in cardiac output, despite a compensatory tachycardia. Right ventricular diastolic pressure increases, with a corresponding increase in right atrial and central venous pressure, ranging from 15 to 40 cm water, the average elevation being 25 to 30 cm water. The venous hypertension produces hepatic enlargement, ascites, peripheral edema, and venous distension, accompanied by a gradual increase in blood volume.

CLINICAL MANIFESTATIONS. Symptoms. The disease is most common in patients in their second or third decade, but patients ranging from two to seventy-eight years have been reported. The youngest patient in our personal series of cases was three years old. The disease is a slowly progressive one with increasing ascites and edema. Fatigability and dyspnea on exertion are common complaints, but dyspnea is rare at rest. Ascites may be unusually severe. The diagnosis is easily confused with cirrhosis.

Physical Findings. Several unusual physical findings are commonly present. There may be striking enlargement of the liver with ascites, often in association with only moderate peripheral edema. Dilatation of peripheral veins is also prominent. Although these findings are the familiar ones of advanced congestive failure from heart disease, with constrictive pericarditis the usual cardiac findings are a heart of normal size without murmurs or abnormal sounds. Atrial fibrillation is present in about one-third of patients, and a pleural effusion in about one-half. The pulse pressure is normally decreased to a variable degree, and a paradoxic pulse, with obliteration of the pulse during deep inspiration, is found in a small percentage of patients.

Laboratory Findings. The venous pressure is regularly elevated to levels between 20 and 40 cm water. The electrocardiogram is not diagnostic but is almost always abnormal, with a low voltage and inversion of T waves. A chest roentgenogram often shows a heart of normal size, but calcification in the pericardium can be seen, often as a linear sheet, in about 50 percent of patients. Fluoroscopy may demonstrate decreased cardiac pulsations.

On cardiac catheterization several characteristic abnormalities are usually detected, although rarely these can also result from diffuse myocardial fibrosis from other causes. There is elevation of the right ventricular diastolic pressure to levels greater than one-third of right ventricular systolic pressure, and a corresponding increase in right atrial pressure. The contour of the right ventricular pressure pulse is characteristically altered, showing an early "dip" in diastole. A similarity of pressures in different cardiac chambers is frequently found, the right atrial pressure, the right ventricular diastolic pressure, the pulmonary artery diastolic pressure, and the pulmonary wedge pressure often being almost identical.

DIAGNOSIS. Once the diagnosis has been suspected from the clinical picture, it can usually be confirmed with findings from the electrocardiogram, chest roentgenogram, and catheterization data. Most diagnostic errors arise from failure to consider constrictive pericarditis, for it is a comparatively rare disease. The most frequent erroneous diagnoses are cirrhosis of the liver and congestive heart failure from other causes.

TREATMENT. Once the diagnosis has been established in a symptomatic patient, pericardiectomy should be performed. The incision may be a sternotomy or a bilateral thoracotomy in the left fifth and right fourth intercostal spaces with oblique division of the sternum. Bilateral thoracotomy provides ready exposure to all areas of the heart. The objective is extensive removal of the constricting pericardium from both ventricles, extending from one phrenic nerve to the other. Usually with displacement of the phrenic nerves laterally, the pericardium can be excised even posterior to the phrenic nerve back to the point of entry of the pulmonary veins, leaving thickened pericardium only behind the posterior portion of the heart. Removal of the pericardium from the atria and the venae cavae is physiologically less important, although we remove most of this pericardium as well. Dissection over the thin-walled atria involves some hazard of perforation and hemorrhage and must be done with caution. Particular care is required over the coronary vessels, leaving a small segment of thickened pericardium if it cannot be satisfactorily mobilized from the underlying coronary arteries.

It is helpful to measure intracardiac pressures by direct needle puncture before and following pericardiectomy. With an extensive pericardiectomy, the characteristic pressure changes present before operation are either eliminated or greatly improved.

Following operation many patients improve immediately with a massive diuresis of edema fluid, but others recover more slowly and require careful restriction of sodium intake with appropriate diuretic therapy for several months before recovery. Atrophy of myocardial muscle fibers compressed by scar tissue has been considered a probable cause of the prolonged convalescence. In the past, inadequate removal of the scarred pericardium was undoubtedly the most frequent cause of a poor result.

PROGNOSIS. The risk of operation varies with the age of the patient and the severity of the disease, but it is in the range of 10 to 12 percent. A good result can be anticipated in 80 to 85 percent of patients, although there is considerable discrepancy in the reports in the literature. In a series of 26 patients reported by Effler, 15 of the 26 obtained substantial improvement from operation while there was a total of nine early and late deaths. Schumacker and Roshe, however, have reported a total of 19 patients with 18 good results. In a long-term follow-up of 78 cases reported by Dalton et al., sustained improvement continuing over many years was found in patients initially obtaining a good result. A group of 40 cases has been reported from Vanderbilt University by Collins et al., including patients originally studied by Blalock and Burwell in 1941. Only 53 percent of 32 patients subjected to operation obtained an excellent result, but this series includes the early operations which are now considered inadequate.

HEART BLOCK AND PACEMAKERS

HISTORICAL DATA. Surgical therapy of complete heart block with an electric pacemaker has evolved with astonishing rapidity in the past 20 years. In 1951 Callaghan and Bigelow developed a transvenous pacemaker which could be used to stimulate the sinoatrial node, and the following year Zoll first described successful treatment of ventricular standstill by external electrical stimulation of the heart through the intact chest wall. In 1958 Lillehei and associates demonstrated that direct cardiac pacing could be performed with an electrode implanted in the left ventri-

cle, but long-term electrical stimulation with such electrodes traversing the chest wall ultimately resulted in infection. Between 1958 and 1962 many investigators contributed to the development of implantable, battery-powered pacemakers, including Chardack, Zoll and Frank, Senning, and Kantrowitz. Glenn has intensively studied radiofrequency stimulation of the heart with a transmitter through the intact chest wall, while Nathan and Center have evaluated pacemakers activated from impulses arising in the atrium, which are subsequently transmitted to the ventricle. Furman and Schwedel, in 1959, described permanent pacing of the heart with a transvenous catheter wedged into the endocardial surface of the right ventricle. Since 1962 modifications of this technique have made it the procedure of choice, with the catheter implanted under local anesthesia and subsequently connected to an implanted pacemaker in a subcutaneous pocket. The great strides made in this field are well illustrated by the fact that as recently as 1957 the first implantable pacemakers were being used. Since 1962 over 10,000 have been inserted.

ETIOLOGY. Complete heart block in elderly patients is usually due to progressive fibrosis of the conduction system. It was formerly thought to be a complication of coronary artery disease or hypertension, but increasing experience has indicated that it may represent an isolated fibrotic disease involving the conduction system. Congenital heart block is very rare, less than 200 patients having been reported in the literature. Heart block from surgical trauma during repair of intracardiac defects has decreased in frequency but still remains a serious postoperative complication. It usually results from direct injury to the bundle of His. Heart block following myocardial infarction is usually transitory in surviving patients. Infections or tumors have been reported, in isolated instances, to cause heart block.

PATHOLOGY AND PATHOPHYSIOLOGY. In normal cardiac conduction the cardiac impulse arises in the sinoatrial node located near the junction of the superior vena cava with the wall of the right atrium. The impulse is propagated through the wall of the right atrium to the atrioventricular (AV) node, lying medial to the ostium of the coronary sinus. From this node it travels along the bundle of His near the annulus of the tricuspid valve to pass through the central fibrous body of the ventricular septum near the junction of the muscular and membranous components. In this area the conduction bundle divides into the right and left bundles, which in turn travel to different areas of the respective ventricles. The most common surgical trauma producing complete heart block occurs during the repair of a ventricular septal defect and also during repair of an ostium primum defect. More rarely it can occur during prosthetic valve replacement of the aortic valve, mitral valve, or tricuspid valve, as there are areas along the annulus of any of these three valves where the bundle of His can be injured. Surgical injuries of either the right or left conduction bundle are usually not of clinical significance.

Heart block, of whatever degree, may seriously impair cardiac output by any of a number of mechanisms. With complete heart block the resulting bradycardia, varying from 25 to as high as 60 beats per minute, may decrease coronary and cerebral circulation. There may be progressive refractory congestive heart failure even with rates as high as 45, marked intolerance to exercise, and even symptoms of cerebrovascular insufficiency with syncope and convulsions. With complete AV dissociation there may be periods of transient ventricular asystole with cessation of cardiac output, syncope, convulsions, and even death if asystole continues. In some patients, rather than standstill, there may be equally disastrous bouts of ventricular tachycardia or ventricular fibrillation. In others there may be only periodic marked accentuation of the bradycardia. With lesser degrees of heart block, although the cardiac rate is usually normal, abrupt transition to complete AV dissociation with any of its complications can occur. Any one episode may be followed by complete recovery with resumption of the pre-attack rhythm, or it may result in death.

Attacks of syncope and convulsions due to sudden alterations of cardiac output from heart block have long been designated as the Stokes-Adams syndrome. Some patients with a low cardiac output from severe bradycardia become disabled with progressive cardiac failure but never develop Stokes-Adams syndrome.

It is a curious and as yet unexplained phenomenon that with ventricular standstill from heart block, mechanical or electric energy delivered to the heart will result in intermittent ventricular contractions. Thus, even rhythmic thumping of the chest wall may result in 1:1 ventricular responses until the ventricles resume their intrinsic rhythmic contractions.

CLINICAL MANIFESTATIONS. Although some patients may be asymptomatic with a rate as low as 30 to 35 beats per minute, most patients have symptoms with a rate less than 45 per minute. Episodic Stokes-Adams attacks are the most frequent disability, between which the patient feels entirely well. During such episodes, there is the sudden onset of syncope, often followed by convulsions. Examination reveals severe bradycardia or cardiac standstill. Recovery depends upon the spontaneous return of cardiac contractions. In milder forms, recurrent syncope for a short period may be the only symptom. Then, the differential diagnosis must consider heart block, aortic stenosis, simple syncope, carotid sinus syndrome, epilepsy, or occlusive arterial disease of the cerebral circulation. When a complete heart block is present, the diagnosis can be quickly established with the electrocardiogram. With an intermittent heart block, continuous electrocardiographic monitoring may be necessary.

With intermittent heart block there may be no definite findings between syncopal attacks. However, certain electrocardiographic findings are suggestive. Bi-bundle branch block, degrees of block less than complete AV dissociation and the Möbius II type, usually signify impending or intermittent AV dissociation. Attempts have been made to induce heart block under controlled conditions to confirm the diagnosis. One method reported by the author involved atrial pacing to rates of 120 or less, which ordinarily does not affect normal conduction.

Some patients become disabled from progressive heart failure simply as a result of inadequate cardiac output. Dramatic improvement, with a prompt diuresis of many liters of fluid, may follow insertion of a pacemaker.

TREATMENT. Physiology of Cardiac Pacemakers. The electrical resistance of the normal heart is 300 to 350 ohms, and the fibrillating threshold to electrical stimulation is at least ten times greater. The efficacy of cardiac pacemakers depends upon the ability of the heart in ventricular standstill to respond to short bursts (2 milliseconds) of small electric voltages, usually less than 7 volts. The current is effective if delivered directly to the heart or through the chest wall. This may be accomplished by having both positive and negative electrodes in or on the heart, the so-called bipolar systems, or by having only one electrode in contact with the heart and the indifferent electrode at a distant site in the body, the unipolar system. The electrodes may be implanted directly into the myocardium (epicardial electrodes) or passed into the right ventricular chamber via a major vein for contact with the endocardium (pervenous endocardial electrodes).

The electric current can be delivered at fixed rates, usually 65 to 72, which quite effectively will override and suppress spontaneous ventricular activity of hearts in complete AV dissociation in which rates are usually 45 or slower. This results in prevention of Stokes-Adams attacks due to ventricular standstill, ventricular tachycardia, or ventricular fibrillation, as well as in marked improvement in cardiac output, as much as 50 to 80 percent. There is frequently an impressive improvement in exercise tolerance, with regression of any overt signs of cardiac failure, and not infrequently an impressive diuresis even in the absence of these overt signs. Despite the fixed rates of stimulation, variations in cardiac output are quite effectively achieved by variations in cardiac stroke volume, so that many patients have tolerated major operative procedures such as prostatectomies, gastrectomies, and aneurysmectomies, and have carried pregnancies to term and successful delivery. Rates higher than 70 to 75 beats per minute have not resulted in significant increases in cardiac output and have been employed only in the rare instances where higher rates were required to suppress attacks of ventricular fibrillation.

Variations of the fixed-rate mode of delivery of the stimulus were sought to correct certain problems which became evident during early pacemaker experience. The most significant of these was a markedly decreased fibrillatory threshold to electric currents under certain conditions such as hypokalemia or during acute myocardial infarction. In patients who either did not have complete AV dissociation at the time of pacemaker implant or who had return of intermittent AV conduction after periods of electrical pacing, the coincidence of the fixed-rate stimulus with the "supernormal phase" of the cardiac cycle might precipitate ventricular fibrillation if the patient sustained an acute myocardial infarct or became hypokalemic. This led to the so-called "demand" pacemaker, which may be of the R-wave-suppressed or R-wave-triggered type. In both, the electrode acts as an element which senses beginning ventricular depolarization. In one the pacemaker output is suppressed, and no artifact appears on the electrocardiogram, while in the other the pacemaker discharge occurs during the refractory period of the heart, and the artifact is seen on the electrocardiogram within the QR segment. This seems to have quite effectively eliminated the problem. However, suppressing the pacemaker discharge when it is not needed does not appear to increase the life expectancy of the pacemaker.

Asynchrony between atrial and ventricular contractions which impair cardiac output, and the limitations of rate imposed by ventricular pacemakers, led to the development by Nathan and associates of the P-wave-activated pacemaker, which senses atrial depolarization and synchronizes the delivery of the ventricular stimulus to coincide with atrial activity. Although this system is more "physiologic," it requires more complex circuitry and implantation of electrodes on the atrium as well as the ventricle via thoracotomy. Significant advantages have not yet been proved; its final evaluation will have to await its availability as a simple unit implanted pervenously.

Selection of Patients for Operation. All asymptomatic patients with acquired heart block should probably have a pacemaker inserted if the cardiac rate is below 45 beats per minute. Patients with rates of 50 to 60 per minute may be safely observed, but the possibility always exists that the first Stokes-Adams attack may be a fatal one. Patients with syncopal episodes from intermittent complete block, even though asymptomatic between attacks, should, after exclusion of other causes of syncope, also receive cardiac pacemakers. Medical therapy of symptomatic complete heart block with myocardial stimulants such as isoproterenol has been associated with a high mortality. In one group of 100 patients treated before pacemakers were developed, 30 percent were dead in 6 months and 75 percent within 5 years. A heart block resulting from acute myocardial infarction usually can be treated by temporarily pacing the heart with an electrode catheter introduced through a peripheral vein and advanced into the right ventricle. The block usually disappears as the patient recovers from the infarction.

Heart block following intracardiac operations is a grave complication, requiring a pacemaker if the block is permanent. Most such problems develop at operation and can be prophylactically treated by leaving an electrode wire in the ventricle before the thoracotomy incision is sutured. Stimulation can be performed through the wire for several days, but prolonged use of the unit is inadvisable because of the risk of infection. It was found by Lillehei and associates, reporting experiences with 40 patients with complete heart block in 1963, that a heart block lasting more than 1 month after operation was almost always permanent. Until that time, some hope remains that the complete block is temporary and may subside with healing of the intracardiac wound.

In some unfortunate patients a complete block may develop several months following a cardiac operation, probably from progressive fibrosis near the conduction bundle. With a cardiac rate less than 50 beats per minute, it is probably wise to implant a permanent pacemaker before the patient leaves the hospital, especially if the

block has persisted longer than 1 month after operation. A study of 20 patients discharged without pacemakers found an appalling mortality of 80 percent in subsequent years. Because of the complications of pacemaker use in a small child, some investigators have cautiously managed a few asymptomatic children without pacemaker implantation with better long-term results than those reported earlier by Lillehei and associates.

Technique of Endocardiac Catheter Pacing. This technique is preferred at present, because the procedure can be performed with little risk under local anesthesia in the cardiac catheterization laboratory. It has become increasingly popular since 1962. A total of 305 patients so treated were reported by Lagergren and associates in 1966, with a 16 percent mortality in the subsequent years. Twenty-one patients over eighty years of age had been treated, with only four subsequent deaths. Furman et al. have described experiences with 38 patients with two postoperative deaths, neither of which was related to cardiac conduction.

When the catheter pacemaker is inserted in the cardiac catheterization laboratory, the right cephalic vein is exposed under local anesthesia, after which the electrode catheter is introduced and advanced into the right ventricle, where, under fluoroscopic control, it is wedged firmly into the trabeculae near the apex of the ventricle (Figs. 19-35 and 19-36). A stylet in the catheter facilitates intro-

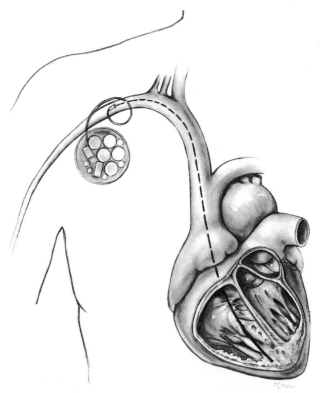

Fig. 19-35. Diagrammatic illustration of transvenous pacemaker. The endovascular electrode is advanced from the subclavian vein to imbed the apex of the electrode near the apex of the right ventricle. Subsequently, the pacemaker unit is implanted in a subcutaneous position on the right anterior chest wall. (*Adapted from Furman et al., Ann Surg, 164:468, 1966.*)

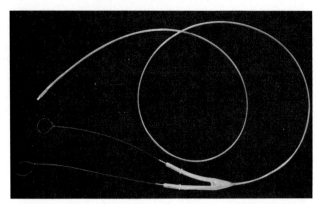

Fig. 19-36. Electrode with stylet wires in position to facilitate insertion. The stylet wires are subsequently removed. (*Photograph supplied by Medtronic, Inc., Minneapolis, Minn.*)

duction and can be subsequently removed. Once the catheter is firmly in place, a subcutaneous infraclavicular pocket is prepared through a separate short incision in which the pulse generator is implanted (Fig. 19-37). We have preferred the Medtronic unit developed by Chardack and associates. The catheter is tied in the cephalic vein, advanced under the intervening skin to the infraclavicular pocket, and connected to the generator, sealing the connections with Silastic adhesive. The incisions are then closed by simple suture (Fig. 19-38). Catheter selection is considered important. Platinum-iridium spring coil catheters measuring 3.2 mm in diameter seem to be an ideal compromise between larger catheters which maintain position well but may produce cardiac tamponade from perforation of the heart and smaller ones which have a higher incidence of displacement.

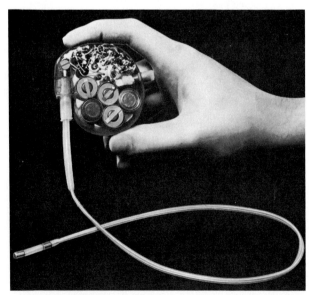

Fig. 19-37. Chardack-Greatbatch pacemaker with the attached transvenous electrode for insertion into the right ventricle. (*Photograph supplied by Medtronic, Inc., Minneapolis, Minn.*)

Complications of this technique have been numerous but have been managed without patient mortality. Imparato and Kim, reporting on a 10-year experience, described 31.5 percent of cases with complications, all of which were successfully managed.

Technique of Direct Myocardial Implantation. When for any reason a transvenous catheter cannot be successfully inserted, a left thoracotomy is performed for direct implantation of the electrodes in the left ventricle. Anesthesia in such patients is a significant risk but can be minimized by the preliminary insertion of an electrode catheter through a peripheral vein into the ventricle, followed by commencement of electrical pacing before anesthesia is induced. Before this technique was routinely adopted, induction of anesthesia often provoked serious arrhythmias, even cardiac arrest or ventricular fibrillation.

A short thoracotomy through the left fifth intercostal space is preferred, with subsequent incision in the pericardium anterior to the phrenic nerve. The pacemaker is placed in a separate subcutaneous pocket below the costal margin, after which the electrodes are brought under the costal margin into the pericardial cavity and buried in the left ventricular muscle, preferably near the base of the heart (Fig. 19-40). The electrodes are composed of platinum-iridium, which has been found preferable to stainless steel. Much care should be taken to avoid acute bends in the electrode wires because of the risk of subsequent flexion and breakage of the wires. Our preference for such units is the helical spring electrodes associated with the Medtronic generator developed by Chardack. Once the implanted pacemaker is functioning properly, the previously inserted transvenous pacemaker is removed.

Temporary Cardiac Pacing. After an acute myocardial infarction associated with a heart block, temporary cardiac pacing is preferably done with an electrode catheter inserted through a peripheral vein. If a catheter pacemaker cannot be quickly inserted, the heart can be stimulated directly through needles implanted subcutaneously over the anterior chest wall.

Postoperative Care. In the immediate postoperative course, the electrocardiogram should be closely monitored both to be certain that the pacemaker is functioning properly and to detect any ectopic rhythms. Such rhythms may appear because of increased myocardial irritability, with a resulting lowering of threshold to electrical stimulation. These ectopic rhythms can be controlled by potassium or procainamide.

Diaphragmatic contractions may occur with either electrode system, either from stimulation of the phrenic nerve or by direct stimulation of the diaphragm. With endocardial systems the catheter tip usually must be repositioned.

Following discharge from the hospital the patients should follow their pulse rates daily. The patient or a member of the family can be taught to count the radial pulse for a full minute and report any variations at once. A transistorized portable radio placed over the pulse generator may sense the rhythmic pacemaker discharge. At present rapid oscilloscopic scanning of the pacemaker artifacts through signals transmitted via the telephone is

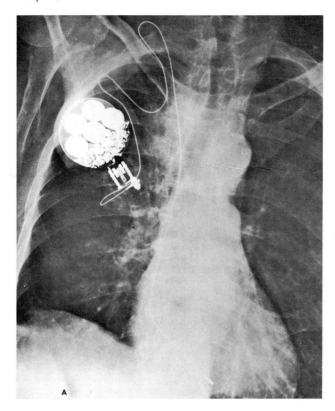

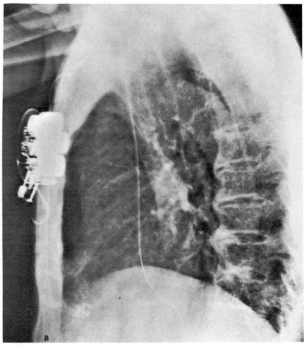

Fig. 19-38. *A.* Chest roentgenogram of a patient with the endocardiac electrode in position and the pacemaker implanted in a subcutaneous pocket on the anterior chest wall. *B.* Lateral roentgenogram showing the position of the endocardiac catheter and the pacemaker unit.

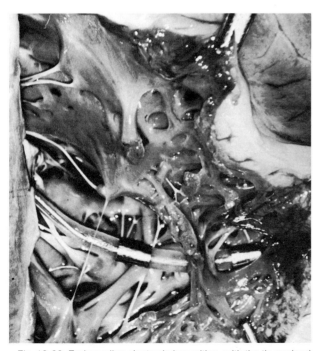

Fig. 19-39. Endocardiac electrode in position, with the tip wedged in the trabeculae lining the right ventricle. (*From W. M. Chardack, A. A. Gage, A. J. Federica, G. Schimert, and W. Greatbatch, The Long-Term Treatment of Heart Block, Prog Cardiovasc Dis, 9:105, 1966. Reprinted by permission of Grune & Stratton, Inc., New York.*)

possible. Battery depletion usually becomes manifest by gradual slowing of the pacemaker discharge rate. Failure with marked acceleration of the rate, the "runaway pacemaker," has been eliminated by changing the internal circuitry. Sudden failure with cessation of all pacemaker output, usually due to circuitry failure, has been virtually eliminated.

At present, most pacemakers require change between the second and third years due to battery depletion. Attempts to prolong their usefulness by use of radioactive isotopic electric generators and variable output have not yet proved to be of value.

PROGNOSIS. In a series of patients reported by Chardack and associates, 55 percent were alive 4 years following implantation of a pacemaker. Since many patients were aged and had other diseases, death was often unrelated to the function of the pacemaker. Zoll et al., one of the earliest investigators of permanent implantation of pacemakers, reported experiences with 77 patients in 1964; there were 16 subsequent deaths, 8 of which were related to the cardiac condition. In at least some of these 8, death was related to an arrhythmia of uncertain cause. These uncertainties emphasize clearly the need for careful long-term observation of patients with pacemakers to detect either the appearance of ectopic rhythms or signs of malfunction of the pulse generator.

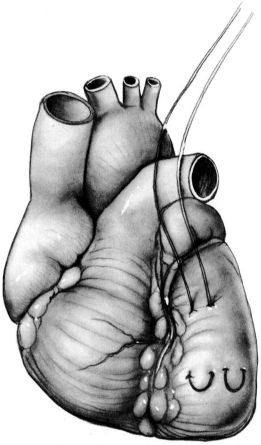

Fig. 19-40. Transthoracic method of implantation of electrodes in the anterior wall of the right ventricle, as developed by Frank, Zoll, and others. The two electrodes are implanted on the anterior wall of the left ventricle. Great care is taken to avoid any kinking of the wires as they are inserted, because of the subsequent danger of breakage from repeated flexion. (*Adapted from Zoll et al., Ann Surg, 160:356, 1964.*)

CARDIAC TRANSPLANTATION, ASSISTED CIRCULATION, AND ARTIFICIAL HEARTS

For certain forms of advanced heart disease, cure seems possible only with cardiac transplantation or the implantation of an artificial heart. This occurs with some complex congenital anomalies, but most commonly with advanced coronary artery disease in which more than 40 percent of the left ventricular muscle mass has been destroyed. Significant experimental progress has been made with both forms of treatment, but ultimate solution remains unclear at this time. Both are active fields of laboratory investigation. Subsequent paragraphs will briefly describe the status of these areas as of late 1972.

Cardiac Transplantation

After Barnard accomplished the first human heart transplant, clinical successes in the United States followed, and

a wave of enthusiasm for transplantation rapidly mounted throughout the world. It was quickly demonstrated that transplantation could be done with an acceptable mortality rate and good initial cardiovascular function. Subsequent experiences demonstrated, however, that the problem of immunologic rejection had been far underestimated and that most patients succumbed from this process within several months. For unknown reasons, probably a fortuitous immunologic match between donor and recipient, a small percentage of patients have continued to do well after cardiac transplantation, and one is now well over 4 years since operation.

However, the procedure has been abandoned in almost all centers except as a research investigation by Shumway and associates. Their experiences are summarized in a report by Dong et al. in late 1972; 42 patients had undergone transplantation, 16 of whom were still alive; 12 of 31 survived 1 year; 7 of 20 survived 2 years; and 2 of 14 survived 3 years. Operations were usually performed for end-stage coronary artery disease and occasionally for idiopathic myopathy. Constant supervision for early signs of cardiac rejection had been mandatory. Immunosuppression included administration of azathioprine, prednisone, and antilymphocyte globulin. In addition, rejection crises were treated with actinomycin D, massive amounts of methylprednisilone, and systemic heparinization. Cardiac function in surviving patients was reasonably good, with 13 patients returning to compensatory work or active housekeeping. No precise correlation had been found between immunologic assays and long-term function.

Until further advances in the immunology of organ transplantation are made, cardiac transplantation will probably remain a research study limited to large centers where constant surveillance of surviving patients is possible.

Assisted Circulation and Artificial Hearts

THEORETIC CONSIDERATIONS. The concept of assisting the failing heart by pumping part or all of the circulation through a heart-lung machine as a parallel circuit is, on first glance, a simple and attractive one. One of the first observations of the possible beneficial effects of assisted circulation was made by Senning, who noted that an injured left ventricle incapable of supporting the circulation after an intracardiac operation might recover if extracorporeal circulation was continued for 30 to 60 minutes. Apparently the injury of the left ventricle was reversible.

Subsequent investigation of this seemingly simple hypothesis encountered many problems: First, attempting to "rest" a contracting left ventricle is a complex undertaking. Unless the left ventricle is decompressed during cardiopulmonary bypass, which requires the insertion of a cannula into the left atrium and left ventricle, blood will continue to accumulate in the left ventricle, which in turn will contract as a closed chamber against closed mitral and aortic valves. Left ventricular systolic pressure must then exceed that produced in the aorta by the extracorporeal pump, as a result of which oxygen requirements of the contracting left ventricle remain near those levels existing before the extracorporeal pump was used. Hence, although most of the circulation may be supplied from an extracorporeal pump, a contracting left ventricle intermittently ejecting a small amount of blood may metabolize a large amount of oxygen, and thus not be significantly "rested."

If a peripheral circulatory bypass is employed, as with a venoarterial circuit, the left ventricle can actually be harmed. Blood pumped into a peripheral artery from the extracorporeal pump may increase work requirements of the ventricle as it contracts and attempts to propel blood through the aortic valve, which is being maintained in a closed position by the pressure generated from the "assist" circulatory device. Electronic synchronization of the natural heart and the artificial heart so that the artificial heart infuses blood during diastole is physiologically of greater benefit.

A second hypothesis—that recovery of a failing heart would be aided by "resting" the heart with assisted circulation—has also been difficult to demonstrate. The most encouraging data are from experiments in which an acute, reversible injury has occurred, such as transient anoxia, where extracorporeal circulation for 30 minutes to 1 hour may permit recovery. With an extensive injury, such as a myocardial infarction, how long extracorporeal circulation would be required is unknown. It seems likely that bypass for several days may be necessary, during which time collateral circulation could develop around the acutely occluded coronary artery.

TECHNIQUES OF ASSISTED CIRCULATION. Intraaortic Balloon Pumping. In the past 2 years the most effective technique for assisted circulation has been intraaortic balloon pumping. A balloon catheter is inserted into a peripheral artery, usually the femoral, and advanced into the thoracic aorta. With electronic synchronization, the balloon is alternately inflated during diastole and deflated during systole. This intermittent inflation is of significant benefit to the peripheral circulation, but careful synchronization is essential. Inflation of the balloon during systole actually may harm the left ventricle as it attempts to open the aortic valve against the pressure generated by the inflating balloon. Careful experimental and clinical studies with balloon pumping have been reported by several investigators, including Goetz and Austen.

Left Heart Bypass. A decade ago Dennis demonstrated the benefits of assisted circulation with left heart bypass, withdrawing blood from the atrium and infusing it into a peripheral artery. Difficulties with closed chest cannulation of the left atrium, however, have thus far greatly limited application of the procedure. Several years ago the author and associates applied left heart bypass in a small group of patients by direct cannulation of the left atrium through a thoracotomy incision and employing perfusion for periods of 3 to 4 hours, but longer periods of perfusion were impractical because of the necessity for thoracotomy. In recent months, at New York University, a special transvenous cannula has been developed by Glassman and associates which permits closed-chest cannulation of the left atrium through a modification of the transseptal puncture technique. First a standard transseptal left atrial puncture is done, introducing the needle and catheter

through the femoral vein. A guide wire is subsequently introduced, after which the special large bore (28 F) catheter is advanced over the guide wire into the left atrium. With this large catheter bypass flow rates as great as 4 liters/minute have been obtained. This technical advance may increase the applicability of left heart bypass, especially as the circulatory support feasible is far greater than that attainable with intraaortic balloon pumping.

Peripheral Bypass. A peripheral bypass may be a venoarterial bypass in which venous blood is withdrawn, oxygenated, and returned into a peripheral artery. As indicated earlier, such perfusion should be synchronized to return blood during diastole. Alternatively, a venovenous bypass can be used, returning the blood from the oxygenator into a peripheral vein. Hill and associates have reported on extensive use of this technique for the treatment of acute pulmonary insufficiency, employing a membrane oxygenator and continuing perfusion for several days.

A number of other techniques have been attempted for assisted circulation, such as counterpulsation or synchronized application of external pressure to the extremities, but none have found widespread clinical use. The main limitation of all techniques is that short periods of assisted circulation seem of little value unless the underlying cardiac injury can be corrected. As myocardial infarction is the most common cause of such injury, there has been an increasing tendency to perform emergency coronary bypass if short periods of assisted circulation are ineffective. Significant data with this approach, however, are not yet available.

ARTIFICIAL HEARTS. The ideal solution to many difficult cardiac problems would be a satisfactory mechanical heart. The National Heart and Lung Institute for the past few years has coordinated a large multidisciplinary program directed toward this goal, studying many engineering, physical, chemical, and hematologic problems. Recent experiences in an attempt to develop a nuclear-fueled support system were summarized by Norman et al. Bernhard has successfully implanted left ventricular bypass pumps in calves for periods of several months. DeBakey and associates, Kolff, Bernstein, Shumacker, and Timmis are leading some of the many groups continuing active investigation in this area.

One major obstacle is the inability to pump blood without the use of heparin. Continuous heparinization results in intractable bleeding, while pumping without heparin results in thromboembolism. Development of a technique which will enable pumps to be used for several days, weeks, even months, without heparin would be a major advance.

Future basic questions concerning long-term assisted circulation include not only indications for its use but how long it should be employed and how benefits can be measured. It probably will be employed primarily for patients with massive myocardial infarction, supporting the circulation for long periods during which collateral circulation may permit recovery. If injury proves irreversible, a decision must be made about either cardiac transplantation or an artificial heart. With myocardial infarction, replacement of the left ventricle rather than the entire heart should be sufficient if cardiac conduction remains intact with a functioning right ventricle.

References

Introduction; Clinical Manifestations

Gibbon, J. H., Jr., Sabiston, D. C., Jr., and Spencer, F. C.: "Surgery of the Chest," 2d ed., W. B. Saunders Company, Philadelphia, 1969.

Hurst, J. W., and Logue, R. B.: "The Heart, Arteries, and Veins," 2d ed., McGraw-Hill Book Company, New York, 1970.

Extracorporeal Circulation

Allen, J. G. (ed.): "Extracorporeal Circulation," Charles C Thomas, Publisher, Springfield, Ill., 1958.

Bahnson, H. T., and Spencer, F. C.: Extracorporeal Circulation, in C. D. Benson et al. (eds.), "Pediatric Surgery," vol. I, Year Book Medical Publishers, Inc., Chicago, 1962.

Boyd, A. D., Tremblay, R. E., Spencer, F. C., and Bahnson, H. T.: Estimation of Cardiac Output Soon after Intracardiac Surgery with Cardiopulmonary Bypass, *Ann Surg*, **150:**613, 1959.

Clowes, G. H. A., Jr.: Extracorporeal Maintenance of Circulation and Respiration, *Physiol Rev*, **40:**826, 1960.

DeWall, R. A., Warden, H. E., Varco, R. L., and Lillehei, C. W.: The Helix Reservoir Pump-Oxygenator, *Surg Gynecol Obstet*, **104:**699, 1957.

Ellison, L. T., Duke, J. F., III, and Ellison, R. G.: Pulmonary Compliance following Open-Heart Surgery and Its Relationship to Ventilation and Gas Exchange, *Circulation*, **35**(*Suppl 1*):217, 1967.

Gibbon, J. H., Jr.: Application of a Mechanical Heart and Lung Apparatus to Cardiac Surgery, *Minn Med*, **37:**171, 1954.

Jones, R. E., Donald, D. E., Swan, H. J. C., Harshbarger, H. G., Kirklin, J. W., and Wood, E. H.: Apparatus of the Gibbon Type for Mechanical Bypass of the Heart and Lungs: Preliminary Report, *Proc Staff Meetings Mayo Clin*, **30:**105, 1955.

McGoon, D. C., Moffitt, E. A., Theye, R. A., and Kirklin, J. W.: Physiologic Studies during High Flow, Normothermic, Whole Body Perfusion, *J Thorac Cardiovasc Surg*, **39:**275, 1960.

Porter, G. A., Kloster, F. E., Herr, R. H., Starr, A., Griswold, H. E., and Kimsey, J. A.: Renal Complications Associated with Valve Replacement Surgery, *J Thorac Cardiovasc Surg*, **53:**145, 1967.

————, Starr, A., Kimsey, J., and Lenertz, H.: Mannitol Hemodilution-Perfusion: The Kinetics of Mannitol Distribution and Excretion during Cardiopulmonary Bypass, *J Surg Res*, **10:**447, 1967.

Sachdev, N. S., Carter, C. C., Swank, R. L., and Blachly, P. H.: Relationship between Post-Cardiotomy Delirium, Clinical Neurological Changes, and EEG Abnormalities, *J Thorac Cardiovasc Surg*, **54:**557, 1967.

Spencer, F. C., Benson, D. W., Liu, W. C., and Bahnson, H. T.: Use of a Mechanical Respirator in the Management of Respiratory Insufficiency following Trauma or Operation for Cardiac or Pulmonary Disease, *J Thorac Cardiovasc Surg*, **38:**758, 1959.

Cardiac Arrest and Ventricular Fibrillation

Joseph, W. L., and Maloney, J. V., Jr.: Extracorporeal Circulation as an Adjunct to Resuscitation of the Heart, *JAMA*, **193:**683, 1965.

Jude, J. R., and Elam, J. O.: "Fundamentals of Cardiopulmonary Resuscitation," F. A. Davis Company, Philadelphia, 1965.

Kouwenhoven, W. B., Jude, J. R., and Knickerbocker, G. G.: Closed Chest Cardiac Massage, *JAMA*, **137:**1064, 1960.

————, Milnor, W. R., Knickerbocker, G. G., and Chestnut, W. R.: Closed Chest Defibrillation of the Heart, *Surgery*, **42:**550, 1957.

Spencer, F. C., and Bahnson, H. T.: Treatment of Cardiac Arrest, in C. D. Benson et al. (eds.), "Pediatric Surgery," vol. I, p. 522, Year Book Medical Publishers, Inc., Chicago, 1962.

Williams, G. R., and Spencer, F. C.: The Clinical Use of Hypothermia following Cardiac Arrest, *Ann Surg*, **148:**462, 1958.

Zimmerman, J. M., and Spencer, F. C.: The Influence of Hypothermia on Cerebral Injury Resulting from Circulatory Occlusion, *Surg Forum*, **9:**216, 1958.

Mitral Stenosis

Bailey, C. P.: The Surgical Treatment of Mitral Stenosis (Mitral Commissurotomy), *Dis Chest*, **15:**377, 1949.

Bryant, L. R., and Trinkle, J. K.: Mitral Valvotomy in the Valve Replacement Era, *Ann Surg*, **173:**1024, 1971.

Cutler, E. C., and Levine, S. A.: Cardiotomy and Valvulotomy for Mitral Stenosis, *N Engl J Med*, **188:**1023, 1923.

Duvoisin, G. E., Brandenburg, R. O., and McGoon, D. C.: Factors Influencing Embolism Associated with Prosthetic Heart Valves, *Circulation*, **35**(*Suppl 1*):70, 1967.

Ellis, L. B., Harken, D. E., and Black, H.: A Clinical Study of 1000 Consecutive Cases of Mitral Stenosis Two to Nine Years after Mitral Valvuloplasty, *Circulation*, **19:**803, 1959.

Gerami, S., Messmer, B. J., Hallman, G. L., and Cooley, D. A.: Open Mitral Commissurotomy: Results of 100 Consecutive Cases, *J Thorac Cardiovasc Surg*, **62:**366, 1971.

Gerbode, F.: Transventricular Mitral Valvulotomy, *Circulation*, **21:**563, 1960.

Harken, D. E., Ellis, L. B., Ware, P. E., and Normal, L. R.: The Surgical Treatment of Mitral Stenosis, *N Engl J Med*, **239:**801, 1948.

Higgs, L. M., Glancy, D. L., O'Brien, K. P., Epstein, S. E., and Morrow, A. G.: Mitral Restenosis: An Uncommon Cause of Recurrent Symptoms following Mitral Commissurotomy, *Am J Cardiol*, **26:**34, 1970.

Kiser, I. O., Hoeksema, T. D., Connolly, D. C., and Ellis, F. H., Jr.: Long-Term Results of Closed Mitral Commissurotomy, *J Cardiovasc Surg*, **8:**263, 1967.

Logan, A., and Turner, R.: Surgical Treatment of Mitral Stenosis with Particular Reference to the Transventricular Approach with a Mechanical Dilator, *Lancet*, **2:**874, 1959.

Morrow, A. G., and Braunwald, N. S.: Transventricular Mitral Commissurotomy: Surgical Technique and a Hemodynamic Evaluation of the Method, *J Thorac Cardiovasc Surg*, **41:**225, 1961.

Nathaniels, E. K., Moncure, A. C., and Scannell, J. G.: A Fifteen-Year Follow-up Study of Closed Mitral Valvuloplasty, *Ann Thorac Surg*, **10:**27, 1970.

Nichols, H. T., Blanco, G., Morse, D. P., Adam, A., and Baltazar,

N.: Open Mitral Commissurotomy: Experience with 200 Consecutive Cases, *JAMA*, **182:**268, 1962.

Olinger, G. N., Rio, F. W., and Maloney, J. V., Jr.: Closed Valvulotomy for Calcific Mitral Stenosis, *J Thorac Cardiovasc Surg*, **62:**357, 1971.

Roe, B. B., Edmunds, L. H., Jr., Fishman, N. H., and Hutchinson, J. C.: Open Mitral Valvulotomy, *Ann Thorac Surg*, **12:**483, 1971.

Selzer, A., and Cohn, K. E.: Natural History of Mitral Stenosis: A Review, *Circulation*, **45:**878, 1972.

Souttar, P. W.: The Surgical Treatment of Mitral Stenosis, *Br Med J*, **2:**603, 1925.

Spencer, F. C., Cortes, L., Marcarenhas, G., Ifuku, M., and Koepke, J.: The Mechanism of Thrombus Formation upon the Starr-Edwards Prosthetic Mitral Valve, *Ann Surg*, **165:**814, 1967.

Starr, A.: Mitral Valve Replacement with Ball Valve Prostheses, *J Thorac Cardiovasc Surg*, **64:**354, 1972.

——— and Edwards, M. L.: Mitral Replacement: Clinical Experience with a Ball Valve Prosthesis, *Ann Surg*, **154:**726, 1961.

———, Herr, R. H., and Wood, J. A.: Mitral Replacement: Review of Six Years' Experience, *J Thorac Cardiovasc Surg*, **54:**333, 1967.

Mitral Insufficiency

Anderson, A. M., Cobb, L. A., Bruce, R. A., and Merendino, K. A.: Evaluation of Mitral Annuloplasty for Mitral Regurgitation: Clinical and Hemodynamic Status Four to 41 Months after Surgery, *Circulation*, **26:**26, 1962.

Braunwald, N. S., and Bonchek, L. I.: Prevention of Thrombus Formation on Rigid Prosthetic Heart Valves by the Ingrowth of Autogenous Tissue, *J Thorac Cardiovasc Surg*, **54:**630, 1967.

Isom, O. W., Williams, C. D., Falk, E. A., Glassman, E., and Spencer, F. C.: Long-Term Evaluation of Cloth-covered Metallic Ball Prostheses, *J Thorac Cardiovasc Surg*, **64:**354, 1972.

Kay, J. H., and Egerton, W. S.: The Repair of Mitral Insufficiency Associated with Ruptured Chordae Tendineae, *Ann Surg*, **157:**351, 1963.

McGoon, D. C.: Repair of Mitral Insufficiency Due to Ruptured Chordae Tendineae, *J Thorac Cardiovasc Surg*, **39:**357, 1960.

Reed, G. E., Tice, D. A., and Clauss, R. H.: Asymmetric Exaggerated Mitral Annuloplasty: Repair of Mitral Insufficiency with Hemodynamic Predictability, *J Thorac Cardiovasc Surg*, **49:**752, 1965.

Spencer, F. C., Reppert, E. H., and Stertzer, S. H.: Surgical Treatment of Mitral Insufficiency Secondary to Coronary Artery Disease, *Arch Surg*, **95:**853, 1967.

Starr, A.: Mitral Valve Replacement with Ball Valve Prostheses, *Br Heart J Suppl*, **33:**47, 1971.

——— and Edwards, M. L.: Mitral Replacement: Clinical Experience with a Ball Valve Prosthesis, *Ann Surg*, **154:**726, 1961.

Wychulis, A. R., Connolly, D. C., and Ellis, F. H., Jr.: Open Mitral Valve Reconstruction: Review of 232 Operations, *Arch Surg*, **101:**332, 1970.

Aortic Stenosis

Angell, W. W., Shumway, N. E., and Kosek, J. C.: A Five Year Study of Viable Aortic Valve Homografts, *J Thorac Cardiovasc Surg*, **64:**329, 1972.

Bahnson, H. T., Spencer, F. C., Busse, E. F. G., and Davis, F. W., Jr.: Cusp Replacement and Coronary Artery Perfusion in Open Operations on the Aortic Valve, *Ann Surg*, **152:**494, 1960.

Bigelow, W. G., Trimble, A. S., Aldridge, H. E., Bedard, P., Spratt, E. H., and Lansdown, E. L.: The Problem of Insufficiency following Homograft Replacement of the Aortic Valve, *J Thorac Cardiovasc Surg*, **54:**478, 1967.

McGoon, D. C., Ellis, F. H., and Kirklin, J. W.: Late Results of Operations for Acquired Aortic Valvular Disease, *Circulation*, **31:**108, 1965.

———, Pestana, C., and Moffitt, E. A.: Decreased Risk of Aortic Valve Surgery, *Arch Surg*, **91:**779, 1965.

Magovern, G. J., Kent, E. J., Cromie, H. W., Cushing, W. B., and Scott, S.: Sutureless Aortic and Mitral Prosthetic Valves: Clinical Results and Operative Technique on 60 Patients, *J Thorac Cardiovasc Surg*, **48:**346, 1964.

Pacifico, A. D., Karp, R. B., and Kirklin, J. W.: Homografts for Replacement of the Aortic Valve, *Circulation*, **45:**I-36, 1972.

Senning, A.: Fascia Lata Replacement of Aortic Valves, *J Thorac Cardiovasc Surg*, **54:**465, 1967.

Starr, A., Edwards, M. L., McCord, C. W., and Griswold, H. E.: Aortic Replacement: Clinical Experience with a Semi-rigid Ball-Valve Prosthesis, *Circulation*, **27:**779, 1963.

Tricuspid Stenosis and Insufficiency

Arbulu, A., Thoms, N. W., and Wilson, R. F.: Valvulectomy without Prosthetic Replacement: A Lifesaving Operation for Tricuspid *Pseudomonas* Endocarditis, *J Thorac Cardiovasc Surg*, **64:**103, 1972.

Braunwald, N. S., Ross, J., Jr., and Morrow, A. G.: Conservative Management of Tricuspid Regurgitation in Patients Undergoing Mitral Valve Replacement, *Circulation*, **35**(*Suppl* 1):63, 1967.

Grondin, P., Lepage, G., Castonguay, Y., and Meere, C.: The Tricuspid Valve: A Surgical Challenge, *J Thorac Cardiovasc Surg* **53:**7, 1967.

Kay, J. H., Maselli-Campagna, G., and Tsuji, H. K.: Surgical Treatment of Tricuspid Insufficiency, *Ann Surg*, **162:**53, 1965.

Spencer, F., C., Shabetai, R., and Adolph, R.: Successful Replacement of the Tricuspid Valve 10 Years after Traumatic Incompetence, *Am J Cardiol*, **18:**916, 1966.

Starr, A., Herr, R., and Wood, J.: Tricuspid Replacement for Acquired Valve Disease, *Surg Gynecol Obstet*, **122:**1295, 1966.

Multivalvular Heart Disease

Starr, A., McCord, C. W., Wood, J., Herr, R., and Edwards, M. L.: Surgery for Multiple Valve Disease, *Ann Surg*. **160:**596, 1964.

Cardiac Trauma

Bahnson, H. T., and Spencer, F. C.: Pericardial Aspiration and the Treatment of Acute Cardiac Tamponade from Penetrating Wounds in the Heart, in J. H. Mulholland, E. H. Ellison, and S. R. Freisen (eds.), "Current Surgical Management," W. B. Saunders Company, Philadelphia, 1957.

Beall, A. C., Jr., Ochsner, J. L., Morris, G. C., Jr., Cooley, D. A., and DeBakey, M. E.: Penetrating Wounds to the Heart, *J Trauma*, **1:**195, 1961.

————, Gasior, R. M., and Bricker, D. L.: Gunshot Wounds of the Heart: Changing Patterns of Surgical Management, *Ann Thorac Surg,* **11:**523, 1971.

Berger, R. L., Loveless, G., and Warner, O.: Delayed and Latent Postcardiotomy Tamponade: Recognition and Nonoperative Treatment, *Ann Thorac Surg,* **12:**22, 1971.

Blalock, A., and Ravitch, M. M.: A Consideration of the Non-operative Treatment of Cardiac Tamponade Resulting from Wounds to the Heart, *Surgery,* **14:**157, 1943.

Bland, E. F., and Beebe, G. W.: Missiles in the Heart: A 20-Year Follow-up Report of World War II Cases, *N Engl J Med,* **274:**1039, 1966.

Boyd, T. F., and Strieder, J. W.: Immediate Surgery for Traumatic Heart Disease, *J Thorac Cardiovasc Surg,* **50:**305, 1965.

Harken, D. E.: Foreign Bodies in and in Relation to the Heart and Thoracic Vessels, *Surg Gynecol Obstet,* **83:**117, 1946.

Holdeger, W. F., Lyons, C., and Edwards, W. S.: Indications for Removal of Intracardiac Foreign Bodies, *Ann Surg,* **163:**249, 1966.

Isaacs, J. P.: Sixty Penetrating Wounds to the Heart: Clinical and Experimental Observations, *Surgery,* **45:**696, 1959.

Spencer, F. C.: Treatment of Chest Injuries, *Curr Probl Surg,* January, 1964.

———— and Kennedy, J. H.: War Wounds of the Heart, *J Thorac Cardiovasc Surg,* **33:**361, 1957.

Sugg, W. L., Ecker, R. R., Webb, W. R., Rose, E. F., and Shaw, R. R.: Penetrating Wounds of the Heart: An Analysis of 459 Cases, *J Thorac Cardiovasc Surg,* **56:**531, 1968.

Tabatznik, B., and Isaacs, J. P.: Post-Pericardiotomy Syndrome following Traumatic Hemopericardium, *Am J Cardiol,* **7:**83, 1961.

Cardiac Tumors

Bahnson, H. T., Spencer, F. C., and Andrus, E. C.: Diagnosis and Treatment of Intracavitary Myxomas of the Heart, *Ann Surg,* **145:**915, 1957.

Crafoord, C.: Case Report, *Int Symp Cardiovasc Surg Henry Ford Hosp,* p. 202, 1955.

Dong, E., Hurley, E. J., and Shumway, N. E.: Primary Cardiac Sarcoma, *Am J Cardiol,* **10:**871, 1962.

Gassman, H. S., Meadows, R., and Baker, L. A.: Metastatic Tumors of the Heart, *Am J Med,* **19:**357, 1955.

Geha, A. S., Weidman, W. H., Soule, E. H., and McGoon, D. C.: Intramural Ventricular Cardiac Fibroma: Successful Removal in Two Cases and Review of the Literature, *Circulation,* **36:**427, 1967.

Gerbode, F., Keith, J. W., and Hill, J. D.: Surgical Management of Tumors of the Heart, *Surgery,* **61:**94, 1967.

Hanfling, S.: Metastatic Cancer to the Heart, *Circulation,* **22:**474, 1960.

Mahaim, I.: "Les Tumors et les polypes du coeur: Étude anatomo-clinique," Masson et Cie, Paris, 1945.

Prichard, R. W.: Tumors of the Heart, *Arch Pathol,* **21:**98, 1951.

Scannell, J. G., and Grillo, H. E.: Primary Tumors of the Heart, *J Thorac Cardiovasc Surg,* **35:**23, 1958.

Spencer, F. C.: The Heart, in T. F. Nealon (ed.), "Management of the Patient with Cancer," p. 537, W. B. Saunders Company, Philadelphia, 1965.

Steinberg, I., Dotter, C. T., and Glenn, F.: Myxoma of the Heart: Roentgen Diagnosis during Life in Three Cases, *Dis Chest,* **24:**509, 1953.

Thomas, K. E., Winchell, C. P., and Varco, R. L.: Diagnostic and Surgical Aspects of Left Atrial Tumors, *J Thorac Cardiovasc Surg,* **53:**535, 1967.

Whorton, C. M.: Primary Malignant Tumors of the Heart, *Cancer,* **2:**245, 1949.

Yater, W. M.: Tumors of the Heart and Pericardium, *Arch Intern Med,* **48:**627, 1931.

Coronary Artery Disease

Buchwald, H., and Varco, R. L.: A Bypass Operation for Obese Hyperlipedemic Patients, *Surgery,* **70:**62, 1971.

Dilley, R. B., Cannon, J. A., Kattus, A. A., MacAlpin, R. N., and Longmire, W. P.: The Treatment of Coronary Occlusive Disease by Endarterectomy, *J Thorac Cardiovasc Surg,* **50:**511, 1965.

Favaloro, R., Effler, D. B., Groves, L. K., Sones, F. M., Jr., and Fergusson, B. J. G.: Myocardial Revascularization by Internal Mammary Artery Implant Procedures, *J Thorac Cardiovasc Surg,* **54:**359, 1967.

Green, G. E., Stertzer, S. H., and Reppert, E. H.: Coronary Arterial Bypass Grafts, *Ann Thorac Surg,* **5:**443, 1968.

Kouchoukos, N. T., and Kirklin, J. W.: Coronary Bypass Operations for Ischemic Heart Disease, *Mod Concepts Cardiovasc Dis,* **41:**47, 1972. *

Provan, J. L., Hammond, G. L., and Austen, W. G.: Flowmeter Studies of Internal Mammary Artery Function after Implantation into the Left Ventricular Myocardium, *J Thorac Cardiovasc Surg,* **52:**820, 1966.

Spencer, F. C.: Surgical Procedures for Coronary Atherosclerosis, *Prog Cardiovasc Dis,* **14:**399, 1972.

————:Bypass Grafting for Preinfarction Angina, *Circulation,* **40:**274, 1972.

————, Green, G. E., Tice, D. A., and Glassman, E.: Surgical Therapy for Coronary Artery Disease, *Curr Probl Surg,* September, 1970.

————, ————, ————, Wallsh, E., Mills, N. L., and Glassman, E.: Coronary Artery Bypass Grafts for Congestive Heart Failure, *J Thorac Cardiovasc Surg,* **62:**529, 1971.

Vineberg, A. M.: Technical Considerations for the Combined Operation of Left Internal Mammary Artery or Right and Left Internal Mammary Implantations with Epicardiectomy and Free Omental Graft, *J Thorac Cardiovasc Surg,* **53:**837, 1967.

Ventricular Aneurysm

Abrams, D. L., Edelist, A., Leuria, M. H., and Miller, A. J.: Ventricular Aneurysm: A Re-appraisal Based on a Study of 65 Consecutive Autopsy Cases, *Circulation,* **27:**164, 1963.

Cooley, D. A., Hallman, G. L., and Henly, W. S.: Left Ventricular Aneurysm Due to Myocardial Infarction: Experience with 37 Patients, *Arch Surg,* **88:**114, 1964.

Effler, D. B., Groves, L. K., and Favaloro, R.: Surgical Repair of Ventricular Aneurysm, *Dis Chest,* **48:**37, 1965.

Schlichter, J., Hellerstein, H. K., and Katz, L. N.: Aneurysm of the Heart: A Correlative Study of 102 Proved Cases, *Medicine,* **33:**43, 1954.

Pericarditis

Berger, R. L., Loveless, G., and Warner, O.: Delayed and Latent Postcardiotomy Tamponade: Recognition and Nonoperative Treatment, *Ann Thorac Surg,* **12:**22, 1971.

Boyle, J. D., Pearce, M. L., and Guze, L. B.: Purulent Pericarditis: Review of Literature and Report of 11 Cases, *Medicine,* **40:** 119, 1961.

Collins, H. A., Woods, L. P., and Daniel, R. A.: Late Results of Pericardectomy, *Arch Surg,* **89:**921, 1964.

Dalton, J. C., Pearson, R. J., and White, P. D.: Constrictive Pericarditis: A Review and Long-Term Follow-up of 78 Cases, *Ann Intern Med,* **45:**445, 1956.

Effler, D. B.: Chronic Constrictive Pericarditis Treated with Pericardectomy, *Am J Cardiol,* **7:**62, 1961.

Holman, E.: The Pericardium, in J. H. Gibbon (ed.), "Surgery of the Chest," chap. 24, 1st ed., W. B. Saunders Company, Philadelphia, 1962.

Shumacker, H. B., and Roshe, T.: Pericardectomy, *J Cardiovasc Surg,* **1:**65, 1960.

Heart Block and Pacemakers

Chardack, W. M., Gage, A. A., Federico, A. J., Schimert, G., and Greatbatch, W.: The Long-Term Treatment of Heart Block, *Prog Cardiovasc Dis,* **9:**105, 1966.

Cheng, T. O.: Percutaneous Transfemoral Venous Cardiac Pacing: A Simple Practical Method, *Chest,* **60:**73, 1971.

Furman, S., Escher, D. J., Solomon, S., and Schwedel, J. B.: Implanted Transvenous Pacemakers: Equipment, Technic and Clinical Experience, *Ann Surg,* **164:**465, 1966.

Genig, S., and Lichstein, E.: Incomplete Bilateral Bundle Branch Block and AV Block Complicating Acute Anterior Wall Myocardial Infarct, *Am Heart J,* **84:**38, 1972.

Glenn, W. W. L.: Cardiac Pacemakers and Heart Block, in J. H. Gibbon (ed.), "Surgery of the Chest," 1st ed, W. B. Saunders Company, Philadelphia, 1962.

Imparato, A. M., and Kim, G. E.: The Trapped Endocardial Electrode: Removal by Prolonged Graded Skin Traction, *Ann Thorac Surg,* **14:**605, 1972.

——— and ———: Electrode Complications in Patients with Permanent Cardiac Pacemakers, *Arch Surg,* **105:**705, 1972.

———, Reppert, E., and Spencer, F. S.: Rapid Atrial Pacing to Produce Heart Block, *Surgery,* **63(1):**198, 1968.

Lagergren, H., et al.: Three-hundred-five Cases of Permanent Intravenous Pacemaker Treatment for Adams-Stokes Syndrome, *Surgery,* **59:**494, 1966.

Langendorf, R., Cohen, H., and Gozo, E. G., Jr.: Observations on Second Degree A-V Block, Including New Criteria for the Differential Diagnosis between Type I and Type II Block, *Am J Cardiol,* **29:**111, 1972.

Lillehei, C. W., Sellers, R. D., Bonnabeau, R. C., and Eliot, R. S.: Chronic Postsurgical Complete Heart Block: With Particular Reference to Prognosis, Management, and a New P-wave Pacemaker, *J Thorac Cardiovasc Surg,* **46:**436, 1963.

Morgan, C. V., Orcutt, T. W., Collins, H. A., and Killen, D. A.: Permanent Cardiac Pacing for Sino Atrial Bradycardia, *J Thorac Cardiovasc Surg,* **66:**453, 1972.

Nathan, D. A., Center, S., Wu, C., and Keller, W.: An Implantable Synchronous Pacemaker for the Long Term Correction of Complete Heart Block, *Am J Cardiol,* **11:**362, 1963.

Parsonnet, J.: Power Sources for Implantable Cardiac Pacemakers, *Chest,* **61:**165, 1972.

Rockland, R., Parsonnet, V., and Myers, G. H.: Failure Modes of American Pacemakers: In Vitro Analysis, *Am Heart J,* **83:**481, 1972.

Von Mour, K., Nelson, E. W., Holsinger, J. W., Jr., and Elliott, R. S.: Hypersensitive Carotid Sinus Syncope Treated by Implantable Demand Cardiac Pacemaker, *Am J Cardiol,* **29:**109, 1972.

Zoll, P. M.: Historical Development of Cardiac Pacemakers, *Prog Cardiovasc Dis,* **14:**421, 1972.

———, Frank, H. A., and Linenthal, A. J.: Four Year Experience with an Implanted Cardiac Pacemaker, *Ann Surg,* **160:**351, 1964.

Cardiac Transplantation, Assisted Circulation, and Artificial Hearts

Austen, W. G.: title? *Ann Surg,* September, 1973.

Bergman, D., and Goetz, R. H.: Clinical Experience with a New Cardiac Assist Device: The Dual-Chambered Intra-aortic Balloon Assist, *J Thorac Cardiovasc Surg,* **62:**577, 1971.

Bregman, D., and Goetz, R. H.: Clinical Experience with a New Cardiac Assist Device; the Dual-chambered Intra-aortic Balloon Assist, *J Thorac Cardiovasc Surg,* **62:**4.

Burns, W. H., Shumacker, H. B., Jr., and Loubier, R. J.: The Totally Implantable Mechanical Heart: An Appraisal of Feasibility, *Ann Surg,* **164:**445, 1966.

Clauss, R. H., Birtwell, W. C., Albertal, G., Lunzer, S., Taylor, W. J., Fosberg, A. M., and Harken, D. E.: Assisted Circulation. I. The Arterial Counterpulsator, *J Thorac Cardiovasc Surg,* **41:**447, 1961.

Dong, E., Jr., and Lower, R. R.: Transplantation of the Heart, in J. C. Norman (ed.), "Cardiac Surgery," Appleton-Century-Crofts, Inc. New York, 1967.

———, Griepp, R. B., Stinson, E. B., and Shumway, N. E.: Clinical Transplantation of the Heart, *Ann Surg,* **176:**503, 1972.

Dowling, J. B., and Drapanas, T.: Uses and Abuses of Autotransfusion, in T. Drapanas and W. Ballinger (eds.), "Practice of Surgery—A Current Review," C. V. Mosby Company, St. Louis, 1974.

Gold, H. K., Leinbach, R. C., Mundth, E. D., Sanders, C. A., and Buckley, M. J.: Reversal of Myocardial Ischemia Complicating Acute Infarction by Intra-aortic Balloon Pumping (IABP), *Circulation, 1973.*

Hall, D. P., Moreno, J. R., Dennis, C., and Senning, A.: An Experimental Study of Prolonged Left Heart Bypass without Thoracotomy, *Ann Surg,* **156:**190, 1962.

Hill, J. D., deLeval, M. R., Fallat, R. J., Bramson, M. L., Eberhart, R. C., Schulte, H. D., Osborn, J. J., Barber, R., and Gerbode, F.: Acute Respiratory Insufficiency: Treatment with Prolonged Extracorporeal Oxygenation, *J Thorac Cardiovasc Surg,* **64:**551, 1972.

Liotta, D., Maness, J., Bourland, H., Rodwell, D., Hall, W. C., and DeBakey, M. E.: Recent Modifications in the Implantable Left Ventricle By-pass, *Trans Am Soc Artif Intern Organs,* **11:**284, 1965.

Norman, J. C., Molokhia, F. A., Harmison, L. T., Whalen, R. L., and Huffman, F.: An Implantable Nuclear-fueled Circulatory Support System: I. Systems Analysis of Conception, Design, Fabrication, and Initial *In Vivo* Testing, *Ann Surg,* **176:**492, 1972.

Okura, T., Tjønneland, S., Fred, P. S., and Kantrowtiz, A.: U-shaped Mechanical Auxiliary Ventricle, *Arch Surg,* **95:**821, 1967.

Schenk, W. G., Delin, N. A., Camp, F. A., McDonald, K. E., Pollock, L., Gage, A. A., and Chardack, W. M.: Assisted Circulation, *Arch Surg,* **88:**327, 1964.

Shumway, N. E., Lower, R. R., and Stofer, R. C.; Transplantation of the Heart, in C. E. Welch (ed.), "Advances in Surgery," vol. II, Year Book Medical Publishers, Inc., Chicago, 1966.

Skinner, D. B., Anstadt, G. L., and Camp, T. F., Jr.: Applications of Mechanical Ventricular Assistance, *Ann Surg,* **166:**500, 1967.

Spencer, F. C., Eiseman, B., Trinkle, J. K., and Rossi, N. P.: Assisted Circulation for Cardiac Failure following Intracardiac Surgery with Cardiopulmonary Bypass, *J Thorac Cardiovasc Surg,* **49:**56, 1964.

Szentpetery, S., Kemp, V. E., Raper, A. J., Robertson, L. W., and Lower, R. R.: title?, *Ann Thorac Surg,* **13:**330.

Chapter 20

Diseases of Great Vessels

by **Frank C. Spencer**

Aneurysms of the Thoracic Aorta
Aneurysms of the Ascending Aorta
Aneurysms of the Transverse Aortic Arch
Traumatic Thoracic Aneurysms
Aneurysms of the Descending Thoracic Aorta
Thoracoabdominal Aneurysms

Dissecting Aneurysms

Wounds of the Great Vessels
Penetrating Injuries
Nonpenetrating Injuries

Obstruction of the Superior Vena Cava

ANEURYSMS OF THE THORACIC AORTA

Aneurysms of the thoracic aorta may be classified in five groups, varying with the anatomic location: (1) ascending aorta; (2) transverse aortic arch; (3) traumatic thoracic aorta, uniformly occurring distal to the left subclavian artery; (4) descending thoracic aorta; and (5) thoracoabdominal. The etiology, disability, and surgical approach all vary with these different types. Hence, each one is discussed separately.

Aneurysms of the Ascending Aorta

Aneurysms localized to the ascending aorta are often due to a degenerative connective tissue disease of the aortic media. This is seen typically as cystic medial necrosis, one manifestation of a generalized disorder in the Marfan syndrome, or as an isolated disease in Erdheim's cystic medial necrosis. Syphilitic destruction of the media of the aorta was formerly a frequent cause of such aneurysms but is now uncommon. Atherosclerotic aneurysms are seldom limited to the ascending aorta, usually evolving as diffuse fusiform lesions involving both the ascending aorta and the transverse arch.

PATHOLOGY. As an aneurysm develops in the proximal ascending aorta, dilatation of the annulus of the aortic valve often develops, stretching the cusps of the aortic valve apart and producing aortic insufficiency (Fig. 20-1). Often cardiac failure from aortic insufficiency is the significant disability, rather than enlargement of the aneurysm with rupture or compression of adjacent structures. Large saccular syphilitic aneurysms can enlarge and erode through the sternum (Fig. 20-2), but these are now rare.

Once aortic insufficiency has resulted from an aneurysm, progression of disability is fairly rapid with death from cardiac failure in 1 to 2 years in many patients unless operation is performed. In the Marfan syndrome, the degenerated wall of the aorta may also rupture and form a dissecting aneurysm. Before surgical therapy was available, most patients with the Marfan syndrome died from one of two complications—either dissecting aneurysm or aortic insufficiency.

CLINICAL MANIFESTATIONS. Patients are often asymptomatic when the diagnosis is made following detection of a mass on a chest roentgenogram performed for other purposes. Expanding saccular aneurysms may cause symptoms from compression of the superior vena cava or the trachea, but compression rarely occurs from fusiform aneurysms. Frequently, the first symptom is due to congestive heart failure from aortic insufficiency. Physical examination usually demonstrates no abnormalities except the aortic diastolic murmur and wide pulse pressure of aortic insufficiency.

DIAGNOSTIC FINDINGS. The diagnosis can be suspected from the chest roentgenogram, disclosing enlargement of the ascending aorta, but aortography is required to establish the exact diagnosis. The aortographic finding of a fusiform aneurysm in the proximal ascending aorta, tapering to an aorta of near-normal diameter at the level of the innominate artery, is virtually diagnostic of cystic medial necrosis (Fig. 20-3).

TREATMENT. Because of the progressive nature of the aortic insufficiency, operation should be performed as soon as possible after the diagnosis is made. The operative procedure must include both correction of the aortic insufficiency and excision of the aneurysm. This, of necessity, involves the use of extracorporeal circulation. If aortic insufficiency is minimal, simple excision of the aneurysm, combined with narrowing of the aortic annulus by suturing the dilated aortic valve ring to a prosthetic graft of smaller diameter, may be adequate. In some patients the aortic insufficiency has been successfully treated by excision of the noncoronary cusp to narrow the aortic annulus, converting the aortic valve to a bicuspid one, but in most patients replacement with a prosthetic valve is the preferable procedure.

At the time of operation, once cardiopulmonary bypass has been started, the aorta can be occluded and the aneurysm excised, the proximal point of division of the aorta usually being a few millimeters distal to the ostia of the coronary arteries. Both coronary arteries should be cannu-

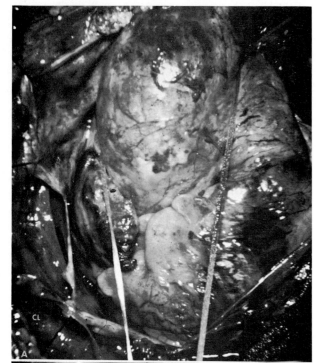

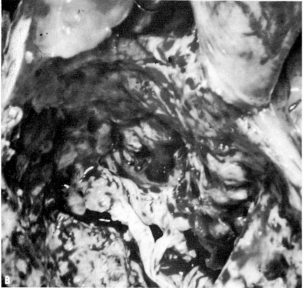

Fig. 20-1. Operative photograph of a patient with a large aneurysm of the ascending aorta. *A*. The aneurysm in the proximal aorta has been isolated and the aorta elevated by encircling umbilical tapes. *B*. Once the aorta has been incised, the incompetent aortic valve is exposed. The aortic insufficiency was produced by dilatation of the aortic annulus.

lated and perfused during the operative procedure. Initially the aortic valve is excised and replaced with a prosthetic valve; we prefer a Starr-Edwards ball-valve prosthesis. Subsequently a short, woven Dacron graft, usually about 10 cm long, is inserted to reestablish aortic continuity. Because the aortic wall is thin from the disease in the media, much care must be taken in performing the

aortic anastomoses to avoid serious or even fatal hemorrhage from the suture lines. Often the suture lines must be buttressed with pledgets of Teflon felt (Fig. 20-4).

Following operation, long-term prognosis depends upon the cause of the aneurysm, usually either the Marfan syndrome or aortic dissection, and also whether insertion of a prosthetic aortic valve was necessary or not (Fig. 20-5). Published long-term results are thus far meager. Experiences with 36 patients were reported by Bloodwell et al. in 1966, with three postoperative deaths and four other deaths in the first 5 months after discharge from the hospital, a combined mortality rate of 20 percent. In 1971 Liotta et al. described experiences with a group of 56 patients with a combined mortality of 17 percent. There were 24 patients with acute aortic dissection with a mortality of 25 percent, and 34 with chronic dissecting aneurysm. In 1972 Shumacker reported experiences with 12 patients, one of whom died from rupture of an abdominal aneurysm 4 months later, but the other 11 remained well. In the discussion of the report by Shumacker, Edwards mentioned experiences with an alternative technique in eight patients in whom a composite graft of an aortic ball-valve prosthesis and a woven Dacron graft was inserted inside the aneurysm and attached to the aortic annulus, after which the wall of the aneurysm was wrapped around the graft and appropriate openings made for connecting the coronary ostia to side openings in the graft. Such a technique may be particularly useful when the aneurysm extends proximal to the ostia of the coronary arteries.

Fig. 20-2. Patient with a large syphilitic aneurysm eroding through the sternum and projecting beneath the skin. Fortunately such lesions are now rare. An attempt at operative extirpation of the lesion was unsuccessful because of hemorrhage.

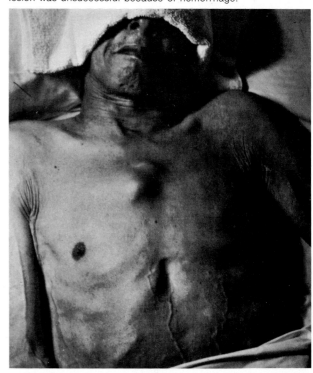

Aneurysms of the Transverse Aortic Arch

Aneurysms of the transverse aortic arch are almost always due to atherosclerosis, rarely syphilis. The diagnosis is usually established by aortography, differentiating the aneurysm from a malignant mediastinal tumor. The degree of involvement of the great vessels arising from the aortic arch also can be determined.

Detailed consideration of the technical management of these aneurysms is beyond the scope of this textbook, but limited pertinent references are listed in the bibliography at the end of the chapter. Because of the complexity of the operative procedure and the high mortality, excision should be attempted only for expanding aneurysms with an obviously impending fatal outcome, usually from tracheal obstruction, unless operation is performed. Surgical excision is a complex undertaking, requiring perfusion of the distal aorta, the great arch vessels, and often the coronary arteries. Hemorrhage and neurologic complications from perfusion of the innominate and carotid arteries have been responsible for an operative mortality often exceeding 60 to 70 percent (Fig. 20-6). Retrograde perfusion of the right brachial artery has been the most satisfactory method of perfusing the right vertebral and right carotid arteries arising from the innominate artery, while perfusion of the left carotid artery has been through direct cannulation. Pressure in the carotid artery should be monitored during perfusion to avoid the extremes of inadequate or excessive perfusion. Surgical techniques have gradually improved and undoubtedly will continue to do so. One remarkable example was published in 1972 by Lefrak et al., who described excision of a massive aneurysm of the aortic arch in a seventy-six-year-old patient which had virtually occluded the trachea. One year later the patient remained well and free of symptoms.

Traumatic Thoracic Aneurysms

ETIOLOGY AND PATHOLOGY. Traumatic aneurysms almost invariably arise from transection of the thoracic aorta associated with closed chest trauma. In those few patients fortunate enough not to succumb from exsanguinating hemorrhage an aneurysm will subsequently develop. If a patient survives longer than 6 to 8 weeks following injury, the risk of acute rupture is small. In a review of the English and French literature between 1950 and 1965, Bennett and Cherry found rupture occurring nine times in a total of 105 aneurysms. The usual course is one of progressive enlargement with compression of adjacent structures.

The aneurysm virtually always arises just distal to the left subclavian artery, opposite the point of insertion of the ligamentum arteriosum. Although a huge aneurysm filling most of the hemithorax may be found, at operation the point of origin is almost invariably found in this area. This localization is a significant one in planning operative therapy, for little disease of the adjacent segments of aorta exists. Reconstruction can usually be done with a short prosthetic graft; occasionally direct anastomosis is possible.

CLINICAL MANIFESTATIONS. Unlike most aneurysms

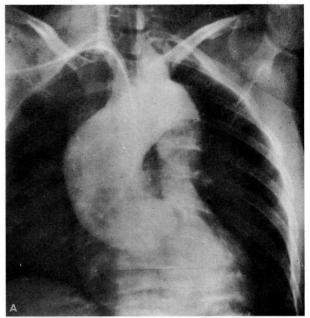

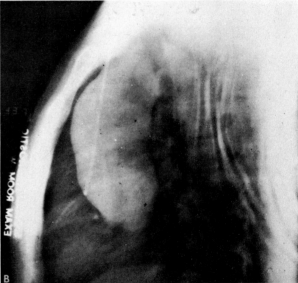

Fig. 20-3. *A.* Posteroanterior view of a thoracic aortogram demonstrating a large aneurysm in the ascending aorta, stopping near the innominate artery. Resection of the aneurysm was successfully performed. The patient was well 5 years following operation. *B.* Lateral view of a thoracic aortogram in the same patient.

from other causes, traumatic thoracic aneurysms enlarge slowly and in some patients have apparently remained stationary for 10 to 20 years, the diagnosis being made in retrospect after finding an asymptomatic aneurysm with a history of closed-chest trauma 10 to 20 years before. A detailed study of the natural "life history" of such aneurysms was reported by Bennett and Cherry in 1967. As the aneurysm enlarges, compression of the left main bronchus with pain, dyspnea, cough, and atelectasis are the predominant complications. Hoarseness from compression

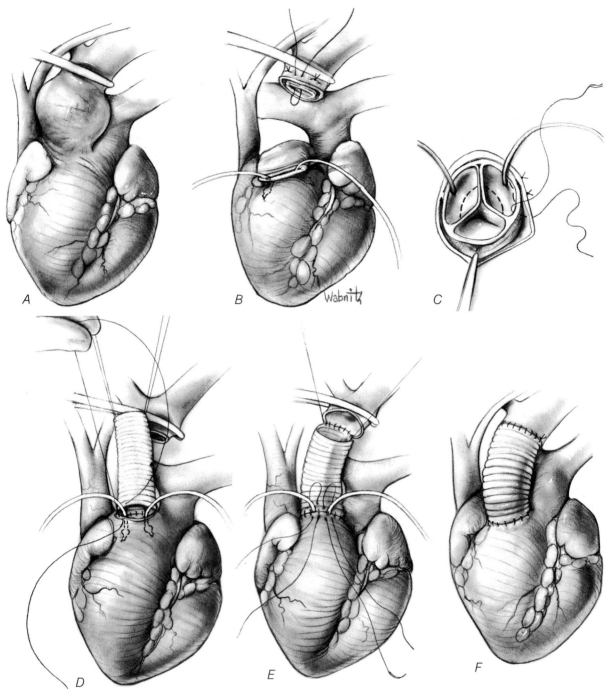

Fig. 20-4. Procedure for excision of dissecting aneurysm of the ascending aorta. A. A dissecting aneurysm of the ascending aorta in a patient with the Marfan syndrome. The lesion had produced acute aortic insufficiency. B. Initially at operation the aneurysm was excised, and the coronary arteries were perfused to support coronary circulation. Distad the dissected wall of the aorta was approximated with interrupted sutures. C. The mechanism of production of aortic insufficiency by an aortic dissection. The area of dissection proceeds proximally to detach the aortic cusps from the aortic wall, permitting them to prolapse into the lumen and cause aortic insufficiency. Prolapse of the right and left coronary cusps is minimized by the location of the coronary artery; hence, dissection of the noncoronary cusp is the most extensive. Reapproximation of the aortic wall may correct the insufficiency. D. Aortic reconstruction is performed with a woven Dacron graft, performing the anastomosis with continuous silk sutures. The disease in the aortic wall results in unusual friability, which may make adequate hemostasis difficult. E. The proximal anastomosis is completed, leaving the coronary cannulae in position. The distal anastomosis is then similarly performed, after which the coronary catheters are withdrawn and aortic is circulation reestablished.

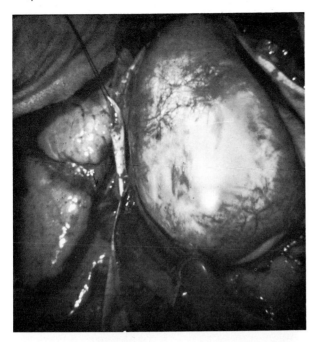

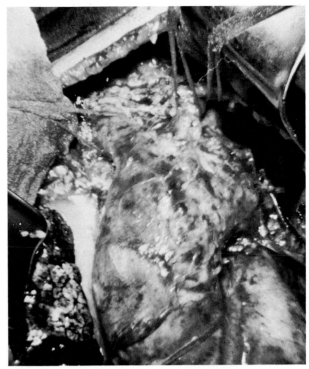

Fig. 20-6. Operative photograph of a patient with aneurysm of the aortic arch. The procedure is a complicated one requiring multiple bypass grafts, temporarily diverting blood through bypass channels to the carotid arteries and distal aorta while the aneurysm is excised and the aortic arch reconstructed.

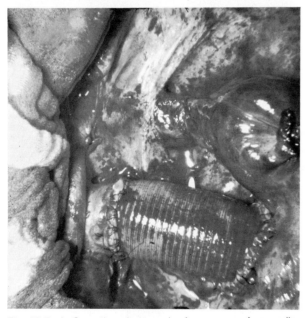

Fig. 20-5. A. Operative photograph of aneurysm of ascending aorta in the Marfan's syndrome. The classic finding is an aneurysm extending down to the aortic sinuses with a thin, glistening wall, developing from the cystic medial necrosis. The aorta classically tapers to a virtually normal diameter near the origin of the innominate artery. B. Operative photograph showing reconstruction of the ascending aorta with a short Dacron graft, stopping just proximal to the level of the left innominate artery.

and distortion of the left recurrent laryngeal nerve may appear. These symptoms usually well precede enlargement of the aneurysm to such a degree that rupture occurs. This course of events is emphasized because of the small risk of rupture, which is in direct contrast to factors governing the surgical policy with the majority of aneurysms from atherosclerosis or syphilis, where the threat of rupture constitutes a major reason for recommending elective excision as soon as possible.

Frequently there are no abnormalities on physical examination unless compression of the main bronchus has produced atelectasis of the left lung. A murmur is usually not heard, and there is no abnormality of peripheral pulses.

DIAGNOSTIC FINDINGS. The chest roentgenogram usually discloses an ovoid density near the left subclavian artery. If an aneurysm has been present for several years, calcification is often visible in the wall. The diagnosis can be established by aortography, which is required to delineate the extent of the aneurysm and to differentiate it from other mediastinal tumors (Fig. 20-7).

TREATMENT. The problem of management of acute rupture of the thoracic aorta, with the risk of exsanguinating hemorrhage, is presented in the section on Wounds of the Great Vessels. Elective excision is recommended for the majority of patients, although probably 20 to 30 percent of aneurysms remain stationary and asymptomatic for many years. Apparently most aneurysms, despite long latent periods of stability, eventually progressively enlarge. When serious associated disease, such as coronary atherosclerosis, is present, observation with serial chest roentgenograms may be safely employed.

Technique of Operation. A left posterolateral thoracotomy through the fourth or fifth intercostal space is used.

Initially the aorta is mobilized and encircled proximal and distal to the aneurysm. Proximal involvement of the left subclavian artery often requires encirclement of the aorta between the left carotid and the left subclavian arteries. This is facilitated by opening the pericardium and dissecting the intrapericardial portion of the aortic arch. The vagus nerve with the recurrent laryngeal nerve should also be mobilized and protected, for the recurrent laryngeal is often adherent to the wall of the aneurysm.

Once the aorta has been encircled proximally and distad and the recurrent laryngeal nerve mobilized as much as possible, further dissection is unnecessary. Some form of aortic bypass should then be established to maintain flow to the distal aorta during aortic occlusion and prevent ischemic injury of the spinal cord and kidneys. Without an aortic bypass, paraplegia has been reported to develop within as short a time as 20 to 25 minutes of aortic occlusion.

The first effective technique of aortic bypass is the left atriofemoral bypass, withdrawing blood through a cannula inserted into the left atrium which in turn is pumped into the distal arterial tree, usually the left iliac, occasionally the distal aorta. Slow rates of 2 to 2.5 liters/minute are required to keep the pressure in the proximal aorta near that before the aorta was occluded, as well as maintain distal aortic pressure between 60 and 75 mm Hg. This technique has been widely used, but has the disadvantage

Fig. 20-7. *A*. Chest roentgenogram following an automobile accident, demonstrating widening of the mediastinum with subcutaneous emphysema. Traumatic rupture of the aorta was not recognized at this time. *B*. Chest roentgenogram 5 months after the injury demonstrated a left upper mediastinal mass. *C*. Posteroanterior view of an aortogram demonstrating a localized thoracic aneurysm. This lesion was excised successfully. *D*. Lateral view of an aortogram in the same patient. *E*. Chest roentgenogram in a different patient 2 years after an automobile accident demonstrated an asymptomatic mass in the upper mediastinum. *F*. Aortography demonstrated a saccular thoracic aneurysm, which was subsequently resected successfully. *G*. Aortogram in the same patient as in *F*. This film demonstrated the size and extent of the aneurysm as additional contrast material flowed freely within the lesion.

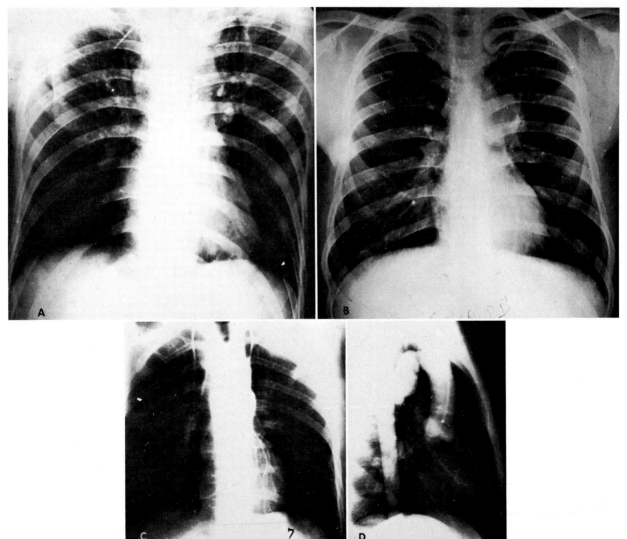

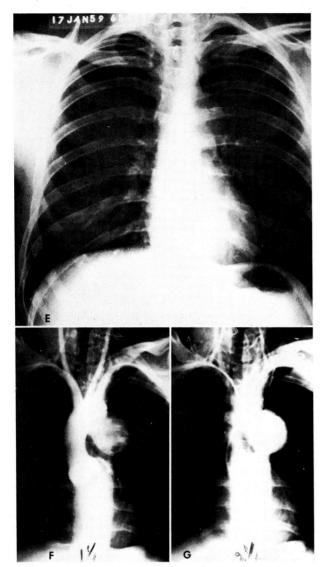

Fig. 20-7 E–G (See legend on facing page.)

entry is frequently normal. Hence, it is unnecessary to excise any significant length of aorta. The inner lining of the aneurysmal sac may be removed, but it is unnecessary and unwise to attempt complete excision, because of vascular adhesions surrounding the wall of the aneurysm. In a few patients direct anastomosis of the ends of the aorta is possible following excision of the aneurysm, but in most patients a 5- to 8-cm segment of woven Dacron graft is inserted to restore arterial continuity.

Convalescence following operation is usually uneventful, and long-term results are excellent. The risk of operation is probably less than 5 percent. One of the largest groups of patients has been reported by Cooley. This included over 60 such lesions without any operative mortality. The low mortality is due both to the young age of many of the patients and also to the localized nature of the aneurysm.

Aneurysms of the Descending Thoracic Aorta

ETIOLOGY AND INCIDENCE. Aneurysms in the descending thoracic aorta may result from atherosclerosis, syphilis, trauma, or a dissection of the aortic wall. Most are due to atherosclerosis and are exceeded only by abdominal aneurysms in frequency of occurrence. They are most frequently found in men in the fifth to the seventh decades. Formerly, saccular aneurysms from syphilis were common, but these are now rare. Dissecting aneurysms and traumatic aneurysms are considered in the accompanying sections.

The majority of atherosclerotic aneurysms are located in the proximal part of the descending thoracic aorta, beginning distal to the left subclavian artery. They extend for varying distances and in some instances can involve the entire descending thoracic aorta. They are generally fusiform (Fig. 20-8), in contrast to syphilitic saccular aneurysms. Their rate of growth is significantly slower than that of abdominal aneurysms, with a less malignant tendency toward rapid enlargement and rupture, but eventual rupture is the outcome in most cases unless other complications of atherosclerosis appear. Syphilitic saccular aneurysms, by contrast, usually rapidly enlarge and rupture, a high percentage rupturing within 2 years after the diagnosis is made. Erosion of bone, commonly seen with saccular syphilitic aneurysms, is unusual with fusiform atherosclerotic aneurysms.

CLINICAL MANIFESTATIONS. In many patients a thoracic aneurysm is found as an asymptomatic mass on a chest roentgenogram made for other reasons. Probably the most common symptoms from enlargement result from compression or erosion of the lung, or compression and obstruction of the left main bronchus with resulting dyspnea and atelectasis. Erosion into the bronchus will produce hemoptysis. Involvement of the left recurrent laryngeal nerve where it encircles the ligamentum arteriosum may lead to paralysis of the vocal cord with hoarseness. In contrast to abdominal aneurysms, where acute rupture may be the first indication of a previously unsuspected aneurysm, such a sequence of events is unusual with a thoracic aneurysm.

of increased bleeding associated with systemic heparinization. Accordingly, there has been an increasing use of different types of temporary shunts inserted between the proximal and distal aorta to avoid the use of heparin. The safety of such shunts was greatly aided by the work of Gott, who developed a method of temporarily binding heparin to the surface of polyvinyl tubes. In 1968 Kahn et al. also reported different techniques for temporary shunts. More recently, Krauss and associates, in 1972, described experiences with the use of temporarily heparinized shunts in eight patients. In all likelihood such shunts will become increasingly popular, for the use of systemic heparinization greatly increases the severity of bleeding at operation.

After the aorta has been opened, the point of origin usually can be identified as a transverse laceration or transection near the point of insertion of the ligamentum arteriosum. The aorta proximal and distal to the site of

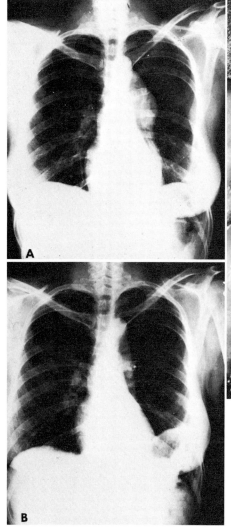

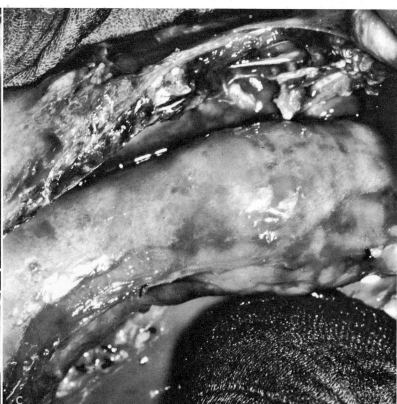

Fig. 20-8. *A.* Chest roentgenogram of a forty-five-year-old patient with a large diffuse aneurysm of the thoracic aorta from atherosclerosis. The aneurysm was excised and the aorta reconstructed with a Teflon graft. *B.* Chest roentgenogram 6 months after operation shows the area of insertion of the Teflon graft. *C.* Operative photograph of atherosclerotic aneurysm demonstrated in the chest roentgenogram seen in *A.*

Physical examination often yields entirely normal findings. Infrequently, a bruit may be heard over the left chest, loudest in the left paravertebral area. Peripheral pulses are frequently normal, unless involvement of the left subclavian artery produces hypotension in the left arm.

DIAGNOSTIC FINDINGS. The diagnosis can usually be suspected from the appearance of the mass in the region of the aorta on the chest roentgenogram. The differential diagnosis includes other conditions producing an opacity on the chest roentgenogram, such as bronchogenic carcinoma, metastatic carcinoma, or rarely esophageal tumors. Laminar calcification may be visible in the wall of the aorta. Aortography is used both to confirm the diagnosis and to delineate the precise extent of the aneurysm. An electrocardiogram and a blood urea nitrogen determination should be routinely obtained, because atherosclerotic disease in other organs, especially the heart and kidney, is frequent.

TREATMENT. In most patients once the diagnosis of a discrete aneurysm has been made, excision should be recommended. With small aneurysms, associated with sig-

nificant coronary or cerebrovascular disease, observation with frequent chest roentgenograms to evaluate the rate of enlargement may be safely employed. Serial observations also may be preferable in some patients with a diffuse fusiform dilatation of the entire thoracic aorta.

The technique of operation is detailed in Fig. 20-9. As mentioned in the section on Traumatic Thoracic Aneurysms, the major hazards are operative hemorrhage and ischemic injury to the spinal cord and kidneys while the aorta is clamped and the aneurysm excised. The different methods for perfusing the distal aorta to protect the spinal cord and kidneys are discussed in that section. Either the conventional left atriofemoral bypass, which has the advantage of simplicity but the disadvantage of systemic heparinization, should be used, or some type of temporary shunt without heparin should be employed, which may be more awkward to insert but avoids the use of systemic heparin. Whatever method of perfusion is employed, it is important to monitor pressure in the distal aorta, keeping mean pressure above 60 mm Hg. Pressure in the proximal aorta is similarly monitored to avoid excessive hypertension which may precipitate left ventricular failure, especially in the presence of preexisting coronary disease.

As with aneurysms elsewhere, an important principal in

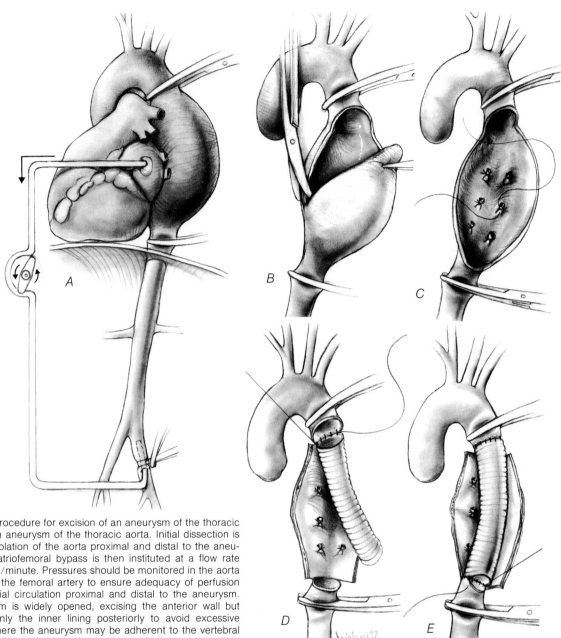

Fig. 20-9. Procedure for excision of an aneurysm of the thoracic aorta. *A.* An aneurysm of the thoracic aorta. Initial dissection is limited to isolation of the aorta proximal and distal to the aneurysm. Left atriofemoral bypass is then instituted at a flow rate near 2 liters/minute. Pressures should be monitored in the aorta and also in the femoral artery to ensure adequacy of perfusion of the arterial circulation proximal and distal to the aneurysm. *B.* Aneurysm is widely opened, excising the anterior wall but removing only the inner lining posteriorly to avoid excessive bleeding where the aneurysm may be adherent to the vertebral column and lung. *C.* Bleeding intercostal arteries may be oversewn from within the lumen of the aneurysm. *D.* A woven Dacron prosthesis is used for reconstruction of the aorta, employing a continuous suture for the anastomosis. *E.* Following completion of the anastomosis the adventitial sac remaining from the aneurysm can be used to partly surround the graft.

minimizing operative hemorrhage is to avoid an attempt to completely excise the aneurysm, especially when the wall is adherent to the lung or vertebral column. Initial dissection should be limited to encircling the aorta proximally and distad. Once aortic bypass has been instituted, the aorta can be occluded with clamps and the aneurysm opened widely. The inner wall then can be removed, suturing the ostia of any patent intercostal vessels but leaving the outer adventitial layers to avoid bleeding. Following

excision of the aneurysm, aortic continuity is reestablished with a vascular prosthesis (Fig. 20-10). Our preference is for woven Dacron prostheses, carefully preclotted, inserted with continuous synthetic sutures. The remaining adventitial wall of the aneurysm then can be wrapped around the prosthesis to further minimize bleeding.

The most serious complication is paraplegia. Fortunately this is rare with adequate aortic bypass. In some instances, however, some degree of spinal cord injury has occurred despite seemingly adequate bypass, probably as a consequence of ligation of intercostal arteries during excision of the aneurysm. As the blood supply to the spinal cord

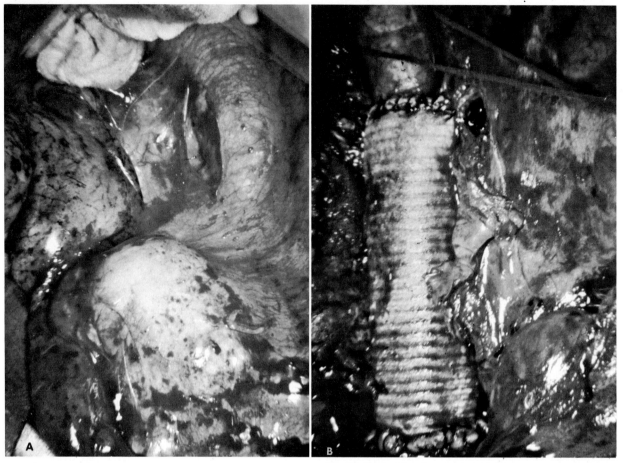

Fig. 20-10. *A*. Operative photograph of saccular syphilitic aneurysm of distal thoracic aorta. *B*. Teflon graft used to restore continuity following excision of a syphilitic aneurysm of the lower thoracic aorta. This graft was used in the patient seen in *A*.

is highly variable, it is impossible to know which, if any, intercostal arteries are vital to spinal cord circulation. Fortunately, with many thoracic aneurysms intercostal arteries arising from the aneurysm have become occluded beforehand by thrombus. Although some patients have tolerated excision of the entire thoracic aorta uneventfully, it is probably wise to limit the degree of excision of adjacent thoracic aorta, even though moderate disease and dilatation are present, especially if large patent intercostal arteries are seen arising from this segment.

Following recovery from operation, the prognosis is favorable and related chiefly to the extent of atherosclerotic disease in other organs. Complications from the prosthetic graft or the adjacent diseased aorta are unusual. With experienced surgical groups, the operative mortality is in the range of 10 to 15 percent. This varies both with the size of the aneurysm and with the age of the patient; for larger aneurysms there is a greater operative risk from hemorrhage. Actually there is only a limited amount of data in the surgical literature concerning excision. It is probable that infrequently performed operations for thoracic aneurysm have a much higher mortality rate. In a report of 237 aneurysms treated at The Johns Hopkins Hospital between 1952 and 1959 by Vasko and associates, there were only eight patients with thoracic aneurysms due to syphilis or atherosclerosis. All survived operation, but

three died within 2 years from further vascular complications. In 1966 Bloodwell and associates described experiences with nearly 400 thoracic aneurysms, but detailed analysis of these cases was not presented. The low mortality reported by Krauss et al. in 1972 in the series of eight patients with seven survivors in whom the temporary heparinized shunt was used indicates the progressive improvement in surgical mortality with improved techniques.

Thoracoabdominal Aneurysms

These aneurysms fortunately are rare, because their excision is a complicated surgical procedure, involving restoration of blood flow to the celiac, superior mesenteric, and renal arteries. Such procedures have usually been performed with multiple bypass techniques to minimize duration of ischemia to different organs, but operative mortality has remained high. More recently some procedures have been performed with a simple left atriofemoral bypass, opening the aneurysm widely and attempting to reestablish flow to different organs with a relatively short period of ischemia.

INCIDENCE AND ETIOLOGY. The rarity of such aneurysms is indicated in the report by DeBakey and associates of experiences with treating over 2,000 aneurysms of the abdominal aorta below the renal arteries, during which less than 50 of these aneurysms above the renal arteries were treated. They are usually due to atherosclerosis, rarely to cystic medial necrosis as in the Marfan syndrome. In the group of 42 patients reported by DeBakey et al., 62 percent resulted from atherosclerosis, and 26 percent were due to syphilis.

CLINICAL MANIFESTATIONS. The rate of enlargement is slow, and excision should be attempted only for expanding aneurysms causing symptoms from compression and displacement of adjacent structures. Often the aneurysm cannot be palpated, because it is concealed in the upper abdomen by the stomach and pancreas. The diagnosis may be suspected from the chest roentgenogram disclosing enlargement of the thoracic aorta near the diaphragm, but aortography is required to confirm the diagnosis.

TREATMENT. Most of the earlier operations have been performed with a multiple bypass technique, inserting an initial bypass graft from the thoracic aorta above the aneurysm to the abdominal aorta below the origin of the renal arteries. From this initial graft, branch grafts are then serially inserted to the celiac artery, superior mesenteric artery, and both renal arteries. Once the grafts have been inserted, avoiding prolonged ischemia of any individual organ, the aneurysm can be opened widely and the inner lining removed. Anastomosis to the right renal artery may be more conveniently performed at this time.

These procedures have been performed through a variety of thoracic and abdominal incisions. A thoracoabdominal incision from a left lateral position has been employed, or a separate midline abdominal incision combined with a left thoracotomy incision.

In recent years Cooley and others have reported the use of left atriofemoral bypass for excision of the aneurysm, establishing bypass and then opening the aneurysm widely, followed by direct anastomoses to the involved visceral arteries with a long straight graft. This technique must be accomplished in a short period of time, however, to avoid significant ischemic injury.

Patients surviving this complex operative procedure have had a fairly good prognosis. In the group of 42 surgically treated patients reported by DeBakey in 1965, 11 died within 1 month of operation, a mortality of 26 percent. There were four deaths subsequently, but the remaining 27 patients were alive without significant disability at the time of the report. The longest individual follow-up was about 10 years (Fig. 20-11).

DISSECTING ANEURYSMS

ETIOLOGY AND INCIDENCE. Dissecting aneurysms are related to degenerative disease of the media of the aorta, the cause of which is unknown. The disease is about three times as common in males as in females and is most frequently seen in patients in the fifth and sixth decades. However, it can occur in almost any age group, one of

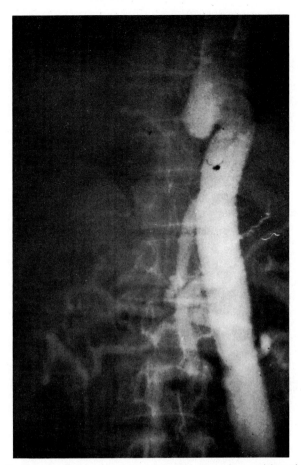

Fig. 20-11. Angiogram of Dacron graft 1 year after excision of thoracoabdominal aneurysm. The graft was inserted between the thoracic aorta, as an end-to-side anastomosis, and the abdominal aorta, not shown in this illustration. Side branches to the superior mesenteric artery, celiac artery, and right and left renal arteries are individually visible.

the youngest patients being only 14 months of age. The most frequently associated factor is hypertension, present in 75 to 85 percent of patients, although the reported incidence has varied widely.

Conditions associated with abnormalities of connective tissue have a greater frequency with dissecting aneurysm. The most common of these is the Marfan syndrome. Before surgical therapy was available, most patients with the Marfan syndrome succumbed either from a dissecting aneurysm or from aortic insufficiency as a result of dilatation of the aortic annulus. Other conditions occasionally associated with dissecting aneurysm include coarctation of the aorta, pregnancy, and kyphoscoliosis. Atherosclerosis is not a definite causative factor. The segment of aorta most frequently involved is different in the two diseases, since dissecting aneurysm usually involves the proximal thoracic aorta while atherosclerosis is most severe near the bifurcation of the abdominal aorta. There is also no known relationship to trauma or syphilis.

Experimentally, dissecting aneurysm can be produced in young rats with a diet containing 50 percent sweet peas, which causes a distinct abnormality of connective tissue, known as *lathyrism*.

PATHOLOGY. The term "dissecting aneurysm" is actually a misnomer, for the pathologic lesion is more accurately described as a "dissecting hematoma," consisting of a hemorrhagic separation of the layers of the aortic wall (Fig. 20-12). The basic lesion is degeneration of the aortic media, often associated with rupture of the vasa vasorum. Most patients also have a tear in the intima of the aorta, establishing a communication between the lumen of the aorta and the hematoma in the aortic wall. Whether the tear in the intima is a primary or secondary event is uncertain. If it is the primary event, superimposed upon underlying disease of the aortic media, the progressive dissection of the aortic wall which follows may result from establishing a communication between the lumen of the aorta and the aortic wall. The alternative hypothesis is that rupture of the vasa vasorum is the primary event, creating an intramural hemorrhage, which secondarily ruptures through the intima to establish communication with the aortic lumen. Rarely no intimal laceration can be found at autopsy, which indicates that rupture of the vasa vasorum was the primary event. The frequency with which tears of the intima are localized either to the ascending aorta or near the ligamentum arteriosum, however, suggests that laceration of the intima is probably the initial event in the majority of patients.

In 60 to 70 percent of patients the dissection originates in the ascending aorta, while in about 25 percent it originates beyond the left subclavian artery near the ligamentum arteriosum (Fig. 20-13). Infrequently it may originate in the aortic arch or at more distal locations in the aorta.

Once a dissection has begun, it may extend progressively to involve all of the thoracic and abdominal aorta as well as many of the arterial tributaries. This occurs in a high percentage of patients. As dissection progresses, branch vessels are sheared off, either becoming obliterated or establishing a communication with the false lumen created by the dissection. Proximally, the coronary arteries may be involved, and frequently one or more aortic valve cusps are detached and prolapse into the lumen, creating aortic insufficiency. More distad the vessels involved may include any tributary of the aorta. Involvement of the carotid arteries may produce neurologic injury. Obstruction of the subclavian arteries produces differences in blood pressure between the two arms. Dissection of intercostal arteries may cause spinal cord injury with paraplegia. Dissection of renal arteries may produce fatal renal insufficiency; in the extremities acute obstruction of the iliac or femoral arteries can result in either claudication or gangrene.

The dissection may terminate fatally at any time by rupture of the false lumen. The usual mode of death is rupture into the pericardial cavity from proximal dissection or rupture into the left pleural cavity. In the extensive review of 425 cases by Hirst et al., 21 percent of the patients died within 24 hours and 74 percent within 2 weeks. Ninety-one percent had succumbed within 6 months. In a group of 50 patients reported from the Massachusetts General Hospital by Austen et al., 45 percent died in the first week, 75 percent in the first month, and 86 percent

Fig. 20-12. *A.* Photograph of dissecting aneurysm of the thoracic aorta operated upon a few days after onset of the dissection. The lung is being separated from the aneurysm. Hematoma in the wall of the dissected aorta is visible. *B.* With a left atriofemoral bypass functioning and the aorta occluded, the aneurysm has been incised. The lacerated edges of the aortic wall from the dissection can be seen. Clot is visible in the wall of the aorta superior to the tip of the metal aspirator.

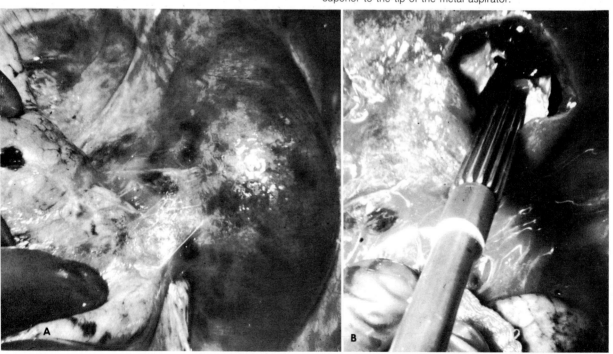

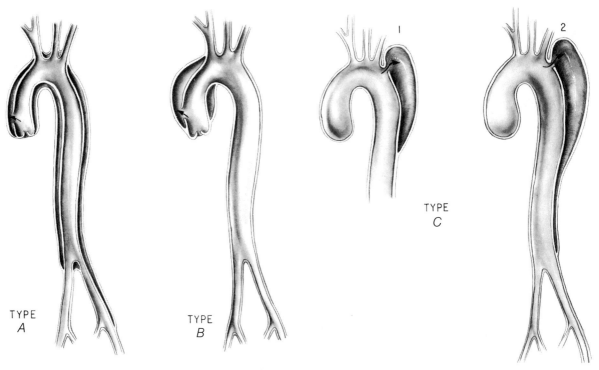

Fig. 20-13. Different types of aortic dissection. *A.* Dissecting aneurysm which begins in the ascending aorta near the aortic valve and extends throughout the aorta down to the external iliac arteries. Unfortunately, this is a common type of dissecting aneurysm. *B.* Dissecting aneurysm limited to the ascending aorta. This is commonly seen in the Marfan syndrome. *C1.* Dissecting aneurysm beginning distal to the left subclavian artery. The localized nature of this aneurysm makes it readily accessible to surgical excision. *2.* Dissecting aneurysm arising distal to the left subclavian artery but extending into the abdominal aorta. Only partial excision of the area of dissection is possible.

within the first year. In evaluating mortality statistics, it is important to differentiate dissections arising in the ascending aorta from dissections arising distal to the left subclavian artery. The former have a much higher mortality rate. In a group of 62 patients reported by Lindsay and Hurst, almost all 40 patients with dissection involving the ascending aorta succumbed within 3 weeks, while in the group of 19 patients in whom the disease began distal to the aortic arch the survival was greater than 50 percent.

In patients who survive with a dissecting aneurysm an endothelial lining of the false lumen, termed a *healed dissecting aneurysm,* may develop and establish a so-called "double-barreled" aorta. A wide variety of bizarre circulatory patterns may be found in such patients. For example, one renal artery may arise from the "false" lumen and the other from the true lumen (Fig. 20-14), or alternatively both renal arteries can arise from the false lumen. In other patients, one iliac artery may originate from the false lumen, and the other from the true lumen.

In the few patients surviving an aortic dissection, rupture of the false lumen back into the true aortic lumen has often been found at the termination of the dissection. This spontaneous "reentry" into the aortic lumen suggested that establishing a communication between the false lumen and the true lumen might terminate the dissecting process. These observations led to the development of the aortic fenestration operation, originally attempted by Gurin and by Shaw, and later extensively used by DeBakey and associates. At the time of introduction of this operation, little else could be offered such patients. Significant benefit from fenestration operations has been meager, however, and the operation has now been almost completely abandoned as more effective methods of therapy have been developed. The failure of development of a reentry area

to protect against external rupture was noted by McCloy and associates. In a group of 22 patients who died from external rupture of a dissecting aneurysm, 11 had developed a point of reentry of the dissection into the aortic lumen, but this had not prevented fatal rupture.

CLINICAL MANIFESTATIONS. The abrupt onset of excruciating pain, almost immediately reaching its peak intensity, is very characteristic of a dissecting aneurysm. A myocardial infarction, by contrast, may gradually develop pain of increasing severity over several minutes. Usually anterior chest pain develops with dissection of the ascending aorta, while back pain is more common with dissection beginning distal to the aortic arch. Pain may be in both the front and back of the chest with dissection of either type, but usually predominant back pain suggests dissection beyond the left subclavian artery. Another significant characteristic of the pain is its tendency to migrate into different areas as dissection extends distad. As might be predicted from the wide variation in the extent of the dissection process, many pain syndromes may occur. Pain may radiate to the neck, the arm, the epigastrium, or the leg. Seldom is pain completely absent, probably in no more than 10 percent of patients.

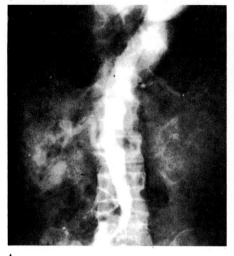

A

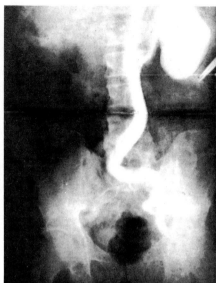

B

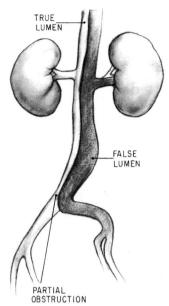

Fig. 20-14. *A.* Aortogram showing an unusual pattern of aortic dissection in which dissection extended from the thoracic aorta into the abdominal aorta, creating two lumens, with the right renal artery arising from one and the left renal artery from the other. Focal stenosis of the right common iliac artery is seen at the lower part of the field producing intermittent claudication, which was the presenting complaint of the patient. *B.* Aortogram performed by a different root opacifies the left kidney and the left common iliac artery. The condition of the dissected aorta is illustrated in the accompanying drawing. Circulation was reestablished by excising the septum between the two channels at the aortic bifurcation. (*Adapted from W. Gryboski and F. C. Spencer, Intermittent Claudication Caused by a Dissecting Aneurysm of the Aorta, South Med J, 58:593, 1965.*)

Syncope occurs in 10 to 20 percent of patients, and some neurologic symptoms are present in 20 to 40 percent. These may result from ischemia of the brain, spinal cord, or a peripheral nerve, depending upon whether a carotid artery, an intercostal artery, or a peripheral artery has been compromised.

Hypertension, often of severe degree, is present in 75 to 85 percent of patients. Often the hypertension with severe vasoconstriction contrasts with the clinical picture of an acutely ill patient, pale, sweating, and in acute distress. An aortic diastolic murmur appears in 20 to 30 percent of patients and is of great diagnostic significance, usually originating from detachment of an aortic valve cusp. Less frequently a pericardial friction rub may be audible due to leakage of blood into the pericardial cavity. Inequality of the carotid or subclavian pulses may be found, caused by unequal compression of these vessels. A variety of neurologic abnormalities may be detected, the most common being either a monoplegia or paraplegia.

DIAGNOSTIC FINDINGS. On the chest roentgenogram a widened mediastinum or a left pleural effusion from extravasation of blood is frequently seen. In some patients, however, the roentgenogram may be completely normal. The electrocardiogram is of particular value in distinguishing dissecting aneurysm from myocardial infarction, but there are no characteristic features of aortic dissection. The most common abnormality is left ventricular hypertrophy from the antecedent hypertension.

Aortography to demonstrate the double lumen created by the dissection is the most definitive diagnostic procedure. In some patients a diagnosis cannot be established by any other technique, especially if there are no abnormal physical findings and the only abnormality is a history of severe back pain. Aortography is probably most safely performed by injection of dye through a catheter into the pulmonary artery.

TREATMENT. The most effective treatment for acute dissecting aneurysm has not yet been determined. The urgency of treatment is well emphasized by the grim mortality statistics, with 40 to 50 percent of patients dying within 2 weeks and the majority of those surviving the first 2 weeks succumbing within 1 year. Only about 10 percent of untreated patients survive beyond this time.

It is important in evaluating different forms of therapy to separate patients with dissections of the ascending aorta from patients in whom the dissection is distal to the aortic arch. The prognosis is much worse with dissections in the ascending aorta, with an acute mortality exceeding 90 percent in some series.

A significant addition to the therapy of dissecting aneurysms was made by Wheat and associates in 1965 when they reported the successful treatment of six patients with antihypertensive drugs. These studies were partly stimulated by observations from the poultry industry that certain flocks of turkeys had a high fatality rate from spontaneous dissecting aneurysm which could be reduced dramatically by adding to the food a small amount of reserpine (0.1 part to 1 million). Wheat et al. noted that their patients often lived a few hours to a few days following onset of the aortic dissection, only to succumb from continued dissection with eventual rupture. Because of the high frequency of hypertension in this group of patients, antihypertensive drugs were utilized to ameliorate the dissecting process. The therapeutic program included the immediate lowering of blood pressure by an intravenous infusion of Arfonad (trimethaphan), combined with the simultaneous administration of reserpine, chlorothiazide (Diuril), and guanethidine (Ismelin). Other investigators employing this form of therapy have substituted methyldopa (Aldomet) for guanethidine. Harris et al. stated that 19 of 21 patients had survived treatment with induced hypotension, 18 of whom were living and well with no progression of the disease. Austen and associates, in contrast, had a 60 percent mortality in patients with acute dissection.

At this time the ultimate role of drug therapy remains uncertain. Although Wheat and associates have obtained an impressively low mortality in their series of patients, others have been unable to duplicate these findings. With improved surgical techniques there has been an increasing tendency to perform early operation, within either a few hours or a few days after onset of symptoms. Data supporting an early operative approach were published in 1970 by Daily et al. and in 1972 by Liotta et al., by Shumacker, and by Najafi and associates.

Although the final role of antihypertensive therapy is uncertain, its value is obvious as emergency therapy in the presence of severe hypertension to slow or reduce by half the dissecting process. Once the patient's condition is stabilized, emergency aortography can be performed to identify the area of dissection. From the location of the dissection, a decision can be made whether to perform emergency operation or not. Operation is simpler if dissection is located distal to the left subclavian artery. At New York University most patients in this category have been operated upon promptly, excising the area of dissection and restoring arterial continuity with a woven Dacron prosthesis (Fig. 20-15 and 20-16). If the dissection extends throughout the thoracic aorta, only the major area of involvement is removed, and the layers of the dissected aorta are sewed together distad before insertion of the prosthetic graft.

When operation is performed upon patients with dissection of the ascending aorta, the preferred treatment is excision of the ascending aorta and reconstruction with a Dacron prosthetic graft. Concomitant aortic insufficiency may be treated by reattachment of the prolapsed aortic valve cusps, occasionally by prosthetic valve replacement (Fig. 20-4). If the dissection has extended into the transverse arch and involves the origin of the great vessels, excision is probably best limited to the ascending aorta, sewing the layers of the dissected aorta together before the prosthetic graft is inserted. The long-term prognosis for these dissected aortas is yet unknown, but data thus far available indicate that prognosis is reasonably good if hypertension is controlled. After months or years, some will probably develop into a localized aneurysm in a manner similar to that occurring with an aorta affected by syphilis, where function continues for several years after injury before a focal aneurysm develops.

Several years ago DeBakey and associates reported an extensive series of 142 patients with a mortality of 20 percent. Austen and associates had a similar mortality of 22 percent in 23 patients, while Harris et al. reported a mortality near 50 percent in 22 patients. According to recent reports, with improved techniques mortality rates have been significantly improved.

WOUNDS OF THE GREAT VESSELS

Penetrating Injuries

Penetrating injuries of the aorta or venae cavae are a frequent cause of death with penetrating chest injuries. Fatal hemorrhage occurs so quickly that only a few patients survive long enough for treatment. Patients alive with such injuries when first seen are usually in profound shock with signs of massive intrathoracic bleeding. Immediate thoracotomy offers the only chance for survival. In some instances this must be employed in the emergency department, often with conditions less than ideal. Once hemorrhage has been stopped, the patient is often transferred to the operating room for more definitive surgical exploration and subsequent closure of the incision. Depending upon the location of the injury, a variety of thoracic incisions have been used, including thoracotomy, median sternotomy, resection of the clavicle to expose the subclavian artery, or a cervicothoracic approach. In all likelihood a median sternotomy should be employed far more frequently than in the past, as was emphasized by Brawley et al. in 1970. Injuries involving the origin of the innominate or left common carotid artery, with cerebral ischemia, may be most safely managed with a temporary shunt. Experiences with shunts for injuries of this type were described recently by Ecker et al.

An unusual type of penetrating injury is one involving the intrapericardial portion of the ascending aorta; development of cardiac tamponade may temporarily control bleeding and allow more time for operation. In 1961 Dively et al. reported successful treatment of three patients with this type of unusual injury and described published experiences with others. Rarely a small penetrating injury may produce a fistula between the aorta and right ventricle, between the aorta and vena cava, or between the aorta and pulmonary artery.

Nonpenetrating Injuries

Traumatic injury of the aorta following blunt trauma is important to recognize, because effective surgical therapy is possible in many patients. Unfortunately the diagnosis is often not considered because of the unusual nature of the lesion. It is a frequent finding at autopsy following a fatal injury, but careful analysis of 171 cases by Parmley et al. emphasized that surgical therapy was possible because 20 percent of the patients lived longer than 30 minutes after injury and several survived for several days before fatal hemorrhage occurred. Only in the past decade has increasing familiarity with the lesion occasionally resulted in early diagnosis and successful therapy.

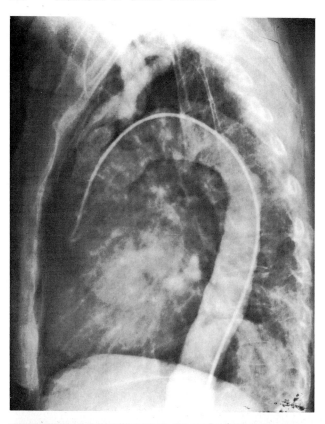

Fig. 20-15. *Opposite.* Thoracic aortogram, performed with a catheter introduced retrograde through the femoral artery, showing a dissecting aneurysm arising distal to the left subclavian artery. The outer channel is faintly visualized as a double density beyond the left subclavian artery. *Lower left.* Operative photograph of dissecting aneurysm arising distal to the left subclavian artery. A clamp is visible on the aorta proximal to the left subclavian artery, which has been encircled with an umbilical tape. The vagus nerve is visible proximally. Laminated clot was found in the lumen of the aneurysm. *Lower right.* Dacron graft inserted to restore aortic continuity following excision of the aneurysm.

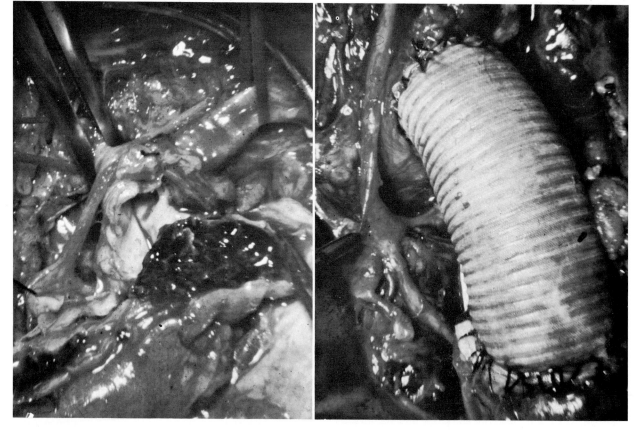

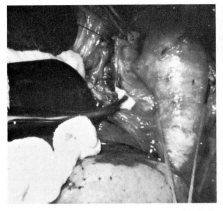 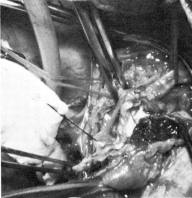 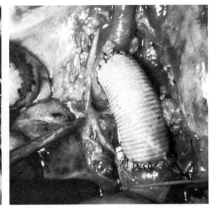

Fig. 20-16. *Left.* Operative photograph of dissecting aneurysm of upper thoracic aorta, starting a few days before operation. The hematoma in the aortic wall is visible. *Center.* With a functioning left atrial bypass, the aorta has been occluded and the aneurysm incised. A tape encircles the left subclavian artery. The vagus nerve with the recurrent nerve encircling the aorta is visible. The aneurysm began in the classic location, just beyond the left subclavian artery. A large thrombus is present in the aortic wall. *Right.* Aortic reconstruction was accomplished with a short woven Dacron graft. The proximal anastomosis is immediately beyond the left subclavian artery.

ETIOLOGY AND PATHOLOGY. A rupture of the aorta is usually produced from a deceleration-type injury, typically in an automobile accident. In 70 to 75 percent of patients the aortic laceration occurs just distal to the left subclavian artery. Apparently the descending thoracic aorta and the aortic arch decelerate at different rates because of differences in anatomic structure, and a transverse tear of the aorta is produced near the site of insertion of the ligamentum arteriosum. The tear may involve part or all of the layers of the aortic wall, varying from laceration of the intima to transection of the aorta with retraction of the two ends. Part or all of the circumference of the aortic wall may be involved (Fig. 20-17). Fatal hemorrhage is prevented in some patients by the adventitia, which has been reported to constitute 60 percent of the tensile strength of the aortic wall.

The next most frequent site of injury is in the ascending aorta near its origin from the left ventricle. Other sites are very unusual and may be produced by various forms of injury, such as direct trauma or vertical deceleration injuries as in a fall from a building. A dissecting aneurysm following trauma is extremely rare.

In patients who do not exsanguinate soon after injury, a hematoma forms in the mediastinum and produces a characteristic roentgenographic appearance due to enlargement of the mediastinum. Disturbances in blood flow through the aorta usually do not occur. Only a few instances of paraplegia appearing after aortic injury from acute interruption of blood flow have been described. Following the acute injury, a latent period is often present before the mediastinal hematoma surrounding the aortic laceration suddenly ruptures into the pleural cavity and causes fatal hemorrhage. The fatal rupture almost always occurs within 4 weeks after injury. Spencer et al. described a few examples of rupture 30 to 90 days after injury.

In patients who survive longer than 2 months after injury a false aneurysm of the aorta gradually develops and may pursue an unusually benign course. Unlike the more common atherosclerotic or syphilitic aneurysms, traumatic aneurysms may remain as asymptomatic mediastinal masses for many years, or even decades, until enlargement occurs. Calcification develops in most such lesions after varying periods of time and may provide the first clue to the diagnosis when first recognized on a chest roentgenogram made for other reasons. Only a moderate amount of data is available about the long-term course of traumatic aneurysms, probably because many have been misdiagnosed as calcified atherosclerotic or syphilitic aneurysms. In 1961, in a detailed review of reported experiences with traumatic aneurysms Spencer et al. found only about 60 reported cases. Apparently most such lesions tend to enlarge after months or years, producing compression of the left main bronchus and the recurrent laryngeal nerve. With such enlargement, symptoms from obstruction of the left bronchus appear and require therapy. Usually enlargement of traumatic aneurysms proceeds slowly for a long period of time before rupture occurs, providing ample time for diagnosis and therapy.

Associated injuries are common. Most patients have fractures of the ribs, and fractures of the extremities occur in about 50 percent of patients, reflecting the severity of trauma producing the aortic injury.

CLINICAL MANIFESTATIONS. Following injury to the thorax, there are usually no symptoms or signs to indicate that an aortic injury has occurred. Dyspnea and chest pain are usually present, but these commonly result from the almost universally present rib fractures and do not aid in recognizing rupture of the aorta. A hemothorax, with varying degrees of shock, is also frequent, but again such findings frequently arise from rib fractures and pulmonary lacerations which do not involve the aorta. A murmur has been present in only a few patients. Rarely, signs of acute obstruction of the aorta, apparently from prolapse of a segment of intima with obstruction of the lumen, have occurred, with weak or absent femoral pulses and even acute paraplegia.

Patients with a traumatic aortic aneurysm who are first seen months or years following injury are often asymptomatic and are evaluated because of the accidental dis-

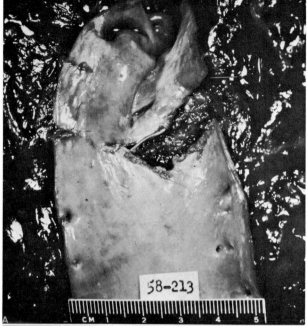

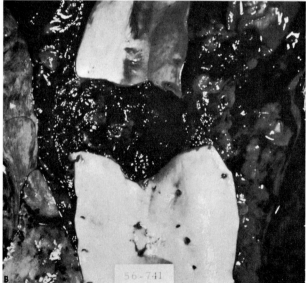

Fig. 20-17. *A.* Transected aorta found at autopsy when the patient was exsanguinated 24 hours following injury. The patient had only minor chest pain before the terminal event. The sharp, transverse laceration of the aorta is the usual finding, resulting from the deceleration forces at the time of injury. *B.* Partial transection of the aorta found at autopsy when the patient was suddenly exsanguinated 3 weeks following an automobile accident. An aortic lesion had not been previously suspected.

covery of a mediastinal mass on a chest roentgenogram. Symptoms, if present, are usually due to compression of the left main bronchus from an expanding aneurysm, causing cough, wheeze, dyspnea, and pneumonia. Compression and paralysis of the left recurrent laryngeal nerve may produce hoarseness. (See the section on Traumatic Thoracic Aneurysms.)

DIAGNOSTIC FINDINGS. The chest roentgenogram provides the best clue to the diagnosis. In acutely injured patients with rupture of the aorta, widening of the mediastinum (Fig. 20-18) is almost invariably present. It is important to realize, however, that this may result from a hematoma arising from some cause other than rupture of the aorta. When widening of the mediastinum is recognized on the chest roentgenogram, serious consideration should be given to performing an emergency aortogram, for only with an aortogram can the diagnosis be firmly established (Fig. 20-19). Postponing aortography may be fatal, for the mediastinal hematoma surrounding the lacerated aorta often ruptures without any warning symptoms. In asymptomatic patients who are seen because of an undiagnosed mediastinal mass, aortography also provides the most definitive means of establishing the diagnosis.

TREATMENT. Thoracotomy should be performed as soon as possible after the diagnosis has been established. A 1961 review of all reported experiences found only one patient who had survived repair of an aortic laceration. In the past decade, fortunately, many patients have been successfully treated, a result of increasing familiarity with the clinical picture combined with the availability of emergency aortography and thoracotomy.

As with thoracic aneurysms, the surgical approach is through a left posterolateral thoracotomy in the fourth intercostal space. Some form of aortic bypass is essential to avoid paraplegia during occlusion of the aorta (Fig. 20-9). This was initially done with the conventional left atriofemoral bypass, but more recently systemic heparinization has been avoided by the use of aortic shunts. An excellent report by Kirsh et al. in 1970 described experi-

Fig. 20-18. Chest roentgenogram of a patient with traumatic rupture of the thoracic aorta, illustrating the characteristic widening of the mediastinum. When this is observed following a chest injury, emergency aortography should be performed to establish the diagnosis of rupture of the thoracic aorta.

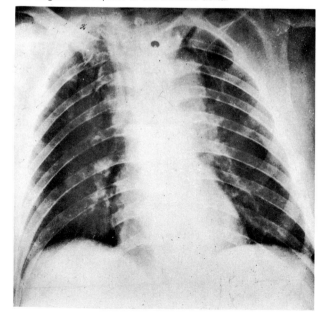

ences with 12 patients over a period of 4 years in whom a simple bypass shunt was used without extracorporeal circulation. Six patients underwent operation within 8 hours of injury and eleven within 48 hours. In all instances direct suture was not possible, and insertion of a prosthetic graft was required. A successful repair was accomplished in 10 of the 12 patients (Fig. 20-20).

OBSTRUCTION OF THE SUPERIOR VENA CAVA

Obstruction of the superior vena cava produces an unusual but distinctive clinical syndrome which can be easily recognized once the diagnosis is considered. Diagnostic errors are surprisingly common, however, partly because of the infrequent occurrence and partly because of a lack of familiarity with the distinctive clinical features.

ETIOLOGY. In 70 to 80 percent of patients superior vena cava obstruction is due to a malignant neoplasm. This was true in 48 of 64 patients described by Effler and Groves and in 90 percent of 60 cases reported by Hanlon and Danis. Usually the neoplasm is a bronchogenic carcinoma of the right upper lobe which is invading the mediastinum. Less frequently seen are primary mediastinal tumors, such as thymoma or lymphoma. Metastatic neoplasms from a distant source are unusual.

In the past, saccular aneurysms were found in about 30 percent of patients with vena cava obstruction, but with the marked decrease in frequency of syphilitic aneurysms, these are now infrequently seen. If superior vena cava obstruction is not due to a malignant tumor, a chronic fibrosing mediastinitis, usually of unknown origin, is the most common cause. Probably many of the cases undiagnosed in the past were due to histoplasmosis. Obstruction from a benign tumor, such as a substernal thyroid, is unusual.

PATHOPHYSIOLOGY. With obstruction of the superior vena cava there is an increase in venous pressure in its tributaries in the arms and head to levels ranging between 200 and 500 cm of water. The degree of increase in venous pressure varies with the rate of development and the site of the obstruction. Obstruction proximal to the site of entry of the azygos vein is more disabling than more distal sites of obstruction in which a patent azygos vein can function as a collateral pathway. Acute obstruction of the vena cava, as during a thoracic operation, can produce fatal cerebral edema within a few minutes. At the opposite extreme are instances where superior vena cava obstruction develops slowly, permitting time for the development of collateral circulation, as a result of which symptoms are mild.

CLINICAL MANIFESTATIONS. With mild obstruction, frequent symptoms are headache, swelling of the eyelids, puffiness of the face, or enlargement of the neck. In males there may be a noticeable increase in collar size. The severity of symptoms is closely related to posture, for the patient quickly notes that his symptoms increase if he bends over or lies down. If obstruction of the vena cava develops rapidly, as with hemorrhage into a rapidly growing neoplasm, more serious symptoms of cerebral conges-

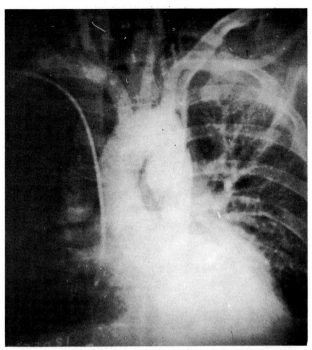

Fig. 20-19. Aortogram demonstrating traumatic rupture of the thoracic aorta distal to the left subclavian artery. The point of rupture can be seen as an irregular border of the thoracic aorta, in association with localized bulging. This angiogram represents the first instance in which emergency aortography was employed to establish firmly the diagnosis of traumatic rupture of the aorta.

tion are present, including drowsiness and blurring of vision. Edema of the vocal cords may produce hoarseness or dyspnea. As the majority of cases are due to a rapidly growing bronchogenic carcinoma, pulmonary symptoms such as cough and hemoptysis are also frequently present. In most patients death results in a few months.

In the minority of patients in whom obstruction is due to a benign process, collateral circulation may enlarge sufficiently to where little disability is present. Prominent features include dilated veins with edema and cyanosis, the degree varying with the degree of stasis. Venous hypertension is manifested by prominence and distension of the veins. Effler and Groves have reported 16 patients with obstruction from a benign process, all of whom eventually developed sufficient collateral circulation to have minimal symptoms; there were no fatalities as a direct result of the chronic venous obstruction. We have observed one child over a period of 15 years in whom the superior vena cava was obstructed following an intracardiac operation for correction of anomalous pulmonary veins entering the superior vena cava. Initially there was serious venous hypertension to levels of 350 cm of water, producing a bilateral chylothorax ultimately controlled by ligation of the thoracic duct. Within a few months, however, all symptoms subsided, and the patient, now a young woman, has participated fully in school athletic activities without any disability.

DIAGNOSTIC STUDIES. Although the clinical picture is characteristic when fully developed, early manifestations

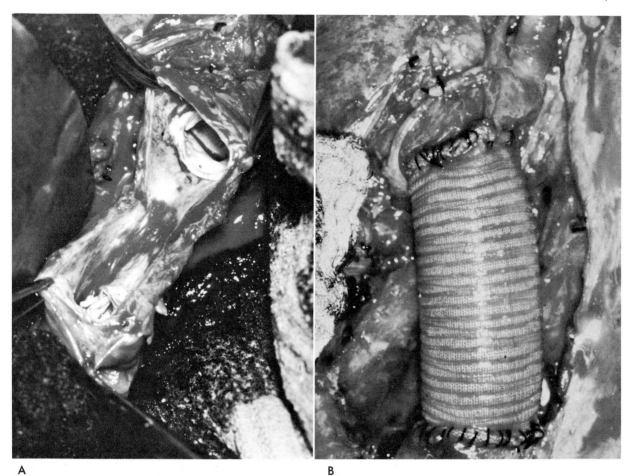

A

B

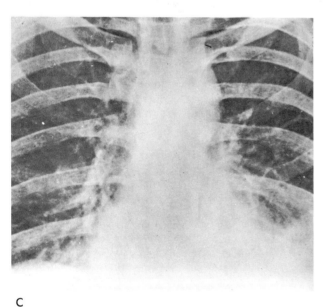

C

Fig. 20-20. *A.* Operative photograph of transection of aorta found approximately 2 weeks following injury. Complete retraction of the two ends of the aorta was found at operation. The patient was asymptomatic *except* for a mass found on the chest roentgenogram. *B.* Aortic reconstruction with a knitted Dacron graft. Postoperative course was uneventful. *C.* Chest roentgenogram 13 days after an automobile accident, showing a localized bulging in the upper mediastinum, subsequently found at operation to represent transection of the thoracic aorta distal to the left subclavian artery.

of the disease, such as swelling of the eyes or headache, may be confused with angioneurotic edema, congestive heart failure, or constrictive pericarditis. The diagnosis can be confirmed by measuring the venous pressure, which is usually in the range of 200 to 500 cm of water. The location and extent of the obstruction can be best outlined by venography. In some patients the underlying disease process is uncertain, although usually signs of a bronchogenic carcinoma are visible on a chest roentgenogram. Bronchoscopy and biopsy may be helpful in confirming the diagnosis. Aortography can be used if necessary to exclude the presence of an aneurysm.

TREATMENT. With a malignant process, there is almost uniform agreement that involvement of the superior vena cava precludes curative surgical resection. Therefore, thoracotomy usually should be avoided. Serious bleeding is often encountered from the venous hypertension, and interruption of collateral pathways may intensify the venous hypertension. If the diagnosis can be established by bronchoscopy, mediastinoscopy, or by biopsy of a supraclavicular node, there is no need for thoracotomy. In some seriously ill patients with a mass in the right upper lung field on the chest roentgenogram, it may be simpler to proceed directly with radiation therapy rather than employ a thoracotomy to confirm an almost obvious diagnosis.

Significant palliation can be obtained by intensive radiation therapy, often in combination with diuretics and chemotherapy. Improvement in symptoms soon occurs, probably from diminution in edema associated with a growing neoplasm. Death from the neoplasm, however, usually occurs within a few months.

With benign obstructions, the report of Effler and Groves clearly indicates that there is no urgency in performing an operation if symptoms are mild. In all likelihood symptoms will improve or subside completely as collateral circulation develops. A number of ingenious attempts have been made to reconstruct an obstructed superior vena cava. Prosthetic grafts have been almost uniformly unsuccessful, with the possible exception of a crimped Teflon graft, which experimentally has given the best results. The most favorable graft is a composite one of autogenous veins, prepared by combining both superficial femoral veins into a graft of larger diameter. Good results lasting for several years have been reported by Hanlon and Danis in three patients in whom such grafts were used.

Rarely a localized granuloma may compress and thrombose the vena cava; patency can be restored by opening the vein and removing the clot. Three such cases have been reported by Pate and Hammon and one such patient by Hanlon and Danis. Other ingenious attempts to bypass the obstructed vena cava, applicable in certain specific instances, have been reported. Cooley and Hallman rotated the azygos vein to provide a bypass route for draining blood directly into the atrium, while Schramel and Olinde reversed the saphenous vein in a subcutaneous tunnel to drain blood from the superior vena cava system to the common femoral vein.

References

Aneurysms of the Ascending Aorta

Bahnson, H. T., and Spencer, F. C.: Excision of Aneurysm of the Ascending Aorta with Prosthetic Replacement during Cardiopulmonary Bypass, *Ann Surg,* **151:**879, 1960.

Bloodwell, R. D., Hallman, G. L., and Cooley, D. A.: Aneurysm of the Ascending Aorta with Aortic Valvular Insufficiency, *Arch Surg,* **92:**588, 1966.

Lefrak, E. A., Stevens, P. M., and Howell, J. F.: Respiratory Insufficiency Due to Tracheal Compression by an Aneurysm of the Ascending, Transverse, and Descending Thoracic Aorta: Successful Surgical Management, *J Thorac Cardiovasc Surg,* **63:**956, 1972.

Liotta, D., Hallman, G. L., Milam, J. D., and Cooley, D. A.: Surgical Treatment of Acute Dissecting Aneurysm of the Ascending Aorta, *Ann Thorac Surg,* **12:**582, 1971.

Shumacker, H. B., Jr.: Operative Treatment of Aneurysms of the Thoracic Aorta Due to Cystic Medial Necrosis, *J Thorac Cardiovasc Surg,* **63:**1, 1972.

Spencer, F. C., and Blake, H. A.: A Report of the Successful Surgical Treatment of Aortic Regurgitation from a Dissecting Aortic Aneurysm in a Patient with the Marfan Syndrome, *J Thorac Cardiovasc Surg,* **44:**238, 1962.

Aneurysms of the Transverse Aortic Arch

Bloodwell, R. D., Hallman, G. L., and Cooley, D. A.: Total Replacement of the Aortic Arch and the "Subclavian Steal" Phenomenon, *Ann Thorac Surg,* **5:**236, 1968.

DeBakey, M. E., Beall, A. C., Jr., Cooley, D. A., Crawford, E. S., Morris, G. C., Jr., and Garrett, H. E.: Resection and Graft Replacement of Aneurysms Involving the Transverse Arch of the Aorta, *Surg Clin North Am,* **46:**1057, 1966.

Lefrak, E. A., Stevens, P. M., and Howell, J. F.: Respiratory Insufficiency Due to Tracheal Compression by an Aneurysm of the Ascending, Transverse, and Descending Thoracic Aorta: Successful Surgical Management, *J Thorac Cardiovasc Surg,* **63:**956, 1972.

Liotta, D., Hallman, G. L., Milam, J. D., and Cooley, D. A.: Surgical Treatment of Acute Dissecting Aneurysm of the Ascending Aorta, *Ann Thorac Surg,* **12:**582, 1971.

Traumatic Thoracic Aneurysms

Bennett, D. E., and Cherry, J. K.: The Natural History of Traumatic Aneurysms of the Aorta, *Surgery,* **61:**516, 1967.

Cooley, D. A.: Discussion of R. J. Stoney, B. B. Roe, and J. V. Redington, Rupture of Thoracic Aorta Due to Closed-Chest Trauma, *Arch Surg,* **89:**840, 1964.

Kirsh, M. M., Vathayanon, S., Kahn, D., Crane, J. D., Anastasia, L., Lui, A. H., Moores, W. Y., Bookstein, J., and Sloan, H.: Repair of Acute Traumatic Rupture of the Aorta without Extracorporeal Circulation, *Ann Thorac Surg,* **10:**227, 1970.

Liotta, D., Hallman, G. L., Milam, J. D., and Cooley, D. A.: Surgical Treatment of Acute Dissecting Aneurysm of the Ascending Aorta, *Ann Thorac Surg,* **12:**582, 1971.

Spencer, F. C., Guerin, P. F., Blake, H. A., and Bahnson, H. T.: A Report of Fifteen Patients with Traumatic Rupture of the Thoracic Aorta, *J Thorac Cardiovasc Surg,* **41:**1, 1961.

Aneurysms of the Descending Thoracic Aorta

Bahnson, H. T.: Definitive Treatment of Saccular Aneurysms of the Aorta with Excision of the Sac and Aortic Suture, *Surg Gynecol Obstet,* **96:**382, 1953.

Bloodwell, R. D., Hallman, G. L., Beall, A. C., Jr., Cooley, D. A., and DeBakey, M. E.: Aneurysms of the Descending Thoracic Aorta: Surgical Considerations, *Surg Clin North Am,* **46:**901, 1966.

Connolly, J. E., Kountz, S. L., and Boyd, R. J.: Left Heart Bypass: Experimental and Clinical Observations on its Regulation with Particular Reference to Maintenance of Maximal Renal Blood Flow, *J Thorac Cardiovasc Surg,* **44:**577, 1962.

Cooley, D. A., Belmonte, B. A., DeBakey, M. E., and Latson, J. R.: Temporary Extracorporeal Circulation in the Surgical Treatment of Cardiac and Aortic Disease: Report of 98 Cases, *Ann Surg,* **145:**898, 1957.

DeBakey, M. E., Cooley, D. A., Crawford, E. S., and Morris, G. C., Jr., Aneurysms of the Thoracic Aorta. Analysis of 179 Patients Treated by Resection, *J Thorac Surg,* **36:**393, 1958.

Gerbode, F., Braimbridge, M., Osborn, J. J., Hood, J., and French, S.: Traumatic Thoracic Aneurysms: Treatment by Resection and Grafting with the Use of Extracorporeal Bypass, *Surgery,* **42:**975, 1957.

Groves, L. K.: Experience with Thirteen Cases of Resection of Aneurysms of the Descending Thoracic Aorta, *Cleve Clin Q,* **28:**176, 1961.

Kahn, D. R., Vathayanon, S., and Sloan, H.: Resection of Descending Thoracic Aneurysms without Left Heart Bypass, *Arch Surg,* **97:**336, 1968.

Krauss, A. H., Ferguson, T. V., and Weldon, C. S.: Thoracic Aneurysmectomy Using the Tedmac Heparin Shunt, *Ann Thorac Surg,* **14:**123, 1972.

Vasko, J. S., Spencer, F. C., and Bahnson, H. T.: Aneurysm of the Aorta Treated by Excision: Review of 237 Cases Followed Up to Seven Years, *Am J Surg,* **105:**793, 1963.

Thoracoabdominal Aneurysms

DeBakey, M. E., Crawford, E. S., Garrett, H. E., Beall, A. C., Jr., and Howell, J. F.: Surgical Considerations in the Treatment of Aneurysms of the Thoraco-abdominal Aorta, *Ann Surg,* **162:**650, 1965.

Garrett, H. E., Crawford, E. S., Beall, A. C., Jr., Howell, J. F., and DeBakey, M. E.: Surgical Treatment of Aneurysm of the Thoracoabdominal Aorta, *Surg Clin North Am,* **46:**913, 1966.

Dissecting Aneurysms

Austen, W. G., Buckley, M. J., McFarland, J., DeSanctis, R. W., and Sanders, C. A.: Therapy of Dissecting Aneurysms, *Arch Surg,* **95:**835, 1967.

Daily, P. O., Trueblood, H. W., Stinson, E. B., Wuerflein, R. D., and Shumway, N. E.: Management of Acute Aortic Dissections, *Ann Thorac Surg,* **10:**337, 1970.

DeBakey, M. E., Henly, W. S., Cooley, D. A., Morris, G. C., Crawford, E. S., and Beall, A. C.: Surgical Management of Dissecting Aneurysms of the Aorta, *J Thorac Cardiovasc Surg,* **49:**130, 1965.

Gryboski, W., and Spencer, F. C.: Intermittent Claudication Caused by a Dissecting Aneurysm of the Aorta, *South Med J,* **58:**593, 1965.

Harris, P. D., Malm, J. R., Bigger, J. T., and Bowman, F. O.: Follow-up Studies of Acute Dissecting Aortic Aneurysms Managed with Antihypertensive Agents, *Circulation,* **35** (*Suppl* 1): I-183, 1967.

Hirst, A. E., Johns, V. J., and Kime, S. W.: Dissecting Aneurysm of the Aorta: A Review of 505 Cases, *Medicine* (*Baltimore*), **37:**217, 1958.

Lindsay, J., and Hurst, J. W.: Clinical Features and Prognosis in Dissecting Aneurysm of the Aorta, *Circulation,* **35:**880, 1967.

Liotta, D., Hallman, G. L., Milam, J. D., and Cooley, D. A.: Surgical Treatment of Acute Dissecting Aneurysm of the Ascending Aorta, *Ann Thorac Surg,* **12:**582, 1971.

McCloy, R. M., Spittell, J. A., and McGoon, D. C.: The Prognosis of Aortic Dissection (Dissecting Aortic Hematoma or Aneurysm), *Circulation,* **31:**665, 1965.

Najafi, H., Dye, W. S., Javid, H., Hunter, J. A., Goldin, M. D., and Julian, O. C.: Acute Aortic Regurgitation Secondary to Aortic Dissection: Surgical Management without Valve Replacement, *Ann Thorac Surg,* **14:**474, 1972.

Schumacker, H. B., Jr.: Operative Treatment of Aneurysms of the Thoracic Aorta Due to Cystic Medial Necrosis, *J Thorac Cardiovasc Surg,* **63:**1, 1972.

Spencer, F. C., and Blake, H. A.: A Report of the Successful Surgical Treatment of Aortic Regurgitation from a Dissecting Aortic Aneurysm in a Patient with the Marfan Syndrome, *J Thorac Cardiovasc Surg,* **44:**238, 1962.

Wheat, M. W., Jr., and Palmer, R. F.: Dissecting Aneurysms of the Aorta, *Curr Probl Surg,* July 1971.

———, ———, Bartley, T. D., and Seelman, R. C.: Treatment of Dissecting Aneurysms of the Aorta without Surgery, *J Thorac Cardiovasc Surg,* **50:**364, 1965.

Wounds of the Great Vessels

Bennett, D. E., and Cherry, D. K.: The Natural History of Traumatic Aneurysms of the Aorta, *Surgery,* **61:**516, 1967.

Blake, H. A., Inmon, T. W., and Spencer, F. C.: Emergency Use of Antegrade Aortography in Diagnosis of Acute Aortic Rupture, *Ann Surg,* **152:**954, 1960.

Brawley, R. K., Murray, G. F., Crisler, C., and Cameron, J. L.: Management of Wounds of the Innominate, Subclavian, and Axillary Blood Vessels, *Surg Gynecol Obstet,* **131:**1130, 1970.

Clarke, C. P., Brandt, P. W. T., Cole, D. S., and Barratt-Boyes, B. G.: Traumatic Rupture of the Thoracic Aorta: Diagnosis and Treatment, *Br J Surg,* **54:**353, 1967.

DeMuth, W. E., Jr., Roe, H., and Hobbie, W.: Immediate Repair of Traumatic Rupture of Thoracic Aorta, *Arch Surg,* **91:**602, 1965.

Dively, W. L., Daniel, R. A., and Scott, H. W.: Surgical Management of Penetrating Injuries of the Ascending Aorta and Aortic Arch, *J Thorac Cardiovasc Surg,* **41:**23, 1961.

Ecker, R. R., Dickinson, W. E., Sugg, W. L., and Rea, W. J.: Management of Injuries of the Innominate and Proximal Left Common Carotid Artery, *J Thorac Cardiovasc Surg,* **64:**618, 1972.

Gerbode, F., Braimbridge, M., Osborn, J. J., Hood, M., and French, S.: Traumatic Thoracic Aneurysm: Treatment by Resection and Grafting with the Use of Extracorporeal Bypass, *Surgery,* **42:**975, 1957.

Jahnke, E. J., Jr., Fisher, G. W., and Jones, R. C.: Acute Traumatic Rupture of the Thoracic Aorta: Report of Six Consecutive Cases of Successful Early Repair, *J Thorac Cardiovasc Surg,* **48:**63, 1964.

Kahn, A. M., Joseph, W. L., and Hughes, R. K.: Traumatic Aneurysms of the Thoracic Aorta: Excision and Repair without Graft, *Ann Thorac Surg,* **4:**175, 1967.

Kirsh, M. M., Vathayanon, S., Kahn, D., Crane, J. D., Anastasia, L., Lui, A. H., Moores, W. Y., Bookstein, J., and Sloan, H.: Repair of Acute Traumatic Rupture of the Aorta without Extracorporeal Circulation, *Ann Thorac Surg,* **10:**227, 1970.

Parmley, L. F., Mattingly, T. W., and Manion, W. C.: Penetrating Wounds to the Heart and Aorta, *Circulation,* **17:**953, 1958.

————, ————, ————, and Jahnke, E. J., Jr.: Non-penetrating Traumatic Injury of the Aorta, *Circulation,* **17:**1086, 1958.

Spencer, F. C., Guerin, P. F., Blake, H. A., and Bahnson, H. T.: A Report of 15 Patients with Traumatic Rupture of the Thoracic Aorta, *J Thorac Cardiovasc Surg,* **41:**1, 1961.

Steenburg, R. W., and Ravitch, M. M.: Cervico-thoracic Approach for Subclavian Vessel Injury from Compound Fracture of the Clavicle: Considerations of Subclavian Axillary Exposures, *Ann Surg,* **157:**839, 1963.

Obstruction of the Superior Vena Cava

Cooley, D. A., and Hallman, G. L.: Superior Vena Caval Syndrome Treated by Azygos Vein–Inferior Vena Cava Anastomosis: Report of Successful Case, *J Thorac Cardiovasc Surg,* **47:**325, 1964.

Effler, D. B., and Groves, L. K.: Superior Vena Caval Obstruction, *J Thorac Cardiovasc Surg,* **43:**574, 1962.

Hanlon, C. R., and Danis, R. K.: Superior Vena Caval Obstruction: Indications for Diagnostic Thoracotomy, *Ann Surg,* **161:**771, 1965.

Pate, J. W., and Hammon, J.: Superior Vena Cava Syndrome Due to Histoplasmosis in Children, *Ann Surg,* **161:**778, 1965.

Schramel, R., and Olinde, H. D. H.: A New Method of Bypassing the Obstructed Vena Cava, *J Thorac Cardiovasc Surg,* **41:**375, 1961.

Chapter 21

Peripheral Arterial Disease

by **Frank C. Spencer and Anthony M. Imparato**

Introduction

Occlusive Disease of the Lower Extremities

Clinical Manifestations
Manifestations of Acute Arterial Occlusion
Manifestations of Chronic Arterial Occlusion
Atherosclerotic Disease of the Lower Extremities
  Aortoiliac Disease
  Femoropopliteal Occlusive Disease
  Tibioperoneal Arterial Disease
  The Diabetic Foot
  Summary of Therapeutic Concepts for Arterial Occlusive Disease of the Lower Extremities

Arterial Embolism

Cardioarterial Embolization
Arterioarterial Embolization

Acute Arterial Thrombosis

Buerger's Disease

Arterial Trauma

Anterior Compartment Syndrome
Traumatic Arteriovenous Fistulas

Congenital Arteriovenous Fistulas

Thoracic Outlet Syndromes

Extracranial Occlusive Cerebrovascular Disease

Abdominal Aneurysms

Ruptured Abdominal Aneurysm

Peripheral Aneurysms

Popliteal Aneurysms
Femoral Aneurysms
Carotid Artery Aneurysms
Subclavian Aneurysms
Visceral Aneurysms
  Splenic Artery Aneurysms
  Renal Artery Aneurysms
Traumatic Aneurysms

Vasospastic Disorders

Raynaud's Disease
Uncommon Vasomotor Diseases
  Livedo Reticularis
  Acrocyanosis
  Erythromelalgia

Frostbite

INTRODUCTION

Progress in vascular surgery has been so rapid since 1950 that it is difficult for a student of medicine at this time to realize that most of the vascular operations commonly performed today scarcely had been considered 25 years ago. For perspective, certain milestones which have contributed to the rapid evolution of this specialty should be mentioned.

Before the close of the nineteenth century, progress in vascular surgery was greatly hampered by the lack of anesthesia and asepsis. A significant advance was recorded by Matas in 1888 when he reported his successful operation upon a patient with a traumatic aneurysm of the brachial artery upon whom endoaneurysmorrhaphy was applied for the first time. Nine years later (1897) Murphy performed the first end-to-end anastomosis in man following excision of an arteriovenous fistula in the thigh. Before embarking upon this significant operation, never before accomplished in man, Murphy performed a total of 34 experiments in dogs, sheep, and calves to evaluate methods of vascular suture. Subsequently, Carrel and Guthrie (1905–1906) developed many of the techniques of vascular surgery which are still in use today. Soon thereafter autogenous vein grafts were successfully used following excision of aneurysms. In 1915 Bernheim used a vein graft in man for the first time in the United States in treating a patient with a syphilitic popliteal aneurysm.

After World War I a curious lag occurred in vascular surgery until the 1940s, when the epochal work of Blalock, Gross, and Craford with tetralogy of Fallot, patent ductus arteriosus, and coarctation of the aorta launched the modern era of vascular surgery. The development of atraumatic vascular clamps by Potts, in conjunction with fine arterial sutures with swaged needles, greatly facilitated the techniques of vascular operations. The introduction of aortic homografts for repair of coarctation of the aorta by Gross stimulated intensive investigation of vascular prostheses. Soon thereafter the successful excision of an abdominal aneurysm with replacement by an aortic homograft was reported by Dubost et al. in 1952, and in the same year Voorhees et al. reported the first use of a cloth material

(Vinyon) as a vascular prosthesis. This pioneering work led within the next 5 years to the development of the presently used vascular prostheses of Dacron and Teflon, with many contributions made by DeBakey, Cooley, Bahnson, and others. The increasing use of arteriography, along with the development of safer opaque media, greatly enhanced further development of reconstructive surgery. In the period between 1955 and 1960 operations for carotid artery stenosis and renal artery stenosis appeared for the first time. With the rapid advances in the field of vascular surgery, associated with similar advances in diagnostic techniques, vascular surgery has become an increasingly important segment of surgical practice.

Peripheral arterial diseases lend themselves to broad classification as occlusive, aneurysmal, and vasospastic. Accordingly, the topics in this chapter are grouped in a sequence representing these three broad categories.

OCCLUSIVE DISEASE OF THE LOWER EXTREMITIES

Clinical Manifestations

HISTORY. As in most areas of surgery, a carefully elicited history is often essential to establish the correct diagnosis. With vascular disease of the extremities the most frequently encountered symptoms are related to pain, changes in color, or ulceration.

Pain may occur abruptly, as with acute arterial occlusion, intermittently with exercise (claudication), or constantly as *rest pain.* Pain of acute onset, typically seen with an arterial embolus, is a specific event that is virtually diagnostic. The pain is confined to the extremity made ischemic by occlusion of the segmental artery and is often followed by paralysis or anesthesia. *Claudication* is one of the most specific symptom complexes in medicine. It is due to inability of the circulation to supply oxygen during exercise, although circulation is adequate at rest. Patients use different adjectives to describe claudication, including "pain," "cramp," "tiredness," or "fatigue." A characteristic feature, however, is that if the patient attempts to continue to use the involved muscle despite the subjective discomfort, he will find that he is unable to do so, because the muscle will no longer voluntarily contract. The onset of the symptom with exercise, with relief by rest, is diagnostic of chronic arterial insufficiency. The location of the discomfort is often diagnostic of the artery involved. Hip claudication occurs with bilateral iliac artery occlusion, thigh claudication with occlusion of the common femoral artery, calf claudication with involvement of the superficial femoral artery, and foot claudication with tibial arterial occlusion.

Rest pain, usually due to tissue necrosis and ischemic neuritis, is a grave symptom, because it indicates far advanced arterial insufficiency, usually terminating shortly in gangrene and amputation of the extremity if arterial reconstruction cannot be performed. It is important to recognize that diabetics may have rest pain due to diabetic neuropathy and not associated with ischemia. Characteristically, patients with ischemic rest pain experience some relief by keeping their feet in the dependent position, while patients with diabetic neuropathy experience no such relief.

Visible changes in *color* in an extremity are usually seen with vasospastic conditions, such as Raynaud's disease, when the patient notices marked changes in color with emotion or with exposure to cold. With chronic occlusive disease the ischemic foot typically develops a reddish purple color in dependency, alternating with pallor on elevation. *Ulceration* is self-evident, but a history of chronic ulceration in the past, at times terminated by amputation of a toe, may be a significant clue to longstanding vascular disease.

Important specific diseases to be noted in obtaining a history include diabetes, heart disease, collagen disorders, or previous trauma. The use of tobacco or other drugs which may influence vascular tone should also be noted.

PHYSICAL EXAMINATION. Physical examination is of paramount importance in assessing the presence and severity of vascular disease. In this regard physical examination is relatively of greater importance than with abdominal or thoracic problems, where laboratory investigations play a more dominant role. Palpation of the peripheral pulses is the most important feature of the examination. In the lower extremity, the femoral, popliteal, posterior tibial, and dorsalis pedis pulses should be noted. It is important to remember that the common femoral artery extends only about 5 cm below the inguinal ligament before bifurcating into the profunda femoris and superficial femoral arteries. In the upper extremity the brachial, radial, and ulnar pulses should be noted. In many patients it is possible to feel the digital pulses at the bases of the phalanges. The integrity of the palmar arterial arches can be tested by the performance of the Allen test. This is done by having the patient make a tight fist, then occluding the radial and ulnar arteries at the wrist and having the patient slowly open the hand. With the hand in a relaxed position, the integrity of the radial artery in the hand is determined by releasing radial compression and noting the return of color. The maneuver is repeated releasing the ulnar artery while the radial remains compressed. The ability to determine definitely the presence or absence of a peripheral pulse is one of the most essential features of an adequate evaluation of the peripheral circulation.

With chronic ischemia, characteristic nutritional changes develop in the feet. These include the loss of hair from the toes, the development of brittle, opaque nails, the appearance of atrophy and rubor in the skin, and atrophy of muscles of the feet with increasing prominence of the interosseous spaces. Hence, a simple glance at a foot can determine the presence or absence of serious vascular disease. The importance of this evaluation is emphasized by the fact that gangrene seldom appears in an extremity with chronic vascular disease until these stigmata of chronic ischemia have appeared.

Characteristic color changes also appear with advanced arterial insufficiency, consisting of a purplish rubor in dependency, changing to pallor when the extremity is elevated. The colors are quite different from the chronic congested extremity with venous insufficiency.

The location of ulcerations offers a major clue to cause, for ulceration from venous insufficiency is virtually unknown below the level of the malleolus. By contrast, most ulcers from arterial insufficiency begin over the toes, corresponding to the most distal parts of the arterial tree. Rarely ischemic ulcers develop on the leg or about the ankle without involvement of the toes, perhaps as a result of local tissue infarction especially after localized trauma.

Palpation of the extremity for temperature and moisture may provide useful information, especially with vasospastic conditions with increased sympathetic tone, where the cool, sweaty extremity affords an important clue to the diagnosis.

Auscultation is of value for certain disorders, particularly arteriovenous fistulas, where detection of the classic continuous murmur quickly establishes the diagnosis. With localized stenotic lesions in peripheral arteries, usually from atherosclerotic plaques, a systolic bruit may be heard, promptly confirming the presence of arterial stenosis.

Estimation of venous filling time is of some value in the diagnosis of arterial insufficiency, but the test is of no value where incompetent valves are present in the venous system. In the absence of varicosities, the test is performed by elevation of the extremities until collapse of the veins has occurred. The extremities are then quickly lowered, and the time required for the veins to fill, usually on the dorsum of the foot or hand, is noted. Normally venous filling will occur within 10 to 15 seconds. Prolonged filling frequently denotes arterial insufficiency. Venous filling times of longer than 1 minute denote a very high degree of arterial compromise.

An oscillometer may be of some value in extremities with edema where peripheral pulses may be difficult to palpate. This instrument consists of a blood pressure cuff attached to a manometer and provides a method for evaluating pulsatile oscillations when the cuff is inflated to just above diastolic pressure. It is of value for specific problems but is tedious and inaccurate for routine use.

LABORATORY EXAMINATION. The most important laboratory examination by far is selective arteriography to outline the location and extent of arterial obstruction. Selection of the appropriate method of examination varies with the disease present, for virtually every artery in the body can now be successfully outlined by appropriate catheter angiography. Percutaneous introduction of the arterial catheter is the most frequently employed technique. Arteriography may not be essential to confirm the diagnosis but is important to evaluate the possibilities of successful therapy. Illustrative angiograms are shown in specific disease sections in this chapter.

Other techniques for evaluating peripheral circulation are of little clinical value and are utilized mostly for investigative studies. These include precise measurements of skin temperature, sweating, plethysmography, and radioactive isotope clearing rates.

Manifestations of Acute Arterial Occlusion

Acute occlusion usually appears without specific warning symptoms. Prompt diagnosis can be made only if the clinical picture is quickly recognized. This is essential for successful therapy, because within 4 to 8 hours after acute occlusion ischemic necrosis in the involved muscles may become irreversible. An additional feature in the pathogenesis of acute arterial occlusion that emphasizes the time factor is the tendency for thrombi to develop in the arteries distal to the point of occlusion where the flow of blood is either decreased or stagnant. This development, superimposed upon the acute obstruction, makes surgical therapy to restore circulation much more difficult. With persisting ischemia, thrombosis finally develops in the venous system as well, making surgical therapy impossible.

The usual causes of acute arterial occlusion are embolism, trauma, or thrombosis. Thrombosis of a previously undiagnosed aneurysm, such as a popliteal aneurysm, is an unusual cause. Each of these is discussed in subsequent sections. Embolism is noteworthy in that it often appears without any previous signs of underlying disease as an acute catastrophe involving an extremity. In many it is the first symptom of serious underlying heart disease: mitral stenosis, atrial fibrillation, or myocardial infarction. Arterial trauma, when occurring as an isolated injury, may be easily recognized, but when complicated with associated fractures or head injuries, the diagnosis may be difficult.

FIVE P's. For emphasis the five prominent features of acute arterial occlusion may be summarized as five p's: *p*ain, *p*aralysis, *p*aresthesia, *p*allor, and absence of *p*ulses.

Pain is present in 75 to 80 percent of patients with acute arterial occlusion, representing the onset of ischemia in the involved tissues. It is absent in some patients, apparently from the prompt onset of complete anesthesia and paralysis. In others, when collateral circulation minimizes the degree of ischemia produced, pain may also be minimal.

Paralysis and paresthesias (or anesthesia) are the most important symptoms in evaluating the severity of arterial occlusion. The importance of these features is based on the fact that the peripheral nerve endings are the most sensitive tissues to anoxia in an extremity. A familiar illustration of the sensitivity of sensory nerve endings to anoxia is the common experience of one's foot "going to sleep" while one sits with the extremity flexed in an unusual position. The sensitivity of striated muscles to anoxia is almost as great as that of nerve endings. Hence, an extremity with paralysis and paresthesia will almost surely develop gangrene, while, conversely, if motor and sensory function are intact even though signs of ischemia are present, gangrene probably will not occur. Hence, the neurologic findings are an important clue both to the urgency of prompt therapy and in the evaluation of the effectiveness of therapy in restoring circulation. Recognition that a paralysed, anesthetic extremity will develop gangrene in most patients within 6 to 8 hours after onset emphasizes the urgency of immediate treatment.

Pallor is a less important symptom, representing varying degrees of decreased circulation. Associated with visible pallor may be the sensation of coldness.

Absence of pulses confirms the diagnosis and localizes the point of occlusion. With uncertainty, as in an edematous extremity, an oscillometer may be of some value in confirming the absence of pulses. When palpation is indeterminate, the presence of neurologic symptoms indicates the urgency of deciding whether arterial occlusion is present. A frequent example is seen in a patient with a swollen extremity with a fracture of the femur in whom swelling of the extremity may make palpation of the pulses difficult. To determine whether or not an associated injury of the femoral artery is present may require arteriography. If neurologic symptoms are present, angiography should be performed on an emergency basis.

Manifestations of Chronic Arterial Occlusion

The picture of chronic progressive arterial ischemia is typically seen with atherosclerosis involving the abdominal aorta and its branches to the lower extremities, including the iliac, femoral, and popliteal arteries. The course of the disease may be a gradual, progressive one, or it may be interrupted with acute episodes of segmental arterial thrombosis or minor traumatic injuries to the toes resulting in gangrene. The disease almost always is due to atherosclerosis with its protean variations. Diabetic patients in general tend to have more distal arterial involvement of the popliteal and tibial arteries. The clinical syndromes are further modified by the not infrequent presence of diabetic neuropathy and by characteristic susceptibility to necrotizing infections. This is more fully discussed in a subsequent section, The Diabetic Foot. In the upper extremities Buerger's disease, Raynaud's disease, and cervical rib are unusual causes of chronic ischemia.

The hallmark of chronic arterial insufficiency is claudication, the pathophysiology of which was discussed earlier. This is a highly specific symptom, virtually diagnostic of chronic arterial insufficiency. Hence, a carefully taken history to establish the presence of claudication is essential to establishing the diagnosis. For a long period of time the only measure of progression of arterial insufficiency is the appearance of claudication with progressively smaller amounts of exercise, usually measured in terms of walking two blocks, one block, or even shorter distances.

An important subsequent feature of progressive arterial insufficiency is the appearance of trophic changes in the feet, including loss of hair from the toes, the appearance of brittle, opaque nails, and atrophy of the skin with the development of rubor in dependency. These objective changes are associated with few symptoms except for an increasing susceptibility to cold. However, their presence in association with claudication indicates a much more advanced state of arterial insufficiency.

The importance of recognizing these changes in management of chronic ischemic disease is the fact that gangrene will readily occur in a foot or hand with advanced trophic changes following trivial trauma, such as trimming of a callus or corn, a blister from improper shoes, or minor exposures to extremes of heat or cold. Thirty to forty percent of patients with gangrene of the extremities ultimately requiring amputation may date the onset of gangrene in a toe to such trivial trauma. Apparently local trauma results in increased metabolic demands and perhaps in regional thrombosis of collateral circulation. The latter may be progressive despite all therapy unless immediate surgical revascularization can be carried out.

The end stages of chronic arterial insufficiency are represented by ischemic rest pain, usually in association with ulceration. Rest pain is due to ischemic neuritis and may be associated with tissue necrosis, often with superficial ulceration. It is seen in its most severe forms in patients with Buerger's disease, probably with superimposed ischemic neuritis. The recognition of ischemic rest pain and its ominous prognosis is of great significance, because unless ulceration or gangrene are already present, they will develop shortly if arterial circulation cannot be improved. Hence, surgical therapy if feasible should be done as soon as possible. Prolonged nonsurgical measures, consisting principally of rest to avoid trauma, vasodilators, and avoidance of tobacco, may be successful in a limited number of patients over a period of many weeks, probably because of the development of additional collateral circulation. In many patients, however, rest pain inevitably progresses to gangrene and amputation unless the occluded vascular bed can be reconstructed.

Fortunately, in the upper extremity, in contrast to the lower extremity, atherosclerosis which progresses to rest pain and gangrene is unusual. Claudication of the arm with exercise may be moderately disabling, but more serious symptoms are uncommon. Rest pain and tissue necrosis when present usually denote digital vessel occlusion either due to embolization from proximal atherosclerotic plaques or end-stage Raynaud's phenomenon.

Atherosclerotic Disease of the Lower Extremities

Atherosclerotic disease of the arteries to the lower extremities may be divided into three large groups, varying with the level of involvement. These are aortoiliac, femoropopliteal, and tibioperoneal. There are distinctive clinical features about each of the categories; more than one area is involved in at least one-third of patients seen. Aortoiliac disease in the fifth and sixth decades is characterized by relatively mild atherosclerosis with aortic occlusion from superimposed thrombosis, but in the seventh and eighth decades atherosclerosis is severe and thrombosis is mild. Isolated femoropopliteal disease is especially frequent in cigarette smokers, while tibioperoneal disease occurs predominantly in diabetics. No matter where the obstruction is located, the physiologic deficit is decreased blood flow to the lower extremities, with symptoms ranging from intermittent claudication to gangrene. Tissue necrosis is more prone to occur with distal arterial disease and occlusive disease which progresses rapidly without time for collateral circulation to develop.

The choice of surgical therapy for the three different types depends upon several variables. These include the natural history of the arterial disease and the severity of the ischemic symptoms; the age and responsibilities of the patient; and the reliability of arterial reconstructive procedures, which varies greatly from one area to another.

AORTOILIAC DISEASE

HISTORICAL DATA. The ischemic syndrome produced by atherosclerotic disease of the bifurcation of the abdominal aorta has been recognized with increasing frequency over the past 30 years. Leriche is credited with emphasizing in the early 1940s the clinical characteristics of occlusion of the abdominal aorta, i.e., claudication, impotence, and absence of gangrene. The development of angiography, pioneered by dos Santos, greatly facilitated diagnosis.

ETIOLOGY AND PATHOLOGY. Some degree of atherosclerosis is almost universally seen at autopsy in the abdominal aortas of patients over sixty years of age, but symptoms from decrease in blood flow do not occur unless the diameter of the aorta has been greatly narrowed by as much as 90 percent. The process may simply be atherosclerosis with intimal thickening and fibrosis, or it may be complicated by ulceration of atherosclerotic plaques with superimposed thrombosis or embolization of portions of atherosclerotic plaques. As in other arteries, the disease often begins at bifurcations where turbulent flow of blood occurs. Hence, disease is often greatest at the aortic bifurcation, the iliac bifurcation, and the bifurcation of the common femoral artery. The disease may extend proximally in the abdominal aorta up to the level of the renal arteries, but fortunately disease proximal to the renal arteries is rare.

Patients are frequently seen in the fifth and sixth decades with thrombosis of the abdominal aorta but only mild atherosclerosis of the common iliac arteries. The thrombus often propagates up to the level of the renal arteries, rarely occluding one renal artery, and extending up to near the superior mesenteric artery. These patients contrast to a curious degree with patients in the seventh and eighth decades who may have unusually severe atherosclerosis but without thrombosis and total occlusion despite advanced stenosis. This variation with age suggests that some unrecognized factor in the younger group may precipitate the thrombotic process.

Fortunately atherosclerosis of the abdominal aorta is virtually always segmental. Proximally it stops at the level of the renal arteries; distad the profunda femoris artery is almost always patent, even though the superficial femoral artery may be occluded. Hence, reconstruction can be done in over 95 percent of patients, directing flow distad into the patent profunda femoris artery. If the superficial femoral artery is occluded, additional reconstruction may be required if tissue necrosis is present, but otherwise simple aortoiliac reconstruction will suffice.

A separate therapeutic consideration is the 10 percent of persons with aortoiliac occlusive disease who have small aneurysms as well. This group must be treated by excision and graft replacement, for aneurysmal dilatation may develop following endarterectomy.

Concomitant coronary or cerebral atherosclerosis occurs frequently, probably in 30 to 50 percent of patients with symptomatic aortoiliac disease. Coronary disease is by far the principal cause of death in the 5-year period following surgical aortoiliac reconstruction.

PATHOPHYSIOLOGY. Aortoiliac disease decreases blood flow to the pelvic viscera and lower extremities. Collateral circulation develops to an extensive degree when the aorta becomes completely occluded. The principal tributaries are through the lumbar arteries, anastomosing distad with the branches of the gluteal arteries and the profunda femoris arteries. Fortunately this collateral circulation is sufficient to prevent ischemia at rest, so symptoms appear only with exercise. In men impotence is frequent because of decreased blood flow through the hypogastric arteries. Claudication is present in the lower extremities, but as blood flow is adequate at rest, the extremity remains well nourished. Only with additional disease in the superficial femoral, profunda femoris, or popliteal and tibial arteries do nutritional changes with ulceration and gangrene appear. Rarely a few patients develop occlusion of the aorta at a rapid rate, before collateral circulation develops; these may show severe ischemic changes in the legs, even though no additional disease is present distad.

CLINICAL MANIFESTATIONS. The classic symptoms are intermittent claudication and impotence of varying severity in males. Claudication may be symmetric or asymmetric, depending upon the pattern of involvement of the iliac arteries. Characteristically with walking, discomfort is felt in the calf, thigh, and buttocks muscles. The symptoms vary in severity from difficulty after walking three to four blocks to inability to walk even indoors. Rest pain, ulceration, or gangrene almost always indicate additional distal disease. This is particularly true in diabetics, where disease of the tibial arteries is common.

Symptoms may remain stable for years and progress only with additional distal atherosclerosis. In some patients the symptoms improve with exercise as collateral vessels enlarge. Conversely, symptoms may worsen, sometimes dramatically, with hypotension secondary to myocardial infarction or cardiac arrhythmias. Impotence is a complex syndrome which may arise from multiple causes. Its presence or absence cannot be relied upon to diagnose aortoiliac disease. Although it may improve after successful arterial reconstruction, the likelihood in any particular patient is unpredictable.

Physical Examination. The principal finding is diminution or absence of the femoral pulses, combined with absence of popliteal and pedal pulses. Pulsations in the abdominal aorta may be palpable if occlusion is limited to near the aortic bifurcation, but these are absent if the abdominal aorta is occluded up to the renal arteries. A systolic bruit is often audible over the aorta or iliac arteries, confirming the presence of atherosclerosis. However, it does not correlate with the degree of stenosis. Nutrition in the extremities is usually normal. With signs of chronic ischemia, such as absence of hair, brittle nails, or rubor, additional atherosclerotic disease in the femoral or popliteal arteries is probably present.

Occasionally patients are seen with aortoiliac disease with acute episodes of severe ischemia of the toes or feet, often with cyanosis and rest pain. The diagnosis may be especially puzzling if the aortoiliac obstruction is not severe. Occasionally pedal pulses are palpable. The syndrome probably arises from arterioarterial embolization of fragments of atherosclerotic plaques or thrombi dislodged from the surface of such plaques. The diagnosis may be suspected if a localized bruit in the abdomen or groin is found.

As multiple areas of atherosclerosis are frequent, particular care should be taken to search for bruits over the carotid or subclavian arteries, as well as to note the adequacy of pulses in the upper extremities.

LABORATORY STUDIES. With the exception of patients experiencing arterioarterial embolization, the diagnosis usually can be established by the history and physical examination. Roentgenograms often show calcification in the wall of the aorta, but as the calcification is in the media, it does not correlate with the degree of flow obstruction. An unsuspected abdominal aortic aneurysm, however, may be outlined by the calcification within its wall. Aortography is performed if surgical reconstruction is being considered. It delineates the proximal extent of the occlusion and may outline the patent arteries beyond the obstruction, especially the profunda femoris vessels.

TREATMENT. Nonsurgical. The need for surgical reconstruction depends upon the severity of the symptoms and the age of the patient. For example, mild claudication in a forty-five-year-old patient whose occupation necessitates frequent walking is a strong indication for operation. By contrast, a retired patient of seventy with angina pectoris and claudication does not require operation. The presence of trophic changes in the feet, rubor, absence of hair, and brittle nails is a useful guide to the risk of gangrene, for gangrene is rare except with acute arterial occlusion as long as trophic changes are absent.

If operation is not recommended, daily exercise to the point of claudication should be encouraged, for this may enhance collateral circulation, as manifested by gradual increase in walking tolerance. If walking is not feasible, a similar exercise can be performed indoors by having the patient raise himself on his toes and then rock back on his heels, repeating the sequence rapidly until calf cramps occur. Following a rest period the exercise is repeated, as often as twenty or more times daily.

Abstinence from tobacco in any form is mandatory. There is reasonable statistical evidence that claudication improves when smoking is stopped and that the risk of gangrene is greater in patients who smoke. The precise mechanism is unknown, but tobacco is a potent vasoconstrictor. Drug therapy with vasodilators may be tried, but unfortunately few patients have had any improvement in the claudication. Alcohol, orally administered, is employed for its peripheral vasodilator effect.

With severe ischemia, one of the most crucial points in management is educating the patient to protect the feet from any form of trauma. This includes extremes of heat or cold, improperly fitting shoes, or vigorous trimming of calluses, corns, or toenails. A familiar tragedy is that a trauma that would be minor in a foot with normal circulation will produce gangrene of a toe in a severely ischemic foot which not only fails to heal but may gradually progress upward to result in a low thigh amputation. Infection associated with unguis incarnatus or dermatophytosis sim-

ilarly may cause decompensation of the circulation with gangrene, probably from an increase in local tissue metabolism.

Therapy directed toward lowering blood lipid concentrations by diet, drugs, or even surgical procedures remains of uncertain benefit. Anticoagulant therapy with heparin or warfarin sodium has not been helpful. The recent exciting discovery that acetylsalicylic acid in small doses strikingly alters platelet aggregation and may thereby prevent intravascular thrombosis is now undergoing clinical evaluation and holds considerable therapeutic promise.

Lumbar Sympathectomy. In patients with trophic changes in the feet not amenable to direct arterial reconstruction, lumbar sympathectomy may be of benefit both in improving symptoms and in protecting from gangrene. Unfortunately, the benefits of sympathectomy are variable and unpredictable. In several reports objective signs of improvement were demonstrated in only 20 to 30 percent of patients, usually consisting of increased circulation in the skin which provides some protection from ulceration. Increased blood flow to the leg muscles, associated with improvement in claudication, is unfortunately rare.

Due to the great variability of the morphologic features of the lumbar sympathetic chain, lumbar sympathectomies should involve near-total denervation, removing the sympathetic chain from the level of the crus of the diaphragm superiorly down to the level of the common iliac inferiorly. Bilateral excisions of the uppermost lumbar ganglia may cause impairment of sexual function, usually disturbances in ejaculation, and must be considered in deciding the extent of bilateral sympathectomy in young men.

Aortic Reconstruction. The two most frequently performed surgical procedures are thromboendarterectomy or a bypass graft, usually with Dacron or Teflon. As mentioned earlier, the almost uniform patency of the profunda femoris vessels makes reconstruction feasible in the vast majority of patients. The risk of operation is between 5 and 10 percent, determined principally by the degree of associated coronary or cerebral atherosclerosis. The superiority of one operative procedure over the other has not been demonstrated. Long-term patency rates after either procedure range from 65 to 90 percent. Though tedious, endarterectomies have been successfully performed from the level of the renal arteries proximally to the profunda femoris vessels distad. Concomitant aneurysmal disease of the aorta is a definite contraindication to endarterectomy. In some instances the procedures are combined, performing an aortofemoral bypass in combination with localized endarterectomy of the common femoral arteries.

The most frequent late complication after bypass procedures are false aneurysms developing at the suture lines, a complication which has decreased sharply in frequency with the routine use of nonabsorbable sutures. The most frequent complication after endarterectomy is a recurrent stenosis from progressive fibrosis and narrowing of the arterial wall.

Preoperative Considerations. An aortogram is usually performed to determine the extent of disease in the external iliac and femoral arteries. As it is not needed to confirm the diagnosis, which is readily made on physical examination, the aortogram is of little value unless the distal circulation is visualized. In some instances the authors perform operative angiograms of the common femoral artery to delineate the extent of disease in the proximal profunda femoris artery, for endarterectomies may be successfully performed down to the midportion of this artery (Fig. 21-1).

Operative Technique. A midline abdominal incision, usually extending from the xiphoid process to the pubis symphysis, is preferred. The intestines are retracted onto the right abdominal wall and placed in a plastic bag, after which the retroperitoneal tissues are incised to expose the aorta proximally up to the level of the left renal vein. Once the proximal and distal extent of arterial disease has been defined, a choice is made between a bypass graft or an endarterectomy.

As mentioned earlier, the presence of small aneurysms in the aorta or common iliac artery are absolute contraindications to endarterectomy. A small external iliac artery or severe atherosclerosis in the external iliac artery has influenced many surgeons to perform a bypass procedure to the common femoral artery because of the technical difficulties with endarterectomy of a small diseased external iliac artery. The availability of arterial strippers, as well as the eversion endarterectomy popularized by Conley, however, has extended the scope of endarterectomy and made the operation more satisfactory in these circumstances.

Thromboendarterectomy. A typical pattern of atherosclerotic involvement is extension of disease proximally to within 2 to 3 cm of the renal arteries and distad into the common iliac arteries, stopping in about 50 percent of patients just beyond the bifurcation of the common iliac arteries. Initially the aorta proximally and the external and hypogastric arteries distad are encircled with cotton tapes. The lumbar and inferior mesenteric arteries are similarly exposed. Fifty milligrams of heparin is then given by intravenous injection before occlusive clamps are applied to avoid thrombus formation during the periods of stasis. External iliac clamps are applied before clamping the abdominal aorta to protect from distal embolization. Incisions are made over the distal common iliac arteries, and cleavage planes between the plaques and media are developed. A longitudinal incision is made into the aorta above the level of the inferior mesenteric artery and an appropriate cleavage plane near the junction of the arterial intima and media identified. Using various techniques, including arterial strippers, the core of atherosclerotic material is freed proximally. Usually by blunt dissection the aortic and iliac cores can be mobilized and removed in one piece. A critical aspect of the operative procedure distad is careful inspection of the intima of the proximal external iliac artery to eliminate ledges of thickened intima by suturing. The caliber of the external iliac arteries may be measured with catheters. A diameter smaller than a #16 F catheter often indicates the necessity of extending the endarterectomy to the common femoral arteries. In the hypogastric arteries, endarterectomy is limited to removal of the occluding material near the ostia, for distal dissection of this artery is usually technically unsatisfactory.

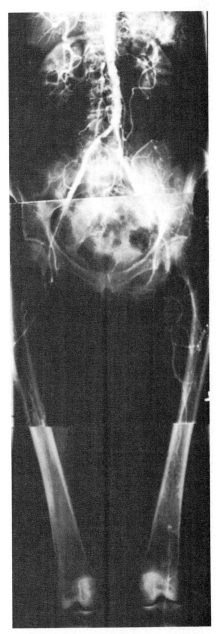

Fig. 21-1. Angiogram illustrating that the profunda femoris artery is usually patent in the presence of aortoiliac occlusive disease. Advanced lesions may be present, however, requiring surgical correction to render the profunda femoris suitable for an outflow tract.

The aortotomy incision is closed with a simple continuous suture of 4-0 or 5-0 Tevdek. The iliac arteriotomies may be closed similarly or with a patch graft of either autologous saphenous vein or a prosthetic patch of knitted Dacron. The choice depends upon both the diameter of the artery and the rigidity of the wall. After the incisions are sutured, the occluding clamps are sequentially removed to permit flushing initially into the hypogastric arteries and subsequently into the external iliacs. Strong pulses should be palpable immediately. Weak or absent pulsations indicate obstruction from either retained plaques or stenotic suture lines, in which case the arteriotomy should be promptly reopened and the obstruction corrected. Occasionally in such circumstances operative angiography is needed.

Once blood flow is restored, heparin is neutralized with protamine, giving 1 to 1.5 mg for each mg heparin used. The posterior peritoneum is sutured over the reconstructed aorta (Fig. 21-2). A concomitant bilateral lumbar sympathectomy is a simple adjunct to the reconstructive procedure but not clearly beneficial. It is more definitely indicated if occlusive disease in distal vessels is significant. When it is performed, the sympathetic chain can be identified by palpation as cordlike nodular structures parallel to the aorta on the left and just under the lateral border of the vena cava on the right.

Bypass Grafting. When a bypass procedure is chosen, a knitted rather than a woven Dacron prosthesis is preferred, because of firmer adherence of the neointima which forms subsequently to the wall of the graft. In some tightly woven prostheses, the neointima remains loose, gelatinous, and relatively nonadherent.

After initial determination of where the occlusive disease stops distad, the femoral arteries are exposed if disease extends to the inguinal ligament. The aorta is then isolated proximally and incised longitudinally for 4 to 5 cm. The anastomosis is simpler if a short segment of aorta is identified and clamped, rather than employing a tangential clamp on the anterior wall, which is particularly awkward if the aorta is small and stiff.

The anastomosis is constructed end to side with a continuous suture of 3-0 or 4-0 Tevdek. The graft then can be clamped adjacent to the anastomosis and flow restored to the iliac vessels. Soft tissue tunnels are then developed by blunt dissection anterior and parallel to the iliac vessels, after which the limbs of the prosthesis are brought through the tunnels, lying parallel to the iliac arteries. If the distal anastomosis is performed to the common femoral artery, the graft is brought beneath the inguinal ligament, and the common femoral is incised near the origin of the profunda femoris artery to be certain that there is no obstruction of flow into either the deep or the superficial femoral artery. A continuous suture of 4-0 or 5-0 Tevdek is used. The graft is placed under slight tension at the time of performing the anastomosis to avoid buckling of the graft when it is distended with arterial pressure after the clamps are removed (Figs. 21-3 and 21-4).

A major technical hazard in bypass grafting is the formation of thrombi in the proximal or distal arterial tree with subsequent embolization into the extremity when blood flow is restored. This can be avoided by carefully flushing the graft and routinely inserting a balloon catheter down the distal arterial tree before the distal anastomosis is completed. As the knitted prostheses are porous, they should be preclotted with blood before insertion.

Antibiotics in large amounts are routinely begun at the start of the operation to have circulating blood levels at bactericidal concentrations during the operation. Antibiotics are repeated at appropriate intervals during long procedures.

Postoperative Care. Peripheral pulses should be closely monitored, for sudden disappearance of a previously palpable pulse usually indicates thrombosis of the graft or an embolus, either of which should be treated by prompt reoperation. Ileus is the most frequent postoperative complication, simply managed by nasogastric suction until adequate peristalsis returns. Antibiotics are given for about 3 to 5 days.

The most catastrophic postoperative complication, fortunately extremely rare, is infection developing around the prosthetic graft. In such circumstances the graft usually must be removed to prevent fatal hemorrhage. This can result in unilateral or bilateral amputation of the extremities unless another graft can be inserted. Probably the best form of management is the temporary insertion of axillary-femoral bypass grafts through long subcutaneous tunnels, followed by removal of the infected retroperitoneal prosthesis. The axillary-femoral grafts, however, often become occluded within 1 to 3 years, so that they are not a satisfactory long-term substitute.

Results and Prognosis. Immediate results of aortoiliac reconstructions are excellent. A nearly 100 percent patency rate can be achieved by meticulous technique and proper selection of operative procedures. The immediate functional results are predictable from the angiographic patterns of arterial involvement and the functional status of patients (Fig. 21-5). Claudication is almost always relieved. If tissue loss with gangrene is present, however, additional reconstructive procedures in the distal arterial tree are needed in about 50 percent of the patients.

Numerous data have been published about the long-term results following endarterectomy or bypass grafting. In general, good to excellent results have been sustained in the majority of patients for at least 5 years after operation. If reconstruction is limited to the aorta and common iliac arteries, the 5-year results are similar for endarterectomy and bypass grafts. In a study of 420 patients, Wylie reported that 108 patients with aortoiliac endarterectomy had a 10-year patency of 90 percent. Kouchoukos et al. reported a series of 206 patients treated either by endarterectomy or bypass grafting, after which the 5-year patency rates were virtually identical, 62 and 63 percent. Szilagyi et al. reported similar results 5 years after operation with patency rates of 89 and 85 percent, respectively, when comparing bypass grafting and endarterectomy. Gomes et al. described good results in 84 percent of 401 patients 5 years after operation, and Garrett et al. reported that in over 3,000 operations performed for aortoiliac disease using bypass grafts in the majority of patients good results approached 90 percent 5 years after operation.

Hence, it is clear from the data available that the procedure chosen for an individual patient must vary with the disease present and the experience of the surgeon. Whichever technique is used, immediate patency rates should approach 100 percent. False aneurysms following the use of bypass grafts have greatly decreased in frequency with the use of synthetic sutures and the avoidance of excessive tension on the suture lines.

The principal cause of late deaths after operation is coronary arterial disease, approximately 12 percent within

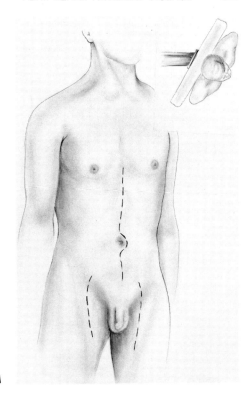

Fig. 21-2. Endarterectomy for atherosclerotic obstruction of the aortoiliac segments. *A.* A midline incision from xiphoid process to pubis symphysis is employed. Rotation of the operating table 30 to 40° to the right side facilitates retraction of the intestines. The thighs should be included in the operative field to permit exposure of the bifurcation of the common femoral arteries. *B.* The intestines are either encased in a plastic bag or covered with moist pads. The retroperitoneal tissues are incised exposing the aorta up to the left renal vein. *C.* The arteriotomy incisions are shown placed according to the distribution of the disease. *D.* Endarterectomy strippers may be used to separate the atherosclerotic cores in the iliac arteries. *E.* Following endarterectomy the distal intima is carefully attached to the arterial wall with vertically oriented interrupted sutures to prevent its dissection when circulation is reestablished. *F.* The multiple arteriotomies are either closed by direct suture or with roof patches of autologous vein or Dacron if the vessels are narrow.

A

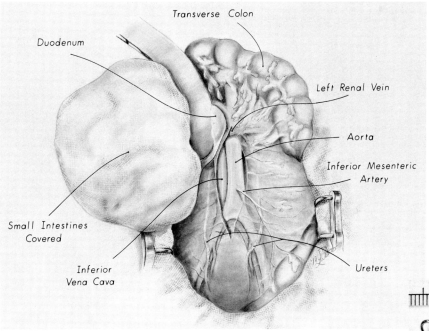

Transverse Colon

Duodenum

Left Renal Vein

Aorta

Inferior Mesenteric
Artery

Small Intestines
Covered

Inferior
Vena Cava

Ureters

B

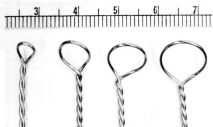

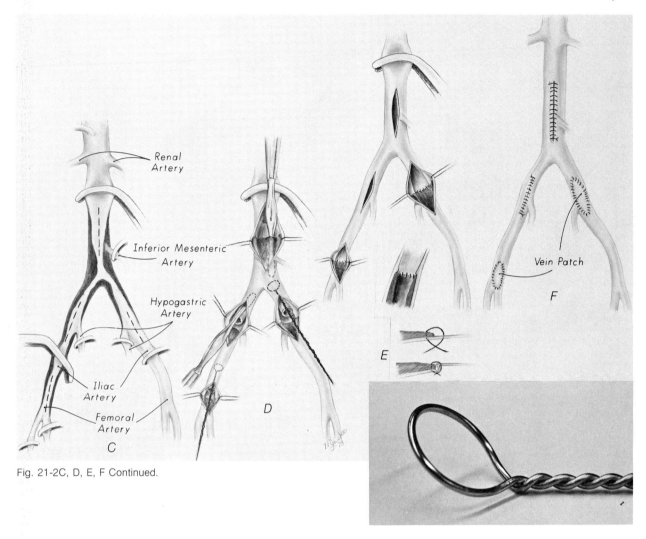

Renal Artery

Inferior Mesenteric Artery

Hypogastric Artery

Iliac Artery

Femoral Artery

C

D

E

F

Vein Patch

Fig. 21-2C, D, E, F Continued.

2 years at New York University. It is hoped that recent advances with coronary bypass operations will improve this poor prognosis.

FEMOROPOPLITEAL OCCLUSIVE DISEASE

PATHOLOGY. The most common site for atherosclerotic occlusion in the lower extremities is the distal superficial femoral artery within the adductor canal. The reason for this unusual localization is unknown but may be related to the anatomic position of the artery as it traverses the adductor foramen to become the popliteal artery. The usual sequence of atherosclerotic occlusion is to extend gradually proximally in the superficial femoral artery until the artery is occluded at its origin from the common femoral. Fortunately, involvement of the profunda femoris artery is infrequent, a complete contrast to the frequency of involvement of the superficial femoral. For this reason atherosclerotic occlusion of the superficial femoral artery alone usually produces claudication but no more serious circulatory impairment.

When more extensive occlusive disease develops, usually from occlusion of the popliteal artery or its branches, the anterior and posterior tibial arteries, more serious circulatory insufficiency appears. With occlusion of this extent, ulceration and gangrene are common. Such diffuse patterns of atherosclerosis are particularly common in diabetic patients.

CLINICAL MANIFESTATIONS. Segmental occlusion of the superficial femoral artery produces claudication in the leg with moderate exercise, but no symptoms at rest. Physical examination finds a normal femoral pulse but absent popliteal and pedal pulses. Rarely pedal pulses are present at rest but disappear with exercise. The nutrition of the foot is normal. If additional occlusive disease is present beyond the femoral artery, claudication is more severe, perhaps associated with rest pain and trophic changes in the foot, and ulceration and gangrene ultimately ensue. Fortunately, the rate of progression of atherosclerotic occlusion is slow in many patients, and the risk of gangrene developing within 5 years in an extremity with claudication as the only symptom is only about 5 percent.

LABORATORY STUDIES. Arteriography is required to determine the segmental nature of the occlusive disease and the consequent possibilities of arterial reconstruction.

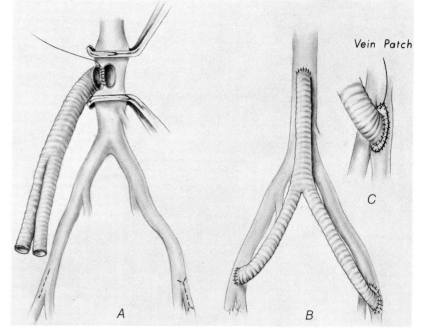

Fig. 21-3. Bypass graft of abdominal aorta. Dissection and exposure are similar to that for endarterectomy procedures. *A.* The proximal anastomosis is performed end to side to the aorta proximal to the point of obstruction. Knitted Dacron is preferred. *B.* The distal anastomoses are performed as end-to-side anastomoses either to the iliac artery proximal to the inguinal ligament or to the common femoral artery at the point of origin of the profunda femoris artery depending upon the degree of atherosclerotic involvement of the external iliac artery. Anastomoses distal to the inguinal ligament are avoided whenever possible to avoid trauma to the prosthesis passing under the inguinal ligament. *C.* A vein roof patch may be employed to facilitate suture of the prosthesis to small arteries.

Adequate visualization of the popliteal artery and its branches is essential (Fig. 21-6). Fortunately, with current techniques, revascularization procedures extended to the popliteal artery are quite satisfactory if the anterior or posterior tibial branches are patent. The peroneal artery, which does not directly contribute to the formation of the pedal arch, is less satisfactory. If all three branches are occluded, under special circumstances reconstructive procedures may be extended down to the pedal arches of the foot. This is discussed under Tibioperoneal Occlusive Disease.

TREATMENT. If claudication is the only symptom, operation is an elective decision, determined from the age and occupation of the patient. As the risk of gangrene with claudication alone is small, this alone does not constitute an indication for operation. Only when trophic changes appear in the feet is operation indicated because of the risk of gangrene. Care to avoid trauma to the foot, described in the section on aortoiliac occlusive disease, is similarly applicable, avoiding even minor trauma or exposure to extremes of heat or cold. Recommendations regarding tobacco, alcohol, exercise, and vasodilator drugs similar to those made for aortic occlusive disease are applicable. In patients able to walk at least one city block, or 300 feet, a vigorous exercise program of walking at least 1 mile daily has resulted in marked improvement in claudication in at least 50 percent of patients within 6 to 12 months.

Sympathectomy. Unfortunately, when claudication is the only symptom, sympathectomy is of little value. It may enhance the development of collateral circulation and thereby lessen the hazard of more serious insufficiency, but this is primarily theoretic. When trophic changes are present, however, and direct arterial reconstruction is not possible because of diffuse occlusive disease, a sympathectomy should be performed. The vasodilating effect of sympathectomy on the vessels of the skin provides some protection from ulceration of the ischemic foot. Statistically the results are disappointing, however, for objective improvement can be demonstrated in little more than 20 percent of patients receiving operation.

Direct Arterial Reconstruction. *Bypass Grafting; Endarterectomy.* The basic principle of arterial reconstruction is that there must be both adequate inflow and adequate outflow of blood from the area of reconstruction. Early operative failures are almost always due either to obvious technical faults or to inadequate inflow or outflow. Most groups have become dissatisfied with bypass prosthetic grafts. Although Crawford and associates reported in 1966 that crimped Dacron prostheses, 8 mm or more in diameter, employed in over 2,500 cases gave adequate long-term function, up to 10 years, in about 75 percent of patients, most others have had less satisfactory results. Szilagyi et al. reported a patency rate of only 40 percent in 193 cases 4 years after operation, and Linton achieved only a 6 percent patency 5 years after operation. These poor results contrast markedly to the excellent results following aortoiliac reconstruction.

The bypass operation with the autologous saphenous vein is used most commonly though not by all groups. Wylie described similar 5-year results following either endarterectomy or vein bypass. At New York University, three different techniques—venous bypass, long endarterectomy procedures with a venous roof patch, and endarterectomy performed through multiple arteriotomies with multiple vein roof patches—had almost identical results 5 to 7 years later. Analysis of the cause of late failures after reconstruction found that about one-third were due to progressive distal atherosclerosis and one-third to intimal proliferation in the areas of arterial reconstruc-

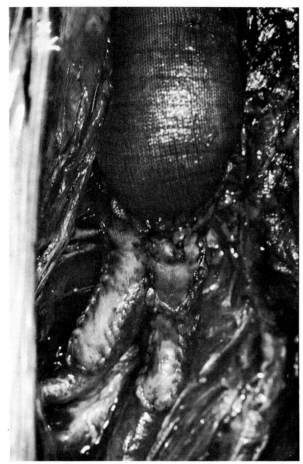

Fig. 21-4. Interposition of vein roof patches over the profunda femoris and superficial femoral arteries facilitates suture of plastic prostheses to the common femoral artery in aortofemoral bypass procedures. •

tion. Tissue specimens were not obtained to determine the cause of failure in the other one-third of the cases.

With prosthetic grafts, failure is due to stiffening of the prosthesis from the ingrowth of fibrous tissue, especially when the graft crosses a joint, as well as extensive scarring about the graft which results in poor adherence of the neointima. Venous bypass is favored if a saphenous or cephalic vein can be dilated to an internal diameter greater than 4 mm. If a suitable vein is not available, endarterectomy with wire strippers and multiple vein roof patches has given comparable results, even in diabetic patients. If, for some reason, this is not possible, usually due to a previous operative procedure, then a long endarterectomy with a long vein roof patch, originally described by Edwards et al., is favored. The least satisfactory choices are either a prosthetic graft, usually Dacron, or a homologous vein (Fig. 21-7).

Other techniques have been proposed but lack substantial experience. This includes carbon dioxide ("gas") endarterectomy, developed by Sawyer et al., bovine heterografts, or autologous tissue tubes prepared with a silicone mandrel.

Bypass Grafting. The technique of bypass grafting is illustrated in Fig. 21-8. It is particularly attractive because of its simplicity and ease of performance. The precision required for obtaining nearly 100 percent immediate patency can best be evaluated by operative angiography. Relatively small imperfections in the anastomotic suture lines or within the body of the graft can lead to deposition of platelet-fibrin aggregates with occlusion within a few hours.

The saphenous vein is carefully removed from the inguinal ligament to the knee, reversed to permit blood to flow in the direction of the venous valves, and then attached with end-to-side anastomoses to the femoral and popliteal arteries proximal and distal to the obstruction. As mentioned earlier, the vein should be at least 4 to 5 mm in diameter. In 15 to 25 percent of patients a satisfactory vein is not available, because of either previous

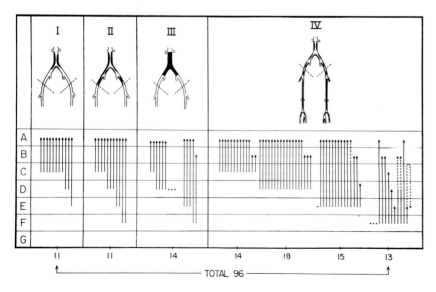

Fig. 21-5. Preoperative angiographic studies provide an excellent index of functional results which can be achieved by aorto-iliacfemoral reconstructions. Functional categories A to D are increasing severities of claudication, while E and F represent rest pain and gangrene respectively. Even in the presence of disseminated distal occlusive lesions and ischemic lesions aorto-iliac reconstructions to the profunda femoris artery resulted in marked improvement.

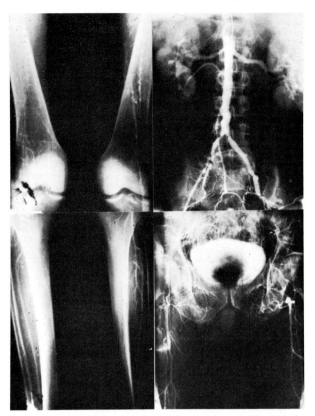

Fig. 21-6. Representative angiographic study required to evaluate patients for arterial reconstruction for claudication. Only in this manner can the inflow and outflow tracts be critically evaluated and arterial reconstructions planned.

surgical removal or anatomic variations. A suitable cephalic vein is an acceptable substitute, though a lot of data are not yet available. Otherwise one of the techniques previously described is used.

Endarterectomy. Since its introduction over 20 years ago, between 1951 and 1953, endarterectomy has been modified several times. A completely open technique, incising the artery throughout its length, removing the atherosclerotic core, and suturing the long arteriotomy, had a very high failure rate. Similarly, closed tehniques with mechanical strippers often failed, usually from leaving loose fragments of intima or atherosclerotic plaque in the lumen. Closure of the long arteriotomy with a vein roof patch, developed by Edwards et al., gave significantly better results. A subsequent modification was the use of multiple vein roof patches to close multiple arteriotomies used for semiclosed endarterectomy. This technique is illustrated in Fig. 21-9. Operative angiography is essential to be certain that atherosclerotic debris has been entirely removed from the lumen.

A technique utilized in some patients is the so-called "in situ" vein graft, in which the saphenous vein is not removed from its bed but is mobilized proximally and distad to be anastomosed end to side to the femoral artery proximally and the popliteal artery or its branches distad. Before the anastomoses are performed, however, the valves in the vein are disrupted by passage of a mechanical instrument along the course of the vein. One limitation of the technique is the production of small arteriovenous fistulas from tributaries of the saphenous vein. Another objection is incomplete disruption of the venous valves with the production of turbulent flow. Some such grafts have been successfully inserted from the common femoral artery proximally to the posterior tibial artery near the ankle, but in general long-term results with the technique have been found unsatisfactory by most groups.

TIBIOPERONEAL ARTERIAL DISEASE

PATHOLOGY. Occlusive disease of the tibial arteries occurs most commonly in patients with diabetes mellitus. It is also seen in patients with Buerger's disease. Some instances of arterioarterial embolism are almost surely incorrectly diagnosed initially and considered as primary occlusive disease of the tibial arteries.

In the diabetic patient there are different patterns of disease which can be recognized, though the reason for development of such patterns is unclear. All tibial arteries may be involved, as well as occlusion of the pedal arches formed by branches of the anterior and posterior tibial vessels. In such instances surgical reconstruction is impossible. In other patients one or more of the tibial arteries may be entirely patent, or there may be proximal occlusion with patent vessels starting at the level of the malleoli. With this pattern of involvement, arterial reconstruction is possible if grafts are extended to the ankles. Unfortunately, in some diabetic patients there is additional disease in the aortoiliac or femoral areas.

CLINICAL MANIFESTATIONS. Occasionally occlusive disease of the tibial arteries merely produces claudication of the foot. Usually, however, there are signs of advanced ischemia. With diabetes there is the additional problem of diabetic neuropathy, difficult to differentiate from ischemic rest pain. Characteristically, ischemic pain is relieved by placing the foot in a dependent position, while that of diabetic neuropathy is not. A frequent problem in the diabetic patient is ulceration on the plantar surface of the foot, secondary to pressure associated with diabetic neuropathy. A more serious problem is a spreading necrotizing infection, with absent pedal pulses. Because of associated ischemia the infection is often refractory to both antibiotic therapy and surgical debridement unless revascularization can be done. This type of progressive, refractory infection may lead to amputation before tissue ischemia per se has caused widespread necrosis. Infection undoubtedly increases the metabolic requirements of the tissue and thereby accentuates the degree of ischemia. A third type of terminal event in the ischemic diabetic foot is soft tissue atrophy to a severe degree, terminating with progressive ischemic dry gangrene of the toes and foot.

LABORATORY STUDIES. Precise angiography is essential to determine the adequacy of the proximal circulation in the aorta and iliac arteries, as well as in the distal arterial tree, especially the small arteries of the ankle and foot. Significant advances in the technique of angiography have permitted excellent delineation of small arterial branches in these areas. Such studies may be done by direct needle puncture of the femoral artery, followed by injection of

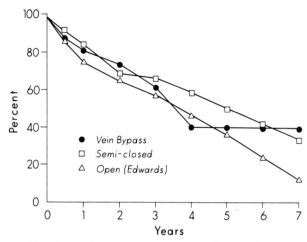

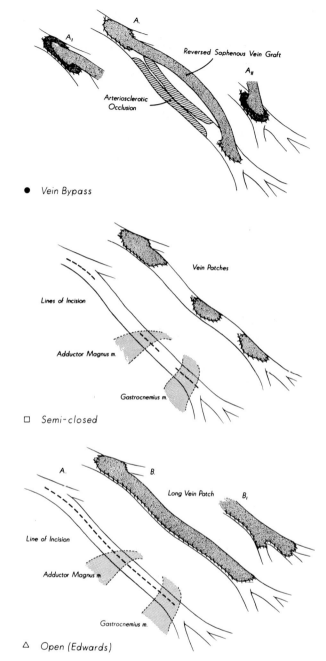

Fig. 21-7. Cumulative patencies of femoropopliteal arterial reconstructions performed by one of three techniques employing only autologous tissue are nearly statistically identical. The three groups are otherwise comparable for indications for operation and grading of severity of involvement of the outflow tracts. Inserts show the three basic techniques employed in reconstructions.

a large bolus (50 ml) of contrast medium with serial films made over a long period of time (Fig. 21-10). An alternative technique is to produce ischemic vasodilation by temporary arterial occlusion with an inflated blood pressure cuff for 5 minutes or longer, injecting the dye immediately after deflation of the cuff. This almost invariably produces excellent opacification of distal vessels.

TREATMENT. Unless the extremity is in jeopardy, arterial reconstructions into the tibial arteries are avoided because of the unpredictable outcome in any particular patient. When a reconstruction fails, amputation is usually necessary because the trauma of surgical dissection usually impairs collateral circulation to a significant degree. If operation is not considered indicated, treatment is primarily directed at careful avoidance of foot trauma, as emphasized in the preceding sections.

Surgical reconstruction may be undertaken if only a single tibial artery remains patent or if the pedal arch is found patent on angiogram, usually seen at the ankle as a communication between the anterior and posterior tibial arteries across the dorsum of the foot.

When a necrotizing infection is present, characteristically extending as a necrotic phlegmon rather than an abscess and requiring debridement as opposed to drainage, therapy is almost hopeless without arterial reconstruction. A combined approach of revascularization into the distal tibial and malleolar vessels, followed soon thereafter by debridement of all infected tissue, has been successful. As a practical guideline, if more than one-half of the sole of the foot has been destroyed, the limb will never be suitable for weight bearing, despite effective arterial reconstruction; so amputation is the primary choice. In all such difficult problems intensive antibiotic therapy for the specific organism involved is essential.

Direct Arterial Reconstruction. Bypass venous grafts, usually the greater saphenous vein, have been effective in

some patients when connected distad to the anterior or posterior tibial arteries at the level of the malleolus. Tyson and Reichle recently described a substantial experience with the technique performed over the last 4 years. Endarterectomy procedures are not feasible in the small vessels of the calf. However, they have succeeded in the proximal portion in the anterior tibial down to where it passes through the tibiofibular interosseous membrane and down the posterior tibial and peroneal arteries for about 2 in. beyond their origins, removing the overlying soleus muscle to expose the vessels in this area.

These procedures are performed by widely exposing the

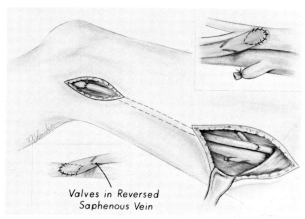

Valves in Reversed
Saphenous Vein

Fig. 21-8. Bypass graft procedure for occlusion of the superficial femoral artery. *A.* Incisions employed for exposure of the major vessels. A proximal incision is made over the saphenous vein from just below the inguinal ligament to the apex of Scarpa's triangle, avoiding undermining of adjacent skin flaps which might result in ischemic necrosis. The distal incision is made on the medial aspect of the popliteal fossa to expose the popliteal artery. The adductor magnus tendon, the site often of most severe superficial femoral arterial involvement, is shown. It is frequently cut to facilitate passing the vein graft from adductor canal to popliteal fossa. *B.* Completed bypass graft of the reversed saphenous vein. The anastomoses are performed end to side to the common femoral and popliteal arteries. The vein is brought either subcutaneously or through the subsartorial canal. Inserts show details of the bevel created in the vein bypass and reversal of the valves. An alternative technique is to leave the saphenous vein in its usual location, without reversal, destroying the valves, accomplishing an in situ nonreversed bypass graft.

bifurcation of the popliteal artery through a long medial incision over the calf and lower thigh, a surgical approach described by Imparato and Kim. The endarterectomy is performed with a longitudinal arteriotomy, followed by endarterectomy and closure of the vessels with venous roof patches up to the level of the distal popliteal artery. If arterial reconstruction proximal to this level is required, a bypass procedure or an endarterectomy can be combined with a distal endarterectomy. Similarly if reconstruction is required distad down to the ankle, the reversed autologous vein bypass technique is employed. Although the arteries at the malleolus are small, with an internal diameter of 1 to 2 mm, the anastomoses can be performed with fine suture material (7-0) and optical magnification. Operative angiography is quite useful when such small anastomoses are performed (Fig. 21-11).

Prognosis. As mentioned earlier, arterial reconstructions in this area are performed only when ulceration and gangrene threaten amputation. Arterial reconstruction is initially successful in about 75 percent of patients, both with reconstruction at the proximal tibioperoneal level and with reconstruction extending down to the malleolus. Immediate failures are almost always due to inadequate outflow tracts. Failures occur invariably if the dorsal arch at the ankle is not complete. When the reconstruction is initially successful, limb salvage is excellent, for the necrotic tissue can be debrided and the wound subsequently closed by skin grafting. If the arterial reconstruction fails before

complete healing is obtained, however, amputation is usually required.

If healing is complete and the arterial reconstruction subsequently becomes occluded, a significant percentage of patients remain with a viable functional extremity. Some reconstructions into the proximal tibial arteries so far have remained patent for as long as 5 to 7 years. Fewer data are available for bypass grafts extending down to the ankle, but the failure rate within 2 years after operation seems to exceed 50 percent.

Lumbar Sympathectomy. Lumbar sympathectomy is often tried in desperation as an alternative to amputation when arterial reconstruction cannot be performed. It also may be combined with reconstruction, although its value in this case cannot be determined. As an isolated procedure, improvement is seldom significant in more than 10 to 20 percent of patients in this group. Occasionally a brilliant result occurs, consisting of relief of rest pain and marked increase in temperature of the foot; unfortunately this is uncommon.

Amputation. Some important guidelines should be emphasized when amputation threatens because of progressive ulceration of the foot: First, an arterial reconstructive procedure may be successful if only one major arterial tributary is patent, a branch of the popliteal artery, the anterior tibial, the posterior tibial, or even the peroneal artery. Second, a foot will remain useful for weight bearing as long as the posterior half, including the heel, is intact. If more than 50 percent of the sole has been lost, however, the foot is probably useless for weight bearing even if arterial reconstruction is successful. With these two guidelines, angiograms should be seriously considered for virtually all patients in whom amputation is being considered. Data published by Dale in 1967 are quite significant in this regard. Of 100 patients threatened by amputation, either because of rest pain (38 percent) or ulceration with gangrene (62 percent), arterial reconstructive procedures were performed in 73 and lumbar sympathectomy in 13. The leg was salvaged in 64, and a minor amputation was possible in 10 others.

Both morbidity and mortality are surprisingly high in patients requiring amputation for peripheral vascular disease. Mortality is related to the advanced age in many and to a rate of severe coronary occlusive disease exceeding 50 percent. Morbidity is primarily related to failure of wound healing from improper selection of the site of amputation. In general, as long as gangrene is limited to a toe, the amputation should be delayed and the ischemic toe permitted to mummify and undergo virtual autoamputation. Delay permits growth of collateral circulation in the more proximal tissues so that wound healing may occur if the toe is allowed to gradually separate over a period of weeks; a definitive amputation often results in failure and extension of the wound onto the foot. A transmetatarsal amputation may be effective in some diabetic patients when infection superimposed upon a gangrenous toe requires operation. This is successful if pedal pulses are palpable but ineffective if gangrene has extended into the forefoot. Foot amputations proximal to the transmetatarsal level are generally unsatisfactory for weight bearing except

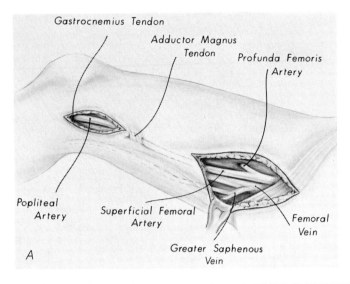

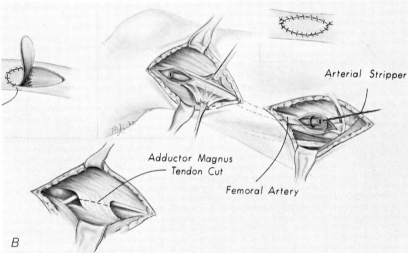

Fig. 21-9. *A.* Femoral popliteal endarterectomy performed by exposing the femoral artery proximally and the popliteal artery distad. *B.* An endarterectomy stripper is used to detach atherosclerotic material via a plane in the media or between media and adventitia. Cutting the adductor magnus tendon facilitates passage of the arterial stripper. The distal intima in the popliteal artery is carefully sutured to prevent detachment and dissection of this free edge when circulation is restored. Arteriotomies are closed with autologous vein roof patches. Angiographic studies are performed to ensure that all debris has been removed, since even minute fragments left behind may result in immediate rethrombosis. Alternative techniques are exposing the entire femoral artery, opening it longitudinally in its entirety and suturing a long roof patch for closure, or utilizing CO_2 intramural injection to accomplish endarterectomy.

for the Syme amputation, which is almost never successful in the presence of peripheral vascular disease.

A fortunate and surprising development in the past few years has been the demonstration by several groups that below-knee amputations can be successfully performed in a high percentage of patients, even in the absence of a popliteal pulse. Preservation of the knee joint greatly facilitates the wearing of a prosthesis. Guidelines are still being sought to determine the likelihood of wound healing if a below-knee amputation is performed in the absence of a popliteal pulse. The degree of skin bleeding is one of the most useful guidelines, though not infallible, that has yet appeared. An attempted below-knee amputation is a significant benefit to the patient if successful but is detrimental if the wound fails to heal and a subsequent above-knee amputation must be performed.

THE DIABETIC FOOT

The foot of the diabetic patient has distinct problems, characteristic of the diabetic state, which can quickly prog-

ress to conditions that threaten both life and limb. Three distinct characteristics can be delineated:

First, the diabetic has an extraordinary susceptibility to infection. This can develop after minor trauma to the toe, the sole of the foot, or the heel. After a seemingly trivial injury, within hours or days a virulent necrotizing infection can appear which rapidly spreads along musculofascial planes. It characteristically begins in an interdigital space, spreads along the plantar fascia, and may continue along tendon sheaths into the muscles of the leg. Frequently the infecting organism is gas-producing and may be of the clostridial group. A life-threatening infection quickly evolves. This same susceptibility to infection manifests itself in the development of carbuncles in the neck and in different types of necrotizing infections of the abdominal wall after elective abdominal operations. These infections often occur with patent major arteries and seemingly are not closely related to local ischemia.

A second peculiarity of the diabetic is diabetic neuropathy. Characteristically this appears as hypalgesia or true

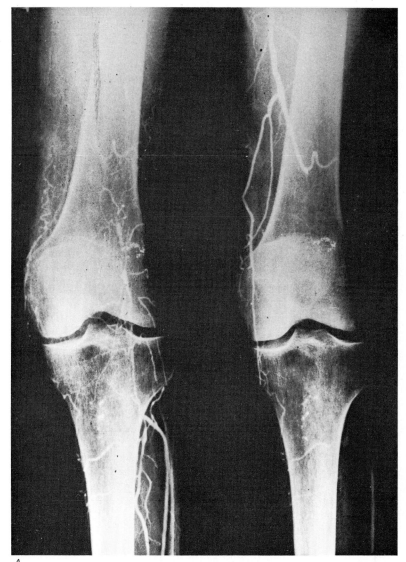

A

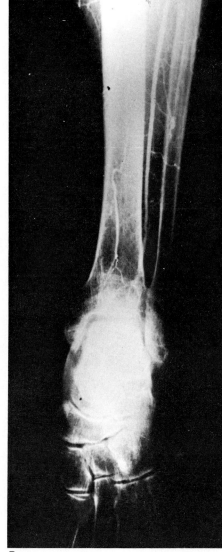

B

Fig. 21-10. Preoperative angiographic studies in the presence of tibial disease. *A.* Angiographic studies routinely performed showing poor visualization of tibial arteries. *B.* Angiograms in the same patient obtained 6 weeks later, when an ischemic lesion developed in the foot, showing patency of the anterior tibial artery. This degree of opacification can be obtained using the ischemic hyperemia technique described in the text.

anesthesia of some portion of the sole of the foot, subsequently complicated by trophic ulcers. These also are unrelated to ischemia and often develop with strongly palpable pedal pulses. The trophic ulcer, anesthetic and painless initially, then becomes a portal of entry for necrotizing infection.

The third peculiarity of the diabetic foot is the type of arterial occlusive disease which typically involves the popliteal artery and its branches down to the pedal arches. The process may be diffuse, or one or more arteries may be spared. Arteries proximal to the popliteal may be nor-

mal or may show a typical "nondiabetic" pattern of atherosclerosis.

CLINICAL MANAGEMENT. Infection. In some unfortunate instances a rampant uncontrolled infection with clostridia may necessitate immediate open amputation through the midcalf or midthigh to prevent death from septic shock. If patients are seen earlier, immediate widespread incision and drainage with debridement of infected tissue may prevent amputation. At an earlier stage, when infection is the dominant process without extensive tissue necrosis, localized debridement combined with intensive antibiotic therapy may be successful. A basic guideline is that all necrotic tissue must be extensively debrided, for simple drainage is hopelessly inadequate in the presence of extensive tissue necrosis, as is radical debridement alone because of the underlying tissue ischemia. In such instances the combination of radical debridement with arterial recon-

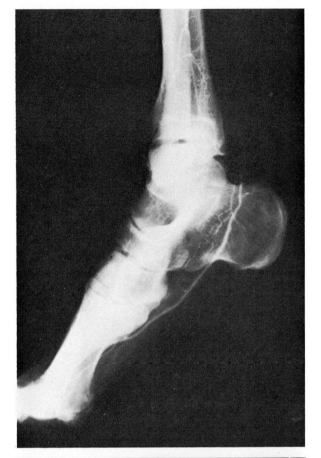

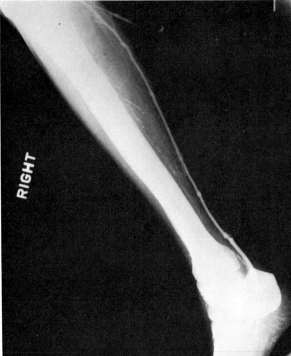

Fig. 21-11. Angiograms obtained in the operating room showing reversed autologous femoral–dorsal pedal bypass graft.

struction down to the ankle may permit salvage of the extremity. These considerations were discussed in the preceding section on tibioperoneal arterial reconstruction.

Gangrene. If gangrene of a toe is present and not complicated by infection, a much more leisurely approach is indicated, quite in contrast to the urgency of therapy if spreading infection is present. As discussed earlier, localized dry gangrene of a toe is best treated by postponing operation, often permitting autoamputation over a period of weeks, during which time the development of collateral circulation may permit wound healing to occur. In all likelihood such instances of gangrene of a digit represent occlusion of a critical digital vessel. This may be followed by the development of enough collateral circulation to salvage the foot, but such circulation requires time to develop.

Trophic Ulcers. A trophic ulcer can be readily recognized by several characteristics. It is usually a sharply demarcated, punched out area on the sole of the foot overlying a pressure point, usually the metatarsal heads. A location over the first or third metatarsal head is particularly common. Often the ulcers are completely anesthetic and hence relatively free of pain until secondary infection develops. Similarly, the pedal pulses may be entirely normal.

Treatment in the majority of patients consists of local cleansing, protection from trauma, and most important of all, avoidance of weight bearing. Reconstruction of shoes to distribute weight differently is often effective. Special types of shoes, such as those lined with lamb's wool, are useful. Effective therapy requires long-term careful periodic observation to readjust the weight-bearing characteristics of the foot so that pressure on the area of ulceration is avoided. Any superimposed infection requires antibiotics and local debridement. As most patients fortunately do not have any vascular occlusion, arterial reconstruction is not needed.

SUMMARY OF THERAPEUTIC CONCEPTS FOR ARTERIAL OCCLUSIVE DISEASE OF THE LOWER EXTREMITIES

Intermittent claudication with normal nutrition in the extremity is a comparatively benign disease in many patients. The risk of gangrene within 5 years is no more than 5 percent. If a patient stops smoking and exercises regularly, claudication may improve to a significant degree within months or years. This, combined with the fact that arterial reconstructions are not curative, indicates that a conservative approach can be applied to many patients with claudication, depending upon the patient's age and occupation.

A quite different approach is indicated when the nutrition of the foot is impaired from chronic ischemia, for the likelihood of ulceration and gangrene within 1 to 2 years is great. In these patients, the possibilities of arterial reconstruction should be carefully investigated by detailed angiography, examining the arterial tree from the abdominal aorta to the pedal arches at the ankle. This has been especially productive when ulceration and gangrene already have appeared and amputation appears imminent.

ARTERIAL EMBOLISM

It has been long recognized that the majority of arterial emboli originate in the heart. The embolus originated from the heart in 86 percent of 426 emboli reported by Darling and associates and in 91 percent of 214 emboli reported by Cranley et al. In the past few years there has been increasing recognition of emboli which originate in atherosclerotic arteries, either fragments of a plaque or thrombi adherent to the surface of an ulcerated plaque which subsequently dislodge. For simplicity in presentation, emboli arising from the heart, constituting the majority of emboli seen, are referred to as *cardioarterial embolization.* As a separate entity, the frequency of which is yet unknown, emboli arising from an atherosclerotic artery and lodging in the distal tributaries are referred to as *arterioarterial emboli.*

Cardioarterial Embolization

HISTORICAL CONSIDERATIONS. Emboli have been long recognized as a cause of acute arterial occlusion resulting in gangrene. Several unsuccessful embolectomies were attempted near the end of the nineteenth century, but the first successful embolectomy is credited to Lahey in 1911. For many years embolectomies performed within 4 to 6 hours after lodging of the embolus were successful, while those performed subsequently had a progressively higher failure rate. Less than 10 years ago a serious proposal was made that emboli which had lodged more than 12 hours previously should not be operated upon. It is now well established that such a viewpoint is erroneous. The difficulties with late operation have been found due to inadequate removal of distal thrombi. With the combination of operative angiography and the balloon catheter developed by Fogarty et al. in 1963, viability can be preserved in well over 90 percent of patients operated upon if operation is performed before the muscles become necrotic, regardless of whether the embolus lodged 3 hours or 3 days beforehand.

INCIDENCE AND ETIOLOGY. In about 90 percent of patients with emboli, the embolus originates in the heart from one of three causes: mitral stenosis, atrial fibrillation, or myocardial infarction. In some patients it is the first sign of previously unrecognized heart disease. Hence, an embolus, though a serious or catastrophic event, is best regarded as a symptom of serious heart disease which must be treated separately.

With mitral stenosis emboli originate from thrombi which have formed in the left atrium because of restriction of blood flow through the stenotic mitral valve. Most such patients also have atrial fibrillation with impaired contractility of the atrium. Atrial fibrillation from atherosclerosis without mitral stenosis can occur and becomes increasingly frequent in older patients. Emboli have been recognized to occur following the spontaneous or induced conversion of fibrillation to sinus rhythm, probably because the contractions of the atrial appendage expel thrombi which have accumulated during the impaired contractility from fibrillation. Emboli following a myocardial infarction originate

from mural thrombi forming over the endocardial surface of the infarct. Their frequency is greatest in the first 2 to 3 weeks following the infarct, and in some patients they are the first sign that an infarction has occurred.

Unusual causes of emboli include a paradoxic embolus in which a thrombus arising in the venous circulation passes through a congenital atrial or ventricular septal defect and lodges in a peripheral artery. Other unusual causes include bacterial endocarditis, mural thrombi in subclavian or popliteal aneurysms, and atrial myxoma. In 4 to 5 percent of patients, despite the most diligent search, the source is never found.

PATHOLOGY. Most emboli ejected from the heart, 70 percent of the 426 emboli reported by Darling, lodge in the arteries of the lower extremities. Unfortunately 20 to 25 percent lodge in the cerebral circulation, usually intracranially, and are surgically inaccessible. Five to ten percent lodge in visceral arteries, the superior mesenteric or renal, and an unknown number lodge in silent areas of

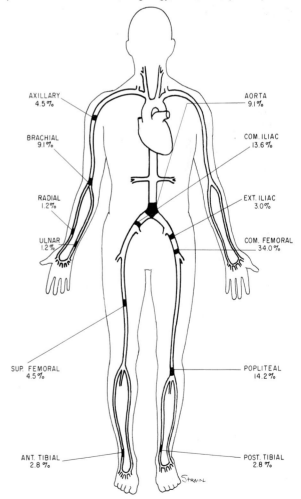

Fig. 21-12. Frequency of involvement of different peripheral arteries by arterial emboli. In the majority of patients arteries in the lower extremity are involved. (*Redrawn from H. Haimovici, Peripheral Arterial Embolism, Angiology, 1:20, 1950.*)

the circulation, such as the spleen, for which clinical signs are obscure.

Emboli usually lodge at bifurcations of major arteries where the diameter abruptly narrows. Common sites are the bifurcation of the abdominal aorta, the common iliac artery, the common femoral artery, and the popliteal arteries (Fig. 21-12). In the upper extremity a similar pattern is found, including the distal subclavian artery and the bifurcation of the common brachial. The severity of the ischemia produced is due both to the abrupt occlusion and the fact that the site of occlusion involves two major arteries whereas an occlusion either immediately proximal or distal to the site of bifurcation would permit collateral circulation through the bifurcation.

PATHOPHYSIOLOGY. The physiologic consequences of an arterial embolus are the immediate onset of severe ischemia of the tissues normally supplied by the occluded artery. Depending upon the artery involved, if untreated, an embolus results in gangrene in about 50 percent of patients. The prominent early symptoms of pain, paralysis, and paresthesia all result from the great sensitivity of peripheral nerves to oxygen deprivation. Striated muscle is secondary only to peripheral nerves in susceptibility to anoxia. Necrosis may appear within 4 to 6 hours after onset of ischemia but varies with a number of factors. These include the size of the artery occluded, the collateral circulation around the site of occlusion, blood pressure, and temperature. If collateral circulation is well developed, necrosis may not appear for 8 to 12 hours; occasionally moderate ischemia is present but necrosis does not develop. The fact that muscle necrosis often begins within 4 to 6 hours is the reason that surgical embolectomy is uniformly successful within 4 to 6 hours but considerably less effective after longer periods of time.

Sluggish flow of blood in arteries distal to the embolus results in secondary thrombosis within the distal arterial tree. This may be a thrombus in continuity with the original embolus, or separate thrombi may develop in areas of severe stasis, varying with the degree of blood flow through collateral circulation. Secondary thrombi further occlude major collateral channels and intensify the ischemia. Effective therapy becomes more difficult because not only the primary embolus but also the secondary thrombus must be removed. Eventually the progressive circulatory stasis is further complicated by extensive venous thrombosis.

CLINICAL MANIFESTATIONS. The five p's discussed earlier under manifestations of acute arterial occlusion, pain, paralysis, paresthesia, absent pulses, and pallor, describe the principal clinical features of arterial embolism. The onset is abrupt in most cases, gradual in a few. In 75 to 80 percent of patients there is severe and unremitting pain, usually referred to the most peripheral portions of the limb. The color may be extreme pallor or mottling from alternate areas of pallor and cyanosis. Sensory disturbances vary from anesthesia to paresthesia. Paralysis may be the most prominent feature; complete paralysis and anesthesia mask the true nature of the disorder, diverting the physician into investigations for neurologic disease while muscle necrosis is occurring.

The neurologic symptoms are the crucial prognostic signs for muscle necrosis usually appearing within 6 to 8 hours after onset unless therapy is effective. Conversely, if motor and sensory function is intact, the extremity will survive even though chronic ischemia may persist.

Physical Examination. The extremity is often pale and cold with collapsed peripheral veins. With less severe degrees of ischemia there may be cyanosis instead of pallor. A temperature level may be detected which coincides with the level at which the color changes. The arterial pulse is absent at the site of occlusion, frequently with accentuation of the pulse immediately proximal to this point. Sensory impairment varies from hypesthesia to anesthesia, and motor disturbances from weakness to paralysis.

The level of occlusion can often be estimated from the color, temperature level, and pulse findings. Ordinarily acute ischemia develops one joint away from the site of occlusion. An iliac embolus produces ischemia at the level of the hip joint, while a common femoral embolus produces ischemia distal to the knee. These, of course, vary with the effectiveness of collateral circulation. Muscle turgor in the ischemic limb is most important. Shortly after the onset of ischemia, the muscles are soft. With continuing ischemia, edema appears, progresses to necrosis, and finally to rigor mortis. Early ischemic edema creates a "doughy" sensation on palpation, termed by some "football calf." The importance of this physical finding is the fact that as long as the muscles are soft to palpation, the extremity can be salvaged with effective embolectomy and thrombectomy, regardless of how long the embolus has been present. Conversely, the presence of stiff muscles warns that necrosis has occurred. This is most clearly apparent in the leg where the muscle tone of the gastrocnemius and soleus group can be easily evaluated. Some limbs with early muscle necrosis can be salvaged by embolectomy and thrombectomy, combined with extensive fasciotomy and later debridement of localized muscle necrosis, but failure is frequent.

An additional important aspect of physical examination is the cardiac examination for underlying heart disease. The cardiac rhythm, murmurs, or friction rubs may provide clues to atrial fibrillation, mitral stenosis, or acute myocardial infarction. Examination of other peripheral arteries for pulses and bruits provides additional clues to underlying cardiac or arterial disease.

LABORATORY STUDIES. A critical decision is whether an angiogram should be performed or not. The diagnosis of acute arterial occlusion can be readily made from the history and physical findings. An electrocardiogram and a chest roentgenogram should both be done to evaluate the presence of heart disease. If performance of angiography delays surgical therapy beyond the 4- to 6-hour "golden period" of therapy, it should be omitted. Intraoperative angiography is one alternative. Angiography is particularly useful where the site of the embolus is uncertain or in distinguishing between arterial embolism and arterial thrombosis superimposed upon an atherosclerotic plaque.

DIAGNOSIS. The condition most easily confused with an

arterial embolus is acute thrombosis of an artery previously diseased with atherosclerosis. The importance of differentiating the two conditions is to determine the method of surgical therapy, for a more extensive operative procedure is required with thrombosis. Certain clinical findings suggest thrombosis rather than embolism. Atherosclerosis is usually seen in an older age group, and often symptoms of chronic ischemia, such as claudication, have been present for some time. The involved extremity may show signs of chronic ischemia such as loss of hair from the toes and atrophy of the skin and nails. The absence of heart disease which could cause an arterial embolus further supports the diagnosis of thrombosis. At times differential diagnosis is difficult or even impossible, because an embolus may occur in an older patient with atrial fibrillation who also has claudication from femoral atherosclerosis. Then, an arteriogram is of great value. With atherosclerosis and secondary arterial thrombosis, diffuse changes of atherosclerosis can be seen throughout the peripheral arteries, often with the development of prominent collateral circulation. By contrast, with embolism, the distal arteries are usually normal except at the site of occlusion.

Rarely, acute extensive thrombophlebitis may be confused with an embolus. Thrombophlebitis may be associated with extensive vasospasm, causing pain and peripheral vasoconstriction with diminished pulses. A bluish extremity, termed *phlegmasia cerulea dolens,* is also characteristic of venous thrombosis. With arterial embolism edema appears only after extensive gangrene has developed.

Even more rarely, acute dissecting aneurysm of the thoracic aorta with obliteration of peripheral pulses may suggest multiple peripheral emboli. A dissecting aneurysm can be suspected because of pain in the chest or back, often with a left pleural effusion.

TREATMENT. Indications for Operation. Because patients with arterial emboli usually have serious heart disease, the operative procedure must be planned with regard to the influence of anesthesia and operation on the heart disease. This is particularly critical when the embolus has resulted from a myocardial infarction. With modern vascular techniques, however, embolectomy can be performed in most patients with minimal trauma, often with local anesthesia. Hence, a decision not to operate because of heart disease should be made only if death is imminent. The reason for this is that failure to remove a peripheral embolus, which subsequently produces gangrene, of necessity requires a major amputation, a much greater surgical stress than simple embolectomy.

As repeated frequently in this chapter for emphasis, the urgency of an arterial embolectomy can be simply estimated from the presence of paralysis and anesthesia. When these are present, muscle necrosis often occurs within 4 to 6 hours. If they are absent, a more conservative approach may be undertaken. However, their absence does not guarantee that claudication will not subsequently develop in the extremity with resumption of normal physical activity.

An unusual indication for nonsurgical therapy occurs with a migrating embolus. An embolus may lodge in a proximal artery, such as the common femoral, then fragment spontaneously within a few hours and migrate distad. Rarely such patients may recover completely, but most remain with significant residual occlusion of peripheral arteries. Peripheral pulses should be unequivocally present before simple observation is continued for a long period of time.

Preoperative Therapy. The prompt intravenous administration of heparin to inhibit the development of thrombi distal to the embolus is the most important therapeutic measure in the treatment of an arterial embolus. Heparin, 50 to 100 mg, is given intravenously and repeated at 3- to 6-hour intervals, depending upon the clotting time, if embolectomy is delayed. Lumbar sympathetic blocks are of dubious value and cannot be safely performed in the presence of systemic anticoagulation. Other measures to influence collateral circulation, such as vasodilator drugs, are of little value.

Operative Technique. For operations on the extremities, local anesthesia can be used in seriously ill patients. Frequently the operative incisions are short, for the location of the embolus can be accurately predicted from the clinical picture. The Fogarty balloon catheter has permitted removal of propagated clot both distal and proximal to the embolus, making possible the entire operative procedure through limited surgical incisions. Frequently, it is possible to perform the entire embolectomy and thrombectomy through incision in the upper thigh over the common femoral artery. Emboli and thrombi can be removed from the aorta and both iliac arteries by a retrograde approach. With emboli at the common femoral bifurcation, it is possible to remove thrombi from the arterial tree down to the ankle through the same incision. Rarely is it necessary to enter the peritoneal cavity for aortoiliac embolectomy and thrombectomy. This should be avoided when possible, for these patients are usually quite ill from their cardiac disease. Many have had a large myocardial infarction which in turn produced an embolus large enough to occlude the abdominal aorta. On other occasions, because of difficulty in passing Fogarty balloon catheters from the common femoral artery into the anterior tibial artery, a separate incision is made at the level of the knee joint to expose the origin of the anterior tibial from the popliteal artery.

In general, surgical incisions are placed directly over the uppermost level of arterial occlusion unless the aortoiliac system is involved, in which case incisions are placed over both common femoral arteries. Once the artery has been isolated proximal and distal to the embolus, 50 mg heparin should be given intravenously. A transverse or a longitudinal arteriotomy is then made in the artery immediately proximal to its bifurcation, where the embolus is usually lodged. The embolus characteristically "pops" out as soon as the lumen is entered and can be recognized by its gray appearance and nonadherence to the arterial wall. Hence, removal is a simple procedure, but removal of thrombi which have formed distad or even proximally may be unusually complex. Fogarty balloon catheters have virtually eliminated the need to make multiple incisions along the course of the arterial tree for the laborious retrograde washing out of thrombi. The preferred technique is to pass the catheter into the distal artery as far as possible, inflate the balloon, and withdraw it in its inflated state. Comparison of the length of the catheter inserted with the length of the extremity indicates how far the catheter has been advanced. Passage of catheters into the aorta for the removal of aortoiliac thrombi is similarly performed. Occasionally it is impossible to pass the balloon catheter into various distal tributaries, either the anterior and posterior tibial in the calf or the radial and ulnar in the forearm. In such instances separate distal incisions are made over these vessels, followed by separate introduction of the catheter into each branch. Dale has used polyethylene catheters to aspirate clot. With these techniques, retrograde flushing of the artery through a distal incision is rarely necessary.

As indicated, the most crucial aspect of the operation is determining the completeness of removal of propagated thrombus. Back-bleeding is a notoriously unreliable indicator. Obviously if there is no back-bleeding, thrombus is still present. Back-bleeding can occur, however, through the nearest arterial branch, while the major artery distad is still occluded. Failure to remove all residual thrombus

usually results in reocclusion (Fig. 21-13). The operative procedure should be continued until, by an appropriate combination of techniques, all pulses are restored at the ankle or wrist, or an operative arteriogram has demonstrated that the arteries are patent. On occasion, restoration of a pulse can be misleading, and bounding pulses may be felt in an artery partly reopened but with persisting distal obstruction.

If severe ischemic injury has been present beforehand, wide fasciotomy of the fascial envelop containing the major muscles may help preserve limb viability. This should be particularly considered if embolectomy has been delayed beyond the golden first 4 to 6 hours and definite change in muscle turgor was palpable before operation.

Postoperative Care. The most important aspect of postoperative care is to be certain that peripheral circulation

Fig. 21-13. Embolic material and secondary clot. The embolic material which was deposited in the heart chambers during active blood flow is gray salmon-colored, of firm consistency, and unattached to the arterial wall. It is composed mainly of fibrin and degenerated platelets. The gelatinous clot which appears homogeneous is secondary stasis clot and was formed when blood flow ceased. It contains all the blood elements.

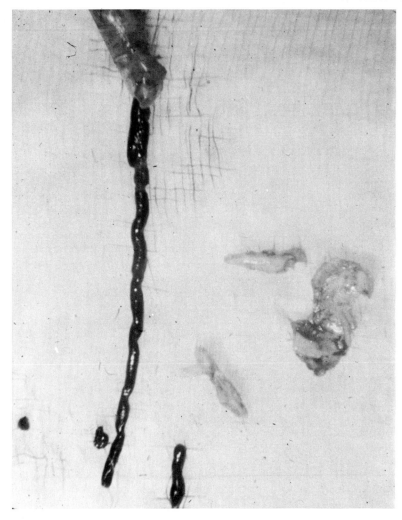
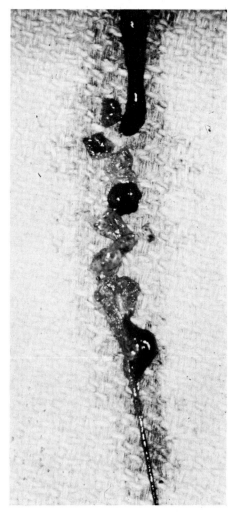

is adequate. A palpable pulse is the best clinical sign. This should be identified immediately after operation and its presence periodically confirmed by palpation. Disappearance of a previously palpable pulse is an indication for either arteriography or immediate reoperation.

The persistence of paralysis and anesthesia following operation is ominous; gangrene is almost a certainty. Conversely, restoration of normal neurologic function indicates adequate circulation for muscle viability. This is particularly reassuring either when pulses cannot be restored or palpation is inconclusive because of edema and swelling.

Anticoagulant therapy should be started with heparin given intravenously within 6 hours after operation, delaying therapy for this short period to prevent bleeding into the wound. Subsequently heparin is given by intravenous injection, 50 mg every 4 to 6 hours, until oral therapy with sodium warfarin is begun 3 to 4 days later. The importance of prompt and continuous anticoagulant therapy cannot be overemphasized, for the arterial embolus is only a symptom of serious heart disease. Recurrence of emboli, each with a 25 to 30 percent likelihood of lodging in the brain, is distressingly common unless the heart disease is effectively treated. Patients with intractable atrial fibrillation should be maintained on permanent anticoagulant therapy. Those with mitral stenosis should have a mitral valvulotomy performed soon. Those with myocardial infarction should receive anticoagulants for several weeks, by which time the endocardial surface of the infarct will have healed and the likelihood of embolism is small.

Antibiotic therapy, usually penicillin or methicillin, generally is started at the time of operation and continued for 2 to 4 days.

PROGNOSIS. The most important feature influencing survival of the extremity following embolectomy is the time elapsing between the onset of the embolus and its removal at operation. As mentioned repeatedly, removal within 4 to 6 hours after onset is almost always associated with an excellent prognosis, having the two great advantages of avoiding muscle necrosis and limiting the secondary thrombus formation beyond the site of embolism. In both of the large series reported by Darling et al. and by Cranley et al. excellent results were obtained in 85 to 95 percent of patients. When more than 6 hours elapsed between embolism and embolectomy, unsuccessful results are much more common. These particularly occur with inexperienced vascular surgeons and limited facilities. The crucial concept is that as long as the calf muscles are "soft" before operation, indicating that muscle necrosis has not occurred, salvage of the extremity should approach 95 percent or higher, regardless of the time interval. However, in delayed cases achieving this goal taxes the resources, skills, and ingenuity of the vascular surgeon to the utmost, for thrombi may have accumulated from the aortic bifurcation to the posterior tibial artery at the ankle and complete removal requires a combination of careful surgical exploration, frequently multiple incisions, and serial operative angiography. If muscle necrosis is present before operation, indicated by a rigid calf muscle, possibilities of limb salvage are small, though these findings are seldom

clear enough to warrant primary amputation. Rarely, a functional extremity may be salvaged in which virtually all the calf muscles are lost from necrosis but a viable foot is preserved.

The crucial long-term feature determining prognosis is the ability to prevent further emboli. Without adequate prophylactic anticoagulation recurrence is dismally inevitable, eventually terminating with fatal or crippling cerebral thrombosis. Vigilance to prevent emboli can be relaxed only when a myocardial infarction has healed or mitral stenosis has been treated by valvulotomy.

In any large series of patients with arterial embolism, death occurs in 25 to 30 percent of patients during that hospitalization. This is almost always due to the underlying heart disease causing the embolus, indicating the gravity of the basic illness. In some instances death is due to either inadequate management of the embolic episode, with the complications of sepsis from gangrene, or to recurrent embolism to the brain or viscera, a result of inadequate anticoagulant therapy.

Arterioarterial Embolization

HISTORICAL CONSIDERATIONS. In the past decade there has been increasing awareness of the entity of arterioarterial embolism to produce ischemic syndromes previously unexplained. With cerebrovascular insufficiency, the ophthalmologic visualization of minute particles of atherosclerotic plaque or platelet fibrin emboli in the retina in association with an ulcerated atherosclerotic plaque at the bifurcation of the carotid artery indicated the genesis of minute emboli. In the lower extremities, sudden onset of toe and foot ischemia, the "blue toe" syndrome, with little or no impairment of peripheral pulses led to the finding that minute emboli were the mechanism, having originated in aortic or iliac atherosclerotic plaques. The occasional finding of peripheral emboli beyond aneurysms has been described periodically. Miles et al. have cited observations suggesting that small emboli in the coronary circulation could come from ulcerated plaques, producing diffuse myocardial scarring from myriads of tiny emboli.

PATHOGENESIS. The basic process seems to be ulceration of an atherosclerotic plaque with discharge of minute fragments of atherosclerotic debris into the circulation. The ulcerated surface may become covered by platelets and fibrin which in turn are intermittently dislodged. How often these are subsequently resorbed is unknown. The emboli may arise from an atherosclerotic artery near the end organ where the emboli lodge or may originate some distance away, occasionally seen when emboli in the toes apparently originate from plaques in the abdominal or thoracic aorta. Repeated embolic episodes are frequent, at times with almost complete recovery from ischemia between each episode; in other patients progressively greater degrees of ischemia occur, ultimately terminating in necrosis.

CLINICAL FINDINGS. A most striking syndrome occurs with emboli from the distal thoracic aorta, the "blue toe" syndrome. There is severe ischemia of the toes and feet, bilaterally, in association with renal failure. Before the pathogenesis was understood, the diagnosis remained an enigma, for pulses often remained palpable even while distal ischemia progressed to gangrene. There is a wide range in severity, from complete clearing of ischemia to progressive occlusion and gangrene.

Similar episodes occur in the cerebrovascular circulation with any combination of neurologic symptoms from the most transient, fleeting symptoms to complete stroke with cerebral infarction. In the upper extremity the subclavian artery is most frequently involved, with repeated attacks simulating Raynaud's phenomenon.

DIAGNOSIS. The diagnosis can be suspected from the combined findings of severe ischemia of a digit with palpable pulses. Determining the source of the emboli is crucial, for many can be corrected surgically, often by simple endarterectomy. Hence, detailed angiographic studies are necessary. The source of the embolus can be estimated by noting the peripheral circulation in other areas, where previous emboli may have lodged. For example, involvement of branches of the profunda femoris artery indicate emboli arising proximal to this level. Similarly in the upper extremity emboli may arise from the subclavian artery or alternatively from lesions located far distad, such as small aneurysms in the palm of the hand. These diagnostic possibilities can be resolved only by precise, extensive angiography.

TREATMENT. When the atherosclerotic plaque can be related to the pattern of distal embolization (Fig. 21-14), arterial reconstruction of the atherosclerotic segment either by endarterectomy or replacement with a prosthetic graft has prevented further embolism. In the carotid system, there is now extensive experience with arterial reconstruction to prevent recurrent ischemic episodes, so-called transient ischemic attacks (TIA). The operation is effective and durable. Similar procedures have been performed in the subclavian artery to prevent TIA in the upper extremity. In the lower extremity experience is still limited, but good results in a series of 10 cases operated upon at New York University have confirmed both the validity of the concept and the surgical approach.

Theoretically emboli from platelet or fibrin aggregates should be inhibited or prevented by anticoagulants, but their effectiveness is yet uncertain. Paradoxically, anticoagulant therapy might prevent healing of an ulcerated plaque and thereby increase the tendency for embolization. This may explain the infrequent clinical puzzle of an embolus developing *after* heparin therapy has been started.

ACUTE ARTERIAL THROMBOSIS

ETIOLOGY AND PATHOLOGY. Acute arterial thrombosis usually occurs in an artery previously narrowed by atherosclerosis. In some patients the process of occlusion is gradual; no acute symptoms appear, but chronic arterial insufficiency slowly becomes more severe. In others, however, sudden thrombosis precipitates acute symptoms, closely mimicking an arterial embolus.

Unusual causes of arterial thrombosis are a cervical rib or repeated occupational trauma, such as operation of a pneumatic tool, the vibrations of which locally injure the arterial wall and produce thrombosis. Very rarely arterial thrombosis develops within a normal artery. This can happen with debilitating infections, especially in infants, usually with diarrhea and dehydration. It may also occur with primary hematologic disorders, such as polycythemia vera.

Iatrogenic thrombosis has become much more common from percutaneous introduction of catheters for cardiac catheterization or selective angiography. Thrombosis develops from detachment of a flap of intima from the arterial wall with subsequent formation of an occluding thrombus. Acute lower extremity arterial thrombosis also has been seen following long periods of immobilization such as in long automobile or plane trips, similar to acute venous thrombosis, which occurs more commonly.

CLINICAL MANIFESTATIONS. When thrombosis occurs suddenly, the findings are similar to those occurring with arterial trauma or embolism: pain, absence of pulses, paresthesias, and paralysis.

The usual question in differential diagnosis is the distinction between an arterial embolus and an arterial thrombosis. Such a distinction cannot always be made with accuracy, but several clues are helpful. A history of claudication in the involved extremity indicates chronic arterial disease. Similarly, examination of the extremity may show the stigmata of chronic arterial insufficiency, including absence of hair and trophic changes in the skin and nails. Significant findings may also be present in the contralateral, asymptomatic extremity. The absence of heart disease commonly associated with an arterial embolus is indirect evidence that thrombosis is the most likely cause.

Before successful techniques of arterial reconstruction were developed, the distinction between arterial thrombosis and arterial embolism in a patient in whom acute arterial occlusion suddenly developed was an important one. Surgical exploration of patients with arterial thrombosis usually was futile, because the underlying cause of the thrombosis, atherosclerotic stenosis of the artery, could not be treated. Futile surgical exploration often made the condition worse through interruption of collateral circulation. With present surgical techniques, differentiation between the two conditions is much less important, because operation is necessary with either if circulation is impaired to such an extent that gangrene is imminent. The main reason for recognizing which condition is present before operation is to anticipate the degree of vascular reconstruction which will be required. Restoration of blood flow in an extremity with chronic occlusive disease, with an arterial thrombosis superimposed upon an artery previously narrowed by atherosclerosis, is much more difficult than the performance of simple embolectomy upon an artery with no intrinsic vascular disease. Patients with arterial thrombosis should have an arteriogram before operation to assess the extent of occlusive disease and to evaluate the patency of the vascular bed beyond the point of occlusion in order to determine where a bypass graft can be inserted distad.

TREATMENT. Operative correction of the arterial occlusion requires both removal of the thrombus and correction

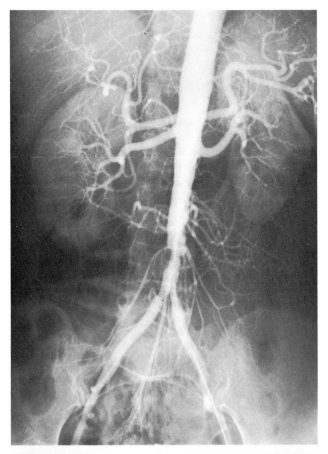

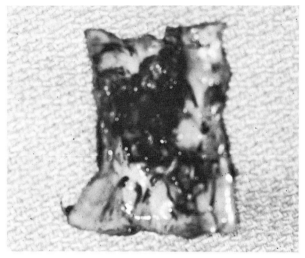

B

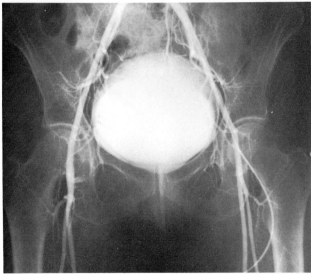

A

Fig. 21-14. Arterioarterial embolization, also known as athero-embolization, in a patient in whom marked ischemia of the toes developed in the presence of palpable pedal pulses. Several attacks occurred with progressive ischemia. *A.* Angiograms showing infrarenal abdominal aortic plaques with occlusion of small calf arteries and no involvement of the renal arteries. *B.* Aortic plaque removed by endarterectomy. There has been no recurrence of embolization since operation.

of the atherosclerotic stenosis. The operative techniques are described in detail in the section on chronic arterial disease. Usually either the atherosclerotic narrowing is removed directly with an endarterectomy, or a bypass graft is inserted around the area of obstruction.

BUERGER'S DISEASE

HISTORICAL DATA. The best descriptive term for Buerger's disease is thromboangiitis obliterans, emphasizing the inflammatory reaction throughout the wall of blood vessels ultimately terminating in thrombosis. It was first described by von Winiwarter in 1879, but attention was focused on the disease by Buerger in a publication in 1908, and further observations were summarized in his monograph in 1924. With the increasing use of arteriography, it has become evident that many conditions clinically diagnosed as Buerger's disease in the past were simply atherosclerosis developing in the second and third decades. A small controversy was initiated by Wessler et al. in 1960, who raised the question whether Buerger's disease actually existed or was simply a misdiagnosis of atherosclerosis in unusual forms. Subsequent studies have indicated that the diagnosis "Buerger's disease" probably was made too frequently in the past, but the disease does indeed exist as a definite clinical entity separate from atherosclerosis. One of the most comprehensive descriptions of the clinical syndrome and its course was by Silbert.

INCIDENCE AND ETIOLOGY. The disease is found most frequently in men between twenty and forty years of age. In a Mayo Clinic series exceeding 500 patients, the youngest patient seen was seventeen years of age. The disease is uncommon in women, only 5 to 10 percent of patients with Buerger's disease being women. It is also rare in Negroes; of 936 cases found in the Armed Forces and analyzed by DeBakey and Cohen, only 2 percent were in Negroes. Initially it was felt that the disease was much more common in the Jewish race; subsequent statistical studies have shown that this frequency has been greatly exaggerated and the incidence is only slightly greater if at all.

Heavy tobacco smoking has been the most significant agent associated with the disease. Well over 95 percent of the patients smoke, often 20 or more cigarettes per day. In a 30-year period, the Mayo Clinic group found only one proved and two probable cases in nonsmokers. Furthermore, there is a peculiar addiction to tobacco, closely resembling the severity of narcotic addiction. Even though patients are repeatedly warned that continued smoking will result in amputation, the majority continue to smoke nonetheless. In the 936 cases analyzed by DeBakey and Cohen, only 10 percent in the 10 years following the diagnosis were reported to have stopped smoking. The progress of the disease, often episodic in character, can also be related to smoking. Resumption of smoking following a period of abstinence has been noted to be associated with exacerbation of the disease.

Although the correlation between smoking and the disease is strong, the mechanism of action is not clear. There are many heavy smokers in the normal population, but the disease is rare, indicating that a direct relationship must represent an abnormal sensitivity of the blood vessels to tobacco. Such a sensitivity, however, cannot be demonstrated with extracts or other methods. Furthermore, most patients have smoked for many years before the disease appears, indicating a delayed onset of reaction, whatever the mechanism is. Finally, it is puzzling that the deleterious action of tobacco does not become evident before actual organic occlusion occurs. If a direct cause-effect relationship existed, an intermediate zone of less clinical severity would be expected to become evident. At present, the strong association with tobacco smoking is beyond question, but the mechanism of action remains uncertain.

Intensive search for an infectious agent or a primary disorder of blood clotting has been unproductive. At present, the basic cause remains unknown.

PATHOLOGY. The disease most frequently occurs in the small arteries of the feet and similarly involves the hands in about 30 percent of patients. Involvement of the hands without concomitant involvement of the feet is almost unknown. Involvement of the larger arteries of the extremity occurs at a later stage. Often a popliteal pulse remains palpable for many years. Occlusion proximal to the arteries of the wrist in the upper extremities is most unusual. Similarly, involvement of visceral arteries is rare.

Involvement of superficial veins, usually as a superficial migratory phlebitis, is a characteristic feature. Large veins, such as the iliac or femoral, are rarely diseased. Involvement of peripheral nerves may occur with inflammatory fibrosis, but this has been overstated in the past, for extensive disease is unusual.

On histologic examination of a small thrombosed artery, the most striking feature is extensive proliferation of endothelial cells and fibroblasts throughout all segments of the arterial wall. This proliferation and fibrosis thicken the wall of the artery and narrow the lumen, but the architecture remains well preserved. Calcification or deposition of lipid, so characteristic of atherosclerosis, is not seen. Inflammatory cells, usually lymphocytes, are frequently

seen, but giant cells, originally emphasized by Buerger, are uncommon. Necrosis of the arterial wall, or abscess formation, is very unusual. The thrombus in the lumen of the occluded vessel often shows an unusual degree of fibroblastic activity with endothelial proliferation and areas of partial recanalization. Recanalization to the extent that effective blood flow is restored in the occluded vessel, however, is unusual. Some have suggested that the unusual histologic reaction to the thrombus indicates a primary antigen in the blood, but such has not been identified.

The characteristic histologic findings in Buerger's disease are felt by most observers to be sufficiently distinct to permit an accurate diagnosis from histologic examination of diseased arteries. In a study of 229 amputated extremities by Kelly a precise retrospective diagnosis could be made solely on the basis of histologic examination. Similar conclusions were reached by McKusick et al.

The gross pathologic features in Buerger's disease are also characteristic of an inflammatory process. The diseased artery is usually surrounded by dense fibrosis, often incorporating the adjacent vein with the artery. Rarely the concomitant nerve is also involved. The fibrotic reaction about the artery contrasts vividly to the usual atherosclerotic artery, where the artery can be separated from the adjacent vein and surrounding soft tissues with little difficulty. In the operating room the inflammatory reaction found around the artery is characteristic of Buerger's disease, although on occasion the inflammatory reaction around thrombosed atherosclerotic arteries can be intense.

The arterial occlusion is often segmental in nature and occurs in acute episodes, alternating with quiescent periods during which the growth of collateral circulation may significantly improve circulation to the ischemic extremity. The severity of the disease is related to the frequency and severity of the acute episodes, counterbalanced by the development of collateral circulation during the quiescent periods.

The disability is primarily the result of ischemia of the distal extremity. Initially this is manifested simply as claudication on exercise, but subsequently trophic changes, postural color changes, and rest pain occur with more advanced ischemia. Eventually ulceration and gangrene of one or more digits appear. Thrombophlebitis, although frequent, is usually superficial and of limited extent, and does not result in significant venous insufficiency.

The rapidity of progression of the disease, as determined by follow-up examinations in 936 patients during a 10-year period after onset of symptoms, was studied by DeBakey and Cohen. There was a 10 percent mortality rate, approximately three times higher than a comparable age group in the normal population, usually from cardiovascular disease. Actual involvement of the coronary or cerebral arteries by a process histologically similar to that found in the extremities was unusual. Postmortem examination usually demonstrated the familiar pattern of atherosclerotic heart disease, suggesting an increased susceptibility to atherosclerosis in patients with Buerger's disease. The incidence of amputation within 10 years following onset of symptoms varied from 20 to 30 percent, while about 40 percent showed some progression of the disease which did not result in amputation. The Mayo Clinic series, in contrast, had a more favorable outlook, in that the 10-year survival was similar to that for patients in the general population, although the amputation rate was near 20 percent.

CLINICAL MANIFESTATIONS. Claudication is usually the first symptom noted. In some, recurring warning attacks of acute superficial phlebitis appear years before claudication. Often this is in the arch of the foot, evolving from occlusion of the posterior tibial and dorsalis pedis arteries. Claudication in the calf is second in frequency, but thigh or hip claudication, so common in atherosclerosis, is unusual. Claudication in the upper extremities is rare, apparently because involvement of the arteries seldom progresses proximal to the wrist.

Pain is often the most prominent feature in Buerger's disease and may result from several causes. Rest pain, as opposed to claudication, is a grave symptom, indicating that ischemia has progressed to such a degree that ulceration and gangrene are imminent. The pain is localized, severe, and may last for hours, preventing sleep. Many patients note that the pain is less with the extremity in a dependent position and may sleep in a sitting position. Pain from ischemic neuritis also may be severe, varying with the distribution of peripheral nerves. Pain may be intensified by infection or phlebitis, either of which can usually be recognized on physical examination. Similarly pain may be intensified from arteriolar spasm, superimposed upon ischemia from organic occlusion of the arteries. In such instances, measures to induce vasodilatation may give significant relief.

Spontaneous variation in color of the extremity may be noted by the patient, usually a rubor appearing in the dependent position. The mechanism of rubor, resulting from oxygenated blood in dilated capillaries, is not certain. It may be due to loss of tone in capillaries from ischemia, resulting in a chronic vasodilated state. In addition the patient often notices that symptoms are worse on exposure to cold, but the sensitivity to cold is not as prominent as that seen in Raynaud's disease.

Physical Examination. The most frequent finding is absence of the posterior tibial and dorsalis pedis pulses in the feet. Often the popliteal pulse is palpable, especially in the early stages of the disease. Absence of the posterior tibial pulse is highly suggestive of the diagnosis, especially when bilateral. In the upper extremity, the radial pulse may be congenitally absent in 5 to 10 percent of patients, but absence of both pulses again is very suggestive of the disease. Signs of chronic tissue ischemia include loss of hair from the digits, atrophy of the skin, brittle nails, and rubor on dependency. In more advanced cases there may be ulceration or gangrene in the digits, often beginning near the nail and involving only the distal portion of the digit. With more extensive disease, gangrene extends into the foot. In the upper extremity, fortunately, extension of gangrene beyond the fingers is rare, and amputation of the hand is almost never necessary.

Edema is also frequently seen with advanced ischemia. It may result from keeping the extremity in a dependent position for many hours in an attempt to relieve rest pain.

Other mechanisms causing edema include abnormal dilatation of the capillaries, producing rubor, and, rarely, significant venous obstruction. Superficial phlebitis involving segments of superficial veins is frequent, but rarely is phlebitis found in the large veins, such as the femoral or iliac. Accordingly, edema on the basis of phlebitis is unusual.

Another helpful distinction from atherosclerosis is the fact that a bruit is virtually never heard over the involved arteries, whereas such a bruit is frequently audible over the iliac or femoral arteries when atherosclerotic plaques are present.

Laboratory Studies. The most significant laboratory examination is arteriography. Plain roentgenograms of the extremity are helpful only if calcification can be demonstrated in the diseased arteries. This virtually excludes the diagnosis of Buerger's disease. The arteriographic findings, as emphasized by McKusick et al., are frequently characteristic. Typically, the intimal lining of the large arteries is smooth, without the characteristic irregularities seen from cholesterol plaques in atherosclerosis. In the small arteries, there are abrupt areas of occlusion, frequently surrounded by extensive collateral circulation. The collateral circulation, which evolves over many years, is unusually tortuous and has been termed "tree root" or "spiderlike." A "corkscrew" deformity also has been noted in peripheral arteries, probably representing partial recanalization of an artery previously occluded by a thrombus. The combination of extensive occlusive disease in small arteries with large vessels which remain smooth and normal in appearance, especially in association with extensive collateral circulation, is highly characteristic of Buerger's disease and is most useful in differentiating it from atherosclerosis (Fig. 21-15).

DIAGNOSIS. Buerger's disease can be differentiated from atherosclerosis without undue difficulty. Other entities with occlusive disease of small arteries, however, closely resemble Buerger's disease. These include diabetes mellitus or popliteal aneurysms, repeated episodes of arterioarterial embolization from proximal atherosclerotic plaques, and different collagen disorders. Patients with any of these may have palpable popliteal pulses, absent pedal pulses, and severe ischemia in the digits. In most of these, however, the upper extremities are not involved. Positive factors supporting the diagnosis of Buerger's disease are its onset in men between the ages of twenty and forty years, a history of migratory phlebitis, strong dependence upon tobacco, usually cigarettes, and frequent involvement of the upper extremities.

Factors suggesting that the disease is not Buerger's disease include diabetes mellitus, palpable popliteal or abdominal aneurysms, audible bruit over a major artery, high blood cholesterol, calcification of peripheral arteries, and onset after forty years of age.

Usually the diagnosis can be made from the history and physical examination. Angiographic studies are needed for confirmation and to define the possibilities of arterial reconstruction. Final proof of the diagnosis may require gross and microscopic examination of the diseased arteries.

TREATMENT. The most important aspect of treatment

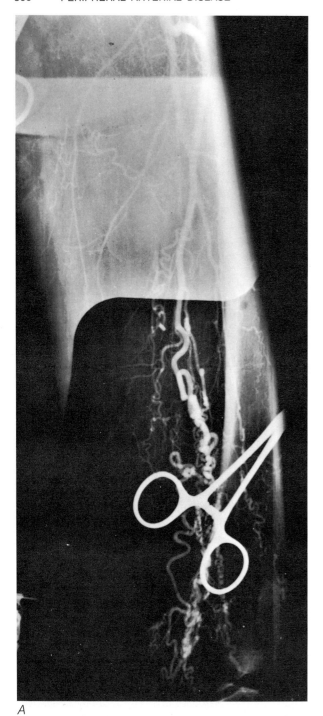

A

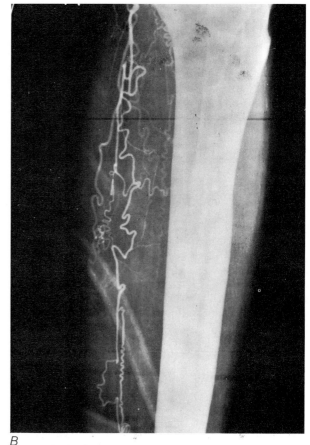

B

Fig. 21-15. *A.* Femoral arteriogram in a patient with Buerger's disease, demonstrating extensive tortuous collateral circulation in the lower thigh which has developed over a period of years as a result of occlusion of the superficial femoral and popliteal arteries. *B.* Angiogram of vessels below the knee, demonstrating the usual tortuosity of small arterial tributaries and illustrating the extensive collateral circulation which may develop with Buerger's disease.

is to have the patient forego the use of tobacco in any form. Simply decreasing the frequency of cigarette smoking is ineffective. The great difficulty in getting the patient to stop smoking cannot be overemphasized, for the pernicious addiction to smoking in this disease closely resembles the tenacity of a heroin addict. In most teaching institutions there are one or more pathetic individuals who have undergone amputation of both legs and most of the fingers of each hand but who are trying to get someone to light

a cigarette for them! The statistical facts cited by DeBakey and Cohen that a 10-year follow-up demonstrated that only 10 percent of patients had stopped smoking completely further indicates the magnitude of the problem. In the experience of one of the authors with a few patients with histologically proved Buerger's disease, almost none stopped smoking completely for a significant period of time.

A sympathectomy should be performed routinely in the

involved extremity to limit the degree of vasospasm which, when superimposed on ischemia from organic occlusion, may precipitate tissue necrosis. The benefit from sympathectomy is difficult to measure because of the episodic characteristics of Buerger's disease, but at least 50 percent of patients significantly benefit from the procedure. Vasodilating drugs, such as alcohol or Arlidin, may be tried but are of less benefit than sympathectomy.

Exposure to extremes of cold or heat should be avoided. Education regarding foot care similar to that described for the atherosclerotic patient is very important. Often gangrene is precipitated by minor trauma to the foot, such as unwise trimming of a callus or wearing tight shoes, which a foot with normal circulation can tolerate uneventfully. The patient must recognize that his foot has to be carefully protected from all forms of even minor trauma permanently if ulceration and gangrene are to be avoided.

Arteriography should be performed to confirm the diagnosis and exclude other forms of smaller arterial occlusions which may require surgical therapy. If a popliteal pulse is absent, it may indicate the possibility of performing local direct arterial reconstruction.

Occasionally patients with Buerger's disease develop atherosclerotic obstruction of major arteries which are surgically accessible to reconstruction. Such a combination of arterial disease is suggested if the popliteal pulse is absent. In these patients arterial reconstruction may be successfully done upon the atherosclerotic disease, with marked circulatory improvement. Direct surgical approach to the vessels primarily involved by Buerger's disease, however, is not possible.

A conservative procedure is indicated when amputation is required. Often the patients are among the younger of the twenty-to-forty age group, and the episodic nature of the disease indicates that conservatism may be rewarded by subsidence of the acute episodes with subsequent partial revascularization by the growth of collateral circulation. As long as gangrene is confined to a toe, amputation should be postponed as long as possible unless rest pain or infection cannot be controlled otherwise. Delaying amputation of a gangrenous digit can permit sufficient development of collateral circulation to allow healing following amputation, whereas amputation soon after gangrene has appeared is often followed by failure of wound healing and the necessity for a more extensive amputation.

Once gangrene has involved the foot extensively, there is little point in delaying amputation, because a functional foot can rarely be obtained if the point of amputation is more proximal than the base of the metatarsal bones. Often a below-knee amputation can be performed, rather than an above-knee, because the popliteal artery is frequently patent.

Long-term anticoagulant therapy has not been of measurable benefit. Therapy with adrenal steroids, so effective for many inflammatory conditions, has similarly not been of consistent value and may aggravate the intimal changes in the tibial arteries.

PROGNOSIS. As stated earlier, 10-year follow-up studies have not agreed upon the prognosis. The Mayo Clinic group have found the survival similar to that of the general population, whereas the group studied by DeBakey and Cohen had a 10-year mortality about three times greater than the normal population. The risk of amputation within 10 years after onset of symptoms is probably near 20 percent, although this varies with the continued use of tobacco as well as the degree to which the ischemic foot is carefully protected. In the few patients who stop smoking completely, progression of the disease may be greatly restricted. A marked advance in therapy would be the discovery of a method by which abstinence from tobacco could be achieved uniformly in this unfortunate group of individuals.

ARTERIAL TRAUMA

HISTORICAL DATA. The feasibility of routinely repairing injured arteries in military casualties was first demonstrated in the Korean conflict in 1952. Earlier attempts in World War II were generally unsuccessful, and rather pessimistic conclusions were reached concerning the possibilities. Following the Korean conflict experiences, injured arteries have been repaired almost routinely, for ligation of major arteries has an overall incidence of subsequent gangrene of about 50 percent. The advances in therapy in the Korean conflict were due to several factors. The most significant was the almost routine prevention of infection in traumatic wounds by extensive debridement, followed by antibiotics and secondary wound closure 4 to 10 days later. Familiarity with techniques of vascular surgical treatment, in combination with the availability of vascular instruments, was also important. The prompt evacuation of wounded men by helicopter, often bringing a wounded patient to the hospital within 2 to 4 hours after injury, also was a significant factor.

ETIOLOGY. Most arterial injuries result from penetrating wounds which partly or completely disrupt the wall of the artery. Nonpenetrating injuries, usually associated with a fracture in an adjacent bone, are less frequent but often have a more serious prognosis, partly related to extensive crushing injury to the wall of the artery and partly due to delay in diagnosis.

PATHOLOGY. Most injuries are either lacerations or transections of the arterial wall. Uncommon injuries include arterial spasm, arterial contusion with thrombosis, and arteriovenous fistula. With lacerations or transections, the extent of injury varies with the type of trauma, which is an important consideration in subsequent debridement and surgical therapy. With clean incised wounds, such as those made by a knife or an icepick, injury to the arterial wall is minimal. In contrast, trauma from a high-velocity missile will disrupt the intima and media for a short distance away from the actual laceration in the arterial wall and requires a wider debridement at the time of surgical repair.

Contusion or spasm often occurs in association with fractures and extensive soft tissue injuries from blunt trauma. The presence of multiple injuries obscures recognition of the arterial injury, especially with extensive comminuted fractures. With such problems arteriography has been found of increasing value. Arterial spasm is an infrequent response to injury in which sustained contraction of the smooth muscle in the wall of the artery may obstruct blood flow and precipitate thrombosis. The cause is obscure. The spasm results from direct muscular contraction rather than a neurogenic stimulus. It occurs most frequently in the brachial artery associated with fracture of the humerus.

Arterial contusion from a blunt injury may be characterized by multiple areas of fragmentation of the arterial wall with intramural hemorrhage. The intima may become detached and prolapse into the lumen, creating an intraluminal obstruction which can be detected only by performing an arteriotomy and inspecting the intima. A serious error occurs when a contusion is misdiagnosed as "spasm." The delay in treatment as a consequence of this diagnostic error can result in gangrene. The well-known Volkmann ischemic contracture of the muscles of the forearm is due to an untreated spasm or contusion of the brachial artery in association with a supracondylar fracture of the humerus.

PATHOPHYSIOLOGY. The severity of the ischemic response following an arterial injury varies with the tolerance of different tissues for anoxia. In the extremity the peripheral nerves are the most sensitive to anoxia; hence, paralysis and anesthesia quickly develop when arterial blood flow is seriously decreased. Striated muscle is almost equally sensitive to anoxia and will usually become necrotic if arterial blood flow is decreased to such a degree that anesthesia and paralysis are present. Skin, tendon, and bone all have a greater tolerance for anoxia and may survive an ischemic injury which has produced irreversible extensive muscle necrosis. This is seen in an extremity in which an arterial repair is performed several hours after injury. The skin may appear viable, but the extremity is anesthetic and paralyzed, and after a period of time will be found to have widespread necrosis of the muscles.

The period of tolerance of striated muscle for ischemia is in the range of 6 to 8 hours. Experimental studies by Miller and Welch found arterial repair successful in about 90 percent of experiments when performed within 6 hours after injury, but the success rate decreased to 50 percent when repair was delayed for 12 hours. Therefore, every effort should be made to complete arterial repair within 6 hours after injury if anesthesia or paralysis are present, indicating a severe degree of anoxia. A definite time limit does not exist, however, beyond which arterial repair is futile, for the importance of the time interval varies with the collateral circulation. The collateral circulation, in turn, varies with the artery injured, with the degree of soft tissue injury which has interrupted collateral circulation, with associated shock, and with ambient temperature. In some patients with little disturbance of collateral circulation, arterial repair may be successfully performed 12 to 15 hours after injury, but in general successful repairs are obtained much more frequently when accomplished within 6 hours after injury.

CLINICAL MANIFESTATIONS. Shock, from loss of blood, is present in over 50 percent of patients with an arterial injury, either as a result of hemorrhage from the injured

artery or because of associated injuries. The degree of shock varies with the severity of the blood loss or the severity of other injuries. When profound shock is present, the severe peripheral vasoconstriction may conceal the presence of an arterial injury until blood pressure has been restored to near-normal levels.

With blunt trauma, multiple organ injuries are commonly present. These include skull fractures, rib fractures, or blunt abdominal injuries. Careful assessment of each injury, with subsequent assignment of priorities in therapy, is a critical part of initial evaluation of the patient.

In the injured extremity, fractures and nerve injuries are commonly present with either penetrating wounds or following blunt trauma. The presence of a fracture or extensive soft tissue injury greatly influences the prognosis of an arterial injury. For example, in one series of arterial injuries the presence of a fracture of a femur in association with an injury of the femoral artery raised the incidence of gangrene from 11 to 55 percent.

In the extremity, the arterial injury frequently produces four abnormal findings, conveniently remembered as four p's: paralysis, paresthesia or anesthesia, loss of pulses, and pallor. Of these four, the neurologic findings, paralysis and paresthesia, are the most important, because, as previously stated, loss of neurologic function indicates a degree of tissue ischemia which will progress to gangrene unless arterial blood flow is improved. Absence of a pulse in the presence of a normal pulse in the contralateral extremity immediately suggests an arterial injury. If serious vasoconstriction is ascribed to hypotension, evaluation of peripheral pulses may be difficult until blood volume is restored. It is important to emphasize, however, that the presence of a peripheral pulse does not exclude an arterial injury. This is frequently seen with a tangential laceration of the wall of an artery which is sealed by a blood clot with preservation of some flow through the arterial lumen.

With penetrating wounds, bright red bleeding, even in small amounts, immediately suggests an arterial injury. In the absence of hemorrhage, a tense hematoma may be palpated around the wound, evolving from extravasation of blood under significant pressure beneath the fascia. Occasionally a systolic bruit may be audible over the wound, or rarely a continuous bruit if an acute arteriovenous fistula has been produced.

It should be emphasized that an arterial injury can be present with virtually no abnormalities in the extremity. Hence, the presence of a penetrating injury near a major artery should alert the physician to the possibility of an arterial injury. In a series of 85 arterial injuries reported by Dillard and associates, the correct diagnosis was delayed in 15 of the patients. Usually the diagnosis is missed if serious hemorrhage is not present or if a peripheral pulse can be felt. In unrecognized cases a secondary hemorrhage from the wound may subsequently develop a false aneurysm, or an arteriovenous fistula may form in the area where the hematoma has formed around the lacerated artery.

With uncertain cases, an arteriogram should be performed. This is of particular value with blunt trauma producing a fracture of the extremity. A critical question in such patients is whether a decreased or absent pulse is due to an arterial injury or to angulation of the artery from the fractured bone.

TREATMENT. Preoperative Considerations. Control of bleeding is the most urgent immediate problem. This can usually be accomplished by tightly packing the wound with gauze and applying a pressure dressing. A large amount of packing may be required, for the efficacy of the packing depends upon compression of the artery between the overlying skin and the underlying bone. Tourniquets are best avoided for most injuries. When used they must be carefully padded to avoid the risk of permanent injury to a peripheral nerve.

Shock, which is present in 50 to 60 percent of patients, should be treated by the rapid infusion of fluids (500 ml every 5 to 10 minutes) until the systolic blood pressure rises to 80 mm Hg, after which additional fluids can be infused more gradually. Usually 1,000 to 2,000 ml of fluid will be required. Blood is preferable, but until the necessary cross matching has been done, Ringer's lactate solution, plasma, or dextran may be used.

Antibiotic therapy should be started promptly and appropriate prophylactic therapy for tetanus begun. Sympathetic blocks and anticoagulant therapy have no significant role in preoperative care.

Operative Technique. An important basic attitude regarding arterial trauma is that almost all injuries can be repaired successfully with available surgical techniques. The prognosis then becomes a question of whether or not the repair was performed before irreversible muscle necrosis developed. The only special instruments required are atraumatic vascular clamps and arterial silk, sizes 4-0 to 5-0, with swaged needles. The surgical incision should be placed to expose the artery proximal and distal to the site of injury in order to avoid hemorrhage when clots are evacuated from the wound. Once proximal and distal control of the artery has been obtained, the hematoma surrounding the injury can be widely opened and the site of injury mobilized. Most injuries are best treated by excision of the injured area followed by end-to-end anastomosis. With injuries from high-velocity missiles, 2 to 4 mm of adjacent arterial wall should be excised. Tangential repairs of lacerations are deceptive in that the suture of the laceration often results in constriction and subsequent thrombosis. Usually excision followed by direct anastomosis is preferable.

With transection of an artery, elastic recoil will separate the two ends of the vessel for 1 cm or more, giving the erroneous impression that a segment of artery has been destroyed. In most instances application of gentle traction on the ends of the artery with vascular clamps will demonstrate that direct anastomosis can be performed. Normally 1 to 2 cm of a peripheral artery can be excised and the vessel ends still approximated after limited mobilization of the two ends. For example, in 180 arterial reconstructions for civilian injuries reported by Patman and associates, grafts were necessary in only 20 patients. Similarly, in a series of 190 arterial reconstructions reported by Morris et al., primary repair was done in 167 patients and vascular grafts in 23. Before the anastomosis is performed,

the degree of back-bleeding from the distal artery should be noted and any blood clots removed with a catheter. The anastomosis should be performed with 4-0 or 5-0 arterial silk, using a continuous suture interrupted in two or three areas to avoid a purse-string effect. Individual sutures should be 1 to 1.5 mm in depth and a similar distance apart. With small arteries, interrupted or horizontal mattress sutures may be employed. Either a continuous over-and-over suture or an everting suture is satisfactory (Fig. 21-16).

A vascular graft is needed only when direct anastomosis cannot be performed because of loss of 2 cm or more of artery; this occurs in about 10 to 15 percent of injuries. An autogenous vein is the preferable graft, reversing the ends of the vein which is employed, usually the saphenous. If for some reason a vein cannot be utilized, a graft of knitted Dacron is preferable. If a prosthetic graft is used, the diameter rarely should be less than 8 mm, for thrombosis occurs much more frequently with smaller grafts.

With contaminated wounds, the best protection from infection following adequate debridement and arterial

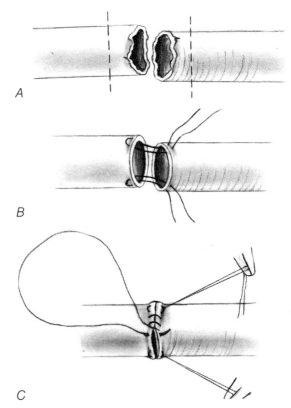

Fig. 21-16. *A.* Repair of traumatic transection of a peripheral artery. Initially the edges of the injured artery are debrided, removing 1 to 2 mm of normal arterial wall, especially if the injury was from a high-velocity missile which would traumatize adjacent segments of arterial wall. *B.* Initially the two ends of the artery are aligned with mattress sutures of 4-0 or 5-0 silk placed about 180° apart. *C.* Anastomosis is then performed with a continuous suture of 4-0 or 5-0 silk, usually as a simple over-and-over suture. Alternatively, an everting suture can be employed. With small vessels, simple interrupted or horizontal mattress sutures can be used to lessen the risk of constriction of the lumen.

reconstruction is approximation of the adjacent soft tissues over the arterial repair and leaving the remaining wound open, to be closed by secondary suture 4 to 7 days later. This technique will almost routinely prevent the development of infection.

Ligation of an injured artery should be performed only for minor arteries, such as a radial or an ulnar artery which is not essential to survival of the limb. Back-bleeding is an inadequate guide to ligation of major arteries, indicating that some collateral circulation is present but not guaranteeing that collateral flow will be large enough to prevent gangrene. In the Korean conflict "good" or "fair" back-bleeding was recorded in 9 of 20 arterial ligations performed in one group of patients, all of which resulted in gangrene.

Arterial spasm, an unusual injury, may be treated by the topical application of 2 to 5% papaverine. Another technique, reported by Mustard and Bull, is the forceful dilatation of the area of spasm by the injection of saline solution into the lumen of the artery. The importance of differentiating spasm from contusion with disruption of the wall of the artery has been mentioned previously. Unless the area of constriction can be satisfactorily corrected, it should be excised and continuity reestablished by direct anastomosis or a vascular graft.

Postoperative Care. Anticoagulant therapy is not recommended after arterial repair, for it provides little protection from thrombosis but does increase the risk of bleeding into the wound. Sympathetic blocks are similarly of little value. The most important consideration following operation is to detect peripheral pulses, which indicate satisfactory restoration of arterial flow. If pulses cannot be detected or if previously palpable pulses disappear, an arteriogram should be performed, or alternatively the site of anastomosis should be reexplored. The important principle to reemphasize is that with modern vascular techniques a traumatic injury of a normal artery can almost always be successfully repaired.

When a femoral artery is repaired hours after injury, ischemic swelling may occur in the leg muscles in the anterior and posterior tibial compartments. The swelling can progress to such an extent that ischemic necrosis results. Prompt fasciotomies over the muscle compartments, decompressing the edematous, turgid muscles, may be of great value.

When an arterial repair is performed several hours after an injury, a peripheral pulse may be restored, but the extremity remains paralyzed and anesthetic. In such patients the skin may be viable, but the status of the underlying muscles is uncertain. Such patients must be carefully observed, because extensive muscle necrosis will result in serious toxic manifestations, with high fever and occasionally renal insufficiency. A decision to amputate such extremities, as opposed to widespread debridement of the necrotic muscles, is a difficult one to make, and each individual case must be evaluated carefully. In some patients the extremity may be salvaged following extensive debridement of necrotic calf muscles, with preservation of a limited but useful foot.

The development of a postoperative infection around the site of arterial repair is a grave complication, because frequently the anastomosis will disrupt with life-threatening hemorrhage. The infection should be treated promptly by widespread drainage, for there is usually inadequate removal of necrotic tissue. If infection involves the arterial reconstruction, ligation of the artery is usually required to prevent fatal hemorrhage or sepsis. Occasionally bypass grafts may be inserted through channels circumventing the area of infection, an anastomosis being performed between the artery proximal and distal to the point of injury. As mentioned earlier, the Korean conflict experiences well emphasized that despite massive contamination, the policy of widespread debridement, followed by secondary wound closure, almost always prevented postoperative wound infections.

PROGNOSIS. With present vascular techniques, arterial reconstruction almost always can be performed successfully if undertaken within 6 hours after injury. In 209 patients with arterial injuries reported by Patman and associates, the amputation rate was 3.8 percent. In another series of 67 arterial reconstructions reported by Dillard et al., only two amputations were necessary. If a vein graft is needed for arterial reconstruction, the long-term patency is probably in the range of 80 to 85 percent, varying with the experience of the surgeon and the circumstances of the injury. If subsequent occlusion of a vein graft does occur, viability of the extremity is rarely jeopardized, although claudication may develop. In such patients a subsequent vascular reconstruction may be performed electively.

Anterior Compartment Syndrome

The anterior tibial compartment syndrome is a progressive neuromuscular disability related to pressure from tissue fluid within the closed anterior tibial compartment.

ETIOLOGY. Any condition which increases the presence of fluid or compromises the outflow of fluid from this closed space may result in augmented pressure and clinical consequences. The swelling continues until the intracompartmental pressure exceeds arterial pressure. The critical structures coursing through the closed compartment and subjected to the effects of the intracompartmental pressure include the tibial artery, the anterior tibial nerve, and the anterior tibial, extensor digitorum longus, perioneus tertius, and extensor hallucis longus muscles. The unyielding walls of the compartment are composed of the tibia, the interosseous membrane, and the anterior crural fascia.

In some cases, there is a readily demonstrable arterial lesion; the syndrome has been associated with arterial trauma, arterial embolism, and acute arterial thrombosis; and it has been a complication of femoropopliteal bypass procedures and also of cardiopulmonary bypass. In a second group of patients, the syndrome is caused by severe exertion, and there is no proved anatomic lesion.

CLINICAL MANIFESTATIONS. In young patients with idiopathic anterior tibial syndrome, a history of marked exertion should be investigated. Characteristically, in most cases, the pain is the first and dominant symptom. Initially, it begins as a dull ache which soon becomes severe and is primarily located over the anterior compartment, where palpation may elicit tenderness. Motion of the leg or foot increases the severity of pain. Subsequently, erythema of the skin over the anterior compartment becomes apparent, and there is measurable increase in the size of the calf. As the syndrome progresses, these signs become more apparent. The dorsalis pedis pulse may be normal, diminished, or absent. Actually, its absence is a late sign and occasionally follows the loss of motor power of the muscles of the anterior compartment. The anterior tibial muscle and the extensor hallucis longus usually become paralyzed first, whereas the extensor digitorum longus loses its function later and is usually the first to return after release of pressure. Loss of the extensor digitorum brevis is an ominous sign. Loss of sensation is confined to the area served by the deep peroneal nerve.

The syndrome must be differentiated from a common condition known as "shin splints." The pain in the latter condition is usually over bone and can be relieved by rest, elevation, and application of cold. There is no associated marked swelling and muscle paresis with shin splints. Other conditions to be differentiated include cellulitis, thrombophlebitis, and stress fractures of the tibia.

TREATMENT. This is directed at decompressing the anterior tibial compartment and should be performed early to avoid anoxic necrosis of the muscle mass. Treatment can be effected with fasciotomy. The skin is incised lateral to the tibial crest over the midportion of the anterior tibial muscle, and the incision is carried through subcutaneous tissue and the fascia. Muscle bellies are then allowed to bulge. The skin may be closed over the bulging muscle or can be left open for secondary closure. A variation of the procedure employs two small incisions, one in the craniad and the other in the caudad portion of the anterior compartment. The fascia is then incised blindly between these two small incisions.

PROGNOSIS. If decompression is performed before muscle necrosis is present, return of function is complete. Thus, in many instances, fasciotomy is indicated prior to total disappearance of the pedal pulse. If fasciotomy is delayed until muscle necrosis occurs or neurologic findings are advanced, total recovery of function is not to be anticipated, and rehabilitation is required.

Traumatic Arteriovenous Fistulas

HISTORICAL DATA. The true nature of an arteriovenous fistula was first recognized by William Hunter in 1764. Previously the lesion had not been distinguished from a traumatic aneurysm. In a careful description of two patients in whom fistulas developed following phlebotomy, he described the typical clinical findings of a thrill, continuous murmur, dilated artery proximal to the fistula, and dilated pulsating veins. He first recognized that the lesion was basically a communication between an artery and a vein. Attempted therapy by proximal ligation of the involved artery, which was frequently effective for traumatic aneurysms, was often disastrous for arteriovenous fistulas, because gangrene resulted. The gangrene developed be-

cause blood flowing through collateral circulation around the ligated artery would flow through the fistula instead of into the distal extremity.

Matas in 1888 established effective therapy with his technique of endoaneurysmorraphy. Directly incising the fistulous sac, followed by suture of the communication between the artery and the vein, was more effective than indirect therapy of proximal and distal ligation of the involved artery and vein. The abnormal physiology of an arteriovenous fistula was carefully analyzed in a scholarly monograph published by Holman in 1937.

Although the collateral circulation which develops with an arteriovenous fistula made it possible to treat such fistulas by excision without gangrene resulting, intermittent claudication was frequently permanent. Consequently, after World War II, reconstruction of the injured artery became the preferable form of treatment.

ETIOLOGY AND PATHOLOGY. An arteriovenous fistula usually results from a penetrating injury which simultaneously injures an artery and an adjacent vein, permitting blood to flow directly from the injured artery into the vein. A fistula may be established immediately, in which case there is little external loss of blood, or the fistula may become apparent days or weeks following injury as clot surrounding the lacerated artery and vein is liquefied.

Unusual forms of arteriovenous fistulas have been reported following different surgical operations. Injury of the iliac artery and vein is a well-recognized, fortunately rare complication of removal of an intervertebral disc. Arteriovenous fistulas have been reported following thyroidectomy, nephrectomy, or even thoracentesis, in all instances representing a concomitant injury of an artery and a vein, sometimes due to simultaneous ligation of artery and vein by the same ligature.

PATHOPHYSIOLOGY. A series of anatomic and physiologic changes begin to evolve when an arteriovenous fistula is produced (Fig. 21-17). The immediate effects are a decrease in blood flow to tissues distal to the lesion and an increase in venous pressure. The peripheral vascular resistance is lowered as a result of blood flowing directly through the newly created arteriovenous shunt. This results in a decrease in systolic and diastolic blood pressure, an increase in heart rate, and an increase in cardiac output.

In the ensuing days, several compensatory events occur as a result of the decrease in peripheral vascular resistance: The blood volume is increased, systolic blood pressure increases with a corresponding increase in pulse pressure, and a decrease in pulse rate occurs. Locally there is the progressive development of extensive collateral circulation around the fistula, because the decreased vascular resistance at the site of the fistula is a very potent stimulus to development of collateral circulation. Within a few weeks the blood flow to the distal extremity may approach normal limits. There is a progressive dilatation of the "fistulous circuit," including the heart, the arteries leading to the fistula, the fistula itself, and the venous channels leading from the fistula to the heart.

In subsequent months or years, additional changes evolve. The artery both proximal and distal to the fistula

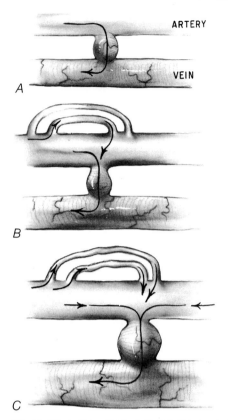

Fig. 21-17. *A.* Immediately following the development of an arteriovenous fistula there is shunting of blood from the artery through the fistula into the vein, from which it returns to the heart. This results in a decrease in peripheral vascular resistance, a fall in diastolic blood pressure, and an increase in heart rate. The venous pressure rises in the involved vein. Peripheral blood flow is decreased in the involved artery. *B.* After several weeks, collateral circulation enlarges around the fistula because of the decreased vascular resistance at the site of the fistula. As the collateral circulation develops, the involved artery and vein also dilate, increasing the amount of blood flowing through the fistula. *C.* After several years, extensive dilatation may develop about a fistula with marked enlargement of collateral circulation. In addition there is enlargement of the artery immediately distal to the fistula, through which blood flows in a retrograde fashion through the fistula toward the heart. The vein may enlarge to marked proportions, creating varicosities in the extremity. Ultimately such progressive dilatation after a period of years may result in congestive heart failure from the increased cardiac output.

may dilate in response to blood flowing through the fistula. The involved veins progressively dilate with marked tortuosity; external rupture with hemorrhage, however, is very rare. Chronic venous congestion may develop in the extremity, causing skin ulcerations resembling those from varicose veins. In growing children, there may be hypertrophy of the involved limb from increased growth of the bones and soft tissues. With large fistulas, involving vessels as large as the iliac artery and vein, continued dilatation of the heart eventually terminates in heart failure. This, however, is an unusual complication with the majority of arteriovenous fistulas, because the volume of blood

shunted is not enough to produce heart failure. Only with large arteries and veins do cardiac symptoms appear.

Two rare complications with arteriovenous fistulas are bacterial endarteritis in the fistula and spontaneous closure. Bacterial endarteritis has been reported in only a few patients and is similar to bacterial endocarditis. Usually with intensive chemotherapy the infection can be controlled or eliminated, after which surgical excision of the fistula should be promptly carried out. A fistula may close spontaneously, occasionally after it has been present for several months. Shumacker reported eight such experiences in 245 patients.

CLINICAL MANIFESTATIONS. A penetrating injury producing an arteriovenous fistula often causes surprisingly few symptoms. External loss of blood can be small, and few disturbances of peripheral circulation develop. Subsequently the patient may be entirely asymptomatic. He is usually aware of a soft mass in the area of the fistula, which transmits a buzzing sensation when the fingers are placed over it. Rarely the patient is totally unaware of the presence of a fistula. In the experience of one of the authors, a fifty-five-year-old patient was admitted for congestive heart failure, presumably due to atherosclerotic heart disease, and was found on physical examination to have a popliteal arteriovenous fistula resulting from trauma many years before. Surgical correction of the fistula promptly eliminated the signs of congestive failure.

In some patients the venous hypertension produces varices with peripheral pigmentation and ulceration from venous insufficiency. Surgical mishaps have resulted from unwise attempts to remove such varices without recognizing their origin.

On physical examination, a soft, diffuse mass is usually palpable and often visible. Dilated veins may surround the area. On palpation a thrill is usually felt, maximal in systole. Auscultation reveals a continuous murmur, loudest in systole, which has been described as a "machinery" murmur, emphasizing the rhythmic rise and fall in intensity and pitch during systole and diastole. It is similar to the murmur of a patent ductus arteriosus. Detection of this classic finding establishes the diagnosis and differentiates the lesion from an arterial aneurysm.

Another significant finding is the demonstration of slowing of the pulse when the fistula is obliterated by digital compression, as evidenced by disappearance of the murmur. This phenomenon, generally known as Branham's sign, was first described by Nicoladoni in 1875. The slowing of the pulse results from the increase in peripheral vascular resistance when the fistula is digitally occluded causing the blood pressure to rise with reflex slowing of the heart rate. The bradycardia results from a neurogenic reflex mediated through pressure-sensitive receptors in the great vessels and carotid sinuses; it can be blocked by atropine.

Usually there are no signs of arterial insufficiency in the extremity. With large fistulas, the pulse pressure is increased, both from an elevation of systolic pressure and a decrease in diastolic pressure. If cardiac enlargement has occurred, a systolic murmur may be audible at the apex of the heart. Usually cardiac failure is found only with fistulas between large vessels, such as the aorta and the vena cava, or when the fistula has been present for many years, allowing time for progressive enlargement of the fistulous opening. In World War II cardiac failure was rarely seen in a collected series of 593 patients treated surgically.

The physical findings are usually sufficient to establish the diagnosis, but if uncertainty exists, an arteriogram readily demonstrates the rapid opacification of adjacent veins and the greatly increased collateral circulation. As the veins fill rapidly, the exact site of the fistula may be obscured unless serial angiograms are obtained. A common problem in differential diagnosis in the cervical area is with a venous "hum," an auscultatory curiosity resulting from flow of blood in the jugular veins. The murmur of a venous hum promptly disappears when intrathoracic pressure is raised by forced expiration against a closed glottis, which will differentiate it from the murmur of an arteriovenous fistula.

TREATMENT. Formerly treatment was delayed for 2 to 4 months to permit the development of collateral circulation in order for the extremity to survive following ligation of the involved artery. Although gangrene virtually never occurred following ligation, claudication frequently resulted, often in as many as 50 percent of patients, despite the abundant collateral circulation. Presently, the majority of patients are treated by division of the fistula and reconstruction of the involved artery, and preferably the injured vein. Excision is performed only for fistulas involving small vessels not essential to normal circulation of the extremity, such as the radial or ulnar arteries. Most fistulas are treated at the time of the arterial injury if the proper diagnosis is made. Otherwise operation is performed within 2 or 3 weeks, after the immediate effects of the injury on the soft tissues have subsided.

Operative Technique. The incision should be placed so as to permit exposure of the artery and vein proximal and distal to the fistula before the fistula is dissected. Once these vessels are isolated and temporarily occluded, the fistulous sac can be incised and the opening directly isolated. Although a large aneurysmal sac may be present, the basic lesion is usually an incomplete laceration of the arterial wall, involving only a short length of artery. A long segment of artery may be incorporated in the wall of the aneurysmal sac, however, which must be freed and mobilized to perform arterial repair. Once the involved vessels have been mobilized, most of the remaining sac may be left, for complete excision is difficult and of little benefit.

In many patients the artery can be repaired by direct anastomosis. In a group of 29 aneurysms and arteriovenous fistulas resulting from civilian injuries reported by Crawford et al., all were treated by end-to-end arterial anastomosis. In 134 fistulas treated by Hughes and Jahnke, an anastomosis was performed in 61, a vessel graft in 23, a lateral repair in 4, and simple division of the fistula in 10.

Repair of the involved vein is indicated if the vein is a large one, such as an iliac or common femoral vein. Permanent edema has been frequent following ligation of such large veins. Repair can often be done by lateral suture.

PROGNOSIS. Convalescence following operation is usually uneventful, and long-term results are excellent if arterial continuity is preserved. Hughes and Jahnke published a 5-year follow-up of 148 such lesions treated during the Korean conflict with satisfactory results in the majority of patients.

CONGENITAL ARTERIOVENOUS FISTULAS

Congenital arteriovenous fistulas are very uncommon lesions. In 1963 Tice et al. estimated that only about 200 cases had been reported in the American surgical literature. In 1956 Coursley and associates reported experiences with 69 patients, and Robertson in a Hunterian Lecture referred to 40 patients.

ETIOLOGY AND PATHOLOGY. As the name indicates, the basic lesion is a congenital abnormality of multiple communications between arteries and veins. A single communication is unfortunately very rare, for the multiplicity of lesions precludes surgical cure in most patients. The extent of the lesion varies from an angiomatous mass localized in a foot or a finger to diffuse involvement of an entire arm or leg. In addition to the presence of multiple lesions, the almost uniform recurrence suggests that a basic defect exists in the peripheral vascular tree as a result of which additional arteriovenous fistulas develop throughout the life of the patient.

The extremities are a common site for such fistulas. When present in childhood, there is increased growth of the affected extremity. Hemihypertrophy of moderate degree was found in over one-half of patients reported by Coursley and associates and also by Robertson. Fortunately, cardiac difficulties from the arteriovenous shunting are uncommon; an increase in heart size has been recorded in only about 15 percent of the patients. The dilated veins associated with the lesions tend to enlarge gradually, causing difficulty from periodic external rupture and bleeding. With involvement of the digits, ischemic pain may occur with gangrene of the tips of the fingers because of shunting of blood proximally through the fistulas.

CLINICAL MANIFESTATIONS. The finding of multiple dilated veins or small angiomas may suggest simple varicosities, but the location of the dilated veins in unusual areas should raise suspicion of congenital arteriovenous fistulas. Detection of a continuous bruit over the lesion establishes the diagnosis, but with some diffuse multiple fistulas involving an entire extremity a bruit may not be audible. In contrast to traumatic single arteriovenous fistulas, it is impossible to obliterate the bruit completely by digital compression. Often a bruit is audible in several widely separated areas, indicating the presence of multiple fistulas.

Occasionally a patient first becomes aware of his condition following an injury, and an error can easily be made by concluding that a traumatic fistula with a single communication is present. Careful inquiry concerning earlier dilatation of the regional veins may give a clue to the correct diagnosis and prevent a long, futile surgical exploration for a single fistula. The finding of multiple bruits which cannot be eliminated by digital compression also suggests a congenital origin. Arteriography is needed to confirm the diagnosis, demonstrating many tortuous arteries with rapid opacification of numerous dilated veins (Fig. 21-18).

TREATMENT. The keynote to therapy is conservatism. Operation should be undertaken only when the lesion is of sufficient size to threaten with ulceration or bleeding, because surgical excision must be considered as palliative in the majority of patients. Only when the lesion is local-

Fig. 21-18. Series of angiograms demonstrating congenital arteriovenous fistulas. *A.* This series of three views shows a popliteal arteriogram in the same patient. The first view is a posteroanterior view which demonstrates the great degree of enlargement of the calf. The next two views are early and late exposures in the arterial phase in a lateral projection. The extensive staining in the late arterial phase is highly suggestive of congenital arteriovenous fistulas. *B.* Arteriogram in the thigh area of a second patient. Note the diffuse staining produced by injection into the profunda femoris vessel. *C.* These two views demonstrate early and late arteriograms in the shoulder area. In this patient the fistulas originate from the circumflex humeral vessels.

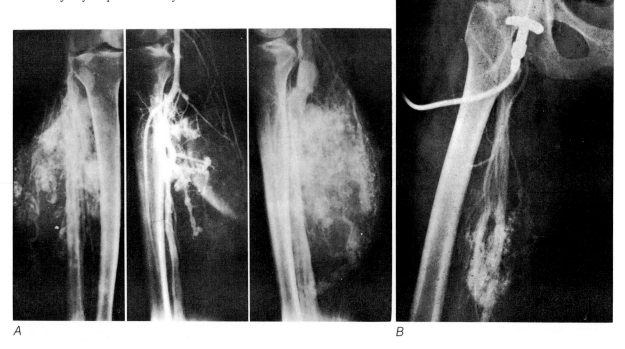

A   *B*

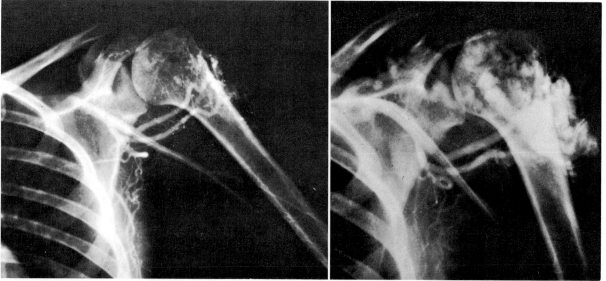

C

ized sufficiently to permit complete excision of adjacent soft tissue is a curative procedure possible. With most lesions, thorough understanding should be reached with the patient beforehand regarding the palliative nature of the surgical procedure.

On the other hand, amputation merely to remove the lesion is unwarranted, for excellent palliation can be obtained for many years by serial surgical procedures to excise all accessible varicosities. Cross et al. has reported eight patients successfully managed with such measures.

At operation, in contrast to traumatic arteriovenous fistulas, a widespread en bloc excision of the soft tissue should be planned, because excision of an isolated fistula is seldom possible. Amputation of one or more digits may be required. Precise arterial control is often impossible; so, a pneumatic tourniquet should be applied proximal to the lesion if possible. In some patients serious bleeding has been encountered which could be controlled only by resection of adjacent bone.

Some of the most difficult lesions to treat are those involving the head and neck. Ravitch and Gaertner described a remarkable patient treated for an extensive recurrence 48 years after the patient was originally operated upon by Halsted. Rosenfeld has described experiences with seven patients which well emphasize the value of conservative therapy. By prolonged, painstaking dissection, the facial nerve was preserved in most of these patients, but resection of the mandible was frequently required (Fig. 21-19).

A lesion operated upon by one of the authors, after several previous surgical procedures had been ineffective, required amputation of an ear to prevent hemorrhage. When the cartilage of the ear was divided adjacent to the skull, numerous large arteries closely adherent to the cartilage were transected. Within a year additional bruits were audible over the head and neck, but fortunately no symptoms were present.

Another area in which lesions generally are not resectable is in the pelvis and flank. One of the authors operated upon one such patient at the Walter Reed Army Hospital in 1958. Previous operation several years before with division of the iliac artery had resulted in only temporary improvement. During a surgical procedure which lasted several hours, numerous large vessels, including the internal iliac artery and vein, were excised and ligated, but it was obvious that a definitive procedure could not be accomplished. Within a week following operation a loud continuous murmur was again audible. Six years later the murmur persisted, but fortunately there was little disability. Such a course emphasizes the value of conservatism with these lesions.

THORACIC OUTLET SYNDROMES

A variety of physical abnormalities have been recognized which constrict or compress the brachial plexus, the

Fig. 21-19. *A.* Large recurrent congenital arteriovenous fistula operated upon by Ravitch 48 years after the lesion had been removed by Halsted. Extensive collateral vessels were found in the neck around tributaries of the external carotid artery. *B.* Operative field following completion of the dissection, indicating the numerous unnamed collateral vessels which had developed over many years, causing recurrence of the lesion. (*Reprinted from M. M. Ravitch and R. A. Gaertner, Congenital Arteriovenous Fistula in the Neck: 48 Year Follow-up on a Patient Operated upon by Dr. Halsted in 1911, Bull Johns Hopkins Hosp, 107:31, 1960.*)

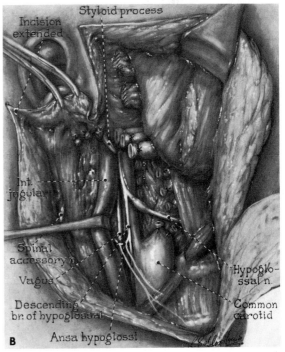

subclavian artery, or the subclavian vein near the first rib and clavicle. Several descriptive terms have been employed, indicating the causative mechanism thought to be present. These include cervical rib, scalenus anticus syndrome, costoclavicular syndrome, and hyperabduction syndrome. The disability is dependent upon which of the major neural or vascular structures is compressed. Regardless of the specific mechanism involved, all such abnormalities may be conveniently grouped together as neurovascular compression syndromes occurring near the thoracic outlet.

HISTORICAL DATA. Cervical ribs have been reported as anatomic curiosities for hundreds of years. They occur in about 0.5 percent of the normal population. Murphy in 1905 described a successful operation upon a patient whose subclavian artery was compressed by a cervical rib. By 1916 Halsted was able to find reports of more than 500 cases of symptoms from a cervical rib. Attention was focused on the scalenus anticus muscle in 1927 when Adson and Coffey observed constriction of the subclavian artery by a scalenus anticus muscle and subsequently proposed that compression by an abnormal scalenus anticus muscle created a syndrome identical to that caused by cervical rib. They also emphasized the role of the scalenus anticus muscle in producing symptoms from a cervical rib, the two structures jointly compressing the brachial plexus between them.

Subsequently the frequency of compression between the clavicle and first rib was recognized and the mechanisms well defined in 1943 by the report of Falconer and Weddel, who named this type of compression the *costoclavicular syndrome.* A short time later, in 1945, Wright observed patients in whom vascular symptoms resulted from hyperabduction and introduced the term *hyperabduction syndrome.*

Some degree of compression of the subclavian artery may be demonstrated in a high percentage of normal individuals in whom no symptoms whatever are present, but it formerly was thought that compression syndromes producing significant disability were rare. Recently, however, since the publication of Roos of a simplified approach to relieve compression syndromes at the thoracic outlet and since the introduction of peripheral nerve conduction velocity determinations, the conditions have been recognized with increasing frequency. It has even been suggested that for certain patients who have thoracic outlet syndromes a diagnosis of angina pectoris is erroneously made. Further experience will be needed to determine the exact frequency of these disorders, for the nerve conduction velocity studies have only recently been developed. The aforementioned transaxillary approach to resection of the first rib, first emphasized by Clagett in 1962, may help define the frequency of the condition more exactly, as removal of the first rib effectively decompresses the thoracic outlet.

REGIONAL ANATOMY. The subclavian artery leaves the thorax by passing over the first rib between the scalenus anticus muscle anteriorly and the brachial plexus and scalenus medius posteriorly. It then passes under the clavicle and subclavius muscle to enter the axilla beneath the pectoralis minor muscle. The subclavian vein has an almost identical course except that it passes anterior to the scalenus anticus muscle. The route of the brachial plexus nearly parallels that of the subclavian artery in the neck, lying posterolaterally between it and the scalenus medius muscle.

A potential area of compression exists in the interscalene triangle between the scalenus anticus anteriorly, the scalenus medius posteriorly, and the first rib inferiorly. Only slightly distal to this area, in the narrow space between the clavicle and the first rib, is another potential site of compression. Finally, in the axilla, where the pectoralis minor tendon attaches to the coracoid process, an area of potential obstruction of the axillary artery exists where it travels around the coracoid process. Lord and Rosati have emphasized that during hyperabduction the axillary vessels and brachial plexus are bent at an angle of approximately 90° in this area.

When a cervical rib persists, there may be in addition either a bony or a ligamentous structure, originating on the lowermost cervical vertebra, coursing between the anterior and medial scalene muscles, passing under the brachial plexus and subclavian artery, and attaching to the first rib.

ETIOLOGY. Although cervical ribs are found in about 0.5 percent of the normal population, only about 10 percent of these produce symptoms. Asymptomatic anomalies of the first rib are also frequently seen. Thus, additional factors other than the presence of a cervical rib or anomalous first rib must contribute to the compression syndrome. Symptoms are very rare in children and most frequently are seen in thin women in the third and fourth decades. An unusually well-developed musculature seems also to predispose to compression. A congenital variation in the anatomy of the head and neck has been suggested by Adson as a predisposing factor, a familiar type of patient being a thin woman with a long, narrow neck. The onset of symptoms in the second and third decade could be due to gradual descent of the shoulder girdle, perhaps from atrophy of the regional musculature.

Local anatomic variations are probably of particular significance. The width of the first rib in individuals in whom we have resected this structure has appeared to be unusually great. The width of the scalene anticus muscle at its insertion into the first rib varies greatly. A wide scalenus anticus muscle, which narrows the space in the interscalene triangle, has often been found at operation in symptomatic patients. Cervical ribs vary from short and rudimentary to completely formed and articulating anteriorly with the first rib. Some incomplete ribs are connected by fascial bands to the first rib which compress the brachial plexus.

Fractures of the clavicle or first rib may subsequently produce a large bony callus, especially if there is poor alignment of the ends of the fractured bone. One patient treated by one of the authors for severe ischemia of the hand was found to have peripheral emboli from a small subclavian aneurysm, produced by fracture of the first rib in an automobile accident.

PATHOLOGY. Disability from compression may be produced in several ways and depends upon which portions of the neurovascular bundle are involved. Compression of the brachial plexus usually causes pain, paresthesias, and a feeling of numbness. Often these symptoms are greatest in the C_8–T_1 distribution, because the ulnar nerve is derived from this most caudad portion of the plexus which rides over the first rib. Muscular weakness, paralysis, or atrophy of muscles are less frequent and appear only in far advanced cases. Vascular symptoms may be intermittent from compression or temporary occlusion of the subclavian artery, producing claudication with exercise, pallor, or a sensation of coldness, numbness, or paresthesia. In chronic cases, a different and more serious mechanism evolves, for intermittent compression and trauma of the subclavian arteries produce atheromatous changes in the artery and, rarely, a poststenotic aneurysm. From either arterial abnormality, emboli may be dislodged into the peripheral circulation and produce ischemia in the hand, even with focal areas of gangrene requiring amputation of digits. Thrombosis of the subclavian artery may eventually result. On occasion Raynaud's phenomenon may occur. Schein and associates found a total of 29 cases of subclavian arterial involvement previously reported. Eleven of these lost part or all of one digit from gangrene, while two required more extensive amputation. Restoration of continuity of the subclavian artery following thrombosis was reported for the first time in a case cited by Schein and associates.

A third group of vascular symptoms are intermittent episodes of vasoconstriction, similar to those seen in Raynaud's disease. The unilateral appearance of the Raynaud's phenomenon, however, almost always suggests a focal disturbance in the blood supply to the involved extremity. Such vasomotor phenomena are uncommon. A possible explanation for this infrequent occurrence has been proposed by Telford and Mottershead, who, on anatomic dissection, found that in 10 to 15 percent of patients the sympathetic innervation of the extremity traveled in a separate cord not incorporated in the main trunks of the brachial plexus. This isolated filament of fibers presumably would be more prone to direct compression and irritation. Finally, intermittent compression of the subclavian vein may cause signs of venous hypertension in the upper extremity with edema and the development of varicosities. The so-called "effort thrombosis," a condition of acute thrombosis of the subclavian vein, may be a result of a neurovascular compression syndrome, but the pathologic mechanisms have not been clearly identified.

CLINICAL MANIFESTATIONS. The symptomatology of the thoracic outlet syndrome depends on whether nerves, blood vessels, or both are compressed. Usually compression of one of these dominates the clinical picture. As reported in a paper by Urschel et al., symptoms of nerve compression manifested by pain and paresthesia were present in all but 6 of 138 patients, the pain usually being of insidious onset, commonly involving the neck, shoulder, arm, and hand with occasional radiation to the anterior chest or parascapular area. Paresthesias in specific nerve distribution occurred in 102 of their patients, the ulnar nerve being involved in 90 percent.

Symptoms of arterial compression were observed less frequently, in about one-quarter of their patients. Thirteen had symptoms of venous compression, including edema, venous distension, and discoloration; only three had the classic effort thrombosis, or Paget-Schroetter syndrome. Raynaud's phenomenon was present in 17 patients, all of whom were women.

Chronic ischemic pain has been observed in three of our patients following embolic occlusion of the radial or ulnar arteries with localized gangrene of one finger in one patient.

Physical Examination. Objective physical signs are more common in patients with vascular compression than in those with neural disorders. In only about 20 percent of patients with nerve compression are objective signs of decreased sensation found; some of these show additional muscle weakness or even atrophy. In the presence of neurologic symptoms at least one of the vascular compression signs can be expected, consisting essentially of loss of radial pulse with either Adson's maneuver, hyperabduction, or hyperextension. In the Adson maneuver, the patient sits with his hands on his knees, inspires deeply, extends his head backward, and turns his chin toward the affected side. Deep inspiration, extension of the neck, and turning of the head all tense the scalene anticus muscle and may decrease or obliterate the radial pulse (Fig. 21-20). Simultaneous auscultation of the supraclavicular space for bruit should be performed. In certain patients, a bruit will appear as the head is turned, reach a peak intensity, and cease as compression is increased to the point of obliterating the radial pulse. In other patients turning the head to the opposite side may demonstrate compression more effectively. The possibility of compression of the neurovascular bundle between the first rib and the clavicle also may be tested by displacing the shoulders backward and downward. The test is considered positive if the radial pulse is obliterated. The hyperabduction maneuver is performed by fully abducting the arm above the head and noting the effect upon the radial pulse.

The signs of arterial compression may be evident by direct physical examination. There may be differences in the qualities of the pulses between the two arms when the subclavian, brachial, radial, and ulnar arteries are compared. A localized supraclavicular bruit may be present. On occasion a particularly wide pulse, denoting a subclavian or axillary aneurysm, is palpable. With mild forms of ischemia there may be only pallor on elevation while in the more severe forms, especially with embolization, there may be atrophy of the skin, brittle nails, or even focal ulceration. In approximately 5 percent of patients frank Raynaud's phenomenon can be induced by application of cold to the extremity. In the approximately 10 percent of patients who have signs of venous obstruction, edema and venous distension are apparent.

In evaluating the maneuvers to detect neurovascular compression, it is important to remember that they are positive in a high percentage of normal individuals. This is particularly true of the costoclavicular compression or the hyperabduction test. A positive result, therefore, does not in itself establish a thoracic outlet syndrome; absence of any positive findings, however, suggests some other diagnosis.

LABORATORY STUDIES. Chest and cervical spine roentgenograms may demonstrate bony abnormalities in as many as one-third of the patients, either as cervical ribs, bifid first ribs, fusion of the first and second ribs, or clavicular deformities either congenital or traumatic.

For diagnosing arterial abnormalities, arteriography may be especially useful in demonstrating intimal irregularities, stenoses, or aneurysms of the subclavian artery. The arteriographic studies are of no value where there is no evidence of arterial compression or occlusion. Venographic studies are useful in patients with signs of venous compression, especially in establishing a differential diagnosis between thoracic outlet compression and other entities which mimic the condition.

The determination of nerve conduction velocities through the thoracic outlet as well as electromyographic determinations have been used to attempt to establish objective criteria for diagnosing neural compression. By applying electrical stimulation to various of the distal components of the brachial plexus and measuring conduction velocities to pinpoint areas of abnormal conduction, it is possible to evaluate sites of involvement of various neural structures. This technique used in conjunction with the specific determination of the ulnar nerve conduction velocity has been employed by Urschel to make diagnoses of thoracic outlet syndromes as well as to establish the differential diagnosis. Where atypical thoracic outlet neural compression syndromes are present, other nerves such as the median and the musculocutaneous can be similarly studied. Differential diagnoses between compression at the thoracic outlet, at the carpal tunnel at the wrist, and at the pronator level are possible. When this is combined with carefully performed electromyographic studies, very specific diagnoses are possible. With increasing experience, correlating the results of electrical studies with postoperative results may permit more precise selection of patients for different types of therapy available.

DIAGNOSIS. Formerly, thoracic outlet syndromes have been erroneously diagnosed on purely clinical criteria, frequently in the presence of neural compression occurring at sites other than the thoracic outlet. Cervical disc disease, arthritis of the cervical spine, and nerve and spinal cord tumors, especially of the extramedullary type, can produce similar symptoms. The most easily diagnosed of the neurologic syndromes is that involving the lowermost portion of the brachial plexus. In this, there are subjective symptoms along the course of the ulnar nerve; relief obtained frequently on moderate abduction at the shoulder joint and a positive vascular compression test confirm the diagnosis. Electrical studies of ulnar nerve conduction velocity,

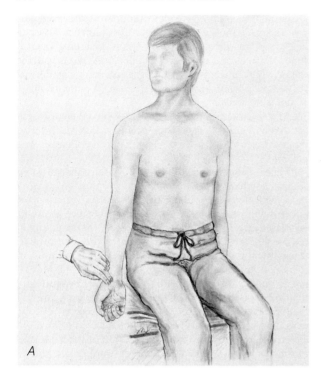

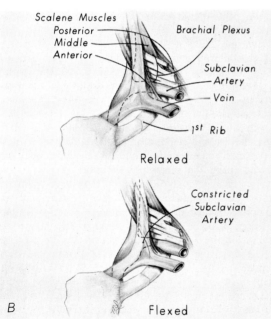

Fig. 21-20. Technique of performance of the Adson test for obstruction of the subclavian artery by the scalenus anticus muscle. *A.* The patient should be seated with his elbows at his sides and his neck extended. During deep inspiration his chin is turned to the affected side, while the intensity of the radial pulse is palpated. All these positions increase the tension on the scalenus anticus muscle. *B.* Course of the brachial plexus and subclavian artery between the scalenus anticus and medius muscles. A localized dilatation of the subclavian artery distal to the scalenus anticus is illustrated. Immediately distal to the scalenus anticus and medius muscles is another potential area of constriction, between the clavicle and the first rib. When the scalenus

anticus muscle is relaxed, there is minimal compression of the subclavian artery. With tension on the scalenus anticus muscle, compression of the subclavian artery results in decrease in the radial pulse, in some patients resulting in disappearance of the pulse. A bruit may become audible in the supraclavicular area as the scalenus anticus muscle is progressively stretched to compress the subclavian artery.

with or without electromyographic studies, can firmly establish the diagnosis. With atypical neural compression syndromes the diagnosis is more difficult in the absence of positive physical signs except for signs of vascular compression during one of the compression maneuvers. An extensive investigation may be required, looking for bony abnormalities in the region of the thoracic outlet and performing nerve conduction and electromyographic studies to establish the probable site of the neural disorder. In many, the diagnosis will be a combination of exclusion of other diagnostic entities associated with positive findings on the specific electrical studies.

Diagnosis of the occlusive vascular disorders is less difficult. Physical findings suggesting arterial or venous compression are usually present. Appropriate angiographic studies may be required to delineate the nature, the specific mechanism, and the indicated therapy.

Diagnosis of the vasospastic disorders (Raynaud's) is clear-cut, but other conditions associated with it must also be considered.

TREATMENT. The treatment can be divided into that for the arterial, venous, and neurologic compressions. Treatment of the arterial compression depends upon the specific entity produced: embolization, stenosis and thrombosis, aneurysm formation, or intermittent vasospasm (Raynaud's). Occlusion of the subclavian artery, if not associated with severe ischemia, may require no therapy except an exercise program to promote development of collateral circulation. With atherosclerotic plaques or aneurysms of the subclavian artery, frequently associated with embolic episodes, therapy should correct the underlying compression mechanism. This usually involves resection of the first rib, preferably by the transaxillary approach, as well as removing the source of emboli. The presence of a thrombus in an aneurysm or ulceration in an atherosclerotic plaque requires resection of the involved artery and replacement, preferably with autologous tissue; composite grafts of saphenous veins have been useful. On occasion direct exposure of the arteries in the arm or forearm is necessary to remove emboli.

The venous occlusions are more difficult to treat, for the compressing mechanism may not be apparent from either physical examination or laboratory studies. It appears clear from results of transaxillary resection of the first rib that the most proximal part of the vein can be decompressed by this procedure, but the roles of the clavicle, the pectoralis minor, and clavipectoral fascia in producing compression cannot be evaluated by this approach. Those patients with effort thrombosis seen within the first day or two of its occurrence should be considered for combined surgical procedures of venous thrombectomy and relief of the compressing mechanism. Anticoagulation therapy then should be used, perhaps for as long as 1 year.

The management of the neural compression syndromes generally involves a conservative, nonsurgical approach. An exercise program designed to strengthen the muscles of the shoulder girdle and lessen the tendency of the shoulder to droop has been of value in some patients with mild to moderate symptoms. A series of such exercises are carefully described by Allen et al. As an example of this approach, fewer than half of a group of 300 patients with thoracic outlet syndromes required surgical intervention. The selection of patients for operation should depend upon the severity of the symptoms, failure to respond to a nonsurgical program, and the specificity of the diagnosis.

Operative Technique. It is important to include the entire extremity in the sterile operative field, permitting manipulation of the extremity in order to define the most likely area of compression. Whether or not a cervical rib is present, the transaxillary approach is favored for its simplicity, the clarity with which the compression mechanisms can be diagnosed, the excellent cosmetic result, and the ease with which cervical ribs together with the first rib can be excised. If vasomotor symptoms are prominent, sympathectomy can be performed through the same transaxillary approach, exposing the third and second thoracic ganglia as well as the lower third of the stellate ganglion; this includes the first thoracic ganglion but avoids the production of Horner's syndrome. If removal of the second and third intercostal nerves with their ganglia is thought necessary, since the demonstration by Skoog that 10 to 15 percent of the sympathetic ganglia to the upper extremity is contained in these nerves, it can be similarly carried out.

The transaxillary approach is performed by making an incision in the lowermost portion of the axilla from the pectoralis major anteriorly to the latissimus dorsi posteriorly (Fig. 21-21). The incision is deepened to the muscles of the chest wall, the serratus anterior and the intercostal muscles coming into view. The dissection is continued upward, avoiding the intercostobrachial nerve, with the arm hyperabducted to raise the neurovascular bundle off the first rib. By gentle dissection, it is possible to outline the scalene muscles and identify the attachment of the cervical rib to the first rib if one is present. The scalene muscles are transected and permitted to retract, and the muscles along the inferior border of the first rib are similarly incised. The first rib and cervical rib usually can be removed in their entirety, including periosteum, from the costochondral junction anteriorly to the posterior angle of the rib. The parietal pleura lies deep to the dissection; care must be taken to avoid puncturing it. If the pleura is punctured, the wound is closed around a catheter in the axilla while the anesthetist expands the lung. This usually suffices to correct the pneumothorax. On occasion it has been necessary to aspirate air from the pleural cavity in the early postoperative period.

If a sympathectomy is indicated, the parietal pleura is stripped from the chest wall attachments and the sympathetic chain exposed, dissected free, and excised.

The postoperative course is usually benign, with the patient ready for discharge by the third postoperative day.

Other approaches have been described for excising the first rib. The posterior approach has been advocated by many but is an operation of greater magnitude. The anterior transthoracic approach has been proposed by others for more extensive exposure. However, most agree that the supraclavicular approach is probably archaic, since it does not permit thorough exploration of the area and easy excision of the first rib, which has become of paramount importance in treatment.

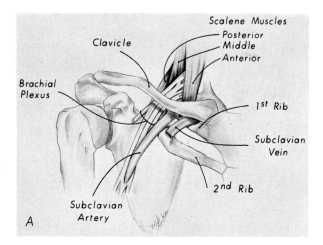

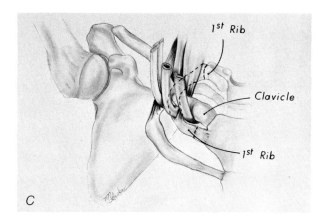

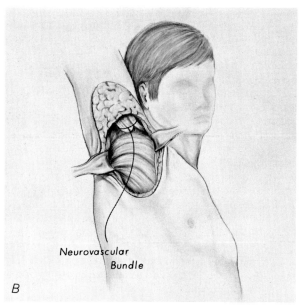

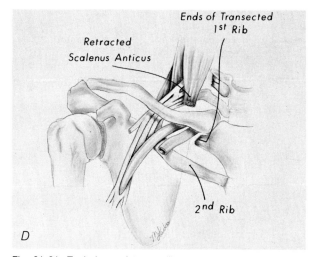

Fig. 21-21. Technique of transaxillary resection of the first rib. *A.* The critical relations of the first rib, clavicle, scalene muscles and neurovascular structures is shown. The lowermost portion of the brachial plexus which gives rise to the ulnar nerve is in contact with the first rib and explains the most characteristic neurologic symptoms usually involving the ulnar aspect of the forearm and fourth and fifth fingers. *B.* Operative incision below the axillary hairline with hyperabduction of the arm which raises the neurovascular bundle out of the operative field. *C.* Effect of hyperabduction in exposing the first rib and scalene muscles, retracting the neurovascular bundle. *D.* Effect of first rib resection, which requires cutting all three scalene muscles, in relieving the compression of artery, vein, and brachial plexus.

PROGNOSIS. The prognosis is dependent upon the specific syndrome present. The arterial compression syndromes can be quite satisfactorily relieved and arterial reconstructions performed with a high degree of precision, although a large series of patients treated with arterial compression has not been reported. In our experience it has been possible to stop embolic episodes and restore circulation to the upper extremity by standard arterial reconstructive procedures. However, patients with Raynaud's phenomena and cervical rib in whom associated sympathectomies have been performed have had variable results. Although immediate effects of sympathectomy have been excellent, relapses have occurred quite abruptly as early as 6 months following operation.

The venous compression disorders also have given variable results. It is not clear at present whether thrombectomy, with or without relief of the venous compression mechanism, is any better than prolonged anticoagulant therapy. Those patients with chronic venous occlusions of the subclavian and axillary veins who have been followed

for years have shown remarkable recovery, with subsidence of edema coincident with the appearance of a prominent venous pattern on the chest wall and little or no resulting disability.

The surgical approach has often changed through the years. Other procedures include scalenotomy performed through the supraclavicular approach, then resection of the clavicle proposed by Lord and Rosati, and now resection of the first rib. Adson, predominantly performing scale-notomy through the supraclavicular approach, reported in 1947 that over a period of 22 years 142 patients had been operated upon with excellent results in about 50 percent and improvement in another 20 to 30 percent. In another series from the Mayo Clinic, Love reported that of 700 patients seen over a 5-year period with a wide variety of thoracic outlet syndromes, only about 3 percent underwent operation. Roos has reported from a wide experience with transaxillary resection of the first rib that 80 to 90 percent of those with predominantly neurologic symptoms obtained complete relief, while approximately 50 percent of those with predominantly vascular symptoms became free of symptoms.

The recent development of electrical conduction studies provides an objective method not only for making the diagnosis but for evaluating the results of therapy. The wide variation in frequency of diagnosis and results with operation from different groups is perhaps due to variation in diagnostic criteria. Urschel emphasized the usefulness of electrical conduction studies; in a series of 300 patients seen between 1946 and 1970, only 138 were operated upon. Seventeen of these had bilateral operations. Employing the electrical conduction studies, 96 percent of patients improved after resection of the first rib. There were only five cases of failure, in two of which a cervical disc subsequently was removed. The most favorable group were those with pain and paresthesia in the distribution of the ulnar nerve, diminution of the pulse by one of the various compression tests, and slowing of ulnar nerve conduction velocity below 60 m/second. Failures following operation were more common in those with atypical pain distributions, often with associated cervical syndromes secondary to whiplash or trauma. Usually, pulse changes with the compression tests were minimal or absent, and there was less slowing of ulnar nerve conduction velocity.

EXTRACRANIAL OCCLUSIVE CEREBROVASCULAR DISEASE

HISTORICAL CONSIDERATIONS. One of the most astonishing but belated findings in the past 20 years is that cerebrovascular disease, frequently termed *stroke,* is due to occlusive disease of the extracranial carotid or vertebral arteries in 50 to 70 percent of patients, not to occlusive disease of the intracranial vessels. As early as 1914 Hunt described infarction in a cerebral hemisphere from occlusion of the extracranial internal carotid artery, with patent intracranial arteries. However, this was thought to be an unusual event, and even as late as 1952 it was assumed to be almost implicit that the majority of strokes were due to intracranial vascular disease and that significant extracranial vascular disease was rare. In large measure this erroneous assumption was due to incomplete postmortem examination. Autopsies included examination of the intracranial arteries and the great vessels at their origin from the aorta, but the bifurcation of the carotid artery in the neck into internal and external carotid arteries was not examined, largely because of the habit of leaving these

vessels intact for the subsequent injection of embalming fluid.

The development of safe techniques for cerebral angiography, combined with careful clinical pathologic studies of the type of vascular disease in large numbers of patients with strokes, led to recognition of the frequency with which stroke syndromes were due to extracranial vascular disease. Classic studies were reported by Fischer between 1951 and 1954 and by Hutchinson and Yates in 1956.

Perhaps the earliest operation for carotid stenosis, and endarterectomy, was reported by Eastcott and Rob in England in 1954. The first significant report in the United States was by Lyons and Galbraith in 1957, which greatly stimulated active surgical investigation. An extensive national cooperative stroke study from 1960 to 1970, in which many universities throughout the country participated, led to a careful understanding of the natural history of the disease and the effect of surgical reconstructive procedures.

ETIOLOGY AND PATHOLOGY. Atherosclerosis is the basic disease in most patients. In a small percentage of patients an arteritis obliterates the great vessels arising from the aortic arch (see Aortic Arch Occlusive Disease in Chapter 20). Fibromuscular hyperplasia occluding the internal carotid artery also has been described but is rare. Trauma, either penetrating or blunt, or even forceful hyperextension of the neck are other rare causes. If patients with stroke syndromes are studied with four-vessel angiography, opacifying both carotid and both vertebral arteries from their origins to their point of entry into the skull, significant extracranial occlusive disease will be found in about 75 percent of the group (Fig. 21-22). The segmental localization is impressive. In the carotid artery, almost all plaques are found at the carotid bifurcation, starting in the distal centimeter of the common carotid and involving the proximal external carotid and the proximal 1 to 2 cm of the internal carotid. Fortunately for surgical reconstruction, and also a striking example of segmental localization of atherosclerosis, the internal carotid beyond the first 1 to 2 cm is usually uninvolved up to its point of entry into the skull, the area of the so-called carotid siphon. Because of the freedom of involvement of this portion, arterial reconstruction almost always can be done if the internal carotid is not thrombosed. Disease in the middle cerebral artery is rare. In the basilar-vertebral system, plaques are usually at the origin of the vertebrals from the subclavian, but disease of the vertebral beyond its origin is unusual. In the basilar artery localized atherosclerosis is more common. Within the thorax, the great vessels are infrequently diseased. The lesions are multiple in more than 50 percent of patients.

Soon after the recognition of the frequency of extracranial vascular disease, it became apparent that simple reduction in cerebral blood flow was not an adequate explanation for many of the neurologic syndromes encountered. As a result of several years of investigation by the National Cooperative Stroke Study, it now seems clear that arterioarterial embolization of fragments of plaque or platelet-fibrin aggregates is probably the most frequent mechanism of neurologic injury (Fig. 21-23). These plaques form on the irregular surface of atherosclerotic

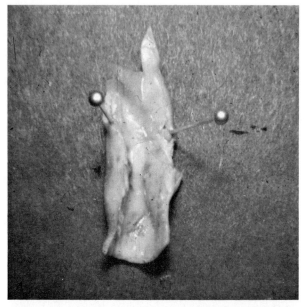

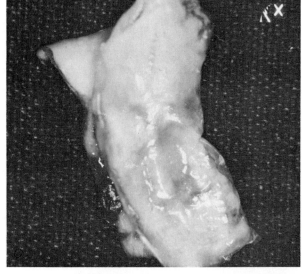

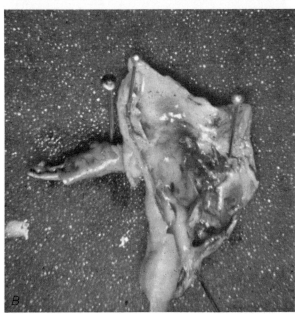

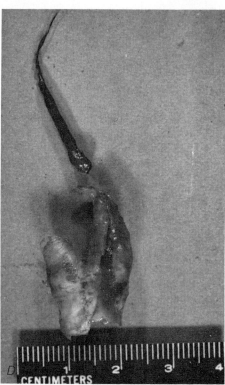

plaques, usually at the carotid bifurcation, and subsequently embolize. Ophthalmologic visualization of these plaques suddenly appearing in the retina during transient ischemic attacks was one of the first clues to the mechanism of the syndrome. The second method for production of symptoms is the obvious one of simple decrease in flow from marked stenosis or occlusion. Because of abundant collateral circulation in the brain, major arteries may become narrowed or occluded without any symptoms whatever unless multiple areas are diseased. As with stenotic lesions in the vascular system elsewhere there is little decrease in blood flow until the cross-sectional area of the vessel is narrowed by more than 75 percent. If collateral circulation is adequate, even complete occlusion may be

Fig. 21-22. Carotid plaque dynamics in the pathogenesis of stroke syndromes are suggested by the variations in the appearances of lesions surgically removed. *A*. Smooth fibrous plaque producing marked stenosis and decreased blood flow. *B*. Ulcerated plaque giving rise to embolization. *C*. Hemorrhage into the wall of a plaque which can result in sudden stenosis or ulceration and subsequent ulceration and embolization. *D*. Total occlusion of an internal carotid artery secondary to thrombosis.

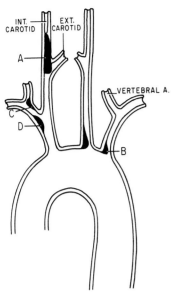

Fig. 21-23. Diagrammatic drawing illustrating the most frequent locations of atherosclerosis in the cerebrovascular circulation. The tendency for focal atherosclerotic plaques to develop at the origin or bifurcation of vessels is shown. Eighty to ninety percent of lesions are found at the bifurcation of the common carotid arteries. Less common sites are the great vessels from the aortic arch, the origin of the vertebral artery, or the origin of the subclavian artery, producing the so-called "subclavian steal" syndrome.

harmless. Routine postmortem studies by Martin and associates of a large group of patients dying from different causes at the Mayo Clinic found that in as many as 40 percent of the patients at least one of the four major extracranial arteries significantly was narrowed or occluded, even though there were no neurologic symptoms before death.

The atherosclerotic plaques removed from the vessels of symptomatic patients have varied greatly in composition and appearance. Some were principally fibrotic, with smooth internal surfaces; others showed advanced degenerative changes, with intramural hemorrhage and little stenosis, but with ulceration of the intimal surface. Plaques with a smooth intimal surface are probably harmless until the cross-sectional area of the artery is reduced to a marked degree. An ulcerated plaque, however, even though the lumen is compromised little, may cause serious or even catastrophic injury from repeated embolization.

CLINICAL MANIFESTATIONS. A great variety of clinical syndromes result from the different patterns of occlusive disease in the carotid, vertebral, and subclavian arteries. These will be only briefly summarized here, for they are described in considerable detail in standard texts of neurology. The classic stroke from unilateral carotid disease is ipsilateral blindness and contralateral hemiplegia. The presence of aphasia depends upon the dominant cerebral hemisphere. The other extreme is the most fleeting focal neurologic defect such as a transient monoplegia, transient hemiplegia, or transient ipsilateral blindness. These episodes, clearing within minutes to hours after an abrupt onset, are termed *transient ischemic attacks*. Between such episodes the patient may be completely well, but unfortunately such attacks often precede a catastrophic stroke. One retrospective study of patients with severe strokes found that almost 75 percent had such premonitory symptoms in the weeks or months before the stroke appeared.

Between the transient ischemic attack on the one hand and the massive stroke on the other, a wide variety of motor and sensory syndromes are seen. Their unilateral localization is strongly suggestive of carotid artery disease. They may be precipitated by hypotension, hypoxia, or changes in position or posture, or they may be unrelated to any known cause.

With disease of the vertebral-basilar system, a number of brainstem symptoms occur. In contrast to carotid disease, the symptoms are often bilateral, involving either both arms or both legs, but may alternate in severity from one side of the body to the other. Tinnitus, dizziness, vertigo, diplopia, and dysarthria are also common. One type of characteristic syndrome is the so-called "drop attack," in which the patient may literally fall to the ground with little or no warning, with or without loss of consciousness, and recover equally rapidly with only residual dizziness or mild ataxia.

Disease of the subclavian artery proximal to the origin of one of the vertebral arteries, more commonly the left, produces the so-called "subclavian steal" syndrome. The proximal obstruction in the subclavian artery decreases the pressure in that artery at the point of origin of the vertebral artery; this results in an actual reversal of flow in the vertebral artery, with blood draining out of the basilar artery into the arm. Although this phenomenon is seen frequently on angiographic studies, production of symptoms from ischemia of the brainstem by exercising the arm is uncommon.

Physical Examination. Examination is directed primarily at determining the presence of any neurologic deficit as well as the pattern of arterial involvement. Palpation of the carotid pulses is useful only for the rare instance of intrathoracic occlusion of the common carotid artery. Separate palpation of the external and internal carotid arteries is impossible because of their location next to one another. Hence, the carotid pulses are normal on palpation in almost all patients with occlusive disease at the carotid bifurcation. However, auscultation over the carotid bifurcation for a bruit is essential. With high-grade stenoses at the bifurcation, a bruit is audible just anterior to the sternocleidomastoid muscle near the level of the angle of the mandible in at least 50 percent of patients with stenosis. Auscultation in the supraclavicular fossae may find bruits from subclavian-vertebral disease. When bruits are detected, they must be differentiated from cardiac valvular lesions, such as aortic stenosis, which produce murmurs transmitted along the great vessels. If occlusive disease of a subclavian artery is present, the blood pressure will be significantly different in the two arms.

Ophthalmodynomometry is a useful screening procedure when there is high-grade stenosis or total occlusion of one of the internal carotid arteries. The technique is simple comparison of the pressure in the retinal arteries of the two eyes; though not quantitative, it is a useful screening technique.

DIAGNOSIS. An important attitude in diagnosis is to consider even transient neurologic symptoms with utmost gravity. Since such symptoms often are the prelude to an atrioventricular (AV) block or paroxysmal tachycardia and may simulate basivertebral insufficiency, the electrocardiogram should be routinely evaluated. The electroencephalogram also may be useful, as some seizure disorders simulate vascular insufficiency syndromes. Other disorders to be considered are Ménière's syndrome, hypersensitive carotid sinus responses, and different metabolic disorders such as transient hypoglycemia.

TREATMENT. General Considerations. Data accumulated from several years of study by the National Cooperative Stroke Study clearly show that effective surgical treatment must be performed before major neurologic deficits are produced from cerebral infarction. Hence, surgical therapy must be basically prophylactic. Operation upon patients with acute strokes is associated with a high mortality, considerably higher than that for patients treated medically. If operation for acute stroke is for an ulcerated plaque which does not narrow the artery, there is little benefit at all to the patient except prevention of subsequent episodes. If a totally obstructed internal carotid artery is reopened, the patient's condition may be exacerbated from edema or hemorrhage developing in the infarct as a result of restoring perfusion pressure. In the following section the surgical approach will be considered for three different groups, carotid lesions, subclavian-vertebral lesions, and aortic arch lesions.

Recently, as the prevalence of arterioarterial embolization in the production of stroke syndromes has become clear, there has been renewed interest in altering the coagulability of the blood. The striking finding of the influence of acetylsalicylic acid on platelet aggregation may be of considerable therapeutic significance. Clinical trials are now in progress to determine the possible value of aspirin in preventing stroke syndromes.

Treatment of Atherosclerotic Disease of the Internal Carotid Artery. Atherosclerosis of the origin of the internal carotid artery is the most common form of extracranial vascular disease. As stated earlier, the disease fortunately is limited only to the first 1 to 2 cm of the origin of the internal carotid and hence is ideal for surgical correction (Fig. 21-24).

When complete occlusion develops in the carotid artery, however, an organized thrombus develops above the atherosclerotic plaque which extends superiorly into the intracranial internal carotid, making successful operation impossible. In approximately 10 percent of patients with complete occlusion, however, the thrombus has not propagaged more than 2 to 3 cm, and surgical removal is still possible.

As stated earlier, the ideal patient for operation is one with transient ischemic attacks without any permanent neurologic abnormality. In such patients operation can be performed under regional cervical block with little risk. Mortality and major neurologic complications are in the

range of 1 to 4 percent. Details of the operation are shown in Fig. 21-25.

The hazards of operation are greater and the likelihood of benefit much less when a stroke has occurred. If the internal carotid has become totally occluded, producing a major neurologic deficit, operation performed within 6 hours after onset of symptoms may produce dramatic recovery. The operative mortality, however, especially with altered states of consciousness, is considerably higher than with elective operations. If operation is delayed much beyond 6 hours after the onset of symptoms, reopening a totally obstructed carotid artery may be followed first by transient improvement, then worsening of symptoms and even death from hemorrhage into the area of infarction precipitated by the restoration of arterial perfusion pressure. It has been suggested by Warren and Triedman that this catastrophe might be prevented by careful avoidance of blood pressure elevation during operation and for some weeks afterward.

If the acute stroke has resulted from embolization of atheromatous debris or platelet aggregates, with occlusion of small intracerebral vessels, emergency operation upon the nonstenosing ulcerated plaque at the carotid bifurcation is neither helpful nor harmful. At a later time such patients perhaps should be considered for operation to prevent future embolization if the permanent neurologic deficit is not severe.

In patients with chronic strokes in whom acute injury weeks or months earlier produced a permanent neurologic deficit indicative of total hemispheric infarction, operation is of little value. A challenging group consists of asymptomatic patients with loud bruits. Thompson et al. have reported a lowered stroke incidence in such patients if angiographic studies revealed significant carotid lesions.

Following endarterectomy of the stenotic carotid artery, the likelihood of long-term patency of the reconstructed artery is excellent. In a group of 100 patients reported by Blaisdell et al., 21 were evaluated by angiography more than 5 years later. There was only one late occlusion, an asymptomatic one found at autopsy. In 1968 Edwards and associates studied 75 patients operated upon 5 to 9 years earlier. Only five of the 75 had subsequently had a stroke. Three of the group had developed recurrent stenosis at the site of endarterectomy, but all experienced successful reoperation.

The effect of prophylactic carotid endarterectomy in altering the incidence of mortality in future stroke has been analyzed in detail by the National Cooperative Stroke Study. Although the results are not completely definitive, certain facts have emerged. If carotid endarterectomy can be performed with mortality and significant complication rates in the range of 1 to 2 percent, overall survival is increased and future strokes are decreased. Strokes in the neurologic area corresponding to the surgically repaired artery are virtually eliminated. Late mortality is primarily due to coronary arterial disease.

Treatment of Subclavian-Vertebral Disease. Stenosis involving only the vertebral artery is infrequent. It is physiologically significant only when bilateral or if one vertebral is congenitally hypoplastic or absent. The disease is fre-

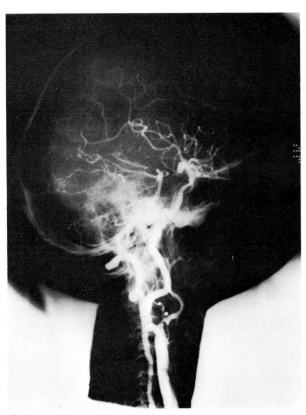

A

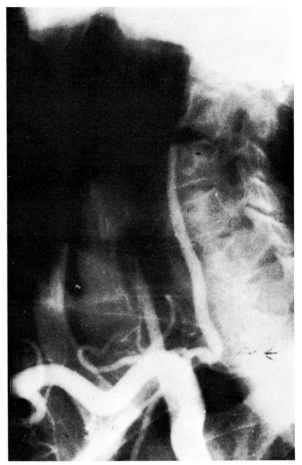

B

Fig. 21-24. Angiographic studies of the cerebral circulation for stroke syndromes should outline the major extracranial as well as the intracranial arteries. This facilitates planning operative procedures and aids in making differential diagnoses of the various causes of stroke syndromes. Cervical carotid and vertebral arteries are outlined by retrograde right brachial arterial injection. *A.* Arrow points to significant lesion in the internal and external carotids. *B.* Arrow points to typical stenotic lesion at the origin of the vertebral with an associated kink.

quently limited to the site of origin of the vertebral from the subclavian. The atherosclerotic plaques in this area usually have a smooth intimal surface, contrasting to the frequency of ulcerated plaques in the carotid artery. In addition, there are frequently tortuous kinks in the first few centimeters of the vertebral artery, which can be shown to result in total occlusion when the head is turned to one side. Symptoms are probably due to decreased flow through the basivertebral system, although embolization cannot be entirely excluded. Concomitant disease in the basilar artery is frequent.

Atherosclerotic stenosis or occlusion of the subclavian artery proximal to the site of origin of the vertebral artery produces the clinical picture termed the subclavian steal syndrome. This abnormality was well defined by Reivich et al. in 1961, following an angiographic description in 1960 by Contorni of retrograde flow in the involved verte-

bral artery. The reduction in pressure in the subclavian artery beyond the stenosis results in retrograde flow from the brainstem down the vertebral artery to the arm; hence the term "subclavian steal." The clinical picture is that of ischemic neurologic symptoms in association with mild ischemia in the involved arm. Diagnosis can be easily made by finding a decreased pulse and blood pressure in the symptomatic arm, often in association with a localized bruit in the supraclavicular space. Serial angiograms after injection of contrast media into the opposite brachial artery or the ascending aorta will demonstrate reversal of flow in the involved vertebral artery by initially opacifying the opposite vertebral artery in a normal fashion, followed by retrograde opacification of the involved vertebral. Although this phenomenon is not infrequent on angiographic examination, clinical symptoms are not common, perhaps because collateral circulation in the brain can readily compensate for the amount of blood diverted away from the brain by the retrograde vertebral flow.

Operations upon the vertebral artery usually can be performed without thoracotomy. Surgical exposure of the subclavian-vertebral junction is obtained through a transverse supraclavicular incision which divides the clavicular head of the sternocleidomastoid muscle and the underlying scalenus anticus muscle. If the stenosing plaque has a

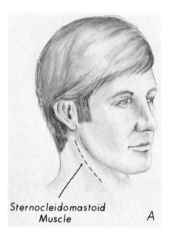

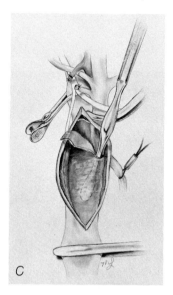

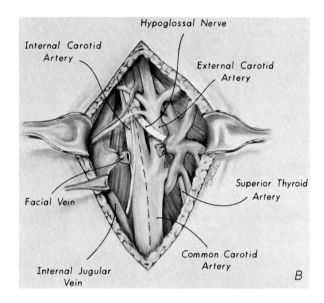

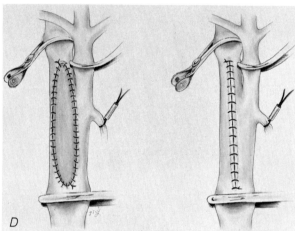

smooth intimal surface, endarterectomy may not be necessary. The artery can be simply widened with a patch angioplasty with autologous saphenous vein. If the vertebral artery is significantly tortuous and redundant, predisposing to kinking, plication can be performed. In approximately 50 arterial reconstructions of the vertebral artery performed at New York University, there has been no neurologic deficit and no evidence of cerebral ischemia during the period of reconstruction.

Operations for the subclavian steal syndrome are seldom necessary. When done, a transthoracic approach to the subclavian artery can be avoided by employing a bypass graft from the ipsilateral common carotid artery to the distal subclavian artery. This is physiologically possible because the common carotid is large enough to deliver sufficient blood to supply both the brain and the upper extremity. On occasion, when the common carotid or innominate arteries are markedly stenotic and not suitable, axilloaxillary bypass grafting has been useful.

Treatment of Aortic Arch Occlusive Disease. In 1962 a report by Crawford et al. stated that during a period of

Fig. 21-25. Technique of carotid endarterectomy. *A.* A skin incision is made anterior to the sternocleidomastoid muscle. *B.* The carotid artery branches are widely mobilized. The internal carotid artery is clamped before widely mobilizing the frequently thrombus-containing bulb, thereby protecting the brain from embolization, which may occur during the dissection. The vagus and hypoglossal nerves are carefully protected. Mobilization of the hypoglossal is facilitated by dividing the sternocleidomastoid artery and vein. A longitudinal arteriotomy is made extending above and below the plaque at the carotid bifurcation. *C.* After division of the intima above the plaque, the plaque can be easily dissected from the underlying media or from the adventitia. The distal intima is carefully inspected and sutured if necessary. *D.* The arteriotomy is either closed primarily with 5-0 Tevdek, or a vein roof patch fashioned from autologous saphenous vein is used to avoid producing stenosis. The technique for restoring flow after completion of the closure is crucial to avoid embolization to the brain. The internal carotid clamp is temporarily removed and reapplied. The common and external carotid clamps are removed, and after 1 or 2 minutes of flushing of the carotid bulb the internal carotid clamp is removed.

100 years since the first clinical description of the aortic arch syndrome by Savory in 1854, only about 90 patients were reported. In the report by Crawford et al., operative experiences with 67 patients in the 4-year period between 1957 and 1961 well indicated the increased recognition of the disease through the widespread use of angiography. Atherosclerosis was the most frequent cause. Formerly syphilitic arteritis was common, but this is now unusual. In the Orient a peculiar arteritis of unknown cause occurs, especially in young women. One eponym referring to this disease, Takayasu's disease, originated from an early description of the clinical syndrome by a Japanese ophthalmologist. An arteritis of this type is rarely seen in the United States.

For several years the occlusive lesions were approached directly with a transthoracic exposure. As the atherosclerotic process was often multiple and diffuse, endarterectomy was seldom possible. Bypass grafts were employed from the ascending aorta proximally to the carotid or subclavian arteries distad. This operative approach is extensive, requiring a thoracotomy incision and separate cervical or supraclavicular incisions.

In more recent years short bypass procedures in the neck establishing grafts from the normal artery to the obstructed artery have become increasingly popular. In a report of 125 patients, Dietrich and his associates expressed a preference for cervical carotid-subclavian bypass rather than the thoracic approach. A left carotid subclavian bypass was employed in 91 patients and a right carotid subclavian bypass in 20. The operative mortality was 5 percent, with good results in the majority of patients. This operative technique avoids an intrathoracic procedure but has the theoretic disadvantage of siphoning blood from a normal artery to a diseased artery. Apparently this theoretic objection is of limited clinical significance, for significant neurologic syndromes have not been produced from the shunting procedure.

ABDOMINAL ANEURYSMS

HISTORICAL DATA. The modern era of treatment of abdominal aneurysms began with the first successful excision of an abdominal aneurysm and replacement with an aortic homograft by Dubost in 1951. Previous therapeutic efforts, such as wiring to promote clotting, wrapping or coating with plastics, and other techniques to induce thrombosis, are now of historic interest only. Following the report of Dubost et al., advances in operative therapy came rapidly, especially those achieved by Cooley, DeBakey and his associates, and Bahnson. Late complications of aortic homografts soon appeared, following which replacement of the aorta with a prosthetic graft was developed. Although nylon was used briefly, Dacron or Teflon has been the preferred reconstruction material since 1957 (Fig. 21-26).

INCIDENCE. Abdominal aneurysms are the most common of the arteriosclerotic aneurysms. With the increasing age of the population, abdominal aneurysms are increasing in frequency, for most patients are in the sixth or seventh decade. Men are affected more frequently than women, in a ratio approximating 10:1.

ETIOLOGY AND PATHOLOGY. The vast majority of abdominal aneurysms are arteriosclerotic in origin. This is probably related to the frequency of involvement of the abdominal aorta by atherosclerosis, and perhaps to mechanical factors creating turbulent flow at the bifurcation of the abdominal aorta. The authors have never seen an abdominal aneurysm arising below the renal arteries from any cause except arteriosclerosis, although they have been reported from syphilis, trauma, the Marfan syndrome, or bacterial endocarditis.

The aneurysms characteristically originate just below the renal arteries and extend beyond the aortic bifurcation into the common iliacs. Fortunately, they seldom involve the external iliac arteries. Small aneurysms may be limited just to the abdominal aorta. The anatomic location of abdominal aneurysms, therefore, makes them accessible to surgical therapy, for a graft can be inserted proximally from the abdominal aorta below the renal arteries to the common iliac arteries distad. The size of abdominal aneurysms varies greatly, small ones 2 to 3 cm in diameter being detected accidentally by aortography while others may enlarge to a diameter of 10 to 15 cm before being discovered accidentally by palpation. The usual course of untreated aneurysms was well documented in the classic report by Estes in 1950. Without treatment there is a 20 percent chance of rupture within 1 year after diagnosis and a 50 percent chance within 4 or 5 years. Complications seldom arise from expanding aneurysms until rupture occurs. Erosion of bone, so common in syphilitic aneurysms, virtually never occurs with abdominal aneurysms. There is usually no impairment of peripheral circulation, although larger aneurysms commonly are composed principally of laminated clot with a small central lumen. Emboli from the shaggy laminated clot lining abdominal aneurysms occur but rarely.

Although aneurysms frequently originate within 1 to 2 cm of the origin of the renal arteries, actual involvement of the origin of the renal arteries in the aneurysm, necessitating reconstruction of the renal arteries during surgical excision, is rare. In a series of over 170 abdominal aneurysms at the Johns Hopkins Hospital, only 3 aneurysms involving the renal arteries were found.

An abdominal aneurysm is often associated with generalized atherosclerosis. In a series of 1,400 patients operated upon by DeBakey and associates, some signs of coronary artery disease were present in 30 percent of the patients, and 40 percent of the patients had some increase in systolic blood pressure. Associated occlusive disease of the carotid arteries was found in 7 percent, of the renal arteries in 2 percent, and of the iliac arteries in 16 percent of the patients. Concomitant clinically significant aneurysms were found in the thoracic aorta in 4 percent, in the femoral artery in 3 percent, and in the popliteal artery in 2 percent of the group.

CLINICAL MANIFESTATIONS. Symptoms. Most patients are unaware of an abdominal aneurysm until a mass is accidentally discovered by the patient or his physician. The importance of careful deep palpation of the abdomen on

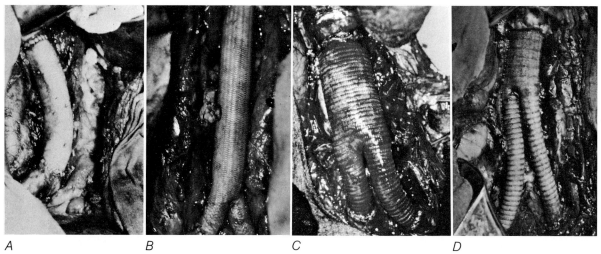

A   B   C   D

Fig. 21-26. Replacement of abdominal aorta. *A.* Aortic homograft inserted following excision of aneurysm of abdominal aorta by Bahnson in 1953. Homografts were among the earliest materials used for arterial grafts but were subsequently discontinued because of late degeneration of the homograft. *B.* Nylon graft used following excision of an abdominal aneurysm in 1954. Nylon was subsequently discontinued because experience found a marked loss in tensile strength 1 year after implantation. (*Courtesy of Dr. Henry T. Bahnson, Department of Surgery, University of Pittsburgh.*) *C.* Operative photograph of knitted Dacron graft inserted following excision of abdominal aneurysm. Dacron has been satisfactorily used since 1967 with excellent long-term results. *D.* Operative photograph of Teflon graft inserted following excision of abdominal aneurysm. Teflon, like Dacron, has given excellent long-term results with large vessels, but with small vessels, such as the femoral artery, results have been less satisfactory.

routine physical examination, outlining the abdominal aorta when possible, is obvious. Occasionally, low back pain caused by an abdominal aneurysm may be diagnosed erroneously as due to an orthopedic condition. The pain apparently arises from tension on retroperitoneal tissues from the aneurysm; erosion of bone almost never happens. Virtually any intraabdominal condition may be simulated by an abdominal aortic aneurysm, such as renal colic, acute appendicitis, diverticulitis, peptic ulcer, pancreatitis, or cholecystitis. Rarely, there is gastrointestinal bleeding. With beginning leakage of the aneurysm or frank rupture momentarily contained retroperitoneally, acute abdominal conditions such as perforated ulcer, hemorrhagic pancreatitis, or generalized peritonitis may be simulated.

Sometimes, sudden vascular collapse with shock is the first indication. Most patients, however, have some premonitory symptoms. The absence of signs preceding fatal rupture is a strong reason for removing most abdominal aneurysms as soon as the diagnosis is made, even though the condition is asymptomatic. Symptoms from an aneurysm are an urgent indication for operation and are sometimes called a *syndrome of impending rupture.*

Physical Examination. On physical examination an abdominal aneurysm larger than 5 cm in diameter can be diagnosed with reasonable certainty. Once the patient has relaxed the muscles of the abdominal wall, careful deep palpation can usually outline the abdominal aorta near the bifurcation, generally slightly inferior to the umbilicus. The aorta may be traced proximally into the upper abdomen, where it is concealed beneath the pancreas and transverse colon. A normal aorta is seldom over an inch in diameter. Careful palpation can usually distinguish the lateral walls of the aorta and hence provide an estimate of the width. Finding a pulsating mass greater than an inch in diameter usually establishes the diagnosis of aneurysm.

Confusion may arise in thin females with diastasis of the rectus muscles in whom the aortic pulsations are abnormally prominent. This is particularly true if an increased pulse pressure is present. Such patients may come to the physician because of concern over the prominent pulsations, and vague tenderness may be elicited in palpating the aorta. Formerly the unwary surgeon was led to perform a laparotomy on such patients because of the prominent pulse. Almost always careful palpation will demonstrate that the aorta is of normal diameter. When palpation is uncertain, aortography may be required to exclude the presence of a small aneurysm. In the majority of patients palpation either establishes or excludes the diagnosis; confirmation by laboratory studies is often superfluous.

During the physical examination, peripheral pulses should be carefully examined, for associated occlusive vascular disease may be present. The presence of a bruit over the bifurcation of the carotid arteries is particularly significant, because an asymptomatic stenosis of a carotid artery can significantly increase the risk of hypotension occurring during operation.

Laboratory Studies. A roentgenogram of the abdomen, including anteroposterior and lateral views, will establish the diagnosis in many patients by demonstrating calcification in the wall of the aneurysm. The lateral view is particularly helpful, for the anterior wall of the aneurysm may be outlined and the distance from the vertebral column used to indicate the diameter of the aneurysm (Fig. 21-27).

Aortography is now used infrequently by most vascular surgeons because of the small but definite risk it entails and because the diagnosis can usually be established by palpation. Formerly, the relationship of the renal arteries

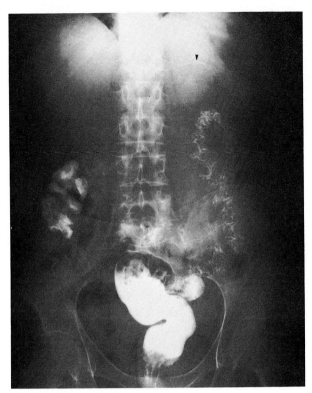

A

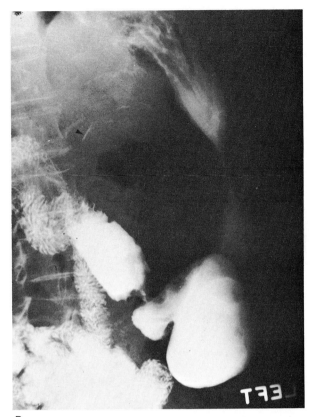

B

Fig. 21-27. X-ray films of the abdomen with the gastrointestinal tract opacified often reveal the calcific rim of abdominal aortic aneurysms quite clearly. The lateral film is most helpful since the thin shadow of the calcification is separated from the shadows of the spinal column. *A.* Anteroposterior view. *B.* Lateral view.

to the aneurysm was considered an important indication for aortography, but accumulated experiences have found renal artery involvement in only about 1 percent of patients. When uncertainty about the diagnosis exists, usually with a small aneurysm, aortography may be needed to differentiate a pulsating mass from an abdominal tumor (Fig. 21-28). For the majority of aneurysms, readily palpable on physical examination and often visible on plain roentgenograms of the abdomen, aortography is not recommended.

TREATMENT. Indications for Operation. Unless disabling cardiovascular disease, such as severe congestive heart failure or a recent myocardial infarction, is present, excision should be recommended for all abdominal aneurysms estimated to be 5 to 6 cm or greater in diameter. Aneurysms smaller than 6 cm rarely rupture, but those 6 cm or larger have an ever-present risk of rupture. The risk of rupture is at least 20 percent within a year after the diagnosis is made, and there is little correlation between the size of the aneurysm beyond 5 to 6 cm, the absence of symptoms, and the tendency to rupture. Operative mortality with a ruptured aneurysm is nearly ten times greater than that for elective excision.

Aneurysms smaller than 6 cm apparently can be safely observed, but such aneurysms are often too small to be detected by palpation and are usually found during laparotomy or on aortography performed for other purposes.

Because of the frequency of associated atherosclerotic disease, an electrocardiogram, chest roentgenogram, and

blood urea nitrogen should be routinely obtained. Renal clearance studies should be performed if there is any likelihood of significant renal insufficiency. A rapid-sequence excretory urogram may be helpful in detecting renal arterial involvement.

Technique of Excision of Abdominal Aneurysms. The operative procedure for excision of abdominal aneurysms is illustrated in Fig. 21-29. Separate from the obvious risk of hemorrhage, avoidable with careful technique, there are several common hazards. These include renal failure, declamping shock, peripheral embolization, and ischemic necrosis of the colon. Renal insufficiency was frequent during early years of experience, but cumulative experience showed that such insufficiency could be virtually eliminated by maintaining the kidney in a diuretic state during operation. This is achieved by adequate hydration, combined with the use of diuretics. A liter of electrolyte solution, usually lactated Ringer's, is infused 1 to 3 hours before induction of anesthesia, and an additional 1 to 2 liters is given during operation. Blood loss is carefully replaced as it occurs. Diuretic agents, such as mannitol, 25 Gm, or furosemide, 20 to 40 mg, are usually given at the start of operation or immediately before the aorta is occluded.

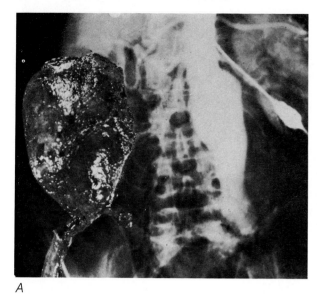

A

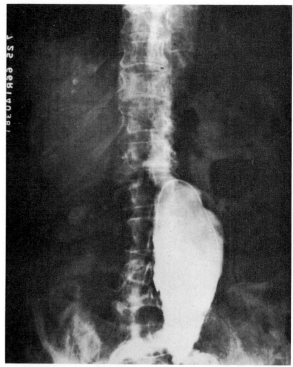

B

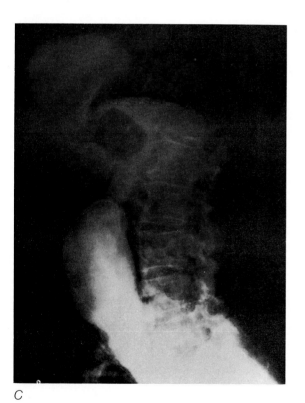

C

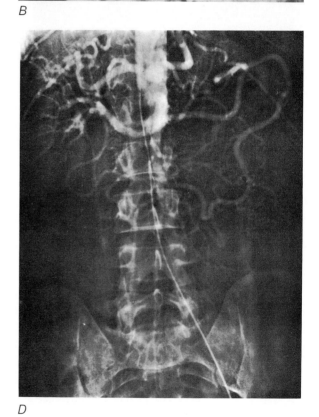

D

Declamping hypotension varies with several factors, such as duration of aortic occlusion, adequacy of blood volume, and degree of collateral circulation to the lower extremities. While the aorta is occluded, the lower extremities are relatively ischemic as a result of which there is pooling of blood in dilated vessels and accumulation of ischemic products of metabolism. If the aorta is unclamped suddenly when ischemia has been severe, profound hypotension, cardiac arrhythmias, and even cardiac arrest can occur. Such problems can be almost completely avoided by different techniques. Hypotension is uncommon if the aorta is occluded for less than 1 hour. With longer periods gradual restoration of the circulation is useful. An effective approach has been as follows: Once the proximal aortic anastomosis and one iliac anastomosis have been completed, flow is restored to that hypogastric artery, permitting gradual reopening of the circulation. When adjustment has occurred, the ipsilateral iliac artery is similarly unclamped while anastomoses are performed on the contralateral side, and the same sequence is repeated. In a series of 202 aortic operations reported by Imparato et al., declamping shock did not occur with this technique, vasopressors were not needed, and sodium bicarbonate was not required.

Distal embolization of atherosclerotic or thrombotic debris can be particularly hazardous, varying with the friability of the contents of the aneurysm. The following guidelines have been useful: The external and internal iliac arteries are mobilized and occluded before the aorta is clamped proximally. At this time 10 to 20 mg heparin is injected into the distal iliac vessels, or 50 mg heparin is given intravenously. Subsequently, as the individual iliac anastomoses are completed, balloon catheters of the Fogarty type are passed into the distal circulation to remove any thrombi which may have occurred. The selective iliac "flush" technique described above has been very effective. Finally, at the conclusion of the operation, the peripheral pulses are examined to be certain that they are the same as before operation.

Ischemic injury of the colon can be avoided by dissecting within the wall of the aneurysm rather than outside it and ligating the inferior mesenteric artery at its origin, carefully avoiding injury to any collateral vessels in the mesentery of the left colon. The technique of removing only the inner portion of the aneurysm, leaving the adventitial sheath, facilitates dissection, avoids injury to adjacent structures such as the vena cava, and provides a soft tissue covering

Fig. 21-28. A. Aortogram showing abdominal aneurysm in the distal aorta. Superimposed on the film is a photograph of a lesion excised at operation, indicating the large laminated clot filling the aneurysm. (*Courtesy of Dr. Henry T. Bahnson, Department of Surgery, University of Pittsburgh.*) B. Anteroposterior lumbar aortogram performed by percutaneous introduction of an arterial catheter, illustrating a large abdominal aneurysm arising in the lower abdominal aorta. Linear calcification of the lower thoracic and upper abdominal aorta is also visible. C. Lateral view in same patient. D. Abdominal aortogram in a patient with atherosclerotic occlusion of the abdominal aorta which has extended up to the level of the renal arteries. The superior mesenteric artery is visible as well as the right renal artery. Extensive collateral circulation has developed, particularly in the left flank.

of the prosthesis to prevent erosion of the duodenum or other structures subsequently. As the inferior mesenteric artery has been ligated, at least one hypogastric artery must be preserved to maintain collateral circulation to the colon through the middle hemorrhoidal arteries. With these guidelines, significant ischemic injury of the colon is very rare, occurring probably only when atherosclerosis has compromised the collateral circulation.

An alternative technique to abdominal aortic aneurysm operation has been a retroperitoneal approach which avoids manipulation of the abdominal viscera. Postoperative recovery is said to be smoother by avoiding the problems of prolonged intestinal atony.

Postoperative Complications. The operative mortality for excision of an abdominal aneurysm is now 5 to 10 percent, varying with the age of the patient and the degree of associated atherosclerosis. Paralytic ileus for 2 to 4 days following operation is the most frequent complication. It is best treated by gastric decompression through a nasogastric tube until bowel function returns. Antibiotic therapy, usually with large amounts of penicillin or methicillin, is begun during operation and continued for 4 to 6 days. In uncomplicated aneurysms, convalescence is usually uneventful once postoperative ileus has subsided.

Following operation particular attention should be given to pedal pulses which were palpable before operation. Absence of a pedal pulse is usually an indication for prompt reoperation, for this is commonly due to embolization of atherosclerotic or thrombotic material during removal of the aneurysm. Renal insufficiency is now infrequent following uncomplicated operations. An unusual but often lethal cause of renal insufficiency is embolic occlusion and infarction of the kidneys from atherosclerotic material dislodged during manipulation of the proximal aorta during operation.

PROGNOSIS. The reported 5-year survival following resection of an abdominal aneurysm has varied from 30 to 60 percent. Fatalities are usually due to cardiac or cerebral complications of atherosclerosis. Complications from the prosthetic graft are unusual. The most frequent of these is development of a false aneurysm, often at the proximal suture line, with subsequent rupture or erosion into the duodenum. This can be minimized by limiting dissection of the proximal aorta at the time that the aneurysm is resected, covering the graft with the adventitia of the aneurysm, and subsequently carefully separating the prosthetic graft from the intestine.

Ruptured Abdominal Aneurysm

CLINICAL MANIFESTATIONS. A ruptured abdominal aneurysm constitutes a grave surgical emergency, for irreversible renal injury develops with great rapidity. The onset is characterized by acute vascular collapse, usually with abdominal or flank pain. With severe collapse, the diagnosis initially may be uncertain, because a stuporous or comatose patient cannot describe pain. Until a pulsating mass is palpated, a frequent erroneous diagnosis is renal colic from a ureteral stone. The diagnosis usually can be established by careful, deep palpation of the abdo-

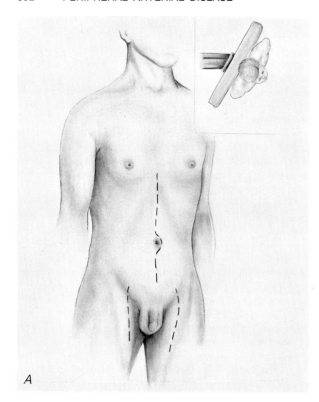

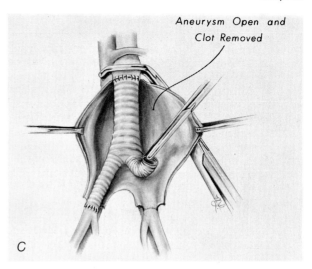

Aneurysm Open and
Clot Removed

C

A

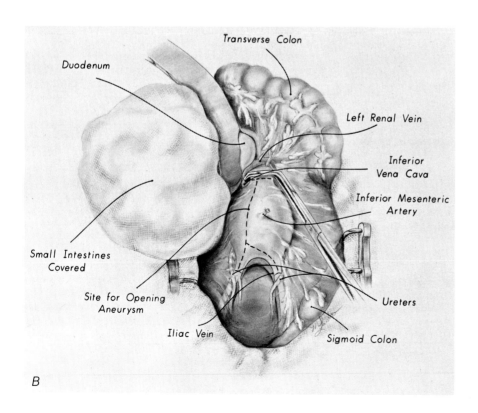

Transverse Colon

Duodenum

Left Renal Vein

Inferior
Vena Cava

Inferior Mesenteric
Artery

Small Intestines
Covered

Site for Opening
Aneurysm

Ureters

Iliac Vein

Sigmoid Colon

B

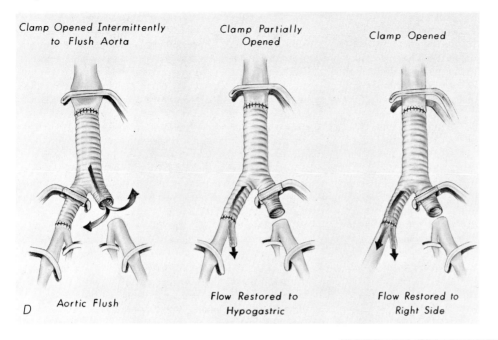

Clamp Opened Intermittently
to Flush Aorta

Clamp Partially
Opened

Clamp Opened

D   Aortic Flush

Flow Restored to
Hypogastric

Flow Restored to
Right Side

Aneurysm Wall Sutured
Over Prosthesis

E

Fig. 21-29. Procedure for substituting aortoiliac bifurcation prosthesis for abdominal aortic aneurysm. *A.* A midline incision extending from xiphoid process to pubis symphysis is usually employed. Insert shows rotation of the table to the patient's right side, which facilitates retraction of the small bowel. *B.* Surgical exposure of vital structures and lines of incision of the aneurysm are shown. *C.* Endarterectomy of the aneurysm wall is performed; the lumbar arteries transfixed with sutures and the prosthesis in place are shown. *D.* Technique for preventing embolization of atherosclerotic debris to the lower extremities and gradually restoring lower extremity circulation to avoid declamping shock. (1) Aorta is flushed through one open limb of the prosthesis. (2) Flow gradually restored to one hypogastric artery and, when the blood pressure has been stabilized, to the ipsilateral external iliac artery. (3) The sequence is repeated on the opposite side. *E.* The remains of the aneurysm wall and the base of the left colon mesentery are carefully sutured over the prosthesis and suture lines to prevent adherence of the bowel and to bolster the suture lines to prevent aorticointestinal fistulas.

men, which should outline a pulsating, ill-defined mass in the epigastrium or flank.

TREATMENT. Operation should be performed as quickly as possible, infusing 500 to 1000 ml of fluid every few minutes until serious hypotension has been corrected. A midline incision is preferred. Proximal control of the aorta generally can be obtained by isolating the aorta above the stomach just below the diaphragm. This should be done initially, because once the posterior peritoneum is incised and the hematoma surrounding the ruptured aneurysm evacuated, massive hemorrhage can occur with exsanguination. The aorta can be safely clamped below the diaphragm for 20 to 30 minutes without serious ischemic

injury to the intestines or liver. Once it has been clamped, the ruptured aneurysm can be widely incised, intraabdominal clots evacuated, and the proximal aorta below the renal arteries isolated, after which a clamp can be applied to the infrarenal aorta and the previously applied clamp below the diaphragm released. Reconstruction is then similar to that with elective excision of an abdominal aneurysm, although excision of the wall of the aneurysm should be limited because of the serious condition of the patient. Unfortunately, despite successful removal of the aneurysm, death results from renal insufficiency in 30 to 50 percent of patients.

The value of prompt excision of ruptured abdominal

aneurysms is reflected by high survival rates if operation is performed within 1 to 2 hours of rupture. If operation is performed 8 to 10 hours after rupture, there is a very high fatality rate from renal insufficiency. The unheralded rupture of asymptomatic aneurysms, with resulting high fatality rates, is the most urgent reason for recommending routine excision of abdominal aneurysms as soon as the diagnosis is made.

PERIPHERAL ANEURYSMS

Aneurysms outside the major body cavities, the skull, thorax, and abdomen, are rare. If traumatic and congenital malformations, considered in different chapters, are excluded, almost all such aneurysms result from arteriosclerosis, for syphilitic aneurysms now are seldom seen. Similarly, mycotic aneurysms associated with bacterial endocarditis are infrequent with present methods of antibiotic therapy. The majority of peripheral arteriosclerotic aneurysms are in the popliteal artery. Infrequent sites include the femoral, carotid, or subclavian arteries. Each of these is considered separately.

The aneurysms in different locations are similar in that they usually occur in men in the fifth to seventh decades, often with hypertension and signs of atherosclerosis in other organs. Multiple aneurysms are frequent. In contrast to abdominal or thoracic aneurysms, where rupture is the greatest threat, peripheral aneurysms infrequently rupture but cause disability due to distal embolization or thrombosis with subsequent ischemia and gangrene of the extremity.

Because of their superficial location, peripheral aneurysms are readily amenable to successful therapy if operated upon electively before embolization and acute ischemia develop in the extremity. Tortuosity of the involved artery often makes it possible to mobilize the artery proximal and distal to the aneurysm and reestablish continuity following excision by end-to-end anastomosis. Continuity also can be established with a short graft, preferably of the saphenous vein. If this is not possible, a knitted Dacron prosthesis is preferred. In 1966 Howell and associates stated that over 400 such aneurysms had been treated at Baylor University during the previous 14 years with serious complications in only 3 percent of the patients. In patients with a distal pulse before operation, distal circulation was restored in all but one.

Popliteal Aneurysms

Almost all popliteal aneurysms originate from arteriosclerosis, usually in men in the sixth or seventh decade. As with other peripheral arteriosclerotic aneurysms, complications of arteriosclerosis in other organs are frequent. Bilateral popliteal aneurysms occur in at least 25 percent of patients. Aneurysms at other sites such as the abdominal aorta also are common. Hypertension is present in 40 to 50 percent of patients.

The aneurysms are often small, 3 by 4 cm, and asymptomatic. Nonetheless they pursue a malignant course of

peripheral embolization with subsequent gangrene of the extremity. The marked tendency to progress rapidly to embolization and gangrene may be related to intermittent compression of the aneurysm by flexion of the knee. In one group of 29 aneurysms reported by Hara and Thompson, 18 progressed to acute ischemic occlusion despite their small size and lack of symptoms preceding acute vascular occlusion. In an extensive study of 100 popliteal aneurysms, Gifford et al. found that only about 20 percent remained free of symptoms within 5 years following diagnosis. In some patients, the tendency for silent aneurysms to embolize is demonstrated by the unheralded development of acute ischemic symptoms from occlusion of the popliteal artery; on subsequent physical examination the aneurysm is discovered.

CLINICAL MANIFESTATIONS. The clinical findings in most patients are characteristic enough to permit an accurate diagnosis. Some patients are unaware of the aneurysm, while others note a vigorous pulse behind the knee joint in a small mass which is otherwise asymptomatic. Rarely, the aneurysm may enlarge sufficiently to cause local pain and tenderness. Actual rupture is unusual.

A pulsating mass is usually found. If the aneurysm is thrombosed, pulsation may be absent, and a mass may or may not be felt. Differential diagnosis must include other cystic tumors about the knee joint, such as Baker's cyst, as well as other causes of tibial arterial occlusion, such as emboli, Buerger's disease, and diabetes mellitus. The presence or absence of pedal pulses should be carefully noted.

Calcification in the wall of the aneurysm is often visible on a roentgenogram. The diagnosis can be confirmed by arteriography, although much of the cavity of the aneurysm may be filled with thrombus (Fig. 21-30).

When a patient is seen with symptoms of acute ischemia in an extremity, such as pain, paralysis, or discoloration, the presence of pedal pulses is of particular importance, because the ischemic symptoms usually result from embolization of thrombotic material from the aneurysm distad into the posterior and anterior tibial arteries.

TREATMENT. Because of the hazard of thrombosis, embolization, and gangrene, operation should be performed as soon as possible after the diagnosis is made even though the aneurysm is small, asymptomatic, and seemingly stable. A retrospective study of gangrene and amputation from popliteal aneurysms which have embolized found no warning signs that such a catastrophe was imminent.

Operative Technique. With the patient in a prone position, an incision across the popliteal crease readily exposes the artery proximal and distal to the aneurysm. An alternative exposure, particularly useful when the femoral artery needs to be exposed for some distance from the popliteal, has been described by Imparato and Kim. An incision is made on the medial aspect of the lower thigh and extended across the knee joint into the upper calf, transecting the muscles inserting into the upper medial tibial plateau as well as the head of the gastrocnemius tendon. Transection of these muscles provides unusually wide exposure and has not resulted in any late impairment of function of the extremity.

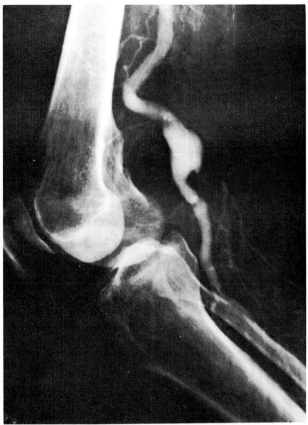

Fig. 21-30. Femoral angiogram indicating the presence of a popliteal aneurysm. Characteristic tortuosity of the involved artery is present. Such tortuosity often makes it possible to establish continuity by direct anastomosis following excision of the aneurysm.

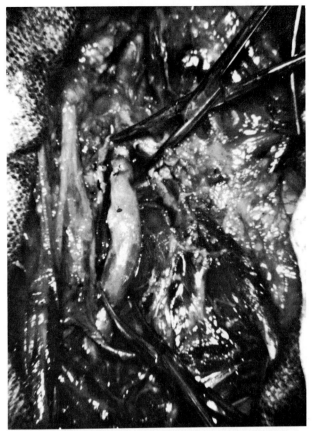

Fig. 21-31. Operative photograph of saphenous vein graft used to restore continuity of the popliteal artery following excision of a popliteal aneurysm. Long-term results of saphenous vein grafts following excision of such aneurysms have been excellent.

Once the artery has been isolated distal to the aneurysm, vascular clamps are applied and the aneurysm widely opened. Any laminated thrombus is removed, as well as the inner lining of the wall of the aneurysm, preserving the adventitial sheath. The origins of the geniculate branches of the popliteal artery are sutured from within the lumen. This technique preserves branches of the popliteal vein which are usually stretched over the wall of the aneurysm, and also the collateral circulation is less disturbed. A small amount of heparin should be given either systemically or into the distal artery at the time that the clamps are applied.

If the aneurysm is small and the popliteal artery tortuous, an end-to-end anastomosis is sometimes possible. Most patients, however, require a short graft, preferably a reversed autologous saphenous vein (Fig. 21-31). Short grafts of knitted Dacron also have been satisfactory. As the anastomoses are completed, the distal popliteal artery is cleared with a Fogarty balloon catheter to remove any laminated thrombus.

In a series of 48 popliteal aneurysms reported by Crichlow and Roberts, a vein graft was used in 21 and a Teflon graft in 14. The 21 saphenous vein grafts remained

of complications. Similar experiences were described by Hunter et al. for 27 patients with a total of 31 aneurysms.

Acute Ischemia. When operation is required because thrombosis has produced severe ischemia with impending gangrene, a different approach is needed. Simple excision of the aneurysm, of course, is futile with the obstructed distal circulation. The major consideration is removal of these distal thrombi followed by restoration of arterial continuity across the occluded aneurysm as in elective procedures. Operative incision and exposure should be planned to permit precise cannulation of the anterior and posterior tibial arteries with balloon-tipped catheters to remove propagated thrombus. Retrograde flushing with saline solution from the posterior and anterior tibial arteries is far less satisfactory than the Fogarty catheter technique. Operative angiography should be available to be certain that all thrombi have been removed. In some patients the distal thrombi have become adherent to the arterial wall and require repeated efforts for removal. If thrombi are not completely removed, as confirmed by angiography, rethrombosis terminating in gangrene and amputation is almost a certainty (Fig. 21-32).

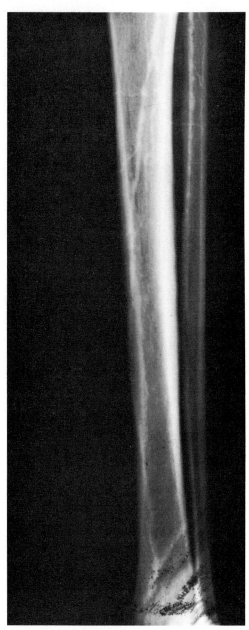

Fig. 21-32. Angiographic study of tibial arteries after surgical repair of popliteal aneurysm showing persistent thrombi in the tibial arteries subsequently removed with Fogarty catheters. Such thrombi almost inevitably lead to occlusion of the tibial arterial outflow tract and may involve the arterial reconstruction itself.

Femoral Aneurysms

INCIDENCE AND PATHOLOGY. Femoral aneurysms are virtually all due to arteriosclerosis, with frequent signs of atherosclerosis in other organs. In one series of 89 patients with 115 aneurysms, 86 of the 89 were men with an average age of sixty-four years. In this large series, 36 percent of the aneurysms were bilateral. At least one other aneurysm was present besides a single femoral aneurysm in 69 per-

cent of the patients. Twenty-eight percent of the group had abdominal aneurysms, and 54 percent had hypertension.

In the femoral artery, the aneurysm was limited to the common femoral in 27 percent and to the superficial femoral in 26 percent, and involved both areas in the remainder. In only 1 percent of the entire group was the aneurysm limited to the profunda femoris artery.

As with popliteal aneurysms, the usual course is that of thrombosis, embolization, and ischemia. Rupture is rare. Of the two events producing ischemia, thrombosis is more common than embolization, in contrast to the usual course of popliteal aneurysms. This occurred in 26 percent of the 89 patients reported by Papas and associates, while rupture occurred only five times. Similar experiences were reported in a smaller series of 12 patients by Tolstedt et al. Eight of the twelve thrombosed, resulting in amputation in each patient.

CLINICAL MANIFESTATIONS. Symptoms usually consist of an awareness of a pulsating mass in the upper thigh until thrombosis or embolization produces ischemic symptoms in the extremity. The diagnosis can often be easily made on physical examination, outlining the pulsating mass in the femoral artery. A roentgenogram may show calcification in the wall of the aneurysm. Arteriography is useful to delineate the relationship of the aneurysm to the profunda femoris artery, as well as to define the patency of the distal circulation.

TREATMENT. Surgical correction should be performed promptly, unless coexisting cerebral or coronary artery disease makes the risk of operation prohibitive. If operation is postponed because of concomitant disease, such decisions should be made with the full realization that a subsequent amputation because of gangrene may entail an even greater operative risk to the patient.

At operation the arteries can be mobilized proximal and distal to the point of aneurysm and the aneurysm excised. Vascular continuity may be restored with either a saphenous vein graft or an 8- or 10-mm knitted Dacron prosthesis. Patency of the profunda femoris artery should be maintained by using a Y-bifurcation graft if necessary. Complications following operation are unusual unless peripheral arterial occlusion has already produced severe ischemic signs. In most patients following operation the prognosis is determined by the coexisting atherosclerotic disease, rather than the femoral aneurysm.

Carotid Artery Aneurysms

INCIDENCE AND PATHOLOGY. The infrequent occurrence of carotid aneurysms has been documented by several reports. Reid found only 12 cases in a 30-year survey at the Johns Hopkins Hospital ending in 1922. At the University of Pennsylvania in a 20-year period ending in 1947, five cases were encountered. Raphael and associates reported six patients seen at the Mayo Clinic in a 25-year period, and Beall et al. in 1962 stated that seven carotid aneurysms had been seen at Baylor University over a period of time during which 2,300 operations for aneurysms had been performed.

Most carotid aneurysms result from arteriosclerosis. As in other arteries, syphilis once was the most common cause but is now rare. Unusual causes include trauma, bacterial infection, or cystic medial necrosis. The most frequent location is in the common carotid artery near its bifurcation into the internal and external carotid arteries. Less frequently aneurysms are localized to the internal carotid. The main hazard from an aneurysm is embolization of thrombotic material into the cerebral circulation with production of cerebral infarcts. Infrequently such aneurysms may enlarge and rupture, but treatment is usually undertaken before this has occurred.

CLINICAL MANIFESTATIONS. Patients are usually seen because of a mass in the neck. Pulsations are often prominent and provide an easy clue to the diagnosis. A more difficult problem arises if pulsations are absent, because of laminated thrombus occupying most of the cavity of the aneurysm. Arteriography is the most definitive laboratory technique, establishing the diagnosis and also defining the relationship of the common and internal carotid arteries to the aneurysm (Fig. 21-33). The differential diagnosis should include prominent pulsations from buckling of the carotid artery, a condition seen in hypertensive women, and other solid tumors of the neck, such as a lymph node or a carotid body tumor.

TREATMENT. Because of the constant risk from cerebral infarction, the aneurysm should be excised as soon as possible. The major consideration in planning operation is protection of the brain from ischemic injury while the carotid artery is occluded during excision. In a review of reported experiences by Raphael and associates, 12 patients were described in whom the aneurysm was excised without any protection of the brain from ischemia. Six of the twelve had a transient neurologic injury, while four developed a permanent neurologic deficit.

The safest surgical technique is excision of the aneurysm under local or regional block anesthesia, keeping the patient awake to assess constantly the tolerance of the brain for temporary occlusion of the carotid artery. If ischemic symptoms develop, an internal shunt may be utilized to maintain cerebral blood flow. Even with a large aneurysm, regional block anesthesia is adequate.

The limited surgical experiences with carotid aneurysms was indicated by the report by Kianouri in 1967, who found a total of 28 patients in whom the aneurysm had been excised and arterial continuity reestablished. The first such report of successful excision of a carotid aneurysm, followed by end-to-end anastomosis, was published by Shea in 1955. Experiences at present indicate that in over one-half of the patients there is sufficient tortuosity and elongation of the carotid artery proximal and distal to the site of involvement of the aneurysm to permit mobilization of the ends of the carotid artery and direct anastomosis (Fig. 21-34). Following excision of the aneurysm with reconstruction of the carotid artery, convalescence has

Fig. 21-34. Carotid aneurysmectomy is possible even when the internal carotid artery is involved in its upper extracranial portion, since the artery can be exposed through lateral neck incisions to the base of the skull. *A.* Internal carotid aneurysm. *B.* Replacement with vein graft.

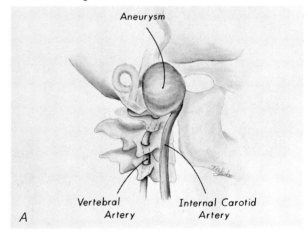

Fig. 21-33. Carotid arteriogram illustrating saccular aneurysm of the internal carotid artery. The internal carotid proximal and distal to the aneurysm is opacified.

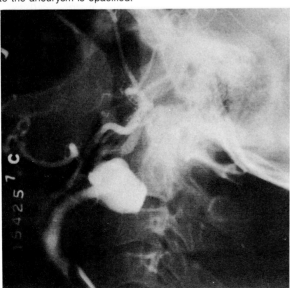

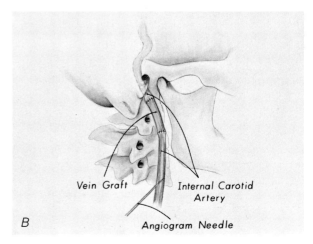

usually been uncomplicated, and long-term results are excellent.

Subclavian Aneurysms

The majority of subclavian aneurysms develop as secondary complications of a cervical rib and are discussed in the section on Thoracic Outlet Syndromes. The extremely rare subclavian aneurysm which results from atherosclerosis is similar to other peripheral atherosclerotic aneurysms, occurring in older men, often with atherosclerotic aneurysms elsewhere. The diagnosis is usually readily made from physical examination. The most important differential diagnosis is from the frequently seen tortuosity of the innominate and subclavian arteries which occurs in hypertensive patients. Careful examination of the bulge will differentiate a true aneurysm from a tortuous vessel. If aneurysm cannot be excluded, an arteriogram should be done. Excision with reconstruction of the involved artery can be easily performed.

Visceral Aneurysms

SPLENIC ARTERY ANEURYSMS

Significant aneurysms of the splenic artery are uncommon. Because of their rarity and unusual manifestations, several detailed reviews have been published. In 1953 Owens and Coffey reported six patients and found a total of 198 cases in previous reports. Of historical interest is the fact that President Garfield in 1881 died from a traumatic aneurysm of the splenic artery 2 months after being shot by an assassin.

INCIDENCE AND PATHOLOGY. A report of unusual interest is that of Bedford and Lodge in 1960 who published findings from 250 consecutive postmortem examinations in older patients. Routine dissection of the splenic artery found 26 aneurysms, an incidence of nearly 10 percent. All had been asymptomatic. Their size was small, ranging from a few millimeters to as large as 2.5 cm; most were near 1 cm in diameter. In the 204 cases reviewed by Owens and Coffey, the average diameter was 3 cm. This great discrepancy between the high autopsy incidence and the rarity of clinically symptomatic aneurysms indicates that small aneurysms are probably of no clinical significance and are usually overlooked.

These aneurysms, like other atherosclerotic aneurysms, occur in older patients with an average age near fifty. Atherosclerosis is present in the splenic artery in over 95 percent of patients. Surprisingly, though, the aneurysms are more frequent in women, in contrast to the overwhelming predominance of the usual atherosclerotic aneurysm in men. In the Owens and Coffey series, 127 patients were women and 63 were men. Bedford and Lodge noted that the aneurysms tended to develop at bifurcations of the splenic artery and suggested that degeneration of the media as well as atherosclerosis might be a predisposing factor.

The aneurysms are usually single and in the main trunk of the splenic artery. Rupture is more likely to occur during pregnancy. The actual risk of rupture is uncertain, for many are recognized only after rupture. Rupture is obviously a grave event, for of 131 symptomatic patients reported by Owens and Coffey 94 died from rupture and only 7 from other causes. In 37 female patients, rupture occurred during late pregnancy.

CLINICAL MANIFESTATIONS. Pain in the epigastrium or left flank is the most frequent symptom, occurring in 93 of 131 symptomatic patients in the Owens series. Other symptoms are nonspecific gastrointestinal symptoms, usually interpreted as due to peptic ulcer. These include nausea, vomiting, dyspepsia, and constipation or diarrhea. Gastrointestinal hemorrhage has occurred in about one-third of patients. For unknown reasons gastrointestinal symptoms may exist for months or years before the diagnosis is made. Perhaps this is fortuitous.

In one patient treated by one of the authors several years ago, acute gastrointestinal bleeding led to the erroneous performance of a subtotal gastrectomy a few days earlier, though an ill-defined mass suggesting an aneurysm was noted. When bleeding returned several days later, reoperation was performed. Recovery eventually ensued after a long and difficult convalescence.

Often rupture is the first sign of the aneurysm, in 46 percent of the patients in one series. A "double" rupture is a significant clinical sequence, recognized in about one-half of patients. The first rupture is hemorrhage into the lesser omental sac; this ceases temporarily but is followed in 1 to 2 days by secondary hemorrhage and exsanguination.

With the small size of the splenic aneurysms, physical abnormalities are usually not found. For unknown reasons, moderate splenomegaly has been reported in 40 to 50 percent of patients. However, a mass has been palpated in only 20 percent, and pulsations or a bruit in 10 percent. Roentgenographic identification of a mass with calcium in the walls suggestive of an aneurysm has been reported in 15 percent of the group.

TREATMENT. Obviously symptomatic aneurysms should be excised as soon as the diagnosis is made, usually with concomitant splenectomy. The widespread use of aortography for investigating many abdominal conditions has disclosed aneurysms smaller than 1 cm which are asymptomatic. Their treatment is uncertain because of the rarity of rupture. On the other hand, it is disquieting to note that rupture without preceding symptoms is the first event in one-half of the patients with splenic aneurysms. From data available, surgical treatment does not seem indicated for asymptomatic aneurysms smaller than 1 cm, but those greater than 3 cm should be excised. Further data are needed to be certain of these guidelines.

RENAL ARTERY ANEURYSMS

INCIDENCE AND PATHOLOGY. Aneurysms of the renal artery are similar to aneurysms of the splenic artery in that recognition has greatly increased with the use of vascular angiography. A collective review in 1957 by Garritano found only 180 patients. Nine years later, Cerny et al. found a total of 345 reported cases and described 25 patients from the University of Michigan alone. In discussing this report, Smith described 17 aneurysms at the Henry Ford Hospital, and Morris described operative experience with 58 patients at Baylor Medical Center. The widespread use of renal angiography to investigate patients with hypertension has been chiefly responsible for the increasing recognition of renal aneurysms. Apparently, about 1 percent of hypertensive patients will be found on angiography to have a small aneurysm of one renal artery.

These aneurysms are equally common in males and females, usually in the fifth and sixth decades, but they have been found in all age groups, even in patients as young as nine months. Anatomically they may be saccular or fusiform. Unusual varieties include a false aneurysm from trauma, a dissecting aneurysm, or an arteriovenous fistula. The saccular aneurysm is apparently congenital, arising from a defect in elastic tissue of the wall of the artery, often near a bifurcation. It varies from 1 to 3 cm in size and often develops extensive eccentric calcification, a so-called "signet ring" on the roentgenogram. It is infrequently associated with hypertension and rarely ruptures. The fusiform aneurysm develops distal to an area of constriction of the renal artery and is basically a poststenotic aneurysm similar to that seen in other parts of the arterial circulation. Because of the proximal stenosis, it is frequently seen with hypertension.

The aneurysms occur with equal frequency in either renal artery, usually in the main renal artery or one of its branches. An intrarenal location is uncommon. In one report, 92 aneurysms were in the main renal artery, 44 were in an extrarenal branch, and 15 were intrarenal.

Rupture has been reported in at least 24 patients with a fatal outcome in 20. Eight of these episodes occurred during pregnancy. Rupture has been recognized only three times in a calcified aneurysm.

CLINICAL MANIFESTATIONS. Abdominal or flank pain has occurred in about 50 percent of the patients but is probably unrelated to the aneurysm. Investigation of the symptom subsequently led to finding the aneurysm.

Hematuria, gross or microscopic, has also been reported in 30 to 40 percent of patients. As expected, hypertension has been frequently seen with poststenotic aneurysms and has been improved or cured in over one-half of these after operation. By contrast, hypertension in one series was present in only 7 of 12 with a saccular aneurysm and improved after operation in only 1 of the 7. A mechanism by which a saccular aneurysm can produce hypertension is not clear except for the rather nebulous possibility of compression or distortion of the renal artery. The association may simply be fortuitous.

There are usually no abnormalities on physical examination. Occasionally a localized bruit is audible. Roentgenographic examination may show signet ring calcification which must be differentiated from calcification of mesenteric lymph nodes or calcification of other visceral arteries. The intravenous pyelogram is abnormal in about one-half of the patients because of ischemia, infarction, or localized pressure defects. Aortography is essential to establish the diagnosis and define the precise location (Fig. 21-35). As mentioned earlier, most aneurysms have been found during aortography performed for other purposes.

TREATMENT. Prompt operation is indicated whenever an aneurysm is found during investigation of a patient for hypertension. With poststenotic aneurysms the aneurysm can be excised and the renal artery reconstructed, with an excellent likelihood of improving the hypertension. With a saccular aneurysm and hypertension, operation is probably indicated to reconstruct the renal artery, although the prognosis for improving the hypertension is less favorable. Of the 25 patients reported by Cerny et al., 20 were operated upon. Unfortunately 9 required a nephrectomy, but there was no operative mortality. In the 17 patients reported by Smith, 5 had successful operations, while 12 with small aneurysms of questionable significance had been

Fig. 21-35. Renal artery aneurysms are frequently saccular, as shown in the angiographic study, and may be associated with arterial hypertension.

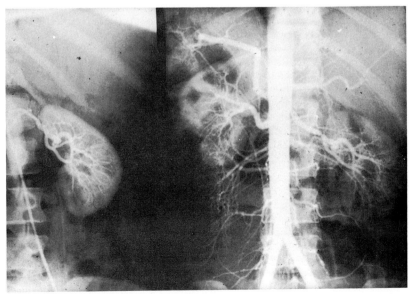
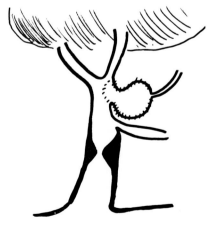

followed for an average of 3 years without complications. Morris stated that reconstructive operations had been performed on 58 patients with renal artery aneurysms, representing about 5 percent of all reconstructive operations upon the renal artery for patients with hypertension. In this group of 58 patients, 8 had previously lost the contralateral kidney, perhaps from complications of an aneurysm in that kidney. In a patient with a small calcified aneurysm without symptoms or hypertension, there probably is little indication for operation, for the risk of rupture is almost negligible. With larger aneurysms, certainly with symptoms present, operation should be performed.

Traumatic Aneurysms

Several milestones in vascular surgery evolved from treatment of traumatic aneurysms produced in military combat. In the second century Antyllus treated an arterial aneurysm by ligature immediately above and below the lesion, followed by incision of the aneurysm, evacuation of the clot, and exteriorization of the cavity. John Hunter, in 1786, electively ligated a femoral artery proximal to a popliteal aneurysm to minimize blood loss during subsequent attempts at extirpation. The anatomic term *Hunter's canal,* referring to the distal third of the superficial femoral artery in the thigh, originated from this surgical episode. In 1888 Rudolf Matas described his operation of endo-aneurysmorraphy, in which the aneurysm was widely opened and the communications into the artery were sutured. This imaginative approach promptly became the standard treatment and was modified little during the next 55 years; even during World War II it was the operation performed for most traumatic aneurysms. Subsequently, as techniques of vascular reconstruction developed, the policy of restoring arterial continuity became preferred.

ETIOLOGY AND PATHOLOGY. A traumatic aneurysm is produced from a tangential laceration of the wall of an artery. Usually continuity of flow through the lacerated artery is maintained. By contrast, injuries that transect an artery often require immediate treatment because of hemorrhage or ischemia in the affected limb and consequently seldom evolve into an aneurysm.

Following the laceration, blood extravasates into adjacent soft tissues to form a hematoma that compresses and seals the point of injury. If the artery is confined within a small space surrounded by fascia, the hematoma may be small enough to escape recognition. Both the patient and the physician are unaware that an arterial injury has occurred. After days or weeks, the blood clot gradually liquefies; then the firm, immobile mass surrounding the artery begins to pulsate. A descriptive term for these lesions was "pulsating hematoma." With the appearance of pulsation, the aneurysm begins to enlarge. This is ominous, for enlargement is progressive and relentless, destroying nerves, even eroding bone, and eventually terminating in rupture and death.

Traumatic aneurysms are often termed *false* aneurysms, as distinguished from *true* aneurysms, for the wall is composed of fibrous tissue rather than components of normal arterial wall, as with arteriosclerotic or syphilitic aneurysms.

As the hematoma enlarges in a recent wound, the tissues are firm, tender, perhaps warm. These findings of redness, tenderness, and heat are, of course, the usual characteristics of an abscess. Occasional vivid reports appear in the surgical literature in which an unsuspecting physician widely incised such a red, tender mass to drain an abscess, with resultant violent hemorrhage.

A similar therapeutic catastrophe occasionally occurs when a traumatic aneurysm stabilizes for years and is subsequently confused with a neoplasm. If the previous history of trauma is not available, the differential diagnosis is difficult, for the aneurysm is partly filled with clot and closely resembles a solid tumor. Attempted biopsy of such lesions, with frightening consequences, has been reported.

Usually there is no disability from a traumatic aneurysm except for the local mass until it enlarges to compress adjacent nerves, causing pain, paresthesias, and eventually paralysis. The peripheral arterial circulation is usually normal. Peripheral embolization of thrombi from the aneurysm is unusual except for the rare aneurysm of the subclavian artery following trauma. Here, intermittent compression by the clavicle may dislodge emboli. One of the authors treated such a patient in whom ischemic symptoms in the arm dominated the clinical picture. Arteriography disclosed a small traumatic aneurysm of the subclavian artery which had developed following an automobile accident some months before.

CLINICAL MANIFESTATIONS. A localized mass is often the only finding. As it enlarges, there is pain or paralysis from compression of nerves. On physical examination the borders of the mass are ill defined because the hematoma surrounding the aneurysm is beneath the deep fascia. Pulsations may or may not be present, depending upon the amount of thrombus in the lumen. A systolic bruit is frequently audible. Peripheral pulsations are normal.

If the mass pulsates, the diagnosis is reasonably certain from the physical findings. Otherwise arteriography is required to differentiate it from a neoplasm or a cyst. On arteriography the full size is not disclosed, as much of the cavity is filled with thrombus.

TREATMENT. Operation should be performed as soon as the diagnosis has been established because of the inevitable outcome of enlargement and rupture. If neurologic symptoms are present, operation should be done urgently, within hours, to prevent irreversible pressure injury of crucial nerves. At operation the incision should be placed to permit exposure of the uninvolved artery proximal and distal to the aneurysm. With these vessels temporarily occluded, the aneurysm can be widely incised, clots evacuated, and the point of origin from the artery identified. Dissection around the aneurysm before it is opened should be avoided; it is unnecessary, complicated, and often dangerous.

With unusually large aneurysms, it is important to remember that there is only one small opening in the wall of the aneurysm, the tangential laceration of the arterial wall from which the aneurysm began. Hence, if the aneurysm is inadvertently entered, this small opening can be digitally occluded to control bleeding while further exposure is obtained. This approach was once employed in desperation during emergency treatment of a badly neglected traumatic aneurysm of the proximal subclavian artery which had involved the brachial plexus and compressed the trachea to a near fatal degree.

Once the aneurysm has been opened and the inner contents removed, the site of communication with the parent artery can be mobilized and the injured area excised. Complete excision of the wall of the aneurysm is unnecessary and should be avoided because of the surrounding dense fibrotic reaction. Once the involved artery has been mobilized, arterial continuity can usually be restored by end-to-end anastomosis or by insertion of a short graft, preferably autologous vein. Ligation should be performed only for small arteries, such as the radial, not essential to normal circulation.

PROGNOSIS. Convalescence after operation is usually uneventful and long-term results excellent. Crawford et al. described experiences with a group of 29 patients with aneurysms or arteriovenous fistulas, all of whom were treated by excision and end-to-end anastomosis with a uniformly good result. Hughes and Jahnke similarly reported continuing good results 5 years after surgical treatment of 67 traumatic aneurysms during the Korean conflict.

VASOSPASTIC DISORDERS

Raynaud's Disease

A syndrome of intermittent vasospasm in the upper extremities without permanent vascular obstruction was described by Maurice Raynaud in 1862. The initial description included several disorders which subsequent observation found were not primary Raynaud's disease, but attention was focused on the disorder by this report. The syndrome described by Raynaud, now termed *Raynaud's phenomenon,* consists of recurrent episodes of vasoconstriction in the upper extremities, initiated by exposure to cold or emotional stress. Three sequential phases classically occur: pallor, cyanosis, and rubor. It is now recognized that Raynaud's phenomenon may exist as a primary disorder, termed *Raynaud's disease,* or may be a secondary manifestation of a more serious vascular disease, often not evident for 1 or 2 years after the initial appearance of the recurrent color changes. The more common disorders associated with Raynaud's phenomenon include Buerger's disease (thromboangiitis obliterans), scleroderma, cervical rib or other thoracic outlet syndrome, and atherosclerosis. It occasionally results from recurrent minor trauma, such as the use of mechanical vibrating tools. Rarely, other collagen diseases, such as periarteritis nodosa or disseminated lupus erythematosus are found. Hence, in the evaluation of a patient the critical decision is to determine whether the disease is primary Raynaud's disease or a secondary manifestation of a more serious disorder. Some suspect that it is always secondary to some other underlying disorder.

ETIOLOGY. The cause of primary Raynaud's disease is unknown. It is much more frequent in women, with a ratio of about 5:1, and appears in over 90 percent of patients before forty years of age. In men, it is usually much less severe in intensity. DeTakats and Fowler observed abnormal electroencephalograms in some patients, suggesting a primary disease in the midbrain, but the existence of a primary neurologic disease has not been established.

PATHOLOGY. The clinical picture of Raynaud's phenomenon is related to the anatomy and physiology of the arteriolar circulation in the dermis. The arterioles penetrate the dermis at right angles with an irregular reticulate pattern and arborize into a capillary network. Some fluctuation in vasomotor tone, as with pallor or blushing, is a normal physiologic variation. In Raynaud's disease, vasospasm occurs with such severity that dermal circulation momentarily ceases, with the production of severe pallor. If the vasospasm is less severe, with slowing but not cessation of the dermal circulation, cyanosis appears, a result of sluggish flow of blood with an increase in the percentage of reduced hemoglobin in the capillaries. When the vasospasm subsides, a reactive hyperemia with vasodilatation develops, probably from the accumulation of tissue metabolites during the anoxic period, producing an unusual redness or rubor.

The basis for the increased tendency of the dermal arterioles to vasoconstriction is unknown. It may be a sensitivity in the arterioles themselves, or possibly may result from hyperactivity of the sympathetic nervous system. Initially the arterioles are normal on histologic examination. With chronic disease, there is progressive hypertrophy of the arteriolar walls and ultimate occlusion. Detailed histologic observation of early phases of Raynaud's disease are not available, because tissue biopsies are seldom performed at this time.

In the majority of patients the episodes of vasoconstriction are precipitated by exposure to cold. In about 25 percent of patients intense emotion, as well as cold, may be the initiating factor. Only rarely is emotion alone the significant stimulus without an abnormal sensitivity to cold.

In most patients the upper extremities are symmetrically involved. Unilateral involvement by Raynaud's phenomenon almost always denotes a proximal mechanical cause, either occlusion of one of the major proximal arteries, recurrent embolization, or neurovascular compression. In 10 to 15 percent of patients the legs are involved as well as the arms. This was found in 51 of 474 patients seen over a period of years at the Mayo Clinic.

With repeated episodes of vasoconstriction and ischemia, trophic changes gradually appear. These include atrophy of the skin with loss of elasticity and hair. The term *sclerodactylia* has been applied to this appearance, since it resembles the changes found in scleroderma in other organs. However, long-term studies by Gifford et al. have demonstrated conclusively that the presence of sclerodactylia in the fingers does not indicate that generalized scleroderma will appear in the future. Focal areas of ulceration develop and leave characteristic scars with healing. Recurrent superficial infections, such as paronychia, may occur. In the more extreme forms of ischemia, gangrene may require amputation of one or more digits, but fortunately gangrene almost never progresses to involve the hands.

CLINICAL MANIFESTATIONS. The patient is usually a young woman who has noted that episodes of cold precipitate vasoconstriction with a repetitive sequence of pallor, cyanosis, and rubor. Several variations in the color phenomena may occur with less severe disease. For example, there may be only cyanosis followed by rubor or only episodes of mild cyanosis.

In addition to the color changes, the patient may have paresthesias and localized pain in the digits. If infection or ulceration is present, pain is more severe. Except for the discomfort in the hands, the patients usually have no other symptoms.

Physical Examination. In the early phases of the disease, the extremities may be entirely normal with peripheral pulses of equal volume. The best index to the severity of the disease is the extent of trophic changes in the fingers, such as atrophy of the skin and nails with loss of hair over the terminal phalanges. In more advanced disease, signs of chronic ischemia are obvious, with punctate scars from healed ulcerations, chronic rubor, and absence of a radial or ulnar pulse.

Arteriography is of value in establishing the diagnosis by revealing the absence of occlusive arterial disease. The most critical examination is demonstration of the vasoconstrictor response to cold. Induction of the characteristic pallor-cyanosis-rubor sequence in both hands following exposure to cold establishes the diagnosis, although it does not differentiate between primary and secondary Raynaud's phenomenon. An electroencephalogram should be obtained to pursue the observation made by DeTakats that abnormal electroencephalographic tracings are present in some patients.

Once the presence of Raynaud's phenomenon has been confirmed, the principal question is whether the vasomotor changes are primary or secondary to some other vascular disease. The possibility of early scleroderma can be evaluated by study of the motility of the esophagus and small bowel. Other blood tests to screen for collagen disorders, such as lupus, should be done. The presence of cervical ribs can be easily determined by roentgenograms of the cervical spine and thorax. Other compression syndromes of the subclavian artery can be detected by performing the maneuvers described under Thoracic Outlet Syndromes. Complete angiographic studies to opacify the arterial circulation from the aortic arch to the small arteries of the hand should be done to exclude the possibility of proximal atherosclerotic plaques producing distal emboli. Occasionally skin and lymph node biopsies are useful.

An important principle in diagnosis is continued observation of the patient over a period of several years. Even after a thorough examination has failed to detect any underlying vascular disease, such a disease may appear in the next 2 to 3 years. In the Mayo Clinic series the diagnosis of Raynaud's disease is simply considered a tentative one for as long as 2 years.

TREATMENT. In the majority of patients the disability is mild. Avoiding cold or other stimuli which precipitate vasoconstriction is adequate. Moving to a warm climate may be considered, but this does not eliminate the attacks. Tobacco certainly should be avoided because of its potent vasoconstrictor action, but this alone does not abolish the syndrome. Various vasodilator drugs have been repeatedly tried, but none have been of consistent benefit. The most recent medications are orally administered methyldopa, employed for patients with ulceration of the fingers and severe pain, and intraarterially administered reserpine. Significant long-term data are not yet available, but one of the authors has used this therapy in some patients, with occasional dramatic and prolonged relief. Therapy for several weeks is required in increasing doses to be effective.

The most effective therapy is cervicodorsal sympathectomy. This is accomplished by removing the first, second, and third thoracic ganglia, preserving the cervical portion of the stellate ganglion to avoid a Horner's syndrome.

The immediate results after sympathectomy in patients with severe vasospasm is quite encouraging, but relapses are common. For this reason, sympathectomy is usually employed only when symptoms are severe and other therapy ineffective. In Gifford's series of 474 patients, only 77 were operated upon; about one-half of these had excellent to good results. DeTakats and Fowler tabulated reports from different groups, including 40 cases of their own, and found an average of 55 percent good results in 424 sympathectomies performed. More radical sympathectomies have not given any better results. Proximally all of the stellate ganglion has been removed, producing Horner's syndrome; distad the fourth thoracic ganglion has been included. Another technical modification has been to include the second and third intercostal nerves with the third ganglion because of the demonstration by Skoog that 10 to 15 percent of sympathetic ganglia to the upper extremity are contained in these two intercostal ganglia. Also there has been considerable discussion about differences in preganglionic and postganglionic sympathectomy. None of these variations have been found significant, however, and the conservative sympathectomy involving the first, second, and third thoracic ganglia is usually performed. Severe trophic changes before operation are unfortunately often associated with a poor result. Patients with scleroderma also obtain little benefit.

Operative Technique. At least four different surgical techniques have been employed at different times for sympathectomy. Originally most were done through a posterior approach, with the patient in a prone position and an incision similar to that for a thoracoplasty. The sympathetic chain was exposed by resecting a short segment of the second or third rib, followed by an extrapleural dissection to isolate the sympathetic chain. In large muscular individuals this approach is quite difficult and provides only limited exposure. It has been virtually abandoned.

A second technique, a supraclavicular approach, provides excellent exposure in patients of small stature with long thin necks. However, in those with short, thick necks, significant trauma to the brachial plexus, resulting in a painful neuritis, may complicate the postoperative course.

An excellent description of the technique was published by Nanson.

Ideal exposure can be obtained by an anterior transthoracic incision, opening the hemithorax in the third or fourth intercostal space. This, of necessity, involves a major thoracotomy, though a simple one. It has been favored by Palumbo, who also emphasized that removal of the lower one-third of the stellate ganglion would adequately sympathectomize the extremity without producing a Horner's syndrome.

In recent years the transaxillary approach has become preferred. This is done through a short incision in the axilla, followed by resection of a short segment of the second or third rib and exposure of the sympathetic chain. Good technical descriptions have been published by Roos and by Kirtley et al. The thoracotomy is of much less magnitude than that through the anterior approach, and the incision is in an inconspicuous location.

PROGNOSIS. The prognosis in most patients with primary Raynaud's disease is good with the exception of the discomfort associated with the abnormal sensitivity to cold. Even in the more advanced forms, tissue loss seldom exceeds the loss of one or more digits. More serious systemic vascular disease does not develop, and although symptoms may continue for many years, there is no known impairment of longevity or health.

Uncommon Vasomotor Diseases

Rare, unusual vasomotor diseases include livedo reticularis and acrocyanosis, which primarily result from vasoconstriction, and erythromelalgia, apparently a result of vasodilatation. The disability with these disorders is usually episodic and mild. Their clinical significance is primarily in differentiating them from more serious underlying disease, such as Buerger's disease, scleroderma, or disseminated lupus erythematosus. Only salient clinical features of these bizarre diseases will be presented here.

LIVEDO RETICULARIS

This unusual vasomotor condition is characterized by a persistent mottled reddish blue discoloration of the skin of the extremities. It is more prominent in the legs and feet than in the hands or arms and only infrequently involves the trunk. Although the severity varies with temperature, becoming worse on exposure to cold, it never entirely disappears spontaneously.

ETIOLOGY AND PATHOLOGY. The cause is unknown, although miscellaneous associated vascular diseases such as hypertension or emotional disorders have been found in different patients.

The pathophysiologic feature apparently is a stenosis of the arterioles which pierce the cutis at right angles and arborize into the peripheral capillaries of the skin. The obstruction of the arterioles, either spastic or organic, therefore affects the peripheral capillary arborizations and accounts for the peculiar reticular nature of the discoloration.

The pathologic changes in the arterioles varies from no visible abnormality to proliferation of the intima, in some

patients progressing to complete occlusion. With severe organic obstruction, focal ulceration of the skin, usually over the lower legs, may occur.

CLINICAL MANIFESTATIONS. Patients with livedo reticularis complain of the persistent reddish blue mottling over the legs and feet, varying somewhat with temperature. Often the cosmetic appearance is the only concern of the patient. In some there are localized symptoms of coldness, numbness, dull aching, and paresthesias. With severe forms and localized tissue ischemia, there may be pain from local ulceration. These symptoms are more prone to appear during the winter in association with cold temperatures.

The diagnosis is usually made from physical examination, with observation of the persistent blotchy discoloration, and a history of prolonged persistence in association with some variation with environmental temperature. Peripheral pulsations are normal, and trophic changes are not present in the digits. Only with more extreme forms are ischemic ulcers present over the lower legs. These usually heal after a short period of time.

TREATMENT. In most patients no treatment is necessary except reassurance regarding the benign nature of the condition. Only one patient is described in the Mayo Clinic series in whom gangrene developed in the legs. Avoiding extremes of cold is beneficial in some patients. Vasodilating agents may be tried, but none has been found of consistent benefit. Sympathectomy should be employed if the disability is severe enough to produce local ulceration. After sympathectomy the discoloration may decrease in extent and remain pink rather than blue. In most patients the disorder is a permanent one, remaining as a moderate cosmetic disturbance, but fortunately with no other disability.

ACROCYANOSIS

Acrocyanosis is a disorder characterized by persistent but painless cold and cyanosis of the hands and feet. The cause and the pathologic and pathophysiologic features are virtually unknown, for the disease consists primarily of persistent color changes. Usually it is confused with Raynaud's syndrome because of the prominent localized cyanosis. Detailed investigation of the pathophysiologic features by Lewis and Landis concluded that the fundamental disorder was a localized abnormality in vasomotor tone in the circulation of the hands and feet. Apparently the basic physiologic condition is a slow rate of blood flow through the skin, the result of chronic arteriolar constriction, which results in a high percentage of reduced hemoglobin in the blood in the capillaries and production of the cyanotic color. Endocrine dysfunction has been found in some patients, but no consistent pattern has been established.

Usually the disorder is found in a young woman who has noted persistent coldness and blueness of the fingers and hands for many years, often with symptoms of less severity in the toes and feet. The abnormalities are more prominent in cold weather, but the extremities are never completely normal. With heat the color may change from deep purple to red, but there are no episodes of blanching, such as occurs with Raynaud's disorder. The peripheral pulses are normal, and there are no trophic changes indicative of chronic tissue ischemia, such as atrophy of the skin, sclerosis, or ulceration.

The principal differential diagnosis is from Raynaud's disease because of the prominent color changes in both disorders. The absence of pallor, as well as the absence of signs of chronic ischemia, are the most useful features. Similarly, the constant presence of the color changes in acrocyanosis, as opposed to the intermittent episodic occurrence in Raynaud's disease, is characteristic.

Usually reassurance is the only treatment needed, with the avoidance of cold temperatures when possible. Sympathectomy can be employed with reasonably good results if the disability is more serious. Prognosis is excellent, with tissue loss virtually never occurring. Usually the color changes remain for many years or permanently.

ERYTHROMELALGIA

This rare disorder is characterized by red, warm, painful extremities. The clinical characteristics were described by S. Weir Mitchell in 1872 and the disorder named by him in 1878. The cause of the primary disease is unknown. Similar phenomena, so-called "secondary erythromelalgia," can occur as a result of hypertension or polycythemia vera.

The basic abnormality is an unusual sensitivity to warmth, for skin temperatures of 32 to 36°C, which produce no effects in normal individuals, will regularly induce the painful burning sensation. The exact temperature at which the distress can be produced varies with different patients but may be a precise one for any individual patient. It was termed by Lewis a "critical point." The increase in temperature is usually a result of vasodilatation with increase in blood flow. The exact basis for the spontaneous vasodilatation with the rise in temperature and the burning sensation is not known.

The disease is equally prevalent in men and women, usually of middle age. The distress may be greater in the summer months, but only a general relationship to extremes of heat or cold may be present. The patient soon learns that exposing the extremities to cold, such as by immersing them in ice water, may abort an attack.

Physical examination usually reveals no abnormalities of the peripheral arteries. The diagnosis is usually established by demonstration of a close relationship between the symptoms and skin temperature. This may be induced by direct application of heat, noting the skin temperature at which distress appears. Erythromelalgia should be differentiated from the painful red but cold extremities which occur with Buerger's disease and also with peripheral neuritis.

Aside from the troublesome symptoms, the disorder is a benign one. Avoiding extremes of heat is one of the most useful therapeutic measures. Acetylsalicylic acid, 0.65 Gm, has been found beneficial in many patients, although the mode of action is uncertain. A trial of therapy with vasoconstrictor drugs, such as ephedrine, should be employed, but consistent value from one drug has not been found.

The disorder is usually a permanent one, but no permanent disability results.

FROSTBITE

Several forms of cold injury have been described, usually varying with the environmental conditions under which exposure occurs. These different syndromes include acute pernio (chilblains), chronic pernio, trench foot, immersion foot, and frostbite. Acute and chronic pernio are focal injuries of the skin and subcutaneous tissue resulting from exposure to cold of moderate intensity, representing an increased susceptibility to cold injury in a particular individual. The disorder is seldom a surgical problem, because the lesions are focal, superficial ones which heal readily. Trench foot and immersion foot are primarily military injuries produced by prolonged exposure to cold in damp surroundings, often with temperatures well above freezing, but in circumstances where there is an element of prolonged immobility. Immersion foot is probably simply the seagoing counterpart of trench foot. Such injuries are rarely seen in civilian practice. For practical purposes frostbite is the type of injury usually encountered and will be discussed in detail. The tissue response in the other disorders mentioned, however, is a similar type of response to cold, modified somewhat with the environmental conditions.

ETIOLOGY. Frostbite results when tissues are exposed to cold for varying periods of time. The severity varies both with the temperature and the duration of exposure. Experimentally, it has been demonstrated that freezing begins in mammalian tissues when the temperature in the deeper parts reaches 10°C and that −5°C is the lowest temperature to which cells may be slowly frozen and still survive. Frostbite injury usually results from exposure over a period of several hours. In the Korean conflict, 90 percent of the cases occurred at temperatures near −7°C after exposure for 7 to 18 hours. A different form of frostbite is produced by acute exposures to below zero temperatures, commonly occurring in airplanes at high altitudes and hence termed "high altitude" frostbite. In such injuries the exposed part is acutely frozen with deposition of ice crystals in the tissues. This unusual form of injury is different from the usual case of frostbite, where a "slow freeze" results.

Several factors influence the injurious effect of cold. Two of the most significant ones are humidity and the presence of wind, both of which accelerate the withdrawal of heat from body tissues. Immobility or occlusive vascular disease also are significant factors, both influencing the rate of peripheral blood flow. Acclimatization has been demonstrated in some persons repeatedly exposed to cold, such as those who live in northern latitudes, and probably is a localized vasomotor adaptation. By contrast, extremities previously injured by cold may remain permanently susceptible to future cold injury, perhaps from an intensified vasoconstrictor response.

PATHOLOGY. The degrees of severity of a frostbite injury have been conventionally grouped into four clinical types:

a first-degree injury consists of edema and redness of the affected part without necrosis; formation of blisters represents a second-degree injury; necrosis of the skin constitutes a third-degree injury; in a fourth-degree injury gangrene of the extremity develops, requiring amputation.

As frostbite occurs, the injured tissue becomes numb and moderately stiff without extensive discomfort. Often the patient is unaware that frostbite is occurring. With subsequent rewarming the tissues become reddened, hot, and edematous. At this time blisters erupt and gangrene gradually appears in the more seriously injured tissues. Edema increases to a maximum within 24 to 48 hours and then gradually is resorbed as gangrenous tissue begins to demarcate. The extent of gangrene is difficult to estimate initially and requires observations for as long as 30 days or more. Fortunately the degree of gangrene is often much less than that initially feared, because the skin may be gangrenous but the underlying tissue viable. For this reason amputation is delayed until the extent of gangrene is definitely known.

Following recovery of the extremity, there is frequently a permanent increase in vasoconstrictor tone resulting in hyperhidrosis, and an abnormal sensitivity to cold. Pain and paresthesias are also common, perhaps as residuals from ischemic neuritis.

It is uncertain whether the fundamental injury from cold results from direct freezing with disruption of cell membranes or whether the injury is primarily an ischemic necrosis from widespread thrombosis of arterioles and capillaries. Certainly vascular occlusion is a prominent feature, whether it is a primary or a secondary event. With exposure to cold, there is severe vasoconstriction, decreasing the rate of blood flow in the chilled extremity, with resulting stasis, sludging of blood, and eventual widespread thrombosis. In clinical experiments, immersion of the arm for 2 hours in water at 13°C decreases blood flow to about 3 percent of normal, while immersion of a finger in water at 7°C stops blood flow altogether. In addition to sludging and capillary thrombosis, there is an increase in capillary permeability, resulting in the formation of edema when blood flow is increased after rewarming.

On histologic examination of the injured tissues, edema, infiltration of inflammatory cells, and deposition of fibrin are prominent findings. Widespread thrombosis of small vessels is frequently seen. In addition focal areas of necrosis may be evident in skin, muscle, and other tissues.

CLINICAL MANIFESTATIONS. Frequently, the patient is unaware that frostbite is occurring. The usual injury occurs with exposure to near freezing temperatures for several hours, often combined with wind, high humidity, damp or wet shoes, or immobility from tightly constricting shoes or confinement in a cramped position. All these factors influence the rate of heat transfer between the extremity and the environment. Initially there may be mild discomfort, but as the extremity becomes numb and somewhat stiff, frequently discomfort is minimal.

When rewarmed, the extremity quickly becomes red, edematous, hot, and painful. This is due to vasodilatation and widespread extravasation of fluid through the walls of capillaries whose permeability has been increased from injury. Edema reaches its peak intensity within 48 hours and then gradually subsides over several days. As described under Pathology, gangrene gradually becomes evident and slowly demarcates over a period of many days. An ominous sign, indicating that gangrene will develop, is the persistence of coldness and numbness in an area while surrounding tissues become edematous, hot, and painful. The persistent coldness and numbness indicate cessation of all circulation with the certain outcome of ischemic necrosis.

Following recovery from frostbite, a high percentage of extremities remain with an increased vasoconstrictor tone, manifested by increased susceptibility to cold, hyperhidrosis, paresthesias, and localized pain.

TREATMENT. Frostbite seldom occurs during exposure to cold if proper precautions are taken. This includes the wearing of dry, insulated, loosely fitting clothing and carefully avoiding long periods of immobility of the exposed extremities. Most cases of clinical frostbite occur in circumstances where exposure to cold inadvertently occurs for long periods of time because of coma from injury, alcohol, or other factors.

Rapid warming of the injured tissue is the most important aspect of treatment. Several studies have clearly demonstrated the advantages of the rapid-rewarming method over any other. The frozen tissue should be placed in warm water, with a temperature in the range of 40 to 44°C. Complete rewarming usually requires about 20 minutes. Higher temperatures are more injurious than beneficial. A frostbitten part should never be exposed to hot water, an open fire, or excessive dry heat, as in an oven, for the loss of sensitivity in the frozen area makes it especially vulnerable to injury. Warming in water is much more rapid than application of warm blankets, which require three or four times as long as the immersion method.

Following rewarming, the injured extremity should be elevated to minimize formation of edema and carefully protected in a sterile environment. Usually it is left exposed but surrounded by a protective cradle. Blisters are opened only when necessary to remove necrotic skin. Antibiotic therapy and tetanus antiserum are routinely given to lessen the risk of infection. Demarcation of gangrenous areas should be carefully observed, often for several weeks, before amputation is performed. Often a gangrenous area which initially appears to involve the foot will gradually regress with the separation of superficial areas of gangrenous skin, ultimately with the loss of one or more digits but preservation of the foot.

The role of sympathectomy has been studied by Shumacker and Kilman and by Golding et al. Both experimental and clinical experiences indicate a beneficial effect from sympathectomy, especially when employed in the first few days after frostbite has occurred. Shumacker and Kilman reported 66 sympathectomies in 38 patients, 24 of which were performed soon after injury. Their experience indicated that sympathectomy should be performed for injuries severe enough to produce necrosis of tissue, both to minimize the extent of necrosis and to prevent the usual late vasomotor sequelae. Golding et al. found in experimental and clinical studies (68 patients) that the proper time for sympathectomy was between 36 and 72 hours after injury. Earlier sympathectomies accelerated the rate of edema formation, while sympathectomies performed following the peak intensity of edema seemed to hasten absorption of edema and minimize eventual tissue necrosis. Sympathectomy is also beneficial in alleviating the late sequelae from cold injury, i.e., paresthesias, coldness, and hyperhidrosis.

If vascular injury is the primary event, therapeutic measures to decrease vasoconstriction or blood clotting, such as sympathectomy or the administration of heparin, should be of routine benefit. The theoretic benefit from sympathectomy is the release of vasospasm, which may precipitate thrombosis in injured capillaries and arterioles. Heparin and dextran have also been given in attempts to lessen the degree of small vessel thrombosis which is such a prominent feature on histologic examination of the injured tissues. Although theoretically plausible, consistent benefit has not been demonstrated from the routine use of either heparin or dextran.

PROGNOSIS. Following recovery from injury, all studies have found a significant percentage of residual disability in the extremity. Simeone evaluated 1,061 limbs 4 months after frostbite while the patients were still in the hospital and found painful feet and hyperhidrosis the most common complaints. Ervasti described similar sequelae in 812 cases of frostbite 5 to 18 years after injury. Orr and Fainer reported that gangrene occurred in only 6 percent of 1,880 cases from the Korean conflict, but some disability remained in 10 to 20 percent of patients.

References

Occlusive Disease: General

Beebe, H. G., Clark, W. F., and DeWeese, J. A.: Atherosclerotic Change Occurring in an Autogenous Venous Arterial Graft, *Arch Surg,* **101:**85, 1970.

Buck, R. C.: Intimal Thickening after Ligature of Arteries: An Electromicroscopic Study, *Circ Res,* **9:**418, 1961.

Cookson, F. B.: The Origin of Foam Cells in Atherosclerosis, *Br J Exp Pathol,* **52:**62, 1971.

Goldenfarb, P. B., Cathey, M. H., and Cooper, G. R.: The Determination of ADP Induced Platelet Aggregation in Normal Men, *Atherosclerosis,* **12:**335, 1970.

Greenhalgh, R. M., Rosengarten, D. S., and Mervart, I.: Serum Lipids and Lipo Proteins in Peripheral Vascular Disease, *Lancet,* **2:**947, 1971.

Hamaker, W. R., Doyle, W. F., O'Connel, T. J., Jr., and Gomez, A. C.: Subintimal Obliterative Proliferation in Saphenous Vein Grafts. A Cause of Early Failure of Aorta to Coronary Artery By-pass Grafts, *Ann Thorac Surg,* **13:**488, 1972.

Honour, A. J., Pickering, G. W., and Sheppard, B. L.: Ultrastructure and Behavior of Platelet Thrombi in Injured Arteries, *Br J Exp Pathol,* **52:**482, 1971.

Imparato, A. M., Bracco, A., Kim, G. E., and Zeff, R.: Intimal and Neointimal Fibrous Proliferation Causing Failure of Arterial Reconstructions, *Surgery,* **72:**1007, 1972.

Kelly, J. P., and James, J. M.: Criteria for Determining the Proper Level of Amputation in Occlusive Vascular Disease: A Review of 323 Amputations, *J Bone Joint Surg [AM],* **39A:**883, 1957.

Lim, R. C., Blaisdell, F. W., Hall, A. D., Moore, W. S., and Thomas, A. N.: Below Knee Amputation for Ischemic Gangrene, *Surg Gynecol Obstet,* **125:**493, 1967.

Marcus, A. J.: Platelet Function, *N Engl J Med,* **280:**1213, 1969.

O'Herman, M. G., and Stahlgren, L. H.: Evaluation of Factors Which Influence Mortality and Morbidity following Major Amputations of the Lower Extremity for Arteriosclerosis, *Surg Gynecol Obstet,* **120:**1217, 1965.

Richards, R. L.: Lumbar Sympathectomy for Chronic Occlusive Arterial Disease, *Am Heart J,* **81:**735, 1971.

Salzman, E. W.: The Limitations of Heparin Therapy after Arterial Reconstructions, *Surgery,* **57:**131, 1965.

Schatz, I. J.: Classification of Primary Hyperlipidemia, *JAMA,* **210:**701, 1969.

Schnetzer, G. W.: Platelets and Thrombogenesis: Current Concepts, *Am Heart J,* **83:**552, 1972.

Scott, H. W., Jr.: Metabolic Surgery for Hyperlipidemia and Atherosclerosis, *Am J Surg,* **123:**3, 1972.

Temes, G., Toth, I., and Török, B.: Structural Changes of Internal Mammary Artery after Transplantation into the Myocardium, *Acta Exp Chir,* **31**(1):2, 1970.

Vlodaver, Z., and Edwards, J. E.: Pathologic Changes in Aortic Coronary Arterial Saphenous Vein Grafts, *Circulation,* **44:**719, 1971.

Wilens, S. L.: The Nature of Diffuse Intimal Thickening of Arteries, *Am J Pathol,* **27:**825, 1951.

Aortoiliac Occlusive Disease

Garrett, H. E., Crawford, E. S., Howell, J. F., and DeBakey, M. E.: Surgical Considerations in the Treatment of Aorto-iliac Occlusive Disease, *Surg Clin North Am,* **46:**949, 1966.

Gomes, M. R., Bernatz, P. E., and Juergens, J. L.: Aortoiliac Surgery: Influence of Clinical Factors on Results, *Arch Surg,* **95:**387, 1967.

Imparato, A. M., Sanoudos, G., Epstein, H. Y., Abrams, R. M., and Beranbaum, E. R.: Results in 96 Aortoiliac Reconstructive Procedures: Pre Operative Angiographic and Functional Classifications Used as Prognostic Guides, *Surgery,* **68:**610, 1970.

Inihara, T.: Endarterectomy for Occlusive Disease of the Aorto-iliac and Common Femoral Arteries: Evaluation of Results of the Eversion Technique Endarterectomy, *Am J Surg,* **124:**235, 1972.

Kouchoukos, N. T., Levy, J. F., Balfour, J. F., and Butcher, H. R.: Operative Therapy for Aortoiliac Arterial Occlusive Disease, *Arch Surg,* **96:**628, 1968.

Lorentsen, E., Hael, B. L., and Hal, R.: Evaluation of the Functional Importance of Atherosclerotic Obliterations in the Aorto-iliac Artery by Pressure-Flow Measurements, *Acta Med Scand,* **191:**399, 1972.

Mannick, J. A., and Nabseth, D. C.: Axillofemoral By-pass Graft: A Safe Alternative to Aortoiliac Reconstruction, *N Engl J Med,* **278:**461, 1968.

May, A. G., Van de Berg, L., DeWeese, J. A., and Rob, C. G.: Critical Arterial Stenosis, *Surgery,* **54:**250, 1963.

Szilagyi, D. E., Smith, R. F., Elmquist, J. G., Gonzalez, A., and Elliott, J. P.: Angioplasty in the Treatment of Peripheral

Occlusive Arteriopathy: A Summary of 12 Years' Experience, *Arch Surg,* **90:**617, 1965.

Wylie, E. J.: Discussion of D. E. Szilagyi, R. F. Smith, and D. G. Whitney: The Durability of Aorto-iliac Endarteriectomy, *Arch Surg,* **89:**827, 1964.

Femoropopliteal Occlusive Disease

Allan, J. S., and Taylor, G. W.: The Relationship between Blood Flow and Failure of Femoropopliteal Reconstructive Arterial Surgery, *Br J Surg,* **59:**549, 1972.

Blumchen, G., Landry, F., Kiefer, H., and Schlosser, V.: Hemodynamic Responses of Claudicating Extremities: Evaluation of Long Range Exercise Program, *Cardiology (Basel),* **55:**114, 1970.

Coffman, J. D., and Mannick, J. A.: Failure of Vasodilator Drugs in Arteriosclerosis Obliterans, *Ann Intern Med,* **76:**35, 1972.

Crawford, E. S., Garrett, H. E., DeBakey, M. E., and Howell, J. F.: Occlusive Disease of the Femoral Artery and Its Branches, *Surg Clin North Am,* **46:**991, 1966.

Dale, W. A.: Autogenous Vein Grafts for Femoropopliteal Arterial Repair, *Surg Gynecol Obstet,* **123:**1282, 1966.

———: Salvage of Arteriosclerotic Legs by Vascular Repair, *Ann Surg,* **165:**844, 1967.

DeWeese, J. A., Barner, H. B., Mahoney, E. B., and Rob, C. G.: Autogenous Vein Bypass Grafts and Thromboendarterectomies for Atherosclerotic Lesions of the Femoropopliteal Arteries, *Ann Surg,* **163:**205, 1966.

Edwards, W. S., Holdefer, W. F., and Mohtashemi, M.: The Importance of Proper Caliber of Lumen in Femoral-Popliteal Artery Reconstruction, *Surg Gynecol Obstet,* **122:**37, 1966.

Fitzgerald, D. E., Keates, J. S., and MacMillan, D.: Angiographic and Plethysmographic Assessment of Graduated Physical Exercise in the Treatment of Chronic Occlusive Arterial Disease of the Leg, *Angiology,* **22:**99, 1971.

Imparato, A. M., Bracco, A., and Kim, G. E.: Femoral-Popliteal Arterial Reconstructions: Comparisons of Autologous Vein By-Pass, Open and Semiclosed Endarterectomy, *Ann Surg,* 1973.

Kaplitt, M. J., Sobel, S., and Sawyer, P. N.: Review of Femoral-Popliteal Reconstruction Utilizing Gas Endarterectomy, *Surgery,* **62:**872, 1967.

Keshishian, J. M., Smyth, N. P. D., and Adkins, P. C.: Clinical Experience with Modified Bovine Arterial Heterograft, *J Cardiovasc Surg,* **12:**433, 1971.

Koontz, T. J., and Stausel, H. C., Jr.: Factors Influencing Patency of the Autogenous Vein Femoropopliteal By-pass Graft: An Analysis of 74 Cases, *Surgery,* **71:**753, 1972.

Linton, R. R.: Discussion in D. E. Szilajyi, R. F. Smith, J. P. Elliott, and H. M. Allen, Long-Term Behavior of a Dacron Arterial Substitute: Clinical, Roentgenologic and Histologic Correlations, *Ann Surg,* **162:**453, 1965.

McCaughan, J. J., Jr.: Surgical Revascularization of 288 Lower Extremities with Occlusive Arterial Disease, *Am Surg,* **33:**628, 1967.

Poliwoda, H.: Treatment of Acute and Chronic Arterial Occlusions with Streptokinase, *Aust Ann Med,* **19**(Suppl 1):25, 1970.

Sawyer, P. N., Kaplitt, M. J., Sobel, S., Golding, M. R., and Dennis, C.: Analysis of Peripheral Gas Endarterectomy in 127 Patients, *Arch Surg,* **97:**859, 1968.

Skinner, J. S., and Strandness, D. E., Jr.: Exercise and Intermittent

Claudication: Effects of Physical Training, *Circulation,* **36:**23, 1967.

Spencer, F. C., and Rienhoff, W. F., III: Reconstructive Surgery for Occlusive Disease of Femoral and Popliteal Arteries, *Surgery,* **54:**709, 1963.

Szilagyi, D. E., Smith, R. F., Elliott, J. P., and Allen, H. M.: Long-Term Behavior of a Dacron Arterial Substitute: Clinical, Roentgenologic and Histologic Correlations, *Ann Surg,* **162:**453, 1965.

Vollmar, J., Frede, M., and Laubach, K.: Principles of Reconstructive Procedures for Chronic Femoro-popliteal Occlusions: A Report of 546 Operations, *Ann Surg,* **168:**215, 1968.

Tibioperoneal Occlusive Disease

Noon, G. P., Diethrich, E. B., Richardson, W. P., and DeBakey, M. E.: Distal Tibial Arterial By-pass: Analysis of 91 Cases, *Arch Surg,* **99:**770, 1969.

Tyson, R. R., and Reichle, F. A.: Femorotibial By-pass for Salvage of the Ischemic Lower Extremity, *Surg Gynecol Obstet,* **134:**771, 1972.

Wheelock, F. C., Jr., and Filtzer, H. S.: Femoral Grafts in Diabetes: Resulting Conservative Amputations, *Arch Surg,* **99:**776, 1969.

Arterial Embolism

Anderson, W. R., and Richards, A. M.: Evaluation of Lower Extremity Muscle Biopsies in the Diagnosis of Atheroembolism, *Arch Pathol,* **86:**535, 1968.

Billig, D. M., Hallman, G. L., and Cooley, D. A.: Arterial Embolism, *Arch Surg,* **95:**1, 1967.

Carvajal, J. A.: Atheroembolism an Etiologic Factor in Renal Insufficiency, Gastrointestinal Hemorrhages and Peripheral Vascular Disease, *Arch Intern Med,* **119:**593, 1967.

Cranley, J. J., Krause, R. J., Strasser, E. S., Hafner, C. D., and Fogarty, T. J.: Peripheral Arterial Embolism: Changing Concepts, *Surgery,* **55:**57, 1964.

Crawford, E. S., and DeBakey, M. E.: The Retrograde Flush Procedure in Embolectomy and Thrombectomy, *Surgery,* **40:**737, 1956.

Dale, W. A.: Endovascular Suction Catheters, *J Thorac Cardiovasc Surg,* **44:**557, 1962.

Darling, R. C., Austen, W. G., and Linton, R. R.: Arterial Embolism, *Surg Gynecol Obstet,* **124:**106, 1967.

Fisher, E. R., Hellstrom, H. R., and Myers, J. D.: Disseminated Atheromatous Emboli, *Am J Med,* **29:**176, 1960.

Flory, C. M.: Arterial Occlusions Produced by Emboli from Eroded Aortic Atheromatous Plaques, *Am J Pathol,* **21:**549, 1945.

Fogarty, T. J., Cranley, J. J., Krause, R. J., Strasser, E. S., and Hafner, C. D.: A Method for Extraction of Arterial Emboli and Thrombi, *Surg Gynecol Obstet,* **116:**241, 1963.

Haimovici, H.: Peripheral Arterial Embolism, *Angiology,* **1:**20, 1950.

Kassirer, J. P.: Atheroembolic Renal Disease, *N Engl J Med,* **280:**817, 1969.

Miles, R. M., Dale, D., and Booth, J. L.: The Dynamics of Peripheral Arterial Embolism, *Ann Surg,* **167:**801, 1968.

Spencer, F. C., and Eiseman, B.: Delayed Arterial Embolectomy: A New Concept, *Surgery,* **55:**64, 1964.

Buerger's Disease

Allen, E. V., Barker, N. W., and Hines, E. A., Jr.: "Peripheral Vascular Diseases," 3d ed., W. B. Saunders Company, Philadelphia, 1962.

DeBakey, M. E., and Cohen, B. M.: Buerger's Disease: A Follow-up Study of World War II Army Cases, Charles C Thomas, Publisher, Springfield, Ill., 1963.

Kelly, P. J.: "Levels of Amputation in Occlusive Vascular Disease: A Clinical and Pathological Study of 319 Amputations," thesis, University of Minnesota Graduate School, Minneapolis, 1955.

Kjeldsen, K., and Mozes, M.: Buerger's Disease in Israel: Investigations on Carboxyhemoglobin and Serum Cholesterol Levels after Smoking, *Acta Chir Scand,* **135:**495, 1969.

McKusick, V. A., Harris, W. S., and Ottesen, O. E.: The Buerger Syndrome in the United States: Arteriographic Observations, with Special Reference to Involvement of the Upper Extremities and the Differentiation from Atherosclerosis and Embolism, *Bull Johns Hopkins Hosp,* **110:**145, 1962.

———, ———, ———, Goodman, R. M., Shelley, W. M., and Bloodwell, R. D.: Buerger's Disease: A Distinct Clinical and Pathologic Entity, *JAMA,* **181:**5, 1962.

McPherson, J. R., Guergels, J. L., and Gifford, R. W., Jr.: Thromboangiitis Obliterans and Arteriosclerosis Obliterans: Clinical and Prognostic Differences, *Ann Intern Med,* **59:**288, 1963.

Silbert, S.: The Etiology of Thromboangiitis Obliterans, *JAMA,* **129:**5, 1945.

Wessler, S.: Buerger's Disease Revisited, *Surg Clin North Am,* **49:**703, 1969.

———, Si-Chun, M., Gurewich, V., and Freiman, D. G.: Critical Evaluation of Thromboangiitis Obliterans: Case against Buerger's Disease, *N Engl J Med,* **262:**1149, 1960.

Arterial Trauma

Dillard, B. M., Nelson, D. L., and Norman, H. G.: Review of 85 Major Traumatic Arterial Injuries, *Surgery,* **63:**391, 1968.

Hughes, C. W., and Cohen, A.: The Repair of Injured Blood Vessels, *Surg Clin North Am,* **38:**1529, 1958.

Miller, H. H., and Welch, C. S.: Quantitative Studies on Time Factor in Arterial Injuries, *Ann Surg,* **130:**428, 1949.

Morris, G. C., Jr., Beall, A. C., Jr., Roof, W. R., and DeBakey, M. E.: Surgical Experience with 220 Acute Arterial Injuries in Civilian Practice, *Am J Surg,* **99:**775, 1960.

Morton, J. H., Southgate, W. A., and DeWeese, J. A.: Arterial Injuries of the Extremities, *Surg Gynecol Obstet,* **123:**611, 1966.

Mustard, W. T., and Bull, C. A.: A Reliable Method for Relief of Traumatic Vascular Spasm, *Ann Surg,* **155:**339, 1962.

Patman, R. D., Poulos, E., and Shires, G. T.: The Management of Civilian Arterial Injuries, *Surg Gynecol Obstet,* **118:**725, 1964.

Spencer, F. C.: Vascular Injury and Arteriovenous Fistula, in "Lewis-Walters Practice of Surgery," vol. XI, chap. 8, W. F. Prior Co., Inc., Hagerstown, Md., 1965.

——— and Grewe, R. V.: The Management of Arterial Injuries in Battle Casualties, *Ann Surg,* **141:**304, 1955.

Anterior Compartment Syndrome

Blum, L.: The Clinical Entity of Anterior Crural Ischemia, *Arch Surg,* **74:**59, 1957.

Carter, A. B., Richards, R. L., and Zachary, R. B.: The Anterior Tibial Syndrome, *Lancet,* **2:**928, 1949.

Getzen, L. C., and Carr, J. E., III: Etiology of Anterior Tibial Compartment Syndrome, *Surg Gynecol Obstet,* **125:**347, 1967.

Leach, R. E., Zohn, D. A., and Stryker, W. S.: Anterior Tibial Compartment Syndrome, *Arch Surg,* **88:**187, 1964.

Mavor, G. E.: The Anterior Tibial Syndrome, *J Bone Joint Surg* [*Br*], **38B:**513, 1956.

Moretz, W. H.: The Anterior Compartment (Anterior Tibial) Ischemia Syndrome, *Am Surg,* **19:**728, 1953.

Traumatic Arteriovenous Fistulas

Crawford, E. S., DeBakey, M. E., and Cooley, D. A.: Surgical Considerations of Peripheral Arterial Aneurysms, *Arch Surg,* **78:**226, 1959.

Creech, O., Jr., Gantt, J., and Wren, H.: Traumatic Arteriovenous Fistula at Unusual Sites, *Ann Surg,* **161:**908, 1965.

Hughes, C. W., and Jahnke, E. J., Jr.: The Surgery of Traumatic Arteriovenous Fistulas and Aneurysms: A Five-Year Follow Up Study of 215 Lesions, *Ann Surg,* **148:**790, 1958.

Shumacker, H. B., Jr.: Arterial Aneurysms and Arteriovenous Fistulas: Report on Spontaneous Cures, in D. C. Elkin, and M. E. DeBakey (eds.), "Vascular Surgery," Office of the Surgeon General, U.S. Public Health Service, 1955.

Spencer, F. C.: Vascular Injury and Arteriovenous Fistula, in "Lewis-Walters Practice of Surgery," vol. XI, chap. 8, W. F. Prior Co., Inc., Hagerstown, Md., 1965.

Congenital Arteriovenous Fistulas

Coursley, G., Ivins, J. C., and Barker, N. W.: Congenital Arteriovenous Fistulas in the Extremities: Analysis of 69 Cases, *Angiology,* **7:**201, 1956.

Cross, F. S., Glover, D. M., Simeone, F. A., and Oldenburg, F. A.: Congenital Arteriovenous Aneurysms. *Ann Surg,* **148:**649, 1958.

Ravitch, M. M., and Gaertner, R. A.: Congenital Arteriovenous Fistula in the Neck: 48 Year Follow-up on a Patient Operated upon by Dr. Halsted in 1911, *Bull Johns Hopkins Hosp,* **107:**31, 1960.

Robertson, D. J.: Congenital Arteriovenous Fistulae of the Extremities: Hunterian Lecture, *Ann R Coll Surg Engl,* **18:**73, 1956.

Rosenfeld, L.: Experiences with Vascular Abnormalities about the Parotid Gland and Upper Neck, *Arch Surg,* **79:**553, 1959.

Spencer, F. C.: Vascular Injury and Arteriovenous Fistula, in "Lewis-Walters Practice of Surgery," vol. XI, chap. 8, W. F. Prior, Co., Inc., Hagerstown, Md., 1965.

Tice, D. A., Clauss, R. H., Kierle, A. M., and Reed, G. E.: Congenital Arteriovenous Fistulae of the Extremities: Observations Concerning Treatment, *Arch Surg,* **86:**460, 1963.

Thoracic Outlet Syndromes

Adams, J. T., and DeWeese, J. A.: Effort Thrombosis of the Axillary and Subclavian Veins, *J Trauma,* **11:**923, 1971.

Adson, A. W.: Surgical Treatment for Symptoms Produced by Cervical Ribs and the Scalenus Anticus Muscle, *Surg Gynecol Obstet,* **85:**687, 1947.

Allen, E. V., Barker, N. W., and Hines, E. A., Jr.: "Peripheral Vascular Diseases," 3d ed., W. B. Saunders Company, Philadelphia, 1962.

Beyer, J. A., and Wright, I. S.: The Hyperabduction Syndrome: With Special Reference to Its Relationship to Raynaud's Syndrome, *Circulation,* **4:**161, 1951.

Clagett, O. T.: Presidential Address: Research and Prosearch, *J Thorac Cardiovasc Surg,* **44:**153, 1962.

Dale, W. A.: Thoracic Outlet Syndrome, *J Tenn Med Assoc,* **64:** 941, 1971.

Falconer, M. A., and Weddell, G.: Costoclavicular Compression of the Subclavian Artery and Vein: Relation to the Scalenus Anticus Syndrome, *Lancet,* **2:**539, 1943.

Kirtley, J. A., Riddell, D. H., Stoney, W. S., and Wright, J. K.: Cervico-sympathectomy in Neurovascular Abnormalities of the Upper Extremities: Experiences in 76 Patients with 104 Sympathectomies, *Ann Surg,* **165:**869, 1967.

Lord, J. W., Jr.: Personal communication, 1968.

——— and Rosati, L. M.: Neurovascular Compression Syndromes of the Upper Extremity, *Ciba Found Clin Symp,* **10:**35, 1958.

Love, J. C.: The Surgical Management of the Scalenus Anticus Syndrome with and without Cervical Rib, in E. V. Allen, N. W. Barker, and E. A. Hines, Jr., "Peripheral Vascular Diseases," 3d ed., W. B. Saunders Company, Philadelphia, 1962.

Nanson, E. M.: The Anterior Approach to Upper Dorsal Sympathectomy, *Surg Gynecol Obstet,* **104:**118, 1957.

Roos, D. B.: Transaxillary Approach for First Rib Resection to Relieve Thoracic Outlet Syndrome, *Ann Surg,* **163:**354, 1966.

——— and Owens, J. C.: Thoracic Outlet Syndrome, *Arch Surg,* **93:**71, 1966.

Ross, J. P.: The Vascular Complications of Cervical Rib, *Ann Surg,* **150:**340, 1959.

Schein, C. J., Haimovici, H., and Young, H.: Arterial Thrombosis Associated with Cervical Ribs: Surgical Considerations: Report of a Case and Review of the Literature, *Surgery,* **40:**428, 1956.

Skoog, T.: Ganglia in the Communicating Rami of the Cervical Sympathetic Trunks, *Lancet,* **2:**457, 1947.

Telford, E. D., and Mottershead, S.: Pressure at the Cervicobrachial Junction: An Operative and Anatomical Study, *J Bone Joint Surg [Br],* **30B:**249, 1948.

Urschel, H. D., Paulson, D. L., and McNamara, J. J.: Thoracic Outlet Syndrome, *Ann Thorac Surg,* **6:**1, 1968.

Wright, I. S.: The Neurovascular Syndrome Produced by Hyperabduction of the Arms, *Am Heart J,* **29:**1, 1945.

Extracranial Occlusive Cerebrovascular Disease

Bahnson, H. T., Spencer, F. C., and Quattlebaum, J. K., Jr.: Surgical Treatment of Occlusive Disease of the Carotid Artery, *Ann Surg,* **149:**711, 1959.

Blaisdell, F. W., Lim, R., and Hall, A. D.: Technical Result of Carotid Endarterectomy: Arteriographic Assessment, *Am J Surg,* **114:**239, 1967.

Cohen, A., Manion, W. C., Spencer, F. C., Czarnecki, S. W., and DeBakey, M. E.: Occlusive Lesions of the Great Vessels of the Aortic Arch, *Arch Surg,* **84:**628, 1962.

Contorni, L.: Il Circolo collaterale vertebro-vertebrale nella obliterazione dell'arteria suclavia alla sue origine, *Minerva Chir,* **15:**268, 1960.

Crawford, E. S., DeBakey, M. E., Garrett, H. E., and Howell, J.: Surgical Treatment of Occlusive Cerebrovascular Disease. *Surg Clin North Am,* **46:**873, 1966.

———, ———, Morris, G. C., Jr., and Cooley, D. A.: Thrombo-obliterative Disease of the Great Vessels Arising from the Aortic Arch, *J Thorac Cardiovasc Surg,* **43:**38, 1962.

Dietrich, E. B., Garrett, H. E., Ameriso, J., Crawford, E. S., El-Bayar, M., and DeBakey, M. E.: Occlusive Disease of the Common Carotid and Subclavian Arteries Treated by Carotid-Subclavian Bypass: Analysis of 125 Cases, *Am J Surg,* **114:**800, 1967.

Edwards, W. S., Bennett, A., and Wilson, T. A. S.: The Long Term Effectiveness of Carotid Endarterectomy in Prevention of Strokes, *Ann Surg,* **168:**765, 1968.

Higgs, W. A., and Bullington, S. J.: Correlation between Opthalmodynamometry and Arteriography in Diagnosing Carotid Arterial Occlusive Disease, *Eye Ear Nose Throat Mon,* **49:**369, 1970.

Imparato, A. M., and Capetillo, A.: Jugular Venous Oxygen Saturation during Extracranial Cerebral Arterial Reconstructions, *Circulation,* **42** (*Suppl* 3):168, 1970.

——— and Lin, J. P. T.: Vertebral Arterial Reconstruction, Internal Plication and Patch Vein Angioplasty, *Ann Surg,* **166:**213, 1967.

———, Kricheff, I., Capetillo, A., and Post, K.: Circulatory Dynamics of the Cerebrovascular System in Surgery for Stroke, *Circulation,* **42:** (*Suppl* 3):94, 1970.

Joint Study of Extracranial Arterial Occlusion as a Cause of Stroke:

I. Fields, W. S., North, R. R., Hass, W. K., Galbraith, J. G., Wylie, E. J., Ratinov, G., Burns, M. H., MacDonald, M. C., and Meyer, J. S.: Organization of Study and Survey of Patient Population, *JAMA,* **203:**955, 1968.

II. Hass, W. K., Fields, W. S., North, R. R., Kricheff, I. I., Chase, N. E., and Bauer, R. B.: Arteriography, Techniques, Sites and Complications, *JAMA,* **203:**961, 1968.

III. Bauer, R. B., Meyer, J. S., Fields, W. S., Remington, R., MacDonald, M. C., and Callen, P.: Progress Report of Controlled Long Term Survival in Patients With and Without Operation, *JAMA,* **208:**509, 1969.

IV. Blaisdell, W. F., Clauss, R. H., Galbraith, J. G., Imparato, A. M., and Wylie, E. J.: A Review of Surgical Considerations, *JAMA,* **209:**1889, 1969.

V. Fields, W. S., Maslenikov, V., Meyer, J. S., Hass, W. K., Remington, R. D., and Macdonald, M.: Progress Report of Prognosis Following Surgery or Non Surgical Treatment for Transient Cerebral Ischemic Attacks and Cervical Carotid Lesions. *JAMA,* **211:**1993, 1970.

Killen, D. A., Foster, J. H., Gobbel, W. G., Jr., Stephenson, S. E., Jr., Collins, H. A., Billings, F. T., and Scott, H. W., Jr.: The Subclavian Steal Syndrome, *J Thorac Cardiovasc Surg,* **51:**539, 1966.

Lyons, C., and Galbraith, G.: Surgical Treatment of Atherosclerotic Occlusion of the Internal Carotid Artery, *Ann Surg,* **146:**487, 1957.

Martin, M. J., Whisnant, J. P., and Sayre, G. P.: Occlusive Vascular Disease in the Extracranial Cerebral Circulation, *Arch Neurol,* **3:**530, 1960.

Millikan, C. H.: The Pathogenesis of Transient Focal Cerebral Ischemia, *Circulation,* **32:**438, 1965.

Ranson, J. H. C., Imparato, A. M., Clauss, R. H., Reed, G., and Hass, W. K.: Factors in Mortality and Morbidity Associated with Surgical Treatment of Cerebrovascular Insufficiency, *Circulation,* **39** (*Suppl* 1):269, 1969.

Reivich, M., Holling, E., Roberts, B., and Toole, J. F.: Reversal of Blood Flow through the Vertebral Artery and Its Effect on Cerebral Circulation, *N Engl J Med,* **265:**878, 1961.

Rosenberg, J. C., and Spencer, F. C.: Subclavian Steal Syndrome: Surgical Treatment of Three Patients, *Am Surg,* **31:**307, 1965.

Ross, R. S., and McKusick, V. A.: Aortic Arch Syndrome, *Arch Intern Med,* **92:**701, 1953.

Santschi, D. R., Frahm, C. J., Pascale, L. R., and Dumanian, A. V.: The Subclavian Steal Syndrome: Clinical and Angiographic Considerations in 74 Cases in Adults, *J Thorac Cardiovasc Surg,* **51:**103, 1966.

Spencer, F. C., and Eiseman, B.: Technique of Carotid Endarterectomy, *Surg Gynecol Obstet,* **115:**114, 1962.

Thompson, J. E., Kartchner, M. M., Austin, D. J., Wheeler, C. G., and Patman, R. D.: Carotid Endarterectomy for Cerebrovascular Insufficiency (Stroke): Follow Up of 359 Cases, *Ann Surg,* **163:**751, 1966.

———— and Patman, R. D.: Endarterectomy for Asymptomatic Carotid Bruits, *Heart Bull,* **19:**116, 1970.

Warren, R., and Triedman, L. J.: Pulseless Disease and Carotid-Artery Thrombosis: Surgical Considerations, *N Engl J Med,* **257:**685, 1957.

Wylie, E. J., Hein, M. F., and Adams, J. E.: Intracranial Hemorrhage following Surgical Revascularization for Treatment of Acute Strokes, *J Neurosurg,* **21:**212, 1964.

Yashon, D., Jane, J. A., and Javid, H.: Long Term Results of Carotid Bifurcation Endarterectomy, *Surg Gynecol Obstet,* **122:**517, 1966.

Abdominal Aneurysms

Bahnson, H. T.: Surgical Treatment of Abdominal Arteriosclerotic Aneurysms, *Surg Clin North Am,* **36:**983, 1956.

Baker, A. G., and Roberts, B.: Long Term Survival following Abdominal Aortic Aneurysmectomy, *JAMA,* **212:**445, 1970.

Creech, O., Jr.: Endo-aneurysmorrophy and Treatment of Aortic Aneurysm, *Ann Surg,* **164:**935, 1966.

DeBakey, M. E., Crawford, E. S., Cooley, D. A., Morris, G. C., Jr., Royster, T. S., and Abbott, W. P.: Aneurysm of the Abdominal Aorta: Analysis of Results of Graft Replacement Therapy One to Eleven Years after Operation, *Ann Surg,* **160:**622, 1964.

Dubost, C., Allary, M., and Oeconomos, M.: Resection of an Aneurysm of the Abdominal Aorta: Re-establishment of the Continuity by a Preserved Human Arterial Graft, with Result after Five Months, *Arch Surg,* **64:**405, 1952.

Estes, J. E., Jr.: Abdominal Aortic Aneurysm: A Study of One Hundred and Two Cases, *Circulation,* **2:**258, 1950.

Imparato, A. M., Berman, I., Bracco, A., Kim, G. E., and Beaudet, R.: Aortic Declamping Shock: Its Prevention, *Surgery,* 1973.

Knowles, P. W., Spencer, F. C., and Steenburg, R. W.: Abdominal Aortic Aneurysm: Successful Excision in a Patient 89 Years of Age, *JAMA,* **178:**661, 1961.

Levy, J. F., Kouchoukos, N. T., Walker, W. B., and Butcher, H. R., Jr.: Abdominal Aortic Aneurysmectomy: A Study of 100 Cases, *Arch Surg,* **92:**498, 1966.

Mehrez, I. O., Nabseth, D. C., Hogan, E. L., and Deterling, R. A., Jr.: Paraplegia following Resection of Abdominal Aortic Aneurysm, *Ann Surg,* **156:**890, 1962.

Nennhaus, H. P., and Javid, H.: The Distinct Syndrome of Spon-

taneous Abdominal Aorto-caval Fistula, *Am J Med,* **44:**464, 1968.

Smith, R. F., and Szilagyi, D. E.: Ischemia of the Colon as a Complication in Surgery of the Abdominal Aorta, *Arch Surg,* **80:**806, 1960.

Szilagyi, D. E., Elliot, J. P., and Smith, R. F.: Clinical Fate of the Patient with Asymptomatic Abdominal Aortic Aneurysm and Unfit for Surgical Therapy, *Arch Surg,* **104:**600, 1972.

Vasko, J. S., Spencer, F. C., and Bahnson, H. T.: Aneurysm of the Aorta Treated by Excision: Review of 237 Cases Followed Up to Seven Years, *Am J Surg,* **105:**793, 1963.

Peripheral Aneurysms: General

Howell, J. F., Crawford, E. S., Morris, G. C., Jr., Garrett, H. E., and DeBakey, M. E.: Surgical Treatment of Peripheral Arteriosclerotic Aneurysm, *Surg Clin North Am,* **46:**979, 1966.

Popliteal Aneurysms

Alpert, J.: Aneurysms of the Popliteal Artery, *J Med Soc NJ,* **67:**791, 1970.

Crichlow, R. W., and Roberts, B.: Treatment of Popliteal Aneurysms by Restoration of Continuity: Review of 48 Cases, *Ann Surg,* **163:**417, 1966.

Edmunds, L. H., Darling, R. C., and Linton, R. R.: Surgical Management of Popliteal Aneurysm, *Circulation,* **32:**517, 1965.

Friesen, G., Ivins, J. C., and Janes, J. M.: Popliteal Aneurysms, *Surgery,* **51:**90, 1962.

Gifford, R. W., Jr., Hines, E. A., Jr., and Janes, J. M.: Analysis and Follow-up Study of 100 Popliteal Aneurysms, *Surgery,* **33:**284, 1953.

Hara, M., and Thompson, B. W.: The Hazards of Popliteal Aneurysms, *Arch Surg,* **92:**504, 1966.

Hunter, J. A., Julian, O. C., Javid, H., and Dye, W. S.: Arteriosclerotic Aneurysms of the Popliteal Artery, *J Cardiovasc Surg,* **2:**404, 1961.

MacCarty, C. S., Janes, J. M., and Allen, E. V.: Treatment of Arteriosclerotic Popliteal Aneurysms by Lumbar Sympathectomy and Extirpation at the Same Operative Session, *Postgrad Med,* **10:**25, 1951.

Spencer, F. C., and Eiseman, B.: Delayed Arterial Embolectomy: A New Concept, *Surgery,* **55:**1, 1964.

Femoral Aneurysms

Crawford, E. S., Edwards, W. H., DeBakey, M. E., Cooley, D. A., and Morris, G. C., Jr.: Peripheral Arteriosclerotic Aneurysm, *J Am Geriatr Soc,* **9:**1, 1961.

Papas, G., Janes, J. M., Bernatz, P. E., and Schirger, A.: Femoral Aneurysms: Review of Surgical Management, *JAMA,* **190:**489, 1964.

Stoney, R. J., Albo, R. J., and Wylie, E. J.: False Aneurysms Occurring after Arterial Grafting Operations, *Am J Surg,* **110:**153, 1965.

Tolstedt, G. E., Radke, H. N., and Bell, J. W.: Late Sequela of Arteriosclerotic Femoral Aneurysms, *Angiology,* **12:**601, 1961.

Carotid Artery Aneurysms

Beall, A. C., Jr., Crawford, E. S., Cooley, D. A., and DeBakey, M. E.: Extracranial Aneurysms of the Carotid Artery: Report of Seven Cases, *Postgrad Med,* **32:**93, 1962.

Kianouri, M.: Extracranial Carotid Aneurysms, *Ann Surg,* **165:**152, 1967.

Paul, R. S., Abadir, A. R., and Spencer, F. C.: Resection of an Internal Carotid Artery Aneurysm under Regional Anesthesia: Posterior Cervical Block, *Ann Surg,* **168:**147, 1968.

Raphael, H. A., Bernatz, P. E., Spittell, J. A., Jr., and Ellis, F. H., Jr.: Cervical Carotid Aneurysms: Treatment by Excision and Restoration of Arterial Continuity, *Am J Surg,* **105:**771, 1963.

Reid, M. R.: Aneurysm in the Johns Hopkins Hospital: All Cases Treated in the Surgical Service from the Opening of the Hospital to January, 1922, *Arch Surg,* **12:**1, 1926.

Sanoudos, G. M., Ramp, J., and Imparato, A. M.: Internal Carotid Aneurysm, *Am Surg,* **39:**118, 1973.

Spencer, F. C.: Aneurysm of the Common Carotid Artery Treated by Excision and Primary Anastomosis, *Ann Surg,* **145:**254, 1957.

Subclavian Aneurysms

Howell, J. F., Crawford, E. S., Morris, G. C., Jr., Garrett, H. E., and DeBakey, M. E.: Surgical Treatment of Peripheral Arteriosclerotic Aneurysm, *Surg Clin North Am,* **46:**979, 1966.

Splenic Artery Aneurysms

Bedford, P. D., and Lodge, B.: Aneurysm of the Splenic Artery, *Gut,* **1:**312, 1960.

Owens, J. C., and Coffey, R. J.: Aneurysm of the Splenic Artery, Including a Report of 6 Additional Cases, *Int Abstr Surg,* **97:**313, 1953.

Renal Artery Aneurysms

Cerny, J. C., Chang, C., and Fry, W. J.: Renal Artery Aneurysms, *Arch Surg,* **96:**653, 1968.

Garritano, A. P.: Aneurysm of the Renal Artery, *Am J Surg,* **94:**638, 1957.

Morris, G. C., Jr.: Discussion of Cerny et al.

Poutasse, E. F.: Renal Artery Aneurysm: Report of 12 Cases, Two Treated by Excision of the Aneurysm and Repair of Renal Artery, *J Urol,* **77:**697, 1957.

Smith, R.: Discussion of Cerny et al.

Traumatic Aneurysms

Crawford, E. S., DeBakey, M. E., and Cooley, D. A.: Surgical Considerations of Peripheral Arterial Aneurysms, *Arch Surg,* **78:**226, 1959.

Dickinson, E. H., Hood, R. H., and Spencer, F. C.: Traumatic Aneurysm of the Innominate Artery, *U.S. Armed Forces Med J,* **3:**1871, 1952.

Hughes, C. W., and Jahnke, E. J., Jr.: The Surgery of Traumatic Arteriovenous Fistulas and Aneurysms: A Five Year Follow-up Study of Lesions, *Ann Surg,* **148:**790, 1958.

Raynaud's Disease

Allen, E. V., Barker, N. W., and Hines, E. A., Jr.: "Peripheral Vascular Diseases," 3d ed., W. B. Saunders Company, Philadelphia, 1962.

Burton, E. E., Jr., et al.: Raynaud's Phenomenon: Treatment with Intraarterial Reserpine, *Cutis (N.Y.),* **9:**464, 1972.

DeTakats, G., and Fowler, E. F.: The Neurogenic Factor in Raynaud's Phenomenon, *Surgery,* **51:**9, 1962.

Farmer, R. G., Gifford, R. W., Jr., and Hines, E. A., Jr.: Raynaud's Disease with Sclerodactylia: A Follow-up Study of Seventy-one Patients, *Circulation,* **23:**13, 1961.

Gifford, R. W., Jr., Hines, E. A., Jr., and Craig, W. McK.: Sympathectomy for Raynaud's Phenomenon: Follow-up Study of 70 Women with Raynaud's Disease and 54 Women with Secondary Raynaud's Phenomenon, *Circulation,* **17:**5, 1958.

Kirtley, J. A., Riddell, D. H., Stoney, W. S., and Wright, J. K.: Cervicothoracic Sympathectomy in Neurovascular Abnormalities of the Upper Extremities: Experiences in 76 Patients with 104 Sympathectomies, *Ann Surg,* **165:**869, 1967.

Nanson, E. M.: The Anterior Approach to Upper Dorsal Sympathectomy, *Surg Gynecol Obstet,* **104:**118, 1957.

Palumbo, L. T.: Anterior Transthoracic Approach for Upper Thoracic Sympathectomy, *Arch Surg,* **72:**659, 1956.

Roos, D. B.: Transaxillary Approach for First Rib Resection to Relieve Thoracic Outlet Syndrome, *Ann Surg,* **163:**354, 1966.

Skoog, T.: Ganglia in the Communicating Rami of the Cervical Sympathetic Trunks, *Lancet,* **2:**457, 1947.

Varadi, D. P., and Lawrence, A. M.: Suppression of Raynaud's Phenomenon by Methyldopa, *Arch Intern Med,* **124:**13, 1969.

Willerson, J. T., and Decker, J. L.: Raynaud's Disease and Phenomenon, a Medical Approach, *Am Heart J,* **82:**572, 1971.

Uncommon Vasomotor Diseases

Allen, E. V., Barker, N. W., and Hines, E. A., Jr.: "Peripheral Vascular Diseases," 3d ed., W. B. Saunders Company, Philadelphia, 1962.

Estes, J. E.: Vasoconstrictive and Vasodilative Syndromes of the Extremities, *Mod Concepts Cardiovasc Dis,* **25:**355, 1956.

Lewis, T., and Landis, E. M.: Observations upon the Vascular Mechanism in Acrocyanosis, *Heart,* **15:**229, 1930.

Frostbite

Ervasti, E.: Frostbites of the Extremities and Their Sequelae: A Clinical Study, *Acta Chir Scand Suppl,* **299,** 1962.

Golding, M. R., Martinez, A., deJong, P., Mendosa, M., Fries, C. C., Sawyer, P. N., Hennigar, G. R., and Wesolowski, S. A.: The Role of Sympathectomy in Frostbite, with a Review of 68 Cases, *Surgery,* **57:**774, 1965.

———, Mendoza, M. F., Hennigar, G. R., Fries, C. C., and Wesolowski, S. A.: On Settling the Controversy on the Benefit of Sympathectomy for Frostbite, *Surgery,* **56:**221, 1964.

Lapp, N. L., and Juergens, J. L.: Frostbite, *Proc Staff Meetings Mayo Clin,* **40:**932, 1965.

Lempke, R. E., and Shumacker, H. B., Jr.: Studies in Experimental Frostbite: VII. An Inquiry into the Mode of Action of Rapid Thawing in Immediate Treatment, *Angiology,* **2:**270, 1951.

Mundth, E. D., Long, D. M., and Brown, R. B.: Treatment of Experimental Frostbite with Low Molecular Weight Dextran, *J Trauma,* **4:**246, 1964.

Orr, K. D., and Fainer, D. C.: Cold Injuries in Korea during Winter of 1950-51, *Medicine (Baltimore),* **31:**177, 1952.

Penn, I., and Schwartz, S. I.: Evaluation of Low Molecular Weight Dextran in the Treatment of Frostbite, *J Trauma,* **4:**784, 1964.

Shumacker, H. B., Jr., and Kilman, J. W.: Sympathectomy in the Treatment of Frostbite, *Arch Surg,* **89:**575, 1964.

Simeone, F. A.: A Preliminary Follow-up Report on Cases of Cold Injury from World War II, in M. I. Ferrer, Cold Injury, *Trans 4th Conf Josiah Macy Jr. Found NY,* 1956, pp. 197-223.

Chapter 22

Venous and Lymphatic Disease

by James A. DeWeese

Venous Thrombosis and Pulmonary Embolism

Etiology
Pathophysiology
Types of Venous Thrombosis
    Superficial Venous Thrombosis
    Deep Venous Thrombosis
Pulmonary Emboli

Venous Insufficiency and Venous Ulcers

Anatomy and Physiology
Etiology of Venous Insufficiency
Symptoms of Venous Insufficiency
Physical Findings
Tests for Venous Insufficiency
Differential Diagnosis
Treatment

Lymphatics and Lymphedema

Anatomy and Physiology of Lymphatic Return
Lymphedema

VENOUS THROMBOSIS AND PULMONARY EMBOLISM

Venous thrombosis is a common direct and indirect cause of morbidity and mortality. During its acute phase, pain and swelling may be incapacitating. The threat of embolization of the thrombus to the pulmonary artery constantly exists. Postthrombotic scarring of the veins may lead to venous insufficiency with chronic discomfort and ulceration. The relatively frequent occurrence of venous thrombosis following operations or trauma arouses the surgeon's interest in the problem. In addition, operative intervention may be indicated to prevent or treat the complications of the thrombosis.

Etiology

Virchow, in the mid 1800s, first recognized three general causes of vascular thrombosis: stasis; injury to the vessel wall; and increased coagulability of the blood. Much more detailed information is now available regarding each of these general causes. Identification of the specific cause for a venous thrombosis seen in a given patient, however, may be very difficult. For example, a patient may present with a deep venous thrombosis following a long car ride, without any history of trauma and without measurable abnor-

malities of coagulation factors. It is currently popular to incriminate stasis of blood as the etiologic agent. However, thousands of people may be in similar positions for equally long periods without developing thrombi. In other words, at the present time the reasons for thrombotic tendencies in certain patients are not known. The situations (as recorded by DeBakey and by Coon and Coller) in which thrombosis is more likely to occur, however, can be identified: following major injuries, following operations, during pregnancy, after previous thrombosis, with cancer, following long periods of sitting or bed rest, with infection, with varicose veins, and in obese females.

The incidences of at least minor thrombosis in these high-risk states have recently been emphasized in the studies of Kakkar. Using a radioiodinated fibrinogen test, venous thrombi were identified in the legs of 27.8 percent of elective surgery patients, in 54 percent of patients with hip fractures, in 3 percent of postpartum women, and in 19 percent of patients with myocardial infarction.

Pathophysiology

Venous thrombosis may be associated with an acute inflammatory response causing pain, local swelling, redness, tenderness, and tachycardia; the syndrome may then be labeled *thrombophlebitis*. Although acute inflammatory changes are present in the vein wall, bacteria are rarely present. The thrombus, on the other hand, may produce no local signs or symptoms and may be loosely attached to a vein wall which microscopically contains only a few chronic inflammatory cells; the condition may then be labeled *phlebothrombosis*. The differentiation of the two types of venous thrombosis, however, is only of academic interest. From a practical viewpoint it is the thrombus which is responsible for the early and late pathologic and physiologic changes, and it is the thrombus which may become a pulmonary embolus.

The thrombus initially causes obstruction of the vein; if the vein is a major one or if many veins are involved, there may be an increase in distal venous pressure. If the pressure in the venous capillaries becomes sufficiently high, water and solutes are not resorbed, and edema occurs. If the pressure becomes higher than local arterial pressures, blood flow ceases and venous gangrene occurs.

Some veins may remain obstructed following thrombosis; others may recanalize. In either case the venous valves are destroyed, leading to chronic venous valvular insufficiency. Thrombi which break loose in the moving venous bloodstream may be swept through the right heart and lodge in the pulmonary arteries as pulmonary emboli.

Although it is not important to differentiate thrombophlebitis and phlebothrombosis, it is important to differentiate superficial and deep venous thrombosis. Thrombi in the superficial veins rarely, if ever, embolize to the lung and can be treated symptomatically unless they propagate into a deep vein. Thrombi in the deep veins frequently embolize, cause permanent damage to the vein, and should be diagnosed early and treated aggressively.

Types of Venous Thrombosis

SUPERFICIAL VENOUS THROMBOSIS

SYMPTOMS. Patients usually complain of aching and swelling localized to a "knot" or "bump" on the leg or arm.

PHYSICAL FINDINGS. The diagnosis can usually be made by palpation of a firm mass or cord along the known course of a superficial vein. In the leg it is helpful to examine the patient in a standing position, since a distended or varicose vein may be palpated above and below the thrombus. In addition, redness, tenderness and *local* induration frequently are present (Fig. 22-1).

DIFFERENTIAL DIAGNOSIS. Insect bites may mimic superficial phlebitis but usually can be differentiated by the history of exposure, the presence of itching, and their lack of relation to the usual anatomic course of the significant superficial veins. Cellulitis or abscesses may at times be difficult to differentiate from thrombophlebitis, but in general, the more marked erythema, tenderness, and finally fluctuance define the diagnosis. The presence of a red lymphatic streak or tender lymphadenopathy may also

Fig. 22-1. Superficial venous thrombosis. There is usually redness, tenderness, and swelling surrounding a palpable, thrombosed superficial vein.

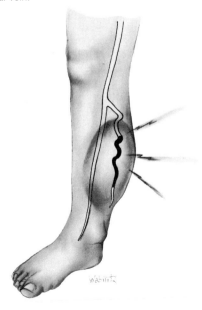

make the diagnosis of infection more obvious. It may be difficult to differentiate a subcutaneous hematoma from a bland thrombus unless a clear-cut history of trauma is present or the site of injury is away from the course of a major vein.

TREATMENT. Nonoperative management is the method of choice in patients with localized disease, since embolization almost never occurs and late morbidity is insignificant. However, superficial venous thrombosis may be present in patients with deep venous thrombosis. The presence of significant distal swelling or of tenderness over the deep veins should make one suspect deep venous thrombosis. A phlebogram may be helpful in ruling out deep-vein involvement.

Nonoperative Management. In general the acute discomfort of the process is over within a few days and symptomatic therapy is adequate. Bed rest is rarely indicated. Hot baths or compresses may be helpful in relieving discomfort. Propagation of the thrombus can usually be prevented by preventing venous stasis. The patient is advised to be either walking with elastic support or lying down with the legs elevated above the level of the heart. Sitting and standing are discouraged. Anticoagulants are not needed. The various enzymatic "clot dissolvers" have little if any effect on the outcome. Expensive and potentially dangerous "anti-inflammatory" drugs do not appear any more effective than aspirin. Antibiotics are not indicated, despite the presence of redness and tenderness, unless a septic cause is obvious.

Operative Treatment. Ligation. Thrombi in the greater saphenous system above the level of the knee may propagate into the common femoral vein, and any evidence of the ascension of such thrombi should be treated by ligation of the vein at the saphenofemoral junction, using local anesthesia. Similarly, the lesser saphenous vein may be ligated in the popliteal fossa.

Excision or Stripping. Veins which are the site of recurrent phlebitis and are stubbornly symptomatic can be ligated at their junctions with the deep system and then excised or in some instances "stripped," as suggested by Herrmann.

DEEP VENOUS THROMBOSIS

The deep veins are hidden within their muscular compartments, and the diagnosis of thrombosis, particularly of the bland type, may be difficult. DeBakey, as well as Barner and DeWeese, have reported that venous thrombosis is recognized prior to death in less than 55 percent of patients with fatal pulmonary emboli. This poor record exists despite the fact that the sources of approximately 85 percent of pulmonary emboli are the veins of the lower extremity, according to the experiences of Byrne and O'Neil, Ravdin and Kirby, and Short.

CLINICAL MANIFESTATIONS. Symptoms. There may be an aching pain, which is aggravated by muscular activity, at the site of a deep venous thrombus. In the presence of a massive thrombosis, there may be an extremely severe aching or cramping pain in the calf and thigh. At other times, however, only a feeling of "heaviness," accentuated by standing, will be noticed. Depending on the site of thrombosis, noticeable swelling may be absent, minimal, or marked. Few, if any, symptoms may be noticed by a patient confined to bed.

Physical Findings. The three signs most frequently described as being useful in the diagnosis of deep venous thrombosis include swelling, tenderness, and Homans' sign. Swelling must be searched for with the aid of a measuring tape; the eye cannot be trusted to tell small or even moderate differences in the size of two extremities. When properly looked for, this sign appears to be the most reliable in making a positive diagnosis of deep venous thrombosis. Tenderness over the thrombosed vein is also usually present if carefully looked for by palpation of the calf, popliteal space, adductor canal, and groin.

Homans was one of the first physicians to emphasize the importance of venous thrombosis in the legs as a source of pulmonary emboli. He popularized a simple test for detecting early thrombosis which is now known as Homans' sign. It is performed by dorsiflexing the foot and is considered positive if the patient complains of calf pain. It is thought that passive elongation of the gastrocnemius and soleus muscles causes irritative pain in the calf when the veins of the calf contain thrombi. Although this test is the easiest to perform, it is unfortunately the least reliable, according to the author's personal experience and to McLachlin et al.

The presence of superficial venous dilatation due to deep vein obstruction is considered by some to be a useful observation, but deep venous obstruction can be more objectively determined by measurement of the venous pressure.

Relation to Site of Involvement. The most frequent site of thrombosis is probably in the veins of the calf, particularly in the venous sinuses of the soleus muscle. Untreated, the thrombi may propagate to involve the femoral vein or even the iliac vein. Actually, however, thrombi that involve the iliac and femoral veins most frequently begin in the valve pockets of those veins and propagate distally, according to Gibbs and to McLachlin and Paterson. The signs and symptoms differ according to the veins involved, and it is worthwhile to consider each of the more common sites individually:

Calf Vein Thrombosis (Fig. 22-2*A*). Although the calf is the most frequent site of thrombosis, diagnosis in this location is probably the one most frequently missed. Calf pain and calf tenderness are usually present, but swelling is present in only 70 percent of cases. If present, the swelling is almost always minimal, the circumference of the involved calf and ankle being less than 1.5 cm greater than the normal limb. Homans' sign may or may not be present. The venous pressure is usually normal, which explains why there is little if any edema.

Femoral Vein Thrombosis (Fig. 22-2*B*). Although combined thrombosis of the calf veins and femoral veins is frequently seen, in some instances the thrombus is localized to the femoral vein. There is usually tenderness in the calf, popliteal region, or adductor canal. Swelling is usually present at the ankle and calf level, as might be predicted from the fact that the venous pressure is usually two to five times normal. Homans' sign may or may not be present.

Iliofemoral Venous Thrombosis (Fig. 22-2*C*). Thrombosis which involves the iliac and femoral veins may also involve the calf veins, but it is frequently sharply localized to the iliofemoral or even iliac level. The left leg is involved two or three times more frequently than the right leg, apparently due to the longer course of the vein, its constriction by the right iliac artery, and the occasional presence of congenital webs at its junction with the vena cava. Iliofemoral venous thrombosis is the most dramatic of the thromboses, since pain, tenderness, and marked swelling of the entire leg are usually present. The venous pressure is considerably elevated, which explains the marked edema and also the bluish discoloration frequently observed during the early course of the process. When pain and cyanosis are present, the process may be termed *phlegmasia cerulea dolens.* This syndrome may progress to venous gangrene secondary to massive thrombosis of all the venous drainage of the part involved. Arterial spasm may also be present in some instances.

Pelvic Vein Thrombosis. Thrombosis of the pelvic veins, including the branches of the internal iliac veins, may be seen in women with pelvic inflammatory disease or in men with involvement of the prostatic plexus. The diagnosis is best made by pelvic or rectal examination plus a high degree of suspicion. Leg signs are not present unless the external and common iliac veins are also involved.

Primary Deep Venous Thrombosis of the Upper Extremity. Although this process of deep thrombosis may be seen in patients with congestive heart failure or with terminal carcinomas, it is more dramatic when it appears in otherwise normal individuals. It has been termed "Paget-Schroetter syndrome," "axillary vein thrombosis," or "effort thrombosis," since it most frequently occurs after some unusual muscular activity of the arm. In otherwise healthy patients, the thrombosis apparently originates in the subclavian vein at the point where the vein can be compressed between the first rib and clavicle. The diagnosis is usually made from swelling of the arm and the presence of tenderness over the axillary vein. Phlebography can confirm the diagnosis and determine the site of the obstruction.

SPECIAL TESTS. Special tests which are helpful in the diagnosis of deep venous thrombosis include (1) phlebography, (2) venous pressure measurements, and (3) noninvasive techniques.

Phlebography. Phlebography provides a means of visualizing the deep veins of the extremities (Fig. 22-3*A,B,C*). It is particularly useful in the patient with equivocal signs or symptoms, since it can provide ancillary evidence for or against the diagnosis of venous thrombosis. It is also helpful in determining the source of pulmonary emboli in patients without significant signs of venous thrombosis. It is helpful in determining the extent of thrombosis in patients who will undergo operative treatment, and it offers an objective means of evaluating any form of therapy.

Since the technique of phlebography was first described

CALF

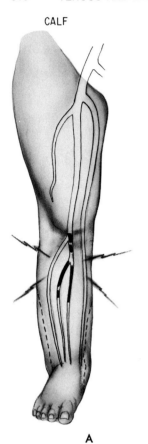

A

FEMORAL

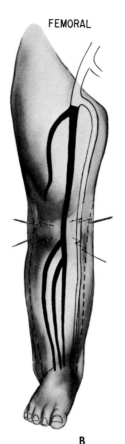

B

ILIO-FEMORAL

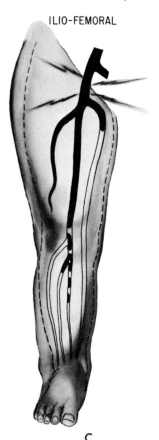

C

Fig. 22-2. *A.* Calf vein thrombosis. Thrombosis is localized to veins of calf and popliteal vein. There is minimal, if any, swelling at level of ankle. Calf pain and tenderness are usually present. Homans' sign may or may not be present. *B.* Femoral vein thrombosis. There is thrombosis of femoral vein and usually associated thrombosis of calf vein. Swelling is usually present and extends to just above level of knee. Popliteal tenderness and calf tenderness may be present. Homans' sign may or may not be present. *C.* Iliofemoral venous thrombosis. There is thrombosis of iliac and proximal femoral vein, and frequently calf veins also are involved. Edema is present from foot to level of inguinal ligament. There is usually tenderness in groin and sometimes popliteal and calf tenderness. Homans' sign may or may not be present.

by Dos Santos and popularized by Bauer, there have been continued improvements in methods. The following technique has been used in over 400 patients with suspected deep venous thrombosis and has been found safe, reliable, and relatively simple to perform.

1. A #21 scalp-vein needle is inserted into a superficial vein on the dorsum of the foot and a slow infusion of saline solution begun to maintain patency of the needle. With experience, a cut-down to expose a vein is rarely necessary.
2. The patient is placed in a semierect position 15 to 45° from the horizontal on a tilt table.
3. A snug rubber tourniquet is placed around the ankle.
4. Over a 1- to 2-minute period, 50 to 100 ml of an angiographic contrast material is injected.
5. Two sets of 14- by 34-in. radiographs are exposed about 30 seconds apart. If the patient was ambulatory prior to the test, he is asked to stand on his toes five times between exposures.

Thrombi are identified as globular or serpentine defects in well-opacified veins. Lack of filling of a vein is considered evidence of venous thrombosis, but only if clots are also seen in the vein, or if the lack of filling of a major vein is associated with visualization of numerous collateral veins at the same level.

Venous Pressure Measurements. Venous pressure is easily measured by inserting a needle into a superficial vein of the foot or ankle and connecting it to a saline solution manometer. The pressure should be compared with those in the other leg and the arm; the test will be positive in the presence of significant venous obstruction only early

in the course of the disease before sufficient collaterals have developed.

Noninvasive Technique. During the past few years, progress has been made in developing noninvasive methods for diagnosing venous thrombosis, i.e., those which require neither incision nor the introduction of needles into the involved extremity. These methods include isotope studies, the Doppler ultrasound technique, and an electrical impedance test, and presently are most valuable in screening patients. The ^{125}I-labeled fibrinogen test is particularly helpful in identifying small areas of thrombosis in the calf, while the Doppler technique is best for identifying significant venous occlusion in the femoral region. However, phlebography may still be necessary in cases where equivocal results are obtained by noninvasive methods, and it

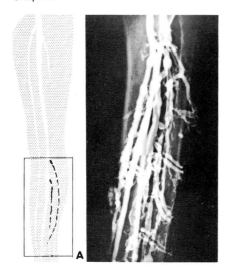
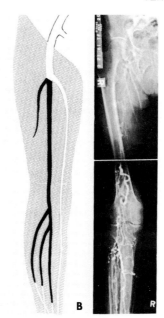
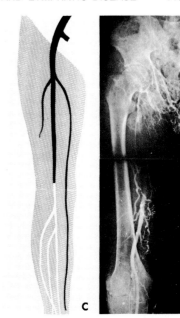

Fig. 22-3. *A.* Phlebogram demonstrating calf throbi. Note areas of relative radiolucency in opaque-filled veins. *B.* Phlebogram demonstrating femoral and calf thrombosis. *C.* Phlebogram demonstrating iliofemoral thrombosis without involvement of calf vein. Note extensive formation of collaterals in upper thigh. (*From J. A. DeWeese and S. M. Rogoff, Surgery, 53:99, 1963.*)

is still recognized as the most definitive test for the diagnosis of deep venous thrombosis.

Isotope Studies. Gomez et al. and Schwartz described methods for the scanning detection of venous thrombi in which radioactive elements are attached to thrombi by either tagged fibrinolytic enzymes or fibrinogen antibodies (Fig. 22-4) Kakkar and Browse more recently reported extensive clinical experience with the use of ^{125}I-labeled fibrinogen to detect venous thrombi.

Human fibrinogen is fractionated from the plasma of a restricted pool of accredited donors to minimize the risk of transmitting viral hepatitis. The fibrinogen is labeled with ^{125}I under sterile conditions and stored at $-20°C$. The patient is given 100 mg of sodium iodide 24 hours before the test to prevent excessive accumulation of the radioactive iodine in the thyroid gland. The test is performed by injecting 100 μCi of the labeled fibrinogen into a femoral vein, and the radioactivity over the legs is measured 2 hours later. Portable bedside equipment is available for this measurement.

The test cannot differentiate thrombi from an inflammatory fibrinous exudate and, therefore, is of no value for patients with superficial thrombophlebitis, recent operative incisions, traumatic wounds, hematomas, cellulitis, active arthritis, or primary lymphedema. In addition, thrombi cannot be accurately diagnosed in the upper thigh and pelvis because of high background counts.

The test is positive only during the active formation or propagation of a thrombus. It is most valuable in detecting the onset of thrombosis in patients at risk, such as during the postoperative period when the test is performed daily

with corroborated accuracy in the range of 90 percent. Test accuracy falls to the 80 percent range when it is used for patients with suspected established deep venous thrombosis.

Doppler Ultrasound Technique. The Doppler ultrasound blood velocity detector emits a sound beam which alters frequency when moving blood cells are encountered. When reflected and detected, the altered frequencies are amplified to drive a loudspeaker or for display on a recorder. Manual compression of the leg augments flow through the veins, producing characteristic "A" sounds for Doppler detection which are hampered or obliterated when venous thrombosis significantly occludes the deep veins.

Sigel et al. have had extensive experience with this technique. The ultrasound method recognized 78.1 percent of new thrombotic venous occlusion corroborated by phlebography. However, the technique cannot differentiate new occlusion from old, and small areas of thrombosis which do not significantly occlude major venous channels cannot be diagnosed.

Electrical Impedance Test. Significant venous obstruction and replacement of blood by thrombi decreases the venous volume changes occurring with respiration. Liquid blood conducts electric currents, and instruments capable of measuring small changes in the electrical resistance of the leg can indirectly assess changes in venous volume. Wheeler et al. have devised an electrical impedance test which uses these principles to detect venous thrombosis indirectly.

Unfortunately, several factors other than patency of the major veins may influence venous volume changes. These include venous tone, extravascular compression which may vary with leg position, and adequacy of the collateral circulation, plus the ventilatory excursion. Dmochowski et al. were able to demonstrate only 53.5 percent test accu-

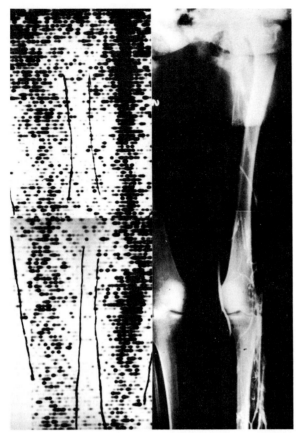

Fig. 22-4. Isotope scan following injection of ^{131}I-labeled anti-fibrinogen. Right leg normal; left leg shows femoral and popliteal thrombus confirmed by phlebography. (*From I. L. Spar, M. I. Varon, R. L. Goodland, and S. I. Schwartz, Arch Surg, 92:752, 1966.*)

racy, and for the present the test must be considered experimental.

DIFFERENTIAL DIAGNOSIS. Superficial venous thrombosis may be associated with deep venous thrombosis. This should be suspected if there is edema other than at the site of thrombosis; if there is calf, popliteal, or groin tenderness; and if Homans' sign is positive. A superficial thrombosis extending to the popliteal space or groin should also arouse suspicion.

A tear of the gastrocnemius or plantaris muscles may mimic a calf vein thrombosis and cause edema, calf tenderness, and a positive Homans' sign. A history of a sharp stinging pain in the calf associated with walking or running and the appearance of ecchymosis over the calf and below the malleoli will usually make the diagnosis of muscle tear obvious. An effusion of the knee joint may produce distal edema and popliteal tenderness but can be differentiated from venous thrombosis by detection of a ballotable patella. A cellulitis in a lymphedematous limb may cause edema of the entire limb and tenderness, but the presence of erythema, high fever, and leukocytosis usually differentiates this condition from an iliofemoral or subclavian vein thrombosis. Phlebography is helpful in differentiating deep venous thrombosis from all these conditions.

TREATMENT. This generally relies on a medical regimen but occasionally requires an aggressive surgical approach.

Nonoperative Treatment. The primary aims of nonoperative therapy are to prevent thrombi which have already formed from embolizing and to prevent new thrombi from forming.

Bed Rest and Elevation. It is generally agreed that bed rest is indicated for approximately 7 days after onset or progression of symptoms to allow thrombi which are present to become firmly adherent to the vein wall. Bed rest prevents the fluctuations of pressure in the deep venous system that occur with walking. Unfortunately, it does not prevent the more marked fluctuations that may occur with straining during defecation, which all too commonly precipitates a fatal pulmonary embolus. Elevation of the legs above the level of the heart to a height equal to the venous pressure in a superficial vein of the foot, if possible, decreases the pressure in the veins and relieves the edema and pain. In addition, the increased rate of flow in the nondistended veins prevents venous stasis and formation of new thrombi. Elastic support is not required with adequate elevation. When ambulation begins, it is limited to walking with elastic support. The elastic support compresses the superficial veins, and, with walking, the rate of flow in the veins is increased and the venous pressure is kept at a minimum, which impedes the development of edema. Standing and sitting are initially forbidden, since the additional hydrostatic pressure in the veins would increase edema and discomfort. Limitation of the amount of standing and sitting may be necessary for periods of 3 to 6 months in patients with extensive iliofemoral venous thrombosis. In this way edema can be reduced until recanalization of the major veins and/or dilation of collaterals has occurred.

Anticoagulation. The propagation of established thrombi may be prevented with anticoagulants such as heparin or one of the coumarin derivatives.

Heparin. Heparin is believed to prevent thrombus formation by reducing platelet adhesiveness, inhibiting the formation of thromboplastin, and acting as an antithrombin to inactivate thrombin. Its effect can be determined by measuring the whole blood clotting time. Propagation of thrombi can be prevented if the clotting time is at least twice normal. Such clotting times can be achieved by the administration of aqueous heparin intravenously, either continuously or every 4 hours in 5,000- to 10,000-unit amounts. Similar results can be obtained by administering 15,000 to 20,000 units of concentrated aqueous heparin (20,000 unit/ml) into the deep fat of the abdominal wall every 12 hours. Heparin therapy is advised for varying lengths of time, but it seems reasonable to use it for a period of 7 days, until the thrombi have become firmly adherent to the vein; the amounts given are then tapered off over a 3- to 5-day period. If the drug is discontinued abruptly, new thrombosis is frequently observed within the next few days. This is described as "heparin rebound" by some but may merely be a return of a pretreatment thrombotic tendency. It is advisable to continue anticoagulant therapy with the coumarin derivatives after discontinuing heparin. Possible complications of heparin therapy are bleeding and arterial emboli. Bleeding is most apt to occur in fresh surgical wounds. If necessary the heparin effect can be reversed by injecting protamine sulfate intravenously in 50- to 100-mg amounts. Platelet emboli have been observed by Roberts et al. in patients receiving heparin, but at this time the mechanism is unknown.

Controlled and comparative studies indicate that heparin therapy is superior to no anticoagulation but that pulmonary emboli may still occur. The incidence of pulmonary emboli in patients with venous thrombosis during treatment with heparin is variously reported as 0.9 to 7.7 percent.

Coumarin Derivatives. The coumarin derivatives may interfere with four factors in the clotting mechanism, but the effect of clinical importance is its reduction of the plasma concentration of prothrombin. Its effect can therefore be determined by measuring the prothrombin time, which must be less than 10 percent of normal to inhibit the propagation of thrombi as effectively as heparin does. This, unfortunately, is the level at which bleeding complications are most likely to occur. However, somewhat higher prothrombin times are apparently able to prevent formation of new thrombi. Coumarin derivatives can be administered orally and at the present time are the drugs of choice for prophylactic therapy or long-term therapy following initial heparin therapy. It appears logical to continue anticoagulation with the coumarin derivatives for approximately 4 weeks after an acute venous thrombosis or pulmonary embolism, since recurrence is most likely within that period. Patients with iliofemoral venous thrombosis may be maintained on therapy for 6 months after the onset, since recurrence is most likely during this period when venous stasis is still being decreased by the enlargement of collaterals.

Other Medications. The administration of fibrinolytic drugs or dextran for the treatment of venous thrombosis shows some promise. At present, however, it would seem best to consider their use experimental until further clinical studies are available.

Operative Treatment. Thrombi can be successfully removed from major veins such as the subclavian, iliac, or femoral. Iliofemoral venous thrombectomy is performed through an incision in the groin, using a local anesthetic (Fig. 22-5), via a femoral venotomy. The iliac system is cleared with forceps and suction applied to polyethylene tubing or long fine catheters with an inflatable balloon on the end. Thrombi can be removed from the femoral vein by the same method plus tight wrapping of the leg with an elastic bandage. The venotomy is then closed with fine arterial suture. In general, venous interruptions are not necessary. Heparin is administered after the operation. The best results are obtained in patients operated on within 1 week of onset and in those in whom the thrombus is segmental in nature as determined by an ascending phlebogram. Care must be taken not to push thrombi into the moving flow of blood in the common iliac vein or inferior vena cava, but pulmonary embolization has rarely if ever occurred during the operation. Despite the use of heparin, thrombosis occasionally recurs, probably secondarily to the

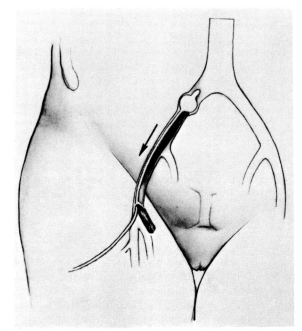

Fig. 22-5. Venous thrombectomy. (*Courtesy of C. Rob and R. Smith.*)

mechanical or inflammatory processes which initiated the thrombosis originally. In general, thrombectomy has successfully decreased the early and late morbidity of massive venous thrombosis, and phlebograms have demonstrated restoration of patent veins with normal valves in at least one-third of patients.

Pulmonary Emboli

INCIDENCE. Complete autopsy studies by Hunter et al. indicate that deep venous thrombi may be found in approximately 50 percent of patients who die in a hospital. Approximately 1 in 5 of these patients demonstrates nonfatal emboli, while 1 in 10 had fatal emboli.

PATHOPHYSIOLOGY. Thrombi, which break loose from their point of origin, pass through the right atrium and ventricle and lodge in the pulmonary arteries. Large thrombi which lodge in major pulmonary arteries may cause immediate death secondary to vasovagal shock, right ventricular failure, and inadequate transfer of oxygen and carbon dioxide in the pulmonary circulation. It is debatable whether small emboli lodging in a lobar or segmental artery can cause death, and if so, by what mechanisms. It is postulated, and supported by some laboratory data, that intense bronchoconstriction and vasoconstriction might explain such an occurrence. Such single small emboli may also result in infarctions. Infection and even abscesses and empyema may ensue. Multiple small emboli may eventually produce enough arterial obstruction to cause pulmonary hypertension and right ventricular failure.

Various autopsy series indicate that the lower extremity (including the iliac veins) is the source of pulmonary emboli in approximately 85 percent of patients. Approximately 10 percent of emboli arise from the right atrium. The remaining 5 percent come from the pelvic veins, vena cava, or upper extremities.

SYMPTOMS. Classically, patients with pulmonary emboli complain of dyspnea, pain, and hemoptysis. The dyspnea is usually the first and may be the only symptom. There may be crushing substernal pain in the presence of a massive embolus lodged in the main pulmonary artery. The pain may be sharp, localized, and stabbing, occurring with breathing, in the presence of a peripheral infarct. This is referred to as *pleuritic* pain. Epigastric pain is occasionally described. Hemoptysis, with coughing up of small flecks or even massive amounts of blood, may occur in the presence of infarction of segments of the lung.

PHYSICAL FINDINGS. Tachycardia is frequently observed, and tachypnea is common. Shock is an ominous sign of a massive embolus. Cyanosis may be present if there is a massive embolus. Splinting of the chest and pleural friction rubs are observed in the presence of peripheral infarcts. Râles may be heard in the region of infiltrates or may be bilateral and bubbling with secondary pulmonary edema. Small pleural effusions are frequently present and sometimes large enough to be recognized on examination.

Less than 50 percent of all pulmonary embolisms found at autopsy had been suspected before death. A retrospective study by Coon and Coller of patients later shown at autopsy to have pulmonary emboli indicates the follow-

Fig. 22-6. Chest x-ray demonstrating peripheral wedge-shaped area of infarction.

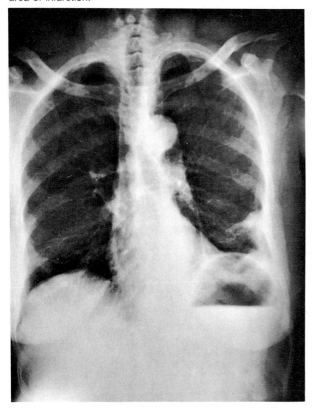

ing frequency of certain signs and symptoms: dyspnea, 58 percent; chest pain, 22 percent; hemoptysis, 11 percent; shock, 28 percent; friction rub, 16 percent. Epigastric pain, cough, fever, and cyanosis are less frequently seen. The classic triad of dyspnea, pain, and hemoptysis was observed in only 3 percent of the patients, and 27 percent appeared to have had no signs or symptoms.

SPECIAL TESTS. Chest X-rays. Since pulmonary emboli do not always cause infarction, the wedge-shaped infiltrate may not be seen (Fig. 22-6). Other signs such as areas of decreased vascularity, dilated pulmonary arteries, or pleural fluid may be found. Stein et al. state that the diagnosis can be suspected from x-rays in approximately 50 percent of patients with pulmonary emboli.

Electrocardiogram. The classic finding of right heart strain is usually not present. However, Henderson reports some significant abnormality concomitant with the acute event in over 60 percent of patients.

Chemical Tests. There is increasing evidence that an elevation of the blood lactic dehydrogenase (LDH) level, as opposed to the serum glutamic oxalacetic transaminase (SGOT) level, is helpful in differentiating pulmonary embolism from myocarial infarction.

Pulmonary Angiograms. Pulmonary angiography probably provides the most effective means of diagnosing pulmonary emboli. It is indicated in patients with unexplained pulmonary infiltrates and in those with recurrent symptoms suggestive of pulmonary emboli. It is most helpful in diagnosing the presence and extent of a massive pulmonary embolus. The procedure may be performed by rapidly injecting a radiopaque material into the right atrium or main pulmonary artery through a catheter threaded into position through a peripheral vein. It can also be performed by the simultaneous rapid injection of a bolus of radiopaque material through needles placed in superficial veins in both arms. Visualization of the significant pulmonary arteries can be obtained by either technique, and occlusion of the arteries can be identified by the lack of filling (Fig. 22-7).

Gas Analysis. Pulmonary arterial obstruction with decreased perfusion of the lung results in a decrease in the alveolar carbon dioxide tension (P_{CO_2}). Therefore, the gradient between the brachial arterial P_{CO_2} and the end-tidal ("alveolar") P_{CO_2}, which is usually minimal, is increased in the presence of significant pulmonary emboli.

Radioisotope Scanning. The rapid intravenous injection of radioactive substances such as [131]I- tagged macroaggregated albumin accompanied by scintillation scanning of the chest may be used to diagnose areas of decreased vascularity in the lung field. Obstruction of the pulmonary arteries by emboli usually results in the appearance of crescent-shaped defects along the lateral borders of the lung (Fig. 22-8).

DIFFERENTIAL DIAGNOSIS. Inflammatory infiltrates of the lung may mimic recurrent pulmonary emboli, particularly on the chest roentgenogram. Significant fever, leukocytosis, and positive sputum cultures usually differentiate the inflammatory from the embolic lesions. Pulmonary edema may result from pulmonary emboli as well as heart disease. The differentiation is easy only in the absence of heart disease or murmurs. It is frequently difficult to differentiate a massive pulmonary embolism from acute myocardial infarction, and in this situation it may be necessary to perform pulmonary angiography to make an accurate diagnosis.

TREATMENT. Venous Interruption. It is generally agreed that interruption of the veins of the lower extremity is indicated if a pulmonary embolus occurs in a patient receiving adequate anticoagulant therapy or in one for whom anticoagulant therapy is contraindicated. In some centers, venous interruptions are even performed prophylactically or instead of administering anticoagulants. The interruption, which can be performed at the femoral vein level if the thrombi are localized in the distal veins, would be the procedure of choice in the desperately ill patient. Phlebography is routinely used in the author's clinic to assist in localizing the thrombi. The interruption should always be performed at the vena cava level in the presence of pelvic vein or iliac vein thrombosis.

Ligation or Division. Ligation or division of the femoral vein is variously performed below the entrance of the deep femoral vein or below the entrance of the greater saphenous vein. The postligation sequelae are less severe if only the superficial femoral vein is ligated. However, the deep femoral vein is also frequently the site of thrombosis, and in such instances ligation of the superficial femoral vein would offer no protection. Donaldson et al. report that approximately 4 percent of patients treated by femoral vein interruption alone develop pulmonary emboli. This is an incidence approximately equal to that following anticoagulation therapy alone.

Ligation or division of the vena cava should be performed just distal to the right renal vein to prevent forming a pocket in which thrombi might develop. The operation requires a general or spinal anesthetic, as opposed to

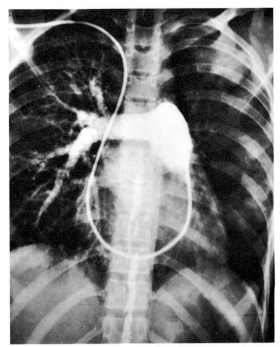

Fig. 22-7. Pulmonary angiogram demonstrating absence of filling of left pulmonary arterial branches, indicative of large embolus obstructing left main pulmonary artery.

femoral vein ligation, which can be performed under local anesthesia. The incidence of pulmonary embolism following this procedure is generally lower than the reported incidence following femoral vein ligation. Its routine use in desperately ill patients, however, can result in an increased mortality rate which may equal that from pulmonary embolism following femoral vein ligation.

The ligation of a vein in which there is distal venous thrombosis usually results in propagation of the thrombus to the site of the ligature. Recurrent phlebitis, pain, edema,

Fig. 22-8. Radioisotope scans following intravenous injection of macroaggregated albumin tagged with [131]I. *A.* Massive pulmonary embolus to right lung. *B.* Small bilateral emboli evidenced by crescent-shaped defects.

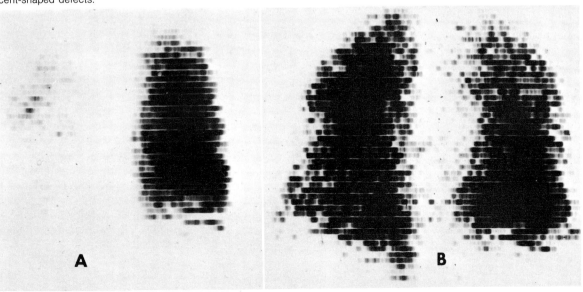

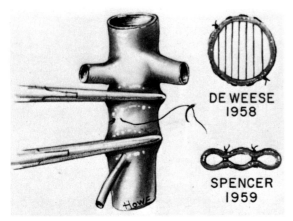

Fig. 22-9. Partial interruption of inferior vena cava: grid and compartmentalization.

and ulceration may ensue. Adams and DeWeese report a 30 to 35 percent incidence of these distressing postligation sequelae.

Partial Vein Interruption. In the hope of preventing post-ligation sequelae, partial interruptions of the femoral vein or inferior vena cava have been performed to allow normal venous flow and yet trap potential pulmonary emboli (Figs. 22-9, 22-10). The methods described include creation of a grid filter of silk sutures [DeWeese], compartmentaliz-ation of the vein with sutures [Spencer et al.], constriction of the vein with a plastic clip [Moretz], and compart-mentalization of the vein with a plastic clip having serrated edges [Miles et al.]. Although thrombosis may occur at the site of the partial interruption or the vein may be occluded by a trapped embolus, the results of such an occurrence would be no worse than if the vein were ligated. Mobin-Uddin et al. devised a filter which can be introduced under

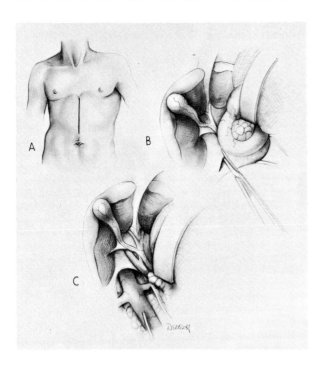

local anesthesia through a small incision into the jugular vein. Under fluoroscopic control, the collapsed filter is passed to the lower vena cava on the tip of a catheter. As the catheter is withdrawn, the filter is dislodged, opens like an umbrella, and is impinged against the wall of the vena cava distal to the renal vein. However, the umbrella can be misplaced or subsequently dislodged, and at present it appears to be ideally suited for the desperately ill patient who requires interruption at the vena cava level.

Comparison of the reported results of all types of vena cava interruption indicates a slightly higher incidence of nonfatal pulmonary emboli following partial interruption than following ligation (6.7 versus 4.1 percent) (Table 22-1). The incidence of fatal emboli following both proce-dures is about 1 percent. However, fatal shock secondary to ligation of the vena cava with sudden decrease in venous return or massive distal venous thrombosis occurred in 2.9 percent of cases, compared to no observed occurrence following partial interruption.

When postoperative vena cavagrams are performed fol-lowing partial interruptions, at least 70 percent are patent, and the incidence of significant late postphlebitic sequelae is only 7 percent following partial interruption compared to 23 percent following ligation. In addition, the large collaterals observed by Parrish et al. following vena cava ligation are capable of transmitting fatal pulmonary emboli from the lower extremities within a few weeks after operation.

Partial interruption of the femoral veins was also found by Adams et al. to be at least as effective as ligation in preventing pulmonary embolism and associated with less late extremity morbidity.

Urokinase Therapy. Urokinase activates the available plasminogen which causes lysis of thrombi. Treatment of pulmonary embolism with materials of high specific activ-ity which are much less toxic and pyrogenic than previ-ously available plasminogen activators was recently evalu-ated in a cooperative study. Twelve-hour urokinase infusion followed by at least 5 days of heparin was more effective than heparin alone in lysing thrombi, as seen by significantly greater improvement in pulmonary arterio-grams, lung scans, and right heart pressure measurements.

Fig. 22-10. Partial interruption of inferior vena cava using ser-rated clip. *A.* Transperitoneal approach is preferred to permit high interruption of vena cava and concomitant ligation of the left spermatic or ovarian veins. *B.* Kocher maneuver. *C.* Vena cava cleared immediately below renal veins. *D.* Clip applied. *E.* Clip closed. *F.* Final position of clip in the immediate infrarenal region to prevent cul-de-sac. (*From J. T. Adams and J. A. DeWeese, Surg Gynecol Obstet, 123:1087, 1966.*)

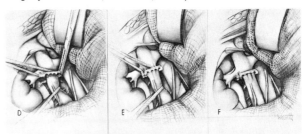

Table 22-1. *Table 22-1.* VENA CAVA INTERRUPTIONS:
COMPARISON OF LIGATIONS AND
PARTIAL INTERRUPTIONS*

	Ligation	Partial interruptions
Operations	1,159	569
Operative mortality	14.0%	10.3%
Fatal emboli	1.3%	0.7%
Fatal shock	2.9%	0
Nonfatal emboli	4.1%	6.7%
Patent vena cava	0†	72.0%†
Disabling symptoms	23.0%‡	7.0%‡

*A summary of 30 reports.
†In patients who had postoperative vena cavagrams.
‡When late follow-up information was available.

Unfortunately, bleeding complications were sufficiently frequent and severe that Sautter et al. felt urokinase therapy to be contraindicated within 10 days of childbirth or any operation within the major body cavity. Severe systemic hypertension, a recent cerebrovascular accident, active gastrointestinal bleeding, renal or hepatic insufficiency, active rheumatic disease, bacterial endocarditis, a history of nephritis, or pregnancy at any stage were also considered contraindications. No significant differences in the rate of pulmonary embolism recurrence or in the 2-week mortality rate were observed. The report concluded that further evaluation of urokinase in the treatment of pulmonary thromboembolism is indicated before specific therapeutic recommendations can be made.

Pulmonary Embolectomy. Approximately 95 percent of patients with a pulmonary embolism massive enough to cause hypotension die. Although most of them die within a few minutes, at least 25 percent live longer than 1 hour. In 1908 Trendelenburg first advocated the emergency removal of large emboli from the pulmonary artery. From 1908 to 1962 only 17 survivors of such a procedure were reported. Since the development of cardiopulmonary bypass, however, pulmonary embolectomies are performed much more frequently. With this technique the main pulmonary arteries can be opened leisurely and emboli removed. Peripheral emboli can also be evacuated by massaging the lung and by the use of catheters to which suction is applied. It may be possible to use a portable temporary cardiopulmonary bypass to sustain desperately ill patients until they can be transported to the operating room. The studies of Sautter et al. suggest that urokinase therapy is preferable to pulmonary embolectomy for patients recovering from shock. Patients with cardiac arrest or unresponsive shock are still candidates for emergency cardiopulmonary bypass and pulmonary embolectomy.

VENOUS INSUFFICIENCY
AND VENOUS ULCERS

There are three conditions of the veins of the lower extremities associated with venous ulcers. These are varicose veins, incompetent perforators, and deep venous abnormalities. Venous ulcers usually appear in the presence of one, two or all three of these conditions, and they are therefore best discussed together. The abnormality common to all is reflux of blood from the deficiency or absence of competent valves.

Hippocrates (460–377 B.C.) is credited with first noting the association between varicose veins and ulcers of the leg and recommending the use of compression bandages in their treatment. However, many centuries elapsed before the role of deep venous abnormalities in the etiology of venous ulcers was appreciated. Gay and Homans demonstrated the relation between postthrombotic changes including the destruction of venous valves, and venous ulcers. More recently Linton and also Dodd and Cockett have emphasized the role of the incompetent perforator in causing ankle ulceration.

Anatomy and Physiology

The veins of the lower extremity consist of superficial veins, deep veins, and perforating veins which join the superficial and deep systems. The superficial veins consist of the greater saphenous and lesser saphenous veins. The greater saphenous vein begins on the dorsum of the foot, passes *anterior* to the medial malleolus, ascends the medial calf and thigh lying close to the deep facia, and enters the common femoral vein in the groin through the fossa ovalis. Several smaller veins join the greater saphenous vein along its course. The important branches, clinically, include the anterior and posterior branches of the lower leg, which enter the major vein in the upper medial calf region, and the lateral and medial branches of the upper leg, which join the saphenous in the upper thigh (Fig. 22-11*A*). The lesser saphenous vein begins posterior to the lateral malleolus, ascends the posterior calf, where it pierces the deep fascia, usually near the popliteal fossa, and enters the popliteal vein (Fig. 22-11*B*).

The deep veins, in general, follow the course of the major arteries and carry the same names. In the lower leg, however, the veins are routinely paired. The paired anterior tibial, posterior tibial, and peroneal veins join to form the popliteal vein in the region of the knee. The popliteal vein passes beneath the adductor tendon, where it becomes the superficial femoral vein and is joined by the deep femoral vein in the upper thigh to become the common femoral vein. The common femoral veins become the external iliac veins as they pass beneath the inguinal ligament and are joined in the pelvis by the internal iliac veins to become the common iliac veins; these veins join to become the inferior vena cava.

There are numerous veins perforating the deep fascia connecting the superficial and deep veins. The most constant and clinically important of these perforators are those posterior and superior to the medial malleoli. These perforators, which usually are three in number, connect the posterior branch of the greater saphenous vein to the paired posterior tibial veins. One perforator usually lies posterior to the medial malleolus, the second is 5 to 10 cm superior to the first, and the third is 5 to 10 cm higher

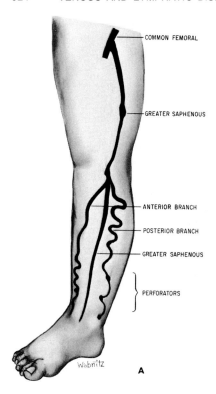

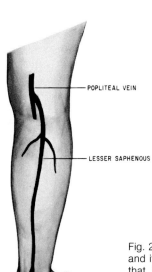

Fig. 22-11. *A.* Usual course of greater saphenous vein and its major branches in lower leg, emphasizing fact that branch varicosities are the ones usually seen. Perforating veins, posterior and superior to medial malleoli, are indicated. *B.* Usual course of lesser saphenous vein in lower leg.

(Fig. 22-11*A*). A similar perforator connects the lesser saphenous and peroneal veins posterior and superior to the lateral malleolus.

Normal veins contain bicuspid valves, which, although sometimes found in other areas, are almost always just distal to major branches. In the upper leg only a few valves are found, whereas in the lower leg they are numerous in both the superficial and deep systems. The valves are oriented to permit flow of blood superiorly in the super-

Fig. 22-12. Orientation of valves and flow of blood in superficial, deep, and perforating veins of lower leg.

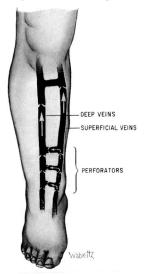

ficial and deep veins. More important is the fact that the valves in the perforators normally allow flow only from the superficial to the deep veins (Fig. 22-12).

There is normally a progressive decrease in mean pressure in the bloodstream beginning in the left ventricle and ending in the right atrium. It is this force from behind, or vis a tergo, that guarantees the continued flow of blood in the venous system. The actual pressure in any one vessel, however, is also dependent on the effect of gravity. In the standing resting position, therefore, the actual pressure in any vein includes a hydrostatic pressure approximately equivalent to the distance between the vein and the heart. The actual pressures in the arteries are also increased by hydrostatic pressure, and venous flow continues.

In addition to vis a tergo, venous return is aided by muscular action and possibly by respiration. Contraction of the calf muscles, for example, squeezes blood from the intramuscular veins into the deep veins. In addition, the veins which pass through the relatively rigid fascial compartment about the muscle are also compressed by the muscle. The combined result is an increase in pressure and flow in the popliteal vein and increased venous return with muscular contraction. During relaxation of the muscles the popliteal venous pressure falls below the resting pressure, and increased emptying of the superficial veins into the deep veins occurs, so that with repeated muscular activity the quantity of blood in the superficial veins decreases and superficial venous pressure decreases to below normal resting pressures. It must be emphasized that these normal variations in venous pressure and flow are dependent upon normal valves. Valves in the calf veins prevent reflux of blood distad when the venous pressure is increased by muscle contraction. Valves in the perforators prevent reflux of blood from the deep into the superficial veins during muscular contraction. The negative intrathoracic pressure which is accentuated by inspiration is believed by some to increase venous return. This positive effect is probably offset by the increased abdominal pressure secondary to descent of the diaphragm, which slows venous return.

Etiology of Venous Insufficiency

The causes of venous insufficiency are varicose veins, incompetent perforators, and deep vein abnormalities.

VARICOSE VEINS. The term *varicose veins* is usually applied to dilated, tortuous, elongated branches of the greater and lesser saphenous veins. These branches are quite superficial and are, therefore, most easily seen. The same changes occur to a much lesser extent in the greater and lesser saphenous veins themselves. The important abnormality in both the branches and the major superficial veins in the incompetency of their valves.

It is not known whether the valvular incompetency is the cause of the dilatation of the veins in varicosities or whether the dilatation of the valvular ring occurs first and causes secondary valvular incompetence. There are probably several causes of varicose veins. The rare presence of varicose veins in very small children without other visible arterial and venous malformations indicates that they may be congenital. The occurrence of severe varicosities in several members of a family suggests that heredity may be important in some cases. The frequent appearance of varicosities during pregnancy is well known, but it is not known whether hormonal influence, increased pelvic venous blood flow, or the mechanical effect of the enlarged uterus is the primary cause of these varicosities. The appearance of varicose veins in patients with congenital or acquired arteriovenous shunts implicates these as causative factors. The appearance of branch varicosities following superficial venous thrombosis indicates that trapping and fragmentation of the valves by the thrombus as it retracts to the wall and becomes organized is of importance in some instances. The predilection of varicose veins for the lower extremities in human beings, as opposed to quadrupeds, and for people in professions requiring long periods of standing indicates that the hydrostatic pressure in the veins of the lower extremities in the standing resting position aggravates and may actually cause varicosities.

INCOMPETENT PERFORATORS. There are numerous perforators between the superficial and deep veins. The largest and most constant are those posterior and superior to the medial and lateral malleoli. Normally these perforators cannot be demonstrated clinically. When their valves are incompetent, however, they become dilated and may form rather large localized dilatations at their junctions with the superficial vein. Defects in the deep fascia of the leg at the site where the dilated perforators pierce the fascia may be palpated. The frequent occurrence of incompetent perforators following deep venous thrombosis suggests that the valvular damage in these instances is secondary to recanalization of the perforators. Incompetent perforators, however, may be found in patients without known previous venous thrombosis but with varicose veins. It is likely, therefore, that the factors which cause venous dilatation and valvular incompetency in the valves of other veins may also cause incompetency of the valves of the perforating veins.

DEEP VEIN ABNORMALITIES. The most common abnormalities of the deep veins result from thrombosis of the veins. Following thrombosis, the major deep veins may become patent by gross recanalization, or they may remain functionally occluded, with only microscopic recanalization. With gross recanalization, the veins have the phlebographic appearance of irregular walled valveless tubes. If the veins remain occluded, numerous dilated collaterals *without apparent valves* are visualized. Examination of the occluded major veins demonstrates only microscopic recanalization. The deficiency or absence of valves and the dilatation of the deep veins is observed also in many patients with complicated varicose vein problems. This suggests that the congenital or familial causes of varicosities may also cause deep vein abnormalities.

Symptoms of Venous Insufficiency

The symptoms most frequently attributed to venous insufficiency of the lower extremities include aching, swelling, and night cramps.

An "aching" discomfort in the lower legs is frequently described by patients with severe venous insufficiency. With lesser degrees of insufficiency, "tenderness" of the legs or a "heaviness" may be described. The discomfort may occur soon after arising in the morning but usually begins after a period of relatively inactive standing or sitting, as experienced by housewives while they are ironing or washing dishes. Salesgirls, secretaries, dentists, and even surgeons may have similar periods of inactive standing. In many women the symptoms are worse just before and during the first part of the menstrual period. The symptoms are relieved by elevation of the legs.

Edema of the lower leg may also occur in venous insufficiency. Although it may occur with varicose veins alone, it is almost always seen in patients with deep venous abnormalities and incompetent perforators. It usually appears during the course of the day and is aggravated by prolonged standing or sitting. It usually disappears or is markedly decreased during a night's sleep.

The explanation for the heaviness, tiredness, and aching is undoubtedly the increase in the weight of the lower extremities secondary to an increase in volume of blood and edema fluid. In a normal individual the erect position is associated with an increased volume of blood in the legs. This volume is increased in venous insufficiency, where dilated veins increase the potential storage space and incompetent valves hinder venous return. Normally the erect position is also associated with an increased amount of interstitial fluid, transferred across the arterial capillary membrane. This fluid is normally resorbed by the venous capillaries or lymphatics. Resorption by the veins is primarily due to the osmotic force exerted by the intravascular protein, but an increase in venous pressure can overcome the osmotic force and prevent resorption. The venous pressure at the ankle in the normal erect individual is sufficient to prevent resorption, and indeed an increase in interstitial fluid is observed. In normal individuals, however, the venous pressure is markedly decreased by the frequent muscular contractions occurring with daily living. The same exercise in patients with venous insufficiency causes lesser decreases in the pressure and hence more significant increases in interstitial fluid (or edema). Lymphatic abnormalities can also decrease the resorption of the interstitial fluid. Such abnormalities may be observed in patients following venous thrombosis.

Night cramps are due to sustained contractions of muscles and most frequently occur in the muscles of the calf and feet. They usually appear after a few hours of sleep. They are relieved by massage or by standing and walking. Night cramps may be associated with a number of other abnormalities besides venous insufficiency. Patients with night cramps secondary to venous insufficiency, however, can be relieved by proper management. The underlying cause of the increased muscular irritability or increased muscular stimulation is unknown.

Physical Findings

The changes which may be observed in patients with venous insufficiency include edema, brawny induration, brownish discoloration, dermatitis, and ulceration.

Edema also may be observed in patients with varicose veins, but it is almost always present to some degree in patients with deep vein pathologic conditions and incompetent perforators. It may be soft and pitting initially and may completely disappear overnight. In the presence of long-standing venous insufficiency, however, the edema becomes more firm and may decrease slowly and minimally with elevation. It then acquires a "woody" feeling, termed *brawny induration*, due to increased connective tissue in the subcutaneous tissue. This scarring may be secondary to excess protein in the interstitial tissue (see section below on lymphedema) or to repeated trauma, infection, and phlebitis.

Fig. 22-13. Venous ulcers of lower leg.

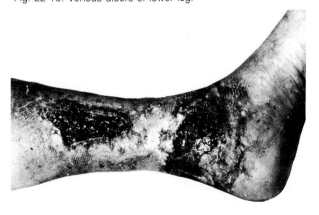

Brown pigmentation of the lower leg is frequently observed in long-standing venous insufficiency, particularly about healed ulcers. It is known to be secondary to hemosiderin in the subcutaneous tissue, presumably derived from the breakdown of extravasated blood.

Various types of dermatitis may be seen in patients with venous insufficiency. Dryness and scaling with some pruritis may be seen over prominent varices, particularly at the ankle level. Although the cause is unknown, this condition is apparently related to the underlying venous abnormalities, since it will disappear with treatment of the venous insufficiency alone. Skin infections secondary to dermatophytosis (athlete's foot) may be seen. The most frequent dermatitis, however, is secondary to local medications. The allergic dermatitis may be particularly difficult to control.

Venous ulcers are almost always found in the lower third of the lower leg and are particularly common posterior and superior to the medial and lateral malleoli (Fig. 22-13). Characteristically they are shallow ulcerations with surrounding rims of bluish discoloration and erythema. They may penetrate to the level of the deep fascia or tendons, but not through them. They can, however, erode veins or even arteries. They may on occasion encircle the leg.

The ulcers may appear spontaneously or follow trivial trauma. The underlying problem, however, is venous insufficiency, a point frequently forgotten by the patient and ignored by the physician treating him. Their occurrence in the ankle region incriminates the high venous pressure of the superficial veins in that region as a prime cause. Further support for this hypothesis is the fact that ulcerations are more common in patients with deep vein abnormalities and incompetent perforators than in patients with varicose veins alone. The high venous pressure results in localized varicosities and edema, with consequent increased deposition of fibrous tissue. A localized area of redness, tenderness, and brawny induration frequently precedes an ulcer. Dodd and Cockett present interesting pathologic material to support the thesis that this preulcer state is due to thrombosis of small end veins in the subcutaneous tissue resulting in fat necrosis. A contusion, laceration, or necrosis of the skin over this area results in a deep ulceration because of the underlying fat necrosis.

Although the above chain of events may occur rapidly after the onset of venous insufficiency, it more commonly occurs several years later. Bauer followed a group of patients with known deep venous thrombosis for several years: ulcers appeared in 20 percent of the patients within 5 years, in 52 percent within 10 years, and in 79 percent at a later date.

Test for Venous Insufficiency

There are a number of tests for diagnosing of venous insufficiency which are also helpful in understanding the pathophysiology of the condition and differentiating the various causes.

PERCUSSION TEST. This test, which is commonly associated with the name of Schwartz, was originally described as a means of determining the incompetency of valves in superficial veins. The saphenous vein is tapped near the saphenofemoral junction and the opposite hand placed over the knee to feel the impulse transmitted through an unbroken column of blood if the valves are incompetent. The percussion of veins may actually be more helpful in other ways. The greater saphenous vein in the thigh usually lies quite close to the deep facia and is neither visible nor palpable, particularly in obese individuals. Percussion of a varix in the region of the knee, with the opposite hand following the expected course of the greater saphenous vein, can confirm the association of the varix with the greater saphenous vein. In addition, once the varicose saphenous vein is found by percussion, its size can be estimated. In a similar fashion the size, position, and importance of the lesser saphenous vein in the popliteal space can be determined by tapping varicosities on the posterior calf.

COMPRESSION TESTS. These tests are usually associated with the name of Trendelenburg. The patient lies down and elevates the involved leg until the superficial veins are collapsed. The saphenous vein is then compressed high in the thigh with the fingers of the hand or with a *tight* tourniquet (part 1). With the hand or tourniquet in place, the patient stands up. The sites of previously noted varicosities are carefully observed for 20 to 30 seconds (part 2). The tourniquet is then removed and the veins again carefully observed. There are four possible results of the test:

1. Negative-negative (Fig. 22-14*A*). In the presence of normal veins there is gradual ascending filling of the superficial veins when the patient stands up; part 1 is negative. With release of compression the gradual filling continues; part 2 is negative.
2. Negative-positive (Fig. 22-14*B*). In the presence of incompetent valves in the greater saphenous vein without incompetent valves in the perforators, part 1 is negative. With release of compression, however, there is rapid reflux of blood from the femoral vein into and down the greater saphenous vein, with rapid distension of the varicosities; part 2 is positive.
3. Positive-negative (Fig. 22-14*C*). In the presence of incompetent valves in the perforators, there is reflux of blood from the deep to the superficial system when the patient stands up. The varices in the region of the perforator becomes rapidly filled, and part 1 is positive. If the saphenofemoral valve is competent, there is no further rapid distension of the veins when the compression is released, and part 2 is negative.
4. Positive-positive (Fig. 22-14*D*). In the presence of incompetent valves in the perforators and also in the greater saphenous vein, filling of the varices occurs on standing, and further rapid filling occurs after the compression is released. Both part 1 and part 2 are positive.

Thus the test can detect the presence of an incompetent saphenous vein and determine the site of incompetent perforators.

VENOUS PRESSURE. The normal standing resting pressure in the saphenous vein at the level of the ankle is slightly higher than the hydrostatic pressure of a column of blood reaching from the tip of the catheter to the level of the right midatrium. There are no significant differences in the standing resting pressures for normal extremities and for extremities with varicose veins, incompetent perforators, or abnormal deep vein valves. With walking or rhythmic contraction of the calf muscles, different venous pressure responses are noted (Fig. 22-15). Normally there is a marked decrease in the saphenous vein pressure with exercise, indicating that the muscular action has increased the flow of blood in the deep veins and allowed increased drainage of blood from the superficial to the deep veins during muscular relaxation. When exercise stops, there is a gradual return of venous pressure to normal levels, indicating that the valves in the deep and the superficial systems are competent, preventing rapid reflux of blood. Extremities with varicose veins demonstrate lesser decreases in venous pressure with exercise and more rapid return to normal levels when walking ceases; that is, some of the effect of the rapid emptying of the superficial veins with exercise is counteracted by reflux of blood from the femoral vein into the saphenous vein with its incompetent valves. When exercise stops, there is rapid reflux of blood down the saphenous vein. In the presence of uncomplicated varicose veins, pressure on the saphenofemoral junction or operative removal of the varicosity can result in a normal venous pressure response. Extremities with postthrombotic veins demonstrate little if any decrease in pressure with exercise. After cessation of exercise the venous pressure rapidly returns to normal. The normal decrease in pressure with exercise is prevented by the reflux of blood back down the abnormal valveless deep veins during muscular relaxation and the propulsion of blood through incompetent perforators during muscular contraction. Ligation of the femoral vein in these patients does not significantly improve the venous pressure response. In the presence of significant obstruction of the deep veins, such as may be seen following a major venous thrombosis or during some pregnancies, the venous pressure actually increases with exercise. Following exercise, the pressure slowly decreases to normal.

FUNCTIONAL PHLEBOGRAPHY. Phlebograms performed with the patient in the semierect position before and immediately after a standard active exercise may demonstrate important pathologic and physiologic abnormalities:

1. The patient lies on a table tilted 60° from the horizontal.
2. A #21 needle is inserted into any superficial vein on the dorsum of the foot and a tourniquet applied snugly to the ankle.
3. Over a 1-minute period, 50 ml of any suitable angiographic contrast material is injected.
4. Radiographs of the entire lower extremity are taken before and after the patient stands on his toes ten times.

Normally, slender veins with prominent valves are visualized, and after exercise little radiopaque material is seen except in the cusps of the valves. In the presence of varicose veins alone, the appearance of the deep veins before and after exercise is usually the same as with normal veins. If the superficial veins are visualized, tortuosity and dilatation of the veins may be seen. Following deep venous thrombosis, the veins may be completely recanalized but valveless. They may also remain obstructed, in which case numerous dilated valveless collaterals are visualized. Following exercise there is poor emptying of the radiopaque material from the deep veins, and increased filling of collateral veins, perforating veins, and superficial veins may be seen. Similar changes and responses to exercise may be seen in patients with dilated valveless deep veins

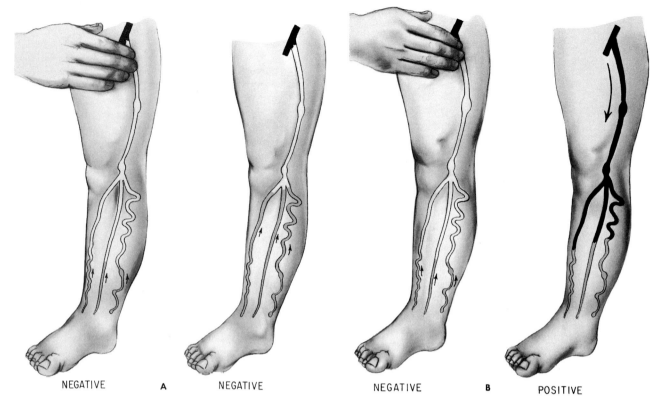

presumably of congenital or familial origin. The poor emptying of the radiopaque dye from the veins and dye reflux through perforators into the superficial veins is another demonstration of the abnormal valvular function seen in patients with venous insufficiency.

Differential Diagnosis

Lymphedema may be confused with the edema of venous insufficiency in the early postthrombotic phase before brawny induration, brownish discoloration, and ulceration occur. Lymphedema, however, generally is of a rubbery consistency and is nonpitting. The edema of congestive heart failure and renal failure is usually bilateral and should also be differentiated by the history and physical examination. Phlebography is particularly helpful in ruling out deep venous thrombosis as a cause of edema.

Venous ulcers almost always occur behind the medial and lateral malleoli. Their positions and associated brawny induration and brownish discoloration generally differentiate them from arterial ulcers, which may occur anywhere on the lower leg, usually have a surrounding blue and then erythematous ring, and are much more painful than venous ulcers. It should also be noted that venous ulcers do not penetrate fascia as arterial ulcers commonly do. A malignant tumor should be suspected in ulcerations of long duration, particularly if they do not respond to proper management.

Treatment

Experience with several hundred patients with venous insufficiency in the author's large vascular clinic indicates

Fig. 22-14. Four possible results of Trendelenburg compression test. Patient has been lying down with leg elevated; he then stands up with compression over saphenofemoral junction. *A.* Negative-negative response, in which there is gradual filling of veins from below over a 30-second period and there is continued slow filling after release of hand. *B.* Negative-positive response. On standing, there is gradual filling of distal veins; on release of compression there is rapid retrograde filling of saphenous vein. *C.* Positive-negative response. With hand in place, filling of superficial varicosities through incompetent perforators occurs; with release of compression there is further slow filling of the veins. *D.* Positive-positive response. On standing with hand in place, there is filling of varices through incompetent perforators. On release of compression there is additional rapid filling of saphenous vein.

that the management of these patients is demanding but rewarding. A single operative procedure is rarely curative except in the mildest cases. Careful education of the patient in the nonoperative management is of utmost importance. In addition, the patients must be seen periodically in order to be sure that they are continuing proper elastic support and periodic elevation.

NONOPERATIVE MANAGEMENT. The nonoperative management of patients with venous insufficiency is based on decreasing the amount of blood sequestration in the veins of the lower extremities and decreasing the venous pressure in the superficial veins.

Elevation of the legs overcomes the hydrostatic pressure in the veins and thereby decreases the pressure and the amount of blood in the dilated valveless veins. It should be emphasized that this is accomplished ideally only when the legs are elevated above the level of the heart, which

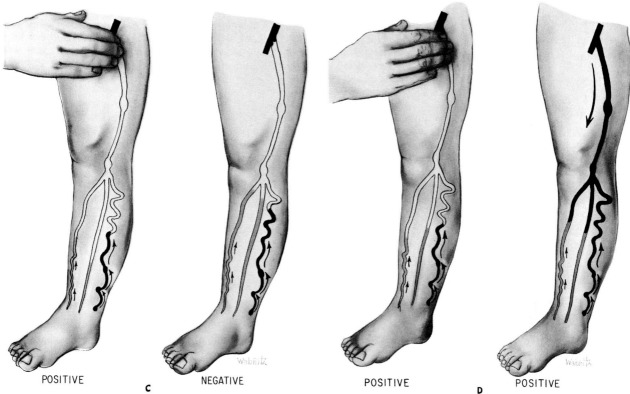

POSITIVE   NEGATIVE   C   POSITIVE   D   POSITIVE

Fig. 22-14 (continued)

Fig. 22-15. Responses in venous pressure of superficial veins at ankle with exercise. In standing position, venous pressure is slightly higher than hydrostatic pressure in column extending from ankle to heart. This pressure is approximately the same for normal persons and for those with venous insufficiency or chronically obstructed veins in which collaterals have formed. With walking, however, normal persons demonstrate rapid decrease in venous pressure and slow return to normal when exercise stops; patients with varicose veins show lesser decrease in pressure with walking but more prompt return to normal following cessation of exercise; patients with postthrombotic veins demonstrate little if any decrease in venous pressure with walking and rapid return to normal; patients with obstructed veins show increase in pressure with walking and slow return to normal.

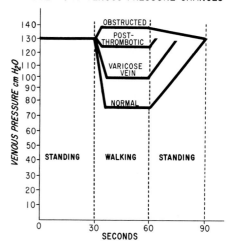

is facilitated by having the patient sleep with the foot of the bed or the foot of the mattress elevated. During the day, the patient should lie on a couch with the feet elevated on pillows. A sitting posture in a chair with the legs outstretched does not provide adequate elevation.

Active exercise, except in the presence of obstruction, also decreases the volume and pressure in the veins of the lower extremities. Walking is excellent exercise. Standing, without muscular contraction, and sitting increase the volume and pressure of the peripheral venous blood.

Compression of the superficial veins also decreases the volume of the venous pool and if strong enough overcomes the venous pressure transmitted through the superficial veins via incompetent perforators. Means of providing compression vary in strength and, in order of increasing effectiveness, include nylon support hose, ordinary cotton elastic stockings, snugly applied Ace bandages, heavy-duty cotton elastic stockings (Truform), specially constructed pressure-gradient stockings (Jobst), Gelucast, Unna's paste, or Elastoplast boots, and canvas boots containing an inflatable rubber bladder (Aeropulse). The goals of any compression therapy are the relief of symptoms and the prevention of measurable evening swelling of the legs. The importance of proper elastic support in accomplishing this goal cannot be overemphasized. Nylon support hose and ordinary cotton elastic stockings are effective only in the management of patients with very mild venous insufficiency. Ace bandages are only as good as the care with which they are applied. The management of patients with moderate to severe insufficiency and particularly those with ulceration demands the use of one of the stronger means of support.

The severity of the venous insufficiency governs the type of therapy prescribed. A patient with mild symptomatic varicosities might find relief of symptoms and edema with ordinary cotton elastic stockings and elevation of the legs whenever there is a choice between lying down and sitting down. A patient with severe venous insufficiency would need more aggressive treatment similar to the "new way of life" described by Luke. The patient may require overnight elevation of the legs, planned periodic elevation of the legs during the day, and strong elastic support. The nonoperative management of patients with venous ulcers is primarily an aggressive management of the venous insufficiency as outlined above. The use of local medications should be avoided unless a definite secondary infection is present. Increasing the local pressure over the ulcer by means of a sponge rubber pad beneath a strong elastic support can usually heal ulcers of silver-dollar size and sometimes larger.

OPERATIVE MANAGEMENT. Surgical treatment may in some instances be curative, but in most instances is merely helpful as an adjunct to the conservative management of venous insufficiency.

Ligation and Stripping of Greater or Lesser Saphenous Veins. The ligation and stripping of the saphenous veins should not be performed unless incompetency of the vein is demonstrated by the Trendelenburg test. The indications for the procedure are (1) moderate to severe symptomatic varicosities, (2) severe varicosities, even though the patient does not admit to symptoms, (3) severe venous insufficiency with recurrent ulcerations, in association with aggressive nonoperative management. Patients with mild varicosities and significant symptoms usually do not benefit from the procedure, and it is usually found that the symptoms are due to some unrelated cause or to deep venous abnormalities. Significant edema rarely accompanies greater saphenous varicosities alone and is not appreciably helped by vein stripping. Treatment of other underlying conditions or the aggressive nonoperative management of deep venous abnormalities is necessary.

The operative procedure (Fig. 22-16) consists of ligation of the greater saphenous vein at its junction with the femoral vein and ligation of its four major branches at the margin of the transverse groin incision. The entire vein is then stripped from its bed by making a separate incision at the ankle, passing a wire within the lumen in a craniad direction the length of the vein, transecting the vein in the ankle, and avulsing the entire vein by pulling on the wire from the groin incision. The branches of the veins break off near their junctions with the saphenous vein, but bleeding is minimal, particularly if the feet are markedly elevated during the operation. As noted before, however, the visible varicosities are usually found in the branches of the vein, and attention must also be directed toward them. Some surgeons prefer to remove the veins through separate incisions at the time of the original operation, others prefer to inject the remaining branches with sclerosing solutions at a later date. These solutions produce a localized phlebitis and thrombosis of the veins. The veins will remain obstructed unless complete recanalization of the lumen occurs.

Following operation, snug elastic stockings are applied, and the foot of the bed is elevated above the level of the heart. During the first week after operation patients are allowed up to walk or allowed to lie in bed with the feet elevated. Sitting is prohibited except for bathroom privileges. During the second week patients find it necessary to elevate the legs during a portion of the day to avoid discomfort. During the third or fourth week after operation they gradually increase their activities to their preoperative level.

Ligation of Incompetent Perforators. Incompetent perforators rarely occur without other types of venous insufficiency. Their ligation, however, may be a valuable adjunct to the nonoperative management of patients with venous insufficiency. It is particularly effective if performed before the patient develops an ulcer. This preulcer state may be

Fig. 22-16. Ligation and stripping of saphenous vein. *A*, Groin incision, showing junction of greater saphenous and femoral veins. Note four major branches of saphenous vein which required ligation and division. *B*, counterincision at knee or ankle to permit stripping of saphenous vein. Additional incisions to permit removal of branch varicose veins.

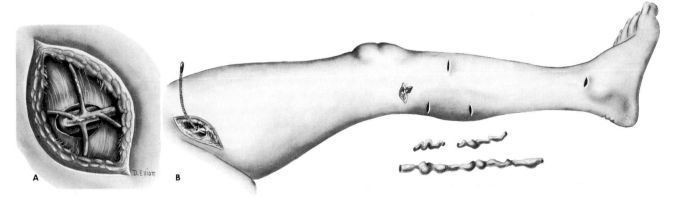

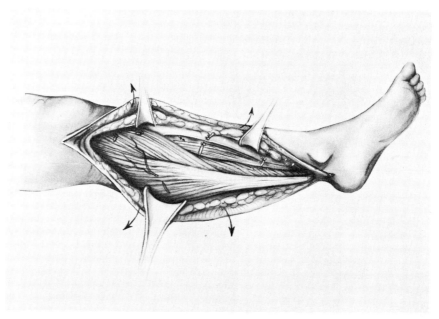

Fig. 22-17. Perforating veins interrupted subfascially. Skin flaps are carefully developed, and the great and small saphenous veins and the subcutaneous tissue, with many communicating veins are excised. (*After D. Silver, J. J. Gleysteen, G. R. Rhodes, N. G. Georgiade, and W. G. Anlyan, Surgical Treatment of the Refractory Postphlebitic Ulcer, Arch Surg, 103:554, 1971. Copyright 1971, American Medical Association.*)

recognized by the presence of telangiectasia, brownish pigmentation, or mild brawny induration behind the medial or lateral malleoli. The operation is also indicated after the nonoperative healing of recurrent ulcers. It should not be performed in the presence of an active infected ulcer.

Various techniques for ligation of the perforators in the lower leg have been described by Linton, Felder and associates, and Dodd and Cockett. Dodd and Cockett point out that the perforators most frequently associated with ulcers are those posterior and superior to the medial and lateral malleoli. Longitudinal incisions are made posterior and superior to the malleoli; then the perforators are interrupted above or below the fascia near their communication with the deep veins (Fig. 22-17). Extensive undermining of the tissue should be avoided, since there is a risk of sloughing of the overlying skin. Ligation of perforators is only an adjunctive measure, and aggressive nonoperative treatment of the underlying deep venous abnormalities is still indicated.

Ligation of the Superficial Femoral or Popliteal Veins. Some surgeons advocate the ligation of the superficial femoral or popliteal veins in the presence of deep venous abnormalities. The procedure was originally advocated to prevent reflux of blood down valveless normal deep veins. However, postoperative phlebograms in patients who have had this type of operation indicate that the obstructed deep veins are only replaced by dilated valveless collaterals. In addition, venous pressure measurements indicate that after such ligations increased venous hypertension occurs.

LYMPHATICS AND LYMPHEDEMA

Anatomy and Physiology of Lymphatic Return

The lymphatic system provides a means of returning certain extravascular materials in the interstitial space to the bloodstream. Normally there is a constant leakage of fluid and protein through the arterial capillary membrane into the interstitial space. The water and solutes can be resorbed by the vascular capillaries; the protein cannot. Proteins, however, can readily enter the lymphatic capillaries. Other materials, including red blood cells, bacteria, and small particulate matter, can also pass through the lymphatic capillary membrane.

The lymphatic capillaries form a superficial plexus within the dermis which covers the whole body surface. Another similar plexus lies in the deep dermis or subdermal region. These join other deeper lymphatics to form larger vessels which, in general, follow the course of the major blood vessels to the neck, where they empty into the bloodstream at the junction of the internal jugular and the subclavian vein. The continuity of the larger lymphatics is interrupted by lymph nodes, which acts as filters and also contribute lymphocytes to the lymph. The lymph vessels contain valves which direct the flow of lymph toward the neck. The movement of the lymph is aided by extrinsic factors such as muscle contraction, arterial pulsations, respiratory movement, and massage.

Information regarding the normal or altered anatomy and physiology of the lymphatics can be obtained from special examinations, including (1) dye injections of the superficial dermal lymphatics, (2) lymphangiography, and (3) analysis of the protein content of edema fluid.

DYE INJECTIONS. Hudack and McMaster introduced patent blue dye, and Butcher and Hoover used 4% direct sky blue dye for the intradermal injection of the human

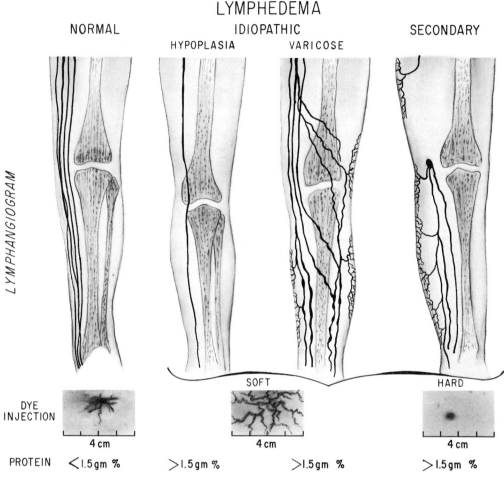

Fig. 22-18. Diagnostic procedures for lymphedema: dye injections, lymphangiograms, and protein analysis.

superficial dermal lymphatics; 0.2 ml is inserted via a 30-gauge needle, and in normal skin a network of very fine intradermal lymphatic capillaries is demonstrated within 30 to 60 seconds after injection (Fig. 22-18).

LYMPHANGIOGRAPHY. Kinmonth demonstrated the feasibility of obtaining radiographs of the lymphatics. Patent blue dye or direct sky blue dye is injected into the subcutaneous tissue of the foot. The dye rapidly enters the lymphatics. Massage of the foot and muscular contractions increase the lymph flow. An incision is then made on the dorsum of the foot and a cannula inserted into a blue-dye-filled lymphatic; 10 ml of radiopaque dye is injected, and x-rays of the entire extremity are made.

Normally the slender lymphatics, unlike veins, appear of uniform caliber throughout their course. Unlike veins, they bifurcate as they proceed proximally. As with veins, slight dilatations at the level of the valves are visualized (Fig. 22-18).

ANALYSIS OF THE PROTEIN CONTENT OF EDEMA FLUID. Edema fluid can be collected by the insertion of a special Southey tube into the subcutaneous tissue. The protein content of peripheral edema fluid secondary to venous, heart, or renal disease is less than 1.5 Gm/ 100 ml. Since the lymphatics are responsible for removal

of protein from the interstitial space, abnormally high levels of protein would reflect abnormal lymphatic function.

Lymphedema

Congenital or acquired abnormalities of the lymphatics may hinder the lymphatic capillaries from absorbing materials such as proteins or prevent the main channels from carrying sufficient quantities of tissue fluid from a limb. The result is an accumulation of plasma protein in the tissue spaces. This protein concentration is of high osmotic pressure, causing absorption of fluid into the extravascular space. Edema, or in other words lymphedema, is the result.

ETIOLOGY. The various types of lymphedema have been outlined by Taylor as follows:

1. Primary lymphedema
    a. Congenital
    b. Lymphedema precox
2. Secondary lymphedema
    a. Neoplastic invasion
    b. Surgical excision
    c. Radiotherapy
    d. Inflammation or parasitic invasion
    e. Motor paralysis

Primary Lymphedema. Primary lymphedema of the lower extremities is caused by abnormal development of the lymph vessels. The edema may be present at birth and is then called *congenital lymphedema*. More frequently the edema appears during the teens and is then termed *lymphedema precox*. It may appear insidiously or may follow minor trauma or infection. Primary lymphedema is about three times more common in females than in males. It involves both legs in about 50 percent of patients.

Secondary Lymphedema. Secondary lymphedema is usually due to obstruction or destruction of normal lymphatic channels. It may, therefore, follow obstruction of the lymphatics by tumor, repeated infection, or parasitic infestation. It may also follow the excision of lymph nodes, as during a radical mastectomy or radical groin dissection. Radiation therapy, particularly for malignant disease, may similarly destroy the lymphatics.

PATHOPHYSIOLOGY. Primary Lymphedema. Kinmonth et al. performed lymphangiograms on 87 patients with primary lymphedema. Aplasia, or the absence of any significant lymphatic trunks in the subcutaneous tissue, was observed in 14 percent of the extremities. Dye injected beneath the skin, however, would travel great distances through dilated dermal vessels. Hypoplasia, a deficiency in size or number of lymphatic vessels, was seen in 55 percent of the extremities. Dye injected subcutaneously in the interdigital webs would frequently appear in the dermal plexus of the dorsum of the foot. Varicose lymphatics which were broader and more tortuous than normal were observed in 24 percent of the patients. Dye injected subcutaneously would frequently appear in dermal lymphatics some distance from the site of the injection. This "dermal backflow" in the lymphatics is assumed to be secondary to incompetency of valves in the lymphatics. It can be demonstrated also by the intradermal injection of dye, when "skip areas" in the filling of the dermal lymphatics is observed. The protein content of the edema fluid of patients with primary lymphedema, studied by Crockett and by Taylor et al., was found to be greater than 2 Gm/100 ml in 41 of 48 patients. It would appear, therefore, that the underlying cause of the edema is the inability of the lymphatic system to remove protein from the interstitial fluid at a normal rate. In primary lymphedema this lymphatic insufficiency may be due to aplasia, hypoplasia, or varicosities of the lymphatic vessels (Fig. 22-18).

Secondary Lymphedema. Lymphangiograms of patients with acquired lymphedema demonstrate the point of obstruction of the lymphatics. The remaining vessels appear normal, but there is considerable dermal backflow of the radiopaque material. Intradermal dye injections demonstrate dilatations and prominence of the dermal lymphatics. The inability of the lymphatics to effectively remove protein from the interstitial fluid can be demonstrated by measurements of the protein content of the edema fluid (Fig. 22-18).

CLINICAL MANIFESTATIONS. Symptoms. The usual symptoms of primary and secondary lymphedema are the same. Edema increases during the course of the day and decreases overnight, but the limb always remains larger. There is gradual increase in the degree of swelling over a period of years. The edema may cause some fatigue and be cosmetically objectionable but in most instances causes no real concern. In others the disability is significant, particularly in those with elephantiasis secondary to filariasis.

Physical Findings. Lymphedema is characteristically a firm, rubbery, nonpitting edema. Early in the course of the disease the edema is somewhat softer, and much of it will disappear overnight with elevation of the legs. With the passage of time the edema may become woody in character. This is a result of an increase of fibrous tissue within the subcutaneous tissue, which is believed to be secondary to the increase in protein-rich edema fluid. Repeated infections will hasten growth of fibrous tissue. Some patients develop small blisters containing edema fluid of high protein content. These blisters may occur on the lower abdomen and upper thigh and contain a milky white fluid with the characteristics of chyle; they are believed to be secondary to reflux from the retroperitoneal lymphatics. Hyperkeratosis of the skin is common in long-standing lymphedema.

COMPLICATIONS. Recurrent Cellulitis and Lymphangitis. The major complication of lymphedema is recurrent attacks of cellulitis and lymphangitis. These attacks may occur without warning or may follow minor injuries or infections in the extremity. They are characterized by an elevated temperature, constitutional symptoms of malaise, nausea and vomiting, and local symptoms of redness, pain, and increased swelling of the involved limb. Beta-hemolytic streptococci are the offending organisms and, if carefully looked for, may be found at the site of minor injuries, in the nose and throat, in blood cultures, or in edema fluid. The protein-rich edema fluid is apparently an excellent culture medium, since the lymphedematous limb is very susceptible to repeated infections. Once the infection starts it spreads rapidly.

Lymphangiosarcoma. A rare but serious complication of lymphedema is the appearance of lymphangiosarcoma. This malignant tumor is most frequently described in patients with lymphedema following a radical mastectomy for breast cancer but is also seen in long-standing lymphedema due to other causes. It is usually first recognized as a bruiselike blue or reddish purple nodule in the skin of the lymphedematous extremity. As the primary lesion enlarges, satellite tumors appear about it. Metastases appear early in the course of the disease, particularly to the lung.

DIFFERENTIAL DIAGNOSIS. The firm, rubbery, nonpitting character of unilateral lymphedema usually differentiates it from the soft, pitting, bilateral edema secondary to heart failure, renal failure, hypothyroidism, or aldosteronism. Some deep cavernous hemangiomas may be confused with lymphedema, but the presence of overlying birthmarks, the sponginess of the hemangiomas, and their decrease in size on elevation usually indicate the correct diagnosis. The edema of an acute postoperative or infectious lymphedema may be confused with deep venous thrombosis, and a phlebogram may be most helpful in establishing the correct diagnosis. The edema of chronic venous insufficiency can usually be differentiated from lymphedema because of its brawniness, overlying brownish discoloration, and telangiectasia. However, lymphedema is commonly a complication of acute thrombophlebitis, and venous insufficiency and lymphedema may coexist. Streptococcal infection should be carefully searched for in the patient with a postphlebitic extremity who is repeatedly admitted to the hospital with high fever and redness, tenderness, and marked swelling of the leg. In the author's experience these cases are usually labeled "recurrent phlebitis" but in actuality are recurrent cellulitis and lymphangitis secondary to lymphedema.

Whenever there is a question of deep venous disease versus lymphedema, a phlebogram may be helpful in establishing the diagnosis of deep venous disease, and the author has found dye injections of the superficial dermal lymphatics helpful in confirming the diagnosis of lymphedema. Lymphangiograms and, in confusing cases, analysis of the protein content of the edema fluid may be necessary to establish the diagnosis.

TREATMENT. Nonoperative Management. The conservative management of lymphedema is directed toward control of the edema and prevention of recurrent infection. Elevation of the involved extremity above the level of the heart will increase lymph drainage by reducing the hydrostatic pressure within the lymph vessels. Patients are therefore instructed to elevate the foot of the bed; they are also instructed to lie down and elevate the extremity whenever they have the opportunity. Massage is also known to increase lymph flow. Special apparatuses are available to accomplish this: one is a cloth sleeve containing a plastic bladder that can be alternately inflated and deflated to produce a rhythmic pneumatic compression of the entire extremity; another is a series of bladders that can be sequentially inflated and deflated to give a massaging effect beginning at the hand or foot and extending to the shoulder or thigh. When the maximal decrease in edema is achieved by these methods, very tight elastic stockings or canvas boots containing an inflatable rubber bladder can be applied. These supports can prevent reaccumulation of edema fluid. In addition they provide a semirigid encasement of the extremity so that muscular action, which causes alterations in the volume of the leg, can produce a massaging effect on the lymphatics. Diuretics may be helpful in reducing the size of the limb temporarily. However, none of the procedures mentioned can completely return the limb to its normal size, particularly in long-standing cases; they can only delay or prevent progression of the process.

The control of the recurrent bouts of infection associated with lymphedema is important. Ideally it should be possible to prevent these by control of edema, local hygiene, avoidance of trauma, and prevention of athlete's foot. These procedures alone are usually not sufficient, however, and the use of prophylactic antibiotics may be indicated. Since the offending organism is almost always the streptococcus, oral penicillin is the drug of choice.

Surgical Treatment. Surgical treatment is indicated for a very small percentage of patients with lymphedema. The indications include excessive edema, when the weight and size of the limb interfere with normal activities, and recurrent bouts of cellulitis. Surgery for cosmetic reasons alone is rarely indicated, since after an effective operation a disproportion in the size of the two limbs will still usually remain, and in addition the scars resulting from the operation may still call attention to the limb.

Numerous surgical approaches to the problem are described, including (1) insertion of silk threads of polyethylene tubing into the subcutaneous tissue in the hope of draining the edema fluid into normal tissue; (2) removal of long strips of fascia in the hope that new anastomoses will form between the superficial and deep lymphatics; (3) construction of pedicle grafts from the involved limb to the trunk in the hope of bypassing obstructed lymphatics; (4) excision of long strips of subcutaneous tissue and deep fascia to reduce the size of the limb; (5) complete excision of all the skin, subcutaneous tissue, and deep fascia from the limb, followed by application of split-thickness skin grafts to the exposed muscle and periosteum, as originally described by Charles.

The Charles procedure is, in the author's opinion, the most effective of the surgical procedures. The size and weight of the limb are effectively reduced, and there is lower incidence of recurrent cellulitis and lymphangitis after removal of the edematous subcutaneous tissue. It should be reemphasized, however, that this, like other treatments for lymphedema, cannot return the limb to a normal appearance.

References

Venous Thrombosis and Pulmonary Embolism

Adams, J. T., and DeWeese, J. A.: Experimental and Clinical Evaluation of Partial Vein Interruption in the Prevention of Pulmonary Emboli, *Surgery,* **57:**82, 1965.

——— and ———: Partial Interruption of the Inferior Vena Cava with a New Plastic Clip, *Surg Gynecol Obstet,* **123:**1087, 1966.

——— and ———: Comparative Evaluation of Ligation and Partial Interruption of the Femoral Vein in the Treatment of Thromoembolic Disease, *Ann Surg,* **172:**795, 1970

———, Feingold, B. E., and DeWeese, J. A.: Comparative Evaluation of Ligation and Partial Interruption of the Inferior Vena Cava, *Arch Surg,* **103:**272, 1971.

———, McEvoy, R. K., and DeWeese, J. A.: Primary Deep Venous Thrombosis of Upper Extremity, *Arch Surg,* **91:**29, 1965.

Allen, E. V., Hines, E. A., Jr., Kvale, W. F., and Barker, N. W.: The Use of Dicumarol as an Anticoagulant: Experience in 2,307 Cases, *Ann Intern Med,* **27:**371, 1947.

Artz, C. P., and Amspacher, W. H.: Evaluation of Various Methods of Administration of Heparin, *Surg Forum,* **3:**530, 1952.

Barner, H. B., and DeWeese, J. A.: An Evaluation of the Sphygmomanometer Cuff Pain Test in Venous Thrombosis, *Surgery,* **48:**915, 1960.

Barritt, D. W., and Jordan, S. C.: Anticoagulant Drugs in the Treatment of Pulmonary Embolism: A Controlled Trial, *Lancet,* **1:**1309, 1960.

Bauer, G.: A Venographic Study of Thromboembolic Problems, *Acta Chir Scand [Suppl],* vol. 84, 1940.

———: Clinical Experiences of a Surgeon in the Use of Heparin, *Am J Cardiol,* **14:**29, 1964.

Brockman, S. K., and Vasko, J. S.: Phlegmasia Cerulea Dolens, *Surg Gynecol Obstet,* **121:**1347, 1965.

Browse, N. L.: The [125]I Fibrinogen Uptake Test, *Arch Surg,* **104:** 160, 1972.

Byrne, J. J., and O'Neil, E. E.: Fatal Pulmonary Emboli: A Study of 130 Autopsy-proven Fatal Emboli, *Am J Surg,* **83:**47, 1952.

Carey, L. C., and Williams, R. D.: Comparative Effects of Dicumarol, Tromexan, and Heparin on Thrombus Propagation, *Ann Surg,* **152:**919, 1960.

Cegelski, F. C., DeWeese, J. A., and Lund, C. J.: Deep Iliofemoral Venous Thrombosis during Pregnancy, *Am J Obstet Gynecol,* **89:**510, 1964.

Cooley, D. A., and Beall, A. C., Jr.: A Technic of Pulmonary Embolectomy Using Temporary Cardio-pulmonary Bypass, *J Cardiovasc Surg (Torino),* **2:**469, 1961.

Coon, W. W., and Coller, F. A.: Clinicopathologic Correlation in Thromboembolism, *Surg Gynecol Obstet,* **109:**259, 1959.

——— and ———: Some Epidemiologic Considerations of Thromboembolism, *Surg Gynecol Obstet,* **109:**487, 1959.

———, Mackenzie, J. W., and Hodgson, P. E.: A Critical Evaluation of Anticoagulant Therapy in Peripheral Venous Thrombosis and Pulmonary Embolism, *Surg Gynecol Obstet,* **106:** 129, 1958.

Cosgriff, S. W.: Thromboembolism, *Am J Med,* **3:**758, 1947.

Crane, C.: Deep Venous Thrombosis and Pulmonary Embolism, *N Engl J Med,* **257:**147, 1957.

———: Femoral vs. Caval Interruption for Venous Thromboembolism, *N Engl J Med,* **270:**819, 1964.

Dale, W. A.: Inferior Vena Caval Ligation for Venous Thromboembolism, *Rev Surg,* **19:**1, 1962.

Deaton, H. L., Anlyan, W. G., Silver, D., and Webster, J.: Thrombosis: Prevention and Treatment, *Surgery,* **49:**130, 1961.

DeBakey, M. E.: A Critical Evaluation of the Problem of Thromboembolism, *Surg Gynecol Obstet,* **98:**1, 1954.

DeWeese, J. A.: Current Status of Plastic Procedures on the Venous System, *NJ Acad Med Bull,* **7:**1, 1961.

———: Thrombectomy for Acute Iliofemoral Venous Thrombosis, *J Cardiovasc Surg (Torino),* **5:**703, 1964.

———, Adams, J. T., and Gaiser, D. L.: Subclavian Venous Thrombectomy, *Circulation,* **41, 42** (*Suppl* II):158, 1970.

——— and Rogoff, S. M.: Phlebographic Patterns of Acute Deep Venous Thrombosis of the Leg, *Surgery,* **53:**99, 1963.

———, ———, Phillips, C. E., Jr., and Pories, W. J.: Deep Venous Thrombosis, *Postgrad Med,* **29:**614, 1961.

DeWeese, M. S., and Hunter, D. C.: A Vena Cava Filter for the Prevention of Pulmonary Embolism, *Arch Surg,* **86:**852, 1963.

Dmochowski, J. R., Adams, D. F., and Couch, N. P.: Impedance Measurement in the Diagnosis of Deep Venous Thrombosis, *Arch Surg,* **104:**170, 1972.

Donaldson, G. A., Linton, R. R., and Rodkey, G. V.: A Twenty-Year Survey of Thromboembolism at the Massachusetts General Hospital, 1939–1959, *N Engl J Med,* **265:**208, 1961.

Edwards, W. H., Sawyers, J. L., and Foster, J. H.: Iliofemoral Venous Thrombosis: Reappraisal of Thrombectomy, *Ann Surg,* **171:**961, 1970.

Engelberg, H., and Berk, M. Z.: Prolonged Anticoagulant Therapy with Subcutaneously Administered Concentrated Aqueous Heparin, *Surgery,* **36:**762, 1954.

Fogarty, T. J., and Krippaehne, W. W.: Catheter Technique for Venous Thrombectomy, *Surg Gynecol Obstet,* **121:**362, 1965.

Fontaine, R., and Tuchmann, L.: The Role of Thrombectomy in Deep Venous Thromboses, *J Cardiovasc Surg (Torino),* **5:**298, 1964.

Gibbs, N. M.: Venous Thrombosis of the Lower Limbs with Particular Reference to Bed-Rest, *Br J Surg,* **45:**15, 1957.

Gomez, R. L., Wheeler, H. B., Belko, J. S., and Warren, R.: Observations on the Uptake of a Radioactive Fibrinolytic Enzyme by Intravascular Clots, *Ann Surg,* **158:**905, 1963.

Hafner, C. D., Cranley, J. J., Krause, R. J., and Strasser, E. S.: A Method of Managing Superficial Thrombophlebitis, *Surgery,* **55:**201, 1964.

Haller, J. A., and Abrams, B. L.: Use of Thrombectomy in the Treatment of Acute Iliofemoral Venous Thrombosis in Forty-five Patients, *Ann Surg,* **158:**561, 1963.

Henderson, R. R.: Pulmonary Embolism and Infarction, *Med Clin North Am,* **48:**1425, 1964.

Herrmann, L. G.: Superficial Venous Thrombosis (Saphenous Thrombophlebitis): Should Treatment be Empirical or Definitive? *J Cardiovasc Surg (Torino),* **5:**239, 1964.

Hughes, E. S. R.: Venous Obstruction in the Upper Extremity (Paget-Schroetter's Syndrome): A Review of 320 Cases, *Int Abstr Surg,* **88:**89, 1949.

Hume, M.: The Relation of "Hypercoagulability" to Thrombosis, *Monogr Surg Sci,* **2:**133, 1965.

Hunter, W. C., Sneeden, V. D., Robertson, T. D., and Snyder, G. A. C.: Thrombosis of the Deep Veins of the Leg, *Arch Intern Med,* **68:**1, 1941.

Jorpes, J. E.: Heparin: Its Chemistry, Pharmacology and Clinical Use, *Am J Med,* **33:**692, 1962.

Kakkar, V.: The Diagnosis of Deep Vein Thrombosis Using the [125]I Fibrinogen Test, *Arch Surg,* **104:**152, 1972.

Lawen, A.: Weitere Erfahrungen über operative Thrombenentfernung bei Venenthrombose, *Arch Klin Chir,* **193:**723, 1938.

Mahorner, H., Castleberry, J. W., and Coleman, W. O.: Attempts to Restore Function in Major Veins Which Are the Site of Massive Thrombosis, *Ann Surg,* **146:**510, 1957.

Mavor, G. E.: Deep Vein Thrombosis, *Postgrad Med J,* **47:**311, 1971.

McLachlin, J., and Paterson, J. C.: Some Basic Observations on Venous Thrombosis and Pulmonary Embolism, *Surg Gynecol Obstet,* **93:**1, 1951.

———, Richards, T., and Paterson, J. C.: An Evaluation of Clinical Signs in the Diagnosis of Venous Thrombosis, *Arch Surg,* **85:**738, 1962.

Miles, R. M., Chappell, F., and Renner, O.: A Partially Occluding Vena Caval Clip for Prevention of Pulmonary Embolism, *Am Surg,* **30:**40, 1964.

Mobin-Uddin, K., McLean, R., Bolooki, H., and Jude, J. R.: Caval Interruption for Prevention of Pulmonary Embolism: Long Term Results of a New Method, *Arch Surg,* **99:**711, 1969.

———, Trinkle, J. K., and Bryant, L. R.: Present Status of the Inferior Vena Cava Umbrella Filter, *Surgery,* **70:**914, 1971.

Moretz, W. H., Rhode, C. M., and Shepherd, M. H.: Prevention of Pulmonary Emboli by Partial Occlusion of the Inferior Vena Cava, *Am Surg,* **25:**617, 1959.

Moser, K. M., Houk, V. N., Jones, R. C., and Hufnagel, C. C.: Chronic, Massive Thrombotic Obstruction of the Pulmonary Arteries: Analysis of Four Operated Cases, *Circulation,* **32:** 377, 1965.

Murray, G.: Anticoagulants, in Venous Thrombosis and the Prevention of Pulmonary Embolism, *Surg Gynecol Obstet,* **84:**665, 1947.

Nabseth, D. C., and Moran, J. M.: Reassessment of the Role of Inferior-Vena-Cava Ligation in Venous Thromboembolism, *N Engl J Med,* **273:**1250, 1965.

Parrish, E. H., Adams, J. T., Pories, W. J., Burget, D. E., and DeWeese, J. A.: Pulmonary Emboli Following Vena Caval Ligation, *Arch Surg,* **97:**899, 1968.

Ravdin, I. S., and Kirby, C. K.: Experiences with Ligation and Heparin in Thromboembolic Disease, *Surgery,* **29:**334, 1951.

Robb, G. P., and Steinberg, I.: Visualization of the Chambers of the Heart, the Pulmonary Circulation, and the Great Blood Vessels in Man, *Am J Roentgenol Radium Ther Nucl Med,* **41:**1, 1939.

Roberts, B., Rosato, F. E., and Rosato, E. F.: Heparin—A Cause of Arterial Emboli? *Surgery,* **55:**803, 1964.

Robin, E. D., Julian, D. G., Travis, D. M., and Crump, C. H.: A Physiologic Approach to the Diagnosis of Acute Pulmonary Embolism, *N Engl J Med,* **260:**586, 1959.

Sautter, R. D., Myers, W. O., and Wenzel, F. J.: Implications of the Urokinase Study Concerning the Surgical Treatment of Pulmonary Embolism, *J Thorac Cardiovasc Surg,* **63:**54, 1972.

Sawyer, R. B., Moncrief, J. A., and Canizaro, P. C.: Dextran Therapy in Thrombophlebitis, *JAMA,* **191:**740, 1965.

Schwartz, S. I.: Diagnosis of Thromboembolic Disease, *J Cardiovasc Surg (Torino),* suppl. issue, VII Congress of International Cardiovascular Society, Philadelphia, Sept. 5–18, 1965.

Sharp, E. H.: Pulmonary Embolectomy: Successful Removal of Massive Pulmonary Embolus with Support of Cardiopulmonary Bypass: Case Report, *Ann Surg,* **156:**1, 1962.

Short, D. S.: A Survey of Pulmonary Embolism in a General Hospital, *Br Med J,* **1:**790, 1952.

Sigel, B., Felix, W. R., Jr., Popky, G. L., and Ipsen, J.: Diagnosis of Lower Limb Venous Thrombosis by Doppler Ultrasound Technique, *Arch Surg,* **104:**174, 1972.

Spencer, F. C., Quattlebaum, J. K., Quattlebaum, J. K., Jr., Sharp, E. H., and Jude, J. R.: Plication of the Inferior Vena Cava for Pulmonary Embolism: A Report of 20 Cases, *Ann Surg,* **155:**827, 1962.

Stein, G. N., Chen, J. T., Goldstein, F., Israel, H. L., and Finkelstein, A.: The Importance of Chest Roentgenography in the Diagnosis of Pulmonary Embolism, *Am J Roentgenol Radium Ther Nucl Med,* **81:**255, 1959.

Templeton, J. Y.: Endvenectomy for the Relief of Obstruction of the Superior Vena Cava, *Am J Surg,* **104:**70, 1962.

Urokinase-Pulmonary Embolism Trial, Phase I Results (A Cooperative Study), *JAMA,* **214:**2163, 1970.

Wacker, W. E. C., Rosenthal, M., Snodgrass, P. J., and Amador, E.: A Triad for the Diagnosis of Pulmonary Embolism and Infarction, *JAMA,* **178:**8, 1961.

Wagner, H. N., Sabiston, D. C., Jr., McAfee, J. G., Tow, D., and Stern, H. S.: Diagnosis of Massive Pulmonary Embolism in Man by Radioisotope Scanning, *N Engl J Med,* **271:**377, 1964.

Wessler, S., and Morris, L. E.: Studies in Intravascular Coagulation: IV. The Effect of Heparin and Dicumarol on Serum-induced Venous Thrombosis, *Circulation,* **12:**553, 1955.

Wheeler, H. B., Pearson, D., O'Connel, D., and Mullick, S. C.: Impedance Phlebography: Technique, Interpretation, and Results, *Arch Surg,* **104:**164, 1972.

Williams, J. R., Wilcox, W. C., Andrews, G. J., and Burns, R. R.: Angiography in Pulmonary Embolism, *JAMA,* **184:**473, 1963.

Williams, R. D., and Zollinger, R. W.: Surgical Treatment of Superficial Thrombophlebitis, *Surg Gynecol Obstet,* **118:**745, 1964.

Zilliacus, H.: On the Specific Treatment of Thrombosis and Pulmonary Embolism with Anticoagulants, with Particular Reference to the Post-thrombotic Sequelae, *Acta Med Scand [Suppl],* **171:**13, 1946.

Venous Insufficiency and Ulcers

Bauer, G.: A Roentgenological and Clinical Study of the Sequels of Thrombosis, *Acta Chir Scand,* **86**(Suppl 74):1, 1942.

DeCamp, P. T., Schramel, R. J., Ray, C. J., Feibleman, N. D., Ward, J. A., and Ochsner, A.: Ambulatory Venous Pressure Determinations in Postphlebitic and Related Syndromes, *Surgery,* **29:**44, 1951.

DeWeese, J. A.: Functional Popliteal Phlebography in the Patient with a Complicated Varicose Vein Problem, *Surgery,* **44:**390, 1958.

———, and Rogoff, S. M.: Clinical Uses of Functional Ascending Phlebography of the Lower Extremity, *Angiology,* **9:**268, 1958.

——— and ———: Functional Ascending Phlebography of the Lower Extremity by Serial Long Film Technique: Evaluation of Anatomic and Functional Detail in 62 Extremities, *Am J Roentgenol Radium Ther Nucl Med,* :841, 1959.

Dodd, H., and Cockett, F. B.: "The Pathology and Surgery to the Veins of the Lower Limb," E. & S. Livingstone Ltd., Edinburgh and London, 1956.

Edwards, E. A., and Edwards, J. E.: The Effect of Thrombophlebitis on the Venous Valve, *Surg Gynecol Obstet,* **65:**310, 1937.

Felder, D. A., Murphy, T. O., and Ring, D. M.: A Posterior Subfascial Approach to the Communicating Veins of the Leg, *Surg Gynecol Obstet,* **100:**730, 1955.

Fell, S. C., McIntosh, H. D., Hornsby, A. T., Horton, C. E., Warren, J. V., and Pickrell, K.: The Syndrome of the Chronic Leg Ulcer: The Phlebodynamics of the Lower Extremity; Physiology of the Venous Valves, *Surgery,* **38:**771, 1955.

Gay, J.: On Varicose Diseases of the Lower Extremities, in "The Lettsomian Lectures of 1867," J. & A. Churchill Ltd., London.

Homans, J.: The Etiology and Treatment of Varicose Ulcer of the Leg, *Surg Gynecol Obstet,* **24:**300, 1917.

Linton, R. R.: The Post-thrombotic Ulceration of the Lower Extremity: Its Etiology and Surgical Treatment, *Ann Surg,* **138:**415, 1953.

Luke, J. C.: The Deep Vein Valves, *Surgery,* **29:**381, 1951.

Myers, T. T.: Results and Technique of Stripping Operation for Varicose Veins, *JAMA,* **163:**87, 1957.

Pollack, A. A., Taylor, B. E., Myers, T. T., and Wood, E. H.: The Effect of Exercise and Body Position on the Venous Pressure at the Ankle in Patients Having Venous Valvular Defects, *J Clin Invest,* **28:**559, 1949.

Schneewind, J. H.: The Walking Venous Pressure Test and Its Use in Peripheral Vascular Disease, *Ann Surg,* **140:**137, 1954.

Scott, W. J. M., and Radakovich, M.: Venous and Lymphatic Stasis in the Lower Extremities: I. A Test for Incompetence in the Perforating Veins; II. A Simple Method of Adequate Control, *Surgery,* **26:**970, 1949.

Staffon, R. A., and Buxton, R. W.: Deep Vein Ligation in the Postphlebitic Extremity, *Surgery,* **41:**471, 1957.

Veal, J. R., and Hussey, H. H.: The Venous Circulation in the Lower Extremities during Pregnancy, *Surg Gynecol Obstet,* **72:**841, 1941.

Warren, R., White, E. A., and Belcher, C. D.: Venous Pressures in the Saphenous System in Normal Varicose and Postphlebitic Extremities: Alterations following Femoral Vein Ligation, *Surgery,* **26:**435, 1949.

Lymphatics and Lymphedema

Brush, B. E., Wylie, J. H., Jr., and Beninson, J.: Some Devices for the Management of Lymphedema of the Extremities, *Surg Clin North Am,* **392:**1493, 1959.

Butcher, H. R. Jr., and Hoover, A. L.: Abnormalities of Human Superficial Cutaneous Lymphatics Associated with Stasis Ulcers, Lymphedema, Scars, and Cutaneous Autografts, *Ann Surg,* **142:**633, 1955.

Charles, R. H.: In A. Latham and T. C. English (eds.), "A System of Treatment," vol. 3, p. 516, J. & A. Churchill, Ltd., London, 1912.

Crockett, D. J.: The Protein Levels of Oedema Fluids, *Lancet,* **2:**1179, 1956.

Gibson, T., and Tough, J. S.: The Surgical Correction of Chronic Lymphoedema of the Legs, *Brit J Plast Surg,* **7:**195, 1954.

Hudack, S. S., and McMaster, P. D.: The Lymphatic Participation in Human Cutaneous Phenomena: A Study of the Minute Lymphatics of the Living Skin, *J Exp Med,* **572:**751, 1933.

Jantet, G. H., Taylor, G. W., and Kinmonth, J. B.: Operations for Primary Lymphedema of the Lower Limbs: Results after 1-9 Years, *J Cardiovasc Surg (Torino),* **2:**27, 1961.

Khodadadeh, M., and Johnson, R.: Lymphangiosarcoma Arising from Postmastectomy Lymphedema, *JAMA,* **186:**1097, 1963.

Kinmonth, J. B.: Lymphangiography in Man: A Method of Outlining Lymphatic Trunks at Operation, *Clin Sci,* **11:**13, 1952.

———, Taylor, G. W., Tracy, G. D., and Marsh, J. D.: Primary Lymphoedema: Clinical and Lymphangiographic Studies of a Series of 107 Patients in Which the Lower Limbs Were Affected, *Br J Surg,* **45:**1, 1957.

Scott, W. J. M., and Radkovich, M.: Venous and Lymphatic Stasis in the Lower Extremities: I. A Test for Incompetence in the Perforating Veins; II. A Simple Method of Adequate Control, *Surgery,* **26:**970, 1949.

Taylor, G. W.: Lymphoedema, *Postgrad Med J,* **35:**2, 1959.

———, Kinmonth, J. B., and Dangerfield, W. G.: Protein Content of Oedema Fluid in Lymphoedema, *Br Med J,* **1:**1159, 1958.

Wakim, K. G., Martin, G. M., and Krusen, F. H.: Influence of Centripetal Rhythmic Compression on Localized Edema of an Extremity, *Arch Phys Med Rehabil,* **36:**98, 1955.

Yoffey, J. M., and Courtice, F. C.: "Lymphatics, Lymph and Lymphoid Tissue," Harvard University Press, Cambridge, Mass., 1956.

Chapter 23

Surgically Correctible Hypertension

by John H. Foster

Physiology and Pathophysiology

Clinical Manifestations

Laboratory Studies

Classification

Pheochromocytoma

Primary Aldosteronism

Cushing's Syndrome

Coarctation of the Aorta

Renovascular Hypertension

Unilateral Renal Parenchymal Disease

Surgical Treatment of Essential Hypertension

Systemic hypertension and its associated cerebrovascular, renal, and cardiovascular sequelae are among the most common causes of crippling illness and death in the world today. Gordon and Devine estimated in the early 1960s that there were 17 million people with hypertension in the United States; current estimates are that 30 million people have hypertension. Although the vast majority of hypertensive patients have essential hypertension, an increasingly significant percentage, estimated to be between 5 and 10 percent of all hypertensive patients, are being found to have a specific underlying lesion which is surgically correctible.

PHYSIOLOGY AND PATHOPHYSIOLOGY

Blood flows through a series of elastic arterial tubes. The peak pressure within arteries, a reflection of ventricular contraction, is referred to as systolic pressure. Residual resting pressure during ventricular diastole accounts for the diastolic pressure. The accepted upper limit of normal blood pressure in the adult is 140/90 mm Hg. The so-called "normal" varies with age as follows: infants, 70/45 mm Hg, early childhood 85/55 mm Hg, and adolescence 100/75 mm Hg.

The factors influencing arterial blood pressure include (1) viscosity of blood, (2) blood volume, (3) cardiac output, (4) elasticity of arterial wall, and (5) peripheral resistance.

An increase in viscosity results in an increase in resistance to blood flow and may give rise to hypertension, as in polycythemia. An increase in the amount of blood or fluid circulating in the vascular system may also result in hypertension, just as a reduction in the blood volume is manifest by hypotension. The cardiac output, which refers to the volume of blood pumped into the vascular system per unit of time, is an important determinant. An increase in output, as in thyrotoxicosis, may cause hypertension, whereas the decrease which accompanies myocardial disease and cardiomyopathies is attended by hypotension. The arterial wall normally relaxes in systole and contracts in diastole; loss of this function, as in rigid arteriosclerotic vessels, results in increased systolic and decreased diastolic pressure. Perhaps the most important determinant in the development of systemic hypertension is the peripheral resistance within the arteriolar segments of the vascular system. Small changes in arterial caliber result in marked changes in resistance and pressure, chiefly the diastolic pressure.

Although each of these factors may influence the blood pressure, the effect depends largely on the modifying influence of the autonomic nervous system and on renal and hormonal contributions. Reflex arcs within the nervous system control the vasomotor tone, cardiac rate, and cardiac output. Proprioceptors or baroreceptors in the aortic wall and carotid sinus participate in the reflex arcs and play an important role in the regulation of blood pressure.

In most cases of hypertension, little is known about the factors which alter the arteriolar tone and caliber. Age, race, and environment are significant but ill-defined factors in essential hypertension. A more precise role has been determined for certain humoral agents in a small percentage of patients. Excessive production of catecholamines such as epinephrine and norepinephrine by the adrenal medulla in cases of pheochromocytoma has been shown to increase small-vessel tone and consequently increase peripheral resistance. Adrenal cortical hormones have also been implicated in clinical hypertension. Aldosterone, the sodium-retaining hormone of the cortex, has been shown to potentiate the rise in blood pressure caused by pressor agents. Excessive secretion of aldosterone is accompanied by retention of sodium and water, with consequent expansion of the blood volume and resultant hypertension. Although sodium seems to have an unquestioned role in human hypertension, the mechanism or locus of its effect is unclear. The volume-expansion effects of sodium are the most obvious. In addition, an increased sodium content of the vascular wall appears to make the blood vessels more responsive to vasoconstrictor agents. Production or accentuation of experimental hypertension by salt feeding is well documented and carries over into the clinical management of hypertensive patients, where salt restriction is commonly advised. However, the relation between aldosterone and hypertension does not seem to be limited to salt retention and volume expansion. In many cases of malignant hypertension of renovascular origin there is an associated hyperplasia of the cortex and increase in aldosterone secretion, and in such cases the urinary excretion of sodium may be high and the blood volume normal.

The role of other adrenocortical hormones in human hypertension is even more obscure. Hypertension is a manifestation of Cushing's syndrome which is associated with excessive production of cortisol. The effects of this hormone on hypertension have not been defined. In Cushing's syndrome, an increase in aldosterone is inconstant, and hyperresponsiveness of blood vessels to pressor amines, which has been related to an increase in glucocorticoids, has not been observed. Androgenic adrenal tumors are also occasionally associated with hypertension, but the mechanism is obscure.

Humoral mechanisms are also involved in the role of the kidney in the production of hypertension, an area of intense interest and controversy for over half a century. In response to the compromising of the arterial blood supply, the kidney releases renin, which by interaction with a serum globulin produces angiotensin I. A plasma enzyme acts to convert angiotensin I to angiotensin II, which is a powerful vasoconstrictor. Angiotensin also stimulates aldosterone production, which, with its resultant sodium and water retention and expansion of blood volume, plays an important role in the production of hypertension. More obscure renal mechanisms which may play a role in the formation of systemic hypertension include the production of antirenins and vasoexciter material (VEM), which may potentiate arteriorlar response to epinephrine, and the excretion or metabolism of circulatory pressor substances.

CLINICAL MANIFESTATIONS

The signs and symptoms of hypertension are rarely to be attributed to the elevated blood pressure per se but rather to the effects of the elevated pressure on a given organ system. Early in the course of hypertension there are usually no signs or symptoms. Headache, weakness, palpitation, and dizziness are among the early symptoms. Epistaxis occurs more frequently in older patients with established hypertension. A history of flushing, sweating, paroxysmal headaches, and episodic hypertension suggests pheochromocytoma. The combination of paresthesia, muscular weakness, transient paralysis, polyuria, and polydipsia is associated with aldosteronism. Urinary tract infection may suggest renal parenchymal disease, and the presence of peripheral vascular disease intensifies suspicion of renal vascular hypertension.

The duration of hypertension and the presence or ab-

sence of visual disturbances, angina, stroke, and myocardial infarction should all be documented, since these provide an index of the severity of hypertension and have prognostic implications.

On physical examination, the finding of a persistently elevated diastolic pressure establishes the diagnosis of systemic hypertension. Vascular changes in the optic fundi, graded on the Keith-Wagener-Barker scale from 0 to 4 for increasing severity, are indicative of general systemic changes and of the degree of hypertension. With all types of hypertension, signs of specific organ involvement may be apparent. These include congestive failure, renal failure, hypertensive encephalopathy, and manifestations of cerebrovascular accident. Certain causes of surgically correctible hypertension are associated with specific findings. Coarctation of the aorta is suggested by decreased femoral pulses and decreased blood pressures in the leg. A loud systolic bruit may be heard over the precordium and posterior chest wall. After the first decade of life, patients have well-developed shoulders and arms, and enlarged collateral arteries are palpable in the musculature of the thorax posteriorly. The finding most suggestive of renovascular hypertension is the presence of a bruit in the upper abdomen. This is most frequently encountered in young females with fibromuscular hyperplasia of the renal artery. Evidence of arteriosclerotic disease of the aorta or of the iliac, femoral, or carotid arteries in hypertensive patients increases the likelihood of similar lesions in the renal arteries.

Cushing's syndrome is associated with the physical findings of central obesity, "buffalo hump," moon face, abdominal striae, ecchymoses, hirsutism, and evidence of osteoporosis. Pheochromocytoma is characterized by sweating, blanching or flushing, syncope, tachycardia, or angina associated with extreme fluctuations in blood pressure. These paroxysms may be induced by painful stimulus, exercise, or palpation of the tumor. The physical manifestations of primary aldosteronism are nonspecific except for those associated with advanced hypokalemic alkalosis, in which a positive Chvostek's sign may be present and carpal spasm may occur when the blood pressure cuff is inflated. Muscle weakness or paralysis also may be noted.

LABORATORY STUDIES

The chest x-ray and electrocardiogram serve as indices for the extent of cardiomegaly and left ventricular hypertrophy. The x-ray may provide the diagnosis in cases of coarctation of the aorta, in which rib notching and the silhouette of a coarcted segment of aorta may be seen. In hyperaldosteronism, the electrocardiogram demonstrates the typical findings of hypokalemia.

Abnormalities demonstrated in routine urine examination such as bacterial growth and proteinuria, accompanied by an elevation of the blood urea nitrogen (BUN) and impaired creatinine clearance, suggest bilateral parenchymal disease. However, these findings do not rule out the possibility of renovascular hypertension. If the urine culture shows bacterial growth, split renal function studies should be delayed until the infection is brought under control.

In pheochromocytoma, a 24-hour urinary output of catecholamines in excess of 200 μg/day and an excretion of the catecholamine metabolite VMA (3-methoxy-4-hydroxymandelic acid) in excess of 7 mg/day are key diagnostic findings. However, certain drugs and foods give false-positive results. The fasting blood sugar level and basal metabolic rate are often elevated. In Cushing's syndrome, the critical determination is an elevated 24-hour urinary output of 17-hydroxysteroids in relation to the daily excretion of creatinine; the fasting blood sugar and glucose tolerance tests often show a diabetic-type response.

In primary aldosteronism, serum electrolyte determinations reveal the potassium to be less than 3 mEq/L and the carbon dioxide more than 30 mEq/L, while the sodium is normal or only slightly increased. The daily urinary potassium excretion exceeds 40 mEq/L, while sodium excretion is normal. The urinary specific gravity is low and there is an alkaline pH. The changes of hypokalemic alkalosis may also occur with secondary aldosteronism related to renovascular hypertension.

CLASSIFICATION

In general, surgically correctible hypertension involves the consideration of diastolic hypertension. Systolic hypertension with normal or decreased diastolic pressure is usually dependent upon cardiac output, and changes in the elasticity of the aortic wall are not commonly associated with pathologic sequelae in the small vessels or target organ systems. Examples of systolic hypertension include arteriovenous fistulas, thyrotoxicosis, and atherosclerosis of the aorta in the elderly patient. Elevation of diastolic pressure is primarily the result of a chronically increased residual resistance in the peripheral vascular bed.

Table 23-1 lists the more important surgically correctible causes of hypertension. Although several entries might be added, those which are included have the greatest practical importance, because of their relative frequency and the lasting benefits which may result from their recognition and treatment. Correction of any of these disease processes may save a patient from a lifetime of antihypertensive drug therapy.

The first three causes listed in the table, i.e., pheochromocytoma, primary aldosteronism, and Cushing's syndrome, are related to abnormalities in the adrenal glands and are discussed in detail in Chap. 37; coarctation of the

Table 23-1. SURGICALLY CORRECTIBLE CAUSES OF HYPERTENSION

Pheochromocytoma
Primary aldosteronism
Cushing's syndrome
Coarctation of the aorta
Renovascular hypertension
Unilateral renal parenchymal disease

Table 23-2. STUDY OF THE HYPERTENSIVE PATIENT FOR EVIDENCE OF A SURGICALLY CORRECTIBLE LESION

History
Physical examination
Roentgenogram of the chest
Electrocardiogram
Laboratory studies:
  Urinalysis, urine culture, and 24-hour urine protein
  Hemogram
  Serum: BUN, creatinine, and cholesterol
  Serum*: CO_2, K, Cl, Na
  Fasting blood sugar and glucose tolerance test
  24-hour urinary excretion of catecholamines†, VMA†, and 17-hydroxy steroids
  24-hour urinary excretion of K and Na
  Creatinine clearance
Special tests:
  Rapid-sequence excretory urogram
  Radioisotope renogram
  Renal arteriography, via aortic injection and selective injection if indicated

If the above studies show or suggest one of the following correctible causes, further procedure is as indicated:

Renal artery stenosis: Split renal function study and renal vein renin assay.
Aldosteronism: Plasma renin activity and aldosterone secretion rates.
Cushing's syndrome: Adrenopituitary function studies.
Pheochromocytoma: Reconfirm results and proceed with operation.
Coarctation of the aorta: Thoracic aortogram.
Unilateral renal parenchymal disease: Split renal function study and renal vein renin assay.

  * Patient should not be receiving diuretic therapy.
  † A number of drugs or foods may cause false-positive results.

aorta is considered in Chap. 18. These causes are briefly summarized in this chapter, with special emphasis on their relation to the diagnostic study of a patient with hypertension.

In September of 1963, at Vanderbilt University Hospital, a careful search was initiated for patients with surgically correctible hypertension. As of July 1, 1972, a total of 1,070 patients with diastolic hypertension had been investigated. In this study, the history, physical examination, and laboratory and special diagnostic studies (Table 23-2) were designed to detect the causes listed in Table 23-1. The results of this study are referred to throughout the chapter. The very low incidence of patients with hypertension secondary to adrenal causes or coarctation of the aorta in this study may be somewhat misleading. In most patients with hypertension secondary to an adrenal pathologic condition the diagnosis of a pheochromocytoma, Cushing's syndrome, or primary aldosteronism is established or strongly suspected before they are referred. Ordinarily such patients are not included in our general study of patients with hypertension; the same is true of most patients with coarctation of the aorta. Therefore the incidence of this condition will be very small, which indeed it is, but not so small as may be indicated.

PHEOCHROMOCYTOMA

Pheochromocytoma is undoubtedly the most dramatic and treacherous of the surgically correctible causes of hypertension. Unfortunately, many reported cases to date have been undiagnosed during the patient's life or have been suspected only at the last minute during a lethal paroxysmal hypertensive crisis and confirmed at autopsy. The incidence of pheochromocytoma even in the hypertensive population is very low. It has been estimated by Barbeau et al. and Kvale et al. that 0.4 to 2 percent of patients with hypertension have a pheochromocytoma. In the 9-year study of 1,070 consecutive hypertensive patients investigated for evidence of a surgically correctible cause, only 3 patients with pheochromocytoma were found at Vanderbilt University Hospital. During that time, approximately 150 patients presented with a clinical picture suggestive of pheochromocytoma which subsequent study failed to confirm.

CLINICAL MANIFESTATIONS AND LABORATORY STUDIES. The clinical manifestations of these neoplasms are related to their secretion of norepinephrine and epinephrine, and the resultant hypertension may be paroxysmal or sustained. It occurs in all age groups, although 80 percent of the reported cases have been in adults. Although pheochromocytoma is rare, the lethal propensities of the tumor in the untreated case and the extremely good result attending well-planned surgical treatment make it important to screen all patients with hypertension for the lesion. From a practical point of view, this can be done by determining the 24-hour urinary excretion of catecholamines (normally less than 100 $\mu g/24$ hours) and of the catecholamine metabolite VMA (usually excreted in the urine in excess of 7 mg/24 hours in patients with pheochromocytoma). This latter test is especially useful in patients taking an antihypertensive drug such as alpha-methyldopa, which interferes with the measurement of catecholamine excretion but does not alter the validity of the VMA determination. Other pharmacologic tests useful in the study

of patients suspected of having pheochromocytoma are discussed in Chap. 37.

Pheochromocytoma should be strongly suspected in all patients who have hypertensive or hypotensive reactions associated with anesthesia, pregnancy, or antihypertensive drug therapy, and in patients with family histories of pheochromocytoma, von Hippel-Lindau syndrome, von Recklinghausen's disease, or Sipple's syndrome. When performing any diagnostic study which may involve painful stimuli or provoke catecholamine release in a patient suspected of having a pheochromocytoma, adequate means of supporting or lowering the patient's blood pressure should be instantly available. Although aortography may demonstrate the location of a pheochromocytoma, the powerful stimulation attending this procedure can precipitate a paroxysmal crisis, and deaths have resulted. It is for this reason that, in the Vanderbilt University Hospital study protocol for hypertensive patients, the catecholamine and VMA levels are routinely determined before aortography if there is any suggestion of a pheochromocytoma in the history or physical examination. Although we formerly believed that aortography should not be done in the patient with a pheochromocytoma, we now believe that with certain precautions it can be done safely and will provide important localizing information. In general the tumor is very vascular, and an intense tumor stain is demonstrated. Obviously if a palpable adrenal mass is present or is demonstrated on an intravenous pyelogram (IVP), aortography assumes less importance. However, many of the tumors are small, 10 percent occur in extraadrenal locations, and 7 to 11 percent are multiple or bilateral.

TREATMENT. Once the diagnosis of pheochromocytoma has been established, the preoperative preparation becomes very important. The use of alpha- and beta-adrenergic blockage in preparing these patients for operation as well as during and after the operation is presented in Chap. 37. These advances have contributed significantly to the greatly lessened operative mortality noted below. Anesthesia for these operations is critical. There is a paramount need for smooth, nonstressful induction, atraumatic tracheal intubation, and avoidance of anesthetics which stimulate catecholamine release or enhance responsiveness to these amines. The operative approach is shown in Fig. 23-1.

During the last decade, reports by Greer et al., by Hume, and by Scott et al. indicate that better understanding of the pharmacologic problems engendered by pheochromocytoma and adherence to a careful plan of treatment have resulted in a reduction of operative mortality from 25 percent to less than 5 percent. Following removal of the tumor, the majority of patients (70 to 75 percent) become normotensive and remain so. About 25 percent of the patients have persistent mild to moderate hypertension, which is thought to be due to hypertensive vascular changes in the kidney.

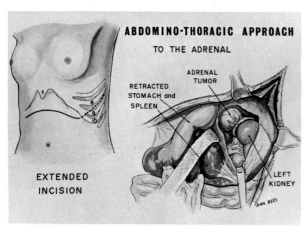

Fig. 23-1. Abdominothoracic approach to the adrenal glands. This approach is preferred in cases of pheochromocytoma and in Cushing's syndrome due to adrenal carcinoma; it allows radical nonmanipulative removal of the adrenal tumor.

PRIMARY ALDOSTERONISM

Primary aldosteronism refers to a syndrome caused by autonomous hypersecretion of aldosterone by hyperplastic adrenal, or by an adrenal adenoma or (rarely) carcinoma. Aldosterone, a mineral corticoid discovered in 1952, regulates extracellular fluid volume by controlling the excretion and resorption of sodium and water by the kidney. It is the most potent sodium-retaining hormone naturally occurring in man. In 1955, Conn described a syndrome of hypertension, hypokalemia, and alkalosis due to overproduction of aldosterone by an adrenal adenoma. Since that time several hundred cases have been reported.

In the vast majority of reported cases of primary aldosteronism, the cause is an adrenal adenoma. Less frequently, bilateral adrenal hyperplasia with or without nodularity has been reported as causing primary aldosteronism. Adrenal carcinoma is rare as a cause of aldosteronism.

CLINICAL MANIFESTATIONS AND LABORATORY FINDINGS. Conn collected 145 cases and found females predominated 3 to 1. Patients have ranged in age from fifteen to seventy-five years, but most have been in the fourth and fifth decades of life. Hypertension is usually present but is rarely severe. However, it may be associated with headache, cardiomegaly, and retinopathy. In the juvenile cases, severe and even malignant hypertension may occur. Symptoms related to the hypokalemia and alkalosis include muscle weakness, often episodic, which sometimes progresses to paralysis. Paresthesias of the hands and feet are common. Frank tetany may occur, with positive Chvostek's and Trousseau's signs. Polyuria and polydipsia are often prominent. Edema is usually absent.

Laboratory findings include hypokalemia (usually below 3 mEq/L), increased serum bicarbonate, normal or increased serum sodium, and elevated serum pH. Urinary potassium exceeds 40 mEq/24 hours, while urinary sodium is normal. Conn has recently stressed the opinion that hypokalemia may be a late manifestation of the disease and has reported cases of primary aldosteronism with persistent normokalemia. In primary aldosteronism, the plasma renin activity is low and the daily aldosterone secretion rates are high. The reasons for these pathophysiologic changes are discussed in detail in Chap. 37.

Primary aldosteronism is to be suspected in any hypertensive patient with the signs and symptoms listed above, especially the patient with hypertension, lack of edema, low serum potassium level, and increased serum sodium and carbon dioxide. Hypokalemia has proved to be the most valuable simple laboratory test. Plasma renin activity is low, usually 100 m μg/100 ml (nanograms) or less. The definitive diagnosis depends on the finding of a low serum renin with an increased urinary aldosterone excretion. The normal range for the latter study is 3 to 17 μg/24 hours, while in patients with primary aldosteronism the excretion rate may be elevated to levels as high as 160 μg/24 hours.

A number of factors influence the serum potassium, aldosterone, and renin levels, two of the most important being salt restriction and diuretic therapy. Thiazide diuretics cause potassium depletion and hypokalemia. A low-salt diet may prevent the hypokalemia and alkalosis of primary aldosteronism. Finally, a low-salt diet may cause a considerable rise in aldosterone and renin secretion. Patients being screened for evidence of primary aldosteronism should therefore be off diuretic therapy and on a liberal-salt diet (200 mEq sodium for 4 to 5 days) if meaningful serum potassium, aldosterone, and renin levels are to be obtained.

Secondary aldosteronism occurs in renovascular hypertension, congestive heart failure, nephrosis, cirrhosis of the liver, and other edematous states. In all these, the urinary sodium level is low as contrasted to normal or high levels in primary aldosteronism, and plasma renin activity is usually high.

At one point in the initial Vanderbilt University Hospital series of 341 patients with diastolic hypertension, 90 consecutive patients were studied for evidence of primary aldosteronism. After the patients had received a high-salt diet for 4 to 5 days, peripheral venous renin activity and aldosterone secretion rates were determined. Any patient with a suggestive elevation of aldosterone secretion or depression of plasma renin activity was readmitted to the hospital and again studied. Of these 90 patients, none proved to have primary aldosteronism due to an adrenal adenoma; one had a marked decrease in aldosterone secretion following removal of the left adrenal gland and 50 percent of the right adrenal. An initial serum potassium of less than 3.5 mEq/L was encountered in 42 of 341 patients. Many of these patients actually turned out to have a syndrome of hypokalemia, suppressed renin levels even with stimulation, normal aldosterone levels, and hypertension which was controlled by aldactone.

Conn's early estimate that 15 to 20 percent of patients designated as having essential hypertension have primary aldosteronism was excessive. Simpler and better methods of renin and aldosterone assays for widespread use will provide the means of answering many of the troublesome questions about this form of surgically correctible hypertension. Treatment and results are discussed in Chap. 37.

CUSHING'S SYNDROME

In 1932, Harvey Cushing described a syndrome consisting of central obesity ("buffalo hump" and moon face), osteoporosis, amenorrhea, hirsutism, abdominal striae, hypertension, and weakness. Cushing's syndrome is presently defined as a constellation of clinical and metabolic disorders which result from a chronic excess of cortisol (hydrocortisone). The source of the excess cortisol may be an adrenocortical tumor or, more commonly, bilateral adrenocortical hyperplasia under the stimulation of ACTH from the pituitary or a nonendocrine ACTH-secreting tumor of the lung, pancreas, or other organ. Untreated Cushing's syndrome is a highly incapacitating and lethal disorder. With early recognition and treatment a favorable outcome may be expected.

PATHOLOGY. The underlying adrenal pathologic condition in Cushing's syndrome is bilateral adrenocortical hyperplasia in 60 to 70 percent of cases. The remainder have adrenocortical tumors, of which two-thirds are adenomas and one-third carcinomas. The incidence of Cushing's syndrome due to nonendocrine ACTH-secreting tumors (ectopic ACTH syndrome) is unknown, but this type probably accounts for fewer cases than do adrenocortical tumors. In cases due to adrenal hyperplasia under the influence of pituitary ACTH, the pituitary may or may not contain an adenoma.

Normal adults excrete 3 to 12 mg of 17-hydroxycorticosteroids (17-OHCS) in 24 hours, while adults with Cushing's syndrome usually excrete in excess of 12 mg/day. However, it is more accurate to relate the daily urinary output of 17-OHCS to the quantity of creatinine excreted per 24-hour period. In this way variation due to body size and to the collection of less than the 24-hour output can be averted. Normal persons usually excrete 3 to 7 mg of 17-OHCS/Gm of creatinine; with Cushing's syndrome more than 7 mg of 17-OHCS/Gm of creatinine is usually excreted.

CLINICAL MANIFESTATIONS AND LABORATORY FINDINGS. Cushing's syndrome is three times as frequent in females as in males. It is found at all ages but is most common in the third and fourth decades. In children it almost always is due to an adrenocortical tumor, usually a carcinoma. The frequency of the various clinical and metabolic manifestations of the syndrome is shown in Table 23-3.

The florid case of Cushing's syndrome may be recognized by the clinical picture alone. However, many patients present only a few of the classic findings. The basic diagnostic study is the measurement of 24-hour urinary excretion of 17-OHCS. If the 17-OHCS output is abnormally elevated, special adrenopituitary function studies as described by Liddle are perfomed to confirm the diagnosis and to determine the underlying pathologic condition. These are discussed in detail in Chap. 37.

In the Vanderbilt University Hospital study of 1,070 consecutive hypertensive patients one patient with Cushing's syndrome was encountered. Interestingly enough, the initial determination of 17-OHCS had been in the normal range. Aortography revealed a tumor of the right adrenal gland. Subsequent 17-OHCS determinations and the other tests of adrenopituitary function indicated that the lesion was an adrenal adenoma, and this was confirmed when the tumor was removed.

TREATMENT. Diagnostic precision is important because appropriate therapy depends on recognition of the under-

Table 23-3. FREQUENCY OF THE MANIFESTATIONS OF CUSHING'S SYNDROME
(61 Cases, Vanderbilt University Hospital, 1954–1964)

Manifestation	Frequency, percent
Central obesity	100
Hypertension	83
Impaired glucose tolerance	83
Protein wasting	77
Osteoporosis	70
Hirsutism	70
Weakness	60
Menstrual aberrations	50
Ecchymoses	47
Edema	33
Striae	27

lying pathologic condition. Before surgical treatment is undertaken, severe metabolic derangements, infections, and complications related to hypertension should be brought under control. The views on treatment expressed here primarily reflect the experience of Liddle's Division of Endocrinology at Vanderbilt University Hospital.

Cushing's Syndrome Due to Adrenal Tumors. The only satisfactory treatment of Cushing's syndrome due to adrenocortical neoplasm is complete surgical removal of the tumor. In cases due to an adenoma, the posterior approach (Fig. 23-2) through the bed of the twelfth rib provides satisfactory exposure. Hayes has advocated bilateral adrenal exploration, because bilateral adenomas are found in about 10 percent of the cases. The most practical approach is perhaps the use of two surgical teams carrying out simultaneous posterior exposure of the two adrenal glands. This approach is less difficult, especially in the obese patient, and is associated with a lower postoperative morbidity than is the transperitoneal approach (Fig. 23-3). Following surgical excision of the adenoma, prompt and permanent regression of the syndrome is to be expected in the overwhelming majority of cases, although the hypertension may take some time to subside completely. An important consequence of "autonomous" production of cortisol by an adrenal tumor is the supression of ACTH production by the pituitary with resultant atrophy of the remaining adrenal tissue. A careful regimen of adrenal substitution therapy (usually hydrocortisone) must be initiated during the operation and continued until it has been demonstrated (by ACTH stimulation tests and 17-OHCS urinary levels) that the remaining adrenal tissue is functionally adequate.

In cases of Cushing's syndrome known or suspected to be due to an adrenocortical carcinoma, a thoracoabdominal incision is preferred so that a radical, nonmanipulative resection can be performed (Fig. 23-1). If preoperative roentgen studies have failed to localize the tumor, the abdominal component of the incision is made first and then extended into the appropriate hemithorax after the tumor has been identified. If the carcinoma can be completely removed, the results are the same as described above for an adenoma; the remarks regarding adrenal substitution therapy also apply. Obviously, if the tumor has metastasized beyond the limits of the resection or if the carcinoma is so extensive as to defy complete excision, the ultimate result is usually poor.

Cushing's Syndrome Due to Ectopic ACTH Syndrome. The only satisfactory treatment of an ACTH-secreting tumor (usually of the lung or the pancreas) is complete surgical removal. This has been accomplished in few cases to date; widespread metastases are usually present by the time the diagnosis is established. Irradiation or chemotherapy has been of little if any benefit in these cases. Bilateral adrenalectomy or therapy with adrenal-inhibiting agents may offer substantial benefit in selected cases, even though it has no influence on the tumor or on ectopic ACTH production.

Cushing's Syndrome Due to Bilateral Adrenocortical Hyperplasia. Treatment is dependent on the severity of the syndrome. If the patient has severe hypertension, osteoporosis, or psychosis, bilateral total adrenalectomy should be performed. The bilateral posterior approach is preferred for the reasons indicated earlier. Patients so treated usually have complete regression of the syndrome. Lifelong adrenal replacement therapy is required. Mild to moderate hypertension persists in about 10 percent of the cases.

If Cushing's syndrome is only mild to moderate and not associated with the severe manifestations listed above, irradiation of the pituitary with 4,000 to 5,000 r should be the initial treatment. Approximately 30 percent of the patients so treated with irradiation will obtain complete and lasting remission of the syndrome. Patients who fail to respond to this form of therapy should have bilateral adrenalectomy.

Patients with sellar enlargement or neurologic deficits attributable to a pituitary tumor should have the tumor removed. Transsphenoidal hypophysectomy employing magnification technique is being used with increasing frequency and success.

In patients treated by bilateral adrenalectomy as the initial therapy evidence of pituitary tumors may develop subsequently. Thorn has reported the incidence as 15 to 20 percent in his experience; in the Vanderbilt University Hospital experience, as reported by Liddle, it had occurred in three of seven cases. Of 11 patients treated by irradiation and then bilateral adrenalectomy, none had developed evidence of a pituitary tumor; of 18 patients treated with irradiation alone, none had developed evidence of a pituitary tumor. This experience would support the belief that pituitary irradiation lessens the incidence of pituitary tumor in patients who have bilateral adrenalectomy.

Finally, mention must be made of subtotal adrenalectomy in the treatment of Cushing's syndrome with bilateral adrenocortical hyperplasia. Subtotal adrenalectomy refers to complete removal of one adrenal and 80 to 90 percent of the other. This procedure had its origin at the time when adrenal steroid substitution therapy was not available. Persistent severe hypertension has been common in patients with hyperplasia who were treated by subtotal adrenalectomy. As Orth has reported, in our experience every patient treated by subtotal adrenalectomy was a treatment failure.

COARCTATION OF THE AORTA

Coarctation of the aorta is to be suspected in all infants, children, and adults with hypertension. The coarctation can occur anywhere in the aorta from the midpoint of the aortic arch down to the aortic bifurcation; however, 98 percent of coarctations are located in the first part of the descending thoracic aorta. The association of coarctation and systemic hypertension has long been known. It was not until 1945, however, that both Crafoord and Gross performed successful surgical correction of the coarctation and demonstrated that this form of hypertension was surgically correctible.

The mechanism of hypertension in coarctation·remains debatable. The explanation that it is caused by mechanical

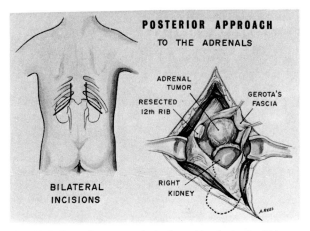

Fig. 23-2. Posterior approach to the adrenal glands. This approach is recommended in cases of Cushing's syndrome due to an adrenal adenoma or bilateral adrenocortical hyperplasia and in primary aldosteronism.

obstruction of the aorta causing increase in resistance to blood flow, with resultant hypertension in the circulation of the arms and head, has never seemed valid, since obstruction of the lower abdominal aorta does not produce hypertension. The experimental studies of Scott and associates have suggested that the coarctation results in reduced renal blood flow and activation of the renal pressor system. Convincing corroborative evidence in patients with coarctation has not yet been presented. Sealy performed angiotensin assays in five patients with coarctation of the aorta and found elevated levels in only two of them.

CLINICAL MANIFESTATIONS AND LABORATORY FINDINGS. The presence of vigorous pulses in the upper extremities and absence or profound decrease in the pulses of the lower extremities provide the basis for prompt recognition of this important cause of hypertension. Decreased blood pressure in the legs, normally 20 to 40 mm Hg higher than in the arms, and a precordial systolic murmur are valuable confirmatory findings. In infants and young children, the blood pressure in the arms may be normal or only mildly elevated. In older children and

Fig. 23-3. Anterior transperitoneal approach to the adrenals for removal of adrenal adenoma or hyperplastic adrenal glands.

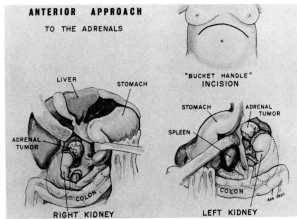

adults, hypertension is the rule. After the first decade of life, the shoulders and arms of a patient with coarctation are often extremely well developed and collateral arterial pulsation can be palpated in the musculature of the posterior thorax. The chest roentgenogram frequently reveals a silhouette of the coarcted segment in the descending thoracic aorta and notching of the ribs due to compensatory changes in the collateral circulation. The electrocardiogram usually shows left axis deviation.

A detailed consideration of coarctation of the aorta is presented in Chap. 18. Suffice it to say that coarctation is an important cause of hypertension which, if not corrected, leads to death in 60 percent of patients before the age of forty years. With surgical treatment, complete remission of the hypertension occurs in 95 percent of patients. In our study of 1,070 hypertensive patients two adults and one teen-ager had coarctation of the thoracic aorta.

RENOVASCULAR HYPERTENSION

Renovascular hypertension may be defined as diastolic hypertension secondary to an occlusive lesion of a main renal artery or segmental renal artery which is sufficiently

Fig. 23-4. Aortogram showing left renal artery stenosis due to atherosclerosis involving orifice and proximal third of the renal artery. Poststenotic dilatation is common with such lesions.

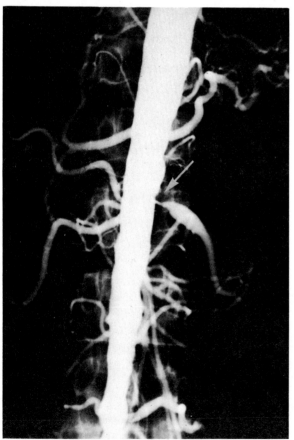

severe to activate the renal pressor mechanism. Interest in renovascular hypertension was initiated by Goldblatt and colleagues in the early 1930s, when they produced persistent hypertension in dogs by constriction of the renal arteries. Thereafter Page, Helmer, and Braun Menendez, with their colleagues, independently described the renin-angiotensin system. For the next two decades attention was focused on the kidney in the etiology of hypertension, although renal artery stenosis was considered to be a relatively uncommon cause of hypertension. Adequate and safe methods of studying renal function and vascular anatomy were not available. Nephrectomy was frequently performed for hypertension with an associated small kidney seen on excretory urography, but remission of the hypertension was observed infrequently. In 1956 Homer Smith reviewed a series of 575 hypertensive patients treated by nephrectomy in which it was observed that only 26 percent were normotensive after 1 year. Smith concluded that nephrectomy should be done only for strict urologic indications and not with any hope of relieving hypertension. At that time vascular surgery was developing rapidly, and new and improved techniques of aortography were being introduced and used with increasing frequency. Renal artery stenosis was seen frequently, and usually in patients with hypertension. The demonstrations by DeCamp and Birchall, Morris et al., DeBakey et al., Dustan et al., and others that normal blood pressure could be restored in many hypertensive patients with obstructive disease of the renal artery by surgical relief of the stenotic lesion initiated the present interest in renovascular hypertension. Refinements in excretory urography and renal arteriography and the development of split renal function studies, isotope renography, better methods of renin-angiotensin assay, and improved surgical techniques followed. All these advances contributed materially to a better understanding of renovascular hypertension and to a better selection of those hypertensive patients who would benefit from surgical treatment.

PATHOLOGY. Arteriosclerosis has been the underlying cause in 60 to 70 percent of the proved cases of renovascular hypertension reported to date. The atherosclerotic lesions usually occur in older patients and more frequently in the male. There is usually an atheromatous plaque situated in the orifice or proximal third of the renal artery (Fig. 23-4). However, the presence of an arteriosclerotic plaque in a renal artery does not necessarily indicate a causal relationship to associated hypertension. Autopsy and arteriographic studies by Eyler et al., Holley et al., and Foster et al. show that over 50 percent of patients after fifty years of age have some degree of arteriosclerotic renal artery stenosis whether they are hypertensive or normotensive. Associated arteriosclerotic disease of other vascular systems is commonly encountered. Bilateral renal artery lesions are present in roughly one-third of patients with renovascular hypertension due to arteriosclerosis (Fig. 23-5). Complete occlusion of a renal artery, with filling of the distal segment of the artery via collaterals, is not uncommon in patients over fifty-five years of age (Fig. 23-6).

Fibromuscular hyperplasia or dysplasia of the renal

artery has been the underlying cause in 20 to 25 percent of the reported cases of renovascular hypertension. Significant series of cases have been reported by Wylie et al., by Hunt et al., by Ernst et al., and by Fry et al. It has usually been observed in young patients, especially women in the twenty-five to forty-five age range. The lesion is characterized by a thickening of the media with a myxomatous-appearing fibrous tissue, which separates and distorts the muscle fibers, and by degenerative and disruptive changes in elastic tissue and smooth muscle. These changes result in lesions of the arterial wall which have been termed *microaneurysms*. Dissecting aneurysms and hematomas have also been observed. The striking feature of fibromuscular hyperplasia is the corrugation of the internal surface of the renal artery caused by alternating zones of hyperplasia and disruption of the media and elastic tissue in the wall of the artery. This corrugation gives the "string of beads" effect seen on renal arteriography (Figs. 23-7 and 23-8).

Earlier it was thought the lesions were unilateral in the majority of cases. However, it has now become apparent that the vast majority are bilateral lesions. The reason for this turnabout is found in the improvements in renal arteriography during the past few years. Selective oblique arteriograms in several projections are demonstrating lesions which previously were undetected. This holds true for both atherosclerotic and fibrodysplastic lesions but most commonly for the latter. Hunt et al. believe that virtually 100 percent of the fibromuscular lesions are bilateral, and our recent experience tends to support this concept. An aortogram in the anteroposterior projection will not suffice to demonstrate many renal artery lesions. The reason for this is shown schematically in Fig. 23-9. The origin of the renal artery may be masked by the aorta in such a projection, and the distal renal artery courses in almost an antero-

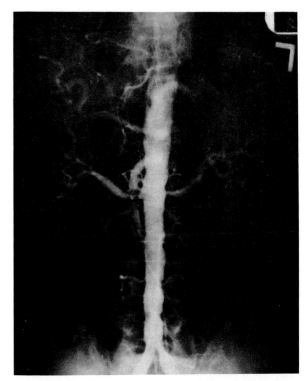

Fig. 23-5. Aortogram showing bilateral renal artery stenosis due to atherosclerosis. About one-third of patients with renovascular hypertension due to atherosclerosis have bilateral lesions.

posterior direction. The lesion is usually located in the middle and distal thirds of the artery, frequently extending into the segmental branches. With multiple renal arteries to one kidney, more than one of the arteries may show fibromuscular hyperplasia. On serial arteriograms over a period of several years, the lesions have been seen to become progressively more severe in some patients.

A variant of fibromuscular hyperplasia called *subadventitial fibroplasia* by McCormack et al. consists of a dense collar of collagen located in the periphery of the media, which is often thinned and disorganized by the fibrous tissue (Fig. 23-10). These lesions also have been most commonly found in females in the twenty-to-forty age

Fig. 23-6. *A.* Aortogram showing complete atherosclerotic occlusion of the left renal artery in a fifty-three-year-old man. Arrow indicates proximal portion of left renal artery which is still patent. *B.* Later film in aortographic series showing filling of the distal portion of the left renal artery via collaterals. Arrow indicates patent distal left renal artery. Lesion is amenable to correction by either bypass grafting or thromboendarterectomy with a patch graft.

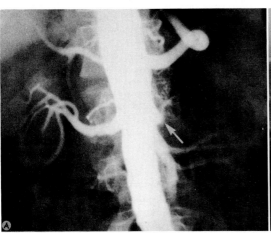

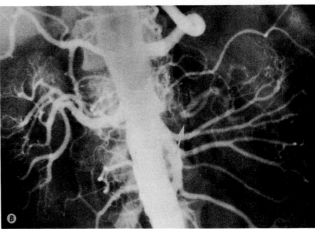

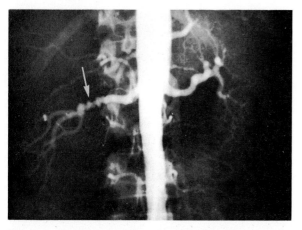

Fig. 23-7. Aortogram showing fibromuscular hyperplasia of the right renal artery with typical "string of beads" effect. Lesions often extend out to or even involve branch arteries. Selective left renal arteriography in this patient showed some lesions which had not been demonstrated by the aortogram.

range. A third variant is the occlusive lesion caused by an intimal fibrous proliferation producing either a discrete short area of stenosis or a long tubular stenosis; this has been called *single mural hyperplasia* (Fig. 23-11). It has been most commonly encountered in the very young patient, less than twenty years of age and as young as four months. Children with unilateral stenosis have been observed by Foster et al. to develop contralateral stenosis in subsequent years.

Harrison and McCormack, and Sheps et al. (1972), have devised a classification of the various fibromuscular lesions which allows recognition on radiograph and has some prognostic implications. These writers feel they can recognize whether the lesion will progress in severity.

The pathogenesis of the fibromuscular dysplasia group of lesions is not known. The lesion does occasionally occur in other arterial systems. Whether it is congenital or acquired is uncertain, and there may be more than one underlying cause. Suggested etiologic factors have been summarized by Hunt et al.; they include congenital anomaly, intrinsic defects in the elastic tissue, Erdheims' medial necrosis, healed arteritis, and abnormal stretching of arteries, especially in pregnancy.

Less common lesions causing renovascular hypertension are renal artery aneurysm, dissecting aneurysm of the renal artery, embolism with segmental infarction, primary thrombosis, and compression of the artery by a fibrous or muscular band (right crus of diaphragm) or a mass. In the author's experience, segmental infarction, presumably due either to an embolus or a segmental artery thrombosis, has been the third most common cause of proved renovascular hypertension.

PATHOPHYSIOLOGY. Reduction or dampening of the arterial pulse pressure in the renal artery beyond the obstruction is thought to be the stimulus which initiates the renal pressor mechanism. The manner in which this is brought about is not entirely understood. Both Crocker et al. and Tobian have shown that patients with renovascular hypertension frequently have hyperplasia and increased cellularity of the juxtaglomerular apparatus (JGA). The JGA surrounds the afferent arteriole of the cortical nephron and is thought to be the source of renin production. These observations have led to the hypothesis that the JGA contains a volume- or pressure-sensing mechanism which responds to reduced pulse pressure by liberating renin. Renin, a proteolytic enzyme, acts on the substrate angiotensinogen, a globulin produced by the liver and found in the α 2-globulin fraction of plasma, to produce a decapeptide which is designated *angiotensin I*. A plasmolytic converting enzyme splits off the last two amino acids from the apparently inert angiotensin I to produce an octapeptide called *angiotensin II*, which is the active pressor agent. Angiotensin II is an extremely powerful vasoconstrictive substance. On a weight basis, it is approximately ten times as potent a pressor agent as norepinephrine. The biologic properties of angiotensin II have been studied extensively, and it appears well established as the active vasoconstrictive factor in renovascular hypertension. Angiotensin II has other effects which are important in producing hyper-

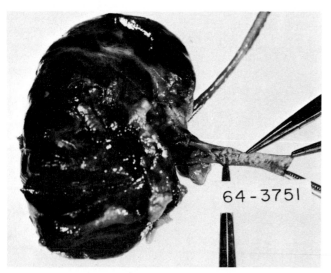

64-3751

Fig. 23-8. Resected right kidney with renal artery opened longitudinally to show fibrous septa forming corrugated internal surface.

tension. It potentiates the circulatory responses to norepinephrine, and it also stimulates secretion of aldosterone by the adrenal cortex. This latter effect may result in potassium depletion, sodium and water retention, and all the other features of aldosteronism in patients with renovascular hypertension. Recent studies by Louis and his associates have cast some doubt about the role the renin-angiotension system plays in the etiology of experimental renovascular hypertension.

CLINICAL MANIFESTATIONS. The incidence of renovascular hypertension in patients with diastolic hypertension is not known. In a study searching for patients with renovascular hypertension at Vanderbilt University Hospital during the years 1963 to 1972, the incidence was 16 percent. However, this cannot be considered a study of diastolic hypertension in unselected subjects, because of the bias introduced by the physician's referral of a patient to the study. At present it is estimated that 5 percent of patients with diastolic hypertension have renovascular hypertension.

There are no unique features in history, physical examination, or routine laboratory determinations which will differentiate renovascular hypertension from essential hypertension, although a number have been suggested. Most of the classic concepts about essential hypertension are based on patients in whom other causes of hypertension were not excluded. Table 23-4 shows a comparison of the clinical findings in a group of 57 patients with proved renovascular hypertension and a group of 260 patients with essential hypertension. These data still pertain to our larger experience with 1,070 hypertensive patients. Every one of these patients had a complete evaluation, including rapid-

Fig. 23-10. *A.* Selective right renal arteriogram of patient with subadventitial fibroplasia; lesion is more disorganized and does not have the regularity of the "strings of beads" effect seen in Fig. 23-7. *B.* Photomicrograph of renal artery with subadventitial fibroplasia. In the upper and lower corners at the right the dense collar of collagen is seen in the peripheral media. Disorganization of the media and intima is also seen.

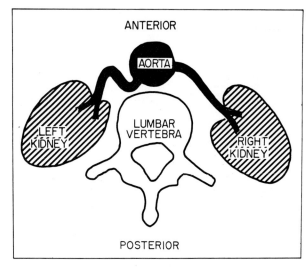

Fig. 23-9. Diagram showing the course of the renal arteries. Lesions in the renal arteries may be masked in the anteroposterior projection. Oblique selective arteriograms are required to demonstrate these lesions.

sequence excretory urography, isotope renography, and renal arteriography. If a renal artery stenosis was found, split renal function study was performed, and in the later period of the study renal vein renin was assayed. The diagnosis of renovascular hypertension was based strictly on a favorable response to surgical treatment, the most critical of diagnostic criteria. In those cases designated as essential hypertension, all tests were normal. Patients with hypertension due to adrenal causes or renal parenchymal disease were eliminated. The reason for the disparate figures under the various clinical observations is that for some patients the pertinent information was not known.

Classic teaching has been that a family history of hypertension suggests essential hypertension, but renovascular hypertension was just as frequently associated with this

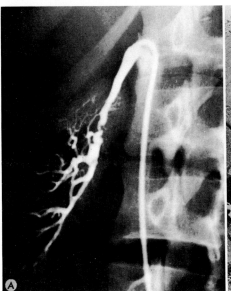
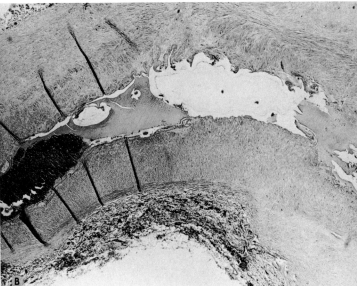

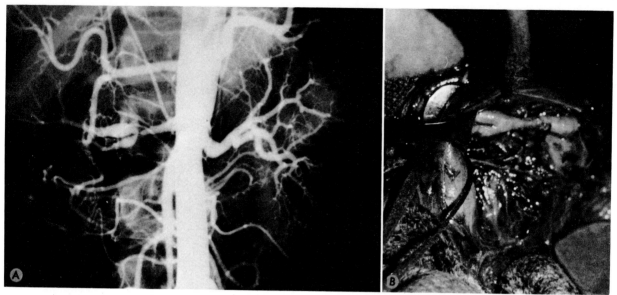

Fig. 23-11. *A.* Aortogram showing single mural hyperplasia of the right renal artery, in an eighteen-year-old girl. *B.* Photograph of the stenosis seen at operation. The vena cava has been retracted to the patient's right to expose the renal artery and the area of stenosis.

observation. A history of recent acceleration of hypertension, recent onset of hypertension, and flank pain or trauma in the hypertensive patient was equally frequent in the two groups. The mean duration of hypertension was but slightly longer in the patient with essential hypertension. Only the finding of an upper abdominal bruit on physical examination provided any differentiation between the two groups, since it was four times more frequent in the renovascular hypertension group. The eye ground changes on fundoscopic examination provided information as to the severity of the hypertension but not as to the origin.

It is commonly stated that hypertension in the young patient is more likely to have a renovascular cause. Figure 23-12 compares patients with renovascular hypertension

and those with essential hypertension by decade of life. Again patients with renal parenchymal disease were eliminated, and the diagnoses of essential hypertension and renovascular hypertension were on the same basis as for Table 23-4. The highest incidence of renovascular hypertension was in the first decade of life, the next highest incidence was in the sixty- to sixty-nine-year age group, and surprisingly few instances were found in patients ten to nineteen years of age. It can only be concluded that renovascular hypertension occurs at all ages. Certainly the very young patient with severe hypertension is a

Table 23-4. CLINICAL FINDINGS IN RENOVASCULAR HYPERTENSION AND ESSENTIAL HYPERTENSION
(Vanderbilt University Hospital, 1963–1966)

	Renovascular hypertension		Essential hypertension	
	Number	*Percent*	*Number*	*Percent*
Family history of hypertension	26/51	51	130/245	53
Recent acceleration of hypertension	7/48	15	31/225	14
Recent onset of hypertension (6 months)	10/50	20	40/230	17
Hypertension associated with history of flank pain, hematuria, or renal trauma	4/57	7	18/260	7
Upper abdominal bruit	22/57	40	24/260	9
Duration of hypertension, years:				
Range	0–23		0–28	
Mean	5.4		6.2	

prime suspect, but so is the older hypertensive patient.

LABORATORY FINDINGS. Routine laboratory determinations provide little help in the detection of renovascular hypertension. Only an occasional patient will have secondary aldosteronism with hypokalemic alkalosis. Tarazi et al. have noted an increased incidence of elevated hematocrit level in patients with hypertension secondary to renal artery stenosis, but this was found in only a small percentage (less than 20 percent) of the patients. The urinalysis, phenolsulfonphthalein excretion, and hemogram or serum electrolyte determinations provide few clues as to the cause of the hypertension. Azotemia occurs with equal frequency in renovascular and essential hypertension. The changes of left ventricular hypertrophy found on the chest x-ray or electrocardiogram are helpful in gauging the severity of the hypertension but not in determining the underlying cause.

SELECTION OF PATIENTS FOR INTENSIVE DIAGNOSTIC STUDY. As the foregoing discussion of the clinical characteristics of renovascular hypertension indicates and as will be seen in the discussion of some of the special screening tests, there is no simple way to predict which patient will be found to have renovascular hypertension. This has led to the author's principle that *any patient with significant diastolic hypertension in whom surgical correction would be recommended if a significant lesion were found should have intensive diagnostic study.* This approach eliminates the mildly hypertensive patient and the patient who is an unacceptable operative risk.

SPECIAL DIAGNOSTIC STUDIES. Rapid-Sequence Excretory Urography. This is a simple variation of the standard intravenous pyelogram described by Maxwell et al. The patient, having been dehydrated, receives a rapid intravenous injection of contrast medium, and roentgenograms are made at 1, 2, 3, 4, 5, 10, 15, and 30 minutes. Contrast medium should appear in the calyceal system of the normal kidney on the 2-minute film. Findings suggestive of renovascular hypertension include (1) unilateral delay in appearance of contrast medium, strongly suggesting renal artery stenosis (Fig. 23-13); (2) decrease in renal length greater than 1.5 cm as compared with the contralateral kidney (Fig. 23-14); (3) unilateral decreased concentration or density of the medium on the early films; (4) ureteral notching due to collateral arterial supply; and (5) unilateral hyperconcentration of the medium on the late films (Fig. 23-15), which is explained by the fact that the kidney with a significant renal artery stenosis displays increased tubular resorption of water and sodium, while the contrast medium is a fixed solute and is not resorbed, thus appearing in hyperconcentration on the late films. (This effect may be accentuated by hydrating the patient or even giving an intravenous infusion of a saline solution of urea, so-called "washout" intravenous pyelography.) This phenomenon is the basis of the split renal function tests described below. A further finding on the urogram, defects in the renal silhouette, may indicate segmental infarction (Fig. 23-16).

The urogram also provides important information re-

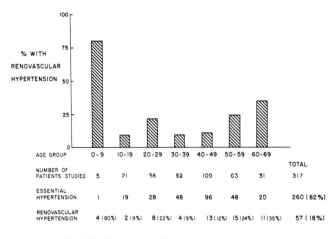

INCIDENCE OF RENOVASCULAR HYPERTENSION AND ESSENTIAL HYPERTENSION
BY DECADE OF LIFE
VANDERBILT UNIVERSITY SERIES 1963-1966

Fig. 23-12. Incidence of renovascular hypertension and essential hypertension in 317 hypertensive patients.

garding renal parenchymal disease, e.g., pyelonephritis and hydronephrosis. However, in the recent analysis by Foster et al. of 122 patients with proved renovascular hypertension, the urogram was judged to be normal in 31 percent of the cases. If, as some have advocated, the urogram had been used to determine whether to proceed with further studies (i.e., arteriography), we would have missed almost one-third of the patients with renovascular hypertension. The fact that one-half the false-negative results occurred in patients with bilateral lesions is of interest but does not alter the fact that they would have been missed. A urogram that is abnormal preoperatively but normal postoperatively is very reassuring. On many occasions we have seen a kidney increase in length by 1.5 to 2.0 cm

Fig. 23-13. Two-minute film from a rapid-sequence excretory urogram. Contrast medium is present in the calyceal system on the right; none is seen on the left. This is strongly suggestive of a left renal artery stenosis.

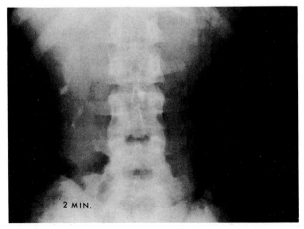

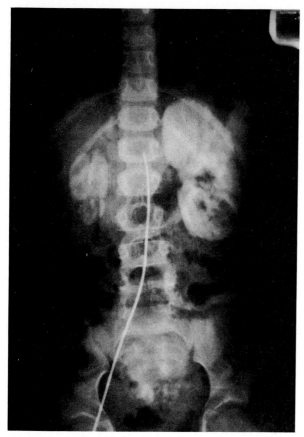

Fig. 23-14. Nephrographic phase of aortogram showing difference in renal size which suggests renal artery stenosis.

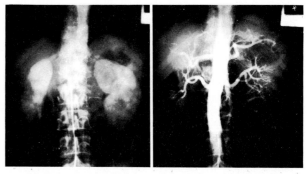

Fig. 23-16. Nephrographic phase of an aortogram showing defect in midportion of the right kidney. This was detected on the excretory urogram. Aortogram shows branch artery to midportion of right kidney completely occluded. Heminephrectomy resulted in remission of hypertension.

by the seventh day following successful operative treatment.

Isotope Renography. The ^{131}I orthoiodohippurate renogram has been widely used in screening hypertensive patients for renovascular hypertension. Tracer doses of the

Fig. 23-15. Late film in excretory urogram showing hyperconcentration of contrast medium in the right renal pelvis, a sign indicative of right renal artery stenosis.

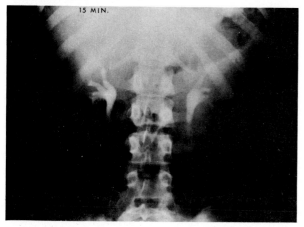

isotope are injected intravenously, and external scintillation counters, placed posteriorly over each kidney, simultaneously record timed uptake and excretion curves. Features characteristic of renal artery stenosis are reduced total height of curve, delayed time to maximal height, and delayed excretion. These abnormalities reflect the degree of reduced renal tubular function and the reduced volume of urine excreted by the ischemic kidney. The test is not specific and must be interpreted with the aid of the excretory urogram. Obstructive uropathy simulates renal ischemia. Pyelonephritis and other parenchymal renal diseases are also responsible for false-positive interpretations in perhaps 20 percent of patients with renovascular hypertension. As with excretory urography, the renogram compares one kidney with the other; hence bilateral renal artery stenosis may not be detected. We have not found the renogram to be particularly helpful in the diagnosis of renovascular hypertension. A triple isotope renogram study is currently being evaluated in the study of patients with hypertension.

Renal Arteriography. If one accepts stenosis of a main or segmental renal artery as part of the definition of renovascular hypertension, renal arteriography becomes the best screening test for renovascular hypertension. Hesitancy to apply arteriography in all patients with diastolic hypertension is related to the fact that the procedure involves a small but definite risk, is expensive, and ordinarily requires that the patient be hospitalized.

A number of methods of obtaining contrast angiographic demonstration of the renal arteries are available. The most widely accepted method is the percutaneous retrograde catheter technique via a femoral artery. Under fluoroscopic control the catheter tip is located in the aorta at the level of the L_1–L_2 interspace; a pressure injector is used to inject the contrast medium, and a rapid film changer is used to obtain serial films. The films will show the aorta, the main renal arteries, the segmental branch arteries, and the entire kidney in the nephrographic phase.

In recent years oblique aortograms and selective renal arteriography, with the catheter tip placed in the renal artery, have been used to obtain additional information. With a catheter selectively placed in a renal artery one

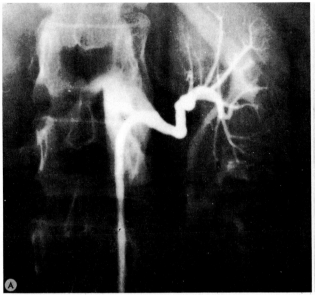

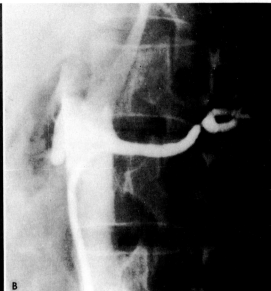

Fig. 23-17. *A.* Left selective renal arteriogram in straight antero-posterior projection; renal artery stenosis is not seen. *B.* Repeat arteriogram with same patient in oblique position shows severe stenosis of distal left renal artery and distal renal artery segment suitable for implantation of an aorticorenal bypass graft utilizing a segment of saphenous vein.

can rotate the patient in various oblique views to demonstrate a severe stenosis which may have appeared to be of questionable significance on straight posteroanterior projection (Fig 23-17). Similarly, in some patients with extensive fibromuscular hyperplasia which on the aortic-injection arteriogram did not appear amenable to surgical correction, a selective arteriogram may show a distal seg-

ment of the renal artery suitable for placement of a bypass graft (Fig. 23-18). Figure 23-9 shows why oblique arteriograms are required in these patients.

In patients with severe arteriosclerotic occlusive disease of the aortoiliac-femoral system it may not be possible or advisable to insert the catheter via a femoral artery. In this situation translumbar aortography or a catheter inserted via an axillary artery may be used to demonstrate the renal arteries.

In the Vanderbilt University Hospital study of 1,070 consecutive hypertensive patients, 1,423 renal arteriograms have been made in the course of initial and followup studies. There have been 10 serious complications (0.7 percent): three massive hematomas, one false aneurysm of the femoral artery, thrombosis of the femoral artery in six patients, and one death following aortic surgery for postaortogram thrombosis of the aorta in a patient with severe atherosclerotic occlusive disease.

Fig. 23-18. *A.* Aortogram showing fibromuscular hyperplasia which appears to extend into branch arteries and precludes satisfactory corrective surgery. *B.* Oblique left renal arteriogram in same patient showing distal segment suitable for implantation of a bypass graft (see Fig. 23-23).

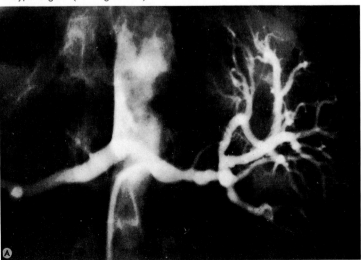

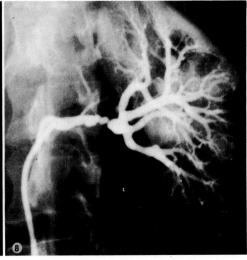

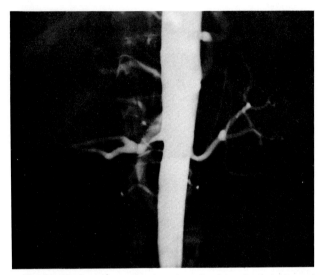

Fig. 23-19. Aortogram showing stenosis of proximal right renal artery due to extrinsic compression of the artery. At operation the right crus of the diaphragm was found to be compressing the artery in this forty-two-year-old man.

Arteriosclerosis is the most common cause of renal artery stenosis, and the lesions are bilateral in about one-third of the cases (Fig. 23-4 and 23-5). The process usually involves the origin and the proximal third of the renal artery; poststenotic dilatation is common with severe lesions. Complete occlusion is not uncommon in patients over fifty years of age; in this circumstance the distal renal artery is usually seen to opacify on the later films via collateral arterial supply (Fig. 23-6).

Fibromuscular hyperplasia is the second most commonly encountered stenosis of the renal artery. The lesion usually involves the middle and distal thirds of the renal artery, and frequently the segmental branch arteries are involved. In women in the twenty-five to forty-five age range the lesion is that of multiple mural hyperplasia with the "string of beads" appearance (Fig. 23-7). In patients under twenty years of age and in the male in general a single mural hyperplasia (intimal hyperplasia) is more common (Fig. 23-11).

Less common lesions causing renal artery occlusion are aneurysm, embolism or thrombosis, and compression by a fibrous or muscular band or mass (Fig. 23-19).

Figure 23-20 shows the frequency of arteriographic demonstration of a renal artery stenosis in 317 hypertensive patients. Stenosis in patients under thirty years of age was almost exclusively due to fibromuscular dysplasia; arteriosclerosis was the predominant lesion in patients over fifty years of age. Between ages thirty and fifty the incidence of arteriosclerosis and fibromuscular dyplasia was about equal. Table 23-5 shows the arteriographic findings in the larger series of 1,070 patients.

A renal artery stenosis found on arteriogram in hypertensive patients does not establish a causal relationship. Two-thirds of patients over sixty years of age had a stenosis, but Fig. 23-12 shows that only half the stenoses were of proved functional significance. At present there are three ways of determining whether a stenosis is functionally significant: renal biopsy and histologic study of the juxtaglomerular apparatus, reninangiotensin assay, and split renal function study. The first (JGA study) is not very practical, and accumulated experience to date is quite limited. From our experience, if either of the latter two studies are positive, a good blood pressure response following operative treatment can be expected in 90 percent of the patients.

Split Renal Function Studies. In normal persons and persons with essential hypertension the two kidneys seldom vary significantly in their handling of water, sodium, or solutes. In renal artery stenosis a functionally ischemic kidney resorbs sodium and water excessively, while fixed solutes appear in the urine in increased concentration. These characteristics of the ischemic kidney led to the development of a number of tests to determine when a given stenosis is functionally significant. All the tests involve catheterizing the ureters, collecting urine specimens for successive controlled periods of time, and analyzing the urine specimens.

The Howard test was the first such test described. A reduction in urine volume of 50 percent and a reduction in urine sodium concentration of at least 15 percent or an increase of urinary creatinine concentration of at least 15 percent from the involved kidney have functional significance. The Rappaport test is based on sodium/creatinine ratios from each kidney. A tubular rejection fraction ration (TRFR) is obtained by multiplying the sodium/creatinine ratio on the left by that on the right. A ratio of less than 0.6 indicates significant left renal artery stenosis, and a ratio of more than 1.6 implicates the right renal artery. When the values are between 0.6 and 1.6, the test is negative. The Birchall test employs an infusion of hypertonic saline solution (0.25 Gm sodium chloride/100 ml/kg body weight in 45 minutes). Sodium/creatinine urinary concentration ratios from the two kidneys are compared. The larger sodium/creatinine ratio is divided by the smaller one; if the resultant value is 2 or more,

Fig. 23-20. Incidence of renal artery stenosis, demonstrated by arteriography, in 317 hypertensive patients.

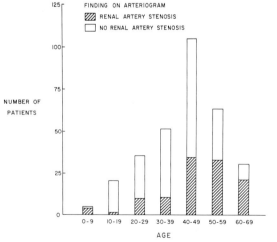

INCIDENCE OF ANGIOGRAPHIC RENAL ARTERY STENOSIS BY DECADE OF LIFE

Table 23-5. RESULTS OF EVALUATION OF
1,070 HYPERTENSIVE PATIENTS

	Renal arteriogram	*Renovascular hypertension**	
Normal	610 (57%)	—	
Renal artery stenosis due to:			
Atherosclerosis	297 ⎫ (43%)	114 ⎫	16%
Fibromuscular dysplasia . .	152 ⎭	51 ⎬ 39%	
Miscellaneous	11	11 ⎭	

*Positive functional tests—split renal function studies or renal venous renin assays.

the test is positive. The smaller ratio indicates the involved kidney. The Stamey test involves osmotic diuresis by means of an intravenous infusion of urea. Para-aminohippurate (PAH), a fixed solute excreted by the kidney but not resorbed by the tubules, is added to the infusion. Functionally significant renal artery stenosis is suggested when the involved kidney shows a 66 percent smaller urine volume and a 100 percent greater PAH concentration than the uninvolved kidney. In the Stamey test one also determines the effective renal plasma flow (ERPF) in each kidney. This is valuable in assessing the function of the contralateral or normal kidney; severely impaired plasma flow usually indicates intrarenal small vessel disease. Table 23-6 shows the results of split renal function studies in patients with functionally significant right renal artery stenosis.

In bilateral renal artery stenosis, the split function studies are frequently difficult to interpret; however, in most cases of bilateral stenosis there is a marked discrepancy in the severity of stenosis on the two sides, and the split function studies demonstrate this functional difference.

The author's experience is limited to the use of the Howard and Stamey tests. The original criteria for the interpretation of these tests were based on a very small number of patients. In the beginning we adhered rigidly to those criteria in selecting patients for operative treatment. However, since 1966 liberalized criteria for a positive test have been used. A recent retrospective study of 41 patients who are unequivocally cured following unilateral

renal arterial surgery revealed that the following criteria seem to suffice for a positive test: (1) consistently lateralizing discrepancies in the triplicate samples; (2) Howard test—25 percent reduction in urine volume and 15 percent increase in creatinine from the involved kidney as compared with the contralateral kidney; and (3) Stamey test—25 percent increase in PAH concentration and 25 percent reduction in urine volume in the affected kidney.

Disadvantages of split renal function studies include patient discomfort and occasional complications secondary to the study, e.g., urinary tract infection, ureteral colic, and, rarely, transient ureteral obstruction secondary to edema. A more frequent problem is technical failure to obtain a satisfactory study in about 10 percent of the patients. This occurs most frequently in the male over fifty years of age with prostatic enlargement which interferes with ureteral catheterization.

Renal Venous Renin Assay. If the renin-angiotensin pressor system is the mechanism through which renal artery stenosis causes renovascular hypertension, assay of these substances should afford an accurate way of detecting the disorder. Reports by Fitz, by McPhaul et al., and by Michelakis et al. support this concept. Renin assays, using a radioimmunoassay technique, are now widely available and have proved to be extremely accurate in demonstrating renovascular hypertension. Peripheral venous renin assays are important in detecting primary aldosteronism or other conditions in which renin secretion is severely depressed. However, for the diagnosis of renovascular hypertension, comparative assays of the renin activity in the individual veins are usually required. In our initial report, Michelakis et al. stated that the criterion for a positive study was a 1.5 renin ratio when comparing the involved and uninvolved kidneys, and we have continued to use this criterion. Ernst and his associates have indicated that a 1.4 ratio is sufficient, and under certain circumstances (e.g., extensive collateralization) even a smaller ratio is significant.

Disadvantages of the renal vein renin assay are few. Thrombophlebitis subsequent to femoral vein catheterization is occasionally encountered. Catheterization of the renal veins under fluoroscopic control is simple and almost always feasible.

Table 23-6. RESULTS OF SPLIT RENAL FUNCTION STUDIES IN
PATIENTS WITH RIGHT RENAL ARTERY STENOSIS

	Right kidney			*Left kidney*			*Serum*		
	Patient 1	*Patient 2*	*Patient 3*	*Patient 1*	*Patient 2*	*Patient 3*	*Patient 1*	*Patient 2*	*Patient 3*
Volume, ml/min	1.6	1.5	2.4	15.2	18.0	23.2			
Na, mEq/L	35.0	43.0	54.0	70.0	93.0	103.0	140.0		
Creatinine, mg/100 ml .	19.0	18.0	16.0	5.0	3.5	3.5	0.67	0.67	0.67
Creatinine clearance, ml/min	55.0	49.0	70.0	138.0	115.0	148.0			
PAH, mg/100 ml	264.0	240.0	216.0	60.0	52.0	48.0	1.84	1.76	1.76
PAH cleared, mg/min . .	4.224	3.600	5.184	9.120	9.360	11.136			
ERPF, ml/min	281	250.0	360.0	605.0	649.0	772.0			
Osmolality, mOsm/kg . .	488	522	532	275	292	309	290	292	299

Relative Value of Split Renal Function Studies and Renal Venous Renin Assays in Renovascular Hypertension. Now that renin assays are fairly widely available, many physicians are using this test alone to determine when a renal artery stenosis is causing hypertension. As mentioned earlier, in our experience when either or both of the tests are positive, a good blood pressure response will follow operative treatment in 90 percent of the cases. We have persisted in using both tests whenever feasible and recommend operative treatment when either is positive. Retrospective analysis of patients who are unequivocally cured following operative treatment of unilateral lesions reveals that about 10 percent had negative or normal split function studies and the same number had negative or normal renin assays. In each of these patients the other test had been positive. There are a number of variables which influence the results of both tests, and these variables are often difficult to control. We think the two tests compliment each other and, in addition, the renal function studies provide valuable information regarding the status of the contralateral, or uninvolved, kidney.

Preoperative Renal Biopsy. Vertes et al. have advocated percutaneous biopsy of the kidney in the assessment of patients with renovascular hypertension. They have correctly noted that there are degrees of intrarenal arterial and arteriolar nephrosis which *may* preclude a beneficial result following corrective surgery. The problem has been to determine when such changes exist. Schacht et al., Baker et al., and Strickler have reported patients with renovascular hypertension and a renal biopsy interpreted as moderate or severe who have been cured or unequivocally improved by corrective surgery. In the future a well-controlled retrospective study of a large group of patients with renovascular hypertension may validate the recommendation of Vertes et al. However, it must also be pointed out that the etiology of hypertension does not follow an "all-or-none" law. Patients with severe renovascular hypertension due to an ischemic kidney may also have an element of hypertension as the result of arteriolar nephrosclerosis. Correction of the renovascular lesion will often change such a patient from the category of malignant hypertension to a mild hypertensive categorized as improved in the results of treatment. This has been observed repeatedly in older patients with complete occlusion of a renal artery.

TREATMENT. Selection of Patients for Surgical Treatment. Patients who have significant diastolic hypertension secondary to a functionally significant rental artery stenosis, as demonstrated by split renal function study or renal vein renin assay, and who present a reasonable surgical risk should have corrective surgical treatment. The consideration of surgical risk is relative. A patient with severe or malignant renovascular hypertension, even though cardiac or central nervous system complications may have already occurred, should have corrective surgical treatment if at all possible because of the extremely poor prognosis if the hypertension is not brought under control. Stamey and others have stated that unless the contralateral, uninvolved kidney has a renal plasma flow of 200 ml/minute or more, as determined by split function study, the patient

will not benefit from corrective surgery. As with Vertes' opinion regarding nephrosclerosis, future analysis of differential renal function studies in a large number of patients may provide accurate prognostic information of this sort. The author and others have seen patients with unilateral renovascular hypertension and contralateral renal plasma flow of less than 200 ml/minute who have been benefited by corrective surgery.

Preoperative Preparation. If at all possible the patient should be off antihypertensive medication for 10 days or 2 weeks before operation. These agents alter the vasomotor system so that when a general anesthetic is administered, profound vasomotor collapse may occur. Reserpine and other *Rauwolfia* drugs are notorious for this effect: it takes 10 to 14 days for patients on reserpine or guanethidine to become free of their effects. However, there are patients in whom the hypertension is so severe that antihypertensive medication must be continued up to and even during the surgical procedure. This has been demonstrated particularly in young children with malignant hypertension secondary to renal artery stenosis. In such instances control of the blood pressure with alpha-methyldopa, a relatively short-acting agent which does not deplete the nerve endings of norepinephrine stores, has been well tolerated, and vasomotor instability has not been a problem. In general, if the anesthetist knows that the patient has been receiving drugs, anesthesia can be administered safely.

Renal artery reconstruction or nephrectomy should not be undertaken after split renal function study or renal arteriography until it has been determined that these procedures have not caused any degree of renal injury. This is rarely a problem after arteriography, but after split renal function study some degree of ureteral edema is not infrequent. If one adds the trauma of a period of renal artery occlusion or removal of functioning kidney tissue, a disastrous result may ensue. Therefore a 2- or 3-day period should elapse between split renal function study and the surgical procedure, during which the patient's urine output and BUN levels should be monitored. If there is evidence of renal or ureteral injury, the operative procedure should be postponed until the patient has fully recovered.

A blood volume deficit of 500 to 1,740 ml is encountered in 31 percent of patients with renovascular hypertension. Preoperatively the blood volume should be determined, and appropriate correction of plasma or red blood cell deficits should be made to avoid postoperative hypotension and attendant thrombotic complications. In the occasional patient with secondary aldosteronism, metabolic aberrations must be corrected preoperatively.

Operative Treatment. In the selection of an operative procedure for renovascular hypertension, preservation of renal tissue is a prime consideration. Nephrectomy should be done only as a last resort. Patients with both fibromuscular and atherosclerotic lesions frequently have progression of insignificant lesions or develop new lesions in the contralateral renal artery. The younger the patient, the more important this consideration becomes. At present about the only indication for nephrectomy is a destroyed, virtually nonfunctioning kidney.

Adequate exposure for reconstruction of the renal arteries can be obtained through either a long midline incision from the pubic symphysis to the xiphoid or a supraumbilical transverse incision extending from flank to flank. When a coexisting lesion of the abdominal aorta, an aneurysm, or occlusive disease requires attention, the midline incision provides better exposure for dealing with the iliac arteries. Previously we performed bilateral renal biopsy and measurement of pressure gradients across the stenosis in every case. The value of these observations was quite limited, and now these determinations rarely are made. Any judgment the value of bilateral renal biopsies must await the report of the pathologists of The Cooperative Study of Renal Arterial Hypertension. They are analyzing biopsy material from several hundred cases. As regards pressure gradients, as Thomas et al. have pointed out, if there is one present, it means the stenosis is significant, but the absence of a gradient is difficult to interpret.

To expose the left renal artery, the entire small bowel is retracted to the right, and the posterior peritoneum overlying the aorta is incised. With appropriate dissection of the surrounding retroperitonal fatty areolar tissue, the left renal vein crossing the aorta is displaced superiorly and the left renal artery exposed. To expose the right renal artery, the inferior vena cava is mobilized and retracted to the right to expose the origin and first portion of the artery. One or more pairs of lumbar veins may be divided in this dissection. To approach the distal right renal artery, the hepatic flexure of the colon and the second portion of the duodenum are mobilized and retracted to the left, and the dissection is carried down to expose the distal right renal vein and artery. This approach is now used in most cases of right renal artery stenosis. It provides the best exposure for an anastomosis between the graft and the renal artery.

The most applicable and most commonly used operative procedure is either a thromboendarterectomy, with or without a patch graft, or some form of bypass graft from the aorta to the renal artery distal to the stenosis (Fig 23-21). Other operative procedures include splenorenal anastomosis, implantation of the renal artery into the side of the aorta; resection of the lesion with end-to-end anastomosis of the renal artery; and interposition of a graft into the renal artery (Fig. 23-22).

When thromboendarterectomy is performed, the remaining renal artery is usually an extremely delicate and thin-walled structure. A patch graft of autogenous vein or Dacron is often required to avoid narrowing of the renal artery lumen by the suture line. Sometimes a thromboendarterectomy can be performed transaortically after the aorta has been occluded above the renal artery, thus avoiding direct handling and suturing of the renal artery. Transaortic endarterectomy in patients with orificial atherosclerotic lesions has been strongly advocated by Wylie and Starney and their associates.

From a practical point of view, the bypass procedure is the most widely applicable. In dealing with a small renal artery, as in most cases of fibromuscular hyperplasia, a segment of saphenous vein or autologous hypogastric artery lends itself well to a precise, delicate anastomosis with the renal artery (Fig. 23-23). If the distal renal artery is

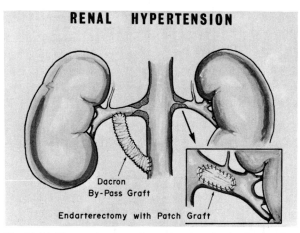

Fig. 23-21. The most commonly employed methods of correcting a renal artery stenosis. Saphenous vein or a Dacron prosthesis may be used for a bypass or patch graft.

large, as is often the case in arteriosclerotic lesions with poststenotic dilatation, a Dacron prosthesis works quite well (Fig. 23-24).

Prior to application of occluding vascular clamps the patient is given 50 mg of heparin intravenously. A mannitol solution is infused intravenously to stimulate osmotic diuresis prior to and during periods of renal artery occlusion. The graft is first anastamosed end to side to the renal artery. This is the more difficult anastomosis and is easier if done first. Occluding vascular clamps are then removed from the renal artery, and a small bulldog clamp is placed across the graft at the anastomotic site. The aortic anastomosis is then done. A recent improvement in technique has been the use of a monofilament polypropylene suture material (Prolene). Previously we had used a braided polyester suture and routinely encountered brisk bleeding from the suture lines requiring administration of 2 or more units of blood and reversal of the heparin with protamine. Since 1971 we have used the polypropylene suture; we have noted minimal anastomotic bleeding, blood transfu-

Fig. 23-22. Various operative procedures available to correct a renal artery stenosis.

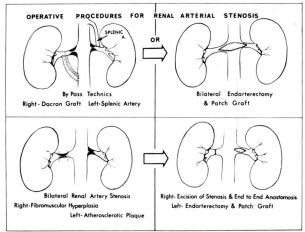

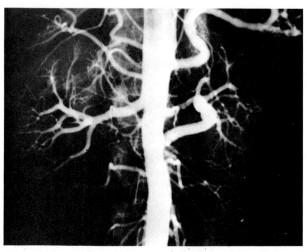

Fig. 23-23. Aortogram showing left aorticorenal bypass graft 1 year after implantation (same patient as Fig. 23-18). The graft is a segment of saphenous vein.

sion rarely has been necessary, and we have not had to give protamine. A review of 38 comparable procedures showed over twice as much blood replacement was required with the braided suture. Examination of the braided suture under the microscope reveals that it is quite porous and has an irregular serrated surface when compared with smooth monofilament material. When the braided suture is pulled through an artery or vein, a sawing effect results which enlarges the hole created by the needle. We believe this is the cause of the greater suture line's bleeding with the braided suture. At any rate the polypropylene suture creates a watertight suture line. It has virtually no drag as it is pulled through the vessel wall. One must take care to avoid a purse-string effect with this suture. For this

Fig. 23-24. Aortogram showing bilateral aorticorenal bypass grafts of crimped Dacron. This aortogram was obtained 4 years after the operation (preoperative aortogram is shown in Fig. 23-5).

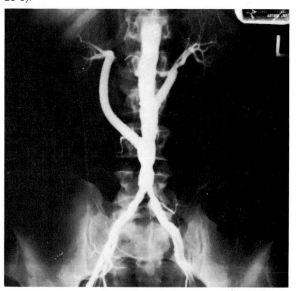

reason the suture line is interrupted in four places, and the arteriotomy is held open widely with traction sutures during the anastomosis.

In constructing an aorticorenal bypass great care must be taken in orienting the course of the graft so as to avoid kinking or twisting. Wylie et al. and Fry and his associates prefer an end-to-end anastomosis between the renal artery and the graft. This technique avoids angulation at the renal artery anastomosis which sometimes causes kinking. If a kink is encountered, the anastomosis must be redone. The best course for the graft from the renal artery to the aorta varies from patient to patient. On the left side the graft usually seems to course better behind the left renal vein. On the right side a retrocaval course usually works best.

If the aortic bifurcation has been resected, because of occlusive disease or aneurysm, and there is a coexisting significant renal artery stenosis, a side-arm bypass graft can be attached in the aortic prosthesis before the graft is interposed between the aorta and iliac arteries and subsequently anastomosed to the renal artery.

Renal transplantation experience has shown that if the vasculature of the donor kidney is washed out and the kidney cooled, tubular necrosis and renal dysfunction are minimized. This technique is now being employed in renal artery reconstructions. When the renal artery is opened, a cannula is inserted and the kidney perfused with 500 ml of a saline solution which has been cooled to 1 to 2°C. The perfusate is collected from the renal vein to prevent its entrance into the systemic circulation. Thereafter the arterial reconstruction is done. This technique produces a core kidney temperature of 16°C. The results with this technique are only preliminary, but they appear to show better tubular function in the early postoperative period, and no complications have attended the procedure. Prior to adoption of this technique, the triple isotope renogram done on the first postoperative day would show normal renal artery blood flow but poor tubular function. With this technique, tubular function appears to be normal or near normal on the first postoperative day. Again, these are preliminary results.

Another perplexing problem has been the patient with renovascular hypertension secondary to stenoses and/or aneurysm in the distal renal artery with extension into the branch renal arteries, usually fibromuscular lesions. A distal renal arterial segment suitable for conventional bypass is not present. In the past for many such patients nephrectomy was performed. However, the propensity for the development of bilateral severe lesions in these patients has dampened any enthusiasm for nephrectomy. In patients with stenoses involving the segmental branch arteries, Fry and his associates adopted a technique of using olive-tipped dilators to dilate these lesions and have presented interesting follow-up arteriographic data supporting the merits of the procedure.

Renal transplantation experience has led to an alternative technique that appears to be applicable in these patients: ex vivo reconstruction of the renal artery. Ota et al., Lim et al., and Belzer as well as others have reported use of this technique. The exact details of the operative procedure have varied from group to group, and the technique is still in the developmental stage. We have employed the procedure in five renal arterial reconstructions, anatomically successful in each instance. The renal artery and vein are divided close to the aorta and vena cava. The kidney is then rotated out on the abdominal wall onto a small operating platform. The ureter has been mobilized to allow this maneuver but has not been divided. The renal vasculature is flushed with 500 ml of a cold (1 to 2°C) saline solution. The artery is then attached to the Belzer apparatus and perfused with an acellular, oxygenated solution. Gravity is used to return the venous effluent to the Belzer pump. Using magnification and 7-0 arterial sutures, the multiple segmental renal artery lesions are repaired. In the case of terminal renal artery aneurysm the branch arteries are implanted into a saphenous vein graft. The artery or vein graft is then implanted into the common iliac artery and the renal vein into the distal vena cava. Ureteral collaterals, in cases of severe stenosis, can lead to significant renal blood flow which appears in the venous effluent. This can be avoided by application of atraumatic Potts ties to the ureteral artery. It is too early to judge this technique, but it appears to be an exciting development in renal artery surgery.

The problem of what to do in case of a severe functionally significant stenosis in one renal artery and a moderate nonsignificant stenosis in the other has not yet been answered objectively. In the opinion of some, performing a bypass on the side with the moderate stenosis adds little time or risk to the operative procedure, may be beneficial in avoiding future problems, and will improve renal blood flow. The evidence supporting this concept at the present time is tenuous.

Postoperative Care. Following renal artery reconstruction the patient is maintained on nasogastric suction and intravenous fluids for 3 to 5 days. Central venous pressure is monitored in the early postoperative period in older patients and in any patient with an impaired myocardial reserve. Most patients have some degree of diuresis following successful repair. In an occasional patient the diuresis may be massive, and severe electrolyte aberrations may ensue if the losses are not replaced. Urine output is monitored hourly via an indwelling catheter, and daily urinary output of sodium, potassium, and chlorides is determined, as are the serum levels of these electrolytes. Significant losses are replaced quantitatively. The patient is weighed daily to gauge fluid balance and to avoid overloading. It is difficult to overemphasize the importance of this simple observation. These patients often have an impaired myocardial reserve, and a fluid overload can result in congestive heart failure, pulmonary edema, and accelerated hypertension.

The blood volume should be determined early in the postoperative period, and the hematocrit should be monitored for several days. Postoperative hypotension and oliguria are usually related to an inadequate blood volume, due either to failure to expand a contracted blood volume preoperatively or to failure to replace operative blood losses.

Severe hypertension in the postoperative period is not an uncommon problem. There are a number of underlying causes: *Hypothermia* with peripheral vasoconstriction is managed by warming the patient and administering Thorazine. *Fluid overload* with increased central venous pressure and weight gain is managed with fluid restriction and judicious diuretic therapy. Finally, a number of patients will have *severe blood pressure elevations* that cannot be explained and must be treated with antihypertensive drugs; alpha-methyldopa is administered intravenously (500 mg every 4 to 6 hours) for several days. If hypertension becomes more severe than it was preoperatively, thrombosis of the reconstruction is to be strongly suspected. An excretory urogram or renogram is helpful in determining whether the kidney is functioning properly; if it is not, renal arteriography should be performed. Thrombosis of a renal artery reconstruction can result in malignant hypertension in a matter of a few days, as reported by Miller and Foster. Revision of the reconstruction or nephrectomy is usually required.

Some degree of transient azotemia is usually observed in patients who have undergone bilateral renal artery operations and in many patients who have had unilateral operation. This is probably due to renal tubular damage secondary to intraoperative renal artery occlusion which has been previously noted, and we are now reluctant to do bilateral simultaneous renal artery reconstructions. The degree of renal injury is usually minor, and with adequate hydration the BUN usually returns to normal by the time the patient is ready for discharge, ordinarily the eighth to tenth postoperative day. Renal failure secondary to tubular necrosis occasionally occurs after surgical treatment of renovascular hypertension. Other postoperative complications that have been recorded are those which might be expected in any seriously ill patient with hypertensive cardiovascular disease: myocardial infarction, congestive heart failure, cerebrovascular accident. Avoidance of hypotension or severe hypertension is the only means of preventing these complications.

RESULTS OF SURGICAL TREATMENT. The bulk of experience with operative treatment of renovascular hypertension has accumulated in the last decade. It is not surprising that there has been considerable variation in classifying the response to surgical treatment. Definition of the term "cure" presents the least problem: adults with documented diastolic hypertension who 3 or more months after surgical treatment have a diastolic blood pressure of less than 90 mm Hg are considered to be cured. It is more difficult to define a cure in children, especially children less than ten years of age.

The blood pressure response in the first 7 to 14 days after operative treatment is not a reliable index to the true response. The combination of the operation and strict bed rest may result in normal blood pressure levels which return to hypertensive levels when the patient resumes normal activity. On the other hand, some patients may remain hypertensive in the early postoperative period and become normotensive several weeks or months later. The greatest problem in defining response to treatment is in patients who are improved by operation but who continue to have a diastolic blood pressure above 90 mm Hg. These patients are largely the elderly, with atherosclerosis, who

Table 23-7. RESULTS OF OPERATIVE TREATMENT
OF RENOVASCULAR HYPERTENSION

Report	Period	Year of report	No. of patients	Cure, percent	Cure and improved, percent	Operative mortality, percent
Michigan	60–61	1962	43	40	82	4.0
Cleveland Clinic	57–61	1963	76	62	78	10.0
UCLA.	59–64	1964	67	37	82	4.0
Baylor	56–64	1966	432	41	81	7.0
Vanderbilt	62–65	1966	35	46	77	6.0
Mayo Clinic*	58–65	1967	100	55	84	0.0
UCSF	52–66	1967	122	37	65	8.0
Virginia	61–67	1968	53	28	75	3.6
Columbia	64–69	1970	40	53	76	2.5
Mayo Clinic†	64–70	1970	46	46	66	6.0
Cooperative Study. . .	61–69	In press	502	47	61	6.8
Vanderbilt‡	62–72	1973	122	70	90	5.4
UCSF§	52–62	1969	41	22	56	15.0
UCSF§	63–68	1969	42	26	74	2.4
Michigan*	61–70	1972	66	62	94	0.0

*None of these patients had simultaneous treatment of extrarenal atherosclerotic vascular lesions.
†All patients had aortic occlusive disease or aneurysm in addition to renal artery stenosis and operative treatment of both.
‡All patients had positive split renal function studies and/or renal venous renin assays.
§Atherosclerotic lesions only.

in addition to a renovascular cause for their hypertension have an underlying essential hypertension or arteriolar nephrosclerosis. "Improvement" has generally been defined as a persistent (i.e., at least 3 months) 20 mm Hg reduction in diastolic pressure. In the future, more rigid criteria for defining improvement should be forthcoming from such groups as The Cooperative Study of Renal Arterial Hypertension, which involves 13 institutions under U.S. Public Health Service sponsorship. The number of patients classified as failures or unimproved after surgical treatment will obviously be influenced by definition of the "improved" category; however, overt failures are quite obvious.

The time lapse between a successful operation for renovascular hypertension and a salutary blood pressure response has been variable. In most patients (perhaps 75 percent) the blood pressure recorded 1 month after operation accurately reflects the ultimate result; but some patients have required 3 months or more to become normotensive. The reasons for this are poorly understood.

Table 23-7 presents a composite view of the response to operative treatment of renovascular hypertension in a number of centers. Methods of selection of patients for operative treatment were varied, as were the criteria used to classify the operative result. The two reports with a 0 percent operative mortality omitted patients with simultaneous treatment of extrarenal atherosclerotic vascular lesions. A similar adjustment of our 1972 series would decrease the number of patients to 106 and the operative mortality to less than 3 percent. The Vanderbilt University Hospital series shows that more than 90 percent of the patients have a good result following operative treatment if the preoperative functional studies were positive. Figure

23-25 shows our yearly incidence of renal artery operations for renovascular hypertension since 1962.

Interest in renovascular hypertension varies widely from one center to another in the United States. In a few institutions the condition is being recognized frequently; however, in most centers it is identified only occasionally or is virtually unknown. There are several reasons for this difference: (1) A prime reason is that in the late 1950s and early 1960s many patients with hypertension and an associated renal artery stenosis had operative treatment but were not benefited. They did not have functional evidence of renovascular hypertension. This experience dampened or extinguished interest in renovascular hypertension. (2) There is widespread belief that renovascular hypertension is a rare condition. Our experience indicates that about 5 percent of patients with diastolic hypertension have renovascular hypertension. By conservative estimate there are at least 30 million patients with hypertension in the United States, or 1.5 million patients with renovascular hypertension. The condition can hardly be considered rare. (3) A multidisciplinary team approach to the study of the patient with hypertension is necessary if patients with renovascular hypertension are to be recognized. The internist is the key physician; if the experience of the 1950s and early 1960s has left him with little interest in renovascular hypertension (Item 1, above) or if he believes renovascular hypertension is rare (Item 2), he will probably treat his hypertensive patients with drugs and not try to find an underlying cause for the high blood pressure. Our group had a slow start, but the medical community has gradually adopted the philosphy of complete study of the patient with hypertension. While we have detailed data on 1,070 hypertensive patients, it is probable that an equal number of hypertensive patients have been evaluated according to the same protocol in our community. This explains the high frequency (16 percent) of renovascular hypertension in the 1,070 patients—many of the patients have been referred after a positive pyelogram or arteriogram.

In the past 15 years there have been tremendous advances in the drug therapy of hypertension. Freis and his associates have presented convincing evidence of the efficacy of antihypertensive drug treatment of hypertension and prevention of the complications attending hypertension. However, drug therapy has many untoward side effects. Most notable is postural hypotension. In many hypertensive patients effective control of the blood pressure is limited to the time spent in the upright position; hypertension during the hours spent in the supine position must be accepted. Control of the supine blood pressure may result in intolerable hypotension in the upright position.

Shapiro and his associates and others have stated that patients with renovascular hypertension who are over fifty years of age should not have operative treatment. From their experience it was felt that the risk is too great and the chance of a good result is too small. They advised drug therapy in this age group. Fifty-two of our patients were over fifty years of age, and 80 percent of them were either cured or improved following operative treatment. The operative mortality (10 percent) was higher in these older patients, but this was primarily because of patients who had simultaneous operative treatment of extrarenal vascular lesions such as an aortic aneurysm or occlusive disease.

A comparative study of drug treatment and operative treatment of renovascular hypertension has not yet been reported. Our group is presently doing such a prospective randomized study, but it is too early to report any results.

Figure 23-25 shows the number of patients a year since 1960 who have had renal artery operations. An analysis of the results of surgical treatment related to the type of renal artery lesion shows that patients with fibromuscular hyperplasia are cured more often (73 percent) than patients with an arteriosclerotic plaque (53 percent), although the improved group of patients contains a higher percentage of patients with arteriosclerosis. If the results of treatment are related to the type of surgical procedure, renal artery reconstruction has resulted in cure in 76 percent, while cure has been effected in 52 percent of nephrectomized patients. However, the nephrectomy series contains a larger proportion of the improved patients.

The severity of arteriolar nephrosclerosis, as determined by study of bilateral renal biopsies, has not correlated well with the response to operative treatment. There is a higher incidence of severe arteriolar nephrosclerosis in the unimproved group and of benign arteriolar nephrosclerosis in the cured group, but there are numbers of patients with severe changes who have been cured and of unimproved patients with benign changes.

Renovascular hypertension due to unilateral stenosis can so severely damage the contralateral kidney that it becomes the more powerful renin-secreting kidney. In this

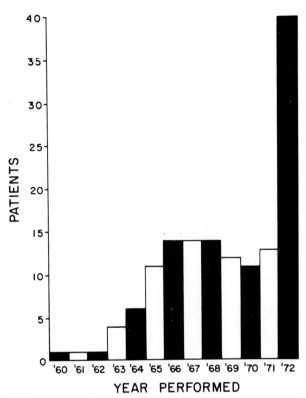

OPERATIONS vs YEAR PERFORMED

Fig. 23-25. Number of patients undergoing operative treatment for renovascular hypertension each year since 1960 at Vanderbilt University Hospital.

condition, the kidney with the renal artery stenosis is protected from the ravages of severe hypertension. Floyer demonstrated this experimentally in the 1950s, and there have been occasional reports providing human confirmation since that time (Thal et al., Marable et al., Morris et al., and others). We have encountered this situation in two patients, one of whom was reported by McAllister et al. Relief of the hypertension requires unilateral arterial reconstruction and contralateral removal of the kidney which has been destroyed by the hypertension (Fig. 23-26). An interesting observation has emerged from the treatment of these patients and of patients with a solitary kidney with renal artery stenosis—their blood pressure returns to normal immediately following successful operative treatment. This is in contradistinction to many patients with renovascular hypertension due to unilateral stenosis in whom it may require days, weeks, or even months before the blood pressure becomes normal. In these patients, as Alpert et al. have shown, it seems likely that the contralateral kidney has been damaged by hypertension. The ultimate result then depends on whether the damage is reversible; if reversible, considerable time may be required.

The reported incidence of thrombosis or stenosis of a renal artery reconstruction has ranged from 15 to 35 percent. In our experience and in that of Ernst et al. and Fry

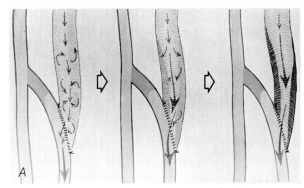

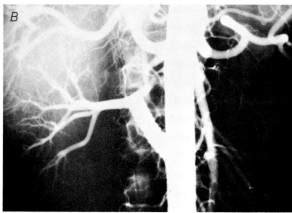

Fig. 23-26. *A.* Dacron graft bypass to right renal artery. *B.* Photomicrograph showing destroyed left kidney which was removed. Arteriolar changes including fibrinoid necrosis are apparent.

et al., thrombosis usually occurs in the first few postoperative days and is due to technical errors in performing the reconstruction. With experience and improved operative technique it has been possible to reduce the frequency of this complication to less than 5 percent. Immediate postrepair arteriograms and flowmeter studies should help reduce this problem further.

Serious postoperative complications have occurred frequently in these patients. Many have compromised cardiac function, and congestive failure and pulmonary edema are common problems unless fluid balance is carefully managed. Table 23-8 lists the complications in 122 patients.

There have been few reported follow-up arteriographic

Table 23-8. POSTOPERATIVE COMPLICATIONS OF OPERATIVE TREATMENT OF RENOVASCULAR HYPERTENSION

Complication	No. of Patients
Congestive heart failure	4
Acute tubular necrosis	4
Intestinal obstruction	2
Aortic suture line disruption	1
Basilar artery thrombosis	1
Hemolytic crisis	1
Bracheal plexus stretch injury	1
Renal arteriovenous fistula	1
Abdominal angina	1

data on aorticorenal bypass. Exceptions are the reports of Kaufman et al. and of Ernst et al. Ernst and Fry and their associates have shown that the saphenous vein, used to construct an aorticorenal bypass, almost routinely undergoes uniform dilatation, sometimes progressing to aneurysmal proportions. We have noted these same changes, and vein graft aneurysm has occurred in 2 of 68 patients 4 to 6 years following implantation (Fig. 23-27). Arteriographic follow-up studies of aorticorenal bypass utilizing hypogastric artery are needed. Ultimately this graft may prove to be superior to the vein graft.

UNILATERAL RENAL PARENCHYMAL DISEASE

There is an ill-defined group of patients with hypertension who have a small atrophic kidney on one side, a normal or hypertrophic contralateral kidney, and no evidence of main or segmental renal artery stenosis on arteriography. The underlying etiologic factors have usually been unilateral pyelonephritis, congenital hypoplasia, radiation fibrosis, or posttraumatic fibrosis. The problem has been to determine when an atrophic kidney is responsible for the hypertension. For 20 years after Goldblatt's original studies, nephrectomy was frequently performed on the basis of hypertension and an associated small kidney. Although these patients were operated on because it was thought they might have a "Goldblatt kidney," remission in the hypertension was observed infrequently. Smith's review in 1956 of 575 patients indicated that only 26 percent were benefited.

A recent 5-year experience with hypertensive patients, involving careful study in search of an underlying cause, indicates that perhaps 5 percent have a small kidney on one side and no evidence of main or segmental renal artery stenosis on arteriography. The involved kidney may be anywhere from 3 to 7 cm shorter than its mate, and the renal cortex of the involved kidney is proportionately thinned. The uninvolved kidney may be normal in length or hypertrophic (less than 13.5 to 14 cm long). Renal artery stenosis can cause these same changes in kidney length. However, in unilateral parenchymal disease the main renal artery and its segmental branches are uniformly small throughout, without evidence of stenosis or occlusion. In unilateral pyelonephritis, calyceal clubbing is usually seen on the pyelogram. There are often areas in the parenchyma which suggest focal atrophy, and there is distortion of the small intrarenal arterial branches. In so-called "congenital hypoplasia" all the structures are small and may be diminutive but have no distortion or other abnormality.

Recent reports by McDonald, by Hickler, et al., and by Crocker et al. indicate that nephrectomy in patients with unilateral renal parenchymal disease has been accompanied by cure or improvement of their hypertension only if there was evidence of an ischemic pattern on split renal function study. The author's experience indicates that an increase in the renal vein renin from the involved side is equally valid. In the case of a totally nonfunctioning kidney, renal vein renin assays may be the only means of

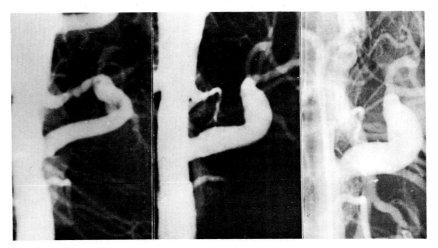

Fig. 23-27. Arteriograms showing a saphenous vein aorticorenal artery bypass 1, 3, and 5 years after implantation. Aneurysmal dilatation is apparent at 5 years.

determining functional significance as regards the hypertension. Hypertension due to unilateral renal parenchymal disease is of unknown pathogenesis but is generally considered to result from activation of the renal pressor mechanism by intrarenal small artery disease.

SURGICAL TREATMENT OF ESSENTIAL HYPERTENSION

During the era 1940 through 1959, before effective antihypertensive drug therapy was available, thoracolumbar sympathectomy or splanchnicectomy was used frequently in the treatment of patients with severe diastolic hypertension. During the latter part of this period, bilateral total or subtotal adrenalectomy alone or in conjunction with thoracolumbar sympathectomy was advocated for control of severe hypertension. The effectiveness of these forms of treatment depends on interrupting the increased peripheral resistance so commonly present in most forms of diastolic hypertension. Beneficial and at times long-lasting results were obtained with these forms of treatment, as documented in reports by Grimson, Smithwick, Zintel, and Jeffers et al. During the following decade these forms of surgical treatment were largely abandoned, being replaced by the use of the potent antihypertensive drugs currently available.

Recently, baropacing of the carotid sinus nerve as a means of decreasing peripheral resistance and thereby lowering the blood pressure has been the subject of experimental and clinical studies reported by Schwartz and Griffith and by Bilgutay and Lillehei. The carotid sinus nerve, a branch of the glossopharyngeal nerve, is the afferent nerve of the carotid baroreceptor reflex and transmits to the medullary vasomotor centers action potentials which originate in the carotid sinus. Under normal conditions, an increase in the intraluminal pressure of the carotid baroreceptor reflexly lowers blood pressure, induces bradycardia, decreases cardiac output, and diminishes venous return. When pressure is lowered in the baroreceptor, the reverse occurs. Chronic neurogenic vasoconstriction is thought to occur when the baroreceptor mechanism loses its efficiency or is "reset" at elevated blood pressure levels. This resetting has been attributed to the development of refractoriness or elevation of the thresholds of the baroreceptors in chronic hypertensive states. McCubbin et al. hypothesized that either the vasomotor centers are altered by hypertension and unable to appreciate afferent stimuli from the baroreceptor organs or there is an adaptation within the baroreceptor, so that an insufficient number of impulses results from the hypertension stimulus. Using electroneurography, they demonstrated that the baroreceptors continued to function in hypertension but that the threshold stimulus required to trigger the receptor was significantly raised. These observations led to Warner's use of electrical stimulation of the carotid sinus nerve to lower systemic blood pressure in the dog. Subsequently, Griffith and Schwartz reported reversal of renal hypertension in dogs by electrical stimulation of the carotid sinus nerve, an observation confirmed by Bilgutay and Lillehei. Chronic electrical stimulation of the carotid sinus nerve as a method of treating hypertension has been applied clinically. The stimulator, or baropacer, was implanted in the neck and connected to the carotid sinus nerve; unilateral stimulation was initially employed, and more recently bilateral stimulation has been used. Schwartz and Griffith have reported encouraging results with treatment of 11 hypertensive patients, and Bilgutay and Lillehei have had favorable experiences with 2 patients.

At present, stimulation of the carotid sinus nerve in the treatment of hypertension must be considered an experimental approach. Two major unresolved questions are whether chronic stimulation will result in fibrosis and destruction of the nerve and whether the baroreceptor system will eventually reset itself so that hypertension will recur. Experience with baropacing continues to accumulate slowly. In addition to controlling hypertension, it has been reported to be useful in management of angina pectoris and paroxysmal supraventricular tachycardia. Recent reports have been summarized by Brest. More study of this method of treatment is needed. It may eventually prove to be a valuable addition to the treatment of hypertension.

Bilateral nephrectomy and renal transplantation for patients with severe essential hypertension and end-stage renal disease are discussed in Chap. 10.

References

Pheochromocytoma

Barbeau, A., et al.: Le Phéochromocytome bilateral: Présentation d'un cas et revue de la littérature, *Union Med Can* **87**:165, 1958.

Greer, W. E. R., Robertson, C. W., and Smithwick, R. H.: Pheochromocytoma: Diagnosis, Operative Experiences and Clinical Results, *Am J Surg,* **107**:192, 1964.

Hume, D. M.: Pheochromocytoma in the Adult and in the Child, *Am J Surg,* **99**:458, 1960.

Kvale, W. F., Roth, G. M., Manager, W. M., and Priesley, J. T.: Present day Diagnosis and Treatment of Pheochromocytoma, *JAMA,* **164**:854, 1957.

Scott, H. W., Jr., Riddell, D. H., and Brockman, S. K.: Surgical Management of Pheochromocytoma, *Surg Gynecol Obstet,* **120**:707, 1965.

Primary Aldosteronism

Conn, J. W.: Primary Aldosteronism: A New Clinical Syndrome, *J Lab Clin Med,* **45**:3, 1955.

———: Plasma Renin Activity in Primary Aldosteronism: Importance in Differential Diagnosis and in Research of Essential Hypertension, *JAMA,* **190**:222, 1964.

———, Cohen, E. L., Rovner, D. R., and Nesbit, R. M.: Normokalemic Primary Aldosteronism: Its Masquerade as "Essential" Hypertension, *JAMA,* **195**:21, 1966.

———, Knopf, R. F., and Nesbit, R. M.: Clinical Characteristics of Primary Aldosteronism from Analysis of 145 Cases, *Am J Surg,* **107**:159, 1964.

Fishman, L. M., and Liddle, G. W.: Effects of Amino-glutethimide on Adrenal Function in Man, *J Clin Endocrinol Metab,* **27**:481, 1967.

Cushing's Syndrome

Cushing, H.: The Basophil Adenomas of the Pituitary Gland and Their Clinical Manifestations, *Bull Johns Hopkins Hosp,* **50**:137, 1932.

Hayes, M.: Operative Treatment of Adrenal Cortical Hyperfunctionary Disease, *Ann Surg,* **154**:33, 1961.

Liddle, G. W.: Tests of Pituitary-Adrenal Suppressibility in the Diagnosis of Cushing's Syndrome, *J Clin Endocrinol Metab,* **20**:1939, 1960.

———: "Cushing's Syndrome: The Adrenal Cortex," Little, Brown and Company, Boston, 1967.

Orth, D. N., and Liddle, G. W.: Results of Treatment on 107 Patients with Cushing's Syndrome, *N Engl J Med,* **285**:243, 1971.

Scott, H. W., Jr., Liddle, G. W., Harris, A. P., and Foster, J. H.: Diagnosis and Treatment of Cushing's Syndrome, *Ann Surg,* **155**:696, 1962.

Thorn, G. W.: Diseases of the Adrenal Cortex, in T. R. Harrison et al. (eds.), "Principles of Internal Medicine," 4th ed., McGraw-Hill Book Company, New York, 1962.

Coarctation of the Aorta

Crafoord, C., and Nylin, G.: Congenital Coarctation of the Aorta and Its Surgical Treatment, *J Thorac Cardiovasc Surg,* **14**:347, 1945.

Gross, R. E., and Hufnagel, C. A.: Coarctation of the Aorta: Experimental Studies Regarding Its Surgical Correction, *N Engl J Med,* **233**:287, 1945.

Sealey, W. C.: Coarctation of the Aorta and Hypertension, *Ann Thor Surg,* **3**:15, 1967.

Scott, H. W., Jr., and Bahnson, H. T.: Evidence for a Renal Factor in the Hypertension of Experimental Coarctation of the Aorta, *Surgery,* **30**:206, 1951.

———, Collins, H. A., and Foster, J. H.: Additional Observations concerning the Physiology of the Hypertension Associated with Experimental Coarctation of the Aorta, *Surgery,* **36**:445, 1954.

Renovascular Hypertension

Alpert, J., Parsonnet, V., and Brief, D. K.: Hypertension and the Solitary Ischemic Kidney, *Ann Surg,* **173**:450, 1971.

Baker, G. W., Jr., Page, L. B., and Leadbetter, G. W., Jr.: Hypertension and Renovascular Disease: A Follow-up Study of 23 Patients, with Analysis of Factors Influencing the Results, *N Engl J Med,* **267**:1325, 1962.

Belzer, F., in discussion of Lim, R. C., Eastman, A. B., and Blaisdell, F. W.: Renal Auto-transplantation: Adjunct to Repair of Renal Vascular Lesions, *Arch Surg,* **105**:847, 1972.

Birchall, R., Barson, H. M., Jr., and Brannon, W.: Contribution of Differential Renal Studies to the Diagnosis of Renal Arterial Hypertension and Emphasis on the Value of U Sodium/U Creatinine, *Am J Med,* **32**:164, 1962.

Braun-Menendez, F., Fasciolo, J. C., Leloir, L. F., Munoz, J. M., and Taquini, A. C.: "Renal Hypertension," translated by L. Dexter, Charles C Thomas, Publisher, Springfield, Ill., 1946.

Crocker, D. W., Newton, R. A., Mahoney, E. W., and Harrison, J. H.: Hypertension Due to Primary Renal Ischemia: A Correlation of Juxtaglomerular Cell Counts with Clinicopathologic Findings in Twenty-five Cases, *N Engl J Med,* **267**:794, 1962.

DeBakey, M. E., Morris, G. C., Jr., Morgen, R. O., Crawford, E. S., and Cooley, D. A.: Lesions of the Renal Artery: Surgical Technic and Results, *Am J Surg,* **107**:84, 1964.

DeCamp, P. T., and Birchall, R.: Recognition and Treatment of Renal Artery Stenosis Associated with Hypertension, *Surgery,* **43**:134, 1958.

Dustan, H. P., Page, I. H., and Poutasse, E. F.: Renal Hypertension, *N Engl J Med,* **261**:647, 1959.

———, ———, ———, and Wilson, L.: An Evaluation of Treatment of Hypertension Associated with Occlusive Renal Arterial Disease, *Circulation,* **27**:1018, 1963.

Ernst, C. B., Bookstein, J. J., Montie, J., Baumgartel, E., Hoobler, S. W., and Fry, W. J.: Renal Vein Renin Ratios and Collateral Vessels in Renovascular Hypertension, *Arch Surg,* **104**:496, 1972.

———, Marshall, F. F., Stanley, J. C., and Fry, W. J.: Autogenous Saphenous Vein for Aortorenal Bypass: A Ten Year Experience, *Arch Surg,* **105**:855, 1972.

Eyler, W. R., Clark, M. D., Garman, J. E., Rian, R. L., and

Meininger, D. E.: Angiography of the Renal Areas Including a Comparative Study of Renal Arterial Stenosis in Patients with and without Hypertension, *Radiology,* **78:**879, 1962.

Fitz, A. E.: Renal Venous Renin (RVR) in Evaluation of Renovascular Hypertension, *Clin Res,* **14:**376, 1966.

Floyer, M. A.: Further Studies on the Mechanism of Experimental Hypertension in the Rat, *Clin Sci,* **14:**163, 1955.

Foster, J. H., Oates, J. A., Rhamy, R. K., Klatte, E. C., Pettinger, W. A., Burko, H. C., Younger, R. K., and Scott, H. W., Jr.: Detection and Treatment of Patients with Renovascular Hypertension, *Surgery,* **60:**240, 1966

——, Dean, R. H., Pinkerton, J. A., and Rhamy, R. K.: Ten Years Experience with the Surgical Management of Renovascular Hypertension, *Ann Surg,* 1973.

——, Klatte, E. C., and Burko, H. C.: Arteriographic Pitfalls in the Diagnosis of Renovascular Hypertension, *Arch Surg,* **99:**792, 1969.

——, Oates, J. A., Rhamy, R. K., Klatte, E. C., Burko, H. C., and Michelakis, A. M.: Hypertension and Fibromuscular Dysplasia of the Renal Arteries, *Surgery,* **65:**157, 1969.

——, Pettinger, W. A., Oates, J. A., Rhamy, R. K., Klatte, E. C., Burko, H. C., Bolasny, B. L., Gordon, R., Puyau, F. A., and Younger, R. K.: Malignant Hypertension Secondary to Renal Artery Stenosis in Children, *Ann Surg,* **164:**700, 1966.

——, Rhamy, R. K., Oates, J. A., Klatte, E. C., Burko, H. C., and Michelakis, A. M.: Renovascular Hypertension Secondary to Atherosclerosis, *Am J Med,* **46:**741, 1969.

Freis, E. D.: The Chemotherapy of Hypertension, *JAMA,* **218:**1009, 1971.

Fry, W. J., Brink, B. E., and Thompson, N. W.: New Techniques in the Treatment of Extensive Fibromuscular Disease Involving the Renal Arteries, *Surgery,* **68:**959, 1970.

Goldblatt, H., Lynch, J., Hanzal, R. F., and Summerville, W. W.: Studies on Experimental Hypertension, *J Exp Med,* **59:**347, 1934.

Gomes, M. R., and Bernatz, P. E.: Aortoiliac Occlusive Disease: Extension Cephalad to Origin of Renal Arteries, with Surgical Considerations and Results, *Arch Surg,* **101:**161, 1970.

Harrison, E. G., Jr., and McCormack, L. J.: Pathologic Classification of Renal Arterial Disease in Renovascular Hypertension, *Mayo Clin Proc,* **46:**161, 1971.

Helmer, O. M.: Presence of Renin in Plasma of Patients with Arterial Hypertension, *Circulation,* **25:**169, 1962.

Hickler, R. B., Birbari, A. E., Howard, F. H., Crocker, D. W., Lauler, D. P., Harrison, J. H., Crane, C., and Vagnucci, A. I.: A Comparison of Unilateral Pyelonephritis and Renal Artery Stenosis Associated with Hypertension, *Am J Surg,* **109:**715, 1965.

Holley, K. W., Hunt, J. C., Brown, A. L., Kincaid, O. W., and Sheps, S. G.: Renal Artery Stenosis: A Clinical-Pathologic Study in Normotensive and Hypertensive Patients, *Am J Med,* **37:**14, 1964.

Howard, J. E., and Connor, T. B.: Use of Differential Renal Function Studies in the Diagnosis of Renovascular Hypertension, *Am J Surg,* **107:**58, 1964.

Hunt, J. C., Harrison, E. G., Jr., Kincaid, O. W., Bernatz, P. E., and Davis, G. D.: Idiopathic Fibrous and Fibromuscular Stenoses of the Renal Arteries Associated with Hypertension, *Proc Staff Meetings Mayo Clin,* **37:**181, 1962.

Kaufman, J. J., Maxwell, M. H., and Moloney, P. J.: Synthetic

Bypass Grafts in the Treatment of Renal Artery Stenosis, *Surg Gynecol Obstet,* **126:**53, 1968.

Kirkendall, W. M., Fitz, A. E., and Lawrence, M. S.: Renal Hypertension: Diagnosis and Surgical Treatment, *N Engl J Med,* **276:**479, 1967.

Lim, R. C., Eastman, A. B., and Blaisdell, F. W.: Renal Autotransplantation: Adjunct to Repair of Renal Vascular Lesions, *Arch Surg,* **105:**847, 1972.

Louis, W. J., Renzini, V., MacDonald, G. J., Boyd, G. W., and Peart, W. S.: Renal-Clip Hypertension in Rabbits Immunized against Angiotensin II, *Lancet,* **1:**333, 1970.

McAllister, R. G., Jr., Michelakis, A. M., Oates, J. A., and Foster, J. H.: Malignant Hypertension due to Renal Artery Stenosis: Greater Renin Release from the Nonstenotic Kidney, *JAMA,* **221:**865, 1972.

McCormack, L. J., Noto, T. J., Jr., Meaney, T. F., Poutasse, E. F., and Dustan, H. P.: Subadventitial Fibroplasia of the Renal Artery: A Disease of Young Women, *Am Heart J,* **73:**602, 1967.

McPhaul, J. J., Jr., McIntosh, D. A., Williams, L. F., Gritti, E. J., Mallette, W. G., and Grollman, A.: Remediable Hypertension Due to Unilateral Renal Disease, *Arch Intern Med,* **115:**644, 1965.

Marable, S. A., Moore, F. T., and Schieve, J. F., Treatment of Hypertension Associated with the Solitary Ischemic Kidney, *N Engl J Med,* **275:**1278, 1966.

Maxwell, M. H., Gonick, H. C., Wiita, R., and Kaufman, J. J.: Use of Rapid-Sequence Intravenous Pyelogram in Diagnosis of Renovascular Hypertension, *N Engl J Med,* **270:**213, 1964.

Michelakis, A. M., Foster, J. H., Liddle, G. W., Rhamy, R. K., and Kuchel, O.: Measurement of Renin in Both Renal Veins and Its Use in Diagnosis of Renovascular Hypertension, *Arch Intern Med,* **120:**444, 1967.

Miller, T., and Foster, J. H.: Rapidly Malignant Hypertension Following Thrombosis of a Reconstructed Renal Artery, *Arch Surg,* **93:**962, 1966.

Morris, G. C., Jr., DeBakey, M. E., Crawford, E. S., Cooley, D. A., and Zanger, L. C. C.: Late Results of Surgical Treatment for Renovascular Hypertension, *Surg Gynecol Obstet,* **122:**1255, 1966.

Ota, K., Mori, S., Awane, Y., and Ueno, A.: Ex Situ Repair of Renal Artery for Renovascular Hypertension, *Arch Surg,* **94:**370, 1967.

Page, I. H.: "The Mosaic Theory of Hypertension: Essential Hypertension," pp. 1–29, Springer-Verlag OHG, Berlin, 1960.

—— and Corcoran, A. C.: Hypertension: Review of Humoral Pathogenesis and Clinical Treatment, *Adv Intern Med,* **1:**183, 1942.

Rappaport, A.: Modification of the "Howard Test" for the Detection of Renal Artery Obstruction, *N Engl J Med,* **263:**1159, 1960.

Schacht, R. A., Zweifler, A. J., and Conway, J.: Renal Artery Stenosis, *N Engl J Med,* **271:**55, 1964.

Scott, H. W., Jr., and Foster, J. H.: Surgical Considerations in Hypertension, *Curr Probl Surg,* July 1964.

Shapiro, A. P., Perez-Stable, E., Scheib, E. T., Bron, K., Montsos, S. E., Bert, G., and Misage, J. R.: Renal Artery Stenosis and Hypertension. Observations on the Current Status of Therapy from a Study of 115 Patients, *Am J Med,* **47:**175, 1969.

Sheps, S. G., Hunt, J. C., and Bernatz, P. E.: Diagnosis of Hypertension Associated with Renal Artery Disease, *Manit Med Rev,* **45:**558, 1965.

———, Kincaid, E. W., and Hunt, J. C.: Serial Renal Function and Angiographic Observations in Idiopathic Fibrous and Fibromuscular Stenoses of the Renal Arteries, *Am J Cardiol,* **30:**55, 1972.

Stamey, T. A.: Renovascular Hypertension—1965, *Am J Med,* **38:**829, 1965.

———, Nudelmon, I. J., Good, P. H., Schwentker, F. N., and Hendricks, F.: Functional Characteristics of Renovascular Hypertension, *Medicine (Baltimore),* **40:**347, 1961.

Strickler, W. L.: Surgical Cure of Malignant Hypertension with Intrarenal Arteriosclerosis, *JAMA,* **194:**119, 1965.

Tarazi, R. C., Frohlich, E. D., Dustan, H. P., Gifford, R. W., Jr., and Page, I. H.: Hypertension and High Hematocrit: Another Clue to Renal Arterial Disease, *Am J Cardiol,* **6:**855, 1966.

Thal, A. P., Grage, G. B., and Vernier, R. L.: Function of the Contralateral Kidney in Renal Hypertension due to Renal Artery Stenosis, *Circulation,* **27:**36, 1963.

Thomas, C. S., Brockman, S. K., and Foster, J. H.: The Variability of Pressure Gradients in Renal Artery Stenosis, *Surg Gynecol Obstet,* **126:**339, 1968.

Tobian, L.: Relationship of Juxtaglomerular Apparatus to Renin and Angiotensin, *Circulation,* **25:**189, 1962.

Vertes, V., Grauel, J. A., and Goldblatt, H.: Studies of Patients with Renal Hypertension Undergoing Vascular Surgery, *N Engl J Med,* **272:**186, 1965.

———, ———, and Stoney, R. J.: Autogenous Tissue Revascularization Technics in Surgery for Renovascular Hypertension, *Ann Surg,* **170:**416, 1969.

Wylie, E. J., Perloff, D., and Wellington, J. S.: Fibromuscular Hyperplasia of the Renal Arteries, *Ann Surg,* **156:**592, 1962.

Unilateral Renal Parenchymal Disease

Crocker, D. W., Newton, R. A., and Harrison, J. H.: Results of Surgical Management of Unilateral Pyelonephritis with Hypertension: Analysis of Twelve Cases, *Am J Surg,* **110:**405, 1965.

Hickler, R. B., Birbari, A. E., Howard, F. H., Crocker, D. W., Lauler, D. P., Harrison, J. H., Crane, C., and Vagnucci, A. I.: A Comparison of Unilateral Pyelonephritis and Renal Artery Stenosis Associated with Hypertension, *Am J Surg,* **109:**715, 1965.

McDonald, D. F.: Renal Hypertension without Main Arterial Stenosis: Function Tests Predict Cure., *JAMA,* **203:**130, 1968.

Smith, H.: Unilateral Nephrectomy in Hypertensive Disease, *J Urol,* **76:**685, 1956.

Essential Hypertension

Bilgutay, A. M., and Lillehei, C. W.: Treatment of Hypertension with an Implantable Electronic Device, *JAMA,* **191:**649, 1965.

Brest, A. N.: Carotid Sinus Nerve Stimulation, *Am J Cardiol,* **26:**328, 1970.

Gordon, T., and Devine, B.: "Hypertension and Hypertensive Heart Disease in Adults, United States—1960–62: Vital and Health Statistics Data from the National Health Survey," U.S. Department of Health, Education, and Welfare, National Center for Health Statistics ser. II, no. 13.

Griffith, L. S. C., and Schwartz, S. I.: Reversal of Renal Hypertension by Electrical Stimulation of the Carotid Sinus Nerve, *Surgery,* **56:**232, 1964.

Grimson, K. S.: Total Thoracic and Partial to Total Lumbar Sympathectomy and Celiac Ganglionectomy in the Treatment of Hypertension, *Ann Surg,* **114:**753, 1941.

Jeffers, W. A., Sellers, A. M., Wolferth, C. C., Ross, A. M., and Blakemore, W. S.: Results of Sympathectomy and Adrenalectomy, *Am J Surg,* **107:**211, 1964.

McCubbin, J. W., Green, J. H., and Page, I. H.: Baroreceptor Function in Chronic Renal Hypertension, *Circ Res,* **4:**205, 1956.

Schwartz, S. I., and Griffith, L. S. C.: "Reduction of Hypertension by Electrical Stimulation of the Carotid Sinus Nerve, Baroreceptors and Hypertension," Pergamon Press, New York, 1967.

———, ———, Neistadt, A., and Hagfors, N.: Chronic Carotid Sinus Nerve Stimulation in the Treatment of Essential Hypertension, *Am J Surg,* **114:**5, 1967.

Smithwick, R. H.: Practical Treatment for Hypertension, Splanchnicectomy, Adrenalectomy, and Nephrectomy, *Postgrad Med,* **34:**32, 1963.

Warner, H. R.: The Frequency-dependent Nature of Blood Pressure Regulation by the Carotid Sinus Studied with an Electric Analog, *Circ Res,* **6:**35, 1958.

Zintel, H. A.: Adrenalectomy versus Sympathectomy: Results of Surgery, in J. H. Moyer (ed.), "Hypertension," p. 695, W. B. Saunders Company, Philadelphia, 1959.

Name Index

Abbott, M. E., 701, 712
Abercrombie, M., 278, 1796
Abrams, D. L., 799, 800
Abrams, H. L., 1788
Ackerman, L. V., 1130, 1132, 1339
Acosta, J., 1244
Adams, J. T., 922, 1313
Adams, W. E., 467
Adelson, E., 29
Adson, A. W., 876, 881
Ahlquist, R. P., 134
Akakura, I., 1036
Albarran, J., 1336
Albers-Schönberg, W., 1751, 1752
Albrecht, M., 143
Albright, F., 1500, 1753
Alfry, A. C., 462
Allen, E. V., 879
Allen, J. G., 19, 32
Allen, T. H., 1021
Allison, P. R., 1038
Alonso-Lej, F., 1224
Alpert, J., 961
Altemeier, W. A., 179, 206, 992, 994
Amatruda, T. T., Jr., 1374
Amerson, J. R., 1182
Amos, D. B., 361
Amyand, C., 1167
Anderson, L. D., 1797
Anderson, N. F., 373
Anderson, R. C., 742
Anson, B. J., 1346, 1349, 1356, 1359
Arnar, O., 403
Arnaud, C. D., 1480, 1498
Artz, C. B., 206
Astrup, P., 72
Atik, M., 983, 994
Attar, S., 29
Auerbach, R., 357
Austen, W. G., 826, 829, 1326
Autio, V., 1306

Bachman, A. L., 1469
Bachrach, W. H., 89
Baclesse, F., 544, 547
Badgely, C. E., 1727
Baez, S., 45
Baffes, T. G., 727
Bahnson, H. T., 716, 791, 840, 887
Bailey, C. P., 480, 759
Bakamijian, V. Y., 1925
Baker, D. R., 1684
Baker, G. W., Jr., 956
Baker, H. W., 538
Baker, J. W., 1136
Baker, R. J., 241
Baragry, R. A., 1796
Barbeau, A., 942
Barcroft, J., 494
Bargeron, L. M., 730
Barker, A. N., 1796
Barnard, C. N., 739, 1527

Barner, H. B., 914
Barnes, J., 462
Barnes, J. P., 237
Barnett, W. O., 982
Barnicot, N. A., 1753
Barratt-Boyes, B. G., 696, 715, 730
Barreras, R. F., 1753
Barrett, N. R., 1038
Barrett, R. J., 1032
Barry, K. G., 41
Bartlett, M. K., 1263
Barton, R. W., 49
Bartter, F. C., 1400, 1477
Barzel, U. S., 1412, 1478
Barzilai, D., 153
Batson, O. V., 529, 1691, 1788
Baue, A. E., 137
Bauer, G., 916, 926
Baxter, C. R., 262
Baylis, S. M., 242, 243
Beahrs, O. H., 1443
Beall, A. C., Jr., 790, 896
Beatson, T. R., 1839
Becker, A., 467, 468
Becker, W. F., 986
Bedford, P. D., 898
Beebe, G. W., 790
Beecher, H. K., 467
Belanger, L. F., 1461
Belsey, R., 1020, 1025
Belzer, F., 958
Benacerrof, B., 361
Bendixen, H. H., 468
Benedict, E. B., 1032
Bennett, D. E., 817
Berg, J. W., 539, 543, 546
Bergentz, S. E., 29, 38
Berger, R. L., 790
Bergofsky, E. H., 1709
Berk, J. L., 26, 44, 152
Berkow, J. W., 1373
Berman, J. K., 221
Berman, L. G., 1123
Bernacki, E., 1476
Bernard, H. R., 172
Bernheim, B. M., 839
Bick, E. M., 1726
Biglieri, E. G., 1398
Bilgutay, A. M., 963
Bill, A. H., Jr., 1531
Biller, H. F., 590
Billingham, R. E., 379
Binkley, F. C., 521
Birchall, R., 946, 954
Bishop, H. E., 1529
Bitene, I., 1719
Black, B. M., 1451, 1452, 1466, 1493
Blackburn, G. L., 24, 28
Blair, O. M., 48
Blaisdell, F. W., 884
Blake, H. A., 706
Blalock, A., 680, 696, 720, 721, 727, 728, 787, 803, 839

Bland, E. F., 739, 790
Bliss, E. L., 480
Block, G. E., 1394
Block, M. A., 1444, 1452
Blomstedt, B., 482
Bloodwell, R. D., 816
Bloom, B. R., 367
Bloom, H. J. G., 535, 546
Blount, S. G., Jr., 709
Blount, W. P., 1808, 1814
Boak, J. L., 367
Bobetchko, W. P., 1719
Bolton, H. E., 480
Bonazzi, 411
Boonstra, C. E., 1487
Boother, R. J., 1788
Border, J. R., 503
Bornside, G. H., 165
Bortin, M. M., 388
Bounous, G., 49
Bowden, L., 1788
Boyd, D. R., Jr., 38, 1305
Boyle, J. D., 801
Boyse, E. A., 363
Braasch, J. W., 1339
Bradham, R.R., 1883
Brailsford, J. F., 1766
Brattstrom, S., 468
Braun-Menendez, F., 946
Braunwald, E., 145, 691, 695
Braunwald, N. S., 771, 785
Braverman, I. B., 690
Brawley, R. K., 829
Brecher, G., 102
Brent, L., 360
Brescia, M. J., 407
Breslow, L., 546
Brest, A. N., 963
Brewer, H. B., Jr., 1464
Brewer, L. A., III, 700
Brief, D. K., 38
Brock, R. C., 685, 721, 732
Broder, G., 38
Brom, A. G., 700, 701
Brown, H., 1286
Brown, J. J., 1397
Brown, P. W., 1831
Browne, J. S. L., 28
Browning, J., 479
Browse, N. L., 917
Brummelkamp, W. H., 169
Bryant, L. R., 771
Buchwald, H., 798
Buckle, R. M., 1485
Buckley, J. J., 470
Buist, N. R. M., 1417
Bull, C. A., 870
Bullough, W. S., 279
Burford, T. H., 470
Burke, J. F., 46, 206
Burnet, F. M., 307
Burnett, C. H., 1489
Burr, A. O., 34

Burr, M. M., 34
Butcher, H. R., Jr., 545, 931
Byrne, J. J., 914

Cahill, G. F., Jr., 19, 86, 87
Calandriello, B., 1727
Calne, R. Y., 404
Cameron, K. M., 1479
Campbell, A. M., 1682
Campbell, E., 556
Campbell, M. G., 737
Canizaro, P. C., 65, 223, 245
Cann, M. S., 45
Cannon, W. B., 137
Canterbury, J. M., 1480
Caplan, B. B., 244
Capper, W. M., 483
Capps, W., Jr., 1882
Carey, L. C., 15
Carlson, L. A., 28
Carnes, W. H., 31
Carpue, J. C., 1920
Carrel, A., 399, 404, 839
Carter, C., 1725, 1726
Carter, D., 49
Carter, R., 1332
Castleman, K. B., 1167
Cattell, R. B., 1273
Catterall, A., 1719
Catz, B., 1456
Celsus, A. C., 1921
Center, S., 803
Cerilli, G. J., 1041
Cerny, J. C., 898, 899
Chaimoff, C., 1233
Chalmers, M. I., 27
Chance, B., 496, 509
Charcot, J. M., 1241
Chardack, W. M., 803, 806
Charles, R. H., 934
Charnley, J., 1864, 1867
Chase, R. A., 1895, 1919
Chatten, J., 1417
Chazan, J. A., 38
Chernov, M. S., 31
Cherry, J. K., 817
Chew, W. B., 373
Child, C. G., III, 1208, 1265, 1290
Chiu, C. J., 49
Clagett, O. T., 876, 1020, 1021, 1034
Clark, D. S., 363
Clark, J. H., 1444
Clark, J. M., 362
Clark, L. C., Jr., 35, 497
Clements, J. A., 468
Clendon, D. R. T., 467
Clermont, H. G., 48
Clowes, G. H. A., Jr., 44, 144
Coalson, J. J., 45
Cobb, J. R., 1708, 1710
Cockett, F. B., 923, 926, 931
Code, C. F., 1009, 1024
Coffey, R. J., 876, 898
Cohen, B., 31
Cohen, B. M., 863, 864, 866, 867
Cohen, I. K., 31, 285
Cohen, S., 1015, 1024
Cohn, I., Jr., 165, 207, 226, 983
Cohn, J. N., 501, 503, 505
Cohn, K. E., 762
Colcock, B. P., 1440, 1455
Cole, W. H., 1448
Cole, W. R., 172
Coley, B., 340
Coller, F. A., 913, 914
Colles, A., 1814
Collier, C., 468
Collier, H. S., 220, 242, 246
Collins, H. A., 803

Collins, J. A., 466
Collins, V. P., 1133
Collins, W. F., Jr., 1631
Collis, J. J., 1025
Colonna, P. C., 1731
Colton, J., 556
Comfort, M. W., 1234
Compere, E. L., 1770
Condie, J. P., 206
Condon, R. E., 1487
Conen, P. E., 463
Congdon, C. C., 388
Conn, J. W., 943, 1375, 1396, 1397, 1399, 1400
Contorni, L., 885
Converse, J. M., 1957
Conway, H., 521
Conway, M. J., 22
Cook, B. H., 49
Cook, W. A., 46
Cooke, A. M., 1761, 1764
Cooley, D. A., 706, 734, 739, 741, 799, 801, 821,
    825, 835, 840, 887
Cooley, E., 545
Coomes, E. N., 1678
Coon, W. W., 913, 920
Coons, A. H., 359, 1443
Cooper, A., 359
Cope, O., 1457, 1466, 1468
Copp, D. H., 1464
Corday, E., 49
Cornell, W. P., 224
Cotton, D. K., 1041
Couch, N. P., 508
Counseller, V. S., 229
Coursley, G., 873
Coventry, M. B., 1691
Crafoord, C., 485, 696, 791, 839, 945
Cramer, L. M., 1895, 1919
Cramond, W. A., 481
Cranley, J. J., 856, 861
Crawford, E. S., 849, 886, 887, 901
Crawford, H. B., 1820
Crenshaw, A. H., 1698
Crichlow, R. W., 895
Crile, G., Jr., 544, 548, 1136, 1444, 1450, 1451
Crocker, D. W., 948, 962
Crockett, D. J., 933
Crockett, K. A., 1415
Crohn, B. B., 1116
Cronin, T. D., 1951, 1961
Cronkite, E. P., 102, 1796
Crosby, W. H., 1291
Cross, F. S., 875, 1020
Crosthwait, R. W., 233
Crowe, H. E., 1709
Culbertson, W. R., 179
Curtiss, P. H., 1849
Curtiss, P. H., Jr., 110
Cushing, H., 120, 943, 993
Cutler, R. E., 1483

Da Costa, J. C., 477
Dahlgren, S., 482
Dahl-Iverson, E., 545
Dahlin, D. C., 1780, 1785
Daily, P. O., 829
Dale, W. A., 853, 860, 1242, 1243, 1882
Dalton, J. C., 803
Dameshek, W., 404
Dammann, J. F., Jr., 679
Danis, R. K., 833, 835
Dao, T. L.-Y., 1394
Daoud, G., 733
Dargan, E. L., 1241
Darling, R. C., 707, 856, 857, 861
Darrach, W., 1737
Dart, D. E., 1834
Davenport, H. W., 981, 1053, 1075
Davie, E. W., 99

Davis, L. E., 89
Day, P. L., 1821
DeBakey, M. E., 827, 829, 840, 863, 864, 866,
    867, 887, 913, 914, 946, 1186
DeCamp, P. T., 946
Deckers, P. J., 340
DeCosse, J. J., 1450
Dehne, E., 1830
Dekker, E. E., 32
Del Guercio, L. R. M., 44, 461, 502, 503
DeLuca, H., 1464
Denham, R. A., 1706
Dennis, C., 1114
Dent, C. E., 1755
DeTakats, G., 901, 902
Devine, B., 939
DeWall, R. A., 753
DeWeese, J. A., 913, 914, 922
Diamonon, J. S., 237
Dieffenbach, J. F., 1920
Dietrich, E. B., 887
Dietz, J. H., Jr., 1967
Dietzman, R. H., 133, 434
Dieulafoy, G., 1073
Dillard, B. M., 868, 870
Dingman, R. O., 1957
Dintsman, M., 1233
Dively, W. L., 829
Dmochowaski, J. R., 917
Doan, C. A., 1290
Dodd, H., 923, 926, 931
Dohlman, G., 1020
Donaldson, G. A., 921
Donaldson, R. M., Jr., 1475
Dong, E., Jr., 792, 808
Doniach, I., 1443
Donnelly, B. A., 1339
Donoghue, F. E., 1039
Donovan, A. J., 240
dos Santos, R., 843
Doty, P., 358
Doublet, H., 1268, 1270
Downing, S. E., 45
Dowson, D., 1865
Dragstedt, L. R., 1063
Drapanas, T., 222, 790
Draper, J. W., 1316
Drucker, W. D., 1389
Drucker, W. R., 26
Dube, O. I., 360
Dubost, C., 839, 887
Dudrick, S. J., 32, 88, 92, 93, 95, 201, 500
Duff, J. H., 44, 1140
Duffy, B. J., 1450
Duke, J. H., Jr., 28
Duke, W. W., 102
Dunbar, J. D., 1330
Dunne, L. R., 1834
Dunphy, J. E., 1238, 1286, 1351
DuPlessis, D. J., 1069
Dustan, H. P., 946
Duthie, R. B., 1675, 1698, 1725, 1726, 1741, 1766,
    1775, 1788, 1791, 1796, 1845
Dutton, R. W., 359
DuVal, M. K., Jr., 1264
Dwight, R. W., 1139

Early, F., 32
Early, P. F., 1716
Eastcott, H. H. G., 881
Ebert, R. V., 123
Ebstein, W., 738
Ecker, R. R., 829
Edeiken, J., 1745
Edgerton, M. T., 1957
Edkins, J. S., 1053
Edmunds, L. H., Jr., 484, 485
Edwards, J. E., 679
Edwards, M. L., 774

Edwards, N. A., 1477
Edwards, W. S., 730, 798, 816, 850, 884
Edynak, E. M., 310
Effler, D. B., 799, 833, 835
Egdahl, R. H., 1, 41, 362, 1389, 1401
Egerton, N., 480
Egerton, W. S., 774
Eggers, G. W. N., 1702
Einheber, A., 49
Eisenstein, A. B., 31
Eitel, G. G., 1316
Elek, S. D., 463
Elliott, D. W., 1260, 1450
Ellis, F. H., Jr., 1009, 1016
Ellison, E. H., 1276, 1277
El-Said, G., 708
Erlandson, M. E., 229
Ernst, C. B., 947, 955, 961, 962
Ervasti, E., 906
Esler, M. D., 1111
Esmarch, J. F. A. v., 1920
Espiner, E. A., 1398
Esser, J. F. S., 1928
Estes, J. E., Jr., 887
Evans, E. B., 1702, 1715, 1812
Eyler, W. R., 946

Fainer, D. C., 906
Fairbank, T., 1767
Falconer, M. A., 876
Fanconi, G., 1758
Favaloro, R., 794
Federman, D. D., 1393
Feinstein, B., 1677
Felder, D. A., 931
Feldman, J. D., 361
Felig, P., 28
Felson, B., 229
Ferencz, C., 733
Ferguson, D. J., 206
Ferguson, A. B., 1709
Fine, J., 137
Fischer, C. M., 881
Fischer, J. E., 1204
Fisher, B., 549
Fishman, L. M., 1396
Fishman, M., 356
Fitz, A. E., 955
Fitz, R., 1167
Fitzgerald, J. B., 220
Fitzsimons, L. E., 244
Flanagan, M. J., 1401
Fleisch, H., 1754
Fletcher, G. H., 547
Flexner, S., 373
Fogarty, T. J., 857
Fogelman, M. J., 216
Foker, J. E., 351
Folger, G. M., Jr., 1407, 1413
Follis, R. H., 1743
Fonkalsrud, E. W., 1276
Foote, F. W., 537, 539, 1452
Foraker, A. C., 339
Forsythe, H. F., 1839, 1840
Fortner, J., 1419
Foster, J. H., 939, 946, 948, 951, 959, 1192
Foulds, L., 1775
Fowler, E. F., 901, 902, 1334
Fox, H. M., 480
Fracchia, A. A., 1394
Frahm, C. J., 690
Frame, B., 1397
Franch, R. H., 689
Frank, H. A., 803
Frantz, C. G., 1738
Frantz, V. K., 537
Fraser, D., 1759
Fraser, T. R., 1368, 1370, 1387
Frazell, E. L., 1450, 1452

Freeark, R. J., 223, 239
Freedman, S. O., 309, 1141
Freund, H. R., 1453
Friderichsen, C., 1485
Friedman, B., 1708
Fry, W. J., 947, 958, 961, 962, 1265, 1331
Frykholm, R., 1678, 1681
Furman, S., 803, 805

Gaarder, A., 98
Gabrilove, J. L., 1392
Gaertner, R. A., 875
Galbraith, G., 881
Galicich, J. H., 1631
Galloway, J. A., 474
Gann, D. S., 84
Ganong, W. F., 4
Garden, R. S., 1819, 1820
Gardner, B., 1136
Garrett, H. C., 1414
Garrett, H. E., 846
Garfield, James Abram, 898
Garritano, A. P., 898
Garvey, F. K., 244
Gary, J. E., 1038
Gassman, H. S., 792
Gasul, B. M., 741
Gavriliu, D., 1027
Gay, B. B., 689
Gay, J., 923
Gaze, R. M., 1676
Gelhorn, A., 1470
Gennard, J. F., Jr., 212, 213
Gentry, J. T., 1725
George, M., 366
George, P. A., 522
Gerbode, F., 706, 792
Gerner, R. E., 339
Gershon-Cohen, J., 530
Gersuny, R., 1928
Geyer, R. P., 35
Gibbon, J. H., Jr., 704, 753
Gibbs, N. M., 915
Gibson, S., 690
Giddings, W. P., 230
Giesecke, A. H., Jr., 202
Gifford, J. H., 482
Gifford, R. W., 1410
Gifford, R. W., Jr., 894, 902
Gilbert, J. W., 687
Gilbertsen, V. A., 325
Gill, K. A., 212
Gillesby, W. J., 1264
Gillies, H. D., 1945
Gillman, T., 279, 280
Gilmour, J. R., 1458, 1706
Giordano, C., 32, 406
Giovannetti, S., 32, 406
Girard, K. F., 207
Girdlestone, G. R., 1857
Gjessing, L. R., 1411
Glass, H. G., 1450
Glass, W. W., 240
Glassow, F., 1355, 1359
Glenn, F., 1240, 1404
Glenn, T. M., 45
Glenn, W. W. L., 732, 803
Goetz, R. H., 809
Gold, D., 546
Gold, P., 309, 1141
Goldberg, M. F., 1470
Goldberg, S. M., 1109
Goldblatt, H., 962
Golden, A., 1498
Golding, M. R., 905
Goldman, J. L., 575
Goldman, L., 1483
Goldner, J. L., 1734
Goldsmith, R. S., 1490

Goldstein, M., 1140
Goldwasser, R. A., 209
Goligher, J. C., 1116, 1140, 1152
Gollan, F., 35
Gomes, M. R., 846
Gomez, R. L., 917
Goodman, A. A., 49
Goodyer, A. V. N., 45
Gordon, G., 1676
Gordon, M., 1261
Gordon, T., 939
Gorer, P. A., 363
Gorfinkel, H. J., 50
Gorlin, R., 684
Gorlin, S. G., 684
Gosney, W. G., 1332
Gould, E. A., 1440, 1455
Goulston, K. J., 1111
Govaerts, A., 361
Gowans, J. L., 355, 367
Graham, E., 1244
Graham, E., 1274
Graham, W. D., 1834
Graham, W. P., 89
Greegor, D. H., 1141
Green, G. E., 794, 798
Greenberg, A. G., 39
Greenberg, R. L., 1961
Greene, N. M., 443
Greenfield, L. J., 45
Greenstein, J. P., 32
Greeves, M. F., 356
Greenwalt, T. J., 124, 126
Greenwood, F. C., 1370
Greer, W. E. R., 942
Gregory, R. A., 1053, 1259
Griffen, W. O., Jr., 1140
Griffith, L. S. C., 963
Griffiths, L. L., 1795
Griffo, Z. J., 468
Grillo, H. C., 277, 278
Grillo, H. E., 793
Grimson, K. S., 1416
Griswold, R. A., 220, 242, 246
Grogan, J. B., 381
Grondin, C., 733
Gross, F., 1380, 1419
Gross, J., 285
Gross, R. E., 696, 700, 701, 704, 716, 720, 734, 735, 839, 945, 1523, 1526, 1528, 1529, 1537
Groves, L. K., 833, 835
Guedel, A. E., 444
Gump, F. E., 41, 146
Gurd, F. N., 48
Guri, J. P., 1690
Guthrie, C. C., 399, 404, 839

Haagensen, C. D., 531, 541, 542, 545, 547
Haas, J., 1726
Habein, H. C., Jr., 1021
Hache, L., 1337
Hackett, E., 1336, 1337
Hagen, W. E., 240
Haglin, J. J., 403
Hahn, L. J., 1332
Haight, C., 1520
Haller, J. A., Jr., 1513
Halligan, E. J., 1317
Hallman, G. L., 835
Halsted, W. S., 324, 875, 876
Halter, B. L., 238
Hamberger, C. A., 1370
Hamman, B. L., 1384
Hammon, J., 835
Handley, R. S., 545
Hanlon, C. R., 727, 728, 833, 835
Hara, M., 894
Hardaway, R. M., 37, 44

Hardy, K. L., 739
Harken, D. E., 762, 774, 790
Harkins, H. N., 221
Harley, H. R. S., 1305
Harness, J. K., 1455, 1456
Harnly, M. H., 521
Harold, Z. H., 1829
Harrington, S. W., 1024
Harris, E. D., 31
Harris, G. W., 4, 390
Harris, H., 1754
Harris, L. D., 1024
Harris, P. D., 829
Harris, R. W., 1798, 1807
Harrison, E. G., Jr., 948
Harrison, J. H., 1414
Harrison, T. S., 1363
Hart, J. T., 1334
Hartmann, W. H., 1413
Hartzell, J. B., 462
Harvey, W., 968
Haskell, Charles M., 297
Hastings, A. B., 72
Haumont, S., 1744
Hawley, P. R., 43
Hayes, M. A., 41, 941
Hazard, J. B., 1413, 1444
Hedgpeth, E. McG., Jr., 46
Heinbecker, P., 1382
Heird, W. C., 33
Heller, E., 1016
Hellstrom, I., 311
Hellstrom, J., 1475, 1476
Helmer, O. M., 946
Hems, G., 534
Henderson, E. D., 1780
Henderson, R. R., 920
Hendrick, J. W., 1443
Henson, S. W., Jr., 1691
Henzel, J. H., 78
Herbst, A. L., 1589
Herman, A. H., 29
Heyman, C. H., 1734
Hibner, R., 482
Hickler, R. B., 962
Hicks, J. H., 1712, 1713
Higgs, L. M., 771
Hill, A. V., 1694
Hill, C. S., 1451
Hill, L. D., 1025
Hillman, D. A., 1483
Hinchey, J. J., 1821
Hinshaw, L. B., 45, 143, 152, 153
Hinton, J. W., 221
Hiott, D. W., 45
Hirabayashi, R. N., 1443, 1450, 1451
Hirsch, C., 1729
Hirsch, P. F., 29, 1464
Hirst, A. E., 826
Hjermann, I., 1411
Hoaglund, F. T., 1675, 1725, 1791, 1845, 1879
Hockaday, J. M., 1676
Hodes, P. J., 1745
Hodges, C. V., 330, 1414
Hodgkinson, A., 1477
Hodgson, A. R., 1714, 1852
Hofmann, W., 89
Holden, W. D., 48, 1882
Holdsworth, F. W., 1841, 1842
Holinger, P. H., 574, 575
Holl-Allen, R. T. J., 1455
Hollander, F., 1068
Hollender, M. H., 480
Holley, K. W., 946
Holloway, C. K., 1474
Holmagyi, D. F. J., 152
Holman, E., 686, 871
Holmes, E. C., 1468
Holmes, J. T., 1107
Holstein, A., 1807

Homans, J., 923
Hoover, A. L., 931
Horowitz, B. G., 1819
Horowitz, H. I., 98
Horwitz, D. L., 29
Hougie, C., 108
Houseworth, J., 479
Howard, J. E., 954, 955
Howe, C. W., 462
Howell, J., 894
Howell, R. R., 1869
Howland, W. S., 125
Hsu, J. M., 31
Hsu, T. H. S., 31
Huang, S., 1413
Huckabee, W. E., 39, 509
Hudack, S. S., 931
Huggins, C., 330, 1394
Hughes, C. W., 901
Hughes, R. K., 700
Hume, D. M., 1, 41, 45, 404, 942, 1363, 1407,
    1413–1415, 1429, 1457, 1477, 1494, 1498
Hummer, C. D., 1736
Hunt, J. R., 881
Hunt, J. C., 947, 948
Hunt, P. S., 1430
Hunt, T. K., 31
Hunter, J., 275
Hunter, J. A., 895, 900
Hunter, S. W., 739
Hunter, W., 871
Hurst, J. W., 827
Huston, J. R., 1414
Hutcher, N., 49
Hutchinson, E. C., 881
Hutter, A. M., Jr., 1393
Huxley, A. F., 1692
Hyman, G., 1714

Imparato, A. M., 806, 839, 852, 894
Ingelfinger, F. J., 1009
Ingle, D. J., 9
Ingleby, H., 530
Inman, V. T., 1802
Interbitzen, T., 373
Iseri, L. T., 1416
Island, D. P., 1374
Ivy, A. C., 102

Jack, E. A., 1714
Jackson, C. E., 1482, 1487
Jackson, J. A., 470
Jackson, P., 1868
Jackson, S. F., 1754
Jacobs, B., 1804
Jacobsohn, D., 390
Jaffe, H. L., 1777
Jagatic, J., 1403
Jahnke, E. J., Jr., 901
James, P. M., Jr., 153
James, D. W., 278
James, H. J., 1204
Jankowski, T., 1476
Janoff, A., 48
Jefferies, W. M., 1384
Jeffers, W. A., 963
Jeghers, H., 1096
Jemerin, E. E., 1032
Jernigan, W. R., 92
Johansen, H., 547, 549
Johnson, E. R., 202
Johnson, W. J., 1498
Johnson, L. C., 1720, 1775
Johnson, L. W., 688
Johnson, S. A., 124, 126
Johnston, R. K., 1316
Johnstone, A. S., 1038
Jones, J. C., 721

Jones, R. C., 125, 204, 207, 216, 220, 237, 243
Jones, R. H., 506
Jones, T. W., 1313
Jordan, G. L., 239, 241, 245, 246
Jordan, H. H., 1872
Joske, R. A., 1032
Jowsey, J., 1462, 1474
Jude, J. R., 759
Judet, H., 387
Jutras, J. A., 1229
Juul-Jensen, P., 411

Kaae, S., 547, 549
Kahn, D. R., 821
Kahn, P., 1401
Kakkar, V., 913, 917
Kaliss, N., 363
Kandalaft, S., 1136
Kaplan, E. B., 1905
Kaplan, E. L., 1429, 1457
Kaplan, M. H., 1443
Kaplan, N. M., 1396, 1397
Karcher, H., 1490
Karlson, K. E., 1114
Kassel, R., 521
Katsilambros, L., 582
Katz, N. M., 481
Katz, R., 128
Kaufman, J. J., 962
Kaufman, L., 506
Kay, J. H., 480, 774
Kayhoe, D. E., 1393
Keiser, H. R., 31, 1478
Keith, A., 1712
Keith, J. D., 739
Keller, J. W., 316
Kellgren, J. H., 1677, 1861
Kelly, A. B., 1038
Kelly, P. J., 864
Kelly, T. R., 1487
Kemph, J. P., 481
Kennaway, E. C., 300
Kennedy, B. J., 549, 551
Kennedy, C. S., 545
Kernohan, J. W., 1646
Kerry, R. L., 240
Kerzner, M. S., 1414
Ketcham, A. S., 463, 590
Khalili, A. A., 1705
Kianouri, M., 897
Kihn, R. B., 1887
Killian, H., 476
Kilman, J. W., 905
Kim, G. E., 806, 853, 894
Kimberg, D. V., 450
Kincaid, O. W., 689
Kinch, R. A. H., 1391
King, J. C., 221
King, M. L., 1440, 1455
King, T., 1683
Kinmonth, J. B., 932
Kinney, J. M., 28, 41, 88, 499
Kinsella, T. J., 1030
Kirby, C. K., 914
Kirklin, J. W., 693, 696, 727, 1034
Kirschner, M. A., 1382
Kirsh, M. M., 832
Kirsner, J. B., 1110
Kirtley, J. A., 903
Kite, J. H., 1733, 1734
Kittle, C. F., 39
Kjellberg, R. N., 1370, 1373
Klatskin, G., 450, 1261
Klein, E., 341, 1327
Klein, L., 1849
Kleinsasser, L. J., 1331
Knaggs, R. L., 1750, 1766
Knickerbocker, G. G., 759
Knisely, M., 1282

Knobil, E., 15
Knoernschild, H. E., 1130
Knopp, L. M., 221
Knowles, R. P., 212
Knox, S. J., 447, 478
Knutson, C. O., 523
Kobold, E. E., 226
Kocher, T., 1429, 1442
Kock, N. G., 990
Koehler, P. R., 1414
Kohatsu, S., 1118
Kokko, J. P., 1396
Konvolinka, C. W., 1450
Koop, C. E., 1529
Kornfeld, D. S., 480
Kouwenhoven, W. B., 759
Kotler, A. N., 207
Kouchoukos, N. T., 846
Kraft, A. R., 1277
Kramer, I. R. H., 181
Kramer, W. M., 537
Krane, S. M., 1762
Krauss, A. H., 821, 824
Kremser, K. H., 475
Krugman, S., 128
Kubicek, W. G., 507
Kuhne, H., 475
Kune, G. A., 240
Kuner, J., 470
Kurzweg, F. T., 467
Kvale, W. F., 942, 1407

Laborit, H., 150, 151
Lack, C. H., 1796
Ladd, W. E., 1529, 1537
LaDue, J. S., 472, 473
LaFave, J. W., 234
Lafferty, J. W., 1470
Lagergren, H., 805
Lahey, F. H., 857, 1020, 1445
Laimer, E., 1010
Lalardrie, J. P., 1958
Lam, S. F., 1714
Landis, E. M., 903
Landman, M. D., 990
Landsmeer, J., 1905
Lane, T. C., 234
Lapiere, C. M., 285
La Roque, G. P., 1355
Lattimer, J. K., 1391
Lauritzen, G. K., 225
Lawrence, A. M., 1410
Lawrence, H. S., 340, 362, 373
Lawson, G., 1922
Lee, R. I., 103
Lees, J. C., 546
Lefer, A. M., 45
Lefer, M. D., 1261
Lefrak, E. A., 817
Lellehei, R. C., 134
LeMesurier, A. B., 1949
Lendvay, P., 1917
Leriche, R., 843
Leslie, J. T., 1806
Lespinasse, V., 244
Lev, R., 49
Levenson, S. M., 27
Levin, E. J., 229
Levine, M., 479
Levinson, S. A., 45
Lewis, A., 477
Lewis, F. J., 690, 704, 733
Lewis, G. B., 1807
Lewis, T., 903
Lewison, E. F., 541
Li, M. C., 336
Lichtenstein, I. L., 1351
Lichtman, A. L., 485
Liddle, G. W., 944, 945, 1385

Likar, L., 741
Lillehei, C. W., 716, 739, 803, 805, 963
Lim, R. C., 958
Lim, R. K. S., 969
Lima, C., 1731
Lindemann, E., 480
Linden, M. C., Jr., 1444
Lindsay, J., 827
Lindsay, S., 1443, 1450, 1451
Linfoot, J. A., 1096
Ling, R. S. M., 1716
Linton, R. R., 849, 931, 1207
Liotta, D., 816, 829
Lipsett, M. B., 1386, 1392
Lipshutz, W., 1015
Little, P. A., 377
Livingston, W. K., 1676
Ljungqvist, U., 29
Lodge, B., 898
Longmire, W. P., Jr., 234, 990, 1224, 1233
Lopez-Mayor, J. F., 463
Lord, J. W., Jr., 876, 880
Lortat-Jacob, J.-L., 1017
Louis, W. J., 949
Louw, J. H., 1527
Love, J. C., 881
Lowe, S. A., 1865
Lower, R. R., 351, 399, 799
Lucas, C. E., 234, 1182
Luft, R., 1373
Luke, J. C., 929
Lynch, C. J., 1796
Lyons, C., 881
Lyons, J. H., Jr., 36, 37

McAlister, W. H., 1414
McAllister, R. G., Jr., 961
McBride, E. D., 1868, 1869
McBurney, C., 1167, 1169
McCance, R. A., 1759
McCarty, D. J., 1870
McClelland, R. N., 220, 245, 992
MacCleod, W. A. J., 1474
McCloy, R. M., 827
McClusky, J. W., 361
McClusky, R. T., 361
McCollough, N. C., 212, 213
McCorkle, H. J., 221
McCormack, C. J., 229
McCormack, L. J., 947, 948
McCubbin, J. W., 963
McDaniel, J. R., 230
McDonald, D. A., 505
McDonald, D. F., 962, 1547
MacDonald, E. J., 522
MacDonald, I., 542
McDonald, J., 222
McDonald, J. C., 1332
McDonald, J. R., 485
MacEwen, G. D., 1736
MacFadyen, B. V., 485
Macfarlane, R. G., 99
McGaw, W. H., 1804
McGeown, M. G., 1477
McGoon, D. C., 689, 693, 712, 736, 737, 774, 779
McGowan, G. K., 1478
McGregor, I. A., 258, 1925
McGuigan, J. E., 1056
McGuire, L. B., 733
McHolick, W., 1684
MacIntosh, D. L., 1857
McKee, G. K., 1864
MacKenzie, I. G., 1730
McKeown, J., 1725
Mackey, W. A., 1240
Mackler, S. A., 1030
McKusick, V. A., 864, 865, 1765
McLachlin, J., 915
McLaughlin, H., 1875

McLean, F. C., 1753
MacLean, L. D., 38, 44
McLeish, W. A., 1413
MacLennan, J. D., 181, 182
McLeod, J. G., 1676
McMaster, P. D., 931
McMinn, R. M. H., 88
McNamara, J. J., 26
McPhaul, J. J., Jr., 955
McVay, C. B., 1356, 1359
McWhirter, R., 544, 547
Madden, J. W., 287, 385, 1136, 1234
Maddock, W. G., 1024
Maggiore, Q., 32
Magnuson, F. K., 482, 483
Mahaim, I., 791
Maher, F. T., 1410
Maier, H. C., 595
Majno, G., 278
Major, S. G., 1334, 1335
Malcolm, J. D., 133
Mallory, G. K., 1039
Mallory, T. B., 475
Malloy, J. P., 41
Malm, J. R., 727
Malt, R. A., 388
Manax, W. G., 462
Manesis, J. G., 1243
Mannick, J. A., 362
Manning, P. C., Jr., 1035
Mannix, H., Jr., 1240, 1404
Mansberger, A. R., 206
Mapother, E. D., 133
Marable, S. A., 234, 961, 1331
Marchetta, F. C., 1450
Marchioro, T. L., 394
Marks, I. N., 1276
Marks, L. J., 1375
Marshall, S. F., 1009
Martin, H., 557, 586
Martin, L. W., 1520
Martin, M. J., 883
Martin, M. M., 1384
Marusic, E. T., 1380
Mathé, G., 338, 341
Matini, K., 994
Massie, W. K., 1820
Masters, Y. F., 49
Matas, Rudolf, 839, 871, 900
Matthewson, C., Jr., 238
Mattsson, O., 1020
Mauney, F. M., Jr., 473
Maxwell, M. H., 951
Mead, J., 468
Meador, C. K., 1375, 1382, 1383
Medina, R. G., 1450
Melby, J. C., 1389, 1391
Melicow, M. M., 1339
Melzack, R., 969, 1666, 1676
Mendeloff, A. I., 1111
Meng, H. C., 32
Menguy, R., 49, 1049, 1259
Mercer, W., 1698, 1766
Merendino, K. A., 234, 771, 1273, 1313
Merendino, K. H., 730
Metchnikoff, E., 143, 373
Metras, H., 402
Meyer, A. C., 544, 548
Meyer, H. W., 541
Meyer, K., 281
Meyer, W., 15
Michelakis, A. M., 955
Mikal, S., 1452
Miles, A. A., 1795
Miles, R. M., 861, 922
Miles, W. E., 1136
Milford, L. W., 1929
Milkman, L. A., 1760
Millar, E. A., 1751

Millard, D. R., Jr., 1949
Miller, E., 545
Miller, H. H., 868
Miller, T., 959
Millesi, H., 1909
Minno, A. M., 1407
Mishell, R. I., 359
Mitchell, G. A. G., 1305
Mitchell, H. H., 1752
Mitchell, S. Weir, 904
Mitchison, N. A., 357, 360
Mixter, C. G., Jr., 1476
Mobin-Uddin, K., 922
Modell, J. H., 35
Moersch, H. J., 467
Mohs, F. E., 520
Molinatti, G. M., 1387
Monaco, A. P., 373
Moncrief, J. A., 253
Moniz, E., 1668
Monks, G. H., 1928
Moon, H. D., 1415
Mooney, V., 1705, 1709
Moore, A., 1705
Moore, F. D., 36, 37, 65, 87, 88, 465, 478
Moore, G. E., 339
Moore, R., 1861
Moore, R. A., 1560
Moore, S. W., 229
Moore, W. S., 1882
Moran, W. H., Jr., 40
Morel-Fatio, D., 1958
Moretz, W. H., 483, 922
Morgan, F. P., 1683
Morley, A. J. M., 1711
Mornex, R., 1372
Morris, G. C., Jr., 869, 899, 900, 946, 961, 1327, 1328
Morrison, E., 1477
Morrow, A. G., 734, 771
Morson, B. C., 1114
Morton, D. L., 297, 308, 338
Morton, J. H., 1345
Moss, G. S., 35
Moss, N. H., 1274, 1276
Motsay, G. B., 143
Mottershead, S., 877
Motulsky, A. G., 1282
Moyer, C. A., 69, 82
Mozden, P. J., 462
Mueller, C. B., 4
Mulhern, L. M., 1444
Mulholland, H. J., 1268, 1270
Muller, G. M., 1729
Muller, M. E., 1799
Muller, W. H., 706
Mulrow, P. J., 1380
Munro, H. N., 27
Munson, P. L., 1464
Murphy, J. B., 360, 839, 876
Murray, J. E., 404, 1957
Mustard, W. T., 726, 727, 730, 870

Nadas, A. S., 679, 691, 692, 701, 722, 728, 733, 739, 742
Naffziger, H. C., 221
Nahas, R. A., 47
Naitove, A., 1330
Najafi, H., 829
Najarian, J. S., 351, 361
Nakayama, K., 1034, 1036
Nance, F. C., 992
Nanson, E. M., 903
Nardi, G. L., 1244
Nash, G., 46
Nathan, D. A., 803, 805
Nathanson, I. T., 569
Natvig, P., 1957
Naylor, B. A., 42

Neely, W. A., 465
Neptune, W. B., 402
Neuhof, H., 1032
Neumann, M. W., 1752
Neumann, W. F., 1752
Neviaser, J. S., 1804
Neville, A. M., 1395
Newcombe, J. F., 278
Newman, P. H., 1684, 1689
Nickerson, M., 134, 151
Nissen, R., 1025
Nivatvongs, S., 1109
Niwayama, G., 733
Noall, M. W., 1130
Nordin, B. E. C., 1763
Norman, J. C., 111, 809
Norris, C. M., 575
Norris, E. H., 1472, 1493
Norström, A., 1754
Nossal, G. J. V., 357
Nourok, D. S., 1413
Nugent, C. A., 1479
Nylin, G., 696, 701

Oberhelman, H. A., Jr., 1118, 1278
Ochsner, A. J., 1173, 1186
Odell, W. D., 1374
Ogden, W. W., 1334
Ogura, J. W., 590
Ohsawa, T., 1009
Old, L. J., 307, 340
Oldham, H. N., Jr., 741
Olinde, H. D. H., 835
Ollodart, R., 206
Ollier, L. L. X. E., 1922
Olsen, A. M., 1016
O'Neil, E. E., 914
O'Rahilly, R., 1738
Orkin, L. R., 45
Ormond, J. K., 1336–1338
Orr, K. D., 906
Orth, D. N., 945
Osborn, J. J., 499
Oschner, A., Jr., 706
Ota, K., 958
Ottinger, L. W., 1326
Owen, E., 1917
Owen, O. E., 21
Owens, G., 13–19
Owens, J. C., 898
Owren, P. A., 102

Pack, G. T., 543, 1339
Page, D., 1922
Page, I. H., 946
Pak, C. Y. C., 1479
Palmer, E. D., 1110
Paloyan, E., 1466, 1476
Papas, G., 896
Parbossingh, I. S., 1412
Park, E. A., 696
Park, W. W., 546
Parker, E. F., 1036
Parkes, J. D., 1204
Parkinson, T., 1414
Parmley, L. F., 829
Paronetto, F., 450
Parrish, E. H., 922
Parrish, H. M., 213, 214
Pate, J. W., 835
Paterson, D. R., 1038
Paterson, J. C., 915
Patman, R. D., 870
Paton, B. C., 735
Payne, R. J., Jr., 1474
Payne, W. S., 1009, 1020
Peacock, E. E., 385
Peacock, E. E., Jr., 275, 285

Peaston, M. J. T., 38
Peckham, G. B., 691
Peltier, L. F., 477
Pemberton, L. B., 462
Pemberton, P. A., 1730
Penn, I., 410, 425, 1231
Penn, J., 279, 280
Pensler, L., 34
Perl, E. R., 1666
Perry, J. F., Jr., 223, 234
Perry, M. O., 199, 220
Persik, S. L., 1456
Peskin, G. W., 124
Peters, R. M., 46, 499
Peterson, T. A., 694
Petrakis, N. L., 534
Petrie, J. G., 1719
Phelps, W. M., 1702
Phemister, D. B., 1849
Phillips, D. G., 1682
Pickles, B. G., 1412
Pierson, J. M., 1257
Pigott, R. W., 1949
Pillemer, L., 43
Pinkerton, J. A., 234
Pitch, Y. H., 340
Platou, E., 1729
Plimpton, C. H., 1470
Polk, H. C., Jr., 463
Pollack, D. J., 1413
Ponsetti, I. V., 1708, 1709
Pontinen, P., 470
Pontoppidan, H., 465
Pool, J. G., 123
Popper, H., 450
Pott, P., 300
Potts, F., 411
Potts, J. T., Jr., 1480
Potts, W. J., 721, 724
Poulantzas, J. K., 240
Poulsen, J. E., 1372
Powers, J. H., 1967
Prendergast, R. A., 361
Price, C. H. G., 1776
Prichard, R. W., 791, 793
Prohaska, J. Y., 1119
Puestow, C. B., 1264
Pygott, F., 467
Pyrah, L. N., 1471, 1476, 1478

Quast, D. C., 245, 246
Quervain, F. de, 1444
Quick, A. J., 98, 103
Quinn, W. F., 482

Rabiah, 1317
Raine, F., 1032
Raju, S., 381
Rand, R. W., 1363
Randall, H. T., 78, 91
Randall, P., 1949
Rankin, F. W., 1334, 1335
Rapaport, A., 954, 1468
Raphael, H. A., 896, 897
Rasmussen, H., 1459, 1478
Rastelli, G. C., 694, 712
Rathbun, J. C., 1759
Ratliff, A. H. C., 1720
Ratnoff, O. D., 99
Ravdin, I. S., 914
Raven, R. W., 1032
Ravitch, M. M., 787, 875, 1530
Ray, B. S., 1369, 1370
Raynaud, Maurice, 901
Rea, W. J., 179
Record, R. G., 1725
Reddi, K. K., 1754
Redding, M., 4

Reed, G. E., 771
Reemtsma, K., 700
Reichle, F. A., 852
Reid, M. R., 896
Reifenstein, E. C., 1753
Reilly, J., 142
Reinikainen, M., 470
Reiss, E., 1480
Reitz, R. E., 1480
Reivich, M., 885
Relman, A. S., 73
Resnick, R. H., 1203
Reverdin, J. L., 1921, 1922
Reynolds, B. M., 1241
Rhinelander, F. W., 1796
Rhoads, J. E., 1274, 1276
Richards, V., 482
Richardson, J. A., 45
Richetts, C. R., 29
Richmond, J., 1414
Riddell, V. H., 1430
Ries, E., 1967
Riley, W. B., Jr., 285
Riordin, D. C., 1738
Ripstein, C. B., 244, 1158
Risser, J. C., 1709
Rob, C. G., 881, 1328
Robbins, G. F., 539, 543, 546
Robert, A., 49
Roberts, B., 895, 919
Robertson, D. J., 873
Robinson, E., 1448
Robinson, R., 1405
Robinson, R. A., 1682, 1742, 1754
Roche, M. B., 1684
Rodkey, G. V., 484
Rogers, W. A., 1840
Rogers, W. R., 471
Roitt, I. M., 1443
Roof, B. S., 1470
Roos, A., 468
Roos, D. B., 876, 881, 903
Ropes, M., 1854
Rosati, L. M., 876, 880
Rose, W. C., 32
Rosenfeld, L., 875
Rosenheim, M. L., 1414
Rosenkrantz, J. G., 1041
Roshe, T., 803
Ross, F. P., 1238
Roth, E. J., 546
Roth, S. I., 1468
Rous, P., 301
Rousselot, L. M., 1138
Rowe, G. G., 1684
Rowe, M. L., 1682
Royster, H. P., 89
Rubin, I. C., 1316
Rubnitz, M. E., 1403
Rudowski, W. J., 127
Ruiz, J. O., 1107
Rumbold, C., 1683
Rush, B. F., Jr., 527, 537, 555
Rushmer, R. F., 497
Rusk, H. A., 1967
Russek, A. S., 52–57n.
Russell, F. E., 213, 215
Russell, P. S., 352
Rutledge, R. H., 1325
Ryan, T. J., 1806
Rydell, W. B., Jr., 237
Ryle, J. A., 968

Sabiston, D. C., 734, 739
Sako, K., 1450
Salter, R. B., 1730, 1798, 1807, 1812
Salzman, E. W., 103, 1263
Samuel, E. P., 1677
Sancassani, D. A., 1921

Sanders, J. W., 1738
Sandison, A. T., 537
Santulli, T. V., 1529
Sapira, J. D., 1413
Sargent, F. T., 229
Sarmiento, A., 1830, 1831
Sarnoff, S. J., 494
Sautter, R. D., 923
Savory, W. S., 887
Sawyer, J. L., 735
Sawyer, P. N., 850
Sayre, G. P., 1646
Scaglietti, C., 1727
Scales, J. T., 1865
Scannell, J. G., 793
Schabel, F. M., Jr., 333
Schacht, R. A., 956, 1397
Schambelan, M., 1402
Schatzki, R., 1038
Schechter, D. C., 1376
Schein, C. J., 877, 1238
Scheller, S., 1729
Schenker, V., 28
Schiebler, G. L., 742
Schimke, R. N., 1413
Schlichter, J., 1709
Schmidt, H. W., 1037
Schonholtz, G. J., 463
Schramel, R., 835
Schrock, T., 234, 245
Schteingart, E., 1374
Schumacker, H. B., 803
Schumer, W., 43, 137, 149, 153, 157
    1177, 1221, 1242, 1243, 1281, 1429, 1879
Schwartz, W. B., 73
Schwedel, J. B., 803
Scothorne, R. J., 358
Scott, H. W., 734
Scott, H. W., Jr., 942, 945
Sealy, W. C., 701, 945
Secarz, E., 359
Seddon, H. J., 1717, 1729
Sedgwick, C. E., 1233, 1450
Seegmiller, J. E., 1869
Seldinger, S. I., 1482
Sellers, R. D., 706
Sellors, T. H., 685
Seltzer, A., 762
Selye, H., 136
Senning, A., 727, 730, 775, 808
Sevitt, S., 475, 1684
Seybold, W. D., 1032
Seymour, R. J., 1391
Shannon, A. E., 123
Shannon, C. E., 497
Shapiro, A. P., 961
Sharp, G. S., 521
Sharp, W. V., 1487
Sharrad, W. J. W., 1703
Shaw, R. S., 1325
Shearer, W. S., 1746
Shepard, R. S., 1709
Sheps, S. G., 948, 1410
Sherman, C. D., 1788
Sherry, S., 101
Shields, R., 1023
Shimaoka, K., 1448
Shimkin, M. B., 302, 546, 548
Shires, G. T., 65, 195, 204, 207, 216, 220, 237, 243
Shires, T., 137
Shocket, W., 1413
Shoemaker, W. C., 153
Short, D. S., 914
Shulman, N. R., 107
Shumacker, H. B., Jr., 736, 816, 829, 905
Shuman, C. R., 474

Shumway, N. E., 727, 808
Siegel, J. H., 143
Siggaard-Andersen, O., 38
Silen, W., 1255
Simmons, R. L., 351, 352, 421
Simonds, R. L., 29
Singer, R. B., 72
Sipple, J. H., 1413
Sjoerdama, A., 31
Skall-Jensen, J., 734
Skandalakis, J. E., 584
Skoog, T., 879, 902, 1949
Slanetz, C. A., 1140
Sloviter, H. A., 35
Small, D. M., 1233, 1234
Smith, G. W., 1682
Smith, H., 946
Smith, H. C., 287
Smith, L., 1810
Smith, R., 899
Smith, R., 1263
Smith, S. S., 544, 548
Smith, W. S., 1729
Smithwick, R. H., 963
Smoak, R. D., 1883
Smyth, F. S., 1483
Snyder, C. C., 212
Sofield, H. A., 1751
Sokolov, A. P., 1054
Solis, R. T., 45
Sommers, S. C., 1111
Souttar, P. W., 762
Sorenson, J., 1479
Sparks, F. C., 297
Spencer, F. C., 677, 690, 716, 749, 815, 831, 839,
    922
Spink, W. W., 43
Spjut, H. J., 1130
Splithoff, C. A., 1683
Spratt, J. S., 1130, 1132
Sproul, E. E., 1469
Stahnke, H. L., 214
Stamey, T. A., 955
Stanbury, S. W., 1498
Stanley, J. C., 1331
Starling, E. H., 134
Starr, A., 771, 774, 785
Starzl, T. E., 372, 373, 398, 410, 425, 1191, 1196,
    1214
Stein, H. D., 31
Steinberg, I., 791
Steindler, A., 1738
Steiner, R. E., 1482
Stemmer, E. A., 32
Stetson, C. A., Jr., 43
Stevens, L. E., 1482, 1483
Stevenson, A. C., 1725
Stewart, F. W., 537, 539, 582
Stewart, R. D., 216
Stewart, S., III, 685
Stewart, W. K., 1392
Stewart, W. R., 1414
Stone, H. H., 1182
Storer, E. H., 967, 1089, 1109, 1167, 1297
Stout, A. P., 1134, 1135
Stowens, D., 1225
Straube, K. R., 1414
Strauch, M., 50
Straus, A. M., 1466
Streeten, D. H. P., 990
Streeter, G. L., 1743
Strickler, W. L., 956
Strohl, E. L., 241
Strott, C. A., 1479
Stuart, F. P., 381
Stubbins, S. G., 1804
Stuck, F. E., 1852
Sturmer, F. C., 237
Suby, H. I., 1337
Sugarbaker, E. D., 545, 549

Sugg, W. L., 790
Sullivan, J. F., 31, 1243
Sullivan, R. C., 1076
Sumner, W. C., 339
Sunzel, H., 1238
Sutherland, A., 480
Sutherland, H. D., 1020
Sutton, G. E., 475
Swan, H., 685, 690
Swanson, L. T., 1957
Swenson, O., 1531
Symington, T., 1395
Szilagyi, D. E., 846, 849

Tabah, E. J., 1339
Tagliacozzi, G., 1919, 1920
Talmage, R. V., 1753
Tandon, R., 689
Tanzer, M. L., 285
Tarhan, S., 473
Tate, J., 1412
Taussig, H. B., 681, 685, 687, 712, 727
Taylor, G. W., 569, 932, 933
Tecimer, L. B., 89
Telford, E. D., 877
Teloh, H. A., 1413
Tennison, C. W., 1949
Terasaki, P. J., 417
Terblanche, J., 1245
Terry, R., 32
Tessier, P., 1957
Thackray, A. C., 545
Thal, A. P., 142, 961, 1268
Thal, E. R., 220, 226, 241
Thiersch, C., 1922
Thomas, G. G., 1237
Thomas, K. E., 791
Thompson, J. E., 884, 894
Thompson, N., 1958
Thompson, N. W., 1455, 1456
Thompson, R. C., Jr., 1882
Thomson, A. D., 1778, 1780, 1781
Tice, D. A., 798, 873
Timmis, H. H., 739
Titchener, J. L., 477–480
Tobian, L., 948
Tollefsen, H. R., 1450
Tolstedt, G. E., 896
Tompkins, R. K., 1277
Tonna, E. A., 1796
Townes, P. L., 1726
Tracy, H. J., 1259
Triedman, L. J., 884
Trimble, C., 47
Trinkle, J. K., 771
Trotter, W. R., 1440
Troup, S. B., 97
Truelove, S. C., 1110
Trueta, J., 1691
Tsuji, H. K., 733
Tubiana, R., 1907
Tucci, J. R., 1385
Turcotte, J. G., 1290
Turnbull, R. B., Jr., 1113, 1134, 1136
Turner-Warwick, R. T., 1778, 1780, 1781
Tuttle, W. M., 1032

Uhr, J. W., 355
Ulfelder, H., 1589
Urban, J. A., 538, 545, 1794

Urist, M. R., 1753
Urschel, H. D., 877, 878, 881
Utz, D., 1571

Vacca, J. B., 738
Vagnucci, A. I., 1384
Van Allen, C. M., 467
Van der Linden, W., 1238
VanGilder, J. C., 1631
Van Slyke, D. D., 494, 497
Varco, R. L., 798
Vasko, J. S., 824
Vaughn, J. H., 366
Veith, F. J., 46
Venes, J. L., 1631
Verdan, C., 1913
Vertes, V., 956
Vigliano, E. M., 98
Vignos, P. J., 1697
Villee, D. B., 1393
Vincent, Y. J., 1771
Vineberg, A. M., 733
Vinson, P. P., 1021
Voitk, A. J., 49
Volkman, 367
Von Euler, U. S., 149, 1375, 1410
Von Graefe, C. F., 1920
Voorhees, A. B., Jr., 839, 1207
Voorhees, M. L., 1417
Vyden, J. K., 49

Waddell, W. R., 1076
Wade, P. A., 1804
Wagner, G., 1485
Wakefield, J. D., 361
Waksman, B. H., 373
Walker, R. M., 1412
Wall, P., 1666
Wall, P. D., 969
Walmsley, T., 1706
Walt, A. J., 1182
Wangensteen, O. H., 325, 982, 1140
Wangensteen, S. L., 45, 153
Ward, G., 557
Warner, H. R., 963
Warren, K. W., 240, 1020, 1273
Warren, R., 884, 1883, 1887
Warren, W. D., 1206
Wasowski, J. R., 234
Watkins, D. F. L., 1237
Watkins, E., Jr., 1456
Watson-Farrar, J., 1864
Watts, G. T., 1263
Waugh, W., 1868
Wear, J. B., 244
Weaver, J. M., 361
Weaver, W., 497
Webb, W. R., 46
Webster, J. P., 1944
Webster, W. P., 111
Weddel, G., 876
Weddell, A. G. M., 1676
Weil, M. H., 38, 43, 153
Weismann, R. E., 1330
Weiss, L., 362
Weiss, P., 279
Weiss, S., 1039
Weissman, S. L., 1829
Welbourn, R. B., 483
Welch, C. E., 484

Welch, C. S., 868
Weldon, C. S., 716
Welin, S., 1130, 1133
Welsh, G. F., 1020
Wermer, P., 1277
Wessler, S., 863
Wheat, M. W., Jr., 470, 828, 829
Wheeler, H. B., 917
Whipple, A. O., 1272, 1275
White, L. P., 522
White, P. D., 103
White, T. T., 1258
Whitty, C. W. M., 1676
Whorton, C. M., 791
Wilensky, A. O., 1332
Wiley, A. M., 1691
Williams, E. D., 1413
Williams, M. H., Jr., 421, 501
Williams, R. D., 221, 229, 316
Willis, R. A., 564
Willis, T., 1013
Wills, M. R., 1478
Wilmore, D. W., 95
Wilson, J. W., 137
Wilson, R. E., 1487
Wilson, R. F., 37, 44, 153, 241, 1268
Wilson, S. D., 1277
Wilson, W. B., 30
Wilt, K. E., 237
Wiltse, L. L., 1684
Winfield, J. M., 462
Winiwarter, F., 862
Winkelstein, C., 478
Wiseman, B. K., 1290
Witebsky, E., 1436
Woldring, S., 508
Wolfe, J. R., 1922
Wolff, W. L., 462
Womack, N. A., 1233
Wood, P., 712
Woodruff, M. F. A., 373, 389
Woodward, E. R., 1025
Wray, J. B., 1796
Wright, A. D., 1368, 1370, 1387
Wright, H. K., 84, 1110, 1134
Wright, I. S., 876
Wright, R. G., 481
Wright, V., 1865
Wroblewski, F., 472, 473
Wulsin, J. H., 206
Wylie, E. J., 846, 849, 947, 958
Wynn, S. K., 1949
Wyrick, W. J., Jr., 179
Wychulis, A. R., 1452

Yannopoulos, K., 1334, 1335
Yater, W. M., 791
Yates, P. O., 881
Yudin, S. S., 1028

Zaks, M. S., 480
Zeavin, I., 685
Zimmerman, L. M., 1346, 1349, 1356, 1359
Zintel, H. A., 963
Zippin, C., 534
Zohman, L. R., 501
Zoll, P. M., 803, 807
Zollinger, R. M., 221, 1276, 1277
Zukoski, C. F., 404
Zweifach, W. B., 49

Subject Index

A bands, 1692
Abbott procedure, 1033
Abdomen:
  abscesses, 1305–1308
  apoplexy, 1331–1332
  gynecologic procedures through, 1624–1650
  pain, 969–973
    (*See also* Pain)
    appendicitis, 1168–1169, 1170
    clinical evaluation, 971–973
    colitis, 1113
    diverticulitis, 1123, 1124
    etiology, 970–971
    gynecologic evaluation of, 1598–1599, 1610
    hematoma, rectus sheath, 1315
    history and, 971–972
    intractable, 969–970
    laboratory procedures and, 973
    location, 971–972
    mesenteric occlusion, 1325
    obstruction of intestine, 983
    peritonitis, 1302
    physical examination and, 973
    referred, 969
    somatic, 969
    visceral, 969
  paracentesis of, 221–222
  rigid, 1303
  trauma of, 220–247
    (*See also* specific organs)
    blunt, 220–223
    penetrating, 223–225
Abdominal aneurysms, 887–894
Abdominal wall, 1313–1316
  desmoid tumor, 1315–1316
  hematoma, rectus sheath, 1313–1315
  hernia, 1345–1360
    anatomy, 1346–1348
    complications, 1350
    definition, 1345–1346
    etiology, 1348–1349
    incidence, 1346
    symptoms and signs, 1349–1350
    treatment, 1350–1360
  injuries, 246–247
    penetrating, 198
  omphalocele and gastroschisis, 1523–1524
  pain, 969
  pedicle flap of, 1928, 1930
Abdominoperineal pull-through for imperforate
  anus, 1539, 1540
Abdominoperineal resection:
  for rectal carcinoma, 1136, 1139
  for villous adenoma, 1128
Abortion, 1605–1606
Abscess, 169
  amebic, 1186–1187
  anorectal, 1152–1153
  appendiceal, 1170
  brain, 722, 1663–1664
  breast, 551
  chest wall, 606
  epidural, 1662

hand, 1899
intraabdominal, 1305–1308
liver, 1184–1187
lung, 630–633
mediastinal, 616
pancreatic, 1269, 1270
pelvic, 1307–1308
pericolic, 1124–1125
perinephric, 1551
perirectal, 1152–1153
pyogenic, 1184–1186
subepithelial, 169
subhepatic, 1307
subphrenic, 1306–1307
Accidents, 195
ACD (acid citrate dextrose), 121
Acetabulum:
  dysplasia of, 1726, 1729, 1730
  fractures and dislocations of, 1835–1837
Acetyl coenzyme A, 19–20
Achalasia, 1013–1017
  clinical manifestations, 1014
  physiologic studies, 1014–1015
  treatment, 1015–1017
Aching, venous insufficiency and, 925
Achlorhydria, gastric cancer and, 1079
Achondroplasia, 1747–1748
Acid-base balance, 70–75
  (*See also* Acidosis; Alkalosis)
Acidity, gastric, 1052–1053, 1056–1057,
  1070–1071
Acidosis, 37–39
  blood transfusion and, 37
  burns and 38–39
  cardiac arrest and, 38
  intravenous alimentation and, 33
  metabolic, 74
  respiratory, 73
    cyclopropane anesthesia and, 446, 447
  rickets and, 1758
  shock and, 37–38, 158
  types of, 36, 71
Acinar cell adenocarcinoma, 582
Aclasis, metaphyseal, 1748–1749
Acne, 516
Acrocyanosis, 903–904
Acromegaly, 1369–1371
  hyperparathyroidism and, 1487
  osteoporosis and, 1765
Acromioclavicular injuries, 1803–1804
ACTH (*see* Adrenocorticotropic hormone)
Actin, 1692, 1693
Actinomycin, 377
  for Wilms' tumor, 1567
Actinomycosis, 187–188
  cecal, 1121
  pulmonary, 639
Acute-phase reactants, 24, 26, 28–29
Adamantinoma, 1786
Addison's disease, 1402–1404
  trauma and, 8
Adenitis, mesenteric, 1332–1334
  appendicitis vs., 1171

Adenocarcinoma:
  appendiceal, 1175–1176
  breast, 535
  colonic, polyps and, 1128, 1130–1131
  endometrial, 1615–1617
  gallbladder, 1244
  gastric, 1080
  pancreatic, 1270
  salivary gland, 582
  small bowel, 1096–1097
  spread of, 315
  vaginal, 1619
Adenocystocarcinoma:
  bronchial, 644
  salivary gland, 570, 571
Adenoids, hypertrophied, 577
Adenoleiomyofibromatosis, 1574
Adenoma:
  adrenal gland, 944, 1382, 1395
  chromophobe, 1372, 1389
  gastric, 1083
  islet-cell, 1274–1276
  liver, 1189
  papillary, 1126–1128
  parathyroid, 665, 1467, 1482, 1496
  pleomorphic, of salivary glands, 566
  salivary gland, 581–582
  thyroid, 1438, 1439
  villous, 1126–1128
Adenomatous polyps, 1128
Adenomyosarcoma, 1567
Adenomyosis, uterine, 1601
Adenosine diphosphate:
  oxygen transport and, 496
  platelet, 98–99, 103
Adenosine monophosphate, glucagon and, 16, 17
Adenosine triphosphate:
  cell metabolism and, 137
  erythrocyte lysis and, 1283, 1287
  liver function and, 48
Adenosis, sclerosing, of breast, 538
ADH (*see* Antidiuretic hormone)
Adolescence, breasts in, 528, 531
Adrenal, 1374–1419
  Addison's disease, 1402–1404
  adenoma, 1051, 1382, 1395
  adrenogenital syndrome and, 1374, 1390, 1392
  aldosterone secretion, 1379–1380
  aldosteronism, 1375, 1395–1402
  amenorrhea and, 1603
  anatomy, 1376–1377
  androgen secretion, 1379–1392
  anesthesia and, 447, 449
  blood supply, 1376
  breast cancer and, 1394–1395
  carcinoma, 1392–1393
  catecholamines, 1404–1407
  cortex, 1374–1375, 1377–1404
    physiology, 1377–1380
  cortisol secretion, 1377–1379
  Cushing's syndrome, 1374–1375, 1380–1390
    (*See also* Cushing's syndrome)
  ectopic tissue, 1375–1376

ectopic-ACTH syndrome and, 1383, 1389
embryology, 1375–1376
estrogen-secreting tumors, 1374, 1392
exogenous corticosteroids and, 7–8
exposure of, 1418
ganglioneuroma, 1419
hemorrhage, 1402
historical background, 1374–1375
hyperplasia, 944–945, 1381–1382
  congenital, 1390–1391
hypertension and, 939–945, 1395, 1396
insufficiency, 8–12, 1402–1404
medulla, 1375, 1404–1419
  physiology, 1404–1407
neuroblastoma, 1417–1419, 1567
nodular dysplasia, 1382–1383
pheochromocytoma, 942, 1407–1417
removal of (see Adrenalectomy)
rests, 1375–1376
  of ovary, 1614
sexual development and, 1393–1394
steroids (see Corticosteroids)
transplants, 390
trauma and, 7–12, 199
virilization and, 1374
zones, 1377
Adrenalectomy:
for aldosteronism, 1401
for breast cancer, 550, 1394
for Cushing's syndrome, 945, 1368, 1388
for hypertension, 1395
for pheochromocytoma, 1415
Adrenergic compounds, 1404–1407
  (See also Epinephrine)
  receptor blockade, 1416, 1417
Adrenergic-corticoid phase, 87
Adrenocorticotropic hormone (ACTH),
  1365–1366
adrenalectomy and, 1389
adrenal hyperplasia and, 1382
adrenocortical insufficiency and, 1403
in adrenogenital syndrome, 1392
afferent nerve stimuli and, 1–2
amenorrhea and, 1603
blood measurements, 1386
cells secreting, 1365
in colitis, 1115, 1120
cord transection and, 6, 7
Cushing's syndrome and, 943, 944, 1368
ectopic secretion of, 1373, 1383, 1389
exogenous corticosteroids and, 7–8
hypopituitarism and, 1368
hypothermia and, 4, 5
in peritonitis, 1301
trauma and, 4, 6, 7–12
Adrenogenital syndrome, 1374, 1390–1392
in adult, 1391–1392
congenital hyperplasia, 1390–1391
postnatal and prepubertal, 1391
Adson maneuver, 877, 878
Aerobic infections, 166, 178, 180
Afferent loop syndrome, 482–483
Afferent nerves:
pain and, 968
sensory pathways, 1676
stimuli, 1–2
Afibrinogenemia, 113
AGM (see Stomach, mucosal lesions)
Air embolism, 684, 758
Airway maintenance, 196, 202
  (See also Tracheostomy)
  burns and, 259–260
  in children, 1515
  foreign bodies and, 627–628
AK (above-the-knee) amputations, 1886–1887
Alanine, 22, 28
Albers-Schönberg disease, 1751–1752
Albright's syndrome, 1749
Albumin, transfusion of, 123
Alcohol:

alimentation mixtures and, 34
anesthesia and, 203
as antiseptic, 190
gastrointestinal bleeding and, 993
Alcoholism:
cirrhosis and, 1197
Mallory-Weiss syndrome and, 1077
oral cancer and, 564
pancreatitis and, 1260, 1264
withdrawal symptoms, 4–5
Aldosterone, 1379–1380
trauma and, 8, 12–13, 15
Aldosteronism, 1395–1402
clinical manifestations and laboratory findings,
  941, 943, 1395–1397
diagnostic tests, 1397–1400
differential diagnosis, 1400–1401
historical background, 1375
pathology, 1395
primary, 942–943
  vs. secondary, 1395, 1398–1399
treatment, 1401–1402
Alimentation:
  (See also Nutrition)
  jejunostomy, 229
  parenteral, 32–34, 35, 91–95
  tube feeding, 89–90
Alkaline phosphatase, 1180, 1191, 1192
bone and, 1742–1743, 1759
in hyperparathyroidism, 1478
Alkalosis, 36–37
hypokalemic, 42
metabolic, 74–75
respiratory, 73–74
types of, 36, 71
Alkylating agents, 331
immunosuppression and, 377
Allergic reactions:
to ALG, 373
to insect bites, 214
to transfusion, 127
Alloantigens, 351–353
Allografts:
bone, 386
bone marrow, 388, 389
in burns, 267–268
cartilage, 386
clinical, 383–390
corneal, 385–386
endocrine, 390
gastrointestinal, 391
immunobiology of, 352–371
kidney, 404–430
liver, 393
lung, 403–404
macrophages and, 356
pancreaticoduodenal, 391
privileged sites for, 381–382
rejection, 354–364
splenic, 389
vascular, 384
Allopurinol, 334
Alpha receptors, 135, 149
Alveolar-arterial oxygen gradient, 465–466, 494,
  498
Alveolar carcinoma, 648
Alveolar ducts of breast, 529–530
Ambulation, 1962
Amebic abscesses of liver, 1186–1187
Amebiasis, 1120–1121
Ameboma, 1121
Ameloblastoma, mandibular, 580
Amenorrhea, 1602–1603
Amino acids:
collagen, 282
growth hormones and, 15
parathyroid hormone sequence of, 1463–1465
parenteral, 32, 33
starvation and, 22, 24
trauma and, 22, 28

Aminoaciduria, pancreatitis and, 1261
p-Aminobenzoic acid, 177
Aminocaproic acid, 115
Aminoglutethimide, 1386–1387
Aminoglycosides, 176
Aminopropionitrile, 284
Aminopterin, 377
Ammonia, 1203–1204
Ammonium, quaternary, 190
Amphotericin B, 177
Ampicillin, 175, 1095
Ampulla of Vater, 1244, 1248
avulsion of, 241
carcinoma, 1270–1271
Amputation, 1879–1892
above-the-knee, 1886–1887
below-the-knee, 1884–1886
  in tibioperoneal atherosclerosis, 853
carpometacarpal level, 1890–1891
conventional, 1881
elbow disarticulation, 1892
finger, 1889–1890, 1914–1917
foot, 1882–1883
  in Buerger's disease, 867
  in tibioperoneal atherosclerosis, 853
forearm, 1891–1892
hand, 1889–1891, 1913–1915
healing of, 1880
hemipelvectomy, 1888
hip disarticulation, 1887–1888
humerus, 1892
indications, 1879
ischemic limbs, 1879
knee disarticulation, 1886
leg, 1882–1888, 1978–1979
open (guillotine), 1881
osteomyoplastic, 1881
postoperative management, 1881–1882
preoperative management, 1880–1881
principles of technique, 1881
prognosis, morbidity, mortality, 1882
rehabilitation and, 1972–1975
site selection, 1879–1880
Syme, 1883–1884
toe, 1882
upper extremity, 1888–1892
for vascular disease, peripheral, 1881
wrist disarticulation, 1891
Amylase:
abdominal trauma and, 221
in intestinal obstruction, 984
pancreatic injury and, 238
in pancreatitis, 1262
Anabolic phase, 88
Anaerobic infections, 166, 179, 181
Analgesics, 1665
in osteoarthritis, 1862
Anaphylaxis, 5
Anaphylotoxin, 140
Anastomotic leak, gastrointestinal, 484
Andrews operation, 1355, 1357
Androgens, 13, 1379, 1595
excesses, 1392
in osteoporosis, 1764
trauma and, 17
Androstenedione, 13, 1595
Anemia:
in blind loop syndrome, 1102–1103
bone disease and, 1772
extracorporeal circulation and, 759
Fanconi's, 1293
gastrectomy and, 1065
gastrointestinal bleeding and, 994
hemolytic, 1284–1285, 1287–1289, 1772
  autoimmune, 1288–1289
Mediterranean, 1287
sickle cell, 1288
Anesthesia, 443–459
arrhythmias and, 470
barbiturate, 451–452

cardiac arrest and, 759
conduction, 454–458
cyclopropane, 446–448
in diabetes, 474
diethyl ether, 448–449
electrocautery and, 444
epidural, 457
epinephrine secretion and, 13
for fracture reductions, 1793–1794
general, 444–454
halothane (Fluothane), 449–450
hypoventilation following, 204
infiltration, 457–458
inhalation, 445–451
intravenous, 451–454
in kidney transplantation, 414
liver function and, 47–48
local, 457–458
methoxyflurane (Penthrane), 450
microcirculation and, 45
narcotics, 452–453
neck wounds and, 217
nerve block, 457–458
nitrous oxide, 445–446
in obstruction, intestinal, operation for, 987
17-OHCS and, 9, 10
in pheochromocytoma surgery, 1416–1417
premedication, 458–459
pulmonary function and, 46–47
relaxants, 453–454
risk, 443
shock and, 203
spinal, 454–457
stimuli from, 3
stomach and, full, 202–203
in thoracic surgery, 602
topical, 457, 458
trauma and, 202–204
vomiting and, 202–203
Aneurysms, 815–829, 887–901
abdominal aortic, 887–894
clinical manifestations, 887–889
prognosis, 891
ruptured, 891–894
treatment, 889–891
aortic, 815–829
(See also Aorta, aneurysms)
apoplexy (abdominal) and, 1331
bone cyst and, 1785–1786
carotid, 896–898
cerebral, 1660–1661
femoral, 896
peripheral, 894–901
popliteal, 894–895
renal artery, 898–900
sinus of Valsalva, 735–736
splenic artery, 898, 1293
subclavian, 898
traumatic, 900–901
ventricular, 799–801
visceral, 898–900
Angina, intestinal, 1327–1328
Angina pectoris, 750
in aortic stenosis, 776
coronary artery disease and, 794, 795
diagnosis of, 795
in mitral stenosis, 764
Angiocardiography in tetralogy of Fallot, 723
Angiography:
abdominal trauma and, 223
in arteriovenous fistula, 874
brain, 1632, 1648–1649, 1655
in Buerger's disease, 866
in cerebrovascular disease, 885
coronary, 795, 796
coronary bypass operation and, 797, 798
in embolism, arterial, 863
face and neck, 560
femoral, 895
hepatic, 1181, 1192

in occlusive disease, 845, 850, 851, 855, 856
parathyroid adenoma, 1482
popliteal, 896
pulmonary, 920
renal, 899, 949, 952–954, 1555
transplants and, 416, 418
thoracoabdominal aortic graft, 825
visceral, 1328, 1329
Angioma:
cardiac, 793
spinal, 1651
Angiomyoneuroma, 518–519
Angiosarcoma, 1786
Angiotensin, 1379, 1399
hypertension and, 940, 948
trauma and, 12
Anions, 66
Ankle, 1831–1833
(See also Foot)
anatomy, 1831
arthritis, 1857, 1868
injuries, 1831–1833
myelodysplasia and, 1703
Annuloplasty, mitral, 774
Annulus fibrosus, 1686
Anoplasty for imperforate anus, 1539
Anorexia, 974–975
Anoxia, 4
cardiac arrest and, 759, 760
diffusion, nitrous oxide and, 445–446
ischemic, 139
polycythemia and, 680
stagnant, 139, 141
in tetralogy of Fallot, 721–722
transposition of great vessels and, 728
Antacids, 1061, 1073
Anterior tibial compartment syndrome, 870–871
Antibiotics, 168–169, 170–178
agents, 172–178
(See also individual agents)
antifungal, 177
in arthritis, 1849
in burns, 263–265
cancer chemotherapy and, 330, 331
complications of, 171
extracorporeal circulation and, 755
in immunosuppression, 377–378
intraperitoneal, 172
modes of action, 170
in peritonitis, 1304
principles of therapy, 170–172
prophylactic, 171–172, 199
in regional enteritis, 1092
in renal failure, 1558
sulfonamides, 177–178
in tuberculous enteritis, 1094
in typhoid enteritis, 1095
in ulcerative colitis, 1114
in urinary tract infections, 1558
wound management and, 206–207
Antibody:
antiglomerular basement membrane
(anti-GBM), 422–423
antilymphocyte globulin and, 373
antisarcoma, 311–312
complement and, 364–365
cytophilic, 367–369
enhancement, 380–381
hemolytic anemia, 1288
humoral, 306–308, 310, 363–364
inhibition of, 379
(See also Immunosuppression)
production, 359, 360
rejection of allograft and, 363–364
specific, 362
structure of, 364
thyroid, 1436, 1443
transfusion purpura, 107–108
tumor, 311–312
Anticholinergics in peptic ulcer, 1061, 1062

Anticoagulants, 118–119
aortic stenosis operation and, 771
arterial embolism and, 859, 861
extracorporeal circulation and, 759
in mesenteric occlusion, 1330
tests for, 104
unsuspected therapy with, 30
for venous thrombosis, 918–919
Antidiuretic hormone, 5, 7, 14–15, 1367
ectopic secretion of, 1374
inappropriate secretion of, 14
peritonitis and, 1301
water and electrolyte metabolism and, 39–41
Antifungal antibiotics, 177
Antigens:
burns and, 256
carcinoembryonic, 309–310, 1141
fetal, 309–310
histocompatibility, 351–353, 380
HL-A, 338, 339, 352, 382
immunogens (see Immunogens)
inheritance of, 352–353
insufficient, 307
modulation, 307
tolerance to, 379–380
transfusion purpura, 107–108
transplantation, 351–353, 409
tumor-specific, 304–312
typing, 382–383
Antihemophilic concentrates, 123
Antihypertensive drugs:
dissecting aneurysm and, 828–829
renal hypertension surgery and, 956
Antilymphocyte globulin, 373–374
Antimetabolites, 331, 337
immunosuppression and, 376–377
Antisepsis, 172, 188–190
Antisera:
histocompatibility typing and, 382
lymphocyte, 373–374
rabies, 210
tumor, 339
Antithyroid drugs, 1440, 1441
Antivenin, 212–214
Antrectomy, 1065–1066
Antrum, pyloric, 1051
gastric secretion and, 1054
Anuria, 1557
renal transplantation and, 415–418
Anus, 1146–1160
abscess, 1152–1153
bleeding, 997
blood supply, 1146
carcinoma, 1159–1160
condyloma acuminatum, 1158
crypts, 1146
examination, 1147
fissure, 1151–1152
fistula, 1153–1155
hemorrhoids, 1149–1151
imperforate, 1531–1533
incontinence, 1155–1156
postoperative, 1149
melanoma, malignant, 1159–1160
neoplasma, 1159–1160
pain, 1149
postoperative care, 1148–1149
pruritus, 1149, 1158
sphincter, 977
stricture, postoperative, 1149
surgical principles, 1148–1149
valves, 1146
warts, 1158
Aorta:
abdominal, 887–894
bypass graft, 844, 846, 849
occlusive disease, 843–847
reconstruction, 844–847, 888, 893
thromboendarterectomy, 844, 845–846
aneurysms, 815–829, 887–894

abdominal, 887–894
ascending, 782, 815–816
coarctation and, 696
descending, 821–824
dissecting, 825–829
thoracic, 815–829
thoracoabdominal, 824–825
transverse, 817
traumatic, 817–821
balloon pumping and, 158, 809
bypass operation, 820–821
coarctation of, 696–701
(See also Coarctation of aorta)
"double-barreled," 827
mesenteric branches, 1320–1322
rupture of, 831
in tetralogy of Fallot, 721
transposition of, 727–730
corrected, 742–743
wounds of, 829–833
Aortic arch:
aneurysm, 817
double, 701–703
occlusive disease, 886–887
right, 701, 703
Aortic-pulmonary anastomosis, 724–726
Aortic-pulmonary window, 734–735
Aorticorenal bypass graft, 958
Aortic valve, 690–696, 768–784
insufficiency, 780–784
aneurysm of aorta and, 815, 818
clinical manifestations, 783
diagnosis, 783–784
etiology, 780
mitral insufficiency with, 787
mitral stenosis and, 787
pathology, 780–781
pathophysiology, 752, 781, 783
treatment, 784
stenosis, acquired, 768–780
clinical manifestations, 775–776
etiology, 775
historical data, 774–775
mitral stenosis with, 787
pathology, 775
pathophysiology, 752, 775
prognosis, 777, 779
treatment, 776–777
stenosis, congenital, 690–696
anatomy, pathologic, 690
clinical manifestations, 691
diagnosis, 691
historical data, 690
hypertrophic subaortic, 694–696
incidence and etiology, 690
laboratory findings, 691
pathophysiology, 690–691
postoperative course, 693
supravalvular, 693–694
treatment, 691–693
ventricular septal defect and, 712–713, 716, 717
Aortography, 697
aneurysms and, 817
abdominal, 888–889, 890
dissecting, 828, 830
sinus of Valsalva, 736
traumatic, 820
celiac artery compression, 1331
diverticulosis coli hemorrhage, 1122
patent ductus arteriosus, 719
pheochromocytoma, 1411
renal artery, 946–950, 952–954, 958
Aortoiliac disease, 843–847
clinical manifestations, 843–844
etiology and pathology, 843
laboratory studies, 844
historical data, 843
treatment, 844–847
Aortoiliac prosthesis, 893
Aortotomy:

in aortic stenosis, 692, 696, 778
in atherosclerosis, 845
in coronary bypass operation, 797
AP reactants, 24, 26, 28–29
Apnea:
alarm, 497
muscle relaxants and, 454
Apocrine glands, 514, 516
Apoplexy:
abdominal, 1331–1332
cerebrovascular, 1650
Appendectomy, 1172–1173, 1174
enteritis laparotomy and, 1094
Appendicitis, 1167–1175
clinical manifestations, 1168–1169
complications, 1170–1171
differential diagnosis, 1171–1172
in the elderly, 1174–1175
epiploic, 1172
etiology and pathogenesis, 1168
historical background, 1167–1168
incidence, 1168
in infants and children, 1173–1174
laboratory findings, 1169–1170
lymphadenitis vs., 1334
pain in, 1168–1169, 1170
prognosis, 1175
treatment, 1172–1173
Appendix, 1167–1176
abscess, 1170
adenocarcinoma, 1175–1176
carcinoids, 1097, 1175
inflammation of (see Appendicitis)
mucocele, 1176
rupture of, 1170–1171, 1302
tumors, 1175–1176
Appetite, loss of, 974–975
Arachnoiditis, spinal anesthesia and, 456–457
Areola, 528
Arm:
(See also Extremities, upper)
amputations, 1888–1892
pain, 1679–1682
paralysis, 1699–1700
prostheses, 1891, 1975
replantation, 387–388, 1892
Arrhenoblastomas, 1614
Arrhythmias, 469–472
aortic stenosis operation and, 771
coronary bypass operation and, 797
extracorporeal circulation and, 757
Arterial disease, 839–906
acrocyanosis, 903–904
aneurysms, 887–901
(See also Aneurysms)
anterior compartment syndrome, 870–871
atherosclerosis (see Atherosclerosis)
Buerger's disease, 863–867
erythromelalgia, 904
embolism, 857–862
(See also Embolism)
fistulas 871–875
congenital, 873–875
traumatic, 871–873
frostbite and, 904–906
livedo reticularis, 903
occlusive, cerebrovascular, 881–887
clinical manifestations, 883–884
diagnosis, 884
etiology and pathology, 881–883
historical considerations, 881
treatment, 884–887
occlusive, of lower extremity, 840–856
acute, 841–842
aortoiliac, 843–847
chronic, 842
clinical manifestations, 840–842
diabetic foot and, 854–856
femoropopliteal, 847–851
tibioperoneal, 851–854

Raynaud's disease, 901–903
thoracic outlet syndromes, 875–881
thrombosis, acute, 862–863
vasospastic, 901–904
Arteries:
(See also specific arteries)
abdominal wall, 1313
adrenal gland, 1376
brain, 1657
brainstem, 1632
breast, 528–529
bypass grafts (see Bypass procedures)
catheterization of, for gastrointestinal
bleeding, 995
chemotherapeutic perfusion through, 325–326
contusion of, 867–868
coronary (see Coronary artery disease)
cutaneous, 1917
diseases of (see Arterial disease)
embolus vs. thrombosis, 862
esophageal, 1011
gallblader, 1222
grafts, 384
implants, 798
infusion of, for head and neck tumors, 585
liver, 1178
of mesentery, 1320–1322
oxygen tension of, 465–466
pancreatic, 1255–1257
parathyroid, 1459, 1494
pelvis, female, 1591, 1592
perfusion therapy for melanoma, 524
pituitary, 1364
spasm, 870
of spleen, 1282, 1283
stomach, 1049
thyroid, 1430
tone regulation, 939–940
trauma, 867–873
aneurysms, 900–901
anterior compartment syndrome, 870–871
arteriovenous fistulas, 871–873
clinical manifestations, 868–869
in fractures, 1786–1787
pathology, 867–868
prognosis, 869
treatment, 869–870
immediate care of, 198
visceral grafts, 1328
Arterioarterial embolism, 861–862
Arteriography (see Angiography)
Arteriolar nephrosclerosis, 960, 962
Arterioles:
in livedo reticularis, 903
pulmonary, 679
in Raynaud's disease, 901
tone of, in shock, 135–136, 137
Arteriosclerosis:
abdominal apoplexy and, 1331–1332
nervous system and, 1657
renal, 946, 954
transplant of heart and, 402, 403
Arteriovenous admixture in shock, 143
Arteriovenous fistulas:
congenital, 873–875
dialysis and, 895–896
traumatic, 871–873
Arteriovenous malformations of cerebrum,
1661–1662
Arthralgia, hyperparathyroidism and, 1487
Arthritis, 1848–1850, 1852–1869
(See also Osteoarthritis)
gonococcal, 1559, 1852–1853
gouty, 1869–1870
hemophilic, 1871–1872
pyogenic (septic), 1848–1850
of hand, 1900, 1905
rehabilitation, 1972
rheumatoid, 1853–1860
clinical manifestations, 1853–1854

Felty's syndrome and, 1292
laboratory findings, 1854
management, 1855–1860
pathology, 1853
roentgenography, 1854–1855
Arthrodesis:
hip, 1731, 1863
knee, 1868
Arthrogryposis multiplex congenita, 1734–1735
Arthroplasty:
hallux valgus, 1868
hand, 1858–1859
hip, 1731, 1863–1864
Aryepiglottic folds, 559
Ascites, 1202
Ascorbic acid, wound healing and, 31
Asepsis, 188–190
Asherman's syndrome, 1594
Askanazy cells, 1443
Aspergillosis, 640
Asphyxia, traumatic, 662–663
Aspiration:
of gastric contents, 202–203
in pneumonia, 633–634
in tracheoesophageal fistula, 1516–1517
hepatic abscess, 1186
intestinal, for obstruction, 986–987, 988–989
pericardial, 789
of synovial fluid, 1847, 1849
Aspirin:
gastric ulcer and, 1070
gastrointestinal bleeding and, 993
Assisted circulation, 808–809
(See also Extracorporeal circulation)
Asthma, tracheal tumors vs., 658
Astrocytomas, 1646
Astrup technique, 72
Atarax, 458
Ataxia, 1695, 1707
cerebral palsy, 1700
Friedreich's, 1703
Atelectasis, 467–469
alkalosis and, 37
clinical manifestations, 468
etiology, 467–468
treatment, 468–469
Atherosclerosis, 793–799, 842–856
aortic aneurysm and, 821
aortoiliac, 843–847
carotid artery, 881–884
coronary artery, 793–799
(See also Coronary artery disease)
cerebrovascular disease and, 881–887
emboli and, 858, 861–862
femoropopliteal, 848–851
lower extremity, 842–856
mesenteric artery, 1360
splenic artery, 898
subclavian artery, 883, 884–886
tibioperoneal, 851–854
vertebral artery, 883, 884–886
visceral artery, 1327
Athetosis in cerebral palsy, 1692
ATP (see Adenosine triphosphate)
Atrial fibrillation, 763, 857
Atrial flutter, postoperative, 471
Atrial septal defects, 704–712
atrioventricular canal, 712
pulmonary vein drainage anomalies, 706–709
ostium primum defect, 709–712
secundum defects, 704–706
transposition of great vessels and, 729
in tricuspid atresia, 730
Atriotomy, mitral stenosis and, 767–770
Atrioventricular block, postoperative, 471–472
Atrioventricular canal, persistent, 712
Atrioventricular dissociation, 804
Atrioventricular node, 803
rhythm, postoperative, 471
Atrium:

enlargement of: in mitral insufficiency, 772
in mitral stenosis, 765
fibrillation, 763, 857
lung transplants and, 402–404
pressure, in mitral stenosis, 763
Atropine, 458–459
Auscultation, 751
(See also Heart sounds)
in arterial occlusion, 841
intestinal obstruction and, 984
Autoclaves, 189
Autografts:
bone, 386
bone marrow, 388–389
in burns, 268
cartilage, 386
endocrine, 389–390
extremity, 387–388
fascial, 385
lung, 402–403
nerve, 385
skin, 1923
vascular, 384
vein, 384
Autoimmune hemolytic anemia, 1288–1289
Autoimmunity:
Hashimoto's disease and, 1443
ulcerative colitis and, 1090–1091
Autonomic nervous system, pain and, 968
Autoregulation, 1658
Axillary nerve injury, 1977
Axillary nodes, 523, 529, 535
Axonotmesis, 1795
Axons, pain and, 1665
Azathioprine, 376
in cardiac transplantation, 401
in colitis, 1117
kidney transplants and, 425
in regional enteritis, 1092
Azotemia:
bleeding and, gastrointestinal, 991
renal artery reconstruction and, 959
in renal failure, 1565
Azulfidine, 1114

B cells, 354, 357, 358
Bacilli, gram-negative, 185–187
Bacitracin, 175
Back pain, 1682–1692
etiologic factors, 1682, 1683
examination, 1683–1684
history, 1683
in osteoporosis, 1763
posttraumatic, 1975–1976
treatment, 1684, 1685, 1688–1689, 1692
Bacteremia, 170, 1558
peritonitis and, 1301
Bacteria:
(See also specific genera)
aerobic, 166, 178, 180
anaerobic, 166, 179, 181
antibiotics for, 174–177
in arthritis, 1841
in burns, 255, 263–265
in cholecystitis, 1236, 1239
in empyema, 615
in hand infection, 1898, 1900
hepatic abscesses and, 1184
indigenous, 166
in intracranial infections, 1662
pathogenic, 167
in peritonitis, 1298, 1300
in prostatitis, 1560
in pulmonary infection, 631
strangulated obstruction and, 982
in subdural empyema, 1663
toxins of, 167
traumatic wounds and, 206
in ulcerative colitis, 1110

in urinary tract infections, 1558
wound infection, 462, 463
Bacterial endocarditis (see Endocarditis, bacterial)
Bacterial shock, gram-negative, 140–144, 157–158
Bactericides, 170, 190
Bacteriophage, allograft immunity and, 356
Bacteriostats, 170
Bacteroides, 157, 186–187, 1184
Bakes dilator, 1243, 1244, 1248
Balloon:
in esophageal physiology tests, 1012
pumping, intraaortic, 809
septostomy, 729
support for circulation, 158
tamponade, 995, 1200
Ball-valve prostheses, 777, 778, 780, 781
mitral, 768
tricuspid, 785
Banking:
blood, 35, 121, 1931, 1933
skin, 1931, 1933
Barbiturates, 451–452, 458
Barium:
in abdominal trauma, 221
in diverticulitis, 1123–1124
in intussusception reduction, 1531
in ischemic colitis, 1119
in obstruction, intestinal, 985
in peptic ulcer, 1059
peritonitis from, 1309
in pneumatosis cystoides intestinalis, 1104
in regional enteritis, 1091–1092
in retroperitoneal tumor, 1340, 1342
in ulcerative colitis, 1114
Baroreceptors, 134, 141, 963
Barr body, 1596
Barrett esophagus, 1038–1039
Bartholin's glands, 1590, 1618
Basal cell carcinoma, 520
lip, 563
vulvar, 1618
Basal metabolic rate, 1436
Base, 70–75
Basilar arteries, 1632
Basilar impression, 1670
Bassini herniorrhaphy, 1355, 1356
BCG in immunotherapy, 340–341
Bee stings, 214
Belching, 1077
Bell's palsy, 1957–1959, 1976
Belsey hiatal hernia repair, 1024, 1028
Bence Jones protein, 1771
Bennett's fracture, 1818
Bentley bubble oxygenator, 754
Benzalkonium chloride, 190
Benzpyrene, 305
Beta-blocking agents, 152
Beta receptors, 134
Betel, 564
Bezoars, 1078
Bicarbonate, 70–74
Bicipital tendonitis, 1875
Bile, 997–1001
composition, 1228
ducts (see Biliary tract; Choledochus)
excretion, 1000–1001, 1228
intraperitoneal, trauma and, 1231–1232
metabolism, 997, 1000
peritonitis, 1308
stasis, 1234
Biliary tract, 1177
atresia, congenital, 1224–1228
clinical manifestations, 1225
differential diagnosis, 1226–1227
incidence, 1224
laboratory studies, 1225–1226
pathology, 1224–1225
treatment, 1227–1228

bleeding into, 1182
bleeding of, 235–236
carcinoma, 1245–1246
cholangiography, 1245
cystic disease, 1224
duct system, 1221
dyskinesia, 1229
extrahepatic, 235–237, 1221–1223
infection, 1240–1243
injury, 235–237, 1232–1233
operations, 1246–1250
    cholecystectomy, 1246–1248
    common bile duct, 1248–1250
    pancreatic pressure relationships with, 1259
roentgenography, 1229–1230
Bilirubin, 997–1001, 1228
hemolysis and, 1226
serum, 1003
Bilirubinuria, 1003
Biliverdin, 1000
Billroth II procedure, 1064–1066
Biological determinism, 541–542
Biopsy:
breast, 538, 542
cancer, 318–320
cervical, 1603
excisional, 319
gastric ulcer, 1076
of head and neck lesions, 560
incisional, 319
for infections, 168
liver, 1004, 1180
lung, 649–651
needle, 319, 1180
renal, 956
    transplantation and, 420
Birchall test, 954
Birth control pills, coagulation and, 29
Bites, 207–216
insect, 214–215
Portuguese man-of-war, 215
rabies and, 207–211
snake, 211–214
spider, 215–216
stingray, 214–215
BK (below-the-knee) amputations, 853,
    1884–1886
Black widow spider, 215
Bladder, urinary (see Urinary bladder)
Blalock-Hanlon technique, 729
Blalock procedure, 725
Blalock-Taussig procedure, 721
Blastomycosis, 188, 640
Blebs, pulmonary, 625–627
Bleeders, evaluation of, 105–107, 756
Bleeding (see Hemorrhage)
Bleeding time, 102
Blind loop syndrome, 482–483, 1065, 1102–1103
Blocking factors, lymphocyte, 311–312
Blood:
banked, 35, 121
coagulation, 29–31, 99–105
    (See also Coagulation)
component therapy, 34–36
factors (see under Factor)
flow (see Hemostasis)
intraoperative replacement of loss, 82
mixed venous unsaturation, 495–503
in pleural cavity, 614
in stool, 1133, 1141
sugar levels, 94, 473
transfusion (see Transfusion)
in urine (see Hematuria)
volume, 123–124
    (See also Transfusion)
    shock and, 135, 147
Blood-gas exchange, 465
Blood-gas studies, 498
in heart disease, congenital, 684
in peritonitis, 1304

pulmonary embolism and, 920
Blood groups:
gastric juice contents and, 1053
renal transplantation and, 409
typing and cross matching, 121–122
Blood pressure:
(See also Hypertension; Hypotension)
abdominal trauma and, 221
arteriovenous fistula and, 861
cyclopropane anesthesia and, 447
Blood urea nitrogen (BUN), 27, 94–95
extracorporeal circulation and, 758
gastrointestinal bleeding and, 991, 994
Blood vessels:
(See also Arteries; Veins; and specific vessels)
cancer spread by, 315, 323
grafts, 384–385
    (See also Bypass procedures)
injuries: cervical, 217–218
    in fractures, 1794–1795
    thoracic inlet, 218–219
response to injury, 98
tumors: of bone, 1785–1786
    of skin, 518–519
"Blue toe" syndrome, 861
Blunt trauma, 220–223
aortic injury in, 829–833
biliary tree, 237
liver injury and, 1181, 1183
of spleen, 1285
unapparent injury and, 198–199
Bochdalek, foramen of, 1040–1041
Body fluids (see Electrolytes; Fluids and
    electrolytes)
Boeck's sarcoidosis, 640–641
Boerhave's syndrome, 1077
Böhler's angle, 1834
Boil, 169
of hand, 1905
Bone, 1741–1772
achondroplasia, 1747–1748
aclasia, metaphyseal, 1748–1749
in acromegaly, 1765
anemia and, 1772
aplasia and dysplasia, congenital, 1738–1739
brittle, 1750–1751
calcification, 1754–1755
calcitonin and, 1753
calcium metabolism and, 1752–1753
cells, 1741
chondroblastoma, 1779
chondroma, 1778–1779
chondrosarcoma, 1780
citrate in, 1742
classification of disorders, 1745–1746
in clubfoot, 1733
collagen, 1754
crystal, 1742
cysts, 1762, 1783–1784, 1785–1786
    hyperparathyroidism and, 1470–1471
densitometry, 1479
developmental disorders, 1747–1752
differential diagnosis of diseases producing
    changes in, 1488
in dwarfism, 1764
dyschondroplasia, 1748
enchondromas, multiple, 1748
enzymes, 1743–1744
epiphysis (see Epiphysis)
Ewing's tumor, 1784–1785
facial, 1633–1634, 1936–1938
fat embolism and, 475
fibroma, 1780
fibrosarcoma, 1781–1782, 1784
fibrous dysplasia, 1749
giant cell tumors, 1782–1783
in gigantism, 1764–1765
grafts, 386–387
    facial contour and, 195
granulomatosis and, 1769–1770

healing, 1796–1797
    vertebral, 1642
hematopoietic system and, 1771–1772
in hip dislocation, congenital, 1726
in Hodgkin's disease, 1768–1769
in hyperparathyroidism, 1470–1471,
    1474–1475, 1479, 1491
hypophosphatasia, 1759
injury, 1795–1797
    (See also Fractures)
in Letterer-Siwe disease, 1770–1771
leukemia and, 1771
losses, head and neck tumors and, 1946
marble, 1751–1752
metabolic diseases, 1752–1766
metastatic tumors, 1788–1790
microradiograph of cross section, 1462
Milkman's syndrome, 1760
mineralization, 1754–1755
mucopolysaccharidoses, 1765–1766
myeloma and, 1771–1772
ossification, 1743–1744
osteitis deformans, 1766–1768
osteogenesis imperfecta, 1750–1751
osteoma, 1776–1777
osteomalacia, 1759–1760
osteopetrosis, 1751–1752
osteopoikilosis, 1752
osteoporosis, 1761–1764
osteosarcoma, 1777–1778
pain, 1677
parathyroid and, 1461–1463, 1470–1471, 1474,
    1753
    osteodystrophy, 1760–1761
phosphorus metabolism and, 1737–1738
pituitary and, 1764–1765
radiography, 1480–1483, 1744–1746
remodeling, 1744
renal transplants and, 426
reticuloses, 1768–1771
reticulum cell sarcoma, 1784, 1785
rickets, 1755–1759
scurvy, 1755
spondylosis, 1674
spotted, 1752
stabilization in poliomyelitis, 1698
thyroid and, 1765
tuberculosis, 1850–1851
tumors, 1775–1785
    biologic properties, 1775–1776
    classification, 1776
    nonosteogenic, 1783–1785
    true, 1776–1785
vitamin D and, 1754, 1755–1756, 1758–1759
water of, 1742
Bone marrow:
anemia and, 1772
Hodgkin's disease and, 1768–1769
multiple myeloma and, 1771
myeloid metaplasia, 1290–1291
reticuloses, 1768–1771
transplant, 388–389
Bougienage, esophageal, 1026
Boutonniere deformity, 1911–1912
Braces, 1970, 1979
in cerebral palsy, 1701
for femoral fracture, 1824–1825
for hemophilic arthritis, 1872, 1873
for scoliosis, 1711
Brachialgia, 1679–1680
Bradycardia, 759–760, 804
Brain, 1631–1633, 1646–1649
abscess, 722, 1663–1664
blood supply, 1657
cardiac arrest and, 760
cyanosis and, 681
death, criteria for, 411–412
edema, 1647
hematoma, 1638–1641
    epidural, 1639–1640

intracerebral, 1640–1641, 1661
  subdural, 1638–1639
hormone secretion and, 5–6
hypoxia and, 494
infections, 1662–1664
injuries, 1634–1635
ischemia, 1659–1660
pain pathways, 967–968
reticular formation, 1631–1632
tumors, 1646–1649
  classification, 1646
  clinical manifestations, 1647
  diagnostic studies, 1648–1649
  evaluation, 1647–1648
  pathophysiology, 1646–1647
  treatment, 1649
Brainstem, 1631–1632, 1646–1647
Branchial anomalies, 1853–1954
Breast, 527–551
  abscess, 551
  adolescent, 528, 531
  alveolae, 529–530
  anatomy and development, 528–531
  areola and nipple, 528
  benign neoplasms, 533, 537–538
  blood supply, 528–529
  cancer, 533–550
    adrenalectomy for, 550, 1394
    biopsy, 538–539, 542
    castration in, 549–550
    chemotherapy for, 337, 550
    classification, 545, 549
    colloid, 540
    death rate, 298
    diagnosis and staging, 536
    differential diagnosis, 537–538
    etiology, 533–535
    histopathology, 539–541
    history, natural, 535–536
    hormones and, 550
    hypophysectomy in, 1373
    incidence, 533
    lobular, mammary, 540
    mammary duct, 539, 540
    medullary, 540
    oophorectomy in, 549–550
    Paget's disease, 539
    papillary, 540
    prognosis, 535–536, 545–549
    radiation therapy, 544, 547–548
    radical mastectomy for, 541–544, 546–547,
      549
    recurrent, 549–550
    sarcoma, 540–541
    simple mastectomy, 544, 547–549
    treatment, 541–545, 549–550
  cyclic changes, 530
  cysts, 537–538
  embryology, 527–528
  examination, 531–533
  fat necrosis, 538
  fibroadenoma, 538
  glandular tissue, 528
  histology, 529–530
  infections, 551
  lactation, 530–531, 551
  lymphatics, 529, 535
  myoblastoma, granular cell, 538
  papilloma, ductal, 538
  plastic surgery, 1952–1955
  in pregnancy, 530–531
  radiography, 532
  sclerosing adenosis, 538
  supernumerary structures, 527, 528
  thermography, 532–533
  thrombophlebitis of, 538
  tuberculosis, 551
Brenner tumor, 1613
Brevicollis, 1728
5-Bromodeoxyuridine, 377

Bromsulphalein test, 994, 1180, 1192, 1200
Bronchi:
  carcinoid of, 642–644
  carcinoma of, 645–649
  foreign bodies in, 627–628
  lymph node erosion into, 634
  mucoid impaction of, 634
  obstruction of, atelectasis and, 467–468
  ruptured, 197, 628
  tumors of, 641–649
Bronchiectasis, 628–630
  bronchiectasia vs., 628
  clinical manifestations, 629
  diagnosis, 629–630
  etiology, 629
  treatment, 630
Bronchoesophageal fistula, 635
Bronchogenic carcinoma, 645–649
Bronchogenic cysts, 665, 666–667
Broncholith, 634
Bronchopleural fistula, 616, 618–619
Bronchoscopy, 601–602, 644
  in burns, 268
Bronchospasm in burns, 269
Bronchospirometry, 600
Bronchotomy, transthoracic, 655
Brooke formula, 262
Bruit:
  in arteriovenous fistula, 872–873
  in thoracic outlet syndrome, 877
Brunner glands, 1051
BSP (see Bromsulphalein test)
Buccal mucosa:
  examination of, 557
  hyperplasia of, 564–565
  tumors, 570–571
Budd-Chiari syndrome, 1197, 1207
Buerger's disease, 863–867
  diagnosis, 865
  historical data, 863
  incidence and etiology, 863–864
  pathology, 864–865
  prognosis, 867
  treatment, 865–867
Buffers, 70
  in shock, 158
Bullae, emphysematous, 625–627
BUN (see Blood urea nitrogen)
Bundle of His, 803
Bunion, 1868–1869
Burkitt's lymphoma, 585
Burns, 253–270
  acidosis in, 38–39
  cardiovascular effects, 44, 256–258
  classification of, 254
  complications, 268–269
  contracture following, 276
  corticosteroids and, 12, 15
  depth of skin destruction, 254–255
  gastrointestinal changes, 258–259, 269
  gastric erosion and, 992–993
  hand, 270
  head, 269–270
  heat transfer and, 253–254
  host defense alterations and, 256
  hypertension in children and, 269
  local results of, 255–256
  nitrogen loss in, 20
  pulmonary function and, 258, 259, 265, 268–269
  renal response, 258
  Rule of Nines, 260, 262
  systemic changes, 256–259
  therapy, 259–268
    airway maintenance, 259–260
    antibacterial, 263–265
    grafting, skin, 267–268, 383–384
    resuscitation, intravenous, 260–263
    sedation, 259
    tetanus prophylaxis, 263
    wound care, 265–267

Bursa of Fabricius, 353
Bypass procedures:
  aortic, 820–821, 825
    abdominal aorta, 844, 846, 849
    aorticorenal, 958
  cardiopulmonary (see Extracorporeal
    circulation)
  for coronary artery disease, 794, 795–798
  femoropopliteal, 849–851, 853
  left heart, 809
  peripheral, 809
  renal artery, 957–958
  small intestine, 1092–1093, 1103, 1105
  visceral arterial, 1328

Calcaneonavicular ligament, 1714
Calcaneus:
  deformity, 1699
  fractures of, 1835
Calcification, 1744, 1754–1755
  aortic valve, 690–691, 777, 779
  bronchial masses, 634
  of cartilage, 1871
  in hyperparathyroidism, 1473
  intracranial, 1640
  of kidney, 1476
  ossification vs. 1745
  pancreatic, 1263
  of pleura, 620–621
  of supraspinatus tendon, 1874–1875
Calcitonin, 1464, 1753
Calcium, 76–77
  bone metabolism and, 1752–1753
  cardiac arrest and, 761
  crystal deposition, 1870–1871
  in gallstones, 1233
  gastrectomy and, 1065
  homeostasis, serum, 1464–1465
  in hyperparathyroidism, 1471, 1477, 1479,
    1480, 1490, 1498
  infusion test, 1479, 1480
  parathyroid and, 1459, 1464–1465, 1472–1474,
    1477–1479
  parenteral administration of, 94
  peptic ulcer and, 1475
  renal damage and, 1471, 1472, 1565–1566
  transplanted kidney and, 425–426
  urinary calculi and, 1561
Calculi:
  gallbladder (see Gallstones)
  urinary, 1561–1564
    composition, 1561–1562
    diagnosis, 1562–1563
    treatment, 1563–1564
Calf vein thrombosis, 915
Calmette-Guérin bacillus vaccine,
    immunotherapy with, 340–341
Caloric requirements, 88
Calories, basal, for weights, 1514
Cancer, 297–343
  (See also Carcinoma; Sarcoma; and specific
    sites involved)
  biochemical changes in, 303
  biopsy for, 318–320
  breast, 533–550
  carcinogens, 300–301
  cell biology, 303–313
  clinical manifestations of, 316–317
  diagnosis, 317–320
  epidemiology, 297–300
  epithelization and, 278–280
  etiology, 300–302
  examination for, 317–318
  gastric, 1078–1082
  geographic factors, 302
  growth rate, 303–304
  hereditary factors, 301–302
  hypopharynx, 576
  immune competence of patients, 310–311

immunobiology of, 304–313
laryngeal, 573–576
lip, 562, 563–564
lung, 645–649
lymphatic extension of, 314–315
metastases, 314–315
    prevention of implantation, 322, 323
    resection of, 325
    routes of, 314–315
    signs of, 316–317
oropharynx, 571–572
prognosis, 342–343
psychologic management of, 343, 480
recurrent, 325
routes for spread of, 314
seeding of cells, 323
sex differences in death rate, 299
smoking and, 302
staging extent of, 320
systemic manifestations of, 316–317, 318
therapy, 321–342
    biologic and pharmacologic factors in,
        331–332
    chemotherapy, 330–337
    choice of, 321
    goals of, 321
    immunotherapy, 337–342
    palliative, 326, 329
    prevention of implantation, 322, 323
    radiation, 326–330
    recurrent cancer, 325
    surgical, 322–326
    types of operations, 323–325
transplants of kidney and, 423–424
vascular spread of, 315
warning signals, 316
Candida albicans:
    shock and, 144
    vaginitis, 1599
Candidiasis, 188
    antibiotics for, 177
Cannulae:
    coronary artery, 779
    radial artery, 499–500
    in shock, 149
Capillaries:
    hemangioma, 518, 566–567
    lymphatic, 931
    oxygen content of pulmonary, 465
    oxygen transport and, 495
    shock and, 135
    skin, 514
Capitellum, fracture of, 1805
Carbenicillin, 175
Carbenoxolone sodium, 1073
Carbohydrate:
    fuel reserves, 86, 87
    liver and, 1179
    trauma and, 24, 26–27, 200
Carbon dioxide insufflation in
    pheochromocytoma, 1411
Carbon dioxide tension:
    acid-base balance and, 37, 39, 72–74
    cerebral flow and, 1658
    extracorporeal circulation and, 754
    head injury and, 1637
    monitoring of, 499
Carbonic acid, 70–71
Carbuncle, 169
    of hand, 1905
Carcinoembryonic antigens, 309–310, 1141
Carcinogens, 300–301, 305–306
    chemical, 300–301
    physical, 301
    tumor-specific antigens and, 305–306
    viral, 301, 305–306
Carcinoids, 1097–1100
    appendiceal, 1175
    bronchial, 642–644
    clinical manifestations, 1098–1099

colorectal, 1141
    diagnosis, 1099–1100
    malignant, 1098
    treatment, 1097–1098, 1100
Carcinoma:
    (*See also* Cancer)
    adrenocortical, 1392–1393
    appendiceal, 1175–1176
    basal cell (*see* Basal cell carcinoma)
    biliary tract, 1245–1246
    bladder, 1572–1574
    bone metastases, 1788–1790
    bronchogenic, 645–649
    cervical, 1602, 1611–1615
    coagulation and disseminated, 30
    colonic, 1113–1114, 1131–1141
    esophageal, 1032–1037
    gallbladder, 1244–1246
    grading of, 314
    liver, 1190–1192
    nasopharyngeal, 577–578
    omental, 1318
    oral, 564, 568–571
    ovarian, 1620–1621, 1622
    pancreatic, 1270–1274
    parathyroid, 1467–1468
    polypoid lesions and, 1129–1131
    prostate, 1550, 1577–1579
    rectal, 1131–1141
    renal, 1570–1572
    in situ, 314
    skin, 519–521
    squamous (*see* Squamous cell carcinoma)
    thyroid, 1448, 1449–1453
    verrucous, 570, 572
Cardia, 1009
Cardiac arrest, 759–762
    acidosis in, 38
    defibrillation for, 761–762
    diagnosis, 760
    drugs and fluids for, 761
    etiology, 759–760
    historical data, 759
    massage for, 760–761
    pathogenesis, 759–760
    prognosis, 762
    treatment, 760–762
    ventilation and, 760
Cardiac glands, 1051
Cardiac massage, 760–761
Cardiac output:
    anesthesia and, 448
    determinations, 494–495, 503–508
    extracorporeal circulation and, 756–757
    mitral stenosis and, 763
    nomogram for, 504
Cardiac tamponade, 197
Cardiac transplantation (*see* Transplantation,
    heart)
Cardinal ligaments, 1590, 1591
Cardioarterial embolism, 857–861
Cardiogenic shock, 144–145, 156, 157
Cardiomyotomy, 1016
Cardiopulmonary bypass (*see* Extracorporeal
    circulation)
Cardiopulmonary measurement cart, 499
Cardiospasm (*see* Achalasia)
Cardiovascular system:
    (*See also* Arteries; Heart; Veins)
    burns and, 256–258
    hyperkalemia symptoms, 75
    hypothyroidism and, 1442
    monitoring, 499–508
    peritonitis and, 1301–1302
    postoperative complications, 469–473
    rehabilitation, 1980
    trauma and, 44–45
    thyrotoxicosis and, 1438
Carotid arteries:
    aneurysms, 896–898, 1661

arteriography, 1648
    brain and, 1657
    endarterectomy, 884, 886
    injuries of, 217–218, 219
    occlusive disease, 881–884
Carotid body tumors, 585
Carotid sinus nerve, 963
Carpal tunnel syndrome, 1859
Carpometacarpal amputations, 1890–1891
Cartilage:
    articular, 1845–1846, 1853
    calcification of, 1871
    costal, 605, 606
    endochondroma, 1779
    knee, 1827–1828
    matrix, 1846
    in nasal plastic surgery, 1924
    pleomorphism in chondrosarcoma, 1781
    transplantation, 386–387
Cascade systems, 364–371
Cast(s), 1800–1801
    brace treatment for femoral fracture,
        1824–1825
    for tarsal navicular epiphysitis, 1721
Castration in breast cancer, 549–550
Catabolic phase, 87–88
Catabolism, trauma and, 200
Catecholamines, 1404–1407
    cyclopropane anesthesia and, 447
    hypertension and, 942
    shock and, 141, 145
    trauma and, 26, 27
Catheter(s):
    alimentation, 92–93
    monitoring, 500–502
    Swan-Ganz, for fluid therapy in shock, 149,
        150
Catheterization:
    in aldosteronism, 1399
    arterial, for gastrointestinal bleeding, 995
    cardiac, 683, 752
        in aortic insufficiency, 783
        in aortic stenosis, 691, 776
        in atrial septal defects, 705
        cardiac arrest and, 760
        in Ebstein's anomaly, 739
        in mitral insufficiency, 773
        in mitral stenosis, 766
        in pericarditis, 802
        in tetralogy of Fallot, 723
        in transposition of great vessels, 729
        in tricuspid atresia, 732
        in tricuspid stenosis and insufficiency, 785
        in ventricular septal defect, 714
    central venous system, 500
    flow-guided, 501–503
    hepatic venule, 1197–1198
    renal arterial, 953
    urinary bladder, 1553, 1557
Cations, 66
Causalgia, 1977
Cautery, 120
Cavernous hemangioma, 518
Cavernous sinus, 1657
Cecostomy:
    complications, 486
    for obstruction, 988
Cecum:
    actinomycosis, 1121
    diverticulitis, 1125–1126
    herniated, 1355
    rotation of, incomplete, 1525
    wounds of, 232
Celiac artery:
    anastomosis in liver transplant, 396
    occlusion, 1330
    stenosis, 1328
Celiac ganglionectomy, 970
Celiac rickets, 1757
Cells:

B, 354, 357, 358
cancer, biology of, 303–313
division, healing and, 279
drug action and life cycle of, 332
efferent pathways of, 366–369
hypoxia and, 496
Kultschitzsky, 1097, 1098
log-, kill hypothesis, 332
lysis of target, 361–362
membrane, mosaic model of, 352
metabolism, 137–138
oxygen transport and, 495–496
pituitary, 1364–1365
population growth, 332
T, 354, 357, 358
Cellular immune response, 306, 310
development of, 353
transplant rejection and, 357–358
Cellulitis, 169
clostradial, 182
of hand, 1904
lymphedema and, 933
Central nervous system:
extracorporeal circulation and, 758–759
infections, 1662–1664
injuries, 4, 1633–1643
pain pathways, 968
response to trauma, 5–7
section of, for pain relief, 1667–1668
thyroid function and, 1433
tumors, 1647
Central venous pressure:
fluid therapy and, 149, 986
monitoring, 500–501
Cephalic tetanus, 184
Cephalic vein, radial artery anastomosis with, 407, 410
Cephalin flocculation test, 1179
Cephalometric speech studies, 1952
Cephaloridine, 174
Cephalosporins, 173
Cephalothin, 174
Cerebellar ataxia, 1703
Cerebellar tonsils, 1632
Cerebellum, hemorrhage of, 1660
Cerebral arteries:
aneurysms, 1660–1661
occlusion, 1659
Cerebral palsy, 1700–1702
clinical manifestations, 1700–1701
etiology, 1700
incidence, 1700
treatment, 1701–1702
Cerebrospinal fluid:
brain tumors and, 1647
head injury convalescence and, 1641
hydrocephalus and, 1654–1656
Cerebrovascular disease, 881–887, 1657, 1658
carotid artery occlusion and, 881–884
orthopedic management, 1704–1705
Cerebrum:
aneurysms of, 1660–1661
angiography, 1648–1649
circulation, 1657–1658
craniosynostosis and, 1656
edema, 1637
hematomas, 1640–1641, 1661
hemorrhage, 1660
ischemia and infarction, 1659–1660
pain pathways in, 968
Cerumen, 534
Cervical blood vessels, injuries of, 217–218
Cervical disc disease, 1672, 1680–1682
clinical manifestations, 1680–1681
etiology, 1681–1682
treatment, 1682
Cervical fractures and dislocations, 1839–1840
Cervical lymph nodes, 584
Cervical mediastinotomy, 1031
Cervical myelopathy, 1681

Cervical rib syndrome, 876
Cervicitis, chronic, 1611
Cervicodorsal sympathectomy, 902–903
Cervicofacial nodes, 523
Cervix, 1590, 1610–1615
anaplasia, 1611–1612
biopsy, 1611
carcinoma, 1602, 1611–1615
diagnosis, 1611
in situ, 1612
invasive, 1612–1613
staging, 1613
therapy, 1612–1615
dilatation and curettage, 1623–1624
eversion, 1611
examination, 1597–1598
polyps, 1610–1611
Chagas' disease, 1145
Chancroid, 1608
Charcot joints, 1873–1874
Charcot-Marie-Tooth muscular atrophy, 1703
Chardack-Greatbatch pacemaker, 806
Charnley-Muller prosthesis, 1866
Charnley prosthesis, 1866
Chemical agents for hemostasis, 120–121
Chemical composition of body fluids, 66
Chemical peritonitis, 1308
Chemodectomas, 585
Chemoprophylaxis, 171–172
Chemotactic factor, 362, 367
Chemotherapy:
(See also Antibiotics)
in aldosteronism, 1401
for cancer, 330–337
as adjuvant to surgery, 329, 330, 333–334
arterial or isolated perfusion, 325–326
biologic and pharmacologic factors, 331–332
of breast, 550
clinical pharmacology, 334–335
guidelines, 335–336
hepatic, 1192
mechanisms of action, 330–331
responsive neoplasms, 336–337
scheduling and combination therapy, 332–333
cholangitis, 1243
in colorectal cancer, 1137–1138, 1140
diarrhea and, 978–979
for head and neck tumors, 585
for hypoparathyroidism, 1456
for melanoma, 524
for prostatic tumors, 1576, 1578
for testicular tumors, 1579
for thyrotoxicosis, 1440, 1441
for tuberculosis, 636–637
Chest:
flail, 197
injuries, 197–198
pain in heart disease, 750
Chest wall, 602–609
abscesses, 606
chondroma, 607
chondrosarcoma, 608
congenital defects, 602
empyema and, 616
Ewing's sarcoma, 608–609
fibrous dysplasia, 607
fractures, rib, 604–605
granuloma, eosinophilic, 607–608
hernias, 604
infection and inflammation, 605–606
metastases, solitary bone, 609
multiple myeloma, 609
osteochondroma, 607
osteogenic sarcoma, 608
osteomyelitis, 605–606
pain, 1684
pectus carinatum, 604
pectus excavatum, 602–604
radiation necrosis, 609

stability, 597
Tietze's syndrome, 606
trauma, 604
tumors, 606–609
Chiari-Frommel syndrome, 1602
Chiari malformation, hydrocephalus and, 1655
Children:
(See also Pediatric surgery)
appendicitis in, 1173–1174
bone disorders in, 1747–1752
cleft lip and palate, 1947–1950
fractures in, 1799
clavicle, 1802–1803
femoral neck, 1821
forearm shaft, 1813–1814
humeral epicondyles, 1810–1811
radial neck, 1808–1809
hand anomalies in, 1895–1896
heart disease in, 677–743
Hirschsprung's disease in, 1145
hydrocephalus in, 1654–1656
hyperparathyroidism in, 1483–1484
hypertension from burns in, 269
lymphadenitis in, 1332–1334
mucoviscidosis in, 634
neck tumors in, 585
neuroblastoma in, 1417, 1419
neurologic malformations in, 1651–1657
peritonitis in, 1298
pheochromocytoma in, 1415
renal transplantation in, 429–430
synovitis, acute, 1873
trachea in, 658
Chlorambucil, 1620
Chloramphenicol, 173, 175–176
in immunosuppression, 378
in regional enteritis, 1095
Chloride, plasma, in hyperparathyroidism, 1478
Chloroquine, 1187
Chlorothiazide, 1202
Chlorpromazine, 150, 151
Cholangiography:
operative, 1230
percutaneous transhepatic, 1003, 1245, 1272
Cholangiojejunostomy, 1227
Cholangiomanometry, 1230–1231
Cholangitis, 1240–1243
acute suppurative, 1241
hepatitis and, 1241–1242
primary sclerosing, 1242–1243
recurrent pyogenic, 1241
Cholecystectomy, 1224
bile duct injury in, 1232
for cholecystitis, 1238, 1239
endocrine response to, 11, 12
for gallstones, 1235, 1236
hormone levels in, 11, 16
postoperative symptoms, 1239–1240
technique, 1246–1248
Cholecystitis, 1236–1240
acalculous, 1240
acute, 1237–1239
chronic, 1239–1240
emphysematous, 1238–1239
Cholecystography, 1229–1230
Cholecystojejunostomy, 1227, 1273
Cholecystokinin, 1054, 1228
Cholecystostomy technique, 1246
Choledochocholedochostomy, 1233
Choledochoduodenostomy, 1224, 1227, 1248–1249
Choledochojejunostomy, 236, 1273
Choledocholithiasis, 1234–1235, 1239
choledochoduedenostomy in, 1248–1249
exploration for, 1248
Choledochostomy, 1235
Choledochotomy, transduodenal, 1248
Choledochus (common bile duct):
anatomy, 1221
carcinoma, 1271

cyst, 1224
function, 1229
operations, 1248–1249
  choledochoduodenostomy, 1248–1249
  choledochotomy, transduodenal, 1248
  decompressive procedures, 1249–1250
  in injury and stricture, 1249
  sphincterotomy, 1248
  stones, 1234–1235, 1239, 1248–1249
  T-tube drainage, 234
Cholelithiasis (see Gallstones)
Cholestasis, 1001
Cholesterol:
  gallstones and, 1233
  intestinal bypass and, 1105
  thyroid function and, 1436
Chondritis, 605
Chondroblastoma, 1779
Chondrocalcinosis, 1870–1871
Chondrodystrophia fetalis, 1747–1748
Chondroitin sulfate, 281, 1765
Chondroma, 1778–1779
  chest wall, 607
  mediastinal, 669
Chondromalacia of patella, 1867
Chondromatosis, synovial, 1872
Chondroosteodystrophy, 1766
Chondrosarcoma, 1780
  chest wall, 608
  mandibular, 581
  mediastinal, 669
Chordae tendineae, 709, 762, 774
Chordee, 1956
Chordoma, 1786
  mediastinal, 667–668
Choriocarcinoma, 1579, 1606
Christmas factor (IX), 99–100, 111–112
Chromaffin cells, 1404, 1407
Chromium, radioactive, in red cell studies, 1285
Chromophobes, 1365, 1372, 1389
Chromosomes:
  hemostatic defects and, 108
  reproductive defects and, 1603–1604
Chvostek's sign, 1500
Chylothorax, 620
Chylous peritonitis, 1309
Cigarette smoking (see Smoking)
Cineradiography, 752
  mitral insufficiency, 773
  urinary tract, 1547
  ventricular aneurysm, 800
Circle of Willis, 1632, 1657
Circulation, assisted, 808–809
  (See also Extracorporeal circulation)
Circulatory collapse (see Shock)
Circumcision, bleeding in, 105
Cirrhosis, 1197
  ammonia and, 1203
  esophagogastric varices in, 1199–1202
  liver transplants for, 394
  surgery in, 1205–1213
Cisterna chyli, cancer spread by, 315
Citrate:
  in bone, 1742
  in transfusions, 121, 127
Clagett-Barrett procedure, 1033
Clark electrode, 498
Claudication, 840, 842
  in aortoiliac disease, 843, 844
Clavicle:
  aplasia, 1736
  fractures of, 1802–1803
Clavicular incisions, 218
Claw hallux deformity, 1691
Cleft lip and palate, 1947–1950
Cleidocranial dysostosis, 1736
Clindamycin, 175
Clitoris, 1632
Clonal selection, 357
Clonorchis sinensis, 1241

Closed-chest massage and defibrillation, 760–761
Clostridial infections, 181–185
  gastrointestinal, 182–183
  tetanus, 183–185
  urogenital, 183
  wound, 181–182
Clot dissolution, 101–102
Clot retraction, 103
Clotting factors, 99–102
  (See also under Factor)
  transfusion and, 121, 124, 125
Clotting time, 103, 105–106
Cloxacillin, 174
Clubbing, cyanosis and, 680
Clubfoot, 1732–1734
Coagulation, 29–31, 99–101
  cascade system, 365
  diagnosis of inherited disorders of, 106
  disseminated intravascular, 114
  dissolution of clot, 101–102
  extracorporeal circulation and, 756
  extrinsic system, 100
  gastrointestinal bleeding and, 994
  hemostasis and, 99–101
  hypercoagulation, 29
  hypocoagulation, 29–31
  liver function and, 1180
  retraction of clot, 103
  tests, 102–105
  time, 103, 105–106
Coagulopathy, consumptive, 114
Coarctation of aorta, 696–701, 945
  anatomy, pathologic, 696–697
  clinical manifestations, 697, 940, 945
  historical data, 696
  hypertension and, 945–946
  incidence and etiology, 696
  laboratory studies, 697–698
  pathophysiology, 697
  postoperative care, 701
  treatment, 698–701, 946
Coccidioidomycosis, 188, 638–639
Coccygeal sinus cyst, 517
Coccygodynia, 1679
Codman Apnea Alarm, 497
Codman's tumor, 1779
Coenzyme A, acetyl, 19–20
Cold injury, 904–906
Cold therapy, 1969
  (See also Hypothermia)
Colectomy, 1134–1135
  epinephrine and, 16
Coley's toxins, 340
Colic, 971, 1550
Colic arteries, 1321
Colic vein, middle, 1256
Colistin, 173, 175
Colitis:
  cystica profunda, 1133
  granulomatous, 1116–1118
    clinical manifestations, 1117
    incidence, 1116
    pathology, 1116–1117
    treatment, 1117–1118
  ischemic, 1118–1119
  pseudomembranous enterocolitis, 1119–1120
  ulcerative, 1110–1116
    clinical manifestations, 1112–1113
    complications, 1113–1114
    diagnosis, 1114
    etiology, 1110–1111
    incidence, 1110
    pathology, 1111–1112
    treatment, 1114–1116
Collagen, 31, 282–286
  of bone, 1461
  calcification and, 1754
  fibroma and, 1780
  joint, 1846
  platelet function and, 98

remodeling of, 284, 285
scar tissue and, 284, 285
sponge, 121
synthesis of, 283, 287
tensile strength of, 284, 287
Collagenases, bone and, 1742
Colles fracture, 1814–1815
Collis gastroplasty, 1028
Colloid:
  in burns, 261
  carcinoma of breast, 540
  osmotic pressure, 67
  for shock, 148
Colomyotomy for diverticulitis, 1124
Colon, 1109–1146
  absorption in, 1109
  adenomas, 1126–1128
  amebiasis, 1120–1121
  ammonia absorption, 1203
  antisepsis for, 172
  arterial supply, 1321–1322
  atresia, congenital, 1526, 1528
  bleeding, 997
  carcinoma, 1131–1141
    chemotherapy, 1137–1138, 1140
    chronic colitis and, 1113–1114
    classification, 1132
    clinical manifestations, 1133
    death rate, 298
    diagnosis, 1133–1134
    early detection, 1140–1141
    etiology, 1131
    incidence, 1131
    metastases, 1132
    operative procedures, 1134–1136
    pathology, 1131–1133
    polyps and, 1129–1131
    prognosis, 1139–1140
    radiation therapy, 1138–1139, 1140
    recurrent, 1140
    sigmoidoscopy for, 1141
  carcinoid, 1141
  defecation and, 977
  diarrhea and, 978
  diverticular disease, 1121–1126
  dysentery, 1120–1121
  endometriosis, 1142–1143
  esophagectomy and, 1035, 1036
  fistulas, 1117
    postoperative, 485
  herniated, 1355
  Hirschsprung's disease, 1531–1536
  infarction, 1325, 1328
  inflammatory disease, 1110–1121
    (See also Colitis)
  injuries of, 230–232
  ischemic, aortic aneurysm and, 891
  leiomyoma and leiomyosarcoma, 1142
  lymphosarcoma, 1141–1142
  megacolon, 1113, 1144–1146, 1531–1536
  mesenteries of, 1318–1319
  obstruction, 983
  polyps, 1126–1131
    (See also Polyps, colorectal)
  resection, 1134–1135
  roentgenography, 1115, 1117, 1119, 1122–1124, 1143
  in tracheoesophageal fistula repair, 1518, 1519
  tumors, 1126–1143
  venous drainage, 1322–1324
  volvulus, 1143–1144
Colonization, 171
Colonoscope, fiberoptic, 1147–1148
Colostomy:
  colorectal cancer and, 1134–1136
  complications, 486
  diverticulitis perforation and, 1125
  for imperforate anus, 1538–1539
  injuries of colon and, 232
  for megacolon, 1533

rehabilitation and, 1981
Coma:
  diabetic, 475
  hepatic, 1201, 1203–1204
Commissurotomy:
  aortic valvular, 691–692
  mitral, 766–767, 771
Common bile duct (see Choledochus)
Complement, 43, 364–365, 367
Complications, postoperative, 461–486
  afferent loop syndrome, 482–483
  anastomotic leak, 484
  arrhythmias, 469–472
  atelectasis, 467–469
  cardiac, 469–473
  dehiscence, 462
  diabetes mellitus, 473–475
  edema, pulmonary, 469
  fat embolism, 475–477
  fistulas, 484–485
  gastrointestinal surgery, 481–486
  hematoma, 464
  hemorrhage, 464, 481–482
    (See also Hemorrhage)
  infection, 462–464
  myocardial infarction, 472–473
  obstruction, 482, 484
  parotitis, 464–465
  psychiatric, 477–481
  respiratory, 465–469
  seroma, 464
  stomal, external, 485–486
  wound, 462–464
Component therapy, 34–36
Compression tests of veins, 927
Computers for monitoring, 499, 504
Concentration changes, 68–70
Conduction anesthesia, 454–458
Conduction studies, 878–879, 881
Condyloma acuminatum, 1158, 1608
Conray, 1553
Consciousness, 1631, 1636
Constipation, 976–978
  clinical evaluation, 978
  etiology, 977
  fecal impaction and, 1145–1146
  megacolon and, 1144–1145
Contraction, wound, 275–278
Contracture, 275–276, 1715–1717
  Dupuytren's, 1715–1716
  in paraplegia, 1978
  scar, 1954
  Volkmann's, 1716–1717
Contusion:
  arterial, 867–868
  nerve, 1647
Convulsions, head injury and, 1640
Cooper's ligament repair, 1355–1358
Copper, wound healing and, 31
Coral snakes, 212, 213
Cori cycle, 19, 23
Corneal transplant, 385–386
Coronary arteries:
  anomalies, 739–742
    fistula, arteriovenous, 741–742
    pulmonary artery origin, 739–741
  in aortic stenosis, 694
  in heart transplant, 403
  in ventricular aneurysm operation, 800
Coronary artery disease, 793–799
  angina pectoris and, 794, 795
  bypass operation, 794
  cardiac arrest and, 759
  etiology and pathogenesis, 794–795
  historical data, 793–794
  operative procedures for, 795–799
  postoperative occlusion, 472–473
Corpus luteum, 1595, 1597
  cysts, 1619
Corrosive esophagitis, 1027–1028

Corrosive gastritis, 1077
Corticoid-withdrawal phase, 88
Corticosteroids, 7–12, 13
  adrenalectomy and, 1388
  anesthesia and, 9, 10, 449
  in burns, 12, 15
  exogenous, 7–8
  immunologic protection and, 43
  in immunosuppression, 378
  in retroperitoneal fibrosis, 1338
  in shock, 152–153
  structure of, 1377
  in thrombocytopenia, 116, 1289
  trauma and, 199
  in ulcerative colitis, 1115
  ulcers from, 49
  urinary, 1384
Corticosterone, 13
Corticotropin-releasing factor, 6, 7, 1377–1379
Cortisol, 7–12, 1377–1379
  in adrenogenital syndrome, 1390
  binding and transport, 1379
  Cushing's syndrome and, 943
  diurnal variations in, 1383–1384
  free, 1386
  hypertension and, 940
  metabolism, 1379, 1380
  pathways for secretion of, 8, 14
  response to ACTH, 1384
  site of defect in, 12
  starvation and, 22
  trauma and, 1, 2, 7–12
Cortisone:
  in hyperparathyroidism, 1479
  in immunosuppression, 378
  for painful shoulder, 1874
Cor triatriatum, 733
Cosmetic surgery, 1954–1956
Costal cartilages, 605, 606
Costoclavicular syndrome, 876
Cough, 600
Coumarin, 118
  for venous thrombosis, 919
Counterpulsion, external, 159
Coxa plana, 1718–1720
Cramping:
  in ulcerative colitis, 1113
  in venous insufficiency, 925
Cranial nerves, carcinoma and, 577
Craniofacial anomalies, 1957
Craniosynostosis, 1656–1657
Craniovertebral abnormalities, 1669–1670
Cranium, 1633–1634
  (See also Skull)
  bifida, 1652
  brevicollis, 1736
Creatinine, 406, 954, 1565
Credé maneuvers, 1980
Crepitus, fractures and, 1792
Cretinism, 1442
  bone disease in, 1765
CRF, 6, 7
Cricopharyngeal myotomy, 1020
  (See also Enteritis, regional)
Crohn's disease, 1110, 1116
Crush syndrome, limb compression and, 1908
Cryosurgery, 120
  hypophysectomy, 1373
Cryotherapy for snakebite, 212
Cryptorchidism, 1562
Crystal deposition disease, 1870–1871
Crystalloids, 149
Cul-de-sac of Douglas, 1591
Curare, 453
Curling's ulcers, 259, 269, 992–993
Cushing's syndrome, 943–945, 1380–1390
  clinical manifestations, 940, 944, 1383
  diagnostic findings, 1383–1386
  differential diagnosis, 1386
  historical background, 1374–1375

incidence, 1383
  laboratory findings, 944
  pathology, 943–944, 1381–1383
  pituitary and, 1368, 1387
  transplants (renal) and, 424
  treatment, 944–945, 1386–1390
    irradiation, 1387
    medical, 1386–1387
    operative, 1388–1389
    postoperative complications, 1389–1390
    preoperative, 1387–1388
Cushing's ulcer, 993
Cutaneous arteries, 1925
Cyanosis, 601, 750
  abdominal, 1325, 1326
  patent ductus arteriosus and, 719
  right-to-left shunts and, 680
  single ventricle and, 737–738
    in tetralogy of Fallot, 722, 723
    in transposition of great vessels, 729
    in tricuspid atresia, 730
    in vasospastic disorders, 902, 903–904
Cyclophosphamide, 332, 377
Cyclopropane, 446–448
Cylindroma, 582, 644
Cyst(s):
  air, 625–627
  appendiceal, 1176
  biliary tract, 1224
  bone, 1470–1471, 1762, 1783–1784, 1785–1786
  breast, 537–538
  bronchogenic, 665, 666–667
  cardiac, 793
  dermoid, 517, 665
  epidermal inclusion, 516
  esophageal, 667, 1037–1038
  ganglia, 516
  hydatid, 640, 1188–1189
  laryngeal, 574
  liver, 1187–1189
  mandibular, 580
  mediastinal, 665–668
  mesenteric, 1334–1335
  nabothian, 1611
  omental, 1318
  oral cavity, 565
  ovarian, 1619–1620
  pancreatic, 1268
  pilonidal, 517
  pleuropericardial, 666
  pulmonary, 615–616, 625–627, 640
  renal, 1571
  rib, 607
  sebaceous, 516–517
  skin, 516–517
  small bowel, 1102
  splenic, 1293
  suprasellar, 1372
Cystadenocarcinoma, pancreatic, 1268
Cystadenoma, salivary gland, 581–582
Cystic adenomatoid malformation of lung, 623
Cystic artery, 1221, 1223
  in hepatic resection, 1194
Cystic duct, 1222–1223
  ligature, in cholecystectomy, 1247
  obstruction, 1234
  stump, postcholecystectomy syndrome and, 1240
Cystic hygroma, 1515–1516
Cystic mastitis, chronic, 537
Cystinosis, 1758
Cystocele, 1599
Cystoduodenostomy, 1224, 1225
Cystogastrostomy, for pancreatic pseudocyst, 1270
Cystolithotomy, 1583–1584
Cystomas, ovarian, 1620
Cystometry, 1556
Cystosarcoma phylloides, 540–541
Cystoscopy, 1553

Cystostomy, 1583–1584
Cystourethroscopy, 1568
Cytology, exfoliative, gastric ulcer and, 1072
Cytophilic antibody, 367–369
Cytosine arabinoside, 332
Cytoxan, 332, 1620

Dandy-Walker syndrome, 1655
o,p′-DDD, 1387
Dead space, physiologic, 465
Death, brain, criteria for, 411–412
Decerebrate rigidity, 1632
Decortication of lung, 619
Decubitus ulcer, 1960, 1978
Defecation, 976–977
  incontinence, 1149, 1155–1156
Defibrillation, ventricular, 761–762
Defibrination, 108, 114
Degenerative disc disease, 1670–1672
Degenerative joint disease (see Osteoarthritis)
Degenerative nervous system disease, skeletal
    deformity and, 1703–1704
Deglutition, 973, 1012
Dehiscence, 462
Dehydroepiandrosterone, 13
Dehydrogenase deficiency, 1390
Del Castillo syndrome, 1602
Delalutin, 1617
Delirium, 478, 481
Demerol, 452
Densitometer, 504, 506
Dental tumors, 580
Dentate line, 1147, 1149
Deoxycorticosterone, 1398–1400
Deoxyribonucleic acid (DNA):
  cancer chemotherapy and, 330
  immunosuppressive drugs and, 376–378
  lymphocyte proliferation and, 359
  radiation and, 374–375
Depo-Provera, 1617
Depressive reactions, 478
Dermabrasion, 1934
Dermal sinus tracts, 1653–1654
Dermatofibrosarcoma, 521
Dermatomyositis, 1039
Dermis, 1922, 1923
  scalp, 1633
Dermoid cysts:
  mediastinal, 665
  of mouth, 565
  of skin, 517
Desensitization for insect bites, 214
Desmoid tumors:
  abdominal wall, 1315–1316
  of muscle, 1787
Desoxycorticosterone, 1381
Detorsion, 1144
Dexamethasone, 1381
  in head injury, 1629
  suppression test, 1384–1385
Dextran:
  coagulation and, 29
  for fat embolism, 477
  in shock, 148
Dextrose solutions, 93
Deyerle plate, 1812
Diabetes, 473–475
  foot in, 854–856
  gangrene in, 855
  insipidus, 17-OHCS in, 12
  insulin therapy, 474
  ketoacidosis in, 474–475
  management, 473–475
  pancreas transplant for, 390–391
  pancreatic cancer and, 1271
  pathophysiology, 473
  "phosphate," 1758–1759
  pituitary and, 1369
  postoperative, 473–475

renal transplant and, 405, 424–425
retinopathy in, 1372–1373
tibial artery disease in, 851
trophic ulcers in, 855–856
Dialysis:
  (See also Hemodialysis)
  BUN changes in, 27
  for hypercalcemia, 1490–1491
  peritoneal, 1297
  in renal failure, 1558
Diaphragm, 597
  crura, 1010, 1011
  eventration of, 1041–1042
  hernias, 1023–1025, 1040–1041
    esophageal hiatal, 1023–1025
    foramen of Morgagni, 1041
    posterolateral (foramen of Bochdalek),
      1040–1041
  respiratory excursion of, 224
  rupture of, 1042–1043
  urogenital, 1592, 1593
Diarrhea, 978–979
  in carcinoid syndrome, 1098
  clinical evaluation of, 979
  consequences of, 979
  in dysentery, 1120
  etiology, 978–979
  jejunostomy tube feeding and, 90
  in pseudomembranous colitis, 1120
  in short bowel syndrome, 1103–1104
  in ulcerative colitis, 1112, 1114
  vagotomy and, 1066
  in Zollinger-Ellison syndrome, 1277
Diastematomyelia, 1653
Diastolic hypertension, 941
Diastolic murmurs, 682
  (See also Murmurs)
Diastolic overloading, 679
Diastolic pressure:
  in aortic insufficiency, 783
  in coronary artery disease, 795
Diazepam, 457, 458
Dibenzyline, 37
DIC, 114
Dicloxacillin, 174
Diet:
  diverticulosis and, 1122
  elemental, 90–91
  gastric cancer and, 1079
  peptic ulcer and, 1060
  urinary calculi and, 1564
Diethyl ether, 448–449
Diethylstilbestrol for prostate tumors, 1576, 1578
Diffusion anoxia, 445–446
Digital pressure, 119
Digitalis:
  cardiac arrest and, 759
  postoperative arrhythmias and, 470–471
  in shock, 152
Digits (see Fingers; Toes)
1,25-Dihydroxyvitamin D₃, 1464, 1465
3,5-Diiodotyrosine, 1431
Dilantin, 1387
Dilatation and curettage, 1623–1624
Dinitrochlorobenzene, 310
Dioctyl sodium sulfosuccinate, 1145–1146
Diphenylhydantoin, 1386, 1387
2,3-Diphosphoglycerate, 34, 42
  red cell, 495
Diphosphopyridine nucleotide, 496
Diplopia, 1939, 1940
Disarticulation (see Amputation)
Discharge, gynecologic, 1607–1608
Disinfectants, 188
Dislocations:
  ankle, 1832
  foot, 1833–1834
  hip, 1835–1837
    congenital, 1726–1731
  knee, 1825–1828, 1829

spinal, 1641–1643, 1839–1842
Disruption of wound, 462
Dissecting aneurysms, 825–829
Disseminated intravascular coagulation, 114
Diuresis:
  renal artery reconstruction and, 959
  in shock, 155
Diverticula:
  colonic, 1121–1126
  duodenal, 1100–1101
  epiphrenic, 1020–1023
  esophageal, 1018–1023
  ileal, 1101
  jejunal, 1101
  Meckel's, 1100, 1522–1523
  parabronchial, 1023
  pharyngoesophageal, 1018–1020
  small bowel, 1100–1101
  thoracic, 667
  traction, 1023
  vesical, 1576
Diverticulitis, 1123–1125
  appendicitis vs., 1171–1172
  cecal, 1125–1126
  clinical manifestations, 1123–1124
  complications, 1124–1125
  fistulas in, 1125
  obstruction in, 1124
  pathogenesis, 1123
  perforation in, 1124–1125
  treatment, 1124
Diverticulosis coli, 1121–1125
  bleeding in, 1122–1123
  complications, 1123–1125
  etiology and pathogenesis, 1121–1122
  incidence, 1121
  inflammation in, 1123–1125
DNA (see Deoxyribonucleic acid)
DNCB, 310, 341
Dog bites, 207–211
Donors, kidney, 408–412
Dopamine, 1404, 1411
Doppler flowmeter, 266
Doppler ultrasound technique, 917
Douglas, pouch of, 1591
Doxycycline, 176–177
DPG, 34, 42
Drainage:
  in appendectomy, 1173
  of common bile duct, 234
  diverticulitis perforation and, 1125
  for duodenal injury, 228–229
  emergency laparotomy and, 206
  empyema, 616–617
  hip joint, 1850
  liver injury and, 233, 234
  for pancreatic injuries, 238
  pancreatic pseudocyst, 1270
  perirectal abscess, 1153, 1154
  in peritonitis, 1304
  pulmonary resection, 653
  subhepatic abscess, 1308
  subphrenic abscess, 1307
  transthoracic, for hepatic abscesses, 1184,
    1185
  vagotomy and, 1066, 1067
Dressings, 290
  graft, 291–292
Drugs:
  (See also Antibiotics; Chemotherapy)
  anesthetic (see Anesthesia)
  immunosuppressive, 376–378
  intoxication from, 203
  liver function and, 47–48
  ulcerogenic, 1070
Drummond, marginal artery of, 1322
Dubin-Johnson syndrome, 1001
Duchenne dystrophy, 1688
Duck embryo vaccine (DEV), 209, 210
Ductus arteriosus, patent, 716–721

anatomy, pathologic, 718
clinical manifestations, 718–719
coarctation and, 696
diagnosis, 719
historical data, 716
incidence and etiology, 716–718
laboratory findings, 719
pathophysiology, 718
postoperative course, 720–721
treatment, 719–720
Duhamel procedure, 1534, 1536
Dukes classification, 1132
Dumping syndrome, 1065
Duodenojejunostomy for intestinal atresia, 1528
Duodenum:
adenocarcinoma, 1096
atresia, congenital, 1527
in biliary tract surgery, 1248–1249
diverticula, 1100–1101
exposure of, 226, 228
fistulas, 227, 484–485
hematoma of, 229
injuries of, 225–229
Kocher mobilization of, 1250, 1267
pancreatic injuries and, 240
pancreatic resection and, 1272–1274
sump drain for, 228–229
transplant, 391
Dupuytren's contracture, 1716–1717
Dwarfism:
achondroplasia and, 1748
osteogenesis imperfecta and, 1750
osteoporosis and, 1764
polydystrophic, 1766
Dye excretion test, hepatic, 1180
Dye injections of lymphatics, 931–932
Dyschondroplasia, 1740
Dysentery, amebic, 1120–1121
Dysgerminoma, ovarian, 1621
Dyskeratosis, 567–568
Dysmenorrhea, 1598
Dysostosis, cleidocranial, 1736
Dysphagia, 973–974
in dermatomyositis, 1039
esophagitis and, 1026
hiatal hernia and, 1024
in neuromuscular disorders, 1039–1040
sideropenic, 1038
Dysplasia:
cervical, 1611–1612
fibrous, of chest wall, 607
hip, congenital, 1726–1731
Dyspnea, 601
heart disease and, 750
in infant, lobar emphysema and, 624–625
in mitral stenosis, 763
pneumothorax and, 612
in tetralogy of Fallot, 722
Dysraphism, spinal, 1702–1703
Dystrophies, muscular, 1696–1697
Dysuria, 1550–1551

Ears:
burns, 270
congenital microtia, 1950–1952
prominent, 1955
Ebstein's anomaly, 738–739
Eccrine glands, 514
Echinococcosis, 1188–1189
of lung, 640
Echocardiography, 507
Echo encephalography, 1648
Edema:
cerebral, 1637, 1647
heart disease and, 750
leg, venous insufficiency and, 925, 926
lymphatic, 932–934
protein content of fluid, 932
Edema, pulmonary, 469

in mitral stenosis, 763–764
transfusion and, 128
Effector molecules, 362, 363
Effusions:
intraperitoneal, 1306
pleural, 613–614
Ehlers-Danlos syndrome, 513
Eisenmenger complex, 713
Elastic fibers of skin, 513
Elbow:
disarticulation, 1892
dislocations, 1811–1812
flexed spastic, 1705
fractures, 1808, 1810–1812
osteoarthritis, 1862
pain, 1679
paralysis, 1699–1700
rheumatoid arthritis, 1860
Electrical conduction studies, 878–879, 881
Electrical impedance test, 917
Electrocardiography, 751
in aldosteronism, 1397
in aortic insufficiency, 783
in aortic stenosis, 776
in atrial septal defect, 710
flow-guided catheterization and, 501, 502
in mitral insufficiency, 773
in mitral stenosis, 766
in myocardial infarction, 472
transplantation of heart and, 401
Electrocautery, 120
anesthesia and, 444
for rectal bleeding, 1148
Electrocoagulation for skin cancer, 520
Electrodes:
gas measurement, 498
pacemaker, 804–806
Electrodesiccation:
for carcinoma of skin, 520
for warts, 517
Electroencephalography, 1648
death and, 411
Electrolytes:
(See also Fluids and electrolytes)
trauma and, 39–42
Electromyography, 1695
Electrotherapy, 1969
Elemental diets, 90–91
Elliptocytosis, hereditary, 1287
Ellsworth-Howard test, 1501
Embolectomy, 859–860
mesenteric artery, 1325–1326
pulmonary, 923
Embolism:
air, 684, 758
aortic aneurysm and, 891
arterial, 857–862
arterioarterial, 861–862
cardioarterial, 857–861
cancer spread by, 314, 323
cerebravascular disease and, 884
fat, postoperative, 475–477
mesenteric artery, 1324
in mitral stenosis, 764
pulmonary (see Pulmonary embolism)
pulmonary insufficiency and, 47
transfusion and, 127–128
Embryoma, 1191
Emesis (see Vomiting)
Emetine, 1187
Emotional trauma, 4
Emphysema, 598
bullae in, 625–627
lobar, of infancy, 624–625
mediastinal, 660
after pneumonectomy, 657
Emphysematous cholecystitis, 1238–1239
Empyema, 615–619
acute, 615
chronic, 619

complications, 616
differential diagnosis, 615–616
necessitans, 616
subdural, 1654–1655
treatment, 616–619
Encephaloceles, 1653
Encephalography, 1655
Encephalopathy, portal-systemic, 1203
Endochondral ossification, 1743
Enchondroma, 1748, 1779
Endarterectomy:
abdominal aorta, 844, 845–846
carotid artery, 884, 886
coronary artery, 798
femoropopliteal, 849–851
renal artery, 957
in tibioperoneal disease, 852
End-diastolic pressure, 795
Endoaneurysmorraphy, 871, 900
Endobronchial tumors, 641–642
Endocardial cushion defect, 709
Endocarditis:
bacterial: arteriovenous fistula
and, 872
mitral insufficiency and, 771
patent ductus arteriosus and, 718, 719
ventricular defect and, 714
rheumatic fever, mitral stenosis and, 762
tricuspid valve, 786–787
Endocrine glands:
(See also individual glands)
gynecologic disorders and, 1593–1597
in hyperparathyroidism, 1486–1487
osteoporosis and, 1762
peritonitis and, 1301
transplantation, 389–391
trauma and, 5–17, 199–200
Endometriomas, 1619
Endometriosis, 1608–1609
colonic, 1142–1143
syncytial, 1606
Endometrium, 1596–1597
carcinoma, 1615–1617
hyperplasia, 1611–1612
Endoscopy:
bladder tumors and, 1573
gastric mucosal lesions and, 1075
hemorrhage and, 994–995
peptic ulcer and, 1060
Endotoxin, hormone secretion and, 3
Endotoxin shock, 43, 45, 140–144, 157–158
Endotracheal intubation, 202, 466–467
Enemas, peritonitis from, 1300
Energy:
metabolism, 19
sources, sensing and, 497
trauma and, 200
Enflurane, 451
Enhancement, immunologic, 308, 380–381
Entamoeba histolytica, 1120
hepatic abscesses and, 1186–1187
Enteritis:
regional, 1089–1094
appendicitis vs., 1172
clinical manifestations, 1091
incidence, 1089
lymphadenitis vs., 1333
pathology, pathogenesis, etiology, 1089–1091
roentgenography, 1091–1092
treatment, 1092–1094
staphylococcal, 181
tuberculous, 1094
typhoid, 1094–1095
Enterobacter aerogenes, 186
Enterocolitis, pseudomembranous, 181, 1119–1120
Enterocutaneous fistulas, 1101–1102
Enterogastrone, 1051, 1055
Enuresis, 1570

Enzymes:
  bone, 1742
  cancer chemotherapy and, 330
  collagenolytic, 285
  liver, 1180
Eosinophilic gastritis, 1077–1078
Eosinophilic granuloma, 1769, 1770
Epidermal inclusion cyst, 516
Epidermis (see Skin)
Epidermization, cervical, 1611
Epidermoid carcinoma:
  anal, 1159–1160
  nasopharyngeal, 577–578
  oral, 570, 572
  salivary glands, 582
Epididymis, 1548–1549
Epididymitis, 1551
Epidural abscess, 1662
Epidural anesthesia, 457
Epidural hematoma, 1639–1640
Epiglottis, 559
  tumors, 572
Epinephrine, 504, 1404–1409
  anesthesia and, 10
  cardiac arrest and, 761
  control cells, 7
  epidural anesthesia and, 457
  lipid metabolism and, 1406
  low-cardiac-output syndrome and, 757
  metabolites of, 1405
  pheochromocytoma and, 1409–1411
  shock and, 134, 141
  tolerance, 147
  urinary, 1407, 1410
Epiphrenic diverticulum, 1020–1023
  clinical manifestations, 1021–1022
  incidence, pathophysiology and anatomy,
    1020–1021
  treatment, 1022–1023
Epiphyseal growth plants, grafts of, 386–387
Epiphysis, 1717–1721
  injuries, 1798–1799
    Köhler's disease, 1720–1721
    Legg-Calvé-Perthes disease, 1718–1720
    Osgood-Schlatter disease, 1720
  ossification, 1743
  remodeling and, 1744
  in rickets, 1756
  in scurvy, 1755
Epiphysitis, 1707–1708, 1717–1721
Epispadias, 1570
Epithelioma, adamantine, 1786
Epithelization, 278–281
Epulis fissurata, 565
Equinus deformity, 1699
Equivalents, 67
Erb's dystrophy, 1696
Erosion, gastric, 1073–1076
Erysipelas, 169, 178–179
Erysipeloid, 179
Erythrocytes:
  2,3-DPG of, 42
  component therapy and, 34, 35
  labeling of, 1284–1285
  packed and frozen, 122–123
  porphyria erythropoietica, 1293
  sickling of, 1288
  spherocytic, 1287
  spleen and, 1283, 1284
Erythromelalgia, 904
Erythromycin, 173, 175
Eschar, 266
Escharotic preparation for skin cancer, 520
Escherichia coli, 186, 1184
  meningitis and, 1653
  peritonitis and, 1300
  shock and, 140
Esophageal speech, 575–576
Esophagitis, 1025–1028
  clinical manifestations, 1026, 1027–1028

  corrosive, 1027–1028
  pathology, 1026, 1027
  reflux, 1026–1027
  treatment, 1026–1027, 1028
Esophagogastrectomy, 1027, 1035
Esophagogastric junction, 1009
  carcinoma, 1034–1035
Esophagogastric varices, 1199–1202
  balloon tamponade in, 996
  bleeding, 993, 996, 1200, 1201
  natural course, 1199–1200
  treatment, 1200–1202
Esophagojejunostomy, 1028, 1081, 1207
Esophagomyotomy, 1016, 1017, 1021, 1022
Esophagopleural fistula, 1031–1032
Esophagoscopy, 1200
  for carcinoma, 1034
Esophagus, 1009–1040
  achalasia, 1013–1017
    clinical manifestations, 1014
    physiologic studies, 1014–1015
    treatment, 1015–1017
  anatomy, 1009–1011
  atresia, 1516–1521
  Barrett, 1038–1039
  benign cysts and tumors, 1037–1038
  blood supply, 1010–1011
  bougienage, 1026
  carcinoma, 1032–1037
    clinical manifestations, 1034
    death rate, 298
    incidence and etiology, 1032
    pathology, 1033
    treatment, 1034–1037
  diverticula, 1018–1023
    epiphrenic, 1020–1023
    parabronchial, 1023
    pharyngoesophageal, 1018–1020
  duplication cyst, 667
  dysphagia and, 973–974
  fistula, 1031–1032
    tracheal, 1516–1521
  hiatal hernia, 1023–1025
    paraesophageal, 1023
    sliding, 1023–1025
  hydrostatic dilation of, 1015
  inflammation, 1025–1028
    (See also Esophagitis)
  injuries of, 219
  Mallory-Weiss syndrome, 1039
  motility disturbances, 1013–1018
    hypermotility, 1017–1018
    hypomotility, 1013–1017
  neuromuscular disturbances, 1039–1040
  perforation, 1029–1033
    clinical manifestations, 1030–1031
    etiology, 1029–1030
    incidence, 1029
    pathophysiology, 1030
    treatment, 1031–1032
  physiology, 1012–1013
  Plummer-Vinson syndrome, 1038
  ring, lower, 1038
  roentgenography, 1014, 1017, 1019, 1030–1031,
    1038
  rupture of, mediastinitis and, 660–661
  scleroderma, 1039
  stricture, 1025–1028
  varices (see Esophagogastric varices)
Essential hypertension, 963–964
Essex-Lopresti method, 1835
Estlander flap, 1944
Estrogens (estrone, estradiol, estriol), 13,
    1594–1595
  in bleeding disorders, 1601
  in breast cancer, 551
  in osteoporosis, 1764
  for prostate tumors, 1576, 1578
  tumor secretion of, 1374, 1392
Ether, diethyl, 448–449

Ethmoid sinus carcinoma, 579
Eventration of diaphragm, 1041–1042
Ewing's tumor, 1784–1785
Exercise, 1967–1968, 1978
Exercise tolerance, 681
Exfoliative cytology, gastric ulcer and, 1072
Exophthalmos, 1441
Exostoses, multiple, 1748
Exotoxins, 167
Expiration, 597–598
Extensor tendon injuries of hand, 1911
External counterpulsion, 159
Extracellular fluid, 66–67
Extracorporeal circulation, 126, 753–759
  anemia and, 759
  anticoagulants and, 759
  aortic aneurysm repair and, 815
  in aortic stenosis operation, 777
  arrhythmias and, 757
  bleeding syndromes and, 756
  cardiac failure and, 756–757
  central nervous system and, 758–759
  coagulation and, 30
  complications, 755–759
  in coronary bypass operation, 795
  fever and, 758
  fluids following, 757–758
  gastrointestinal disturbances and, 759
  heart transplantation and, 400
  historical data, 753
  low-cardiac-output syndrome, 756–757
  oxygenators, 753
  perfusion, 753–755
    risk of, 755
    technique of, 753–754
    termination of, 754
    trauma from, 755
  physiology, 753–755
  postoperative care, 755–759
  priming solutions, 753
  pumps, 753
  renal function and, 758
  respiratory insufficiency and, 757
Extracorporeal irradiation, immunosuppression
    and, 372–373
Extradural tumors, 1650–1651
Extramedullary tumors, 1651
Extremities:
  lower (See also Leg; and specific areas and
    structures)
    amputations, 1882–1888
    in cerebral palsy, 1702
    fractures and joint injuries of, 1819–1835
    occlusive disease of, 840–856
    in poliomyelitis, 1698–1699
    prostheses, 1973–1974
    stroke and, 1705
  upper (See also specific areas and structures)
    amputations, 1888–1892
    in cerebral palsy, 1702
    fractures and joint injuries, 1802–1819
    pain, 1679–1682
    in poliomyelitis, 1699–1700
    prostheses, 1975
    replantation, 387–388
    stroke and, 1705
    venous thrombosis of, 915
Exudate, 168
Eye:
  allografts in anterior chamber of, 381
  reconstructive procedures for, 1958
Eyebrow reconstruction, 1925, 1945, 1954–1955
Eyelid:
  injury, 1943
  reconstructive procedures, 1958

Face:
  bones of, 1633–1634
  composite tissue transplant to, 1928

examination of, 557, 560
fractures, 1936–1938
lifting, 1956
paralysis, 1957–1967, 1976
rehabilitation and, 1976, 1981
scars, 1954
soft tissue losses, skin grafts for, 1948
trauma, 289, 1935–1944
Facial nerve:
  parotidectomy and, 587
  repair, 1957
  salivary gland tumors and, 583–584
Factitial proctitis, 1159
Factor II, 113
Factor V (proaccelerin), 112
Factor VII (proconvertin), 100, 112–113
Factor VIII, 100, 109–111
  arthritis and, 1871
  component therapy and, 35
  hypocoagulation and, 30
Factor IX (Christmas), 99–100, 111–112
Factor X (Stuart-Prower), 100, 113
Factor XI (PTA), 99, 112
Factor XII (Hageman), 99, 365
Factor XIII (fibrin-stabilizing), 101
Fallopian tubes, 1590
  infertility and, 1605
  operations, 1625–1627
  tumors, 1622–1623
    bleeding and, 1602
Fallot, tetralogy of (see Tetralogy of Fallot)
Familial polyposis, 1128–1129
Fanconi syndrome, 1293
  rickets and, 1758
Fascia:
  autograft of, 385
  contracture of, 1715
  hernias and, 1346, 1347, 1354
Fasciitis, necrotizing, 179
Fascioscapulohumeral dystrophy, 1696
Fasting, 21–22
  (See also Starvation)
Fat(s):
  biopsy, scalene, 649
  embolism, postoperative, 475–477
  fuel reserves, 86–87
  metabolism: epinephrine and, 1406
    glucagon and, 16
    liver and, 1179–1180
  necrosis of breast, 538
  in short bowel syndrome, 1104
  trauma and, 25, 27, 200
  tumors, of skin, 519
Fatigue, heart disease and, 750
Fatty acids, 19–20
  deficiency, hyperalimentation and, 34
  shock and, 138
Fecaliths, appendicitis and, 1168, 1170
Feces, 976–977
  (See also Stool)
  impaction of, 1145–1146
Feeding (see Alimentation; Nutrition)
Feet (see Foot)
Felon, 1899–1900
Felty's syndrome, 1292
Female reproductive tract, 1589–1593
  (See also Gynecologic disorders:
    and specific structures involved)
  anatomy, morphologic, 1590–1593
  chronologic developmental physiology,
    1596–1597
  embryologic development, 1589–1590
  external genitalia, 1590
  infertility, 1605
  inherited defects, 1603–1604
  injuries, 245–246
  internal genitalia, 1590–1591
  pelvic environment, 1591–1593
  urethritis, 1561
Feminizing tumors, 1392

Femoral artery:
  aneurysms, 896
  aortic anastomosis with, 846
  injury, 870
Femoral hernia, 1347, 1357
Femoral nerve injury, 1977
Femoral vein:
  interruptions, 922
  ligation, 921, 931
  thrombosis, 915
Femoropopliteal disease, 848–851
  clinical manifestations and pathology, 848
  pathology, 848
  treatment, 849–851
Femur:
  amputation through, 1887
  arthroplasty, 1864
  fractures, 1819–1825
    cast-brace treatment, 1824–1825
    in children, 1821
    intertrochanteric and subtrochanteric, 1822
    neck, 1819–1821
    prosthesis for, 1821
    reduction and fixation, 1820
    shaft, 1822–1825
    Steinmann pin for, 1824
    supracondylar, 1825
  in hip dislocation, congenital, 1726, 1730
  necrosis of, renal transplants and, 426
  osteotomy, 1863
  shortening of, 1738–1739
  tumors of, 1778, 1782, 1783
Ferguson operation, 1355, 1357
Fertilization, 1589, 1597, 1605
Fetal antigens, 309–310
α-Fetoglobulin, 309
α-Fetoprotein, 310, 1191
Fetus:
  achondroplasia in, 1747–1748
  osteogenesis imperfecta in, 1750
  position, deformities from 1725–1726
Fever, 461
  in appendiceal rupture, 1171
  extracorporeal circulation and, 758
  in peritonitis, 1298, 1302
  trauma and, 4
Fiberoptic colonoscopy, 1131, 1147–1148
Fiberoptic oximetry, 505
Fibrillation, 759–762
  atrial: emboli from, 857
    in mitral stenosis, 763
  ventricular, 759–762
    in aortic stenosis, 690
    etiology, 759–760
Fibrin, allografts and, 365
Fibrinogen, 29, 99, 101, 104
  component therapy and, 35
  inherited abnormalities, 113–114
  labeled, 917
  transfusion of, 123, 124
Fibrinogenopenia, 30
Fibrinolysin, overproduction of, 30–31
Fibrinolysis, 101–102, 108, 114–115
  tests of, 104
Fibroadenoma, breast, 538
Fibroepithelial polyp, oral, 565
Fibroids, uterine, 1601, 1609–1610
Fibroma:
  bone, 1780
  cardiac, 793
  mesenteric, 1335
  oral, 565, 566
Fibroplasia, renal artery, 946–948, 954
Fibrosarcoma, 1781–1782
  hepatic, 1192
  of muscle, 1786–1787
  periosteal, 1784
  of skin, 521
Febrosis:
  mammary duct cancer and, 540

  in regional enteritis, 1090
  retroperitoneal, idiopathic, 1336–1338
  of sphincter of Oddi, 1243–1244
  vein graft, 798
Fibrositis, 1690
Fibrous dysplasia, 1749
  chest wall, 607
Fibrous mediastinitis, 661–662
Fibula, absence or dysplasia of, 1738
Fick principle, 503
Fingers:
  (See also Hand)
  amputations, 1889–1890, 1914–1917
  clubbing of, cyanosis and, 680
  extra, 1896
  fractures, 1818–1819
  mallet, or dropped tip, 1912
  replantation of severed, 1915, 1917
  in skin grafting, 1928
  tendon rupture, 1859
  webbed, 1895–1896
Fingernail infection, 1899
Finney pyloroplasty, 1065, 1066
Fissure, anal, 1151–1152
Fistula:
  in ano, 1153–1155
  aorticopulmonary, 734–735
  arteriovenous, 871–875
    coronary, 741–742
    dialysis and, 407–408
    pulmonary, 623
    splenic, 1196
  bronchoesophageal, 635
  bronchopleural, 616, 618–619
  cholecystoenteric, 1236
  colocutaneous, 1125
  coloenteric, 1125
  diverticulitis, 1125
  duodenal, following injury, 227
  in enteritis, 1091
  enterocutaneous, 1101–1102
  esophageal, 1031–1032
  gastrocolic, 1065
  in granulomatous colitis, 1117
  orocutaneous, 1945, 1947
  pancreatic, traumatic injury and, 241
  portal hypertension and, 1196
  small bowel, 1101–1102
  tracheoesophageal, 635, 1516–1521
Fistulotomy, anal, 1154, 1156
Five P's, 841
Flagellar immunogens, 355
Flail chest, 197
Flatfoot, 1713–1715, 1734
Flexor tendon injuries of hand, 1912–1913
Flexor tenosynovitis, 1902
Flow-guided catheterization, 501–503
Flowmeter for cardiac output, 507
Fluids and electrolytes, 65–86
  acid-base balance, 70–75
  ADH release and, 39–41
  anatomy of body fluids, 65–68
  in burns, 257, 260–263
    Brooke formula for, 262
  calcium abnormalities, 76–77
  cardiac arrest and, 759, 761
  chemical composition of compartments, 66
  in children, 1514–1515
  classification of changes, 68–78
  colloids, 147–148
  composition changes, 70–78, 81–82
  concentration changes, 68–69, 80–81
  crystalloids, 148–149
  distributional changes, 68
  extracellular fluid, 66–67
  extracorporeal circulation and, 757–758
  intestinal obstruction and, 980–982
  intracellular fluid, 66
  intraoperative, 82
  kidney transplantation and, 414–415

magnesium abnormalities, 77–78
mixed volume and concentration
    abnormalities, 69–70
normal exchange, 78–79
osmotic pressure, 67–68
pancreas and, 1257–1259, 1262
parenteral administration of, 79, 93–94
Parkland formula for, 262
in peptic ulcer, 1062
in peritonitis, 1300–1301, 1303
postoperative, 82–86
potassium abnormalities, 75–76
preoperative, 80–82
rate of fluid administration, 81
in renal failure, 1565–1566
salt gain and losses, 78–79, 84–85
in shock, 147–149
sweat and, 514–515
"third space" loss, 80
total body water, 65–66
volume changes, 68, 80, 84
water exchange, 78
Fluke, liver, 1241
Fluorocarbons, oxygen transport and, 35
Fluorohydrocortisone, 1381
5-Fluorouracil, 337
    in breast cancer, 550
    in colorectal cancer, 1138, 1140
    in hepatic carcinoma, 1192
    in ovarian cancer, 1621
Fluothane, 449–450
Fluroxene, 451
Flutter, atrial, postoperative, 471
Foley catheter for duodenal injury, 227
Folic acid antagonists, 377
Follicle-stimulating hormone, 6, 7, 1593,
    1597
    trauma and, 17
Follicular carcinoma of thyroid, 1451
Foot, 1712–1715
    amputations, 1882–1883
        in Buerger's disease, 867
        in tibioperoneal atherosclerosis, 853
    arches, 1712
    arthritis, 1857
    cerebral palsy and, 1702
    claw, 1699
    club, 1732–1734
    deformities, 1712–1715
    diabetic, 854–856
    drop, 1672
    flat, 1713–1715, 1734
    fractures and dislocations, 1833–1835
    immersion, 516, 904
    Köhler's disease, 1720–1721
    mechanics of, 1712–1713
    myelodysplasia and, 1703
    osteoarthritis, 1868–1869
    paralysis, 1698–1699
    strain, 1715
    trench, 516, 904
Footwear, 1714
Foramen:
    of Bochdalek, 1040–1041
    magnum, 1632–1633, 1655
Foramen:
    of Morgagni, 1041
    ovale, patent, 686, 687, 689
Forane, 451
Forbes-Albright syndrome, 1371
Forearm:
    amputations, 1891
    contracture, 1716–1717
    fractures, 1813–1814
    lacerations, 1912–1913
    spastic, 1697
Foreign bodies:
    airway, 627–628
    gastric, 1078
    in heart, 790

peritonitis and, 1309
small bowel, 1101
Fractures, 1791–1842
    acetabulum, 1837
    anesthesia for reductions, 1793–1794
    ankle, 1832–1833
    Bennett's, 1818
    bone injury, 1795–1797
    calcaneus, 1834–1835
    capitellum, 1813
    casts, plaster, 1800–1801
    in children, 1799
        (See also Children, fractures in)
    clavicle, 1794–1795
    closed vs. open reduction, 1799
    Colles, 1814–1815
    comminuted, 1792, 1811, 1823, 1834
    defense and demolition stage, 1796
    definitions, 1792
    delayed union of, 1797
    diagnosis, 1792
    elbow, 1808, 1810–1812
    epiphyseal plate injuries, 1798–1799
    evaluation of patient, 1793
    facial, 1936–1938
    femur, 1819–1825
    foot, 1833–1835
    forearm, 1813–1814
    greenstick, 1792, 1813
    hand, 1817–1819
    healing and regeneration, 1796–1797
    hip, 1837–1839
    humerus, 1806–1811
    immediate management of, 198, 1793
    lower extremity, 1819–1835
    mandibular, 1941
    maxillary, 1940–1941
    metacarpal, 1817–1818
    metatarsal, 1835
    navicular (wrist), 1816–1817
    nerve injuries and, 1795
    nonunion of, 1797
    nose, 1941
    open, 1794
    patella, 1828–1829
    pathologic, 1797
    pelvic, 1837–1839
    phalangeal (foot), 1835
    phalangeal (hand), 1818–1819
    radius, 1808–1809, 1813–1815
    rehabilitation from, 1972
    rib, 604–605
    shoulder dislocation and, 1806
    skull, 1634
    Smith, 1815
    spinal, 1839–1842
    stress, 1797–1798
    talus, 1833–1834
    tibia, 1829–1831
    traction for, 1801–1802
    ulna, 1809, 1813
    upper extremity, 1802–1819
    vascular injury and, 1794–1795
    vertebral, 1641–1643
    wrist, 1816–1817
    zygoma, 1939–1940
Freckles, 522
Fredet-Ramstedt operation, 1521, 1522
Freezing, organ, 434–435
Friedreich's ataxia, 1703
Frostbite, 904–906
Fructose, 34
FSH, 6, 7, 17, 1593, 1597
Fuel composition of man, 20
Fuel reserves, body, 86–87
Fundoplication, 1025, 1029
Fungal infections, 187–188
    actinomycosis, 187–188
    antibiotics for, 177
    blastomycosis, 188

candidiasis, 144, 177, 188, 1607
coccidioidomycosis, 188
histoplasmosis, 188
of lung, 638–640
shock and, 144
Funnel chest, 602–604
Furuncle, 169, 170
Fusobacterium, 187

Gait disturbances, 1706–1707
Galactosamine, bone and, 1741
Galactosemia, 1226
Galea, 1625
Gallbladder, 1221–1250
    anatomy, 1221–1223
    anomalies, 1223–1228
    bile secretion, 1228
    biliary atresia, 1224–1228
    carcinoma, 1244–1246
    cholangiomanometry, 1230–1231
    cholecystectomy, 1246–1248
    cholecystostomy, 1246
    common duct operations, 1248–1250
    cystic disease, 1224
    diagnosis of disease of, 1229–1231
    duct injuries, 1232–1233
    inflammation, 1236–1244
    injuries, 236–237
    motor dysfunction, 1229
    operations, 1246–1250
    physiology, 1228–1229
    retrograde dissection of, 1248
    roentgenograms, 1229–1230, 1237, 1239, 1240,
        1242, 1245
    stones (see Gallstones)
    trauma, 1231–1233
    tumors, 1244–1246
Gallstones, 1233–1236
    asymptomatic, 1234
    choledocholithiasis, 1234–1235
    composition of, 1233
    cystic duct obstruction by, 1234
    formation of, 1233–1234
    ileus, 541–542
    pancreatitis and, 1260
    pheochromocytoma and, 1414
Gamma globulin:
    in burns, 263
    serum hepatitis and, 128
Ganglia, 516
Ganglioneuroma, 1419
Gangrene:
    amputation for, 1882, 1884, 1886
    in Buerger's disease, 867
    diabetic foot, 856
    femoropopliteal disease and, 848–849
    gas, 182
    gastrointestinal resection and, 482
    ischemic colitis and, 1118–1119
    lung, 631
    progressive synergistic, 179–180
Gardner's syndrome, 1129
Gas:
    blood, measurement of, 498
    exchange, 465, 493, 498, 600
    gangrene, 182
    intestinal, 982, 984
    pleural, 611
    sterilization, 189
Gastrectomy:
    afferent (blind) loop syndrome following,
        482–483
    endocrine response to, 11
    fistulas following, 484–485
    partial, 1064–1066
    in portal hypertension, 1205
    stomal obstruction following, 482
    subtotal, 1081
    total, 1081

Gastric arteries, 1049
Gastric juice, 1052–1054
    (*See also* Stomach, secretion)
Gastrin, 1052, 1054
Gastritis, 1077–1078
    atrophic, 1079, 1083
    cancer and, 1079
    corrosive, 1077
    eosinophilic, 1077–1078
    gastric ulcer and, 1069–1070
    hemorrhagic, 1075
    hypertrophic, 1078, 1083
Gastrocolic fistula, 1065
Gastrocolic ligament, 1281
Gastrocolic trunk, 1256
Gastroduodenal artery, 1049
Gastroenteritis, acute, appendicitis vs., 1171
Gastroenterostomy, 1064, 1066
Gastroepiploic artery, 1049
Gastroepiploic vein, 1256
Gastroesophageal reflux, 1024, 1026–1027
Gastroileostomy, inadvertent, 483–484
    anastomotic leak, 484
    arterial supply, 1320–1322
    burns and, 258–259, 269
    clostridial infections of, 182–183
    complications of surgery of, 481–486
    extracorporeal circulation and, 759
    fistulas, 484–485
        (*See also* Fistula)
    gangrene, postoperative, 482
    hemorrhage, 481–482, 991–997
        (*See also* Hemorrhage, gastrointestinal)
    hyperkalemia symptoms, 75
    hyperparathyroidism and, 1473
    manifestations of disease, 967–1004
        anorexia, 974–975
        bleeding, 991–997
        constipation and diarrhea, 976–979
        dysphagia, 973–974
        ileus, 990–991
        jaundice, 997–1004
        nausea and vomiting, 975–976
        obstruction, 979–991
        pain, 967–973
    mechanical postoperative problems, 988–990
    secretions, composition of, 76
    transplants, 391
    trauma and, 48–49
    venous drainage, 1322–1324
Gastrojejunal fistulas, 484
Gastroscopy, 1072
Gastroschisis, 1523–1524
Gastrosplenic ligament, 1281
Gastrostomy:
    feeding, 90
    for tracheoesophageal fistula, 1517
Gaucher's disease, 1293
Gelfoam, 120, 233
Genetic factors:
    adrenal hyperplasia and, 1390
    in cancer, 301–302
        breast, 533
        gastric, 1079
    in clubfoot, 1732
    hemostatic defects and, 108
    histocompatibility and, 352–353
    in hyperparathyroidism, 1483
    peptic ulcer and, 1057, 1070
    polyposis and, 1128–1129
    reproductive defects, female, 1603–1604
    in sexual development disorders, 1393, 1394
Genitourinary tract:
    (*See also* Kidney; Urinary bladder; *and* other
        portions)
    anatomy, 1547–1549, 1590–1593
    anorectal surgery and, 1149
    calculi, 1561–1564
    diagnosis, 1549–1555
    examination, 1551–1552

female (*see* Female reproductive tract)
infections, 1558–1561
    acute, 1558–1560
    appendicitis vs., 1171
    chronic, 1560–1561
    clostridial, 183
    gonorrheal (*see* Gonococcal infections)
    lymphogranuloma venereum, 1159
injuries, 1580
instrumentation, 1553
operations, 1580–1587
    rectal cancer involving, 1136
secretions, 1552–1553
Gentamicin, 157, 173, 176
Genu recurvatum, congenital, 1732
Genu valgum, 1711
    in rickets, 1757
Genu varum, 1712
Geographic factors in cancer, 302
GH, 15–16, 22
Giant cell granuloma, gingival, 565–566
Giant cell tumor of bone, 1782–1783
Gibbs-Donnan equation, 67
Gigantism, 1369–1371
    digital, 1896–1897
    osteoporosis and, 1764–1765
Gillies operation, 1958, 1959
Gingivae:
    cancer of, 569–570
    fibroma of, 566
    granuloma of, 565–566
Girdlestone pseudarthrosis, 1857
Gliomas, 1646, 1651
Glisson's capsule, 1194
Globulin:
    α_2-AP, 28
    antilymphocyte, 373–374
    gamma (*see* Gamma globulin)
    synovial fluid, 1838
Glomerular filtration rate, high-output renal
    failure and, 86
Glomerulonephritis, renal transplantation and,
    405, 421–422
Glomus tumor, 518–519
Glottis, 559
Glove powder peritonitis, 1308–1309
Glucagon, 16, 1259
    in shock, 152
    starvation and, 22
Glucocorticoids, 13, 1377
Glucocorticosteroids in shock, 153
Gluconeogenesis, 19, 22, 26, 28
Glucosamine, bone and, 1741
Glucose:
    excess, in diabetes, 473
        (*See also* Diabetes)
    glucagon and, 16
    intravenous, 32
    starvation and, 20–24
    trauma and, 26
Glucose-6-phosphate deficiency, 1287
Glucuronic acid, bone and, 1741
Glycerol, 27
Glycogen, 19, 20
    storage disease, portacaval shunt for, 1214
Glycoproteins, AP-reactant, 28–29
Goiter, 1445–1449
    benign metastasizing, 1451
    clinical manifestations, 1439, 1446–1447
    diagnostic findings, 1447
    diffuse (nonnodular), 1447–1448
    endemic, 1446
    etiology, 1438, 1445–1446
    familial, 1446
Goiter, intrathoracic, 664–665, 1454–1455
    lymphadenoid, 1443–1444
    multinodular, 1438, 1439, 1448
    pathology, 1446
    sporadic, 1446
    treatment, 1447–1449

Goldstein technique, 1710
Gompertzian growth, 332, 333
Gonadal dysgenesis, 1604
    mixed, 1394
Gonadotropins, 6, 1366, 1593–1594
    cells secreting, 1365
    ectopic secretion of, 1374
    human chorionic, 1593–1594
    urinary, total, 1594
Gonococcal infections (gonorrhea), 1608
    arthritis, 1852–1853
    proctitis, 1158–1159
    urethritis, 1559
Goodsall's rule, 1154
Gout, 1869–1870
    hyperparathyroidism and, 1487–1488
Graafian follicle, 1595, 1597
    cysts, 1619
    rupture, appendicitis vs., 1172
Grafting (*see* Skin grafting; Transplantation)
    bypass (*see* Bypass procedures)
    nerve, 1644
Graft-versus-host reaction, 355
    bone marrow transplantation and, 388
    cellular interactions in, 357–358
Gram-negative microorganisms, 185–187
    bacteremia, 1558
    shock (*see* Shock, endotoxin)
Gram-positive microorganisms:
    antibiotics for, 174–177
    shock and, 144
Granuloma:
    eosinophilic, 607–608, 1769, 1770
    gingival, 565–566
    inguinale, 1608
    pyogenicum, 566
    regional enteritis and, 1090, 1091
    venal caval obstruction by, 835
Granulomatosis:
    histiocytic, 1769
    lipoid, 1769–1770
Granulomatous colitis, 1116–1118
Granulosa-theca cell tumor, 1622
Graves' disease, 1437–1438, 1439
    clinical manifestations, 1439
    diagnosis, 1439
    treatment, 1441
Griseofulvin, 177
Groin dissection for melanoma, 523–524
Groin hernia, 1345, 1346–1348, 1354–1358
Ground substance, 281–282, 1741
Growth hormone, 15–16, 1366–1367
    acromegaly and gigantism and, 1369–1371
    starvation and, 22
Guillain-Barré syndrome, 1679
Gums (*see* Gingivae)
Gunshot wounds, 225
GVH reaction (*see* Graft-versus-host reaction)
Gynecologic disorders, 1589–1630
    appendicitis vs., 1172
    cervical cancer, 1611–1615
    embryology and, 1589–1590
    endocrinologic factors, 1593–1597
    endometriosis, 1608–1609
    examination, 1597–1598
    fallopian tube tumors, 1622–1623
    infections and discharges, 1607–1608
    morphologic anatomy and, 1590–1593
    operations, 1623–1630
        dilatation and curettage, 1623–1624
        ectopic pregnancy, 1625
        hysterectomy, 1627–1630
        incisions, 1624–1625
        salpingo-oophorectomy, 1625–1627
    ovarian tumors, 1619–1622
    psychiatric complications in, 480
    symptoms, 1598–1607
        bleeding, 1601–1603
        hirsutism and masculinization, 1603
        incontinence, 1599–1601

in inherited defects, 1603–1604
pain, 1598–1599, 1610
in pregnancy, 1605–1607
in reproductive capacity, 1605
uterine, 1609–1617
vaginal, 1619
venereal disease, 1608
vulvar, 1617–1619
Gynecomastia, 531, 1961

H zone, 1692
H-2 alloantigens, 351–352
Hageman factor (XII), 99, 365
Hair transplants, 1924, 1925
Hairline injuries, 1943
Hallux, claw, 1699
Hallux valgus, 1868–1869
Halothane, 449–450
liver function and, 48
in pheochromocytoma surgery, 1416
Halsted operation, 1355, 1357
Hamartoma:
liver, 1189
pulmonary, 642
Hamster cheek-pouch graft, 381–382
Hand, 1895–1917
abscess, 1899
amputations, 1889–1891, 1913–1914
arthritis, 1900, 1905
rheumatoid, 1854–1855, 1857
arthroplasty, 1858–1859
atrophy of muscles of, 1704
burns of, 270
congenital abnormalities, 1895–1897
Dupuytren's contracture, 1715–1716
enchondromas, 1779
felon, 1899–1900
fractures and dislocations, 1817–1819
grooves, circumferential, 1896
incisions, 1907, 1916
infection, 1897–1901, 1904–1905
injuries, 1901–1917
clinical manifestations, 1901–1907
treatment, 1907–1913
ligaments, 1905–1907
macrodactyly, 1896–1897
missing parts, 1896
muscular function, 1904–1905
nerves, 1904, 1908–1911
pain, 1679, 1917
palmar space infections, 1900, 1905
paralysis, 1700
paronychia, 1899, 1905
postoperative care, 1917
rehabilitation, 1975
spastic, 1705
syndactyly, 1895–1896
tendons, 1900, 1901, 1911–1913, 1975
tenosynovitis, 1900, 1905
wringer injury, 1907–1908
Hand-Schüller-Christian disease, 1769
Haplotype, 352
Harrington rod, 1710, 1711
Hartmann's pouch, 1222
Hashimoto's disease, 1443–1444
Head:
burns, 269–270
congenital anomalies, 1947–1954
examination of, 557–560
hematoma, 1638–1641
epidural, 1639–1640
intracerebral, 1640–1641, 1661
subdural, 1638–1639
hemorrhage, 1637–1638
injuries, 1633–1641
ADH secretion and, 14
brain, 1634–1635
care of, 1635–1637
facial (see Face)

scalp, 1633
skull, 1633–1634
postoperative care of, 590–591
soft tissue losses, 1945–1946
tumors, 555–591
(See also specific areas)
chemotherapy for, 585–586
diagnosis, 557–561
historical background, 555–557
hypopharynx, 576
larynx, 573–576
lip, 561–564
mandible, 579–580
nasal cavity and paranasal sinuses, 578–579
nasopharynx, 576–578
operations for, 586–591
oral cavity, 564–571
oropharynx, 571–572
plastic surgery, 1936–1938
salivary gland, 580–584
Headaches, spinal anesthesia and, 456
Healing, 31–32, 275–294, 1920
amputation, 1880
bone, 1642, 1796–1797
catalyst for, 290
collagen and, 282–286
contraction and, 275–278
epithelization and, 278–281
ground substance and, 281–282
lag phase of, 277, 286
secondary, 287
sequence of events in, 286–287
Heart, 677–743, 749–810
(See also specific diseases)
acquired disease, 749–810
catheterization, 752
clinical manifestations, 749–752
electrocardiography, 751
history, 749–750
multivalvular, 787
pathophysiology, 752–753
physical examination, 750–751
radiology, 751–752
aortic insufficiency, acquired, 780–784
aortic-pulmonary window, 734–735
aortic stenosis, 690–696, 774–779
arrest (see Cardiac arrest)
artificial, 809
assisted circulation, 808–809
atrial septal defects, 704–712
block, 803–807
etiology, 803
historical data, 803
pathology and pathophysiology, 803–804
prognosis, 807
treatment, 804–807
ventricular septal defect and, 716
carcinoid syndrome and, 1098–1099
catheterization, 683
(See also Catheterization, cardiac)
coarctation of aorta, 696–701
complications, postoperative, 469–473
conduction, 803, 804
congenital disease, 677–743
classification, 678
complex malformations, 727–732
examination, clinical, 681–684
infant care, 684–685
left-to-right shunts, 679–680, 704–721
obstructive lesions, 678, 685–704
pathophysiology, 678–681
rare malformations, 732–743
right-to-left shunts, 680–681, 721–727
coronary artery anomalies, 739–741
coronary artery disease, 793–799
cor triatriatum, 733
Ebstein's anomaly, 738–739
electrical resistance of, 804
emboli from, 857–861
extracorporeal circulation and, 753–759

failure: in aortic stenosis, 690, 691, 776
extracorporeal circulation and, 756–757
mesenteric infarction and, 1327
myocardial ischemia and, 794
in tetralogy of Fallot, 722
transposition of great vessels and, 728
trauma and, 788
in ventricular septal defect, 713
fibrillation, 759–762
foramen ovale, patent, 686
foreign bodies, 790
massage, 760–761
metastatic neoplasms of, 792
mitral insufficiency, 771–774
mitral stenosis, 733–734, 762–771
monitoring, 499–508
murmurs (see Murmurs)
myxoma, 791–792
output (see Cardiac output)
pacemakers, 803–807
patent ductus arteriosus, 716–721
pericarditis, 801–803
acute pyogenic, 801–802
chronic constrictive, 802–803
pheochromocytoma and, 1413
psychiatric complications in operations on, 480–481
pulmonic stenosis, 685–690
rehabilitation, 1980
resuscitation, 760–762
rhabdomyoma, 793
rings, vascular, 701–704
sarcoma, 792–793
septal defects (see Atrial septal defects;
Ventricular septal defects)
single ventricle, 737–738
sinus of Valsalva, ruptures aneurysm of, 735–736
size and shape, 682, 764
sounds, 682
in aortic insufficiency, 783
in aortic stenosis, 776
in atrial septal defects, 705, 710
in hypertension, 940
in mitral insufficiency, 772
in mitral stenosis, 764–765
in pulmonic stenosis, 687
in tricuspid atresia, 732
in ventricular septal defect, 714
tamponade, 197, 756, 788, 789
tetralogy of Fallot, 721–727
transplants (see Transplantation, heart)
transposition of great vessels, 727–730
corrected, 742–743
trauma, 787–790
tricuspid atresia, 730–732
tricuspid stenosis and insufficiency, 784–787
truncus arteriosus, 736–737
tumors, 790–793
valves: aortic, 690–696, 768–784
mitral, 733–734, 762–774
multivalvular disease, 787
pulmonic, 685–690
tricuspid, 730–732, 784–787
ventricular aneurysm, 799–801
ventricular septal defects, 712–716
Heartburn, 1024
Heart-lung machines (see Extracorporeal circulation)
Heat:
exhaustion, 516
in physical therapy, 1968–1969
transfer, burns and, 253–254
Heberden's nodes, 1861
Hegar dilators, 688, 691
Heidenhain pouches, 1051, 1052
Heinecke-Mikulicz pyloroplasty, 1065, 1066
Heller esophagomyotomy, 1016
Hemangiofibroma, juvenile nasopharyngeal, 577

Hemangioma:
  bone, 1786
  capillary, 518, 566–567
  cavernous, 518, 623
  immature, 518
  lip, 562
  liver, 1189–1190
  lymphedema vs., 933
  mediastinal, 669
  oral, 566–567
  sclerosing, 518
  skin, 518
  small bowel, 1095
Hemangiopericytoma, 519, 521
Hemarthrosis, 109, 110
Hematemesis, 991, 994
  esophagogastric varices and, 1200
Hematobilia, 235, 1182
Hematoma:
  abdominal wall, 247
  in aneurysm, traumatic, 900
  dissecting, 826
  epidural, 1639–1640
  intracerebral, 1640–1641, 1661
  intramural, 229
  intramural, in hemophilia, 109, 111
  mediastinal, 660, 831, 832
  pancreatic, 1266
  rectus sheath, 1313–1315
  retroperitoneal, 242–243
  subcutaneous, postoperative, 464
  subscleral, 1939
Hematuria, 1549
  trauma and, 198
Hemicolectomy, 1134
Hemiotruncus, 737
Hemipelvectomy, 1888
  for cancer, 325
Hemodialysis:
  fistulas and, arteriovenous, 407–408
  indwelling cannulas, 407
  peritoneal dialysis vs., 1313
  renal transplant and, 406–408
Hemoglobin:
  component therapy and, 34–35
  hemolysis and, 127
  oxygen transport and, 495
  in peritonitis, 1300
  phosphates, 42
  preoperative therapy and, 82
  in sickle cell disease, 1288
  in thalassemia, 1287
Hemolysis:
  biliary atresia and, 1226
  burns and, 256
  transfusion and, 107, 126–127
Hemolytic anemia, 1284–1285, 1287–1289, 1772
Hemolytic jaundice, 1000, 1002
Hemoperitoneum, 1309
Hemophilia, 109–111
  arthritis in, 1871–1872
  transfusion in, 123, 124
  unsuspected, 30
Hemopneumothorax, 612
Hemopoietic stem cell, 353
Hemopoietic tissues, transplantation of, 388–389
Hemoptysis, 601
  in bronchiectasis, 629
  heart disease and, 750
  in lung cancer, 646
  in mitral stenosis, 763
  in pulmonary embolism, 920
Hemorrhage:
  adrenal, 1402
  aortic injury and, 829
  arterial injury and, 868, 869
  biliary tract, 235–236
  coagulation and, 29
  corticosteroids and, 9
  diverticulosis coli and, 1122–1123

endoscopy in, 994–995
esophagogastric varices, 992, 1200, 1201
evaluation of, during or after surgery, 107–108
extracorporeal circulation and, 756
gastrointestinal, 481–482, 991–997
  in burns, 269
  consequences of, 991
  definitions, 991
  diagnosis, 994–996, 997
  etiology, 992–994, 996–997
  lower, 996–997
  Mallory-Weiss syndrome, 1039
  mucosal lesions, acute, 1075, 1076
  transplanted kidney and, 425
  upper, 992–996
gynecologic, 1600–1604, 1611
hand injury, 1907
hemophiliac, 109–111
  arthritis and, 1871–1872
hiatal hernia, 993
intracranial, 1637–1638, 1660
intrathoracic, 788, 790
liver, 234, 235, 1182, 1193
local procedures for, 119–121
menstrual (see Menstruation)
multiple transfusions and, 30
peptic ulcer, 992, 995, 1061, 1067
petechial, fat embolism and, 476
pressure techniques for, 119–120
rectal, postoperative, 1148–1149
rectus sheath, 1313–1315
resuscitation and, 196–197
retinopathy, 1372–1373
retroperitoneal, 242–243, 1331
scalp, 1633
shock and, 133–138
small bowel tumors and, 1095
stress ulcer, 992
thyroid wound, 1454
trauma and, 2
uterine fibroids, 1609–1610
wound, postoperative, 464
Hemorrhoid(s), 1149–1151
  clinical manifestations, 1150
  etiology, 1149–1150
  prognosis, 1151
  treatment, 1150–1151
Hemorrhoidal arteries, 1322
Hemorrhoidal veins, 1323
Hemorrhoidectomy, 1150–1151
Hemostasis, 97–129
  biology of normal, 97–102
  chemical agents for, 120–121
  clinical defects, 108–119
  evaluation of risk, 105–108
  inheritance of defects, 108–109
  local, 119–121
  mechanical procedures for, 119–120
  schematic representation of, 98
  tests, 102–105
  thermal agents for, 120
Hemostat, 119
Hemothorax, 197, 614
Henderson-Hasselbalch equation, 71
Henle's loop, hyperparathyroidism and, 1471
Henoch-Schönlein purpura, appendicitis vs., 1172
Heparin, 118
  aortic aneurysm repair and, 821, 822
  in aortic endarterectomy, 846
  in cardioarterial embolism, 859, 861
  defibrination syndrome and, 114
  in extracorporeal circulation, 753, 754, 756
  for fat embolism, 477
  iatrogenic hemostasis and, 108
  prothrombin time and, 103
  rebound phenomenon, 756
  renal hypertension operation and, 957
  for venous thrombosis, 944–945
Hepatectomy, 1191

Hepatic artery, 1178, 1183, 1259
  anomalies, 1223–1224
  anastomosis in liver transplant, 396
  ligation of, in portal hypertension, 379
  –portal venous fistula, 1196
  in resection of liver, 1194
  rupture, 1332
Hepatic ducts, 1221, 1223
  carcinoma, 1245
Hepatic function (see Liver)
Hepatic venous system, 1178, 1184, 1197
Hepatic venule catheterization, 1197–1198
Hepaticocholedochostomy, 1233
Hepaticojejunostomy, 1224
  neonatal, 1226
  serum, 128–129
Hepatitis:
  cholangitis and, 1241–1242
Hepatofugal circulation, 1198–1199
Hepatopetal circulation, 1196, 1198
Hepatorenal syndrome, 1182
Hepatosplenomegaly, renal tumors and, 1571
Heredity (see Genetic factors)
Herellea vaginicola, 186
Hermaphroditism, 1391, 1394, 1604
Hernias:
  abdominal wall, 1345–1360
  anatomy, 1346–1348
  bilateral, 1357–1358
  chest wall, 604
  complications, 1350
  definition of, 1345–1346
  diaphragmatic, 1023–1025
  diverticulosis coli, 1121
  etiology, 1348–1349
  femoral, 1347, 1358
  groin, 1345, 1346–1348, 1354–1358
  hiatal, 1023–1025
    hemorrhage, 993
  incisional, 1358–1359
  inguinal, 1346–1348, 1355–1357
  interparietal, 1345
  intervetebral disc, 1671–1672, 1686–1689
  lumbar, 1345
  mesenteric, 1320
  paraesophageal, 1023
  pelvic, 1599–1601
  pleural, 611–612
  Richter's, 1350
  scrotal, 1347
  sliding, 1345, 1346, 1352–1353, 1355
    hiatal, 1023–1025
  Spigelian, 1345
  strangulated, 1345, 1351
  symptoms and signs, 1349–1350
  treatment, 1350–1360
  umbilical, 1348, 1358
  ventral, 1345, 1358–1359
Herniorrhaphy, 1350–1360
Hesselbach's triangle, 1346–1347, 1354, 1355
Hessing braces, 1872, 1873
Heterozygous bleeding disorders, 108
Hexachlorophene, 189
5-HIAA, 1098–1100
Hiatal hernia, 1023–1025
Hidradenitis suppurativa, 516
Hidradenomas, 1618–1619
Hilar duct carcinoma, 1245–1246
Hilar lymphadenopathy, 663
Hill's hiatal hernia repair, 1025, 1026
Hilus cell tumors, ovarian, 1622
Hip:
  arthritis, 1857
  arthrodesis, 1863
  arthroplasty, 1863–1864
  cerebral palsy and, 1700
  disarticulation, 1887–1888
  dislocation, 1835–1837
  dislocation, congenital, 1726–1731
    clinical manifestations, 1727–1728

differential diagnosis, 1728
pathogenesis, 1726–1727
prognosis, 1729
treatment, 1729–1731
drainage, posterior, 1850
femoral osteotomy, 1863
forces across, 1864
myelodysplasia and, 1703
osteoarthritis, 1862–1867
osteochondritis, 1718–1720
paralysis, 1699
prostheses, 1865–1867
pyogenic, 1849
replacement, 1864–1867
tuberculosis of, 1852
Hippuran, renal transplants and, 416, 418
Hippurate, 1555
Hirschsprung's disease, 1145, 1531–1536
clinical manifestations, 1532
diagnostic studies, 1532–1533
pathology, 1531–1532
prognosis, 1534–1536
treatment, 1533–1534
Hirsutism, 1603
Histalog, gastric secretion and, 1056
Histamine, 14
in pheochromocytoma, 1410
tests, 1060, 1880
Histiocytic granulomatosis, 1769
Histocompatibility antigens, 351–353, 380
kidney transplantation and, 408–409
matching, 382–383
Histoplasmosis, 188, 638
HL-A antigens, 338, 339, 352, 382
Hodgkin's disease, 1291–1292
bone changes in, 1768–1769
mediastinum and, 666
staging extent of, 320
Hofmeister gastrectomy, 1064
Hollander insulin test, 1060
Homans' sign, 915
Homografts (see Allografts)
Homovanillic acid, 1405, 1411
Homozygous bleeding disorders, 108
Hormones:
(See also individual hormones)
adrenal, 1377–1380
daily secretion of, 13
endotoxin effects on, 3
gastric function and, 1053, 1057
hypothalamic control of, 5–6
pituitary, 1364–1367
skin absorption of, 514
starvation and, 936
thyroid, 1431–1432
trauma and, 1–2, 5–17
Host defense:
burns and, 256
foreign cell graft and, 388
immunotherapy and, 337
Hot packs, 1969
Houston's valves, 1146
Howard test, 954, 955
Howell-Jolly bodies, 1283
Howship's lacunae, 1782
Hubbard tank, 1968
Huhner's test, 1605
Human chorionic gonadotropin, 1593–1594
Humerus:
amputation through, 1892
chondroblastoma of, 1780
dislocations, 1804–1806
fractures of, 1806–1811
Humoral antibody, 363–364
Hunter's canal, 900
Hunter syndrome, 1766
Hurler syndrome, 1765
Hürthle cells, 1451
Hutchinson freckle, 522
Hyaluronic acid, bone and, 1741

Hydatid cysts, 1188–1189
of lung, 640
Hydatidiform moles, 1606
Hydration, 41
Hydrocele, 1551, 1579
Hydrocelectomy, 1585
Hydrocephalus, 1654–1656
Hydrochloric acid of stomach, 1053–1054
Hydrocortisone:
for idiopathic thrombocytopenic purpura, 116
in shock, 152
Hydrolases, acid, bone and, 1742
Hydronephrosis, 1569–1570
Hydrotherapy, 1968–1969
Hydroxyandrostenedione, 13
17-Hydroxycorticosteroids, 1596
in amenorrhea, 1603
anesthesia and, 9, 10
in burns, 12, 15
in Cushing's syndrome, 944
in diabetes insipidus, 12
endotoxin effects on, 3
immobilization and, 4
immunologic protection and, 43
nerve impulse effect on, 11
suppression of, 1385
trauma and, 24, 25, 199
5-Hydroxyindole acetic acid, 1098–1100
Hydroxypregnenolone, 13
Hydroxyproline, 282, 1461, 1478, 1741
5-Hydroxytryptamine (see Serotonin)
Hydroxyzine, 458
Hygroma:
cystic, 1515–1516
subdural, 1639
Hymen, imperforate, 1604
Hymenoptera bites, 214
Hypaque, 1553
Hyperabduction syndrome, 876
Hyperacidity, 1056–1057, 1070
Hyperalimentation (see Alimentation)
Hyperammonemia, 1203
Hyperbaric therapy, 169
Hyperbilirubinemia, 998–999
congenital, 1226
Hypercalcemia, 77
differential diagnosis of, 1488–1490
in hyperparathyroidism, 1465, 1472–1473, 1487
crisis, 1473–1474, 1490–1491
metastases to bone and, 1789
peptic ulcer and, 1475
Hypercalcinuria, differential diagnosis of, 1488, 1489
Hypercoagulation, 29
Hyperglycemia, 24, 26
in diabetes, 473
hyponatremia and, 85
parenteral feeding and, 95
Hyperhidrosis, 515
Hyperinsulinism, 1274–1276
Hyperkalemia, 75
renal failure and, 1565
Hyperkeratosis:
laryngeal, 574
lip, 562–563
oral cavity, 567
Hyperlipemia, pancreatitis and, 1261
Hypermagnesemia, 78
Hypernatremia, 69
therapy for, 80–81, 85
Hyperparathyroidism, 1466–1499
adenomas and, 1467, 1482
alkaline phosphatase in, 1478
arthralgia in, 1487
bone biopsy and densitometry in, 1479
calcification in, 1473
calcium levels in, 1471, 1477, 1479, 1480, 1490, 1498
carcinoma and, 1467–1468
in children, 1483–1484

chloride levels in, 1478
clinical manifestations, 1471–1477
cortisone administration in, 1479
crisis, hypercalcemic, 1473–1474, 1490–1491
diagnostic findings, 1477–1483
differential diagnosis, 1488–1490, 1762
ectopic, 1469–1470
endocrinopatheis, multiple, 1486–1487
familial, 1483
frequency of entities producing, 1466
gastrointestinal symptoms, 1473
gout, pseudogout in, 1487–1488
historical background, 1457
hydroxyproline in, 1478
hyperplasia and, 1468–1469
hypertension and, 1476
incidence, 1471–1472
kidney function and, 1471, 1472–1473, 1476
calculi and, 1564
mental changes in, 1473
muscle weakness and, 1473
osteodystrophy and, 1760–1761
pancreatic beta cell tumor and, 1486–1487
pancreatitis and, 1476
pathology, 1466–1471
peptic ulcer and, 1475–1476, 1487
phosphate levels in, 1477–1478, 1479, 1498
physical findings, 1477
plasma PTH in, 1479–1480
in pregnancy, 1484–1486
primary, 1466–1496
roentgenography, 1480–1482
secondary, 1497–1498
skeletal changes, 1470–1471, 1472, 1474–1475, 1491
squeeze test in, 1480
symptoms, 1472–1477
hypercalcemia related, 1472–1474
PTH direct action and, 1474–1476
renal damage and, 1476
urinary calcium related, 1474
tertiary, 1498–1499
treatment, 1490–1496
of crisis, 1490–1491
mediastinal exploration, 1495–1496
operative technique, 1491–1495
postoperative complications, 1496
tumors and, 1467–1470
nonparathyroid, 1469–1470
Zollinger-Ellison syndrome and, 1475, 1487
Hyperpituitarism, osteoporosis and, 1764–1765
Hyperplasia:
endometrial, 1615–1616
oral cavity, 564–565, 567
parathyroid, 1468–1469
renal artery, 946–948, 954
Hyperpyrexia, malignant, 454
Hypersensitivity, dinitrochlorobenzene, 310
Hypersplenism, 1283, 1290
functional abnormality in, 1284
portal hypertension and, 1202–1203
primary, 1290
secondary, 1290
Hypertension, 939–964
adrenalectomy for, 1395
aldosteronism and, 942–943, 1396
burns and, in children, 269
cerebral hemorrhage and, 1660
classification, 941
clinical manifestations, 940
of coarctation, 697, 945–946
Cushing's syndrome and, 943–945
dissecting aneurysm and, 828, 829
essential, 963–964
hormones and, 939–940
hyperparathyroidism and, 1476
laboratory studies, 940–941
pheochromocytoma and, 942, 1408, 1409, 1414
physiology and pathophysiology, 939–940
portal, 1196–1214
(See also Portal hypertension)

Hypertension, pulmonary, 679, 753
   in mitral stenosis, 763
   in ventricular septal defect, 713
  renovascular, 946–962
   (*See also* Renovascular hypertension)
  tamponade and, 789
  transplanted kidney and, 425
Hyperthyroidism:
  clinical manifestations, 1438–1439
  pituitary, 1372
Hypertrophic subaortic stenosis, 694–695
Hyperuricemia, gout and, 1869
Hyperventilation, alkalosis and, 37, 73
Hypocalcemia, 76
  parathyroidectomy and, 1496
Hypocalcemic agents, 1491
Hypocapnia, 47
Hypocoagulation, 29–31
Hypofibrinogenemia, acquired, 114–115
Hypogastric arteries, 845, 1591
  transplantation of kidney and, 415
Hypoglycemia, 24, 27
  GH release and, 15
  islet-cell tumor and, 1275
  trauma and, 4
Hypokalemia, 75–76
  aldosteronism and, 943
  metabolic alkalosis and, 74
Hypomagnesemia, 77, 1460
Hyponatremia, 41–42, 69
  postoperative management of, 84–85
  postthyroidectomy, 1456–1457
  therapy for, 80–81
Hypoparathyroidism, 1457, 1500
  parathyroidectomy and, 1496
Hypopharynx, 576
Hypophosphatasia, 1759
Hypophosphatemia, intravenous alimentation
  and, 33
Hypophyseal artery, 1364
Hypophysectomy:
  for acromegaly, 1370
  for carcinoma, 1373
   of breast, 550
  for diabetic retinopathy, 1372
  in hypopituitarism, 1368
Hypophysis (*see* Pituitary)
Hypopituitarism, 1367–1368
Hypoplasia, lung, 622
Hypoprothrombinemia, 30
  inherited, 113
Hypospadias, 1570, 1962–1964
Hypotension:
  aortic occlusion and, 891
  barbiturates and, 451–452
  halothane anesthesia and, 449
  liver transplantation and, 397
  mesenteric infarction and, 1327
  pheochromocytoma and, 1414–1415
Hypothalamus:
  hormone control by, 5–6
  median eminence of, 6–8
  releasing factors, 1593–1594
Hypothermia, 120
  ACTH and, 4, 5
  in amputations, 1880
  in esophagogastric varices, 1200
  liver transplants and, 397
  storage of organs and, 433
Hypothyroidism, 1442–1443
  bone disease and 1765
Hypoventilation:
  atelectasis and, 467
  postoperative, 204, 465–466, 467
  resection of lung and, 657–658
Hypovolemia:
  acidosis and, 38
  gastrointestinal function and, 49
  perforated ulcer and, 1063
  in peritonitis, 1301

  resuscitation and, 196
  trauma and, 2
Hypoxia:
  cellular, 496
  monitoring and, 494, 508
  organ storage and, 432
  surgical, 46, 47
Hysterectomy, 1627–1630
  vaginal, 1599–1600

Icterus index, 1003, 1237
Ileal conduit, 1581–1583
Ileitis:
  "backwash," 1111
  terminal (*see* Enteritis, regional)
Ileocecal nodes, 1332
Ileocolic artery, 1321
Ileocolostomy, 1093
Ileofemoral vein thrombosis, 915
Ileoproctostomy, 1116, 1118
Ileostomy, 1116, 1118
  complications, 485–486
Ileum:
  adenocarcinoma, 1096
  arteries of, 1321
  atresia, congenital, 1526, 1528, 1529
  bleeding, 996
  carcinoids, 1097
  diverticula, 1100, 1101
  fistulas of, postoperative, 485
  in intestinal bypass operations, 1105
  Peutz-Jeghers syndrome and, 1096
  regional enteritis, 1090–1094
  short bowel syndrome and, 1103–1104
  urinary diversion and, 1581–1583
Ileus, 990–991
  adynamic, 990, 1301clinical manifestations,
   990
  gallstone, 1235–1236
  meconeum, 1529
  paralytic, 990, 991
  spastic, 990
  treatment, 990–991
  vascular occlusion, 990
Iliac arteries, 843–847, 1591
Iliac vein, transplantation of kidney and, 414
Ilioinguinal nerve, 1354
Immersion foot, 516, 904
Immobilization, 4
Immune apparatus, 353–354
Immunity:
  afferent arc of, 355
  efferent arc of, 359, 366–369
  expression of, 359–364
  induction of, 355–359
Immunization:
  rabies, 209–210
  tetanus, 184
Immunogens:
  flagellar, 355
  graft release of, 355
  lymphocyte recognition of, 356–357
  processing of, 355–356
Immunoglobulins:
  burns and, 256
  structure of, 364
  thyroid, 1436, 1439
  transplant rejection and, 356–357
Immunology, 304–333, 352–371
  allograft, 352–371
  cellular interactions, 357–358
Immunology:
  competence, 310–311, 359
  enhancement, 308, 380–381
  histocompatibility antigens and, 351–353
  indifference, 307
  molecular cascade systems and, 364–371
  morphologic changes of lymphocyte and,
   358–359

  neoplastic specificity, 305–306
  protective mechanisms, 42–44
  rejection of allograft and, 354–364
  rejection, tumor-specific, 306–307
  surveillance, 307–308
  tolerance, 307–308, 379–380
  of tumors, 304–313
  ulcerative colitis and, 1090–1091
Immunosuppression, 307, 371–379
  antilymphocyte globulin, 373–374
  drugs, 376–378
  kidney transplants and, 415, 416, 422–426
  liver transplants and, 1196
  lymphoid tissue extirpation and, 372
  radiation and, 374–376
   extracorporeal, 372–373
  thoracic duct drainage and, 372
  thymectomy and, 372
  in ulcerative colitis, 1115
Immunotherapy for cancer, 337–342
  active, 338
  nonspecific, 340–342
  passive and adoptive, 339–340
Impedance, electrical, 917
Impetigo, 169
Imuran, 376
Inandione, 118
Incisions:
  bilateral subcostal, 1418
  collar, 1453
  emergency laparotomy, 205
  gynecologic, 1624–1625
  hand operations, 1907, 1916
  hernias, 1358–1359
  low transverse abdominal, 1583
  lumbar, 1581
  McBurney, 1173
  midline abdominal, 1582
  neck, 218, 219, 586
  parathyroidectomy, 1492
  Pfannenstiel, 1624, 1625
  scrotal and inguinal, 1585–1587
  subcostal transabdominal, 1212
  thoracoabdominal, 1212
  thyroidectomy, 1453, 1454
Incisura of tentorium, 1632–1633
Inclusion cyst, epidermal, 516
Incontinence, 1550, 1599–1601
Indicator-dilution curves, 504, 506
Indocyanine green dye, 504
Infantile hydrocephalus, 1654–1656
Infantile osteogenesis imperfecta, 1750
Infants (*see* Children; Pediatric surgery)
Infarction:
  cerebral, 1659–1660
  intestinal, 1325, 1327, 1328
  mesenteric, 1325–1327
  myocardial (*see* Myocardium, infarction of)
  of omentum, idiopathis segmental, 1317–1318
Infections, 165–190
  (*See also* specific infections)
  aerobic, 166, 178, 180
  anaerobic, 166, 179, 181
  antibiotic therapy, 168–169, 170–178
  antifungal antibiotics, 177
  asepsis and, 188–190
  biliary tract, 1240–1243
  chemoprophylaxis, 171–172
  chest wall, 605–606
  classification of, 166
  clostridial, 181–185
  colonic, 1110–1121
  contamination vs., 168, 182
  diagnosis, 167–168
  emergency laparotomy and, 206
  exudate from, 168
  gallbladder, 1236, 1239
  gram-negative microorganisms, 175–177,
   185–187
  gram-positive microorganisms, 174–177

gynecologic, 1607–1608
hand, 1897–1901, 1904–1905
hyperbaric therapy, 169
indigenous microorganisms and, 166
intestinal antisepsis and, 172
intraperitoneal antibiotic therapy, 172
kidney transplants and, 421, 423
mycotic, 187–188
nervous system, 1662–1664, 1679
pleural effusion and, 614
pulmonary, 628–640
rectal, 1158, 1159
secondary or opportunistic, 171
skin degerming and, 189–190
small bowel, 1094–1095
staphylococcal, 180–181, 206
sterilization and, 189
stimuli from, 3
streptococcal, 178–180
sulfonamides, 177–178
surgical therapy, 168
urinary tract, 1558–1561
wound, postoperative, 462–464
Infertility, 1605
Infiltration anesthesia, 457–458
Infrared radiation, 1968
Infundibular stenosis, 686
    tetralogy of Fallot and, 726, 727
    ventricular septal defect and, 714
Infundibulum, gallbladder, 1222
Inguinal dissection for melanoma, 523–524
Inguinal hernias, 1346–1348, 1355–1357
Inguinal orchiectomy, 1585–1586
Inhalation anesthesia, 445–451
Inheritance (see Genetic factors)
Injuries (see Trauma; Wounds)
Innominate osteotomy, 1730
Innovar, 452
Inspiration, 597–598
Insulin, 1260
    for diabetes, 474
    excessive, 1274–1276
    peptic ulcer and, 1061
    starvation and, 22
    trauma and, 5, 17, 18, 26
Intensity duration curves, 1695
Intermittent positive-pressure breathing, 46, 467
    muscle relaxants and, 453
Interphalangeal joints, 1818, 1854, 1856–1858
    amputations, 1890
    muscles, 1904, 1906
Interstitial pulmonary tumors, 642
Intervertebral discs, 1670–1672, 1686–1689
Intestine:
    angina, 1327–1328
    atresia, 1526–1528
    gas, 982, 984
    infarction and ischemia, 1325, 1327, 1328, 1331
    intussusception, 1530–1531
    large, 1109–1160
        (See also Anus; Cecum; Colon; Rectum)
        anorectal surgery, 1146–1160
        antisepsis, 172
        diverticular disease, 1121–1126
        inflammatory disease, 1110–1121
        megacolon, 1144–1146
        neoplasms, 1126–1143
        volvulus, 1143–1144
    malrotation, 1525–1526
    obstruction, 979–991
        clinical manifestations, 983–985
        closed-loop, 983
        diverticulitis and, 1124
        etiology, 980
        ileus, 990–991
        incidence, 980
        intubation for, 986–987
        laboratory findings, 984
        management, 985–991
        Meckel's diverticulum and, 1100

mesenteric tumors and, 1335
operative procedures for, 987–989
pathophysiology, 980–983
postoperative care, 989–990
roentgenography, 984–985
simple mechanical, 980–982
strangulated, 982–983
small, 1089–1105
    (See also Duodenum; Ileum; Jejunum)
    adenocarcinoma, 1096–1097
    afferent (blind) loop syndrome, 482–483,
        1102–1103
    blood supply, 1321, 1322
    bypass operations, 1092–1093, 1103,
        1105
    carcinoids, 1097–1100
    diarrhea and, 978
    diverticula, 1100–1101
    fistula, 485, 1101–1102
    foreign bodies, 1101
    inflammatory diseases, 1089–1095
    injuries to, 229–230
    neoplasms, 1095–1100
    obstruction, 483
    Peutz-Jeghers syndrome, 1096
    pneumatosis cystoides intestinalis, 1102
    regional enteritis, 1089–1094
    short bowel syndrome, 1103–1105
    transplantation of, 391, 392
    tuberculous enteritis, 1094
    typhoid enteritis, 1094–1095
    ulcer, 1101
Intracellular fluid, 66
Intracerebral hematoma, 1640, 1661
Intracranial hemorrhage, 1637–1638, 1660
Intracranial infections, 1662–1664
Intradural tumors, 1651
Intramural hematoma, 229
Intraperitoneal antibiotics, 172
Intraperitoneal effusions, 1306
Intrathoracic pressure, pulmonary resection and,
    655–656
Intravenous alimentation, 32–35, 91–95
Intravenous anesthesia, 451–454
Intravenous component therapy, 34–36
Intravenous resuscitation in burns, 260–263
Intrinsic factor, gastric, 1053
Intubation:
    endotracheal, 202, 466–467
    for intestinal obstruction, 986–987
    nasogastric, 199, 1076–1077
Intussusception, 1530–1531
    appendicitis vs., 1172
    "chronic," 1096
In utero position, deformities from, 1725–1726
Iodine:
    in cholecystography, 1229
    metabolism, 1431
    protein-bound (see Protein-bound iodine)
    radioactive: in pulmonary embolism, 920
        thyroid and, 1434–1435, 1440
        in venous thrombosis, 917
Iodocholesterol, 1399
Iodohippurate, 952
Iodophors, 190
Iodothyronines, 1432
IPOP (immediate postsurgical prostheses), 1881
IPPB (see Intermittent positive-pressure
    breathing)
Ischemia:
    anoxia, 139
    aortoiliac, 843–847
    arterial emboli and, 857, 858
    in arterioarterial embolism, 861
    cerebral, 1659–1660
    cerebrovascular disease and, 883
    colitis, 1118–1119
    colonic, aortic aneurysms and, 891
    contracture and, 1716–1717
    intestinal, 1325, 1327, 1331

kidney, 954
limb, amputation and, 1879
myocardial, 794, 798
peripheral arterial occlusion and, 840
popliteal aneurysm and, 895
in Raynaud's disease, 901
spinal, 1679
in tibial artery disease, 851
Island pedicle flaps, 1926, 1928
Islet-cell tumors, 1274–1278
Isogravimetric perfusion, 147, 148
Isoniazid, 1094
Isoproterenol, 151–152
Isotopes (see Radioisotopes)

Jaboulay pyloroplasty, 1065, 1066
Jaundice, 997–1004
    evaluation and management, 1001–1004
    hemolytic, 1000, 1002
    history and, 1001
    injury of bile ducts and, 1232–1233
    laboratory studies, 1002–1003
    neonatal, 1225, 1226
    obstructive, 1001
    in pancreatic carcinoma, 1271, 1272
    physical examination, 1001–1002
    roentgenography in, 1003
Jaw:
    (See also Mandible)
    adamantinoma of, 1786
Jejunoileal bypass, 1105
Jejunostomy, 90, 229
    Witzel, 90
Jejunum:
    adenocarcinoma, 1096
    arteries of, 1321
    atresia, congenital, 1527, 1528
    bleeding, 24
    choledochal anastomosis with, 236
    diverticula, 1101
    fistulas of, postoperative, 485
    pancreatic anastomosis with, 239
    Peutz-Jeghers syndrome, 1096
    Roux-en-Y procedures (see Roux-en-Y
        procedures)
Johnson procedure, 1033
Joints, 1845–1875
    (See also specific joints)
    acromioclavicular, 1803–1804
    anatomy, 1845–1847
    ankle, 1831–1833, 1857, 1868
    arthritis (see Arthritis; Osteoarthritis)
    arthroplasty, 1858, 1863–1864, 1868
    cartilage, 1845–1846
    Charcot, 1873–1874
    collagen, 1846
    contracture, 1715
    crystal deposition disease, 1870–1871
    degenerative disease (see Osteoarthritis)
    density of tissue, radiographic, 1745
    elbow, 1808, 1810–1812, 1862
    examination, 1847–1848
    gait disturbances and, 1707
    gout, 1869–1870
    hemophilia and, 109, 110, 1871–1872
    hip, 1835–1839
    interphalangeal, 1818, 1854, 1856–1858, 1890,
        1904
    knee, 1825–1829, 1856–1857, 1867–1868
    metatarsophalangeal, 1854–1857, 1858
    mucin clot test, 1848
    neuropathic, 1704, 1873–1874
    pain, 1678
    pulmonary osteoarthropathy, 1873
    rehabilitation for, 1972
    roentgenography, 1847, 1850–1851, 1854
    shoulder, 1874–1875
    sternoclavicular, 1802
    synovial lesions, 1872–1873

synovial membrane and fluid, 1846–1848
thumb, 1859–1860, 1862
transplant of, 387
tuberculosis, 1850–1852
wrist, 1862
Jugular vein catheterization, 500
Jugular vein injury, 218, 219
Juvenile bone cyst, 1783–1784
Juvenile polyps, 1126
Juxtaglomerular apparatus, hypertension and, 948
Juxtaglomerular hyperplasia, 1400
Juxtaintestinal nodes, 1332

Kallikreins, 45, 1099
Kanamycin, 172, 173, 176, 207
Kantor, string sign of, 1092
Kaposi's sarcoma, 521
Kay-Shiley disc prosthesis, 772
Kegel exercises, 1599
Keloid, 517–518
Keratosis, 517
Kerley lines, 766
Ketamine, 453
Ketoacidosis, diabetes and, 474–475
Ketones, 27
in diabetes, 473, 474–475
fasting and, 21
17-Ketosteroids, 596
in adrenogenital syndrome, 1391, 1392
in amenorrhea, 1603
Kidney, 1547–1555
ADH release and, 39–41
anatomy, 1547
arteriography, 1555
arteriosclerosis, 946, 954
biopsy, 420, 956
burns and, 258
carcinoma, 1570–1572
congenital conditions, 1567, 1569–1570
cortisol and, 9
cyst, 1571
extracorporeal circulation and, 758
failure, 1564–1566
acute, 1564–1566
in burns, 261–262
chronic, 1566
high-output, 85–86, 450
hyperparathyroidism and, 1498
laboratory findings, 1565
shock and, 50
transplantation and, 415
treatment, 1565–1566
freezing for storage, 434
function studies, 954–955, 956
hyperparathyroidism and, 1471, 1472–1473, 1476
hypoxia and, 494
infections, 1551
ischemia, 954
liver injury and, 1182
lumbar nephrectomy, 1580–1581
necrosis, acute papillary, 1559
osteodystrophy, 1757–1759
parathyroid hormone and, 1465
pelvic tumors, 1571–1572
phosphate resorption, 1479
physical examination, 1551
polycystic disease, 1571
potassium excretion by, 75
pyelography, 1553–1555
renography, 1555
shock and, 145
sodium excretion, 79
stones, 1561–1564
hyperparathyroidism and, 1476
trauma and, 49–50, 1580
transplants (see Transplantation, kidney)
tuberculosis, 1561

tubular necrosis, acute (see Tubular necrosis, acute)
tumors, 1570–1572
unilateral parenchymal disease, 962–963
volume deficits and, 70
Wilms' tumor, 1567
xenografts, 431–432
Kinases, 101, 115
Kinin, 143, 366, 1099
Kininogen, 143
Klebsiella pneumoniae, 186
Klinefelter's syndrome, 1393
Klippel-Feil syndrome, 1736
Knee, 1825–1829
amputations: above, 1886–1887
below, 853, 1884–1886
through, 1886
arthritis of, 1856–1857
arthrodesis, 1868
calcification, 1871
cerebral palsy and, 1702
deformities, 1711–1712
dislocation, congenital, 1732
dislocation of patella, 1829
fracture of patella, 1828–1829
instability, 1856–1857
ligamentous injuries, 1825–1828
meniscus injuries, 1827–1828
myelodysplasia and, 1703
osteoarthritis, 1867–1868
paralysis, 1699
prosthesis, MacIntosh, 1857
synovectomy, 1856
synovial fluid, 1847
Knock-knee, 1711
Kocher maneuver, 1250, 1267
Köhler's disease, 1720–1721
Kraurosis, 1617
Kultschitzsky cells, 1097, 1098
Küntscher's technique, 1823–1824
Kyphosis, 1685, 1707–1708

Labia majora, 1590
Lacerations, 288
Lacrimal duct injury, 1943
Lactation, 530, 531, 551
persistent, 1371, 1372
prolactin and, 1366
Lactate, oxygen transport and, 495, 496
Lactic acid:
acidosis and, 38
alkalosis and, 37
shock and, 137
Lactose in galactosemia, 1226
Lag phase of healing, 277, 286
Laminectomy, 1672
metastatic tumors and, 1789, 1790
Laminography of head and neck, 570
Landouzy-Dejerine dystrophy, 1652
Langer's foramen, 528
Laparotomy:
corticosteroid secretion and, 10, 11
emergency, 205–206
drains, 206
infection, 206
incisions, 205
suture, 205–206
for stab wounds, 224
Laplace's law, 1326
Laryngeal mirror, 559
Laryngeal nerve:
parathyroids and, 1459, 1494
thyroid and, 1430, 1455–1456
Laryngectomy, 575, 576
partial, 590
rehabilitation and, 1981
total, 588–590
Laryngoscopy, 558–560
Larynx, 573–576

examination of, 558–560
injuries of, 219
resection of, 558–560
tumors, 573–576
benign, 574–575
classification, 573
diagnosis, 573–574
incidence and etiology, 573
malignant, 575–576
pathology, 573
Lathyrism, 284
LATS (long-acting thyroid stimulator), 1436, 1437
Lavage, peritoneal, 223
Lawrence's transfer factor, 340
Laxatives, peritonitis from, 1300
Lecithin, gallstones and, 1233
Left-to-right shunts, 679–680, 704–721
Leg(s):
amputations, 1882–1888, 1978–1979
braces, 1979
cervical myelopathy and, 1681
edema, 925, 926
length discrepancy, 1707
length equalization in poliomyelitis, 1698
limping and, 1706–1707
pain, 840, 951
prostheses, 1886, 1887, 1889, 1973–1974
veins, 923–925
(See also Veins, thrombosis; Venous insufficiency)
Legg-Calvé-Perthes disease, 1718–1720
Leiomyoma:
colorectal, 1142
esophageal, 1037
small bowel, 1095
uterine, 1609–1610
Leiomyosarcoma:
colorectal, 1142
gastric, 1082
uterine, 1617
Lentigo maligna, 522
Letterer-Siwe disease, 1769, 1770–1771
Leukemia:
bone disease and, 1771
death rate, 298
splenectomy for, 1291
Leukocytes:
abdominal trauma and, 221
in appendicitis, 1169
hepatic abscess and, 1184
infections, and, 168
intestinal obstruction and, 984
in myeloid metaplasia, 1291
in periotonitis, 1298, 1303
polymorphoneuclear, allograft rejection and, 367, 371
transfusion and, 123
typing, 382–383
ulcerative colitis and, 1111
Leukoparakeratosis, 1603
Leukopenia, 1290
Leukoplakia, 567, 1617
Leukorrhea, 1607–1608
Levarterenol, 150
Levator ani muscles, 1592
Levin tubes, 221, 227
LH, 6, 17
Lidocaine, 458, 471
Ligaments:
ankle, 1824
calcaneonavicular, 1714
Cooper's, 1355–1358
hand, 1905–1907
knee, 1825–1828
ovarian and uterine, 1590–1591
Poupart's, 1355–1358
Ligamentum arteriosum, coarctation of, 696, 698
Ligation:
in arterial injury, 870

of hemorrhoids, 1150
transesophageal, 1201, 1206
venous, 921, 930–931
Ligatures, 119
Lignac-Fanconi syndrome, 1758
Limb girdle dystrophy, 1696
Limb replantation, 387–388
Limping, 1706–1707
Lincomycin, 173, 175
Lingual gland, 580, 581
Lingual thyroid, 1431
Linoleic acid, 34
Lip, 561–564
    benign tumors, 562
    biopsy, 560
    cancer, 562, 563–564
    cleft, 1947–1950
    etiology of tumors of, 561–562
    hyperkeratosis, 562–563
    mucous cysts, 565, 566
    plastic surgery of, 1943, 1944, 1947–1950
    V excision of, 587
Lipase, fat embolism and, 477
Lipids:
    (See also Fats)
    liver and, 1179
Lipoid granulomatosis, 1769–1770
Lipoid pneumonia, 633
Lipolysis, glucagon and, 16
Lipoma:
    cardiac, 793
    mediastinal, 668
    mesenteric, 1335
    skin, 519
Liposarcoma, 1787
    antigen, 312
    immunotherapy, 338
    mesenteric, 1335
Lipuria, embolism and, 477
Livedo reticularis, 903
Liver, 1177–1217
    abscesses, 1184–1187
    adenoma, 1189
    amebic abscesses, 1186–1187
    anatomy, 1177–1178
    anesthesia and, 47–48
    angiography, 1181
    ascites, 1202
    bile metabolism and, 997–1001
    biliary drainage, 1177
    biopsy, 1004, 1180
    blood supply, 1178, 1198, 1323–1324
    carbohydrates and, 1179
    carcinoma, 1190–1192
    cirrhosis, 1197
    coagulation and, 1180
    coma, 1201, 1203–1204
    cortisol and, 9
    cysts, 1187–1189
    dearterialization, 325
    dye excretion, 1180
    enzymes, 1180
    failure, 1215–1216
        transplants and, 394, 395
    fatty acid oxidation in, 19–20
    function, 1178–1180
    glycogen, 19, 23, 1214
    halothane effects on, 450
    hamartoma, 1189
    hemangioma, 1189–1190
    hematobilia, 1182
    hemorrhage, 1182, 1193
    hemostatic disorders and, 117
    hepatorenal syndrome, 1182
    hilar duct carcinoma, 1245–1246
    hydatid cysts, 1188–1189
    hypersplenism and, 1202–1203
    intravenous alimentation for, 32–33
    jaundice and (see Jaundice)
    lipids and, 1179–1180

metastatic neoplasms, 1192–1193, 1417
obstructive jaundice, 1001
peptic ulcer and, 1057
portacaval shunt, 1208, 1214
portal hypertension (see Portal hypertension)
proteins and, 1179, 1203
pyogenic abscesses, 1184–1186
radiography, 1189, 1191, 1198
regeneration of, 275
resection, 233–235, 1193–1196
rupture, 1181
scintillation scanning, 1180–1181
segmentectomy, 1193–1196
shock and, 48
spaces above and below, 1305
thyroid and, 1433
transplants (see Transplantation, liver)
trauma, 47–48, 232–235, 1181–1184
tumors, 1189–1193
vascular injuries, 1183–1184
Liver fluke, 1241
Lobar emphysema of infancy, 624–625
Lobectomy:
    hepatic, 1193
    prefrontal, 1668
    pulmonary, 648–649, 651–658
        postoperative care, 655–658
        precautions during, 652–653
        technique, 652–655
Locomotion disturbances, 1706–1707
Log-cell kill hypothesis, 332
Long-acting thyroid stimulator, 1520–1521
Looser's zones, 1759
Loxoscelism, 215–216
Lumbago, 1690
Lumbar arteries, atherosclerosis of, 843
Lumbar disc disease, 1671–1672, 1686–1689
Lumbar hernias, 1345
Lumbar nephrectomy, 1580–1581
Lumbar puncture, 1636, 1637
Lumbar sympathectomy, 844, 853
Lumbrosacral disorders, 1689–1690
Lumpectomy, 547
Lunate, dislocations of, 1817
Lung(s), 622–658
    abscess, 630–633
    actinomycosis, 639
    adenoid cystic carcinoma, 644
    agenesis, 622
    air cysts, 625–627
    arterial anomalies, 622–623
    aspergillosis, 640
    benign tumors, 642–643
    biopsy, 649–651
    blastomycosis, 640
    blood supply, 598
    bronchiectasis, 628–630
    bronchotomy, 655
    burns and, 258, 259, 265, 268–269
    calcified mass, 634
    cancer, 645–649
        clinical manifestations, 646–647
        death rate, 298
        diagnosis, 647–648
        differential diagnosis, 648
        pathology, 645
        smoking and, 302
        treatment, 648–649
    carcinoid, 642–644
    clinical manifestations of disease, 600–601
    coccidioidomycosis, 638–639
    collapse (see Atelectasis)
    compliance, 498
    congenital malformations, 622–625
    congestion, congenital heart disease and, 679
    cryptococcosis (torulosis), 640
    cysts, 615–616, 623, 625–627
    dead space, physiologic, 465
    decortication, 619
    diagnostic operative procedures, 649–651

drainage, 653
edema, 128, 469
embolism (see Pulmonary embolism)
emphysema, 598, 624–627, 660
fistulas, 635
foreign bodies, 627–628
function, 599–600
gangrene, 631
hamartoma, 642
hernias, 604, 1040–1041
histoplasmosis, 638
hydatid cysts, 640
hyperlucent, 623
hypoplasia of, 622
inflammation and infection, 628–640
interstitial tumors, 642
intrapleural pressure and, 611
lymph nodes, 598–599, 634, 640
lymphangiectasis, 624
margins, 597
mediastinoscopy, 650
metastases to, 648, 649, 1566
mucoid impaction, 634
mucoviscidosis, 634
mycotic infections, 638–640
nocardiosis, 639–640
nodule, solitary, 641
oxygen transport in, 493–494
peptic ulcer and, 1057
pleural cover of (see Pleura)
pneumonia, 633–634
postoperative care, 655–658
rehabilitation, 1974
resection, 651–655
rupture, 628
sarcoidosis, 640
sarcomas, 644
segmental resection, 653
sequestration, 622
shock and, 46, 146, 466
tidal volume, 465
transplantation, 402–404
trauma, 627–628
tuberculosis, 635–638
tumors, 641–649
vascular anomalies, 622–624
"Vietnam," 148–149
wedge resection, 653–655
Lupus erythematosus, renal transplant for, 405
Luschka, ducts of, 1223
Luteinizing hormone, 6, 1593, 1597
    trauma and, 17
Luteotropic hormone, 1366, 1593
Lymph nodes:
    axillary, 523, 529, 535
    biopsy, 319, 650
    breast, 529, 535
    bronchial erosion by, 634
    cervical cancer spread, 1612–1613
    colorectal cancer and, 1132, 1140
    excision of, 324
    Hodgkin's disease and, 1292
    lung cancer metastases of, 645
    mediastinal, 650, 666–669, 1023
    melanoma and removal of, 523
    mesenteric, 1324, 1332–1333
    metastases, 314–315
    neck, 558, 578, 584
    pulmonary, 640
    retroperitoneal, 1339
    supraclavicular, 584
    thymus and, 353–354
    transplantation, 389
    vulvar cancer spread, 1618
Lymphadenectomy, pelvic, 1627–1630
Lymphadenitis, mesenteric, 1332–1334
Lymphadenoid goiter, 1443–1444
Lymphangiectasia in regional enteritis, 1090
Lymphangiectasis, pulmonary, 624
Lymphangiography, 932

Lymphangioma, 519
  mediastinal, 668–669
  mesenteric, 1335
Lymphangiosarcoma, 933
  mesenteric, 1334
  of skin, 521
Lymphangitis, 169
  lymphedema and, 933
Lymphatic system, 931–934
  anatomy and physiology, 931–932
  anorectal, 1147
  bone disease and, 1768–1769
  breast, 529, 535
  cystic hygroma, 1515–1516
  dye injection of, 931–932
  esophageal, 1011
  gallbladder, 1244
  gastric cancer spread, 1080
  liver, 1202
  lungs, 598–599, 624
  pancreatic, 1259
Lymphedema, 932–934
  clinical manifestations, 933
  differential diagnosis, 933–934
  etiology, 932–933
  pathophysiology, 933
  treatment, 934
  venous insufficiency vs., 928
Lymphocytes:
  antilymphocyte globulin and, 373–374
  blocking factors, 311–312
  effector molecules released by, 362
  immunogen recognition by, 356–357
  immunotherapy with, 339–340
  lysis (in vitro) of target cells, 361–362
  mixed cultures of, 352–353, 362, 363, 383
  morphologic changes, 358–359
  proliferation and differentiation of, 359
  recruitment of, 362
  rejection and, 354–364
  specifically immunized, 360–363
  T and B cells, 354, 357, 358
  transformed, 355
  tumor destruction by, 307, 311–312
  typing, 382–383
Lymphogranuloma venereum, 1159
Lymphoid tissue:
  immunosuppression by extirpation of, 372
  transplantation of, 388–389
Lymphoma:
  Burkitt's, 585
  gastric, 1082
  rectal, 1141
  staging extent of, 320
  thyroid, 1450
Lymphopathia venereum, 1608
Lymphosarcoma:
  colorectal, 1141–1142
  mediastinal, 666
  nasopharyngeal, 578
  splenectomy for, 1291
Lysis of target cells, 361–362
Lysosomes, liver cell, 48

McBride procedure, 1868–1869
McBurney incision, 1173
MacIntosh prosthesis, 1857
McKee-Farrar prosthesis, 1866
Mackenrodt ligaments, 1590
McMurray test, 1828
Macrodactyly, 1896–1897
Macrogenitosomia praecox, 1390, 1391
Macrophages:
  allografts and, 356, 367
  tumor destruction by, 307
Madelung's deformity, 1737–1738
Mafenide in burns, 263–265
Magnesium, 77–78
  deficiency, 77

excess, 78
  parathyroid and, 1460–1461
Malleolar fractures of ankle, 1832–1833
Mallett finger, 1818
Mallory-Weiss syndrome, 993, 1039, 1077
Mammary artery, internal, 528
  coronary anastomosis with, 798
Mammary duct cancer, 539, 540
Mammary gland (see Breast)
Mammary lobules, cancer of, 540
Mammary tumor virus, 308
Mammary lymph nodes, internal, 529
Mammary ridge, 527
Mammography, 532
Mammoplasty, 1960–1963
  augmentation, 1961–1963
  reduction, 1960–1963
Manchester-Fothergill operation, 1599
Mandible, 1941, 1956–1957
  fibroma of, 1781
  resection, 586–587
  tumors of, 579–580
Marble bones, 1751–1752
Marfan syndrome, 781, 782, 818, 819, 825
Marginal artery of Drummond, 1322
Marginal ulcer, 1056, 1068
Maroteaux-Lamy syndrome, 1766
Marrow (see Bone marrow)
Marshall-Marchetti procedure, 1600
Marsupialization, 1270
Masculinization, 1391, 1603
Massage, 1963
Mast cells, 1111
Mastectomy, radical, 541–544, 546–547, 549
  rehabilitation following, 1980–1981
Mastectomy, simple, 544, 547–549
Mastitis, chronic cystic, 534
Matrix formation, 1754
Maxilla, 1940–1941, 1956–1957
  swelling of, early, 559
Maxillary sinus polyps, 578
Maxillectomy, 587–588
Maxillomandibular relationship, distorted,
  1956–1957
MDF, 45, 138
Meatal stenosis, 1568
Meckel's diverticulum, 1100, 1522–1523
  appendicitis vs., 1171–1172
Meconium ileus, 1529
Median arcuate ligament syndrome, 1330–1331
Median nerve injury, 1977
Median nerve palsy, 1910
Mediastinitis, 660–662
  acute, 660–661
  chronic, 661–662
  fibrous, 661–662
  treatment, 661
Mediastinoscopy, biopsy and, in lung cancer, 650
Mediastinotomy, 661, 1031
Mediastinum, 660–669
  abscess, 616
  asphyxia and, traumatic, 662–663
  bronchogenic carcinoma and, 646, 648
  bronchogenic cysts, 667
  chondroma and chondrosarcoma, 669
  chordoma, 667–668
  cysts, 665–668
  diverticula, 667
  emphysema, 660
  esophageal duplication, 667
  hemangioma, 669
  hematoma, 660
    from aortic injury, 831, 832
  in infancy, 668
  inflammation of, 660–662
  lymph nodes, 1023
  lymphadenopathy, 663, 666–669
  meningocele, 669
  neurogenic tumors, 668, 669
  parathyroid adenoma, 665

  in parathyroidectomy, 1495–1496
  pheochromocytomas, 669, 1416
  pleural effusion and, 614
  pleuropericardial cyst, 666
  pulmonary resection and, 655–656
  thoracic duct lesions and, 663
  thymic lesions, 665–666
  thyroid masses, 664–665
  tumors, 663–669
    anatomy, 663–664
    anterior, 665–666
    clinical manifestations, 664
    costovertebral region, 669
    in infancy, 668–669
    nonspecific location, 668
    posterior, 666–668
    superior, 664–665
    treatment, 664
    vena caval obstruction and, 662
Meditarsus adductus, 1725, 1726
Medullary carcinoma of breast, 540
Medulloblastoma, 1638
Megacolon, 1144–1146
  acquired, 1145
  congenital, 1145
  fecal impaction and, 1145–1146
  toxic, 1113
Meigs' syndrome, 614, 1622
Melanoma, 521–525
  of anus, 1160
  BCG for, 340–341
  prognosis, 525
  treatment, 522–525
Melanophore-stimulating hormone, 1365–1366
  cells secreting, 1365
  ectopic secretion of, 1374
Melena, 991
Meleney's gangrene, 179–180
Meleney's ulcer, 180
Melorheostosis, 1752
Mendelson's syndrome, 633–634
Meningeal artery, middle, 1639
Meningiomas, 1646, 1651
Meningitis, 1653
Meningocele, 1653, 1703
  intrathoracic, 669
Meningococcal septicemia, 1402
Menopause, 1597
  breasts in, 531
    cancer of, 550
  osteoporosis and, 1708
Menstruation, 1596–1597
  amenorrhea, 1602–1603
  bleeding disorders, 1601–1603
  dysmenorrhea, 1598
  pain, 1598
  pregnancy and, 1605
Meperidine, 452
  in pancreatitis, 1263
  in shock, 151
6-Mercaptopurine, 334, 376
Mesenchymoma, hepatic, 1192
Mesenteric arteries, 1178, 1320–1322
  embolism, 1324
  occlusion, 1324–1326, 1328–1329
    inferior, 1328–1329
    superior, 1324–1326
  rupture, 1331
  thrombosis, 1325
  trauma of, 1332
  vena caval shunt with, 1210–1213
Mesenteric nodes, 1324
  inflammation of, 1332–1334
Mesenteric veins, 1322–1324
  occlusion, 1329–1330
  trauma of, 1332
Mesentery, 1318–1336
  anatomy, 1318–1324
  angina, 1327–1328
  apoplexy, 1331–1332

arcuate ligament syndrome, 1330–1331
attachments of, 1319
circulation, 1320–1324
cysts, 1334–1335
infarction, 1326–1327
lymphatic system, 1324
inflammation of, 1332–1334
panniculitis, 1334
tumors, 1334–1336
vascular disease, 1324–1332
Mesocolon, 1319
Mesothelioma:
cardiac, 792
pleural, 621
Metabolic acidosis, 74
Metabolic alkalosis, 74–75
Metabolism:
anesthesia and, 448
bile, 997–1001
bone, 1752–1766
calcium, 76–77, 425–426
cell, 137–138
diarrhea and, 978
energy, 19
gout and, 1861
intravenous alimentation and, 33
iodine, 1431
liver transplantation and, 397–398
monitoring of tissue, 508–509
pancreaticoduodenectomy and, 1273–1274
pancreatitis and, 1261
pheochromocytoma and, 1410
storage of organs and, 432–433
thyroid and, 1432–1434, 1436
trauma and, 17–42, 199–202
Metacarpals:
in amputations, 1890–1891
fractures, 1817–1818
Metachromasia, 281
Metaphyseal aclasis, 1748–1749
Metaphysis, aneurysmal bone cyst and, 1783
Metaplasia, myeloid, 1290–1291
Metaraminol, 150
Metastases:
bone, 609, 1788–1790
cardiac, 792
cervical cancer, 1612–1613
colorectal cancer, 1132, 1140
from hepatic tumors, 1191
to liver, 1192–1193
pulmonary, 645, 648, 649
to spinal cord, 1649–1650
of thyroid, 1452–1453
Metatarsal amputation, 1883
Metatarsal fractures, 1835
Metatarsophalangeal joints, 1854–1858
Methicillin, 174
Methimazole, 1440
Methotrexate, 335, 336, 377
Methoxyflurane, 450
3-Methoxytyramine, 1405
Methylcholanthrene, 304
Methyl-2-cyanoacrilate, 120
Methylprednisolone:
in cardiac transplantation, 401
in shock, 153–155, 156
Methysergide, 1337, 1338
Metopirone, 1379, 1385–1386
Metyrapone, 1379, 1385–1386
Microaneurysms, renal, 947
Micrococcus pyogenes, 1119–1120
Micrognathia, 1956
Microsurgery, 1931
Microtia, congenital, 1950–1952
Migration inhibitory factor, 362, 366–367
Mikulicz's disease, 582
Miles procedure, 1136
Milk, breast cancer and, 534–535
Milk-alkali syndrome, hyperparathyroidism vs.,
1489

Milk line, 527
Milk sinus, 529
Milkman's syndrome, 1760
Milliequivalent, 67
Millimole, 67
Milliosmole, 67
Mima polymorpha, 186
Mineralization, 1754–1755
Mineralocorticoids, 13, 1377
Mirror, laryngeal, 559
Mitochondria, oxygen transport and, 495–496
Mitogenic factor, 362
Mitomycin C, 340, 377–378
Mitral insufficiency, 771–774
anatomy, pathologic, 771–772
aortic disease with, 787
atrial septal defect and, 709, 712
clinical manifestations, 773–774
etiology, 771
historical data, 771
pathophysiology, 772–773
prognosis, 774
treatment, 774
Mitral stenosis, 762–771
aortic insufficiency and, 787
aortic stenosis with, 787
clinical manifestations, 763–766
congenital, 733–734
diagnosis, 766
emboli from, 857
etiology, 762
historical data, 762
laboratory studies, 765–766
pathology, 762–763
pathophysiology, 752, 763
physical examination, 764–765
prognosis, 770–771
symptoms, 763–764
treatment, 766–770
open commissurotomy, 766–767
replacement of valve, 767–770
tricuspid disease with, 787
Miyagawanella, 1159
Molecular cascade systems, 364–371
Molecules, effector, 362, 363
Moles, 67, 522
hydatidiform, 1606
Monilia vaginitis, 1607
Moniliasis, 188
Monitoring, 491–509
cardiovascular, 499–508
cardiac output determination, 494–495,
503–508
cart, 499
concepts, physiologic, 492–496
metabolism, tissue, 508–509
oxygen, 492–494, 498
respiratory, 497–499
sensing, physiologic, 497
ultrasound in, 507
3-Monoiodotyrosine, 1431
Monostotic fibrous dysplasia, 1749
Monteggia's deformity, 1812
Montgomery's tubercles, 530
Morgagni, foramen of, 1041
Morgagni, rectal columns of, 1146
Morison's pouch, 1307
Morphine, anesthetic use of, 452
Morquio-Brailsford syndrome, 1766
Moschcowitz procedure, 1158, 1357
Motor nerve fibers, 1694
Mouth (*see* Oral cavity)
Mucin clot test, 1848
Mucocele, appendiceal, 1176
Mucoepidermoid carcinomas, 582
Mucoid impaction of bronchi, 634
Mucolytic agents, 468–469
Mucopolysaccharides:
bone and, 1741–1742
healing and, 281

Mucopolysaccharidoses, 1765–1766
Mucosa:
anal canal, 1146
buccal (*see* Buccal mucosa)
in colitis, ulcerative, 1112
diverticulosis coli, 1121
gallbladder, 1228
gastric, 992, 993, 1069–1070, 1074–1076
Mucous cysts, oral, 565
Mucoviscidosis, 634, 1523
Mucus, gastric, 1051–1052
Mullerian ducts, 1590
remnants, 1620
Multiple myeloma (*see* Myeloma, multiple)
Multiple transfusion syndrome, 30
Mumps orchitis, 1552
Murmurs, 681–682, 751
in aortic insufficiency, 783
in aortic stenosis, 691, 776
in arteriovenous fistula, 872
in atrial septal defect, 705, 710
diastolic, 682
in mitral insufficiency, 772
in mitral stenosis, 765
in patent ductus arteriosus, 718, 719
physical examination and, 681–682
systolic, 681–682
in tetralogy of Fallot, 723
in transposition of great vessels, 728
in tricuspid atresia, 732
in tricuspid stenosis and insufficiency, 785
in ventricular septal defect, 714
Muscle, 1692–1705
anatomy, 1692
atrophy and wasting in hand, 1704
cerebral palsy, 1700–1702
contraction, 1692–1694
contracture, 1715
definitions of function, 1693
degenerative nervous system diseases,
1703–1704
dystrophies, 1696–1697
electrical diagnosis and assessment of
denervation, 1695
electromyography, 1695
eyelid, paralysis of, 1958
hand, 1904–1905
inflammatory diseases, 1697
intrinsic diseases, 1695–1697
myelodysplasia, 1702–1703
myotonias, 1697
neuromuscular junction, 1694
pain, 1677–1678
paralysis and spasticity, 1694–1705
pelvic organ support, 1592, 1599
poliomyelitis, 1697–1700
potentiometric monitoring of, 508
rectus abdominis, 1313–1315
reeducation, 1967–1968
relaxants, 453–454
stroke management, 1704–1705
tone, 1694–1695
tumors, 1786–1788
wounds, 204–205
Musculocutaneous nerve injury, 1977
Musculoskeletal disorders, 1677–1721,
1775–1790
(*See also* Bone; Joints; Muscle; Vertebral
column)
rehabilitation for, 1971–1976
renal transplants and, 426
tumors, 1775–1790
Myasthenia gravis:
esophagus and, 1040
thymic lesions and, 666
Mycobacterium tuberculosis, 1094, 1298, 1561
Mycotic infections, 187–188
(*See also* Fungal infections)
Myelodysplasia, 1702–1703
Myelography, 1688

Myeloid metaplasia, 117, 1290–1291
Myeloma, multiple:
  bone disease and, 1762, 1771
  of chest wall, 609
  hyperparathyroidism vs., 1489
  osteodystrophy vs., 1753
Myelomeningoceles, 1652–1653, 1703
Myeloproliferative diseases, 116–117
Myeloschisis, 1703
Myenteric ganglia, 1531, 1534
Myoblastoma:
  granular cell, 538
  oral, 567
Myocardial shock, 144–145
Myocardium:
  contusion of, 790
  cyclopropane and, 447
  depression of, in shock, 45, 138
  electrode implantation in, 804, 806
  infarction of, 794
    emboli from, 857
    postoperative, 472–473
  ischemia: in aortic stenosis, 775
    in coronary atherosclerosis, 794, 798
Myodesis in amputation, 1886–1887
Myodystrophia fetalis, 1734–1735
Myoglobin, 495, 997
Myonecrosis, 179, 182
Myosin, 1692, 1693
Myositis, 1697
Myotonias, 1040, 1697
Myxedema, pituitary, 1442
Myxoma, cardiac, 791–792

Nabothian cysts, 1611
Nafcillin, 174
Narcotics:
  in anesthesia, 452–453
  withdrawal, 4–5
Nasal cavity tumors, 578–579
Nasogastric intubation:
  gastric distension from, 1076, 1077
  in trauma, 199
Nasolabial fold, 1944
Nasopharyngeal tube feeding, 89–90
Nasopharyngoscopy, 560
Nasopharynx, 576–577
  benign lesions, 576–577
  examination of, 560
  malignant lesions, 577–578
Nausea, 975–976
Nauta-Glees staining, 1666
Navicular:
  tarsal, epiphysitis of, 1720–1721
  of wrist, fractures of, 1816–1817
Neck:
  arteriovenous fistula of, 875
  branchial anomalies, 1953–1954
  cystic hygroma, 1516
  examination of, 558
  inflammatory swelling, 584
  lymph nodes, 558, 578, 584
  penetrating wounds of, 216–220
  radical dissection of, 586–587, 1981–1982
  short, congenital, 1736
  soft tissue losses, 1945–1946
  thyroglossal duct anomalies, 1952–1953
  torticollis, 1736–1737
  tumors, 584–591
  venous distension, 750
  webbed, 1736
Necrosis:
  amputation and, 1879, 1883
  arterial emboli and, 858
  papillary, acute, 1559
  tibial artery disease and, 851–852
Necrotizing fasciitis, 179
Needle biopsy, 319, 1180
Neisseria gonococcus, 1608

Nembutal, corticosteroids and, 10, 11
Neomycin, 176
Neoplasms, 297–343
  (See also Tumors; and specific names of
    tumors)
  benign, 313
  biopsy of, 318–320
  classification of, 313–314
  clinical manifestations of, 316–317
  etiology, 300–313
  geographic factors, 302
  growth rates of, 303–304
  hereditary factors, 301–302
  immunobiology of, 304–313
  malignant (see Cancer; Carcinoma)
  pathology of, 313–315
  resection of, 323–325
  routes for spread of, 314
Nephrectomy:
  lumbar, 1580–1581
  transplantation and, 412–414
Nephrocalcinosis, hyperparathyroidism and,
  1476
Nephrosclerosis, arteriolar, 960, 962
Nephrotomography, 1555
Nerve(s):
  afferent, 1–2, 968, 1676
  autotransplants, 385
  block, 457–458
  conduction tests, 878–879, 888, 1695
  cranial, carcinoma and, 577
  gallbladder, 1222
  grafts, 1644
  of hand, 1904, 1908–1911
  injuries, 1643–1646, 1976–1978
    evaluation, 1644
    in fractures, 1795
    functional recovery from, 1644–1645
    neck, 219–220
    peripheral, 1643–1646
    treatment, 1644
  motor, 1693, 1694
  pancreatic, 1257
  peripheral, pain and, 1666–1667, 1678–1679
  renal, 1547
  replantation of extremity and, 387
  root compression, 1681
  sensory, 968, 1676
  trigeminal, 1667
  urinary bladder, 1556
Nervous system, 1631–1673
  anesthetic complications, 456–457
  axial skeleton abnormalities, 1669–1673
  brain tumors, 1646–1649
  central (see Central nervous system)
  cerebrovascular disease and, 883
  degenerative disease, 1703–1704
  embryology, 1652
  evaluation of, in trauma, 197–198
  gait disturbances and, 1707
  general considerations, 1631–1633
  head injury, 1633–1641
  intracranial infections, 1662–1664
  malformations, 1651–1657
    craniosynostosis, 1656–1657
    dermal sinus tracts, 1653–1654
    hydrocephalus, 1654–1656
    spina bifida and cranium bifida, 1652–1653
  pain, 1664–1669
    pathways, 967–968
  peripheral injuries, 1643–1646
  rehabilitation, 1976–1980
  spinal cord injuries, 1641–1643
  spinal cord tumors, 1649–1651
  sympathetic (see Sympathetic nervous system)
  thoracic outlet syndrome and, 877, 878–879
  vascular diseases, 1657–1662
    anatomy, 1657
    aneurysms, 1660–1661
    arteriovenous malformations, 1661–1662

  cerebral and cerebellar hemorrhage, 1660
  clinical manifestations, 1658–1659
  congenital lesions, 1660–1662
  etiology, 1657
  physiology, 1657–1658
  transient ischemia and cerebral infarction,
    1659–1660
Neural compression syndromes, 878, 879
Neurapraxia, 1795
Neurilemmomas, 519, 1786
Neuroblastoma, 1417, 1419
  adrenal, 1567
  mediastinal, 668
  pheochromocytoma vs., 1411
Neurofibroma:
  chest wall, 606
  pheochromocytoma and, 1412–1413
  retroperitoneal, 1341
  spinal, 1651
Neurogenic bladder dysfunction, 1550,
  1556–1558, 1569, 1979
Neurogenic tumors of mediastinum, 669
Neurologic surgery, 1631–1673
  (See also Brain; Nerves; Nervous system;
    Spinal cord)
Neuromas, 519
  of hand, 1909–1910
  lip, 562
Neuromuscular disorders, esophagus and,
  1039–1040
Neuromuscular junction, 1694
Neuron(s):
  motor, 1691, 1693
  pain, 968, 1165–1667
Neuronapraxis, 1602
Neuropathic joints, 1873–1874
Neutropenia, splenic, 1290, 1292
Neutrophils, 1283
Neurotmesis, 1795
Nevus, 521, 522
Newborn (see Children; Pediatric surgery)
Nipples, 528
  abnormalities, 527–528
  Paget's disease of, 539
Nissen fundoplication, 1025
Nitrogen:
  ammonia, 1203, 1204
  balance, 87–88
  blood urea (See Blood urea nitrogen)
  loss, 20, 26, 27–29, 515
  mustard, 1620
  requirements, 88
  sweat loss of, 515
Nitrosoureas, 331
Nitrous oxide, 445–446
Nocardiosis, 639–640
Nocturia, 1550
Nodular dysplasia, adrenal, 1382–1383
Nodular glycogenic degeneration, 793
Nomograms for cardiac output, 504
Norepinephrine, 13–14, 1404–1409
  anesthesia and, 10
  control cells, 7
  pheochromocytoma and, 1409–1411
  urinary, 1409, 1410
Nose:
  (See also Nasopharynx)
  cosmetic surgery, 1945, 1955–1956
  fractures, 1941
No-touch isolation technique, 1134, 1135
Nucleic acids (see Deoxyribonucleic acid;
  Ribonucleic acid)
Nucleus pulposus, 1671, 1686
Nutrition, 86–95
  anabolic events and, 88
  catabolic events and, 87–88
  cirrhosis and, 1197
  elemental diets, 90–91
  esophageal fistula and, 1032
  fuel reserves and, 86–87

gastrostomy tube feeding, 90
indications for support, 89, 92
jejunostomy tube feeding, 90
methods of feeding, 89–95
nasopharyngeal tube feeding, 89–90
osteoporosis and, 1762
parenteral alimentation, 32–34, 35, 91–95
requirements, base-line, 88–89
rickets and, 1755–1759
scurvy and, 1755
starvation and, 87
   (See also Starvation)
surgery, trauma, sepsis and, 32–34, 87–88
Nystatin, 177

Obstruction, intestinal (see Intestine,
   obstruction)
Obturator sign, 1169
Occipital bone, 1669–1670
Occupational therapy, 1969–1971
Ocular muscular dystrophy, 1696
Oddi, sphincter of (see Sphincter of Oddi)
Odontogenic tumors, 579–580
Odontoid process, 1670
Odynophagia, 973
17-OHCS (see 17-Hydroxycorticosteroids)
Oliguria:
   ADH release and, 39
   renal failure and, 1564, 1565
      high-output, 85–86
   renal transplantation and, 415–418
   in shock, 155
   trauma and, 50
   water requirements and, 85
Ollier's disease, 1748
Ombrédanne orchiopexy, 1586–1587
Omentum, 1316–1318
   cysts of, 1318
   infarction of, 1317–1318
   torsion of, 1316–1317
   tumors of, 1318
Omovertebral mass, 1735
Omphalocele, 1523–1524
Omphalomesenteric duct persistence, 1522
Oncology, 297–343
   (See also Cancer; Carcinoma; Tumors;
      specific tumors)
Oophorectomy in breast cancer, 549–550
Oral cavity, 564–571
   benign lesions of, 564–567
   biopsy of, 560
   carcinoma, 568–571
   cysts, 565
   etiology of lesions of, 564
   examination of, 557–558
   fibroma, 566
   floor tumors, 569
   granuloma, 565–566
   hemangioma, 566–567
   hyperkeratosis, 567
   hyperplasia, inflammatory, 564–565
   incidence of lesions of, 564
   myoblastoma, 567
   pathology, 568
   polyps, 565
Orbital floor injury, 1940
Orchiectomy, inguinal, 1585–1586
Orchiopexy, transseptal, 1586–1587
Orchitis, mumps, 1552
Organ preservation for transplantation, 432–435
Organs of Zuckerkandl, 1404, 1415–1416
Orocutaneous fistula, 1945, 1947
Oropharynx:
   dysphagia and, 973
   examination of, 559
   tumors, 571–572
Orthopedic deformities, congenital, 1725–1739
Orthopedic surgery:
   in cerebral palsy, 1702

in clubfoot, 1733–1734
fractures (see Fractures)
in hip dislocation, congenital, 1729–1731
hip replacement, 1864–1867
in osteoarthritis, 1862–1869
in pes valgus, 1854
in rheumatoid arthritis, 1855–1859
for scoliosis, 1720–1721
in Sprengel's shoulder, 1735
in stroke, 1704–1705
in wryneck, 1736–1737
Orthotics, 1702
Oscillometer, 841
Osgood-Schlatter disease, 1720
Osler-Rendu-Weber syndrome, 1095
Osmolal discriminant, 38
Osmolar concentration, 70
Osmole, 67
Osmotic pressure, 67–68
Osseomucoid, 1741
Ossification, 1743–1744
   calcification vs., 1745
Osteitis deformans (see Paget's disease)
Osteitis fibrosa, 1760
   hyperparathyroidism and, 1470–1471
Osteoarthritis, 1860–1869
   of ankle and foot, 1868–1869
   cervical compression vs., 1681
   clinical manifestations, 1861, 1867, 1868
   of hip, 1862–1867
   of knee, 1867–1868
   pain, 1677
   pathology, 1860–1861
   primary and secondary, 1861
   spinal, 1690
   of thumb, 1862
   treatment: conservative, 1861–1862
      orthopedic, 1862–1869
   wrist, elbow, shoulder, 1862
Osteoarthropathy, hypertrophic pulmonary,
   1873
Osteoblasts, 1741, 1743, 1776
   tumors and, 1777, 1778
Osteoblastic prostatic carcinoma, 1578
Osteochondral grafts, 387
Osteochondritis, 1717–1721
Osteochondroma, 1778
   chest wall, 607
Osteoclastoma, 1782–1783
Osteoclasts, 1741, 1776
   hyperparathyroidism and, 1461, 1462, 1470
Osteocytes, 1461, 1741
Osteodystrophy:
   parathyroid, 1760–1761
   renal, 1498, 1757–1758
Osteogenesis imperfecta, 1750–1751
   differential diagnosis, 1762
   roentgenography in, 1480–1481
Osteogenic sarcoma, chest wall, 608
Osteogenic tumors of mandible, 580
Osteoma, 1776–1777
Osteomalacia, 1759–1760
   differential diagnosis, 1762–1763
      hyperparathyroidism vs., 1444
      osteodystrophy vs., 1761
Osteomyelitis:
   empyema and, 616
   of skull, 1662
   spinal, 1691–1692
   of sternum, 605–606
Osteomyoplastic amputations, 1881
Osteon, 1744
Osteopathia condensans disseminata, 1752
Osteopathia striata, 1752
Osteopoikilosis, 1752
Osteoporosis, 1462–1463, 1761–1764
   clinical manifestations, 1762, 1763
   etiology, 1761–1763
   osteodystrophy vs., 1761
   pathology, 1763

senile, 1708
treatment, 1764
Osteosarcoma, 1777–1778
Osteosclerosis, 1751–1752
Osteotomy:
   in congenital hip dislocation, 1730, 1731
   femoral, 1863
   in rickets, 1757
Ostium primum defect, 709–712
   anatomy, pathologic, 709
   clinical manifestations, 710
   diagnosis, 711
   laboratory findings, 710–711
   pathophysiology, 709–710
   treatment, 711–712
Outflow block syndrome, 394
Ovarian hormones, trauma and, 17
Ovaries, 1590, 1619–1622
   adrenal rest tumors, 1622
   amenorrhea and, 1602
   arrhenoblastomas, 1622
   Brenner tumor, 1621
   carcinoma, 1620–1621, 1622
      death rate, 298
   cystomas, 1620
   ovary, cysts, 1619–1620
   dysgerminoma, 1621
   granulosa-theca cell tumor, 1622
   hilus cell tumors, 1622
   Meigs' syndrome, 1622
   salpingo-oophorectomy, 1625–1627
   struma ovarii, 1622
   teratoma, 1621
   tumors, 1619–1622
Ovulation, 1597, 1601, 1605
Oxacillin, 174
Oxidative phosphorylation, 496
Oxycel, 120, 233
Oxygen:
   alveolar-arterial gradient, 465–466, 494, 498
   cyanosis and, 680
   gastric dilatation and, 1076–1077
   hyperbaric, 169
   inspired concentration, 465, 466
   low-cardiac-output syndrome and, 756–757
   measurements of, 465–466
   mixed venous unsaturation, 495, 503
   monitoring, 492–494, 498
   nitrous oxide anesthesia and, 446
   organ storage and, 433
   respiratory alkalosis and, 73
Oxygen:
   shock and, 143, 155–156
   tension, 465–466, 492–494, 498
      cerebral flow and, 1658
      extracorporeal circulation and, 754
   in tetralogy of Fallot, 722
   toxicity, 47
   transfusion and, 124
   transport, 492–496
      component therapy and, 34–35
   trauma and consumption of, 24
   wound healing and, 31
Oxygenators, 753, 754
Oxytetracycline, 173, 176
Oxytocin, 5, 7, 1367

PABA, 177
Pacemakers, 803–807
   demand, 804
   direct myocardial, 806
   endocardiac catheter, 805–806
   historical data, 803
   physiology of, 804–805
   postoperative care, 806
   selection of patients for, 805
   temporary, 806
   ventricular septal defect and, 716
Pacinian organs, 1676

Paget's disease, 1766–1768
  clinical manifestations, 1767
  differential diagnosis, 1762
    hyperparathyroidism vs., 1489
    osteodystrophy vs., 1761
  etiology, 1766
  osteosarcoma in, 1778
  pathology, 1766–1767
  of pelvis, 1578
  treatment, 1768
Pain, 967–973, 1664–1669, 1675–1692
  abdominal, 969–973
    (See also Abdomen, pain)
    apoplexy, 1331
    clinical evaluation, 971–973
    etiology, 970–971
  anatomy and physiology, 1665–1666,
    1675–1676
  appendicitis, 1168–1169
  in arterial occlusive disease, 840–842
  back, low, 1682–1692
    (See also Back pain)
  bone, 1677
  brachial, 1679–1680
  cervical compression syndrome, 1680–1682
  characteristics, 1676
  chest, in heart disease, 750
  chest wall, 1692
  convergence, 969
  diverticulitis, 1123, 1124
  gynecologic, 1598–1599, 1610
  hand, 1917
  hematoma, rectus sheath, 1316
  history, 971–972
  joint, 1678
  mesenteric lymphadenitis, 1333
  mesenteric occlusion, 1325
  menstrual, 1556
  muscle and tendon, 1677–1678
  in omental torsion, 1317
  osteoarthritis, 1861–1862
  pathways, 967–968, 1667, 1676
  pattern theory of, 967, 1677–1679
  peptic ulcer, 1058–1059
  peripheral nerve, 1678
  in peritonitis, 1302
  pulmonary, 601
  rectal, 1159
  referred, 969
  retractable, 969–970
  in retroperitoneal fibrosis, 1337
  sciatica, 1685–1686
  sensory end organs and, 1676
  shoulder, 1874–1875
  sites, 1676–1677
  somatic, 969
  specificity theory of, 967
  sphincter of Oddi fibrosis, 1244
  in spinal tumor, 1650
  splenic trauma, 1286
  stimuli, 1675–1676
  surgical relief of, 1666–1669
    central nervous system section, 1667–1668
    peripheral pathway section, 1666–1667
    response alteration, 1668
    stimulation for suppression, 1668–1669
    vasomotor reflex arc section, 1668
  tissue patterns, 1677–1679
  upper limb, 1679–1682
  urinary calculi, 1562, 1563
  urination, 1550–1551
  uterine fibroids, 1610
  in venous thrombosis, 914
  from vertebral column, 1678–1679
  visceral, 969
Palate:
  cleft, 1947–1950
  hard, 558
  soft, 557–558
  tumors, 570, 572

Palmar space infections, 1900, 1905
Palpitation, 750
Palsy:
  cerebral, 1700–1702
  facial nerve, 1957–1959
  median nerve, 1910
  radial nerve, 1911
Pancoast tumor, cervical compression vs.,
    1681–1682
Pancreas, 1255–1278
  abscess, 1269, 1270
  anatomy, 1255–1257
  annular, 1257
  blood supply, 1255–1257
  calcification, 1263
    carcinoma, 1270–1274
    clinical manifestations, 1271
    death rate, 298
    diagnosis, 1272
    laboratory studies, 1271–1272
    pathology, 1270–1271
    treatment and prognosis, 1272–1274
  cysts, 1268
  ductal system, 1255
  duodenal injuries and, 240
  endocrine, 1259–1260
  enzymes, 1258, 1259
  exocrine, 1257–1259
  exposure of, 1266
  fistula, traumatic injury and, 241
  hematoma, 1266
  hyperinsulinoma, 1274–1276
  inflammation (see Pancreatitis)
  intrabiliary pressure relationships, 1259
  islet-cell tumors, 1274–1278
  juice, 1257–1259
  lymphatic drainage, 1257
  mobilization of, 1267
  nerve supply, 1257
  peptic ulcer and, 1057–1058, 1068
  physiology, 1257–1260
  pseudocyst, 241, 1268–1270
  reflux from, gallstones and, 1233
  resection, 1273–1274
  roentgenograms, 1257, 1262, 1269, 1270
  shock and, 146
  transection of, traumatic, 239
  transplants of, 390–391
  trauma, 237–242, 1264–1268
    clinical manifestations, 1264–1265
    complications, 241
    diagnosis, 237–238
    mechanisms of injury, 1265
    morbidity and mortality, 241–242, 1268
    treatment, 238–241, 1266–1268
  tumors, 1270–1278
    in hyperparathyroidism, 1486–1487
    ulcerogenic, 1276–1278
  Zollinger-Ellison syndrome, 1276–1278
Pancreatectomy, 1276
  distal, for injuries of pancreas, 238–239
Pancreatic arteries, 1255–1256
Pancreatic duct, 1221, 1255, 1272
  accessory, 1255
  injuries of, 239
  jejunal anastomosis with, 1273
Pancreaticoduodenal arteries, 1255, 1321
Pancreaticoduodenal transplants, 391
Pancreaticoduodenectomy, 1272–1274, 1276
  for penetrating trauma, 240
  technique, 1273–1274
Pancreaticojejunostomy, 1264–1265, 1273
  for traumatic injuries, 239
Pancreatitis, 1260–1265
  acute, 1260–1263
    alcoholism and, 1260–1261
    clinical manifestations, 1261–1262
    complications, morbidity, mortality, 1263
    etiology, 1260
    gallstones and, 1260

    laboratory studies, 1262
    metabolic factors, 1261
    postoperative, 1261
    treatment, 1262–1263
  chronic, 1263–1265
    clinical manifestations, 1264
    laboratory studies, 1264
    treatment, 1264–1265
  hyperparathyroidism and, 1476
  renal transplants and, 426
Pancreozymin, 1258, 1259
Pancytopenia, 1290
Panniculitis, mesenteric, 1334
Papanicolaou smear, 1611
Papilla of Vater, 1255
  fibrosis or stenosis of, 1243–1244
Papillary adenomas, 1126–1128
Papillary carcinoma:
  of breast, 540
  of thyroid, 1450–1451
Papillary cystadenoma lymphomatosum,
    581–582
Papillitis, ampulla of Vater, 1244
Papilloma:
  ductal, of breast, 538
  laryngeal, 547–575
Pappenheimer bodies, 1283
Pappenheimer isogravimetric perfusion
    technique, 147, 148
Para-aminomethylbenzene, 263n.
Para-aminosalicylic acid, 1094
Parabronchial diverticulum, 1023
Paracentesis:
  trauma and, 221–222
  unapparent injury and, 198
Paraesophageal hernia, 1023
Parahemophilia, 112
Paralysis, 1694–1705
  arm, 1699–1700
  in arterial occlusion, 841
  dystrophies, 1696–1697
  eyelid, 1958
  facial, 1957–1959
  foot, 1698–1699
  hand, 1700
  hip, 1699
  knee joint, 1699
  motor, 1694
  poliomyelitis, 1697–1700
  scoliosis and, 1709
  ulnar nerve, 1910–1911
  urinary bladder, 1557
Paralytic ileus, 990, 991
Paranasal sinuses:
  examination of, 558
  intracranial infection from, 1662–1663
  tumors, 578–579
Paranoid psychosis, 478
Paraplegia:
  bladder dysfunction in, 1557
  epinephrine and norepinephrine in, 17
  rehabiltation in, 1978–1979
Parasympathetic nervous system, pain and, 968
Parasympatholytics, 458–459
Parathormone, 1753
  (See also Parathyroid hormone)
Parathyroid, 1457–1501
Parathyroid adenoma, 665, 1467, 1482, 1496
  anatomy, 1458–1459
  blood supply, 1459, 1494
  bone formation and, 1461–1463, 1470–1471,
    1474, 1475
  calcitonin and, 1464
  calcium metabolism and, 1459, 1464–1465,
    1472–1474, 1477–1479
  carcinoma, 1467–1468
  chief cell hyperplasia, 1468–1469
  embryology, 1457–1458
  historical backgroung, 1457
  hormone (see Parathyroid hormone)

hydroxyproline and, 1461, 1478
hyperparathyroidism, 1466–1499
  (*See also* Hyperparathyroidism)
hyperplasia, 1468–1469
hypoparathyroidism, 1457, 1500
in kidney transplants, 1498
laryngeal nerve and, 1459, 1494
magnesium metabolism and, 1460–1461
operative technique, 1491–1496
osteodystrophy, 1760–1761
peptic ulcer and, 1058
phosphorus metabolism and, 1459–1460,
  1477–1478, 1479
physiology, 1459–1465
pseudohypoparathyroidism, 1500–1501
pseudopseudohypoparathyroidism, 1501
roentgenography, 1480–1486
squeeze test, 1480
transplants, 389, 390
tumors, 1467–1470
vitamin D and, 1464
Parathyroid hormone, 1463–1464, 1753
  amino acid sequence, 1463–1465
  calcium levels and, 1465
  infusion test, 1479
  maternal crossover of, 1485
  osteodystrophy and, 1760–1761
  plasma measurements, 1479–1480
  renal effects of, 1465
  symptoms relating to, 1474–1476
  tumors producing, 1469–1470, 1488
Parathyroidectomy, 1490–1496
  renal transplants and, 426
Parenteral alimentation, 32–34, 35, 91–95
Parenteral solutions, 79, 201
Paresthesia in arterial occlusion, 841
Parietal cells, 1051, 1053
Parkland formula, 262
Paromomycin, 176
Paronychia, 1899, 1904
Parotid duct injury, 1935–1936, 1943
Parotid gland, 580, 581
Parotidectomy, 587
Parotitis, postoperative, 464–465
Paroxysmal ventricular tachycardia,
  postoperative, 471
Partial thromboplastin time (PTT), 29, 103–104,
  106
Patella:
  chondromalacia, 1867
  dislocation, 1827
  fractures of, 1828–1829
  osteosarcoma of, 1777
Patent ductus arteriosus (*see* Ductus arteriosus,
  patent)
Patterson-Kelly syndrome, 1038
Pavlov pouches, 1051, 1052
Payne-DeWind bypass, 1105
PBI (*see* Protein-bound iodine)
P_{CO_2} (*see* Carbon dioxide tension)
Pectinate line, 1147
Pectoral artery, 528
Pectus excavatum, 602–604
Pediatric surgery, 1513–1540
  (*See also* Children)
  adrenogenital syndrome, 1390–1391
  airway maintenance, 1515
  appendicitis, 1173–1174
  biliary atresia, 1224–1228
  cystic hygroma, 1515–1516
  emphysema, lobar, 624–625
  esophageal atresia, 1516–1521
  fluid and electrolyte replacement, 1514–1515
  gastroschisis, 1523–1524
  hernia, 1349
    foramen of Bochdalek, 1040–1041
    inguinal, 1358
    umbilical, 1348
  Hirschsprung's disease, 1531–1536
  imperforate anus, 1537–1539

intestinal atresia, 1526–1528
intraoperative management, 1513–1514
intussusception, 1530–1531
malrotation of intestine, 1525–1526
Meckel's diverticulum, 1522–1523
meconium ileus, 1529
neurologic malformations, 1651–1657
omphalocele, 1523–1524
omphalomesenteric duct persistence, 1522
postoperative management, 1514
preoperative care, 1513
psychiatric complications in, 479
pyloric stenosis, 1521
rectal prolapse, 1536–1537
tracheoesophageal fistula, 1516–1521
umbilical anomalies, 1348, 1521–1525
urachus, 1524–1525
urologic disorders, 1566–1570
volvulus, midgut, 1525–1526
Wilms' tumor, 1567
Pedicle tissue transfers, 292–294, 1924–1930
  design of flap, 1930
  distant flaps, 1928–1930
  local flaps, 1925–1928
PEEP (positive end-expiratory pressure
  ventilation), 467
Pelvic abscesses, 1307–1308
Pelvic environment, female, 1591–1593
Pelvic exenteration for cancer, 324, 1136
Pelvic inflammatory disease, 1608
Pelvic lymphadenectomy, 1627–1630
Pelvic vein thrombosis, 915
Pelvis:
  (*See also* Hip)
  dislocations, 1835–1837
    congenital, 1726–1731
  fractures, 1837–1839
  surgical anatomy of, 1626
Pendred's syndrome, 1449
Penetrating wounds, 216–220, 223–225, 235–237
  (*See also* Wounds, penetrating)
Penicillin, 173, 174
  in gonococcal arthritis, 1853
  in gonorrhea, 1559
  for hand infection, 1899
Penicillinase, 174
Penis, 1548
  anomalies, 1567–1568, 1569
  carcinoma, 1580
  hypospadias, 1962–1964
Pentagastrin stimulation test, 1060
Penthrane, 450
Pentothal, 451
PEP/LVET, 506–507
Pepsin, 1057
Pepsinogen, 1053
Peptic ulcer, 1055–1074
  appendicitis vs., 1172
  bleeding, 992, 995, 1062, 1067–1068
  dumping syndrome and, 1065
  duodenal, 1055–1069
    clinical manifestations, 1059
    diagnosis, 1059–1060
    diathesis, 1055–1069
    gastric ulcer vs., 1069
    management, 1061–1069
    pathogenesis, 1056–1058
  endocrine disorders and, 1057–1059
  endoscopy, 1060
  gastric, 1068–1074
    cancer vs., 1072–1073, 1079
    clinical manifestations, 1071
    diagnosis, 1072–1073
    duodenal ulcer vs., 1069
    etiology, 1070–1071
    trauma and, 49
    treatment, 1073, 1076
  gastric analysis, 1060, 1073
  hereditary factors, 1057, 1071
  hyperacidity and, 1057, 1071

hyperparathyroidism and, 1475–1476, 1487
indications for surgery, 1061–1063
intractability, 1062
liver disease and, 1057
marginal, 1056, 1068
pain, 1058–1059
pancreatic disease and, 1057, 1276–1278
parathyroid glands and, 1058
pepsin's role, 1057
perforation, 1062–1063, 1068
peritonitis from ruptured, 1302
pulmonary disease and, 1057
pyloric obstruction, 1062, 1068
roentgenography, 1059, 1072
steroid therapy and, 1404
subtotal gastric resection for, 1064
treatment, 1060–1068, 1076
  long-term, 1061
  surgery, 1064–1068
  vagotomy, 1066–1067
Zollinger-Ellison syndrome and, 1057–1058,
  1069
Percussion test for venous insufficiency, 926–927
Percutaneous absorption, 514
Perforators, incompetent, 925, 930–931
Perfusion:
  extracorporeal circulation, 753–755
  organ storage and, 432–433
  ventilation and, 598–599
Periampullary carcinoma, 1270–1274
Pericardial sarcoma, 792
Pericardiectomy, 802–803
Pericardiotomy syndrome, 758, 797
Pericarditis, 801–803
  acute pyogenic, 801–802
  chronic constrictive, 802–803
  empyema and, 616
Pericolic abscess, 1124–1125
Perineal anoplasty, 1539
Perineal prostatectomy, 1584
Perinephric abscess, 1559
Perineum, female, 1590
Periosteum, 1745
Peripheral aneurysms, 894–901
Peripheral arterial disease (*see* Arterial disease)
Peripheral nerve injuries, 1643–1646
Perirectal abscess, 1152–1153
Peritoneal dialysis, 1297
Peritoneal lavage, 223
Peritoneal tap (*see* Paracentesis)
Peritoneum, 1297
  (*See also* Peritonitis)
  anatomic spaces and, 1306
  rectum and, 1146
Peritonitis, 1297–1309
  abscesses and, 1305–1308
  appendiceal rupture and, 1170–1171
  appendicitis vs., 1172
  barium, 1309
  bile, 1232, 1308
  cardiovascular system and, 1301–1302
  chemical, 1308
  clinical manifestations, 1298, 1302–1303
  chylous, 1309
  diagnostic studies, 1298, 1303
  endocrine response to, 1301
  enemas and, 1300
  etiology, 1299
  fluid shifts in, 1300–1301
  foreign bodies and, 1309
  glove powder, 1308–1309
  hemoperitoneum and, 1309
  idiopathic, 1298
  ileus in, 1301
  laxatives and, 1300
  pain in, 1302
  pathogenesis, 1299–1300
  pathophysiology, 1300–1302
  pericolic abscess and, 1124–1125
  pneumoperitoneum and, 1309

primary, 1298–1299
prognosis, 1304–1305
pseudomyxoma peritonei, 1309
respiratory system and, 1302
secondary, 1299–1305
toxic absorption in, 1301
treatment, 1303–1304
tuberculous, 1298–1299
Pernio, 904
Peroneal muscle atrophy, 1703
Peroneal nerve injury, 1977
Peroneal spastic flatfoot, 1713
Peroxisomes, 496
Pes planus and valgus, 1713, 1734
Petechial hemorrhage, fat embolism and, 476
Petit's triangle hernia, 1345
Petrosphenoidal syndrome, 577
Peutz-Jeghers syndrome, 1096
Pfannenstiel incision, 1624, 1625
pH:
    buffer system and, 70–71
    in alkalosis and acidosis, 36, 38
    gastric juice, 1053, 1054
    in heart disease, congenital, 684
    hypoxia and, 508
    muscle surface, 508
    oxygen transport and, 496
    of sweat, 515
    trauma and, 3
    urinary calculi and, 1564
Phalangeal amputations:
    foot, 1882–1883
    hand, 1889–1890
Phalangeal fractures:
    foot, 1835
    hand, 1818–1819
Pharyngoesophageal diverticulum, 1018–1020
Pharyngostomy, 1517, 1518
Pharynx:
    injuries of, 219
    laminogram of, 562
    swallowing and, 1012
Phenothiazine, 151
Phenoxybenzamine, 44, 151
Phentolamine, 1410, 1416
Phenylalanine mustard, 1620
Pheochromocytoma, 942, 1407–1417
    acid-base balance and, 39
    bilateral, 1415
    of bladder, 1416
    in children, 1415
    cholelithiasis and, 1414
    clinical manifestations and laboratory studies,
        940, 942
    diagnostic findings, 1410–1411
    familial relationships, 1412
    heart disease and, 1413
    historical background, 1375
    hypertension and, 1408, 1409
    hypotension, shock, sudden death and,
        1414–1415
    incidence, 1407–1408
    intrathoracic and mediastinal, 1416
    localization, 1411
    malignant, 1408
    mediastinal, 669
    neurocutaneous syndromes and, 1412–1413
    in pregnancy, 1412
    renovascular hypertension and, 1414
    signs and symptoms, 1409–1410
    thyroid carcinoma and, 1413–1414
    treatment, 942, 1416–1417
    of Zuckerkandl organs, 1415–1416
Phimosis, 1567–1568
Phlebitis:
    (See also Thrombophlebitis)
    in Buerger's disease, 864
    mesenteric, 1330
Phlebography, 915–916
    venous insufficiency and, 927–928

Phlebothrombosis, 913
Phlegmasia cerulea dolens, 859, 915
Phlegmon, periappendiceal, 1170
Phosphatase:
    alkaline (see Alkaline phosphatase)
    bone and, 1742–1743
Phosphate:
    deprivation test, 1479
    diabetes, 1758–1759
    hemoglobin, 42
    in hyperparathyroidism, 1459–1460,
        1477–1478, 1479, 1498
    parenteral administration of, 94
    tubular resorption of, 1479
Phosphorus, bone metabolism and, 1753–1754
Phosphorylation, oxidative, 496
Phrenic artery, 1376
Phrenoesophageal membrane, 1010
Physical therapy, 1967–1969
    for cerebral palsy, 1701
    in rheumatoid arthritis, 1855–1856
Physiologic monitoring (see Monitoring)
Pigeon breast, 604
Pigment, bile, 997–1001
Pigmented lesions of skin, 521–525
Pigmented spots of lip, 562
Pigmented villonodular synovitis, 1872
Pilonidal cyst, 517
Pinworms, vaginal, 1607
Pitressin in esophagogastric varices, 1200
Pituitary, 1363–1374
    acromegaly and, 1369–1371, 1765
    adenomas, 1372
    adrenocortical insufficiency and, 1403
    anatomy, 1364–1365
    anterior lobe hormones, 1365–1367
    bone disease and, 1764–1765
    breast cancer and, 1373
    cell types, 1364–1365
    Cushing's syndrome and, 1368, 1387
    cysts, 1372
    disorders, 1367–1372
    dwarfism and, 1764–1765
    ectopic hormones and, 1373–1374
    embryology, 1363–1364
    gigantism and, 1369–1371, 1764–1765
    historical background, 1363
    hyperthyroidism and, 1372
    hypopituitarism, 1367–1368
    lactation persistence and, 1371–1372
    myxedema, 1442
    physiology, 1365–1367
    posterior lobe hormones, 1367, 1374
    prostate cancer and, 1373
    removal of, 1368
        (See also Hypophysectomy)
    in retinopathy, diabetic, 1372–1373
    vascular supply, 1364
pK, 71
PK test, 1605
Placenta:
    hormone secretion, 1593
    polyp, 1606
Plasma:
    chemical composition of, 66
    fresh frozen, 35
    hemophilic transfusion, 109–110, 111
    pooled, 123
    protein, 19, 28
    substitutes, 35
    thromboplastin component, 99
    volume, 66–67
        (See also Hypovolemia)
    burns and, 257
Plasma membrane, antigens on, 352
Plasmin, 101, 365–366
Plasminogen, 101, 107
Plastic surgery, 1919–1964
    bone losses, 1946
    branchial anomalies, 1953–1954

cleft lip and palate, 1947–1950
decubitus ulcer, 1960
dermabrasion, 1934
ear, 1950–1952, 1955
eyebrow reconstruction, 1925, 1943,
    1954–1955
facial, 1935–1944, 1954–1959
    contour defects, 1956–1957
    cosmetic, 1954–1956
    paralysis, 1957–1059
    trauma, 1935–1944
head and neck, 1944–1954
    congenital anomalies, 1947–1954
    tumors, 1944–1946
historical background, 1919–1920
hypospadias, 1922–1964
lip, 1943, 1944, 1947–1950
mammoplasty, 1960–1963
mandible, 1941, 1956–1957
maxilla, 1940–1941, 1956–1957
microsurgery, 1931
nose, 1941, 1945, 1955–1956
scar placement and correction, 1933–1934, 1954
skin grafting, 1921–1931
    (See also Skin grafting)
soft tissue losses, 1945–1946
tattooing, 1934–1935
thyroglossal anomalies, 1952–1953
tongue, 1944
wound management, 1920–1921
zygoma, 1939–1940
Platelets, 98–99
    adenosine diphosphate, 98–99, 103
    allograft rejection and, 368, 371
    component therapy and, 35
    estimation and count of, 102–103
    factor 3, 103
    splenic sequestration, 1283
    tests of function of, 102–103
    thrombocytopenia and, 115, 1289
    transfusion and, 107–108, 123, 124
Platybasia, 1669–1670
Pleura, 610–621
    absorption and transudation, 611
    anatomy, 610
    calcification of, 620–621
    chylothorax and, 620
    effusion, 613
    empyema and, 615–619
    esophageal fistula with, 1031–1032
    gases, 611
    hemothorax and, 614
    herniation, 611–612
    intrathoracic pressure after pneumonectomy,
        655–656
    Meigs' syndrome, 614
    mesothelioma, 621
    physiology, 610–611
    pneumothorax, spontaneous, 612–613
    thoracentesis and, 613–614
    tuberculosis and, 619–620
    tumors, 621
Pleurisy, serofibrinous, 619
Pleuropericardial cyst, 666
Pleuroperitoneal canal hernias, 1040–1041
Plummer-Vinson syndrome, 1038
Pneumatocele, 604, 625–627
Pneumatosis cystoides intestinalis, 1102
Pneumococcal empyema, 615
Pneumocystis carinii, 634
Pneumoencephalography, 1640
    nitrous oxide and, 446
Pneumomediastimun, 660
Pneumonectomy, 651–658
    postoperative care, 655–658
    precautions during operation, 651–652
    technique, 652–655
    for tuberculosis, 637
Pneumonia, 633–634
    aspiration, 633–634

burns and, 259, 265, 268–269
  lipoid, 633
  staphylococcal, 633
Pneumonitis, radiation, 609
Pneumoperitoneum, 1309
  roentgenography and, 221
Pneumotachygraph, 498, 499
Pneumothorax, 197
  spontaneous, 612–613
Podophyllum, 1158
Poietins, 353
Poisons, 4
Poliomyelitis, 1697–1700
  clinical course, 1698
  treatment, 1698–1700
Pólya operation, 1064
Polycystic disease:
  of kidney, 1571
  of liver, 1187–1188
Polycythemia, cyanosis and, 680
Polycythemia vera, 116–117
Polydactyly, 1896
Polymorphonuclear leukocytes, allograft
  rejection and, 367, 371
Polymyxin B, 173, 175
Polyostotic fibrous dysplasia, 1749
Polyp(s):
  cervical, 1610–1611
  colorectal, 1126–1131
    adenocarcinoma, polypoid, 1128
    adenomatous, 1128
    familial polyposis, 1128–1129
    Gardner's syndrome, 1129
    juvenile, 1126
    malignant potential of, 1129–1131
    villous adenoma, 1126–1128
  endocervical or endometrial, 1601
  gastric, 1082–1083
  juvenile, 1126
  laryngeal, 574
  mucous, 1126
  nasal, 578
  oral, 565
  Peutz-Jeghers, 1096
  retention, 1126
Polypropylene suture, 957
Poly-X syndrome, 1604
Pontocaine, 447
Popliteal artery:
  aneurysms, 894–895
  arteriovenous fistula, 874
Popliteal vein:
  ligation, 931
  thrombosis, 916
Porphyria erythropoietica, 1293
Port wine hemangioma, 518
Portacaval shunt, 1205–1208
  for glycogen storage disease, 1214
  technique, 1208
Portal hypertension, 1196–1214
  anatomy, pathologic, 1198–1199
  ascites and, 1202
  coma and, 1201, 1203–1204
  esophagogastric varices and, 1199–1202
  etiology, 1196–1197
  hypersplenism and, 1202–1203, 1290
  pathophysiology, 1197–1198
  surgery of, 1204–1214
    gastrectomy and, 1205
    ligation, transesophageal, of varices,
      1204–1205
    portacaval shunt, 1208
    pressure-reducing procedures, 1205–1213
    selection of patients, 1207–1208
    selection of procedure, 1206–1207
    splenorenal shunt, 1208–1210, 1213
    superior mesenteric–inferior vena cava
      shunt, 1210–1213
Portal venous system, 1178, 1323
  isotopic evaluation of, 995

in liver transplants, 392–393, 397
  pressure, 1197
  (See also Portal hypertension)
Portuguese man-of-war, 215
Positive end-expiratory pressure ventilation
  (PEEP), 467
Postcholecystectomy syndrome, 1239–1240
Postoperative complications (see Complications,
  postoperative)
Posture, 1705–1715
  foot and ankle deformities, 1712–1715
  gait disturbances, 1706–1707
  knee deformities, 1711–1712
  spinal deformities, 1707–1711
Potassium:
  abnormalities, 75–76
  acid-base balance and, 37, 39, 42
  in aldosteronism, 1397–1401
  in burns, 261
  cardiac arrest and, 759
  in diabetes, 475
  hypertension and, 943
  liver transplants and, 398
  parenteral administration of, 93, 94
  preoperative therapy, 81
  in renal failure, 1565
  in stomach, 1052
  vomiting and, 976
Potassium chloride ulcers, 1101
Potts aortic-pulmonary anastomosis, 726
Pott's disease, 1851–1852
Poupart's ligament, 1355–1358
Power mower wounds, 205
Pouch of Douglas, 1591
Powder peritonitis, 1308–1309
PPT, 103–104
Precordium, inspection and palpation of, 750–751
Prednisolone, formula of, 1381
Prednisone, 1095, 1445
  in cardiac transplantation, 401
  formula of, 1381
Preejection period/left ventricular ejection time
  ratio, 506–507
Pregnancy, 1605–1607
  abdominal apoplexy in, 1331
  abnormal growth, 1606–1607
  amenorrhea and, 1602
  breasts in, 530–531
  cervical carcinoma in, 1615
  coagulation and, 29
  ectopic, 1598, 1606
    appendicitis vs., 1172
    operation for, 1625
  frog test for, 1594
  hyperparathyroidism in, 1484–1486
  osteomalacia in, 1759
  pheochromocytoma in, 1412
  traumatic uterine injuries in, 246
  trophoblastic disease, 1606–1607
Pregnenolone, 13
Premature contractions, 472
Prepuce, redundant, 1567–1568
Pressure sores, 516
Proaccelerin, 112
Procidentia, 1536
Proconvertin, 100, 112–113
Proctalgia fugax, 1159
Proctitis:
  factitial, 1159
  gonococcal, 1158–1159
Proctosigmoidoscopy, 1147
Profunda femoris arteries, 843–845
Progesterone, 13
  secretion of, 1595
Progestin, 13
Prognathism, 1957
Prolactin, 1366
  persistent lactation and, 1371–1372
Prolene, 957
Propranolol, 152

Propylthiouracil, 1440
Prostaglandin, 366
Prostate, 1548
  bleeding after surgery of, 107
  carcinoma, 1550, 1577–1579
    chemotherapy for, 336
    death rate, 298
    hypophysectomy in, 1373
  examination, 1552
  hypertrophy, benign, 1574–1577
  infections, 1560–1561
  resection, 1576–1577, 1584–1585
  secretion, 1553
  tumors, 1574–1577
Prostatectomy, 1576–1577, 1584–1585
  open, 1577
  perineal, 1584
  retropubic, 1584–1585
  suprapubic, 1584
  transurethral, 1576–1577
Prostatitis, 1560–1561
Prostheses:
  for aorta, 829, 888, 893
  aortic valve, 775, 777, 778, 780–782, 784
  arm, 1891, 1975
  atrial septal defect, 705–706, 708
  ball-valve, 768, 777, 778, 780, 781, 785
  breast, 1961, 1963
  bypass (see Bypass procedures)
  Canadian Syme, 1884
  femoral head, 1821
  hip, 1865–1866
  immediate postsurgical (IPOP), 1881
  knee, 1857
  leg, 1886, 1887, 1889, 1973–1974
  mitral valve, 768–769
  for opposition loss, 1970
  rehabilitation and, 1971, 1973–1975
  for spastic hand, 1970
  tricuspid, 785
  wrist, 1971
Prosthetics, 1970
Protamine sulfate, 108
Protein:
  Bence Jones, 1771
  burns and, 257
  C-reactive, 28
  calcium and, 1459
  catabolism, 87–88
  in edema fluid, 932
  fuel reserves, 86, 87
  liver and, 1179, 1203
  loss in trauma, 27–29
  muscle, 1692, 1693
  pancreatic juice and, 1258
  plasma, 19, 28
  requirements, 88
  storage, 28
  starvation and, 20–22
  trauma and, 24, 27–29, 201
  tube feeding of, 91
Protein-bound iodine, 1433–1434
  in amenorrhea, 1603
  thyroid and, 1431, 1433, 1440
Proteolysis, 101–102
Prothrombin:
  consumption, 104
  liver synthesis of, 1180
  time, 29, 100–101, 103
Prothrombinase, 100
Pruritus ani, 1158
  postoperative, 1149
Pseudarthrosis, 1857
  congenital, of tibia, 1732
Pseudocyst, pancreatic, 241, 1268–1270
Pseudoepitheliomatous hyperplasia, 567
Pseudogout, 1487–1488, 1870–1871
Pseudohemophilia, 111
Pseudohermaphroditism, 1390–1392, 1394, 1604
Pseudohypoparathyroidism, 1500–1501

Pseudomembranous enterocolitis, 181, 1119–1120
Pseudomonas aeruginosa, 185–186
 burns and, 255–256
 shock and, 157
Pseudomyxoma peritonei, 1309, 1620
Pseudopseudohypoparathyroidism, 1501
Pseudotruncus, 736
Psoas sign, 1169
PSP excretion, 1575
Psychiatric complications, 477–481, 1970
 in brain injuries, 1640
 of cancer patient, 343, 480
 hepatic coma and, 1203
 prefrontal lobotomy for, 1668
 ulcerative colitis and, 1111
Psychosis:
 postperfusion, 759
 postoperative, 478
PTA, 99, 112
PTC, 99
Pubic fractures and separations, 1838
Pull-through procedures:
 abdominoperineal, for imperforate anus, 1539, 1540
 for Hirschsprung's disease, 1534–1535
 rectal operation, 1136
Pulmonary arteriovenous shunting, alkalosis and, 37
Pulmonary artery:
 anomalies, 622–623
 aortic fistula with, 734–735
 catheterization, 501
 coronary artery arising from, 739–741
 emboli, 919–923
 in resection of lung, 654
 stenosis, 689–690
 transplant of lung and, 402
 transposition of, 727–730
  corrected, 742–743
 in tetralogy of Fallot, 724–726
 in tricuspid atresia, 731, 732
Pulmonary arterioles, 679
Pulmonary disease (*see* Lung)
Pulmonary embolism, 919–923
 amputations and, 1882
 differential diagnosis, 920–921
 fat, postoperative, 475–477
 incidence, 919
 pathophysiology, 919–920
 physical findings, 920
 special tests for, 920
 treatment, 921–923
 urokinase therapy, 922–923
Pulmonary function, 599–600
 burns and, 258, 259, 265, 268–269
 tests, 600
 trauma and, 46–47
Pulmonary hypertension (*see* Hypertension, pulmonary)
Pulmonary insufficiency:
 liver transplantation and, 395
 posttraumatic, 46–47
 shock and, 145
Pulmonary osteoarthropathy, 1873
Pulmonary veins:
 anomalous drainage of, 706–709
 cor triatriatum and, 733
 transplant of lung and, 403, 404
Pulmonic stenosis, 685–690
 anatomy, pathologic, 685–686
 clinical manifestations, 687
 diagnosis, 688
 historical data, 685
 incidence and etiology, 685
 laboratory findings, 687–688
 pathophysiology, 686–687
 treatment, 688–689
Pulse, 750
 abdominal aorta, 843

amputation healing and, 1880
 in aortic stenosis, 775
 in arterial occlusion, 841
 in Buerger's disease, 865
 volume, 507
Pump-oxygenator:
 (*See also* Extracorporeal circulation)
 cardiac trauma and, 790
 intraaortic balloon assist, 158
Puncture wounds, 205
Purines, 376–377
Puromycin, 378
Purpura:
 Henoch-Schönlein, appendicitis vs., 1172
 idiopathic thrombocytopenic, 115–116, 1289–1290
 thrombotic thrombocytopenic, 1290
 transfusion, 107–108
Pyelography, 1553–1555, 1571, 1580
 retroperitoneal fibrosis, 1338, 1340, 1341
Pelophlebitis, 1330
Pyeloplasty, 1569
Pyeloureterography, 1555
Pyemia, 170
Pyloric glands, 1050
Pyloric obstruction, duodenal ulcer and, 1062, 1067–1068
Pyloric stenosis, congenital, 1521
Pyloromyotomy, 1521, 1522
Pyloroplasty, 1065, 1066
 in short bowel syndrome, 1105
Pyogenic arthritis, 1848–1850
Pyogenic osteomyelitis, 1691–1692
Pyrimidine, immunosuppression and, 377
Pyrophosphate, bone metabolism and, 1754
Pyrroles, 1293
Pyruvate, 137–138, 1742
Pyruvate-kinase deficiency, 1287

Quadriplegia, rehabilitation in, 1978–1979
Quaternary ammonium compounds, 190
Quick test, 103, 106

Rabies, 207–211
 confirmed cases in U.S., 208
 diagnosis, 207–209
 epidemiology, 207
 incidence, 207
 prophylaxis, 209–210
 treatment, 210–211
Rad, 326
Radial artery:
 cannula for monitoring, 499–500
 cephalic vein anastomosis with, 407, 410
Radial nerve injury, 1977
Radial nerve palsy, 1911
Radiation, 326–330
 for breast cancer, 544, 547–548
 carcinogenic effects of, 301
 for cervical carcinoma, 1614–1615
 for colorectal cancer, 1138–1139, 1140
 complications from, 327–328
 in Cushing's syndrome, 1387
 dosage, 326, 327
 for esophageal carcinoma, 1036
 extracorporeal, 372–373
 historical notes, 556–557
 immunosuppression by, 374–376
 indications for, 328–329
 infrared, 1968
 local effects of, 328
 for lung cancer, 649
 mechanism of action, 326–327
 necrosis of chest wall from, 609
 palliative, 329
 postoperative, 329–330
 preoperative, 329
 for retroperitoneal tumors, 1341

sensitivity vs. curability, 327
 sterilization, 189
 surgery combined with, 329, 330
 ultraviolet, 1969
Radicular cyst, 580
Radiography (*see* Roentgenography)
Radioisotopes:
 brain studies, 1648
 in Cushing's syndrome, 1387
 fluid and electrolyte studies, 981
 in parathyroid adenoma, 1482–1483
 in pituitary disorders, 1368, 1370
 portal circulation studies, 995
 in renography, 952, 1555
 scanning (*see* Scanning)
 in splenic studies, 1284–1285
 in thrombosis, 917
 thyroid studies, 1434
 thyrotoxicosis therapy, 1440
Radiosensitivity vs. radiocurability, 327
Radioulnar synostosis, 1737
Radium in cervical cancer, 1614
Radius:
 absence of, 1738
 fractures of, 1808–1809, 1813–1815
 metastasis to, 1789
 subluxation of, 1812
Rana pipiens test, 1594
Ranula, 565
Rappaport test, 954
Rathke's pouch, 1364
Rattlesnake bites, 212, 213
Rebound phenomenon, anticoagulants and, 118
Recklinghausen's disease, 1749, 1760–1761
Reconstructive surgery (*see* Orthopedic surgery; Plastic surgery; Skin grafting)
Rectocele, 1599
Rectosigmoid junction:
 cancer, 1134, 1136
 lymphoma, 1141
Rectum:
 abdominoperineal resection and, 1136
 abscess, 1152–1153
 anal lesions and (*see* Anus)
 anatomy, 1146
 bleeding from, 997, 1133, 1160
  postoperative, 1148–1149
 blood supply, 1146
 carcinoids, 1097, 1141
 carcinoma, 1131–1141
  chemotherapy, 1137–1138, 1140
  classification, 1132
  clinical manifestations, 1133
  diagnosis, 1133–1134
  early detection, 1140–1141
  etiology, 1131
  incidence, 1131
  metastases, 1132
  operative procedures, 1136–1137
  pathology, 1131–1133
  prognosis, 1139–1140
  radiation therapy, 1138–1139, 1140
  recurrent, 1140
  sigmoidoscopy for, 1141
 defecation and, 977
 examination of, 1133, 1142, 1303
 factitial proctitis, 1159
 fecal impaction, 1145–1146
 gonococcal proctitis, 1158–1159
 inflammation, 1158–1159
 injuries of, 230–232
 leiomyoma and leiomyosarcoma, 1142
 lymphogranuloma venereum and, 1159
 lymphoma, 1141
 lymphosarcoma, 1141–1142
 pain, 1149, 1159
 peritoneal reflection of, 1146
 polyps, 1126–1131
  (*See also* Polyps, colorectal)
 postoperative care, 1148–1149

proctalgia fugax, 1159
prolapse, 1156–1158, 1530–1531
pull-through operation for, 1136
surgical principles, 1148–1149
tumors, 1126–1143
ulcerative colitis, 1111
Rectus sheath hematoma, 1313–1315
Red cells (see Erythrocytes)
Redox potential measurements, 508
Reflexes, preanesthetic medication and, 458
Reflux, gastroesophageal:
esophagitis and, 1026–1027
hiatal hernia and, 1024
tracheoesophageal fistula and, 1516–1517
Regional enteritis (see Enteritis, regional)
Regitine, 1410, 1416
Rehabilitation, 1967–1982
ambulation, 1968
amputation, 1881–1882, 1972–1975
back pain and, 1975–1976
cardiac surgery, 1980
colostomy and ileostomy, 1981
electrotherapy, 1969
exercises and muscle reeducation, 1967–1968
facial paralysis, 1976
fractures, 1972
hand surgery, 1975
head-injured patient, 1640–1641
heat in, 1968–1969
joint disabilities, 1972
laryngectomy, 1981
massage in, 1969
mastectomy, radical, 1980–1981
maxillofacial surgery, 1981
musculoskeletal problems, 1971–1976
neck dissection, radical, 1981–1982
nervous system diseases, 1976–1980
occupational therapy, 1969–1971
paraplegia or quadriplegia, 1978–1979
physical therapy, 1967–1969
(See also Physical therapy)
principles, 1967
psychiatric problems, 1970
pulmonary operations, 1980
spinal cord injury, 1642–1643
uropathy in, 1979–1980
Rejection, transplant (see Transplantation,
rejection)
Relaxants, 453–454
Renal arteries, 1547
aneurysms, 898–900
bypass graft operation, 957–958
exposure of, 957
fibroplasia, 946–948, 954
single mural hyperplasia of, 948
stenosis, 946, 947, 954, 955, 958
transplantation and, 415
unilateral parenchymal disease and, 962
Renal disease (see Kidney)
Renal osteodystrophy, 1498
Renal veins, 1547
transplantation and, 414
Renin:
in aldosteronism, 1398
hypertension and, 948
assay, renal venous, 955–956
pheochromocytoma and, 1414
trauma and, 12
Renography, 1555
isotope, 952
transplant function and, 416
Renovascular hypertension, 946–962
clinical manifestations, 949–950
diagnostic studies, 951–961
arteriography, 952–954
biopsy, 956
function studies, split, 954–955, 956
isotope renography, 952
renin assay, 955–956
urography, rapid-sequence, 951–952

laboratory findings, 951
pathology, 946–948
pathophysiology, 948–949
pheochromocytoma and, 1414
renal parenchymal disease and, 962–963
treatment, 956–962
operative, 956–959
postoperative, 959
preoperative, 956
results, 959–962
Reproductive tract, female (see Female
reproductive tract; Gynecologic disorders;
and specific structures)
Respiration, 597–598, 600
acid-base disturbances and, 73–74
anesthesia and, 444–445, 446, 448, 456
monitoring of, 497–499
mouth-to-mouth, 760
support of, 466–467
Respiratory acidosis, 73
Respiratory alkalosis, 73–74
Respiratory disease (see Lungs)
Respiratory complications, 465–469
extracorporeal circulation and, 757
failure, postoperative, 465–467
high-output, 46
lobectomy and, 656–657
in peritonitis, 1302
pleuroperitoneal hernia and, 1040
spinal anesthesia and, 456
Resuscitation, 196–198
cardiac, 760–762
intravenous, in burns, 260–263
Reticular activating system, 1624
Reticular formation, 6, 1631–1632
Reticulin, 1741
Reticuloendothelial system, 42, 43
bone disease and, 1768–1771
spleen and, 1283
Reticuloses, 1768–1771
Reticulum cell sarcoma, 1784, 1785, 1787
splenectomy for, 1291
Retinopathy, diabetic, 1372–1373
Retroperitoneum, 1336–1341
bleeding, 1331
hematoma, 242–243
hemophilic, 109
fibrosis, idiopathic, 1337–1338
clinical manifestations, 1337–1338
etiology, 1336–1337
pathology, 1337
treatment, 1338
tumors, 1339–1341
clinical manifestations, 1339–1340
pathology, 1339
treatment, 1340–1341
Rets, 326
Retzius, space of, 1600
Rh factors, 121–122
Rhabdomyoma, cardiac, 793
Rhabdomyosarcoma of muscle, 1787
Rheumatic fever:
aortic stenosis and, 775
aortic insufficiency and, 780
mitral stenosis and, 762
tricuspid stenosis and insufficiency and, 784
Rheumatoid arthritis, 1853–1860
Rheumatoid factor, 1854
Rhinoplasty, 1955–1956
Rhizotomy, 1667
Rhytidectomy, 1956
Rib(s):
(See also Chest wall)
anomalies, 602
cervical, 876
chondroma of, 1779
empyema and, 616
fibroma of, 1781
fibrous dysplasia of, 607
fractures, 604–605

osteopetrosis, 1751
Ribonucleic acid (RNA):
cancer chemotherapy and, 330
immune, 340
immunosuppressive drugs and, 376–378
recruitment of lymphocytes by, 362–363
Richter's hernia, 1350
Rickets, 1755–1759
celiac, 1757
clinical manifestations, 1756–1758
hypophosphatasia, 1759
pathology, 1756, 1757
renal osteodystrophy, 1757–1758
treatment, 1756–1757
Riedel's (struma) thyroiditis, 1445
Right-to-left shunts, 680–681, 721–727
Ring, lower esophageal, 1038
Ring prosthesis, 1866
Ringer's lactate solution, 35
acidosis and, 74
in burns, 262
in shock, 149
Rings, vascular, 701–704
Risus sardonicus, 183–184
RNA (see Ribonucleic acid)
Roentgenography:
abdominal aneurysm, 889, 890
abdominal trauma and, 221, 224, 226
adrenal gland, 1386, 1411
aortic, 820, 822, 832, 834
(See also Aortography)
appendicitis, 1169–1170
biliary tract disease, 1229–1230
bone disorders, 1744–1745, 1749, 1751,
1756–1761, 1763, 1768, 1770
fractures, 1793, 1797–1800, 1803–1809,
1811–1824, 1829–1836, 1840–1841
tumors, 1777–1783, 1785, 1787–1789
brain, 1648–1649, 1664
breast, 532
cephalometric speech studies, 1952
chest wall, 603, 607–610
colonic disease, 1115, 1117, 1119, 1122–1124,
1143
diarrhea, 1021
esophageal, 1014, 1017, 1019, 1030–1031, 1038
face and neck, 560–561, 1936–1938
foot, 1721
gallbladder, 1229–1230, 1237, 1239, 1240, 1242,
1245
hand, 1897, 1912
heart disease, 682–683, 751–752
aortic stenosis, 691, 776
coarctation of aorta, 697
coronary arteriography, 795, 796
mitral insufficiency, 773
mitral stenosis, 764, 765
pacemakers, 807
patent ductus arteriosus, 719
sinus of Valsalva aneurysm, 736
tetralogy of Fallot, 682, 723
transposition of great vessels, 683, 729
tricuspid prosthetic valves, 786
trivalvular disease, 788
ventricular aneurysm, 799, 800
ventricular septal defect, 714
hemorrhage, gastrointestinal, 995–996
hip, 1701, 1719, 1728, 1731
Hirschsprung's disease, 1532
hyperparathyroidism, 1480–1486
imperforate anus, 1538
intestinal atresia, 1527
intestinal obstruction, 984–985
intussusception, 1531
jaundice, 1003
joints, 1847, 1849, 1851, 1852, 1854, 1855,
1860–1862, 1870–1872, 1874
liver, 1189, 1191, 1198
lung, 623–627, 629–633, 635–641, 643–650,
656–658

embolism, 476, 920, 921
kidney transplant, 416, 418, 424, 425
lymphatic, 932
mediastinum, 662–663, 665–669
mesenteric, 1328, 1329, 1331, 1336
pancreas, 1257, 1262, 1269, 1270
peptic ulcer, 1059, 1071–1072
pituitary disorders, 1371
pleura, 611–613, 615, 617, 619–622
pneumatosis cystoides intestinalis, 1104
regional enteritis, 1091–1092
retroperitoneal, 243, 1338, 1340, 1341
sella turcica, 1386
spleen, 1284, 1286
subphrenic abscess, 1306
tracheoesophageal fistula, 1518
skull, 1480–1483, 1636, 1648–1649
small bowel tumors, 1096
spinal cord, 1650
in trauma, 199, 221, 224, 226
urinary tract, 1553–1555, 1559, 1562–1563,
    1567–1569, 1572–1576, 1578–1579
vertebral column, 1680, 1685, 1688–1690, 1708,
    1710
Roger's disease, 712
Rokitansky-Aschoff sinuses, 1239, 1240
Rongeur for stenotic excision, 692, 694
Rosenthal's syndrome, 99, 112
Rotator cuff lesions, 1874–1875
Round ligaments, 1590, 1591
Roux-en-Y procedures:
    in biliary tract decompression, 1227
    for biliary tract injury, 236
    for choledochal cyst, 1224, 1225
    esophagojejunostomy, 1028, 1207
    marginal ulceration and, 1056
    for pancreatic pseudocysts, 1270
    pancreaticojejunostomy, 239
Rovsing's sign, 1169
Rubella, heart disease and, 677
Rumpel-Leede test, 102

Sacralization, 1689–1690
Salicylazosulfapyridine, 1114
Salivary glands, 580–584
    adenocarcinoma, 582
    adenomas, 566
    carcinoma, 570, 582
    cysts, 565
    enlargement, asymptomatic, 582
    inflammation, postoperative, 464–465
    injuries of, 220
    Mikulicz's disease, 582
    mixed tumors, 581, 582–583
    papillary cystadenoma lymphomatosum,
        581–582
    tumors, 580–584
        benign, 581–582
        differential diagnosis, 583
        incidence, 581
        malignant, 582–583
        natural history, 583
        prognosis, 584
        treatment, 583–584
Salivary sodium/potassium ratio, 1398
Salmonella, 186, 1094–1095, 1171
Salpingitis isthmica nodosa, 1622
Salpingo-oophorectomy, 1625–1627
Salt:
    burns and, 257, 261
    gain and losses, 78–79
    intraoperative management of, 82
    postoperative management of, 84–85
Sanfillipo syndrome, 1766
Santorini, duct of, 1255
Saphenous vein(s):
    in bypass operations, 795, 849, 850
    ligation for venous insufficiency, 930
    percussion test, 927

popliteal artery graft with, 895
renal artery anastomosis with, 957
thrombi of, 914
Sarcoidosis:
    Boeck's, 640–641
    hilar lymph node, 663
    hyperparathyroidism vs., 1489
    regional enteritis and, 1091
    splenic, 1292–1293
Sarcoma, 314
    antibodies, 311
    breast, 540–541
    cardiac, 792–793
    esophageal, 1033
    Ewing's, 608–609, 1784–1785
    lung, 644
    osteogenic, 608, 1777–1778
    parosteal, 1778
    resection, 323, 325
    reticulum cell, 1291, 1784, 1785, 1787
    of skin, 521
    spread of, 315
    synovial, 1787
    thyroid, 1452
    uterine, 1617
Scab, 286
Scalene fat pad biopsy, 649–650
Scalenus anticus syndrome, 876
Scalp, 1633
    transplant of hair-bearing, 1924, 1925
Scanning:
    abdominal trauma and, 223
    adrenal, 1399
    brain, 1648
    liver, 1180–1181
    for pulmonary embolism, 920, 921
    spleen, 1284
    thyroid, 1435
Scapula:
    fractures of, 1804
    high, congenital, 1735
Scara's fascia, 1346
Scars:
    collagen in, 284, 285
    hypertrophy, 292
    maturation of, 289
    placement and correction, 289–290, 1933–1934,
        1954
Scheie syndrome, 1766
Scheuermann's disease, 1707–1708
Schilling test, 1103
Schimmelbusch's disease, 537
Schmorl's nodules, 1671, 1686
Schwann cells, autotransplants and, 385
Schwartz percussion test, 926–927
Sciatic nerve injury, 1977
Sciatica, 1685–1686
Scintillation scanning (see Scanning)
Sclerodactylia, 901
Scleroderma, esophageal, 1039
Sclerosing adenosis of breast, 538
Sclerosing carcinoma of hilar ducts, 1245–1246
Sclerosing cholangitis, primary, 1242–1243
Sclerosing hemangioma, 518
Scoliosis, 1683, 1708–1711
    classification, 1708
    idiopathic, 1709–1710
    postural, 1708
    structural, 1708–1709
    treatment, 1709–1710
Scopolamine, 458–459
Scribner shunt, 407
Scrotum:
    examination of, 1551
    hernias, 1347
    hydrocelectomy, 1585
Scuderi "sizzle" test, 477
Scurvy, 1755
Sebaceous cyst, 517
Seborrheic keratosis, 517

Secretin, 1051, 1258, 1259
Secundum defects, 704–706
Segmental resection, pulmonary, 653
Segmentectomy, hepatic, 1193–1196
Sella turcica, 1386
Semen analysis, 1553, 1605
Seminal vesicles, 1548
Sengstaken-Blakemore tube, 1200
Senile kyphosis, 1708
Senile osteoporosis, 1708, 1761, 1762
Sensing, physiologic, 497
Sensory end organs and pathways, 1676
Sensory function of skin, 514
Sensory nerves of hand, 1904
Sensory neurons, pain and, 968
Septal defects (see Atrial septal defects;
        Ventricular septal defects)
Sepsis:
    abortion and, 1605–1606
    burn wound, 256
    coagulation and, 29
    colorectal operations and, 1140
    lung changes and, 47
    metabolism and, 24
    nutrition and, 87–88, 95
    pancreatic injury and, 241
    transfusion and, 127
Septic arthritis, 1848–1850
Septic shock, 44–45, 140–144, 157–158,
        1605–1606
Septicemia, 170
    hepatic abscess and, 1184
    meningococcal, 1402
    peritonitis and, 1301, 1305
Septostomy, balloon, 729
Sequestration, pulmonary, 622
Seroma, postoperative, 464
Serosa:
    diverticulitis perforation, 1124–1125
    in ulcerative colitis, 1111
Serotonin:
    carcinoid and, 1098, 1099
    ulcerative colitis and, 1111
Serous cavities, cancer spread by, 315
Serratia marcescens, 186
Sertoli-Leydig cell tumors, 1622
Serum:
    antirabies, 210
    antitumor, 339
    antivenin, 212–214
    prothrombin, 104
    transaminases, 1180
    typing histocompatibility of, 382–383
Serum hepatitis, 128–129
Seton for fistula in ano, 1155, 1157
Severinghaus electrode, 497, 498
Sexual development, 1393–1394
    adrenogenital syndrome and, 1390–1392
SGOT and SGPT, 1180
Sheehan's syndrome, 1602
Shin splints, 871
Shock, 133–159
    acidosis and, 37–38
    anesthesia and, 203
    arterial injury and, 868
    beta-blocking agents for, 152
    buffers for, 158
    cardiac injuries and, 789
    cardiogenic, 144–145, 156, 157
    cardiovascular function in, 44–45
    cart, 504–505
    cell metabolism in, 137–138
    coagulation in, 29
    crystalloids for, 149
    digitalis for, 152
    endotoxin, 43, 45, 140–144
    experimental observations of, 134–142,
        144–145
    fluid therapy for, 147–148, 149
    gastrointestinal function and, 48–49

glucagon for, 152
glucocorticosteroids for, 153
hemodynamics, 134–137
hemorrhagic, 134–138
isoproterenol for, 151–152
kidney and, 50, 145
liver function and, 48
lung and, 46, 146, 466
mechanical circulatory support, 158–159
myocardial infarction and, 472
pancreas and, 146
perforated ulcer and, 1062
in peritonitis, 1301
pheochromocytoma and, 1414
protocol for, 155–158
resuscitation and, 196–197
reversible, 135
septic, 44–45, 140–144, 157–158
    abortion and, 1605–1606
stimuli inducing change from, 3
sympathetic nervous system and, 136, 138, 141
tolerance to, 147
traumatic, 134–138, 156
treatment of, 147–159
vasoconstriction and, 135–137, 140
vasopressor therapy for, 150–151
Short bowel syndrome, 1103–1105
Shoulder:
dislocations, 1802, 1804–1806
fracture-dislocations, 1806
frozen, 1704
motion, 1802
osteoarthritis, 1862
painful, 1874–1875
paralysis, 1699
Sprengel's, 1735
Shunts:
aortic, 821
dialysis, 408
left-to-right, 679–680, 704–721
portacaval, 1205–1208, 1214
    in liver transplants, 392, 393
right-to-left, 680–681, 721–727
shunt, splenorenal, 1201, 1205, 1209–1210,
    1213
superior mesenteric–inferior vena cava,
    1210–1213
in shock, 143
traumatic arteriovenous, 871
ventriculoatrial, for hydrocephalus, 1655
Sickle cell disease, 1288
Sigmoid colon:
carcinoma, 1124, 1134
diverticulitis, 1123
mesentery, 1319
volvulus, 1144
Sigmoidoscopy, 1147
colorectal cancer and, 1141
colorectal polyps and, 1130–1131
in ulcerative colitis, 1114
Silver nitrate in burns, 263
Silver sulfadiazine, 265
Sinoatrial block, postoperative, 472
Sinus arrhythmia, postoperative, 471–472
Sinus of Valsalva, ruptured aneurysm of,
    735–736
Sinus venosus, 707, 708
Sinuses:
(See also Paranasal sinuses)
tumors of, 578–579
Skeletal changes in hyperparathyroidism,
    1470–1471, 1472, 1474–1475, 1491
Skeletal disorders (see Bone; Vertebral column;
    and specific structures
Skeleton:
axial, abnormalities of, 1669–1673
metastatic tumors of, 1788–1790
Skene's glands, 1590
Skin, 513–525
absorption through, 514

banking, 1931, 1933
blood supply, 514, 1925
burn destruction of, 254–255
contraction of, 275–278
cysts, 516–517
degerming of, 189–190
epithelization, 278–281
functions, 513–516
grafts (see Skin grafting)
hidradenitis suppurativa, 516
insensible water loss, 515
physical properties, 513
pressure sores, 516
sensory function, 514
structure, 1922–1923
sweat secretion, 514–515
tattooing, 1934–1935
tension lines of, 1933
tensile strength, 513
thermoregulation, 515–516
thyrotoxicosis and, 1438
transplants, 383–384
    (See also Skin grafting)
tumors, 517–525
benign, 517–519
carcinoma, 520–521
fat, 519
keloid, 517–518
keratosis, 517
malignant, 519–521
melanoma, 521–525
neuromas, 519
pigmented lesions, 521–525
vascular, 518–519
warts, 517
Skin grafting, 290–294, 1921–1931
autografts, 268, 383, 1931
bipedicle flap, 1926, 1928
bipetal (bilobed) flap, 1926, 1928
in burns, 267–268, 383
composite, 1923–1924
delay principle, 293, 1930
design of flap, 1930
distant flaps, 1928–1930
dressing, 291–292
facial soft tissue losses and, 1948
free, 290–291
full-thickness, 291, 1923
historical background, 1921–1922
homografting, 267–268
interpolation, 1926, 1927
island flap, 1926, 1928
local flaps, 1925–1928
pedicle, 292–294, 1924–1930
rotation, 1926, 1927
split-thickness, 291, 1923
take, 290
transposition, 1926, 1927
V-Y advancement, 1925
xenografts, 1933
Z-plasty, 1925–1926, 1934, 1949
Skull, 1633–1634
anatomy, 1633–1634
craniosynostosis, 1656–1657
fracture, 1634
osteomyelitis, 1662
roentgenography, 1480–1483, 1636, 1648–1649
Small intestine (see Duodenum; Ileum;
    Intestine, small; Jejunum)
Smith fracture, 1815
Smoking:
aortoiliac disease and, 844
atelectasis and, 468
Buerger's disease and, 864, 866
cancer and, 302
    laryngeal, 573
    lip, 562
    lung, 645
    oral, 564
Snakebites, 211–214

Social service, 1971
Sodium:
aldosterone and, 1379, 1397, 1398
in burns, 261
concentration, 68–69
–creatine ratio, 954
pain and losses, 78–79
parenteral administration of, 79, 93
postoperative management of, 84–85
in renal failure, 1565
therapeutic correction of, 80–81
water metabolism and, 41–42
Sodium bicarbonate, 70–74
cardiac arrest and, 761
in resuscitation, 74
vomiting and, 976
Sodium colistimethate, 1120
Solutions:
hyperalimentation, 93–95
priming, for extracorporeal circulation, 753
Somatotropin (see Growth hormone)
Spasticity, 1694–1705
cerebral palsy, 1700
flatfoot, 1713
prosthesis for hand, 1970
in stroke, 1705
Speech, laryngectomy and, 575–576
Spermatic cord, hernias and, 1346, 1354, 1355
Spermatocele, 1551
Spherocytosis, hereditary, 1287
Sphincter:
anal, 1146
    incontinence and, 1149, 1155–1156
esophageal, 1012–1013, 1014
of Oddi, 1228
    fibrosis or stenosis, 1243–1244
vesical, 1599
Sphincteroplasty, anal, 1156
Sphincterotomy:
anal, 1152
transduodenal, 1244, 1248
Spider bites, 215–216
Spina bifida, 1652–1653, 1702–1703
Spinal anesthesia, 454–457
Spinal cord:
compression, 1680–1682
decompression, 1642
dermal sinus tracts, 1653–1654
diastematomyelia, 1653
electrical stimulation of, 1668
infection, 1679
injuries, 1641–1643, 1840–1841
myelomeningoceles, 1653–1654
pain and, 1666, 1667
puncture, lumbar, 1636, 1637
syringomyelia, 1703, 1704
tumors, 1649–1651
Spinal dysraphism, 1702–1703
Spine (see Vertebral column)
Spinnbarkheit phenomenon, 1597
Spinothalamic pathway, 1665
Spironolactone, 1398, 1401
Splanchnic circulation, liver transplantation and,
    392, 393, 396
Splanchnic pain, 969
Splanchnicectomy, 969, 1667
Spleen, 1281–1294
accessory, 1281
anatomy, 1281–1282
autoimmune hemolysis and, 1288–1289
blood supply, 1281–1282, 1283
cysts and tumors, 1293
diagnostic considerations, 1284–1285
ectopic, 1293
spleen, elliptocytosis and, 1287
enlargement (see Splenomegaly)
Fanconi syndrome, 1293
Felty's syndrome, 1292
Gaucher's disease, 1293
hemolytic anemias and, 1287–1289

Hodgkin's disease and, 1291–1292
hypersplenism, 1283, 1290
immunologic role of, 354, 357
injuries, 242
leukemia and, 1291
ligaments, 1281
mobilization of, 1267
myeloid metaplasia and, 1290–1291
physiology and pathophysiology, 1282–1284
porphyria erythropoietica, 1293
portal hypertension and, 1198, 1202–1203
removal of (see Splenectomy)
reticulum cell sarcoma and, 1291
roentgenography of, 1286
rupture, 1285–1286
sarcoidosis, 1292–1293
sickle cell disease and, 1288
size, 1284
spherocytosis and, 1287
thalassemia and, 1287–1288
thrombocytopenic purpura and, 1289–1290
transplantation, 389
for hemophilia, 111
Splenectomy, 1293–1294
in Hodgkin's disease, 1291–1292
for hypersplenism, 1290
palliative, 1291
in portal hypertension, 1205
for ruptured spleen, 1286
for spherocytosis, 1287
technique, 1293–1294
Splenic arteries, 1282
aneurysms, 898, 1293
rupture, abdominal apoplexy and, 1331
fistula, 1196
Splenic flexure:
cancer, 1134
ischemia, 1118
mesentery, 1319
Splenic pulp manometry, 995, 1200, 1285
Splenocolic ligament, 1281
Splenomegaly:
portal hypertension and, 1202–1203
roentgenography in, 1284
Splenoportography, 1191, 1198
Splenorenal ligament, 1281
Splenorenal shunt, 1201, 1205, 1209–1210, 1213
Splenosis, 1286
Splints, 1970
clubfoot, 1733
emergency, 1793
for hip dislocation, congenital, 1729
in rickets, 1756–1757
Spondylitis, tuberculous, 1851
Spondylolisthesis and spondylolysis, 1640–1641
Spondylosis, 1673, 1690
Sprengel's shoulder, 1735
"Sprung back," 1689
Sputum, 601
abscess of lung and, 632
Squamous cell carcinoma, 520
of cervix, 1611
of floor of mouth, 569
of lip, 563
of paranasal sinus, 579
vaginal, 1619
Squamous metaplasia of cervix, 1611
Stab wounds, 223–224
of gallbladder, 1231
of heart, 787–788
of pancreas, 1265
Stable factor, 112
Staging extent of tumors, 320
Stagnant anoxia, 139
Stamey test, 955
Staphcillin, 174
Staphylococcal infections, 180–181
in burns, 265
enteritis, 181
of hand, 1898, 1899

of kidney, 1559
osteomyelitis, 1691
pericarditis, 802
pneumonia, 633
pseudomembranous enterocolitis, 1119–1120
of wounds, 206, 463
Staphylococcus aureus, 180, 181, 1184
antiseptics for, 189
shock and, 140
Staphylococcus epidermidis, 180
Starling's law, 135
Starr-Edwards valve prosthesis, 768–769, 772, 778, 780–782
Starvation, 87
hormones and, 22–24
osteomalacia in, 1759
trauma and, 4, 19–24
Steam sterilization, 189
Steatorrhea:
gastrectomy and, 1065
osteomalacia and, 1759–1760
in short bowel syndrome, 1104
Steinmann pin, 1824
Sterilization, 189
Sternberg–Reed cells, 1291
Sternoclavicular joint injuries, 1802
Sternocleidomastoid muscle, radical neck dissection and, 586
Sternotomy, median, 218
Sternum:
anomalies, 602
empyema and, 616
Steroids, 7–12, 13
antivenin and, 213
diabetes, transplanted kidney and, 424–425
gynecologic disorders and, 1594–1597
metabolism, 1595
neplasms and, 331
normal values, 1384
ulcers from, 49, 1404
Stilbestrol in breast cancer, 551
Stimuli:
painful, 1675–1676
traumatic, 1–5
Stingrays, 214–215
Stings, 214–215
Stitches, removal of, 289
Stokes–Adams attacks, 804, 805
Stoma, obstruction of, postoperative, 482
Stomach, 1049–1083
acidity, 1053, 1057–1058, 1070
adenocarcinoma, 1080
adenomas, 1083
anatomy, 1049–1050
aspiration of contents of, pneumonia from, 633–634
benign tumors, 1082
bezoars, 1079
blood supply, 1049
burns and erosion of, 992–993
cancer, 1079–1083
clinical manifestations, 1080
death rate, 298
etiology, 1079–1080
incidence, 1079
pathology, 1080–1082
prognosis, 1083
treatment, 1082–1083
ulcer vs., 1073, 1079
diarrhea and, 978
dilatation, 1077
fistulas, postoperative, 484–485
foreign bodies, 1079
full, anesthesia and, 202–203
function, 1050–1055
glands, 1051
inflammation, 1078–1079
injuries of, 225
leiomyosarcoma, 1082
lymphoma, 1082

Mallory-Weiss syndrome, 1078
mucosal lesions, 992, 993, 1074–1076
anatomy, pathologic, 1075
clinical manifestations, 1076
diagnosis, 1076
etiology, 1075
hypersecretion and, 1075
treatment, 1076–1077
mucosal resistance, 1053, 1070, 1074–1075
musculature, 1050
polyps, 1083
prolapse of mucosa, 1078
pyloric stenosis, congenital, 1521
reflux from, 1024, 1026–1027
in tracheoesophageal fistula, 1516–1517
resection, 1064
secretion, 1051–1055
analysis, 1060–1061, 1072
composition of, 1052–1054
duodenal ulceration and, 1055–1056
histology, 1051–1052
hyperacidity, 1056–1057, 1070–1071
methods of studying, 1052
regulation of, 1054–1055
ulcerogenic tumors of pancreas and, 1276–1278
tumors, 1079–1083
ulcer, 1054–1055, 1069–1076
(See also Peptic ulcer)
volvulus, 1079
Stool:
black, tarry, 991
blood in, as cancer sign, 1133, 1141
diarrheic, 979
(See also Diarrhea)
villous adenoma and, 1127
Strain:
foot, 1715
lumbosacral, 1689
shoulder, 1874–1875
Strangulation:
in hernias, 1345, 1351
intestinal obstruction and, 982–983
in volvulus, 1144
Strawberry mark, 518
Streptococcal infections, 178–180
in burns, 265
erysipelas, 178–179
erysipeloid, 179
gangrene, progressive synergistic, 179–180
Meleny's ulcer, 180
myonecrosis, 179
necrotizing fascilitis, 179
patent ductus arteriosus and, 718
pericarditis, 802
Streptokinase, 101, 115
Streptomycin, 173, 176, 1094
Streptozotocin, 1275
Stress fractures, 1797–1798
Stress incontinence, 1599–1601
Stress ulcers, 992
trauma and, 49
String sign, 1092
Stroke, 1658
(See also Cerebrovascular disease)
orthopedic management of, 1704–1705
spasticity in, 1705
Struma ovarii, 1622
Stuart-Prower factor (X), 100, 113
Subarachnoid hemorrhage, 1554, 1661
Subclavian arteries, 876–881
aneurysms, 898
atherosclerosis, 883, 884–886
coarctation of aorta and, 699, 700
retroesophageal, 702, 703
in tetralogy of Fallot, 724, 725
thoracic outlet syndrome, 876–881
Subclavian steal syndrome, 883
Subclavian vein catheterization, 92–93, 500
Subcostal transabdominal incision, 1212

Subcutaneous tissue, 513
  (*See also* Skin)
  abscess of hand, 1899
  arthritis and, 1853
  cysts, 516
  tumors, 518, 519
Subdiaphragmatic infection, 614
Subdural empyema, 1662–1663
Subdural hematoma, 1638–1639
Subhepatic abscess, 1307
Subhepatic space, 1305
Submaxillary gland, 580–581
Subphrenic abscess, 1306–1307
Subphrenic space, 1305
Succinylcholine, 453–454
Sulfamylon, 263n.
Sulfonamides, 177–178
  in burns, 265
Sump drains, 228–229, 1304
SU-9055, 1386
Superinfection, 171
Superior mesenteric–inferior vena cava shunt,
  1210–1213
Superior vena cava syndrome, 662
Suprahepatic space, 1305
Supraspinatus tendonitis, 1874–1875
Supravalvular aortic stenosis, 693–694
Supraventicular paroxysmal tachycardia,
  postoperative, 471
Surgicel, 120
Surveillance, immune, 307–308
Suture(s):
  closure of wounds, 288
  cosmetic result of, 1920–1921
  emergency laparotomy, 205
  hemostatic, 119
  for liver wounds, 233
  polypropylene, 957
  through-and-through closure, 205–206
SV-40 virus, 305
Swallowing, 973–974, 1012
  gastriodilatation and, 1077
Swan-Ganz catheter, 149, 150, 502
Sweat gland carcinoma, 520–521
Sweat secretion, 514–515
  sodium loss in, 79
Swenson's pull-through procedure, 1534–1535
Syme amputations, 1883–1884
Sympathectomy:
  in aortoiliac atherosclerosis, 844
  in Buerger's disease, 866–867
  in femoropopliteal atherosclerosis, 825
  in frostbite, 905–906
  in hypertension, essential, 1033
  in Raynaud's disease, 902–903
  in tibioperoneal atherosclerosis, 853
Sympathetic nervous system:
  cyclopropane anesthesia and, 446–447
  ileus and, 990
  pain and, 968
  shock and, 137, 138, 142
  spinal anesthesia and, 454–457
Sympathoadrenal response, 138
Syncope:
  in aortic stenosis, 776
  dissecting aneurysm and, 828
  heart block and, 807, 808
Syndactyly, 1895–1896
Synostosis, congenital radioulnar, 1737
Synovectomy:
  knee, 1856
  metatarsophalangeal, 1858
Synovial membrane and fluid, 1845–1848
  lesions, 1872–1873
  sarcoma, 1787
Synovial sheaths of hand, 1901
Synovitis:
  acute, of hip in childhood, 1873
  pigmented villondular, 1872
  rheumatoid, 1853, 1855, 1857

Syphilis, 1608
  aortic aneurysms and, 815, 816, 821, 824
  oral cancer and, 564
Syringomyelia, 1703–1704
Systolic hypertension, 941
Systolic murmurs, 681–682
  (*See also* Murmurs)
Systolic pressure, 683–684

T cells, 354, 357, 358
Tachycardia, postoperative, 471
Talipes equinovarus, 1703, 1732–1734
Talus:
  injuries, 1833–1834
  vertical, 1734
Tamponade, balloon, 995
  for esophagogastric varices, 1200
Tamponade, cardiac, 197
  diagnosis of, 789
  extracorporeal circulation and, 756
  trauma and, 788, 789
Tarsal epiphysitis, 1720–1721
Tattooing, 1934–1935
Taussig-Bing syndrome, 728
Technetium scan of spleen, 1284
Telangiectasia:
  hemostatic risk evaluation and, 105
  lip, 562
  small bowel tumors vs., 1095
Telepaque, 1230
Temperature:
  in heart disease, congenital, 684
  trauma and, 4
Temporal lobe hematoma, 1640
Tendon(s):
  autografts, 385
  hand, 1900, 1901, 1911, 1913, 1975
  rupture of, 1859
  pain, 1677–1678
  reflexes, 1695
  transfer in poliomyelitis, 1698
Tendonitis:
  bicipital, 1877
  supraspinatus, 1874–1875
Tenosynovitis:
  of hand, 1900, 1905
  of wrist, 1859
Tenotomy, adductor, 1702
Teratoma, 314
  cardiac, 793
  mediastinal, 665
  ovarian, 1621
Testes, 1549–1550
  orchiectomy, inguinal, 1585–1586
  orchiopexy, transseptal, 1586–1587
  torsion of, 1552
  tumors, 1552, 1579–1580
  undescended, 1570
Testosterone:
  in breast cancer, 550
  trauma and, 17
Tetanus, 183–185
  clinical manifestations, 183–184
  complications, 184
  immunization, 184
  prophylaxis, 184–185, 263
  treatment, 184
Tetracaine, 457
Tetracyclines, 173, 176–177
  bones studies with labeled, 1462
Tetralogy of Fallot, 721–727
  acyanotic, 714
  anatomy, pathologic, 721
  clinical manifestations, 723
  diagnosis, 723–724
  historical data, 721
  incidence and etiology, 721
  laboratory findings, 723
  pathophysiology, 721–723

  postoperative course, 727
  roentgenogram, 682
  treatment, 724–727
Thal procedure, 1033
Thalamus, pain and, 1665, 1666
Thalassemia, 1287–1288
THAM, 158
Thermal agents for hemostasis, 120
Thermal dilution, 505
Thermography, 509
  breast, 532–533
Thermoregulation, skin in, 515–516
Thiazides, hypercalcemia and, 1490
Thiobarbiturates, 451–452
Thiopental, 451–452
Thomsen's disease, 1697
Thoracentesis, 613–614
  for empyema, 616
Thoracic artery, lateral, 528
Thoracic disc hernia, 1672
Thoracic duct, 598–599
  cancer spread by, 315
  cannulation for esophagogastric varices, 1200
  immunosuppression and, 372
  injuries of, 220
  lesions, 663
Thoracic inlet, penetrating wounds of, 216–220
Thoracic nerve injury, 1977
Thoracic outlet syndromes, 875–881
  anatomy, regional, 876
  clinical manifestations, 877–878
  diagnosis, 878–879
  etiology, 876
  historical data, 876
  laboratory studies, 878
  pathology, 876–877
  prognosis, 880–881
  treatment, 879
Thoracoabdominal aneurysms, 824–825
Thoracoabdominal incision, 1212
Thoracolumbar fractures and dislocations,
  1840–1842
Thoracostomy for empyema, 617–618
Thoracotomy:
  aortic injury and, 829
  cardiac injuries and, 790
  in hemothorax, 614
  in pneumothorax, 613
  pulmonary resection and, 652
Thorax, 596–602
  anatomy, 596–597
  anesthesia in surgery, 602
  diverticula, 667
  meningocele, 669
  pathophysiology, 597–602
Throat (*see* Oropharynx; Pharynx)
Thrombasthenia, 99
Thrombectomy, venous, 919
Thrombin, 101
  allografts and, 365, 366
  time, 104
Thromboangiitis obliterans (*see* Buerger's
  disease)
Thrombocytes (*see* Platelets)
Thrombocytopenia, 115–116
  detection of, 102–103
  hemostasis and, 106–108
  idiopathic purpura, 115–116, 1289–1290
  thrombotic purpura, 1290
  transfusion purpura and, 107–108
  treatment, 115–116, 1289–1290
    transfusion of platelets for, 123, 124–125
  types of, 115
Thrombocytosis in polycythemia vera, 116
Thromboelastogram, 105
Thromboendarterectomy (*see* Endarterectomy)
Thrombophlebitis, 913
  of breast, 538
  emboli and, 859
  transfusion and, 128

Thromboplastin, 29, 99
  generation test, 104
  time, partial, 103–104, 106
Thrombosis:
  abdominal aortic, 843
  anticoagulation for, 918–919
  arterial, 858, 862
    (See also Buerger's disease)
  hemorrhoid, 1150
  kidney transplants and, 425
  mesenteric artery, 1325
  mesenteric vein, 1329–1330
  omental infarction and, 1317–1318
  operatiive treatment for, 919
  in polycythemia vera, 116
  popliteal artery, 895
  venous, 839–845
    (See also Veins, thrombosis)
Thrombosthenin, 99
Thrombotest, 104–105
Through-and-through closure, 205–206
Thumb:
  absence of, 1896, 1897
  amputations, 1914
  arthritis of, 1859
  osteoarthritis, 1862
Thymectomy, immunosuppression and, 372
Thymocytes, immunogen interaction with,
    357–358
Thymol turbidity test, 1179
Thymosin, 358
Thymus:
  immune apparatus and, 353–354
  transplantation, 389
  tumors of, 665–666
Thyrocalcitonin, 1464
Thyroglossal duct anomalies, 1952–1953
Thyroid, 1429–1457
  adenoma, 1438, 1439
  anatomy, 1430–1431
  anomalies, 1430–1431
  blood supply, 1430
  carcinoma, 1448, 1449–1453
    pheochromocytoma and, 1413–1414
  chemotherapy, 1440
  evaluation of disease of, 1434–1436
  exophthalmos, 1441
  function tests, 1434–1436
  goiter, 1438, 1439, 1445–1449, 1454–1455
  Graves' disease, 1437–1438, 1439
  hemorrhage, wound, 1455
  historical background, 1429
  hormones, 571, 1431–433, 1435
  hyperthyroidism, 1438–1439
  hypoparathyroidism and, 1456–1457
  hypothyroidism, 1442–1443
  inflammation, 1443–1445
  iodine metabolism and, 1431, 1433, 1440
  laryngeal nerve and, 1430, 1455–1456
  lingual, 1431
  lymphoma, 1452
  mediastinum and, 664–665
  metabolism and, 1432–1434, 1436
  metastases to, 1452–1453
  physical examination and, 558
  physiology, 1431–1434
  radioactive isotope studies, 1434–1435
  radiotherapy, 1440
  regulation of, 1432–1436
  resection, 1440–1441
    (See also Thyroidectomy)
  rests, 1430–1431
  Riedel's disease, 1445
  sarcoma, 1452
  scanning, 1435
  storm, 1455
  surgery, 1453–1457
  T4 and T3, 1432, 1433, 1435
  thyrotoxicosis, 1436–1441
  transplants, 389

tumors, 1449–1453
  uptake and urinary excretion, 1434–1435
Thyroid-stimulating hormone, 6, 7, 16–17, 1367,
    1431, 1433
  cells secreting, 1364–1365
  ectopic secretion of, 1374
Thyroidectomy, 1387–1391
  complications, 1455–1457
  for carcinoma, 1450, 1451
  for intrathoracic goiter, 1454–1455
  subtotal, 1440–1441
  technique, 1453–1455
  wound hemorrhage, 1455
Thyroiditis, 1443–1445
  acute, 1443
  Hashimoto's, 1443–1444
  Riedel's (struma), 1445
  subacute, 1444–1445
Toyrotoxicosis, 1436–1441
  clininical manifestations, 1438–1439
  diagnostic findings, 1439
  etiology and pathology, 1437–1438
  osteoporosis, 1762–1763
  treatment, 1439–1441
Thyrotropin-releasing factor, 6
Thyroxin, 16–17
Tibia:
  amputation through, 1885–1886
  epiphysitis of tubercle, 1720
  fractures of, 1829–1831
  pseudoarthrosis, congenital, 1732
Tibial compartment syndrome, 870–871
Tibiofibular diastasis, 1832
Tibioperoneal arterial disease, 851–854
Tic douloureux, 1667
Tidal volume, 465
Tietze's syndrome, 606
TNM system, 320, 573
Tobacco smoking (see Smoking)
Toes:
  amputation, 1882
  arthritis, 1857
  ischemic, 861
  osteoarthritis, 1868–1869
Tolerance, immunologic, 307–308, 379–380
Tomography in bronchogenic carcinoma, 646
Tongue:
  biopsy, 560
  carcinoma, 568
  examination of, 557
  hairy, 557
  tumors, 572, 1944
Tonsil(s), 571–572
  cancer, 571–572
  examination of, 557–558
Topical anesthesia, 457, 458
Torkildsen procedure, 1655
Torticollis, 1736–1737
Torus, 558
Tourniquet:
  in amputations, 1881, 1889
  for hand, 1897–1898
  for snakebite, 212
  test, 102
Toxemia, 170
Toxic megacolon, 1113
Toxins:
  bacterial, 167
  Coley's, 340
  pancreatitis and, 1261
  strangulated obstruction and, 982
Trace elements:
  hyperalimentation and, 34
  wound healing and, 31
Trachea, 658–660
  in adults, 658–659
  in infancy and childhood, 658
  injuries of, 219
  opening in (see Tracheostomy)
  stenosis of, 659

Tracheoesophageal fistula, 635, 1516–1521
Tracheostomy, 659–660
  in burns, 259–260
  in children, 1515
  extracorporeal circulation and, 757
  head and neck operations and, 590
  postoperative care, 660
  technique, 659–660
  for ventilatory support, 467
Tracheotomy, facial trauma and, 1935
Traction, 1801–1802
  diverticula, 1023
  for humeral fracture, 1810
  vertebral, 1642
Tranquilizers, 453, 458
Transcellular water, 67
Transducers, 497–499
Transesophageal ligation, 1201, 1206
Transfer factor, 362
Transfusion, 121–129
  acidosis and, 37
  allergic reactions, 127
  bacterial sepsis, 127
  banked blood, 121
  citrate toxicity, 127
  clotting factors, 124
  complications, 126–129
  concentrates, 123
  embolism and, 127–128
  extracorporeal circulation and, 126, 756
  fibrinogen, 113
  fresh whole blood, 121, 122
  frozen red cells, 122–123
  hemolytic reactions, 107, 126–127
  in hemophilia, 109–110, 111
  hemostasis and, 107
  hepatitis transmission, 128–129
  indications for, 123–126
  intraperitoneal, 1297
  massive, 125–126
  methods, 126
  multiple, syndrome, 30
  oxygen-carrying capacity and, 124
  packed red cells, 122
  platelets, 123
  pooled plasma, 123
  purpura, 107–108
  replacement therapy, 121–126
  selective therapy, 124–125
  single-unit, 125
  tetralogy of Fallot and, 727
  thrombophlebitis and, 128
  trauma and, 196
  typing and cross matching, 121–122
  volume replacement, 123–124
Transmetatarsal amputations, 1883
Transphalangeal amputation, 1882–1883
Transplantation, 351–435
  allografts (homografts), 381–383
    (See also Allografts)
  antigens, 351–353, 409
  autografts (see Autografts)
  bone, 386–387
  bone marrow, 388–389
  cartilage, 386–387
  clinical, 383–430
  corneal, 385–386
  endocrine, 389–391
  extremity, 387–388
  fascia, 385
  freezing of organs for, 434–435
  gastrointestinal, 391
  hair, 1924, 1925
  heart, 399–402
    historical background, 399
    postoperative care, 401
    rejection, 401
    selection of patients, 399–400
    results, 401–402
    technique, 400

hemopoietic and lymphoid tissues, 388–389
histocompatibility matching, 382–383
immunogen release in, 355
immunosuppression and, 371–379
kidney, 404–430
  acute tubular necrosis and, 417–418
  anuria and oliguria in, 415–418
  in children, 429–430
  complications, 415–426
  death, brain, criteria of, 411–412
  hemodialysis and, 406–408
  immunosuppression in, 415, 416, 422–426
  multiple, 430
  nephrectomy in, 412–414
  organ harvest, 412
  parathyroid and, 1498
  posttransplant care, 1492–1493
  recurrent disease and, 1499–1501
  registry, 426–429
  rejection of, 369–371, 417, 418–421
  results, 426–430
  selection of donors, 408–412
  selection of recipients, 404–406
  technique, 414
  work-up of recipient, 406
liver, 391–399, 1196
  clinical, 394–399
  complications, 396–398
  experimental, 391–392
  heterotopic, 393–394, 396
  indications, 394–395
  metabolism and, 397–398
  orthotopic, 392–393, 395–396
  postoperative care, 398
  precautions, 395
  rejection, 398
  results, 398–399
  technique, 395–396
lung, 402–404
lymph node, 389
nerve, 385
pancreas, 390–391
privileged sites for, 381–382
rejection, 354–364, 369–371, 398, 401, 417,
    418–421
  antibody role in, 363–364
  cellular interactions and, 357–358
  immunoglobulins and, 356–357
  integrated view of, 369–371
  macrophages and, 356
  molecular cascade systems and, 364–371
  morphologic lymphocyte changes in,
    358–359
  polymorphonuclear leukocytes and, 367–371
  prevention of, 371–383
  radiation and, 374–376
  specifically immunized lymphocyte role,
    360–363
skin, 383–384
spleen, 111, 389
storage of organs, 432–435
tendon, 385
thymus, 389
tumor, 304–308
  immunotherapy and, 340
  tumor-specific antigens and, 305
vascular, 384–385
xenografts, 430–432
Transposition of great vessels, 727–730
  anatomy pathologic, 728
  clinical manifestations, 728–729
  corrected, 742–743
  diagnosis, 729
  historical data, 727
  incidence and etiology, 727–728
  laboratory findings, 729
  pathophysiology, 728
  treatment, 729–730
Transversalis fascia, 1346, 1347, 1354, 1356
Trauma, 1–50, 195–247

abdominal, 220–247
abdominal wall, 246–247
acid-base balance and, 36–42
acidosis in, 37–39
ACTH-cortisol in, 7–12
adrenal insufficiency in, 8–12
afferent nerve stimuli from, 1–2
airway adequacy and, 196, 202
aldosterone in, 8, 12–13
alimentation mixtures for, 32–34, 35
alkalosis in, 36–37
anaphylaxis from, 5
anesthesia and, 3, 45, 46, 202–204
aneurysms from, 817, 900–901
anoxia and, 4
antidiuretic hormone and, 14–15
aorta and, 829–833
  aneurysms from, 817–821
arterial, 867–873
asphyxia in, 662–663
biliary tree, extrahepatic, 235–237
bites and stings, 207–215
blunt, 198, 220–223, 237
carbohydrate metabolism and, 26
cardiac, 787–790
cardiovascular function and, 44–45
catabolic response to, 200
central nervous system and, 4, 5–7
chest injuries, 197–198, 604
coagulation in, 29–31, 35
colon, 230–232
component therapy for, 34–36
diaphragmatic, 1042–1043
duodenum, 225
emotional, 4
endocrine changes in, 5–17, 199–200
energy metabolism and, 19
from extracorporeal circulation, 755
epinephrine and norepinephrine in, 13–14
facial, 1935–1944
fat metabolism and, 27
female reproductive organs, 245–246
fractures (see Fractures)
FSH-LH and, 17
gallbladder, 1231–1233
gastrointestinal function and, 48–49
genitourinary tract, 1580
GH and, 15
glucagon and, 16
gunshot wounds, 225
hand, 1925–1941
head, 1633–1641
healing of wound, 31–32
hemorrhage and hypovolemia from, 2
hepatic function and, 47–48
hernias and, 1348
hormone secretion in, 5–17, 22–24
hypoglycemia and, 4
immediate care for, 198
immobilization after, 4
immunologic protective mechanisms, 42–44
infection and, 3
insulin and, 5, 17, 18, 26
liver, 232–235, 1181–1184
local wound factors, 2–3
lung, 628
  pulmonary function and, 46–47
metabolic changes in, 17–42, 199–202
nerve, peripheral, 1643–1646
nutrition and, 32–34, 35, 87–88
organ system changes, 44–50
ovarian hormone secretion, 17
oxygen transport and, 42
pancreatic, 237–242, 1265–1268
penetrating injuries, 216–220, 223–225,
    235–237
peritonitis from, 1299
pH and, 3
plasma substitutes for, 35
poisons, 4

  protein metabolism and, 27–29
  renal function and, 49–50
  renin in, 12
  resuscitation in, 196–198
  retroperitoneal hematoma, 242
  shock from, 3, 37, 44–45, 48–50, 134–138, 156
  small bowel, 229–230
  spinal cord, 1641–1643
  spleen, 242, 1285–1286
  stab wounds, 223–224, 787–788, 1231, 1265
  starvation and, 4, 19–24
  stimuli inducing change, 1–5
  stomach, 225
  temperature and fever and, 4
  testicular hormones and, 17
  therapeutic considerations, 32–36
  TSH-thyroxin and, 16–17
  unapparent injury, 198–199
  vascular response to, 98
  visceral blood vessels, 1332
  water and electrolyte metabolism in, 39–42
  withdrawal symptoms, 4–5
  wound management, 204–207
    (See also Wounds)
  vena cava, inferior, 243–245
Trench foot, 516, 904
Trendelenburg test, 927, 1727
Trichomonas vaginalis, 1607
Tricuspid atresia, 730–732
  anatomy, pathologic, 730
  clinical manifestations, 731–732
  diagnosis, 732
  laboratory findings, 732
  pathophysiology, 730–731
  treatment, 732
Tricuspid stenosis and insufficiency, 784–787
  clinical manifestations, 784–785
  diagnosis, 787
  Ebstein's anomaly and, 738, 740
  etiology, 784
  mitral stenosis with, 787
  pathology and pathophysiology, 784
  treatment, 785–787
Tricuspid valve, atrial septal defect and, 709, 712
Triethylenethiophosphoramide, 1137
Trigeminal nerve injury, 1942–1943
Trigeminal neuralgia, 1667
Triglycerides, 19
Trivalvular disease, 787
Tromethamine, 158
Trophoblastic disease in pregnancy, 1606–1607
Tropocollagen, 282
Trousseau's sign, 1500
Truncus arteriosus, 736–737
Trypanosoma cruzi, 1145
Trypsin, 1258
Tryptophan, 1098
TSH (see Thyroid-stimulating hormone)
T-tube drainage of common bile duct, 234, 1248
Tube feeding, 89–90
Tuberculosis, 635–638
  of bones and joints, 1850–1852
  of breast, 551
  historical background, 635–636
  of hip, 1852
  pelvic infection, 1608
  pleura in, 619–620
  renal, 1561
  spinal, 1851–1852
  sternal, 606
  treatment, 636–638
Tuberculous enteritis, 1094
Tuberculous mesenteric adenitis, 1333
Tuberculous peritonitis, 1298–1299
Tubular necrosis, acute: burns and, 258
  renal failure and, 1565
  shock and, 50
  transplants and, 417–418
Tumors, 297–343
  (See also Cancer; Carcinoma; specific tumors)

antibodies, 311
antigens, 304–312
appendiceal, 1175–1176
biology and pharmacology, 331–332
biopsy of, 318–320
brain, 1646–1649
breast, 533–550
cardiac, 790–793
chest wall, 606–608
colonic, 1126–1143
desmoid, 1315–1316
doubling time, 303–304
embolism, 323
enhancement of, 308
esophageal, 1032–1038
estrogen-secreting, 1392
feminizing, 1392
gastric, 1078–1083
gynecologic, 1601–1602, 1609–1623
head, 555–591, 1944–1946
hereditary factors, 301–302
hormone-secreting, 1373–1374
immunology of, 304–313
lung, 641–649
mandibular, 579–580
mesenteric, 1334–1336
musculoskeletal, 1777–1790
neck, 584–591, 1944–1946
necrosis, 316
oral cavity, 564–571
oropharynx, 571–572
pleural, 621
radiosensitivity of, 328
rectal, 1126–1143
resection, 323–325
retroperitoneal, 1339–1341
skin, 517–525
small intestine, 1095–1100
spinal cord, 1649–1651
spontaneous regression of, 308
thyroid, 1449–1453
TMN system for, 320
transplantation of, 304–308, 423–424
urologic, 1570–1580
vaccine, 338
Turner's syndrome, 1393–1394, 1604
Typhoid enteritis, 1094–1095
Typhoid fever, appendicitis vs., 1171

Ulcer(s):
arterial occlusion and, 840, 841
Curling's, 259, 269, 992–993
Cushing's, 993
decubitus, 1960, 1978
marginal, 1056, 1068
Meleney's, 180
peptic (see Peptic ulcer)
potassium chloride, 1101
in regional enteritis, 1091
small bowel, 1101
steroid, 49
stress, 49, 992
trophic, 856
venous, 923, 926, 928
Ulcerative colitis, 1110–1116
(See also Colitis, ulcerative)
Ulcerogenic drugs, 1070
Ulcerogenic tumors of islets, 1276–1278
Ulna:
absence of, 1738
fractures of, 1809, 1813
Ulnar nerve:
conduction velocity, 878–879
paralysis, 1910–1911
Ultrasound:
monitoring and, 507
for thrombosis, 917
Ultraviolet, 1969
Umbilical hernia, 1348, 1358

Umbilical vein, 1198
Umbilicus:
congenital anomalies of, 1521–1525
Meckel's diverticulum, 1522–1523
omphalocele and gastroschisis, 1523–1524
omphalomesenteric duct persistence, 1522
Unconsciousness, 198, 1636, 1638
Urachus, 1524–1525
Urate crystals, 1869
Urea, 28
nitrogen, blood (see Blood urea nitrogen)
Uremia:
hemodialysis and, 406
high-output renal failure and, 86
Ureter:
anatomy, 1548
calculi, 1562, 1563
appendicitis vs., 1172
colic, 1542
ectopic orifice of, 1570
radiography for, 1555
retroperitoneal fibrosis and, 1337
trauma, 1580
tumors, 1572
Ureterocele, 1569
Ureteroileostomy, cutaneous, 1581–1583
Ureterolysis for retroperitoneal fibrosis, 1338
Urethra, 1548
discharge from, 1552–1553
stenosis, 1568
valves, 1568–1569
Urethritis, 1559
Urethroplasty, 1963, 1964
Uric acid:
gout and, 1869
stones, 1562, 1564
Urinalysis, 1552
Urinary bladder, 1556–1558
anatomy, 1548
calculi, 1562
cystostomy, cystolithotomy, 1583–1584
diverticulum, 1576
exstrophy, 1570
incontinence, 1550
injury, 1580
innervation, 1556
instrumentation, 1553
neck obstruction, 1568–1569
neurogenic dysfunction, 1550, 1556–1558,
1569, 1979
paralysis, 1557
pheochromocytoma of, 1416
physiology, 1556
prostate hypertrophy and, 1575
retention, 1549–1550
sliding hernia and, 1355
tumors, 1572–1574
ureteroileostomy and, 1581–1583
Urinary tract (see Genitourinary tract; Kidney;
Urinary bladder; Urology; other specific
parts)
Urination:
colorectal surgery and, 1140
frequency, 1550
incontinence, 1550, 1599–1601
nocturia, 1550
pain in, 1550–1551
retroperitoneal fibrosis and, 1337
urgency, 1550
Urine:
in aldosteronism, 1397–1398
bilirubin in, 1003
blood in (see Hematuria)
in burns, 261
calcium in hyperparathyroidism, 1474
catecholamines, 1407, 1410
corticosteroids, 1384
diversion, 1581–1583
gonadotropin assay, 1594
in hypertension, 940–941

protein loss in, 27
in prostatitis, 1560
in renal failure, 1565
high-output failure, 85–86
residual, 1575–1576
retention of, postrenal, 1549–1550
sodium loss in, 79
steroids, 1596
sugar level, 94
volume, replacement of, 83
Urobilinogen, 1003, 1228
Urography, rapid-sequence, 951–952
Urokinase, 101, 115
for pulmonary embolism, 922–923
Urology, 1547–1587
(See also Genitourinary tract; Kidney;
Urinary bladder, other specific structures)
anatomy, 1547–1549
calculi, 1561–1564
diagnosis, 1549–1555
genital secretions, 1552–1553
history, 1549–1553
instrumentation, 1553
physical examination, 1551–1552
special studies, 1553–1555
urinalysis, 1552
function of bladder, 1556–1558
infections, 1558–1561
acute, 1558–1560
chronic, 1560–1561
injuries, 1580
neoplasms, 1570–1580
operative procedures, 1580–1587
pediatric, 1566–1570
renal failure, 1564–1566
Uterosacral ligaments, 1591
Uterus, 1590, 1609, 1617
adenomyosis, 1601, 1610
anomalies, 1591
benign disorders, 1609–1611
carcinoma, 1611–1617
death rate, 298, 299
cervical disorders, 1610–1615
chemotherapy for tumors of, 336
endometritis, 1610
fibroids, 1601, 1609–1610
fundal disorders, 1609–1610, 1615–1617
hysterectomy, 1627–1630
injuries, 245–246
polyps, 1601, 1610
sarcomas, 1617

Vaccination, rabies, 209–210
Vaccine, tumor, 338
Vagina, 1590
absence of, 1604
bleeding from, 1611
(See also Menstruation)
dilatation and curettage through, 1624–1625
discharge from, 1607–1608
examination, 1142, 1597–1598
hysterectomy through, 1599–1600
infections, 1607–1608
malignant tumors, 1619
pessaries, 1600–1601
Vagotomy:
for peptic ulcer, 1066–1067
in short bowel syndrome, 1105
Vagus nerve:
cardiac arrest and, 760
esophagus and, 1011
gastric secretion and, 1054
Valium, 457, 458
Valsalva, sinus of, 735–736
Valves:
anal, 1146
cardiac:
aortic, 690–696, 768–784
in artrial septal defect, 709, 712

mitral, 762–774
multivalvular disease, 787
pulmonic, 685–690
tricuspid, 730–732, 784–787
prostheses (see Prostheses)
venous, 925
Valvulotomy, 688–689
Vancomycin, 174
Vanilmandelic acid, 1405, 1410–1411
Van Slyke device, 503
Varices, esophagogastric (see Esophagogastric
varices)
Varicocele, 1551
Varicose veins, 923, 925
Vascular disease (see Arteries; Cardiovascular
system; Heart, Nervous system, vascular
diseases; Veins)
Vascular permeability factor, 362
Vascular rings, 701–704
Vascular tumors of skin, 518–519
Vasoconstriction:
anesthesia and, 447, 448
baroreceptors and, 963
injury and, 98
pulmonary, in mitral stenosis, 763
in Raynaud's disease, 901
regulation of, 939–940
shock and, 135–137, 140
skin circulation, 514
in thoracic outlet syndrome, 877
Vasodilatation:
aortic insufficiency and, 783
spinal anesthesia and, 455
Vasodilators, 151
Vasomotor reflex, 1668
Vasopressin in esophagogastric varices, 1200
Vasopressor therapy, 150–151
Vasospastic disorders, 901–904
acrocyanosis, 903–904
erythromelalgia, 904
livedo reticularis, 903
Raynaud's disease, 901–903
Vater (see Ampulla of Vater; Papilla of Vater)
Veins:
breast, 529
catheterization of, for monitoring, 500
compression tests of, 927
decompression techniques in liver
transplantation, 392, 393
grafts, 384, 400
in coronary bypass operation, 795, 797
intracranial hematomas and, 1638–1641
ligation or division for pulmonary emboli, 921
ligation and stripping of, 914, 930
of mesentery, 1322–1324
percussion test of, 926–927
spinal anesthesia and, 455–456
thrombosis, 913–919
deep, 914–919, 925
differential diagnosis, 914, 918
electrical impedance test, 917
etiology, 913
isotope studies, 917
noninvasive methods for, 916–917
pathophysiology, 913–914
phlebography for, 915–916
physical findings, 914, 915
pressure measurements, 916
sites of involvement, 915
superficial, 914
symptoms, 914–915
treatment, 914, 918–919
valvular incompetence, 925
varicose, 923, 925
Vena cava:
inferior: injuries of, 243–245
interruption of, for pulmonary embolism,
922
ligation of, for pulmonary embolism, 921
in liver transplants, 392, 393, 397

superior mesenteric shunt with, 1210–1213
superior: obstruction of, 662–663, 833, 835
pulmonary artery anastomosis with, 732
roentgenography of, 683
Venous compression disorders, 879, 880
Venous filling time, 841
Venous insufficiency, 923–931
anatomy and physiology, 923–925
differential diagnosis, 928
etiology, 925
lymphedema vs., 933
physical findings, 926
symptoms, 925–926
tests for, 926–928
treatment, 928–931
Venous pressure, 500–501, 986
in shock, 149
thrombosis and, 916
venous insufficiency and, 927, 929
Venous return in shock, 140
Ventilation (see Respiration)
Ventilation/perfusion ratio, 466, 598–599, 600
Ventilatory support, 466–467
Ventricles of heart:
aneurysms, 799–801
arrhythmias (see Arrhythmias)
assisted circulation and, 808–809
coronary artery disease and, 795
defibrillation of, 761–762
diastolic overloading of, 679
ejection time, 506–507
failure (see Heart, failure)
fibrillation (see Fibrillation, ventricular)
hypertrophy of: in aortic insufficiency, 781
in aortic stenosis, 775
obstruction to emptying of, 678, 685–704
septal defects (see Ventricular septal defects)
single, 737–738
subaortic stenosis and, 694–695
tachycardia, 471
in tetralogy of Fallot, 721, 726
in tricuspid atresia, 730, 731
Ventricular septal defects, 712–716
anatomy, pathologic, 712–713
clinical manifestations, 714
historical data, 712
incidence and etiology, 712
laboratory findings, 714
pathophysiology, 713–714
postoperative course, 716
in tetralogy of Fallot, 721, 726
in transposition of great vessels, 729
treatment, 714–716
Ventriculoatrial shunt for hydrocephalus, 1655
Ventriculotomy, 688, 715, 726
Venules, tone of, in shock, 135–137
Verdan's zones, 1913
Verruca vulgaris, 517
Verrucous carcinoma, 570, 572
Vertebral arteries, 1657
injury, 218
occlusive disease, 883, 884–886
radiography, 1648
Vertebral column, 1669–1673
abnormalities of, 1669–1673
anatomy, 1669
cervical disease, 1672, 1680–1682
cervical injuries, 1839–1840
chordoma, 1786
craniovertebral border, 1669–1670
degenerative disease, 1670–1671, 1679
epiphysitis, 1707–1708
fractures and dislocations, 1641–1643,
1839–1842
herniated discs, 1671–1672
ischemia, 1679
kyphosis, 1707–1708
lumbar disease, 1671–1672, 1686–1689
metastases to, 1789–1790
osteoarthritis, 1690

osteoporosis, 1763
Paget's disease of, 1767
pain arising from, 1678–1679
pathophysiology, 1669
posture and, 1707–1711
pyogenic osteomyelitis, 1691–1692
scoliosis, 1708–1711
spondylolisthesis and spondylolysis,
1684–1685
spondylosis, 1673, 1690
thoracolumbar injuries, 1840–1842
tuberculosis, 1851–1852
tumors, 1678–1679, 1690–1691
wedge compression injury, 1841
"Vest over pants" repair, 1358
Videodensitometry, 506
"Vietnam lung," 148–149
Villous adenoma, 1126–1128
Vinca alkaloids, 331, 337
Vineberg procedure, 798
Virilization, 1390–1392
Virulence, 167
Viruses as carcinogens, 301, 305–306
Vis a tergo, 924
Visceral blood vessels:
chronic occlusion of, 1327–1328
rupture, spontaneous, 1331–1332
trauma to, 1332
Visceral pain, 969
Vistaril, 458
Vital capacity, 600
Vitamin A in wound healing, 31
Vitamin B12, 1052
in blind loop syndrome, 1102–1103
Vitamin C:
requirements, 89
scurvy and, 1755
trauma and, 31, 201
Vitamin D:
bone and, 1754–1756, 1758–1759
parathyroid and, 1464
poisoning, hyperparathyroidism vs., 1489
scurvy and, 1755
Vitamin K:
anticoagulant therapy and, 118–119
liver function and, 1180, 1193
in wound healing, 31
Vitellointestinal duct, 1521–1522
VMA, 942
Vocal cords (see Larynx)
Vocal nodules, 574
Vocational therapy, 1969–1971
Volkmann's contracture, 1716–1717
Volvulus, 1143–1144
cecal, 1144
gastric, 1078
midgut, 1525–1526
sigmoid, 1143–1144
Vomiting, 975–976
anesthesia and, 202–203
in atresia of intestine, 1527
of blood, 991, 994
esophageal perforation and, 1030
Mallory-Weiss syndrome and, 1039
obstruction and, 983
in pancreatitis, 1261
in pyloric stenosis, 1521
Von Recklinghausen's disease, 1760–1761
Von Willebrand's disease, 111
Vrolich's disease, 1750
V-Y advancement, 1925, 1926
Vulva, 1617–1619

Wallerian degeneration, autotransplants and, 385
Warfarin, 759, 771
Warthin's tumor, 581–582
Warts, 517
anal, 1158
Water, 39–42

(*See also* Fluids and electrolytes)
ADH release and, 39–41
of bone, 1742
burns and loss of, 255
exchange, 78
insensible loss of, 41, 78, 515
postoperative patterns of, 41–42
sodium loss replaced by, 84–85
total body, 65–66
transcellular, 67
weight and, 65–66
Waterhouse-Friderichsen syndrome, 12, 1402
Weber-Christian disease, 519
Wedge compression fracture, 1841
Wedge excision of tongue, 1945
Wedge resection, pulmonary, 653–655
Weight, body, fluids and, 66
Wertheim hysterectomy, 1627–1630
Wheal, 514
Wheeze, 600–601
  tracheal tumors and, 658
Whipple's triad, 1275
Whirlpool bath, 1968
Wilms' tumor, 1567
  chemotherapy for, 336–337
Window, aortic-pulmonary, 734–735
Wirsung, duct of (*see* Pancreatic duct)
Withdrawal symptoms, 4–5
Witzel jejunostomy, 90
Wolffian duct remnants, 1619–1620
Woodward method, 1033
Wooky operation, 1037
Wounds, 275–294
  (*See also* Trauma)
  aortic, 829–833
  burn, 265–268
  care of, 287–290

chemoprophylaxis for, 172
chest, 197–198
clostridial infection of, 181–182
closure of, 288, 1920–1921
collagen and, 282–286
complications, postoperative, 462–464
contraction of, 275–278
dehiscence, 462
"dog ears," 1934, 1935
dressings, 290
epithelization of, 278–281
fracture (*see* Fractures)
ground substance and, 281–282
gunshot, 225
healing of 31–32, 275–294, 1920
  sequence of events in, 286–287
heart, 787–790
infection, 462–464
local care of, 204–205
local factors, metabolic response to, 2–3
neck, 216–220
penetrating, 216–220, 223–225, 235–237
  of aorta, 829
  arterial injury, 867, 868
  arteriovenous fistula and, 871, 872
  of pancreas, 1265
  of spleen, 1285
  stab, 223–224, 787–788, 1231, 1265
power mower, 205
puncture, 205
skin grafts for, 290–294
thyroid, 1455
Wringer injury, 1907–1908
Wrist:
  in cerebral palsy, 1702
  disarticulation, 1891
  dislocations, 1817

fractures, 1816–1817
lacerations, 1912–1913
Madelung's deformity, 1737–1738
osteoarthritis, 1862
pain, 1679
splint for rheumatoid arthritis, 1856
tenosynovitis, 1862
Wryneck, congenital, 1736–1737

Xenografts, 430–432
  cartilage, 386
  skin, 1933
Xeroradiography, 532
X-rays (*see* Roentgenography)
Xylocaine, 458
  in fracture reduction, 1793

Y-plasty for anal fissure, 1153
Yttrium, radioactive, 1368, 1370, 1387

Z line, 1692
Zephiran chloride, 190
Zinc, wound healing and, 31
Zinc sulfate turbidity, 1179
Zollinger-Ellison syndrome, 1057–1058, 1068,
  1276–1278
  hyperparathyroidism and, 1475, 1487
Zona glomerulosa and fasciculata, 1377
Z-plasty, 1925–1926, 1934
  for cleft lip, 1949
Zuckerkandl, organs of, 1404
  pheochromocytoma of, 1415–1416
Zygoma, 1939–1940